Robert J. Wityk

Feb 28, 1984

Infectious Diseases

Infectious Diseases

THIRD EDITION

A Modern Treatise of Infectious Processes

edited by ***Paul D. Hoeprich,*** *M.D.*

Professor of Medicine and Pathology
Departments of Internal Medicine and Pathology
School of Medicine
University of California Davis Medical Center
Sacramento, California

with 122 contributors

HARPER & ROW, PUBLISHERS

PHILADELPHIA

Cambridge
New York
Hagerstown
San Francisco

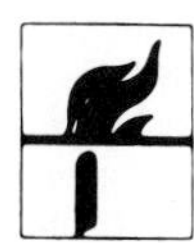

1817

London
Mexico
São Paulo
Sydney

Acquisitions Editor: John DeCarville
Sponsoring Editor: Sanford Robinson
Manuscript Editor: Don Shenkle

Indexer: Sandra King

Art Director: Maria Karkucinski
Designer: Patrick Turner
Production Coordinator: George V. Gordon
Compositor: York Graphic Services, Inc.
Printer/Binder: Halliday Lithograph

3rd Edition

1 3 5 6 4 2

Library of Congress Cataloging in Publication Data
Main entry under title:

Infectious diseases.

Bibliography: p.
Includes index.
1. Communicable diseases. I. Hoeprich, Paul D.
RC111.I5129 1983 616.9 82-9339
ISBN 0-06-141197-3 AACR2

The authors and publisher have exerted every effort to ensure that drug selection and dosage set forth in this text are in accord with current recommendations and practice at the time of publication. However, in view of ongoing research, changes in government regulations, and the constant flow of information relating to drug therapy and drug reactions, the reader is urged to check the package insert for each drug for any change in indications and dosage and for added warnings and precautions. This is particularly important when the recommended agent is a new or infrequently employed drug.

To Our Families

Contributors

Aaron D. Alexander, Ph.D.

Chapter 76
Professor and Chairman, Department of Microbiology, Chicago College of Osteopathic Medicine, Chicago, Illinois

Jeffrey D. Band, M.D.

Chapter 126
Associate Professor, Department of Medicine, Wayne State University School of Medicine, Hutzel Hospital Medical Unit, Detroit, Michigan

Alan G. Barbour, M.D.

Chapter 123
Rocky Mountain Laboratories, National Institute of Allergy and Infectious Diseases, National Institutes of Health, Hamilton, Montana

Arthur L. Barry, Ph.D.

Chapters 9, 10, 12
President and Scientific Director, Clinical Microbiology Institute, Tulatin, Oregon

Roberto G. Baruzzi, M.D.

Chapter 109
Professor Titular, Departamento de Medicina Preventiva, Escola Paulista de Medicina, São Paulo, Brasil

Blaine Beaman, Ph.D.

Chapter 1
Associate Professor, Department of Medical Microbiology, School of Medicine, University of California, Davis, California

John V. Bennett, M.D.

Chapter 126
Director, Bacterial Diseases Division, Bureau of Epidemiology, Centers for Disease Control, Atlanta, Georgia

F. William Blaisdell, M.D.

Chapters 154, 155
Professor and Chairman, Department of Surgery, School of Medicine, University of California, Davis, California

Dane R. Boggs, M.D.

Chapter 7
Professor and Chief, Division of Hematology, Department of Medicine, University of Pittsburgh School of Medicine, Pittsburgh, Pennsylvania

William R. Bowie, M.D.

Chapter 55
Assistant Professor, Department of Medicine, University of British Columbia, Vancouver, British Columbia, Canada

Philip S. Brachman, M.D.

Chapter 104
Director, Epidemiology Program Office, Centers for Disease Control, Atlanta, Georgia

Abraham I. Braude, M.D., Ph.D.

Chapter 52
Professor, Departments of Medicine and Pathology, School of Medicine, University of California, San Diego, La Jolla; Director, Microbiology Laboratory and Head, Division of Infectious Diseases, University Hospital, San Diego, California

George F. Brooks, M.D.

Chapter 152
Professor, Departments of Laboratory Medicine, Medicine, and Microbiology and Immunology, School of Medicine; Chief, Microbiology Section, Clinical Laboratories, University of California, San Francisco, California

Donald E. Campbell, M.D.

Chapter 91
Assistant Professor, Department of Pediatrics, Emory University School of Medicine, Atlanta, Georgia

Charles C.J. Carpenter, Jr., M.D.

Chapters 61, 65
Professor and Chairman, Department of Medicine, Case Western Reserve University, Cleveland, Ohio

Robert S. Chang, M.D., D.Sc.

Chapters 1, 77
Professor, Department of Medical Microbiology, School of Medicine, University of California, Davis, California

Denny G. Constantine, D.V.M., M.P.H.

Chapter 124
Public Health Veterinarian, Infectious Disease Section, California Department of Health Services, Berkeley, California

Sebastian Conti, M.D.

Chapter 158
Clinical Assistant Professor of Surgery, Department of Surgery, University of California, Davis, California

Henry G. Cramblett, M.D.

Chapter 166
Acting Vice President for Medical Affairs, Ohio State University; Dean, College of Medicine; Professor, Departments of Pediatrics and Medical Microbiology, College of Medicine, Ohio State University, Columbus, Ohio

D. Joseph Demis, M.D., Ph.D.

Chapter 106
Clinical Professor, Department of Dermatology, Albany Medical College; Director, Dermatology Research Associates, Albany, New York

Robert H. Demling, M.D.

Chapter 157
Associate Professor, Department of Surgery, Harvard Medical School; Director, Longwood Area Trauma–Burn Center, Boston, Massachusetts

Hugh C. Dillon, Jr., M.D.

Chapters 24, 101
Professor, Departments of Pediatrics and Microbiology, School of Medicine, University of Alabama, Birmingham, Alabama

Ralph L. Doherty, M.D.

Chapter 122
Director, Queensland Institute of Medical Research, Herston, Brisbane, Australia

W. Christopher Duncan, M.D.

Chapters 8, 15, 102
Associate Professor, Department of Dermatology, Baylor College of Medicine, Houston, Texas

David T. Durack, M.D., D. Phil.

Chapter 134
Professor, Department of Medicine; Chief, Division of Infectious Diseases, Duke University Medical Center, Durham, North Carolina

John E. Edwards, Jr., M.D.

Chapter 128
Associate Professor, Department of Medicine; Chief, Division of Infectious Diseases, Harbor-UCLA Medical Center, Torrance, California

Theodore C. Eickhoff, M.D.

Chapter 3
Professor, Department of Medicine, University of Colorado; Director, Department of Internal Medicine, St. Luke's Hospital, Denver, Colorado

Sydney M. Finegold, M.D.

Chapters 32, 47, 53, 82, 83, 84, 85, 125
Chief, Infectious Diseases Section, Department of Medicine, Wadsworth Veterans Administration Hospital; Professor, Department of Medicine, School of Medicine, University of California, Los Angeles, California

Neil M. Flynn, M.D.

Chapter 19
Assistant Professor, Department of Internal Medicine, School of Medicine, University of California Davis, Sacramento, California

Vincent A. Fulginiti, M.D.

Chapter 121
Professor and Head, Department of Pediatrics, University of Arizona, Health Sciences Center, Tucson, Arizona

George Goldsand, M.D.

Chapter 38
Associate Professor, Department of Medicine and Director, Division of Infectious Diseases, University of Alberta, Edmonton, Alberta, Canada

Wendell H. Hall, M.D., Ph.D.

Chapter 138
Professor, Departments of Medicine and Microbiology, University of Minnesota Medical School; Infectious Disease Section, Veterans Administration Medical Center, Minneapolis, Minnesota

Scott B. Halstead, M.D.

Chapter 89
Professor and Chairman, Department of Tropical Medicine and Medical Microbiology, University of Hawaii, Honolulu, Hawaii

H. William Harris, M.D.

Chapters 34, 36
Professor of Clinical Medicine, Department of Medicine, New York University, School of Medicine, New York, New York

Charles L. Hatheway, M.D.

Chapter 127
Microbiologist-in-Charge, Anaerobe Foodborne Disease Laboratory, Bacteriology Division, Centers for Disease Control, Atlanta, Georgia

Paul D. Hoeprich, M.D.

Chapters 4, 6, 7, 9, 16, 17, 18, 19, 20, 25, 31, 37, 39, 41, 48, 51, 97, 103, 106, 119, 120, 134
Professor of Medicine and Pathology, Deparments of Internal Medicine and Pathology, School of Medicine, University of California Davis Medical Center, Sacramento, California

King K. Holmes, M.D., Ph.D.

Chapters 55, 56
Chief, Division of Infectious Diseases, United States Public Health Service Hospital; Professor, Department of Medicine, University of Washington, Seattle, Washington

Richard B. Hornick, M.D.

Chapters 60, 62, 63, 64, 139
Professor and Chairman, Department of Medicine, University of Rochester School of Medicine, Rochester, New York

Calderon Howe, M.D.

Chapter 141
Professor and Head, Department of Microbiology, Louisiana State University Medical Center, New Orleans, Louisiana

George L. Humphrey, D.V.M.

Chapter 124
Chief Public Health Veterinarian, Infectious Disease Section, California Department of Health Services, Berkeley, California

Carolyn Coker Huntley, M.D.

Chapters 78, 111
Professor, Department of Pediatrics, Bowman Gray School of Medicine, Winston-Salem, North Carolina

D. Geraint James, M.A., M.D., F.R.C.P.

Chapter 168
Consultant Physician and Dean, Royal Northern Hospital; Consultant Ophthalmic Physician, St. Thomas' Hospital, London, England

Burton Janis, M.D., D.V.M.

Chapters 94, 95
1818 West Northern Lights Boulevard, Anchorage, Alaska

Karl M. Johnson, M.D.

Chapter 90
Program Director, Hazardous Viruses, United States Army

Medical Research Institute of Infectious Diseases, Fort Detrick, Frederick, Maryland

Henry Earl Jones, M.D.

Chapter 107
Professor and Chairman, Department of Dermatology, Emory University School of Medicine, Atlanta, Georgia

M. Colin Jordan, M.D.

Chapter 75
Associate Professor, Department of Medicine, School of Medicine, University of California, Davis; Chief, Infectious Diseases Section, Martinez Veterans Administration Hospital, Martinez, California

Kerrison Juniper, Jr., M.D.

Chapters 66, 67
Professor, Department of Medicine, and Chief, Division of Gastroenterology, Southern Illinois University, School of Medicine, Springfield, Illinois

Irving G. Kagan, Ph.D.

Chapter 150
Assistant Director for Laboratory Science, Division of Parasitic Diseases, Centers for Disease Control, Atlanta, Georgia

Rudolph H. Kampmeier, M.D.

Chapters 57, 58
Emeritus Professor, Department of Medicine, Vanderbilt University, School of Medicine, Nashville, Tennessee

Mohammed Y. Khan, M.D., Ph.D., F.R.C.P.(C)

Chapter 138
Assistant Professor, Department of Medicine, University of Minnesota Medical School; Director, Department of Infectious Diseases, Hennepin County Medical Center, Minneapolis, Minnesota

Sidney Kibrick, M.D., Ph.D.

Chapters 74, 86, 87, 88, 93
Emeritus Professor, Department of Pediatrics and Microbiology (Virology), Boston University School of Medicine, Boston, Massachusetts

Pedro Lavalle, M.D.

Chapter 110
Professor, Medical Mycology, Universidad Autonoma de Mexico; Chief, Medical Mycology Service, Centro Dermatologico Pascua, Mexico City, Mexico

Ruth M. Lawrence, M.D.

Chapters 6, 20, 35, 50, 77
Associate Professor, Department of Medicine; Chief, Division of Infectious Diseases, Texas Tech University Medical School, Lubbock, Texas

Louis Levy, M.D., Ph.D.

Chapter 105
Visiting Associate Professor, Department of Comparative Medicine and Medical Ecology, The Hebrew University–Hadassah Medical School, Jerusalem, Israel

Chien Liu, M.D.

Chapters 9, 21, 22, 23, 26, 27, 28, 30
Professor, Departments of Medicine and Pediatrics; Director, Division of Infectious Diseases, School of Medicine, University of Kansas, Kansas City, Kansas

Alberto T. Londero, M.D.

Chapter 42
Professor, Departamento de Microbiologia e Parasitologia, Seccae do Micologia Medica e Veterinaria, Universidade Federal de Santa Maria, Santa Maria, RS, Brasil

Benjamin Luft, M.D.

Chapter 129
Post-doctoral Fellow, Department of Immunology and Infectious Diseases, Palo Alto Medical Research Foundation, Palo Alto, California

Philip E.C. Manson-Bahr, M.D., F.R.C.P.

Chapter 147
Consulting Physician, Ministry of Overseas Development; Senior Lecturer in Clinical Tropical Medicine, London School of Hygiene and Tropical Medicine, London, England

Luis F. Marcopito

Chapter 109
Departamento de Medicina Preventiva, Escola Paulista de Medicina, São Paulo, Brasil

S. Michael Marcy, M.D.

Chapters 74, 86, 87, 88, 93
Associate Clinical Professor, Department of Pediatrics, University of Southern California, School of Medicine; Consultant, Children's Hospital of Los Angeles, Los Angeles; Staff Pediatrician, Kaiser Foundation Hospital, Panorama City, California

Philip D. Marsden, M.D.

Chapters 11, 46, 112, 130, 148
Professor of Tropical Medicine, Universidade de Brasilia, Faculdade de Clencias de Saude, Brasilia, D. Federal, Brasil

Allen W. Mathies, Jr., M.D., Ph.D.

Chapter 68
Professor, Department of Pediatrics; Dean, University of Southern California, School of Medicine, Los Angeles, California

John H. McClement, M.D.

Chapters 34, 36
Professor, Department of Medicine, New York University School of Medicine, New York, New York

Edwin M. Meares, Jr., M.D., F.A.C.S.

Chapter 49
Professor and Chairman, Division of Urology, Department of Surgery, Tufts University School of Medicine; Chairman, Department of Urology, New England Medical Center; Urologist-in-Chief, Department of Urology, New England Medical Center Hospital, Boston, Massachusetts

Marian E. Melisch, M.D.

Chapter 165
Associate Professor, Department of Pediatrics, John A. Burns School of Medicine, University of Hawaii, Kapiolani–Childrens Medical Center, Honolulu, Hawaii

Richard D. Meyer, M.D.

Chapter 33
Associate Professor, Department of Medicine, School of Medicine, University of California; Director, Division of Infectious Diseases, Cedars–Sinai Medical Center, Los Angeles, California

J. Donald Millar, M.D., D.T.P.H.

Chapter 92
Assistant Surgeon General, Director, Center for Environmental Health, Centers for Disease Control, Atlanta, Georgia

Louis H. Miller, M.D.

Chapter 145
Head, Malaria Section, Laboratory of Parasitic Diseases, National Institute of Allergy and Infectious Diseases, National Institute of Health, Bethesda, Maryland

Thomas P. Monath, M.D.

Chapter 73
Director, Vector-Borne Diseases Division, Bureau of Laboratories, Fort Collins, Colorado

J. Glenn Morris, M.D., M.P.H., T.M.

Chapter 127
Research Fellow, Division of Infectious Diseases, Center for Vaccine Development, School of Medicine, University of Maryland, Baltimore, Maryland

Stephen A. Morse, M.D.

Chapter 56
Professor, Department of Microbiology and Immunology, Oregon Health Sciences University, Portland, Oregon

James W. Mosley, M.D.

Chapter 2
Professor, Department of Medicine, University of Southern California, Acute Communicable Disease Control, Department of Health Services, Los Angeles, California

Kenneth E. Mott, M.D., M.P.H.

Chapter 136
Medical Officer, Schistosomiasis and Other Helminthic

Infections, World Health Organization, Geneva, Switzerland

Ralph L. Muller, Ph.D.

Chapter 80
Senior Lecturer, Department of Medical Helminthology, London School of Hygiene and Tropical Medicine, London, England

Maury E. Mulligan, M.D.

Chapters 53, 125
Staff Physician, Infectious Disease Section, Department of Medicine, Wadsworth Medical Center; Assistant Professor, Department of Medicine, School of Medicine, University of California, Los Angeles, California

Andre J. Nahmias, M.D., M.P.H.

Chapter 91
Professor, Department of Pediatrics, Chief, Infectious Disease and Immunology Division, Emory University, School of Medicine, Atlanta, Georgia

James H. Nakano, Ph.D.

Chapter 92
Viral Exanthems Branch, Virology Division, Bureau of Laboratories, Centers for Disease Control, Atlanta, Georgia

John D. Nelson, M.D.

Chapter 164
Professor, Department of Pediatrics, The University of Texas Southwestern Medical School, Dallas, Texas

James C. Niederman, M.D.

Chapter 137
Clinical Professor, Department of Epidemiology and Public Health, Yale University School of Medicine, New Haven, Connecticut

Sheila M. Nolan, M.D.

Chapters 16, 17
Research Fellow in Infectious Diseases, Department of Internal Medicine, School of Medicine, University of California Davis, Sacramento, California

John W. Osebold, Ph.D.

Chapter 14
Professor, Department of Microbiology, School of Veterinary Medicine, University of California, Davis, California

Masao Okumoto, M.A.

Chapters 160, 161, 162, 163
Specialist in Ophthalmic Microbiology, Francis I. Proctor Foundation, University of California, San Francisco, California

H. Bruce Ostler, M.D.

Chapters 160, 161, 162, 163
Research Ophthalmologist, Francis I. Proctor Foundation, University of California, San Francisco, California

Gary D. Overturf, M.D.

Chapter 119
Associate Professor, Department of Pediatrics, School of Medicine, University of Southern California; Director, Communicable Disease Service, Los Angeles County-University of Southern California Medical Center, Los Angeles, California

Richard H. Parker, M.D.

Chapter 135, 142, 144, 151
Chief, Section of Infectious Diseases, Medical Service, Veterans Administration Hospital; Associate Professor, Department of Medicine, Howard University, Washington, D.C.

Zbigniew S. Pawlowski, M.D.

Chapter 69
Medical Officer, Parasitic Diseases Programme, World Health Organization, Geneva, Switzerland

George J. Pazin, M.D., M.S.

Chapter 52
Associate Professor, Department of Medicine, Division of Infectious Diseases, School of Medicine, University of Pittsburgh, Pittsburgh, Pennsylvania

Peter L. Perine, M.D., M.P.H.

Chapter 54
Associate Professor, Department of Epidemiology, School

of Public Health and Community Medicine, University of Washington, Seattle, Washington

Fred E. Pittman, M.D.

Chapter 167
Professor, Department of Medicine, Medical University of South Carolina; Chief, Section of Gastroenterology, Veterans Administration Medical Center, Charleston, South Carolina

Jack D. Poland, M.D.

Chapter 140
Chief Medical Epidemiologist, Bureau of Laboratories, Vector-Borne Diseases Division, Fort Collins, Colorado

Vincent G. Pons, M.D.

Chapter 152
Assistant Clinical Professor, Departments of Medicine and Neurosurgery, School of Medicine, University of California, San Francisco, California

C. George Ray, M.D.

Chapter 149
Professor, Departments of Pathology and Pediatrics, University of Arizona College of Medicine, Tucson, Arizona

Jack S. Remington, M.D.

Chapter 129
Professor, Department of Medicine, Division of Infectious Diseases, Stanford University School of Medicine; Chief, Department of Immunology and Infectious Diseases, Division of Allergy, Palo Alto Medical Research Foundation, Palo Alto, California

Michael G. Rinaldi, Ph.D.

Chapters 1, 9, 39
Adjunct Assistant Professor, Department of Microbiology, Montana State University, Bozeman, Montana

William S. Robinson, M.D.

Chapters 70, 71, 72
Professor, Department of Medicine, Stanford University School of Medicine, Stanford, California

Allan R. Ronald, M.D.

Chapter 48
Professor and Head, Departments of Medical Microbiology and Clinical Microbiology, Health Sciences Center, University of Manitoba, Winnepeg, Manitoba, Canada

Judith G. Rose, M.D.

Chapter 53
Chief of Clinical Imaging, Wadsworth Medical Center; Adjunct Assistant Professor, Department of Radiology, School of Medicine, University of California, Los Angeles, California

Andrew H. Rudolph, M.D.

Chapter 59
Associate Professor, Department of Dermatology, Baylor College of Medicine; Chief, Dermatology Service, Veterans Administration Hospital, Houston, Texas

Trenton K. Ruebush II, M.D.

Chapter 146
Medical Entomology Research and Training Unit/Guatamala, Centers for Disease Control, Atlanta, Georgia

Peter M. Schantz, V.M.D., Ph.D.

Chapter 79
Veterinary Epidemiologist, Parasitic Diseases Branch, Bureau of Epidemiology, Centers for Disease Control, United States Public Health Service, Atlanta, Georgia

Arthur D. Schwabe, M.D.

Chapter 169
Professor, Department of Medicine; Chief, Division of Gastroenterology, School of Medicine, University of California, Los Angeles, California

Alexis Shelokov, M.D.

Chapter 170
Professor, Department of Epidemiology, School of Hygiene and Public Health, Johns Hopkins University, Baltimore, Maryland

Margarita Silva-Hutner, Ph.D.

Chapter 110
Professor, Department of Dermatology, College of Physicians and Surgeons, Columbia University, and Director, Mycology Laboratory, Columbia Presbyterian Medical Center, New York, New York

Stewart Sell, M.D.

Chapter 5
Professor, Department of Pathology, University of California, San Diego School of Medicine, La Jolla, California

Charles B. Smith, M.D.

Chapters 132, 133
Professor, Department of Internal Medicine, University of Utah College of Medicine; Chief, Department of Medicine, Veterans Administration Hospital, Salt Lake City, Utah

David H. Smith, M.D.

Chapter 29
Professor and Chairman, Department of Pediatrics, University of Rochester Medical Center, Rochester, New York

Peter B. Smith, Ph.D.

Chapter 13
Chief, Clinical Bacteriology Branch, Bureau of Laboratories, Centers for Disease Control, Atlanta, Georgia

Paul M. Southern, Jr., M.D.

Chapter 143
Associate Professor, Departments of Pathology and Internal Medicine, The University of Texas Health Science Center, Dallas, Texas

Spotswood L. Spruance, M.D.

Chapter 123
Associate Professor, Department of Internal Medicine, University of Utah College of Medicine, Salt Lake City, Utah

†Died November 11, 1980.

Mario L. Tarizzo, M.D.†

Chapter 159
Programme Manager, Prevention of Blindness, World Health Organization, Geneva, Switzerland

Jerold H. Theis, D.V.M., Ph.D.

Chapter 1, 9
Associate Professor, Department of Medical Microbiology, School of Medicine, University of California, Davis, California

John P. Utz, M.D.

Chapters 40, 43, 44, 108, 153
Professor, Department of Medicine, Georgetown University, School of Medicine, Washington, D.C.

Kenneth L. Vosti, M.D.

Chapter 24
Professor, Department of Medicine, Stanford University School of Medicine, Stanford, California

San-Pin Wang, M.D., Dr. Med. Sci.

Chapter 54
Professor, Department of Pathobiology, University of Washington, School of Public Health and Community Medicine, Seattle, Washington

Thomas H. Weller, M.D.

Chapter 81
Emeritus Professor, Department of Tropical Public Health, Harvard School of Public Health, Boston, Massachusetts

Herbert A. Wenner, M.D.

Chapter 118
Professor, Department of Pediatrics, University of Missouri–Kansas City; Chief, Infectious Diseases Section, Children's Mercy Hospital, Kansas City, Missouri

L. Joseph Wheat, M.D.

Chapter 100
Assistant Professor, Department of Medicine, School of Medicine, Indiana University, Indianapolis, Indiana

Arthur C. White, M.D.

Chapter 100
Professor, Department of Medicine; Director, Division of Infectious Diseases, School of Medicine, Indiana University, Indianapolis, Indiana

Roger W. Williams, Ph.D.

Chapters 113, 114, 115, 116, 117, 131
Professor of Public Health (Medical Entomology), Division of Tropical Medicine, College of Physicians and Surgeons and School of Public Health, Columbia University, New York, New York

Charles L. Wisseman, M.D.

Chapters 9, 96, 98, 99,
Professor and Chairman, Department of Microbiology, School of Medicine, University of Maryland, Baltimore, Maryland

Bruce M. Wolfe, M.D.

Chapter 156
Associate Professor, Department of Surgery, School of Medicine, University of California, Davis, Sacramento, California

Lowell S. Young, M.D.

Chapter 45
Professor, Department of Medicine, Center for the Health Sciences, University of California, Los Angeles, California

Preface

*During the years since the publication of the second edition of Infectious Diseases: A Modern Treatise of Infectious Processes, the continuing vigor of inquiry and endeavor in infectious diseases has been manifested by the recognition of "new" diseases (*e.g., *legionellosis, campylobacteriosis, antomicrobic-associated enterocolitis caused by toxinogenic* Clostridium difficile, *toxic shock syndrome); documentation of the rise in resistance to antimicrobial agents in cholera, gonorrhea, malaria, tuberculosis, and even in the pneumococcus (!); the eradication of smallpox; the introduction of new antimicrobics—mostly evolutionary products such as the newer penicillins, cephalosporins and aminocyclitols, and some novel compounds such as the penems, carbapenems, and monobactams; and the development of new (hepatitis B vaccine) and improved (rabies vaccine) immunogens. Furthermore, there appears to be a strong association between viral infections and certain malignant neoplastic diseases in humans: Epstein–Barr virus and both Burkitt's lymphoma and nasopharyngeal carcinoma; hepatitis B virus and hepatocyte carcinoma. Despite these changes, the impact of infectious diseases is enormous.*

For example, in the United States alone, the burden, according to the National Health Interview Survey of 1980, amounted to 53,580,000 cases of acute infective and parasitic diseases (24.6 per 100 population), yielding 205,806,000 days of restricted activity, 110,921,000 days of bed disability, 24,620,000 days lost from work (among persons 17 years of age or older), and 30,169,000 days lost from school (among persons 6 to 16 years in age). An important factor in such morbidity is the persisting increase in the numbers of patients who develop infectious diseases secondary to underlying, noninfectious diseases that diminish natural defenses and require nonspecific therapies that often aggravate incapacities of host defenses. Possibly also contributory is the increasing proportion of aged persons in the population. It is hoped that these factors have been appropriately weighed in this edition.

The preparation of a new edition of Infectious Diseases offered an opportunity to fill omissions, record advances, and correct errors. To these ends, all chapters were revised, and eight chapters were added: Chapter 5, Immunopathology of Infectious Diseases; Chapter 33, Legionnaires Disease; Chapter 42, Paracoccidioidomycosis; Chapter 72, Non-A, Non-B Hepatitis; Chapter 109, Jorge Lobo's Disease; Chapter 110,

Chromoblastomycosis; Chapter 146, Babesiosis; and Chapter 165, Kawasaki Syndrome.

Nevertheless, as in prior editions, shortcomings will be apparent to readers according to their special interests and particular needs. Such faults should not be attributed to contributors, reviewers, or the publisher, but are the editor's alone.

Paul D. Hoeprich, M.D.

Preface to the First Edition

Infectious diseases remain leading causes of morbidity and mortality throughout the world primarily because known measures of control and therapy are not applied. In technically advanced countries, the pestilences of antiquity no longer occur. Yet, even in these areas infectious diseases remain important contributors to illness and death. For example, according to the National Health Interview Survey, in the United States in 1969 there were 49,310,000 cases of acute infective and parasitic diseases (25 per 100 population). As a result, there were 199,701,000 days of restricted activity, 99,713,000 days of bed disability, and 21,164,000 days lost from work.

Among clinical specialty areas, that of infectious diseases is remarkable in being non-systemic in orientation. The specialist in infectious diseases must be prepared to deal with involvement in any organ, system, or region of the body. In assessing illness, he must be capable of taking into account age, sex, and genetic constitution; nutritional, hormonal, and metabolic status; the consequences of trauma, surgery, and other physical or chemical agents; and the effects of neoplastic, degenerative, and hypersensitive states. In this requirement, the specialty of infectious diseases becomes the last disciplinary domain of general medicine. It is to subserve these broad requirements that this volume was conceived. The aim is synthesis of information rather than encyclopedic assemblage of ideas and data. Students of medicine are the intended audience—primarily the predoctoral and newly fledged physician-in-training, but hopefully also the postresident physician-in-practice.

In the first three sections of the book, the sequence of discussion that is subsequently employed in the rest of the book with specific diseases is applied to the general problem of infectious diseases. Section I surveys the attributes of infectious agents; the field of epidemiology, particularly as it relates to infectious diseases; factors bearing on the occurrence and development of infectious diseases, and their manifestations. Although this section concludes with a general approach to the care of patients with infectious diseases, laboratory findings are so important to the diagnosis and treatment of infectious diseases that all of Section II is devoted to laboratory examinations. Because antimicrobic and anthelminitic agents are also vital to the control of infectious diseases, they are considered in Section III, along with other measures traditionally thought to be preventive.

Specific infectious diseases are then approached from the point of view of the system that is involved. This approach is consistent with the facts of clinical life. A patient comes to see a physician because of a sore throat, not because of infection caused by Streptococcus pyogenes *of Lancefield's Group A or because the respiratory tract is a classic portal for entry of* S. pyogenes.

The sequence of consideration of organ systems is based on frequency of infection. The respiratory tract is the most commonly infected of all the organ systems, and accordingly, respiratory tract infections are taken up first (Sections IV–VII). Other systems follow in approximate descending order of frequency of involvement.

However, there are infectious diseases that are almost always multisystem in extent. Moreover under suitable circumstances, nearly all infections may be general rather than localized to one organ or system. As a practical accommodation, the major discussions of infectious agents that have notable capacity for multisystem infection are given in connection with the system most often afflicted. Usually, this is the system affording the portal of entry of the etiologic agent, although it may be the most common site of localization by sign and/or symptom, or as localized in lesions demonstrable by gross or microscopic examinations.

The pattern of discussion of each infectious disease is uniform: etiology, epidemiology, pathogenesis and pathology, manifestations, diagnosis, prognosis, therapy, and prevention. Considerable emphasis is placed on epidemiology and pathogenesis because this is the path to understanding the host-parasite interactions that are overt as infectious diseases.

At the end of most chapters, a concluding section is devoted to questions yet unanswered. Problems that can be named represent, at best, only the interface between that which is known and the vastness yet unknown. The act of naming, however, requires a forward-facing attitude.

Discussion of infections caused by some protozoal and metazoal parasites are included. Rapid, global air travel and the worldwide involvement of the United States require such inclusive coverage.

Section XXIV, the last in the book, takes up several clinical entities that have attributes of infectious diseases but which have not been proved to be caused by living agents. Notable among omissions in this section is cancer. Leukemias, cancer of the breast, and sarcomas are the leading candidate malignancies for viral causation—mainly on the basis of analogy with observations of laboratory animals and certain RNA viruses. DNA viruses of the herpes group have also been implicated in human cancers. However, there is at present no proof of causation of any human cancer by a viral or other infectious agent.

Other omissions or abbreviated treatments of particular infectious diseases will be apparent to readers—in accord with their special interests and needs. Similarly, topics have been included that will appear to be superfluous to some readers. These faults are not attributable to contributors, reviewers, or the publisher, but are the editor's alone.

Acknowledgments

I am obliged most deeply to the contributors who—often with patience and forebearance—literally made this book possible. Many contributed to the first, the second, and now the third editions. The debt to such stalwarts is triply great.

For lack of space, many richly deserved acknowledgments of aid cannot be made individually. Citations of sources of illustrations and data, and references to published works are included and constitute at least token expressions of appreciation for such help.

The essential secretarial assistance of Mrs. Carol A. Edwards and Mrs. Mary Lou Mangum is gratefully acknowledged.

Several colleagues gave generously of their thoughts and time in discussing ways to improve this book and in reviewing typescript: Drs. Stuart H. Cohen, Sheila M. Nolan, and Michael G. Rinaldi.

The illustrations in color of the first edition—generously made possible through grants-in-aid from Burroughs Wellcome Company, Hoffman-LaRoche Incorporated, Eli Lilly and Company, Winthrop Laboratories, and Wyeth Laboratories—are incorporated in the third edition, as are the two pages of illustrations in color that were added to the second edition through the generous support of Schering Laboratories and the Upjohn Company.

In the course of the three years that the third edition has been in preparation, many persons on the staff of the Medical Department of Harper & Row have worked on it. Their able and patient assistance is gratefully acknowledged.

Contents

Section VI

PARENCHYMAL RESPIRATORY INFECTIONS

Section VII

PLEURAL INFECTIONS

Section VIII

INFRARENAL GENITOURINARY TRACT INFECTIONS

Section XII

INFECTIONS OF THE DIGESTIVE GLANDS

Section XIII

INFECTIONS OF THE PERITONEUM

Section XIV

INTEGUMENTARY INFECTIONS

Of all the diseases
to which man is heir, those
—known in etiology
—possible of cure
—capable of prevention
are, for the most part,
caused by infectious agents.

Color Plates

Plate 31-1. (*A*) Photomicrographs of Gram-stained smears of authentic specimens of lower respiratory tract secretions/exudates obtained from patients with pneumonias by transtracheal aspiration. (*1*) Pneumonia caused by *Mycoplasma pneumoniae.* (*2*) Pneumonia caused by *Streptococcus pneumoniae.* (*3*) Pneumonia caused by *Candida albicans.* (*B*) Oropharyngeal lesions. (*1*) Pharyngeal diphtheria. (Courtesy of R. V. McCloskey, MD) (*2*) Inflamed orifice of Stenson's duct in mumps parotitis. (*3*) Prodromal measles with Koplik's spots. (*C*) Drawings of photomicrographs of smears of urethral exudates from men with urethritis. (Jacobs NF, Kraus SJ: Gonococcal and non-gonococcal urethritis in men. Ann Intern Med 82:7–12, 1975) (*1*) Gonococcal urethritis—intracellular and extracellular gram-negative diplococci. (*2*) Equivocal smear—extracellular gram-negative diplococci and bacili. (*3*) Nongonococcal urethritis—gram-positive cocci, gram-negative bacilli, and no gram-negative diplococci. (*D*) Photomicrographs of gram-stained smears of sediment obtained by centrifuging cerebrospinal fluid obtained from patients with meningitis. (*1*) Meningitis caused by *Haemophilus influenzae.* (*2*) Meningitis caused by *Neisseria meningitidis.* (*3*) Meningitis caused by *Streptococcus pneumoniae.*

Color Plate 31-1

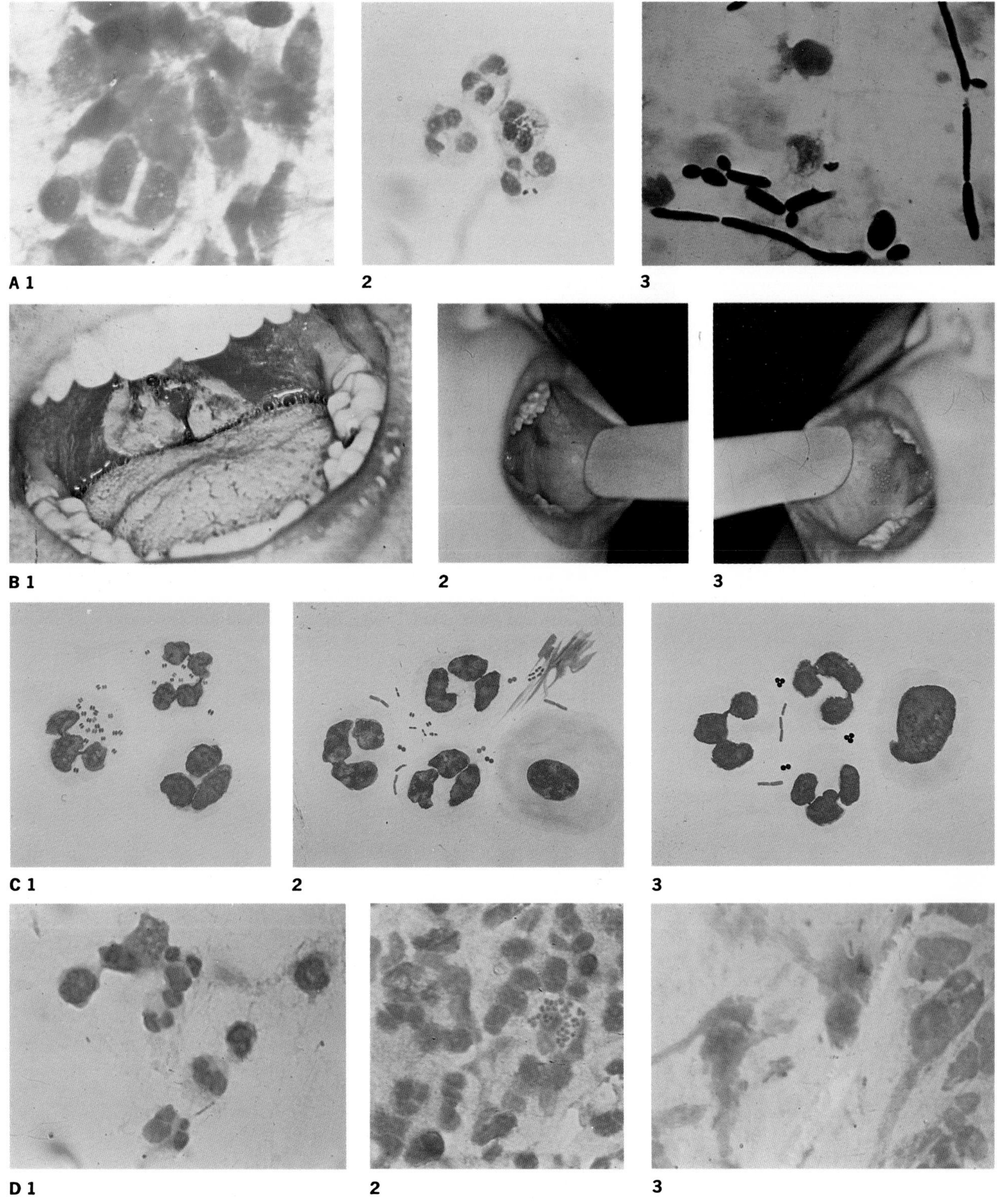

Plate 32-1. (*A*) Necrotizing pneumonia. Gram-stained smear of percutaneous transtracheal aspirate. Filamentous, pleomorphic gram-negative bacilli with swollen areas on the filaments *(Fusobacterium necrophorum)* are predominant. Next most prevalent are very small gram-negative coccobacilli *(Bacteroides melaninogenicus).* Also present are a few gram-positive diplococci *(Peptostreptococcus).* (Courtesy of John G. Bartlett, M.D.) *(B)* Necrotizing pneumonia. Gram-stained smear of a percutaneous transtracheal aspirate. Slightly pleomorphic gram-negative bacilli *(Fusobacterium* spp.*)* predominate. The long chains of cocci proved to be microaerophilic streptococci on culture. There were small numbers of somewhat elongated cocci *(Peptococcus* spp.*)* (Courtesy of John G. Bartlett, M.D.) *(C)* Aspiration pneumonia without cavitation. Gram-stained smear of percutaneous transtracheal aspirate. The large gram-positive bacilli at the bottom center of the field proved to be *Clostridium perfringens* on culture. A number of destained gram-positive cocci *(Peptococcus* spp.—appearing gram-negative) are present; two pairs lie just below the center of the field. *(D)* Peritonitis secondary to perforated duodenal ulcer. Gram-stained smear of peritoneal fluid. The large, broad gram-positive bacilli are characteristic of *Clostridium perfringens,* as recovered in culture. *(E)* Subphrenic abscess. Gram-stained smear of pus. The large, broad gram-negative bacilli were *Clostridium perfringens* (all gram-positive anaerobes tend to destain). The thin, delicate gram-negative filaments were *Fusobacterium nucleatum* (much more commonly found in infections above the diaphragm). Also present are two kinds of short, regular gram-negative bacilli—*Bacteroides fragilis* and *Escherichia coli.* *(F)* Appendiceal abscess. Gram-stained smear of pus. Three different kinds of gram-positive bacilli predominate in the smear. The pleomorphic rods were *Clostridium ramosum.* The other gram-positive anaerobic bacilli were *Clostridium perfringens* and *Eubacterium lentum.* Small numbers of gram-negative bacilli *(E. coli, B. fragilis, B. melaninogenicus,* and *Fusobacterium mortiferum)* were recovered, and some gram-positive cocci are present (microaerophilic cocci and *Peptostreptococcus* were recovered). *(G)* Pelvic abscess. Gram-stained smear of pus. Gram-positive cocci occurring singly and in pairs are predominant (microaerophilic streptococci were grown). Also present are a few slightly pleomorphic gram-negative bacilli (*B. fragilis* on culture). *(H)* Anaerobic myositis. Gram stain of muscle imprint preparation from patient pictured in Figure 156-1. *Clostridium septicum* was isolated from the amputated forequarter.

Color Plate 32-1

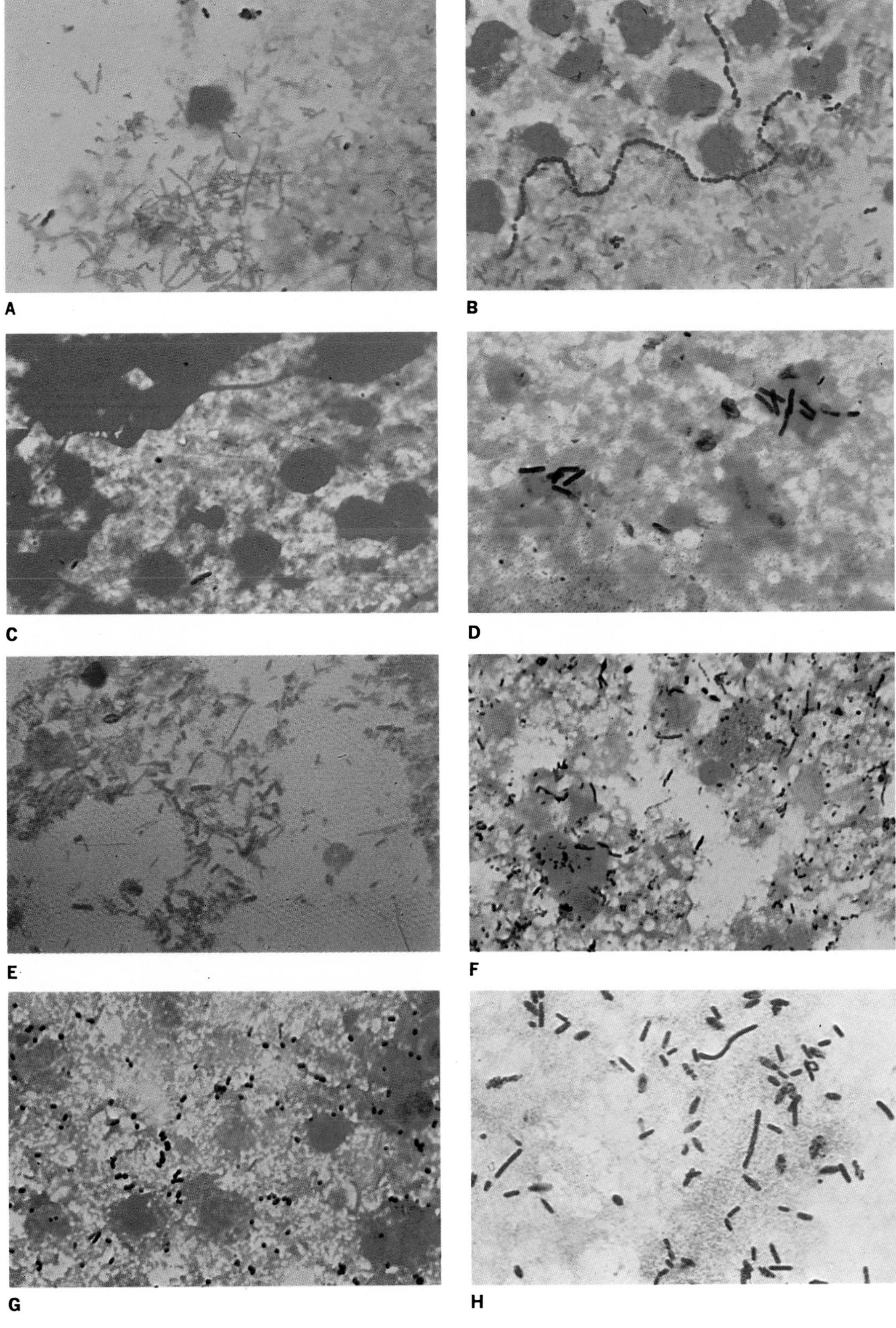

A B C D E F G H

Plate 52-1. (*A*) Gram stain of drop of uncentrifuged fresh urine (*Escherichia coli,* 1.7 × 10^6/ml). (Original magnification approximately × 1500) (*B*) Leukocyte cast, pyelonephritis (No stain; original magnification approximately × 400) (Nutley NJ: Urine Under the Microscope. Hoffmann-La Roche) (*C*) Leukocyte cast, chronic pyelonephritis (Peroxidase stain, original magnification approximately × 400) (*D*) Leukocyte cast, chronic glomerulonephritis (peroxidase stain, original magnification approximately × 400) (*E*) Leukocyte cast, disseminated lupus erythematosus (Peroxidase stain, original magnification aproximately × 400) (*F*) Erythrocyte cast as seen in acute hemorrhagic glomerulonephritis (Sternheimer–Malbin stain, original magnification approximately × 400) (*G*) Streptococcal impetigo contagiosa involving the leg of a child who had acute hemorrhagic glomerulonephritis.

Color Plate 52-1

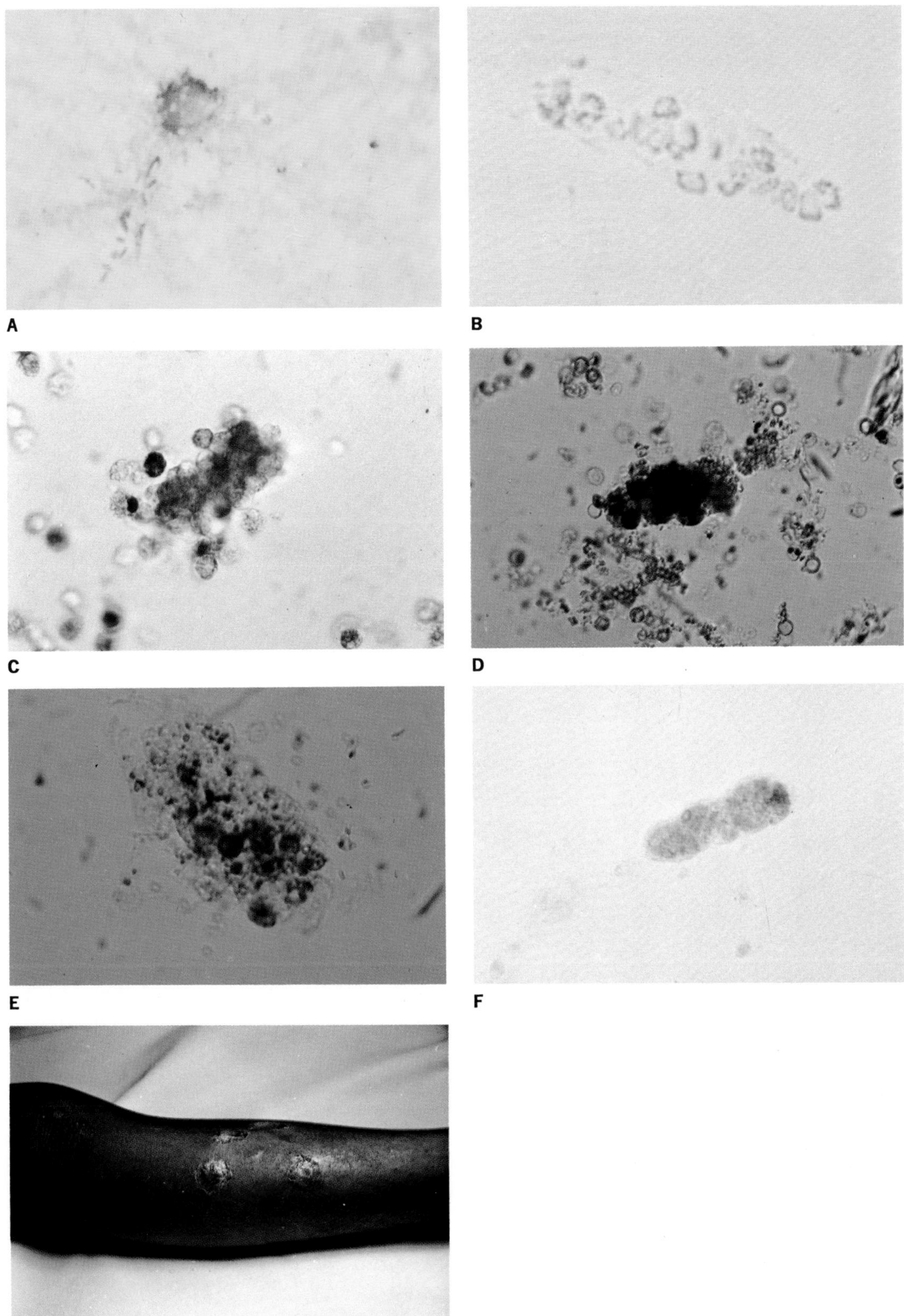

Plate 68-1. The eggs and larvae of some of the important enteric and enteric-associated parasites of humans as they appear in clinical specimens.

Color Plate 68-1

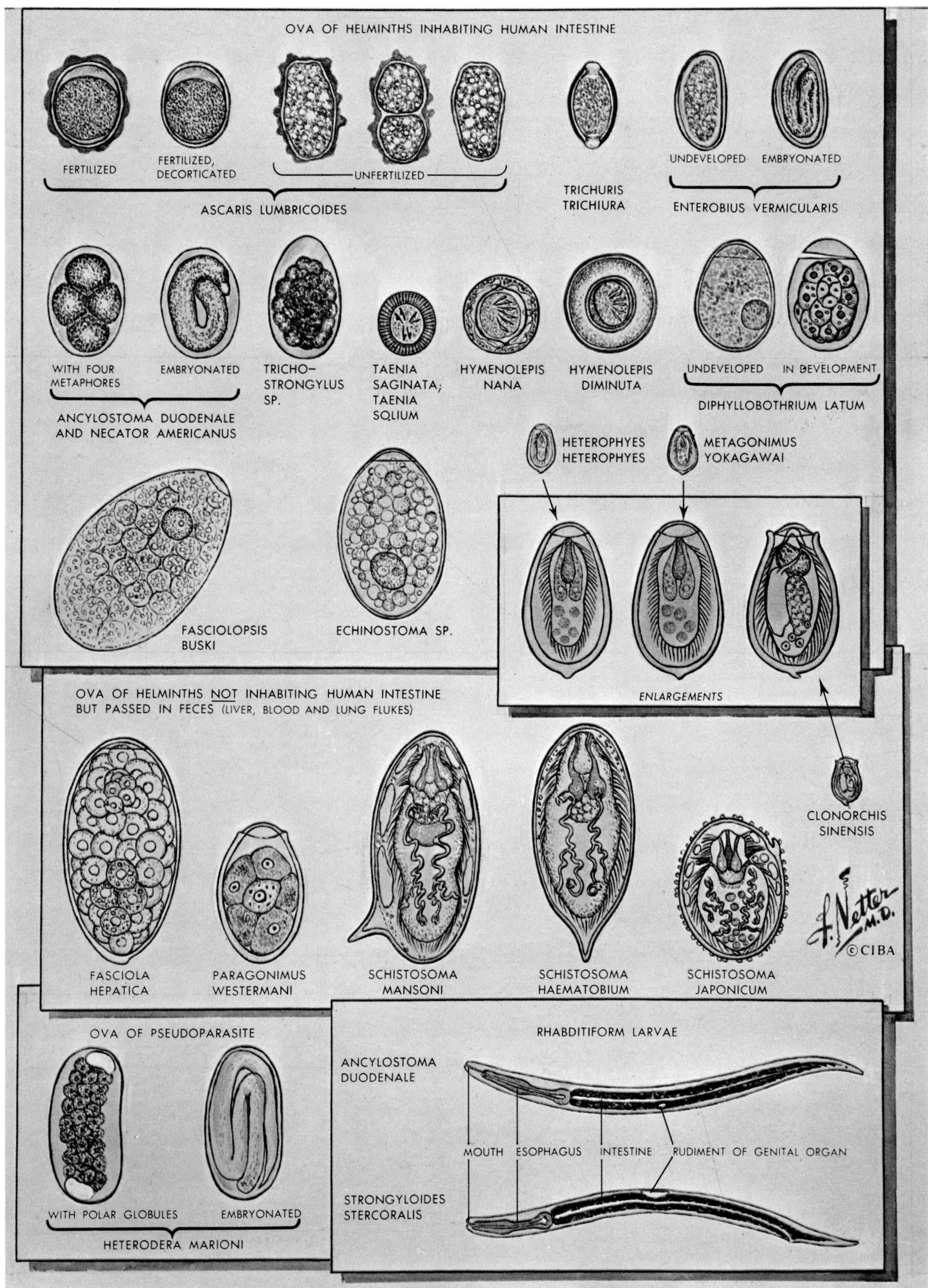

Plate 91-1. Lesions caused by herpes simplex virus (HSV) in man. (*A*) Gingivostomatitis (HSV 1), the most common clinically manifest herpetic infection of children. Herpetic lesions on the thumb probably resulted from thumb sucking. (*B*) Labial herpes (HSV 1) with iris lesions of erythema multiforme, a feature of every recurrence. (*C*) Eczema herpeticum (HSV 1), recurrent despite high titers of neutalizing antibodies in the serum. An underlying Wiskott–Aldrich syndrome was also responsible for thrombocytopenia manifest in the hemorrhagic nature of the lesions. (*D*) Penile herpes (HSV 2) with typical clusters of vesicles; this patient's consort had herpetic cervicitis. (*E*) Herpetic cervicitis (HSV 2) with ulcerations. In most cases, there are no characteristic lesions. (*F*) A multinucleated giant cell in Papanicolaou cervicovaginal smear with intranuclear inclusion bodies (HSV 2). (*G*) Neonatal herpes (HSV 2) with chorioretinitis and encephalitis in an infant born to a woman with genital herpes around the time of delivery. (*H*) Numerous intranuclear inclusions in brain in fatal herpetic encephalitis.

Color Plate 91-1

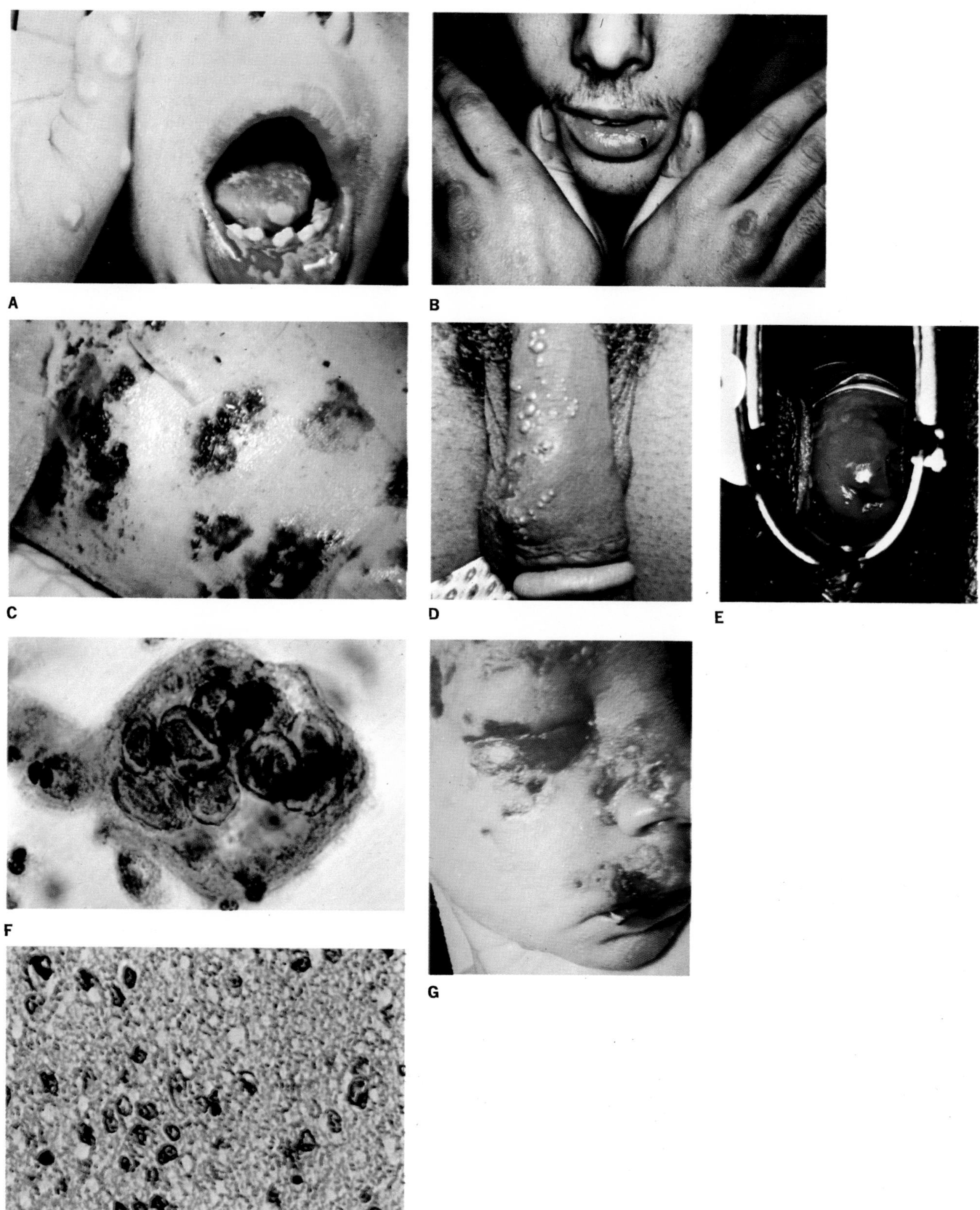

Plate 92-1. (*A*) The skin lesions of smallpox mature as a single crop. In this patient, pustulation was underway 6 days after onset of the rash. (*B*) Pustules, all in the same stage of development, are round, smooth-edged, and deep in the skin. (*C*) The lesions of chickenpox evolve in 24–28 hours; lesions in all stages of development are present in a single area of skin. (*D*) The skin lesions of monkeypox are remarkably similar to those of smallpox. (*A, B,* and *D* courtesy of the World Health Organizations; *C* courtesy of the Centers for Disease Control)

Color Plate 92-1

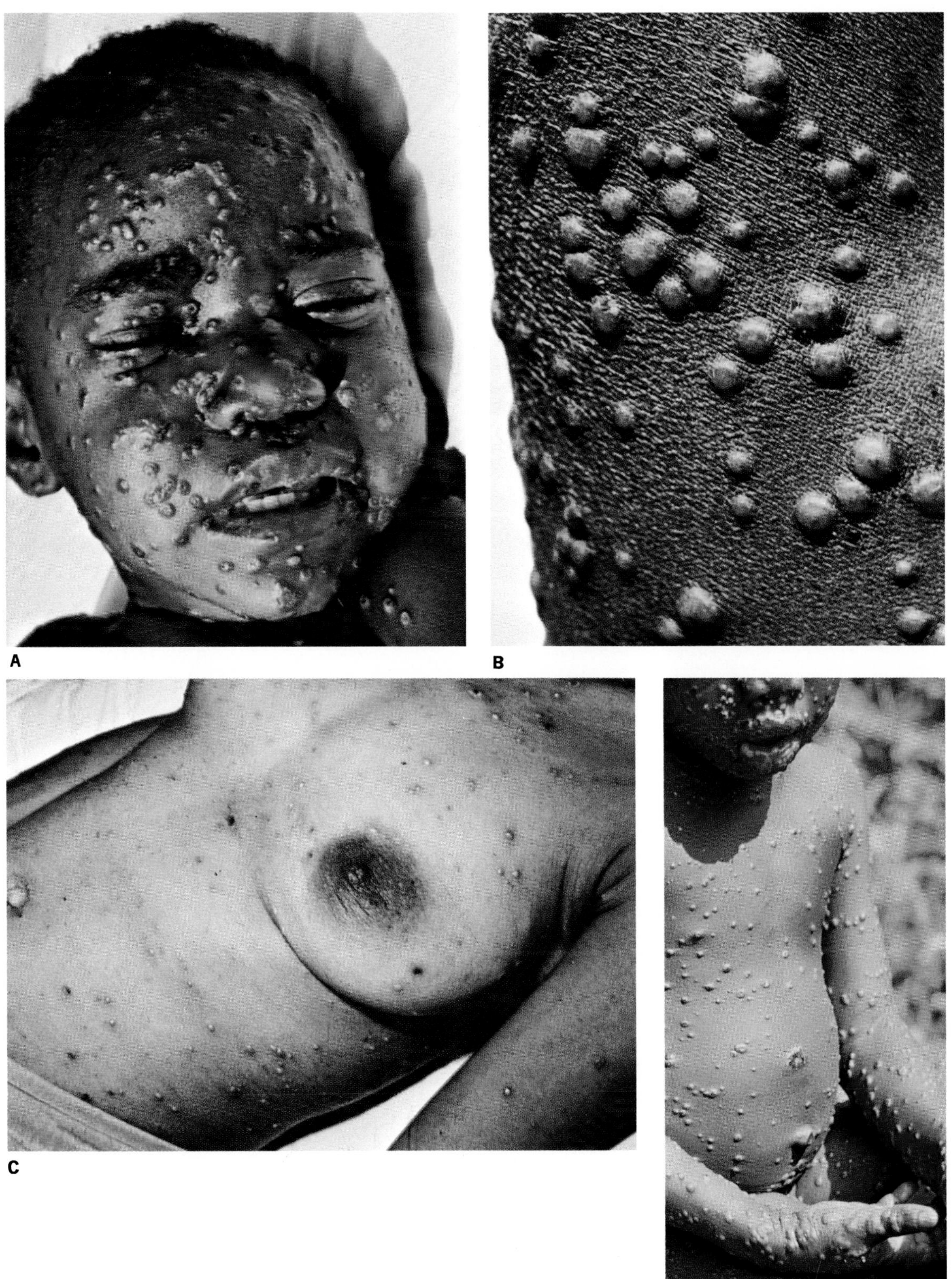

A B C D

Plate 92-2. (*A*) Successful primary vaccination evolves over a 2-week period. (*B*) Late revaccination often elicits a reaction of delayed hypersensitivity in 24–72 hours, regardless of the potency of the vaccine. If viral replication occurs (potent vaccine), the classic skin lesion evolves over a 1- to 2-week period after vaccination. (Courtesy of the Centers for Disease Control)

Color Plate 92-2

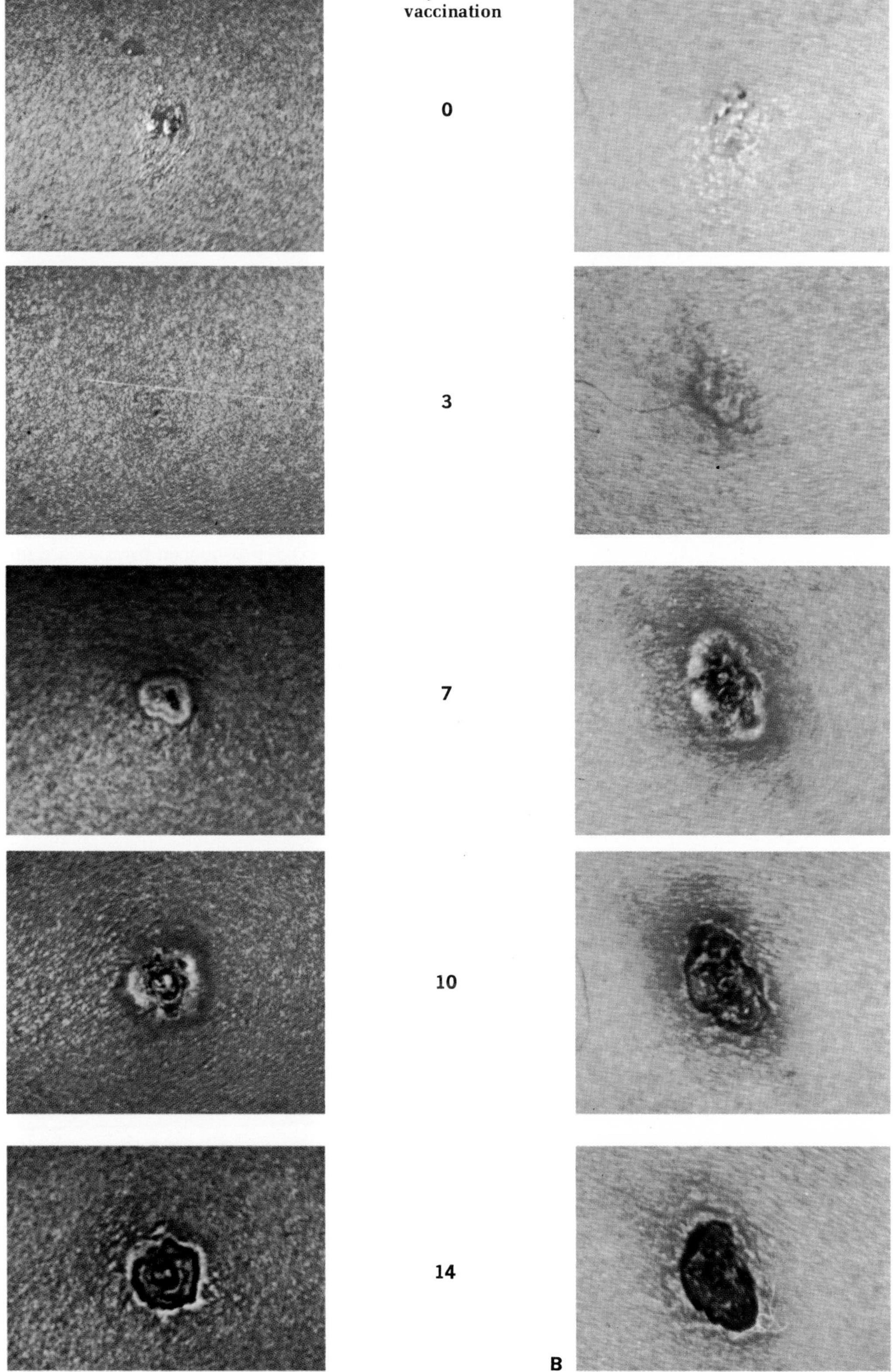

Plate 145-1. Diagnosis of malaria by thin blood film. Students and even some experienced microscopists prefer thin blood films to thick smears for malaria diagnosis. Four species of malaria are identified by alterations in infected red cells and by the morphology of asexual and sexual erythrocytic stages. Giemsa-stained parasites consist of blue cytoplasm, red nucleus and brown to black malarial pigment, hemozoin. (*A–D*) *Plasmodium falciparum.* Usually only ring forms are found in peripheral blood. Although rings are observed in all malarias, the tenuous nature of the cytoplasm and the double nuclei in *P. falciparum* are characteristic. The novice may overlook these fine rings. Appliqué forms, rings adherent to the red cell membrane, are commonly observed in *P. falciparum*. Mature rings that contain thicker cytoplasm are also present. Multiple invasion of red cells is more common than in other malarias, in part because falciparum malaria has the highest parasitemia. Mature trophozoites and schizonts are lacking in peripheral blood except during high parasitemia, when all stages may be observed. The patient whose blood film is shown in (*C*) had a 30% parasitemia, renal failure, jaundice, and cerebral malaria. Note two rings in same field as the schizont. Red cells containing asexual forms are not enlarged but may be discolored and contain a few red dots, Maurer's clefts. After the first week of infection, characteristic crescent- or banana-shaped gametocytes are found in the blood smear (*D*) (*E–H*) *Plasmodium vivax*. Infected red cell is larger than surrounding erythrocytes and has eosinophilic stippling. Note Schüffner's dots. Although Schüffner's dots may not always be evident, characteristic enlargement and paling of the erythrocyte will still be observed (*F*). Ring form may be difficult to distinguish from *P. falciparum* (*E*), but careful search of thick and thin blood films should demonstrate other stages, even in a synchronized infection. Trophozoite cytoplasm is more ameboid than in *P. malariae* or *P. ovale* (*F*). Mature schizonts contain 12 to 14 merozoites (*G*), whereas the number of schizont merozoites of *P. ovale* never exceeds 16. Round gametocyte is similar to *P. ovale* and *P. malariae;* however, Schüffner's dots and enlarged red cell differentiate it from *P. malariae* (*H*). (*I–L*) *Plasmodium malariae.* Erythrocytes that contain parasites are unchanged. The ring may be confused with *P. falciparum,* but other stages are usually present. The cytoplasm of trophozoites is compact and may extend in a band across red cell (*I*). However, the cytoplasm may be more rounded or irregular (*J*). Schizonts are easily differentiated from *P. vivax* and *P. ovale* by lack of Schüffner's dots (*K*). Mature schizonts contain 6 to 12 merozoites, occasionally in a rosette around central malaria pigment. As in *P. vivax,* the gametocytes are round (*L*). *M–O. Plasmodium ovale.* Infected red cell contains Schüffner's dots and may be oval in shape (*M*) with fimbriated edges (*M* and *O*). The trophozoite cytoplasm is compact (*M*) and mature schizont contains 6 to 16 merozoites (*N*). Gametocytes are round (*O*). (*P*) Platelet on a red cell, which is identified by a characteristic halo around the platelet; may be confused with a malaria parasite. (Colorplate by LH Miller and I Nathan) (Giemsa stain, original magnification approximately × 1350)

Color Plate 145-1

Plasmodium falciparum

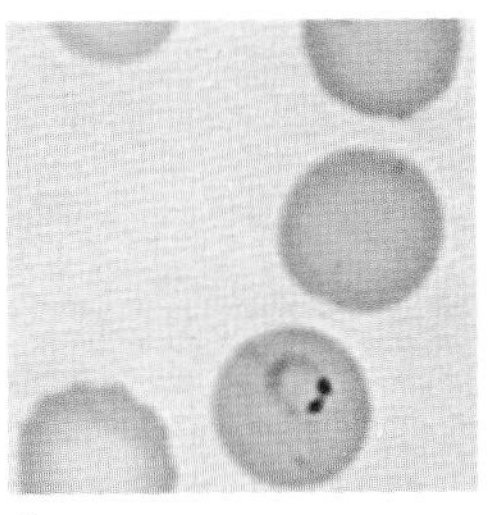
A

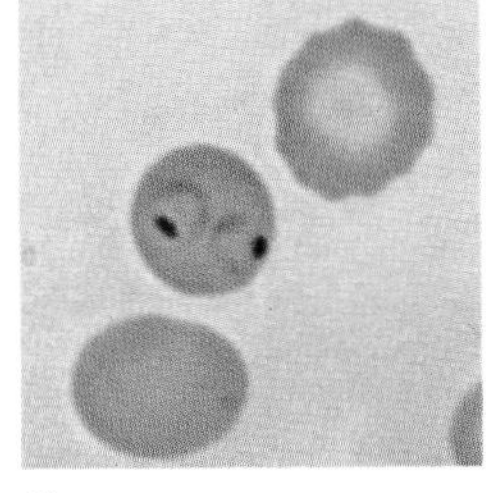
B

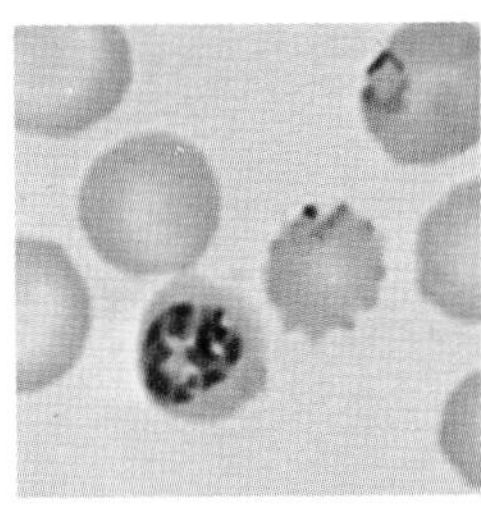
C

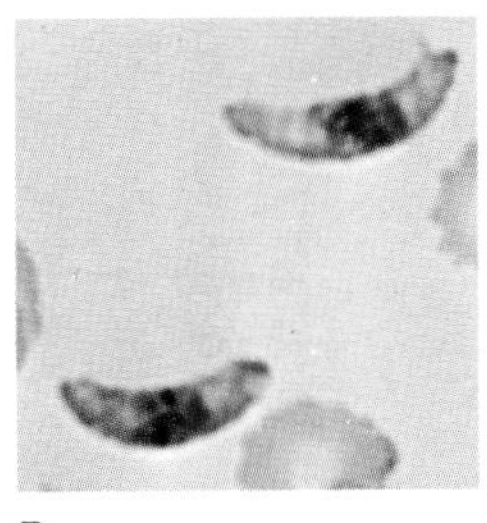
D

Plasmodium vivax

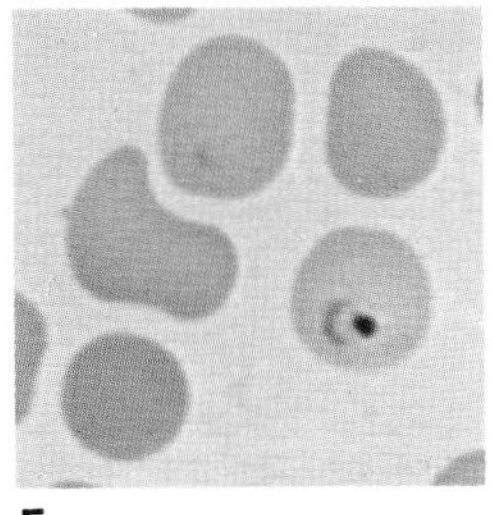
E

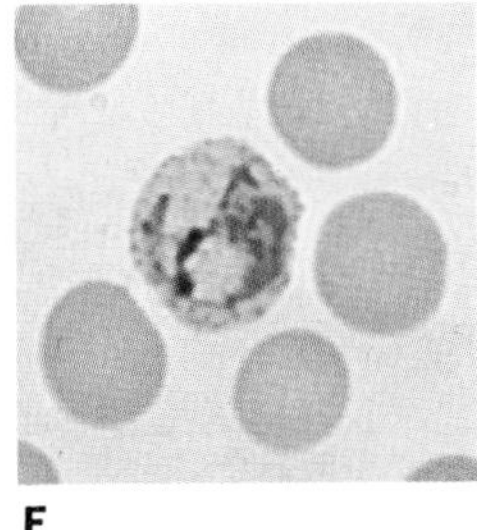
F

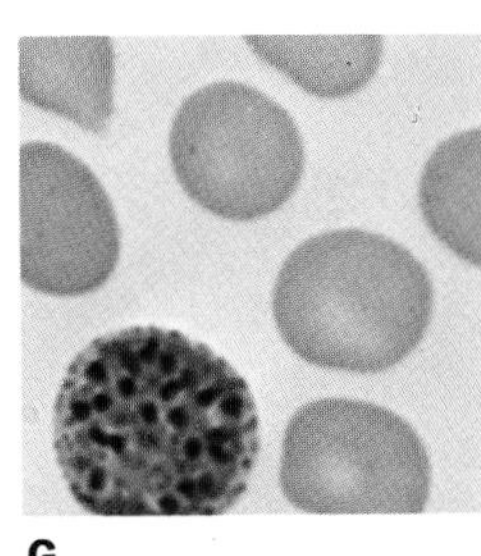
G

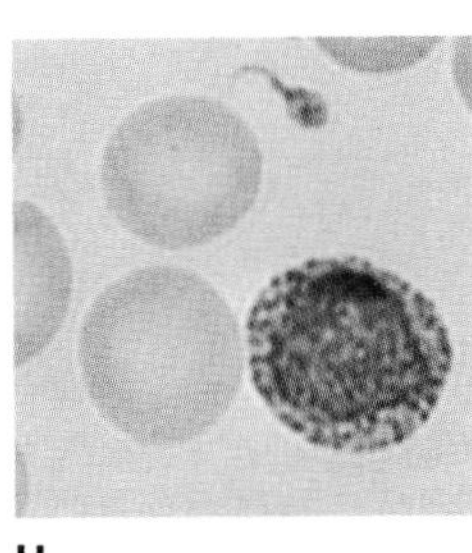
H

Plasmodium malariae

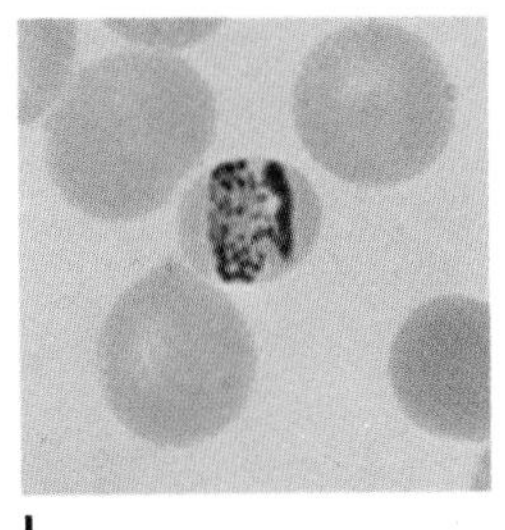
I

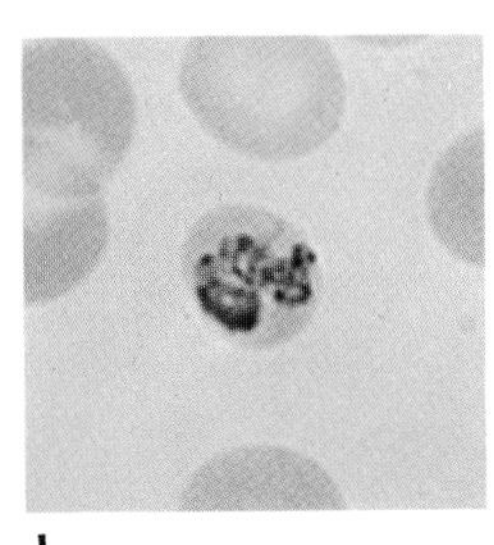
J

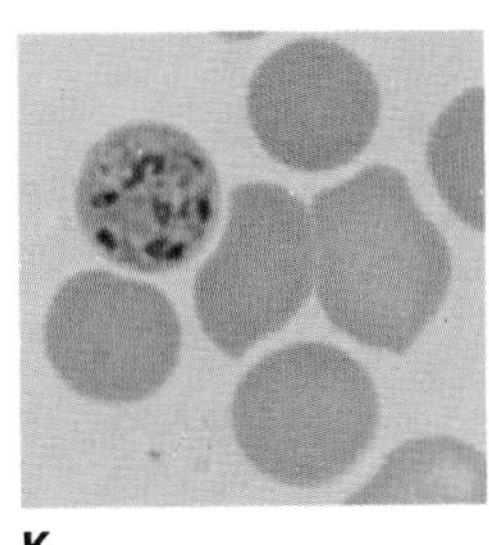
K

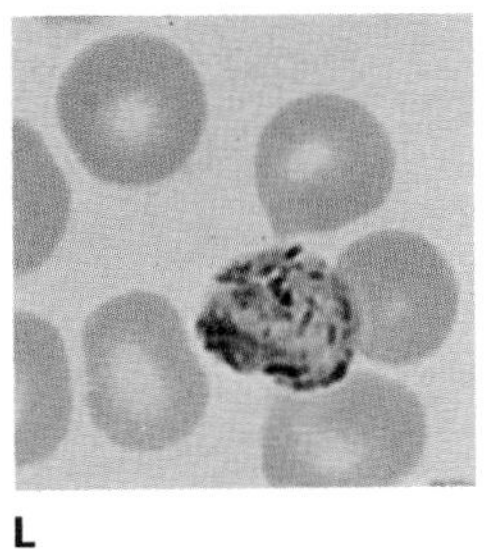
L

Plasmodium ovale

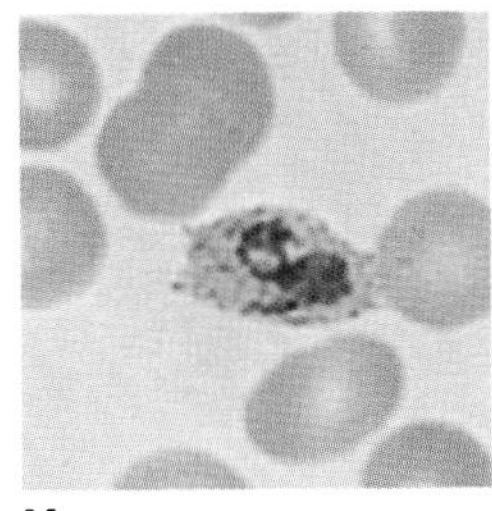
M

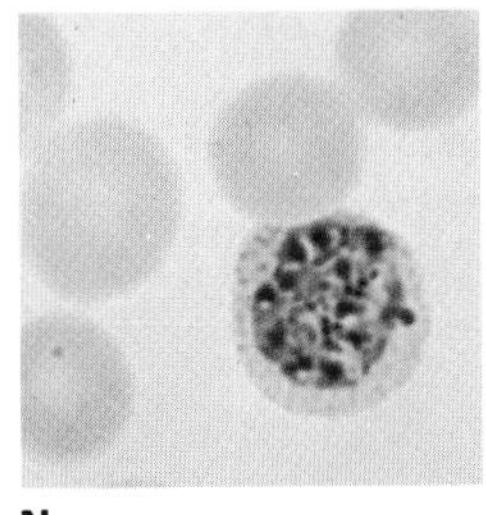
N

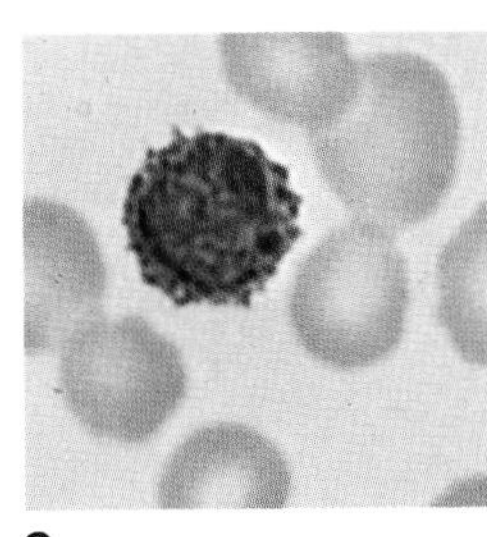
O

Platelet on RBC

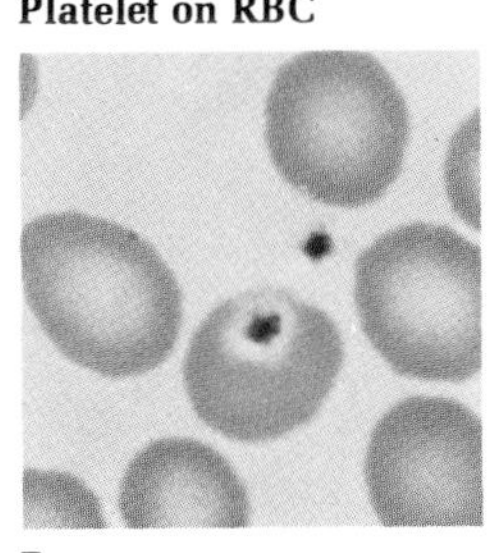
P

Infectious Diseases

Section I

General Considerations

ROBERT S. CHANG
BLAINE L. BEAMAN
MICHAEL G. RINALDI
JEROLD H. THEIS

Attributes of Infectious Agents

1

Infectious agents are environmental organisms that are capable of multiplying in or on the host and provoking responses in the host. The host responses to an infectious agent may be immunologic, inflammatory, or degenerative. A typical example is the influenza virus. After deposition on the respiratory epithelium of a susceptible host, the virus multiplies within epithelial cells, elicits specific immunologic responses, induces degeneration of the infected cells, and provokes inflammation at the site of infection. A less typical example is *Clostridum botulinum.* This bacterium induces botulism through the action of a powerful neurotoxin. Generally, adult humans acquire botulism through the ingestion of preformed botulinal toxin; since multiplication of *C. botulinum* within the host is not a prerequisite for the development of the disease, botulism is usually not infectious. However, in two special circumstances, botulism is an infectious disease as a result of absorption of toxin elaborated during multiplication of *C. botulinum* within the host: in adults when traumatically inoculated *C. botulinum* proliferates deep in wounds; in infants when ingested *C. botulinum* proliferates in the gut.

It is not known how many environmental agents are infectious for humans. A rough estimate would place the number in the thousands. Students of medicine often find it difficult to learn and retain information fundamental to working with infectious agents. In large part, this difficulty stems from the great number and the heterogeneity of these agents. Also, the lack of a sound basis for defining species and the difficulty of establishing phylogenetic relationships among species are contributory and aggravating factors. Finally, there is the constantly changing classification, including the tendency to apply commemorative or exotic names that convey no insight into the nature of microorganisms as, for example, *Francisella tularensis and Coxiella burnetii.* There is a distinct need for a rational scheme of classificaton and nomenclature that can serve as a framework for the organization of present knowledge and additional information as it is acquired.

In this chapter, infectious agents of humans are arbitrarily placed in groups and subgroups arranged in a sequence of increasing complexity of organization proceeding from acellular, through unicellular, to multicellular parasites (see list below). In describing the characteristics of these groups, emphasis is placed on those aspects pertinent to identification, pathogenesis, and intervention.

Acellular

Prions

Prions are small proteinaceous infectious agents resistant to inactivation by most procedures that

INFECTIOUS AGENTS THAT PARASITIZE HUMANS, ARRANGED IN ORDER OF INCREASING COMPLEXITY OF ORGANIZATION

Acellular
- Prions (<5 nm)
- Viroids (<5 nm)
- Viruses (20 nm–200 nm)

Unicellular
- Prokaryotic cells (200 nm–2000 nm)
  - Chlamydias
  - Mycoplasmas
  - Rickettsias
  - Bacteria
- Eukaryotic cells (>2000 nm)
  - Fungi
  - Protoza

Multicellular
- Helminths
- Arthropods

modify nucleic acids. That is, their chemical characteristics fit neither viroids nor viruses, but underscore the requirement of a protein for infection—without excluding the possible presence of a small bit of nucleic acid within the particle. The term was coined for the scrapie agent. However, the "unconventional viruses" that cause transmissible virus dementia (Creutzfeldt–Jakob disease) and kuru share many characteristics with the scrapie agent, and it is quite possible that they are also prions. Little is known of how prions replicate and induce disease.

Viroids

Viroids are low-molecular-weight nucleic acids that have the properties of infectious agents. One well-characterized viroid, the potato spindle tuber viroid, consists of a naked molecule of RNA with a molecular weight of only about 10^5 daltons. Except for its length, this viroid is morphologically indistinguishable from other nucleic acids (Fig. 1-1).

Many attributes of viroids can be deduced from the fact that they are naked molecules of RNA with low molecular weights. Being small in size, viroids are much more resistant to inactivation by ultraviolet and ionizing radiation than are all other infectious agents. Having no protein, viroids are less susceptible to inactivation by heat and formalin than are all other infectious agents. Pure, natural nucleic acids are not immunogenic; viroids do not provoke specific immune responses in the host.

Assuming that the dogma of nonoverlapping of the genetic code is correct, the genome of a viroid such as the potato spindle tuber viroid can code for at most 95 amino acids. A polypeptide with only 95 amino acids is unlikely to have RNA replicase activity. Because the host cell does not have RNA replicase and cannot synthesize RNA from RNA, it is difficult to visualize how a viroid replicates within the host cell. Presumably, viroids replicate by a unique process that is different from all other forms of life.

Since viroids do not provoke specific immune responses in the host, infections caused by viroids should progress inexorably. There is as yet no direct proof that viroids induce diseases in humans.

Fig. 1-1. Electron micrograph of a viroid (potato spindle tuber viroid). Scale line = 200 nanometers. (Sogo JM, Koller T, Diener TO: Virology 55:74, 1973)

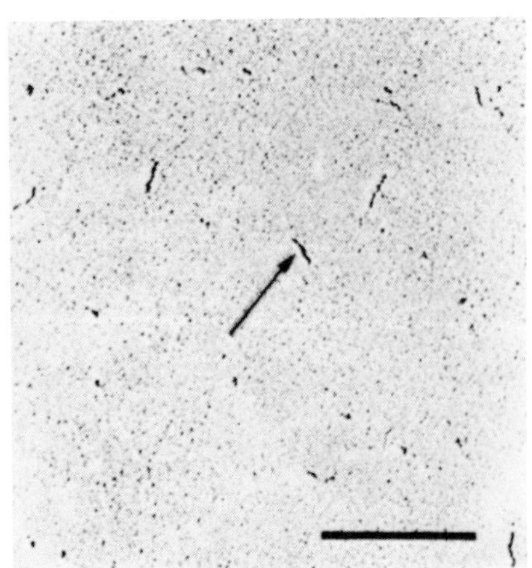

Viruses

GENERAL CHARACTERISTICS

Viruses are a heterogenous group of submicroscopic, subcellular, filterable agents that vary from 20 nm to 200 nm in size and consist of a central core of nucleic acid wrapped in a coat of protein that may, in turn, be surrounded by a lipoprotein membrane. The nucleic acid of an individual virus is of one type only, either DNA or RNA, with RNA much more common among viruses pathogenic for humans. Energy-generating and biosynthetic mechanisms are lacking in viruses; therefore, viral replication requires the active participation of host cells.

Constancy of size and form is an essential characteristic of any population of organisms, and viruses qualify as organisms in this respect. However, with viruses, such constancy is generally a property of a "species" or group of viruses, and the different groups vary widely in size and shape. Hence, size and shape are important characteristics in classifying viruses. The smallest virus, such as the adenosatellite virus, measures only about 20 nm in diameter; the largest, such as the poxviruses, measure about 250 nm × 350 nm. Many so-called species of virus are spherical; others are shaped like rods, bricks, bullets, or tadpoles.

The structural components of a virus particle (virion) consist of the following: (1) a central core of nucleic acid (nucleoid); (2) a protein coat (capsid); and (3) an outermost lipoprotein membrane (envelope), which is found only in certain groups of viruses. The nucleoid and the capsid are often referred to as the nucleocapsid. Analysis of the structure of a virus particle shows the following three basic symmetries: cubic (also known as icosahedral or spherical), helical, and complex (Figs. 1-2, 1-3). Nucleocapsid symmetry is also important in the classification of viruses.

The capsid of the simplest viruses (*e.g.,* RNA bacte-

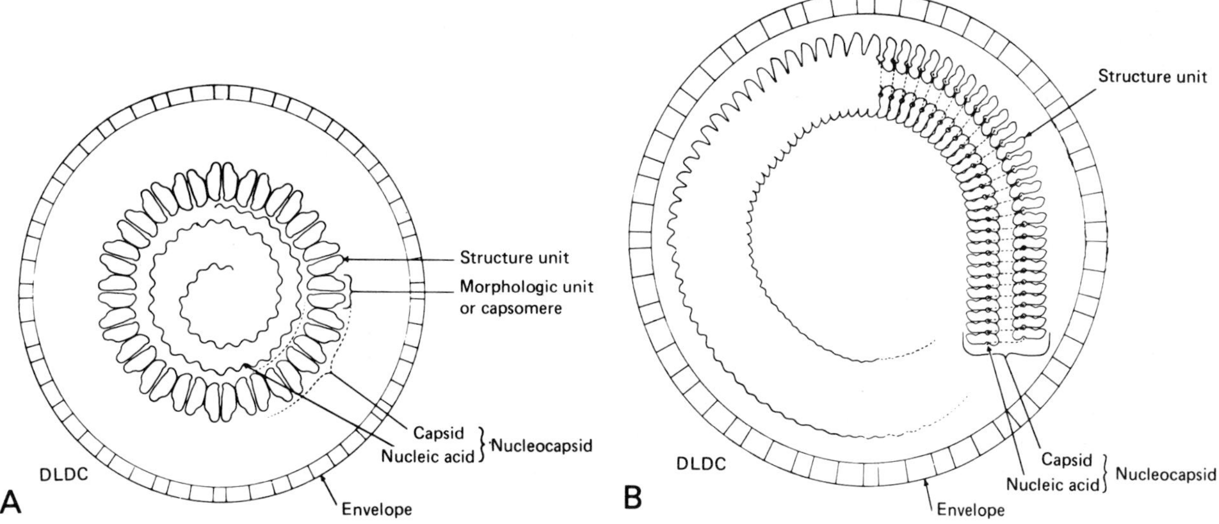

Fig. 1-2. Viruses in cross section. *(A)* Virus with spherical, cuboidal, or icosahedral symmetry. *(B)* Virus with helical symmetry. (Casper DLD, Dulbecco R, Klug A, Lwoff A, Stoker MGP, Lournier P, Wildy P: Cold Spring Harbor Symp Quant Biol 27:50–51, 1962)

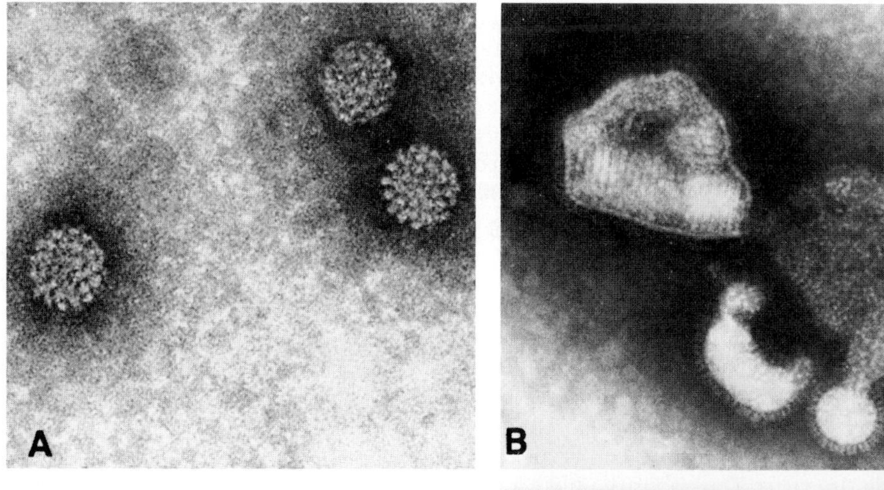

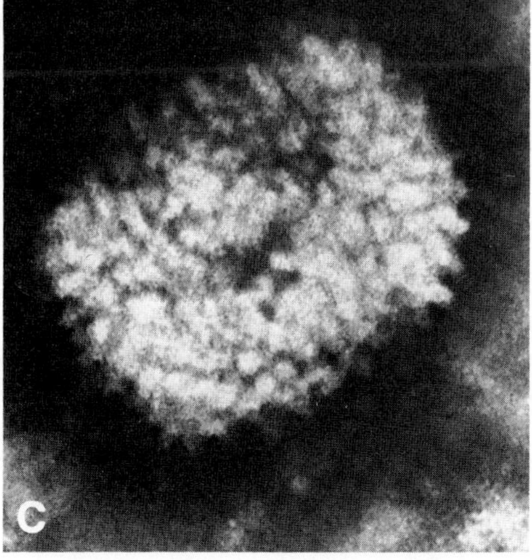

Fig. 1-3. *(A)* Human wart virus (cubic symmetry, nonenveloped). *(B)* Influenza virus (helical symmetry, enveloped). *(C)* Vaccinia virus (complex symmetry). (Madely CR: Virus Morphology. Baltimore, Williams & Wilkins, 1972)

riophages) is made up of one or more varieties of polypeptides (structural units) that fold and attach to one another to form morphologic units (capsomeres), which aggregate into capsids (Figs. 1-2, 1-3*A*). The number of capsomeres is believed to be constant for each virus with cubic symmetry (*e.g.,* 252 for the adenovirus and 32 for the poliovirus) and is an important criterion in the classification of viruses.

Many larger viruses (>70 nm) also contain internal proteins, some of which have polymerase activity that is essential for the replication of viral genes. Smaller viruses do not contain polymerases within the virion.

The nucleic acids of small viruses may be rendered free of other components through chemical extraction. These "naked" nucleic acids are still capable of initiating a cycle of viral replication. In contrast to the whole virus, the naked viral nucleic acid is (1) not neutralized by specific antibody; (2) extremely sensitive to nucleases that are ubiquitous in most biologic environments; (3) able to initiate a cycle of replication in certain host cells ordinarily insusceptible to the whole virus; and (4) low in efficiency of infection. As a corollary, the protein coat (capsid) of a virus (1) determines serologic specificity; (2) protects the nucleic acid from enzymatic degradation in biologic environments; (3) controls host specificity; and (4) increases the efficiency of infection. The nucleic acid of the smallest virus consists of one molecule of polynucleotide with about 3000 nucleotides, which have the capacity of coding for three polypeptides.

The outermost lipoprotein membrane of the enveloped viruses is essential for the attachment to, and penetration of, host cells. Removing the envelope renders the virus (nucleocapsid) noninfectious. The envelope also contains important viral antigens.

The key difference between a large complex virus and the simplest prokaryotic cell is the lack of ribosomes in the virus. Thus, a virus, unlike a prokaryotic or eukaryotic cell, cannot synthesize its own proteins.

REPLICATION

Purified suspensions of viruses do not glycolyze, respirate, or synthesize. The virus can only provide the genetic material for viral replication, and the host cell provides the biosynthetic and energy-generating mechanisms. Thus, virus replication requires the active participation of the host cell.

Unlike obligatory intracellular prokaryotic or eukaryotic parasites, which maintain their morphologic integrity during multiplication, virus multiplication involves the disassembly of the virion into components, the synthesis of viral components, and the assembly of newly synthesized components into progeny virions.

The replication of poliovirus in cultures of primate cells has been studied in considerable detail, and it is described here to illustrate virus multiplication. The replication process may be conveniently described in the following three phases: (1) initiation of infection; (2) synthetic phase; and (3) maturation and release.

Initiation of Infection. This phase consists of the following three steps: attachment, penetration, and uncoating

Attachment. Viruses attach to the host cell surface through physical contact with specific viral receptors. The configurations of the attachment site of a virus and the viral receptor on the cell surface are complementary. Once viruses are attached they can no longer be removed by washing the host cells, but the viruses remain susceptible to inactivation by specific antiserum. The process of attachment is independent of temperature. Cells without receptors for a specific virus are not susceptible to infection by that virus; this fact may explain, in part, the tissue tropism of certain viruses. Specific antibodies inactivate viruses primarily by preventing viruses from attaching onto viral receptors of the host cell.

Penetration. The optimum temperature for penetration by most viruses is approximately 37°C. It is not known how a virus penetrates a cell, but pinocytosis may play a role. Once inside host cells, viruses are insusceptible to the action of antibodies. For a brief time after penetration, intact virus particles can be recovered through disruption of host cells.

Uncoating. Following penetration, the virion is uncoated through the separation of the capsid and nucleoid as a result of the action of host cell enzyme(s). Cell disruption no longer yields infectious virions. The naked viral gene is now within the cell and is ready to enter into the synthetic phase.

Synthetic Phase. The central goals of the synthetic phase are the production of many copies of viral genomes and viral messenger RNA (mRNA). Host ribosomes will then translate viral mRNA into viral proteins, including capsid proteins. When the two viral components (genome and capsid proteins) reach critical concentrations, the components will assemble into virions.

The genome of poliovirus is a single strand of RNA

that can also serve as mRNA; because the host cell does not have RNA replicase (an enzyme for synthesizing RNA using RNA as a template), the logical first step in the synthetic phase must be the translation of the poliovirus genome by host ribosomes into viral proteins. Among the newly formed viral proteins is the RNA replicase, which then synthesizes many copies of the viral genome. This synthesis is achieved by forming several copies of RNA complementary in base sequences (minus strand) to the viral genome, and then many copies of plus strands (identical to the viral genome) using minus strands as templates.

Virus-specific polymerases are suitable targets for antiviral chemicals because it is theoretically possible to devise a chemical that will inactivate virus-specific, but not host-specific, polymerases. For intervention in the sequence of RNA virus replication, the ideal target for antiviral antimicrobics would be the RNA-dependent RNA polymerase (RNA replicase) because this enzyme has no function and is not present in uninfected host cells. Unfortunately, a chemical capable of specifically inhibiting RNA replicase has not yet been discovered.

Although the translation of viral mRNA depends entirely on the translating mechanism of the host cell, there must be significant differences between the translation of viral mRNA and host mRNA. This follows from the fact that interferons induce virus-inhibitory protein(s) in the host cell, which interfere with the translation of viral mRNA. At therapeutic concentrations, interferons inhibit the growth of all viruses to varying degrees, but they exert inconsequential interference with cellular functions.

Maturation and Release. The formation of a complete virion from its components is known as maturation. From experiments with bacterial viruses, maturation occurs by self-assembly. That is, simply mixing the viral components (capsid proteins and viral genomes) in sufficiently high concentrations *in vitro* automatically results in the formation of virions. Hence, it is surmised that poliovirions form automatically when the intracellular concentrations of capsid proteins and RNA reach critical levels.

Progeny virions are released when the infected cell disintegrates. Under optimal conditions *in vitro,* a cell releases several thousand progeny virions within 4 hours after infection by poliovirus.

Replication of other viruses is generally similar to that described for the polioviruses. However, if the nature of the viral genome is different, the pathway of viral mRNA formation is also different. Also, if a virus is enveloped, the process of penetration, maturation, and release differs significantly from that of the nonenveloped polioviruses.

The genome of influenza virus is a minus single-strand RNA that cannot serve as the virus mRNA. It must first be transcribed into the plus strand. This critical step is achieved through preformed RNA replicase, which is an essential component of the virion.

The genome of DNA viruses is transcribed in two distinct stages: early and late. Early genes are transcribed by the host's enzymes and yield virus-specific polypeptides, some of which are essential for the transcription of late genes. Late genes are transcribed only after early gene products have reached a sufficiently high concentration. The replication of viral DNA depends on products of late genes. Under certain circumstances, the transcription of late genes may be inhibited. For example, when a B-lymphocyte is infected by the Epstein–Barr virus, the early viral genes are transcribed by the host cell's enzymes, but the transcription of late viral genes is blocked by host factors of unknown nature. This results in a lymphocyte that contains a few copies of the viral genome and virus-specific antigens (products of early genes), which is incapable of releasing progeny viruses. Interestingly, this infected lymphocyte has also acquired the capability of rapid and persistent multiplication *in vitro,* a characteristic not shared by uninfected B-lymphocytes.

The maturation of an enveloped virus involves the additional step of formation of a lipoprotein envelope around the nucleocapsid. The host cell membrane at the replicating site is modified by the replacement of host proteins with viral proteins and by the aggregation of another viral protein (M protein) on its inner surface. The nucleocapsid then buds through the modified membrane, which becomes the viral envelope. By this process, progeny virions may be released without cell death, although the infected cell may be recognized by the host's immune system as a foreign cell because of virus-specific proteins on its surface.

CLASSIFICATION

Hundreds of viruses are infectious for humans. A meaningful scheme of classification is exceedingly important for the purpose of identifying relationships and as an aid in memorizing important characteristics. Three schemes of classification, based on epidemiologic, clinical, or basic characteristics, have been proposed. Unfortunately, no single scheme has proved satisfactory for students of infectious diseases. Despite many shortcomings, a classification scheme that relates to basic characteristics of the virion appears to have gained increasing acceptance. Viruses are placed in groups or families according to morphology (size, shape, and symmetry of nucleocapsid; the presence of an envelope; and the number of capsomeres) and the chemical nature of genomes (DNA or RNA; single- or double-stranded; plus or minus strands). After viruses are grouped into families, biologic and antigenic characteristics common to each family are used for further classification.

There are 15 recognized families or groups of viruses that are infectious for humans (Table 1-1 and Fig. 1-4). Attempts to devise Linneaen binomial names for viruses have not gained wide acceptance. Consequently, both vernacular and group names are used (Table 1-2). Thus, smallpox vaccine contains the vaccinia virus (vernacular name), which is a poxvirus (family name); also, polioviruses (vernacular) are picornaviruses (family).

Unicellular

Infectious unicellular microorganisms may be divided into two broad groups according to their structural complexity and intracytoplasmic compartmentalization. Chlamydias, mycoplasmas, rickettsias, and bacteria are prokaryotic, whereas fungi, protozoa, and algae are eukaryotic.

With cell diameters that are usually less than 1 μm, prokaryotic cells are generally smaller than eukaryotic cells. However, there is considerable variation in size among different species, and both size and shape are influenced by the environment. The fundamental differences between prokaryotic and eukaryotic cells are summarized in Table 1-3.

Prokaryotes

The lumping of prokaryotes together as bacteria is favored by their common lack of a discrete nucleus. Further, the microbiologist may view the differences between *Chlamydia trachomatis* and *Excherichia coli* as being no greater than the differences between *E. coli* and *Mycobacterium leprae.* Yet, the chlamydias, mycoplasmas, rickettsias, and bacteria differ in medically important ways with regard to epidemiology, pathogenesis, pathology, clinical manifestations, laboratory diagnosis, prognosis, and therapy. Hence, some separation, some distinction among these prokaryotic pathogens is warranted.

CHLAMYDIAS

Common characteristics of the *Chlamydia* spp. include (1) particle size of 250 nm to 500 nm in diameter; (2) obligatory intracellular parasitism with multiplication by means of a unique developmental cycle; (3) production of characteristic cytoplasmic

Table 1-1. *Characteristics of the 15 Families of Viruses Infectious for Humans*

Family Name	Genome*	Morphology			
		SIZE†	SHAPE	SYMMETRY	ENVELOPE
Poxvirus	DNA,DS,±	150×250	Brick	Complex	?
Herpesvirus	DNA,DS±	150	Round	Icosahedral	Yes
Adenovirus	DNA,DS,±	80	Round	Icosahedral	No
Papovavirus	DNA,DS,±	50	Round	Icosahedral	No
Parvovirus	DNA,SS,?	20	Round	Icosahedral	No
Paramyxovirus	RNA,SS,−	200	Round	Helical	Yes
Orthmyxovirus	RNA,SS,−,F	100	Round	Helical	Yes
Rhabdovirus	RNA,SS,−	70×175	Bullet	Helical	Yes
Picornavirus	RNA,SS,+	25	Round	Icosahedral	No
Togavirus	RNA,SS,+	30–90	Round	Icosahedral	Yes
Retrovirus	RNA,SS,+,F	100	Round	?	Yes
Reovirus	RNA,DS,±,F	70	Round	Icosahedral	No
Bunyavirus	RNA,SS,?,F	100	Round	Helical	Yes
Coronavirus	RNA,SS,?	100	Round	?	Yes
Arenavirus	RNA,SS,?,F	50–300	Round	?	Yes

* DS = double-stranded; SS = single-stranded; + = plus strand; − = minus strand; ± = plus and minus strand; ? = data on whether the strand is plus or minus is unavailable; and F = the genome is fragmented (*i.e.,* consists of several molecules of nucleic acids).

† Approximate size in nanometers (generally, nonenveloped viruses show a greater constancy in size than enveloped viruses).

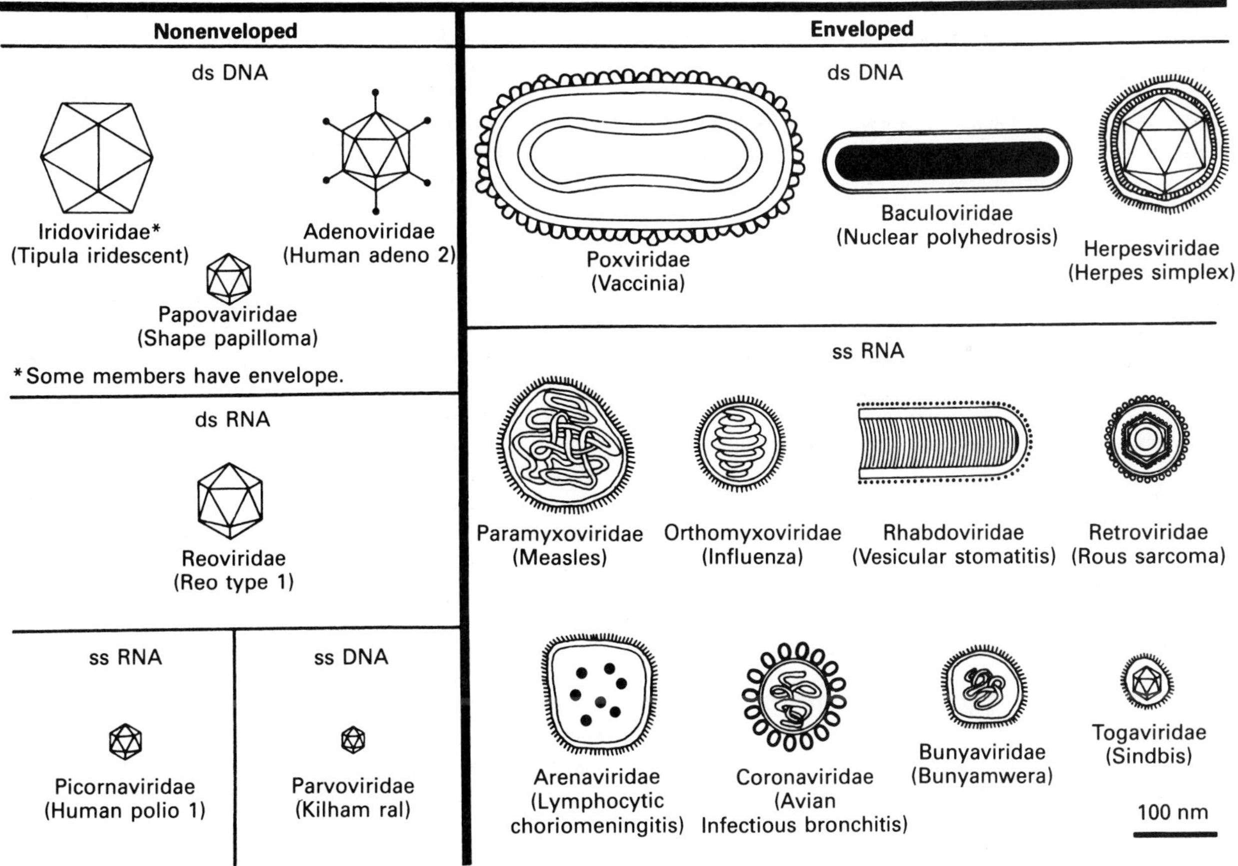

Fig. 1-4. Diagrams of the 17 families of animal viruses. (Mathews REF: Intervirology 12:158, 1979)

inclusions in susceptible host cells; (4) susceptibility to antimicrobics such as sulfonamides, chloramphenicol, and tetracycline; and (5) possession of group-specific, complement-fixing antigens. Individual members are identified by their virulence for different hosts, by the pathology produced, and by the possession of specific antigens.

A typical cytoplasmic inclusion, which is pathognomonic of infection by *Chlamydia* spp., consists of a colony of small (elementary bodies) and large (reticulate bodies) particles in varying proportions. The small particles measure 250 nm to 500 nm in diameter; the large particles may attain the size of 1 μm. In electron micrographs of air-dried, chromium-shadowed preparations, the small and large particles are further distinguished by a central dense body found only in the small particles. The small particles are specialized to enable a brief extracellular existence that permits them to invade new host cells. The genetic material of the small particles is sequestered, and they cannot multiply without first reorganizing into large particles. The large particles are vegetative forms specialized for intracellular multiplication by binary fission. They survive poorly outside the host cells and rarely invade new cells. The growth cycle consists of the entry of small particles into susceptible cells by pinocytosis, reorganization into large particles, replication by binary division, conversion into small particles, and exit from host cells. The growth cycle lasts approximately 30 hours for *Chlamydia psittaci* in cultured human cells.

The chlamydial particles contain DNA, RNA, proteins, lipids, and carbohydrates. Peptidoglycan, a component characteristic of bacterial cell walls, is also found in *Chlamydia* spp.

The *Chlamydia* spp. are capable of synthesizing folic acid, lysine, and muramic acid (compounds that the host cell cannot synthesize). Presumably, enzymes for the synthesis of nucleic acids and proteins are present. Energy-generating mechanisms are, how-

Table 1-2 *Vernacular and Family Names of the More Important Viruses Pathogenic for Humans*

Virus Family	Vernacular Names
Adenovirus	Adeno and its 34 serotypes
Arenavirus	Lymphocytic choreomeningitis, Lassa
Bunyavirus	California encephalitis
Coronavirus	Corona (infectious bronchitis?)
Herpesvirus	Herpes simplex, varicella-zoster, cytomegalo, Epstein–Barr
Orthomyxovirus	Influenza
Papovavirus	Papilloma (wart), SV40
Paramyxovirus	Measles, mumps, parainfluenza, respiratory synticial, NDV
Parvovirus	Adeno-associated
Picornavirus	Polio, Coxsackie, echo, rhino, hepatitis A (?)
Poxvirus	Vaccinia, variola (smallpox), molluscum contagiosum
Reovirus	Rota (diarrhea), reo
Retrovirus	Oncornavirus (species pathogenic for humans not yet identified)
Rhabdovirus	Rabies, vesicular stomatitis
Togavirus	Rubella, yellow fever, equine encephalitis, St. Louis and Japanese B encephalitis, dengue

ever, absent in this group, and they must depend on the host cell for an adequate supply of high-energy compounds to carry out biosynthetic processes. On this basis, it has been suggested that the *Chlamydia* spp. are energy parasites.

Two species, *Chlamydia trachomatis* and *Chlamydia psittaci,* are differentiated by the compactness of the chlamydias in the cytoplasmic inclusion, the presence or absence of glycogen in the matrix of the inclusion, and inhibition of growth in the yolk sac by sulfadiazine, 1 mg per embryo (*C. trachomatis*—compact, glycogen-positive, and inhibited by sulfadiazine). The two species share a major common antigen, and there are numerous serotypes within each species. In human, *Chlamydia* spp. cause trachoma, inclusion blennorrhea, lymphogranuloma venereum, psittacosis (ornithosis), nongonorrheal urethritis, and pelvic inflammatory disease.

MYCOPLASMAS

Mycoplasmas are the smallest living entities that can grow independent of host cells on artificial culture mediums. Some are smaller than the larger viruses and pass through filters with an average pore size of 150 nm. They are gram-negative organisms without cell walls; as a result, they are pleomorphic and fluid, and they are insusceptible to antimicrobics that affect the integrity of bacterial cell walls. Some species contain sterols in their cell membranes and are susceptible to polyene antimicrobics. The growth of mycoplasmas on nutrient agar enriched with animal serum, sterols, and yeast extract leads to the development of colonies with a characteristic fried-egg appearance. When stained with Giemsa or Dienes stain, the small, individual granules that make up such colonies are barely visible with the compound light microscope. One species of *Mycoplasma* is definitely pathogenic for humans—*M. pneumoniae,* the cause of primary atypical pneumonia; *Ureaplasma urealyticum* may cause nongonococcal urethritis.

RICKETTSIAS

Those pathogenic microorganisms commonly referred to as rickettsias are small, plemorphic, gram-negative bacteria. There are three genera: *Rickettsia, Coxiella,* and *Rochalimaea.*

Rickettsia spp. are obligatory intracellular parasites, have a cell membrane that is usually permeable to such cofactors as purine nucleotides and coenzyme A, require an arthropod vector for perpetuation in nature and for transmission to the human host, lose viability rapidly in most extracellular environments, and generally produce in humans a severe infection with exanthematous eruptions. The medically important species are *R. rickettsii, R. prowazekii, R. mooseri, R. akari,* and *R. tsutsugamushi,* respectively the etiologic agents of Rocky Mountain spotted fever, epidemic typhus, murine typhus, rickettsialpox, and scrub typhus.

Coxiella spp. is also an obligatory intracellular parasite but has none of the attributes listed for *Rickettsia* spp. It remains infectious for weeks in most extracellular environments. There is only one species, *Coxiella burnetii,* the etiologic agent of Q fever.

Rochalimaea spp. are capable of extracellular growth. There is only one important species, *Rochalimaeal quintana* (also frequently referred to as *Rickettsia quintana*), the etiologic agent of trench fever.

Rickettsia diseases are uncommon in the United States. However, they must be considered in the differential diagnosis of acute exanthematous diseases because specific antimicrobial treatment is available for all rickettsial infections and because mortality rates for certain rickettsial diseases are extremely high. Moreover, effective methods for the elimination of endemic foci are available for several rickettsial diseases.

Table 1-3. *Differences Between Prokaryotic and Eukaryotic Organisms*

	Prokaryotes	Eukaryotes
Relative size (diameter)	0.2 μm–2.0 μm	>2.0 μm
Nuclear membrane	−	+
Chromosomes/cell	One	More than one
Histone-bound DNA	−	+
Mitotic division	−	+
Nucleolus	−	+
Cytoplasmic ribosomes	(70 S)	(80 S)
Organellar ribosomes	−	(70 S)
Mitochondria	−	+
Chloroplasts	−	Plants
Structured outer coat (not membrane)	(Cell wall) +/−	Plants (Cell wall)
Endoplasmic reticulum	−	+
Golgi apparatus	−	+
Membrane-bound —structured cilia or flagella	−	+ (If present)
Simple flagella (not membrane-bound)	+	−
Cytoplasmic streaming	−	+/−
Ameboid movement	−	+/−
Phagocytosis and pinocytosis	−	+/−
Storage inclusion bodies	+	+ (Membrane-bound)
Microtubules	− (may be some exceptions)	+
Mesosomes	+	−
Centrioles	−	+
Sterols in membrane	− (Except some mycoplasmas)	+
Lysosomal structures	−	+
Peptidoglycan in cell wall	+	−

BACTERIA

Because most bacteria have a specific shape that remains relatively constant, their morphology is useful in recognizing and differentiating them. Bacteria that are spherical in shape are called cocci; those that are rodlike are referred to as bacilli; and spiral or helical forms are known as spirilla or spirochetes. Within these morphologic groupings, there are several subgroups that permit further differentiation (see list below). However, determining the size and shape of bacteria is not sufficient to distinguish one species from another. Rather, it is the sum total of many biologic and physiological characteristics that permits the speciation of bacterial isolates. Such precise identification may be quite time consuming. In many clinical situations, therapeutic decisions must be made promptly—before species identification can be accomplished. Direct microscopic examination of suitably stained, properly collected, appropriate clinical specimens may provide useful preliminary data. Gram's stain and acid-fast stains are particularly important in differentiating bacteria; both types of stains are discussed in Chapter 9, Microscopic Examinations.

BACTERIAL MORPHOLOGY

Streptobacillus: bacilli that always divide in a longitudinal fashion but remain attached to one another; form chains of bacilli

Streptococcus: cocci that divide in a single plane but remain attached to one another; form chains

Tetracoccus: cocci that divide in two planes perpendicular to each other; form sheets of cells. Characteristically, these sheets will take on a tetrad arrangement (four cocci in a plane); for example *Gaffkya,* which cause arthritis, meningitis, endocarditis, and abscesses.

Diplococcus: cocci that divide in two planes and then break apart; appear as pairs of cocci; for example *Streptococcus pneumoniae* (gram-positive) and *Neisseria gonorrhoeae* (gram-negative)

Sarcina: anaerobic cocci that divide in three planes, forming cubes of cocci

Staphylococcus: cocci that divide randomly in all planes and in all directions; form grapelike clusters; for example *Staphylococcus aureus*

Coccobacillus: bacilli having a plump, ovoid appearance (not really bacillus and not really coccus)

Fusiform Bacillus: rods that are especially prominent in the mouth of humans. They are very large bacilli with tapered ends—spindle shaped; for example *Fusobacterium* spp.

Filamentous Bacillus: rods that become very long

Branched Filamentous Bacillus: long filaments with lateral branches that are still only a single bacterium

Pleomorphism: bacteria that can take on many

shapes; for example, *Corynebacterium diphtheriae*

Spheroplasts: spherical-shaped cells that result from partial removal of the cell wall of bacteria in a hypertonic environment. They are osmotically fragile and gram-negative—whether derived from gram-negative or gram-positive bacteria.

Protoplast: osmotically fragile, spherical-shaped cells that result from complete removal of the cell wall of bacteria in a hypertonic environment

Structure. The structure of bacterial cells has been subjected to study virtually continuously since the microscope was invented. In addition to electron microscopy, various other physical and chemical methods have been employed as they became available. A synthesis of this information follows.

Cell Walls and Capsules The cell wall is the outermost structure surrounding the bacterial cell. It serves as a physical barrier that gives both rigidity and shape to the cell. Because of the strength of the wall, bacteria are relatively resistant to osmotic lysis, and they survive in a wide range of environmental conditions that are lethal to eukaryotic cells that lack a cell wall. The walls of bacteria are structurally complex and their composition differs in gram-negative and gram-positive cells (Fig. 1-5). Gram-negative bacteria possess a cell wall that appears to have several layers when observed in cross section with the electron microscope. There is a thin, basal peptidoglycan layer (also referred to as murein or mucopeptide), which may be less than 10 nm thick and constitutes less than 15% of the dry weight of the cell wall. Associated with this basal layer are proteins and lipoproteins linked to the outer portion of the wall, which consists of a membrane composed of phospholipids, proteins, and lipopolysaccharide (endotoxin). In contrast, gram-positive cells usually possess a relatively thick peptidoglycan layer (20 nm–80 nm), which may represent 50% or more of the mass of the cell wall. The walls of gram-positive bacteria are more variable in composition, but they generally have less lipid and no endotoxins (lipoplysaccharides). Many species of gram-positive bacteria have proteins and polysaccharides within their cell walls, and most have considerable quantities of teichoic acids, that is, polymers of glycerol or ribitol phosphate. These teichoic acids are not present in the cell walls of gram-negative bacteria.

The peptidoglycan polymer consists of a backbone of alternating units of N-acetylglucosamine connected by a β-1,4 linkage to N-acetylmuramic acid. Oligopeptides are covalently linked to the muramic acid moiety, and these peptides (usually consisting of l-alanine, d-glutamic acid, a diamino-acid such as lysine or diaminopimelic acid, and d-alanine) are cross-linked to form a rigid polymer.

The cell walls of bacteria are exceedingly important structures. For example, the endotoxin of gram-negative cells engenders a remarkable variety of reactions in the host, notably, adverse effects on the cardiovascular system. The cell walls of some bacteria are responsible for the pathology induced in the host, including delayed hypersensitivity (*e.g., Mycobacterium* spp.). Many cell wall components are important surface antigens that play major roles in host–parasite relationships, including the provocation of immunity. Some cell wall components, such as the M protein of *Streptococcus pyogenes,* are important virulence factors. Further, cell wall structures vary from one species of bacteria to another so that they can be used for taxonomic and serologic identification of bacterial pathogens. Finally, chemicals (*e.g.,* the penicillins) that interfere with cell wall synthesis or integrity are uniquely effective antibacterial agents because host cells do not have comparable structures.

Most, if not all, bacteria grown under proper conditions are surrounded by a layer of gelatinous, poorly defined material referred to as a *slime layer.* If this material is organized, displays a definite border, and is shown to have a specific chemical composition, it is called a *capsule.* Among pathogenic bacteria, the presence of a capsule, as with *Streptococcus pneumoniae,* is often associated with virulence—the capsule renders engulfment by phagocytes difficult. Most bacterial capsules are polysaccharides. An exception is the d-glutamyl polypeptide capsule of *Bacillus anthracis.* The antigenic characteristics of capsules are useful for serodifferentiation of strains and for serodiagnosis. Some capsules are immunogenic and may be used to provoke protective immunity.

Cytoplasmic Membrane and Periplasmic Space The region just internal to the cell wall appears as a transparent zone when fixed material is sectioned and observed with an electron microscope (Fig. 1-5). This region is the periplasmic space, and it is rich in both acid and alkaline phosphatase as well as in many exoenzymes necessary for breaking down larger molecules for use by the cell. They cytoplasmic membrane lies just beneath the periplasm. It is a three-layered structure (unit membrane) that resembles

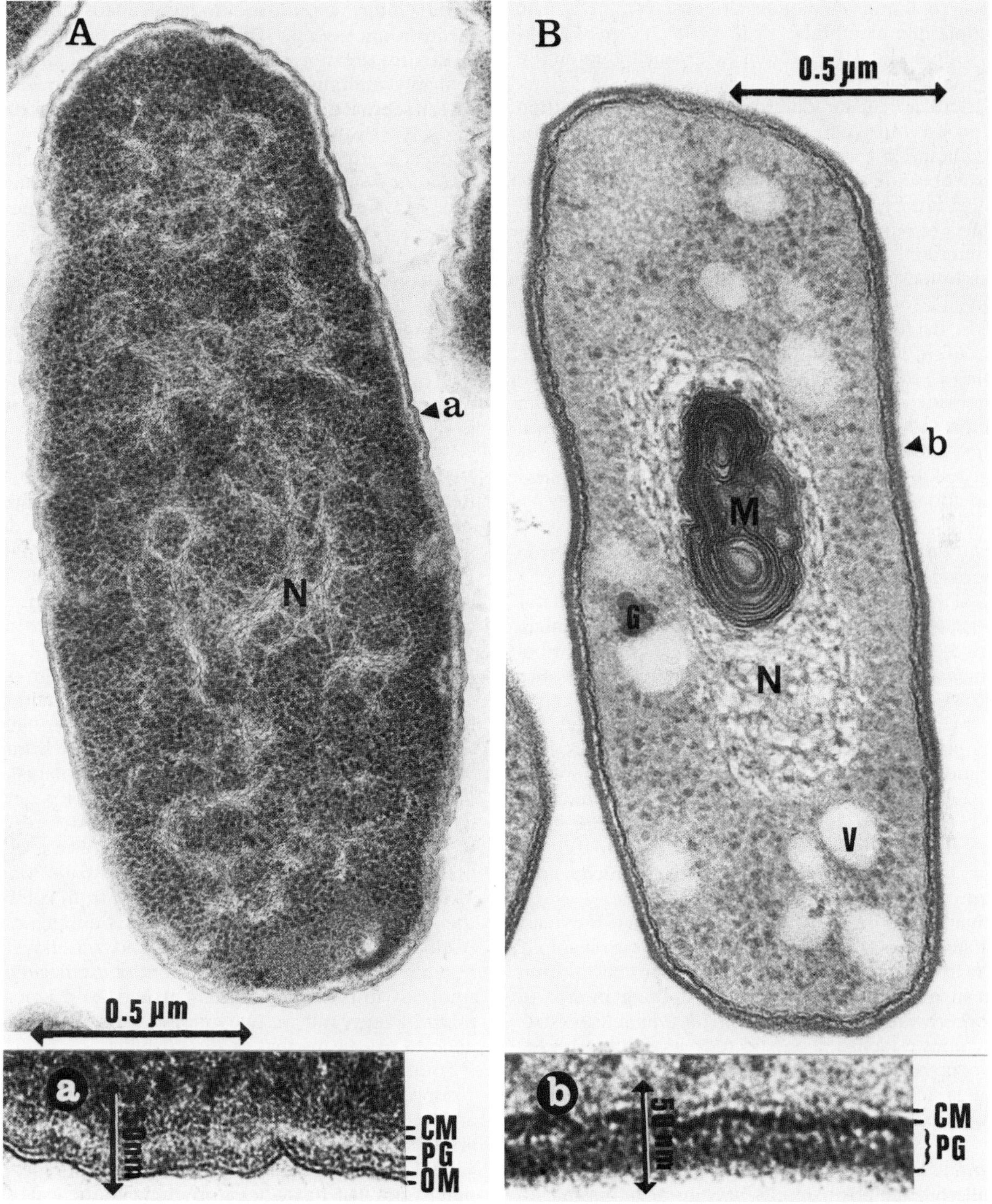

Fig. 1-5. Ultrastructural profiles comparing gram-positive and gram-negative bacteria. *(A)* Electron micrograph of a thin section of gram-negative bacillus. Insert *a* is an enlargement of a portion of the wall. *CM* = cytoplasmic membrane, *PG* = peptidoglycan region, *OM* = outer membrane (possesses the lipopolysaccharide [endotoxin]). *(B)* Electron micrograph of a thin section of a gram-positive bacillus. *M* = mesosome, *N* = nuclear region, *V* = lipid vacuole, *G* = phosphate inclusion granule. Insert *b* is an enlargement of a portion of the wall. *CM* = cytoplasmic membrane, *PG* = peptidoglycan region (compare insert *a* with *b*).

the cytoplasmic membrane of eukaryotic cells. The cytoplasmic membranes of bacteria consist of about 40% lipid and 60% protein, with small amounts of carbohydrates.

There are major differences in the composition of prokaryotic and eukaryotic cell membranes. The membranes of eukaryotic, but not of prokaryotic (except some mycoplasmas), cells contain sterols, which are believed to confer toughness. The membranes of eukaryotic cells contain lecithin and polyunsaturated fatty acids. In contrast, the cytoplasmic membranes of bacteria generally do not possess lecithin and contain saturated or monounsaturated fatty acids. Bacterial membranes have several important functions, including the following: (1) osmoregulation; (2) transport of molecules from the outside to the inside of the cell; (3) excretion of material from within the cell; (4) electron transport for cell respiration and energy production; (5) cell wall synthesis and cell division; and (6) participation in the replication and separation of chromosomes.

Cytoplasm and Nuclear Region Under the electron microscope, bacterial cytoplasm appears to be granular. The granules are ribosomes, which account for about 40% of the dry weight of the cell and contain 60% RNA and 40% protein. Although bacterial ribosomes are smaller (70 S) than eukaryote ribosomes (80 S), they also function in protein synthesis. Most of the bacterial ribosomes are associated with the cytoplasmic membrane. Unlike eukaryotic cells, bacteria do not have an endoplasmic reticulum.

Bacteria do not have a membrane-bound nucleus, and they have no nucleolus. Instead, the DNA appears as a fine, fibrillar network within the cell (Fig. 1-5) to form a nuclear region (also called *nucleotid*), which is the bacterial chromosome.

Bacteria normally exist and reproduce asexually by means of fission; therefore, they are haploid. However, during rapid growth, nuclear division runs ahead of cell division, thereby resulting in two or more chromosomes per cell. The uninucleate state becomes established only in resting cells after cessation of bacterial growth. Discrete sets of chromosomes rich in histones and mitotic structures are not found in bacteria.

Intracytoplasmic Membranes Many bacteria, particularly gram-positive cells, have intracytoplasmic invaginations of the cytoplasmic membrane (Fig. 1-5). These infoldings increase the surface area of the cell membrane and are called *mesosomes.* Their structure may be tubular or lamellar, or a combination of both depending upon growth conditions, age of the culture, and the method used to fix the cell for electron microscopy. The specific functions of these structures are not clearly established, but they are probably multifunctional. They may play an active role in septum formation and cell wall production during cell division. The DNA has been shown to be anchored to the mesosome during DNA replication, and mesosomes may function in separating newly formed DNA replicas prior to cell division. Some investigators believe that mesosomes may be a bacterial equivalent to mitochondria, and mesosomes may be involved in the transport of molecules into or out of the cell. Apparently, some bacteria do not possess mesosomes (gram-negative cells frequently lack these structures), and mesosomal structure (electron micrography) can be dramatically altered by fixation procedures. Thus, the true nature of mesosomes is not completely established.

Inclusion Bodies Many bacteria produce specific types of inclusions that are food- or energy-storage structures. In medically important bacteria, they include lipid bodies (usually composed of poly-β-hydroxybutyric acid), metachromatic granules (composed of inorganic metaphosphate), glycogen, and starch.

Flagella and Pili Both gram-positive and gram-negative bacteria are capable of vital movement by means of hairlike appendages called *flagella.* These structures are aggregates of a specific protein subunit (flagellin) arranged in a helical pattern. The flagellum is a coiled helix, and the length as well as the periodicity of the helix is characteristic of each species of bacteria. The flagellum originates beneath the cytoplasmic membrane from a hooklike basal body. Movement of the bacterial cell results from rotating the flagellum. The protein flagellin is antigenically distinct for each bacterial strain, and antibody frequently immobilizes the movement of the flagellum. Antibody to the flagellum may be used in diagnostic microbiology, and antibody may enhance host resistance to organisms that possess flagella.

Some gram-negative bacteria possess hairlike projections called *pili,* which are smaller in diameter and shorter in length than flagella. Like flagella, pili are composed of protein subunits and originate from a basal body beneath the cytoplasmic membrane. Pili differ from flagella by being straight (nonhelical) and more numerous around the cell. The specific functions of pili are not completely defined; however, some gram-negative bacteria have a specialized pilus referred to as the *sex pilus.* This structure occurs only in donor cells, and it forms a bridge between the donor and the recipient. Apparently, DNA is transferred through this structure from one bacteria to another. Pili may also be involved in bacterial attachment to the surface of host cells, and these structures appear to be associated with the virulence of some bacteria *(e.g., Neisseria gonorrhoeae).* Pili are not usually recognized in gram-positive bacteria; however, *Actinomyces viscosus* and some *Corynebacterium* spp. appear to be exceptions.

Classification. Although complete identification of pathogenic organisms as to genus and species is always desirable, at times this is a complex and time-consuming task. There are, however, a few readily determinable attributes of bacteria that are minimal observations of every isolate from clinical materials. These include the size and morphology of the organism (see list entitled Bacterial Morphology, above); the staining properties (Gram's stain, acid-fast stain), motility (few cocci are motile), capsulation, spore formation, and oxygen tolerance. The oxygen tolerance is critical in recognizing and recovering bacteria from clinical specimens. Some bacteria will grow only in the complete absence of molecular oxygen—the strict anaerobes. Facultatively anaerobic organisms will grow either in the absence or in the presence of molecular oxygen. Microaerophilic bacteria prefer to grow in the presence of reduced amounts of molecular oxygen, whereas strict aerobes grow only in the presence of molecular oxygen.

Under conditions of depleted nutrients, endospores are formed by certain bacteria. The clinically important genera are *Bacillus* (aerobic, spore-forming rods) and *Clostridium* (anaerobic, spore-forming rods). Endospores are more refractile and less easily stained than vegetative cells; they are significantly more resistant to heat, drying, and chemical agents. Thus, endospores serve as a survival mechanism.

Most medically important bacteria fall into one of nine major groupings. Examples of specific pathogens are listed below.

MAJOR GROUPINGS OF MEDICALLY IMPORTANT BACTERIA

Gram-positive cocci

- Anaerobic—*Streptococcus* spp.
- Facultative—*Staphylococcus aureus, Streptococcus pyogenes, Streptococcus pneumoniae,* other *Staphylococcus* spp., and *Streptococcus* spp.
- Aerobic—*Micrococcus* spp.

Gram-negative cocci

- Anaerobic—*Veillonella* spp.
- Facultative—none
- Aerobic—*Neisseria meningitidis, Neisseria gonorrhoeae,* other *Neissera,* and *Branhamella* spp.

Gram-positive bacilli

- Anaerobic, spore-forming—*clostridium botulinum, Clostridium tetani, Clostridium perfringens,* other *Clostridium* spp.
- Anaerobic, nonspore-forming—*Atinomyces israelii* and other *Actinomyces* spp.
- Facultative—*Corynebacterium diphtheriae* and other *Corynebacterium* spp.
- Aerobic, spore-forming—*Bacillus anthracis* and other *Bacillus* spp.
- Aerobic, nonspore-forming—*Nocardia asteroides,* other *Nocardia* spp., aerobic Actinomycetes

Gram-negative bacilli

- Anaerobic, nonmotile, and nonspore-forming—*Fusobacterium* spp.; *Bacteroides* spp.
- Facultative—coliforms (*Escherichia coli, Klebsiella* spp., *Enterobacter* spp., *Proteus* spp., *Shigella* spp., *Salmonella* spp.), *Versinia pestis, Vibrio cholerae*
- Aerobic—*Pseudomonas aeruginosa, Francisella tularensis, Hemophilus influenzae* and other *Hemophilus* spp., *Bordetella pertussis, Brucella* spp., *Legionella pneumophila* (also shares some properties with Rickettsiae)

Acid-fast bacteria

- Aerobic—*Mycobacterium tuberculosis, Mycobacterium leprae,* and other *Mycobacterium* spp.; *Nocardia asteroides* and other *Nocardia* spp.
- Facultative—none
- Anaerobic—none

Slender spiral-shaped, gram-negative rods (Spirochetes)

Thin, corkscrew-shaped cells that are too slender to be visualized in a normal light microscope without darkfield or phase-contrast microscopy. Stained by immunofluorescent antibody or by silver impregnation techniques. Not cultivatable on ordinary culture media for bacteria—

Treponema pallidum (Other *Treponema* spp. can be cultivated *in vitro.*)
Thin, spiral-shaped cells that are too slender to visualize without special techniques (*e.g.,* darkfield microscopy). Grow in peptone broth supplemented with serum—*Leptospira* spp.
Slender, loosely coiled spiral-shaped cells, gram-negative, grow in liquid medium supplemented with blood, arthropod vector—*Borrelia* spp.

Eukaryotes

FUNGI

Fungi are (1) eukaryotic, (2) achlorophyllous, (3) heterotrophic, (4) obligatory or facultative aerobes, (5) capable of sexual and asexual reproduction, and (6) composed morphologically of yeasts (unicellular ovoids or spheres 3 μm–8 μm in diameter) or of hyphae (branching filaments 2 μm–10 μm in diameter). Typically, the outermost layer is a cell wall containing chitin or cellulose together with many other complex molecules. Some species grow only as molds (*i.e.,* a mass of intertwining strands of hyphae), others only as yeasts, and still others both as molds and as yeasts depending on environmental conditions (*i.e.,* they exhibit dimorphism). Many of the fungi that are pathogenic for humans are dimorphic. Both the classification and identification of fungi are based primarily on morphology.

Classification A current classification of fungi is given in the list below. The majority of the medically important fungi are classified as Fungi Imperfecti, a form division that includes the asexual forms (anamorphs) of Ascomycota and Basidiomycota. Although the name Deuteromycota has been applied to this group, it should not be used because it implies a category equivalent to the other four divisions. Within the Fungi Imperfecti, three anamorph classes are recognized; of these, the Blastomycetes (yeasts) and the Hyphomycetes (molds) accommodate almost all of the medically important fungi. Like the anamorph division Fungi Imperfecti, these classes are morphodemes, not taxa. Even though they are given taxonomic names, they are not mutually exclusive groups; that is, a single species may have anamorphs referable to two or even all three classes, plus a telemorph (sexual form) in the Ascomycota or Basidiomycota.

CLASSIFICATION OF THE FUNGI

Superkingdom: Eukaryota
- Kingdom: Mycota (fungi)
- Division: Mastigomycota—lower fungi (no human pathogens reported)
  - Zygomycota—lower fungi (*Rhizopus arrhizus;* Fisher, 1892)
  - Ascomycota—higher fungi (*Petriellidium boydii* [Shear], Malloch, 1970)
  - Basidiomycota—higher fungi (*Filobasidiella neoformans;* Kwon–Chong, 1975)
- Form Division: Fungi Imperfecti—asexual forms (anamorphs) of higher fungi
- Form Class: Blastomycetes—asexual yeasts (*e.g., Candida albicans* [Robin], Berkhout, 1923)
- Form Class: Hyphomycetes—asexual molds (*e.g., Aspergillus fumigatus;* Fresenius, 1863)

Reproduction. Molds grow by apical extension and branching of the hyphae. In addition, they form asexual and sexual spores. Asexual spores produced by members of the form division Fungi Imperfecti are properly termed *conidia.* They are formed at the tips or sides of hyphae in various ways. Other types of asexual propagules are formed by thickening of hyphal walls (chlamydoconidia) or by fragmentation of the hyphae (arthroconidia). Many fungi of the division Zygomycota reproduce asexually by the development of a sac (sporangium), which contains the spores (sporangiospores) that arise from progressive cleavage. Each asexual propagule is a reproductive unit and presumably functions to facilitate aerial dissemination.

The prevailing asexual reproductive growth in yeasts is through budding, with resultant production of blastoconidia. Some fungi reproduce asexually through the formation of endospores from spherules, a process distinct from conidiation by most molds and yeasts.

Sexual reproduction involves the fusion of two haploid cells into a diploid zygote and the meiotic division of the zygote into haploid cells. This process allows for genetic recombination. In most species, it is the haploid cells that undergo prolonged vegetative growth. (The diploid state is transient.) In other species, the opposite is true. The end product of sexual reproduction is the sexual spore. There are three morphologic types: (1) zygospores (large, thick-walled spores); (2) ascospores (generally four to eight spores within a saclike structure called an ascus); and (3) basidiospores (spores formed on the surface of a specialized clubshaped cell, the basidium). The morphology of sexual spores is an important characteristic in the classification of fungi.

Imperfect fungi are those species that do not have a demonstrable sexual reproductive phase; they are not known to form sexual spores. Most of the fungi pathogenic for humans are imperfect.

Fungal Diseases Fungal diseases are termed *mycoses.* They may be classified as superficial (*e.g.,* pityriasis versicolor); cutaneous (*e.g.,* dermatophytosis); subcutaneous (*e.g.,* sporotrichosis); systemic or deep (*e.g.,* coccidioidomycosis); and "opportunistic" (*e.g.,* aspergillosis). It must be recognized that the clinical forms of mycoses all blend into each other; for example, a deep mycosis such as coccidioidomycosis may become manifest with cutaneous lesions, and a primarily subcutaneous mycosis such as sporotrichosis may disseminate to become a systemic disease.

Among the most common infectious diseases of human are dermatophytic infections (ringworm; see Chap. 107, Superficial Fungus Infections of the Skin). Moreover, as mycological awareness and acumen expand, fungi are recognized as entities that must be dealt with because of the increasing prevalence and severity of human mycoses. This is especially so with a population of patients found in contemporary medicine who exhibit defects in host defense mechanisms such as disorders of the skin–mucosal barriers, phagocytosis, chemotaxis, antibody-mediated immunity, and cell-mediated immunity. Such patients serve as fertile ground for virtually any fungus to initiate infection, and they have ushered in the age of the "opportunistic" mycoses.

The exact mechanism(s) through which fungi damage tissue is not known. Toxic products (*e.g.,* aflatoxin) may be responsible in some instances. Hypersensitivity reactions to fungi and fungal products appear to account for some of the clinical manifestations.

PROTOZOA

Protozoa of medical importance are unicellular, nonphotosynthetic, eukaryotic cells that lack cell walls. Pathogenic species vary in size from about 2 μm *(Leishmania donovani)* to about 50 μm *(Balantidium coli)* in diameter. Their classification and identification are based primarily on morphology. Especially important are the organelles of locomotion and the nuclear morphology. Sites of infection within the host and the vector are also useful in identifying intracellular protozoa. Table 1-4 lists medically important species and their characteristics.

Mechanisms by which protozoa damage host tissues have not been firmly established. Possible mechanisms include the following: (1) the release of lytic enzymes from surface-active lysosomes of extracellular protozoa; (2) the destruction of parasitized host cells through multiplication of intracellular protozoa; (3) toxicity of disintegration products from protozoa or host cells; and (4) the host's immune response.

Multicellular

Helminths

The classification and identification of helminths depends on the morphology of adult worms, larvae, and ova. Medically important helminths are listed in Table 1-5.

The consequences of helminth infections vary from the subclinical to severe disease, depending on the species of helminth, the helminth load (the total number of helminths supported within the body of the host), and the host defenses. The mechanism through which helminths damage the host varies from species to species. Hookworms, which attach to intestinal mucosa and feed on blood, produce anemia and hypoproteinemia in long-standing infections. Migrating larval nematodes, such as *Ascaris lumbricoides,* produce pneumonia as the larvae migrate through the lungs. The larvae of *Toxocara canis* induce granulomas in the liver, the kidneys, and the eyes. In schistosomiasis, it is the ova that stimulate granulomatous tissue responses.

Arthropods

Arthropods are important medically because they infest the human skin or serve as vectors in the transmission of other pathogens. Only those arthropods that infest human skin qualify as infectious agents. Arthropods capable of infecting humans are the scabies mite *(Sarcoptes scabiei),* the head and body louse *(Pediculus),* and the crab louse *(Pthirus pubis).* Clinical manifestations are primarily the consequence of hypersensitivity to these arthropods or their products. Characteristics of these arthropods are listed in Table 1-6.

Table 1-4. Major Groups of Medically Important Protozoa

Class	Genus	Characteristics
Zoomastigophora (possessing flagella; reproducing asexually by symmetrical binary fission)	*Trypanosoma*	Arthropod-borne Extracellular or intracellular Possess a single flagellum and undulating membrane when extracellular in vertebrate host
	Leishmania	Arthropod-borne Intracellular Lack flagella in vertebrate host Develop in the macrophage–lymphocyte system, i.e., multiorgan sites
	Giardia	Contaminative transmission through cysts Trophozoites have two nuclei and four pairs of flagella No undulating membrane Extracellular in lumen of small intestine
	Trichomonas	Veneral transmission No cyst stage Trophozoites have four anteriorly directed flagella and one posteriorly directed flagellum that is fused in an undulating membrane Extracellular in vagina and urethra (both sexes)
Rhizopodea (locomotion by pseudopodia; reproduction asexual by simple binary fission)	*Entamoeba*	Contaminative transmission through cyst Trophozoites are uninucleate with fine chromatin granules on inside of nuclear membrane Invasive and extracellular Found in large intestine and, transmitted by way of the portal system, in the liver
	Naegleria	Normally free living in soil Contaminative transmission through fresh water by either trophozoite or transient flagellated stage Cyst stage very resistant to drying Invasion of brain by way of nasal passages Nucleus of trophozoite has large, dense nucleolus circumscribed by a clear zone
	Acanthamoeba	Normally free living in soil May cause meningoencephalitis, acute inflammation of internal organs, granulomas, corneal ulcers, transient diarrhea Differentiation of trophozoites:

	Acanthamoeba	*Naegleria*
Plasma membrane	Spiny projections	Smooth contour
Distance travelled per minute	$<$ 2 body lengths	$\geqslant$ 2 body lengths

Class	Genus	Characteristics
Telosporea (no visible organelles of locomotion on most stages in life cycle; male gametes possess a flagellum; sexual as well as asexual means of reproduction. Some are Arthropod borne; others involve contaminative or food chain transmission. Obligatory intracellular parasites for most of life cycle)	*Isospora*	Contaminative transmission by oocysts containing sporozoites in food or water Obligatory intracellular asexual reproduction in epithelium of small intestine Sexual stage also in small intestine Sporulation may occur in lumen of gut or in external environment. Oocysts passed in feces measure 20μm–23μm × 10μm–19 μm
	Sarcocystis	Contaminative and food chain means of transmission, depending on species

Table 1-4. (continued) Major Groups of Medically Important Protozoa

Class	Genus	Characteristics
Telosporea (continued)	*Sarcocystis (continued)*	Tissue cysts in beef and pork responsible for food chain infections, which develop in epithelial cells of intestine Oocysts from unknown definitive host responsible for contaminative transmission Skeletal and cardiac muscle tissue of human invaded by sporozoites following ingestion of oocysts
	Toxoplasma	Congenital, contaminative, and food chain means of transmission Oocysts produced by felines, passed in feces Common sources of meat known to contain tissue cysts include beef, pork, mutton, and horse. Pregnant female acquiring infection may have parasitemia, leading to congenital infection of fetus
	Plasmodium	Arthropod borne Initial development in humans in hepatocytes followed by invasion of erythrocytes Gametocytes taken up by mosquitoes during feeding Sexual stage in mosquitoes
Piroplasmea (reproduce asexually only)	*Babesia*	Transmitted during feeding of infected ticks; normal hosts are nonhuman animals In humans, develop in erythocytes; infected erythrocytes ingested by ixodid ticks during feeding Asexual reproduction in ticks, with transovarial or transstadial transmission

Table 1-5. Major Groups and Characteristics of Medically Important Helminths

Phylum	Class	Genus	Characteristics
Platyhelminthes	Trematoda (Leaflike, nonsegmented, most flattened dorsoventrally. Possess a digestive tract that ends blindly. Monoecious except for one group. All have gastropod as first intermediate host. All have asexual reproduction in first intermediate host.)	*Schistosoma*	Sexes separate Live in blood vessels draining portions of digestive tract or urinary bladder Ova stimulate major reaction in tissues of infected host (ova may reach liver or lungs accidentally)
		Clonorchis	Two intermediate hosts Certain freshwater fish contain infective metacercariae, which are able to survive freezing temperatures and pickling in brine Adult fluke in bile ducts of liver Related genera found in intestinal lumen
		Paragonimus	Two intermediate hosts Fresh water crustaceans contain metacercariae Young fluke migrates through peritoneal cavity to lungs Most lesions are in diaphragmatic lobes Ova of fluke in both sputum and feces

Table 1-5. *(concluded) Major Groups and Characteristics of Medically Important Helminths*

Phylum	Class	Genus	Characteristics
Platyhelminthes (*continued*)	Cestoda (Ribbonlike, flattened dorsoventrally. No digestive tract. All monoecious. Use Arthropods and vertebrates as intermediate hosts, depending on species. Only a few have asexual reproduction in intermediate host.)	*Taenia*	Food chain transmission Intermediate infective stage in beef or pork, depending on species Humans only definitive host, also capable of supporting intermediate stage in the case of *T. solium* Adult tapeworm in small intestine Larvae in muscles or central nervous system
		Hymenolepis	Contaminative type transmission *H. nana* does not require separate intermediate host; ova directly infective to humans Adult tapeworm in small intestine
		Echinococcus	Contaminative-type of transmission Ova passed in feces of canine Intermediate form only found in humans; liver, lungs most commonly involved Asexual reproduction within hydatid cyst
		Diphyllobothrium	Two intermediate hosts required Fish, the second intermediate host, contain the form infective to humans. Predatory fish may serve as carrier hosts. Position of adult tapeworm in the small intestine may affect the likelihood of causing megaloblastic anemia.
Nematoda (Round worms. Possess an oral opening and anus; are pseudocoelomate, have sexes separate, and are transmitted by contaminative, food chain or vector-borne lifecycles.)	Aphasmida (lacking caudal chemoreceptors)	*Trichinella*	Food chain transmission primarily via pork or bear meat Develops to maturity in small intestine; larvae encyst within muscle cells
		Capillaria	Food chain transmission Adults in liver or small intestine, depending upon species
		Trichuris	Contaminative transmission by embryonated ova Adults in colon, caecum, rectum
	Phasmida (caudal chemoreceptors present)	*Strongyloides*	Skin penetrated by infective larvae or autoinfection by infective larvae in colon Adults found in small intestine, but may disseminate to liver and lungs in heavy infections
		Ancylostoma and *Necator*	Skin penetrated by infective larvae Mature worms in small intestine suck blood
		Trichostrongylus	Contaminative transmission via infective larvae ingested with vegetation Mature worms live in small intestine No migration through lungs
		Angiostrongylus	Normally lung worms of rats Humans become involved by eating

Table 1-5. (continued) Major Groups and Characteristics of Medically Important Helminths

Phylum	Class	Genus	Characteristics
Nematoda (continued)		*Angiostrongylus* (continued)	the intermediate hosts, which are slugs, snails, and small crustaceans. In humans the worms are found in the brain.
		Enterobius	Contaminative transmission by embryonated ova Ova become infective within 6 hours of being deposited on perianal region by female worm. Female worms live in caecum and colon.
		Ascaris	Contaminative transmission by embryonated ova Larvae migrate through lung. Mature worms live in small intestine.
		Wuchereria and *Brugia*	Arthropod-borne filarial worms Mature worms are found in afferent lymphatic vessels, often near their junction with lymph nodes. First stage larvae (microfilariae) are found in blood stream and may be nocturnally periodic. Microfilaria retain shell membrane as a sheath.
		Onchocerca	Arthropod-borne filarial worm Adults found in subcutaneous nodules. First-stage larvae (microfilaria) accumulate in dermis near epidermal junction. Microfilariae are unsheathed.
		Loa loa	Arthropod-borne filarial worm Adults migrate throughout the subcutaneous tissue. Microfilariae are in the blood stream and are sheathed.

Table 1-6. Characteristics of Certain Medically Important Arthropods

Phylum	Class	Genus	Characteristics
Arthropoda (invertebrates with bilateral symmetry, jointed appendages and a chitinous exoskeleton)	Arachnida (Two segments to body; a fused head and thorax, called the cephalothorax, and an abdomen. Lacking antennae, adults with four pairs of legs)	*Sarcoptes*	Burrowing mites Live in stratum corneum of epidermis Close contact with infected individual major means of transmission
	Insecta (Invertebrates with distinct head, thorax, and abdomen. Adults have three pairs of legs attached to thorax.)	*Pediculus*	Head and body lice pass entire lifecycle on host Body louse is vector of typhus rickettsia and relapsing fever spirochete.
		Pthirus	Pubic louse, but also found in armpits, eyebrows, eyelashes, beard, and mustache. Pass entire life cycle on host

Bibliography

Books

ALEXOPOULOS CJ, MIMS CW: Introductory Mycology, 3rd ed. New York, John Wiley & Sons, 1979, 613 pp.

DAVIS BD, DULBECCO R, EISEN HN, GINSBERG HS: Microbiology, 3rd ed. New York, Harper & Row, 1980, 1,355 pp.

DIENER TO: Viroids and Viroid Diseases. New York, John Wiley & Sons, 1979, 252 pp.

KRIER JP (ED): Parasitic Protozoa, Vols 1–4. New York, Academic Press, 1977

MCGINNIS MR: Laboratory Handbook of Medical Mycology. New York, Academic Press. 1980, 661 pp.

STANIER RY, ADELBERG EA, INGRAHAM JL: The microbial World, 4th ed. Englewood Cliffs, NJ, Prentice-Hall, 1976, 894 pp.

Journals

GADJUSEK DC: Unconventional viruses and the origin and disappearance of kuru. Science 197:943–960, 1977

MATTHEWS REF: Classification and nomenclature of viruses. Third Report of the International Committee on Taxonomy of Viruses. Intervirology 12:129–296, 1979

PRUSINER SB: Novel proteinaceous infectious particles cause scrapie. Science 216:136–144, 1982

JAMES W. MOSLEY

Epidemiology

2

Epidemiology as a general discipline has been and still is variously defined. The differences among definitions reflect differences in emphasis or approach among epidemiologists and are of relatively little practical importance. Nevertheless, it is conceptually helpful to have some knowledge regarding its scope as a science. For such a purpose, one may use a broad delimitation close to the etymologic meaning. Most, if not all, phases of medical activity to which the term *epidemiology* is applied are encompassed by defining it as *the study of medically significant occurrences, usually but not necessarily diseases, in human populations.*

Although our present concepts are quite broad, epidemiology historically began as the study of epidemics of communicable diseases. Even before the availability of microbiologic techniques for demonstrating etiologic agents, investigation of factors common to case clusters pointed to mechanisms of transmission and also to ways of control. Especially noteworthy were Snow's study of cholera and Budd's study of typhoid fever, both in the 1850s, some 30 years before either causative bacterium was isolated in the laboratory. More recently, purely through epidemiologic study of the 1933 epidemic of St. Louis encephalitis, Leake correctly identified the mechanism of transmission and even the characteristics of the mosquito vector. It is not surprising, therefore, that epidemiology has been closely identifed with microbiology and infectious diseases. In fact, until recently there was a tendency to define epidemiology largely in terms derived from study of the host–parasite balance—that is, as the ecology of disease.

Advances in the control of infectious diseases—through epidemiologic insights, improved conditions of living, treatment with antimicrobics, and artificial immunization—have made more obvious a tardiness in discovering and applying preventive approaches to the chronic, noninfectious diseases. As a consequence, both epidemiologists and clinicians have shifted their attention to the latter. Indeed, the need to uncover the etiologic factors in chronic processes of obscure or complex etiology justifies the enthusiastic application of epidemiologic techniques. That the epidemiologic approach is useful for noninfectious diseases is, however, not a recent discovery. The classic example, Goldberger's identification of the origin of pellagra in nutritional deficiency, dates back some 65 years.

The recent emphasis on noninfectious diseases should not be construed as an indication that most problems in the epidemiology of infectious diseases have been solved. Many apparent vagaries of microbial agents in the human host remain unexplained. Moreover, some presumed explanations, based on superficial evidence and analogies, have been found wanting when resurgence of an infection forced reconsideration. Finally, it appears that some chronic, supposedly noninfectious diseases may, in fact, be caused by microbial agents, especially viruses. Subacute sclerosing panencephalitis, progressive multifocal leukoencephalopathy, kuru, and Jakob–Creutzfeldt disease may be forerunners of what will become a large group of diseases to be recognized as communicable.

Besides the historical ties to infectious diseases and microbiology, epidemiology has also been closely allied to statistics. As a science particularly concerned with rates and the comparison of rates, epidemiology was the earliest field of medicine in which statistical methods were used extensively. In addition, a number of vital statisticians have become epidemiologists as a result of exploring ramifications of data concerned with morbidity and mortality. There is some tendency, consequently, to confound these separate disciplines. Epidemiologic investigations are sometimes called "statistical studies" if statistical techniques are used extensively in evaluating the findings. The latter label is no more or less appropriate than the term *logical* when the rules of correct reasoning are applied.

Epidemiologic Activities

There are several kinds of epidemiology, simply in terms of how epidemiologic information is obtained and used (Table 2-1). Recognition of this fact results in an operational description of epidemiology that is particularly pertinent to infectious diseases while it is applicable to all of medicine.

Descriptive Epidemiology

The simple delineation of a disease in a population, or any other phenomenon of epidemiologic interest, is essential to our understanding of it. The descriptive epidemiologist, like the clinician approaching a series of hospitalized patients, characterizes cases with respect to such attributes as sex, age, and socioeconomic status. Unlike the clinician, however, the epidemiologist is interested in *all* cases in the community, and expresses rates in terms of the total population or subgroups of the population rather than just in terms of patients at a particular hospital. In addition, the descriptive epidemiologist examines other features—secular trend, seasonal distribution, and differences in rate by geographic area—that the clinician usually does not include in his analyses.

The descriptive study of a disease is often the first step in the epidemiologic approach, especially if its etiology is complex or poorly defined. For this purpose, the epidemiologist ordinarily utilizes readily available data concerning cases (morbidity reports or death certifications) and the population in which cases occurred (census data). The initial effort is followed by periodic review, the frequency of which depends on the rapidity with which the trend or distribution changes. In contrast to the approach in surveillance (see Surveillance, below), there is no attempt to detect immediate changes. In fact, many of the data (*e.g.,* information on deaths) are not available on a contemporaneous basis.

For some communicable diseases, especially those that are not notifiable or have a low mortality rate, neither morbidity reports nor death certificates can serve as indices. In such circumstances the descriptive epidemiologist must turn to survey techniques. If the disease has a reasonably distinctive clinical picture or is one for which a diagnostic test is widely available, admissions to hospitals in the community may provide a means of case identification. Many factors, however, besides the mere occurrence of the disease influence the relative frequency of hospitalization and the particular hospitals to which patients with that diagnosis are admitted. Alternatively, if the disease is characterized by a high ratio of subclinical to clinical cases and an appropriate test is available, the epidemiologist may survey for immunity. Results of serologic procedures or skin testing, especially when analyzed by sex, age, occupation, and residence, provide one of the most comprehensive pictures of *past* infection for a community.

Although reliable delineation of diseases is primary to descriptive epidemiology, inferences concerning etiologic or epidemiologic determinants may be provided by the coincidence of secular trends, seasonal distributions, or particular concentrations of cases with respect to sex, age, or other characteristics. Thus, in Figure 2-1, the coincidence of midsummer peaks of maximum frequency of occurrence of encephalitis either caused by arboviruses or of unknown etiology is striking. Coincidence, however, is no more than suggestive and must be confirmed through other data and other approaches. This point is illustrated by the imputation of an etiologic relationship between type A hepatitis and Down's syndrome from relative synchrony in annual fluctuations in Melbourne. Observations elsewhere have shown no such concordance in levels.

Finally, in relation to medicine generally, descriptive epidemiology is gaining great importance in the planning of medical facilities and health care. It seems obvious that the prevalence and distribution of diseases should be taken into account in determining hospital and clinic locations, staffing, and equipment.

Surveillance

Traditionally, the lexicons of health and law corresponded in defining surveillance as the careful observation of persons considered potentially dangerous to the community. For example, the unvaccinated person arriving in the United States from a smallpox-infected country was placed under surveillance—that is, he had to report periodically to the local health department throughout the 14-day interval after his last potential exposure. In the past 30 years, however, surveillance has come to encompass a number of other techniques aimed at quickly detecting situations representing a threat to the public health.

In 1951, Belois in Greece responded to the need for a different strategy of surveillance created by the conjunction of a marked decrease in malaria after several years of residual spraying with DDT, and the threat of emergence of DDT-resistant anopheline

Table 2-1. *Comparison of Three Kinds of Applied Epidemiologic Activities*

	Descriptive	Surveillance	Field
Stimulus	Usually no specific stimulus other than *general* need for information	Usually the *threat* of a *specific* event of sufficient public health importance that a mechanism for detecting it as early as possible is needed	Usually the *occurrence* of a *specific* event of sufficient importance to require an investigation to supply needed information
Aim	Determining the distribution of a disease in a population, and monitoring for changes in distribution	Monitoring of a disease for a particular change in behavior of unusual public health significance	Explanation of the specific occurrence or circumstance
Data collection	Usually utilizes data already collected, but surveys may be necessary to define numerators and/or denominators	Organized in advance of the specific event for which surveillance is maintained	Organized after the occurrence becomes known
Quality of data collected	Usually recognized to be incomplete and to include some diagnostic inaccuracies, although effort is made to minimize such errors	Crude data are acceptable if they deviate significantly and predictably from the usual whenever the event occurs.	Usually a great effort is made to ensure that data are accurate.
Duration	An intermittent activity	A continuing activity as long as the threat of the particular event is sufficient to justify the effort	Limited to the time necessary to determine what happened and why
Contemporaneity	Analyses usually 1 to several years late, because data are not available earlier	Uses data as contemporaneous as possible; lag is no more than 1 to several weeks.	Planning and execution usually to follow the occurrence by no more than a few days to several weeks, at least with respect to communicable diseases
Indices utilized	As many as possible, such as sex, age, residence, socioeconomic status	Usually just one index serves as indicator of the threatened event.	As many as are necessary to understand what happened
Timeliness of reports	Usually neither current nor regular	Regular and as current as possible—to inform those collecting the data of utilization, and of the occurrence of the specific event	Usually at an interval of weeks to years following the event, after analyses have exhausted the potentials of the data
Consequences	Usually involve evolutionary changes in public health approaches or medical practice	Detection of change results in immediate investigation and appropriate action.	Corrective action to prevent future recurrences

mosquitoes. Rather than routine spraying of all houses, emphasis was placed on visits of canvassers who inquired about cases of fever. When found, the canvassers took blood smears to examine for malaria parasites. In this way, a new focus was usually detected before appreciable spread could occur and spraying could be limited to localities where a true danger existed. This strategy proved successful, and

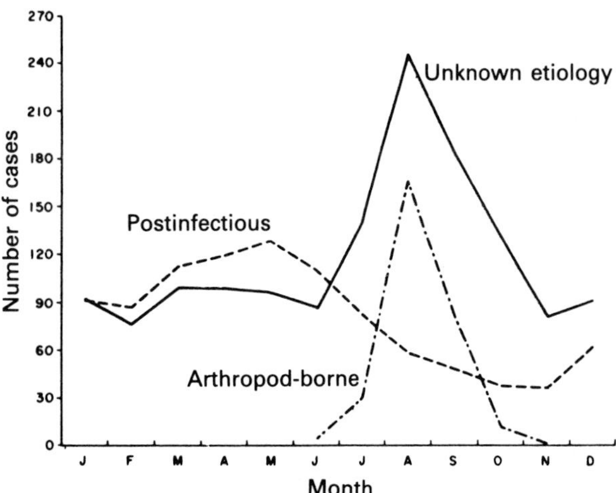

Fig. 2-1. Seasonal distribution of reported encephalitis cases in the United States in 1965. Cases of unknown etiology showed an abrupt midsummer peak coincident with that of cases ascribed to arboviruses. (Morbid Mortal Week Rep 15:266, 1966)

has since been adopted as a routine part of malaria control when the incidence of the disease falls to a low level.

In the United States, surveillance became established as a special epidemiologic procedure in 1955. A few weeks after inactivated poliomyelitis vaccine (IPV) came into widespread use, cases of paralytic disease began to occur among recipients. Shortly thereafter, cases were also recognized among contacts of those vaccinated. Epidemiologic, and then virologic, evidence indicated live, neurovirulent virus was present in a few lots of vaccine in sufficient amounts to cause infection. A poliomyelitis surveillance program was set up, involving a partnership of state and local health departments with federal agencies. Each case of paralytic disease was investigated with special reference to whether the patient had received IPV and, if so, what batch and at what interval before onset. Information from the entire country was compiled by the Centers for Disease Control (then the Communicable Disease Center) and rapidly disseminated to physicians and officials concerned with the vaccination campaign. Through immediate monitoring, paralytogenic batches of IPV were identified, enabling the continued use of safe vaccine, thereby protecting hundreds of thousands of children against naturally acquired infection.

It should be noted that the initial purpose of poliomyelitis surveillance was not epidemiologic analysis of the disease but determination of the vaccination status of each case. This was accomplished by simple verification of the presumptive diagnosis and a few questions concerning epidemiologic and vaccination background. Once the initial problems concerning the safety of IPV were resolved, the same surveillance mechanism was available to monitor IPV potency, and later, the safety of oral poliovirus vaccine when that material became available.

A third disease for which surveillance is applicable is influenza. The number of deaths attributed to pneumonia and influenza fluctuates seasonally but is sufficiently regular to enable prediction of the probable total in any week (Fig. 2-2). Against this projected level of expected deaths, the surveillance officer plots the actual number of deaths in 122 cities located throughout the United States. When immunity to a given contemporary strain of type A influenza falls to a sufficiently low level, a wave of influenza moves through the community causing an increase in the actual number of deaths above that expected—as demonstrated by the excess mortality from $A_2(H_2N_2)$ influenza virus in 1967–1968. When an antigenically new strain of influenza virus appears, there is usually a much greater excess mortality, as exemplified by the higher peak caused by the appearance of the Hong Kong variant (H_3N_2) in 1968–1969. Monitoring the progression across the United States of new variants of influenza virus by means of excess mortality provides short-term warning to at least some communities prior to their involvement in any new waves. On brief reflection, however, it will be obvious that a much earlier warning is necessary if influenza vaccine is to be modified to elicit antibodies that will protect against the antigens of new strains prior to anticipated epidemics. Accordingly, the World Health Organization has established world-wide surveillance through a group of collaborating laboratories. At these laboratories, new influenza virus isolates from geographically representative outbreaks are compared with previously prevalent strains to detect an antigenic "drift" or a major shift.

From these examples, as well as from Table 2-1, it should be apparent that surveillance is a distinct, practical epidemiologic approach. The physician contributes vitally to surveillance by reporting to the health department new cases of diseases for which preventive measures are applicable—diptheria, tetanus, hepatitis, and measles, among others. Diseases for which preventive measures do not seem applicable, for example, infectious mononucleosis and herpes zoster, are not reportable in most states.

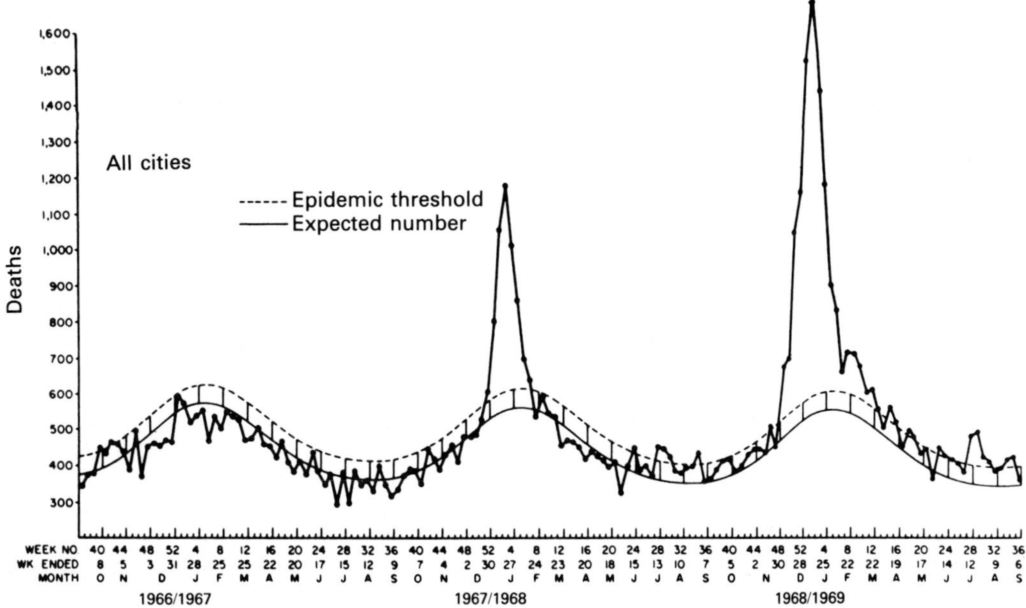

Fig. 2-2. Number of deaths certified as due to pneumonia and influenza each week in 122 cities of the United States. Through this kind of surveillance, the epidemics caused by two variants of influenza virus in 1967–1968 and 1968–1969 were clearly evident. (Morbid Mortal Week Ann Suppl 48, 1969)

Field Epidemiology

Field investigation of epidemics is carried out for the purpose of taking corrective measures to prevent further spread or to prevent recurrences. It consists, therefore, of the application of existing information to unknown situations.

Whereas surveillance activities are organized in anticipation of particular events—to detect their occurrence—the field investigation is organized after an unusual occurrence becomes known. Because he often arrives after cases have passed their peak, the field epidemiologist is sometimes called "the hero of the descending limb of the epidemic curve."

The existence of an unusual occurrence may become known through a variety of circumstances: routine morbidity reporting, special surveillance procedures, and formal or informal inquiries or complaints to the health department. As would be expected, field investigations usually (but not necessarily) represent a response to an epidemic occurrence. Field investigation of *each* case or suspected case of some diseases is warranted: the internationally quarantinable diseases (plague, yellow fever, cholera, and smallpox), rabies, anthrax, malaria, and unusual protozoal and helminthic infections.

Roueché has vividly portrayed the excitement of field investigations, also describing accurately the investigative process. The steps that are followed fall into a general pattern: (1) verification of diagnoses by review of accumulated clinical and laboratory data, and submission of appropriate materials (throat cultures, feces, serums, smears of vesicular fluids) for immediate testing if laboratory facilities are available; (2) search for additional unreported or unsuspected cases, to define the extent of the problem; (3) confirmation of the existence of an epidemic through review of the previous experience of the community and consideration of the possibilities of either unusual diligence in reporting or the occurrence of a number of misdiagnoses; (4) evaluation of mechanisms of transmission with respect to the specific situation, taking into account the temporal and geographic distribution of cases, as well as their demographic characteristics; and (5) collection of specific information to verify tentative hypotheses—which often involves showing that the rate of infection is significantly higher in persons exposed to a suspected mode of transmission than in those not exposed.

The alert, thorough field epidemiologist will often find an epidemiologic situation not covered by existing information. Thus, the opportunity for new contributions is very great. In reality, field epidemiology is not only an application of, but also an avenue to, research.

Clinical Epidemiology

This term was introduced to describe the opportunity available to clinicians to understand disease by looking beyond the patient to his family, his home, his occupational milieu, and the segment of the community in which he lives and works. An early example was Zenker's 1860 investigation of the inn at which a girl with trichinosis had worked. Recognition of similar illnesses in others led to the examination of pork, the ingestion of which was common to all patients. Thus, the major mechanism for transmission of *Trichinella spiralis* to humans was established.

A more recent example occurred in 1955. On the basis of the three cases of type A hepatitis in persons who were casually acquainted, clinicians in Gothenberg, Sweden, suspected a common vehicle. The three patients had attended a party several weeks earlier, as had several additional persons also hospitalized within the next several days with hepatitis. By questioning *all* guests, whether ill or well, about foods consumed at the party, raw oysters were incriminated as the vehicle. This bit of alert clinical epidemiology uncovered part of the first large-scale epidemic in which the vehicle was recognized to be a bivalve.

Although the opportunity to make new observations is afforded to all clinicians by their patients, relatively few physicians have sufficient time to pursue such leads outside their offices or the hospital. The physician, in the course of taking each history, should nevertheless explore the epidemiologic background with the patient *and* his family. This is not only indicated clinically for the assistance it provides in diagnosis, but also because of public health and preventive aspects. Even if the physician himself cannot follow the case into the setting in which the patient acquired the infection, such followup by the health department is routine for many communicable diseases. Where the implications are sufficiently grave, the local health department may be assisted by appropriate personnel from state health departments and the Public Health Service's Centers for Disease Control.

Two additional epidemics of shellfish-associated hepatitis in 1964 provide examples of the latter points. Recognition in the United States of this epidemiologic entity in 1961–1962 resulted in establishment of a surveillance mechanism based on the relative numbers of reported cases among children and adults. During a bivalve-borne epidemic, the preponderance of cases shifts from children to adults; this surveillance mechanism, however, proved to be relatively insensitive. The first clues to both of the 1964 epidemics were calls to city health departments occasioned by the simultaneous hospitalization of three and five cases, respectively, in New Jersey and Connecticut. The epidemiologic history obtained by alert clinicians initiated investigations that substantiated clam-associated outbreaks.

Hospital Epidemiology

In demonstrating the role of the physician in the spread of infection, Joseph Lister and Oliver Wendell Holmes may be said to have originated hospital epidemiology. Adoption of the principles of antisepsis resulted in temporary abatement of a major problem, but physicians themselves and the techniques used in hospital and clinic manipulations of patients have continued to provide new mechanisms for nosocomial infections. (see Chap. 3, Nosocomial Infections). During the 1920s, 1930s, and early 1940s, jaundice was a frequent complication of diseases as diverse as diabetes mellitus (after administration of insulin and capillary puncture for blood glucose were introduced), rheumatoid arthritis (with the introduction of gold therapy), and venereal diseases (with the introduction of arsenical therapy). By the mid-1940s, enough information about the transmission of type B hepatitis was available to identify the common denominator as ineffective procedures for sterilization of equipment used in parenteral therapies.

The advent of antimicrobics, immunosuppressive agents, and cancer chemotherapy ushered in a new era of hospital-acquired infections. Physicians, nurses, and patients became carriers of strains of *Staphylococcus aureus* resistant to antimicrobial agents. Equipment such as that used for respiratory assistance was found to be contaminated with gram-negative bacilli, including *Pseudomonas* spp. Nosocomial infections are so difficult to control and the mechanisms for infection with resistant bacteria are so diverse that a hospital epidemiologist and hospital infections committee have become standard components of hospital staffs.

Analytic Epidemiology

Epidemiologic activities that have as their primary purpose the uncovering of new information about the determinants of disease are called *analytic epidemiology.* These determinants may be either primary (*i.e,* sufficient) causes or secondary (*i.e.,* contributory) causes, such as environmental or host factors and conditions facilitating or damping communicability. In general, the analytic epidemiologist uses three techniques of investigation: the actuarial survey, the retrospective study, and the prospective study. Although largely employed at present in the investigation of chronic diseases presumed to be noninfectious, these tools are also useful in the study of infectious diseases. All three approaches, for example, have been applied in attempts to define the significance to humans of the reservoirs of toxoplasmosis and to determine the mechanisms of transmission.

The bases for actuarial surveys—the assessment of the relative risk of the disease in various populations and subpopulations—are often the results obtained by the descriptive epidemiologist. From surveys, it may appear that persons with certain exposures or characteristics are more (or less) likely to have the disease. In other instances, the frequency distribution of characteristics (such as age, sex, or race) in a clinical series of cases may be consistent with a preponderance worthy of further investigation. Because of coincidence and bias, associations can be accepted as no more than the stimulus for further, potentially fruitful work. The relation of two variables (such as socioeconomic status and the incidence of a particular illness) can then be determined in a number of other populations, or at different points in time in the same population. The more nearly concurrent the variations, the more plausible becomes the association. There are, however, obvious limitations. Groups, whether in different communities or at different points in time, almost never differ in only the tentatively identified independent variable. In addition, concurrent variation may signify dependence of both variables on a third. The actuarial approach, therefore, provides evidence that is often helpful, sometimes misleading, and always presumptive.

The retrospective study begins with a group of patients with the disease under investigation, and one or more groups of persons without that disease. The relative frequency of prior exposure to one or more factors thought to be primary or secondary determinants is then assessed. Possible biases that could account for a difference are taken into account, and an attempt to negate or minimize them is made by matching or stratifying the controls. Unfortunately, the operation of unidentified biases sometimes results in spuriously significant differences in proportions. As a result, "retrospective" as a descriptive adjective has acquired a pejorative connotation. This attitude is by no means justified, as retrospective studies have yielded, and will continue to yield, valuable and reliable information. To avoid the implications mentioned, the more accurate term *case control* has been proposed as a substitute for "retrospective."

The prospective study begins with populations or subpopulations respectively having and lacking a suspected exposure or determinant. After an appropriate interval of time, the relative frequency of the presumed outcome is assessed. Consideration of this definition should make it obvious that the prospective study may be entirely "retrospective" in terms of the time at which exposure took place and its effect became manifest. "Prospective" implies neither identification of the exposed population at the moment of exposure, nor continuous observation until the effect becomes discernible. For some questions, however, definition of populations at the time of exposure (or nonexposure) may be necessary for reliable classification. Similarly, for some investigations continuous observation, perhaps using special or sophisticated diagnostic procedures, may be necessary to identify reliably those evidencing the effect. For other purposes, this is *not* so. To avoid the confusion inherent in the term "prospective," the substitute term *cohort study* has been proposed, implying only a uniform group moving forward in time to meet its fate. "Cohort study" also avoids the automatic, and perhaps unjustified, upgrading in estimation now attached to prospective studies. A well-designed retrospective study can give more reliable results than a poorly designed prospective study. The major difficulty with a cohort study is maintaining the entire population under observation. Losses from the cohort can distort the results as seriously as bias in case selection can mar a retrospective study.

In general, all three analytic approaches are used in investigating the role of a suspected determinant of a disease. In terms of ease of completion, the first studies are likely to be actuarial, then retrospective, and finally prospective studies. These techniques have provided much valuable information in the past and will undoubtedly continue to do so.

Experimental Epidemiology

It should be obvious from the foregoing discussion that epidemiology is usually an observational rather than an experimental science. The epidemiologist "controls" variables by analyses of subpopulations and standardizations of rates rather than by deliberate manipulation of circumstances themselves. Certain situations are sometimes described as "unplanned experiments" when they help answer particular epidemiologic questions. Such a manner of speaking, however, ignores the fact that the alert, prepared field epidemiologist can almost always learn something new about the behavior of a disease from any investigation of its occurrence.

Nevertheless, the experimental approach, using groups of laboratory animals or even human subjects as models for populations, is sometimes appropriate or necessary. This avenue was first exploited in the 1920s and 1930s by Topley and Greenwood in England, and Webster in the Unted States. Subsequently a number of other investigators have made contributions, although work in this area has been less extensive than appears to be justified by its potential.

Epidemics obviously represent a set of complex interactions between a variety of factors: microbial virulence, with its influence on the ratio of subclinical or mild infections to those producing obvious or severe disease; microbial infectivity, the ease of transmission from one host to another; host resistance, especially that related to nonspecific factors; herd immunity, the ratio of susceptibles to immunes in the population; the rate of entry of new susceptibles; the extent and character of host aggregations; and environmental influences, such as humidity and temperature. The potential contribution of each can be studied only when others are held constant. Unfortunately, the greatest problem in extrapolating from such studies is knowing the relative role of each when all are operative together. Experimental studies using volunteers are feasible if the disease is mild, as in rhinovirus infections, or of great importance when no alternative approach is available, as was the case in World War II with viral hepatitis. The availability of live poliovirus vaccines has made possible experimental infection with a nonvirulent microorganism in circumstances under which mechanisms and extent of transmission can be assessed.

A resurgance of interest in the experimental approach, especially using animal models, should enable closer approximations to actual conditions in the community. In this way, new light may be shed on the many factors influencing infections in the community.

Epidemiologic Definitions

In relation to communicable disease, the epidemiologist has traditionally been especially concerned with mechanisms of transmission and reservoirs in which the infectious agent is maintained. The situation with respect to some diseases is simple. Measles (see Chap. 86, Measles), for example, has only the human as host, expresses itself as an overt, clinically characteristic illness in most instances, is transmitted easily by the respiratory route, and has no carrier state. Other agents have complex "ecologies." Tularemia (see Chap. 139, Tularemia), for example, is primarily a sylvatic (rodent) infection with man infected only incidentally, but through a variety of mechanisms. The latter include contact with infected animals, both domestic (sheep) and wild; arthropod vectors (wood ticks and deerflies); and ingestion of drinking water contaminated by rodents.

It is impossible to summarize the infinite variety of epidemiologic mechanisms exhibited by infectious diseases. An introduction to epidemiologic concepts and terminology is necessary, however, as a background for the remaining chapters of this book. The Glossary of Epidemiologic Terms (at the end of this chapter) provides a set of definitions for this purpose.

The Epidemiologic History

Exploration of the epidemiologic background of the patient's major problem is an essential part of any initial medical evaluation. The epidemiologic history, however, assumes particular importance whenever the illness is thought to be infectious. A positive or strongly suggestive epidemiologic history can be very helpful in differential diagnosis, supplying evidence in support of other clinical and laboratory features. Diagnoses may be considered that would not have been thought of unless the history of potential exposure was elicited. Identification of a source or vehicle of infection may be helpful in the diagnosis of other, less typical illnesses in patients with similar exposures, or may point to prophylactic measures if exposed individuals have not yet become ill. Finally, identification of a source or vehicle of infection may lead to corrective measures that will prevent others from becoming infected.

As in eliciting any other portion of the medical history, a given set of questions about possible sources of infection should be covered. The questions, however, should neither be asked in a perfunctory manner nor by rote. The goal is not to obtain a set of positive or negative answers to a checklist, but to obtain valid, useful replies from the patient. Particularly important questions should be asked several times, using different ways of phrasing the inquiry, to make certain the patient understands. Illness creates anxiety and often a certain sense of guilt, however unjustified from an objective point of view. The patient may feel he needs to screen some activity until he is certain that the physician will not be critical of him for it, even though that activity when subsequently disclosed seems in no way reprehensible to the physician. Questions should be posed neutrally so that the patient does not anticipate the reply the physician wants or expects.

In evaluating the patient epidemiologically, differential diagnoses must be kept in mind constantly. The categories of exposure in which one is most interested vary greatly with the type of illness, as well as the particular agents capable of causing it. The patient with nausea, vomiting, and diarrhea is likely to have a different background than the patient with a stiff neck and muscular weakness. Taking the history of an illness requires a well-informed physician whose mind is constantly exploring the ramifications of each statement of the patient.

Finally, it is important to realize that the epidemiologic history, as is true for any other part of the history, does not end with questioning the patient at the time of admission. Relatives, especially family members accompanying the patient on admission or visiting him subsequently, should be asked about significant exposures. Additionally, the epidemiologic history should be repeatedly reconsidered as new leads are exposed by the physical examination, the laboratory data, and the patient's course. Repetition of questions after the patient's initial anxieties have subsided often results in actual rather than ritualistic "communication." Also, with increasing rapport, the patient is often willing to disclose information about which he was initially reticent.

Table 2-2 outlines the epidemiologically important areas to be covered in talking with the patient, and also, the epidemiologic considerations with respect to agents capable of producing disease compatible with the patient's illness. Of these two aspects, the former is much more important than the latter because the individual patient may be an exception to the "usual" circumstances under which the agent produces disease.

Table 2-2. *Potential Exposures of the Patient and Epidemiologic Characteristics of Infectious Agents Considered in Differential Diagnosis*

Potentially important exposures of the patient	Epidemiologic considerations with respect to agents capable of producing the patient's illness
1. Known exposure to a similar illness	1. Sex predilection
2. Place of residence	2. Age predilection
3. Membership of the household	3. Seasonal prevalence
4. Pets	4. Incubation period
5. Occupation or daily activity	5. Ratio of subclinical infections to cases
6. Place of work or school	6. Distribution in the community and surrounding area
7. Avocational exposures	7. Reservoirs in or adjacent to the community
8. Travel	8. Vector distribution, prevalence, and range
9. Vaccination status	9. Current prevalence in the community
10. Illicit exposures	10. Existence and prevalence of agents outside the community in areas visited by the patient

Known Exposure to a Similar Illness

The likelihood of obtaining a history of exposure to an antecedent illness similar to the patient's depends on several factors. Such a history will be obtained only for agents transmissible directly from human to human, and not for those transmitted indirectly through a vehicle or acquired from a nonhuman source. The extent of direct transmission from human to human varies greatly with the agent, and sometimes with the form of the infection (*e.g.,* the difference in human-to-human infectivity of pneumonic and bubonic plague) (see Chap. 140, Plague).

The ratio of subclinical infections (temporary infections and the carrier status) to clinical cases varies from agent to agent. Measles virus (see Chap. 86, Measles) produces relatively few subclinical cases; type 2 poliovirus (see Chap. 121, Poliomyelitis) produces few cases of paralytic disease.

Some agents produce a characteristic illness; others are capable of a variety of manifestations. Chickenpox virus (see Chap. 93, Varicella and Herpes Zoster) produces either chickenpox itself or herpes zoster; coxsackieviruses (see Chap. 149, Coxsackievirus and Echovirus Infections), on the other hand, produce a wide variety of syndromes, including aseptic meningitis, encephalitis, pleurodynia, pericarditis, gastroenteritis, and herpangina. With agents that produce a spectrum of manifestations, the clinician and epidemiologist should seek a history of exposure not only to a similar illness but also to diseases compatible with the clinical potential of the suspected agent.

Identified contact is helpful in many ways beyond providing a probable source of infection. The interval from contact to onset (*i.e.,* the incubation period) provides one clue for identification of the agent. In addition, disease in the person initially ill may have advanced to clinically diagnostic features not yet present in the subsequent case. Finally, therapeutically important information, such as susceptibility to antimicrobial agents, may already be available.

Residence

The physician usually identifies the general segment of the community in which the patient lives but seldom considers epidemiologic implications in other than socioeconomic terms. Place of residence, however, is important in other ways. Is it in an area of the city where certain illnesses are currently or continuously prevalent? Does it imply possible exposure to rats, flies, lice or bedbugs? Does it imply such good sanitation and low population density that exposure to enteric or even respiratory agents may have been delayed until a later than usual age? Is it in a newly developed housing tract where wildlife harboring potential pathogens may have been disturbed (a common situation for infections with California encephalitis virus)? Does it border wooded or forested areas into which the patient may have wandered, or from which feral animals may emerge in proximity to the house? Are there domestic animals such as chickens, cattle, horses, or pigs on the premises or on adjacent property?

Membership of the Household

The patient with an infectious illness is often asked about similar illness at home, but exploration seldom goes beyond this. Who are the other household members? Does their work or daily activity, such as school, expose them to potential sources that may have led to covert infections? Has a household member received oral poliovirus immunization? Has a household member been hospitalized (with exposure to nosocomial *Staphylococcus aureus*) or been transfused (with potential exposure to type B hepatitis)?

Pets

The family pet, and those of neighboring households, is a source of pleasure, companionship, and, on occasion, of disease. This is especially true when the home is near creeks or woods where the pet may be exposed to a sylvatic reservoir. The dog can expose household members to rabies (see Chap. 124, Rabies), visceral larva migrans (see Chap. 78, Visceral Larva Migrans), leptospirosis (see Chap. 76, Leptospirosis), and Rocky Mountain spotted fever (see Chap. 96, The Spotted Fevers); the cat, to rabies (see Chap. 124, Rabies), cat-scratch fever (see Chap. 166, Cat Scratch Fever), and murine typhus (see Chap. 98, The Typhus Fevers); the parrot, to psittacosis (see Chap. 30, Nonbacterial Pneumonias); and the turtle, to salmonellosis (see Chap. 63, Nontyphoidal Salmonelloses). Exposure to pets may also occur at work—a cat or dog may be kept at a place of business for a variety of reasons, and contact with such animals at lunchtime or coffee breaks may be as great as with a similar pet at home. Cases of primate-associated hepatitis were seen in persons having no professional contact with the animals but who handled them as an amusement during lunch periods. "Petting zoos" must also be considered, although animals at most such institutions are carefully supervised by veterinarians.

Occupation or Daily Activity

Potential occupational exposures usually receive some consideration but are seldom thoroughly explored. Those whose work brings them into contact with *sick persons* obviously have the greatest hazard: physicians, nurses, students in either profession, paramedical personnel, and laboratory workers. Even work in a building where patients are housed or specimens are processed is potentially dangerous, especially when ventilation systems are poorly designed or special instruments such as high-speed homogenizers and centrifuges are in use. Extensive contact with the general *public* probably also increases the hazard of exposure, especially to respiratory-transmitted agents; examples include salespeople, waiters and waitresses, dentists and dental hygienists, and schoolteachers. Some occupational groups are exposed to human wastes: sanitation workers, sanitary engineers, garbage workers, and some construction workers. Exposure to animal reservoirs may also be occupational: veterinarians, animal handlers, pet-store workers, taxidermists, field biologists, and even geologists and archeologists.

Apart from obviously occupational exposures, daily activity may also be epidemiologically significant in other ways. School attendance is obvious; potential exposures should be explored not only with the patient and patient's mother (fathers are seldom epidemiologically helpful in relation to their children's illnesses), but also by telephoning the teacher or school nurse. Less obvious but no less important may be other groups such as scouts, athletic teams, or other extracurricular gatherings.

The nonworking mother may also have significant exposures that neither she nor the physician may consider unless there has been contact with an obviously similar illness: volunteer work for the Red Cross, at hospitals or institutions for the retarded, or with children through school activities.

Most occupations, school attendance, and many other daily activities involve a trip from and to the home. In most instances, this is not epidemiologically significant, but car pools and school buses may be, and children do take detours through vacant lots and wooded areas.

Place of Work or School Attended

Inquiry about the kind and actual place of work, not just the occupation and name of the company, can occasionally be helpful. A place of work or a school may take the individual into a community or into proximity to an enzootic focus that would not otherwise have been appreciated.

Avocational Exposures

Of avocational pursuits, the epidemiologically most hazardous, at least with respect to diversity of agents, is hunting. Aside from the hazard of a concealed position in areas in which arthropods often sustain enzootic cycles, the contact with freshly killed animals poses possible exposure to plague (see Chap. 140, Plague), tularemia (see Chap. 139, Tularemia), and leptospirosis (see Chap. 76, Leptospirosis). Consuming the meat of bears and other carnivores can transmit trichinosis (see Chap. 150, Trichinosis).

Sporotrichosis (see Chap. 108, Sporotrichosis) occurs among rose fanciers; histoplasmosis (see Chap. 40, Histoplasmosis) and ornithosis (see Chap. 30, Nonbacterial Pneumonias), among pigeon raisers. Any hobby, therefore, must be considered for its epidemiologic potenital.

Travel

The mobility of the population, for both business and pleasure, has ended the era in which the physician could be epidemiologically parochial. The traveler who returns from Africa with falciparum malaria (see Chap. 145, Malaria) or trypanosomiasis (see Chap. 130, African Trypanosomiasis) is only the most flagrant example (and also, fortunately, the most uncommon). International travel poses a small but definite hazard of disease not encountered in this country, especially when it is to less commonly visited areas where tourist accommodations may be inadequate. A greater hazard is attached to residence in such areas, although the physician in this country is more likely to see chronic rather than acute infections in such persons.

Travel in the United States implies exposures that might not be seen in the patient's own community. Camping carries a very small but definite risk of plague (see Chap. 140, Plague), Colorado tick fever (see Chap. 123, Colorado Tick Fever), Rocky Mountain spotted fever (see Chap. 96, The Spotted Fevers), rabies (see Chap. 124, Rabies), tularemia (see Chap. 139, Tularemia), and California encephalitis (see Chap. 122, Viral Encephalitides). Venezuelan encephalitis (see Chap. 122, Viral Encephalitides) is now enzootic in southern Florida and Texas. Although only a few indigenous illnesses attributable to this agent have been recognized, it is now possible for an infection acquired during a visit to the Everglades National Park to become manifest in Iowa, and its nature thereby go unsuspected. During the epidemics of clam-associated hepatitis (see Chap. 70, Hepatitis A) in the northeastern United States, cases were reported in traveling businessman from the Midwest.

Vaccination Status

Because no vaccine is entirely effective, prior vaccination against one or more of the agents considered in the differential diagnosis is of only relative importance. Passive immunization with human serum and mass immunization with a variety of vaccines using a multiple-dose-per-syringe technique has occasionally resulted in hepatitis (see Chap. 71, Hepatitis B). The possibility cannot yet be excluded of unsuspected, yet undetected, "passenger" viruses in cell lines used for producing an increasing number of viral vaccines. Despite the best efforts of manufacturers and regulatory agencies, agents capable of inducing infections or neoplastic diseases could contaminate these materials.

Illicit Exposures

Illicit exposures, either sexual or to drugs, are of increasing epidemiologic importance, but they are one of the areas of the history least reliably covered. This is due not only to the reluctance of the patient, but also (perhaps more important) to the unease of the physician. Only if the physician feels no embarassment and approaches the subject with clinical objectivity, can he hope to obtain the data he needs to help the patient.

Epidemiologic Responsibilities of the Clinician with Respect to Communicable Diseases

Cultures

It has been, and unfortunately remains, common to treat febrile patients, especially when seen in the office rather than the hospital, without taking appropriate cultures for definitive laboratory diagnosis. With potent, broad-spectrum antimicrobics, the patient is usually cured, and the practitioner feels justified in having saved time and expense. Unfortunately, an occasional patient receives too little antimicrobial therapy to eradicate the infection, but enough to make subsequent diagnosis difficult. Incompletely treated bacterial meningitis has emerged as a new and vexing form of "aseptic meningitis" (see Chap. 119, Acute Bacterial Meningitis). Initially unsuspected tuberculosis (see Chap. 34, Pulmonary Tuberculosis) may be missed, or the nontuberculous patient may be unnecessarily sentenced to long-term treatment with agents that have potential for toxicity. As is emphasized throughout this book, there are highly practical and entirely rational grounds for obtaining cultures before specific treatment is given.

Culturing of suspected bacterial (and viral) infection, even when the infection is not severe or appears likely to respond, also has preventive and public health aspects. Prophylactic measures to prevent the infection in contacts, some of whom could contract the infection in a more severe form, may be indicated. In addition, it is increasingly important to monitor the frequency of occurrence of certain agents to enable the application of broader preventive measures. To an increasing extent, reports of specific laboratory isolations, rather than of clinical illness, are being used for surveillance. This is the result of the variety of clinical syndromes for which some agents may be responsible, or the variety of serotypes that may produce the same manifestations. Salmonellal surveillance especially depends on this mechanism, and it is increasingly important on a national scale. An infected worker or a contaminated ingredient may result in the sudden emergence of a new *Salmonella* serotype or unusual prevalence of any given serotype, not just in one community but in many states if the product (such as powdered milk) is widely (and spottily) distributed.

The clinician should insist on prompt reporting of laboratory results and availability of consultative help from the health department's epidemiologist and laboratory director.

Prophylaxis

The family practitioner, or the specialist in the absence of a true family physician, must consider the advisability of prophylactic measures for exposed persons in the household of the patient. These may be advisable in general terms. For example, all members in the household of a clinical case should receive oral poliovirus vaccine when poliomyelitis occurs, or immune globulin on exposure to type A hepatitis (see Chap. 20, Immunoprophylaxis of Infectious Diseases). In other situations, some measures may be required only for certain individuals—for example, attempted prophylaxis of rubella using immune globulin in the susceptible woman who is pregnant. Prophylactic measures for protection of contacts outside the household, if appropriate, are usually undertaken by the health department. For such attempts at protection to be successful, it is obviously necessary that the health officer be informed promptly.

Isolation of the Patient

For household members, transmission to susceptibles is likely to have occurred by the time the diagnosis is made in the patient; therefore, precautions, such as boiling dishes, are generally too late. The physician, however, has responsibility for instituting measures to prevent exposure of persons not already in contact wth the patient. If the patient remains at home, the physician may need to restrict visitors, depending on the probability of persistent infectiousness, as well as routes and ease of transmission. In the hospital, isolation procedures should protect staff and visitors without imposing more restrictions than are necessary. Each precautionary measure imposes a barrier to adequate patient care. Both the Centers for Disease Control and the American Hospital Association issue, and revise periodically, recommendations based on available microbiologic and epidemiologic evidence. These are contained in the booklets entitled *Isolation Techniques for Use in Hospitals* and *Infection Control in the Hospital.* These guidelines need not be exceeded.

Some hospitals have a policy of refusing admission to patients with infections feared to be highly communicable. Thus, the pregnant woman who develops measles at term is often inconveniently (and sometimes belatedly) referred to a public facility accepted by the community as the modern equivalent of a pest house. There is no justification for such actions by professionals whose training routinely involves instruction in protecting other patients and themselves.

Reporting

Although sometimes considered merely a nuisance by the practicing physician, prompt reporting of communicable diseases is an invaluable surveillance mechanism for the physician himself, public health officials, and the entire community. In return for his cooperation, the physician is entitled to summaries of the community's *total* experience, and periodic analyses of trends (see below).

Sources of Contemporaneous Information Concerning Trends in Infectious Diseases

In any community, the prevalence of various infectious diseases is usually changing, although the extent of that change differs with the characteristics of the infectious agent and the population. When the level of infection is high, knowledge of that fact can lead the physician to order the most appropriate tests early in the work-up, to suspect the correct diagnosis in atypical illnesses, and to recognize mild cases that would otherwise remain undiagnosed. Even for uncommon agents, knowing that sources of potential infection exist in the community or in an area visited by the patient can be very helpful.

Through the problems presented by other patients in his practice and through the exchange of information with colleagues, the physician is usually aware of epidemic occurrences and sometimes of unusual infections. This is more likely in small communities than in urban and suburban areas. In addition, the prevalence of intrastate, interstate, and international travel leads to potential exposures that the patient would not encounter within the area in which he lives. Accordingly, the physician has a continuous need for contemporaneous information about trends in the occurrence of infectious diseases. Fortunately, a variety of sources of such data are available.

Weekly or monthly bulletins are published by most state health offices, and by some large city and county departments. The numbers of recently reported infections are summarized by county, district, or community. The totals for each disease during a given period are usually compared with those for the immediately preceding interval and also for the comparable period during the prior year. This format provides the physician at a glance with an idea of the level and trend of notifiable diseases in his immediate area. Additionally, these bulletins often include analyses of statewide or local patterns over longer periods, and provide details of investigations of epidemics or cases of infections of unusual interest. Such publications are usually sent without charge to any physician requesting them.

A similar bulletin covering communicable diseases throughout the United States is the *Morbidity and Mortality Weekly Report* (MMWR). It is issued by the Centers for Disease Control, United States Department of Health and Human Services, Atlanta, Georgia. The MMWR summarizes *by state* the number of cases of reportable infections that occurred during the preceding week throughout the nation, and total cases for the more important diseases for the year to date. More importantly, it provides comprehensive summaries of national and regional trends on a quarterly or annual basis and much information on important occurrences of infectious diseases anywhere in the United States and abroad. The present mobility of the American population makes such information important to each practitioner.

In addition to MMWR, a series of surveillance reports covering individual diseases in considerable detail is published by the Centers for Disease Control. These include poliomyelitis and other enteroviral diseases, the infectious encephalitides, measles, rubella, viral hepatitis, salmonellosis, shigellosis, leptospirosis, rabies, and psittacosis.

For international trends, especially of the quarantinable diseases (smallpox, yellow fever, plague, and cholera), the World Health Organization's Weekly Epidemiological Record is useful. It is, however, of primary interest to industrial or other physicians responsible for supervising health care of Americans abroad or advising about prophylactic measures for overseas travel.

Bibliography

Books

FOX JP, HALL CE, ELVEBACK LA: Epidemiology: Man and Disease. New York, Macmillan, 1970, 339 pp.

FOX JP, HALL CE: Viruses in Families: Surveillance of Families as a Key to Epidemiology of Virus Infections. Littleton, PSG Publishing, 1980, 441 pp.

LILIENFELD AM (ed): Times, Places, and Persons: Aspects of the History of Epidemiology. Baltimore, Johns Hopkins University Press, 1980, 160 pp.

MORRIS JN: Uses of Epidemiology, 3rd ed. Edinburgh, Churchill Livingstone, 1975, 318 pp.

MCNEILL WH: Plagues and Peoples. Garden City, NY, Anchor Press/Doubleday, 1976, 340 pp.

PICKLES WN: Epidemiology in Country Practice. Bristol, John Wright & Sons, 1939, 110 pp.

ROUCHE B: Annals of Epidemiology. Boston, Little, Brown & Co, 1967, 307 pp.

Journals

IPSEN J JR: Social distance in epidemiology: Age of susceptible siblings as the determining factor in household infectivity of measles. Hum Biol 31: 162–179, 1959

LANGMUIR AD: The surveillance of communicable diseases of national importance. N Engl J Med 268: 182–192, 1963

LILIENFELD DE: Definitions of epidemiology. Am J Epidemiol 107:87–90, 1978

STEWART GT: Epidemiological approach to assessment of health. Lancet 2:115–119, 1970

Glossary of Epidemiologic Terms

Epidemic: A level of disease that is above the usual for the population or community. Applicability of the term therefore depends on the disease in question, its past history in the particular area, and factors such as seasonality that influence the relative number of cases. "Epidemic" in common parlance implies a sudden and unexpected increase rather than a level merely numerically above the mean, especially when the latter can be anticipated on the basis of secular cycles. Although technically correct in the latter situation, the epidemiologist's use of "epidemic" publicly may depend on whether he wishes to foster some community action, such as a vaccination campaign, or allay apprehension.

Outbreak: The sudden, unexpected occurrence of disease, usually focally or in a limited segment of the population, without necessary reference to the usual level in the total community. Although the public health implications may be no different from those of an epidemic, the community regards an outbreak as less serious.

Endemic: Pertaining to the persistance of an infectious agent within a human population at a more or less constantly low level or without large increases manifest as overt clinical cases. The word implies that the reservoir is in the human population, and this term should not be applied to intermittent spillover from enzootic and epizootic foci.

Hyperendemic: Pertaining to persistence of an infectious agent in a human population at a very high level. When truly applicable, most infections must be clinically inapparent or exist in long-term carriers. The term is most commonly used with respect to enteric agents in an area with poor sanitation, and it has a pejorative connotation.

Prosodemic: Pertaining to infections that maintain themselves in human populations by a variety of mechanisms of transmission. Applied originally by Winslow to typhoid fever and more recently by Mosley to type B hepatitis.

Sporadic: Said of a case of a disease when apparently related neither to other cases in terms of common exposure, nor to increased prevalence of the agent in a human or other reservoir population

Epizootic: A level of infection or disease above the usual for a nonhuman population of vertebrates

Enzootic: Pertaining to peristence of infection or disease in a nonhuman population of vertebrates

Prevalence: The number of occurrences or cases of a disease in a specific population *at a given point* in time

Incidence: The number of occurrences or cases of a disease in a specific population *during a specified interval* of time. Data are usually given on an annual basis, even if accumulated over a shorter period; intervals other than annual must be specified. If the event or disease is not one that begins and ends within the period used in the definition, consideration is restricted to new or newly identified cases.

Attack rate: The number of *overt* cases of a disease in a specified population during a specified interval. This term is ordinarily used when the cases occur in an epidemic setting and have been well defined through investigation.

Morbidity rate: The number of overt cases of a disease in a specified population during a specified interval. The term is commonly used when the cases have been identified by physicians' reports and refer to a general population or the entire community

Case fatality rate: The number of deaths due to a disease in a well-identified group of cases

Death-to-case ratio: The number of deaths due to a disease in a group of cases not necessarily representing all clinically overt instances of disease. The death-to-case ratio is most commonly used to indicate the relation between deaths attributed to a given cause on certification and cases identified through physicians' reports.

Mortality rate: The number of deaths due to a disease in a general population or a community (that is, not just among cases)

Vector: Although the term can be defined more broadly, it is commonly used for arthropods that transmit infectious agents from man to man or from animal to man. Transmission may be mechanical—that is, the microbial agent contaminates the proboscis or other parts of the insect—or biologic, if the agent replicates in the arthropod.

Source: The milieu from which the agent was derived immediately prior to producing infection

Vehicle: A medium through which an infectious agent is conveyed to man, most commonly used with reference to drinking water or food. A source of infection is capable of sustaining replication of the agent; a vehicle is not.

Fomes (*pl.* fomites): An inanimate object in the environment of a patient, or one that has been in contact with a patient (such as clothes and bed linen), capable of sustaining the viability (etymologically, of keeping warm) of an infectious agent

Carrier: The individual who continues to harbor an infectious agent either following recovery from the illness it induced, or for a period more prolonged than expected in an asymptomatic infection. The term "temporary carrier" is sometimes used for an asymptomatic infection that persists as long as the usual clinically overt case, but a distinction seems preferable. Carrier implies that the individual is or may become the source of infection for others.

Reservoir The host or hosts on which the infectious agent depends for survival or perpetuation. It may be human (as for measles virus), nonhuman (as for *Francisella tularensis*), or environmental (as for *Clostridium tetani*).

THEODORE C. EICKHOFF

3 Nosocomial Infections

Infections that occur in an institutional setting (*e.g.,* hospitals, convalescent centers, nursing homes are nosocomial infections. The term nosocomial (Greek, *nosos,* disease + *komeion,* to attend to → nosokomeion, hospital) is preferable to hospital-acquired because the latter may imply a culpability that does not necessarily exist.

Most descriptive studies of nosocomial infections exclude infections that may be incubating at the time of admission to an institution, that is those that become apparent during the first 48 or 72 hours after entry. At the other end of the scale, some infections that are acquired during institutional care become apparent only after discharge (*e.g.,* surgical wound infections or cutaneous infections in neonates) and may be missed unless there is follow-up after leaving the hospital.

History

Nosocomial infections have undoubtedly existed ever since sick people were first gathered together for care. Medical writings of the 18th and 19th centuries report wound infection rates as high as 50% or more—presumably, infections caused primarily by streptococci and staphylococci. In the mid-19th century, Semmelweiss in Austria and Holmes in the United States wrote vividly of the astonishing rates of puerperal fever in lying-in hospitals, infections most likely caused primarily by group A streptococci. During World War I and II, nosocomial infections were usually caused by streptococci and staphylococci. The introduction of penicillin abated streptococcal but had only temporary effect on staphylococcal nosocomial infections. The predominant staphylococci were resistant to penicillin and became resistant in turn to a succession of antimicrobics introduced during the decade beginning in 1945.

Thus, nosocomial infection during the 1950s was synonymous with staphylococcal infection. Multiple drug resistance in certain bacteriophage groups of staphylococci was associated with a remarkable ability to persist in the hospital environment and in hospital personnel, and to spread from patient to patient. Outbreaks of pustular disease in neonates, surgical wound infections, and pneumonias were common in hospitals and were caused principally by multi-drug-resistant staphylococci.

During the 1960s, epidemic staphylococcal infection in hospitals began to subside—for reasons which remain as poorly defined as those that led to

Table 3-1. Prevalence and Incidence of Nosocomial Infections in Several Hospitals in the United States, 1970—1980

Hospitals	Prevalence* (%)	Incidence†
Boston City Hospital, 1970	12.0	
Boston City Hospital, 1973	15.0	
Latter-Day Saints Hospital, 1971	8.5	
Latter-Day Saints Hospital, 1979	6.9	
University of Virginia, 1972–75		7
Virginia Hospitals, 1974–77		3.3
NNIS Hospitals, CDC, 1970‡		3.1
NNIS Hospitals, CDC, 1979‡		3.3

* *Prevalence:* Proportion at any given time of hospitalized patients with nosocomial infection.

† *Incidence:* Rate of nosocomial infection per 100 admissions or discharges.

‡ National Nosocomial Infection Study, 71–87 hospitals.

its emergence. At the same time, there was a striking and progressive increase in the frequency of infection caused by gram-negative bacilli and, more recently, by fungi.

The predominance of infection caused by gram-negative bacilli continued and stabilized in the 1970s; 60% or more of all nosocomial infections were caused by gram-negative bacilli in that decade. Of other secular trends in the etiology of nosocomial infection in the 1970s, none was note save a gradual increase in the frequency of infection caused by methicillin-resistant staphylococci.

Current patterns

Representative reports of the incidence and prevalence of nosocomial infections are presented in Table 3-1. Data from hospital surveillance programs regarding incidence are generally believed to be about 75% sensitive; thus, the adjusted or true incidence of nosocomial infection is about 5% to 8%. According to detailed analyses of surveillance data, the incidence is lower in small community hospitals than in large teaching and tertiary-care hospitals. If the estimate of a 5% overall national rate is accurate, then there are 1.9 million nosocomial infections per year in the United States. The direct cost of nosocomial infections is probably well over 2 billion dollars annually.

The distribution of nosocomial infections by site of infection varies but little among diverse kinds of hospitals (Table 3-2). Urinary tract infections regularly account for one third or more of all nosocomial infections.

Table 3-2. Clinical Distribution of Nosocomial Infections in Several Hospitals in the United States

	% of infections		
Site of Infection	BOSTON CITY HOSPITAL 1973	NNIS HOSPITALS 1975–1978	LATTER-DAY SAINTS HOSPITAL (SALT LAKE CITY) 1979
Respiratory tract	29	16	15
Urinary tract	33	38	34
Surgical wounds	17	27	17
Skin and subcutaneous tissues	15	6	2
Other	7	13	32

Table 3-3. Distribution of Putative Pathogens in Nosocomial Infections Reported from Several Hospitals in the United States

	% of infections		
Putative Pathogens	BOSTON CITY HOSPITAL 1973	LATTER-DAY SAINTS HOSPITAL (SALT LAKE CITY) 1979	NNIS HOSPITALS 1978
Staphylococcus aureus	14	7	10.3
Staphylococcus epidermis	-	-	3.6
Streptococcus pneumoniae	2	-	0.8
Nonenterococcal *Streptococcus* spp.	6	4	2.1
Enterococci	12	11	9.0
Escherichia coli	14	14	18.8
Klebsiella and *Enterobacter* spp.	18	18	12.0
Proteus spp.	12	2	7.1
Serratia spp.	-	4	2.1
Pseudomonas aeruginosa	10	18	7.8
Others	12	22	26.4

The distribution of pathogens found in several recent studies is shown in Table 3-3. Staphylococcal infections continue to occur in hospitalized patients, but about two thirds of nosocomial infections are caused by enteric gram-negative bacilli and enterococci, pseduomonads, and fungi such as *Candida albicans.*

Until recently, most descriptive studies of nosocomial infection have given relatively little attention to nosocomial viral infections. The most important and serious of these include hepatitis B, rubella, and the herpes group of viruses. Enteroviral infections, including poliomyelitis, and infections of the respiratory tract, such as influenza and respiratory syncytial virus infections, also occur as nosocomial infections.

Host Factors

Because of their adverse effects on host defense mechanisms, many technologic advances of life-saving value have played a major role in shaping the present character of nosocomial infections.

These include immunosuppressive drugs such as the glucosteroids, invasive diagnostic techniques such as angiography, cancer chemotherapy with ionizing irradiation or cytotoxic drugs, and prolonged and complex surgical procedures for example the insertion of prosthetic valves, grafts, shunts, and joints. Other successes of modern medical care have increased both the numbers of patients and the life spans of individual patients with serious diseases that are noninfectious but crippling of host defenses, for example Hodgkins's disease. Such compromised hosts are at increased risk of clinical infection by elements of the ordinarily innocuous indigenous microflora.

Examples of major clinical determinants, or risk factors, in nosocomial infections are shown in the list below. The mechanisms by which these determinants serve to increase the risk of nosocomial infections is usually quite apparent, but a few merit more detailed comment.

EXAMPLES OF CLINICAL DETERMINANTS OF NOSOCOMIAL INFECTIONS

Age

The very young and the very old

Anatomic determinants

Surgery
Burns or other trauma
Foreign bodies, *e.g.,* urethral, IV and intraarterial catheters; trachesostomy and endotracheal tubes; artificial grafts, shunts, valves, and prostheses; sutures
Structural bronchopulmonary disease
Structural genitourinary tract disease

Metabolic Determinants

Diabetes mellitus, acidosis, renal failure

Decreased numbers of function of neutrophils

Acute leukemia, chronic granulomatous disease, drug-induced granulocytopenia, acidosis

Diminished or defective immunoglobulin synthesis, or rapid loss of immunoglobulins

Multiple myeloma, immunosuppressive drug therapy, nephrotic syndrome, burns

Defective cell-mediated immune mechanisms

Immunosuppressive drugs, cytotoxic drugs, disease states involving alteration of T-lymphoctye function; *e.g.,* Hodgkins disease; advances malignancies

Antimicrobic therapy

Age *per se* is probably a major risk factor only in the infant, particularly if premature, and in the elderly. Anatomic risk factors act by impeding normal clearance or drainage mechanisms, as in the case of strutural abnormalities of the genitourinary or bronchopulmonary tracts. Some foreign bodies, such as urinary or intravenous (IV) catheters, not only impair local tissue defenses, but also provide a direct portal of entry for microorganisms; others do not communicate with body surfaces (*e.g.,* prostheses or sutures) but interfere with cellular defenses by providing refuges inaccessible to phagocytes.

Leukocyte function is impaired in acidosis, whether systemic or local. Hypotension and shock resulting from any cause is regularly accompanied by systemic acidosis, and reduced tissue perfusion from any cause is regularly accompanied by local acidosis in the hypoperfused area. Thus the increased risk of infection in shock, congestive heart failure (CHF), renal disease, vascular insufficiency, and a variety of seemingly unrelated states may all result in part from the deleterious effect of decreased pH on leukocytic function.

Antimicrobial therapy is often overlooked as a major determinant of nosocomial infections. Generally, without adverse reactions such as severe dermatitis, bone marrow depression, or renal failure with an associated acidosis, antimicrobics given in normal doses appear to have little direct effect on host defense mechanisms. However, two interdependent effects of antimicrobics profoundly shape the character of nosocomial infections: (1) suppression of those elements of the microflora of the host that are susceptible to the prescribed drug(s) and (2) proliferation of those elements of the microflora of the host that are resistant to the prescribed drug(s). These effects are clinically evident in the gastrointestinal and upper respiratory tracts, the vagina, and the skin. The broader the spectrum of the drug(s), the more severe the perturbations of the indigenous microflora. Thus, it is no accident that most of the bacteria regularly associated with nosocomial infections (*e.g.,* staphylococci and gram-negative bacilli) are capable of acquiring resistance to many drugs in a relatively short time. There is little evidence that multi-drug-resistant staphylococci or enteric gram-negative bacilli are more virulent than their drug-susceptible counterparts; there is abundant evidence that multi-drug-resistant bacterias have a distinct survival advantage in hospitalized patients exposed to the selective pressures of antimicrobic therapy.

Epidemiology

Exogenous and Endogenous Infections

Exogenous nosocomial infections are caused by microorganisms acquired from a source outside the patient, that is, from a source within the institutional environment. This could be personnel, other patients, or some inanimate part of the hospital environment, such as air, food, water, medication, fluids, and disposable devices (*e.g.,* needles, syringes, catheters).

Endogenous nosocomial infections are caused by microorganisms derived from the patient's own microflora (see Table 4-1). Usually some event or process has occurred that predisposes the patient to infection by his own indigenous microflora, and thus endogenous infections usually result from an alteration of the existing balance between host microflora and host defense mechanisms.

There is a third category: exogenous acquisition followed by endogenous infection. The host first acquires the microflora of the institution as part of his own indigenous microflora. Then, given an event or process that suppresses the host's defense mechanisms, endogenous nosocomial infection occurs. However, the infection is not caused by the host's original susceptible microflora, but by the drug-resistant microflora characteristic of the institution. It is likely that many nosocomial infections fall into this category.

Endemic and Epidemic Nosocomial Infections

It is not always apparent whether a given nosocomial infection arose from an endogenous or an exogenous source. Hence, it is more useful to consider nosocomial infections as endemic or epidemic, depending on whether or not the infection is part of a definable outbreak. In general, endogenous infection is endemic in nature, and exogenous infection may be endemic or epidemic, depending on whether transmission occurs within the hospital. It is estimated that about 5% of all nosocomial infections are epidemic, that is, outbreak-related.

Reservoirs and Routes of Transmission

In Table 3-4 are shown examples of some of the more common reservoirs and routes of transmission of microorganisms that regulary cause nosocomial infection. Several generalizations may be made, though it must be borne in mind that exceptions always occur. In general, nosocomial infections caused by the group A *Streptococcus pyogenes* and *Staphylococcus aureus* are associated with people; that is, other patients or personnel of the institution who either have an overt infection or are asymptomatic but disseminating carriers. Transmission is usually by direct contact, although airborne infection can occur.

Epidemiologically, the enterococci, as components of the intestinal microflora, are the same as the enteric gram-negative bacilli. Although both are usually associated with endogenous infection, there are a number of exceptions. For example, diarrhea caused by *Escherichia coli* may be spread by indirect contact from infant to infant or by direct contant from carrier personnel to infants in newborn nurseries. A number of outbreaks of klebsiellal and proteal infections in hospitals have been traced to exogenous sources, including both the inanimate environment and hospital personnel. Furthermore, the mixed exogenous–endogenous category of nosocomial transmission usually involves infections caused by these enteric bacteria.

Nosocomial infections caused by aerobic gram-negative bacilli that are not ordinarily part of the host microflora, such as *Enterobacter agglomerans, Serratia* spp., *Pseudomonas* spp. and *Flavobacterium* spp., should be considered exogenous in origin unless proved otherwise. As a group, these bacteria have a remarkable ability to survive and even multiply in moist areas such as nebulizers for anesthesia and respiratory support equipment, humidifiers in isolettes, and in liquids containing minimal nutrients (*e.g.,* solutions for IV infusion) and antiseptic agents (*e.g.,* benzalkonium chloride), and thus cause outbreaks.

The epidemiologic patterns of nosocomial infections associated with intense immunosuppression are not yet well defined. Examples include infections caused by viral agents (Chap. 75, Cytomegalovirus Infections; Chap. 93, Varicella and Herpes Zoster), bacteria (Chap. 33, Legionnaires Disease; Chap. 37, Nocardiosis; Chap. 51, Listeriosis), fungi (Chap. 39, Candidosis; Chap. 44, Aspergillosis), and protozoa (Chap. 45, Pneumocystosis; Chap. 129, Toxoplasmosis). Apparently, these are often endoge-

Table 3-4. Examples of Reservoirs and Routes of Transmission of Nosocomial Pathogens

Microorganism	Reservoir*	Route of Transmission*
Group A *Streptococcus pyogenes*	Patients and personnel	Contact; may be airborne
Staphylococcus aureus	Patients and personnel	Contact; rarely airborne
Clostridium perfringens	Host flora	Endogenous infection
	Contaminated supplies	Contact
Escherichia coli	Host flora	Endogenous infection
	Patients and personnel	Contact
Klebsiella spp.	Host flora	Endogenous infection
	Contaminated liquids and supplies	Contact
Proteus supp.	Host flora	Endogenous infection
	Asymptomatic personnel	Contact
Pseudomonas aeruginosa	Host flora	Endogenous infection
	Contaminated liquids and supplies	Contact
	Infected patients	Contact or airborne
Pseudomonas cepacia	Contaminated liquids and supplies	Contact
Serratia spp.	Contaminated liquids and supplies	Contact
Enterobacter agglomerans	Contaminated liquids and supplies	Contact
Candida albicans	Host flora	Endogenous infection
	Contaminated liquids and supplies	Contact
Hepatitis B virus	Blood secretions, or excretions of infected patients or carrier personnel	Contact; rarely airborne
Influenza virus	Infected patients or personnel	Contact or airborne

*Patients and personnel may include those with overt infection, or asymptomatic but disseminating carriers. *Host flora* is known to be modified by disease or therapy during hospitalization. *Contaminated supplies* may include instruments (*e.g.,* catheters), equipment (*e.g.,* respiratory assistance), or apparatus (*e.g.,* tonometers). Hospital flora may be acquired by contact (touch, food, water) or by inhalation. *Contaminated liquids* include preparations for parenteral injection, peroral administration, irrigation, instillation, topical application, and cleaning and disinfection. *Contact* includes direct and indirect touch, food, water, and large droplets. *Airborne* includes small particles and droplet nuclei that remain suspended in air, travel more than several feet, and enter the lower respiratory tract by inhalation.

nous in origin, emerging to cause overt infections only under the intense selective pressure of antimicrobial therapy or intense immunosuppression. Nevertheless, there is substantial evidence in support of exogenous sources of some nosocomial aspergillosis, and of most, if not all, nosocomial Legionnaires disease.

Prevention

The first step in the control of nosocomial infections is a surveillance program designed to identify and define patterns of occurrence of nosocomial infections within each institution. Although there are a number of methods for obtaining such information on a current basis, the use of a nurse–epidemiologist has gained wide popularity.

Whatever the method, it is critically important that the persons charged with this responsibility be reliable and motivated in carrying out their duties. An effective surveillance program should (1) provide information on nosocomial infections as they occur; (2) identify outbreaks of nosocomial infections early in their course so that appropriate investigations and preventive measures may be undertaken; (3) eliminate unnecessary or wasteful procedures used for the control of nosocomial infections; and (4) provide a continuing reminder to physicians and hospital personnel of the importance of measures to minimize nosocomial infection.

There is general agreement that 50% or more of nosocomial infections are simply not preventable with current knowledge, whereas 20% to 25% are preventable. Reasonably, surveillance efforts should be focused on the areas within the hospital where most of the preventable infections occur. These are the procedure-related and the device-related (urinary, IV, arterial catheters) infections that tend to occur in high-risk areas such as nurseries, intensive care units, other special care units (such as dialysis and oncology), and surgical suites.

Data collection alone will neither prevent nor control nosocomial infections. Specific measures are necessary for the control of infected patients, personnel, the environment, and problem areas and procedures.

Control of Infected Patients

Appropriate isolation of infected patients is an important means of limiting the spread of infectious agents within the hospital. Problems encountered with the implementation of isolation techniques in most hospitals usually fall into one of two extremes that should be avoided: (1) adherence to unnecessarily complicated isolation procedures, the isolation of patients whose infection does not merit isolation, or the failure to take patients out of isolation when the condition no longer requires it; and (2) casual observation of isolation techniques by all personnel or repeated failures by one or more persons to observe isolation protocols, thus rendering the entire effort ineffective.

Control of Personnel

Hospitals must protect personnel from acquiring infections within the hospital and patients from acquiring infections from personnel. To that end, most large hospitals maintain employee health programs aimed at protecting personnel by periodic skin testing, administering immunizing agents, and other preventive programs. The preventive value of simple hygienic measures such as hand washing must be continuously stressed to all personnel *including* physicians and nurses. Routine screening of healthy personnel for carriage of potential nosocomial pathogens such as staphylococci or streptococci has not been an effective approach to control. However, personnel known to have a communicable infectious disease should be restricted from direct contact with patients.

Control of the Environment

The hospital environment has received a great deal of attention from microbiologists and sanitarians whose goal is the prevention of nosocomial infections. Unfortunately, the resultant reports deal primarily with the enumeration of bacteria on environmental surfaces and their reduction by germicides and disinfectants; such data often bear little relation to the actual occurrence of nosocomial infections. Meaningful standards for permissible levels of microbial contamination of air, surfaces, or fomites do not yet exist, and it has been impossible to relate data on environmental contamination in hospitals to the occurrence of prevalence of nosocomial infections. Accordingly, microbiologic sampling programs within the hospital environment have been useful only within the context of specific epidemiologic investigations.

However, there is some evidence that very stringent environmental control, such as in laminar air flow rooms, may be of some use in minimizing temporarily the risk of infection in certain highly vulnerable patients, such as patients with acute leukemia undergoing remission-induction chemotherapy.

Problem Areas and Procedures

The problem areas that merit special attention in hospitals include surgical suites, nurseries, and intensive care units. Special procedures that should be given particular attention include the management of catheters (both vascular and urinary) and respiratory support apparatus. Techniques that minimize the risks of nosocomial infections associated with these high-risk procedures are well documented, but must be aggressively applied with continuous surveillance to assure compliance.

Another aspect of environmental control relates to the wide variety of supposedly sterile disposable materials distributed commercially. Serious infections have resulted from the use of contaminated items the manufacturer claimed were sterile: antiseptics for urinary tract catheterization, IV fluids, and IV catheters. The detection of such problems requires careful epidemiologic study, coupled with an appreciation of the many ways in which contamination of sterile products may occur both in manufacture and in use.

Approach to the Investigation of Hospital Outbreaks

The study of a cluster of unusual infections or a nosocomial epidemic is to the hospital epidemiologist as the diagnosis of a fever of unknown origin is to the clinician. That is, hypotheses must be constructed and data obtained to prove or disprove them. The following points are useful as guidelines:

1. The character of the outbreak must be defined. Information about the sites and kinds of infections must be collected. Risk factors, particularly those common to all infected patients, must be identified. Have the infections occurred throughout the hospital, on one ward, or one service? Are all infections of a specific kind, such as postoperative wound infections?
2. If risk factors or potential sources of infection are common to all infected patients, it is useful to do a case control study to determine the significance of the suspected risk factor. A significant association of a particular risk factor with the outbreak under study should then provide direction for further microbiologic investigation.
3. The nature of the infecting organism is often a helpful clue to possible reservoirs or routes of transmission.
4. Identification of the pathogen under study in

personnel or in the environment does not establish that person or item as the source for spread of the outbreak. Both personnel and environment may have become contaminated by infected patients. The significance of personnel who are carriers or environmental contamination can be interpreted only in the light of epidemiologic data.

Problems for the Future

Full delineation of the problems requiring additional investigation to control nosocomial infections would encompass most of the research areas of the broad field of infectious diseases and immunology. However two points are specifically concerned with nosocomial infections:

1. The cost-effectiveness of nosocomial infection control programs and recommendations. Knowing that many nosocomial infections simply cannot be prevented, can infection control activities be focused more sharply, so that resources are not wasted trying to prevent infections that are simply not preventable? The cost of hospital health care continues to rise at a rate that society may find intolerable. It is thus critically important to evaluate the cost effectiveness of widely recommended, but unproven, infection control procedures.
2. The enhancement of host defense mechanisms. Preventive techniques directed at enhancing host defense mechanisms appear promising, but are not yet to the point at which implementation on a broad scale can be recommended. For example, the use of antibody directed against core glycolipid in the treatment of bacteremic illness caused by aerobic gram-negative bacilli shows promise; if it is useful in therapy, would it also be preventive in high-risk, hospitalized patients? Enhancement of host defense mechanisms in the severely neutropenic patient, by granulocyte transfusion, also has shown some promise; however, it is very expensive, and not optimally effective. Enhancement of cell-mediated immune mechanisms by immunostimulatory drugs is a potentially exciting possibility.

Bibliography

Books

BENNETT JV, BRACHMAN PS (eds): Hospital Infections. Boston. Little, Brown & Co., 1979, 542 pp.

DIXON RE, BRACHMAN PS, BENNETT JV (eds): Isolation Techniques for use in Hospitals: Atlanta, 2nd ed. PHS Publication No. 76-8314. Center for Disease Control, 1975. 104 pp.

Infection Control in the Hospital, 4th ed. Chicago, American Hospital Association, 1979, 242 pp.

Journals

BRITT MR, SCHLEUPNER CJ, MATSUMIYA S: Severity of underlying disease as a predictor of nosocomial infection: Utility in the control of nosocomial infection. JAMA 239:1047–1051, 1978

DIXON RE (ed): Symposium on nosocomial infections, Parts I, II, and III. Am J Med 70:379–473, 631–744, 899–986, 1981

EICKHOFF TC: Standards for hospital infection control. Ann Intern Med 89:829–831, 1978

FREEMAN J, ROSNER BA, MCGOWAN JE JR: Adverse effects of tion. J Infect Dis 138:811–819, 1978

FREEMAN J, ROSNER BA, MCGOWEN JE JR: Adverse effects of nosocomial infection. J Infect Dis 140:732–740, 1979

GREEN JW, WENZEL RP: Postoperative wound infection: A controlled study of the increased duration of hospital stay and direct cost of hospitalization. Ann Surg 185:264–268, 1977

GROSS PA, NEU HC, ASWAPOKEE P, VAN ANTWERPEN C, ASWAPOKEE N: Deaths from nosocomial infections: Experience in a university hospital and a community hospital. Am J Med 68:219–224, 1980

HALEY RW, SCHABERG DR, CROSSLEY KB, VON ALLMEN SD, MCGOWAN JE JR: Extra charges and prolongation of stay attributable to nosocomial infections: A prospective interhospital comparison. Am J Med 70:51–58, 1981

MCGOWAN JE JR, BARNES MW, FINLAND M: Bacteremia at Boston City Hospital: Occurrence and mortality during 12 selected years (1935–1972), with special reference to hospital-acquired cases. J Infect Dis 132:316–335, 1975

MCGOWAN JE JR, FINLAND M: Infection and antibiotic usage at Boston City Hospital: Changes in prevalence during the decade 1964–1973. J Infect Dis 129:421–428, 1974

MCGOWAN JE JR, PARROTT PL, DUTY VP: Nosocomial bacteremia: Potential for prevention of procedure-related cases. JAMA 237:2727–2729, 1977

STEVENS GP, JACOBSON JA, BURKE JP: Changing patterns of hospital infections and antibiotic use. Arch Intern Med 141:587–592, 1981

WENZEL RP, OSTERMAN CA, HUNTING KJ, GWALTNEY JM JR: Hospital-acquired infections. I. Surveillance in a university hospital. Am J Epidemiol 103:251–260, 1976

WENZEL RP, OSTERMAN CA, TOWNSEND RT, VEAZEY JM JR, SERVIS KH, MILLAR LS, CRAVEN RB, MILLER GB JR, JACKSON RS: Development of a statewide program for surveillance and reporting of hospital-acquired infections. J Infect Dis 140:741–746, 1979

PAUL D. HOEPRICH

Host–Parasite Relationships and the Pathogenesis of Infectious Disease

4

Parasitism

The earth teems with life forms as remarkable in their diversity as in their numbers. Over the eons, as life evolved to the forms we know, inevitably there occurred myriads of interactions that contributed to continuing differentiation and selection of species. Special requirements of environment developed and fixed more or less permanent associations between life forms as necessary to the maintenance of particular species. In general, the larger, stronger species, in supporting and providing for the smaller, weaker species, became hosts to these dependent life forms—the parasites. The host–parasite relationship is in fact an extremely common biologic phenomenon.

The ideal of parasitism is actually commensalism, a relationship in which no injury is dealt to either participant by the other. Commensals live and reproduce, carrying out in full the activities unique to each participating life form, none apparently adversely affected by the others. Examples of medical relevance are the mycoplasmas, bacteria, spirochetes, fungi, protozoa, and metazoa that are commonly resident on or in humans without causing disease (Table 4-1). Such microorganisms are not to be confused with those only transiently present, finding the human an inhospitable environment because of factors such as temperature, nutrients, metabolism, immune reactions, and resident microbiota. There are, in addition, interactions beyond commensalism, termed mutualism, in which the relationship is mutually beneficial; for example, the human enteric bacteria which synthesize vitamin K.

The parasites of primary medical importance are those that are less sophisticated—parasites that have not attained the Nirvana of commensalism, for they have the capacity to injure the human host. Injury to the host is disadvantageous to both the host and the parasite. Should the host die, the parasite must also unless transfer to another host is accomplished. If the host survives, it often does so by mobilizing defenses that eliminate the parasite entirely.

Table 4-1. *Microorganisms Commonly Found on Healthy Human Body Surfaces*

Species or group	**Skin** GENERAL	FEET	EXTERNAL AUDITORY CANAL	CONJUNCTIVA	**Upper Respiratory Tract** NASAL PASSAGE	NASOPHARYNX
Mycoplasmas						
Bacteria						
Gram-positive cocci						
Staphylococcus epidermidis	**85–100*** 2–6/cm²		**27–100**	**37–94**	**90**	++
Staphylococcus aureus	**5–24**[§]		**12–20**	**0–30**	**20–80** **2–100**[a]	++
Anaerobic micrococci	±					
Streptococcus mitis; undifferentiated α and γ streptococci	± to 0		**0.2–23**	**0.3–1**	±	**24–99**
Streptococcus hominis (salivarius)						+
Enterococci or group D *Streptococcus* spp.						
Streptococcus pyogenes (usually group A unless noted)	**0–4**			**0.3–2.5**	**0.1–5**	**0–9**
Anaerobic *Streptococcus* spp.						
Streptococcus pneumoniae			+	**0–5**	**0–17**[j]	**0–50**
Gram-negative cocci						
Branhamella catarrhalis; other nonpathogenic *Neisseria* spp.				**2.3**	**12**	**10–97**
Neisseria meningitidis						+
Veillonella alcalescens						+
Gram-positive bacilli						
Lactobacillus spp. Aerobic *Corynebacterium* spp.	**55** 5/cm²		**86**	**3–83**	**5–80**	+
Propionibacterium acnes	**45–100** 6/cm²				+	
Mycobacterium spp;	+				±	±
Clostridium perfringens						
Clostridium tetani						
Other *Clostridium* spp.						
Eubacterium limosum						
Bifidobacterium bifidum						
Actinomyces bifidus						
Actinomyces israelii						
Leptotrichia buccalis						
Aerobic gram-negative bacilli						
Enterobacteriaceae	±		**4–8**	**2.1**		**21–23**
Escherichia coli						±
Enterobacter spp.			**0.1–0.4**			±
Klebsiella spp.			+	**0.1**		±
Proteus mirabilis; other *Proteus* spp.			**0.2–1**	**0.4**		

	Mouth			Intestine			Genitourinary Tract		
		SALIVA–TOOTH SURFACES			FECES				
OROPHARYNX–TONSIL	PREDENTULOUS		GINGIVAL CREVICE	UPPER LEVELS	INFANT	ADULT	EXTERNAL GENITALIA	ANTERIOR URETHRA	VAGINA
+		+				+	+	±	+
30–70	+	**75–100** 1–4/ml			**31–59**‡	+ 2–4/g	+	++	**3**
35–45		+ **(16–35)**‖		+	**10–93**[a]	**30–50**§		±	**5–15**
+		+		+					+
100	++	**100** 6–8/ml	**100** 6/mg	 +	**14–32**	+	+	±	**10–21** **47–50**[b]
++	**100**	**100** 7/ml	++	+	**0–6**	+			
+[c]	+	**4–22**[d]		+	**87** 6–9/g	**100** 3–8/g	+	**2–10**	**30–90**
8–66[e]		**12–68**[f] 3–6/ml[f]			**0.7–19**[g]	**16**[h]			**5–20**[i]
+	+	++	++ 6/mg			+	+		**30–60**
7	+	**26**							±
98		**95–100** 5–7/ml	+					+	+
0–15									
+	+	**100** 6–8/ml	+						+
	 +	**95**[k] 0–6/ml		 +		**20–60**[k] −7 g			**50–75**
50–90		**59**			**10–21**	**6**	+	+	**45–75**
	±								
±						+	+	±	
		±		++	**13–19**	**25–35**			**0–10**
						1–35			
						5–25			**15–30**
						30–70			**5**
						30–70			**10**
					15–60[l] 90[m] 7–11 g[m]				**25–75**
+		+	+						±
		++ 0–3/ml	++						
 +	 +	**65** 0–3/ml			**86–100** 7–9/g	**100** 5–8/g	 +	 +	**15–40**[b] **3–10**
		4.2		++	**67–99**	**100**		+	+
±		**31**			**28–52**	**40–80**			**6**[b]
+		**52**		++	**19–48**	**40–80**		+	
+	+				**48**	**5–55** −6/g		 +	+[b]

Table 4-1. *Microorganisms Commonly Found on Healthy Human Body Surfaces* **(Continued)**

Species or group	Skin: GENERAL	Skin: FEET	Skin: EXTERNAL AUDITORY CANAL	CONJUNCTIVA	Upper Respiratory Tract: NASAL PASSAGE	Upper Respiratory Tract: NASOPHARYNX
Pseudomonas aeruginosa			**0–1.3**			
Alcaligenes faecalis			**1.1–1.6**	±		
Moraxella lacunata				±	+	±
Acinetobacter calcoaceticus				±		±
Hemophilus influenzae				**0.4–25**	**12**	**43–90**
Hemophilus parainfluenzae						**5**
Hemolytic Hemophilus spp.						+
Hemophilus vaginalis						
Anaerobic gram-negative bacilli						
Bacteroides fragilis (5 subspecies)						+
Bacteroides melaninogenicus (3 subspecies)						
Bacteroides oralis (2 subspecies)						
Fusobacterium nucleatum						
Fusobacterium necrophorum						
Curved bacteria						
Selenomonas sputigena						+
Campylobacter sputorum						+
Treponema denticola						
Treponema refringens						
Fungi						
Candida albicans	±	±				
non-*albicans Candida* spp.	**1–15**	+	+			
Torulopsis glabrata						
Pityrosporon ovale	**100**[p]					
Pityrosporon orbiculare	++					
Dermatophytes		**2–41**				
Protozoa						
Entamoeba gingivalis						
Entamoeba coli						
Endolimax nana						
Dientamoeba fragilis						
Iodamoeba buetschlii						
Trichomonas tenax						
Trichomonas hominis						
Trichomonas vaginalis						
Giardia lamblia						
Chilomastix mesnili						
Enteromonas hominis						
Retortamonas intestinalis						
Metazoa						
Demodex folliculorum	+					

$^{\pm}$ to 0, rare; ±, irregular or uncertain (may be only pathologic); +, common; ++, prominent.

*Boldface values (*e.g.,* **30–60**) = range of incidence in percent, rounded, in different surveys. Values given with units (*e.g.,* 3–6/ml) = range of concentrations expressed as $\log_{10}$:6 = >5 × 10^5 < 5 × 10^6.

† + in newborn; more common in school children than in adults.

‡ Predominant first day; decreasing during first month.

§ Associated with nasal carriage.

	Mouth			Intestine			Genitourinary Tract		
					FECES				
OROPHARYNX–TONSIL	PREDENTULOUS	SALIVA–TOOTH SURFACES	GINGIVAL CREVICE	UPPER LEVELS	INFANT	ADULT	EXTERNAL GENITALIA	ANTERIOR URETHRA	VAGINA
±					+	**3–11**		+	
		±			**0–2.1**	+		±	
							±	±	
3–97		**25–100**							
20–35		**25**				±		**5**	+
77		+							+[b]
								±	+
+		+	+	+		**100**	+		±
						7–10/g			
+		+	+			**100**	+		
			6/mg						
+		+	+			**100**			
+	+	**15–90**	+			**100**	+		
		3–5/ml	4/mg						
+			+			**100**			±
	±	+	+			+?	+		
	±	+	+						+
+			**60–88**	+	**18**[b]	**28**	+		
+		+	6/mg						
6–28		**5–50**	**15–40**		+	**1–3**	+	±	**30–50**
		0–5/ml				0–4/g			
±		**1–4**				**1–12**		±	**4–6**[o]
		+				+	+	±	+
+			**0–72.6**						
						8.0–32.1[q]			
						9.3–16.0			
						0.2–5.9			
						1.4–5.0			
+			**4.0–33.8**						
						0.3–4.1			
								+	**10–25**
						2.9–14.7			
						17.6[b]			
						0.4–6.1			
						0.1–3.2			
						0.1–1.3			

‖Percent of strains isolated.
[a]In infants and children; highest in hospital nursery infants.
[b]Children.
[c]In newborn.
[d]More common below age 20.
[e]More common in school children.
[f]Associated with presence in throat.
[g]"Hemolytic": Lancefield group not given.
[h]Groups B, C, F, and G; no A.
[i]Children; usually group B.
[j]More common in children.
[k]Especially in dental caries.
[l]Bottle-fed infants.
[m]Breast-fed infants.
[n]After the second week.
[o]*Candida stellatoidea*, principally.
[p]Especially scalp and nasal folds; also other skin areas.
[q]Values in this column are for North America and western Europe.

(Rosebury T: *Microorganisms Indigenous to Man.* New York, McGraw-Hill, 1962)

However, here, as with most biologic phenomena, there is no sharp, abrupt distinction, but rather a gradation, a spectrum of parasitic competence. Thus, some microorganisms are able to injure the host only when some predisposing, otherwise unrelated injury has occured; for example, cystitis arising from displacement of *Escherichia coli* into the urinary bladder by passage of a catheter through the urethra. Other parasites engender overt infectious disease infrequently compared with covert infection that is subclinical but does evoke a specific antibody response (poliomyelitis). Some parasites quite predictably cause overt infectious disease that typically culminates in the elimination of the parasite (measles). The extreme in parasite-mediated injury to the host verges on predation and is the ultimate in clumsy incompetence on the part of the parasite when death of the host is the usual outcome; for example, pneumonic plague (*Yersinia pestis,* Chap. 140, Plague). In all fairness, it should be added that usually the human is not the preferred or definitive host for these particularly lethal parasites.

The ultimate in ecologic specialization among parasites of medical importance may be represented by cytophilism—a preference for dwelling inside the cells of the host. Indeed, some infectious agents (*e.g.,* viruses, chlamydias, and rickettsias) are obligate intracellular parasites, for they cannot reproduce or long survive in any other environment. Others *(e.g., Salmonella typhi)* are facultative, growing either inside or outside cells, although a human host appears to be required for survival of the parasites. Still others may be intracellular or extracellular as parasites and may also be capable of a free-living nonparasitic existence *(e.g., Coccidioides immitis).* Finally, there are parasites that typically do not survive inside cells, for example, *Streptococcus* spp.

An obvious mode of entry into cells is phagocytosis, a process that results in enclosure of the parasite in a phagolysosomal vacuole. Survival requires either resistance to lysosomal agents *(e.g., Mycobacterium leprae)* or inhibition of transfer of lysosomal agents into the phagocytic vacuole (*e.g., Chlamydia* spp.)

Nonphagocytic entry into host cells generally does not elicit a hostile reaction and often appears to ensure a welcome. The mechanisms involved are often highly selective. Indeed, the restriction of some parasites to certain hosts probably reflects specific physicochemical requirements of both parasite and host surfaces for interaction. Thus, influenza viruses attach to specific receptor sites that are particularly plentiful on the cells of the mucous membrane of the human tracheobronchial tree. The enveloped herpes simplex virus fuses with the cell membrane to clear a passage for the entry of the nucleocapsid into the host cell (Fig. 4-1*A*). With some viruses, the intact virion penetrates the host cell, perhaps without requiring a specific portal.

The merozoites of *Plasmodium* spp. enter erythrocytes when the anterior (paired organelles) end of the parasite contacts the erythrocyte membrane. This causes invagination and then interiorization (Fig. 4-1*B*); specific receptors in the red cell membrane appear to be necessary to the interaction, for example, the Duffy blood group determinants may be receptors for *Plasmodium vivax.* After entry of a merozoite, the erythrocyte either regains its normal shape, becomes spherical, or lyses.

The advantages to intracellular residence are several. If the parasite is incomplete, that is, lacks energy-generating systems (rickettsias) or replicative abilities (viruses), exploitation of the machinery of the host cell is critical to survival. In addition, an intracellular environment is a haven from the host's immune defenses and phagocytic cells and from some antimicrobics. However, a host cell can support only a limited number of parasites, and indiscreet replication of the parasite kills the host cell. Unless there is spread through cell membranes to adjacent uninfected cells—as is usual for the herpesviruses—the parasite will then be exposed to the extracellular defenses of the host.

Infection and Infectious Disease

Infection is the establishment of a host–parasite interaction; because it requires only the presence of a parasite on or in a host, it is extremely common. When clinically manifest injury to the host results from this interaction, an overt infectious disease has occurred. At the other extreme, the parasite is present in the host and proliferates at least enough to maintain its numbers, but it does so with no evidence of having incited any reaction at all in the host; colonization has been suggested to describe this common situation (*e.g., Staphylococcus aureus* on the nasal mucosa). Between colonization and overt infectious disease lie covert or subclinical infections—all those instances in which the host–parasite interaction does not cause noticeable deviation from good health but does cause sufficient injury to the host to provoke a response specific for the parasite. These relationships are summarized in Fig. 4-2.

A given parasite, when hosted by a given species, does not always provoke identical disease in all infected individuals. As infectious diseases occur in nature, there is variation in the inoculating dose of the

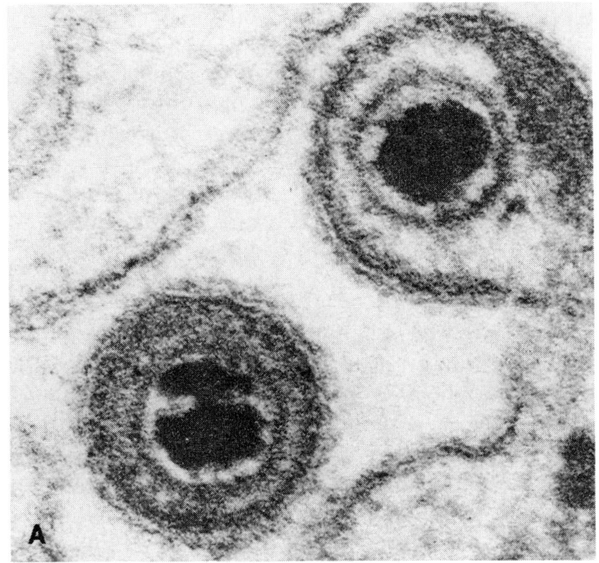

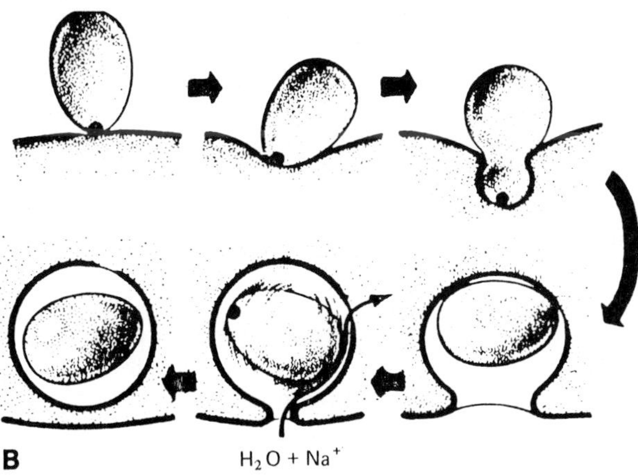

Fig. 4-1. Nonphagocytic entry of parasites into host cells. (*A*) Fusion of herpes simplex viruses with host cell membrane. (Morgan C. Rose HM, Nednis B: J Virol 2:507–516, 1968) (*B*) Progression of entry of a merozoite into an erythrocyte. (Dvorak JA, Miller LH: Science 187:748–750, 1975)

parasite. There are also variations within species, with regard to both the virulence of the parasite and the resistance of the host. Yet, the spectrum of intensity of interaction between host and parasite can be broadly delimited for given species. Typhoid fever may be a very severe disease with a high mortality; infection is usually clinically evident (Chap. 64, Typhoid Fever). Polioviruses, on the other hand, usually parasitize without producing clinical disease, and death is uncommon (Chap. 121, Poliomyelitis). With most infectious agents, the number of clinically inapparent infections vastly outstrips the number of apparent illnesses, a fact of great importance to the dissemination and persistence of parasitic microorganisms.

When the conjunction of host and parasite is a chance phenomenon that results in an infectious disease, an *accidental infection* has occurred. Into this category fall most of the infectious diseases that afflict previously well persons between neonatal and geriatric groups. With accidental infections, the host–parasite relationship is one of conflict. Typically, the issue is decided quickly and usually is influenced in favor of the host by the availability of powerful chemotherapeutic agents. Prevention of accidental infection, either by chemoprophylaxis or immunoprophylaxis, is frequently practical. The parasites involved are not normally either components of the endogenous microbiota or of commensal interactions; thus, the occurrence of such infections truly represents the accident of the host encountering a specific parasite. Pneumococcal pneumonia is just such a disease. The requirements are a nonimmune human who happens to inhale live *Streptococcus pneumoniae* borne on droplet nuclei that happen not to be trapped by nasopharyngeal–tracheobronchial–bronchiolar respiratory components but successfully lodge in the alveolar ducts and alveoli (Chap. 31, Bacterial Pneumonias).

More numerous by far, particularly in the very

Fig. 4-2. An interaction between host and parasite may result in infection, which consists of colonization and infectious disease. Infectious disease may be either covert (subclinical) or overt (symptomatic).

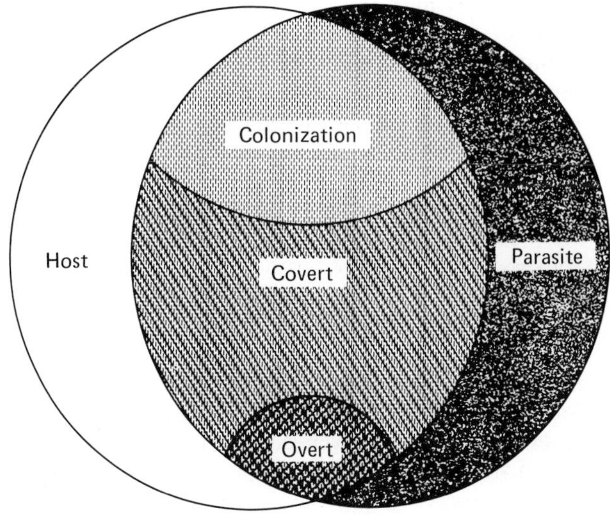

young and in the old, are infections that are conditioned in occurrence by some existing abnormality of the host: that is, *obligatory infections.* Abnormalities of many kinds oblige infection, ranging from anatomic (urethral stricture), metabolic (diabetes mellitus), neoplastic (bronchogenic carcinoma), collagen vascular (disseminated lupus erythematosus), therapeutic (ionizing radiation), devitalized tissue (ischemic necrosis), to unknown (hypogammaglobulinemia). The infections that result may be abrupt in onset and may run a severe course, leading even to death. More commonly, a smoldering, sullen chronic truce is the outcome. Chemotherapeutic agents may be limited value, and generally neither chemoprophylaxis nor immunoprophylaxis is possible. The parasites involved usually are elements of the endogenous microbiota or bear a quasi-commensal relationship to the host. Acute cholecystitis complicating cholelithiasis and caused by *E. coli* is an example of an obligatory infection.

In addition to accidental and obligatory infections, there are other categories of infectious diseases. Thus, infections are spoken of as being either *localized* or *generalized.* Actually, these are relative terms. Although localized refers to focal infection, as attested by signs or symptoms of disease, inapparent or potential involement elsewhere is always a distinct possibility. Staphylococci in a furuncle are localized to the furuncle, yet the whole host may experience fever and malaise. If staphylococcal osteomyelitis develops, it is evident that localization has been only partially successful. Mumps at one time was thought of as a viral disease typically localized to the parotid glands; now it is known that involvement of the parotids is consequent to viremia secondary to replication in the mucosa of the upper respiratory tract (Chap. 74, Mumps).

The course of infectious diseases may be acute or chronic. Generally, the parasites that are least well adapted to the human host, those that most rapidly and most often kill the human host, are those that incite the most acute and violent reaction; for example, plague pneumonia. Conversely, accomplished parasites, because they do not cause rapidly lethal injury, also provoke less reaction as they become established in the host; for example pulmonary tuberculosis. These terms, *acute* and *chronic,* are useful generalizations. However, there are many examples of acute infections that become chronic: acute osteomyelitis that persists as chronic osteomyelitis. Chronic infections may become acute—acute pyelonephritis flaring forth from the coals of a chronic pyelonephritis.

Cycle of Parasitism

With all parasites, regardless of whether or not the incursion results in disease, a uniform sequence of events must take place. The parasite must gain access to the host; establish itself, either at the locale of entry, remotely, or generally; and leave the host. Although it is apparent that all these events occur, the ways in which they come about are often obscure.

Access

There is no mystery about means of access when an inoculum of a parasite is injected into the host; for example, arthropod vectors and contaminated needles, syringes, and injectable medicines. However, most infections occur through the mucous membranes, or much less frequently, through the skin. In the former situation, potential parasites usually must survive in the presence of a resident microbiota that is rich both in variety and numbers; for example, the upper respiratory tract and the digestive tract. Beyond survival, there is the necessity for penetration through an epithelial barrier. The facilitating effect of minor, even microscopic, injuries to the epithelium is apparent. However, of greater importance may be the interaction between specific host cell surface components and particular surface structures of the parasite.

Establishment

Regardless of how a parasite succeeds in reaching the host's tissues, it must proliferate in order to cause disease—that is, the internal milieu of the host must be nutritionally suitable, and the parasite must be able to withstand the various defenses mounted by the host (Chap. 6, Resistance to Infection). Human tissues are nutritionally adequate to support the growth of a wide variety of microorganisms. However, there are variations from one parasite to another, one human to another, and one organ, tissue, and cell type to another that are sufficient to cause a preference for hosts, organs, and tissues by particular parasites. The bases for such preferences are not clear. For example, why in nature are typhoid fever and hepatitis A solely diseases of humans? When respiratory droplet exposure of humans to *Corynebacterium diptheriae, Streptococcus pneumoniae,* or *Neisseria meningitidis* leads to disease, why are the illnesses likely to be pharyngitis, pneumonia, and meningitis, respectively? With a few parasites, some insight into localization has been developed. Thus the 33°C temperature optimum for growth of *Mycobacterium marinum* corresponds to the clinically observed limitation of lesions (Chap. 36, Nontuberculous Mycobacterioses). The growth stimulatory effect of erythritol for *Brucella* spp. is reflected in growth to high densities in tissues containing this substance (Chap. 138, Brucellosis).

For most pathogens, neither the rate nor extent of replication in the human is accurately known. When studied in experimental animals, the generation time is usually much longer than it is *in vitro*—for example, 8 to 10 hours for *Salmonella typhimurium* in the mouse compared with 30 minutes in broth.

Egress

Egress from the host typically occurs through the portal of entry. However, with some parasites, multiple paths of egress may be achieved; for example, polioviruses in oropharyngeal secretions and in the feces.

Attributes of Parasites

A *pathogen* is a parasite that is capable of causing disease. Among pathogens, the degree of pathogenicity varies—that is, a pathogen may be slightly to highly virulent. For example, both *Staphylococcus aureus* and *Streptococcus pyogenes* (of Lancefield's group A) are pathogenic for man; the latter microorganisms are more virulent in that the application of around 10^7 streptococci to the mucosa of the normal oropharynx causes a pharyngitis, whereas pharyngeal application of virtually any number of staphylococci does not cause illness.

Virulence can be altered. Many generations' growth in unusual, bland, or even inhospitable environments frequently results in attenuation of virulence. Thus, Bacille Calmette–Guérin (BCG), a strain of *Mycobacterium bovis,* was rendered avirulent by the manifold repetition of subcultures on artificial culture mediums. It is still pathogenic for humans, causing the formation of tubercles at the site of inoculation and engendering delayed hypersensitivity; however, it remains localized to the site of inoculation (noninvasive) and does not cause progressive disease in normal hosts. Similarly, measles virus was attenuated by repeated passages in tissue cultures.

The reverse effect, enhancement of virulence, may occur when an infectious agent survives in the dangerous environment of the living host. Survival and replication in a hostile environment require affirmation of pathogenicity and are properly viewed as the selection of spontaneously occuring mutants. An example is the disappearance of bacilli that are susceptible to phagocytosis early in the course of plague in humans (Chap. 140, Plague).

Invasiveness, the ability to spread from a portal of entry, is another important characteristic of parasites. By itself, invasiveness does not guarantee virulence or even pathogenicity. *Treponema pallidum* is a classic example of a highly invasive parasite that is capable of passing through apparently unbroken mucous membrane. However, it does not produce clinical disease as it invades, and about one-third of those who contract syphilis seem to suffer no ill effect as a consequence (Chap. 59, Syphilis).

Pathogenesis

When parasites gain entry into a potential host, time must elapse before clinical illness can begin. This time is known as the *incubation period* and is of variable duration with rather definite, often characteristic, limits for a given host–parasite system. During the incubation period, dissemination of the parasite can take place and lead to inoculation of a preferred or target organ. Proliferation of the parasite, either in a target organ, throughout the body, or at the locus of entry, implies more than nutritional compatibility, especially if an infectious disease is provoked.

Generally, three modalities of disease causation are invoked: (1) invasion of the tissues of the host through inflammatory mobilization of phagocytic cells and a variety of humoral substances; (2) intoxication by specific substances elaborated by the parasite that are capable of injuring the cells of the host—even at sites distant from the parasite; and (3) induction of hypersensitivity; that is, an inappropriate, exaggerated immune response. However, these processes seldom operate in isolated, pure form (Table 4-2).

Table 4-2. *Spectrum of Pathogenetic Host–Parasite Interactions*

Disease	Invasiveness	Intoxication	Hypersensitivity
Botulism	0	++++	0
Tetanus	+	++++	0
Diphtheria	++	++++	0
Staphylococcosis	+++	++	±
Pneumococcosis	++++	0	0
Streptococcosis	++++	++	++
Tuberculosis	+++	0	++++

Invasiveness

The growth of parasites in the tissues of the host, without the liberation of recognized toxins, could conceivably lead to ill effects in the host. Depletion of nutrients locally by rapidly proliferating parasites might theoretically harm vicinal host tissues. This is unlikely to be a critical matter in view of the biochemical versatility of mammalian cells and the quantitative resources of the host. However, competition for space may produce disease; for example, hypoxemia consequent to blockage of gas exchange by obliteration of alveolar spaces in infectious pneumonias. Local ill effects have also been attributed to waste products said to arise from parasites. Similarly, it has been suggested, but not proved, that dead or dying parasite and host cells might be sources for substances injurious to other host cells.

Successful invasion implies either a failure to elicit host defense mechanisms or an ability to inhibit such defenses. For example, the phagocytosis of microorganisms is hampered by the presence of surface and capsular components that are intrinsically noninjurious to phagocytes. The capsular polysaccharides of pneumococci (Chap. 31, Bacterial Pneumonias), the M protein and hyaluronic capsule of *Streptococcus pyogenes* (Chap. 24, Streptococcal Diseases), the poly-*d*-glutamic acid capsule of *Bacillus anthracis* (Chap. 104, Anthrax) and the Vi antigen of *Salmonella typhi* (Chap. 64, Typhoid Fever) appear to be such substances.

Actively antiphagocytic substances are produced by some bacteria, for example, the leukocidins of some strains of *Staphylococcus aureus* and *Streptococcus pyogenes,* and the toxin(s) of some strains of *B. anthracis.* In addition, virulent strains of some kinds of bacteria (*Mycobacterium* spp., *Neisseria* spp., *Brucella* spp., some *Staphyloccus aureus, Listeria monocytogenes, Erysipelothrix insidiosa, Francisella tularensis, Y. pestis, Haemophilus ducreyi, Salmonella* spp.) some fungi (*Coccidioides immitis*), all pathogenic *Chlamydia* spp., rickettsias, viruses, as well as many spirochetes and protozoa, remain unaffected by the lethal and digestant factors of the intraphagocytic milieu.

Perhaps *Streptococcus pneumoniae* provides the purest example of a parasite with marked powers of invasion and high virulence, but with no apparent capacity to intoxicate and little potential for induction of hypersensitivity. The vigorous, neutrophil-rich inflammatory response and the severe systemic illness characteristic of pneumococcal infection are not reproduced by injection of either dead pneumococci or cell-free filtrates of broth cultures of pneumococci. Actual growth of *Streptococcus pneumoniae* in the host is necessary to produce disease (Chap. 31, Bacterial Pneumonias). Characteristically, recovery from infection caused by pneumococci—for example, pneumococcal pneumonia—is complete, with no residual anatomic or physiologic evidence of damage. This speaks for the lack, or very minor role, of hypersensitivity in the pathogenesis of pneumococcal infections.

There is no doubt of the pathogenicity or invasiveness of *Streptococcus pyogenes* for humans (Chap. 24, Streptococcal Diseases). Serious illness is engendered—the "blood poisoning" classic in the past—and there is a vigorous host response. Yet, other pathogenetic mechanisms are operative. Of the many toxins elaborated in cultures, only the erythrogenic toxins are clearly active *in vivo* as the cause of the scarlatinal rash. However, it is not established that persons parasitized by *Streptococcus pyogenes,* which elaborates erythrogenic toxins, are sicker than persons whose illness is caused by nonproducers of erythrogenic toxins. Furthermore, immunity to erythrogenic toxins and to the other known toxins does not protect against infection by *Streptococcus pyogenes.* Hypersensitivity evoked by *Streptococcus pyogenes* appears to be involved in the pathogenesis of the nonsuppurative complications, hemorrhagic glomerulonephritis, and rheumatic fever. Both the timing of occurrence and the restriction to only certain persons infected with *Streptococcus pyogenes* are consistent with hypersensitivity as the pathogenetic mechanism.

Proliferation of *Staphylococcus aureus* in the tissues of the host calls forth a marked neutrophilic cellular response and is attended by inflammation. However, invasive disease is not common except in the very young and in adults disabled by some nonstaphylococcal disease. The mature, healthy adult characteristically localizes staphylococci and suffers some tissue destruction in the process—the necrotic core of a furuncle is an example. Such tissue destruction is in keeping with some degree of hypersensitivity. *Staphylococcus aureus* elaborates several toxins. Although cell-free filtrates of broth cultures of staphylococci do provoke marked inflammation localized to the site of injection and also result in prostration if large doses are given intravenously, the profound illness of staphylococcal sepsis is not thereby reproduced. Indeed, only two extracellular products of staphylococci are unequivocally associated with intoxication of the host: the enterotoxins, which must be ingested preformed to cause disease (Chap. 60, Gastroenterocolitis Syndromes), and the pyrogenic exotoxin(s) that have been implicated in toxic shock syndrome (Chap. 50, Infections of the Female Genital Tract).

Intoxication

Although many infectious agents produce demonstrable toxic substances, it is unusual for toxins to be the sole determinants of diseases. Notable exceptions are diphtherial, tetanal, botulinal, and other clostridial (gas gangrene) toxins, staphylococcal enterotoxins, and the enterotoxins of *Vibrio cholerae* and certain strains of *Escherichia coli.* Several of these toxins have been purified and even crystallized. Although the details of biochemical interactions are not discussed here, it is noteworthy that these are the most powerful of poisons to humans and other mammals (Table 4-3).

Botulism is so absolutely a disease of intoxication that it scarcely qualifies as an infectious disease. *Clostridium botulinum* rarely grows on or in the human. The actual cause of botulism—botulinal toxin—is almost always elaborated outside the human body and causes the disease when ingested (Chap. 127, Botulism). From observation of functional neuropathology, the toxin appears to affect nerve endings primarily, blocking nerve impulses; there is also evidence of central action. However, botulinal toxin leaves no morphologic trace of its action.

Tetanus is quite clearly an infectious disease (Chap. 126, Tetanus), for some vegetative growth of *Clostridium tetani* within the body of the host is essential to elaboration and absorption of the tenanal toxin. Also a neurotoxin, tetanal toxin is extraordinarily potent and provokes no detectable anatomic lesion. There is no spread of the bacilli from the site of traumatic inoculation, and there is no element of hypersensitivity.

Table 4-3. *Toxicity of Several Poisons*

Toxin	Weight of Animal Killed by 1 μmole (kg)	Animal
Strophanthin	3.6	Rabbit
Ricin	1,120	Mouse
Cobra venom	90,000	Mouse
Clostridium perfringens,		
α-toxin	40,000	Mouse
Diphtherial toxin	245,000	Guinea pig
Tetanal toxin	120,000,000	Guinea pig
Botulinal toxin		
Type A	1,200,000,000	Guinea pig
Type B	72,000,000	Guinea pig

In diphtheria (Chap. 25, Diphtheria), intoxication is undoubtedly the primary cause of disease. Diphtherial toxin is a much less potent poison than either botulinal or tetanal toxins, and anatomic evidence of its effect is demonstrable. Death of mucosal cells subjacent to areas of growth of diptheria bacilli and remote effects (necrosis of myocardial and renal tubular cells, demyelination of axons) bear testimony to the lethal effect of interference with protein synthesis by toxin. However, there is an element of bacterial virulence in diphtheria. This is most clearly evident in the mild clinical illness that results when humans are parasitized with nontoxinogenic *Corynebacterium diphtheriae.*

Other toxins clearly contribute to pathogenesis, but are not the primary determinants of disease. The α-hemolysin of *Staphylococcus aureus,* erythrogenic toxins of *Streptococcus pyogenes,* and lethal toxins of *Bacillus anthracis* fall into this category. Aflatoxin, produced by *Aspergillus flavus* growing on animal foods, has been implicated as a cause of abortion, death, and neoplasia in sheep and cattle.

A number of toxins that are detectable in the laboratory may be of pathogenetic significance. Examples include the neurotoxin of *Shigella dysenteriae* and the lethal toxins of *Pseudomonas aeurginosa.* Toxic effects have also been observed from the experimental injection of influenza viruses and in experimental rickettsial infections.

The endotoxins of gram-negative bacteria cause fever, diarrhea, abortion, prostration, and death in shock on injection into experimental animals. Although endotoxins may contribute to the pathogenesis of infections caused by gram-negative bacteria, it is quite clear that other factors are critical to the establishment of such infections.

Hypersensitivity

Hypersensitivity, as it relates to the pathogenesis of infectious diseases, refers either to reactions associated with humoral and cellular elements (Arthus phenomenon, atopy, anaphylaxis) or to reactions involving only sensitized cells of the host (delayed, tuberculin-type hypersensitivity). Immunoglobulin mediation of injury implies union of antigen with antibody *in vivo.* If the complex is formed locally, as by subcutaneous injection of antigen into a hypersensitive animal, an intense, localized inflammation results in which thrombosis and necrosis of arteriolar, capillary, and venular endothelium may occur. This is the *Arthus phenomenon.* Although tissue injury results, even to the extent of necrosis and sloughing, the reaction can be viewed as protective to the animal, for systemic distribution of the antigen is prevented. The rhinitis, conjunctivitis, and nasal congestion of hay fever are less violent, less injurious consequences of a localizing antigen–antibody reaction in which release of histamine appears to be an important link in pathogenesis.

Anaphylaxis can be elicited by the rapid flooding of a hypersensitive animal with an excess of antigen. Both humoral and cellular components of the immune process are involved. Injection of antigen–antibody complexes, near equivalence, but with a slight excess of antigen, may initiate anaphylactic shock. However, this does not mean that anaphylaxis is solely the result of reaction between circulating immunoglobulins and antigen. Isolated organs from a hypersensitive animal, for example, the guinea pig uterus, when washed free of excess antibody, manifest anaphylactic reactions with detectable release of histamine when exposed to antigen, presumably as a result of antibody retained on the cells. Histamine (to some extent, also serotonin, heparin, proteases, and perhaps other polypeptide substances) appears to be implicated in the pathogenesis of anaphylactic shock. Not only is histamine released during anaphylactic shock, but also the clinical picture of shock can be mimicked by the injection of histamine. Drugs that block the action of histamine also suppress the manifestations of shock. The primary effect in anaphylaxis is violent contraction of smooth muscles. However, the clinical result varies according to the anatomic nature of the species observed and remains constant within a given species. Thus, in humans, though there is often difficulty in breathing and there may be involuntary urination and defecation, the prominent, life-threatening feature of anaphylaxis is usually shock.

Delayed (cellular) hypersensitivity results in tissue damage through inflammation in which mononuclear cells predominate. Tissue destruction is brought about both by lysosomal activity and by perivascular aggregation of mononuclear cells that compromise the blood supply. The Koch phenomenon is an example. In the normal guinea pig, the subcutaneous deposition of live *Mycobacterium tuberculosis* evokes little reaction at the site of injection until 10 to 14 days have passed, although the bacilli have spread and multiplied enormously. Local induration then becomes apparent, progressing to necrosis with the formation of an indolent ulcer. In contrast, inflammation develops 1 to 2 days after subcutaneous injection of either live or dead *M. tuberculosis* into a guinea pig with tuberculosis. Necrosis and ulceration quickly develop; however, healing is prompt and regional nodes are not involved.

The classic infectious disease wherein hypersensitivity is the host–parasite interaction of primary pathogenetic importance is tuberculosis (Chap. 34, Pulmonary Tuberculosis). *Mycobacterium tuberculosis* does not produce detectable toxins. It is invasive, particularly in the young and in certain racial groups. In the nonhypersensitive person, *M. tuberculosis* survives and multiplies within phagocytes; proteins derived from tubercle bacilli (tuberculin) are innocuous on injection. When hypersensitivity is established, however, tuberculin is lethal to the host cells. It is in the hypersensitive host that systemic manifestations of illness occur and the tissue destruction characteristic of tuberculosis takes place. However, hypersensitivity alone is not sufficient to cause disease. Indeed, BCG does not cause tuberculosis in humans even after intradermal or subcutaneous inoculation, although such inoculation engenders hypersensitivity. Helminthic and fungal parasitization also result in disease chiefly through initiation of hypersensitivity.

Bibliography

Books

BROCK TD: Principles of Microbial Ecology. Englewood Cliffs, NJ, Prentice–Hall, 1966. 306 pp.

MUDD S (ED): Infectious Agents and Host Reactions. Philadelphia, WB Saunders, 1970. 626 pp.

ROSEBURY T: Microorganisms Indigenous to Man. New York, McGraw–Hill, 1962. 435 pp.

SKINNER FA, CARR JG (EDS): The Normal Microbial Flora of Man. London, Academic Press, 1974. 264 pp.

SMITH T: Parasitism and Disease. New York, Hafner, 1963. 196 pp.

VAN HEYNIGEN WE: Bacterial Toxins. Oxford, Blackwell Scientific Publications, 1950. 133 pp.

Journals

BROCK TD: Microbial growth rates in nature. Bacterial Rev 35:39–58, 1971

FREDERICKSON AG, STEPHANOPOULOS G: Microbial copetition. Science 213:972–979, 1981

HANKS JH: Host-dependent microbes. Bacteriol Rev 30:114–135, 1966

SMITH H: Biochemical challenge of microbial pathogenicity. Bacterial Rev 32:164–184, 1968

STEWART SELL

Immunopathology of Infectious Diseases

5

The specific immune reactivity of hosts to infectious agents may lead not only to protection but also to disease by causing symptoms, and lesions in the tissues. The purpose of this chapter is to define specific immune effector mechanisms, to describe how these mechanisms may contribute to and cause disease, and to illustrate the interplay of protective and destructive mechanisms through the use of examples of specific infectious diseases.

Specific Acquired Immunity

The system of reactivity to foreign agents and substances that brings forth unique products from the lymphoid organs is known as specific acquired immunity. It is one of the mechanisms that enable humans to resist a wide variety of potentially infectious agents. Other mechanisms of resistance include nonspecific, inherent characteristics such as temperature, pH, metabolic products, and the nature of the external surfaces of the body (see Chap. 6, Resistance to Infection).

Specific acquired immunity occurs naturally following recovery from an infectious disease. The primary infection results in the acquisition of new reactive systems, which have the capacity to recognize the infectious agent, or a product of the infectious agent, and to limit or to prevent the consequences of a subsequent attack.

The importance of specific acquired immune mechanisms is illustrated by persons in whom immune reactions are depressed or absent. Such immune-deficient individuals are unable to protect themselves against a variety of infectious agents that are usually limited to causing mild effects or no serious symptoms in persons with normal immune capacity.

Specific acquired immune mechanisms are mediated by two major systems: humoral antibody (immunoglobulin system) or specifically reactive lymphocytes (cellular system). Humoral antibody is generally effective against organisms that exist extracellularly, whereas cellular immunity is active against intracellular parasites. A number of accessory systems involving inflammatory cells or proteins play an important role in the complete expression of immune mechanisms initiated by humoral antibody or sensitized lymphocytes.

In this chapter, the role of the effector phase of the immune response in evoking the manifestations of infectious diseases will be emphasized. The protective role of immune effector mechanisms will be mentioned only to illustrate and to contrast more vividly the destructive capacity of immune effector mechanisms.

Accessory Systems of Immune Reactions

Before discussing the immune effector mechanisms that depend upon specific recognition of antigen, several nonantigen-specific accessory systems that are activated by antigen-specific reactions will be described briefly. These accessory systems contribute substantially to the events that are set in motion upon reaction of antigen with antibody or reactive cells *in vivo.*

Complement

The complement system consists of 20 or more serum proteins that are essential for some inflammatory reactions associated with infection. The activation of the various components of complement is achieved by a series of cleavage reactions and molecular aggregations. Three stages of the activation process may be identified: recognition, activation, and attack. A detailed scheme of complement activation is presented in Figure 5-1.

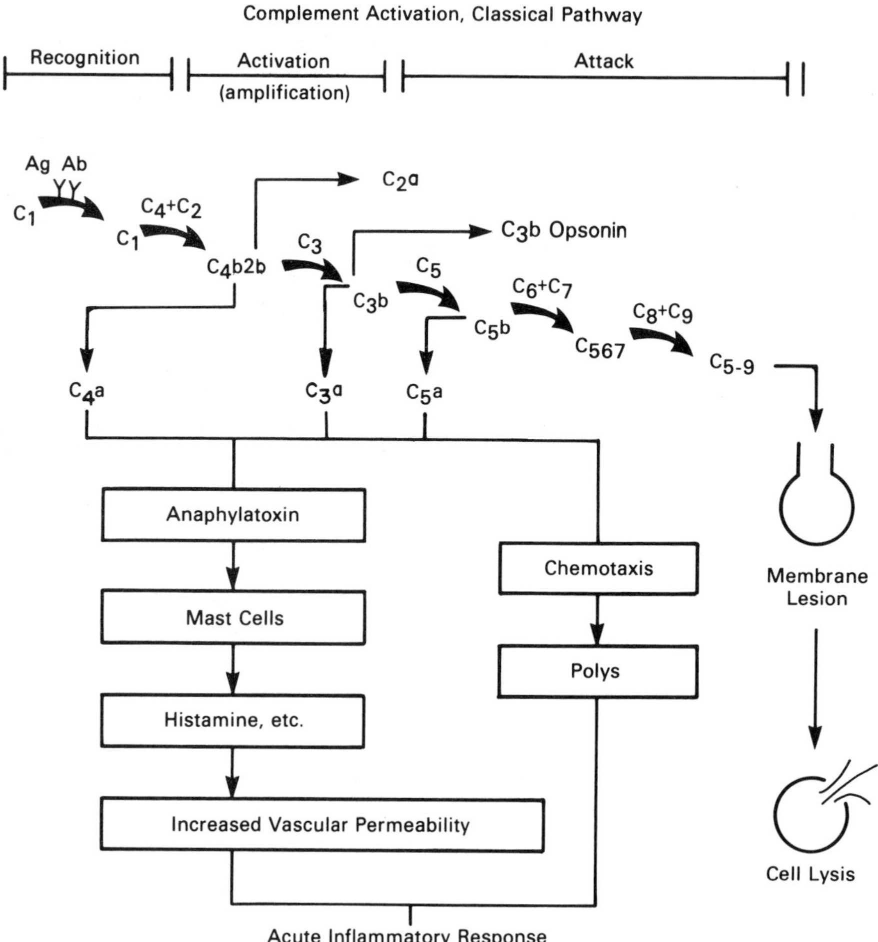

Fig. 5-1. The classical pathway of activation of complement. Following reaction of antibody with antigen, a cascade of reactions of the components of complement is activated. C_1 functions as a recognition unit for the altered F_c of two IgC or one IgM molecule; C_2 and C_4 function as an activation unit leading to cleavage of C_3. C_3 fragments have a number of biologic activities: C_3a is anaphylatoxin, and C_3b is recognized by receptors on macrophages (opsonin); C_3b also joins with fragments of C_4 and C_2 to form C_3 covertase, which cleaves C_5. C_5 reacts with C_6 through C_9 to form a membrane attack unit that produces a lesion in cell membranes through which intracellular components may escape (lysis).

Several of the products that arise from cleavage of complement activate inflammatory processes. C3a and C5a cause contraction of endothelial cells resulting in gaps in capillary walls through which the liquid and formed elements of the blood pass out into the tissues. These same components of complement are also chemotactic for polymorphonuclear leukocytes, stimulating the development of acute inflammatory reactions.

Complement may also be activated by nonimmune mechanisms through an alternate pathway that involves a different system of proteins—the properdin system. The properdin system behaves much like components C1, C2, and C4 to activate C3 and set off the interaction of the remaining components of complement. In this manner, endotoxins produced by various infectious organisms may mimic the effects of complement-mediated immune specific reactions.

Polymorphonuclear Neutrophils

The polymorphonuclear neutrophil is a major effector cell in inflammatory reactions initiated by immune complex activation of complement. Fragments C3a and C5a attract and activate polymorphonuclear cells in sites where antibody–antigen reactions have taken place. In an attempt to phagocytize and digest the immune complexes, these cells may release digestive lysosomal enzymes into the adjacent tissue, particularly if the antibody–antigen complex is deposited on a structure such as vascular basement membrane. Digestion of tissue by lysosomal enzymes results in characteristic changes known as firbrinoid necrosis.

Mast Cells and Pharmacologic Mediators

Another accessory system is provided by tissue mast cells or circulatory basophils, which have receptors for one class of humoral antibodies, IgE. Mast cells contain intracellular membrane-delineated structures (granules) filled with pharmacologic mediators such as histamine, serotonin, slow-reacting substance, and eosinophilic chemotactic factors of anaphylaxis (ECF-A). Mast cells become coated passively with antibody of the IgE class. Upon reaction with the appropriate antigen, granule and cell membranes fuse to form a portal for the extracellular release of mediators. The mediators act on smooth muscle and endothelial cells to produce immediate constriction. Some of the consequences of this constriction include bronchial asthma and edema. In addition, certain mediators, for example, ECF-A, lysosomal enzymes, platelet activating factors, fatty acids, and inflammatory peptides, produce a delayed inflammatory phase, recruiting cells to the site of the reaction. The mast cell is the major effector cell of anaphylactic or atopic reactions (see below).

Macrophages

Macrophages function as an amplifying or accessory system for several immune mechanisms. They may engulf (phagocytize) and destory cells coated with antibody and complement (C3b, opsonin). Macrophages (1) appear later than polymorphonuclear cells in sites of acute inflammation initiated by antibody and complement; (2) are enlisted into sites of inflammation by lymphokines that have been activated by reaction with antigen released from specially sensi-

Table 5-1. *Mechanisms of Immune Injury*

Mechanism	Immune Reactant	Accessory Component	Skin Reaction	Protective Function	Examples of Protection	Pathologic Mechanism	Disease States
Neutralization	IgG antibody			Inactivate toxins	Tetanus; diptheria	Inactivation of biologically active molecules or cell surface receptors	Insulin-resistant diabetes; myasthenia gravis; hyperthyroidism (LATS)
Cytotoxic or Cytolytic	IgM > IgG antibody	Complement; Macrophages		Kill bacteria	Bacterial infections	Cell lysis or phagocytosis (opsonization)	Hemolytic anemias; vascular purpura; transfusion reactions; erythroblastosis fetalis
Toxic complex	IgG antibody	Complement; Polymorphonuclear leukocytes	Arthus: peaks in 6, fades by 24 hr	Mobilize neutrophils to sites of infection	Bacterial and fungal infections	Polymorphonuclear leukocyte infiltrate—release of lysosomal enzymes	Glomerulonephritis; vasculitis; arthritis; rheumatoid diseases
Anaphylactic	IgE antibody	Mast cells; Mediators; End organ cells	Cutaneous anaphylaxis: peaks in 15–30 min, fades in 2-3 hr. Hives	Opens vessels to deliver blood components to sites of inflammation	Helminthic infections	Bronchoconstriction, edema, shock	Anaphylactic shock; hives; asthma; hay fever; insect bites
Delayed hypersensitivity	T_K and T_D cells	Lymphokines; Macrophages	Delayed (tuberculin): peaks in 24–48 hr.	Kills organisms, virus infected cells	Viral, fungal, mycobacterial infections	Mononuclear cell infiltrates, target cell killing	Viral skin rashes; graft rejection; autoallergic diseases; demyelination
Granulomatous	T_D cells	Macrophages (epithelioid and giant cells)	Granulomas (weeks)	Isolation of infectious agents	Leprosy; tuberculosis	Replacement of tissue by granulomas	Sarcoidosis; berylliosis; tuberculosis

tized T-lymphocytes (T_D cells); and (3) may accumulate and occupy space if they are unable to digest phagocytized antigen (granulomatous reactions). Although macrophages do not recognize antigens, they are activated or attracted by antibody or lymphocytes that do recognize or react with antigens. Moreover, macrophages also have cell surface receptors for antibody–antigen complexes and will engulf immune complexes and clear such complexes from the circulation.

Immune Effector Mechanisms

Understanding immune effector mechanisms is greatly aided by a mechanistic classification according to six major immune effector mechanisms (Table 5-1). Four are mediated by immunoglobulin antibody: namely, neutralization, cytotoxic, immune complex, and anaphylactic. Two are mediated by specifically sensitized cells: namely, delayed or cellular, and granulomatous reactions.

Although these immune mechanisms may be supposed to have arisen to protect and preserve the individual, they may in fact contribute to or actually cause disease; the terms allergy and hypersensitivity are then applied to connote that the immune mechanisms are immunopathologic.

Neutralization or Inactivation

Neutralization or inactivation occurs when antibody reacts with an antigen that provides a vital function (Fig. 5-2). Such an antigen may be a soluble, circulating molecule—a hormone or an enzyme, or a cell surface receptor for a biologically active molecule. The reaction of antibody with soluble molecules causes alteration of tertiary structure of the molecule so that it becomes biologically inactive or is cleared from the circulation by the reticuloendothelial system as an immune complex. Antibody reacting with cell surface receptors may block the ability of the molecule to function as a receptor or cause loss of the receptor from the cell surface by modulation (capping or endocytosis). In some instances, reaction of antibody may actually stimulate cells by mimicking the effect of the biologically active molecule that normally reacts with the receptor. For example, antibodies to insulin may produce diabetic states by inhibiting insulin activity, whereas antibodies to thyroid-stimulating hormone receptors (long-acting

Fig. 5-2. Inactivation or activation of biologically active molecules. Reaction of antibodies with enzymes or other biologically active molecules may result in loss of biologic function. The antigenic determinants of an enzyme are usually located on parts of the molecule other than the substrate binding site. Inactivation by reaction with antibodies may occur by alteration of the tertiary structure of the enzyme affecting the substrate binding site or activity of the enzyme molecule, or by increased catabolism of the enzyme–antibody complex. Antibodies may also cause blocking or modulation of cell surface receptors so that the cell is refractory to stimulation. In some instances, reactions of antibody with cell surface receptors result in stimulation.

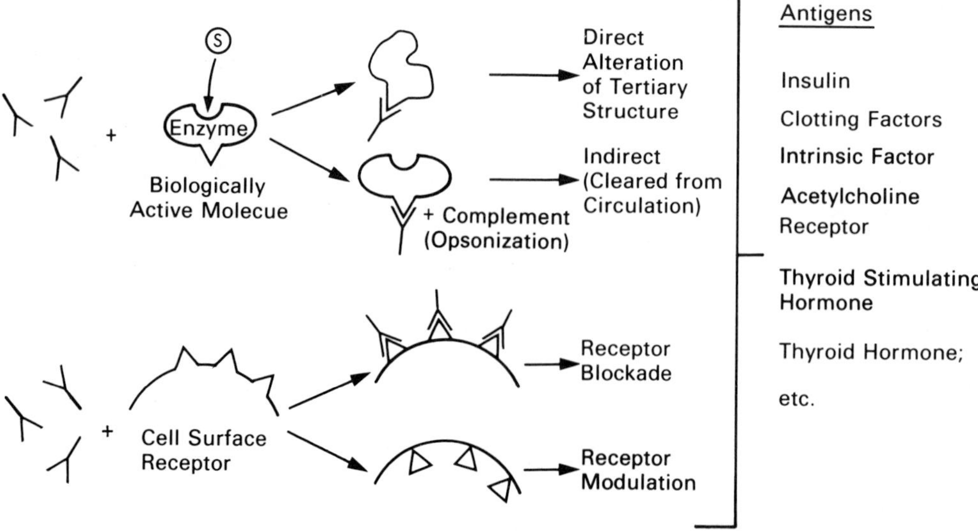

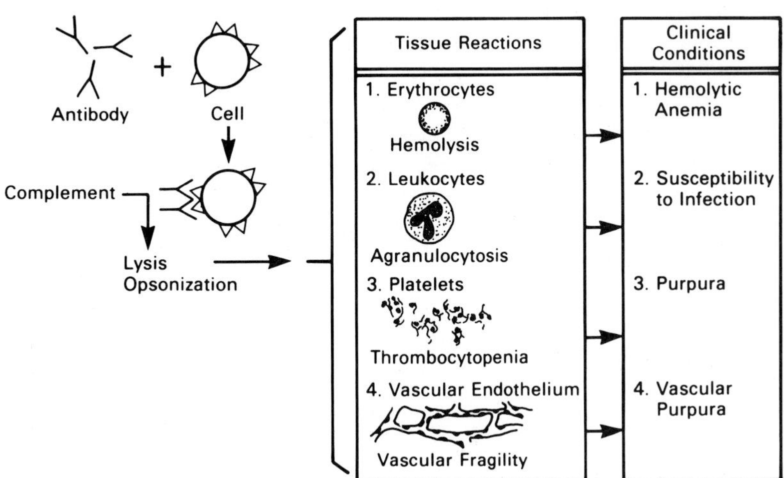

Fig. 5-3. Cytotoxic or cytolytic reactions. These reactions most often affect cellular elements in intimate contact with circulating plasma, such as erythrocytes, leukocytes, platelets, or vascular endothelium. Circulating humoral antibody reacts with antigens present on cell membranes, activating the complement system. Through action of the complement system, the integrity of cell membranes is compromised and the cell is lysed, or the altered cell is subject to phagocytosis.

thyroid stimulator, LATS) may mimic the activity of thyroid-stimulating hormone (TSH) and produce hyperthyroidism by stimulating the elaboration of thyroid hormone.

The protective role of neutralization reactions is important and varied. Perhaps the most obvious protective function is the ability of antibody to neutralize toxins such as diptherial, tetanal, and choleraic toxins. The goal of immunization using diptherial and tetanal toxoids is to produce antibody that will neutralize the effects of the respective toxins. Antibodies to cell surface receptors or to the structures on the surfaces of infectious agents (*e.g.,* the cell surface receptors of the cholera vibrio for intestinal epithelial cells; the receptors of *Neisseria gonorrhoeae* for urothelial cell surfaces) may prevent interaction of the parasite with host cells and prevent infection. Antibodies of the IgG class are most important for blocking the receptors of bloodborne infectious agents, whereas, IgA (secretory immunoglobulin) antibodies are most important for blocking adherance to epithelial cells.

Cytotoxic or Cytolytic Reactions

The reactions of antibodies with cell surface antigens, such as red blood cell antigens (ABO, Rh), result in activation of complement at the cell surface (Fig. 5-3). Destruction of the cell follows, either by alteration of cell membrane permeability or by opsonization (coating of the cell by antibody and certain components of complement that render the cell susceptible to phagocytosis).

The clinical effect of cytolytic reactions depends upon the cell involved. Cytolytic reactions more commonly affect cells in suspension in the circulation, such as red cells (hemolytic anemia), white cells (granulocytopenia), or platelets (thrombocytopenia), than cells in solid tissues.

Cytolytic reactions are protective when the activities of the complement system, such as lysis or opsonization, are brought to bear or infectious organisms. This mechanism is active in many bacterial infections and may result in destruction of bacteria directly on activation of phagocytosis so that clearance of infectious agents from the blood stream is enhanced.

Immune Complex Reactions

The reaction of complement-fixing antibody (usually IgG) with soluble circulating antigens or with tissue antigens, such as the basement membrane antigens of the kidneys or lungs, initiates an inflammatory reaction involving infiltration of tissues with polymorphonuclear cells (Fig. 5-4). Most circulating antibody–antigen complexes are opsonized by complement and are then cleared by the reticuloendothelial system. However, when there is an excess of antigen, immune complexes are not readily cleared but are deposited in small vessels or on the glomerular basement membrane and initiate inflammation (vasculitis and glomerulonephritis). Antigen excess complexes have a tendency to become localized in organs where the vascular basement membrane is not completely covered by endothelial cells (glomeruli, alveoli, synovia, and choroid plexus). The activation of complement products C3a and C5a by immune complexes may result in constriction of endothelial cells, thus permitting immune complexes to deposit in vessels usually covered by endothelium. In addition, C3a and C5a have chemotactic activity, which attracts polymorphonuclear leukocytes to sites of activation of complement. The neutrophils may damage tissues

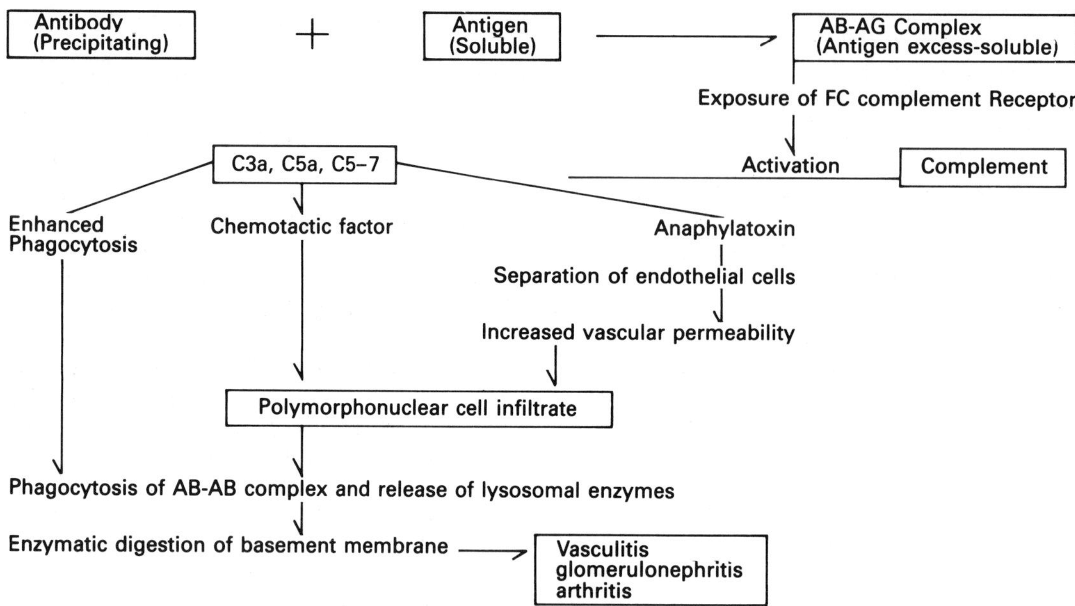

Fig. 5-4. Immune complex reactions. Circulating antibody, usually of the IgG class, reacts with soluble antigen to form intravascular immune complexes. If the complexes are in antigen excess they will not be cleared well by the reticuloendothelial system but will deposit in tissue sites. Exposure of the IgG receptor site for complement results in fixation and activation of complement and formation of active components of complement, which cause separation of endothelial cells, attraction of polymorphonuclear leukocytes, and activation of phagocytosis by polymorphonuclear cells. Release of lysosomal enzymes from polymorphonuclear cells results in digestion and fibrinoid necrosis of vessel walls, glomerular basement membranes, or the synovium of joints.

by digestion when lysosomal enzymes are released as immune complexes are engulfed and digested.

The acute inflammatory reaction initiated by immune complexes can be elicited in the skin of animals with circulating IgG antibody by injection of the antigen into the skin—the Arthus reaction. The reaction reaches a maximum about 6 hours after injection of antigen and consists of swelling and redness at the site of injection. Central hemorrhage or necrosis may occur if the reaction is severe. The reaction is caused by the formation of antigen–antibody complexes in the skin. The complexes form in the wall of small vessels, where the injected antigen reacts with antibody released from the circulation. The serum proteins of the complement system are activated, polymorphonuclear cells invade the vessel walls, and fibrinoid necrosis of the vessel walls occurs.

A number of other lesions are caused by the deposition of immune complexes in tissues. Glomerulonephritis may follow the deposition of circulating immune complexes on or within the glomerular basement membrane. An acute arthritis may result from immune complex deposition in the synovia. Transient glomerulonephritis and arthritis are frequently associated with the recovery phase of many infections. Rheumatoid arthritis is caused by the chronic activation of complement by autoantibodies to immunoglobulin, reacting with immunoglobulin in the joint space. Systemic lupus erythematosus is caused by anti-DNA—DNA immune complexes depositing in vessels, glomeruli, synovia, and other sites. It is postulated that the autoimmunization responsible for these diseases may be initiated by an infectious disease.

The protective function of immune complex reactions lies in mobilization of inflammatory cells at sites of acute infection. The reaction of specific antibody with an infectious organism is an exquisitely precise and accurately focused defense mechanism: Complement is activated on the surface of the offending organisms, resulting in opsonization and chemotaxis of polymorphonuclear cells. This mechanism is the major defense against extracellular bacteria, such as staphylococci and streptococci.

Anaphylactic or Atopic Reactions

Anaphylactic reactions result when antigens react with IgE antibodies passively bound to mast cells (Fig. 5-5). Mast cells have two important properties with regard to anaphylactic reactions. First, they bear surface receptors for IgE, and second, their cytoplasm is filled with granules containing a number of biologically active molecules. Upon reaction of antigens with IgE antibody attached to mast cells, the mast cells degranulate, releasing the biologically active molecules into the surrounding milieu. These substances cause constriction of endothelial cells and contraction of smooth muscle cells, leading to extravasation of intravascular fluids (edema) and eventually to shock. Cutaneous anaphylaxis is a skin reaction that is elicited by injection of antigen (allergen). The anaphylactic reaction reaches a maximum in about 15 to 30 minutes, fades by 6 hours, and consists mainly of edema (wheal and flare reactions). This is the test used by allergists to determine hypersensitivity in humans with allergic symptoms. In the lung, constriction of the smooth muscles of the airways and increased mucous secretion cause difficulty in breathing (asthma). Anaphylactic reactions or atopic diseases include asthma, hay fever, anaphylactic shock, food allergy, and reactions to insect stings and snake bites. The nature of an anaphylactic reaction depends upon a number of variables, including route of exposure, dose, and individual susceptibility. The intensity of an anaphylactic reaction depends upon the state of activation of the target organs—which may be modified by pharmacologic means. Epinephrine decreases the sensitivity of end organs to mediators. In addition, the reactivity of end organs may be influenced by the autonomic nervous system. Sympathetic stimulation decreases reactivity, whereas parasympathetic stimulators increase reactivity. Through the autonomic system, the emotional state of the reactive individual may influence the severity of an anaphylactic reaction.

Anaphylactic reactions may actually be protective. The opening of vessels at sites of reaction provides access for plasma proteins and cells. Severe constriction of gastrointestinal smooth muscle results in diarrhea and purging the gut of parasites. Sneezing and coughing help to remove infectious or toxic agents from the respiratory tract. Because the reactions are often sudden and very uncomfortable, they serve to warn an individual to avoid areas where exposure to potentially damaging agents might occur.

Delayed Hypersensitivity

Delayed hypersensitivity occurs when specifically sensitized lymphocytes that have receptors for antigens react with the antigen in tissue (Fig. 5-6). The nature of the cell surface receptor is not clearly

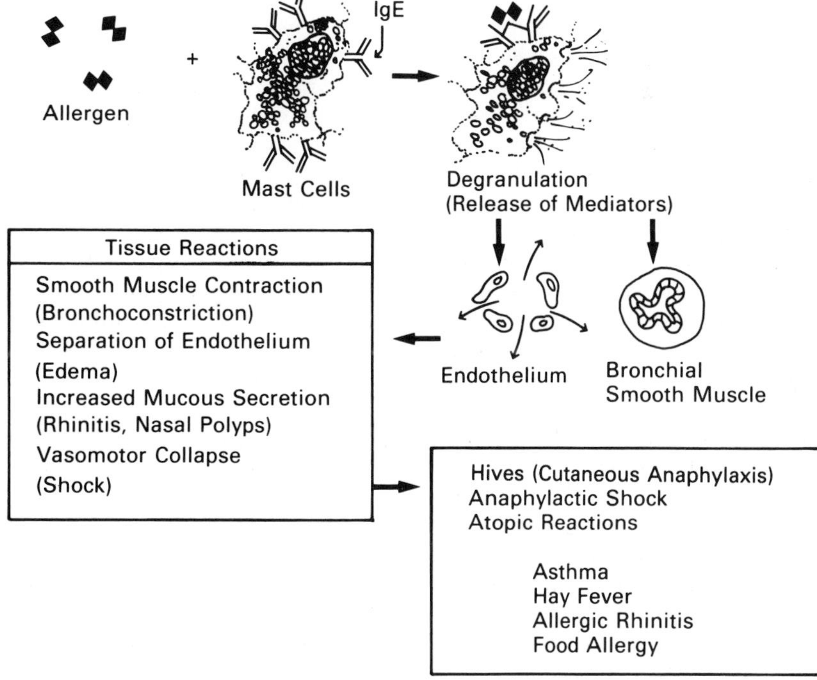

Fig. 5-5. Atopic or anaphylactic reactions. Reaction of antigen (allergen) with reaginic antibody (IgE) fixed to effector (mast) cells causes release of pharmacologically active agents stored in cytoplasmic granules (degranulation of mast cells). These released mediators cause contraction of endothelial cells and bronchial smooth muscle cells and produce tissue changes of edema and bronchoconstriction. The reactions may be acute (anaphylactic) or chronic (atopic), depending on the nature of exposure to the eliciting allergen.

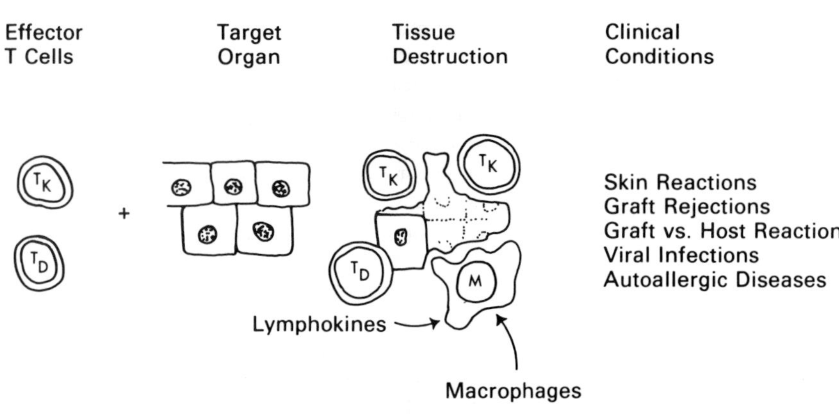

Fig. 5-6. Delayed hypersensitivity (cellular) reactions. Specifically modified T-lymphocytes containing a mechanism capable of recognizing antigen are the initiators. TK cells may kill target cells directly, whereas TD cells release mediators that in turn act to influence nonsensitive cells to participate in the reaction.

known, but it is believed to immunoglobulinlike, perhaps mimicking a part of an immunoglobulin molecule. The lymphocytes that effect delayed hypersensitivity reactions belong to at least two subpopulations of the T cell class, TD and TK cells. TD cells react with antigens and release a variety of mediators (lymphokines), which mainly act on macrophages to attract them, induce phagocytic activity, and enhance digestive capacity. TK cells react directly with antigens on the surface of target cells and cause their destruction (cytotoxicity).

The term delayed is used because characteristically the reaction in the skin requies 24 to 48 hours to reach a peak, in contrast to the Arthus (6 hours) and cutaneous anaphylactic reactions (15 minutes); the term hypersensitivity is applied because the sensitized animal demonstrates an increased sensitivity to the antigen upon challenge, in comparison with the unimmunized animal. The characteristic lesion of delayed hypersensitivity is a perivascular and diffuse mononuclear cell infiltrate. TD lymphocytes reacting with antigen in tissues are activated to release lymphokines, which in turn attract and activate macrophages. Phagocytosis and digestion by macrophages are directly responsible for tissue destruction. Some examples of delayed hypersensitivity reactions are the tuberculin skin test, contact dermatitis (poison ivy, poison oak), viral exanthems (measles), tissue graft rejection, and a number of autoallergic diseases.

The protective functions of delayed hypersensitivity reactions are mainly directed against intracellular parasites, such as viruses, fungi, and mycobacteria. Delayed reactions are particularly important in eliminating virus infections when the viral antigens are expressed on the cell surface. In addition, lymphocyte activation of macrophages may be effective in infections in which intracellular parasites escape digestion after phagocytosis by macrophages. In diseases such as tuberculosis, leprosy, and trypanosomiasis, macrophages that have been activated by lymphokines may no longer provide a favorable environment for the infecting microorganism.

Granulomatous Reactions

A granulomatous reaction is a space-occupying collection of mononuclear inflammatory cells. Granulomatous reactions may be considered a variant of delayed hypersensitivity in which the antigen is poorly catabolized and remains as a chronic irritant. In the early stages of development, the lesion resembles a delayed hypersensitivity reaction. However, instead of the macrophages digesting and clearing the antigen, a prolonged accumulation of macrophages and lymphocytes occurs (Fig. 5–7). The macrophages undergo a change that is recognized histologically as epitheloid cells, which are organized into ball-like clusters of cells known as granulomas. In addition to epitheloid cells, multinucleated giant cells, lymphocytes, and fibroblasts are frequently seen. The major disease-producing mechanism is the gradual replacement of normal cells. The space-occupying lesions may become so extensive that the normal function of the organ is lost. Diseases in which granulomatous reactions play a major part are tuberculosis, leprosy, mycoses, sarcoidosis, Wegener's granulomatosis, regional enteritis, and berylliosis.

The protective function of granulomatous hypersensitivity is to isolate infectious organisms that may resist other immune mechanisms. The offending organisms are encased by the granulomatous tissue and sequestered from causing disease.

Immunopathologic Mechanisms in Infections

The participation of immunopathologic mechanisms in immune responses to infectious agents is quite varied and complicated. A given infectious agent may activate more than one mechanism at the same time or sequentially. Immune effector mechanisms may be (1) directed specifically against the infectious agent, (2) part of autoallergic reactions stimulated by infectious processes, or (3) aimed at unrelated factors, such as nonpathogenic fungi or drugs used to treat infectious diseases. A few examples of the immune effects of responses to the specific agents of the many infectious diseases considered in this book will be discussed in this chapter.

Postinfectious Autoallergic Diseases

Antibodies or cells reactive to components of the tissues of the host are frequently found during or after a variety of infectious states. Autoantibodies may be incidental findings without evidence of tissue damage (autoimmunization), but in some instances autoantibodies may produce tissue damage (autoallergy). Autoimmunization may occur as a result of at least four mechanisms: (1) There may be antigenic determinants that are common to the infectious agent and the host's tissue; (2) antigenic components of the host, which are normally sequestered from the host's immune system, may be released as a result of the infection; (3) molecular components of the host may become altered during an infectious condition so that natural tolerance is broken not only to the altered molecules but also to the native molecules; and (4) the infectious process may perturb mechanisms that normally control the immune response (*e.g.,* T cell suppression, idiotype network) so that immune responses occur that are directed against normally nonimmunogenic molecular components of the host. Autoallergic reactions are responsible for a number of different diseases, some of which are associated with infections (Table 5-2). Because the preceding infection is not always obvious, it has been suggested that subclinical viral infections may be antecedent to diseases such as diabetes mellitus, myasthenia gravis, and thyroiditis.

Autoallergic Blood Diseases

Autoallergic hemolytic anemia is caused by autoantibodies that destroy red blood cells. Reaction of antibodies with red blood cells results in activation of complement and destruction of red cells by phagocytosis in the liver and spleen or by direct lysis of the cells. Different types of autoantibodies have been identified. Cold-reacting autoantibodies to red cells (Donath–Landsteiner antibodies) may appear after viral infections or in patients with syphilis or other chronic infectious diseases. Paroxysmal cold hemoglobinuria (the appearance of dark red urine after exposure to cold) results from intravascular hemolysis by cold-reacting autoantibodies. Demonstration of the antibody requires (1) mixing the patient's serum with red cells at 4°C to permit binding and (2) warming the mixture to 37°C. The disease is caused by IgC antibodies to erythrocytes that bind only in the cold. Cold agglutinin disease is caused by an IgM antibody that may appear after infection with mycoplasmas; intense hemagglutination occurs in the

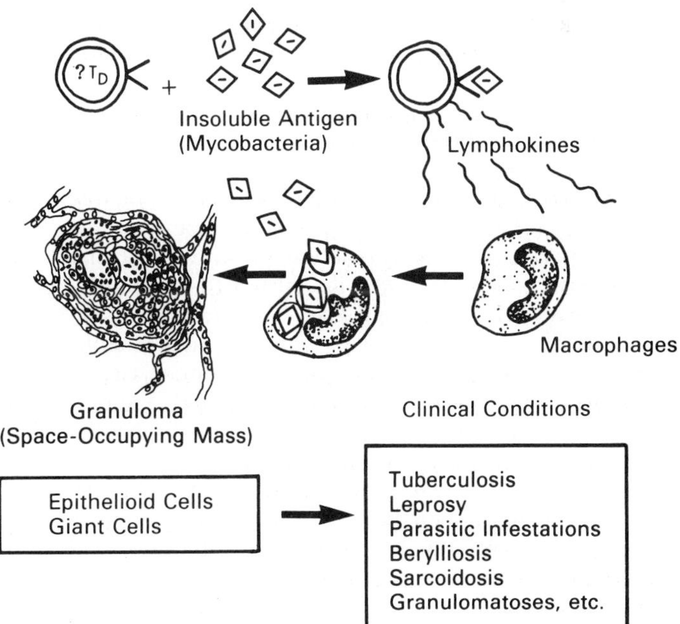

Fig. 5-7. Granulomatous reactions. Granulomatous hypersensitivity reactions may be identified morphologically by the appearance of reticuloendothelial cells (including histiocytes, epithelioid cells, giant cells, and in some instances lymphocytes) arranged in a characteristic round or oval laminated structure called a granuloma.

Table 5-2. *Relation of Experimental Autoallergic Diseases to Human Diseases*

		Histologically Similar Disease in Humans	
EXPERIMENTAL DISEASE	TISSUE INVOLVED	ACUTE MONOCYCLIC	CHRONIC RELAPSING
Allergic myasthenia gravis	Acetylcholine receptors		Myasthenia gravis
Experimental allergic nephritis	Glomerular membrane	Acute glomerulonephritis	Chronic glomerulonephritis
Allergic encephalomyelitis	Myelin (CNS)	Postinfectious encephalomyelitis	Multiple sclerosis
Allergic neuritis	Myelin (PNS)	Guillain–Barré polyneuritis	
Phacoanaphylactic endophthalmitis	Lens		Phacoanaphylactic endophthalmitis
Allergic uveitis	Uvea	Postinfectious iridocyclitis	Sympathetic ophthalmia
Allergic orchitis	Germinal epithelium	Mumps orchitis	Nonendocrine chronic infertility
Allergic thyroiditis	Thyroglobulin	Mumps thyroiditis	Subacute and chronic thyroiditis
Allergic sialadenitis	Glandular epithelium	Mumps parotitis	Sjögren's syndrome
Allergic adrenalitis	Cortical cells		Cytotoxic contraction of adrenal
Allergic gastritis	Gastric mucosa		Atrophic gastritis

cold—not hemolysis, as is caused by Donath–Landsteiner antibodies.

Autoantibodies to other blood cells may also be found following infectious conditions and are responsible for such disorders as acute idiopathic thrombocytopenic purpura (autoantibody to platelets following measles or other viral infections) and acute agranulocytosis (autoantibody to polymorphonuclear leukocytes.

Glomerulonephritis

Glomerulonephritis is an inflammation of the renal glomeruli caused either by deposits of circulating immune complexes on the basement membrane or by direct binding of autoantibodies by glomerular basement membrane antigens. Although glomerulonephritis may occur transiently following many infections, it is commonly associated with cutaneous infections caused by nephritogenic strains of Group A B-hemolytic streptococci (see Chap. 101, Streptococcal Skin Infections and Glomerulonephritis). Leakage of plasma proteins, erythrocytes, and leukocytes into the urine results from digestion of the glomerular basement membrane by lysosomal enzymes from polymorphonuclear leukocytes attracted and activated by immune complexes and complement. The temporal onset of acute glomerulonephritis corresponds to the time when circulating antibodies to streptococcal antigens appear in the serum. Examination of the kidneys by specific labeling techniques may demonstrate the presence of immunoglobulins, complement, and streptococcal antigens in the affected glomeruli.

Rheumatic Fever

Rheumatic fever is an acute systemic sequel to infections caused by Group A B-hemolytic streptococci (see Chap. 24, Streptococcal Diseases). The lesions are believed to result from the formation of immune complexes between antibodies produced to streptococcal antigens, which crossreact with antigens present in the tissues of the host. Antibodies to a number of streptococcal antigens are found in the serum (Table 5-3). Because antistreptococcal M protein antibodies crossreact with heart muscle, they may be responsible for the carditis; T cell cytotoxic activity for myocardial cells may also play a role. That is, rheumatic myocarditis may be caused by the activity of autoantibody, autosensitized cells, or both. The chorea of rheumatic fever has been associated with autoantibodies to basal ganglia, which can be absorbed with streptococcal cell walls. Other lesions of rheumatic fever are most likely the result of immune complex formation, in particular, erythema marginatum (vasculitis in the dermis) and glomerulonephritis. Rheumatic nodules are most likely the result of vasculitis caused by the deposition of immune complexes containing antigens resistant to degradation, leading to accumulation of macrophages and the formation of granulomas.

Malaria

Although the role of immune mechanisms in the pathogenesis of malaria (see Chap.145, Malaria) is incompletely understood, IgG antibodies appear to play an important part through the formation of immune complexes. In endemic areas, natives develop resistance to malarial strains that is associated with specific humoral antibodies. Neonates in endemic areas are resistant as a result of placentally transferred maternal antibody. A peak of susceptibility occurs at about 1 year of age. However, infection at this age is less severe than in persons who first contract infections as adults. Malaria organisms exist primarily within erythrocytes during an established infection. Some of the major manifestations of malaria (anemia, fever, nephritis, and vasculitis) appear to be associated with antibody-mediated immunopathologic mechanisms. The erythrocytes of patients with malaria become coated with IgG and have an increased susceptibility to phagocytosis and destruction by splenic macrophages. Although this reaction may help eliminate infected cells, it also contributes to the anemia. During malarial paroxysms, parasites are released from intracellular (intraerythrocyte) locations, resulting in the formation of immune complexes in antigen excess; the occurrence of glomerulonephritis, the nephrotic syndrome, and multiple vasculitides are presumed to be consequences. Finally, the preoccupation of macrophages with erythrophagocytosis may contribute to the immunosuppression observed in association with malaria.

Trypanosomiasis

African trypanosomiasis (see Chap. 130, African Trypanosomiasis) is characterized by fluctuating waves of parasitemia and a prominent polyclonal B cell response. There is marked hyperplasia of B cell (follicular) areas of lymph nodes and spleen, hyperplasia of T cell areas, marked elevations of serum IgM (up to 20 times normal), and a number of parasite-unrelated antibodies, including rheumatoid factor, autoantitissue reactivity, LE factor, and heterophile antibody. These activities, as well as antibody to trypanosomal antigens, are responsible for a variety of immune complex mediated lesions that are not major components of the disease. The following are of greater importance: (1) an apparently decreased ability to respond to an antigenic challenge with a specific antibody response; (2) a marked general depression of cellular immune responses; and (3) a decreased reticuloendothelial clearance. Proposed mechanisms causing these immune abnormalities include loss of controlling T cells, or polyclonal activation of B cells by the infection. Although a specific antibody response eliminates the dominant population of trypanosomes, antigenic variants are able to repopulate the blood, and the disease continues. If the condition is untreated, trypanosomes invade the central nervous system and parasitemia remains high until death occurs.

Allergic Bronchopulmonary Aspergillosis (Mucoid Impaction Syndrome)

Anaphylactic reactions to fungal or bacterial antigens are not uncommon and may be responsible for some

Table 5-3. *Antibodies in Rheumatic Fever*

Steptococcal Antigens	Host Tissues	Lesions
Streptolysin O		
Streptokinase		
Hyaluronidase →	Cartilage →	Arthritis
Group A Carbohydrate →	Heart Valves →	Endocarditis (Valvulitis)
Cell Walls →	Basal Ganglia →	Chorea
M Protein →	Heart Muscle →	Myocarditis
	Immune Complexes →	Vasculitis
		Erythema Marginatum
		Rheumatic Nodule
		Glomerulonephritis

After Sell S: Immunology, Immunopathology and Immunity, 3rd ed. p. 265. Hagerstown, Harper & Row, 1980

acute asthmatic attacks and dermal reactions. For example, several laundry detergents contain enzymes from *Bacillus subtilis,* which may elicit acute allergic reactions. A more serious problem is allergic reaction to fungi in the tracheobronchial flora *(e.g., Aspergillus fumigatus).*

The syndrome of allergic bronchopulmonary aspergillosis (See Chap. 44, Aspergillosis) includes wheezing, fever, occasional expectoration of golden brown plugs that contain mycelia, systemic eosinophilia, elevated serum IgE concentrations, and the presence of antibodies to *Aspergillus* spp. in the serum. The syndrome is caused by prolonged anaphylactic reactions to aspergillal antigens. Allergic aspergillosis most likely begins with the inhalation and trapping of aspergillal conidia in the viscous secretions present in the bronchi of an asthmatic. The spores germinate and form mycelia; antigens released from mycelia react with IgE on mast cells in the bronchial walls, resulting in greatly increased mucous secretion and bronchospasm. Allergic bronchopulmonary aspergillosis differs from other forms of asthma in that the supply of inciting antigen is continuously replenished by replication within the bronchi and bronchioles.

Influenza

The immune response to infection with influenza viruses (see Chap. 28, Influenza) is essentially protective and plays little, if any, role in the pathogenesis of lesions. There is inflammation and desquamation of the ciliated, goblet, intermediate, and basal cells of the tracheobronchial epithelium, in which influenza viruses replicate. The systemic effects of the disease are most likely caused by the release of toxic products from virus-infected epithelial cells and from release of leukocyte pyrogens from polymorphonuclear leukocytes or macrophages that become disrupted after reaction with viruses.

The major mechanism of damage appears to be direct viral cytotoxicity or viral depletion of essential components of cells, as the main pathological and clinical events occur quite soon after infection. The specific protective effect of the immune response depends primarily on the production of antibody to the influenza hemagglutinin—by preventing the attachment of viruses to host cells; antineuraminidase may also help by preventing the release of viruses from infected cells. In addition, viruses may be destroyed by lysis or may be opsonized by activation of complement through reaction of antibody with the virus envelope. Infected cells may be killed by antibody-dependent, cell-mediated lysis, by direct lysis through sensitized T cells, or by release of lymphokines and activation of macrophages. Although the role of specific immune reactants in the production of lesions appears to be minimal, temporary immune suppression due to direct action of virus on T cells, B cells, or nonspecific inflammatory cells may contribute to increased susceptibility to pulmonary infection. However, the denuding of the epithelial lining of the airways, inhibition or loss of ciliary activity, and increased mucous secretion with blockage of the airways are probably more important.

The Common Cold

The possible contributions of atopic hypersensitivity to the symptoms of the common cold are not clearly understood. Most colds are the result of infection with one of a large number of different viruses (see Chap. 21, The Common Cold). The usual manifestations of the common cold are similar to those that occur in seasonal allergic rhinitis (hay fever). Therefore, it would seem likely that most of the symptoms of the common cold could be caused by an IgE-directed, mast cell-mediated system. However, there is little or no direct evidence to support immune mechanisms. In fact, eosinophiles are not prominent in the mucous secretions, and the concentrations of IgE are not increased. Viruses may produce a direct effect on epithelial or mast cells, or they may initiate inflammatory reactions through activation of complement by the alternate pathway or the kallikrein system. On the other hand, the presence of IgA in external secretions is believed to be an extremely important immune-specific mechanism of protection against viral upper respiratory infections.

Smallpox and Viral Exanthems

Smallpox, once a devastating disease of man, has been effectively eliminated by a global immunization program (see Chap. 92, Smallpox and Other Poxvirus Infections). Immunization is accomplished by dermal inoculation of an antigenically similar, but essentially nonpathogenic, virus. The result of immunization is establishment of delayed hypersensitivity, which is responsible for long-lasting immunity to the smallpox virus. The cellular reaction cures the patient of the virus infection by destruction not only of viruses but also of host cells infected with virus. Such a reaction is obviously beneficial if the infected cells can be replaced by regeneration of normal cells.

The contribution of specific immune sensitivity to the lesion produced by vaccination was recognized in 1907 when Von Pirquet observed that the local lesion following smallpox inoculation consisted of two stages. For the first 8 days there is a vesicular lesion—presumably due to growth of the virus; from 8 to 14 days, an indurated, erythematous reaction takes place—corresponding to the development of delayed hypersensitivity. Similar lesions appear at the same time on different parts of the body even if the other areas are inoculated at different times. Infective virus disappears from lesions when the delayed reaction is maximal.

Similar reactions are most likely responsible for other viral exanthems (measles, varicella); that is, lymphocytes and macrophages invade and cause destruction of epithelial cells. Healing occurs when the infected cells have been eliminated and noninfected cells regenerate. Severe, lasting disease occurs in situations where delayed reactions kill vital cells that do not regenerate or that regenerate poorly. Viral infection of nerve cells (postvaccinial encephalomyelitis) is illustrative; the infected nerve cells that are destroyed by cellular immune reactions to viral antigens are irreplacable. Thus, immune elimination of virus-infected cells produces lasting, sometimes fatal secondary effects. A similar situation may be responsible for death of liver cells in chronic active hepatitis.

Immune Reactions in Virus-Related Encephalomyelitis

The pathogenesis of viral infections of the central nervous system of mice as related to the role of the immune response is shown in Table 5-4. In the example of lymphocytic choriomeningitis (LCM), lesions are caused by cellular immune reactions to virus antigens on neurons. If the virus is administered to neonatal animals, they will not develop delayed hypersensitivity but will become tolerant. If delayed hypersensitivity to LCM virus is suppressed by administration of drugs or antilymphocyte serum, the symptoms and central nervous system (CNS) lesions of LCM do not develop. However, these mice may develop immune complex glomerulonephritis as a result of production of humoral antibody to LCM and the formation of antibody–antigen complexes.

In contrast, mouse hepatitis virus produces demyelination by direct infection of oligodendrocytes, which results in plaques of demyelination. There is little or no evidence for a destructive role of the immune response. Immunosuppression leads to more severe lesions and increased mortality. Thus, in mouse hepatitis virus encephalomyelitis the immune response is protective, and depression permits more extensive virus-mediated tissue destruction.

Theiler's myelitis is an immune mediated inflammation that occurs 1 to 3 months following infection. Immunosuppression increases the level of virus production but prevents demyelination. Demyelination is the result of postinfectious autosensitization to myelin similar to that produced in experimental allergic encephalomyelitis.

Experimental allergic encephalomyelitis is induced by immunizing an animal to its own myelin (Fig. 5-8). Paralysis of the hind legs occurs within 1 to 3 weeks and is associated with local perivascular accumulation of mononuclear inflammatory cells around small veins. The mononuclear cells invade the white matter and produce focal areas of demyelination. Phagocytosis and digestion of myelin are carried out by macrophages activated by reaction of specifically sensitized lymphocytes with myelin antigens.

These examples in mice are reflected in the relationship between viral infections and immune responses in viral encephalitides in humans (Table 5-5). The viral encephalitides of humans (see Chap. 122, Viral Encephalitides) are grouped clinically into acute, postinfectious, latent, slow, and chronic. In acute viral encephalitides, viral infection of host nerve cells destroys the cells directly. Loss of neuronal function may be caused by destruction of the cells (lytic) or by deviation of neuronal function to provide for virus replication. The immune response is protective and will prevent virus-mediated destruction. Autoimmunization to myelin following relatively mild viral infections or vaccination may lead to cell mediated immune destruction of myelin. For example, the use of rabies vaccines made from animal brains or preparations containing neural tissues may rarely result in postimmunization encephalomyelitis, whereas vaccines from nonneural tissue cultures have not been associated with this complication of rabies immunization. The course of the disease and the nature of the lesions are essentially the same as those seen in animals with experimental allergic encephalomyelitis. The end stage or chronic form of allergic encephalomyelitis is considered by many to be multiple sclerosis, but definite proof of such a relationship is lacking.

Destruction of brain cells may result when a viral infection that has been held to a subclinical state by the immune system erupts into activity because of

Table 5-4. *Role of Immune Response in the Pathogenesis of Viral Encephalitis in Mice*

Disease	Role of Immune Response
Lymphocytic choriomeningitis	Cellular destruction of neurons expressing viral antigens
Hepatitis virus encephalitis	Viral destruction of infected cells leading to demyelination
Theiler's virus myelitis	Postinfectious autoallergy to myelin

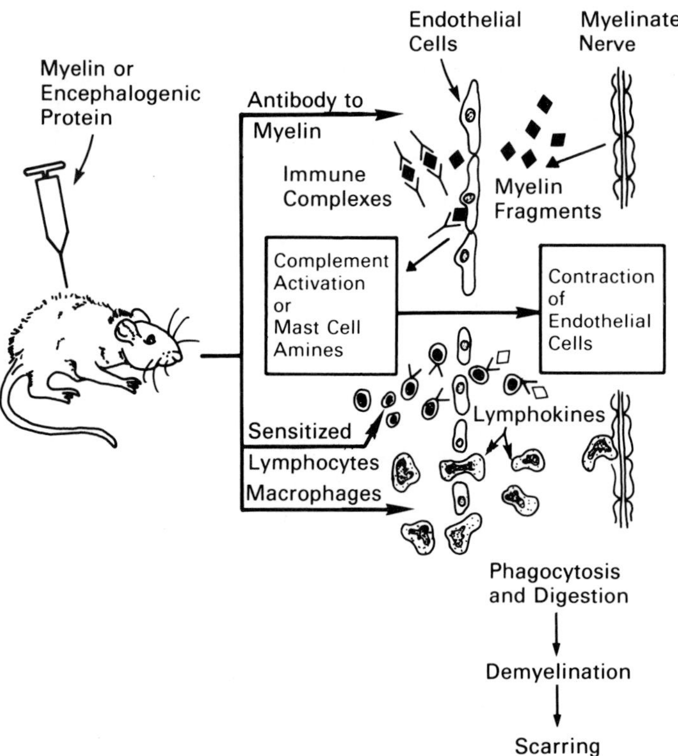

Fig. 5-8. Possible pathogenic events in experimental allergic encephalomyelitis. Immunization of experimental animals with myelin or encephalogenic protein results in production of humoral antibody and specifically sensitized cells, which together lead to demyelination by macrophages. Antibody reacting with myelin released into the circulation through capillaries in the white matter (*i.e.,* myelinated areas of brain and spinal cord) activates either anaphylatoxin (complement) or mast-cell (IgE) degranulation. Contraction of endothelial cells opens up gaps in the walls of small blood vessels. Sensitized small lymphocytes move into white matter, react with myelin antigen, and release lymphocyte mediators. Macrophages, attracted and activated by these mediators, phagocytose and digest antibody-coated myelin or myelin affected by reaction with sensitized lymphocytes. If zones of demyelination are large, fibrosis will occur and permanent loss of function will result.

immunosuppression. For example, progressive multifocal leukoencephalopathy occurs in patients whose state of immunity is depressed by leukemia or lymphoma. Slow virus disease is caused by a gradual loss of neuronal function, presumably owing to prolonged intracellular virus multiplication in the absence of evidence of an immune response. Chronic encephalomyelitis occurs in association with chronic measles infections in which the humoral immune response is prominent but the cellular immune response is low. It is possible that the relative lack of a delayed hypersensitivity response may permit prolonged replication of a defective virus. In summary, lesions of the brain may be caused by direct destruction of infected cells by viruses, induction of autoallergy to myelin, or inadequate protection because of suppression of immune reactivity, no immunity, or inappropriate immunity.

Table 5-5. *Viral Encephalitides of Humans*

Type	Examples	Mechanism
Acute	Poliomyelitis, rabies, herpes simplex	Virus destroys infected cells; immune response is protective.
Postinfectious	Vaccina, mumps, measles, rabies	Delayed hypersensitivity reaction destroys myelin (autoallergic).
Latent	Progressive multifocal leukoencephalopathy	Failure to maintain adequate immunity permits progressive viral multiplication.
Slow	Kuru; Creutzfeldt–Jakob disease	Infection persists; there is no immune response.
Chronic	Subacute, sclerosing panencephalitis	Inappropriate immune response results in lack or protection.

Table 5-6. *Immunologic Characteristics of Leprosy*

CHARACTERISTICS	Form of Leprosy		
	TUBERCULOID	BORDERLINE	LEPROMATOUS
Mycobacterium leprae in tissues	− or ±	+ or ++	++++
Formation of granulomas	++++	+++	−
Infiltration with lymphocytes	−++	−	−
Lymph node morphology			
Paracortical lymphocytes	++++	++	−
Paracortical histocytes	−	++	++++
Germinal center	+	++	++++
Plasma cells	−	+	+++
Lepromin test	+++	−	−
Delayed hypersensitivity, % with			
Dinitrochlorobenzene	90	75	50
Hemocyanin	100	100	100
Antimycobacterial antibodies (% with precipitins in serum)	11–28	82	95
Autoantibodies in serum (%)	3–11		30–50
Immune complex disease (erythema nodosum leprosum)	−	±	+++

Key: − to ++++ indicates extend of the observation noted.
After Sell S: Immunology, Immunopathology and Immunity, 3rd ed. 6.361. Hagerstown, Harper & Row, 1980

Leprosy

The clinical manifestations of leprosy (see Chap. 105, Leprosy) are determined by the immune response of the patient (Table 5-6). Indeed, the protective function of granulomatous reactivity is exemplified by the spectrum of leprosy. The high resistance of tuberculoid leprosy is associated with delayed hypersensitivity and the formation of granulomas, whereas the low resistance characteristic of lepromatous leprosy is associated with the presence of humoral antibodies. When a patient with lepromatous leprosy responds to chemotherapy, there is acquisition of delayed hypersensitivity reactivity: The skin lesions become swollen and erythematous; the macrophages lose their cytoplasmic bacilli and become epithelioid.

Patients with humoral antibodies may display immune complex reactions, as exemplified by the lesions of erythema nodosum. Crops of tender red nodules appear in the skin and persist for 24 to 48 hours. Consisting of foci of fibrinoid vascular necrosis infiltrated with polymorphonuclear leukocytes, the lesions are typical of immune complex vasculitis and are similar to the Arthus reaction. There may also be systemic reactions in the form of arthritis, inflammation of the eyes, pain along the nerves, fever, and proteinuria. In lepromatous leprosy, there is also a high incidence of autoantibodies, including antinuclear factor, rheumatoid factor, antithyroid antibodies, and false positive serologic tests for syphilis.

Tuberculosis

Infection with *Mycobacterium tuberculosis* (see Chap. 34, Pulmonary Tuberculosis) results in circulating antibody, delayed hypersensitivity, generally increased macrophage activity, and granulomatous hypersensitivity. There is little or no evidence that humoral antibody is protective. That immunity is provided by the granulomatous reaction is supported by finding singular lesions at autopsy, namely, the Ghon complex—a small granuloma at the periphery of the lung that is associated with healed granulomas in the bronchotracheal lymph nodes at the hilus of the lung. This finding, in association with the observation that many patients with primary tuberculosis recover without chemotherapy, supports the conclusion that granulomatous reactivity is beneficial. However, an opposite view holds that granulomatous reactivity contributes to the pathogenesis of tuberculosis and is not a protective response. Viable tubercle bacilli may be found within granulomas, where they are protected from the defenses of the host. However, intragranuloma bacilli are isolated and kept from dissemination, and, if the reaction is adequate, the macrophages that make up the granuloma will eventually destroy the tubercle bacilli. Yet, there may be breakdown of granulomas releasing live *M. tuberculosis* to fuel dissemination. Such failures of the granulomatous reaction do not discredit the generally protective nature of the response.

On the other hand, a major feature of tuberculosis is the replacement of normal tissue (usually the lung) with multiple, space-occupying granulomas. In other words, a gain in protection is balanced by a loss of function—the doubleedged sword of immunopathology.

Schistosomiasis

Schistosomiasis is a disease caused by infection with trematodes that live as adult worms in the blood (see Chap. 81, Schistosomiasis).

Both the minor and the major symptoms of schistosomiasis result from immune effector mechanisms. Swimmers itch is a pruritic, papular rash that occurs at sites of penetration of cercariae from the intermediate host (snail). In a sensitized person, both immediate and delayed immune mediated skin reactions occur at these sites. These reactions not only are responsible for swimmers itch but also to a large extent limit the penetration and development of the cercariae.

Acute schistosomiasis is a relatively rare syndrome of fever, eosinophilia, splenomegaly, lymphadenopathy, and urticaria that may occur in primary infections at the time of the initial systemic release of eggs. The symptoms are believed to be caused by immune complex and anaphylactic reactions. Glomerulonephritis due to immune complexes may occur in patients with schistosomiasis presumably as a result of IgG or IgM antibody reactions to schistosomal antigens.

The major destructive lesions of schistosomiasis are caused by cellular reactions to eggs or miracidia trapped in the liver and urinary tract. The lesions consist of granulomas, which surround eggs; if the number of granulomas are sufficiently great, they may obstruct the portal blood flow in the liver and cause hepatosplenomegaly. Isolated eggs will evoke a granulomatous reaction when injected into sensitized animals, and this capacity can be transferred to normal animals by lymphoid cells but not by humoral antibody. In the urinary bladder there is marked thickening and fibrosis of the bladder wall. In some instances, obstruction of the ureters causes hydronephrosis. Again, the cause is granulomatous reactivity to eggs in the bladder wall. Presumably, if such granulomatous reactions did not occur, the lesions typical of the disease would not occur. It is theoretically possible that a host–parasite relationship could be established whereby transient release of eggs without tissue damage might occur if there were no specific immune response in the host, but the effects of the passage of myriads of miracidia through the patient in the absence of granulomatous reactivity could be even worse.

Filariasis

Filaria are worms with complex lifecycles. They invade humans or other animals as definitive hosts, and insects as intermediate hosts (see Chap. 112, Cutaneous Filariais, and Chap. 148, Lymphoreticular Filariasis). All of the seven filariids known to infect humans may evoke allergic reactions (Table 5-7); however, only three cause serious disease: *Wuchereria bancrofti, Brugia malayi,* and *Onchocerca volvulus.*

The manifestations of filariasis clearly reflect the state of immune responsiveness of the host (Table 5-8). It is remarkable that chronic, asymptomatic filaremia may be associated with specific hyporesponsiveness to filarial antigens. It is a host–parasite relationship that permits prolonged production of microfilaria, which are cleared from the circulation by the lungs, liver, and spleen without evoking symptoms.

Table 5-7. *Some Helminths That Produce Allergic Reactions in Humans*

Species	Site of Infection	Immune Effector Mechanism	Distribution
Wucheria bancrofti	Lymphatic	Multiple	Tropics
Brugia malayi	Lymphatic	Multiple	Southeast Africa
Onchocerca volvulus	Subcutaneous	Cellular	Africa; South and Central America
Loa loa	Subcutaneous	Anaphylactic	Africa
Dipetalonema perstans	Subcutaneous	Anaphylactic	Africa; South America
Dracunculus medinesis (nonfilarial)	Connective tissue	Anaphylactic	Tropics

Table 5-8. *Relationship of Manifestations to Immune Effector Mechanisms in Lymphatic Filariasis*

Disease State	Immune Manifestation
Asymptomatic microfilaremia	Tolerance
Occult filariasis	IgG antibody
Tropical eosinophilia	Anaphylactic; ? immune complex
Filarial fever	? Immune complex; ? delayed hypersensitivity
Lymphadenitis	Delayed hypersensitivity
Lymphatic obstruction	Granulomatous

In occult filariasis, there are neither symptoms nor microfilaria in the blood. IgG antibodies may be responsible for the rapid, apparently complete clearance of organisms from the blood.

However, immune responses that apparently cure the infection may actually lead to disease. Thus, filarial fevers are an indication that an immune response has been activated, most likely involving immune complexes. The manifestations of tropical eosinophilia—attacks of bronchial asthma with interstitial inflammation of the lungs—are consistent with an IgE response and the formation of immune complexes. A cellular (granulomatous) response is implicated in the pathogenesis of lymphadenitis and lymphatic obstruction.

The development of the more benign host—parasite relationships may be determined by exposure to the parasite in childhood. When previously unexposed adults are infected, there is a tendency to develop acute inflammation with pain, urticaria, angioedema, and marked lymphangitis, which disappear without sequellae if exposure is terminated. However, if exposure continues, the disease progresses rapidly from temporary to permanent lymphatic obstruction. Thus, continued exposure to the organism in sensitized individuals is required for the development of lymphatic obstruction by granulomas formed around killed microfilaria. However, something special about the immune response of residents of endemic regions who contact filaria early in life results in less frequent and less severe manifestations of disease. In some as yet unknown way, the immune response of such persons is either specifically suppressed or is restricted to IgG antibody production, resulting in an asymptomatic carrier state or occult filariasis; adults from outside the endemic area tend to produce IgE antibody or cellular hypersensitivity when infected. This intriguing host–parasite relationship clearly deserves further study.

Syphilis

The host–parasite relationship in syphilis has been the subject of considerable study for over 100 years. The evolution of the chancre, the first clinical manifestation (see Chap. 59, Syphilis), follows closely the pattern of a delayed hypersensitivity reaction in the skin. It is initiated by sensitized T cells reacting with antigen and is resolved by phagocytosis and digestion of organisms by macrophages.

The skin lesions of secondary syphilis appear to be delayed hypersensitivity reactions at sites of dissemination and replication of *Treponema pallidum.* The cellular reaction is similar to that of primary lesions, although plasma cells may be more prominent. The lesions heal spontaneously, and the patient enters latency.

In latent syphilis there is no clinical evidence of infection. However, some *T. pallidum* survive the immune attack of the host and remain viable. There does not appear to be any abnormality of the immune system; indeed, persons with latent syphilis are resistant to reinfection; that is, they are immune. The destructive lesions characteristic of tertiary syphilis are granulomatous reactions (gummas), which occur in areas where spirochetes apparently persist during latency, for example, brain, skin, bone, or viscera. As no differences in immune potential distinguish patients who develop tertiary disease and those who do not, it is known why some patients move from latency to tertiary disease. Development of tertiary lesions could result either from an increased state of hypersensitivity causing more intense inflammation or from a decreased state of reactivity permitting organisms to proliferate and initiate a destructive reaction.

Hypersensitivity Pneumonitis (Extrinsic Allergic Alveolitis)

Hypersensitivity pneumonitis is an interstitial inflammatory disease of the lung caused by inappropriate reactivity to antigens inhaled as a result of environmental exposure. The antigens involved appear to be of animal or plant origin, and they include noninfectious organisms that grow in decaying organic matter such as fungi and thermophilic actinomyces (Table 5-9). Acute episodes may resolve without residua, but repeated exposures may cause noncaseating granulomas or interstitial pulmonary fibrosis leading to irreversible damage.

The disease occurs in only a small number of exposed individuals, presumably those who develop hypersensitivity, but the severity and course are clearly dependent on the intensity and frequency of exposure. The acute form of the disease is character-

Table 5-9. *Hypersensitivity Pneumonitis Produced by Fungi and Thermophilic Actinomycetes*

Antigen	Antigen Source	Disease
True Fungi		
Aspergillus clavatus	Moldy Barley	Malt Worker's Lung
Aspergillus clavatus	Moldy Cheese	Cheese Washer's Lung
Cryptostroma corticale	Moldy Maple Logs	Maple Bark Lung
Graphium spp.	Moldy Wood Dust	Sequoiosis
Pullularia spp.	Moldy Wood Dust	Sequoiosis
Alternaria spp.	Moldy Wood Pulp	Wood Pulp Worker's Lung
Mucor stolonifer	Moldy Paprika Pods	Paprika Slicer's Lung
Cryptostroma corticale	Maple Bark	Maple Bark Lung
Penicillium casei	Moldy Cheese	Cheese Worker's Lung
Thermophilic Actinomycetes		
Micropolyspora faeni	Moldy Hay	Farmer's Lung
Thermoactinomyces vulgaris	Moldy Sugar Cane	Bagassosis
Thermoactinomyces sacchari	Moldy Compost	Mushroom Worker's Lung
Thermoactinomyces candidus	Contaminated Air Conditioners	Air Conditioner Lung
Thermoactinomyces viridis	Cattle	Fog Fever
	Moldy Cork	Suberosis
	Vineyards	Vineyard Sprayer's Lung

After Sell S: Immunology, Immunopathology, and Immunity, 3rd ed, p 364. Hagerstown, Harper & Row, 1980

ized by cough, chills, fever, and breathlessness, occurring in a 24-hour period. If unrecognized, the disease may progress to chronic dyspnea, fatigue, anorexia, and wasting as the functional capacity of the lung is lost. Removal from exposure early in the course of the disease usually prevents progression to death. An atopic mechanism appears to be unlikely, as neither IgE nor eosinophils are elevated, and anaphylactic or atopic symptoms are not features of the disease. Immune complex-mediated inflammation has been implicated. Many patients do have specific IgG antibody to presumptive antigens, and vasculitis has been observed in some cases. However, the lesions are more consistent with cellular immune reactions. Hypersensitivity pneumonitis is an example of an immune-mediated disease set off by noninfectious microorganisms; it is a situation in which the immune response has gone awry.

Drug Allergy

The immune reactions to various chemotherapeutic agents may be classified into one or more of the six mechanisms listed in Table 5-1. Any or all of these mechanisms may be set in motion by exposure to penicillin. Breakdown products of penicillin arise spontaneously or through catabolism, bind to proteins of the host, and function as haptens. Because at least three antigenically different products may be formed, there may be different immune responses to different antigens goint on at the same time, triggering more than one type of effector mechanism to the same hapten antigen. Many of these reactions are manifested in the skin as exanthematous rashes, uriticaria, angioedema, cutaneous vasculitis, contact dermatitis (delayed hypersensitivity), erythema multiforme, purpura, and exzema. Systemic reactions may include hemolysis, glomerulonephritis and vasculitis, anaphylactic shock, and systemic cellular reactions.

Summary

Immune responses provide specific, essential, protective mechanisms against infectious diseases. At least six different mechanisms may be identified. However, these mechanisms are not only responsible for cure of most infectious diseases but they may also in some instances be responsible for manifestations of the disease (Table 5-10). In some cases, immune effector mechanisms are responsible for lesions that otherwise would not occur.

Table 5-10. *Protective and Destructive Immune Reactions*

Immune Effector Mechanism	Protective Function "Immunity"	Destructive Reaction "Allergy"
Neutralization	Diptheria; tetanus; cholera; endotoxin neutralization; blockage of virus receptors	Insulin resistance; pernicious anemia; myasthenia gravis; hyperthyroidism
Cytotoxic	Bacteriolysis; opsonization	Hemolysis; leukopenia; thrombocytopenia
Immune complex	Acute inflammation; opsonization; polymorphonuclear leukocyte activation	Vasculitis; glomerulonephritis; serum sickness; rheumatoid diseases
Anaphylactic	Focal inflammation; increased vascular permeability; expression of intestinal parasites	Asthma; urticaria; anaphylactic shock; hay fever
Delayed Hypersensitivity	Destruction of virus infected cells; tuberculosis; syphilis; immune surveillance of tumors	Contact dermatitis; autoallergies, viral exanthemus; postvaccinal encephalomyelitis
Granulomatous	Isolation of infectious agent in granuloma leprosy; tuberculosis; helminths; fungi	Beryllosis; sarcoidosis; tuberculosis; filariasis; schistosomiasis

After Sell S: Introduction to symposium on immunopathology: Immune mechanisms in disease. Human Pathol 9:24, 1978

Bibliography

Books

SELL S: Immunology, Immunopathology, and Immunity, 3rd ed. Hagerstown, Harper & Row, 1980. 521 pp.

STOLLERMAN GH: Rheumatic Fever and Streptococcal Infection, New York, Grune & Stratton, 1975. 336 pp.

Journals

BAKER-ZANDER S, SELL S: A histopathologic and immunologic study of the course of syphilis in the experimentally infected rabbit: demonstration of long-lasting cellular immunity. Am J Pathol 101:387–414, 1980

LAMPERT PW: Autoimmune and virus-induced demyelinating diseases. Am J Pathol 91:176–198, 1978

MANSFIELD JM: Immunobiology of African trypanosomiasis. Cell Immunol 39:204–210, 1978

MOLLER G (ED): The immune response to infectious diseases. Transplant Rev 19:1–254, 1974

OTTESEN EA: Immunopathology of lymphatic filariasis in man. Immunopathol 2:373–385, 1980

SWEET C, SMITH H: Pathogenicity of influenza virus. Microbiol Rev 44:303–330, 1980

TURK JL, BRYCESON ADM: Immunological phenomena in leprosy and related diseases. Adv Immunol 12:209–266, 1971

WARREN KS: The pathology, pathobiology, and pathogenesis of schistosomiasis. Nature 273:609–612, 1978

RUTH M. LAWRENCE
PAUL D. HOEPRICH

6 Resistance to Infection

Both specific and nonspecific factors contribute to the host's ability to resist infectious agents. Specific factors are restricted in effect to particular parasites and depend for their evocation on each person's unique experience. As the goal of immunization procedures, specific resistance has been intensively studied. Because discussion of prevention is uniformly a part of each chapter that deals with a particular infectious disease, only a general overview of specific resistance is given here.

Traditionally, the study of infectious diseases has been little concerned with nonspecific resistance—the host factors present and operative in the normal person at, or soon after, birth. This inborn, native or innate resistance is effective against many parasites and is the qualitatively identical legacy of all individuals of a species.

Nonspecific Factors

Nonspecific resistance is on the whole more essential to survival than are specific factors. Our bodies have everything necessary for the growth of all kinds of microorganisms. Our immediate environment, on and in our skin and mucous membranes, teems with potential parasites that are kept from invading principally by nonspecific factors. It is the suppression of nonspecific factors that prepares for the occurrence of obligatory infections (Chap. 4, Host–Parasite Relationships and the Pathogenesis of Infectious Diseases).

Anatomic Barriers

The skin provides both an anatomic and a chemical barrier. Its most external layer, the stratum corneum, is inhospitable to bacterial growth because of its low water content, and fatty acids in sebum inhibit the growth of many microorganisms. Constant desquamation also aids in reducing the bacterial population. When large areas of skin are damaged, as in extensive burns, these important host defenses are lost, and infection is nearly inevitable.

The respiratory tract is protected from microbial access in a variety of ways. As air passes through the nose and a subsequent series of bifurcating tubes, turbulent flow is assured, and most inhaled organisms impinge on the respiratory epithelium and never reach the lungs. The mucus blanket and cilia of the respiratory epithelium trap inhaled particles and constantly move them cephalad. When secretions are profuse, cough is stimulated and effects removal of particles. Local antibody (IgA), lysozyme, and lactoferrin in respiratory secretions are additional defenses.

Although the epithelium of the gastrointestinal tract lacks cilia, it possesses a mucus layer to trap ingested microbes. Gastric acid is very toxic to most bacteria. Peristalsis aids in the removal of organisms, and the intestinal secretions contain antibody (IgA), bile salts, lysozyme, glycolipids and glycoproteins that prevent proliferation and adherence of organisms. Finally, components of the gut flora interact to restrict each other from overproliferation.

The anatomy of the urinary tract prevents ready ascent of perineal microorganisms into the bladder. Microorganisms trapped in the mucous layer of the bladder may then be engulfed by bladder cells. Urine of low pH and very low or very high osmolality prevents bacterial multiplication.

Therapies

Advances in both nonmedical and medical areas have, as part of the price of progress, posed some threat in the way of compromising the effectiveness of nonspecific resistance factors. For example, ionizing radiations are most often lethal to cell populations that are actively reproducing. Among other tissues, the generative layers of the mucosa lining the gastrointestinal tract are particularly susceptible;

thus, one of the consequences of irradiation is disruption of the enteric mucosa. Numerous ports of entry are opened to the infectious agents present in the lumen of the gut (Table 4-1).

Many modern therapies preserve persons who have noninfectious diseases for eventual infection. Typically, the therapy for the fundamental noninfectious disease process is not curative and is only partially successful, because normal operation of nonspecific resistance factors is not achieved. Thus, before insulin was available, persons with diabetes mellitus died of metabolic imbalance. With insulin, glucose metabolism is ameliorated and life is preserved. However, even with insulin, diabetics are notably susceptible to infections—staphylococcal, urinary tract, and tuberculosis. Acute leukemias and modern antileukemic therapy, and our aged and aging population are other examples.

Heritable and Developmental Factors

Not only have technical, social, and economic changes forced concern with nonspecific resistance, but also it has become apparent that some persons were shortchanged in their complement of nonspecific factors. Such persons display a marked, unusual susceptibility to infections, chiefly with gram-positive cocci. There is failure to develop immunity with the injection of diphtherial toxoid, and neutropenia or other blood dyscrasias occur. A marked deficiency in plasma gamma globulins is characteristic of this disease and hence the name agammaglobulinemia (actually, hypogammaglobulinemia is more accurate). Ancillary findings include lymph node hypoplasia and a high degree of tolerance for skin homografts. Although a markedly decreased ability to synthesize humoral antibodies is characteristic of this disease, persons with hypogammaglobulinemia do become specifically immune to the common viral diseases of childhood, except infectious hepatitis. Hypogammaglobulinemia occurs as a sex-linked hereditary defect virtually limited to males, and as an acquired illness in adults who have some other disease (lymphoma, sarcoidosis, extensive renal loss of proteins, increased protein catabolism, or decreased protein synthesis).

Failure of the thymus-derived cells of the immune system to develop also predisposes to certain infections. An example is congenital thymic aplasia (DiGeorge's syndrome) in which affected children have failure of T-lymphocyte function and develop chronic mucocutaneous candidosis and other fungal, viral, and protozoan (*Pneumocystis carinii*) infections. B-lymphocyte function is normal in these children, and transplants of fetal thymus have restored immune function. Damage to the anlage of the fetal thymus *in utero* appears to be the origin of the disorder.

There are other, less well-defined, but definite, heritable nonspecific defense mechanisms. Although specific with regard to the parasite, these mechanisms are present and effective in persons who were never exposed to the parasite in question. Species immunity is one such form of nonspecific resistance; humans do not become infected with the virus that causes hoof-and-mouth disease of cattle; cows do not contract gonorrhea. Racial immunity is less clearcut in being primarily qualitative: the tuberculosis mortality of blacks and American Indians is 3 to 4 times higher than that of whites. Coccidioidomycosis uncommonly disseminates in whites, whereas dissemination is not uncommon in more intensely pigmented peoples (for example, Filipinos and blacks). Leprosy, rheumatic fever, and malaria are other infections in which racial resistance appears to vary.

Hormonal Factors

The incidence and mortality of nearly every infectious disease has been considered in the light of possible influence from puberty, menstruation, pregnancy, and sexual senility. The views are conflicting, but on the whole the male is more vulnerable than the female to infectious hazards, even as he is to most other vicissitudes of life.

Pregnancy renders women more vulnerable to dissemination of coccidioidomycosis from its primary pulmonary location. The reasons for this are unknown, but there are intriguing preliminary studies indicating that some estrogenic hormones promote growth of the fungus *in vitro*.

Either a deficiency or an excess of adrenocorticosteroids appears to decrease resistance to infection by virtually any kind of parasite. Latent infections appear to be lighted up by large doses of glucosteroids, an effect most difficult to assess because pharmacologic dosage is always undertaken as treatment of a noninfectious process that, in and of itself, commonly predisposes to infection. The concentrations of glucosteroids required are always supraphysiologic and uniformly cause, among other effects, depletion of the mass of lymphoid tissue, decrease in the efficiency of the reticuloendothelial (macrophage) clearing mechanisms, and inhibition of the formation of granulation tissue. The inflammatory response is suppressed, a serious loss when the threat is acute invasion by a parasite. However, suppression of the inflammation associated with allergic reactions and hypersensitivity may be life saving.

Aging

The incidence of infection is increased at both extremes of age, reflecting primarily immaturity and senescence of the immune system. Advancing age also brings about structural and degenerative changes in vital organ systems that may predispose to infection.

Nutrition

Nutrition is intuitively known to be important in resistance to infection. It is perfectly obvious that a well-fed animal is more resistant than a malnourished animal; historically, war, famine, and pestilence have followed each other through the ages. In addition to the fact that controlled experiments in humans are not possible, work with nonhuman animals has been hampered by failures to observe many critical factors such as the caloric adequacy and amino acid balance of diets, and the genetic purity of the species under study. However, there is evidence that severe depletion of protein so impairs protein synthesis and phagocytosis that a generally increased vulnerability to bacterial infections results; for example, kwashiorkor. Of the various B vitamins, deficiency in biotin has been most convincingly shown to result in increased susceptibility to infection; however, biotin is so widely distributed in foodstuffs that deficiency probably never approaches predisposing significance in humans. The squamous metaplasia that results from vitamin A deficiency may cause breaks in the continuity of the epithelium so that invasion by parasites is made easy. Further examples rest on less secure grounds; however, the circumstantial evidence of epidemiology associates increased occurrence of tuberculosis with malnutrition.

On the other hand, deficiency of certain nutrients, such as iron, may actually be protective against some infections. Free ionic iron is known to increase the virulence of many bacterial species. Liberation of heme-containing compounds or saturation of serum-iron-binding proteins increases the availability of ionic iron in the host and has been experimentally shown to increase susceptibility to a number of bacteria, including *Escherichia coli, Pseudomonas aeruginosa,* and *Clostridium* spp. The effect of iron replacement on infection is demonstrated by increased susceptibility to amebiasis and malaria when iron deficiency is corrected. Both fever and inflammation cause a decrease in the concentration of serum iron, and this may help to inhibit bacterial replication.

Fever

Fever commonly occurs with infection, and nonspecific resistance value to the host has been claimed for fever. This is supported by the laboratory observation that the usual strains of type 3 capsulated *Streptococcus pneumoniae* are unable to produce progressive infection in the rabbit after intradermal injection—in definite contrast with *S. pneumoniae* of other types. As fever develops after injection, not only is the growth of type 3 pneumococci inhibited, but also decapsulation occurs and phagocytosis is accomplished. However, mutant type 3 strains that can grow at 39.5°C (103°F) are fully virulent for the rabbit.

It is difficult to be certain that fever has a useful function in the human host with an infection. On review of the hospital records of patients with pneumococcal pneumonia and patients wtih gonococcemia seen many years ago, before specific chemotherapy was available, no evidence was found that the outcome of the infection was influenced by the height or the duration of fever. Yet invasion by some parasites that are sensitive to elevated temperatures, for example, *Treponemea palidum* and *Neisseria gonorrhoeae,* may not cause fever. Moreover, induced fever is therapeutically valuable in the treatment of tertiary syphilis and gonococcal urethritis, although fever therapy has fallen into disuse since penicillin has become available.

In one lower vertebrate, the desert iguana, fever improves the survival rate of animals infected with *Aeromonas hydrophila.* As ectotherms, iguanas regulate body temperature by seeking differing environmental temperatures. When fever was prevented by maintaining a low ambient temperature or by giving antipyretics, mortality increased from ≥ 10% to 75% and 100% respectively. Such a clear-cut effect has not been seen in mammals, but it is evident that fever can result in increased activity of lymphocytes and in increased phagocytic activity of leukocytes.

The other side of the coin, reduction of fever as part of the treatment of an infectious disease, has been advocated to mitigate the stress of fever. Diminution of the work of the heart and reduction of the need for oxygen should result as the fever falls. In addition, febrile convulsions in children are successfully managed by lowering the body temperature.

Induction of actual hypothermia might be expected to go even further toward ameliorating the catabolic and toxic effects of infectious diseases. However, with hypothermia there is also depression of phagocytosis and antibody production. The therapeutic ideal might be the attainment of euthermia—a state most reasonably achieved by cure of the infection.

Secretions

Many nonspecific, antiinfectious properties are associated with various fluids of the body. Secretions elaborated by the skin and by the mucous membranes are alleged to contain substances that have antibacterial effects. The apparent bactericidal action of skin secretions may relate to the presence of lipids, fatty acids, and lactic acid.

The mucus secreted by the cervix uteri of some women is actually bactericidal—an effect that is least pronounced at the time of ovulation. Inhibition of bacterial migration may be all that is achieved by the cervical mucus of other women.

The tissue and body fluids of many animals contain lysozyme, an enzyme that splits sugars from the peptidoglycan polymers that form the cell walls of bacteria. Bacteriolysis is the usual result of the action of lysozyme, particularly with gram-positive bacteria. Human nasal secretions, saliva, tears, and intestinal mucus all contain lysozyme.

Blood platelets are a source for β-lysin, which is bactericidal for gram-positive bacteria.

Alpha-1-antitrypsin is present in respiratory tract secretions. Because it inhibits bacterial enzymes, as well as the enzymes contained in the lysosomal granules of leukocytes, α-1-antitrypsin reduces tissue injury from both bacteria and leukocytes.

Endotoxins

Using appropriate chemical techniques, complex lipopolysaccharide-protein substances may be prepared from some gram-negative bacteria. These substances, referred to as endotoxins, display a rather bewildering array of biologic activities. The effects on injection into mammals vary with the dose and previous experience of the animal. A large dose given intravenously causes peremptory emptying of the stomach, colon, and urinary bladder, and a fall in the blood pressure that may lead to lethal shock. Smaller doses provoke less in the way of immediate systemic reaction but can cause a profound granulocytopenia, rigors, and fever. With the attainment of fever, there is an outpouring of leukocytes into the blood. Certain kinds of neoplasms undergo necrosis on systemic injection of endotoxins. Because of these many effects, endotoxins are also called bacterial pyrogens and tumor-necrotizing substances; if obtained from certain gram-negative bacilli, they are identical with O antigens. Another consequence of the injection of endotoxins is heightened resistance to infection with several varieties of gram-negative bacilli, *Mycobacterium* spp., and viruses. No influence has been demonstrated with gram-positive bacteria. Exacting conditions of dose, route of administration, and timing are required for exhibition of the resistance-increasing effect of endotoxins. The degree of protection is not great and is readily overcome by increasing the challenge dose of the parasite. Other colloidal substances, zymosan, xerosin, colloidal sulfur, and thorium dioxide, also have similar resistance-increasing effects. The injection of endotoxins also causes chemotaxis of neutrophils and monocytes; changes in blood concentrations of lysozyme, adrenocorticosteroid hormones, glucose, and lactic acid; the activation of fibrinolysin; and the inhibition of allergic reactions.

Interference

From nonspecific modification of infection by substances derived from bacteria, it is but a short step to interactions between infectious agents parasitizing the same host. When two or more infectious agents interact in such a way that one is dominant and the other is suppressed, interference is said to have occurred. Clinical observations date back to the 18th century—smallpox was invariably a mild disease when acquired by a child with yaws. Inoculation of vaccinia virus led to the amelioration of whooping cough. In a patient with active herpetic lesions, vaccinia virus often failed to replicate after inoculation. These examples imply interference by nonspecific mechanisms because the parasites are quite unrelated and share no common antigens. Also, in experimental infections, interference can be demonstrated so soon after infection that no opportunity has been provided for the elaboration of antibody.

INTERFERON

It is probable that at least some of the instances of interference just cited are actually the result of interferons—low-molecular-weight (generally 20,000–30,000) glycoproteins that are nonantigenic in homologous species and have a specific activity of 10^9 units/mg protein. They are elaborated by infected cells and protect noninfected cells from cytophilic parasites. Interferons resemble antibodies in that they prevent infection, however, interferons differ markedly from antibodies. 1. Interferons display broad antiviral activity against both RNA and DNA viruses by binding to specific receptors on the host cell surface and inducing the production of enzymes by the cell. These enzymes subsequently inhibit the translation of viral messenger RNA into viral protein. 2. They act intracellularly in a characteristic species-specific fashion to inhibit nonviral intracellular parasites (chlamydias, rickettsias, bacteria, fungi, and protozoa) as well as viruses. 3. They are synthesized and liberated by vertebrate cells *in vivo* and *in vitro* in reponse to (a) cytophilic pathogens; (b) microbial extracts (viral nucleic acids, rickettsial extracts, bacterial endotoxins and exotoxins, and fungal nucleic acids); (c) plant extracts (phytohemagglutinin and pokeweed mitogen); and (d) synthetic polyanions (polycarboxylates, polyphosphates, polysulfates, and polythiosulfates), polynucleotides (polyriboinosinic and polyribocytidilic acids), and certain low-molecular-weight *bis* basic organic compounds. 4. Interferons lack toxicity to normal cell functions (energy metabolism and synthesis of macromolecules), yet inhibit rapidly dividing cells, including tumor cells. 5. Speed of elaboration is high—interferons are released from infected cells at about the same time that virus is produced. Although primarily prophylactic, interferons may also limit the spread of viral infections by protecting cells from being infected in the area of release of virus.

Because interferons are nonspecific, there is considerable interest in evaluating their utility in prevention and therapy. Thus far, production of interferons from human leukocytes in quantities adequate for evaluation has been accomplished primarily in the central, national blood bank of Finland. In limited trials, there was a salutory clinical effect in immunocompromised patients with disseminated herpes zoster. However, the situation in Finland is unique, and there is little hope for volume production of interferons from human leukocytes. Production from human diploid cells grown in culture is under study. The systemic use of natural or synthetic inducers has not proved feasible because of hyporeactivity and adverse reactions in the recipients. Local application of interferon appears to be of value in herpes simplex keratitis and avoids the side-effects of fever, pain at site of injection, and nausea and vomiting that can occur with parenteral administration.

Inflammation

Inflammation is a nonspecific response engendered by injury from physical agents, foreign organisms, and immune reactions. The hallmark of inflammation is dilation and increased permeability of the minute blood vessels, that is, inflammation is the reaction of the living microcirculation and its contents to injury.

Direct injury to cells, as may be caused by toxins elaborated by microorganisms, is reflected by increased permeability of the injured vascular endothelium. Initially, it is a relatively meager response, but it is soon amplified greatly by the release and elaboration of several humoral mediators of the inflammatory response from the killed or injured cells (Table 6-1). Gaps form between vascular endothelial cells through which plasma proteins escape. Granulocytes and monocytes may also leave vascular channels by amoeboid oozing between endothelial cells; erythrocytes are lost from the circulation only if the inter-endothelial junctions have gapped wide enough to permit passage. Such effects are most pronounced in the venules and the venular capillaries, although the lymphvascular endothelium also becomes more porous as a part of such secondary injury. These are the early, potentially reversible (by antihistamines, symphathomimetic amines) phases of the inflammatory response; they are attributable to histamine, serotonin, leukotrienes (formerly called slow reacting substance of anaphylaxis—SRS-A), kinins, prostaglandins, and the early components of complement. Irreversible effects, that is, a compounding of the original injury, are more reasonably associated with lysosomal enzymes, and the late components of complement.

Table 6-1. *Humoral Mediators of Inflammation*

Mediator	Chemical class	Source
Early		
Histamine, Serotonin	Amine	Basophils, macrophages, platelets
Leukotrienes (LTC_4, LTD_4, LTE_4—formerly called slow-reacting substance of anaphylaxis)	Lipid	Leukocytes
Kinins	Peptides	Plasma proteins
Prostaglandins	Lipids	Many cell types
Intermediate		
Plasmin	Enzyme	Plasminogen (liver)
Hageman factor (Factor XII)	Enzyme	Unknown
Complement	Proteins	Reticuloendothelial cells
Late		
Lysosomal enzymes	Proteins	Granulocytes, monocytes, macrophages
Lymphokines	Proteins	Lymphocytes

The utility of the inflammatory response to the host is attested by the marked, rapid spread of an experimental infection—for example, *S. pneumoniae* injected intradermally—when inflammation is prevented by systemic, pharmacologic dosage with glucosteroids or by the concomitant injection of neutral, high-molecular-weight polysaccharides. The salutary effect of the inflammatory response derives from provision of (1) leukocytes in great numbers; (2) plasma proteins—nonspecific and specific humoral agents, fibrinogen that on conversion to fibrin aids in localization of the infectious process while acting as a matrix for phagocytosis; and (3) increased blood and lymph flow that dilutes and flushes toxic materials while causing a local increase in temperature.

In the early stages of inflammation, the exudate is alkaline, and neutrophilic polymorphonuclear leukocytes predominate. As lactic acid accumulates, presumably from glycolysis, the pH drops, and macrophages become the predominant cell type. Lactic acid and antibodies in the inflammatory exudate may inhibit parasites, but the major antiinfectious effect of the inflammatory response is attributable to phagocytic cells.

Phagocytosis

It is advisable to recall at the outset that several aspects of resistance to infection are cell-mediated. These include antibody production and repair of injury, as well as the removal of parasites and their products. Only the removal function is considered here. The cells involved are ubiquitous, abounding in blood, lymph, and connective tissue. They are among the most primitive cells of the postnatal vertebrate. In varying degrees, they possess an embryonic ability to develop into other cells of connective tissue. Phagocytic ability is retained—a primordial function akin to feeding, as emphasized by Metchnikoff—and many of these cells elaborate potent digestive enzymes.

There are two overlapping categories of phagocytic cells: the blood-and lymph-borne, or circulating, leukocytes and the noncirculating phagocytes of the reticuloendothelial system. Granular leukocytes—the microphages of Mechnikoff—and monocytes are the phagocytically capable white blood cells. Of these, the neutrophils are the most efficient phagocytes and are characteristically the predominant cell of the acute inflammatory response (Tables 7-1 and 7-2). Eosinophilic granulocytes are less competent phagocytes and are somewhat specialized in displaying great affinity for antigen–antibody complexes. Monocytes are not part of the initial inflammatory response.

The reticuloendothelial system, as envisioned by Aschoff, is widely distributed throughout the body and is integrated by the common characteristic of noncirculating phagocytic cells. There are sessile macrophages consisting of (1) endothelial cells (very actively phagocytic) of the liver, spleen, lymphoid tissue, bone marrow, adrenal cortex, and anterior pituitary; and (2) reticulum cells (less actively phagocytic) of the spleen, lymphoid tissue, and thymus. In addition, there are wandering macrophages, also called connective tissue histiocytes, or clasmatocytes, which may be derived from, or give origin to, blood-borne monocytes. They are found in connective tissue throughout the body and so are admirably situated for mobilization.

Phagocytosis secures removal of parasites, their products, and inanimate particles by engulfment and digestion. However, there are microorganisms that are engulfed but survive, and even multiply, within the phagocytes; for example, *Mycobacterium tuberculosis* in monocytes. Phagocytized particles that are not lysed are simply stored, and when a particle-laden phagocyte comes to death, a fresh phagocytic cell apparently takes up the burden. Particles too large for a single cell to engulf may be enclosed in giant cells formed by the fusion of several macrophages. Some bacteria, after phagocytosis, kill the phagocyte; for example, strains of *Streptococcus pyogenes* in neutrophils.

Normal neutrophil function requires the integration of several complex processes, including chemotaxis, phagocytosis, degranulation, and oxidative metabolism. Defects in any of these operations can result in impaired host defense.

Chemotaxis is the process by which phagocytes are attracted to the areas where microbial invasion has occurred. Many of the substances that are potent chemoattractants are the same as those involved in the inflammatory response (Table 6-1). Whether generated through the classical or through the alternative pathway, component C5a of complement is the major chemotactic factor in normal serum. Substances elaborated by microorganisms, proteins of the kinin and coagulation pathways, and products of arachidonic acid metabolism (leukotrienes) are also important chemoattractants. Chemotactic factors appear to react with surface receptors on the phagocytes, setting off a series of membrane events that result in directed locomotion. Stimulated phagocytes stick to each other and to vascular endothelium and leave the circulation to reach sites of tissue injury. Diapedesis—passage between intact endothelial cells—requires locomotor capacity plus the ability to change shape by membrane deformation, as bestowed by the action of actin and myosin filaments and microtubules in the cytoplasm.

Once attracted to the site of injury, the phagocyte begins the complex series of events of phagocytosis. Receptors in the phagocytic surface interact with antibody or C3b on the particle to be ingested, and the membrane of the phagocyte invaginates as pseudopods form that close around the particle to create a phagocytic vacuole, which then separates from the cell membrane. Granules in the cytoplasm fuse with the membrane of the phagocytic vacuole to release their contents into the vacuole. Azurophilic granules release lysozyme, myeloperoxidase, and hydrolytic enzymes. Secondary granules release lysozyme, lactoferrin and vitamin B_{12} binding proteins. These substances assist in the killing and degradation of bacteria. If they escape from the phagocytic vacuole, they will also attack host cells.

Bacterial killing during phagocytosis is associated with a surge of aerobic metabolic activity that yields potent oxidizing agents. Oxygen consumption increases as molecular oxygen is transformed to superoxide anion, O_2^-, which is then converted to hydrogen peroxide. The hydrogen peroxide then reacts with myeloperoxidase and halide to effect bacterial killing. Other oxidizing radicals formed by the reaction of the hydrogen peroxide and O_2^- assist in killing. Bacterial killing can take place under anaerobic conditions, but the process is less well understood.

Mononuclear phagocytes are stimulated by contact with lymphocyte products (lymphokines) and with microorganisms. They are the primary defense against facultative and obligate intracellular organisms and contain the necessary metabolic machinery for oxidative and nonoxidative killing.

Esoinophils play a role in defense against certain helminths. They respond to chemotactic factors released by mast cells. Enzymes present in the eosinophil modulate many of the substances of inflammation (leukotrienes, platelet activating factors, histamine), and localization of eosinophils at the site of immediate hypersensitivity reactions may be important in local control of the reaction. In addition, eosinophils can interact with antibody-coated larval stages of helminths (especially schistosomes) resulting in damage to the parasite. Major basic protein (MBP), an arginine-rich protein of the eosinophilic granule, is toxic to both helminths and host cells.

Disorders of Phagocytosis

A defect in any phase of the complex process of phagocytosis can result in increased susceptibility to infection. Chemotaxis is abnormal in a number of conditions. Deficiency of C_3, the critical component for both the classical and the alternative pathways of complement activation, is associated with recurrent infections. Several drugs may affect neutrophil mobility, for example, alcohol, aspirin, and chloramphenicol. Colchicine inhibits locomotion and pseudopod formation, and causes dysfunction of microtubules, thereby interfering with chemotaxis and phagocytosis. Another disorder in which there is abnormal microtubular function is Kartagener's syndrome (recurrent sinus and respiratory infection with situs inversus). Affected males have immotile cilia and sperm because of deficiency of a protein of the microtubules. Abnormal formation of neutrophilic granules is a characteristic of the Chediak–Higashi syndrome (skin and respiratory infections, pancytopenia, hepatosplenomegaly, partial albinism, adenopathy, and neuropathy). Microtubule assembly is abnormal, and defective chemotaxis, adherence, and fusion of granules also occur.

Lack of the respiratory burst in neutrophils results in failure of bacterial killing. This defect is seen in chronic granulomatous disease in which bacteria are ingested normally by leukocytes but are not killed. Patients with this disorder have severe, recurrent infections with pyogenic bacteria.

Function of the Spleen

Splenectomy predisposes to overwhelming bacterial infections. *Streptococcus pneumoniae* is the most common pathogen, but infections with *Haemophilus influenzae, Staphylococcus aureus* and *Neisseria* spp. have also been reported. Without the spleen, the liver must take over the clearance of bacteria; it is a less efficient organ for intravascular clearance, perhaps because of the relatively rapid blood flow past its macrophages as compared with the spleen. In addition, high titers of opsonizing antibodies are required for efficient hepatic clearance of bacteria. This may be the major factor in the increased susceptibility to infections characteristic of asplenia, since splenic function appears to be essential to formation of humoral antibodies. This is evidenced by the fact that splenectomy impairs the response to pneumococcal capsular polysaccharides. Moreover, splenectomized patients have a deficiency of tuftsin, a tetrapeptide produced in the spleen, which stimulates the phagocytic activity of the polymorphonuclear leukocytes and macrophages, increases the production of IgM, and augments the activation of the alternative pathway of complement.

Specific Factors

Specific factors of value to the host in resistance to infection are the results of immune processes—that is, the provocation of either the synthesis of immunoglobulins, the development of cellular immunity, or both. Implied, then, is a finite lapse of time from the receipt of antigenic stimuli until the fruits of immune processes can be harvested to benefit the host. That is, in nature specific factors become operative only after the fact of infection. Once acquired, specific factors are primarily of value in the prevention of recurrences of the corresponding specific diseases. The kinds of infections in which specific resistance factors are important are those that result from accidental encounters between the host and specific parasites (Chap. 4, Host–Parasite Relationships and the Pathogenesis of Infectious Diseases and Chap. 5, Immunopathology of Infectious Diseases).

The development of specific factors by the host may also aid in recovery from infection. The earliest immunoglobulin produced in response to infection is IgM, which is normally followed in about 10 days by the production of IgG. IgG is an important opsonizing factor for a number of gram-positive and gram-negative bacteria. By binding through its Fab portion to the capsular antigens of pneumococci, *H. influenzae, Klebsiella pneumoniae,* and other gram-negative bacilli and through its Fc portion to membrane receptors of neutrophils, it provides a bridge to assist in phagocytosis. Both IgG and IgM can react with microbial antigens to activate C3, another important opsonin. The crisis that occurs around the sixth to eighth day in untreated pneumococcal lobar pneumonia coincides with the appearance of antibody specific for the capsular polysaccharide of the infecting type of *S. pneumoniae.* Continued elaboration and absorption of diphtherial toxin provide a ready avidity for combination with newly synthesized antitoxin because the toxin that has already penetrated cells, causing illness, is beyond neutralization. Augmentation of intoxication is thereby halted.

The provision of exogeneous specific antibody, in the same way as autologous antibody, supplements nonspecific factors and aids in the recovery of the host. However, with the availability of antimicrobial chemotherapeutic agents, the treatment of infectious diseases with heterologous specific antibody has virtually ceased. On the other hand, prophylactic use continues and is discussed in Chapter 20, Immunoprophylaxis of Infectious Diseases.

In addition to therapeutic and prophylactic values, specific factors have pathogenetic potential in the form of hypersensitivity (Chap. 4, Host-Parasite Relationships and the Pathogenesis of Infectious Diseases, and Chap. 5, Immunopathology of Infectious Diseases.) However, the protective aspect of the Arthus phenomenon in preventing dissemination of antigen in the hypersensitive host bears reiterating. The Koch phenomenon, including cellular hypersensitivity, can also be considered to convey resistance to generalized infection at the smaller cost of localized tissue injury.

The specificity of antigen–antibody reactions is very well documented. It is also recognized in diagnosis and therapy and has medicolegal status; for example, distinguishing human from nonhuman blood stains. Yet, there are many situations in which an amazing lack of specificity is prominent. For example, the "antigen" commonly used in the serologic diagnosis of syphilis is an extract of beef heart (Chap. 59, Syphilis). Agglutination reactions involving certain strains of *Proteus vulgaris* are of great use in the diagnosis of rickettsial diseases (Chap. 96, Spotted Fevers). A remarkably high titer of anti-blood group A antibody is characteristic in the person suffering from cutaneous larva migrans (Chap. 111, Cutaneous Larva Migrans). Usually referred to as "cross-reactions" and shrugged off as inexplicable, freak occurrences, these are in fact phenomena of very great informing importance. They tell us that the ways in which antigens and antibodies may react are finite.

Immunoglobulins formed by the stimulus of one antigen can be shown to react with another antigen, utterly unrelated in the biologic sense of origin from a life form of a different phylum. It follows that the antigens have reactive sites of similar chemical nature that are also of comparable spatial distribution so that combination of either antigen with one kind of immunoglobulin is possible. An excellent example of the experimental demonstration of this kind of rationalization is afforded by studies with the type 2 pneumococcal capsular polysaccharide (S II). Knowledge of the structure of S II is quite accurate in terms of monosaccharide components and is of limited precision regarding the arrangement of these components in the polysaccharide macromolecule. However, it was possible to predict the structure of other polysaccharides of unrelated origin through reactivity with anti-S II (Table 6-2).

Table 6-2. *Extend of Cross-Reaction Between Some Nonpneumococcal Polysaccharides and Anti-Type 2 Pneumococcal Antiserum*

	Anti-S II Antibody N_2 Precipitated (%)	**Structure in Common With S II**
Type 2 polysaccharide	100	
Gum arabic	40	D-Glucuronic acid with free carboxyl groups
Gum ghatti	25	
Glycogen (oyster)	2	D-Glucose as branch points
Jellose	2	
M. tuberculosis C fraction	2	L-Rhamnose
Karaya gum	4	

Quite unlike cross-reactions are situations in which antibodies are demonstrable in the very person who suffers from an infectious disease caused by the agent with which his antibodies are specifically reactive. Recurrent clinical infection with herpes simplex viruses is a case in point (Chap. 91, Infections Caused by Herpes Simplex Viruses), as is chronic and recurrent staphylococcal furunculosis (Chap. 100, Staphylococcal Skin Infections). Although specifically reactive antibodies can be demonstrated in serums from such patients, lesions recur over periods of weeks, months, or even years. With recurrent boils, it was once popular to inject subcutaneously a vaccine prepared by heat-killing staphylococci cultured from the patient's lesions—so-called autogenous vaccine therapy. With judicious selection of the doses of vaccine, in some patients a rapid subsidence of the infection resulted without undue systemic reaction. Concomitantly, the phagocytic efficiency of the blood leukocytes increased, often quite markedly, and the titer of humoral antibodies was sometimes increased. When effective, autogenous vaccines apparently suppress delayed hypersensitivity, releasing inhibition of phagocytosis. Autogenous vaccines are rarely used at present—as much because there is uncertainty of dose and of effectiveness as because of the availability of antimicrobics.

Another kind of immunomodulation important in recovery from an acute infection is seen in Epstein–Barr (EB) virus infectious mononucleosis (Chap. 137, Infectious Mononucleosis). EB virus initially infects B cells. This is followed by the appearance of T cells, which are suppressive and cytotoxic to the infected B cells and inhibit their outgrowth. The new T cells have surface markers that are comparable to mature thymus-derived cells. They are believed to be a major factor in the self-limiting nature of infectious mononucleosis.

Bibliography

Books

GRIECO MH (ed): Infections in the Abnormal Host. New York, Yorke Medical Books, 1980. 1035 pp.

WEISSMANN G (ed): Mediators of Inflammation. New York, Plenum Press, 1974. 205 pp.

Journals

ASCHOFF L: Das reticulo-endotheliale system. Ergeb Inn Med Kinderheilkd 26:1–118, 1924

BERNHEIM HA, BLOCK LH, ATKINS E: Fever: Pathogenesis, pathophysiology, and purpose. Ann Intern Med 91:261–270, 1979

BERNHEIM HA, KLUGER MJ: Fever: Effect of drug induced antipyresis on survival. Science 193:237–239, 1976

BULLEN JJ: The significance of iron in infection. Rev Inf Dis 3:1127–1138, 1981

BUTTERWORTH AE, DAVID JR: Eosinophile function. N Engl J Med 304:154–156, 1981

DAVID JR, VADES MA, BUTTERWORTH AE, AZEVEDO DE BRITO P, CARVALHO EM, DAVID RA, BINA JC, ANDRADE ZA: Enhanced helminthotoxic capacity of eosinophiles from patients with eosinophilia. N Engl J Med 303:1147–1152, 1980

DEWAELE M, THIELEMANS C, VAN CAMP BKG: Characterization of immunoregulatory T cells in EBV-induced infectious mononucleosis by monoclonal antibodies. N Engl J Med 304:460–462, 1981

DENSON P, MANDELL GL: Phagocytic strategy vs microbial tactics. Rev Inf Dis 2:817–838, 1980

ELSBACH P: Degradation of microorganisms by phagocytic cells. Rev Inf Dis 2:106–128, 1980

GABIG TG, BABIOR BM: The killing of pathogens by phagocytes. Ann Rev Med 32:313–326, 1981

GAILIN JI: Abnormal phagocyte chemotaxis: Pathophysiology, clinical manifestations, and management of patients. Rev Inf Dis 3:1196–1220, 1980

GARDNER ID: The effect of aging on susceptibility to infection. Rev Inf Dis 2:801–810, 1980

HEIDELBERGER M, ADAMS J: The immunological specificity of type II pneumococcus and its separation into partial specificities. J Exp Med 103:189–197, 1956

HIRSCH MS, SWARTZ MN: Antiviral agents (second of two parts). N Engl J Med 302:949–953, 1980

HOSEA SW, BROWN EJ, HAMBURGER MI, FRANK MM: Opsonic requirements for intravascular clearance after splenectomy. N Engl J Med 304:245–250, 1981

KEUSCH GT: Specific membrane receptors: Pathogenetic and therapeutic implications in infectious diseases. Rev Inf Dis 1:517–529, 1979

MILLS E, QUIE PG: Congenital disorders of the function of polymorphonuclear neutrophiles. Rev Inf Dis 2:505–517, 1980

ROSENTHAL AS: Regulation of the immune response-role of the macrophage. N Engl J Med 303:1153–1156, 1980

SMITH DT: Autogenous vaccines in theory and practice. JAMA 125:344–350, 1970

SPIRER Z, ZAKUTH V, DIAMANT S, MONDORF W, STEFANESCU T, STABINSKY Y, FRIDKIN M: Decreased tuftsin concentrations in patients who have undergone splenectomy. Br Med J 2:1574–1576, 1977

TAUBER AI: Current views of neutrophile dysfunction: An integrated clinical perspective. Am J Med 70:1237–1246, 1981

WEISSMANN G, SMOLEN JE, DORCHAK HM: Release of inflammatory mediators from stimulated neutrophiles. N Engl J Med 303:27–34, 1980

WEKSLER ME: The senescence of the immune system. Hosp Pract 16:53–64, 1981

PAUL D. HOEPRICH
DANE R. BOGGS

Manifestations of Infectious Diseases

7

The manifestations of infectious diseases are protean, as a consequence of the immense variation in the nature of infectious agents (Chap. 1, Attributes of Infectious Agents) and as a result of the possibility of involvement of any organ system of the body. Yet there are manifestations of infection that are quite commonly part of the clinical picture and are unrelated in occurrence either to specific infectious agents or to localization of the infectious process. In addition to such general manifestations of infectious diseases, responses that relate to particular organs or organ systems are discussed. Cutaneous manifestations are considered separately in Chapter 8, Cutaneous Manifestations of Infectious Diseases.

General Manifestations

Affect

Humans appear to be continuously informed by myriads of internal sensors on the state of their internal environment. The reports are subliminal when all is well. Often, the earliest notifications of diseases, be they infectious or noninfectious, are nonspecific. Thus, illness often begins simply as malaise—the person does not feel well. Listlessness, inability to concentrate, lack of drive, uneasiness, light-headedness, weakness, myalgias, arthralgias, headache, and anorexia are also among such nonspecific manifestations.

If the illness becomes more severe, the patient may be toxic. Usually, this connotes more nearly objective findings: flushed facies, dehydration, fever, confusion, and even delirum. If the illness is protracted, loss of body weight may become prominent.

Metabolism

In acute infectious diseases, a catabolic response accompanies the onset of clinical illness. The magnitude of the losses of nitrogen, potassium, magnesium, and phosphorus parallels the severity of the illness. Both a decreased dietary intake and a hypermetabolism consequent to fever contribute to the catabolism of infection.

Fever

Fever—a body temperature in excess of 37.8°C (100.2°F) orally or above 38.4°C (101.2°F) rectally—is a cardinal manifestation of disease, and it is properly viewed as indicative of an infectious process until the disease is proved to be noninfectious. The febrile response to infectious agents is apparently elicited by mechanisms operative with other causes of fever. Thus, there is a diminished loss of body heat through the reduction in both cutaneous circulation and sweating. At the same time, there may be increased production of heat by rigors. These events are mediated by hypothalamic temperature regulatory centers that are provoked to demand an abnormally high body temperature in response to endogenous pyrogens (EPs), and perhaps directly by substances elaborated by pathogenic microorganisms.

Granulocytes appear to be the primary source of EPs, although monocytes, and possibly tissue macrophages, also elaborate EPs. Experimentally, the production and release of EPs can be stimulated by bacterial endotoxins, phagocytosis of various substances (infectious agents, antigen–antibody complexes), pinocytosis, and certain metabolites of steroidal hormones. As obtained from granulocytes, endogenous pyrogens appear to be proteins, possibly lipoproteins. Because both granulocytes and monocytes from humans generate EPs, it is presumed that the pathogenesis of fever in humans is much the same as that in nonhuman animals.

Fever often varies in magnitude during the day in a pattern that is basically an exaggeration of the normal diurnal variation in body temperature. That is, in the normal person the temperature is maximal in the late afternoon–early evening and is minimal about 12 hours later, a pattern that is the inverse of that of endogenous corticosteroid release. Similarly, fevers tend to be highest in the late afternoon and lowest in the early morning. Night sweats simply represent defervescence through diaphoresis at the time the temperature ordinarily drops to its diurnal low point.

Patterns of fever, as derived from charting temperatures versus time, have become formalized with a nomenclature and clothed in a lore. Thus, fever may be *sustained* (little variation during the day, as in typhoid fever, tularemia, and rickettsioses); *remittent* (never normal, but varying 0.5°C (1°F) or more during the day, as in typhoid fever, tuberculosis, scrub typhus, and falciparum malaria); *intermittent* (the temperature becoming normal at least once each day, as in tuberculosis, nonfalciparum malarias, and abscesses); *double quotidian* (two returns to normal each day, with two maxima, as in miliary tuberculosis, gonococcal endocarditis, and kalaazar); *septic* (widely, irregularly varying temperature, as in disseminated tuberculosis, malaria, and abscesses): or *relapsing* (periods of days of fever separated by days of normal temperature, as in tuberculosis, especially if extrapulmonary; malaria; and brucellosis). Although such patterns may bear a statistically valid association with particular etiologic agents, in the individual patient the fever curve is generally of little diagnostic aid. Many causes for fever (noninfectious as well as infectious) yield identical patterns as well as multiple patterns, and there is very great variation from patient to patient.

There are, however, several truisms regarding fever that are clinically sound. (1) The vigor of the febrile response diminishes with age—from maximal responsiveness in young children to minimal response in the aged. (2) Convulsions with fever indicate intracranial infections, if intracranial hemorrhage can be excluded, and excepting infants in whom there is no localizing significance. (3) Hyperthermia—temperatures in excess of 41.2°C (106°F)—is rarely caused by an infection; exceptions include bacterial meningitis and viral encephalitis. (4) Fever blisters (*herpes febrilis*) are common with pneumoccocal, streptococcal, and rickettsial infections, and with malaria. Although common in meningococcal meningitis, fever blisters are infrequent in meningococcemia and rare in typhoid fever. (5) Fever with severe sweating is characteristic of sporadic treatment with aspirin, pulmonary abscesses, bacterial endocarditis, and tuberculosis. (6) Fever is typically preceded by a single chill in pneumococcal pneumonia, streptococcal infections, osteomyelitis, tularemia, plague, leptospirosis, typhus, and influenza. Repeated chills are common in the occasional administration of aspirin and usual in the course of fevers caused by bacteremias (as in acute pyelonephritis, biliary tract obstruction, intravascular infections such as staphylococcal endocarditis, and bacterial phlebitides in the liver, pelvis, and venous sinuses of the brain); infections of the hematopoietic–lymphoreticular system (as in malaria, brucellosis, and rat-bite fever); and collections of pus. (7) Drug fevers do not usually produce symptoms, and the temperature typically remains elevated, fixed at a relatively constant level.

THERAPY

In the adult, fever itself is not ordinarily cause for antipyretic therapy because hydration and the administration of codeine and sedatives usually make the patient comfortable. Moreover, the course of the fever is a valuable indicator of the adequacy of specific treatment of the infection. Children subject to febrile convulsions and adults with hyperpyrexia may benefit from judicious reduction of temperature. Whatever measures are employed, they must not provoke discomfort, cutaneous vasoconstriction, shivering, or rigors. Aspirin or other antipyretic agents (phenacetin is said to be more effective than aspirin) reduce fever, but must be given frequently and regularly, for example, every 2 to 3 hours, to avoid distress from alternating episodes of diaphoresis and chills. Removal of body heat is efficiently accomplished by sponging with tepid water; cutaneous vasoconstriction is avoided and water has a higher heat of vaporization than does ethanol. Cooling blankets or mattresses are quite effective but must not be applied so zealously that the patient is reduced to shivering and hypothermic misery.

In addition to minimizing discomfort and avoiding seizures, reduction of fever has been rationalized as a way to decrease the stress of infection. The requirement for oxygen should decrease, catabolism should abate, and the demands on the cardiovascular system should be moderated as the temperature comes down. Moreover, it is quite difficult to prove that fever per se is beneficial to the host. Only two parasites are known that cannot survive temperatures tolerated by humans: *Treponema pallidum* and *Neisseria gonorrhoeae;* at one time, fever therapy was used with good clinical effect in the treatment of neurosyphilis and the gonorrheal urethritis.

Because fever generally provides no advantage to the host, it is reasonable to inquire if hypothermia might be useful. From experimental work, it appears that the ill effects of toxins such as tetanal toxin are reduced by hypothermia. It might also be supposed that the rate of growth of pathogenic microorganisms would be slowed. In experimental animals, however, such possible gains are outweighed by losses in defense mechanisms: phagocytosis is decreased and antibody production falls off. The relatively few, random applications of hypothermia to humans with infectious diseases are difficult to evaluate because desperately ill patients were treated and there were no controls. In short, while euthermia may be preferable to fever, hypothermia may be disadvantageous in patients with infectious diseases.

FEVER OF UNDETERMINED ORIGIN

Fever of undetermined origin (FUO) is an arbitrary designation of considerable clinical importance because the term connotes the institution of a series of complex, expensive, even painful and dangerous diagnostic investigations. Designation as an FUO requires documentation of fever persistent for at least 3 weeks without discovery of the cause of the fever after in-hospital application of the history and physical, laboratory, radiographic, and scanning examinations. Insistence on these criteria is essential to eliminate a host of self-limiting causes of fever, such as viral infections. Although the resolution of the problem of FUO is a stimulating challenge to the physician, it must be kept uppermost in mind that the game is in deadly earnest for the patient, because death is the outcome in about one-third of patients with FUO. Overall, in the western world, roughly equal numbers of the final diagnoses fall into each of the following categories: infection, neoplasia, collagen–vascular, miscellaneous but identified, and unsolved disease. The range of specific diseases that might be manifest as FUO is enormous. As a consequence, there is no single approach to solving the problem. However, a few principles and some additional points merit presentation:

1. The temptation to invoke the esoteric should be resisted, because an unusual manifestation of a common disease is much more likely to be the cause of fever than is a rare disease.
2. The fourth dimension of patient evaluation—that is, continued observation—must be applied assiduously. The utility of the history and physical, laboratory, radiographic, and scanning examinations is not dissipated in a single application. Patients, their relatives, friends, and associates will recall significant information on repeated questioning. Physical findings may change—the appearance of a rash, a palpable spleen, or a new cardiac murmur. Serial determinations of antibody titers, the outgrowth of blood cultures—all may require time for diagnostic change. Repeated radiographic studies, particularly with computer assistance, as well as radionuclide and ultrasound scanning examinations, may give insight into functional and morphologic changes.
3. The presence of fever must be documented. Manipulation of the thermometer to register an abnormally high temperature is a well-known trick of malingerers and neurotics. Wide, erratic swings in fever that ignore the diurnal pattern of temperature, the lack of corresponding changes in pulse rate, and the absence of sweating at the times of supposed defervescence are useful clues, particularly in patients with multiple complaints and few findings.
4. Both prescribed and social drug intake must be thoroughly reviewed. A sustained fever may be the sole evidence of allergy to a drug; typically, the patient is not as ill as his temperature might indicate. Drugs that commonly provoke fever include the penicillins, the sulfonamides, isoniazid, para-aminosalicylic acid, iodides, thiouracil, barbiturates, and quinidine. Fevers from drug use that are nonallergic in origin may arise from self-use of contaminated equipment and drugs, and from tissue injury at the site of infection.
5. Several infectious diseases offer diagnostic difficulties while manifesting fevers of undetermined origins. Tuberculosis must still head the list and should be thought of automatically in blacks, Mexican–Americans, and American Indians. Several of the Enterobacteriaceae—such as *Salmonella* spp.—may cause occult fevers. Abscesses, particularly when retroperitoneal, pelvic, subdiaphragmatic, hepatic, or perinephric, can be very difficult to detect. Although pararectal abscesses are not uncommon in patients with leukemia or diabetes mellitus, examination of the rectum is required for detection. Infective endocarditis may occur with little evidence of heart disease, particularly in the aged. Infectious mononucleosis is notable among viral diseases, and toxoplasmosis among protozoal diseases, as possible causes for FUO in young adults.
6. Although fever may occur during the course of any kind of neoplastic process, neoplasms of lymphoid and myeloid tissues are especially likely to yield fever. Other neoplasms commonly associated with FUO involve the kidneys, stomach, colon, liver, lungs, and bones. Necrosis of tumor tissue is common but is not a prerequisite for fever.
7. Of all the collagen–vascular diseases, scleroderma and dermatomyositis are least likely to

be associated with fever. On the other hand, fever is prominent at some time in virtually every patient with disseminated lupus erythematosus. Temporal arteritis is most frequent in the elderly and may cause fever.

8. FUO has been associated with a variety of hepatic diseases, acute pancreatitis, regional enteritis, atrial myxoma, head trauma, heat stroke, and sarcoidosis.
9. Biopsy procedures and exploratory surgical operations are of decided diagnostic utility when (a) indirect methods have been applied, repeatedly when possible, without yielding a specific diagnosis; (b) there are clinical or laboratory indicators of a high probability of diagnostic yield from the invasive procedure to be undertaken; or (c) rapid deterioration of the patient's condition makes diagnosis particularly urgent. Computed tomography (CT) scanning is especially valuable. Lymphangiography, ultrasound, and radionuclide scanning are often useful.
10. Therapeutic trials should be undertaken with reluctance because the course of an FUO is not predictable and very few therapies are restricted in effect to a single etiologic agent or specific disease process. Isoniazid plus ethambutol is specifically antituberculous; however, the coincidence of apparent response with spontaneous improvement of a nontuberculous process cannot be excluded.
11. Some patients with unsolved FUO eventually recover spontaneously. Others go to their death, the origin of the fever unknown even after postmortem examination.

Hematologic

Leukocytosis

Quantitative and qualitative changes in blood leukocytes accompany most infectious diseases, but the kind of abnormality varies from one kind of infection to another (see list below). Normal values for blood leukocytes and relative phagocytic efficiency are listed in Table 7-1. The two major components of host defense against invasion by microorganisms are the phagocytic and immune systems (Chap. 6, Resistance to Infection). Thus it is not unexpected that circulating representatives of these systems would frequently be affected by infection.

During the initial phase of an acute bacterial infection, neutrophilia and eosinopenia are usual; lymphopenia may also be present. Blood neutrophils normally are distributed between circulating and marginated pools of cells. Approximately half circulate freely, and half are stuck to, or roll along, the walls of capillaries or postcapillary venules. As an inflammatory response develops (Chap. 6, Resistance to Infection), neutrophil margination increases, there is diapedesis of cells into the tissues, and a poorly defined humoral control substance increases in con-

LEUKOCYTE RESPONSES IN INFECTIOUS DISEASES

Neutrophilia
Usual in a large variety of acute, local, and general infections caused by bacteria, spirochetes, rickettsias, viruses, protozoa, and helminths. Nearly always absent in uncomplicated salmonelloses (including typhoid fever), tuberculosis, and fungal, chlamydial, some rickettsial, and many viral infections.

Neutropenia
Frequent in salmonelloses, brucellosis, pertussis, and some rickettsial, viral, and protozoal infections.

Eosinophilia
Typical of helminthic infections with invasion of tissues; not uncommon in intestinal helminthic and protozoal infections. Seen in scarlet fever.

Monocytosis
Common in tuberculosis, brucellosis, syphilis, and some rickettsial and protozoal infections. Seen also in convalescence from acute bacterial infections.

Lymphocytosis
Classic in pertussis. Seen also in tuberculosis, brucellosis, syphilis, and many rickettsial and viral infections. Also prominent during convalescence from acute bacterial infections.

Table 7-1. *Blood Leukocytes of Normal Humans*

Leukocyte	Number Per mm^3	Relative Phagocytic Efficiency*
Neutrophils		
Segmented and band	2000–7000	100
Metamyelocyte	rare	83
Myelocyte	0	54
Myeloblast	0	0
Eosinophils	0–700	32
Basophils	0–150	0
Monocytes	200–900	50
Lymphocytes	1500–4000	0

*Judged on the basis of phagocytosis of *Streptococcus pneumoniae.*

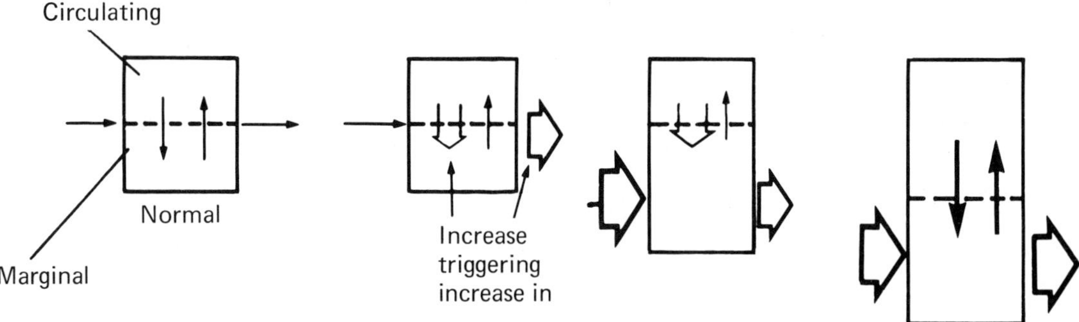

Fig. 7-1. Blood neutrophil response to inflammation.

centration in the blood. This neutrophil-releasing factor produces an accelerated rate of release of segmented and band-form neutrophils from a bone marrow granulocyte reserve containing 10 to 15 times as many functionally mature neutrophils as are normally present in the circulating blood. Because this huge reserve may readily be released into the blood, enormous numbers of phagocytes are available to the inflamed area. As release accelerates, the marginal pool expands initially, followed by expansion of the circulating pool to produce the characteristic neutrophilia in the venous blood (Fig. 7-1). Segmented cells are released in preference to bands, but as release accelerates, a greater than normal proportion of bands is released, producing a "shift to the left." Factors resulting in retention of immature cells within the bone marrow are poorly understood, but relate, at least in part, to the ease with which cells can be deformed enough to pass through small pores that are created within marrow endothelial cells. A few metamyelocytes may be released during infection, but release of still less mature neutrophils (myelocytes, promyelocytes, and myeloblasts) is unusual unless there is intrinsic disease of the bone marrow.

However, the release of immature neutrophils may occasionally accompany extreme leukocytosis, simulating the picture if chronic myeloid leukemia (CML); this has been termed a *leukemoid reaction.* Other infections in which a CML-like leukemoid reaction may occur include diphtherial, meningococcal, and tuberculous infections. A blood picture suggesting acute myeloblastic or monoblastic leukemia is said to be produced by tuberculosis; however, reports of the blood returning to normal with antituberculosis therapy are not available. Differentiation of activated lymphocytes (as are common in infections such as varicella, measles, whooping cough, and infectious mononucleosis) from the cells of acute lymphoblastic leukemia often requires great skill in blood cell morphology. Eosinophilia may occasionally be so marked with helminthic infections that eosinophilic leukemia is suspected.

Although the initial source of additional blood neutrophils is the marrow reserve, increased neutrophil production is also stimulated by an undefined mechanism in bacterial infection. Increased production persists seemingly for as long as a continuing supply of neutrophils is demanded by the infected site(s). The rate of use of neutrophils in an exudate in which there is persistent infection is quite high, that is, there is a continuing rapid turnover of neutrophils within the exudate. Thus, with chronic infections, such as abscesses or empyemas, there is continued neutrophil migration from the blood to the exudate, that is, a chronically increased blood neutrophil turnover is established and is usually accompanied by persistent neutrophilia and hyperplasia of the immature neutrophil production pool of the bone marrow.

The mechanism of the neutropenia that characterizes certain infectious diseases (see list on p. 88) is cryptic. However, in malaria it has been shown that the marginal pool is increased in size even though the circulating pool is modestly decreased. This may be true in certain other diseases as well, because neutropenia does not appear to indicate a poor prognosis in salmonellosis, brucellosis, or pertussis, that is, there is no shortage of phagocytes if the marginal pool is expanded.

However, the development of neutropenia is a poor prognostic sign in several pyogenic bacterial infections, for example, pneumococcal pneumonia. Such neutropenia represents exhaustion of the blood pools and of the marrow granulocyte reserves. Although neutropenia from excessive use of phagocytes may occur occasionally in a patient who initially had a normal neutrophil system, it is much more common in cases in which the marrow reserve was reduced in size when the infection began. This is most commonly the result of treatment with cancer chemotherapeutic agents or of intrinsic diseases of the marrow such as acute leukemia, but it may also be the result of alcoholism, diabetes mellitus, and shock.

The two kinds of neutropenia can often be differentiated by microscopic examination of smears of the peripheral blood. With hyperutilization, bands, often with vacuoles, toxic granulation, and Döhle bodies, predominate, whereas the neutrophilis are predominantly segmented and lacking morphologic abnormality in the cryptic neutropenias of the infections listed on p.000.

Eosinopenia is so frequent in the beginning of severe bacterial infections that ease of demonstration of eosinophils in a blood smear should raise doubts about the diagnosis. Although it is generally assumed that eosinopenia is the result of increased glucosteroids, this has been shown not to be the case in experimental infections in rodents. As infections improve or become chronic, eosinophils return to the blood and may even increase to eosinophilic levels.

The role of the eosinophil in host defense remains to be clarified. It is a fairly able phagocyte (Table 7-1), and eosinophils may accompany neutrophils into any exudate. However, there are chemotactic factors, including antigen–antibody complexes, that selectively attract and are engulfed by eosinophils. Eosinophilia and increased eosinophil production are classically associated with helminthic infections. The response is secondary to the host's immune reaction to the parasite; it is not a response to the parasite *per se.* Thymic lymphocytes react to helminthic antigens to mediate increased production of eosinophils. In general, the degree of helminth-induced eosinophilia is roughly proportional to the severity of the infection, but eosinophilia may be present with completely asymptomatic infections such as ascariasis.

Basophilia is not a response to an infectious process. Indeed, even in leukemoid reactions, basophils are not increased.

Blood monocyte levels are highly variable in infection, but are most often elevated in active chronic infections such as tuberculosis. The blood monocyte is a rather immature cell, the blood-borne precursor of the tissue macrophage. There is no marrow reserve of monocytes; as monocytes are demanded by exudates, blood monocyte turnover is increased, and it is not unusual to see a monocytopenia with acute bacterial infections. However, the rates of production, turnover through the blood, and influx into exudates may all be accelerated without causing an increase in the numbers of monocytes in the blood. Although blood monocytes are less efficient phagocytes than are neutrophils (Table 7-1), their phagocytic funtion improves as they mature into macrophages.

Even as blood lymphocytes are often decreased with acute bacterial infections, they are often increased during chronic infections, particularly in stable or healing tuberculosis. An increased number of large, activated blood lymphocytes is often observed in viral infections, for example, infectious mononucleosis. These cells are in an active generative cycle and represent part of the proliferative immune response to the parasitic antigen: bone marrow-derived B cells that mature into plasma cells for production of circulating immunoglobulins; and thymus-derived T cells, the direct effectors of cellular immunity (delayed hypersensitivity). The immunoglobulins arising from the B cells sustain immunity to specific infections and aid phagocytosis by providing opsonins. T cells play a major role in modifying tuberculosis and salmonellosis, as well as fungal, viral, rickettsial, and protozoal infections, by secreting a group of toxins and mediators known as lymphokines.

Anemia

It is probable that virtually all infections influence the erythroid system. However, the effect of short-lived infections on the numbers of circulating red blood cells is usually of no consequence in view of the normal erythrocyte life span of 120 days. With prolonged infection (or prolonged active inflammatory disease of any type), anemia usually develops. At least three mechanisms contribute to the anemia.

1. Production of erythropoietin, the hormone controlling red cell production, is not increased appropriately as anemia develops. Anemias of such diverse causes as iron deficiency and leukemia, or idiopathic aplastic anemia, result in increased production of erythropoietin in direct proportion to the degree of anemia; there is no such increase in the anemia of infection and, consequently, erythropoiesis is not increased to the degree appropriate to the severity of the anemia.
2. The delivery of iron to developing normoblasts is compromised: the concentrations of serum iron and of transferrin, the iron transport protein, are reduced. There is, effectively, a deficiency in the supply of iron for hemoglobin synthesis. Consequently, moderate degrees of microcytosis and hypochromia may be present. However, iron stores are quite adequate or may even be increased. The relative iron deficiency is the result of the reduced ease with which iron can be

released from reticuloendothelial cells to transferrin.

3. There is also a modest reduction in red cell survival, but the anemia is not primarily hemolytic because compensation for the shortened red cell survival would require only a modest increase in cell production. The anemia of infection develops gradually and usually stabilizes at a non-life-threatening hemoglobin concentration. Since there is no evidence that the anemia makes the infection worse, it should be monitored but ignored. Treatment of the anemia is synonymous with treatment of the infection, and in most instances there is no justification for transfusion.

Progressively severe anemia may develop in certain chronic infections, such as untreated bacterial endocarditis. In this disease, the progressively enlarging spleen adds the factor of hypersplenism (sequestering and destroying red cells in an enlarged spleen) to the anemia of infection.

The very rapid development of an anemia during an infection signifies one of three things: the patient is bleeding; the infection itself directly destroys red cells (*e.g.,* malaria—Chap. 145, Malaria, infection with *Clostridium perfringens*—Chap. 156, Gas Gangrene); or there is an underlying, preexisting hemolytic process. Patients with an underlying hemolytic process, such as sickle cell anemia or hereditary spherocytosis, have very short red cell survival times that are partially or, in the case of the latter disease, completely compensated by a marked increase in red cell production. During or after an infection, erythrocyte production often decreases, as reflected in a falling reticulocyte concentration. Because of the short red cell survival time, anemia may develop precipitously or rapidly increase in severity. With the potential hemolytic disease inherent in deficiency of glucose-6-phosphate dehydrogenase (G6PD), either the infection or drugs used to treat the infection (*e.g.,* sulfonamides or primaquine) can precipitate hemolysis. Hemolysins are elaborated by many kinds of bacteria, but only the α-toxin of *Clostridium perfringens* (an α-lecithinase that causes lysis of the lipoprotein cell membranes of erythrocytes) has been unequivocally associated with intravascular hemolysis *in vivo* (Chap. 156, Gas Gangrene). Intraerythrocyte parasitization is clearly the destructive mechanism responsible for the anemias of malaria (Chap. 145, Malaria) and bartonellosis (Chap. 144, Bartonellosis). Hemolysis may be consequent to cold agglutinins—infection with *Mycoplasma pneumoniae* (Chap. 30, Nonbacterial Pneumonias)—or may occur with infectious mononucleosis (Chap. 137, Infectious Mononucleosis) or with infection by the *Chylamydia* spp. that cause ornithoses (Chap. 30, Nonbacterial Pneumonias).

Erythrocyte Sedimentation Rate

The rate at which erythrocytes agglomerate and settle out of anticoagulated blood—the erythrocyte sedimentation rate (ESR)—is increased in a variety of diseases. Many factors affect ESR, the most important of which are the concentrations of fibrinogen, and α-2 and α-1 globulins in the plasma; increased concentrations yield an increased ESR. Although the test has great sensitivity as an indicator of organic disease, it lacks specificity. Any disease that evokes an inflammatory response engenders an increased ESR. Neoplastic processes, collagen-vascular diseases, dysproteinemias, a variety of renal diseases, and pregnancy also cause an increase in ESR.

Coagulation

The concentrations of various factors important in coagulation may be altered in infection. Perhaps the two most common changes are increased levels of platelets and fibrinogen. Even though thrombocytosis is often present, infection also accelerates the rate at which platelets are lost from the blood. The magnitude of loss may be so great that effective platelet transfusion may become impossible in thrombocytopenic patients with serious infections.

The only common serious coagulation problem that develops in association with infection is *disseminated intravascular coagulation* (DIC). The major clinical manifestations of this disorder are sudden onset of hemorrhagic phenomena or thromboembolic phenomena. DIC occurs as an acute or chronic process, but for all practical purposes only the acute form accompanies infections. Virtually any kind of infection, including a variety of viral, rickettsial, bacterial, mycotic, and protozoal infections, may cause DIC. It is perhaps most common in sepsis caused by gram-negative bacteria. There are also numerous and varied noninfectious causes of DIC (Fig. 7-2)

The pathogenesis of DIC is complex and incompletely understood. The multiple and interrelated factors that can initiate DIC also activate normal coagulation mechanisms of platelet adhesion and aggregation, as well as the contact and tissue-factor-activated pathways. For example, in meningococcemia, thromboplastin may be released from vascular endothelium injured so as to expose collagen; platelets adhere to the collagen, and there is aggregation and contact activation. It has been postulated that endotoxin released during sepsis from gram-negative bacilli enters the circulation and plays a role in DIC. Also controversial is the role of shock in initiating

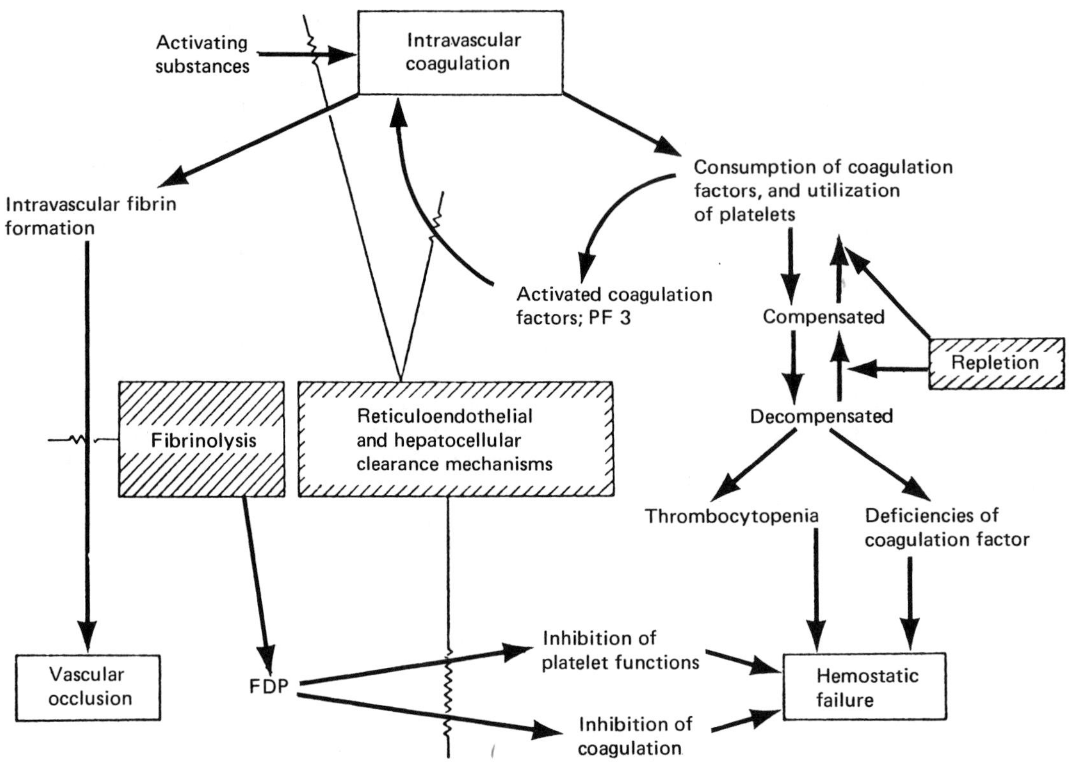

Fig. 7-2. Infectious diseases are among the many pathologic processes that generate substances that activate the intravascular coagulation of blood. Compensatory mechanisms (*hatched blocks*) are inadequate to halt coagulation so long as activating substances continue to be produced. (Wintrobe MM. Lee GR, Boggs DR, Bithell TC, Athens JW, Foerster J: Clinical Hematology, 7th ed. Philadelphia, Lea & Febiger, 1974)

DIC. However, there is no question that shock makes DIC more severe, as does any factor abetting hypoperfusion.

In DIC, forces that activate coagulation are so intense or so continuous that normal compensatory mechanisms are overwhelmed. As a result, there is persistent or recurrent elaboration of thrombin within the circulation; as with normal coagulation, thrombin generation becomes autocatalytic. Fibrinogen, platelets, and other coagulation factors are used, and fibrin is formed in the circulation. This, in turn, activates the fibrinolytic system, which produces large amounts of fibrin degradation products (FDPs). FDPs, in turn, inhibit coagulation, form defective fibrin polymers, impair platelet function, and constrict the pulmonary vasculature. The normal FDP clearing function of the reticuloendothelial system may become impaired. The outcome of DIC depends on the balance between the various pathologic processes and the compensatory system designed to correct them; fibrin formation versus fibrinolysis, coagulation factor production versus destruction, FDP production versus clearance.

The bleeding that accompanies DIC also is multifactorial. Thrombocytopenia and hypofibrinogenemia are common, and the thrombocytopenia is often severe enough to produce hemorrhagic phenomena. When these deficiencies are combined with the multiple anticoagulant properties of FDPs and reduced levels of other coagulation factors, life-threatening hemorrhage often results. Thromboembolic episodes result from the formation of loose intravascular fibrin and fibrin–FDP aggregates.

Laboratory diagnosis of DIC depends on multiple tests since there is no single, completely reliable examination. Schistocytes (fragmented red cells resulting from collision with fibrin strands) and thrombocytopenia may be seen on examination of blood smears. The latter, when confirmed by platelet counting, is usually in the range of 20,000 to 80,000/mm^3. Rapid, accurate tests are available for the detection of abnormal concentrations of FDPs in the plasma, using staphylococcal clumping, red cell hemagglutination inhibition, and latex agglutination systems. If the platelet count is normal and excessive FDPs are not found, the diagnosis of DIC is questionable. Fibrinogen levels are usually decreased; however, this factor is often increased during infection, and the decrease with the onset of DIC may bring the concentration to normal limits in some patients. Levels of other coagulation factors are quite variable with DIC, but factors V, VIII, and XIII are usually decreased. Even the stable factors (VII, IX, X, XI) may be decreased. Hypoprothromobinemia is more common and more profound in DIC caused by infection than in DIC initiated by other illnesses.

Successful treatment of DIC in the infected patient depends more upon successful treatment of the infection and of ancillary factors such as shock than upon treatment directed specifically against DIC. The decision to use heparin in the treatement of DIC must be carefully weighed in each case; heparin therapy is not of proven benefit in septic DIC. It must be given intravenously. If intermittent injection is used, the dose is 100 units/kg body wt every 4 hours; for continuous infusion, a loading dose of 100 units/kg body wt should be followed by 400 to 475 units/kg body wt/day (the lower dose for older women). If there is improvement in laboratory parameters within 24 hours (*e.g.,* increases in fibrinogen, factors II, V, and VIII, and platelets—not every patient responds promptly with an increase in platelets), treatment should be maintained at this level until there is correction of DIC. The dose should then be adjusted to maintain a controlled state of hypocoagulability, and treatment should be continued as long as FDPs are detectable in the serum.

Monitoring the degree of anticoagulation induced by heparin is difficult in any case, and the difficulty is compounded in DIC by the abnormalities that were present when therapy was started. If the partial thromboplastin time (PTT) was normal, it may be followed; if it was abnormal, the effect of heparin can be estimated from changes in the coagulability of whole blood. There are two important limitations to use of the clotting time to regulate the dose of heparin (*i.e.,* a dose that maintains the clotting time at 2½ times normal 3½ hours after injection): (1) gross nonuniformity in the methods of testing (literally dozens of variations in technique have been described) makes for gross nonuniformity in results; and (2) an inordinate amount of time is required (if the control is 10 min, the desired therapeutic clotting time will be 30 min). In contrast, the activated coagulation time of whole blood (ACT test) is a carefully standardized, simple, rapid test (normal range: 70–120 sec) that enables precise control of heparin therapy. When the test is carried out exactly as originally described by Hattersley in standard diatomite tubes (Becton–Dickenson #3206, XF 534), the 4-hourly dose of heparin should be adjusted to yield an ACT of 140 to 180 sec 3½ hours after the preceding dose. Monitoring fibrinogen concentrations is often useful in determining the course of DIC, with or without heparin therapy. However, the overall course of the patient must be carefully monitored without total reliance on any single test.

There is no evident role for the coumarin anticoagulants in DIC. Antifibrinolytic agents, such as ϵ-aminocaproic acid, are probably contraindicated as they may increase the chance of fatal thromboembolism in patients with DIC. Replacement therapy (infusion of platelets and fibrinogen) is somewhat controversial. If heparin is used, replacement therapy is necessary only when thrombocytopenia or hypofibrinogenemia is very severe. If replacement is undertaken and heparin is not given, monitoring for deleterious effects such as a rising creatinine or decreasing pO_2 should be employed.

Acute-Phase Reactants

Acute tissue injury from virtually any cause, including infectious diseases, will result in a rapid increase in the concentrations of several proteins in the serum, including α-1-antitrypsin, haptoglobin, ceruloplasmin, α-1-glycoprotein, C-reactive protein (CRP). The overall significance of the acute-phase reactants is the same as an elevated ESR; namely, they are indicators of organic disease. However, they differ from each other, and from ESR in several ways, including speed of appearance and rate of decline. Because CRP rises more rapidly and is a more reliable indicator of disease than are the other acute-phase reactants, it has received particular attention.

C-Reactive Protein

CRP was so named when it was discovered in 1930 in the serums of patient with pneumococcal pneumonia because it precipitated the C polysaccharide present in the cell walls of *Streptococcus pneumoniae.* However, CRP was soon shown to appear in the serum in virtually any disease, infectious or noninfectious, in which an inflammatory response or tissue destruction has occurred. That is, CRP is not humoral antibody. However, it is immunogenic, and methods for detection depend on the reaction of CRP with specific antibody, as may be raised in goats by injection of purified CRP. Nephelometry, for example, laser-beam nephelometry, offers sensitivity, speed, and accuracy in the quantitative determination of CRP in body liquids by measuring the scattering of light by immune complexes. Thus, it has been shown that within 4 to 6 hours after injury the concentration of CRP in the serum rises exponentially from normal values of about 2 mg/dl. In damaged tissues, deposited CRP may be detected by specific immunofluorescence.

Regardless of the incitant, CRP is an homogeneous gamma globulin consisting of five subunits linked to form two pentamers with a molecular weight of about 120,000. It is synthesized rapidly and in large quantities by hepatocytes.

The functions of CRP are not fully understood. When it binds to phosphocholine determinants of pneumococcal C-polysaccharide, it functions as an opsonin and may activate complement by the classical pathway. Through binding with damaged host cell membranes and activating complement, CRP may contribute to the inflammatory response.

Cardiovascular

Pulse

When there is fever, the pulse rate is usually increased—about ten beats per minute per 0.5°C (1°F). With some infections, the rate is characteristically slower than would be predicated: salmonelloses including typhoid fever, tularemia, Legionnaire's disease, brucellosis, bacterial meningitides complicated by increased intracranial pressure, mycoplasmal pneumonia, rickettsialpox, ornithoses, mumps, infectious hepatitis, Colorado tick fever, and dengue. A disproportionately slow pulse rate is also encountered with factitious fever and in patients with cancers, or patients with atrial fibrillation who have received therapeutic doses of cardiac-active glycosides.

Blood Pressure

HYPOTENSION

Hypotension without shock is not uncommon in the course of severe infections. Although there is a valid assocation with bacteremia, hypotension also occurs in patients who have serious underlying, noninfectious diseases. Also, abrupt defervescence caused by the administration of an antipyretic, such as aspirin, may result in hypotension.

SHOCK

Septic shock is the shock syndrome (acute circulatory dysfunction associated with general hypoperfusion) complicating infectious disease. It is second in frequency only to cardiogenic shock in causing shock-associated deaths in hospital.

PATHOGENESIS

Unfortunately, it has become almost automatic to label septic shock gram-negative shock or endotoxin shock. In common with many terms that leap easily to the tongue, these labels have a midleading aura of implied knowledge of pathogenesis, diagnosis, and even therapy. The phrases have dual roots. There is the association of septic shock with bacteremias caused by gram-negative bacteria in about two-thirds of the patients in whom this complication develops in hospital. Moreover, the commonly studied experimental model is shock induced by the intravenous injection of endotoxins—protein–lipopolysaccharide complexes that overlie the rigid mucopeptide framework of the cell walls of many kinds of gram-negative bacteria. Although the various endotoxins are diverse in specific bacterial origin (*e.g., Escherichia coli, Yersinia pestis,* and *Neisseria gonorrhoeae*) and in chemical structure (*E. coli* 0 antigen is identical with *E. coli* endotoxin), there is qualitative identity in biologic activity. The property of induction of shock on intravenous injection into mammals is one such activity. However, this laboratory experiment should not be construed as proof that endotoxins are the cause of septic shock. In the first place, as septic shock occurs in the United States, about one-third of the patients have infections caused by gram-positive bacteria. Moreover, rickettsial, chlamydial, viral, protozoal, and even metazoal infections may be complicated by shock. Second, the doses of endotoxin used experimentally appear to be very high in terms of the actual body burden of bacteria in the usual infection. Moreover, in experimental models, the dose of endotoxin is delivered IV as a bolus, whereas in patients endotoxin is probably released slowly over relatively long periods, when bacteriolytic therapy is not given. Third, in volunteers, the induction of tolerance to endotoxin by repetitive IV injections failed to prevent the clinical manifestations of experimentally induced typhoid fever. Finally, there has been extraordinary difficulty in detecting what may be trace quantities of endotoxinlike substances in the blood of patients with septic shock—the very patients in whom the concentration of endotoxin ought to be maximal.

Overall, gram-negative bacteria predominate as causes of septic shock. *Escherichia coli* is the most frequent, with *Klebsiella* spp., *Enterobacter* spp., *Proteus* spp., *Pseudomonas* spp., and *Bacteroides* spp. following in approximate descending order of occurrence. As is evident from this listing, the sites of infection are usually the urinary, intestinal, biliary, and female genital tracts. Nonspecific, predisposing afflictions are quite common: diabetes mellitus, cirrhosis of the liver, burns, neoplastic diseases, and therapies (surgery, irradiation, antimitotic and antimetabolic drugs, glucosteroids, and blood transfusions). Quite in keeping with these facts is the predominance of males over 40 years of age and females 20 to 45 years of age. When bacteremia is caused by gram-negative bacteria, shock intervenes in about one-fourth of the patients; of these, 50% to 80% die in shock.

Although frequently associated with septic shock, septicemias are not prerequisites. Intoxication with clostridial or diphtherial toxins may cause shock. Other examples include direct invasion and destruction of vital organs (viral myocarditis, bulbar poliomyelitis, and tuberculosis of the adrenals); obstruction or ischemia of vital organs (cardiac tamponade from an acute pyogenic pericarditis) and acute systemic hypersensitivity reactions (rupture of an echinococcus cyst).

Regardless of the specific etiologic agent—organ–system localization or failure of localization of the infection, or predisposing noninfectious disease or therapy—the critical event in septic shock is stagnation of blood in the microcirculation. Capillary blood flow is preserved to the last in the brain and the heart. Although reduced flow is tolerated by some tissues, the lungs, liver, kidneys, digestive tract, and skin are vulnerable. In these sites particularly, as the microcirculation becomes inadequate, local tissue anoxia may be aggravated by metabolic acidosis (lactic, pyruvic) and a rising intracapillary pressure that causes the escape of liquid into the extravascular space. Anoxia, acidosis and edema are mutually self-perpetuating. If they are not reversed, death of tissues and extravasation of blood result.

TREATMENT

Although in the past the outcome of treatment of septic shock has been poor, there is reason to expect that prompt, constant attention to the patient will improve the results significantly. Initially, care must center on the cardiovascular needs of the patient. Although surveillance of the circulating blood volume and the cardiac output through serial measurements of the central venous pressure (CVP) and the pulmonary artery wedge pressure (PAW) is indubitably valuable, the physician should pay heed to two sensitive clinical indicators of the adequacy of tissue perfusion, namely, the mental status, and the urine flow. If blood pressure and cardiac output values are below normal but the patient is alert and oriented and is excreting urine, there is no shock. However, if the CVP and the PAW are too low and the clinical picture is confirmatory of shock, plasma, or alternatively, packed blood cells plus plasma plus platelets, as necessary, should be injected in 50- to 200-ml portions given over 10 minute periods. Measurement of the pressures after each dose, that is, at 10 minute intervals, will guard against overloads as the desired pressures are attained: a CVP of 10 cm to 15 cm of 0.9% NaCL solution, and a PAW of 14 to 18 mm Hg. If volume therapy is insufficient—low arterial pressure; poor perfusion of the brain (confusion, somnolence), kidneys (oliguria), and extremities (coldness, pallor)—dopamine should be given. In septic shock, doses of 20 μg/kg of body weight/min injected intravenously as a dilute solution (*e.g.,* 400–800 μg/ml in 5% glucose in lactated Ringer's solution) are generally adequate to ameliorate hypoperfusion. In some patients, larger doses may be necessary; however, increases in pulmonary vascular resistance, shunting, and cardiac arrythmias may sometimes occur when higher doses must be given for long periods. An alternative that may be useful in such patients consists of moderate doses of dopamine plus either dobutamine or low doses of 1-norepinephrine.

Next in primacy to cardiovascular function is the treatment of the infection. The detection and treatment of DIC should then occupy the physician.

Adequate surgical therapy is essential. There must be drainage of abscesses, debridement of infected sites of ischemic necrosis, excision of foci of anaerobic cellulitis, removal of the products of conception in septic abortions, and withdrawal of foreign bodies. Treatment with antimicrobics fails unless appropriate surgical measures are vigorously applied.

Usually, neither the exact etiology nor the susceptibility to microbial agents is known when therapy is begun. Clues enabling the selection of agents can often be derived from a knowledge of the site, or sites, of infection and the associated or predisposing conditions. The physician must remain alert to the possible need to alter the regimen of treatment as the results of cultures and susceptibility studies become available.

Potentially bactericidal agents with a high probability of effectiveness against the enteric gram-negative bacilli should virtually always be used because these bacteria are so frequently associated with septic shock. Gentamicin, tobramycin, or netilmicin should be given in a dose of 5 to 6 mg/kg body wt/day, IV, as three equal portions, 8-hourly, after a loading dose of 2 mg/kg body wt. Because these drugs depend on renal excretion for elimination from the body, and because patients with septic shock frequently have diminished urine formation, decision regarding dosage after the first 8 hours of treatment should be based on measurements of the concentrations of these drugs in the serum. As shock improves, renal function also improves, and serial measurements will be necessary for adjustment of the dose.

When it is probable that gram-positive bacteria are involved, different or additional antimicrobics are necessary. One of the penicillinase-resistant penicillins should be given intravenously. Nafcillin is virtually as active as penicillin G against *S. pneumoniae* and group A *Streptococcus pyogenes* and is excreted in the bile as well as the urine—thus, the hazard of toxicity is smaller if there is depressed renal function than it is with penicillin G or methicillin. Cephalothin is fully equivalent to the penicillinase-resistant penicillins; although there is relatively little hazard of toxicity with cephalotin, intravenous injection virtually always provokes a florid thrombophlebitis, and the drug is rapidly catabolized. Hence, cefazolin is preferable. With nafcillin, a loading dose of 50 mg/kg body wt (0.13 mEq Na^+/kg body wt) should be given IV in the first hour of treatment; a daily dose of 200 mg/kg body wt/day (0.46 mEq Na^+/kg body wt/day), IV, as six equal portions, 4-hourly, is adequate for maintenance. With cefazolin, the loading dose is 25 mg/kg given IV in the first hour of treatment; the maintenance dose is 100 mg/kg body wt/day, IV, as four equal portions, 6-hourly.

If nonsporulating anaerobes are likely to have caused the septic shock, chloramphenicol succinate should be used. The loading dose of 25 mg/kg body wt, given IV in the first hour of therapy, should be followed by 75 mg/kg body wt/day, IV, as four equal portions, 6-hourly. Chloramphenicol is effective against all bacteria of this group (Chap. 32, Necrotizing Pneumonias and Lung Abscesses); accordingly, it is the agent of choice despite the remote but definite possibility that it may cause bone marrow aplasia.

Clindamycin is a useful alternative to chloramphenicol, although it may cause colitis, and some strains of anaerobic cocci and *Clostridium* spp. are resistant to it. A loading dose of 10 mg/kg body wt, injected IV, should be followed by 20 to 25 mg/kg body wt/day, IV as four equal portions, 6-hourly.

Metronidazole is another alternative. Excepting the *Actinomyces* spp. and some strains of anaerobic cocci, it is generally active against anaerobic bacterial pathogens. Moreover, it penetrates into all body water. Since it is quantitatively absorbed from the gut, the IV and PO dosage is the same: if renal function is normal, 15 mg/kg body wt to load, followed by 7.5 mg/kg body wt 6-hourly (not to exceed a 4 g/day total dose).

Shock may complicate rickettsial infections and is also an indication for treatment with chloramphenicol (Chap. 96, Spotted Fevers) in the dosage previously given. The tetracyclines should not be used in patients with shock because life-threatening hepatotoxicity may result.

Malaria associated with shock has been treated with intravenously injected quinine. DIC is a not uncommon complication of malaria with shock (Chap. 145, Malaria).

Because glucosteroids are antagonistic to the inflammation of hypersensitivity reactions, their use in the treatment of septic shock has been rationalized in part on this basis. Additional salutary effects attributed to pharmacologic concentrations of glucosteroids include increased cardiac output (positive inotropism); decreased peripheral arteriolar resistance; and the potentiation of vasopressor amines. In experimental endotoxin shock in dogs, dexamethasone appeared to be the most effective glucosteriod. Even though shock in humans differs in many important ways from that induced with endotoxin in dogs, dexamethasone may cause less distortion of electrolyte balance than comparably antiphlogistic quantities of cortisol or other glucosteroids. The dosage of dexamethasone advocated for the treatment of septic shock is 3 mg/kg body wt initially, followed by 2 to 3 mg/kg body wt/day, all by IV injection. There is lack of agreement as to the value of giving such supraphysiologic quantities of glucosteroids in the treatment of septic shock; administration for 3 days neither improved nor worsened the outcome.

Renal

Proteinuria

In normal persons, small amounts of plasma proteins pass through the glomeruli. Because most of such filtered protein is reabsorbed in the proximal convoluted tubles, very little (less than 200 mg every 24 hours) appears in the urine. However, the reabsorptive capacity of the tubules is finite and apparently exceeds only slightly the maximum that is passed by normal glomeruli. Clearly, then, either an increase in glomerular permeability or a decrease in tubular reabsorptive capacity (or both) could lead to an abnormally high urinary concentration of protein.

Febrile proteinuria—the mild, transient proteinuria that occurs with fever of virtually any cause—is most likely the result of an increase in the amount of protein that passes through the glomerular membrane. That is, with the stress of fever, there is a nonspecific, transient increase in glomerular permeability to protein.

There are, however, infections associated with actual structural and functional changes in kidneys that may be permanent and may be manifested by proteinuria. Immunologic mechanisms are important in poststreptococcal (*S. pyogenes*) glomerulonephritis (Chap. 101, Streptococcal Skin Infections and Glomerulonephritis) and the nephritis of chronic streptococcal (*viridans* group *Streptococcus* spp.) endocarditis (Chap. 134, Infective Endocarditis)—a process apparently distinguishable from the focal glomerulonephritis secondary to renal lodgment of microemboli. Although hypersensitivity may also be important in the pathogenesis of renal involvement with syphilis and brucellosis, actual parasitization of the kidneys probably occurs in these diseases. In malaria complicated by black-water fever (Chap. 145, Malaria), massive hemolysis has usually occurred. DIC may be present, and there may be an element of hypersensitivity.

Glucosuria

Nonspecifically, presumably as a consequence of the stress of infection, there may be transient failure of tubular reabsorption of glucose. The glucosuria that results is not ordinarily intense in a previously normal person.

Azotemia

With many infections, particularly if they are severe and are the result of intracellular parasitism, the load of nitrogenous products of catabolism delivered to the kidneys is extraordinarily great. That is, there is prerenal azotemia. Ordinarily, the serum creatinine concentration is normal in such patients. Renal disease preexistent to the infection may be associated with hyperkalemia as well as azotemia: the serum creatine is usually elevated.

Oliguria

Hypotension, particularly if it devolves into shock, may result in diminished renal perfusion with blood. A decreased renal blood flow is manifested as a decrease in the output of urine and progressively severe azotemia.

Hepatic

Some degree of hepatic dysfunction occurs in many infectious diseases, even if the actual localization of the infectious agent is not in the liver. There may be no more than anorexia or loss of taste for cigarettes or coffee. In severe infection—for example, pneumococcal lobar pneumonia before the availability of specific antibacterial agents—jaundice was not uncommon and was regarded as ominous. More recently, staphylococcal and gram-negative bacillary infections have been most frequently associated with jaundice, now an uncommon manifestation of infection but still indicative of a poor prognosis. Intrahepatic cholestasis secondary to hepatocellular dysfunction is the usual finding. Morbid changes are few, often no more than Santee granules or the presence of a few giant cells.

Infections that cause massive hemolysis (malaria, bartonellosis, and gas gangrene) may also cause jaundice. The liver is so overloaded with heme pigments released intravascularly that jaundice results.

A number of infectious agents characteristically localize in the liver and damage it, either by parasitizing hepatic cells (hepatitis A, hepatitis B, non-A, non-B hepatitis, infectious mononucleosis, cytomegalovirus, and yellow fever); by creating space-occupying lesions (granulomas of tuberculosis, brucellosis, and schistosomiasis; syphilitic gummas; amebic abscesses; and echinococcal cysts); or by provoking cholangitis (clonorchiasis). Jaundice is usual and if persistent may cause itching. In addition, there will be abnormally high concentrations of the transaminases (glutamic-oxaloacetic and pyruvic-oxaloacetic) with acute hepatitis. Intrahepatic obstruction causes moderate elevation of serum alkaline phosphatase. Computed tomography and radio-nuclide scans are often of value in detecting space-occupying lesions of the liver. In prolonged and severe involvement of the liver, bleeding may result from the inadequate synthesis of prothrombin.

Brain

Manifestations of brain involvement can be arranged in a sequence of progressively serious import: anxiety, confusion, delirium, stupor, convulsions, and coma. The actual presence of the infectious agent in the tissues of the brain is not a prerequisite to the evocation of such manifestations. Thus, the nonspecific toxicity of an infection such as pneumoccocal pneumonia may include delirium. Convulsions are a classic complication of bacillary dysentery in young children. In general, the severity of manifestations of cerebral malfunction related to infections localized elsewhere is directly proportional to the severity of the infection. The mechanisms of mediation are often obscure. However in a few diseases a pathogenesis has been suggested: microemboli in infective endocarditis and sludging of a parasite-laden erythrocytes in the blood vessels of the brain in cerebral malaria.

Actual invasion of the brain by infectious agents that produce disease is, of course, manifested by varying degrees of cerebral dysfunction.

Bibliography

Books

BOGGS DR, WINKELSTEIN A: White Cell Manual, 3rd ed. Philadelphia, FA Davis, 1975. 75 pp.

KLUGER MJ: Fever. Princeton, NJ, Princeton University Press, 1979. 195 pp.

SCHWARTZ HR: Septic Abortion. Philadelphia, JB Lippincott, 1968. 153 pp.

WICHER K: C-reactive protein. In Rose NR, Friedman H (eds): Manual of Clinical Immunology, 2nd ed. Washington, DC. American Society for Microbiology, 1980. pp. 605–611.

WINTROBE MM, LEE GR, BOGGS DR, BITHELL TC, ATHENS JW, FOERSTER J: Clinical Hematology, 8th ed. Philadelphia, Lea & Febiger, 1981. 2021 pp.

WOOD WB: The pathogenesis of fever. In Mudd S (ed): Infectious Agents and Host Reactions. Philadelphia, WB Saunders, 1970. pp 146–162.

Journals

ASKENASE PW, ATWOOD JE: Basophils in tuberculin and "Jones –Mote" delayed reactions of humans. J Clin Invest 58:1145, 1976

BASS DA: Behavior of eosinophil leukocytes in acute inflammation. I. Lack of dependence on adrenal function. J Clin Invest 55:1229, 1975

BEISEL WR, SAWYER WD, RYLL ED, CROZIER D: Metabolic effects of intracellular infections in man. Ann Intern Med 67:744–779, 1967

BOGGS DR: The kinetics of neutrophilic leukocytes in health and in disease. Semin Hematol 4:359–385, 1967

BRAYTON RG, STOKES PE, SCHWARZ MS, LOURIA DB: Effect of alcohol and various diseases on leukocyte mobilization, phagocytosis and intracellular bacterial killing. N Engl J Med 282:123–128, 1970

CARTWRIGHT GE, LEE GR: The anemia of chronic disorders. Br J Haematol 1:147–152, 1971

CLINE MJ, LEHRER RI, TERRITO MC, GOLDE DW: Monocytes and macrophages: Functions and diseases. Ann Intern Med 88:78–88, 1978

EMERSON WA, ZIEVE PD, KREVANS JR: Hematologic changes in septicemia. Johns Hopkins Med J 126:69–76, 1970

FAHRLANDER H, HUBER F, GLOOR F: Intrahepatic retention of bile in severe bacterial infections. Gastroenterology 47:590–599, 1964

HARRISON TS, CHAWLA RC, WOJTALIK RS: Steroidal influence on catecholamines. N Engl J Med 279:136–143, 1968

JOYCE RA, BOGGS DR: Visualizing the marrow granulocyte reserve. J Lab Clin Med 93:101–110, 1979

KLASTERSKY J, CAPPEL R, DEBUSSCHER L: Effectiveness of betamethasone in management of severe infections. N Engl J Med 284:1248–1250, 1971

KLASTERSKY J, KASS EH: Is suppression of fever or hypothermia useful in experimental and clinical infectious diseases? J Infect Dis 121:81–86, 1970

MCGILL MW, PORTER PJ, KASS ED: The use of a bioassay for endotoxin in clinical infection. J Infect Dis 121:103–112, 1970

MEURET G: Disorders of mononuclear phagocyte sytem. Analytical review. Blut 34:317–328, 1977

MOLD C, NAKAYAMA S, HOLZER TJ, GEWURZ H, DUCLOS TW: C-reactive protective against *Streptococcus pneumoniae* infection in mice. J Exp Med 154:1703–1708, 1981

PETERSDORF RG, BENNETT IL JR: Factitious fever. Ann Intern Med 46:1039–1062, 1957

SPERO JA, LEWIS JH, HASIBA U: Disseminated intravascular coagulation: Findings in 346 patients. Thromb Haemost 43:28–33, 1980

TUMULTY PA: The patient with fever of undetermined origin: A diagnostic challenge. Johns Hopkins Med J 120:95–106, 1967

WEINSTEIN L, KLAINER AS: Management of emergencies. IV. Septic shock: Pathogenesis and treatment. N Engl J Med 274:950–953, 1966

ZUCKER–FRANKLIN D: Electron microscopic studies of human granulocytes: Structural variations related to function. Semin Hematol 5:109–132, 1968

W. CHRISTOPHER DUNCAN

Cutaneous Manifestations of Infectious Diseases

8

One of the most challenging and frequently rewarding problems in medicine is presented by the febrile patient with a rash. Although many illnesses of this kind are clearly not infectious in cause (*e.g.,* drug eruptions) or are viral in nature and not yet amenable to chemotherapy, others are caused by rickettsial, bacterial, or fungal agents for which specific treatment is available. The importance of the skin as an early mirror of systemic infections cannot be overemphasized. Delays in treatment of many infectious diseases may allow irreversible pathophysiologic changes to take place that may result in death despite the administration of large amounts of appropriate antimicrobics.

Lesions of the skin may result directly from inoculation; an example is anthrax (see Chap. 104, Anthrax). They may result indirectly by hematogenous spread (*e.g.,* meningococcemia; see Chap. 119, Acute Bacterial Meningitis), lymphogenous spread (suppurating lymph nodes in tularemia; see Chap. 139, Tularemia), or contiguous spread (see Chap. 100, Staphylococcal Skin Infections, and Chap 101, Streptococcal Skin Infections and Glomerulonephritis). A primary vascular basis of skin lesions may be accidental, as with lodged infected microemboli (see Chap. 134, Infective Endocarditis), or may reflect the key pathogenetic event, as the intraendothelial proliferation of rickettsias (see Chap. 96, Spotted Fevers, Chap. 97, Rickettsialpox, Chap. 98, The Typhus Fevers, and Chap. 99, Scrub Typhus). Thus, the rashes of infectious diseases may involve the epidermis as well as vascular and extravascular structures of the dermis.

The skin is capable of responding in only a limited number of ways. Although some lesions or rashes are unique to a particular pathogen, others are common to a number of etiologic agents.

Classification of skin lesions on a morphologic basis has proved to be the most practical and convenient approach for sorting out the large number of clinicopathologic manifestations and providing a means of communication. Thus, certain definitions are necessary. A *macule* is a circumscribed area of abnormal skin color without elevation or depression relative to the surrounding skin; a *papule* is a solid lesion, generally considered to be less than 1 cm in diameter, which is elevated above the plane of the surrounding skin; a *plaque* is an elevated lesion that occupies a relatively large surface area (greater than 1 cm in diameter) and is frequently formed by a confluence of papules; a *nodule* is a palpable, solid, round or ellipsoidal lesion which lies deeper in the skin than a papule, *i.e.,* in the dermis or subcutaneous tissue; a *vesicle* is a circumscribed, elevated lesion less than 0.5 cm in diameter that contains liquid; *ulcers* are lesions in which there has been destruction of the epidermis and upper papillary dermis.

Certain diagnostic procedures can be utilized to assist in the prompt diagnosis of rashes. A Tzanck smear can be made by scraping the base of a vesicle and staining with Giemsa's, Wright's, or Papanicolaou's stain to differentiate the herpes simplex (see Chap. 91, Infections Caused by *Herpes Simplex* Viruses) and herpes zoster-varicella (see Chap. 93, Varicella and Herpes Zoster) viruses from the poxviruses (see Chap. 92, Smallpox and Other Poxvirus Infections); only with the former group will multinucleated giant cells be seen. In the septicemias, Gram-stained smears of scrapings from early lesions will sometimes demonstrate the causative bacteria. The darkfield examination (see Chap. 9, Microscopic Examinations) will confirm the diagnosis of primary and secondary syphilis.

A cutaneous biopsy is easily and quickly obtained by using the cutaneous punch, and in most cases suturing will be unnecessary. Most pathology laboratories can prepare a hematoxylin and eosin or Gram-stained tissue specimen in 3 to 4 hours.

The more important cutaneous lesions of infectious origin are presented in Table 8-1.

Table 8-1. Cutaneous Manifestations of Infections and Infestations

Causative agent	Disease	Site	Specific characteristics
		MACULOPAPULAR RASHES	
Viruses			
Arboviruses (group A)	Various		Scarlatiniform maculopapules
Coxsackie, types A5, A10, A16	Multiple clinical pictures	Begin on face and neck; descent to trunk	Maculopapules, some vesicular or urticarial
EB (Epstein–Barr)	Infectious mononucleosis	Trunk	Evanescent macules, especially on trunk, may resemble measles; palatine enanthema
Echo, types 4, 6, 9, 11, 16, 18	Multiple clinical pictures	Face and trunk; may involve extremities	Maculopapules
Measles	Rubeola, "hard measles"	Upper lateral neck, hairline; then upper body, lower body, and distal extremities	Maculopapules, tending to blotchy confluence, palatine enanthema and Koplik's spots
Rubella	German measles	Frontal and retroauricular, then spreading over body and limbs	Evanescent pink macules, sometimes pinpoint, sometimes confluent
Presumed viral; not isolated	Exanthema subitum, roseola infantum	Trunk, extending to proximal arms and neck; prominent on buttocks	Discrete, small macules or maculopapules
Presumed viral; not isolated	Erythema infectiosum, fifth disease	Cheeks, then extensor surfaces of arms and thighs, buttocks	Red, confluent maculopapules, as butterfly erythema or "slapped cheek" appearance
Presumed viral; not isolated	Gianotti–Crosti syndrome	Face, neck, buttocks, limbs; can be seen on palms and soles, but spares trunk and mucous membrane	Rounded erythematous papules, often purpuric, but never confluent; hepatitis without jaundice in 95% of cases
Chlamydias			
Chlamydia psittaci	Psittacosis	Trunk	Faint macules; occasionally erythema nodosum or erythema multiforme
Rickettsias			
R. akari	Rickettsialpox	Initial papule at site of mite bite (often unnoticed); generalized	Initial papulovesicle becomes an eschar; later, generalized papules surmounted by small vesicles which heal in a few days
R. mooseri	Endemic, murine typhus	Axillae extending to trunk; sparse on extremities and face	Maculopapules
R. prowazekii	Epidemic typhus	Sides of trunk, spreads centrifugally but spares the palms, soles, and face	Pink macules about 5 mm diameter; during second week become deeply red and often purpuric
R. quintana	Trench fever	Trunk	Red macules
R. rickettsii	Rocky Mountain spotted fever	Distal extremities, moving centripetally to trunk, scalp, palms, and soles	Macules, then maculopapules, then petechiae
R. tsutsugamushi	Scrub typhus	Trunk; may extend to extremities	Red macules (ulcerated papulovesicle at site of inoculation)

(continued)

Table 8-1. (continued) *Cutaneous Manifestations of Infections and Infestations*

Causative agent	Disease	Site	Specific characteristics
Bacteria			
Erysipelothrix insidiosa	Erysipeloid	Fingers or hands	Reddish purple nodules at site of trauma, slowly extending in arciform configuration
Listeria monocytogenes	Listeriosis	Trunk and legs	Red macules that undergo central necrosis with formation of pustules
Salmonella spp.	Typhoid fever; salmonellosis	Abdomen, chest	Evanescent erythematous macules (rose spots); may yield *Salmonella* spp.
Streptococcus pyogenes (Group A)	Scarlet fever	Erythematous skin with accentuation in flexor creases	Pinhead sized red papules, imparting sandpaperlike texture to skin; circumoral pallor, also palatine petechiae (abacterial)
	Erythema marginatum (with acute rheumatic fever)	Trunk and extremities; occasionally proximal hands and face	Rapidly spreading, ringed eruption, sometimes with raised margins that coalesce into annular patterns; may be urticarial
	Erysipelas	Face, extremities	Bright red, edematous, (peau d'orange) tender plaque; extensions may have vesicles or bullae; portal of entry may not be evident
Staphylococcus aureus	Toxic shock syndrome	Trunk, extremities	Erythematous macular rash, sometimes resembling sunburn. May be scarlatiniform. Desquamation—peeling of palms and soles—in convalescence.
Mycobacterium leprae	Lepromatous leprosy	Widespread, symmetric; face, extremities, buttocks, but spares warmer parts of body	Shiny, ill-defined symmetric macules; diffuse infiltration; plaques and nodules; erythema nodosum
	Tuberculoid leprosy	Buttocks, posterolateral aspect of extremities, back, face	Hypopigmented, scaling macules with raised border; well-defined margins; anesthetic
Streptobacillus moniliformis	Rat-bite fever (streptobacillary)	Palms, soles, lower extremities	Discrete morbilliform maculopapules, petechiae, or purpuric eruption
Spirillum minus	Rat-bite fever (spirillary)	Trunk and extremities; frequently on palms and soles	Reddish purple macules
Treponema pallidum	Syphilis (secondary)	Generalized, including palms and soles	Scaly maculopapules, papules in anogenital area; painless mucosal erosions
Treponema carateum	Pinta	Exposed parts	Primary papule; secondary erythematous macules that become depigmented and hyperkeratotic

(continued)

Table 8-1. (continued) *Cutaneous Manifestations of Infections and Infestations*

Causative agent	Disease	Site	Specific characteristics
Fungi			
Pityrosporum orbiculare, Malassezia furfur	Tinea versicolor	Upper trunk (unusual below waist), neck, proximal upper extremities	Whitish or brown, "branny" scaling maculopapules
Dermatophytic fungi			
Trichophyton spp; *Microsporum* spp.; *Epidermophyton floccosum*	Tinea circinata, tinea capitis, tinea cruris, tinea pedis	Trunk, scalp, groin, feet	Erythematous macule becoming papular, annular, or confluent, scaling or vesiculated; pruritic; hair loss from scalp
Protozoa			
Plasmodium spp.	Malaria	Generalized	Urticarial rash in chronic malaria; conjunctival ecchymoses; generalized Addisonian hyperpigmentation
Toxoplasma gondii	Acquired toxoplasmosis	Generalized, but sparing palms and soles	Erythematous macules, purpura, and ecchymoses
Metazoa			
Trichinella spiralis	Trichinosis	Face, especially lids and conjunctiva, hands and feet	Urticaria most commonly; generalized maculopapular or petechial rash later
Necator americanus	Hookworm disease	Toes, toe clefts, and soles	Papules, papulovesicles, or bullae; ankles frequently swollen with an accompanying urticaria
Ancylostoma braziliensis and other hookworms; also *Strongyloides stercoralis*	Creeping eruption or cutaneous larva migrans	Exposed skin	Transient red papule, becoming erythematous zig-zag serpiginous lesion; may be one or many; very pruritic
Strongyloides stercoralis	Strongyloidiasis	Area of contact with ground	Evanescent blotchy red papules or urticaria; also a creeping eruption (larva currens)
Schistosoma spp.	Swimmer's itch	Parts of body exposed to infected water	Transient erythema followed by discrete pruritic papules, then vesiculation
Wuchereria bancrofti, Brugia malayi	Filariasis	Legs, scrotum; upper extremities, breasts	Erythema and edema over involved lymphatic vessels early; late urticaria, swellings similar to erythema nodosum
Onchocerca volvulus	Onchocerciasis	Back, buttocks, pelvis, thighs	Papules, eczematous rash with lichenification; depigmentation
Pediculus humanus	Body lice	Opposite seams in clothing, belt line, axillae	Pruritic red maculopapules
Phthirus pubis	Crabs	Pubic hair; rarely eyebrows or lashes	Pruritic, minute, red macules; bugs or nits on hair; red spots in underwear
Pulex irritans	Flea bites	Feet; exposed skin	Pruritic papules and urticaria; frequently central pustule (sterile)

(continued)

Table 8-1. **(continued)** *Cutaneous Manifestations of Infections and Infestations*

Causative agent	Disease	Site	Specific characteristics
Sarcoptes scabiei	Scabies	Sides of fingers, finger webs, wrists, elbows; genitalia in men, nipples in women	Threadlike burrows, erythematous papules, becoming vesiculated in folds, pruritic at night; folliculitis anterior thighs and buttocks (abacterial)
Trombicula irritans	Chigger bites; trombiculiasis	Lower extremities upward; concentration where clothing constricts	Pruritic papules which appear 18 to 24 hours after exposure
		VESICULAR OR BULLOUS	
Viruses			
Herpes simplex	Cold sores, gingivostomatitis, vulvovaginitis, balanitis, keratoconjunctivitis	Anywhere(!); sensory nerve involvement may occur, producing deep pain, *e.g.*, along sciatic nerve	Grouped vesicles on an erythematous plaque
Coxsackie A16; other group A coxsackie viruses	Hand-foot-and-mouth disease	Margins of palms and soles; dorsa of hands and feet; buttocks; lips and buccal mucosa	Vesicular lesions surrounded by red areola
Orf	Orf, ecthyma infectiosum (contagiosum)	Dorsal right index finger; other exposed sites	History of contact with infected sheep; papule becoming nodular with red center, white middle ring, and red halo (target stage); then develops crust
Varicella-zoster	Herpes zoster, shingles	Dermatomal distribution; unilateral	Painful vesicles from red papules
	Varicella, chickenpox	Trunk, proximal extremities; less prominent over neck, face, and distal extremities; mucous membranes of mouth and vulva	Pruritic maculopapules, vesicles, pustules; discrete, erupting in crops
Variola group	Smallpox, variola	Begins distal extremities, face; extends centripetally	Macules, papules, vesicles, pustules, crusts in sequence, single crop; umbilicated; all lesions in same stage of development
Vaccinia	Alastrim	Distal extremities; spreads centripetally	Similar to smallpox, but milder
	Vaccinia, cowpox	Inoculation site	Local papule, vesicle, pustule, crust; may spread, resembling smallpox or chickenpox
Bacteria			
Streptococcus pyogenes (group A) and/or *Staphylococcus aureus*	Impetigo	Extremities, face	Vesicles that become pustular, crusted; pruritic; bullous variety caused by *Staphylococcus aureus,* phage type 71
Staphylococcus aureus	Staphylococcal scalded skin syndrome	Periorofacial, neck, axillae, groin, generalized (successively). Mucosal involvement is rare.	Scarlatiniform; then large flaccid bullae Marked cutaneous tenderness

(continued)

Table 8-1. ***(continued)*** *Cutaneous Manifestations of Infections and Infestations*

Causative agent	Disease	Site	Specific characteristics
		PETECHIAL OR HEMORRHAGIC	
Viruses			
Arboviruses (group B) and tacaribe-lymphocytic choriomeningitis	Dengue; epidemic Argentinian and Bolivian hemorrhagic fever	Inner arms, upper chest, shoulders, neck and palate	Morbilliform becoming petechial; purpura may occur on extremities late
Rickettsiae			
Rickettsia prowazekii	Epidemic typhus	Sides of trunk, spreads centrifugally, but spares palms, soles, face	Macules becoming hemorrhagic during second week
Bacteria			
Bacillus anthracis	Anthrax, malignant pustule	Exposed skin; face, neck, hands, or arms	Papule, becoming bullous and then forming a central hemorrhagic, crusted ulcer surrounded by edema and vesicles; relatively slight regional node involvement
Neisseria meningitidis	Meningococcemia	Generalized	Maculopapules, petechiae, purpura, or ecchymoses; contain meningococci
Neisseria gonorrhoeae	Gonococcemia	Extremities, frequently over tender joints; fingers	Relatively few hemorrhagic pustules; difficult to culture *N. gonorrhoeae* from pustules
Yersinia pestis	Plague	Generalized	Macular erythema, petechiae, or ecchymoses; may contain *Y. pestis*
Streptococcus spp., other bacteria, fungi, rickettsiae	Infective endocarditis	Oropharynx, conjunctiva retina	Petechiae, splinter hemorrhages (abacterial); erythematous macules (Janeway spots); painful papules of fingers and toes (Osler nodes; may contain infectious agent)
Metazoa			
Cimex lectularius et hemipterus	Bedbug bite	Face, neck, hands, or arms	Bites often two or three in a line
Latrodectus mactans	Black widow spider bite	Buttocks, scrotum, hands, arms	Painful, swollen, and purpuric at site of bite; two red puncta may be seen
		PUSTULAR	
Viruses—see smallpox and chickenpox			
Bacteria			
Staphylococcus aureus	Furunculosis, boils	Face, neck, arms, wrists, fingers, buttocks, and anogenital area	Follicular inflammatory nodule, becoming pustular and then necrotic; tenderness is invariable
Propionibacterium acnes and *Staphylococcus epidermidis*	Acne	Face, upper back, chest	Inflammatory papules, pustules, and cysts

(continued)

Table 8-1. (continued) *Cutaneous Manifestations of Infections and Infestations*

Causative agent	Disease	Site	Specific characteristics
		ULCERATIVE	
Chlamydiae			
Lymphogranuloma venereum	Lymphogranuloma venereum	Penis, labia	Small, usually single ulceration; accompanying adenopathy
Bacteria			
Corynebacterium diphtheriae	Cutaneous or wound diphtheria	Extremities, face	Nonspecific, often impetigo or ecthymalike; in tropics, a shallow ulcer with firm border, with or without eschar
Calymmatobacterium granulomatis	Granuloma inguinale	External genitalia, pubis	Nodule which breaks down to form a painless ulcer with sharply defined overhanging edge
Francisella tularenis	Tularemia	Site of inoculation	Ulcerated nodule with prominent regional adenopathy
Haemophilus ducreyi	Chancroid	Genitalia: preputial orifice, frenulum; fourchette, inner labia minora	Sharply circumscribed, painful, shallow, ragged ulcer; removal of pus reveals vascular granulation tissue which bleeds easily
Treponema pallidum	Syphilis (primary chancre)	Genitalia, rectum, extragenital sites	Ulcer with indurated border and regional adenopathy
	Bejel	Oral mucous membranes; moist perigenital areas	Oral mucosal ulcerations; condylomata lata
Treponema pertenue	Yaws	Site of inoculation anywhere on body	Papule which ulcerates, giving rise to large ulcer with round papillomatous or vegetative surface
Mycobacterium kansasii		Site of inoculation; usually extremities	Granulomatous ulcer with lymphangitic or "sporotrichoid" proximal adenopathy
Mycobacterium marinum	Swimming-pool granuloma	Knees, elbows	Papule which ulcerates; becomes granulomatous; rarely "sporotrichoid"
Mycobacterium tuberculosis	Primary tuberculosis of skin	Site of inoculation	Papule or nodule that may ulcerate; accompanying regional adenopathy (primary complex)
Mycobacterium ulcerans	Buruli ulcer	Site of inoculation; usually arms or legs	Deep, destructive ulceration
Fungi			
Sporothrix schenckii	Sporotrichosis	Hands, arms, legs	Nodules at site of inoculation and along lymphatic vessels that may ulcerate
Candida albicans	Cutaneous candidosis moniliasis, thrush, vaginitis, paronychia	Intertriginous areas, mouth	Erythematous, exudative lesions of mucosa and skin; "satellite" pustules

(*continued*)

Table 8-1. (continued) *Cutaneous Manifestations of Infections and Infestations*

Causative agent	Disease	Site	Specific characteristics
Protozoa			
Leishmania braziliensis, Leishmania mexicana	American leishmaniasis, chiclero ulcer, espundia	Exposed skin	Red papule, ulcerates sometimes after vesiculation; on ears (chiclero ulcer), or advancing destructive mucocutaneous lesion of mouth and nose (espundia)
Metazoa			
Loxosceles spp.	Necrotic arachnidism, brown spider bite	Hands, arms, lower extremities	Painful; site of bite is white with red halo; vesiculates and becomes necrotic, leaving gaping ulcer (resembles "levarterenol slough")
		NODULAR	
Viruses			
Milker's nodule	Milker's nodules	Fingers, hands	Papules, becoming nodules
Molluscum contagiosum	Molluscum contagiosum	Exposed areas on children; pubic area and genitalia of adults	Flesh colored to pink, umbilicated papules
Bacteria *Streptococcus pyogenes* (rheumatic fever) *Mycobacterium tuberculosis* *Francisella tularensis* Fungi *Coccidioides immitis* *Histoplasma capsulatum*	Erythema nodosum	Shins, other extensor extremities	Tender, erythematous nodules
Bacteria			
Mycobacterium leprae	Erythema nodosum leprosum	Widely distributed, but predominant on extremities and face	Erythematous nodules or plaques 1 cm to 5 cm in diameter; occurs in patients with lepromatous leprosy; rarely in borderline
Mycobacterium tuberculosis	Lupus vulgaris	Head and neck; extremities; uncommon on trunk	Reddish brown, flat, soft plaque, some scaling may be present; enlarges slowly
Protozoa			
Leishmania tropica	Oriental sore	Face; other exposed parts	Furuncle-like nodule which ulcerates; red raised area around the ulcer enlarges for 2 to 3 months; heals, leaving a scar

Bibliography

Books

BRAVERMAN IM: Skin Signs of Systemic Disease. Philadelphia, W B Saunders, 1970

CONANT NF, SMITH DT, BAKER RD ET AL: Manual of Clinical Mycology, 3rd ed. Philadelphia, W B Saunders, 1971

FITZPATRICK TB, ARNDT KA, CLARK WA, EISEN AZ, VAN SCOTT ES., VAUGHAN JH (eds): Dermatology in General Medicine. New York, McGraw-Hill, 1971

ROOK A, WILKINSON DS, EBLING FJG: Textbook of Dermatology. Oxford, Blackwell Scientific Publications, 1972

Section | *II*

Laboratory Examinations

PAUL D. HOEPRICH
ARTHUR L. BARRY
MICHAEL G. RINALDI
CHARLES L. WISSEMAN
JEROLD H. THEIS
CHIEN LIU

9 *Microscopic Examinations*

It is the speed and ease with which useful information can be developed that makes microscopic examination of exudates (pus, sputum, swabbings, fibrin membranes), body liquids (urine, cerebrospinal fluid, serous fluid, synovial fluid, tissue juice), and tissues (blood, bone marrow, imprints, scrapings, snips) essential to the care of patients ill with infectious diseases. The powerful, potentially curative remedies available to the physician are often sharply limited in effectiveness to specific groups of parasites; etiologic diagnosis is essential. However, the course of many infectious diseases may be dismayingly rapid, and antimicrobial therapy cannot be delayed until culture and susceptibility studies are completed or rising titer serodiagnosis is possible. Prompt microscopic examination of carefully collected specimens that originated in or were associated with the infectious process is often the adjunct to the history and physical examination that enables the informed choice of antimicrobics for therapy.

Gram's Stain

Almost 90 years ago, Dr. Hans Christian Gram described a staining method that enabled him to distinguish bacteria in sections of mammalian tissues. With other staining methods, bacteria were difficult to see because they took on the same color as the cells, debris, and fibrin in the tissue sections. Gram treated sections with aniline–gentian violet, followed by an iodine–potassium iodide solution, and then decolorized with alcohol (ethanol) in order to remove the dye from the tissue cells, debris, and fibrin without decolorizing the bacterial cells. It was later shown that with Gram's staining method some bacteria characteristically retained the blue color (gram-positive) whereas other bacteria were consistently decolorized by the alcohol treatment (gram-negative). Over the years, Gram's staining technique has undergone innumerable modifications, and the variety of methods now in use are all classed under the generic name *Gram stain*.

The quality and purity of the stains available has greatly improved, and crystal violet (a specific chemical compound, hexamethylpararosanilin) is now generally used as the primary stain. Because crystal violet is a basic compound, nonionic diffusion into cells is favored by an alkaline milieu. Thus, in an acid environment, as is commonly encountered in many clinical specimens, gram-positive bacteria tend to lose their gram-positive quality. For this reason, the crystal violet solution must be alkaline for reliable staining. However, alkaline solutions of crystal violet are relatively unstable; hence, alkalinization is best accomplished at the time of staining, commonly by the addition of sodium bicarbonate solution.

The iodine–potassium iodide solution is also relatively unstable (exposure to heat and light favor reduction of iodine to iodide—the solution becomes less intensely brown to colorless). This is important because it is the iodine that is crucial to the Gram stain. Iodine forms a complex with crystal violet inside cells. The complex is somewhat soluble in ethanol and the ease of removal of the complex with ethanol is a reflection of fundamental structural differences between gram-negative and gram-positive cells (see Chap. 1, Attributes of Infectious Agents). Cells are gram-negative if the cell wall is permeable to the "solubilized" complex, whereas cells are gram-positive if the cell wall is impermeable.

Removal of the iodine–crystal violet complex is termed *decolorization;* it can be accomplished by flooding with ethanol, a mixture of ethanol and acetone, or with acetone. By itself, acetone acts very rapidly, and gram-positive bacteria are too easily decolorized. Ethanol alone acts more slowly, and gram-negative bacteria may not be decolorized completely. Accordingly, a 1:1 (V/V) mixture of ethanol–acetone is a reasonable compromise.

Safranin is most commonly used as the final "counterstain." Cells from which the iodine–crystal violet complex was leached by the ethanol–acetone take up safranin and are stained pink.

Method

The best method for performing a Gram stain depends somewhat on the microorganisms to be stained, the matrix in which they are suspended, and the personal prejudices of the investigator carrying out the stain. The following method has proved to be a practical, reliable technique for staining most clinical specimens.

Procedure

1. Prepare a thin, uniform smear on a clean glass slide and allow it to dry in air without heating. Swabs should be rolled with firm pressure over a small area on the slide. With liquids such as urine or cerebrospinal fluid, 1 drop should be placed in the center of the slide and allowed to dry without being spread. Thick, purulent material, such as sputum, must be spread evenly, avoiding excessively thick areas.
2. Pass the bottom of the dried slide through a gas flame several times in order to kill the bacteria and fix them to the slide.
3. Flood the slide with crystal violet solution; immediately add 2 to 3 drops of the sodium bicarbonate solution and mix by tilting or blowing on the slide. Let it stand 30 to 60 seconds.
4. Tilt the slide to decant the stain, and flush off the crystal violet with iodine. Flood the slide with iodine, and let it stand 30 to 60 seconds.
5. Decolorization is the most critical step of the whole procedure. Tilt the slide to spill the iodine solution, and run acetone-alcohol solution over the slide, held at a long axis tilt of about 15°, until no further blue color comes from the thin portions of the smear. Do not try to decolorize the thick parts of the smear because this only results in overdecolorizing the thin areas, which are the only areas that can be examined satisfactorily.
6. Immediately wash the slide under gently running, cool tap water to remove the acetone-alcohol, stopping the decolorizing process.
7. Flood the slide with safranin; let it stand 15 to 30 seconds and then gently wash with tap water.
8. Wipe the back of the slide to remove any excess stain; set aside to dry *without* blotting the smear.

Reagents

1. Crystal violet solution
   - **a.** Stock crystal violet solution
     - crystal violet 5 g
     - 95% ethanol 100 ml
   - **b.** Working crystal violet solution
     - stock crystal violet 20 ml
     - distilled water 80 ml
2. Sodium bicarbonate solution
   - $NaHCO_3$ 5 g
   - thimerosal (1 : 1000) 10 ml
   - distilled water 90 ml
3. Iodine solution
   - Iodine crystals 2 g
   - 1N NaOH 10 ml
   - distilled water q.s. ad. 100 ml
4. Acetone-alcohol
   - Equal parts, acetone and 95% ethanol
5. Safranin
   - **a.** Stock safranin solution
     - safranin O 2.5 g
     - 95% ethanol 100 ml
   - **b.** Working safranin solution
     - stock safranin 10 ml
     - distilled water 80 ml

Limitations

The timing of each step is not critical and can vary from a few seconds to 5 minutes. Actually, the reagents can be applied in sequence essentially as rapidly as the manipulations of staining permit. Decolorization is the most critical step. The tendency is to overdecolorize so that gram-positive bacteria appear to be gram-negative. The acetone-alcohol should be allowed to run over the slide until blue color does not run from thin areas. The slide should then be rinsed in running water to remove the decolorizing reagent. Once the slide is stained, it should be allowed to dry in air before it is examined; in an emergency, it can be blotted dry with absorbent paper. *Even very gentle blotting removes some of the smeared specimen from the stained slide.*

Applications

Virtually all clinical specimens should be examined microscopically to evaluate the proportion of different microorganisms and the kinds of cellular elements that are present. Gram's method is the most appropriate staining procedure for such smears. If properly stained, the cellular elements will be light pink to red (all mammalian cells are gram-negative), and the bacteria will be stained either dark blue (gram-positive) or red (gram-negative). If fungi are present, they will invariably be gram-positive. Some gram-positive bacteria tend to lose their ability to retain the blue color much more readily than others, especially in clinical specimens and old cultures on aritificial mediums. Although gram-positive bacteria sometimes appear to be gram-negative, the reverse should never occur. In clinical specimens there are frequently many artifacts that closely resemble bacteria and can easily mislead the inexperienced observer. See Figures 31-5, 32-1, and 52-4.

Acid-Fast Staining

Both infectious agents and host cells will be permeated by basic fuchsin (rosanilin and pararosanilin, respectively: triaminodiphenyltolylcarbinol and triaminotriphenylcarbinol) when heated for a time while exposed to the dye in the presence of phenol. However, *Mycobacterium* spp., some *Nocardia* spp., hair, certain lipofuscin pigments, and some waxes will retain the dye despite exposure to solutions of strong mineral acids (*i.e.,* they are acid fast). The property of acid fastness is apparently conferred by certain lipids, which are unusual both in kind and abundance, (*e.g.,* the unsaponifiable wax fraction of *Mycobacterium* spp.). Among acid-fast bacteria there is a descending order of retentivity of basic fuchsin: *Mycobacterium tuberculosis,* other pathogenic *Mycobacterium* spp., saprophytic *Mycobacterium* spp., *Nocardia* spp.

The classic acid-fast staining procedure is the Ziehl–Neelsen method. It is applicable to rapid, microscopic diagnosis and is reliable even when used only occasionally. Although fluorescent staining of *Mycobacterium* spp. with the fluorochrome dyes rhodamine and auramine enables more rapid detection of acid-fast bacilli, this method is too difficult and time consuming for use in any setting but a clinical laboratory processing large numbers of specimens. Other proved but less-often-used methods include Kinyoun's stain and blue-light fluorescence.

With the Ziehl–Neelsen method, *Mycobacterium* spp. are distinctly red bacilli, 1.0 μm to 5.0 μm long by 0.3 μm to 0.6 μm wide. Uneven staining, either with polar granules or distributed granules to give a beaded appearance, is common with *M. tuberculosis,* whereas other *Mycobacterium* spp. tend to take up the stain more evenly. Uneven staining is quite common with *Nocardia* spp. Other microorganisms, leukocytes, and debris stain blue.

Method

PROCEDURE FOR *MYCOBACTERIUM* SPP.

1. Fix smears either by gentle heating over a gas flame or on an electric slide warmer (2 hours at 65°C).
2. Place a piece of filter paper cut to the size of the smear on each slide.
3. Flood slides with basic carbol fuchsin solution and heat to steaming; heat intermittently to maintain steaming for 5 minutes, adding carbol fuchsin as needed.
4. Remove the filter paper strips and wash the slides in tap water.
5. Decolorize with acid-alcohol until no more color appears in the washings.
6. Wash with tap water.
7. Counterstain with aqueous methylene blue for 30 seconds.
8. Wash with tap water and dry in air or over gentle heat.

PROCEDURE FOR *NOCARDIA* SPP.

1. The only change from the procedure for *Mycobacterium* spp. is the use of aqueous HCl instead of acid-alcohol solution for decolorization. Strains of *Nocardia* spp. that are acid-fast are weakly resistant to decolorization relative to *M. tuberculosis.*

REAGENTS FOR ZIEHL–NEELSEN STAIN

1. Basic carbol fuchsin solution
   Dissolve 3.0 g of basic fuchsin in 100 ml of 95% ethyl alcohol.
   Add 10 ml of this solution to 90 ml of 5% aqueous phenol.

2a. Acid-alcohol (for use with *Mycobacterium* spp.)
   Add 3.0 ml of concentrated HCl to 97 ml of 95% ethanol.

2b. Aqueous HCl (for use with *Nocardia* spp.)
   Add 3.0 ml of concentrated HCl to 97 ml of distilled water.

3. Methylene Blue
   Dissolve 0.3 gm of methylene blue in 100 ml of distilled water.

Limitations

Because smears must be examined using the oil-immersion objective, only a limited area of a slide can be observed in the usual 20 to 30 minutes/slide inspection; it is not uncommon for the microscopist to miss rare acid-fast bacilli. On the other hand, detection of just 1 or 2 acid-fast bacilli after diligent search calls for verification by examination of a second smear.

Concentrates of either gastric aspirates or feces from adults should not be examined microscopically because of the high frequency of ingestion of acid-fast bacilli in foods. However, the examination of such specimens is worthwhile in newborn and neonatal infants.

Colorblind persons may find picric acid a more useful counterstain than methylene blue for differentiating acid-fast microorganisms.

Applications

Choice portions (*e.g.*, purulent flecks) of any clinical specimen that is suspected of containing either *Mycobacterium* spp. or *Nocardia* spp. should be smeared on slides for staining. Concentration of specimens by centrifuging liquids (*e.g.*, cerebrospinal fluid) and digesting exudates (*e.g.*, sputum) is often helpful.

Staining Methods for Fungi

The microscopic examination of tissues, secretions, or other clinical specimens for fungi requires the use of direct mounts of unfixed specimens and stained sections of tissues. Direct mounts may be treated with 10% potassium hydroxide (KOH), lactophenol cotton blue (LPCB), Gram stain, nigrosin stain, India ink, periodic acid-Schiff stain (PAS), and Giemsa stain. Fixed tissue sections are usefully stained with hematoxylin and eosin (H and E), Gomori's methenamine silver stain (GMS), Gridley's fungus stain, Mayer's mucicarmine stain, and Masson–Fontana stain.

Methods

DIRECT MOUNTING PROCEDURES

1. Potassium hydroxide. A 10% KOH preparation is used to clear clinical material of mammalian cells and nonmycotic debris so that fungi can be seen more readily. An equal volume of permanent blue–black fountain pen ink may be added to the KOH solution to stain fungal cell walls (blue). Dimethyl sulfoxide (DMSO) may be added to the KOH (40% V/V) to aid the clearing of nail tissues and thick skin scrapings.
   a. A drop of 10% KOH is placed on a clean, microscope slide.
   b. Tissue fragments, sputum, pus, scrapings, or other clinical materials are placed in the KOH and teased apart.
   c. A glass coverslip is placed over the clinical specimen and the preparation is allowed to clear at room temperature. To speed the clearing process and expel air bubbles; the slide may be passed through a flame.
   d. Observe the specimen while wet, reducing the light intensity if a bright-field microscope is used. Alternatively, phase-contrast microscopy may be used.
   e. The clearing action of KOH continues and eventually even fungi are completely destroyed.
2. Lactophenol cotton blue.
   a. A drop of LPCB is placed on a clean, microscope slide and the clinical material is placed in the stain.
   b. A coverslip is placed over the specimen and pressed down firmly to eliminate air bubbles.
   c. The specimen is examined, looking for blue-stained fungi.
3. Gram stain. The treatment of specimens and the staining procedure are exactly the same for fungi as for bacteria. All fungi are gram-positive.
4. Nigrosin stain. The capsules of yeastlike fungi (some species of the genera *Candida* Berkhout, 1923; *Cryptococcus* Kützing emend. Phaff and Spencer, 1969; *Rhodotorula* Harrison, 1927; *Torulopsis* Berlese, 1894; and *Trichosporon* Behrend, 1890) are detectable, without the artifactual interference that may obfuscate the use of India ink, by using nigrosin as a relief stain that provides a homogeneous background. Confusing precipitates and particulates are avoided, as are errors from the haloing of leukocytes sometimes seen in India ink preparations—attributed to repulsion of the colloidal carbon particles by the leukocytes.
   a. Place a loopful of nigrosin stain 3 mm in diameter on a clean slide.
   b. Add and mix a 3-mm-diameter loopful of the specimen to be examined—the suspended "sediment" collected by centrifugation of CSF, or a touch pickup from a yeastlike colony.
   c. Cover with a coverslip, reduce the intensity of the light, and examine the preparation (45 × objective) for the presence or lack of encapsulated yeast forms.
5. India ink. The capsules of certain yeast-fungi may also be demonstrated using India ink. Neither the fungal cell nor its capsule are stained; the ink provides a dark background (colloidal suspension of carbon particles), which reveals the transparent capsules by contrast.

   a. Make certain there are no artifacts or other agglutinating particles in the ink by examining a simultaneously prepared control.
   b. Place a 3-mm loopful of India ink on a clean microscope slide.
   c. Add to the ink a 3-mm loopful of the clinical specimen (sediment collected by centrifugation if CSF) or a small portion of the yeast colony to be examined.
   d. Cover with a coverslip, reduce the intensity of the light of the microscope, and examine the preparation for the presence or lack of capsules and the size and the shape of the yeast cells.

6. Periodic acid-Schiff stain. When KOH preparations fail to demonstrate fungi, the PAS technique should be used because it offers increased sensitivity.
   a. For dermatologic specimens, spread a very light film of albumin fixative on a clean microscope slide using a clean finger. For other specimens, prepare a smear as usual and allow it to air dry.
   b. Using a teasing needle, work fragments of the clinical specimen into the film of albumin.
   d. The slide is placed on a warmer for 2 to 3 hours (drying time may be reduced by passing the slide through a flame, but overheating must be avoided).
   d. Staining procedure:
   slide → absolute ethanol, 1 minute → drain, place in periodic acid, 5 minutes → wash in running water, 2 minutes → basic fuchsin, 2 minutes → wash in running water, 5 minutes → dehydrate, 70%, 80%, 95%, 100% ethanol, 2-minute intervals → xylene, 2 minutes → mount with Permount → examine by bright field microscopy; fungi are stained a pink purplish red.

7. Giemsa stain. This technique is used to demonstrate the parasitic form (yeast cells) of *Histoplasma capsulatum* Darling, 1906 variety *capsulatum* Kwon–Chung, 1975 inside cells. The intracellular organisms stain light to dark blue and are surrounded by a halo of transparency, which is a staining artifact and not a capsule.
   a. Smear clinical material onto a clean slide and fix by gentle heating.
   b. Staining procedure:
   slide → 100% methanol, 1 minute → drain, air-dry → 10–15 drops of Giemsa stain, 1 minute → cover stain with 1.5 ml of distilled, buffered (pH 6.8) water, 5 minutes → wash, distilled water, air-dry → examine by bright-field microscopy; fungi stain dark blue.

Tissue Stains Procedures

Directions for the preparation of tissue sections and the particulars of staining methods are readily available in manuals and are not considered here. Examination of stained tissues sections is often the most valuable, and sometimes the only method available for the detection and presumptive identification of mycotic agents. Sections cut from frozen tissues, as well as those obtained by biopsy or at autopsy, are suitable.

1. Hematoxylin and eosin. Many fungi can be seen with hematoxylin and eosin (H and E); however, some are not stained at all, and others are stained poorly or not at all unless the fungi were viable at the time of fixation. A major benefit of the H and E stain is the demonstration of histopathology, which may provide important clues leading to the eventual detection of a fungus.

2. Gomori's methenamine silver nitrate stain. An excellent stain for screening purposes, this method is widely used and is recommended for all mycotic agents. Fungi are stained brown–black.

3. Gridley's fungus stain. Fungi, mucin, and elastic tissue (and little else) are stained purplish red on a yellow background. It is a very useful method for screening tissues suspected of containing fungi.

4. Mayer's mucicarmine stain. Because the heteroacidic mucopolysaccharide capsular material of *Cryptococcus* spp. stains deep rose to red, the nuclei stain black, and the background is yellow, this stain is very useful for differentiating cryptococci from other fungi of similar size and appearance.

5. Masson–Fontana stain. A staining technique utilized mainly for the detection of melanin, this stain has now been found to be almost specific for cryptococcal pathogens. Cryptococci stain dark brown–black and the background is pink. No other fungal pathogens (either systemic or opportunistic) are stained with this method.

Reagents

1. Potassium hydroxide
   a. 10% KOH

Potassium hydroxide	10.0 g
Distilled water q.s. ad	100.0 ml

   Mix; keep the mixing vessel cool while the KOH dissolves.

b. 10% KOH plus DMSO

Potassium hydroxide	10.0 g
Dimethyl sulfoxide	40.0 ml
Distilled water	60.0 ml

Mix the DMSO and the distilled water in a chemical fume hood. Add the KOH and cool while it is dissolving.

2. Lactophenol cotton blue

Phenol, concentrated	20.0 ml
Lactic acid	20.0 ml
Glycerol	40.0 ml
Cotton blue	0.05 g
Distilled water	20.0 ml

Dissolve the cotton blue in the distilled water; add the phenol, lactic acid, and glycerol.

3. Gram stain. See previous section in this chapter.
4. Nigrosin stain

Nigrosin powder	10 g
Formalin (10% HCHO V/V in distilled water) buffered by the addition of sufficient sodium acetate to bring the pH to 7.5	100 ml

Heat in boiling water bath for 30 minutes with occasional swirling. Restore volume to 100 ml with buffered formalin; mix. Filter twice through double-thickness filter paper.

5. India ink

India ink (*e.g.,* Parker 51)	15.0 ml
Thimerosal, aqueous, 1 : 1000	3.0 ml
Tween 80, aqueous, 1 : 1000	0.1 ml

Mix and filter.

6. Tissue stains. Reagents and procedures used in tissue staining for fungi are described in the references listed at the end of this chapter.

Limitations

As with all infectious diseases, microscopic examinations for fungi should be, whenever possible, corroborated by specific and definitive cultural studies. Interpretatons of microscopic examinations must always be carried out cautiously and critically because many artificts may be confused with fungi. Many kinds of pathogenic fungi have a similar appearance in direct mounts of clinical specimens. Care must be taken not to confuse two different pathogenic agents, or a pathogenic with a saprobic fungus. It may be very difficult, or impossible, to identify a specific fungus in tissues (*e.g.,* moniliaceous). Septate hyphae in a skin scraping only affirm the presence of a fungus; the organism is not identified and it is not categorized as an etiologic agent or a saprobe. Two different fungi may look identical in tissue specimens viewed microscopically—this is particularly true with the ever-increasing number and kinds of fungi capable of inciting opportunistic infections in humans.

When tissue sections stained for fungi are examined, the preceding admonitions remain in force. Also, a single etiologic agent can evoke a wide range of tissue reactions, and many dissimilar fungi can cause similar tissue responses; a specific etiologic diagnosis cannot be made unless a fungus is actually identified in tissues.

All specimens should be examined promptly after collection, and all procedures should be done according to the directions outlined. The use of microscopic examinations in clinical mycology can offer rewarding results when the techniques are carried out properly and as experience is gained.

Applications

Pus, exudates, blood, bone marrow, cerebrospinal fluid, other body fluids, hair, nails, skin scrapings, sputum, tissues, and urine may be examined microscopically either by direct wet mounts or tissue sections stained for the presence of fungi.

These techniques have greatly stimulated the interest and enthusiasm of the clinician and the laboratorian in searching for etiologic agents.

Giménez Stain

The Giménez modification of the Macchiavello method has replaced the latter in most laboratories for staining rickettsias because of greater reliability and reproducibility if carried out meticulously according to directions on *thin* smears. Using the Giménez method A, all rickettsias, except *Rickettsia tsutsugamushi,* stain red. *Rickettsia tsutsugamushi* may be stained a red black with Giménez method B, which uses a different mordanting and destaining procedure. It is important that smears are thin and that heat fixation is gentle.

Methods

METHOD A—PROCEDURE FOR ALL RICKETTSIAS EXCEPT *RICKETTSIA TSUTSUGAMUSHI*

1. Air dry a thin smear.
2. *Gently* heat-fix the back of slide.
3. Filter dilute carbol basic fuchsin onto slide; let stand 1–2 minutes.
4. Gently wash *back* of slide with tap water.

5. Apply aqueous malachite green (0.8%) for 6–9 seconds
6. Gently wash with tap water.
7. Reapply malachite green for 7 seconds or as needed with some types of smear, as judged by microscopic examination (low to high power) of the washed wet smear.
8. Gently wash with tap water.
9. Air dry.

METHOD B—PROCEDURE FOR *RICKETTSIA TSUTSUGAMUSHI*

1. Air dry thin smear.
2. *Gently* heat fix back of slide.
3. Filter dilute carbol basic fuchsin onto slide; let stand 3 minutes.
4. Gently wash back of slide with tap water.
5. Apply 4–6 drops of 4% ferric nitrate solution. Wash off immediately and thoroughly with tap water.
6. Apply 0.5% fast green for 15–30 seconds.
7. Gently wash with tap water.
8. Air dry.

REAGENTS

1. Carbol basic fuchsin
   a. For 10% basic fuchsin, measure into graduated cylinder 10 g dry basic fuchsin. Dilute to 100 ml with 95% ethyl alcohol. Basic fuchsin must have at least 95% total dye content. Smaller amounts do not stain. It may be necessary to test several different lots of basic fuchsin before one is found that gives good results. Some lots of basic fuchsin manufactured by the national Aniline Division, Allied Chemical Co., have been suitable.
   b. For 4% aqueous phenol, melt phenol crystals (ACS) in 56°C water bath. Add 10 ml of the liquefied 100% phenol to 240 ml distilled water.
   c. Stock solution of carbol basic fuchsin
      100 ml 10% basic fuchsin
      250 ml 4% phenol
      650 ml distilled water
      Place at 37°C for 48 hours before use. The solution may be stored at least 10 months at room temperature without losing its staining properties.
   d. Dilute working solution of carbol basic fuchsin (made fresh daily)
      4 ml stock carbol basic fuchsin
      10 ml dilute buffer (made daily)
2. Buffers
   a. Stock buffer solutions
      0.2 M NaH_2PO_4
      24.0 g diluted to 1000 ml with distilled water
      (27.6 g $NaH_2PO_4 \cdot H_2O$)
      0.2 M Na_2HPO_4
      28.40 g diluted to 100 ml with distilled water.
   b. Dilute working buffer solutions
      pH 7.45—made fresh daily

3.5 ml	0.2 M NaH_2PO_4
15.5 ml	0.2 M Na_2HPO_4
19 ml	distilled water
38 ml	Total

3. Aqueous malachite green oxalate (0.8%)
   0.8 g malachite green oxalate in 100 ml distilled water.
4. Aqueous ferric nitrate (4%)
   4 g $Fe(NO_3)_3 \cdot 9H_2O$ in 100 ml distilled water.
5. Aqueous fast green (0.5%)
   0.5 g fast green in 100 ml distilled water

Limitations

The constitution of the reagents and the staining procedure must be carried out exactly as described. The method gives good results only with very thin smears. Well-separated infected cells stain satisfactorily but, as in slide cultures, even confluent monolayers pose some problems of destaining and differentiation; thicker areas of smears are impossible to stain adequately. Method B may give satisfactory results with *R. tsutsugamushi,* but the results are sometimes variable. With some materials, it may be necessary to resort to the Giemsa stain, especially for intracellular organisms.

Applications

The Giménez stain can be applied to any tissue suspected of harboring rickettsias—yolk sac smears, exudates, tissue cultures (see above), impression smears of tissues, organs or biopsy specimens but not sections—always provided the smear is thin. A properly stained *thin* smear shows brightly stained red rickettsias against a green background of cell debris (as in yolk sac smears) or host cell cytoplasm. Improperly destained yolk sac smears may show confusing small particles. Thicker specimens may retain varying degrees of basic fuchsin so that the counterstained background may range from blue to reddish (unsatisfactory). Cytoplasmic granules in human polymorphonuclear leukocytes, but not in murine neutrophils, tend to retain the red basic fuchsin stain and may cause confusion.

The Giménez stain is also suitable for *Chlamydia* spp. However, some investigators prefer a modified Macchiavello method.

Macchiavello Stain (Modified)

With slight modification, the Macchiavello stain is quite satisfactory for *Chlamydia* spp. A major requirement to achieving a useful preparation is a thin smear of the test material on a slide.

Method

PROCEDURE

1. Air dry *thin* smear.
2. Fix with 70% ethyl alcohol for 1 minute; dry.
3. *Filter* 0.5% basic fuchsin onto smear and leave for 5 minutes.
4. Rinse in lukewarm tap water.
5. Decolorize in dilute citric acid a few seconds.
6. Rinse with lukewarm tap water.
7. Apply aqueous methylene blue (1%) 1–2 seconds.
8. Rinse with lukewarm water.
9. Air dry.

Length of staining and decolorization time may be varied according to the type of material on the smear.

REAGENTS

1. **Basic Fuschsin.** Stock Basic Fuchsin (5%): finely grind 5 g basic fuchsin powder in a mortar, and dissolve in 100 ml 95% ethanol. The basic fuchsin powder must have at least 95% total dye content. (The product of National Aniline Division, Allied Chemical Co. is suitable.)
   Dilute 0.5% Basic Fuchsin (for staining): dilute 5% stock basic fuchsin 1 : 10 with distilled water.
   Make up fresh after 48 hours.
2. **Aqueous Methylene Blue (1%).** Dissolve 1 g methylene blue powder in 100 ml distilled water.
3. **Citric Acid.** Stock Citric Acid (50%): dissolve 50 g citric acid in 100 ml distilled water.
   Dilute Citric Acid: dilute 2–3 drops of stock 50% citric acid to 50 ml with lukewarm tap water in a Coplin jar.

Limitations

The reagents must be made up as specified and used as described. Fixation of smears with 70% ethanol is particularly important. Smears of blood or of sputum are so rarely productive that staining for *Chlamydia* spp. is not recommended.

Applications

The elementary bodies of *Chlamydia* spp. stain a deep red. They are 280 nm to 450 nm in diameter and are located in the cytoplasm of infected cells. Impression smears of infected tissues (biopsy specimens of lung, liver, spleen, esthiomene) are suitable, as are exudates. Yolk sac and tissue culture cells are also appropriate specimens.

Romanowsky-Type Staining For Microorganisms

The use of methylene blue and eosin to stain blood cells dates back to the early 1890s and the work of the Russian protozoologist D. L. Romanowsky. Subsequently, several other workers used these same dyes to develop techniques still applied in laboratories all over the world as stains bearing the originator's name—Giemsa, Leishman, and Wright stains. All of these stains are combinations of eosin, methylene blue (tetramethylthionine), azure B (trimethylthionine), and azure A (dimethylthionine). When dissolved in water, all components form positively charged, basic dye ions that combine with negatively charged nucleic acids. The azure B and A components are metachromatic stains, and azure B in particular plays an important part in providing the reddish to purple staining effect seen in protozoan and leukocyte nuclei, respectively. At the same time, methylene blue reacts well with RNA, giving a blue color to the cytoplasm of protozoa, lymphocytes, and monocytes. Eosin imparts a pink color to the granules of eosinophilic leukocytes and the cytoplasm of erythrocytes. In addition, eosin adds a reddish color to protozoan nuclei. Thus, the full Romanowsky effect is obtained through the combined action of all the component dyes.

Of the many Romanowsky-type stains available, Giemsa and Wright stains have been chosen for detailed presentation. They are widely used and are quite satisfactory for staining blood smears, impression smears, and tissue sections.

Smears

METHODS

PREPARATION OF SMEARS

1. Thin blood films
   a. Mix blood samples in ethylenediaminetetraacetic acid (EDTA) anticoagulant thoroughly as soon as drawn.
   b. Transfer a small drop of well-mixed blood to the center of a 22-mm square, No. $1\frac{1}{2}$ thickness coverslip, previously dusted by a few

strokes with a No. 6 camel hair brush. The drop that forms when a vertically held, thin, wooden applicator stick is dipped into the blood sample is the correct amount to make a thin smear.

c. Another dusted coverslip of the same dimensions is then placed over the second compressing the blood drop. The edges of the second coverslip should be oriented *before* being placed on the drop so that the sides of the lower coverslips are brought into apposition, the blood between them spreads out toward the edges. Just before the spreading ceases, the two coverslips are pulled across each other with rapid, wrist action to produce two thin smears on the opposing surfaces.

d. The blood films may be allowed to dry at ambient temperature, or are quickly heat dried by moving them carefully over a gas flame.

2. Bone marrow aspirates
   a. Compress a fleck between coverslips, as for blood.
   b. Pull smears, as for blood.
   c. Air dry or heat dry, as for blood.
3. Impression smears
   a. Blot gently a fresh-cut surface of the tissue to be studied (liver, spleen, kidney, adrenal, lymph node) to remove excessive liquid.
   b. Gently touch the "dried," cut surface to a clean glass slide—too heavy a hand will yield too thick a preparation.
   c. Air dry or *gently* heat to hasten drying; for example, on a slide warmer.

PROCEDURES

1. Giemsa stain
   a. Fix smears for 5 minutes in absolute methyl alcohol—Columbia staining jars (coverslips) and Coplin jars (slides) are convenient.
   b. Prepare diluted Giemsa stain in staining jars by adding 1 drop of Giemsa stock stain per ml of .1 M phosphate buffer at pH 6.8 to 7.0.
   c. Drain excess methanol from fixed smears and place in diluted stain for 30—60 minutes. The exact timing depends on what is being sought and is a matter of personal preference. For example, leukocytes are usually well stained in 30 minutes, whereas erythrocytes are often too pale. For parasites within blood cells, longer staining improves contrast.
   d. Rinse in phosphate buffer. When thoroughly dried (in ambient air), coverslips should be mounted smear side down using a synthetic, xylene-miscible medium (*e.g.,* Permount).
2. Wright stain
   a. Fixation of smears in absolute methyl alcohol (5 minutes) is necessary only when staining will be delayed for some time after smears are made.
   b. Add Wright blood stain to smear (about 0.5 ml per coverslip, 1 ml per slide) and let stand for 1 minute.
   c. Add twice as much buffer (.1 M phosphate, pH 6.0 to 6.5) as stain; allow to react for 3–5 minutes.
   d. Pour off stain. Rinse with buffer until thinnest portion of smear is pink.
   e. Dry on bibulous paper. Mount coverslips smear side down, using a synthetic, xylenemiscible medium such as Permount.

REAGENTS

1. Giemsa stain
   a. Absolute methyl alcohol, reagent grade.
   b. Geimsa stain stock solution—various commercial suppliers.
   c. Phosphate buffer (.1 M): either purchase as preweighed packets (*e.g.,* PHydrion Buffers) or make up: 23.3 g Na_2HPO_4
      4.4 g NaH_2PO_4
      distilled water to make
      1000 ml
2. Wright stain
   a. Absolute methanol, reagent grade.
   b. Wright stain—various commercial suppliers.
   c. Phosphate buffer (0.1M): either purchase as preweighed packets (*e.g.,* PHydrion Buffers) or make up using: 23.3 g Na_2HPO_4
      4.4 g NaH_2PO_4
      distilled water to make
      1000 ml

Limitations

GIEMSA STAIN

The pH and the duration of staining must be carefully monitored for best results. Thick smears do not stain adequately. The diluted, working stain should be renewed each day. Simply decant used stain from the jar and refill with fresh, diluted stain.

WRIGHT STAIN

The pH is critical and must be kept between 6.0 and 6.5 for good staining. At pH 6.0, erythrocytes are pink; at 6.5; they are yellow pink. Above pH 6.5, red cells take on a grayish yellow color that gives the smear a muddy appearance and reduces contrast. Smears should be thin for best results.

Applications

Although intracellular microorganisms will stain using either the Giemsa or Wright method, many workers prefer the Giemsa stain citing heightened contrast as the basis for preference.

Tissue Sections

Exposure to neutral buffered formalin for 24 hours is the preferred fixation for tissues to be stained with either Giemsa or Wright stain. Zenker's-fixed tissues must be treated to remove the mercuric chloride.

A major problem is the thickness of sections. If sections are no thicker than 5 μm and the stain is applied for 24 hours, there will generally be sufficient penetration of the stain. The pH must be stabilized for adequate staining. Mordanting in buffer at pH 6.8 before staining is recommended.

The use of Romanowsky stains on tissue sections is of particular value in differentiating types of inflammatory cells. Moreover, both intracellular and extracellular microorganisms are more readily detected in a wide variety of tissues. Thus, protozoa have a reddish purple nucleus with light blue to blue pink cytoplasm. Rickettsias stain blue to purple.

The nuclei of host cells are light to dark blue, and collagen fibers are pink, as is the cytoplasm of leukocytes, erythrocytes, and connective tissue elements. The granules of polymorphonuclear leukocytes stain a variety of colors characeristic of the type: eosinophils are bright pink, basophils are dark purple, and neutrophils are light violet.

Thionine–Eosin Staining Technique for paraffin Sections

As the supply of hematoxylin became scarce, alternative nuclear stains were examined as possible substitutes. Thionine in combination with eosin has proved to be an excellent general histologic stain with the additional value of staining leukocyte granules, mast cells, and protozoa similarly to Romanowsky stains. A dark green dye, thionine (aminophenthiazin [$NH_2 \cdot C_6H_3(NS) \cdot C_6H_3NH_5$*]) gives a purple color in aqueous solution, and had a color index number of 52000.

Methods

PREPARATIONS OF TISSUE SECTIONS

1. Fix tissue in neutral buffered formalin.
2. Impregnate with paraffin and imbed using standard techniques.
3. Cut sections at 5 μm or less for best results.

*Chroma-Brüler Biological Stains, Roboz Surgical Instruments, 810 18th Street, NW, Washington, DC, 20006

PROCEDURE

1. After the usual deparaffin treatment and hydration, wash in three separate changes of distilled water for 3 minutes each.
2. Stain in eosin B for 5 minutes.
3. Rinse in two or three changes of distilled water and drain excess water off slides before placing in thionine.
4. Place slides in thionine solution for 30–60 minutes.
5. Rinse in two changes of distilled water.
6. Dip slides briefly 4–5 times in each of two changes of *absolute* ethanol.
7. Complete dehydration in a third absolute ethanol for 60–90 seconds.
8. Clear in toluene or xylene and coverslip.

REAGENTS

1. Thionine stain
   One g of thionine in 2 liters of distilled water and 2 ml glacial acetic acid. This stain has a fairly long shelf life (2–3 months) and can be reused.
2. Eosin B
   One g of eosin B in 400 ml 50% ethanol and 1 ml glacial acetic acid.

Immunofluorescence

As it is applied to the study of infectious diseases, fluorescence microscopy always implies use of immunologic reagents that have been labeled with fluorescent moieties (see Chap. 14, Immunologic Diagnosis). Thus, immunofluorescence combines the advantages of microscopic sensitivity and immunologic specificity, giving biologists a powerful tool for the localization of immune reactants. Properly applied, immunofluorescence has been a valuable aid in the elucidation of the pathogenesis and diagnosis of many infectious diseases.

Methods

There are two bases to immunofluorescence microscopy: antigen–antibody reactions are immunologically specific; and conjugation of antibody or antigen with fluorochromes does not alter either immunologic specificity or reactivity. Although either antigen or antibody can be labeled, in practice antibodies are conjugated with fluorochromes; for example, fluorescein isothiocyanate. This follows because antigen molecules are usually multivalent, are less often available in either concentrated or pure form, and are present in smaller concentrations in actual situations suitable to immunofluorescence. Under ultraviolet light, the fluorescein-labeled antibody molecules, after reacting with appropriate antigens, emit a yellow green color enabling visualization of the antigen–antibody complex under the fluorescence microscope.

Two methods, direct and indirect, may be used for staining antigenic materials.

DIRECT

Antigenic materials such as bacterial smears, tissue smears, or tissue sections are first fixed and dried on a slide. Appropriate fluorescent antibody solutions are then layered over the smears or sections for about 30 minutes at room temperature. Under these conditions, the labeled antibody molecules will be fixed to the antigens. After washing off the excess antibody solution, the smear or section is mounted under a coverslip and examined.

INDIRECT

Staining of Immunoglobulins. Immunoglobulins are themselves antigenic. Accordingly, antihuman IgG, IgM, and IgA antiserums are prepared by hyperimmunizing rabbits or goats; the resultant immunoglobulins are then labeled with fluorescein isothiocyanate.

For testing, acute or convalescent human serums, in proper dilutions, are first layered onto smears or sections. After reaction and removal of excess serum by washing, the rabbit or goat antihuman globulin fluorescent conjugate is applied. Following reaction, washing, and mounting, the slide is ready for examination.

Staining of Complement. Many antigen–antibody complexes fix various components of complement. Antiguinea pig complement fluorescent conjugate can be prepared just as labeled antihuman globulin is made. For use, acute or convalescent serums from patients to which guinea pig complement had been added are layered on smears. This is followed by staining with fluorescent anticomplement conjugate.

Limitations

Both the direct and indirect methods of immunofluorescence microscopy have been used successfully in the examination of clinical specimens. The direct method is simpler to use, requires less time for staining, and in some instances gives better resolution of antigenic localization than the indirect method. However, separate, specific labeled antiserums are required that correspond to every antigen that is to be sought. This is a serious limitation to the direct techniques.

The indirect method requires as a minimum only two fluorescent antibody solutions—antihuman immunoglobulin and antiguinea pig complement. Also, because the patient's serums for testing can be diluted serially, the indirect immunofluorescence test can be used to measure the titer of antibody. However, the indirect method tends to give more nonspecific staining and, in certain instances, less optimal resolution of specific fluorescence.

Applications

Although immunofluorescence is of indubitable use in diagnosis, it is not at this time a routine procedure, either for the physician's office or for the hospital clinical laboratory. Competently trained persons who make frequent use of immunofluorescence are required for correct interpretation of the test. Moreover, the commercial fluorescent conjugate reagents presently available are not well standardized. However, most state public health laboratories offer fluorescent antibody (FA) tests for certain problems such as the diagnosis of rabies and serologic tests for syphilis.

In bacterial infections, the direct FA test has been applied to early identification of group A β-hemolytic streptococci, the plague bacillus, and *Legionella pneumophilia.* Smears of cerebrospinal fluid from patients with acute bacterial meningitis have also been examined by FA staining. Detection of the gonococcus in cervical smears has also been reported. More important is the demonstration that the fluorescent treponemal antibody-absorption (FTA-ABS) test is more specific and more sensitive than the treponema pallidum immobilization test and the conventional VDRL test for the diagnosis of syphilis.

Laboratory diagnosis of viral and rickettsial infections by isolation or serologic studies is timeconsuming. Using FA staining to demonstrate specific viral antigens in infected cells enables rapid diagnosis to be made. By examining nasal smears from patients thought to have acute epidemic influenza, the laboratory can give a type-specific confirmatory diagnosis of influenza within 1 hour. Similarly, by FA examination of urinary smears from patients with measles (rubeola), a confirmatory diagnosis can be accomplished during, and even before, the appearance of morbilliform rash. In some illnesses involving the central nervous system, such as subacute sclerosing panencephalitis (Dawson's disease) and encephalitis caused by herpes simplex viruses, FA diagnosis from biopsy specimens of the brain can be rapidly accomplished. For diagnosis of rabies, FA staining of imprint smears from animal brains has become a standard procedure in most state public health laboratories.

This test not only gives a rapid diagnosis but also has proven to be specific and sensitive.

For identification of viral isolates, FA staining of tissue cells from primary isolation passages materially speeds up the identification of myxoviruses, polioviruses, and varicella-zoster virus. The indirect FA technique has been used successfully in serologic diagnosis and antibody titrations for a number of infections such as scrub typhus, rubella, and varicella.

Special Optical Methods for Examining Unstained Specimen

Dark-field, phase-contrast, and interference-contrast microscopy are three methods for examining unstained specimens that have application in diagnostic work. All are optical methods for increasing image contrast, and hence they enable the observer to detect objects so small they would otherwise remain invisible. Increased contrast should not be confused with resolving power, an entirely different concept that has finite limits imposed by the wave length of the light used and the numerical aperture of the substage condenser.

The dark-field is the most powerful means of enhancing contrast available in light microscopy. The basic principle is exclusion of all direct light from the objective of the microscope. This is accomplished by a specially designed substage condenser with a central stop that prevents any light from passing directly into the objective lens. Only light from the periphery of the condenser reaches the specimen on the slide. Only that portion of light that is diffracted or reflected from the surface and edges of the specimen so that it enters the lens of the objective is available for visual detection. With this type of illumination, the field is completely dark and the specimen is a bright object against a black background.

Phase contrast depends on retardation of either the direct beam or the reflected beam of light. The result is either anoptral contrast (the specimen appears light with respect to the darker background and hence is similar in final result to dark field) or dark-phase contrast (the specimen appears darker than the background). Specially manufactured objectives and substage condensers are required. There are differences between the systems of the various manufacturers, and the user must become thoroughly familiar with the instrument available to him for best results.

The interference-contrast technique most easily adapted to routine biological work is that developed by Nomarski. Both Reichert and Zeiss optical companies manufacture interference-contrast equipment based on the Nomarski principal, and their manuals should be consulted for specific details on equipping a microscope with interference optics in lieu of purchasing one of their microscopes.

Methods

DARK-FIELD MICROSCOPY

The usual bright-field objectives are used for dark-field illumination. The special dark-field substage condenser selected must produce a sufficiently wide dark cone so the shortest focal length objective used with the system can be accommodated. Special oil-immersion objectives are available that have iris diaphragms built into them so that the outer field margin can be closed down to exclude any direct light. Methods of converting bright-field substage condensers to dark-field condensers by adding an opaque disk at the level of the iris diaphragm are usually adequate only for low-power dark-field microscopy. For high-power dark-field microscopy, however, a substage condenser of considerably higher numerical aperture must be used; this usually necessitates the use of a special substage condenser.

PHASE-CONTRAST MICROSCOPY

Alignment of the light source and phase rings is absolutely essential if the best contrast formation is to be achieved—the manufacturers' instructions are explicit and appropriate. For convenience in changing magnifications, the objectives should be point-centered in the objective slide at the manufacturing plant and should not be moved from this exact sequence in the slide. Thus, the user can center the highest power objective with the corresponding phase ring in the substage condenser, after which all other objectives should be properly centered with their corresponding substage phase rings.

INTERFERENCE-CONTRAST MICROSCOPY

The important distinction between phase-contrast and interference-contrast microscopy revolves around the means by which the light rays are altered in phase amplitude. In phase contrast, refractive differences within and on the surface of the *specimen itself* are taken advantage of in order to alter the light rays, whereas in interference contrast the beam of light is optically split before it reaches the specimen. As a result, the edge effects which often produce halos in phase-contrast, are not apparent in the interference-contrast technique. Such halos are often objectionable in viewing specimens and are very difficult to eliminate when doing photomicroscopy with phase contrast. On the other hand, with interference-contrast microscopy the absence of these halos makes the photomicrographs much clearer and sharper in appearance (Fig. 9-1*A* and *B*).

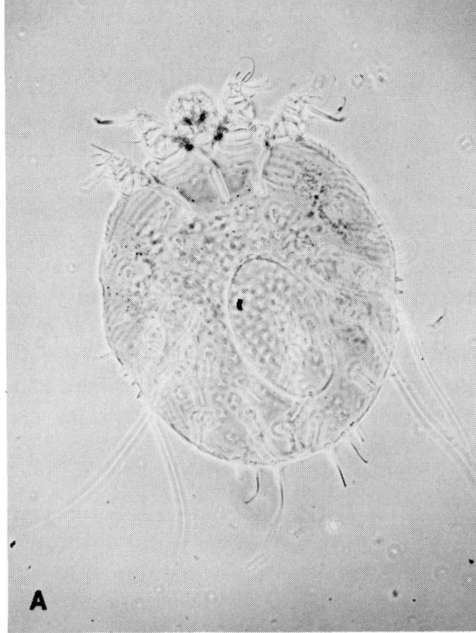

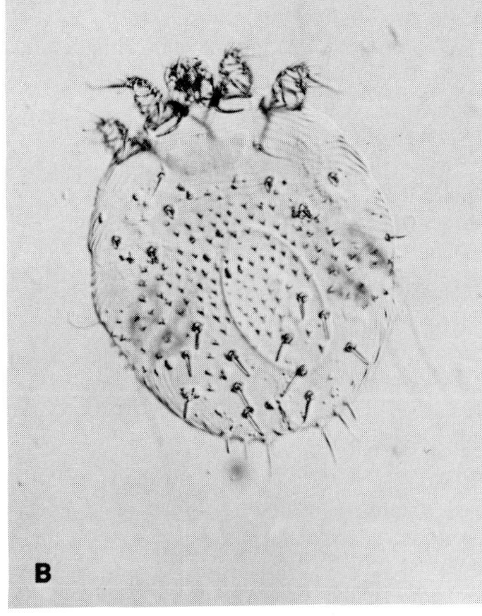

Fig. 9-1. *Sarcoptes scabei,* adult female, unstained. *(A)* Phase contrast. *(B)* Interference contrast. (Original magnification × 100)

Limitations

DARK-FIELD MICROSCOPY

Dark-field microscopy is extremely wasteful of light. Not only does the stop arrangement of the substage prevent most of the light from reaching the specimen, but also there is even further reduction because only the light reflected or diffracted from the specimen is available for visual perception or photographic recording. Usually, this does not present difficulties with visual observation, especially in a room where one can reduce all extraneous light. However, photography under dark-field conditions requires considerably longer exposure times than are normally feasible.

Selection of a light source is critical, particularly if photography is contemplated. Because discussion of the relative merits of the sources and systems of illumination that have been devised is beyond the scope of this chapter, the interested reader should consult a text devoted to the subject.

The slides used for dark-field work should be as clean as possible for grease, lint, dust motes, glass specks, and scratches all reflect or diffract light into the objective and hence detract from the image contrast of the specimen. Again, the observer can tolerate or tune out such background more readily than photographic recording. New slides should be used, but even they may require special washing in distilled water and treatment for a few minutes with strong acids such as 12 M sulfuric acid before a final rinse and drying with a lintless towel readies them for use. Slides properly cleaned can be prepared well in advance of use and will remain dust free if stored in closed slide boxes. Coverslips must also be clean and free of scratches. The thickness may be critical if objectives are corrected for specific coverglass thickness; No. 1½ thickness is best because variation in thickness is within the limits of accommodation of the corrected objectives.

PHASE-CONTRAST MICROSCOPY

Phase-contrast methods are considerably less wasteful of light than dark-field microscopy. Nevertheless, at high magnifications light may be insufficient for brief exposures. Hence, selection of a light source is again quite important.

A thin specimen, certainly no more than 5 nm thick, is best in phase microscopy. Thick specimens provide interfering, internal surfaces that deviate light rays; the pattern of transmission is interrupted and the quality of the image is greatly reduced. Cleanliness in handling the slides, and particularly in handling the phase condenser and objectives, is essential to exclude skin oils, grease, and dirt. A special aqueous mountant medium containing gelatin may be useful in reducing the refractive index between the specimen edges and the medium itself. If this refractive index is too great, the internal detail of the specimen will be blurred.

INTERFERENCE-CONTRAST MICROSCOPY

The quartz halogen lamp is a very good light source for this type of microscopy. Specimens may be a good deal thicker than those providing optimal phase-contrast images and still provide excellent interference-contrast images. In addition, because of the lack of the edge effect, dust particles and extraneous material in the background will not readily produce halos with interference-contrast optics.

Application

DARK-FIELD MICROSCOPY

Dark-field microscopy is particularly valuable when liquid specimens are examined for spirochetes and protozoa. Microorganisms in motion show up very well. Unstained tissue scrapings and tissue sections can also be examined to advantage.

PHASE-CONTRAST MICROSCOPY

In general, phase-contrast illumination has the same application as the dark-field method. The internal structure of unstained cells, small arthropods, and worms is readily studied by phase contrast, enabling identification on morphologic grounds.

INTERFERENCE-CONTRAST MICROSCOPY

Although the viewer can often ignore halos and bright flares when viewing a phase image, the flat film field on which the image is projected in photomicroscopy is not able to do so. Thus, interference-contrast offers an advantage over phase-contrast microscopy in the taking of photomicrographs in which a three-dimensional relief is desirable.

Bibliography

GRAM STAIN

Books

CRUICKSHANK R (ED): Medical Microbiology, 11 ed. Edinburgh, E & S Livingstone, 1969. pp 647–653.

LILLIE RD, STOTZ EH, EMMEL VM: H. J. Conn's Biological Stains, 9th ed. Baltimore, Williams & Wilkins, 1977, 692 pp.

Journals

Austrian R: The Gram stain and etiology of lobar pneumonia, an historical note. Bacteriol Rev 24:261–265, 1960

ACID-FAST STAINING

Books

LILLIE RD, STOTZ EH, EMMEL VM: H. J. Conn's Biological Stains, 9th ed. Baltimore, Williams & Wilkins, 1977, 692 pp.

RUNYON EH, KARLSON AG, KUBICA GP, WAYNE LG: Mycobacterium. In Lennette EH, Spaulding EH, Truant JP (eds): Manual of Clinical Microbiology, 2nd ed. Washington DC, American Society for Microbiology, 1974. pp 148–174.

Journals

KUBICA GP, DYE WE: Laboratory methods for clinical and public health. Mycobacteriology Public Health Service Publication 1547:23–26, 1967

TRUANT JP, BRETT WA, THOMAS W JR: Fluorescence microscopy of tubercle bacilli stained with auramine and rhodamine. Henry Ford Hosp Med Bull 10:287–296, 1962

STAINS FOR FUNGI

Books

AL-DOORY Y: Laboratory Medical Mycology. Philadelphia, Lea & Febiger, 1980. pp 68–84, 376–388.

EMMONS CW, BINFORD CH, UTZ JP, KWON-CHUNG KJ: Medical Mycology, 3rd ed. Philadelphia, Lea & Febiger, 1977. pp 58–60, 541–569.

LUNA LG (ED): Manual of Histologic Staining Methods of the Armed Forces Institute of Pathology, 3rd ed. New York, McGraw-Hill, 1968. pp 158–160, 228–232.

MCGINNIS MR: Laboratory Handbook of Medical Mycology. New York, Academic Press, 1980. pp 100–102, 523–587.

RIPPON JW: Medical Mycology. The Pathogenic Fungi and the Pathogenic Actinomycetes. Philadelphia, W. B. Saunders, 1974. pp. 555–559.

Journal

HILL WB JR, KWON-CHUNG KJ: A new special stain for the histopathological diagnosis of cryptococcosis. Abstr Ann Meet ASM Paper F 77, page 332, 1980

GIMENEZ STAIN

Journals

GIMENEZ DF: Staining rickettsiae in yolk sac cultures. Stain Technol 39:135–140, 1964

ROMANOWSKY-TYPE STAINING

Books

GURR E: Staining Animal Tissues: Practical and Theoretical. London, Leonard Hill Books, 1962. pp 446–447.

THOMPSON SW: Romanowsky-type staining technics. Wright's stain, Giemsa's stain, May–Grünwald Giemsa stain. Methods for the microscopic demonstration of morphologic components of animal tissues. In Selected Histochemical and Histopathological Methods. Springfield, Charles C Thomas, 1966. 757–763.

IMMUNOFLUORESCENCE

Books

CHERRY WB, GOLDMAN M, CARSKI TR: Fluorescent Antibody Techniques in the Diagnosis of Communicable Diseases. U.S. Public Health Service Bulletin No. 729, Department of Health, Education and Welfare. Washington DC, U. S. Government Printing Office, 1961

LIU C: Fluorescent antibody technics. In Lennette EH, Schmidt NJ (eds): Diagnostic Procedures for Viral and Rickettsial Infections, 4th ed. New York, American Public Health Association, 1969. pp 179–204.

SPECIAL OPTICAL METHODS FOR EXAMINING UNSTAINED SPECIMEN

Books

BAKER JR: The blood dyes. In Principles of Biological Microtechnique. New York, John Wiley & Sons, 1958. pp 262–372.

LOVELAND RP: Special methods of illumination. In Clark W (ed): Photomicrography, a Comprehensive Treatise, Vol II. New York, John Wiley & Sons, 1970. pp 527–554.

ARTHUR L. BARRY

10 Clinical Specimens for Microbiologic Examinations

In order to identify the etiologic agent(s) involved in infectious diseases, the microorganisms present at the site of the infection must be isolated. Yet, the recovery of microorganisms from an infected site is not unequivocal evidence of a causative role because a variety of potentially pathogenic microorganisms normally reside on the surfaces of the human body. Isolation and identification must be followed by categorization as (1) a member of the normally resident microbiota, (2) a component of the transient microbiota contaminating a body surface, (3) a totally extraenous contaminant introduced at the time the specimen was collected, or (4) the actual pathogen responsible for the infection. Clearly, a knowledge of both the qualitative and quantitative character of the microbial residents of a given site is essential. In addition, there must be full awareness that both the numbers and kinds of microorganisms finally recovered from a given site depends largely on the methods used to collect specimens and transport them to the laboratory, as well as on the methods used to process the specimens in the laboratory.

General Considerations

In the modern, busy hospital or clinic, the extremely critical processes of collecting specimens and transporting them to the clinical microbiology laboratory is all too frequently left to assistants who have not been adequately trained. Inappropriate specimens or materials collected and transported without the application of necessary precautions may result. Use of even the most precise and exhaustive laboratory examinations with inadequate clinical materials can only produce grossly misleading results. The conscientious laboratory worker will refuse to accept specimens that are obviously unsatisfactory. But unfortunately, the adequacy of clinical specimens cannot always be judged from gross appearances alone. The cellular elements observed in a direct smear of the specimen often provide a useful hint; for example, a urine specimen often provide a useful hint; for example, a urine specimen that contains large squamous epithelial cells, few polymorphonuclear leukocytes, and a mixture of bacteria such as is ordinarily found in the external urethra or vagina, is contaminated. Specimens from areas known to contain a variety of microorganisms as part of the normal flora should be viewed with suspicion when only a sparse growth is detected. Specimens from sites that are normally sterile should not yield a heavy growth of a mixture of several types of microorganisms. When this does occur, external contamination should be suspected. For these reasons, most clinical specimens should be examine microscopically for microorganisms and cultured using at least one general nutrient medium so that the density of the microbial flora will be revealed. A semiquantitative estimate of the amount of growth carried out according to the scheme presented in Fig. 10-1 is helpful in evaluating the adequacy of the specimen and the significance of potential pathogens that are recovered. The specimen is inoculated onto a small area about the size of a quarter and then streaked with a sterile bacteriologic loop over the four overlapping areas, as outlined in Fig. 10-1. Each type of colony is then reported on a

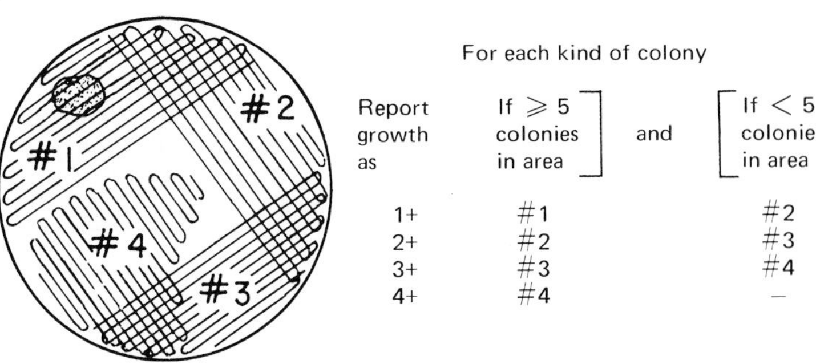

Fig. 10-1. Definition of terms for a semiquantitative estimate of the amount on a nutrient agar medium. Plates are inoculated and then streaked with a sterile loop. The loop is not flamed again until the entire plate is streaked. After appropriate incubation, different types of colonies are evaluated on a 1 + to 4 + scale, as defined. Care must be taken to avoid misinterpreting the swarming growth of *Proteus* spp. Neither anaerobes nor fastidious microorganisms can be evaluated unless the requisite media and conditions of incubation have been met.

1+ to 4+ basis, according to the area in which five or more isolated colonies are observed. Of course, the growth of anaerobes and fastidious microorganisms may not be accurately quantitated. Also, when two or more different kinds of microorganisms are present in large numbers in a given specimen, small numbers of yet another kind will be difficult to detect unless highly selective mediums are utilized. Generally, with properly collected specimens, pathogenic bacteria are among the predominant flora, and minor components of the microbial flora are usually not involved in the infectious process. The common practice of inoculating several highly selective mediums will certainly increase the probability of recovery of potential pathogens, but the significance of such isolates may not be clear. *Salmonella* spp., *Shigella* spp., *Neisseria gonorrhoeae,* and *Mycobacterium tuberculosis* are commonly encountered exceptions that are significant in any kind of clinical specimen, regardless of the numbers recovered. In the latter two cases, respectively, highly selective mediums and concentration methods should always be used, and semiquantitative information is less significant. In summary, the adequacy of a particular clinical specimen can be evaluated by considering the gross appearance of the material, the cellular elements observed in a stained smear, and qualitative and quantitative estimates of the different kinds of microorganisms recovered.

All clinical specimens must be collected in clean, sterile containers that are free from inhibitory materials such as residual detergents. The containers must be properly sealed in order to avoid either desiccation or contamination of the specimen. An unnecessarily hazardous situation is created if the outer portion of the container and the accompanying request form are contaminated.

It is absolutely essential that the specimen be carefully and completely identified and that the appropriate information be recorded on the proper request forms. Any condition, circumstances, or situation that will require special procedures should also be noted on the request form. Indeed, for optimal results, close cooperation between the clinician and laboratory personnel is absolutely essential.

Except in emergencies, specimens should be collected during the normal working hours of the laboratory so that fully qualified microbiologists will be available to process the specimens. This is particularly important when special procedures are to be performed. Whenever possible, the initial diagnostic specimen should be collected before antimicrobial therapy is initiated.

Anaerobic Cultures

The surfaces of the human body, especially the mucous membranes, contain large numbers of aerobic and anaerobic microorganisms which may cause or contribute to deep infectious processes. The expensive, time-consuming procedures involved in the isolation and identification of anaerobic bacteria are warranted only with those specimens not contaminated with anaerobes resident on the body surfaces. Methods for collecting specimens for anaerobic cultures from various anatomic sites are summarized in Table 10-1.

Because some anaerobes are sensitive to brief exposure to atmospheric oxygen and to desiccation, care must be taken in the collection and transportation of specimens to the laboratory. In general, material appropriate for anaerobic cultures is best obtained using a needle and syringe—applicator swabs are rarely adequate. Aspirated material should be processed as soon as possible after collection because it often contains mixed flora, including faculta-

Table 10-1. Clinical Materials Warranting Routine Examination for Anaerobic Bacteria in Addition to Aerobic Microorganisms

Anatomic Site	Specimens Appropriate for Anaerobic Cultures, Provided That Proper Collection and Transport Systems Have Been Used	Specimens Likely to Be Contaminated and Thus Inappropriate for Anaerobic Cultures
Pulmonary	Transtracheal aspirates Thoracentesis fluids Direct needle puncture aspirates of lung infiltrates or abscesses	Coughed sputums Tracheal tube suctioning Bronchoscopic aspirates Nasopharyngeal, throat or mouth swabs
Urinary	Suprapubic aspirate of bladder urine	Voided urine Catheterized specimens
Abscesses	Needle and syringe aspirate of closed abscesses after decontamination of surface	Swab from surface of abscess or swab after incision and drainage
Sinus tract, Wound drainage	Aspirate into syringe through IV catheter introduced as deeply as possible through decontaminated skin orifice	Swab from external portion of sinus tract or of drainage through external orifice
Uterine	Aspirate into syringe through IV catheter passed through the cervical os under direct visualization	Vaginal or cervical swabs
Others	Blood, cerebrospinal fluid (brain abscess), joint fluid, and biopsy specimens collected with ordinary care	Superficial wounds, feces or rectal swabs

tive microorganisms which grow faster than obligate anaerobes. After expelling all air bubbles and inserting the top of the needle into a sterile rubber stopper, the specimen should be carried directly to the laboratory in the syringe. Because air gradually diffuses through the wall of a plastic syringe, no more than 30 minutes should elapse before the specimen is processed. Alternatively, the material may be injected into tubes or vials that have been flushed with oxygen-free CO_2 or N_2 before sterilization; care must be taken to avoid injecting air along with specimen. Blood and other normally sterile body fluids may be inoculated directly into bottles containing reduced liquid culture mediums.

Applicator Swabs

Many clinical specimens are conveniently collected by gently but firmly rubbing swabs over the surface of the infected site. If the surface to be cultured is relatively dry, the swab should first be moistened in nutrient broth or sterile 0.9% NaCl solution, without preservatives.

Ordinary cotton swabs may contain materials that inhibit a number of different microorganisms. Pernasal swabs are often prepared by attaching a small amount of cotton to the end of a metal wire; metallic ions can inhibit certain bacteria. The adhesive used to attach cotton to the end of an applicator stick may be toxic to certain bacteria. The cotton itself may also contain toxic materials such as unsaturated fatty acids. To neutralize the inhibitory activity of the cotton, swabs may be treated with serum, charcoal, or polyvinyl alcohol, after boiling in a phosphate buffer. A simpler alternative is to replace the cotton with less toxic, synthetic fibers made of polyester or calcium alginate. Calcium alginate is doubly advantageous because fibers dislodged during the sampling process will be absorbed by the body tissues and fluids and will not initiate a foreign body reaction; and calcium alginate is completely soluble in sodium salts of numerous organic acids such as glycerophosphate, hexametaphosphate, thioglycollate, enabling concentration and quantitation of swab specimens. Alginate swabs are also less absorbent, that is, less material is actually picked up on the swab, and the material remains on the outer portion of the swab, where it is readily exposed to the deleterious effects of desiccation.

Because of all the preceding considerations, and because a larger sample increases the probability of success in isolation of the responsible pathogen, alternatives to swab collection of specimens should be made use of whenever possible. Pus or serous exudate aspirated directly into a syringe provides a more satisfactory specimen for examination. Similarly, actual feces is preferable to a rectal swab when enteric pathogens are sought.

Transport Mediums

A number of systems have been devised to reduce the effect of desiccation on swabs and to dilute inhibitory substances in the swabs or in the clinical material itself. Nutrient broth is not satisfactory in that commensals may multiply in the broth and overgrow less hardy pathogens. Amies' modification of Stuart's transport medium is quite useful because it is nonnutritive, buffered with phosphate, provides a reducing environment (thioglycolic acid), and contains a small amount of agar. Overgrowth from coliforms is minimized, and both oxygen-sensitive and fastidious bacteria survive. Although most such transport or holding mediums were originally designed to ensure survival of gonococci, other microorganisms also survive quite well. Some kind of holding medium certainly must be used when there will be an excessive delay in transport to the laboratory, especially when specimens are to be delivered by mail. Although transport mediums are useful, they remain second-best to processing clinical material immediately after it is collected. Moreover, because of the agar in transport mediums, stained smears are usually unsatisfactory.

A significant number of viable cells are lost from the swabs and remain in the holding medium, especially with the less absorbent calcium alginate swabs (Table 10-2). There will be some decrease in the number of viable cells as swabs are allowed to stand in holding medium; however, the loss of viability is much greater without holding medium. Specimens that contain relatively few microorganisms will certainly fail to yield any growth if the swabs are left dry 2 to 4 hours, whereas the number of positive cultures will increase if the swabs are kept in a transport medium. Even more specimens will be positive if appropriate mediums are properly inoculated at the time the specimen is collected, but this is generally impractical in hospitals or large clinics. There are currently available special selective mediums in kit form that enable the direct beside inoculation of specimens likely to yield particular pathogens; for example, a urethral exudate containing *N. gonorrhoeae.* These kits are appropriate when excessive delay in transporting specimens to the laboratory cannot be avoided, as in office practice.

Upper Respiratory Tract

Various parts of the upper respiratory tract may be cultured for different reasons. Because there is a resident microbiota that varies both qualitatively and quantitatively according to the region sampled (Table 10-3), the results of cultures must be interpreted with due allowance for the normal ecology of

Table 10-2. *Effect of a Transport Medium on the Recovery of Viable Bacteria From Two Kinds of Swabs (Number of Viable Cells Recovered From One Swab – Average of Triplicate Tests)**

Hours at Room Temperature	Haemophilus influenzae		Streptococcus pneumoniae		Streptococcus pyogenes		Neisseria gonorrhoeae		Clostridium sordellii	
	DRY	AMIES†	DRY	AMIES†	DRY	AMIES†	DRY	AMIES†	DRY	AMIES†
Cotton swabs 0	3×10^6		1×10^5		3×10^6		7×10^5		2×10^7	
2	< 10	5×10^5	< 10	2×10^4	1×10^4	1×10^6	2×10^2	1×10^4	9×10^5	1×10^6
4	< 10	3×10^5	< 10	2×10^4	1×10^3	9×10^5	< 10	3×10^3	< 10	1×10^5
24	< 10	2×10^5	< 10	9×10^3	< 10	1×10^6	< 10	10	< 10	5×10^4
Calcium Alginate swabs 0	4×10^6		4×10^5		3×10^6		1×10^6		2×10^7	
2	2×10^3	2×10^5	5×10^2	3×10^4	5×10^4	2×10^5	< 10	5×10^3	8×10^4	3×10^6
4	< 10	2×10^4	< 10	6×10^3	2×10^4	2×10^5	< 10	2×10^3	< 10	3×10^6
24	< 10	9×10^3	< 10	4×10^2	< 10	7×10^4	< 10	< 10	< 10	2×10^6

*Triplicate swabs were saturated with 0.025 ml of each of four 10 × dilutions of a phosphate buffered (pH 7.2) saline suspension of the test bacteria; after the indicated holding time, the entire surface of a blood or chocolate agar plate was streaked, and the number of viable cells recovered from each type of swab was calculated. Approximately 60% of the inoculum could be recovered from the swabs at time 0.

†Amies' transport medium without charcoal (Difco). A liquid version of this medium mechanically removed approximately 4% of the bacteria from cotton swabs and 44% from the less absorbent calcium alginate swabs.

Table 10-3. *Resident Microbiota of the Upper Respiratory Tract†*

Region	Microorganisms per ml	
	AEROBIC	ANAEROBIC
Nose*	10 to 10^4	10^2 to 10^5
Saliva	10^7 to 10^8	10^8 to 10^9
Teeth*	10^6	10^6
Gingival scrapings*	10^7	10^7

* Washings

† Nonpathogens (normal flora, commensals): *Streptococcus* spp. α-hemolytic, nonhemolytic, anaerobic; *Staphylococcus epidermidis; Branhamella* spp.; diphtheroids.

Potential pathogens: *Streptococcus pyogenes; Staphylococcus aureus; Haemophilus influenzae; Streptococcus pneumoniae; Neisseria meningitidis; Candida albicans; Klebsiella* spp.

the region or origin of the specimen. Interpretation may be quite difficult. For example, infants, children, uncooperative adults, and comatose patients who have a lower respiratory tract infection will not, or cannot, provide sputum for examination. Because the nasopharyngeal flora may change to correspond with that of the diseased lower respiratory tract, nasopharyngeal swab cultures are often collected from such patients. If a thin wire or flexible plastic pernasal swab is used, the isolation of *Staphylococcus aureus* may or may not be significant because *S. aureus* normally inhabit the nose. However, when a particular pathogen is sought that is not a normal resident—for example, *Bordetella pertussis*—the nasopharyngeal swab is by far the best method of obtaining a specimen for culture. The swab is passed gently through the nose and firmly forced into the nasopharynx, where it is rotated, then gently removed and placed into a transport medium. Because freshly prepared agar culture medium must be inoculated for the isolation of *B. pertussis* (see Chap. 29, Whooping Cough), the laboratory must have advance warning.

Throat swab cultures should be taken under direct visualization with good lighting. Areas of exudation, membrane formation, or inflammation are choice sites; otherwise, the tonsillar crypts should be rubbed vigorously with the swab. Requisitions must specify the microbial agent or the disease that is suspected—for example, diphtheria or streptococcal pharyngitis—because different laboratory procedures are required for different specific pathogens.

If streptococcal pharyngitis is suspected, throat swabs may be inoculated onto sterile filter paper, which is allowed to air dry before being enclosed in a sterile foil pack preparatory to mailing to the laboratory. When rapidly dried on filter paper, *Streptococcus pyogenes* can survive at ambient temperatures for prolonged periods; if left to dry on cotton or calcium alginate swabs, however, they will die. Placing swabs in a holding medium assures survival.

For the recovery of viral agents, the patient should be instructed to gargle with a nutrient broth. The resultant throat washings are then sent to the virus laboratory. If there will be a delay, the specimen should be held at or below $-40°C$ and mailed in a container packed in dry ice.

Lower Respiratory Tract

Sputum is a heterogenous material of varying consistency and appearance that is dejected from the lungs, bronchi, and trachea through the mouth. Although the lower respiratory tract is normally sterile, sputum specimens are heavily contaminated with saliva and nasal secretions. Unfortunately, most of the bacteria commonly associated with pulmonary infections (see Chap. 31, Bacterial Pneumonias) can also be found as members of the normal microbiota of the oropharynx, a location from which they may contaminate expectorated specimens of sputum. For that reason, recovery of bacterial pathogens from a single specimen of sputum cannot be accepted as having unequivocal diagnostic implication. In general, the more significant pathogens are present in relatively large numbers, and the normal microorganisms contributed by the oropharynx are usually found in relatively small numbers. For this reason, attempts to quantitiate the different types of microorganisms in a freshly collected sputum specimen may have very real clinical significance. Of course, exhaustive quantitative studies of inadequately collected sputum specimens are not only a waste of time but are also dangerously misleading.

An excessive number of squamous epithelial cells in expectorated sputum indicated contamination with oropharyngeal secretions, and thus the quality of a sputum specimen may be judged objectively by examining a stained smear of an appropriate portion of the specimen. Through use of the scoring system described in Table 10-4, it is possible to identify specimens which are clearly unsuitable for bacteriologic examination; a second specimen should be requested without delay. If anything, this scoring system is too conservative because some contaminated specimens will be accepted for bacteriologic examination. Rejection of all expectorated sputum specimens with more than 10 squamous epithelial cells per low-power (× 100) field would probably eliminate contaminated specimens.

Table 10-4. *Scoring System for Screening Gram-Stained Smears of Expectorated "Sputum" (low-power [100×] magnification)*

Squamous Epithelial Cells (SqE)		**Inflammatory Cells (IC)**	
AVERAGE NO./FIELD	SCORE	AVERAGE NO./FIELD	SCORE
>25	−3	>150	+3
16–25	−2	76–150	+2
5–15	−1	1–75	+1

Add the negative score for SqE and positive score for IC. If the total score is a negative value (SqE predominate), the specimen is rejected and a second specimen is requested.

To collect a specimen of sputum, the patient should be instructed to cough up material from deep in the lungs and expectorate into a sterile, wide-mouth jar. This should be done under direct supervision, preferably when the patient first awakens in the morning. If the sputum is scanty, the collection of a satisfactory specimen may be facilitated by lowering the head of the patient's bed for a few minutes. Stimulation of the cough reflex by exposure to an aerosol mist of warm hypertonic saline solution may be useful. Once collected, the specimen should be sent to the laboratory with a minimum of delay, as the complex microbial flora will undoubtedly change *if* the specimen is allowed to stand.

Because sputum is a heterogenous collection of material, the most appropriate portion must be selected for culture. Purulent or bloody flecks should be selected because they are more likely to have originated in the lungs. Unfortunately, selection of several different flecks from the same specimen can yield as many different results, and thus some workers have attempted to treat the mucopurulent material with one of several mucolytic agents so that the specimen can be homogenized and a single aliquot then cultured. Others have attempted to reduce the number of microorganisms contributed by saliva through washing a choice fleck with several changes of sterile saline solution before culturing. Such a procedure is time consuming and may present a hazard to the laboratory personnel. At present there is no simple, completely satisfactory method for recovery of bacterial pathogens from expectorated sputum.

Specimens collected through a tracheal catheter or bronchoscope are more likely to contain material from the lower pulmonary tree, but they may also be contaminated with the microbial flora of the upper respiratory tract. Moreover, with the latter procedure, a local anesthetic agent invariably becomes mixed with the specimen, and may reduce microbial outgrowth. Recently, a plugged catheter containing a brush has been used successfully to collect pulmonary specimens free of contaminants through the flexible fiberotopic bronchoscope.

Material without anesthetics can be collected from the lower tract without contamination from the upper respiratory tract by inserting a needle through the skin of the neck and the cricothyroid membrane into the trachea. A small, sterile, plastic catheter is passed through the needle, and exudate is aspirated directly from the tracheobronchial tree (see Fig. 31-4). Such transtracheal aspirates are also suitable for anaerobic culture and may provide a clear-cut diagnosis, whereas the cultures of expectorated sputum can be very misleading. Collecting a percutaneous transtracheal aspirate is often the best way out of the diagnostic dilemma presented by repeated cultures of expectorated sputum.

When a bacterial pathogen cannot be recovered from the sputum of patients with active pneumonia, viruses, *Chlamydia* spp., *Coxiella burnetii,* or *Mycoplasma pneumoniae* may be responsible (see Chap. 30, Nonbacterial Pneumonias). These pathogens can be recovered from sputum, but the rather specialized procedures that are required are so slow and cumbersome that a positive isolation cannot ordinarily be accomplished early enough to influence the therapy. However, identification of the responsible agent will be important in handling the disease as it spreads through the patient's family or community.

When acid-fast bacilli are sought (see Chap. 34, Pulmonary Tuberculosis; Chap. 35, Extrapulmonary Tuberculosis; and Chap. 36, Nontuberculosis Mycobacterioses), a large volume of sputum should be processed by digestion and concentration, procedures that remove contaminating microorganisms. A series of three, fresh, early-morning specimens are ordinarily collected and held in the refrigerator to be pooled or processed individually, provided there is at least 5 ml to 10 ml of sputum per specimen. Alternatively, it is still common practice to instruct the patient to collect all the sputum expectorated during a 24-hour period or until a total of 50 ml is obtained. The entire specimen is then concentrated after digestion and decontamination. However, such specimens have generally remained at the bedside during the collection period, and contaminating bacteria and fungi will have multiplied within the specimen. As a result, the cultures are more likely to be overgrown with contaminating bacteria, unless excessively harsh decontamination procedures that will also reduce the numbers of viable acid-fast bacteria have been applied. While categoric statements concerning the relative merits of fresh, early-morning specimens versus 18- to 24-hour collections are not justified, there is certainly no place for 48-hour or 36-hour sputum collection. Two early-morning specimens plus one 18- or 24-hour collection are probably a reasonable compromise. If the volume of sputum is under 10 ml, three 12- to 24-hour pooled specimens may be more rewarding. When stained smears of the concentrated material from these initial specimens are all negative for acid-fast bacteria, and if the patient's condition warrants further study, an additional series of specimens should be collected.

In patients who are unable to cooperate in the collection of sputum, *M. tuberculosis* may be recovered from the gastric contents because such patients tend to swallow sputum as it is produced. Ordinary bacteria do not survive the acidic conditions of the stomach, and even tubercle bacilli can only withstand very short exposure to such an environment. For this reason, gastric washings should be collected early in the morning while the patient is fasting, and the acid should be neutralized as soon as the specimen is collected. Because gastric contents often contain saprophytic mycobacteria that are also acid-fast, in many laboratories smears are not prepared from concentrates of gastric aspirates. This rule should not apply to specimens from pediatric patients.

Unless otherwise indicated, a thoracentesis should be performed whenever pleural fluid has accumulated. A culture of the aspirated fluid usually reveals the pathogen involved (see Chap. 47, Empyema). Such fluid should always be examined for both aerobic and anaerobic pathogens.

Eye

The relatively small numbers of microorganisms normally present in the conjunctival sac consist chiefly of diphtheroids and anaerobic lactobacilli. The conjunctiva owes its comparative freedom from bacteria in part to the actively bacteriolytic enzyme, lysozyme, and partly to the continual flushing activity of normal tears. For the etiologic diagnosis of conjunctivitis, material can be collected by retracting the lower lid and stroking the conjunctiva with a sterile swab. Specimens from a corneal ulcer can also be obtained by scraping the ulcer with a swab, bacteriologic loop, or similar sterile instrument. Smears should be prepared and examined for inclusion bodies if a viral agent is suspected, and a Gram stain should be prepared if a bacterial infection is suspected. Appropriate mediums should also be inoculated promptly in order to recover the etiologic agent. Speed is important because the small specimens also contain inhibitors. Holding mediums should not be used because they will further dilute the already small specimen, reducing the opportunity to recover the pathogen.

Lower Intestinal Tract

Rectal swabs are often helpful in identifying the cause of acute bacterial diarrhea when fecal specimens cannot be collected readily. However, because rectal swabs may not yield enteric pathogens, specimens of feces should be submitted when obtained. Some enteric pathogens are quite vulnerable to desiccation. Accordingly, a transport-holding medium especially compounded for enteric materials should be used when there will be a delay in processing rectal swabs or feces.

Swabbing lesions of the wall of the rectum or sigmoid colon during proctoscopy or sigmoidoscopy is much more likely to be productive than is blind rectal swabbing. For example, the superficial colonic ulcers of shigellosis are often accessible to direct swabbing through the sigmoidoscope (see Chap. 62, Shigellosis). Material taken directly from the rather classic ulcers produced by *Entamoeba histolytica* can be examined directly for motile trophozoites; motility is rapidly lost at room temperature, and the specimen must be examined immediately (see Chap. 11, Diagnostic Methods for Protozoa and Helminths, and Chap. 66, Amebiasis). Similarly, material from duodenal aspirates, sputum, ulcers, and abscesses can be examined for parasites. In all cases, prompt, exhaustive microscopic examination of specimens is essential for accurate diagnoses.

Feces

Feces should be passed directly into a clean, waxed cardboard container that is fitted with a tight cover so that the outside will not be contaminated. Feces passed into a sterile bedpan can be transferred to an appropriate container; however, such specimens may be rendered unsatisfactory by residual soap, detergents, or disinfectants in the bedpan, or may be contaminated with urine. If a sample is transferred from a bedpan, it should include any pus, blood, mucus, or formed elements that may have been passed, and should include representative samples of the first, last, and middle portion of the feces. If bacterial pathogens are sought, the specimen should be cultured as soon as possible, because *Shigella* spp. readily die off with a delay in transit.

If viral isolation is to be attempted, the specimen

should be frozen and kept below −40°C until it can be processed. Serum samples should be collected at the same time and again 2 to 3 weeks later in order to detect an increase in circulating antibodies specific for any viral agents recovered from the feces. A rise in antibody titer must be demonstrated in order to establish the significance of isolation of a viral agent from the feces of the same patient.

Genital Tract

For the diagnosis of gonorrhea in the male (see Chap. 56, Gonococcal Infections), either exudate from a urethral discharge or prostatic fluid can be collected directly onto two swabs. In the female, urethral or cervical swab specimens are more satisfactory than vaginal material. Cervical specimens should be collected through a speculum inserted without lubricant, and with care to avoid contaminating the swab with vaginal contents. At least two swabs should always be collected, one to prepare smears for Gram staining and the other for culture. If the appropriate medium cannot be inoculated immediately, the swabs must be transported in a holding medium. In unusual circumstances, it may be necessary to culture the endometrium, the vaginal orifice, or the rectum. With such heavily contaminated specimens, a selective medium such as that described by Thayer and Martin should be used. Because other microorganisms may be involved in the infectious process, a less selective nutrient medium should also be inoculated. However, in a large, busy venereal disease clinic a single cultured using Thayer–Martin medium is practical and sufficient.

Specimens relevant to vaginitis are best collected by swabbing the mucosa high in the vaginal canal under direct visualization (see Chap. 50, Infections of the Female Genital Tract). Cultures of the external vaginal orifice are not helpful. For diagnosis of trichomoniasis, the swabs should be placed in a small volume of sterile saline solution and sent directly to the laboratory. This material should be examined within 10 to 15 minutes because trichomonads lose their motility on standing, becoming very difficult to identify. *Trichomonas vaginalis* may be cultured by inoculating an appropriate medium; this is the most useful method for detecting asymptomatic carriers. Prostatic fluid or urethral discharge from the male may also be examined for trichomonads in the same way.

For the diagnosis of primary syphilis, fluid expressed from the base of the chancre is examine using dark-field microscopy (see Chap. 9, Microscopic Examinations, and Chap. 59, Syphilis). Vigorous scraping from the base of the chancre is imperative to obtain accurate results. Observation of both morphology and motion is essential to diagnosis; motion is seen only on immediate examination of warm material. The microscopic examination should be carried out in a darkened room immediately adjacent to the patient examination room, or the patient should be brought to the laboratory where the dark-field microscope is set up. Because the dark-field microscope must be properly aligned before it can be used, arrangements should be made before the specimen is collected. It may be possible to identify *Treponema pallidum* in dried smears prepared from primary chancres by using fluorescein-tagged antiserum. Thus, clinics unable to perform dark-field microscopy may prepare smears and simply mail them to central laboratories equipped to carry out fluorescence microscopy.

Chancroid (see Chap. 57, Chancroid) is difficult to diagnose by culture because the etiologic agent, *Haemophilus ducreyi,* is rather fastidious and is usually accompanied by a variety of other less fastidious, rapidly growing bacteria.

Granuloma inguinale (see Chap. 58, Granuloma Inguinale) is usually diagnosed by histologic demonstration of Donovan bodies in biopsy specimens. In practice, isolation of the etiologic agent is rarely attempted.

Urine

Voided urine is often contaminated by bacteria from the urethra and from the external genitalia (see Chap. 48, Urethritis and Cystitis, and Chap. 49 Bacterial Prostatitis and Recurrent Urinary Tract Infections). However, carefully collected, midstream-voided specimens generally contain fewer than 10,000 bacteria/ml, whereas with infection, the etiologic agent is normally present in numbers greater than 100,000/ml. This fact forms the basis for quantitative urine bacteriology, which is valid only when extreme caution is taken to minimize contamination during the collection procedure. Because of the inherent risk of infection following urethral catheterization, a clean-voided, midstream specimen, or urine aspirated directly from the urinary bladder via percutaneous suprapubic puncture (see Chap. 48, Urethritis and Cystitis) is preferred for examination.

The collection of clean-voided specimens must be supervised by an adequately trained individual. The foreskin of the male must be completely retracted before the glans penis is cleansed with sterile cotton balls or gauze sponges soaked in a mild detergent, such as benzalkonium chloride. In the female, the labia must be separated, exposing the urethral orifice so that the urethral area can be swabbed repeatedly over a 2- to 3-minute period with several changes of cotton balls or gauze sponges. This is followed by a thorough rinsing with warm, sterile water, which eliminates the possibility of contaminating the specimen with the detergent and helps to stimulate the patient's desire to urinate. With the labia still separated, the patient begins to void into a bedpan or commode. *Without stopping the stream,* after 20 ml to 25 ml has been passed, a specimen is caught in a sterile container as the urine passes through the air. The initial 20 ml to 25 ml washes out most of the bacteria resident in the urethra. It cannot be overemphasized that urine passed into a bedpan, regardless of preparation of patient or pan, is *not* suitable for culture. Ambulatory females should be encouraged to stand astride a bedpan placed on a chair while urinating. This will help to keep the labia separated, thus reducing the possibility of contamination with microorganisms of the external genitalia. Recumbent female patients must lie with knees bent and legs spread. After careful preparation, the labia should be held apart as the patient voids into a bedpan placed just below the patient's buttocks.

With infants or other patients who are unable to cooperate, plastic bags may be attached after careful preparation. The bags should then be watched so that the urine specimen can be collected immediately after it is voided. If the patient has not voided within 30 minutes after the collecting apparatus has been attached, it should be removed, the patient rescrubbed, and a new collection device attached.

When an indwelling catheter is in place, the draining tube should not be separated in order to collect a specimen, and the urine in the collection bag should not be utilized for culture. Rather, the catheter may be punctured with a needle, after being cleaned with an alcohol sponge, and urine aspirated directly into a syringe.

Because urine itself can serve as a culture medium, contaminating microorganisms will multiply if the urine is allowed to stand at room temperature, thus producing exceptionally large numbers of contaminants. For this reason, urine specimens must be processed in the laboratory within 30 minutes after collection. If this is not possible, the specimen may be refrigerated for as long as 4 to 6 hours with no significant change in bacteriuria. If transferred to sterile tubes containing buffered glyceroboric acid, most urine specimens may be held at room temperature for 12 to 24 hours without a significant change in the number of microorganisms (Table 10-5). However, the number of viable bacteria may be reduced upon standing in the refrigerator or in boric acid transport tubes if the patient is receiving antimicrobics or if the *p*H of the urine is extremely low or high. For that reason, all specimens should be cultured within 4 to 6 hours after collection; otherwise the degree of bacteriuria might be falsely reduced.

When the acid-fast bacilli are being sought in the urine, the first morning voiding should be collected in a sterile container, provided that at least 90 ml of urine is passed. Such fresh specimens are superior to 24-hour collections, which will be heavily contaminated with non-acid-fast bacteria that may survive the decontamination procedures used to recover acid-fast bacilli. At least three successive, daily specimens are required in order to rule out tuberculosis of the urinary tract. Because of the high frequency of saprophytic acid-fast bacilli in urine specimens, acid-fast smears are not routinely examined in most laboratories.

Lesions Involving Epithelium

Both a resident and transient microflora are potential contributors to specimens from lesions involving the epithelium, or specimens collected by incision or puncture of the skin. The transients are multitudinous in kinds, reflecting the continual exposure of the body surfaces to the variety of microorganisms present in the environment. Additional determinants include the personal hygiene of the individual and other local environmental conditions such as the amount of moisture of different areas of the body. Fortunately, healthy skin appears to have an effective self-disinfecting mechanism, which will result in the rapid disappearance of living microorganisms implanted on it.

The resident flora consists of only a few species of bacteria that seem to multiply freely in the skin and its appendages. In the sweat glands, aerobic *Staphylococcus epidermidis* and *Micrococcus* spp. are prominent, but in the sebaceous glands the anaerobic *Propionobacterium acnes* predominates. In most areas of the skin, the anaerobic flora outnumbers the aerobic flora of at least 10 to 1. External forces have little effect on the resident flora, and they persist even when the surface of the skin appears to be sterile. Sweating will result in a temporary increase in the number of staphylococci on the surface of the skin from the resident flora of the sweat glands.

The number of viable microorganisms of the transient flora can be reduced markedly by simply washing the skin or by applying an effective antiseptic. The composition of the transient flora actually re-

Table 10-5. *Survival of Microorganisms in Urine Samples Held at Room Temperature in Two Transport Systems, Compared to Refrigeration for 24 and 48 Hours*

Storage System and Sampling Interval†	Number of Viable Cells Recovered From Seeded Urine Samples* Containing									
						STREPTOCOCCUS			*STAPHYLOCOCCUS*	
	ESCHERICHIA COLI	*KLEBSIELLA* SPP.	*ENTEROBACTER* SPP.	*SERRATIA* SPP.	*PSEUDOMONAS* SPP.	*FAECALIS*	*VIRIDANS*	*PYOGENES*	*AUREUS*	*EPIDERMIDIS*
Refrigeration										
0 hours	2×10^4	7×10^3	2×10^4	4×10^4	4×10^4	6×10^4	4×10^4	1×10^4	5×10^4	3×10^4
24 hours	7×10^3	5×10^3	2×10^4	4×10^4	4×10^3	4×10^4	1×10^4	2×10^4	2×10^4	1×10^4
48 hours	1×10^3	$<1 \times 10^3$	1×10^4	3×10^4	$<1 \times 10^3$	2×10^4	5×10^3	3×10^3	1×10^4	3×10^3
Glyceroboric Acid ‡										
0 hours	2×10^4	6×10^3	1×10^4	2×10^4	2×10^4	1×10^4	3×10^3	1×10^4	2×10^4	4×10^4
24 hours	1×10^3	2×10^3	1×10^4	2×10^4	3×10^4	3×10^4	1×10^4	1×10^4	3×10^4	1×10^4
48 hours	1×10^3	$<1 \times 10^3$	1×10^4	2×10^4	$<1 \times 10^3$	1×10^4	1×10^3	$<1 \times 10^3$	1×10^4	3×10^3
Boric Acid §										
0 hours	1×10^4	7×10^3	2×10^4	4×10^4	1×10^4	2×10^4	4×10^4	8×10^3	3×10^4	4×10^4
24 hours	1×10^3	1×10^3	2×10^4	4×10^4	1×10^4	3×10^4	1×10^4	5×10^3	2×10^4	2×10^4
48 hours	$<1 \times 10^3$	$<1 \times 10^3$	3×10^3	1×10^4	$<1 \times 10^3$	1×10^4	1×10^3	1×10^4	3×10^3	3×10^3

*Sterile urine from five patients were pooled and aliquots seeded with different bacterial strains.

†Duplicate subcultures performed at 0, 24- and 48-hour intervals, using a 0.001 ml calibrated loop.

‡Urine Culture Kits: Becton Dickinson (Rutherford, NJ).

§Urine Specimen Kits: Sage Products, Inc. (Cary, IL).

flects the microorganisms within the person's immediate environment. Potential pathogens such as *S. aureus* are often found on the healthy skin of persons who carry staphylococci in their anterior nose, or who have infected lesions elsewhere on the body. Similarly, *S. pyogenes* can be recovered occasionally from the healthy skin, especially on individuals with streptococcal infections or those in close contact with infected individuals. Thus, microorganisms recovered from the intact skin immediately adjacent to a local infection often include the etiologic agent along with other potential pathogens unrelated to the infection. It also follows that the transient flora may serve as an important vehicle for transmission of infectious agents from one individual to another, especially if good personal hygiene is not practiced.

Although the skin cannot be completely sterilized with antiseptics, the transient flora can be removed or markedly reduced in numbers. If specimens are to be collected by excision, incision, or puncture through the epithelial layer, the surface of the skin most certainly should be prepared by treatment with an effective antiseptic. The number of contaminating microorganisms can be reduced but never completely eliminated. If the scalpel or needle happens to pass through one of the glands of the skin, the specimen will be contaminated with the resident flora of that appendage. It is for this reason that coagulase-negative staphylococci and anaerobic diphtheroids are the most common contaminants found in blood cultures.

Wounds

Pus obtained from previously undrained abscesses contains the etiologic agent in relatively large numbers, permitting microbiologic diagnosis by examining the pus collected after incision and drainage. However, contamination of such specimens with the patient's own transient skin flora undoubtedly gives rise to results that are difficult to interpret. At the time a closed abscess is to be incised and drained, the pus should be aspirated directly into a sterile syringe and sent to the laboratory for bacteriologic examination.

Deep, suppurative lesions often communicate with the surface of the body through fistulas or sinus tracts, and samples of the exudate or pus that drains out are often submitted for examination. Unfortunately, the microbial flora of the sinus tract is not always the actual cause of the underlying, deep lesion. Furthermore, deep abscesses are often caused by anaerobic microorganisms that may not survive even brief exposure to atmospheric oxygen, or they are readily overgrown with contaminating aerobic microorganisms.

In actinomycosis, the pus draining from the lesions often contains small macroscopic granules, frequently referred to as "sulfur granules." These granules actually are a mass of branching filaments with a peripheral zone of swollen bodies arranged radially. The color and size of these granules may vary considerably, but they are generally about 1 mm or less in diameter and are gray to yellow. If the pus is collected in a sterile tube containing water, after shaking, the granules sink to the bottom. A large volume of pus can be processed, yielding granules washed free of contaminating material. Microscopic and cultural techniques can then be applied. A draining sinus tract can be covered with several thicknesses of gauze that are left in place until saturated. Granules in the discharge are trapped within the first few layers of gauze and can be picked out for further identification.

When there are large areas of devitalized tissue—for example, extensive burns or decubiti—a variety of microorganisms will become implanted and will multiply in the superficial necrotic tissue. As systemically administered antimicrobics are unlikely to penetrate into such areas, topical application is often employed. Cultures obtained by swabbing from the surfaces of such lesions generally yield mixtures of bacteria that frequently change from day to day. Repeated culture and susceptibility testing will not only overtax the resources of the clinical laboratory but also may have little influence on the final outcome of the lesion. Such qualitative assessment is of potential value primarily for detecting invasive pathogens such as *Streptococcus pyogenes*, or toxinogenic bacteria such as *Corynebacterium diphtheriae*.

Quantitation of the bacterial load of necrotic material, e.g., burn wound eschar, appears to be useful. If the bacterial density is $\geqslant 10^4$/g, healing may be compromised; with $\geqslant 10^6$/g, bacteremia becomes increasingly probable.

Biopsy Material

Biopsies and other tissue specimens should be submitted for the cultural identification of microbial pathogens. The specimen should be cut in two immediately on collection. One portion should be placed in a clean sterile tube or bottle without formalin or other fixatives, and the other portion should be fixed in neutral formalin so that it can be processed for histologic examination. For culture, tissues should be thoroughly macerated and finely ground to liberate any microorganisms that may be within the tissues. Conical, ground-glass tissue grinders, driven by a constant, slow-speed electric motor, are suitable. Such devices must be used in a contagion hood because infectious aerosols may form during grinding. The laboratory procedures should be suitable for recovery of the wide variety of pathogens that could be involved as etiologic agents and must include bacteria (acid-fast and nonacid-fast), fungi, and viruses. Viral antigens may be demonstrated directly within tissue sections by fluorescent antibody methods, but relatively few clinical laboratories have access to the large number of specific antiserums needed to carry out such procedures.

Exudates and Transudates

Fluids that collect in pericardial, pleural, peritoneal, and synovial spaces must be aspirated with the utmost precaution to avoid introducing microorganisms and to avoid contamination of the specimen. The material should be placed in a sterile tube or bottle and examined as soon as possible. A sterile anticoagulant such as sodium oxalate or heparin is useful to help prevent the formation of clots, which might trap microbial pathogens or interfere with chemical and cytologic examinations to be performed on the same specimen. Frankly purulent fluid should be examined directly without centrifugation because stained smears will usually reveal the etiologic agent—to be identified definitively by culturing on appropriate mediums. If the fluid is transparent or hazy, it should be centrifuged and the sediment examined using stained smears and cultures.

Cerebrospinal Fluid

Because irreversible damage to the central nervous system can evolve rapidly in acute bacterial meningitis, appropriate therapy must be initiated immediately; thus, rapid, precise diagnosis is of the utmost importance. The differentiation of acute purulent bacterial meningitis from nonbacterial meningitis is the first diagnostic goal. The presumptive identification of the bacterial pathogen is next in importance because the antimicrobial chemotherapeutic agent to be used depends on the pathogen involved. The collection and examination of the cerebrospinal fluid (CSF) are described in Chapter 119, Acute Bacterial Meningitis. Generally, in meningitis caused by pyogenic bacteria, microorganisms are readily found in Gram-stained smears; also, there is a polymorphonuclear pleocytosis, an increased concentration of protein, and a markedly decreased concentration of glucose. In tuberculous or fungal meningitides, microorganisms are difficult to demonstrate in smears, lymphocytes predominate, the glucose is moderately reduced, and the protein is elevated in concentration.

Because of the crucial need for information, the CSF should not be stored. If delay in examination is absolutely unavoidable, the CSF should *not* be refrigerated. *Neisseria meningitidis* are particularly fragile and will die off in the cold. Moreover, some bacteria will replicate in CSF at 37°C so that storage in the incubator is preferable when examination must be delayed. However, if the patient was given antimicrobics before the CSF was collected, bacteria may die off in storage.

Exhaustive microscopic examination of gram-stained smears will most often reveal gram-negative intracellular diplococci (*N. meningitidis*); grampositive, lance-shaped diplococci (*Streptococcus pneumoniae*); plump gram-negative bacilli (*Escherichia coli*); or small gram-negative bacilli (*Haemophilus influenzae*). Because bacteria are usually not abundant in smears, each slide must be examined at least 30 minutes before it is reported as negative. Because of the variety of artifacts that can resemble bacteria, a great deal of experience is required to obtain reliable results. Information from stained smears must be correlated with the known frequency of occurrence of particular bacterial pathogens as a function of age of the patient and of predisposing factors—for example, the presence of an atrioventricular shunt predisposes to infection with *Staphylococcus epidermidis*. When certain kinds of bacteria are present in large numbers in the CSF, serodiagnosis can be carried out directly by means of the quelling reaction (group A and C *N. meningitidis, S. pneumoniae, H. influenzae*), precipitin test (as for quelling and *Cryptococcus neoformans*), fluorescence microscopy, and counterimmunoelectrophoresis. Unfortunately, only large hospital laboratories can justify the maintenance of the stocks of antisera and control bacteria requisite to reliable serodiagnosis. In all cases, definitive diagnosis must be based on cultures. Although strict aseptic technique is followed in collecting the CSF, skin contaminants and air contaminants are occasionally introduced, especially when difficulty is encountered in performing the lumbar puncture. This should be kept in mind when interpreting positive cultures that contain microorganisms not normally associated with bacterial meningitis.

Occasionally, a diagnosis of tuberculous meningitis can be supported by examining smears stained by an acid-fast technique, but the number of bacilli is often quite small and negative results are not uncommon. If a pellicle forms on the CSF, bacilli are likely to be trapped in it. Commonly, there is no pellicle, and smears should be built of several layers of the specimen deposited in an area of less than 1 sq cm by allowing 1 drop to dry before superimposing the next. In this way it is possible to carry out microscopic examination of the solids from a large volume of CSF. Although the CSF is usually centrifuged, the fatty tubercle bacilli may be sedimented or may remain in the supernatant liquid. Consequently, the entire specimen should be examined, some by smear, the remainder by culture. The larger the specimen, the better the chance of recovering the pathogen.

Of the fungi that cause meningitis, *C. neoformans* is easiest to recognize (see Chap. 120, Cryptococcosis). The characteristic capsules are readily demonstrated by microscopic examination of wet mounts of CSF mixed with diluted India ink (see Chap. 9, Microscopic Examination). During therapy, intact cryptococci may be observed in India ink preparations although cultures may be negative. In the absence of identifiable yeast cells, cryptococcal antigen can be identified by appropriate serologic techniques. By following the titers of cryptococcal antigens and antibodies in the spinal fluid, the progress of the disease can be monitored during therapy.

The diagnosis of coccidioidal meninigitis is rarely confirmed by the examination of smears or by cultures of the spinal fluid—that is, spherules are rarely found in the CSF (see Chap. 41, Coccidioidomycosis). Detection of antibodies in the serum and spinal fluid is helpful, but few clinical laboratories are equipped to perform such tests.

Viral meningoencephalitis (see Chap. 118, Viral Meningitis), is often diagnosed by ruling out other etiologic agents. Many of the viral agents involved can be cultured from the spinal fluid, but the procedures are rather expensive and time consuming. Because of the nature of the work involved, the final recovery of the virus will be delayed well beyond the point where the information can help in the treatment of the individual patient. For these reasons, virus isolations are rarely attempted in clinical laboratories, but rather the specimen is usually forwarded to a research or public health center equipped to perform the necessary tests. Several milliliters of CSF should be collected in a sterile, tightly sealed tube and immediately frozen, preferably at −70°C. The specimen can then be shipped in an insulated container packed with enough Dry Ice to keep the CSF frozen. Serum collected at the acute and convalescent stages of illness must also be submitted; if virus is not isolated, a rise of titer of antibodies will be the sole clue to etiology.

Blood

With the febrile patient who is severely ill and the patient suspected of having infective endocarditis or other intravascular infections, culture of the blood is one of the most important procedures that can be performed. The isolation and identification of an infectious agent from the blood not only have obvious diagnostic significance, but also provide an invaluable guide for selecting the most appropriate antimicrobial agent for therapy. In healthy individuals, transient bacteremias may occur occasionally when bacteria from the oral cavity or gastrointestinal tract enter the blood stream. Normally, such bacteria are quickly removed by the reticuloendothelial system, and blood from healthy individuals is ordinarily sterile. However, specimens of blood are not infrequently contaminated from exogenous sources during collection and inoculation into culture mediums. The most common contaminants are *S. epidermidis, Micrococcus* spp., and anaerobic diphtheroids, presumably from the flora resident on the patient's skin. Previously, blood cultures containing such bacteria could be disregarded automatically as being contaminated. Now, however, there are many patients with compromised host defenses in whom serious, life-threatening infections are caused by such "nonpathogenic" microorganisms. Accordingly, any positive blood culture has serious diagnostic implications, and the blood must be collected with every possible precaution. Preparation of the skin with an ineffective antiseptic such as aqueous benzalkonium chloride is a common source of error. The most effective preparation involves degreasing the skin before application of 2% tincture of iodine, or an iodophor preparation, keeping the skin wet continuously for at least 2 minutes before the venipuncture is performed. Parameters of thyroid function may be disturbed, and there is a small but definite risk of serious skin reactions.

1. Select the most appropriate site for venipuncture and cleanse and degrease the skin with 70% to 95% isopropanol (or 70% ethanol) by scrubbing with two separate sponges. Use additional sponges if visible dirt is not removed with the first scrubbing.
2. With a sterile cotton-tipped applicator, apply 2% tincture of iodine or iodophor preparation to the venipuncture site, painting a concentric pattern beginning at the site of the proposed skin puncture. Keep the puncture site wet for approximately 2 minutes using a sterile sponge soaked with the iodine solution.

3. Apply a tourniquet and relocate the vein to be punctured but *do not touch* the skin of the proposed site of needle entry. Remove the iodine with either 70% ethanol or 70% to 95% isopropanol, following the pattern of application.
4. Perform the venipuncture and withdraw 12 ml to 15 ml of blood into a sterile syringe.
5. The outer portion of the needle is presumed to be contaminated with bacteria from deep within the skin. It should therefore be removed from the syringe and carefully replaced with a clean, sterile needle.
6. Inject an amount of blood equal to 10% of the volume of two kinds of broth culture mediums, being careful to avoid contamination of the rubber diaphragm on the tops of the bottles.
7. Gently invert both bottles to ensure adequate mixing and anticoagulation.
8. Carefully remove all traces of iodine left on the patient's skin by wiping with alcohol sponges.
9. One bottle is vented to replace the residual vacuum with air so that strict aerobes such as *Pseudomonas* spp. can grow. This is done by puncturing the diaphragm with a sterile, cotton-plugged needle, allowing the pressure to equilibrate. The other bottle is not vented, and is suitable for the recovery of anaerobes. The bottles are placed in the incubator and examined frequently for 7 to 14 days; at least two subcultures are routinely made to detect microorganisms that may be present without yielding visible growth.

If the patient is receiving a penicillin, adding penicillinase to the culture medium may inactivate the penicillin in the patient's blood. However, there is little published work that unequivocally demonstrates the value of such a procedure. The patient's blood is diluted at least tenfold when added to a broth medium, and thus the concentration of penicillin is markedly reduced, perhaps sufficiently to preclude inhibition of any viable bacteria present in the blood when the specimen was collected. Because a low concentration of penicillin might be inhibitory, the use of penicillinase is advocated, although the clinical importance of such very susceptible bacteria may be questioned. However, the actual concentration of penicillins in the blood at the time of culture is usually not known and may be very high. Moreover, the presence of any viable bacteria, even if very susceptible, is of great importance in a disease such as bacterial endocarditis. Adding penicillinase, however, carries the risk of contamination, adds to the cost of culturing, and may be pointless if other antimicrobial agents were used in therapy.

In summary, the routine addition of penicillinase to all blood cultures on the assumption that the patient may have been exposed to penicillin before the blood was collected is not justified. Blood should, of course, be cultured before antimicrobics are given. However, some situations require the culturing of blood during penicillin therapy. In such cases, blood should be collected when the concentration of penicillin would be expected to be lowest. Penicillinase should be added immediately after the blood is inoculated, using strict aseptic precautions. A second aliquot of the penicillinase solution should be separately inoculated into broth to document the sterility of the preparation.

The minimum number of bacterial cells that can initiate growth is a function of the volume of the inoculum of blood and the culture medium that is used. Concentration of microorganisms by sedimentation or filtration is possible but is not practical in a large, busy clinical laboratory.

The culture medium should be capable of supporting rapid growth of all possible pathogens, including the more fastidious genera and the various anaerobes. No single medium fulfills all these requirements. In addition, for quality control purposes, at least two kinds of medium should be used. The broadly nutritive Columbia broth formulation is suitable for aerobic and microaerophilic microorganisms; the highly reducing thioglycolate broth is often used for recovery of strict anerobes.

For the culture of blood from pediatric patients, mediums may be supplemented with peptic digest of blood to supply growth factors required by *Haemophilus influenzae*. Because this supplement must be added aseptically to the sterile broth, another possibility for contamination is provided. Ideally, all blood cultures should be incubated in the presence of 5% to 10% ambient CO_2. If *Brucella abortus* is sought, CO_2 is required, and the laboratory should incubate and observe such cultures for at least 21 days before reporting negative results. The culture mediums selected for use should be put up in bottles or flasks fitted with screw caps with wide skirts that will minimize the possibility of contamination.

Microorganisms may grow undetected in clots or may fail to grow when trapped within clots. Clearly, an anticoagulant is necessary. Sodium citrate has been used but is said to inhibit the growth of certain microorganisms. Sodium polyanethol sulfonate is heat-stable; in a concentration of 25 mg to 50 mg /100 ml of medium, it is an effective anticoagulant that also inactivates complement and leukocytes without exerting adverse effects on fungi and most bacteria.

Growth of bacteria in blood cultures is usually apparent within the first 24 hours of incubation. However, some bacteria, particularly anaerobes and fungi, take longer to grow out. Therefore, blood cultures must be incubated for 7 to 14 days before being reported as negative. Antimicrobial therapy cannot be withheld during this time; as long as an adequate number of cultures has been collected beforehand, therapy should be started.

The number of specimens and the interval between venipunctures depend on the clinical situation. In acute septic shock, two or three separate venipunctures performed over a short period generally suffice. However, in chronically ill patients who may have infective endocarditis, cultures taken at 6- to 8-hour intervals for 2 to 3 days may be necessary. In proven bacterial endocarditis, 90% to 95% of the positive blood cultures will be obtained in the first five or six specimens. Special efforts to achieve etiologic diagnosis in the remaining 5% to 10% of patients are justified because the rational design of therapy requires study of the causative agent *in vitro*.

The significance of a microorganism recovered from a blood culture is not always easy to determine because occasional contamination is practically impossible to avoid. In general, contamination should be suspected if (1) a common component of the skin flora is recovered and the clinical history of the patient does not warrant consideration of a "nonpathogen" as being significant; (2) a mixture of several kinds of bacteria is recovered; and (3) growth is found in only one of the several specimens from separate venipunctures. Accordingly, blood should always be collected from two or three separate venipunctures, and each sample should be inoculated into two broth mediums and a simple pour plate.

Spirochetal infections, such as leptospirosis or relapsing fever, can occasionally be diagnosed by phase-contrast examination of anticoagulated blood. Stained smears of the blood are also of value in these spirochetoses, as well as in malaria and trypanosomiasis. Inoculation of blood into experimental animals is also indicated for laboratory diagnosis of these infectious agents.

Viruses, Chlamydias, and Rickettsias

The most appropriate specimens for isolation of viral, chlamydial, or rickettsial agents depend on the nature of the illnesses. Success in isolation depends largely on the care with which the specimen is collected and transported to the laboratory. In general, the material should be collected as early as possible in the acute phase of the disease, because these agents tend to disappear relatively rapidly after the onset of symptoms. Specimens should be collected so as to minimize bacterial contamination because tissue cultures, embryonated eggs, and laboratory animals will be inoculated. Vesicle fluid is preferably collected in a syringe or capillary pipet and immediately diluted in an equal volume of skim milk or tissue culture medium. All specimens should be frozen and stored at $-70°C$ until cultures are initiated. If Dry Ice is used, care should be taken to enclose the specimen in hermetically sealed glass vials to avoid toxic accumulation of CO_2.

Because a major effort is expended in isolating and identifying viral, chlamydial, and rickettsial agents, the laboratory deserves full and complete cooperation in obtaining the specimens and clinical information. The latter is quite critical because the culture system to be inoculated depends primarily on the particular agent that is suspected. The all too common throat swab for "virus culture" can only be roundly condemned.

Acute and convalescent serums should be routinely obtained whenever specimens are submitted for isolation. A rise in titer of antibody specific for an isolate is proof of etiologic relationship.

Bibliography

Books

BARRY AL, SMITH PB, TURCK M: ASM Cumitech No. 2, Laboratory Diagnosis of Urinary Tract Infections. Washington DC, American Society for Microbiology, 1975. 8 pp.

BARTLETT RC: Medical Microbiology: Quality, Cost and Clinical Relevance. New York, John Wiley & Sons, 1974. pp 24–31.

BARTLETT RC, ELLNER PD, WASHINGTON JA: ASM Cumitech No. 1, Blood Cultures. Washington DC, American Society for Microbiology, 1975. 6 pp.

FINEGOLD SM, SHEPHERD WE, SPAULDING EH: ASM Cumitech No. 5, Practical Anaerobic Bacteriology. Washington DC, American Society for Microbiology, 1977. 14 pp.

ISENBERG HD, SCHOENKNECHT FD, VON GRAVENITZ A: ASM Cumitech No. 9, Collection and Processing of Bacteriological Specimens. Washington DC, American Society for Microbiology, 1979. 22 pp.

JAWETZ E: Diagnostic Tests in Infections. Disease-A-Month. Chicago, Year Book Medical Publishers, August, 1963. 39 pp.

ROSEBURY T: Microorganisms Indigenous to Man. New York, McGraw–Hill, 1962. 435 pp.

SMITH DT, MICROBIOLOGIC ECOLOGY AND FLORA OF THE HUMAN BODY. IN SMITH DT, CONNANT NF, WILLETT HP (EDS): Zinsser's Microbiology, 14th ed, pp 185–195. New York, Appleton–Century Crofts, 1968

SONNENWIRTH AC (ed): Bacteremia; Laboratory and Clinical Aspects. Springfield, Charles C Thomas, 1973. 106 pp.

WILSON GS, MILES AA: The normal distribution of bacterial flora of the human body. In Topley and Wilson's Principles of Bacteriology, 5th ed. London, Edward Arnold Co. pp. 246–248.

Journals

AMIES CR: A modified formula for the preparation of Stuart's transport medium. Can J Public Health 58:296–330, 1967

BARRETT-CONNOR E: The nonvalue of sputum culture in the diagnosis of pneumococcal pneumonia. Am Rev Respir Dis 103:845–848, 1971

BARRY AL, FAY GD, SAUER RL: Efficiency of a transport medium for the recovery of aerobic and anaerobic bacteria from applicator swabs. Appl Microbiol 24:31–33, 1972

HOEPRICH PD: Etiologic diagnosis of lower respiratory tract infections. Calif Med 112:1–8, 1970

MURRAY PR, WASHINGTON JA: Microscopic and bacteriologic analysis of expecterated sputum. Mayo Clin Proc 50:339–344, 1975

MURRAY PR, HAMPTON CH: Recovery of pathogenic bacteria from cerebrospinal fluid. J Clin Microbiol 12:554–557, 1980

STUART RD, TOSHACK SR, PATSULA M: The problem of transport of specimens for culture of gonococci. Can J Public Health 45:73–83, 1954

YRIOS JW, BALISH E, HELSTAD A, FIELD C, INHORN S: Survival of anaerobic and aerobic bacteria on cotton swabs in three transport systems. J Clin Microbiol 1:196–200, 1975

PHILIP D. MARSDEN

11 Diagnostic Methods for Protozoa and Helminths

Morphologic examination is quintessential to the etiologic diagnosis of diseases caused by protozoa and helminths. For the correct diagnosis of such diseases, the physician must be as competent in using the microscope and laboratory procedures to find parasites as in defining and interpreting clinical manifestations at the bedside. As in all infectious diseases, a firm diagnosis rests on finding the infectious agent.

Although a variety of procedures may be employed, diagnostic success is directly proportional to the amount of time and care spent in examining specimens. Serologic tests are at best only secondary aids in diagnosis because they indicate exposure to antigens and give little clue to the actual state of the disease. Culture methods are of limited value in the diagnosis of protozoal and helminthic diseases.

Protozoa

Blood and Tissue Protozoa

Of the Romanowsky stains (see Chap. 9, Microscopic Examinations), there is little to choose between the Wright, Giemsa, and Leishman formulations for staining protozoa found in the blood. Both thin and thick films should be prepared.

Thin films are made in the same way as those that are used for studying blood cell morphology. They must be fixed with methyl alcohol before staining. They are adequate when parasitemia is heavy and are required for species identification.

Thick films are useful when protozoa are few. To make a thick film, a drop of blood is spread with the corner of another slide, using a circular motion. It should be possible to read newsprint through the resultant film (see Fig. 145-6). After drying in air, the film is stained directly without prior fixation, because one of the actions of the aqueous stain is to dehemoglobinize the film. Only leukocytes, platelets, and parasites remain discrete in a field that was originally many red cells thick.

Both thin and thick films can be stained with aqueous Giemsa stain (see Chap. 9, Microscopic Examinations). The chromatin of protozoa stains reddish purple; the cytoplasm, a gray blue. The pH must be stabilized at 7.2 for demonstration of Schüffner's dots and other intracellular inclusions.

MALARIA

Malaria films illustrate the importance of always looking at a population of parasites before deciding on the species present. Also, since many films have uneven staining characteristics, selected portions of the slide should be examined. For example, in films of blood from a Peace Corps worker from West Africa, small, thin, hairlike rings were seen with double chromatin dots, and there was multiple parasitization of cells—undoubtedly *Plasmodium falciparum.* However, a larger trophozoite was also seen, which contained a much larger chromatin dot. Further search in another part of the film revealed Schüffner's dots associated with this large trophozoite. Several schizonts were subsequently found with 8 to 12 merozoites. Thus, the diagnosis was a double infection with *P. falciparum* and *Plasmodium ovale* (only ring forms and gametocytes are usually found in the peripheral blood in malaria caused by *P. falciparum,* but all forms are present in malaria caused by the other three species). Such multiple infections are uncommon in nonimmune persons, but detection has an important bearing on therapy (see Chap. 145, Malaria). If initial blood films are negative, films should be taken again during a febrile attack. Parasites will be present if the fever is caused by malaria. In immune persons, repeated blood film examinations may be needed to detect parasites; when found, they are not necessarily responsible for symptoms. The indirect malarial fluorescent antibody test reflects exposure to malaria antigens. The test may be useful in clinical practice as an indicator of past exposure or for screening potential blood donors. Neither culture of human malaria parasites nor animal inoculations are feasible routine procedures.

TRYPANOSOMIASIS

Trypomastigotes (trypanosomes) are rarely present in large numbers in the blood of humans (see Chap. 136, American Trypanosomiasis, and Chap. 130, African Trypanosomiasis). Nevertheless, fresh liquid blood should always be examined because movement of the morphologically distinct trypomastigotes disturbs the red blood cells, making the protozoa easy to see. Although various methods for concentrating trypomastigotes in the blood have been described, none has been generally adopted. A simple, useful technique involves examination of the layer of leukocytes that separates and lies between the erythrocytes and serum on centrifugation of blood; thick and thin films should be prepared and stained (Giemsa). Observing the kinetoplast, nucleus, and flagellum enables species identification, a matter of some importance in areas of South America, where *Trypanosoma rangeli* and *Trypanosoma cruzi* coexist (see Chap. 136, American Trypanosomiasis).

In African trypanosomiasis (see Chap. 130, African Trypanosomiasis), exudate from lymph nodes and cerebrospinal fluid (CSF) can be stained or examined directly for trypomastigotes. High levels (16 times normal) of 19S immunoglobulins (IgM) are found in the serum and CSF in this infection and are of diagnostic value. An indirect fluorescent antibody test has been developed that is sensitive, specific, and suitable for the early detection of CNS involvement. Culture of African trypanosomes is too difficult for routine use, but animal (rats) inoculation may be successful with *Trypanosoma rhodesiense.*

Trypanosoma cruzi may be cultured on Novy–MacNeal–Nicolle (NNN) medium (a saline agar with 10% defibrinated rabbit blood), especially in acute infections in which mouse inoculations are usually positive. In chronic infections, the serology and xenodiagnosis are most helpful. Recently, fluorescent antibody and indirect hemagglutination tests have been developed. However, the complement fixation test is still widely used, although there are difficulties in its standardization. A positive test is said to indicate active disease; however, many immunologists recommend the use of all three tests on the same specimen. Serologic test results should be confirmed by a reference laboratory. Xenodiagnosis is positive in 20% to 40% of patients with a positive serology. Clean reduviid bugs (usually *Triatoma infestans* or *Rhodnius prolixus*) are allowed to feed on the patient; 30 days after feeding, live flagellates are sought in wet mounts prepared from feces dejected by bugs that had fed on patients with undetectable parasitemia.

LEISHMANIASIS

For diagnosis of cutaneous leishmaniasis, aspirates from the base of the sore are prepared with Giemsa stain. Usually, the longer the history of the lesion, the more difficult it is to find the protozoa. A skin test using an extract of cultured flagellates (Montenegro test) is frequently positive in cutaneous and mucocutaneous leishmaniasis. In visceral leishmaniasis, bone marrow or splenic aspirates should be examined for amastigotes. All amastigotes look alike; for a firm diagnosis a nucleus and a rodshaped kinetoplast should be clearly seen in an oval protozoan measuring about 1.5 μm in length (see Chap. 147, Leishmaniasis).

Leishmania spp. from all sources can be cultured on NNN medium. The promastigotes develop in the water of condensation after 1 to 6 weeks, depending on the density of the inoculum; cultures should be examined weekly. Hamsters are susceptible to cutaneous and visceral leishmaniasis but take months to develop lesions. Material containing *Leishmania donovani* should be injected intraperitoneally. Material from cutaneous and mucocutaneous leishmaniasis should be injected into the nose and feet of the hamster. Amastigotes can be recognized in formalin-fixed biopsy specimens (liver or skin) but are more difficult to identify than in Giemsa-stained smears.

TOXOPLASMOSIS AND PNEUMOCYSTOSIS

Toxoplasma gondii are best isolated by inoculating infected tissues into hypercorticoid mice with subsequent examination of the peritoneal exudate. Usually, the diagnosis depends on the demonstration of significant titers of antibody by the dye test, fluorescent antibody test, or complement fixation test (see Chap. 129, Toxoplasmosis). *Pneumocystis carinii* can be seen in Giemsa-stained smears of lung biopsies or on silver staining of such tissue (see Chap. 45, Pneumocystosis). A serologic test using pneumocystis-infected lung as antigen is under investigation.

ENTERIC PROTOZOA

The most effective examination for trophozoites of *Entamoeba histolytica, Balantidium coli,* and motile flagellates (see Chap. 66, Amebiasis, and Chap. 67, Nonamebic Protozoal Enteritides) involves the microscopic study of a drop of warm, fresh feces diluted with buffered saline. When there is diarrhea, and particularly if blood and mucus are present, amebic trophozoites may be found. On standing, motility is soon lost, and the trophozoites begin to disintegrate. If immediate examination is not possible, a small portion of the specimen should be preserved in polyvinyl alcohol (PVA) fixative by adding one part of feces to three parts of fixative, either in a vial or directly on a slide. Fixed specimens are preserved for months and can be stained for examination at any time. However, the diagnostically useful active motility of trophozoites is lost, because it can only be observed in saline wet mounts prepared from a fresh specimen.

Concentration destroys trophozoites but should be used to detect cysts. The following formalin–either concentration technique is satisfactory in providing a concentration of more than 20 times:

1. Emulsify 1 g to 2 g feces in 7 ml to 10 ml 10% formalin–saline solution. Strain through a mesh gauze (40 mesh) into a centrifuge tube.
2. Add 3 ml ether and shake vigorously for 1 min.
3. Centrifuge, regulating acceleration so that 2000 rpm is attained in 2 min, then turn off.
4. Four layers are apparent in the tube: ether at the top, stained yellow with fat; a plug of vegetable debris; formalin solution; and sediment. The debris is loosened with a swab stick at the interface between the two liquids. The supernatant is poured off, andd the inside of the tube is wiped clean. The deposit is suspended and examined microscopically.

The number of specimens of feces that should be examined varies according to the clinical situation. Less than half of all infections with *E. histolytica* will be discovered if only one specimen is examined; 90% accuracy can be obtained if six or more specimens are properly examined. Generally, two or three specimens per day, followed by one or two purged specimens, are required to rule out the presence of amebas. In the absence of diarrhea, a saline cathartic (buffered phosphate soda or sodium sulfate) should be given, and two or three specimens should be sent to the laboratory for immediate examination. Although administering a cathartic may increase the number of positive examinations, postpurge specimens will be negative; thus, two or three stools should be examined before purging the patient. In addition, trophozoites may be destroyed and cysts may be distorted in specimens containing antidiarrheal medications (bismuth, kaolin), nonabsorbable antacids, antimicrobics (sulfonamides, antiprotozoal drugs), barium sulfate or other heavy metal compounds, oils, magnesium hydroxide, and ingredients of enemas such as tapwater, soap irritants, and hypertonic solutions. Other diagnostic procedures should be postponed until enteric protozoal infection has been ruled out.

Cultivaton of fecal protozoa is time consuming and impractical, either for routine work or for survey purposes, but a variety of mediums are available. The Cleveland–Colliers formula (liver infusion agar with a saline–horse serum overlay and added rice starch) is suitable. Such cultures are maintained at 37°C and examined after 24 and 48 hours for trophozoites. Permanent mounts of pathogenic protozoa stained with iron–hemotoxylin are useful for species identification and as a permanent record. Because preparation is time consuming few laboratories attempt it routinely.

Serologic tests aid in the diagnosis of invasive, extraintestinal amebiasis, as in liver abscess. These tests include indirect hemagglutination, indirect fluorescent antibody, complement fixation, and gel diffusion. Improved, bacteria-free antigens have recently become available.

Helminths

In the invasive stages of helminthic infections, or when the helminths remain in close contact with the host tissue, eosinophilia is often present. Infections with helminths are usually diagnosed by detecting the eggs or larvae produced, because these are specific in size, morphology, and location (blood, subcutaneous tissue, stool, or urine). Some indication of the number of adult worms that are present can be derived from the number of eggs or larvae.

Blood and Tissue Helminths

TRICHINOSIS

Once the larvae of *Trichinella spiralis* have settled in the muscles, the best diagnostic procedure is biopsy of either the gastrocnemius or deltoid muscle. The specimen can be crushed between two slides to reveal the encysted larvae, or it can be digested overnight in pepsin and dilute hydrochloric acid, and the larvae recovered by sedimentation in a tube. A month after onset of the infection, either the complement fixation test or the bentonite flocculation test is a reliable diagnostic aid (see Chap. 150, Trichinosis).

FILARIAE

The appearance of the guinea worm presents little difficulty in diagnosis. Living, coiled embryos can be observed in the uterine discharge following the application of water (see Chap. 112, Cutaneous Filariasis).

Examination of a fresh drop of blood under the low-power objective will reveal considerable agitation of the blood corpuscles by the relatively large microfilariae (200 μm to 300 μm). However, the specific morphology of the five common blood microfilariae of man—*Loa loa, Wuchereria bancrofti, Brugia malayi, Dipetalonema perstans,* and *Mansonella ozzardi* (see Chap. 112, Cutaneous Filariasis)—can only be recognized by staining to reveal the sheath and nuclei. Giemsa stain can be used, but the sheath stains better with Delafield's hematoxylin or Mayer's acid hemalum. *Dipetalonema perstans* and *M. ozzardi* are smaller than the other three microfilariae and are unsheathed. It is doubtful that they cause disease in humans. The time of day the blood is obtained for examination is important in view of the different periodicities of the different filariae. In parts of West Africa, multiple infections occur with *L. loa, W. bancrofti, D. perstans,* and *Onchocerca volvulus.* To concentrate microfilariae, 1 ml blood can be laked in 9 ml 1% formalin and the deposit examined after centrifugation. Even more effective is collecting microfilariae on a clear plastic filter (5 μm average pore size) followed by staining and microscopic examination. When 5 ml blood is filtered, there is a gain in sensitivity sufficient to obviate the need for nocturnal specimens.

The two filariae that involve the subcutaneous tissues —*O. volvulus* and *Dipetalonema streptocerca*— are detected by finding microfilariae in skin snips. A small coneshaped fold of skin is raised by inserting a pin into the epidermis, and this is cut off with a scalpel or razor blade. The snip itself is bloodless, avoiding the possibility of contamination with coexistent blood microfilariae. Snips should be taken from skin rashes or sites of irritation. Six snips are usually taken, two each from the shoulders, buttocks, and shins. Infection with *D. streptocerca* is quite uncommon and is readily recognized by the crooked tail of this microfilaria.

ENTERIC HELMINTHS

Usually, enteric helminths are recognized by their eggs (see Chap. 68, Intestinal Nematodiasis; Chap. 69, Intestinal Cestodiasis; Chap. 80, Liver Fluke Infection; and Chap. 81, Schistosomiasis). Exceptions to this rule are the larvae of *Strongyloides stercoralis* and segments of tapeworms. Because the egg output for most enteric helminths is relatively large, eggs are often detected on a direct smear. The formalin–ether method of concentration should also be used for concentrating helminth eggs. However, certain eggs, such as infertile ascaris and schistosoma eggs, do not concentrate as well as hookworm, trichuris, and fertile ascaris eggs.

It is important to quantitate the output of helminth ova in the feces because this indicates the worm load, which in turn is related to symptoms. Kato's thick smear technique has been shown to be adequate as a quantitation technique for the diagnostic laboratory. A smear of 50 mg feces is cleared with glycerin, and all the eggs on the slide are counted. Other methods for estimating worm load for specific helminths include filtering the feces for schistosoma eggs or diluting a weighed portion of feces before counting the eggs in an aliquot. Stoll's method is used mainly for hookworm: 3 g feces is emulsified in a special flask in 42 ml water or 0.1 N sodium hydroxide (to soften hard lumps). After standing, shaking with glass beads produces a uniform fine emulsion; 0.15 ml (equivalent to 0.01 g feces) is then pipetted onto a glass slide, and all the eggs are counted. From the number of eggs per gram of feces, the total quantity of feces, the egg output per female worm, and the sex ratio of the species population, it is possible to calculate the approximate worm load.

Certain enteric helminths call for special diagnostic techniques. Cestode segments may be stained with India ink or eosin and crushed between two slides to enable identification based on the number of uterine branches.

The eggs of *Enterobius vermicularis* are often successfully collected on gummed cellophane tape. A short piece of tape is applied to a glass slide or a wooden tongue depressor, sticky side out. Early in the morning, the tape is applied, adhesive side down, to the unwashed area where the anal canal joins the perianal skin. The tape is then transferred, sticky side down, to a clean glass slide, which is labeled and then sent to the laboratory for microscopic examination. In the laboratory, a few drops of xylene under the tape removes air bubbles and dissolves artifacts that may resemble pinworm eggs. Somewhat more satisfactory results can be obtained using special anal swabs coated with a warm, melted mixture of petrolatum and paraffin (4:1) and placed in sterile culture tubes. These prepared swabs are given to the patient with instructions to brush the swab lightly over the skin surrounding the anus and then to insert the swab about one-quarter inch into the anus. One swab should be used on each of two consecutive mornings upon awakening, before the child arises from bed. Both swabs are then brought to the laboratory for examination. The tubes are filled with a small amount of xylene and, after a few minutes standing, the petrolatum–paraffin mixture will dissolve. The swabs are then discarded, the tubes are centrifuged, and the sediment is examined for ova. Because the material has been concentrated, the yield of positive examinations is improved. In addition, the anal swab eliminates the discomfort that may result from the use of cellophane tape and reduces the possibility of infecting personnel who handle the specimens.

Schistosoma eggs may be detected in biopsied specimens of rectal mucosa even though they cannot be found in the feces. Six superficial biopsies should be taken and examined for eggs after crushing between two slides (see Chap. 81, Schistosomiasis).

Strongyloides stercoralis may be very difficult to detect because the number of larvae in the feces is quite variable. The Baermann funnel technique is helpful. A portion of the fecal specimen is placed on a wire gauze just touching the surface of the water (at 45°C) in a large funnel. The larvae pass into the water and collect at the bottom of the funnel. After an hour or more, the lower 10 ml water is centrifuged and the sediment is examined for larvae.

Filter paper culture is useful for both strongyloids and hookworms. Fecal matter is smeared at one end of a filter paper strip, and the clean end is dipped into a little water in a test tube. Larvae accumulate in the water and can be identified.

Other Helminths

For helminth eggs and larvae in the sputum, mix equal volumes of sputum and 3% sodium hydroxide, centrifuge at high speed, and examine a wet mount of the sediment. To examine urine for eggs of *Schistosoma haematobium,* a 24-hour collection should be left undisturbed for several hours before the bottom 20 ml is removed and centrifuged. In this way, a very light infection can be detected. With heavy infections, a calculation of egg output can be made after counting the eggs in a known volume of urine (see Chap. 81, Schistosomiasis).

Bibliography

Books

ABADIE SH, MILLER JH, WARREN LG, SWARTZWELDER JC, FELDMAN, MR: Helminths. In Lennette EH, Spaulding EM, Truant, JP (eds): Manual of Clinical Microbiology, 2nd ed. Am Soc Microbial, 1974. pp 617–635.

BELDING DL: Textbook of Parasitology, 3rd ed. New York, Appleton-Century Crofts, 1965. 1139 pp.

BROOKE MM: Intestinal and Urogenital Protozoa In Lennette EH, Spalding EM, Truant JP (eds): Manual of Clinical Microbiology, 2nd ed. Am Soc Microbiol, 1974. pp. 582–601.

FIELD JW: The Microscopical Diagnosis of Human Malaria. I. A Short Description Atlas of Thick Film Diagnosis. Studies from the Institute for Medical Research. Federation of Malaya No. 28, 1948. 113 pp.

FIELD JW, SHUTE PG: The Microscopic Diagnosis of Human Malaria. II. A Morphological Study of the Erythrocytic Parasites. Studies from the Institute for Medical Research. Federation of Malaya No. 24, 1956. 247 pp.

SHUTE PG, MARYON M: Laboratory Techniques for the Study of Malaria. London, J & A Churchill, 1966. 111 pp.

TAYLOR AER, BAKER JR: The Cultivation of Parasites in Vitro. Dorking, England, Alard & Son, 1968. pp. 1–369.

Journals

DENNIS DT, MCCONNELL E, WHITE GB: Bancroftian filariasis and membrane filters: Are night surveys necessary? Am J Trop Med Hyg 23:257–262, 1976

ARTHUR L. BARRY

Antimicrobial Susceptibility Testing

12

A variety of laboratory procedures have been used to determine either the activity of an antimicrobial agent against various microorganisms, or to test the susceptibility of a particular microorganism to a number of antimicrobial agents. Susceptibility tests, as such procedures are collectively known, are now commonly employed to aid the selection of the most effective therapeutic agent(s) for treating a particular infectious disease. It may be said that such *in vitro* tests are really quite artificial because they do not take into account the important role played by the host defense mechanisms, and they do not consider the effects that the drug may have on the cells and tissues of the host. However, the fact remains that *in vitro* susceptibility tests are invaluable when interpreted in the light of our knowledge of the disease process under treatment and of the pharmacologic properties of the drug(s) to be used. Susceptibility tests are now routinely performed in most clinical laboratories, but the accuracy and precision of the techniques as actually applied often leave something to be desired. Furthermore, the microorganisms and the antimicrobial agents routinely selected for susceptibility testing often have little relevance to the clinical problem at hand. The purpose of this chapter is to review some of the practical problems involved in performing susceptibility tests in the clinical microbiology laboratory.

Role of the Clinical Microbiology Laboratory

Isolation and identification of the etiologic agent(s) of an infectious disease are the first requirement of rational antimicrobial chemotherapy. If this requirement is met, there will be few occasions to criticize susceptibility tests because patients appear to respond to treatment with an antimicrobic to which isolates from the patient are resistant, or vice versa.

Appropriate specimens must be collected for culture *before* treatment with antimicrobial agents is begun. Antimicrobial therapy can exert powerful selective pressures on the resident microbiota. As a consequence, relatively resistant commensals—actually of little or no pathogenic significance—may come to predominate in specimens collected after therapy is in force. The danger is that such microorganisms may erroneously be assumed to be etiologic agents and be tested for susceptibility, although they are in fact unrelated to the disease process under treatment. Such a diagnostic-therapeutic trap is especially likely to be set when cultures are not taken until several days of treatment with broad-spectrum antimicrobial drugs has proved to be unsuccessful.

Much time and effort can be wasted in performing elaborate susceptibility tests with microorganisms that actually bear little relationship to the infectious process being treated. For this reason, clinical laboratories must judiciously select isolates that ordinarily require susceptibility testing. To accomplish this, the busy clinical laboratory must establish some general rules that are applied to all specimens. However, such rules can never take into account the variety of extenuating circumstances that may influence the final decision on testing. In this, as in other areas of clinical microbiology, it is essential for clinicians and microbiologists to work together, especially when unusual clinical problems exist.

Indications for Performing Susceptibility Tests

Once the microbiologic diagnosis has been made, the laboratory is often requested to determine the *in vitro* susceptibility of the pathogen to a variety of antimicrobial agents. Such tests are particularly important when the pathogen has been identified as *Staphylococcus aureus,* a member of the family Enterobacteriaceae or *Mycobacterium tuberculosis,* because these bacteria are particularly liable to be resistant to one or more of the commonly used antimicrobics. On the other hand, some microorganisms are uniformly susceptible to an effective antibiotic, and testing is therefore unnecessary. For example, group A *Streptococcus pyogenes* may safely be assumed to be susceptible to penicillin G; *in vitro* susceptibility tests are indicated only with isolates recovered from patients with documented allergy to penicillin. *Streptococcus pneumoniae* with decreased susceptibility to penicillin G have been isolated in the United States. Consequently, isolates from serious infections should be tested using discs loaded with 1 μg oxacillin. Isolates of both *Hemophilus influenzae* and *Neisseria gonorrhoeae* should be screened for β-lactamase activity before assuming they are susceptible to the penicillins. With these latter three pathogens, a few simple screening tests are sufficient; additional susceptibility tests are rarely necessary.

Other microorganisms are uniformly resistant to certain antimicrobial agents, and susceptibility tests are justified only for educational purposes or to help confirm the laboratory identification of genus and species. For example, *Pseudomonas aeruginosa* is relatively resistant to most antimicrobics except for the polymyxins, gentamicin, tobramycin, amikacin, sisomycin, netilmycin, carbenicillin, and ticarcillin.

In some cases, the disc diffusion method of testing that is generally used does not yield appropriate information. For example, enterococci are relatively resistant to the penicillins and quite resistant to streptomycin and kanamycin by disc testing. However, a combination of penicillin or ampicillin with streptomycin or gentamicin is preferred for treatment when a bactericidal effect is required, as in enterococcal endocarditis. The disc diffusion technique is not adaptable to assessment of combinations of antimicrobics and does not permit determination of a lethal end point. Also, the disc diffusion method is inappropriate for measuring the susceptiblitiy of *Neisseria gonorrhoeae* to penicillin; an agar dilution method should be used for such a determination. In actual practice, susceptibility tests are rarely needed to guide the treatment of either streptococcal or gonococcal infections.

When a specimen contains a mixture of different kinds of bacteria of doubtful pathogenicity and a firm bacteriologic diagnosis cannot be established, susceptibility tests should be performed only after consultation with the attending physician. Reporting susceptibility tests on indiscriminately selected bacterial isolates tends to encourage antimicrobial treatment that has no sound basis. Some institutions regularly test all staphylococci, enteric bacilli, and pseudomonads without considering either the source or the relative numbers of bacteria in the specimen. Such potential pathogens are frequently present simply as part of the normally resident microbiota and if eliminated by specific chemotherapy, the patient will be vulnerable to colonization with more resistant microorganisms, which in turn may then initiate a second infection (superinfection).

When dealing with specimens that are normally sterile or with material containing a known pathogen *(e.g., M. tuberculosis),* the decision on whether susceptibility tests should be performed is usually quite simple. With specimens that usually contain a mixture of different kinds of microorganisms, the decision is often difficult, if not impossible. In general, only those microorganisms of a mixture should be tested that are present in predominant numbers in a specimen in which, ordinarily, they are a minor component of the microbial flora.

Selection of Antimicrobics to be Tested Routinely

Because of the ever-increasing number of antimicrobial agents that are available, the selection of drugs to be tested on a routine basis has led to some confusion. In order to simplify the routine test, the number of drugs must be sharply limited. On the other hand, the laboratory report should include information about all the drugs that may be of interest to the physicians of that particular insitution. Laboratory directors are continually faced with requests to add more and more drugs to their routine protocol. The agents reported as part of their routine susceptibility test will profoundly influence the use of different chemotherapeutic agents within an institution. Consequently, after consultation with the appropriate clinical staff, a laboratory may elect to withhold a toxic or ineffective drug from routine testing in order to limit use of the agent within that institution.

Clearly, the agents routinely tested against gram-positive cocci should differ from those tested against gram-negative bacilli. In addition, the nature of the specimen should influence the kind of antimicrobics that are tested. For example, nitrofurantoin and nalidixic acid are limited in use to the treatment of urinary tract infections and need not be used to test microorganisms recovered from specimens other than urine.

Certain drugs should not be tested, because there is good reason to believe that the results of *in vitro* tests may be irrelevant. For example, *in vitro* tests with methenamine mandelate should not be performed because the activity of this drug *in vivo* depends on the attainment of a urinary pH of 5.0 or less, and *in vitro* test conditions bear no relationship to the situation in the urine, the only possible site of antibacterial activity in the patient.

Antimicrobics are usefully classified into groups with similar modes of action; drugs within each group often demonstrate complete or partial cross resistance. Although there may be significant differences in the pharmacologic properties of such drugs, there is little value in testing more than one representative from each group. The following guidelines can be used for selecting agents to be tested routinely.

PENICILLINS

It is advisable to test *Staphylococcus aureus* against a penicillinase-labile penicillin (benzylpenicillin, *i.e.,* penicillin G) and against a penicillinase-stable penicillin (nafcillin or oxacillin). Methicillin is a poor choice because of its instability, and neither cloxacillin nor dicloxacillin should be used. Ampicillin, carbenicillin, and ticarcillin should not be tested against staphylococci because of their lesser activity and similar susceptibility to penicillinase as compared with benzylpenicillin.

The gram-negative bacilli should be tested against ampicillin. Carbenicillin, ticarcillin, mezlocillin, or piperacillin should be included in the battery of drugs tested against *Pseudomonas* spp. and selected Enterobacteriaceae.

CEPHALOSPORINS

The routine battery of drugs should include cephalothin as the representative of the "first generation" of cephalosporins. Occasionally, isolates that are resistant to cephalothin are susceptible to other cephalosporins. Accordingly,discs loaded with other cephalosporins should be available for use in testing when the isolate was obtained from a patient in whom an alternative antimicrobic cannot be used (*e.g.,* a patient allergic to penicillins). Also, a representative cephamycin (*e.g.,* cefoxitin), a second generation cephalosporin (*e.g.,* cefamandole) and a third generation cephalosporin (e.g., moxalactam or cefoperazone) should be tested routinely if these drugs are used regularly within the institution.

TETRACYCLINES

Tetracycline hydrochloride is the preferred representative of the tetracycline family of drugs for routine susceptibility tests. Microorganisms that are susceptible to tetracycline should be susceptible to the other tetracyclines. However, those isolates that are resistant to tetracycline hydrochloride might be inhibited by clinically obtainable concentrations of doxycycline or minocycline. For that reason, minocycline and doxycycline discs should be held in reserve for testing the occasional tetracycline-resistant isolate for which an acceptable alternative therapeutic agent is not readily available. Discrepancies between the three tetracyclines occur most frequently with *Acinetobacter* spp. and with tetracycline-resistant strains of *Staphylococcus aureus.*

AMINOCYCLITOLS

Streptomycin, neomycin, kanamycin, gentamicin, tobramycin, amikacin, sisomicin, and netilmicin are all related antimicrobics. Although cross resistance occurs, exceptions are frequent enough to warrant separate testing with selected isolates. Gentamicin or tobramycin should be tested routinely because they are currently preferred for parenteral therapy. Alternative aminocyclitols may be held in reserve for testing gentamicin-resistant isolates. The selection of the most appropriate aminocyclitols to be tested routinely will depend primarily on the institutional policy of usage of these potentially toxic drugs. Only those agents that are actually used frequently should be included in the routine battery of first-line drugs.

The drugs listed in Table 12-1 represent a compromise between the various considerations previously listed. With a few judicious deletions and additions, this list of drugs should fulfill the requirements for routine use in most clinical laboratories. A secondary battery of drugs could be held in reserve for use when therapeutic problems arise with individual patients. Tests with bacteria not listed in Table 12-1 are indicated only under special circumstances; the selection of drugs and the method of testing should be individualized.

Direct Susceptibility Tests

As long as pure cultures are available, complete, definitive identification of pathogens is not required before susceptibility tests are performed. In actual practice, colonies are selected from the primary agar plates and are subcultured so that both susceptibility tests and identification procedures may be carried out simultaneously. This process ordinarily requires 36 to 48 hours, an excessive period to delay treatment. Once the specimen is collected, therapeutic agents are usually selected on the basis of previous experience with similar infections, and treatment is modified as laboratory data become available. In an effort to obtain more rapid results, inoculation of sus-

Table 12-1. *Suggested Battery of Antimicrobics for Routine Susceptibility Testing of Clinical Isolates*

Gram-positive Cocci		**Gram-negative Bacilli**	
STAPHYLOCOCCUS SPP.	ENTEROCOCCUS	ENTEROBACTERIACEAE	OTHER
Penicillin G	Penicillin G	Ampicillin	Amikacin
Nafcillin	Ampicillin	Cephalothin	Tobramycin
Cephalothin	Erythromycin	Kanamycin	Carbenicillin
Erythromycin	Tetracycline	Gentamicin	Mezlocillin
Clindamycin	Nitrofurantoin*	Tetracycline	Piperacillin
Chloramphenicol	Vancomycin	Chloramphenicol	Polymyxin B
Tetracycline		Nitrofurantoin*	Kanamycin†
		Nalidixic Acid*	Chloramphenicol†
		Sulfonamide*	Tetracycline†
		Trimethoprim-sulfamethoxazole	Sulfonamide*†

* Only for isolates from urinary tract infections.

† Indicated for testing pseudomonads and other nonfermentative gram-negative bacilli, excluding *Pseudomonas aeruginosa.*

ceptibility tests directly with clinical specimens has been advocated. When this is done, the result must be recognzed as tentative because many critical variables—such as the density of the inoculum and the influence of competing microorganisms—cannot be controlled in direct tests. In fact, the direct test may be dangerously misleading if the specimen contains more than one kind of microorganism because the results may simply reflect the presence of the relatively resistant members of the normal microbial flora rather than the susceptibility of an actual, specific pathogen. When the pathogens can be selected from cultures, standardized susceptibility tests must be repeated with pure cultures; useful preliminary results can be obtained as early as 4 to 5 hours after the test plates are inoculated.

Disc Diffusion Techniques

In most clinical laboratories, susceptibility tests are performed by a disc diffusion technique. In general, agar plates are inoculated with a pure culture and antimicrobic-containing discs are then applied to the agar surface. After overnight incubation, the plates are examined. When there is a large clear zone of inhibition around a disc, the microorganism is said to be susceptible to the drug in that disc; if there is no zone of inhibition, the microorganism is said to be resistant to that drug. The amount of drug in the disc cannot be equated to the concentration of drug required to inhibit growth of test microorganism. The actual concentration of drug in the agar adjacent to the disc varies considerably during the first few critical hours of incubation. Techniques that depend on the presence or absence of any zone of inhibition around a disc are unreliable and inaccurate because resistant microorganisms may occasionally produce small zones of inhibition, and susceptible strains will produce much larger zones of inhibition. Using high-content discs, the minimum zone size produced by susceptible microorganisms and the maximum zone diameter produced by resistant microorganisms were defined. Because different drugs diffuse at different rates, it was necessary to establish different zone standards for each drug. Interpretive standards for antimicrobics in current use are listed in Table 12-2.

In the past, the accuracy of the disc method was open to considerable criticism, largely because the method had not been standardized and because the need for adequate controls had not been fully appreciated. This situation was markedly improved in 1968, when a carefully standardized technique that can be controlled adequately was introduced. With this method, the inoculum is prepared by adjusting the turbidity of a broth culture to match that of a $BaSO_4$ standard. Because this critical step is often thought too cumbersome for routine work, more expedient but less reliable modifications have been made without substantiation of adequacy. This situation led to the development of an agar-overlay method that is significantly easier to read and simpler to perform. The overlay technique is applicable only to tests with the common, rapidly growing pathogens—the very microorganisms with which suscep-

Table 12-2. *Zone Diameter Interpretive Standards and Approximate MIC Correlates*

		Zone Diameter (nearest whole mm)			Approximate MIC Correlates	
ANTIMICROBIAL AGENT	DISC CONTENT	RESISTANT	INTERMEDIATE	SUSCEPTIBLE	RESISTANT	SUSCEPTIBLE
Amikacin	30 μg	≤14	15–16	≥17	>16 μg/mL	≤12 μg/mL
Ampicillin*, when testing gram-negative enteric organisms and enterococci	10 μg	≤11	12–13	≥14	≥32 μg/mL	≤8 μg/mL
Ampicillin*, when testing staphylococci and penicillin G-susceptible microorganisms	10 μg	≤20	21–28	≥29	Penicillinase†	≤0.2 μg/mL
Ampicillin*, when testing *Haemophilus* spp.	10 μg	≤19		≥20	≥2 μg/mL	<2 μg/mL
Carbenicillin, when testing *Proteus* spp. and *Escherichia coli*	100 μg	≤17	18–22	≥23	≥32 μg/mL	≤16 μg/mL
Carbenicillin, when testing *Pseudomonas aeruginosa*	100 μg	≤13	14–16	≥17	≥256 μg/mL	≤128 μg/mL
Cephalothin‡	30 μg	≤14	15–17	≥18	≥32 μg/mL	≤8 μg/mL
Cefamandole	30 μg	≤14	15–17	≥18	≥32 μg/mL	≤8 μg/mL
Cefoxitin	30 μg	≤14	15–17	≥18	≥32 μg/mL	≤8 μg/mL
Chloramphenicol	30 μg	≤12	13–17	≥18	≥32 μg/mL	≤8 μg/mL
Clindamycin	2 μg	≤14	15–16	≥17	≥2 μg/mL	≤1 μg/mL
Erythromycin	15 μg	≤13	14–17	≥18	≥8 μg/mL	≤2 μg/mL
Gentamicin	10 μg	≤12	13–14	≥15	>8 μg/mL	≤6 μg/mL
Tobramycin	10 μg	≤12	13–14	≥15	>8 μg/mL	≤6 μg/mL
Kanamycin	30 μg	≤13	14–17	≥18	≥32 μg/mL	≤8 μg/mL
Methicillin§, when testing staphylococci	5 μg	≤ 9	10–13	≥14	—	≤4 μg/mL
Mezlocillin	75 μg	≤12	13–15	≥16	≥256 μg/mL	≤64 μg/ mL
Oxacillin or Nafcillin	1 μg	≤10	11–12	≥13	—	≤1 μg/mL
Penicillin G‖, when testing staphylococci	10 units	≤20	21–28	≥29	Penicillinase†	≤0.1 μg/mL
Penicillin G‖, when testing other microorganisms	10 units	≤11	12–21#	≥22	≥32 μg/mL	≤2 μg/mL
Piperacillin	100 μg	≤14	15–17	≥18	≥256 μg/ mL	≤64 μg/ mL
Tetracycline**	30 μg	≤14	15–18	≥19	≥16 μg/mL	≤4 μg/mL
Vancomycin	30 μg	≤ 9	10–11	≥12	—	≤4 μg/mL
Sulfonamides††	250 μg or 300 μg	≤12	13–16	≥17	>256 μg/mL	≤128 μg/mL
Trimethoprim-sulfamethoxazole††	1.25 μg 23.75 μg	≤10	11–15	≥16	≥8/152 μg/mL	≤2/38 μg/mL
Nitrofurantoin††	300 μg	≤14	15–16	≥17	≥128 μg/mL	≤32 μg/mL
Nalidixic Acid††	30 μg	≤13	14–18	≥19	≥32 μg/mL	<16 μg/mL

*Class disc for ampicillin, hetacillin, and amoxicillin.
†Resistant strains of *Staphylococcus aureus* produce penicillinase.
‡Class disc for the first-generation cephalosporins.
§Class discs for penicillinase-resistant penicillins.
‖Class disc for benzylpenicillin, phenoxymethylpenicillin, and phenethicillin.
#Intermediate category includes some microorganisms, such as enterococci, and certain gram-negative bacilli that may cause systemic infections treatable with high dosages of benzylpenicillin but not of phenoxymethylpenicillin or phenethicillin.
**Class disc for the tetracyclines.
††Use only for testing isolates from urinary tract infections.

tibility tests are most relevant. Both disc diffusion techniques have been standardized by the National Committee for Clinical Laboratory Standards (NCCLS). The reader is urged to refer to the most recent NCCLS document and to the original references before attempting to perform either of these disc diffusion tests. Attempts to modify these standardized techniques are discouraged unless the proposed changes have been carefully evaluated in terms of accuracy and precision.

If carefully performed, the disc diffusion technique can provide precise and accurate results, but it does have certain limitations that are not always fully appreciated: (1) The disc diffusion technique has been standardized primarily for microorganisms that grow rapidly on the standard medium. Microorganisms with a prolonged generation time cannot be tested accurately be the disc diffusion method. (2) The disc test does not measure the bactericidal activity of a drug. (3) Combinations of two or more antimicrobial agents cannot be assayed. (4) Although microorganisms that are classified as being resistant by the disc diffusion technique may not be affected by concentrations of the drug that are normally attainable in the serums of patients, exceptionally high dosage may bring about a cure. A broth or agar dilution technique should be employed for more exact definition of the concentration required to inhibit growth or exert a lethal effect, to study combinations of antimicrobics, and to test fastidious microorganisms.

Dilution Tests

A series of Petri plates with an agar medium, or test tubes with a liquid medium, are prepared with varying concentrations of the antimicrobics to be tested. Tests in liquid medium (*i.e.,* broth dilution tests) may be adapted to the microtitration technique, using plastic trays with rows of small wells rather than racks of test tubes. The inoculum consists of a standardized suspension of the microorganism to be tested made up from overnight growth in the same medium used for testing. After incubation, the lowest concentration of drug required to inhibit the growth of the microorganism is determined by examining each agar plate or tube for macroscopic evidence of growth. Inhibition simply reflects failure of replication, a "static" effect. The result is referred to as the minimal inhibitory concentration (MIC). Actual killing of microorganisms usually requires a higher concentration than the MIC. With broth-dilution tests, the minimal lethal concentration can be determined by subculturing to antimicrobic-free agar from tubes showing no visible growth after overnight incubation. The lowest concentration of drug from which viable microorganisms can no longer be recovered is then expressed as the minimal lethal concentration (MLC). If combinations of two or more drugs are to be tested, tubes of nutrient broth are prepared with varying concentrations of each agent. After overnight incubation, the tubes with no visible growth are subcultured in order to determine the MLC of the different combinations of antimicrobial agents.

In principle, such antimicrobic dilution tests are quite simple, but the results are significantly affected by several procedural details. Standardized methods for determining MIC values have been proposed by the NCCLS. Even when these standardized methods are carefully followed, there will be some variability in MICs obtained when a single strain is repeatedly tested in the same or different laboratories. In general, a testing system is considered to be adequately controlled if 95% of the repeated MIC determinations are no more than ± 1 doubling dilution from the mode.

Two of the most critical variables are the broth culture medium and the density of the inoculum. Various components of commonly used culture mediums adversely affect some drugs—for example, para-aminobenzoic acid-sulfonamides, D-alanine-cycloserine, and ergosterol-amphotericin B. Generally, the apparent antimicrobial activity of an agent is inversely related to the size of the inoculum.

The clinical significance of differences in MICs or MLCs remains a matter of conjecture. Very few clinical studies have attempted to evaluate different dilution techniques for susceptibility testing in terms of prediction of clinical response to treatment with a particular chemotherapeutic agent. Microorganisms inhibited by concentrations of an antimicrobial agent that are well below those ordinarily obtained at the site of an infection should be susceptible to therapy, whereas strains requiring concentrations of the drug well above the concentrations normally attained in tissues are resistant. The interpretation of *in vitro* tests with microorganisms showing MICs at these two extremes will rarely be affected by variations in method. Technique is more critical with the relatively uncommon microorganisms that exhibit MICs between these two extremes. Many investigators consider a microorganism to be susceptible only if the MIC is at least two to four times below the average blood concentration.

In the special case of infections involving the urinary tract, an MIC below concentrations usually attained in the urine has been equated with susceptibility by some workers. Others hold that the average blood concentration is a better yardstick, particularly if there is a pyelonephritis. Critical clinical trials are necessary to settle this question.

Disc Versus *Dilution Tests*

Through automation it is now practical for clinical laboratories to provide quantitative susceptibility data (*i.e.,* to determine MICs, routinely). This is a departure from the disc test, which estimates MIC categories and provides an interpretive report (susceptible, resistant, or indeterminant). The interpretive standards for the disc test are in fact developed by comparing MICs to the usual blood level obtained with the normal dosage of an antimicrobial agent. When the concentration of drug available at the site of infection can be increased either by physiologic concentration or by utilizing modified dosage schedules, the qualitative interpretation of the disc test may not be appropriate. Furthermore, disc test results cannot be interpreted reliably when zones of inhibition fall into the intermediate category. Although the technology for routine, quantitative susceptibility testing is available, there is serious questions about whether many physicians utilize quantitative susceptibility data appropriately. To optimize utilization, the laboratory report should include some type of interpretive guidelines.

In order to interpret the results of antimicrobial agent susceptibility tests, the technologic variables affecting the precision and accuracy of the various procedures in use must be considered. The information obtained from such *in vitro* tests must then be applied with an awareness of the shortcomings in our knowledge of the clinical pharmacology of various drugs and the important but often poorly defined role played by the host's defense mechanisms. When performed with care and interpreted with caution, antimicrobial susceptibility tests can provide information that will help guide the selection of the most appropriate therapeutic agent. On the other hand, susceptibility tests cannot be used as a substitute for good diagnostic microbiology, sound clinical judgment, and experience.

Bibliography

Books

BARRY AL: The Antimicrobic Susceptibility Test: Principles and Practices. Philadelphia, Lea & Febiger, 1976, 236 pp

GARROD LP, LAMBERT HP, O'GRADY F: Antibiotic and Chemotherapy, 4th ed. Edinburgh, Churchill Livingstone, 1973, 546 pp

LORIAN V: Antibiotics in Laboratory Medicine. Baltimore, Williams & Wilkins, 1980, 737 pp

SCHOENKNECHT FD, SHERRIS JC: New perspectives in antibiotic susceptibility testing. In Dyke SC (ed): Recent Advances in Clinical Pathology, pp. 272–292. Edinburgh, Churchill Livingstone, 1972

Journals

BARRY AL: A system for reporting quantitative antimicrobic susceptibility test results. Am J Clin Pathol 72:864–868, 1979

BARRY AL, EFFINGER LJ: Accuracy of the disc method for determining antimicrobic susceptibility of common gram negative bacilli. Current Microbiol 2:305–309, 1979

BARRY AL, GARCIA F, THRUPP LD: An improved single disc method for testing the antibiotic susceptibility or rapidly growing pathogens. Am J Clin Pathol 53:149–158, 1970

BARRY AL, JOYCE LJ, ADAMS AP, BENNER EJ: Rapid determination of antimicrobial susceptibility for urgent clinical situations. Am J Clin Pathol 59:693–699, 1973

BAUER AW, KIRBY WMM, SHERRIS JC, TURCK, M: Antibiotic susceptibility testing by a standardized single disc method. Am J Clin Pathol 45:493–496, 1966

ERICSSON HM, SHERRIS JC: Antibiotic sensitivity testing. Report of an international collaborative study. Acta Pathol Microbiol Scand[B] 217:1–90, 1971

MATSEN JM, KOEPCHE MJH, QUIE JG: Evaluation of the Bauer-Kirby-Sherris-Turck single-disc diffusion method of antibiotic susceptibility testing. Antimicrob Agents Chemother 169:445–453, 1970

NCCLS Subcommittee on Antimicrobial susceptibility Tests: Approved Standard M2-A2, 2nd ed. Performance Standards for Antimicrobial Disc Susceptibility Tests. Villanova, National Committee for Clinical Laboratory Standards, 1979, 17 pp

NCCLS Subcommittee on Antimicrobial Dilution Susceptibility Tests: Proposed Standard M7-P. Standard Methods of Dilution Antimicrobial Susceptibility Tests for Bacteria Which Grow Aerobically. Villanova, National Committee for Clinical Laboratory Standards, 1980, 31 pp

Rules and Regulations: Antibiotic Susceptibility Discs: Fed Regist 37:20525–20529, 1972

Rules and Regulations: Antibiotic Susceptibility Discs—Correction. Fed Regist 38:2576, 1973

PETER B. SMITH

13 Bacteriophage Typing

Bacteriophage typing is an application to diagnostic microbiology of a dictum of nature; namely, parasitism. Bacteriophages are, in fact, viruses parasitic on bacteria. Those used in typing are inept parasites because they kill (lyse) their bacterial hosts, thus terminating the cycle of parasitism.

Typing is accomplished by exposing pure cultures of bacteria to a collection of bacteriophages to determine which of the phages will lyse the cultures. The phages are chosen because of their various host ranges, which are generally unrelated to biochemical or metabolic capabilities and have no apparent connection with antigenic characteristics. Thus, comparison of patterns of lysis by phages enables the determination of unique relationships among strains of bacteria. When an appropriate collection of phages is used, identical or closely related strains of bacteria show identical or very similar patterns of lysis, whereas unrelated strains exhibit quite dissimilar lytic patterns. Phage typing has been applied most effectively to *Staphylococcus aureus* and *Salmonella* spp., and with varying degrees of success to *Pseudomonas aeruginosa, Streptococcus pyogenes, Mycobacterium tuberculosis,* some species of *Shigella* and *Klebsiella* and a few other bacterial species. In all cases, the basic principle is the same, but some details of the procedures vary according to the microorganism under examination. The following description of phage typing of staphylococci illustrates the general procedure.

A collection of 23 basic staphylococcal typing phages is used: phages 29, 52, 52A, 79, 80, 3A, 3C, 55, 71, 6, 42E, 47, 53, 54, 75, 77, 83A, 84, 85, 94, 95, 96, and 81. Each phage is used in an appropriate dilution known as the routine test dilution (RTD), which is the highest dilution that just fails to give confluent (complete) lysis when a series of tenfold dilutions of the phage is spotted on a lawn of its propagating strain of staphylococcus growing on agar. To ensure that the typing phages conform to accepted standards, it is necessary to test them periodically on the propagating strains of staphylococci. Any variations resulting either from mutation of the phages or of the propagating strains may produce patterns of lysis that differ radically from the standards. Methods of propagating and titrating the phages, and criteria for acceptable standards of both the phages and propagating strains, have been established by an international subcommittee.

Procedure for Typing

The *Staphylococcus aureus* culture to be tested is grown for 4 to 5 hours in broth and then used to seed the entire surface of an agar plate so as to produce a uniform, confluent lawn of bacterial growth. Small drops (about 0.01 ml) of the RTD of each phage are then placed at spaced intervals on the seeded agar, and the plate is incubated at 30°C overnight. Susceptibility of the culture to the phages is shown by the development of areas of lysis ranging from small, discrete plaques to confluent lysis (Fig. 13-1) at the site of deposition of one or more phages.

All lytic reactions, from 50 plaques to complete lysis, are regarded as significant. The pattern of lysis, or phage type, is reported in terms of phages that produce significant lysis. For example, a strain of *S. aureus* lysed only by phage 71 is reported as being of phage type 71; a strain lysed by phages 80 and 81 is reported as phage type 80/81; or a strain lysed by several phages might be reported as phage type 6/47/53/54/75/83A.

The establishment of a phage-typing service in a small clinical laboratory usually is not feasible, because maintenance and control of the typing phages and their propagating strains are expensive in terms of time, personnel, and facilities. Considerable experience is required in handling the phages and in reading and interpreting the results. This experience is

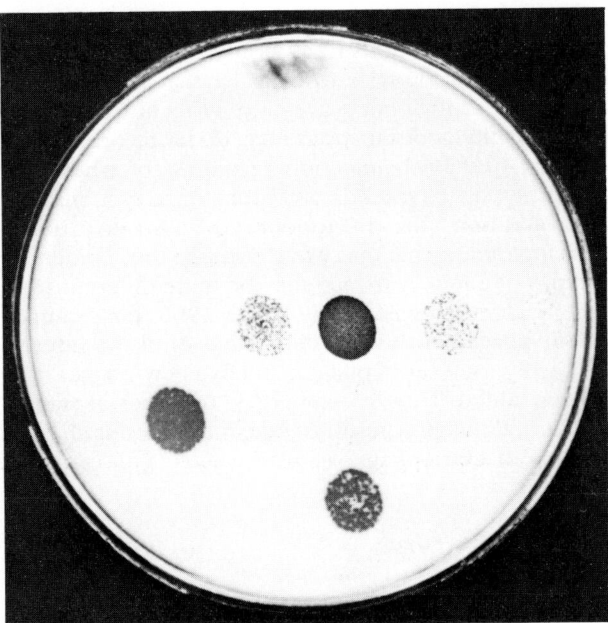

Fig. 13-1. A culture of *Staphylococcus aureus* that has been phage typed. Three lytic areas show complete or confluent lysis; other areas show 50 or more plaques.

not readily acquired by performing occasional tests. For larger laboratories with adequate facilities, starter sets of the phages and propagating strains are available under certain specified conditions from the National Reference Laboratory at the Centers for Disease Control in Atlanta, Georgia.

Application of Phage Typing

Phage typing is primarily an epidemiologic tool. It is of greatest value when used to supplement investigations of the origin and spread of infection. Phage typing does not generate information of diagnostic or therapeutic significance, and for this reason it is not recommended as part of the routine examination of randomly isolated cultures in the clinical laboratory.

Preferably, phage typing should be restricted to the examination of cultures suspected of having a common origin. Thus, typing is indicated when an unusual incidence of infections occurs and when it is important to determine the source and routes of dissemination of the offending microorganism. Hospital-acquired infections are classic examples. A search for the source of the infection will involve a series of cultures from possible carriers (including, particularly, the medical and nursing personnel who are in most frequent and direct contact with the patients) and from suspected or potential vectors and fomites. The resulting set of cultures, presumed to be related epidemiologically, is then submitted to phage typing. By comparison of the phage-typing patterns of the cultures, it becomes possible to identify and characterize the responsible strain and to determine which individuals, vectors, or fomites may have been involved in the spread of the infection. Usually, it is advisable to type all cultures of an epidemiologic set at the same time, under identical test conditions. Therefore, when an outbreak of infection is suspected and when it is anticipated that phage typing may be helpful in tracing its origin, the physician should so advise the bacteriologist, who can then save the relevant isolates as pure cultures.

Phage typing has been widely applied in the investigation of staphylococcal infections such as postoperative and neonatal infections, and staphylococcal food poisoning. The investigation of an outbreak of staphylococcal pyoderma among newborn infants is illustrative. When the outbreak occurred, cultures were taken of the skin lesions, of the anterior nose and the hands of the attending personnel, and of various medications used in the nursery. *Staphylococcus aureus,* phage type 52A, was isolated from the lesions of all infected infants, from the nose and skin of one nurse, and from a jar of ointment. Some of the other attendants in the nursery also harbored coagulase-positive staphylococci in their noses or on their skin, but none of these strains proved to be of phage type 52A. In addition, phage typing of staphylococci isolated from nasal cultures of the infants revealed that all of those with pyoderma and some who were healthy had been colonized by *S. aureus,* phage type 52A.

When phage typing is not available in the individual laboratory, the usual practice is to submit the cultures to a reference laboratory for typing. This may be the National Reference Laboratory or the laboratories of certain state departments of health that are equipped to perform the test. Often a state laboratory not so equipped will forward cultures for typing to the National Reference Laboratory.

Cultures submitted for typing should be accompanied by all relevant epidemiologic data; this is of material assistance in the interpretation of the results of phage typing. Only coagulase-positive cultures of staphylococci should be submitted, for coagulase-negative strains are not susceptible to lysis by the basic typing phages.

A problem of interpretation arises from the fact that even related cultures isolated in a given epidemic situation sometimes show variations in their typing patterns. These variations are usually insignificant in short-lived epidemics, such as staphylococcal food poisoning, but in prolonged outbreaks the variations may become extreme and make interpretation of phage-typing results quite difficult. The assessment of the relationships in a set of cultures therefore cannot be based solely on the observed typing patterns. Interpretation of the results must take into account all available information concerning the source of the cultures, the circumstances of their isolation, and the precise question that the typing is required to answer.

Criteria have been established, on the basis of the experience of many workers, for the interpretation of lytic patterns. It is obviously necessary to have close cooperation between the physician, who is acquainted with the immediate circumstances of the situation, and the bacteriologist, who is familiar with the problems of interpretation of phage-typing patterns.

Although the phage type or pattern of staphylococci does not indicate any specific degree of virulence,there have been some associations noted between certain patterns and specific conditions or syndromes. For example, methicillin-resistant staphylococci are often typable with phages 83A, 84, or 85 (group III); impetigo and other skin infections, including "scalded skin" syndrome, are most often caused by staphylococci that react with phages 3A, 3C, 55, or 71 (group II); staphylococcal toxic shock syndrome has most often been associated with strains that type with phage 29 (group I). However, there are exceptions to all of these associations, and it would not be wise to consider that certain phage types of staphylococci are more virulent than others. Any staphylococcal strain may, under favorable conditions, establish infection regardless of whether it can be phage typed or what the phage type may be. In addition, the bacteriophages used for typing change somewhat every few years, so the "epidemic" types of a few years ago may be quite different from those predominant today. Since 1960, for example, four phages have been eliminated from the internationally used set of phages, and five new phages have been added. Thus, a comparison of trends in staphylococcal phage types must take into account changes in the bacteriophages used.

Bibliography

Journals

ASHESHOV EH, ROUNTREE PM: Report of the subcommittee on phage-typing of staphylococci to the international committee on systematic bacteriology. Int J Syst Bacteriol 25:241–242, 1975

BLAIR JE, WILLIAMS REO: Phage typing of staphylococci. Bull WHO 24:771–784, 1961

Operation of the CDC National Reference Center for bacteriophage typing of staphylococci. Health Lab Sci 2:212, 1965; JAMA 191:33, 1965

THOMSOM WK: Identification of bacteria by bacteriophage. Med Serv J Can 22:351–360, 1966

JOHN W. OSEBOLD

Immunological Diagnosis

14

Immunologic tests are generally employed to establish the current or remote presence of an infectious agent in a patient, to identify an infectious agent that has been isolated from a patient, and to determine the immunological responses of the patient. Optimal use of immunologic testing is made by the physician who knows what studies are appropriate, how to collect specimens for examinations, and how to interpret the results of the tests.

Specimens for Examination

Kinds of Specimens

Any body fluid or tissue that may contain antibody or antigen may be studied serologically: whole blood, serum, pleural fluid, peritoneal fluid, joint fluid, cerebrospinal fluid (CSF), bone marrow, mucosal secretions, extracts of tissues (as in the Ascoli test for anthrax, plague, or tularemia), or tissues for fluorescent antibody tests. The source of the specimen must be carefully labeled—for example, ventricular, cisternal, or lumbar CSF—because valid comparison of consecutive measurements can be made only between specimens identical in origin.

Sufficient quantities of the specimens are essential. Whereas 10 μl serum may suffice for a counter immunoelectrophoresis (CIE) test, 0.5 ml is needed for a macroscopic tube agglutination test. Whenever possible, approximately 5 ml of each specimen should be submitted so that a portion can be saved by freezing for comparison with a later paired specimen.

The time interval between an early (acute) and a late (convalescent or chronic) specimen must be sufficient to allow for the development of a significant change in titer—that is, a fourfold or two-serial dilution increment. The time interval varies (1) with etiologic agent—for example, 5 days with *Mycoplasma pneumoniae,* 7 days in typhus fever, and 3–4 weeks in coccidioidomycosis; (2) with the kind of antibody being measured—in rubella the hemagglutination inhibition titer rises more rapidly than either neutralizing or complement fixation (CF) titers (possibly a reflection of the temporal variation in the variety of immunoglobulin, *e.g.,* IgM or IgG); and (3) with specific antimicrobial therapy—4–6 weeks in treated rickettsioses and chlamydial infections.

Skin testing can stimulate production of humoral antibodies; for example, with the antigens of *Histoplasma capsulatum* and *Brucella* spp. Accordingly, serum collected later than 3 to 4 days after skin testing may not yield valid results. However, this is not an omnipresent effect.

Preservation and Transport of Specimens

Blood should be collected aseptically and preferably as a fasting specimen to avoid lipemia. The requirement of the testing laboratory for whole blood or serum must be known beforehand. In some instances whole blood may be submitted to the serology laboratory, but hemolysis occurring before or during transportation may yield an unsatisfactory specimen for CF and other tests.

Despite aseptic measures, the separated serum may become contaminated. Various preservatives may be used to minimize microbial growth (Table 14-1). However, some preservatives may influence directly the outcome of serologic tests. For example, *in vitro* viral neutralization tests may be invalidated by inactivation of the virus by a preservative such as thimerosal.

Drying is effective in minimizing contamination without use of a preservative. Whole blood or serum may be placed on filter paper and dried in air; serum can be lyophilized for preservation and transportation.

Specimens should be transported in sterile screw-capped tubes. If these are not available, sterile corks, coated by submerging in hot paraffin for 1 min, may be used.

Table 14-1. *Preservatives for Fluids to Be Used in Serologic Tests*

	Final Concentration (W/V) in Specimen	
Thimerosal	0.01%–0.02%	(1:10,000–2:10,000)
Phenol	0.5%	(5:1000)
Tricresol	0.5%	(5:1000)
Sodium azide	0.01%–0.1%	(1:10,000–1:1000)
Thymol	0.1%	(1:1000)
Phenylmercuric borate	0.02%	(2:10,000)

Immunologic Tests

The hallmark of immunologic reactivity is the specificity of the reactions concerned. Yet, paradoxically, several serodiagnostic tests depend on cross reactivity, that is, reaction of antibodies with an antigen or hapten that is not actually derived from the antigen that engendered the antibody response in the patient. The flocculation tests used in diagnosis of syphilis are examples, because the "antigen" of the test, cardiolipin, is derived from dried, defatted beef heart (see Table 14-2 for other examples). Semiquantitative interpretation of the results of cardiolipin-based tests have long been used to follow the course of syphilis and assess the impact of therapy. Recently, tests that make use of specific treponemal antigens have been adapted to yield semiquantitative results, which may prove to be equally valuable. It is only when serial dilutions of a specimen are tested that a semiquantitative assessment can be rendered, yielding the titer of a serum.

The antigens employed include: toxins liberated from bacteria (diphtheria); soluble antigens produced in cultures, filtrates, or autolysates (histoplasmosis, coccidioidomycosis, staphylococcal enterotoxin, botulinal toxin); soluble extracts obtained by chemical extraction (streptococci); soluble substances remaining partially attached to bacterial cells (pneumococcal capsule); cellular components of cells (flagellar and 0 antigens of gram-negative enteropathogenic bacteria); whole bacterial cells (*Brucella* spp., tularemia bacilli); soluble or virus-bound viral antigen (mumps virus); and viral particles (influenza). Some tests require heating the serum at 56°C for 30 min, to inactivate complement.

Antigen-antibody reactions may occur in an inapparent manner, detectable only indirectly as in the neutralization tests (primary reactions), or in an apparent manner with visible manifestations as in agglutination tests (secondary reactions).

Precipitin Test

The precipitin test involves the direct interaction of a soluble antigen with its corresponding antibody (precipitin) to yield a visible precipitate. The reaction is influenced by the concentration of reactants, the pH (optimally near 7.0 in many systems), the presence of electrolytes, and the temperature (the reaction is accelerated at higher temperatures—*e.g.,* 37°C—but more precipitate may develop in the cold). As little as 3 μg to 5 μg of antibody nitrogen may be detected. With pure antigens, the precipitin test can provide a precise, quantitative measurement of antigen-antibody interaction. Usually, however, the antigens are relatively crude. Yet quantitation is possible. A ratio of antigen to antibody that provides the maximum yield of precipitate is termed equivalence. An excess of antigen or an excess of antibody leads to a smaller amount or to no visible precipitate. Frequently, a constant amount of serum (antibody) is exposed to varying quantities of antigen so that a

Table 14-2. *Nonspecific Serologic Tests*

Disease	Diagnostic Test	Antigen-Hapten
Syphilis	Nontreponemal, reagin Wassermann, VDRL, Kahn, and others	Cardiolipin
Infectious mononucleosis	Heterophil agglutination Ox (beef) cell hemolysins	Sheep erythrocytes Beef erythrocytes
Mycoplasmal pneumonia	Cold hemagglutinins Streptococcus MG	Human group O erythrocytes Streptococcus MG (viridans group) washed cells
Rickettsial diseases	Weil–Felix	*Proteus vulgaris* O antigen of strains OX2, OX19, OXK
Various inflammatory or necrotizing states	C-reactive protein	C-reactive protein

range of proportions of reactants is provided; equivalence is indicated by maximum yield of precipitate.

Precipitin reactions are sometimes carried out by layering the antigen solution over the serum and observing some hours later for a ring or layer of precipitate—indicative of the site where the reactants have, by diffusion, achieved an optimal ratio. In some precipitin tests, antigen and serum are mixed and observed for a button or sediment.

Immunodiffusion (agar gel precipitin test) enables the visualization of multiple antigen-antibody systems precipitating in an agar-gelled, aqueous medium with diffusion of reactants bringing them together in optimally reactive proportions. In addition to appropriate pH and osmolality, inclusion of a preservative (thimerosal, sodium azide) is desirable.

Counterimmunoelectrophoresis (CIE) represents an important variation of the agar gel diffusion test. Serum and antigen are placed in apposed wells as in immunodiffusion, but passage of an electric current through the agar (purified agar or agarose) substrate brings reactants together rapidly. The negatively charged antigen moves toward the anode, the antibody globulin toward the cathode; hence, counterelectrophoresis. This confluence results in a detectable precipitation reaction in a much shorter time than the usual precipitin or immunodiffusion test. As a result, CIE can be extremely useful when a rapid diagnosis is needed, as in meningitis. CIE can be used to detect antigen, which may permit a diagnosis before antibody is produced in detectable amounts. Thus, the presence of the capsular antigen of *Haemophilus influenzae* or *Neisseria meningitidis* in the CSF or of group B streptococci in the serum of a neonate can be established within 30 min to 90 min.

Agglutination Test

The aggregation of suspended particulate antigen (or particles coated with antigen) on mixing with its corresponding antibody (agglutinin) constitutes the agglutination test. It is similar to the precipitin test except that the antigen is insoluble and is visible from the start. Depending on the modification used, approximately 0.0002 μg to 20 μg of antibody nitrogen can be detected.

The quantity of antigen is usually maintained constant and the serum serially diluted, allowing determination of the antibody titer. Antigens include: whole, killed bacterial cells, for example, *Bordetella pertussis* and *Brucella* spp.; and inert particles, such as bentonite (0.3 μm to 0.5 μm in diameter), latex polystyrene particles (0.81 μm), or erythrocytes coated with soluble antigen (sensitized). The latter antigens provide tests of considerable sensitivity, for the agglutination of sensitized erythrocytes enables one to detect as little as 0.001 μg antibody nitrogen. Latex particle agglutination, usually associated with diagnosis of rheumatoid arthritis, has been applied in some infectious diseases; for example, in early histoplasmosis and coccidioidomycosis. The flocculation of latex particles and bentonite particles has been applied to the serodiagnosis of trichinosis. Latex particles coated with antibody may be used to detect cryptococcal antigen in serum or CSF.

Agglutination of antigen-sensitized erythrocytes (called passive hemagglutination to distinguish the test from the hemagglutination of erythrocytes by their corresponding isoagglutinins) is applied more often in research than in diagnosis (*e.g.,* toxoplasmosis). Although polysaccharide antigens readily adsorb to erythrocytes, the adherence of protein antigens usually requires pretreatment of the erythrocytes with tannic acid or pyruvic aldehyde plus formaldehyde. Protein antigens can be prepared for linkage to erythrocytes by treatment with bisdiazotized benzidine or chromic chloride.

Hemadsorption and Hemagglutination Inhibition

Far more widely applied than passive hemagglutination is the hemagglutination inhibition (HI) test. Viral and other particles of many kinds can adsorb to human group 0 or chicken erythrocytes, bringing about agglutination. The capacity of a patient's serum to prevent agglutination of the erythrocytes by prior reaction with the virus provides a measure of antiviral antibody. Such tests are applicable with influenza, measles, rubella, and adeno-, echo-, pox-, and other viruses, and with *Mycoplasma pneumoniae* and *Bordetella pertussis.*

Flocculation

The aggregation (flocculation) of suspended particles or droplets of antigen or hapten has wide use, particularly in the serodiagnosis of syphilis. In such tests as the Venereal Disease Reserach Laboratory (VDRL) test, and the Kahn, Hinton, and Kline tests, globules of cardiolipin (emulsified with cholesterol and lecithin) are clumped by serum from patients with syphilis (and from patients with several nonsyphilitic conditions). As little as 0.1 μg antibody (reagin) nitrogen per ml can be detected by this method. Such flocculation tests can be used qualitatively but are even more useful as quantitative measures of changes in the level of reagin.

Complement Fixation (CF) Test

The multicomponent system present in serum and known as complement (C′) can combine with an antigen-antibody complex. When the antigen is resident on or in a component of a cell, lysis of the cell usually results. This property of C′-dependent antigen-antibody interaction is made use of in the classic CF test through hemolysis. Actually, hemolysis is an indirect indicator that is distinct from the antigen-antibody system being tested for (Table 14-3). The end point is precise because it depends on detecting hemolysis by the naked eye or photometrically. It is a relatively sensitive test because amounts as small as 0.05 μg antibody nitrogen can be detected. Moreover, it is adaptable to the use of soluble antigens (mumps, influenza, coccidioidal, histoplasmal, toxoplasmal, rickettsial, mycoplasmal), emulsions (the cardiolipin antigen used in syphilis flocculation tests), and particulate antigens (viruses, *Histoplasma capsulatum* yeast cells, rickettsias, chlamydias).

The technique and performance of the CF test, however, are complicated because of the several reagents that must be carefully assayed. In addition to serum or other body fluids for testing and specific antigen, other essential reagents must be on hand: sheep erythrocytes, antisheep cell hemolysin (produced in rabbits), guinea pig serum (as the source of complement). With so many reagents, several controls are needed in each test: the specimen and antigen, tested separately, must not show anticomplementary activity—that is, they must not by themselves bind or destroy C′ and thus inhibit the indicator hemolytic system. The hemolytic system control lacks the specimen and antigen, and it is used to indicate that hemolysin and C′ are sufficiently active. The red blood cell control, simply a suspension of sheep erythrocytes in saline, makes a decision possible regarding the fragility and tendency to spontaneous hemolysis of these cells.

Of all the pitfalls that can beset the CF test, the occurrence of anticomplementary activity in the specimen submitted for examination is of most direct concern to the physician. Anticomplementary activity may result from improper preservation and contamination of the specimen. Occasionally, former or current narcotic addicts yield, for unknown reasons, anticomplementary sera. The various procedures recommended for the removal of anticomplementary activity are not practical in a busy laboratory. One alternative is to carry out an anticomplementary titration—that is, serial dilutions of the specimen without addition of antigen are set up in parallel with the complete test system. Thus, if the anticomplementary titration results in the binding of C′ by the specimen alone at a dilution of 1:4, and the test system (specimen + antigen) binds C′ at a serum dilution of 1:32, the CF test is presumed to be positive.

Recent advances in both theoretical and experimental knowledge of the CF test enable the design and selection of a variation that is suitable for testing the antigen-antibody system of interest. For all methods, the test serum (or other body fluid) is first heated at 56°C for 30 min to inactivate intrinsic C′. Ca^{++} and Mg^{++} must be present. There are variations in the time and temperature of the C′ binding step, and in the volume of serum and reagents employed.

The Kolmer method is a classic test, although several modifications of it have been developed. In this test, the serum-antigen mixture (0.2–0.5 ml each) is permitted to bind C′ in the refrigerator for approximately 18 hours. A gain in sensitivity results, as compared with a more rapid modification in which binding occurs during 2 hours at 37°C.

A more recent micromodification requires much smaller quantities of serum and reagents (0.025 ml to 0.05 ml). The results appear to be comparable to those with the usual, larger scale tests.

Owing to the vagaries of the CF test, it is important to test consecutive serum specimens simultaneously in order to determine whether a significant change in titer has occurred. It is usually inappropriate to compare titers obtained in different laboratories or by different methods. Thus, if serial titers from a given patient are to be followed, the specimens should be submitted to one laboratory. Although the complexities of the test may appear formidable, once established, the CF test can be extremely valuable in diag-

Table 14-3. *Complement-Fixation Test*

Fixation of complement (positive test)

Test system:

Serum (Ab) + antigen (Ag) + C′ → Ab-Ag (with C′ bound)

Hemolytic system:

Hemolysin (H) + erythrocytes (RBC) → No hemolysis

No fixation of complement (negative test)

Test system:

Serum (no Ab) + antigen (Ag) + C′ → Ag + C′

Hemolytic system:

Hemolysin (H) + erythrocytes (RBC) + C′ → H-RBC (with C′ bound) → hemolysis

nosis and prognosis. Indeed, it may be the only useful test available in some infectious diseases (*e.g.,* psittacosis-ornithosis).

Neutralization

Neutralization tests imply inactivation of a biologically active agent by contact with specific antibody. A viable bacterium can be affected adversely, as in the *Treponema pallidum* immobilization (TPI) test. In this test an observer seeks to detect an immobilizing effect on actively motile treponemes exposed to a serum specimen.

Viral neutralization tests are widely used, but they must be carefully standardized for each viral agent and each test system. An attempt is made to quantitate the capacity of a given specimen (antibody) to nullify the effects of a virus using susceptible experimental animals, embryonated eggs, or cell cultures. A quantity of virus with a known effect on the susceptible system is usually mixed with dilutions of the specimen, and the mixture is then inoculated into the susceptible animal, embryonated egg, or cell culture. The method is complicated by possible variations in the end point, in the use of animals (variation in age, sex, and genetic constitution), in routes of inoculation, time and temperature of incubation of virus-serum mixtures, and other factors. It should be noted that not all antiviral antibodies are neutralizing antibodies.

Neutralization of toxin can also be studied in an intact animal or *in vitro*. The Schick test constitutes a neutralization test carried out in the skin of the human (see Chap. 25, Diphtheria). Neutralization is used in assessing the potency of diphtheria antitoxin by injecting mixtures of toxin and antitoxin intradermally into guinea pigs. Since monkey kidney cells in tissue culture are damaged by diphtheria toxin, protection against such damage by serum from humans or experimental animals provides a means of quantitating antitoxin content. Variations of these methods may be adapted for other bacterial exotoxins.

Immunofluorescence—Fluorescent Antibody (FA)

The immunofluorescence—fluorescent antibody (FA) test was described in 1941 and has been widely applied in diagnostic and experimental serology (see Chap. 9, Microscopic Examinations). The FA method can be used for the demonstration of a specific antigen or infectious agent, as well as for demonstrating the presence of a specific antibody.

It is not practical to list the great number of systems in which the FA method has been used. Yet, the method is of striking utility in the serodiagnosis of syphilis with the fluorescent treponemal antibody-absorption (FTA-ABS) test (see Chap. 59, Syphilis), in rapidly identifying rabies virus in brain tissue (see Chap. 124, Rabies), and in differentiating an upper from a lower urinary tract origin of bacteriuria.

Radioimmunoassay

This extremely sensitive method involves competition between labeled and unlabeled antigen for combining sites on antibody. It has been applied to a limited extent with infectious agents (*e.g.,* hepatitis B) (see Chap. 71, Hepatitis B [Serum Hepatitis]).

Enzyme-Linked Immunosorbent Assays (ELISA)

The applications of the enzyme-linked immunosorbent assay (ELISA) method are increasing rapidly because of high sensitivity, low expense, and speed of testing. Assays may be made for antibody or antigen. The immunosorbent step is the primary or enabling reaction; it consists of the covalent attachment of macromolecules to materials such as cellulose and polyacrylamide. Thus, in the indirect assay for antibody, the wells of polystyrene microhemagglutination plates are sensitized by passive adsorption with the test antigen. After washing, the serum sample is added; if antibodies are present, they will bind to the immobilized antigen. The wells are again washed, and an enzyme-labeled antihuman immunoglobulin conjugate is added. The conjugate reacts with antibodies bound to test antigen. The enzymes horseradish peroxidase or alkaline phosphatase are commonly linked to antibodies by glutaraldehyde or periodate treatment. The presence of bound enzyme is then detected by adding the appropriate substrate, which leads to the formation of a colored compound following enzymatic action. Reactions are read visually or spectrophotometrically.

ELISA tests may have the sensitivity of radioimmunoassays, and they do not carry the health risks associated with the use of radioactive isotopes. The immunodiagnosis of many infectious diseases, caused by all classes of agents, may be enhanced by applications of this very adaptable method.

Additional Serologic Procedures

Unique serologic methods of limited applicability have been employed in a variety of infections:

> The Sabin-Feldman dye test for toxoplasmosis depends on the ability of specific antibodies to block the uptake of alkaline methylene blue into the cytoplasm of *Toxoplasma gondii* (see Chap. 129, Toxoplasmosis).

The capsular swelling (quellung) test for *Haemophilus influenzae, Streptococcus pneumoniae,* and *Neisseria meningitidis* (serogroups A and C) can be carried out directly in CSF by the addition of specific antisera.
Sheep erythrocytes sensitized with extracts of leptospiras are lysed in the presence of C′ and the serum of a patient with leptospirosis.

Bacteriolytic or bactericidal antibodies and opsonic effects of sera are demonstrable, but they provide no advantage over the more conventional methods discussed previously.

Interpretation of Results

As with any laboratory findings, the results of serologic studies must be interpreted in the light of all the data about the patient—clinical and laboratory. Positive serologic findings do not necessarily indicate either active infection or the need for therapy. For example, antibodies detectable in the cord blood or venous blood of a newborn child probably reflect the transplacental transfer of maternal antibodies. On the other hand, the presence of IgM specific for rubella virus is evidence of a congenital rubella infection in the neonate. The titer of histoplasmal complement-fixing antibodies often increases following a positive histoplasmin skin test in a person who actually does not have active histoplasmosis.

The necessity for at least two specimens of serum from a single patient cannot be overemphasized. An "acute" serum may be negative and fail to assist in the diagnosis. A later serum (a "convalescent" specimen if taken during recovery and a "chronic specimen if collected while the infection continues) is important not only in diagnosis but also in providing prognostic assistance. The time interval between paired specimens varies 1 to 6 weeks to allow for rises in titer significant in the diagnosis of active infection.

Complications of serologic procedures should also be recognized. Some of these, such as the occurrence of prozone reactions in brucella agglutination tests, may be due to the presence of an interfering or blocking antibody. Prozone reactions may also occur in agglutination tests when there is an antibody excess in low dilutions of high-titered serums. The possibility also exists that a patient's serum may contain sufficient antigen to provide an antigen excess which, when added to that supplied in setting up the test, gives a prozone reaction in the lower dilutions of serum.

Cross reactions may be confusing. Immunization against typhoid fever, tularemia, or cholera sometimes induces antibrucella antibodies in diagnostic titers. Other serologic cross reactions occur between typhoid fever and other salmonelloses, histoplasmosis and coccidioidomycosis, cat-scratch fever and chlamydial (psittacosis) antigen, and syphilis and nonsyphilitic diseases (biologic false-positive).

Prior immunization must be considered when interpreting serologic results. Typhoid immunization may induce O, H, and Vi agglutinins depending on the type of vaccine employed. The presence of O antibodies, which may be relatively short-lived, may indicate typhoid fever, whereas anti-H agglutinins at a relatively high titer may be a legacy of typhoid vaccination 1 to 5 years earlier.

Various intercurrent conditions may exert profound effects on serologic responses. The primary immunologic (immunoglobulin) deficiency diseases such as congenital (Bruton's) agammaglobulinemia and Swiss type agammaglobulinemia are rare, but they must be kept in mind. Several immune deficiency states secondary to neoplastic disorders—for example, chronic lymphocytic leukemia or multiple myeloma—may yield selective immunologic deficiencies sometimes reflected in inadequate serologic responses. Finally, subnormal serologic responses may be associated with therapies such as pharmacologic doses of glucosteroids, irradiation, and administration of alkylating and antimetabolic compounds.

Tests for Components of the Immunologic Response

Complement

Assays for components of complement (C′) may be useful when low concentrations of C′ contribute to inadequate immunologic defense of the patient. Complement may be depressed in processes associated with extensive binding of antibodies by persisting antigen, as occurs in malaria, chronic bacterial endocarditis, hepatitis B (serum hepatitis), and septicemia. Such reactions *in vivo* require all nine components of the classic complement pathway. Fresh serum, or serum stored at −70°C, can be used to determine the titer of complement in 50% hemolytic units of C′ (CH_{50}) by testing serum dilutions against sensitized erythrocytes. Normal serum contains approximately 20 to 24 CH_{50}/ml.

Extensive complement reactivity can lead to depletion of the early-acting components. Single radial immunodiffusion (SRD) assays for Clq, C3, and C4 may be used to detect C′ components down to the level of 2.5 μg/ml.

The importance of the alternative complement pathway for natural resistance to many bacteria, viruses, and metazoan parasites now seems established. The mechanism operates without antibody and engages the participation of C3 through C9, the late-reacting components. Single radial immunodiffusion assays can be made for factor B (C3 proactivator) and properdin, two required serum proteins of this system, although useful interpretations regarding concentrations require further research.

Assays for Cell-mediated Immunity

Two subsets of T lymphocytes are active in cell-mediated immunity in infectious diseases. *In vitro* tests to detect their presence in the efferent limb of immunity include assays for migration inhibitory factor and cytotoxic T lymphocytes.

MIGRATION INHIBITORY FACTOR

The assay for migration inhibitory factor (MIF) reflects release of lymphokines from specifically sensitized lymphocytes following contact with antigen; MIF is essentially a correlate of delayed-type hypersensitivity (DTH) as detected *in vivo* by skin testing. Resistance to many facultative intracellular microorganisms depends upon conversion of macrophages to a special activated state, which is presumed to be mediated by some lymphokine. While the true nature of the effector lymphokine has not yet been determined, its presence usually appears concurrently with the DTH state. The mechanism is important in resistance to the bacterial genera *Mycobacterium, Salmonella, Brucella,* and *Listeria,* and to many protozoan and viral agents (*e.g.,* measles, rubella, parainfluenza I).

In the direct system for assay of MIF, mononuclear cells collected from the patient's blood are utilized as the source of the specifically sensitized T cells. The test cells are mixed in a ratio of 1:3 with oil-induced peritoneal exudate cells from normal guinea pigs. The guinea pig macrophages serve as indicator cells. The cell mixtures are drawn into capillary tubes and are then packed with gentle centrifugation. Capillary tubes are broken at the interface of cells and medium. The tubes containing cells are attached to the surfaces of coverslips in specially designed chambers. A top coverslip completes the chamber, which is then filled with medium containing test antigen (*e.g.,* tuberculin PPD or virus antigen obtained from frozen and thawed virus-infected cells). The antigen will induce lymphokine release from specifically sensitized T cells, and the MIF will inhibit migration of the guinea pig macrophages. Four replicates of the tests are run and compared to a like number of chambers that permit macrophage migration in the absence of antigen. The migration areas are determined by optical projection of the chamber image on a surface, where the areas are drawn and then measured by planimetry. The following formula is used to calculate the percent of migration inhibition:

$$\%\,\text{Inhibition} = 1.0 - \frac{\text{Test area}}{\text{Control area}} \times 100$$

Twenty percent or more inhibition is scored as a positive test.

An agarose microdroplet procedure is a variation of this test, which is more sparing of test materials. Also, an indirect test may be used wherin the human lymphocytes are incubated for 2 days in the presence of antigen to induce lymphokine release. Supernatant fluid from such cultures can then be added to culture chambers containing guinea pig macrophages, which function as indicator cells.

CYTOTOXIC T LYMPHOCYTES

The assay for cytotoxic T lymphocytes (CTL) detects a subset of T cells that react specifically with antigen on target cells to cause lysis of the cells. These T cells are sometimes called T killer cells or Tk cells. The function of CTLs is especially important in virus infections in which virus-specified antigens appear on the surfaces of infected cells. The spread of viruses is prevented if host cell lysis occurs before mature virions are formed. It has been found in animal studies that this form of target cell attack is most efficient when both the CTL and its target share the same histocompatability antigens. However, several laboratories run assays with human CTLs, disregarding histocompatability restriction; in those tests the target cells are chosen without regard to the incompatability of cellular antigens. Target cell lysis may be observed morphologically, but the assays are best determined by the release of radiolabeled cytoplasmic constituents. The lymphocytes in heparinized blood from the patient are concentrated to a purity of approximately 90% lymphocytes to provide CTLs. Target cells may be purchased commercially or prepared in the laboratory. Tissue culture cells are infected with the appropriate virus and incubated; when 90% of the cells exhibit surface viral antigen, they are harvested and cryopreserved in the presence of dimethyl sulfoxide. The cells are thawed on the day of testing, and both infected and control target cells are radiolabeled with ^{51}Cr. On microtiter plates, the wells are inoculated with 5×10^3 labeled target cells followed by 5×10^5 lymphocytes from the test suspension. This gives a 100:1 ratio of lymphocytes to target cells. It should be noted here that the number of CTLs to a given antigen is a small portion of the total lymphocytes. The spleen cells of immunized animals contain about 1% or 2% CTLs. The cell mixtures are incubated for varying periods, depending upon the virus system under test. The supernatant fluid from the cultures is collected manually or by an automated sample harvester. The test fluids are read by gamma counting in a spectrometer. Specific immune release of the isotope is calculated by subtracting the percentage of ^{51}Cr released in the control target cells from that released by infected cells.

LYMPHOCYTE ACTIVATION

Lymphocyte activation assays may also be determined, but the results are subject to considerable variation, depending upon the stage of the infection. This test measures antigen-induced lymphocyte transformation; as such, it is not strictly a cell-mediated immune test, because both T and B cells participate. Specifically sensitized lymphocytes respond to the antigen by undergoing blast transformation. This can be quantitated by the uptake of [^{3}H]- thymidine, which is used in DNA synthesis. The test is a rather general measure of the afferent lymphoproliferative limb of immunity and is read as a Stimulation Index. Samples are counted in a liquid scintillation spectrometer, and the counts per minute (CPM) reading in test antigen samples is divided by the CPM in control samples.

Human Leukocyte Antigens (HLA) in Infectious Diseases

The major histocompatability complex (MHC) in man is coded on the sixth chromosome. The gene products are alloantigens on the surfaces of nucleated cells, and tests for their presence are usually made on lymphocytes and macrophages. Thus, it is common practice to employ human leukocyte antigens (HLA) typing for the detection of the HLA haplotypes that occur in each individual. The tests are useful to determine histocompatability prior to tissue transplantation, and, in addition, some associations between HLA antigens and disease have been reported. In more than 30 clinical conditions, a statistically significant association has been found between the presence of certain HLA antigens and a disease state. Many of these associations are seen in diseases of uncertain cause. Table 14-4 lists infectious or possibly infectious diseases in which HLA associations have been made.

The procedure of HLA testing depends on detecting MHC glycoprotein antigens on cell surfaces by complement-dependent cellular cytotoxicity using a battery of known antibody reagents arising in the serum of multiparous women, or following blood transfusions and immunization procedures. The mononuclear cell fraction obtained from the blood of the patient can be used directly to detect inherited sets of allelic antigens coded by loci A, B, C.

Typing for antigens coded by the D locus is more difficult, since the distribution of these antigens is more restricted. The DR (D-related) antigens that appear on the surfaces of B lymphocytes can be detected by serologic means when purified B lymphocytes are used as antigens. The D series of antigens have been detected by the mixed lymphocyte culture reaction (MLC), since they do not participate readily in serologic tests. It is not clear what the relationship is between the D antigens revealed by cellular typing and the DR antigens detected by serologic typing. Cellular typing by the MLC reaction is laborious and time consuming. In that procedure, increased DNA synthesis is measured in T cells stimulated by contact with cells bearing incompatible D antigens. The MLC reaction procedure will continue to be important for work in tissue transplantation, but the serologic detection of DR antigens is becoming more important in relating HLA to disease.

To perform the tests for DR antigens, B cells are prepared from a mononuclear cell suspension to which carbonyl iron is added to facilitate the elimination of macrophages. After ingesting the iron, the macrophages can be removed by passing the cells over a magnet. The lymphocyte suspension is then added to tissue culture flasks, after the bottom surfaces have been coated with goat antihuman $F(ab')_2$. The Ig-bearing B cells adhere to the bottom surface, and then nonadherent T cells are washed away. Purified B cells are then eluted with human serum. The test is performed as follows:

1. Purified B cells are added to wells in a tray ($\simeq$2000 cells per well).
2. Selected anti-DR reagents are added to sensitize the lymphocytes.
3. Rabbit complement is added.
4. The numbers of lysed cells are observed after adding trypan blue, a dye that stains only the lysed cells.

Population studies and family studies are used to gather evidence linking the HLA system to disease susceptibility or resistance. At this time, the basis for associations between HLA and disease are only speculative. Associations most often involve the B and D series of antigens, which suggests linkage to the nearby immune response (Ir) genes. The Ir genes are of great importance in defense against infections. Susceptibility might be enhanced if there is molecular mimicry of HLA antigens by certain microbial antigens. Molecular mimicry could also lead to the breaking of self tolerance and give rise to processes such as virus-induced autoimmunity; the abnormal

Table 14-4. *Some Associations Between HLA and Infectious or Possibly Infectious Diseases*

Disease	Etiology	HLA Antigen	No. of Studies	No. of Patients Investigated	Relative Risk	Significance (P)
Recurrent Herpes labialis	Herpes simplex virus	A1	2	292	2.7	$<10^{-10}$
Tuberculosis	*Mycobacterium tuberculosis*	B8	1	46	5.1	$<10^{-6}$
Leprosy	*Mycobacterium leprae*	Type of leprosy (lepromatous, tuberculoid) apparently linked to HLA in family studies				
Multiple Sclerosis	Measles virus?	Dw2	9	932	4.1	$<10^{-10}$
Reiter's Syndrome	?	B27	9	341	37.0	$<10^{-10}$
Ankylosing Spondylitis	?	B27	29	2022	87.4	$<10^{-10}$
Juvenile diabetes	Coxsackie virus?	Dw4	2	232	4.0	$<10^{-10}$

After Svejgaard A. In Rose NR, Friedman H (eds): Manual of Clinical Immunology, 2nd ed. Washington DC, American Society for Microbiology, 1980

reactivity of patients with multiple sclerosis to measles virus might conceivably be illustrative. It is also possible that certain HLA factors could serve as virus receptors. Further research is required to unravel bases for the associations of HLA and disease.

Bibliography

Books

BENNETT CW: Clinical Serology. Springfield, Charles C Thomas, 1977, 304 pp.

CHERRY WB, GOLDMAN M, CARSKI TR: Fluorescent Antibody Techniques. Public Health Service Publication No. 729, US Dept of Health, Education and Welfare. Washington DC, US Government Printing Office, 1960, 73 pp.

FRIEDMAN H, LINNA TJ, PRIER JE: Immunoserology in the Diagnosis of Infectious Diseases. Baltimore, University Park Press, 1979, 193 pp.

GOLDMAN M: Fluorescent Antibody Methods. New York, Academic Press, 1968, 303 pp.

LENNETTE EH, BALOWS A, HAUSLER WJ, TRUANT JP: Manual of Clinical Microbiology, 3rd ed. Washington DC, American Society for Microbiology, 1980, 1044 pp.

Manual of Tests for Syphilis. Public Health Service Publication No 411, US Dept of Health, Education and Welfare. Washington DC, US Government Printing Office, 1969.

MÜLLER-EBERHARD HJ, SCHREIBER RD: Molecular biology and chemistry of the alternative pathway of complement. In Kunkel HG, Dixon FJ (eds): Advances in Immunology, Vol 29. New York, Academic Press, 1980

PEACOCK JE, TOMAR RH: Manual of Laboratory Immunology. Philadelphia, Lea & Febiger, 1980, 228 pp.

ROCKLIN RE, BENDTZEN K, GREINEDER D: Mediators of immunity: Lymphokines and monokines. In Kunkel HG, Dixon FJ (eds): Advances In Immunology, Vol 29. New York, Academic Press, 1980

ROSE NR, FRIEDMAN H: Manual of Clinical Immunology, 2nd ed. Washington DC, American Society for Microbiology, 1980, 1105 pp.

RYDER LP, ANDERSEN E, SVEJGAARD A: HLA and Disease Registry, 3rd report. Copenhagen, Munksgaard, 1979, 61 pp.

ZINKERNAGEL RF, DOHERTY PC: MHC-restricted cytotoxic T cells: Studies on the biological role of polymorphic major transplantation antigens determining T-cell restriction-specificity, function, and responsiveness. In Kunkel HG, Dixon RJ (eds): Advances in Immunology, Vol. 27. New York, Academic Press, 1979

Journals

BRANDT BL, WYLE FA, ARTENSTEIN MS: A radioactive antigen-binding assay for *Neisseria meningitidis* polysaccharide antibody. J Immunol 108:913–920, 1972

HIRATA AA, STALL WT: Reproducible passive hemagglutination procedure with high sensitivity using the double aldehyde treated cells. Proc Soc Exp Biol Med 130:343–345, 1969

NAGEL JG, TUAZON CU, CARDELLA TA, SHEAGRAN JN: Teichoic acid serologic diagnosis of staphylococcal endocarditis. Ann Intern Med 82:13–17, 1975

NORDEN CW, MICHAELS RN, MELISH M: Effect of previous infection on antibody response of children to vaccination with capsular polysaccharide of *Haemophilus influenzae* type B. J Infect Dis 132:69–74, 1975

OSEBOLD JW, PEARSON LD, MEDIN NI: Relationship of antimicrobial cellular immunity to delayed hypersensitivity in listeriosis. Infect and Immun 9:354–362, 1974

RAIZMAN RE, NEVA FA: Detection of circulating antigen in acute experimental infections with *Toxoplasma gondii*. J Infect Dis 132:44–98, 1975

RYTEL MW: Rapid diagnostic methods in infectious diseases. Adv Intern Med 20:37–60, 1975

W. CHRISTOPHER DUNCAN

15 Skin Tests

Skin tests related to infectious diseases have in common the intradermal deposition of relatively specific biologic agents. These agents are termed sensitins when they have the capacity to elicit a skin reaction in a sensitized host but cannot engender such sensitivity (*e.g.,* tuberculin) and immunogens when they can set in motion an immune response and may evoke a skin reaction (*e.g.,* pneumococcal capsular polysaccharide). Useful in diagnosis, epidemiologic studies, and occasionally in prognosis, skin tests may also be applied to determine the presence of circulating antibodies—diphtheria antitoxin in the Schick test (see Chap. 25, Diptheria), antierythrogenic toxin in the Dick test (see Chap. 24, Streptococcal Diseases), and type-specific antipneumococcal antibody in the Francis test (see Chap. 31, Bacterial Pneumonias). Such tests exemplify immediate hypersensitivity (IH) reactions. In addition to specific humoral antibodies, expression of IH requires the presence and activity of specific kinds of cells, for example, mast cells. Other situations in which testing for IH is utilized include protozoan and helminthic infections.

More frequently, skin testing is used to detect delayed hypersensitivity (DH), also known as bacterial allergy, allergy of infection, tuberculin type hypersensitivity, and specific cell-mediated hypersensitivity. Although generally thought of in relation to infectious processes, DH has critical significance to the rejection of allografts, the development of manifestations in some autoimmune diseases, and possibly, the defense against cancer. In contrast to the humoral immune response, the manifestations of delayed hypersensitivity cannot at present be measured quantitatively.

Delayed hypersensitivity can be transferred from a reactive to a nonreactive person by means of thymic origin or T lymphocytes, or by transfer factor. Transfer factor is dialyzable peptide or polynucleotide of less than 10,000 mol wt derived from sensitized peripheral blood lymphocytes. On injection, adoptive transfer of hypersensitivity results and persists in man for many months. The phenomenon of transfer factor must be clearly distinguished from passive transfer of IH by means of humoral antibody.

The mediators of cellular immunity are collectively known as lymphokines. Certain reactions demonstrable *in vitro* correlate with the DH reaction. Migration inhibition factor (MIF) can be shown *in vitro* to affect normal monocytes and peritoneal exudate macrophages causing them to (1) become sticky, adhere to the walls of capillary tubes, and fail to migrate; (2) survive longer; and (3) enter an activated state. Other reactions include (1) the macrophage agglutination tests; (2) the production of lymphotoxin, a lymphocyte derived substance toxic for certain target cells; and (3) stimulation of lymphocytes in culture by the specific antigen to yield lymphoblastlike cells with increased synthesis of DNA. Thus far, however, none of these tests has provided a practical substitute for the determination of DH by skin tests. Indeed, the *in vitro* and cutaneous tests are not invariably wedded to each other.

Anergy, as may be seen in disseminated coccidioidomycosis, has generally been associated with a poor prognosis. Some immunologic deficiency states—for example, failure of development of the thymus—preclude the development of DH.

Delayed hypersensitivity has often been closely linked to intracellular infections, but this may not be an absolute requirement for the development of DH. Despite frequent association or juxtaposition of cellular-delayed hypersensitivity and cellular immunity, the association of DH with resistance to reinfection is not proved.

The induction of DH has usually been related to a protein antigen. However, other molecular species can induce DH. Contact hypersensitivity is similar to the delayed allergy of infection and is induced by the application of small, nonprotein molecules to the skin; for example, picryl chloride. Certain polysaccharides have been shown to induce DH. Moreover, DH-reactive substances derived from fungi contain a substantial proportion of polysaccharide, albeit in association with nitrogenous (amino-acid-containing) components. It is possible, however, that antibody induced by some nonprotein antigens—for example, a polysaccharide—can combine with an excess of homologous antibody and can then induce DH.

Experimentally, the development of DH occurs as early as the fourth day after administration of antigen. However, in infectious diseases the development of DH is probably related both to the nature of the antigen and the incubation period. There is considerable variation in the time of appearance of cutaneous DH, a fact important to skin testing. Thus, the demonstration of the conversion to reactivity is diagnostic of a recent infection with the agent from which the test substance was derived.

The utility of DH as a diagnostic, prognostic, or epidemiologic test is limited to just a few infectious diseases (Table 15-1).

Bacterial Infections

Tuberculosis

The tuberculin reaction is considered the prototype of the DH skin reaction. The incubation period of tuberculosis is 4 to 6 weeks (see Chap. 34, Pulmonary Tuberculosis) and DH to tuberculin becomes demonstrable 2 to 10 weeks after infection occurs. Positive skin reactions with tuberculin are not diagnostic tests for current infection. Allergies of infection are generally persistent through life or remain persistent long after the infection has disappeared. Conversion of the skin test from negative to positive indicates that the person has acquired a tuberculous infection. Generally, it is assumed that infection with *Mycobacterium tuberculosis* has occurred, although infection with *Mycobacterium bovis, Mycobacterium kansasii,* and *Mycobacterium marinum* may also engender DH with reactivity to tuberculin. Currently, about 7% of the population of the United States is reactive to tuberculin; however, the reaction rate among children as they begin school is only

Table 15-1. *Nature and Application of Skin Tests for Infectious Diseases*

Disease	Delayed Hypersensitivity	Immediate Hypersensitivity	Diagnosis	Prognosis	Surveys and Case Finding	Evaluation	Available Commercially
Tuberculosis	+		+	+	+		Yes
Other mycobacterioses	+	+					No
Leprosy	+		+	+			No
Brucellosis	+		+		+	Not very useful	No
Tularemia	+					Useful before antibody production	No
Streptokinase—streptodornase (SK—SD)	+					Used to determine capacity to mount DH reaction	Yes
Blastomycosis	+					Not useful	No
Coccidioidomycosis	+		+	+	+	Should be applied very selectively	Yes
Cryptococcosis	+				?	Not adequately developed	No
Paracoccidioidomycosis	+		+			Not well developed	No
Candidosis	+					Not useful	Yes
Trichophytosis	+	+				Not useful	Yes
Toxoplasmosis	+				+		No
Leishmaniasis	+	?	+			Value not established	No
Echinococcosis	+	+				DH response appears more specific	No
Trichinosis	+	+				Not useful	No
Filariasis	+					Of certain usefulness	No
Schistosomiasis		+	+			Useful in adults but not in children	No
Paragonimiasis		+				Specific and sensitive; not widely used	No
Clonorchiasis		+				Good sensitivity, but cross reaction in paragonimiasis	No
Lymphogranuloma venereum (Frei test)	+					Not useful	No
Cat-scratch fever	+		+		+		No
Mumps	+						Yes

around 0.2%. Therefore, the tuberculin test has little value as a screening test in the United States. Cutaneous DH to tuberculin is long-lasting, but it may wane with advancing age, be diminished during viral diseases such as measles, mumps, and smallpox, or decline temporarily following immunization against these diseases. Sensitivity may also fade during diseases that cause a high fever, sarcoidosis, treatment with glucosteroids and immunosuppressive agents. Indeed, early treatment of tuberculosis may lead to loss of sensitivity to tuberculin.

Materials for Testing. Two separate materials prepared from *M. tuberculosis* may be used in the tuberculin skin test: old tuberculin (OT) and purified protein derivative (PPD). The latter is obtained by the addition of trichloroacetic acid or neutral ammonium sulfate to bacteria-free filtrates (OT) of cultures of *M. tuberculosis.* Although PPD is thought to be more nearly pure, both OT and PPD contain nucleic acids and polysaccharides. The active principal appears to be heat stable but not immunogenic, and repeated skin testing in man does not sensitize. However, a recall effect may result from repeated testing in persons who are already sensitive to similar bacterial antigens. The currently available material for intracutaneous (Mantoux) testing today is PPD, stabilized in solution with the addition of an antiadsorbent (polysorbate 80 or Tween 80) and calibrated to contain 5 TU (Test Units) in each 0.1 ml. Current lots of PPD are standardized for biologic activity against Purified Protein Derivative-Seibert (PPD-S), a bulk lot prepared in 1940 and used as a reference. The relationship between units of PPD and OT is shown in Table 15-2.

Methods of Testing. Three multiple puncture tests are currently available: the Heaf, Tine, and Mono-Vac. All use concentrated tuberculin, but there is no way to standardize the amount of tuberculin that is introduced. They are useful only as screening tests. All positive reactions should be confirmed with an intradermal Mantoux test.

Jet injection makes use of a jet gun with a special nozzle to deliver 5 TU tuberculin intracutaneously in 0.1 ml under high pressure. However, unless the gun is precisely calibrated and properly applied, it often fails to deliver the recommended dose. This test has little use in the United States.

Intracutaneous injection, the Mantoux test, is the most reliable tuberculin test available. It should always be used in high-risk situations and to confirm positive multiple-puncture tests. It is performed by the intracutaneous injection of 0.1 ml PPD, usually containing 5 TU (0.0001 mg), into the skin of the volar or dorsal surface of the forearm. The injection is made with a short (½ in), bluntly beveled, 26- or 27-G needle with a glass or plastic syringe. The injection should be made just beneath the surface of the skin with the needle bevel upward. A discrete wheal 6 mm to 10 mm in diameter should be produced. If the injection is too deep and no wheal appears, the test should be immediately reapplied at a site at least 5 cm away. The test is read at 48 to 72 hours by measuring the maximum transverse diameter of induration in millimeters. The test should be read by someone skilled in its interpretation. Good lighting and careful palpation of the test site are essential.

Nontuberculous Mycobacterial Infections

If 5 TU PPD yields 6 mm to 9 mm induration, the reaction may possibly be caused by previous infection and sensitization with so-called atypical mycobacteria (see Chap. 36, Nontuberculous Mycobacterioses). Differential skin testing with multiple antigens in diseases caused by atypical mycobacteria is practically never of value in establishing which par-

Table 15-2. *Intradermal (Mantoux) Tuberculin Skin Test*

Test (Strength)*	International Tuberculin Units (TU)	PPD* mg/0.1 ml	OT: DILUTION	OT: MG/0.1 ml DOSE †
First	1	0.00002	1:10,000	0.01
Intermediate (usual test dose)	5	0.00010	1:2,000	0.05
Second	250	0.00500	1:100	1.00

* Biologic activity equivalent of listed quantities of PPD-S (Purified Protein Derivative-Standard)
† Dry weight assuming 1000 mg/ml concentrated OT (old tuberculin)

ticular *Mycobacterium* spp. was responsible for the disease, because high cross reactivity (low specificity) is exhibited by these antigens. Such special sensitins (PPD-Y: group I, *M. kansasii;* PPD-G: group II, scotochromogens; PPD-B: group III, Battey bacilli; and PPD-F: group IV, *M. fortuitum*) are not available for general use. Bacteriologic identification, therefore, remains essential to the etiologic diagnosis of nontuberculous mycobacterioses.

Leprosy

The lepromin reaction is not a diagnostic test for leprosy (see Chap. 105, Leprosy); many nonleprous persons have a positive lepromin reaction. The time course of development of DH in leprosy is not known, largely because the incubation period is not precisely known. Lepromin, the skin test reagent, is prepared from cutaneous nodules excised from patients with lepromatous leprosy. Following autoclave sterilzation, the material is triturated in saline containing phenol and filtered. Thus, substances derived from human tissue and from *Mycobacterium leprae* are present. Lepromin is not obtainable commercially, but it is prepared by individual leprologists. Recently, lepromin derived from the armadillo (lepromin-A) has been prepared and tested and appears to be a promising alternative to human-derived lepromin (lepromin-H).

The Mitsuda reaction to lepromin is a nodular response (granuloma) that becomes apparent after 7 days and reaches a peak about 3 weeks after injection. Reactivity to lepromin in a patient with leprosy is characteristic of either tuberculoid leprosy or disease which is becoming tuberculoid; it is, therefore, a good prognostic sign. Failure to react to lepromin is characteristic of lepromatous leprosy or indicative of devolution and is, therefore, a bad prognostic sign. Interestingly, patients with lepromatous leprosy also display impairment of DH response to other antigens and have a depressed lymphocyte response to phytohemagglutinin (PHA).

Brucellosis

Delayed hypersensitivity as elicited by Brucellergen (a nucleoprotein and/or protein material derived from *Brucella* spp.) may be useful in epidmiologic surveys, but is of limited diagnostic value. The test is most helpful when it is negative because it helps to exclude brucellosis from a list of possibilities (see Chap. 138, Brucellosis). A positive test may persist after infection has subsided, however, and falsely negative tests may occur. In addition, the material is antigenic. A specific, active protein that has recently been isolated from *Brucella* spp. may prove useful for testing.

Tularemia

Delayed hypersensitivity usually develops within the first week of tularemia and can be detected before agglutinins can be found in the serum (see Chap. 139, Tularemia). Either a protein extract of *Francisella tularensis* or phenolized, killed whole cells can be used for the intradermal test. A skin test antigen consisting of a phenolized vaccine diluted 1:1000 will give a positive reaction in more than 90% of patients within the first 7 days of infection. It is not commercially available, however.

Diphtheria

Susceptibility to diptherial toxin is tantamount to susceptibility to diphtheria (see Chap. 25, Diphtheria), and can be determined by the Schick test. The Schick test dose is diphtherial toxin, diluted in 0.9% NaCl solution so that 0.1 ml contains 1/50 of a minimal lethal dose for a guinea pig. The dose of 0.1 ml is injected intracutaneously in volar forearm. A positive reacton is characterized by an inflammation appearing after 24 to 36 hours and persisting for 4 days or longer. The presence of as little as 1/500 to 1/250 of a unit of antitoxin per milliliter of blood will neutralize the injected toxin and no reaction will occur. Therefore, a negative reaction signifies that sufficient antitoxin is present to protect against diphtheria. A control test always should be performed on the opposite arm using a portion of the diluted toxin which has been inactivated by heating to 60°C for 15 min. If the allergic response to the control material parallels that to the toxin in size and duration of reaction, the test is recorded as a negative Schick. If, however, the reaction to the unheated toxin is at least 50% larger and persists longer than the reaction to the control, the individual is both susceptible to the toxin and allergic to the contaminating substances which are not destroyed by heating; a combined reaction or positive Schick is recorded.

The test is most often used to determine the immune status of adults or children who have not received diphtherial toxoid and are presumed to be susceptible to diphtheria. There is only a limited need for the test in the United States.

Streptococcosis

Streptokinase-streptodornase (SK-SD), enzymes produced by group *A Streptococcus pyogenes,* is useful in determining the capacity of an individual to develop a DH reaction (see Chap. 24, Streptococcal Diseases). That is, the intradermal injection of 5000 to 10,000 units is of about the same value as oidiomycin or mumps antigen.

Delayed hypersensitivity is also demonstrable with the M protein of group A streptococci, but it is not a clinically useful test. The Schultz-Charlton test (injection of antitoxin to erythrogenic toxin) may assist in differentiating scarlet fever from rashes caused by viruses or drugs.

Fungal Infections

Coccidioidomycosis

The majority of individuals who live in endemic areas will acquire coccidioidomycosis (see Chap. 41, Coccidioidomycosis) and will, therefore, have a positive skin test. The intradermal injection of 0.1 ml 1:1000 coccidioidin, prepared from mycelial growth of *Coccidioides immitis*, is the preferred method of testing. There may be an immediate reaction which can be ignored. Readings should be made 24, 48, and 72 hours after injection. The skin test becomes positive ($\geq$ 5 mm induration) in 87% of patients in the first week of clinical illness and in 99% after the second week of illness. If there is no reaction, the test should be repeated 2 to 3 weeks after the onset of illness to detect conversion to reactivity. Documentation of conversion in a person who has been in an endemic area is virtually diagnostic of coccidioidal infection. Although a skin test with 1:100 dilution may aggravate or precipitate the occurrence of erythema nodosum, coccidioidal infection is not worsened or exacerbated. Patients with primary coccidioidomycosis and erythema nodosum are extremely sensitive to coccidioidin and may react to 0.1 ml of a 1:10,000 dilution. Anergy develops in many patients with disseminated coccidioidomycosis, and a small fraction of patients with old pulmonary cavities fails to react to 1:100 coccidioidin; some patients may react to the 1:10 reagent. Sensitivity persists for years but wanes in some individuals. Coccidioidin neither sensitizes humans nor induces coccidioidal antibodies, although it may provoke antibodies to yeast phase *Histoplasma capsulatum*. Indeed, reactivity to cocciciodin may be evident in persons sensitized by infection with *H. capsulatum*, and probably also with *Blastomyces dermatitidis*. Patients with hypersensitivity to coccidioidin may react to histoplasmin and blastomycin, but to a lesser degree. It is desirable, therefore, in doubtful cases, to perform skin tests with all three antigens simultaneously.

Recently, a skin test sensitin prepared from cultured spherules of the fungus, a morphologic form more akin to the spherules characteristically present in the tissues in coccidioidomycosis, has been tested. This appears to have a lower cross sensitivity with histoplasmin and may be more sensitive than standard coccidioidin.

Histoplasmosis

In areas where histoplasmosis is endemic (see Chap. 40, Histoplasmosis), positive skin tests to histoplasmin may be found in 80% of the adult population. Intradermal injection of histoplasmin does not sensitize or induce humoral antibodies in humans not previously infected with *H. capsulatum*. However, skin testing with the usual 1:100 antigen may, in histoplasmin-sensitive individuals, induce or increase the titer of complement-fixing antibodies to the mycelial phase antigens of *H. capsulatum*, even in the absence of active histoplasmosis. The skin test is read after 48 hours, and another reading at 72 hours is advisable. Allergy usually appears during the second or third week of the illness and 1 to 2 weeks before the appearance of a positive serologic test. Although serum obtained at the time the skin test is applied or read yields valid results, subsequent serologic studies may be increased in titer simply as a result of the skin test. A yeast phase histoplasmin, currently undergoing extensive evaluations, does not induce significant changes in complement-fixing antibody in histoplasmin-reactive subjects. Coccidioidin rarely gives a cross reaction. Blastomycin, however, frequently causes a reaction about 50% as large as that caused by histoplasmin.

Blastomycosis

Blastomycin and a heat-killed, whole yeast vaccine are available for skin testing. The whole yeast vaccine appears to be more sensitive, but results are contradictory. Skin tests do not always correlate with complement fixation tests (see Chap. 43, Blastomycosis).

Candidosis

A positive or negative skin test to oidiomycin is of no help in the diagnosis of infections caused by *Candida albicans* (see Chap. 39, Candidosis). Because *C. albicans* is a normal inhabitant of the human body, reactivity is virtually uniform in man. The test may be helpful in individual patients because the clinical course and management depends to some extent upon whether or not the patient is hypersensitive to the yeast. The test is frequently employed as part of a battery of skin tests to determine immunocompetence.

Sporotrichosis

Heat-killed yeast phase of *Sporothrix schenckii,* or the polysaccharide antigen, may be used to detect DH to this fungus (see Chap. 108, Sporotrichosis). Experience with these materials has been limited however.

Trichophytosis

Skin testing with trichophytin yields positive DH reactions in a large proportion of the population. Although the test is of no help in the diagnosis of dermatophytosis, a positive reaction establishes the capacity of a patient to exhibit DH. An immediate wheallike reaction may occur in a few patients: atopic individuals, patients infected with *Trichophyton rubrum* and patients with recurrent erysipelaslike eruptions caused by a dermatophyte.

Protozoan Infections

Toxoplasmosis

The toxoplasmin skin test may become positive only several weeks, months, or even years after infection (see Chap. 129, Toxoplasmosis). Perhaps the earliest documented conversion of the skin test was 4 months after a laboratory-acquired infection. Thus, the test may be of more use as an epidemiologic tool than in diagnosis. However, many persons known to be infected fail to react to the skin test. Toxoplasmin is available only for experimental use in the United States. As prepared from the peritoneal fluid of infected mice or from guinea pig kidney cell cultures, the material is neither standardized nor even partially purified. Substances of murine or guinea pig origin are included along with qualitatively and quantitatively undefined material from *Toxoplasma gondii.* Toxoplasmin should not be used in the usual clinical situation.

Leishmaniasis

Delayed hypersensitivity to a suspension of phenolized flagellate leishmanial microorganisms—the leishmanin (Montenegro) test—persists for life in a large proportion of persons who have had any form of leishmaniasis (see Chap. 146, Leishmaniasis). Although the test is negative in active kala-azar, it becomes positive in nearly all those who recover. The test becomes positive during active infection with *Leishmania mexicana* (approximately 6 weeks), *Leishmania tropica,* and *Leishmania braziliensis* (approximately 3 months).

Helminthic Infections

Echinococcosis

The skin test (Casoni) is carried out by intradermal injection of hyatid (cyst) fluid, or a derivative thereof, obtained from man or other animals (particularly sheep) infected with *Echinococcus granulosus* (see Chap. 79, Larval Cestodiasis). It can not be used to rule out a diagnosis of hydatid disease, because many cyst carriers do not have a detectable immune response. Although the skin test, when properly controlled, is approximately as sensitive as most serologic tests, it is much less specific. The antigen is not available commercially.

Trichinosis

Both IH and DH can be demonstrated by intradermal testing in trichinosis (see Chap. 150, Trichinosis). The significance of DH is unknown. Only preparations containing 10 μg to 20 μg nitrogen per ml fail to yield an excessively high rate of false negatives. The test is of limited usefulness as a diagnostic tool because as many as 35% of persons in endemic areas give a positive reaction. Reactivity persists for at least 5 years after infection; thus, a positive test indicates either previous or current infection. About the third week after infection, 85% to 90% of infected persons give an IH reaction. Therefore, a negative skin test may be useful in excluding possible trichinosis. Commercial skin test antigen is not available.

Filariasis

Although hypersensitivity may be integral to the pathogenesis of filariasis (see Chap. 112, Cutaneous Filariasis, and Chap. 148, Lymphoreticular Filariasis), presently available sensitins are, at best, group specific. Standardization of antigens is needed.

Schistosomiasis

Sensitization to *Schistosoma* spp. develops 4 to 8 weeks after infection and persists many years (see Chap. 81, Schistosomiasis). Immediate hypersensitivity can be detected by intradermal injection of a sensitin derived from adult schistosomes. The test is specific, save for cross reactivity with other trematodes and *Trichinella spiralis.* It is useful in adults, but not in children.

Paragonimiasis

Fractionation of adult *Paragonimus westermani* has yielded a sensitin that provokes intense IH reactions in individuals infected with *P. westermani* (see Chap. 46, Paragonimiasis). This sensitin elicits no response in normal persons or those infected with *Clonorchis sinensis.* Extensive testing has not been carried out.

Clonorchiasis

Intradermal injection of a protein extracted from adult *Clonorchis sinensis* elicits an IH reaction (see Chap. 80, Liver Fluke Infection). Although it is a sensitive test, there is cross reaction in patients with paragonimiasis. However, a greater reaction results when homologous antigen is used.

Viral Infection

Mumps

Delayed hypersensitivity to intradermally injected inactivated mumps virus vaccine (see Chap. 74, Mumps) may indicate prior or present infection and is, therefore, not effective as a diagnostic agent. Reactions may be related to the egg substrate on which the antigen is prepared. The test is used primarily as part of a battery of skin tests for determining immunocompetence.

Cat-Scratch Disease

The precise nature of the agent of cat-scratch disease (CSD) is not clear (see Chap. 166, Cat-Scratch Fever). The skin test of CSD is carried out with material prepared from pus aspirated from a lymph node of a patient with CSD. After fractional sterilization and treatment by freezing and thawing, the material is diluted and tested for sterility. It must be frozen until used. There is no commercially available antigen, and each new antigen must be tested in both known positive and known negative reactors prior to use. Intradermal injection of 0.1 ml should elicit a reaction of 5 mm or more 36 to 48 hours after injection. Cutaneous sensitivity may appear from the onset of adenitis, but it may be delayed 2 to 3 weeks. Ninety-four percent of patients who have the clinical picture of CSD are reported to react positively to the skin test, but false positive reactions are known to occur in 4 to 8% of the general population with higher percentages in relatives of infected persons and in veterinary workers.

Varicella-Zoster

Results of skin tests with antigen prepared from varicella virus have correlated well with a history of chicken pox and antibody titers in control populations. However, as many as 68% of leukemics in remission and other immunosuppressed children with a history of chickenpox may have negative skin tests; therefore, the skin test alone cannot be used to assess susceptibility to varicella. Future modifications in the skin test material may improve its sensitivity in immunocompromised individuals.

Bibliography

Books

BARRATT JT: Cell-mediated hypersensitivity. In Textbook of Immunology. St. Louis, C.V. Mosby, 1974. pp. 281–305.

BRICOUT F: Mumps. In Debre R, Celers J (eds): Clinical Virology. Philadelphia, W B Saunders, 1970. pp 275–284.

GOBLE FC: South American trypanosomiasis. In Jackson GJ, Herman R, Singer I (eds): Immunity to Parasitic Animals, Vol. II. New York, Appleton-Century Crofts, 1970. pp 597–688.

PARK BH, GOOD RA: Principles of Modern Immunobiology: Basic and Clinical. Philadelphia, Lea & Febiger, 1974. 617 pp.

STABUER L: Leishmaniasis. In Jackson GL, Herman R, Singer I (eds): Immunity to Parasitic Animals, Vol. II. New York, Appleton-Century Crofts, 1970. pp 739–765.

Journals

BARRETT-CONNOR E, DAVIS CF, HAMBURGER RN, KAGAN I: An epidemic of trichinosis after ingestion of wild pig in Hawaii. J Infect Dis 133:473–477, 1976

EDWARDS PQ, FURCOLOW ML, GRABAU AA, GRZYBOWSKI S, KATZ J, MACLEAN RA: Current indications for the use of atypical mycobacterial skin test antigens. Am Rev Resp Dis 102:486, 1970

LAWRENCE HS: Transfer factor and cellular immune deficiency disease. N Engl J Med 283:411–419, 1970

LEVIN S: The fungal skin test as a diagnostic hindrance. J Infect Dis 122:343–345, 1970

LEVINE HB, GONZALEZ-OCHOA A, TEN EYCK DR: Dermal sensitivity to coccidioides immitis. A comparison of responses elicited in man by spherulin and coccidioidin. Am Rev Resp Dis 107:803–818, 1973

LEVINE HB, SCALARONE GM, CAMPBELL GD, GRAYBILL JR, KELLY PC, CHAPARAS SD: Histoplasmin-CYL, a yeast phase reagent in skin test studies with humans. Am Rev Respir Dis 119:629–636, 1979

MACLEAN RA: Tuberculin testing antigens and techniques. Chest 689:455S–459S, 1975

MADDISON EE, KAGAN IG, ELSDON-DEW R: Comparison of intradermal and serologic tests for the diagnosis of amebiasis. Am J Trop Med Hyg 17:540–547, 1968

MORGILETH AM: Cat-scratch disease: Nonbacterial regional lymphadenitis: The study of 145 patients and a review of the literature. Pediatrics 42:803–818, 1968

MYERS WM, KVERNES S, BINFORD CH: Comparison of reactions to human and armadillo lepromins in leprosy. Int J Lepr 43:218–225, 1975

REMINGTON JS, BARNETT CG, MEIKEL M, LUNDE MN: Toxoplasmosis and infectious mononucleosis. Arch Intern Med 110:744–753, 1962

SBARBORO JA: Editorial: Skin test antigens: An evaluaton whose time has come. Am Rev Respir Dis 118:1–5, 1978

SCHANTZ PM: Casoni skin test for hydatid disease. N Engl J Med 293:408, 1975

STEELE RW, MYERS MG, VINCENT MN: Transfer factor for the prevention of varicella-zoster infection in childhood leukemia. N Engl J Med 303:355–359, 1980

Section III

Control of Infectious Diseases

SHEILA M. NOLAN
PAUL D. HOEPRICH

16 Environmental Factors

Control of infectious diseases (1) requires recognition of the cause, source, and mode of transmission of organisms and (2) assumes capability to eliminate the cause or source or to disrupt the transfer of infectious agents to hosts. Manipulation of host susceptibility, as with immunization, has resulted in enormous reduction of morbidity and mortality from diseases such as diphtheria and tetanus and, over the last decade, has completely eradicated smallpox. However, manipulation of the environment has had an even greater impact on the control of infectious diseases by advances in sanitary engineering and other modes of environmental hygiene. Often, such measures provide the only feasible approach to prevention of many infectious diseases that are not currently amenable to immunoprophylaxis (*e.g.,* malaria).

Consideration of environmental factors in infectious diseases properly includes examination of microenvironments of infected loci within the host, as well as extrinsic environments within which organisms reside and multiply before establishing themselves in hosts. An understanding of these factors aids in delineating the epidemiology and provides a basis for anticipating and interpreting the clinical manifestations of infectious diseases. For example, the optimal growth temperature of an infectious agent dictates not only its location and survival in the extrinsic environment, but also its predeliction for physiologically compatible regions of the host and its ability to deploy its pathogenic armamentarium within the host. Thus, organisms with optimal growth at temperatures below 37°C (the agents of leprosy, syphilis, Rocky Mountain spotted fever, the dermatophytoses, sporotrichosis) produce initial lesions in the cooler regions of the skin. Appreciation of the role of ambient temperature in the pathogenesis of disease can direct the search for possible natural reservoirs of the causative agent. For detailed discussion of these and other microenvironmental factors, see Chapter 4, Host–Parasite Relationships and the Pathogenesis of Infectious Diseases, and Chapter 6, Resistance to Infection.

Sanitary Engineering

Sanitary engineering contributes so vitally to the prevention of water-borne and food-borne infectious diseases that only catastrophe, in causing a breakdown of protection, brings home the effectiveness of these engineering measures. For example, in 1933 some 800 cases of acute amebic dysentery originated in two Chicago hotels. Basement food preparation and ice storage areas had been contaminated from flooding with mixed sewage and storm water drainage after torrential rainstorms. In addition, the plumbing was antiquated and there were water–sewer line cross connections.

Water Supply

The rarity of cholera and typhoid fever in the United States, and the infrequency of bacillary and amebic dysentery are all testimony to the effectiveness of water treatment in halting spread of these infections. The measures used are many. Water is obtained from sources as remote from humans and human habitation as is practicable—for example, mountain wilderness catchment areas and deep wells. It is stored, secure from humans and other animals, preferably in covered reservoirs. Treatment often includes (1) aeration, which removes dissolved carbon dioxide, aids in solution of oxygen, and decreases objectionable tastes and odors; (2) coagulation of soluble (iron, manganese) and colloidal (bacteria, finely divided solids) materials, which may occur spontaneously, but is generally augmented by the addition of crude aluminum sulfate; (3) sedimentation of coagulated materials by gravity settling; and (4) filtration through beds of fine sand. Disinfection by chlorination commonly follows before delivery to the human consumer through adequate plumbing. Removing Ca^{++} and Mg^{++}—that is, softening the water—has no effect on microbial contaminants.

Bacteriologic analysis is an integral part of the surveillance of culinary water. Testing determines (1) the total number of viable bacteria per unit volume (plate count)—an index of organic content—and (2) the number of coliform bacteria per unit volume (coliform count)—an indicator of contamination by excreta. The varieties of coliforms present also give some indication of the source of contamination, because coliforms originating in humans and other animals can be distinguished from soil varieties. Isolation of fecal kinds of *Streptococcus* spp., *Clostridium* spp., or *Pseudomonas* spp. also indicates excretory pollution of water. Standards generally refer to coliform counts on the reasonable assumption that as contamination with excrement becomes more intense, the probability of contamination with pathogens also rises. In the United States, drinking water standards define requirements for (1) sites in the water system to be sampled, (2) frequency of sampling, (3) size of samples, and (4) methods for culturing. In general, if coliform bacteria are isolated from three or more 10-ml samples or if four or more coliforms are present in a 100-ml sample collected at a given site, the water is substandard.

Whether fulfillment of these standards following treatment necessarily renders water free of pathogens is unclear. Certain enteroviruses may survive chlorination, but the numbers may be insufficient to threaten community health. An epidemic of waterborne giardiasis in Camas, Washington occurred in 1976 and *Giardia* cysts were recovered from the chlorinated and filtered municipal water supply. Inadequate anicillary treatment (flocculation and sedimentation) may have been a factor in this outbreak. Adequately treated water may become contaminated with potential pathogens through the distribution process, as is demonstrated by the discovery of *Legionella pneumophila* throughout the water delivery systems of at least two hospitals plagued by nosocomial Legionnaires' disease. Entry of the organism into the water supply is presumably followed by multiplication and concentration in sediments at faucets and showerheads throughout the facilities.

Water that is microbiologically safe may not be potable because of chemical quality—for example, it may contain dyes, phenols, pesticides, metallic ions, detergents, or alkalis.

Sewage Disposal

In its broadest terms, sewage is water burdened with excrement and ablutional and industrial wastes. It is obnoxious and is an everpresent hazard to health. With proper management, neither direct contamination nor vector contamination of water or food supplies from sewage can occur. The mechanical aids to this task (the sewerage system) serve to mitigate offense, while providing the greatest possible efficiency in biologic processing of sewage to release the carrying water for other uses. The essential biologic agents of sewage treatment are saprophytic microorganisms acting in septic tanks, in filtration systems, and in activated sludge processes. Not all pathogenic microorganisms are killed in sewage treatment, but their numbers are reduced to the point that chlorination of effluent water renders the water suitable for industrial use.

The number of microorganisms in sewage is enormous. The kinds vary from place to place and from time to time, with enteric nonpathogens predominating—*Proteus* spp., coliforms, fecal kinds of *Streptococcus,* and *Clostridium* spp. Pathogens may include *Salmonella* spp., *Shigella* spp., *Mycobacterium tuberculosis,* and enteroviruses. Sewage treatment achieves both a decrease in numbers of microorganisms and, of major importance, a change in the kinds present. Although pathogenic bacteria are not absolutely eliminated by treatment, the effect is to reduce their numbers greatly, replacing them with saprophytic varieties. Unfortunately, even in the United States, modern sewage treatment is not universal, illustrating the occasional ascendancy of cupidity over knowledge.

Garbage

Garbage in homeowners' garbage cans and in the city dump is a threat to health because it is a source of food for pests (rats) and a breeding place for arthropod vectors (flies and mosquitoes). Probably the most satisfactory method for disposal of garbage avoids separate storage, collection, and transport by grinding and flushing it into sewage lines for eventual disposal along with sewage. If storage of garbage is necessary, it must be in tightly covered containers. Garbage collection in closed trucks at least twice a week in warm climates is best followed either by incineration or by thorough cooking, preferably with superheated steam, if it is to be used as hog food. Burying garbage may be adequate if the garbage is well compacted in a trench suitably deep (6–8 ft) and if it is covered to a depth of at least 2 ft with sandy soil. Decomposition proceeds anaerobically and may require many years for completion. On the other hand, the composting of garbage aims at rapid, aerobic decomposition through the maintenance of high water content (50–60%) and aeration.

Dumping at sea is convenient, but it is deplorable. Not only is the littering and contamination of beach and shore front areas a visible consequence, but underwater contamination of marine life can also become medically and economically detrimental to man, since edible species with commercial value are involved (*e.g.,* clams).

Special Environments

Hospitals and medical laboratories present special problems in sanitary engineering because of the augmented risk of infectious diseases for both the internal population of patients and employees and the external community if appropriate waste disposal is neglected. The exigencies of infection control must be taken into account in the design of hospital ventilation and air conditioning systems, water distribution lines, laundry and housekeeping facilities, and special areas such as intensive care units and operating suites. Laboratories and pharmacy preparation areas should be adequately equipped with hoods and clean areas to avoid accidental infection of staff or patients. All infectious wastes should be sterilized prior to disposal, and less hazardous materials bagged and incinerated in specifically designated facilities.

Food Preservation

Refrigeration

Refrigeration ranks with water and sewage treatment as a technical advance effective in the prevention of infection through the gastrointestinal tract. Chilling prevents food spoilage by markedly slowing the growth of microorganisms; it is economically salutary, of course. In addition, small numbers of potentially pathogenic fungi and bacteria are prevented from multiplying to densities capable of causing disease on ingestion. Thus, a few enterotoxin-producing *Staphylococcus aureus* organisms in a potato salad kept refrigerated until served do not multiply and do not produce enough toxin to cause food poisoning.

Freezing

Freezing foods as a method of preservation generally has no effect in reducing the numbers of pathogenic microorganisms. Indeed, freezing effectively preserves many kinds of microorganisms. For example, a wild rabbit that was the source of tularemia in the hunter who shot and dressed it led to tularemia in a sibling who 6 weeks later removed the rabbit from a home freezer, cut it up, and cooked it. However, multiplication of microorganisms is prevented by freezing, ordinarily preventing the production of an infectious inoculum. Also, freezing is lethal to some parasites, for example *Toxoplasma gondii, Trichinella spiralis.*

Pasteurization

Pasteurization of milk reduces microbial populations to a harmless size if the burden of microorganisms is not too great to begin with. Determination of the number of bacteria per ml of milk—the standard plate count (SPC/ml)—is a legally accepted basis for judging the sanitary quality of milk and milk products. Raw milk to be pasteurized is not acceptable if it contains more than 200,000 bacteria per ml; after pasteurization the count should not exceed 30,000 per ml. As with water, the number of coliform bacteria per unit volume is a better indicator of the degree of contamination than is the total bacterial count. The usual standard specifies fewer than 10 coliforms per ml in three of four samples of milk as delivered for human consumption.

Pathogenic microorganisms may be contributed to milk from the udder—*Mycobacterium* spp., *Brucella* spp., *Streptococcus* spp., and *Coxiella burnetii.* Other pathogens—*Salmonella* spp., *Shigella* spp., *M. tuberculosis, Staphylococcus* spp., *Streptococcus pyogenes* group A, and *Corynebacterium diphtheriae*—are inoculated into milk from humans during collection, transfer, and storage operations. The vegetative forms of pathogenic microorganisms are relatively heat susceptible. However, it must be remembered that the thermal death of microorganisms follows the classic killing curve. That is, there will be viable microorganisms after pasteurization—the larger the number before heating, the larger the number surviving the heat. It is essential to successful pasteurization that the contamination of milk before heating be kept as low as possible. Continuous surveillance is necessary to make certain that only healthy animals and humans are involved and that there is prompt cooling to 5°C to 10°C (40°F to 50°F) immediately after collection, during storage, and after pasteurization.

An almost infinite number of combinations of heat and time brings about the thermal death of microorganisms in milk. Two combinations are in general use: heating to 65°C (not less than 145°F) for 30 minutes—the *low temperature holding (LTH) method*—and heating to 72°C (at least 161°F) for 15

Table 16-1. Some Parasites of Wild Animals That Also Cause Infectious Diseases in Humans

Parasite	Primary host(s) [Vectors]	Diseases in	
		NONHUMAN HOST(s)	HUMAN HOST(s)
Arboencephaloviruses (Chap. 120) Eastern	Small birds, ducks, horses [mosquitoes]	No apparent disease; horses die	Encephalomyelitis
Western	Birds, squirrels, snakes, horses [mosquitoes]	No apparent disease; horses die	Encephalomyelitis
Venezuelan	Rodents, horses [mosquitoes]	No apparent disease; horses die	Encephalitis
St. Louis	Birds [mosquitoes]	No apparent disease	Encephalomyelitis
California	Rabbits, hares, squirrels, deer, horses, cows [mosquitoes]	No apparent disease	Encephalitis
Japanese B	Birds, pigs, horses, cattle [mosquitoes]	No apparent disease; domestic animals may die	Encephalitis
Murray Valley	Birds [mosquitoes]	No apparent disease	Encephalomyelitis
Tick-borne encephalitis	Rodents, birds [ticks]	No known apparent disease	Encephalitis
Russian spring–summer encephalitis	Small mammals, birds [ticks]	No known apparent disease	Encephalitis
Arenaviruses (Chap. 90)	Rodents, nonhuman primates [ticks, mites, mosquitoes]	No apparent disease; death	No clinical disease; malaise, fever, shock, meningitis, encephalitis
Rabies virus (Chap. 124)	Weasel-skunk, civet-ferret families with bats, foxes, skunks most important; dogs; cats, cattle	No apparent disease; death with paralysis	Excitation, paralysis, death
Yellow fever virus (Chap. 73)	Nonhuman primates [mosquitoes]	No apparent disease; death	Yellow fever
Colorado tick fever virus (Chap. 123)	Squirrels, chipmunks, mice, porcupines [ticks]	No apparent disease	Fever, malaise, leukopenia
Ornithosis chlamydias (Chap. 30)	Psittacine birds, pigeons, poultry	No apparent disease; death	Fever, cough, pneumonia
Rickettsia mooseri (Chap. 98)	Rats [fleas]	No apparent disease	Murine typhus
Rickettsia rickettsii (Chap. 96)	Rabbits, squirrels, rats, mice, groundhogs [ticks]	No apparent disease	Rocky Mountain spotted fever
Rickettsia akari (Chap. 97)	Mice [mites]	No apparent disease	Rickettsialpox
Coxiella burnetii (Chap. 30)	Wild ungulates	No apparent disease	Q fever
Brucella spp. (Chap. 138)	Wild ungulates	No apparent disease; abortion	Brucellosis
Francisella tularensis (Chap. 139)	Rabbits, squirrels, rats, skunks, bears, muskrats, coyotes, cats, dogs, swine, sheep, cattle [ticks, deerflies, mosquitoes]	No apparent disease; lymphadenitis, septicemia	Tularemia
Yersinia pestis (Chap. 140)	Rats, mice, prairie dogs, squirrels, marmots, rabbits, gerbils [fleas]	No apparent disease; death	Bubonic, pneumonic, septicemic plague

Table 16-1. (continued) *Some Parasites of Wild Animals That Also Cause Infectious Diseases in Humans*

Parasite	Primary host(s) [Vectors]	Diseases in	
		NONHUMAN HOST(s)	HUMAN HOST(s)
Pseudomonas pseudomallei (Chap. 141)	Rats, mice, rabbits, ruminants, dogs, cats, nonhuman primates	No apparent disease; death	Pulmonary abscesses, septicemia
Streptobacillus moniliformis (Chap. 142)	Rats, squirrels, weasels, turkeys	No apparent disease	Fever, rash
Listeria monocytogenes (Chap. 51)	Wild mammals, birds, domestic mammals	No apparent disease; death	Meningitis, abortion
Leptospira spp. (Chap. 76)	Rats, mice, opossums, skunks, racoons, wildcats, foxes, dogs, shrews, bandicoots, cattle, swine—almost all mammals	No apparent disease; abortion, hemorrhage, nephritis	Weil's disease, nephritis, hepatitis, conjunctivitis
Borrelia spp. (Chap. 143)	Rodents, porcupines, opossums, armadillos [soft ticks]	No apparent disease; death	Relapsing fever, hemorrhage
Spirillum minus (Chap. 142)	Rats, mice, cats	No apparent disease	Fever, rash
Leishmania spp. (Chap. 147	Rodents, carnivores [sandflies]	No apparent disease; skin ulcers	Chronic skin ulcerations, mucocutaneous lesions, kala-azar syndrome
Trypanosoma cruzi (Chap. 136)	Armadillos, bats, rodents, opossums, nonhuman primates, dogs, cats [triatomes]	No known apparent disease	Skin rash, myocarditis, conjunctivitis, myositis, neurologic dysfunctions
Trypanosoma gambiense et rhodesiense (Chap. 130)	Wild ungulates [tsetse flies]	No apparent disease; death in coma	Meningoencephalitis
Pneumocystis carinii (Chap. 45)	Rodents, nonhuman primates, sheep, goats, dogs	No known apparent disease	Plasma cell pneumonia
Diphyllobothrium latum (Chap. 69)	Fresh-water fish, bears, dogs, cats	No known apparent disease	Tapeworm infection
Hymenolepis nana et diminuta (Chap. 69)	Mice, rats	Tapeworm infection	Tapeworm infection
Trichinella spiralis (Chap. 150)	Wild carnivores	No known apparent disease	No apparent disease; death
Fasciola hepatica (Chap. 80)	Snails, fish, cattle, sheep	No apparent disease; death	Acute hepatitis, cholecystitis, cirrhosis
Schistosoma spp. (Chap. 81)	Snails, rodents	No apparent disease; death	Colitis, hepatitis, cystitis
Dracunculus medinensis (Chap. 112)	Wild carnivores, nonhuman primates [water fleas]	No known apparent disease	Skin ulcers
Brugia spp. (Chap. 148)	Nonhuman primates, wild carnivores, rodents [mosquitoes]	No known apparent disease	Lymphadenopathy, lymphedema

Table 16-2. Parasites of Domestic Animals That Also Cause Infectious Disease in Man

Parasite	Primary Host(s) [Vectors]	Diseases in NONHUMAN HOST(s)	Diseases in HUMAN HOST(s)
Cat-scratch fever (Chap. 166)	Cats, dogs	No known disease	Lymphadenitis with suppuration
Cowpox (Chap. 92)	Cattle, horses	Papulovesiculopustular lesions of skin of udder and teats	Papulovesiculopustular skin lesions
Newcastle disease	Poultry	Respiratory, gastrointestinal, central nervous system	Conjunctivitis
Milker's nodules (pseudocowpox) (Chap. 92)	Cattle	Ulcers and granulomas of udder	Papulovesiculogranulomatous skin lesions
Orf (contagious ecthyma)	Sheep, goats	Pustular lesions of mouth, vulva, eye	Papulovesiculogranulomatous skin lesions
Vesicular stomatitis	Cattle, swine, horses	Ulceration of oral mucosa, feet, and teats	Fever, chills, headache, myalgia
Rabies virus (Chap. 124)	Dogs, cats, cattle	No apparent disease; death with paralysis	Excitation, paralysis death
Ornithosis chlamydias (Chap. 30)	Pigeons, poultry	No apparent disease; death	Fever, cough, pneumonia
Coxiella burnetii (Chap. 30)	Sheep, cattle, goats [ticks]	No disease; rickettsemia	Headache, fever, pneumonia
Bacillus anthracis (Chap. 104)	Cattle, horses, sheep, goats, swine, dogs, cats	Sudden death, systemic disease, gastrointestinal affliction	Malignant pustule, gastroenteritis, pneumonitis
Erysipelothrix insidiosa (Chap. 103)	Swine, fowl, sheep	Porcine erysipelas, polyarthritis, speticemia, endocarditis	Erysipeloid
Listeria monocytogenes (Chap. 51)	Sheep, cattle, rabbits, goats, guinea pigs, chickens, horses, rodents, birds	Meningoencephalitis, abortion, myocarditis, septicemia, ophthalmitis	Leptomeningitis, fetal listeriosis, oculoglandular infection
Mycobacterium bovis (Chap. 34)	Cattle, horses, swine, cats, dogs	Pulmonary, lymph nodes, udder, gastrointestinal tuberculosis, spondylitis	Primarily gastrointestinal, lymph node, bone, pulmonary tuberculosis
Streptobacillus moniliformis (Chap. 142)	Fowl	No apparent disease	Fever, rash
Pseudomonas mallei	Horses, mules, asses, cats	Nodular pneumonia, farcy, lymphadenopathy	Granulomatous to pustular lesions, skin and subcutaneous; septicemia
Pasteurella multocida	Fowl, cattle, sheep, swine, goats, horses, mice, rats, rabbits	Hemorrhagic septicemia, pneumonia	Skin ulcer, osteomyelitis, sinusitis, pleuritis, leptomeningitis
Brucella spp. (Chap. 138)	Cattle, goats, swine, sheep, horses, mules, dogs, cats, fowl, deer, buffalo, rabbits	Abortion, lameness, mastitis, granulomas, abscesses	Fever, malaise, lymphadenopathy, bacteremia, splenomegaly, osteomyelitis

Table 16-2. (continued) *Parasites of Domestic Animals That Also Cause Infectious Disease in Man*

Parasite	Primary Host(s) [Vectors]	Diseases in	
		NONHUMAN HOST(s)	HUMAN HOST(s)
Salmonella spp. (nontyphoidal) (Chap. 63)	Fowl, swine, cattle, sheep, horses, dogs, cats, rodents, reptiles, birds, cattle	No apparent disease; enteritis, septicemia, puerperal fever	Gastroenteritis, focal infection, septicemia
Vibrio fetus	Sheep	Metritis, infertility, placentitis, abortion	Placentitis with abortion, endocarditis, bacteremia
Sporothrix schenckii (Chap. 108)	Horses, mules, dogs, cats, mice, rats	Granulomas of extremities	Ulcerative, lymph-vascular, skin, subcutaneous lesions
Microsporum spp. (Chap. 107) *Trichophyton* spp. (Chap. 107)	Dogs, cats, horses, cattle, rodents	Alopecia, dermatitis	Alopecia, dermatitis
Trypanosoma cruzi (Chap. 136)	Dogs, cats [triatomes]	No known apparent disease	Skin rash, myocarditis, conjunctivitis, myositis, neurologic dysfunctions
Balantidium coli (Chap. 67)	Pigs, monkeys	No apparent disease in swine, colitis in monkeys	Colitis
Toxoplasma gondii (Chap. 129)	Cats, dogs, sheep, catle, swine	Stillbirth, congenital defects, CNS lesions	Stillbirth, congenital defects, retinochoroiditis
Ancylostoma canium *Uncinaria stenocephala*	Dogs, cats	Anemia, dysentery, hypoproteinemia, edema, stunted growth, death of pups	Itching, erythema of skin, Löffler's syndrome
Toxocara canis et cati (Chap. 111)	Dogs, cats	Diarrhea, granulomas in kidneys and other viscera, weight loss and stunted growth of young	Granulomas in liver, skeletal muscle, lungs, brain
Dipylidium caninum	Dogs, cats	No apparent or known disease; chronic enteritis	Abdominal discomfort
Trichinella spiralis (Chap. 150)	Swine, cattle, horses, dogs, cats, rabbits, rats, mice, bears, boars	No apparent or known disease	Chemosis, conjunctivitis, myositis, skin rash
Taenia saginata (Chap. 69)	Cattle	No apparent or known disease	Abdominal pain, diarrhea, weight loss
Taenia solium (Chap. 69)	Swine	No apparent or known disease	Abdominal pain, diarrhea, weight loss, cysticercosis
Diphyllobothrium latum (Chap. 69)	Dogs, cats	No apparent or known disease	Tapeworm infection
Dirofilaria immitis, D. tenuis	Dogs, racoons [mosquitoes]	Cardiopulmonary granulomata, subcutaneous nodules	Pulmonary nodules, subcutaneous granulomata of face, trunk or arms
Echinococcus granulosus (Chap. 79)	Dog	No apparent or known disease	Space occupying cysts in liver, lungs; anaphylaxis
Echinococcus multilocularis (Chap. 79)	Dog, wild canines	No apparent disease	Noncapsulated, extensive cysts of liver, lungs

Table 16-3. *Parasites of Humans Occasionally Transferred to Nonhuman Animals and Subsequently Transferred Back to Humans*

Parasite	Nonhuman Host(s)	Diseases in	
		NONHUMAN HOST	HUMAN
Corynebacterium diphtheriae (Chap. 25)	Cattle	Ulcers on teats, mastitis	Diphtheria
Staphylococcus aureus (Chap. 100)	Cattle	Furunculosis, mastitis	Furunculosis
Streptococcus pyogenes (Chaps. 24, 101)	Cattle	Mastitis	Pharyngitis, scarlet fever
Mumps virus (Chap. 74)	Dogs	Parotiditis	Mumps
Infectious hepatitis (Chaps. 70, 71, 72)	Nonhuman primates	Hepatitis	Hepatitis

seconds—the *high temperature, short time (HTST)* or *flash method.* Alkaline phosphatase, normally present in milk, is inactivated by heat. The consequent reduction in the capacity of this enzyme to liberate phenol from phosphoric-phenyl esters is measured by the phosphatase test. The proper pasteurization of milk is indicated when less than 1 μg phenol per ml of milk is liberated.

Antimicrobial agents used in the treatment of cattle may be secreted into milk, adding to the load of nonmicrobial contaminants such as pesticides and radioactive elements. The quantities of antimicrobial agents are generally quite small and may only be significant to highly hypersensitive persons.

Canning and Chemical Preservation

Processing of foods for canning by heating in hot water under high pressure is an effective method of food preservation. Solid and liquid food may also be protected from microbial decomposition (or enzymatic changes that predispose to spoilage) by the addition of chemical preservatives. A wide variety of compounds is used for this purpose in the food industry; the commonest agents are acids, salts, and sugars.

Veterinary Infections

Veterinarians and physicians are jointly involved with infectious agents capable of causing zoonoses—diseases of nonhuman animals that are transmissible to humans. There are some 86 zoonotic diseases of major significance and a further 81 zoonotic diseases of minor significance to public health. This is a cumbersome plethora that can be reduced by weeding out duplications, eliminating instances of unproved transmission, and considering only zoonoses of importance in the Americas and Europe or of particular medical interest. Zoonotic parasites can be categorized according to host preference for (1) wild animals (Table 16-1), (2) domestic animals (Table 16-2), or (3) either humans or nonhuman animals (Table 16-3). Distinct survival value accrues to parasites that exhibit catholicity in hosts. The world-shrinking technologic advances and unceasing exploitation of natural resources, however remote, have doubtless aided in the emergence of parasites from wild to domestic to human hosts. The transfer of jungle yellow fever is an example (Chap. 73, Yellow Fever).

Zoonoses are discussed below under the heading of the clinical entity, or entities, that they occasion in humans. Although not all pathways of interchange of parasites between humans and nonhuman animals are known, it is apparent that control of many infectious diseases of humans requires first, or concomitantly, control in nonhuman animals. In addition, it is probable that as yet undefined zoonotic diseases exist that pose infectious risks for humans. A case in point is Lyme disease, a multisystem disease recognized in the last decade, which may result in serious cardiac and neurologic residua in humans (Chap. 151, Septic Arthritis). The role of nonhuman animal viruses in human disease also presents fertile territory for speculation and investigation.

Vector Control

Vector control consists in destroying or denying access of carriers of infectious agents to noninfected, potential hosts. Most vectors of medical importance are arthropods; indeed, some 1000 species have such status. With several vector-borne agents, the burden of parasites sometimes becomes so great that the vector succumbs—for example, certain filarial larvae in mosquitoes, *Plasmodium* spp. in mosquitoes, and *Francisella tularensis* in ticks. In general, however, the invariably lethal effect of *Rickettsia prowazekii* on human lice is an exceptional case; in the usual vector–agent relationship little harm is done to the arthropod. In addition, some very important vertebrate reservoirs function alone or along with arthropods in transmitting parasites to humans. In describing the historic impact of typhus, Zinsser detailed such an interrelationship.

Control measures are mechanical, chemical, or biologic. Concerted application of all available means will probably eliminate some infectious diseases altogether (*e.g.,* epidemic typhus). With others, the reservoir is so enormous, in numbers of hosts and in their distribution, that elimination does not appear possible (sylvatic plague). Control measures in these situations are directed at preventing the access of vectors to humans.

Mechanical Measures

Mechanical efforts are directed at altering the physical environment to the disadvantage of vectors. Draining swamps and eliminating puddles of water remove the loci necessary for the reproduction of certain of the Diptera. The proper disposal of garbage sharply limits food supplies that could support large numbers of flies, rats, and other vermin. Barriers to vectors can be erected by using insect-proof screening and by rat-proofing houses. The environment can be made favorable to predators of vectors (*e.g.,* protection of certain birds). Mechanical abrasion of the chitinous exoskeleton of fleas and cockroaches by the use of silica aerogel compounds has been reported useful in homes and other buildings.

Chemical Measures

Chemical control of vectors has been synonymous with poisoning—the application of toxicants. Although naturally occurring and synthetic toxicants are employed, relatively few classes of chemical compounds are represented (Table 16-4). Moreover, no toxicant now in use takes advantage of the unique features of arthropods, such as the chitinous exoskeleton, the trehalose enzymes, and the lack of pathways for synthesis of steroids. Available toxicants are broadly poisonous—to all arthropods and other forms of life. Such nonselectivity is a major drawback to the application of toxicants. Even though generally less toxic to vertebrates than to arthropods, toxicant use may be intense enough, or repeated often enough, to produce morbidity and even mortality in nonarthropods. Within the animal body, some toxicants—for example, 1,1,1,-trichloro-2-2-bis (*p*-chlorophenyl) ethane or DDT—are deposited in lipids and persist without degradation for long periods. Thus, birds, fish, frogs, and shrews that eat arthropods killed or weakened by intoxication may accumulate slowly metabolized toxicants. Falling prey themselves, these insectivores will yield up to their predators accumulated stores of toxicants. Sterility in eagles has been ascribed to DDT acquired in this way. Fears about the carcinogenic potential of DDT and related compounds for humans have sharply circumscribed use in many areas. In cases for which DDT is effective (for example, elimination of rabies-infected bats from infested habitations), the relative risks must be weighed and decision to use this or any other hazardous toxicant must be accompanied by stringent precautions to avoid excessive environmental contamination.

The use of toxic chemicals has met in arthropods another difficulty—that of resistance. A given application of a toxicant does not always kill all the target arthropods. The survivors may have greater resistance to the action of the toxicant than their deceased fellows. A single gene mutation is involved in some instances; for example, organophosphate and DDT resistance. When mutant-associated, the quality of resistance breeds true and exalts to the point of rendering the toxicant useless in vector control. For example, houseflies ordinarily display a topical LD_{50} of 3.6 μg of diazinon (an organophosphorus compound) per gram; resistant flies have an LD_{50} of 133 μg per gram. At least 240 insect species are known to have developed resistance to various insecticides.

In general, chemical vector control agents are inefficient when the target population is of low density or is scattered.

Biologic Measures

Knowledge of the hormonal regulation of insect growth and metamorphosis has advanced to the state summarized in Fig. 16-1. A hormone released from the brain of the newly hatched insect larva sets off production and release of (1) juvenile hormone (JH) from the corpus cardiacum and corpus allatum and (2) ecdysone from the prothoracic gland. JH must be *present* for larval maturation, and it must be *absent* for metamorphosis into the sexually mature adult. Ecdysone induces molting, thus allowing for growth, and initiates pupation for the final stage larva, thus allowing for metamorphosis. Continued application of JH to immature insects should prevent pupation/metamorphosis; since an essential, normal hormone

Table 16-4. Some Properties of Substances Used in the Control of Vectors

Substance	Source	Action	Resistance	Specificity
Arsenicals	Synthetic	Toxicant; poisoning sulfhydryl enzymes	None	Poor; affect all aerobes
Fluorides	Synthetic	Toxicant; inhibits tissue respiration	None	Poor; affect all aerobes
Sulfur formulations	Nature, synthetic	Toxicant	None	Poor
Nicotine	Nature	Toxicant; cholinergic effect	None	Poor; toxic to mammals
Rotenone	Nature	Toxicant; inhibits coupled oxidation: reduction, $NADH_2$: cytochrome b	Little	Quasi-selective: toxic to fish, less toxic to mammals
Pyrethrum	Nature	Toxicant	Little	Moderate
Petroleum oils	Nature	Toxicant; prevent normal gas exchange	None	Poor; phytotoxic
Dinitrophenols	Synthetic	Toxicant; decrease O_2 uptake	None	Poor; phytotoxic
Organophosphorus compounds (parathion, malathion, paraoxon, demeton, diazinon, diisopropylfluoro-PO_4, tetraethylpyro-Po_4 dichlorvos, ronnel, dicapthon)	Synthetic	Toxicant; inhibit cholinesterase	Widespread, through aliesterase	Poor; toxic to many nonarthropods
Chlorinated hydrocarbons				
DDT	Synthetic	Toxicant; interfere with nerve transmission	Widespread, through dehydrochlorinase	Poor; toxic to many nonarthropods
BHC, lindane, aldrin, dieldrin, endrin, heptachlor, chlordane, toxophene)	Synthetic	Toxicant; interfere with nerve transmission	Occurs; mechanisms not known	Poor; toxic to many nonarthropods
Carbamates	Synthetic	Toxicant; inhibits cholinesterase and aliesterase	Occurs; mechanisms not known	Poor; toxic to many nonarthropods
Repellents	Arthropods, plants, synthetic	Repel arthropods; mechanisms unknown	Not known	Excellent; limited to arthropods
Attractants	Arthropods	Attract arthropods; sex, food, fellows	Not known	Excellent; limited to arthropods
Chemosterilants	Synthetic	Mutagenic	Not encountered	Poor; afect all life forms
Hormones	Synthetic	Deregulate growth	Not encountered	Excellent—to species levels
Rodenticides				
Coumarin derivatives	Synthetic	Anticoagulant; competitive inhibition of vitamin K	Not known	Poor; affects all mammals
Hydrogen cyanide	Synthetic	Toxicant; inhibits Fe-enzymes	Not known	Poor; affects all aerobes
Strychnine	Nature	Toxicant; convulsant	Not known	Poor; affects all vertebrates
Thallium salts	Nature	Toxicant; paralytic	Not known	Poor; affect all aerobes

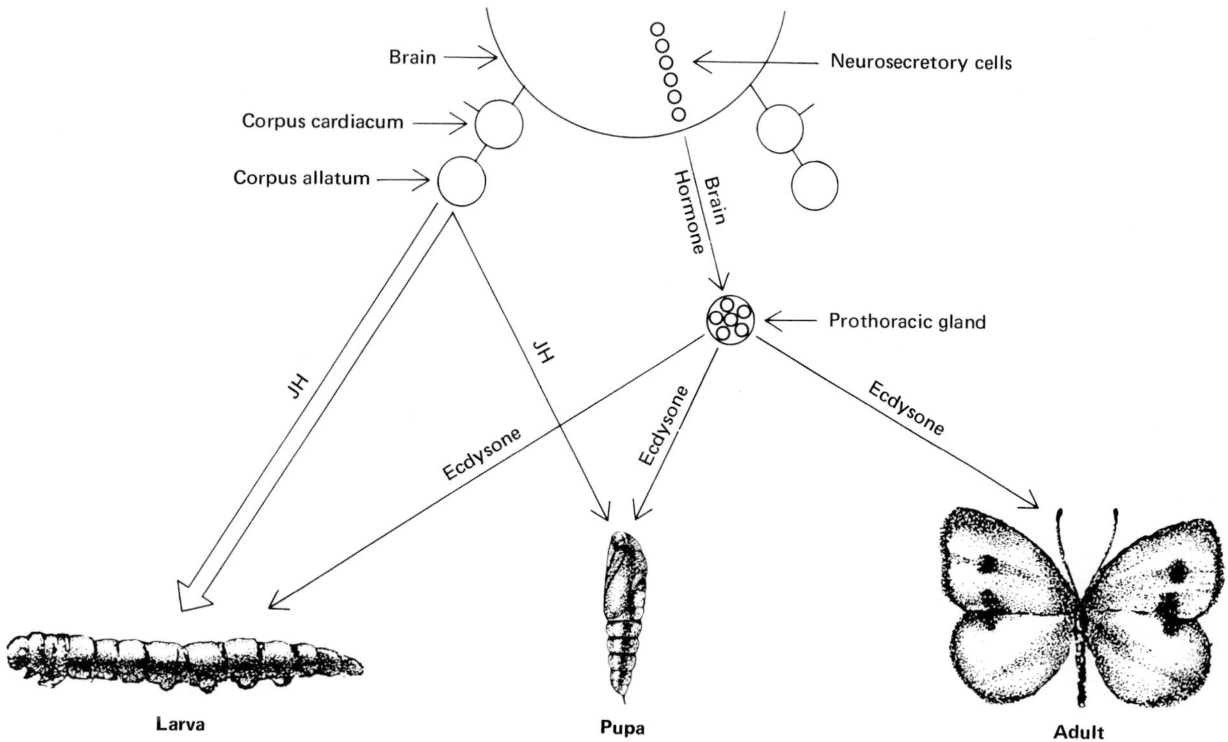

Fig. 16-1. Hormonal control of insect metamorphosis. (Courtesy of Morton Grosser, Ph.D., Zoecon Corporation, Palo Alto, CA)

is involved, insects should neither have nor be able to develop a defense against excess JH. Both premises—activity and lack of resistance—were confirmed using juvenile hormone extracts of insects.

The discovery that conifers and other plants elaborate compounds that mimic insect hormones was additionally remarkable in illustrating selectivity to the level of the insect species affected. Synthetic compounds with JH activity have been prepared with potencies in excess of 1 ng per insect. However, to obtain such potency, application to the vulnerable larval insect stages is required. Coupling a synthetic, JH-active compound with a toxicant, for example, pyrethrum, appears to result in synergy—augmented JH activity and a rapid onset of control. Also, stable formulations have been devised, for example, activity in feces passed by cattle fed a synthetic JH preparation and transmission of enough active drug from exposed male to female insect at mating to sterilize the eggs subsequently deposited. If selectivity for insects harmful to humans is assured, the promise of nontoxic hormonal insect control, as illustrated in successful field trials of mosquito control in California, may be realized.

Purely biologic measures to control arthropods have been studied with growing vigor as the limitation of toxicants—nonselectivity and resistance—become increasingly important. The exploitation of parasites and predators of medically important arthropods is one such measure of biologic control. Of the more than 1500 pathogens, parasites, and predators of medically important arthropods, not all are even potentially useful in vector control. Problems of introduction, distribution, and maintenance must be solved and estimates of effectiveness are yet to be made. High selectivity is characteristic of biologic agents—*Beauvaria* fungi attack muscid flies and ixodid ticks; the wasp *Polistes olivaceus* preys on muscid flies; the larvae of syrphid flies are voracious feeders on aphids; nuclear polyhedrosis and granulosis viruses have efficacy and specificity for arthropods important in human and veterinary medicine.

Birds are the best known of the vertebrate predators of arthropods; however, the provision of nesting places and the protection of birds from predators are measures not proved to augment the consumption of arthropods by birds. Fish consume larval and pupal forms of mosquitoes. Amphibians and reptiles eat insects at ground and pond level. Also, there are mammalian insectivores: bats, deer mice, red-backed voles, and masked shrews.

Natural repellents are substances of unknown chemical constitution produced by arthropods and plants that discourage animals from attacking. The oils of pine trees and cotton plant seedlings are examples. Man-made repellents such as dimethyl phthalate, dibutyl phthalate, benzyl benzoate, *N,N*-diethyl-*m*-toluamide (DEET), and *N,N*-diisopropyl-*p*-toluamide have been used to prevent the attachment of certain trombiculid larval vectors of scrub typhus with some success. As yet, arthropods do not appear to develop resistance to repellents.

Attractants are elaborated by some kinds of arthropods and by plants. Arthropodous attractants are usually species specific. Ants liberate attractants called trail substances from abdominal glands. Many attractants are sex lures of great potency—a male *Bombyx mori* (adult silkworm) will respond to airstreams containing 200 molecules of female sex attractant per ml. Plant attractants are usually food lures. The value of these substances to vector control lies in their potential for luring large numbers of arthropods into traps where they can be killed or sterilized.

Sterilants cause failure of reproduction through interference with oogenesis or spermatogenesis; cessation of production of live gametes; and induction of multiple, lethal mutations either expressed in crippled gametes or lethal to the zygote if fertilization occurs. The result is called autocidal control. Sterilants, in contrast to toxicants, can be applied with selectivity and have lasting effectiveness. The latter point is important: survivors of toxicants mate normally and produce another generation that may be resistant to the toxicant. The fertile fraction of an arthropod population exposed to a sterilant must compete with the sterile fraction in mating; therefore, the sterile population must outnumber the nonsterile to ensure a low probability of fertile matings. This is true even in species that mate several times prior to laying eggs. Autocidal control may be induced by physical (gamma irradiation) or chemical means. Successful reduction of screwfly (the larval form is the cattle screwworm) populations in some parts of the southeastern United States was achieved in the late 1970s by the release of flies sterilized by irradiation. However, a resurgence of the screwfly, now relatively resistant to the previously effective autocidal program, has occurred recently, apparently owing to a genetic modulation among the population (probably induced by the creation of a selective advantage for previously existing genetic subtypes that then reinvaded, aided by altered ecologic conditions). Irradiation is also limited by the requirement for laboratory rearing of arthropods and the inevitable small percentage of animals that escapes sterilization. Chemosterilants have greater promise because they can be applied in nature in conjunction with attractants.

The most effective chemosterilants are antimitotic drugs—radiomimetic, antineoplastic agents. Aziridine derivatives, such as 1,2-tris (1-aziridinyl) phosphine oxide (Tepa), are effective chemosterilants of arthropods and were at one time used with good effect in the treatment of a variety of neoplastic diseases in man. Like other highly reactive alkylating agents, tepa causes gross reduction in the size of ovaries and testes, with necrosis of germinal epithelium. Inactivation of these compounds is rapid, particularly at elevated temperatures and at an acid pH. There is no problem with undesirable residues; indeed, the compounds are difficult to use because of instability. They are usually fed, but some are effective on contact. Antimetabolities—for example, the antifolic agent methotrexate—are also active chemosterilants, usually acting against just one sex (methotrexate sterilizes female, but not male, houseflies). Full exploitation of sterilants to control arthropod vectors of infectious diseases is yet to be accomplished.

Biologic control measures, then, are attractive primarily because of their selectivity and efficiency. In general they produce effects more slowly than do chemical control methods, and in some instances they must be combined with chemical measures to achieve the desired result (in some autocidal control programs, for example, chemicals must be sprayed by hand to kill preexisting larvae that would hatch from the ground). Biologic control is most effective when based on the most complete ecologic information and if it is integrated with other pest management practices.

Rodents

For centuries, rodent reservoirs of infectious diseases have been attacked by trapping and poisoning. Because the rodents are still with us, it appears that such measures only make room for young rodents to grow up. Perhaps, as Zinsser predicted, rats will not disappear until they become esteemed as a table delicacy. The essential element of control is alteration of the environment so that shelter and food are denied to rodents. That is, all buildings, commercial and domestic, must be made rodent-proof. All food must be kept under rodent-proof conditions—food for humans and animals, raw and processed, fresh and stored, as well as garbage, sewage, and industrial wastes that can nurture rodents. Of poisons, the anticoagulant coumarin derivatives offered a large safety factor in dosage requirement and time necessary for effect, along with good antirodent potency. However, in the late 1950s rats with resistance appeared, bred out, and spread across the world. Because the recently developed poison difenacoum is active against warfarin-resistant rats, control may again be aided by poisoning. In closed areas, such as ships, gassing with hydrogen cyanide is very effective.

Isolation

Persons with contagious diseases are isolated to halt the direct and indirect spread of the responsible infectious agents. Because isolation is applicable only after a disease is clinically recognized as contagious, cutting off continued spread from an identified source is the best that can be accomplished. Measures for isolation of hospitalized patients with communicable diseases that need not be exceeded are described in United States Public Health Service Publication No. 2054. Reverse or protective isolation is also described, that is, precautions that can be taken to prevent direct or indirect spread of infectious agents from apparently normal persons to persons peculiarly susceptible to infection as a consequence of other diseases, accidents, or trauma. Specific isolation techniques, of course, are rationally based on knowledge of the nature of the infection and, most particularly, the route of transmission and the environmental factors influencing transmission.

The isolation unit should be a private room equipped with its own toilet facilities, or at least with hot and cold running water. A two- to four-bed unit can be used for several patients with the same kind of infection. All isolation units must be provided with soap and hand scrub brush (not for patient use), paper towels, step-on refuse can with disposable plastic liner, distinctively marked linen hamper, plastic covers on mattresses and pillows, and a supply of masks, gowns, and gloves, as required, on a table outside the door to the unit.

The exact details of isolation procedures vary from hospital to hospital, but the principle of halting the spread of infectious agents is the common denominator that must never be lost sight of in a web of ritual. Isolation procedures are effective only when they are practiced by *everyone* having to do with care for the patient. Cooperation is best based on understanding and encouraged by adoption of the simplest procedure that will be effective.

Persons who have had contact with those subsequently identified as having a contagious disease may be quarantined—that is, restricted by legal decree to their dwelling place for a period corresponding to the longest usual incubation period of the contagious diseases to which they were exposed. Over the years, as knowledge of the cause, means of spread, pathogenesis, and specific treatment of infectious diseases has grown, procedures for isolation have become more rational, and the imposition of quarantine has relaxed. In virtually all instances, state laws govern these matters, often with outmoded statutes.

Reporting

Reporting the occurrence of an infectious disease is the duty of the physician responsible for the care of the patient. Others may report, but the physician's diagnosis is a weighty factor toward setting in motion epidemiologic effort, such as case finding and determining the source of an outbreak (Chap. 2, Epidemiology). Prompt reporting is particularly important when a disease is highly contagious, as in some of the hemorrhagic fevers, or when an unidentified common-source vehicle threatens large numbers of people. The afflicted person may need to be isolated, contacts must be identified if a need for vaccination, chemoprophylaxis, or quarantine exists, and the source of the infection must be determined.

Notification of the local public health agency—for example, the city health department—usually by telephone, generally fulfills the physician's responsibility. Dissemination of the report to county, state, national, and international levels is accomplished by the agency first notified. The functions of politically identifiable public health organizations often overlap and sometimes coincide with areas of interest of voluntary health organizations.

Remaining Problems

The persistence of noxious vectors (rodents) or those that cannot readily be eradicated because of density and range of population (ticks) demands continued efforts to develop effective, environmentally benign methods of pest control. Promising steps in this direction include the concept of competitive, hypovirulent strains introduced into the natural population and the potential use of other organisms as destructive parasites of bacterial, fungal, and protozoal pathogens. In addition, governments at all levels, health institutions, and other appropriate organizations must learn the lessons derived from the eradication of smallpox: the elimination of infectious diseases requires the coordinated, single-minded cooperation of agencies across national boundaries and the acknowledgment of those goals as public-health priorities by all involved (and uninvolved) nations.

On-going investigation into the causes of newly appearing diseases is necessary in order to identify the natural reservoirs and possible vectors as exemplified by Lyme disease and Legionnaires disease. In this vein, continued support for basic investigations into the physical properties of microorganisms will yield a better understanding of potential natural environmental niches and pathogenetic mechanisms.

The identification of means by which environmental factors influence infectious diseases is far from complete—witness the recognition in animal models of the invidious effects of anxiety, noise, and other environmentally induced stresses on immune responses. This research may yield unexpected results in the etiology or pathogenesis of some infectious diseases.

Urgent strategies for the prevention of environmental catastrophes leading to increased prevalence and incidence of infectious diseases must be sought. The profligate use of chemicals has already resulted in the development of resistant populations of disease vectors as well as microbial pathogens. Heedless exploitation of the global environment by humans has produced ecological disruptions that have shifted the equilibrium of host–parasite–vector relationships demonstrably in the past and may continue to do so. The ultimate ecologic disaster, nuclear war, would result in recrudescence of infectious diseases long-controlled and the development of epidemic disease on a scale unequalled since the plagues of the 14th century. Best estimates are that deaths from communicable diseases among the survivors of a nuclear war (if any) would approach 20% to 25%. Those whose aim is disease prevention must consider how best to prevent this among all other potential man-made diseases.

Bibliography

Books

GILMOUR D: Biochemistry of Insects. New York, Academic Press, 1961. 343 pp.

Isolation Techniques for Use in Hospitals. Public Health Service Publication No. 2054. Washington DC, U.S. Government Printing Office, 1970. 87 pp.

KOREN H: Environmental Health and Safety. New York, Pergamon Press, 1974. 315 pp.

MECOND CP: The Zooanthroponoses as occupational diseases in the United States. In Comparative Medicine in Transition: School of Public Health, University of Michigan. Baltimore, Lord Baltimore Press, 1960. 499 pp.

Rat-borne Disease: Prevention and Control. Atlanta, U.S. Public Health Service, Communicable Disease Center, 1949. 292 pp.

SCHWABE CW: Veterinary Medicine and Human Health, 2nd ed. Baltimore, Williams & Wilkins, 1969. 713 pp.

Standard Methods for the Examination of Water and Wastewater, Including Bottom Sediments and Sludges, 12th ed. New York, American Public Health Association, 1965. 744 pp.

ZINSSER H: Rats, Lice and History. Boston, Little, Brown & Co., 1935. 301 pp.

Journals

ABRAMS HL, VON KAENEL WE: Medical problems of survivors of nuclear war: Infection and the spread of communicable disease. N Engl J Med 305:1226–1232, 1981

ANAGNOSTAKIS SL: Biological control of chestnut blight. Science 215:466–471, 1982

BATRA SWT: Biological control in agroecosystems. Science 215:134–139, 1982

DYKES AC, JURANEK DD, LORENZ RA, SINCLAIR S, JAKUBOWSKI W, DAVIES R: Municipal waterborne giardiasis: An epidemiologic investigation: Beavers implicated as a possible reservoir. Ann Intern Med 92:165–170, 1980

EVANS JR, LASHMAN HALL K, WARFORD J: Health care in the developing world: Problems of scarcity and choice. N Engl J Med 305:1117–1127, 1981

JACOBSON M: Chemical insect attractants and repellents. Annu Rev Entomol 11:403–422, 1966

JENKINS DW: Pathogens, parasites and predators of medically important arthropods. Bull WHO (Suppl) 30:1–150, 1964

OPPENOORTH FJ: Biochemical genetics of insecticide resistance. Annu Rev Entomol 10:185–206, 1965

Public Health Service drinking water standards, 1946 Public Health Rep 61:371–384, 1946

Report of a Special Committee: Amebiasis outbreak in Chicago. JAMA 102:369–372, 1934

RICHARDSON RH, ELLISON JR, AVERHOFF WW: Autocidal control of screwworms in North America. Science 215:361–370, 1982

RILEY V: Psychoneuroendocrine influences on immunocompetence and neoplasia. Science 212:1100–1109, 1981

RODBARD D: Role of regional body temperature in the pathogenesis of disease. N Engl J Med 305:808–814, 1981

RUTSTEIN DD: Controlling the communicable and the man-made diseases. N Engl J Med 304:1422–1424, 1981

STAAL GB: Insect growth regulators with juvenile hormone activity. Annu Rev Entomol 20:417–460, 1975

STOUT J, YU VL, VICKERS RM, ZURAVLEFF J, BEST M, BROWN A, YEE RB, WADOWSKY R: Ubiquitousness of *Legionella pneumophila* in the water supply of a hospital with endemic Legionnaires' disease. N Engl J Med 306:466–468, 1982

TULLY JG, ROSE DL, YUNKER CE, CORY J, WHITCOMB RF, WILLIAMSON DL: Helical mycoplasmas (Spiroplasmas) from *Ixodes* ticks. Science 212:1043–1045, 1981

WELLS LF JR, GIRARD KF: DDT, bats and rabies. N Engl J Med 297:390–392, 1977

WILLIS JH: Morphogenetic action of insect hormones. Annu Rev Entomol 19:269–291, 1974

SHEILA M. NOLAN
PAUL D. HOEPRICH

Sterilization and Disinfection 17

Reduction or total removal of microbial populations is necessary to prevent transmission of infectious diseases by ingestion, injection, inhalation, or contact transfer of microorganisms during diagnostic or therapeutic procedures and to prevent deterioration of foodstuffs and other products susceptible to microbially mediated decomposition. These goals are accomplished by one of two processes: (1) *Sterilization* (rendering organisms incapable of reproduction), which denotes destruction of all forms of microbial life, including spores; (2) *Disinfection* (removal of potential pathogens), which may be either *high level,* resulting in the death of all vegetative microorganisms, or *low level,* implying a more limited process in which total bacterial numbers are reduced, and certain disease-causing organisms are eliminated. Topical application of disinfectants (referred to in this setting as *antiseptics*) may yield an intermediate level of disinfection when used on areas difficult or impossible to sterilize, such as the skin. Akin to low level disinfection is the process of *sanitization* (making something healthful), a poorly-defined term of heterogeneous intent generally indicating the use of disinfectant chemical agents in conjunction with cleaning, the aim of which is simply to reduce to variably specified "safe" levels the total reservoir of microorganisms on large areas such as floors, utensils, and equipment.

The choice of either sterilization or disinfection as a means of controlling infectious agents depends on both the relative need for complete sterility and the suitability of the process for the item that is to be treated. Invasive procedures such as surgery, venipuncture, or the insertion of a prosthesis all present stringent requirements for sterility, but the limits of physical tolerance preclude the use of rigorous methods to sterilize the skin preoperatively. Surgical instruments, needles, and prostheses, therefore, should be sterile, but the skin can be, at best, disinfected.

Sterility and varying degrees of disinfection are dictated by the ability of microorganisms to survive the sterilizing process. It is biologically axiomatic that the number of viable individuals remaining in a population exposed to a destructive agent is an exponential function of the duration of exposure. In relation to infectious diseases, this means, in theory, that not every organism originally present in the material subjected to a sterilization procedure is killed. In practice, the probability that actual sterilization will occur is made as high as possible within the limits of time and the fragility of the material to be treated. When heat can be applied, the probability of zero survivors—that is, actual sterility—can be made very high (Fig. 17-1). However, if a brief application of benzalkonium chloride is the most rigorous procedure that is tolerable, the probability of survival of microorganisms is very high.

Although many microorganisms are very susceptible to environmental influences—for example, *Treponema pallidum* and influenza viruses—many are extraordinarily hardy, such as the spores of bacteria and fungi, and the lipid-free viruses such as the enteroviruses. Critical evaluation of procedures for sterilization and disinfection has enabled recognition of the enormous capacity for persistence of viability intrinsic to different microorganisms; accordingly, testing has extended far beyond the use of only typhoid bacilli and staphylococci. Contemporary standards for testing sterilization procedures include assessment of efficacy against tubercle bacilli, enteroviruses, and bacterial and fungal spores. As bacterial spores are the agents most resistant to destruction, any procedure that kills them can be assumed to result in sterility.

Physical Agents

Heat

With a sufficient input of energy, the vital macromolecules of any form of life will be denatured. The application of heat energy is most efficiently accom-

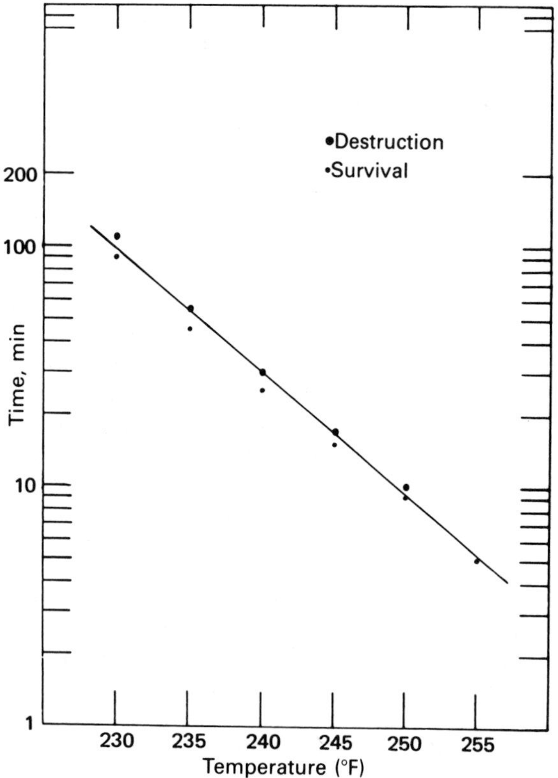

Fig. 17-1. Thermal death time curve of bacterial spores exposed to wet heat. (Pflug IJ, Schmidt CF: Disinfection, Sterilization and Preservation, pp 63–105. Philadelphia, Lea & Febiger, 1968)

plished in a wet environment; the steam autoclave is an extremely reliable and efficient device for applying wet heat. No form of life can survive exposure to saturated steam under pressure—that is, 10 to 15 minutes at 121°C. Sterilization does not result, however, unless the autoclave is properly packed with objects that are appropriately wrapped and positioned. Also, suitable controls are necessary to monitor exposure of all objects to the hot steam. However, cutting instruments are dulled and thermolabile substances and equipment can be destroyed in the steam autoclave. Moreover, tight interstices (the space between plunger and barrel of glass syringes), finely divided powders, oils, fats, and greases are not reliably penetrated by steam.

Sterilization by dry heat is slower than by moist heat—1 to 3 hours at 160°C—but it is also effective against spores, as well as other microorganisms. The denaturative effect of dry heat is probably augmented by oxidation. An electric oven, fitted with a fan to ensure even heating, is necessary. Instruments with cutting edges (including needles), oils, greases, powders (not more than 5 mm–6 mm deep), and glass syringes are best sterilized using dry heat.

If disinfection of heat-sensitive materials is acceptable, as with respiratory assistance and anesthesia equipment (usually contaminated with nonsporulating gram-negative bacilli), pasteurization offers the advantages of low cost, and minimal hazard to personnel and equipment. The washed objects are immersed in water heated to 77°C for 30 minutes. Care in drying is necessary to prevent contamination; a heated, filtered, forced air drying chamber is ideal.

Irradiation

Under the proper conditions, irradiation with photons—gamma rays, x-rays, or ultraviolet (UV) light—is capable of sterilizing. Because UV light will not penetrate most substances, it has been evaluated extensively only for sterilization of surfaces, air, and some liquids. Conclusions about the value of UV (220 nm–300 nm wavelength) irradiation of air have been conflicting, but the passage of air and some liquids directly over the UV source (thereby ensuring maximum intensity of exposure) can effect sterilization. Smooth surfaces of small, confined areas can also be sterilized by this technique. Very rapid flow rates of thick, murky layers of fluid compromise the effectiveness of UV light, as does increased distance from the source. On the other hand, satisfactory disinfection of water or buffer solutions contaminated with sewage not known to contain spores has been demonstrated following exposure of 1 to 2 liter volumes of the liquid in clear glass to direct sunlight for periods of 1 to 2 hours. This has been attributed to solar irradiation in the near-UV range and has implications for the establishment and maintenance of safe oral rehydration solutions (or simply potable water) in circumstances in which more sophisticated means of sterilization are not available. UV and near-UV light is hazardous to personnel: prolonged unprotected exposure of skin may cause burns, and irreversible retinal injuries may occur even at apparently safe distances from the source.

Irradiation with high-velocity electrons (Van de Graaff or microwave accelerator) can be applied to sterilize prepackaged heat-labile materials. The equipment is bulky and expensive, and beams of accelerated electrons have a limited range of penetration. However, electron irradiation, when applicable, is very well suited to industrial, assembly-line technology.

Electrohydraulic Shock and Ultrasound

Electrohydraulic shock (the delivery of a high-voltage discharge under the surface of a liquid) is capable of sterilizing liquids. So is ultrasound. Neither method appears likely to displace heat as a routine measure for sterilization. Ultrasound, however, is used as a practical adjunct to other methods of sterilization by aiding in mechanical disruption and removal of adherent particulate matter prior to the use of chemical agents or heat, thereby ensuring that efficient and complete sterilization will occur.

Filtration

When fluids containing heat-labile substances must be sterilized, fungi, bacteria, spirochetes, and protozoa can be removed by filtration. Two general classes of filters are in use: (1) depth filters—tortuous channels, adsorption, and electrostatic forces add to a sieving effect (filters made of unglazed ceramics, fritted glass, or asbestos pads); (2) screen filters—primarily a sieving effect provided by membranes (typically, cellulose esters) about 150 μm thick with an average pore size of 0.22 μm. Ease of use, reliability, and minimal interaction with the fluid undergoing filtration have led to increased use of membrane filters.

Particles smaller than the actual maximal pore size of a given filter may be retained, apparently as a function of charge, entrapment in the interstitial mazes of the filter, and adherence to larger particles. In this way, even macromolecules and essential nutrients may be removed, particularly by the depth filters. However, filtration cannot be relied on to remove viruses, chlamydias, rickettsias, or mycoplasmas. Although liquids are more often sterilized by filtration than gases, the principles and devices are the same for both fluids.

Chemical Agents

General considerations influencing the usefulness of chemical disinfectants or sterilants are antimicrobial potency and spectrum; potential for residual, or substantive on-going antimicrobial effect; activity in the presence of organic material; chemical stability (shelf life); and risk of adverse effects on the health of personnel and patients or other users of the disinfected material.

Liquids

Soaps have only slight antibacterial activity. Their value to disinfection lies in their efficiency as detergents.

Bichloride of mercury and other inorganic salts of mercury should no longer be used as disinfectants. More effective and less corrosive agents are now available. Organic compounds of mercury have limited disinfectant activity and are applied either topically as antiseptics or as preservatives, for example, thimerosal.

Chlorine and chlorine compounds that yield HOCl on hydrolysis are effective agents. They are quite unstable and corrosive and are inactivated by organic matter. But they are inexpensive and are used principally as sanitizers, for example, in water treatment (see Chap. 16, Environmental Factors).

Iodine preparations are not consistently sporicidal but otherwise are good disinfectants with a broad range of antimicrobial action. Solution in aqueous ethanol augments antimicrobial activity and tissue irritation without mitigating skin staining. Iodine may be combined with surfactants or with nonsurfactant polymers (povidone iodine) in iodophor preparations, with resultant reduction in tissue irritation. However, because iodophors owe their activity to free or available iodine, a preparation that provides at least 2% available iodine is required to equal the germicidal potency of 2% iodine tincture (USP XIX). For the same reason, the activity of the complexed iodine solutions may be inhibited by the presence of organic matter in or on the material to be disinfected, and may vary with time because of changes in the stability of the complexes and the rate of release of unbound iodine. Hypersensitivity to iodine (fever, generalized rash) is rare, but may be engendered by any of the available preparations. Metabolic acidosis in burn patients has been associated with the use of povidone iodine as a topical agent, and evidence that iodine can be absorbed from the peritoneal cavity suggests that its use as an intraoperative wound disinfectant should be proscribed.

Phenols are also inefficient sporicides, but they are generally active germicides that display residual activity after deposition. Soaps decrease the killing action of phenols, whereas organic matter does not interfere with their potency. Neutral detergents and an acid pH increase their activity. Phenol itself is no longer used because the substitution of certain alkyl or aromatic groupings and halogenation, especially *para* to the phenolic–OH, yields derivatives with much greater activity; for example, 2-chloro-4-phenylphenol, *p*-tert-amylphenol. Mixtures of such substituted phenols compounded with detergents are widely used for wet-mopping and cleaning in hospitals because of their immediate effectiveness and residual activity. The halogenated bis-phenols are also used extensively as skin cleansers because of their effect in reducing the resident flora, which may be due to their residual antibacterial activity. However, concern over toxic effects of percutaneously absorbed 2,2′-methylene bis(3,4,6-trichlorophenol)—hexachlorophene—has largely limited its use to hand-washing only. The potential toxicity of 1,1′-hexamethylene bis(5-*p*-chlorophenyl biguanide)—chlorohexidine—is incompletely delineated, though it appears slight, since little percutaneous absorption occurs.

Ethanol (70%–90% by weight) and isopropanol (90%–95% by volume) lack only sporicidal activity as germicides. Both are rapidly active, and they increase the speed and overall effectiveness of many other agents, for example, iodine and quaternary ammonium compounds. With continued use, defatting of the skin may lead to roughening, an effect that is more pronounced with isopropanol.

The quaternary ammonium compounds that are characterized by long chain alkyl or heterocyclic substituents are highly active against many kinds of bacteria. They are cationic detergents that are odorless, colorless, stable, nontoxic, and noninjurious to tissues in the concentrations ordinarily used. There is no useful residual effect after application, and activity is diminished in the presence of organic matter. The quaternary ammonium compounds are inactivated by soaps, possibly as a result of direct interaction of a cationic with an anionic moiety. They are notably inactive against *Mycobacterium tuberculosis* (and other acid-fast bacteria), most *Pseudomonas* spp., *Enterobacter* spp., and *Serratia* spp., as well as some strains of *Klebsiella* spp. Moreover, they are neither sporicidal, fungicidal, nor virucidal. In short, the quaternary ammonium compounds are used far too extensively as antiseptics. They are, however, probably effective as sanitizers.

Formalin (37% formaldehyde in water) as a 20% solution in either ethanol (70% by volume) or isopropanol (95% by volume) is very actively germicidal. Spores, fungi, tubercle bacilli, and viruses are killed. However, such formalin preparations are very difficult to use. Formaldehyde vapors are released and irritate the nose and eyes; skin sensitization develops quite commonly. There is also concern about the carcinogenic potential of formaldehyde preparations.

Glutaraldehyde, a dialdehyde that is a chemical entity quite distinct from formaldehyde, dissolves in water to yield an acid solution that is stable but not remarkably active. When alkalinized, solutions become germicidal but lose activity, since the glutaraldehyde polymerizes at a rate directly proportional to pH and temperature. A 2% solution buffered at pH 7.5 to 8.5 (with $NaHCO_3$) retains the ability to kill vegetative bacteria in 2 minutes, hyphal fungi in 5 minutes, *M. tuberculosis* and enteroviruses in 10 minutes and bacterial spores within 3 hours, for as long as 2 weeks if stored at room temperature. Newer preparations (1) employ variations in the pH of the activated glutaraldehyde compound to prolong shelf life and (2) offer combination with phenate buffer to produce a relatively stable, synergistically acting solution of exceptionally broad spectrum and high potency. Even though there is no obnoxious vapor, buffered glutaraldehyde is a contact irritant to the skin, mucous membranes, and eyes. It is noncorrosive and apparently does not harm instruments having lenses or anesthesia equipment.

An important cautionary note must be appended to any discussion of liquid chemical disinfectants about their unfortunate recently emerging role as purveyors, rather than preventers, of infectious diseases. Bacteria, particularly gram-negative organisms such as *Psuedomonas* spp. and *Serratia marcescens,* can multiply in both full strength and diluted solutions of several classes of liquid disinfectants, including the quaternary ammonium compounds and the bis-phenols. This usually results from failure to sterilize contaminated storage and dispenser bottles before refilling them. Patients may become infected directly or through the use of improperly disinfected supplies, developing wound and skin infections, urinary tract infections, pneumonias, and septicemias. Also, the involved microbial population may become increasingly tolerant to the disinfectant on continuous exposure. The importance of establishing procedures that prevent the development and selection of bacteria resistant to disinfectants cannot be overstressed.

Gases

At one time, formaldehyde was highly regarded as a gaseous sterilant. It is, in fact, effective only when the relative humidity is near saturation and the temperature is 20°C (70°F) or higher. Penetration into tightly fitting equipment, crevices, or porous materials is quite poor. Prolonged aeration for several days may be required to dissipate residual formaldehyde.

Ethylene oxide (EtO) is the sporicidal agent of choice for sterilizing fragile and heat-labile materials, as well as complex apparatus (respiratory assistance equipment, cardiac bypass pump–oxygenator units). It can be bought premixed with either carbon dioxide (90%) or Freons (88%) so that the hazards of fire and explosion are avoided. Although the CO_2 mixture requires the use of a high-pressure reducing valve system, the Freons are soluble in many kinds of plastics and actually increase the uptake of EtO by some materials; for example, polyvinyl chloride. The gas penetrates very well and objects to be sterilized may be packaged in a form suitable for shelf storage. Sterilization is effected by 4 to 12 hours of exposure to EtO (100–500 mg per liter, 30%–50% relative humidity, 25°C–40°C). However, 12 to 24 hours of aeration will be necessary to ensure dissipation of dissolved EtO from plastics and especially articles made of rubber. This is quite important because EtO has a vesicant action on skin and mucous membranes. Certain multiple-dipped items such as spiral-latex-reinforced endotracheal tubes should not be sterilized in EtO because intramural blisters or layer separation may occur in the tubing and pose a threat to the lives of patients during anesthesia if the NO_2 in the anesthetic gas mixture distends the blisters, leading to complete airway obstruction. (Such items should not be subjected to steam sterilization with vacuum, for similar reasons.) The lethal action of EtO appears to involve alkylation through reaction with–SH, COOH,–NH, or $-NH_2$ and –OH groupings of proteins. Such groupings of other compounds are also attacked because the nutritional adequacy of animal diets and the activity of streptomycin are destroyed by exposure to EtO.

Betapropiolactone (βPL) is neither flammable nor explosive; it is a pungent, colorless liquid at room temperature and pressure. As a gas, it does not penetrate as well as EtO, but it is much more rapidly dissipated after use than is formaldehyde. It is much more active than EtO—1 to 2 mg per liter (at a relative humidity of 75% at 25°C–30°C)—and it kills bacterial spores within 2 hours. It also acts through alkylation. Betapropiolactone is toxic to humans, but at concentrations higher than those needed for sterilization.

Peracetic acid (PAA) has been widely used as a disinfectant spray. It is corrosive (as an acid and oxidant), but is an effective germicide. As a gas, PAA is sporicidal at a concentration of 1 mg per liter (80% relative humidity, 25°C) within 1 hour. The decomposition products, acetic acid and oxygen, are readily dissipated.

Disinfection of the Skin

Elimination of all elements of the cutaneous microflora is not possible without destroying the skin. However, thorough washing and the application of disinfectants eliminate transient bacteria and reduce the numbers of the more superficial resident bacteria (chiefly *Staphylococcus epidermidis*), leaving the deep resident bacteria (*S. epidermidis* and *Propionibacterium acnes*) largely intact (Fig. 17-2).

Removal of the transient bacterial flora from the hands is paramount in controlling the spread of nosocomial infections within hospitals, particularly in high-risk areas (*e.g.,* intensive care units, neonatal nurseries). Colonization of the hands of medical and nursing personnel with nosocomial pathogens, usually gram-negative bacilli and *Staphylococcus aureus,* can be demonstrated and represents a major factor in the transmission of these organisms between patients. Thorough hand-washing, employing only soap, water and friction, is sufficient in all but high-risk areas. The addition of disinfectant washes and scrubbing poses a potential problem, however, in that repeated use of agents that can cause drying, chapping, and irritation of the skin may lead to dermatitis; dermatitic skin cannot be satisfactorily disinfected.

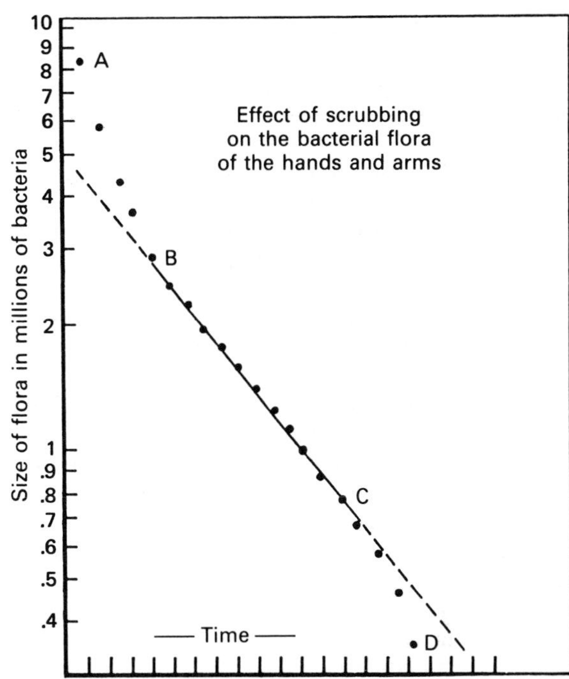

Fig. 17-2. Effect of scrubbing on the bacterial flora of the hands and arms. *AB* corresponds to transients, *BC* to superficial resident flora, *CD* to deep resident bacteria. (Price PB: The Becton, Dickinson Lectures on Sterilization, 1957–1959. Jersey City, 1959)

Three sequential steps are necessary for maximal disinfection in preparing the skin for invasive procedures such as surgical operations, insertion of percutaneous vascular catheters, or lumbar puncture: (1) Scrubbing with soap. For best effect, scrubbing with a brush should be carried out for at least 7 minutes. (2) Application of an alcoholic iodine preparation by rubbing. Gauze squares should be used, and the skin should be kept wet for 5 minutes. Either 2% iodine in 70% ethanol (w/w), 2% iodine +2.5% KI in 50% ethanol, or an iodophor that provides 2% available iodine in 70% (w/w) ethanol can be used. (3) Removal of the iodine by brisk scrubbing using gauze with either ethanol (70%–90%, w/w) or isopropanol (90%–95% by volume).

Remaining Problems

Limitations imposed on existing methods of sterilization and disinfection, whether of efficacy, applicability (relative injury to material being treated), reliability, or economy, remain a stimulus for the development of improved technologies. Implicit in this endeavor is the need for a better understanding of the mechanisms by which microorganisms can resist killing.

Consolidation of standards for sterility and the methods used to evaluate achievement of the standards is a pressing, if not urgent, need. At least two major regulatory agencies (the Environmental Protection Agency and the Food and Drug Administration) are responsible for setting and directing testing methods for standards in the United States, and actual testing criteria have been developed by a number of governmental, professional, and industrial organizations. International standardization of definitions and evaluation methods should be sought. Shortcomings of currently accepted evaluation methods include lack of standard conditions for the testing of disinfectants; imprecision in definitions and variable or lacking standards for such poorly defined concepts as sanitization; failure to include in standard tests criteria for some clinically important pathogens such as hepatitis B virus; and universal disagreement or uncertainty about the necessity of guidelines for disinfection of certain types of medical equipment such as endoscopes and bronchoscopes.

With particular reference to infectious diseases, the value of disinfection in preventing the spread of infection is, curiously, often poorly documented. There is a continuing need for well-designed studies that attempt to correlate clinical benefit with (bio)-chemical achievements of sterilization and disinfection procedures.

Bibliography

Books

BLOCK SS (ed): Disinfection, Sterilization, and Preservation, 2nd Ed, 1049 pp. Philadelphia, Lea & Febiger, 1977

BORICK PM (ed): Chemical Sterilization. Stroudsburg, Dowden, Hutchinson & Ross, 1973. 352 pp.

PRICE PB: The Becton, Dickinson Lectures on Sterilization, 1957–1959. Jersey City, Becton, Dickinson, 1959. 123 pp.

Journals

ACRA A, KARAHAGOPIAN Y, RAFFOUL Z, DAJARI R: Disinfection of oral rehydration solutions by sunlight. Lancet 2:1257–1258, 1980

ALLEN HF: Sterilization of instruments and materials with beta-propiolactone. JAMA 172:1759–1763, 1960

AXON ATR, BANKS J, COCKEL R, DEVERILL CEA, NEWMANN C: Disinfection in upper-digestive-tract endoscopy in Britain. Lancet 2:1093–1094, 1981

DIXON RE, KASLOW RA, MACKEL DC, FULKERSON CC, MALLISON GF: Aqueous quaternary ammonium antiseptics and disinfectants: Use and misuse. JAMA 236:2415–2417, 1976

EHRENKRANZ NJ, BOLYARD EA, WIENER M, CLEARY TJ: Antibiotic-sensitive *Serratia marcescens* infections complicating cardiopulmonary operations: Contaminated disinfectant as a reservoir. Lancet 2:1289–1291, 1980

KAUL AF, JEWETT JR: Agents and techniques for disinfection of the skin. Surg Gynecol Obstet 152:677–685, 1981

LEACH ED: A new synergized glutaraldehyde-phenate sterilizing solution and concentrated disinfectant. Infect Control 2:26–30, 1981

LEERS W–D: Disinfecting endoscopes: How not to transmit *Mycobacterium tuberculosis* by bronchoscopy. Can Med Assoc J 123:275–280, 1980

LOFFER FD: Disinfection versus sterilization of gynecologic laparoscopy equipment: The experience of the Phoenix Surgicenter. J Reprod Med 25:263–266, 1980

PORTNER DM, HOFFMAN RK: Sporidical effect of peracetic acid vapor. Appl Microbiol 16:1782–1785, 1968

RENDELL–BAKER L: A hazard alert: Reinforced endotracheal tubes. Anesthesiol 53:268–269, 1980

STEERE AC, MALLISON GR: Handwashing practices for the prevention of nosocomial infections. Ann Intern Med 83:683–690, 1975

PAUL D. HOEPRICH

Antimicrobics and Anthelmintics for Systemic Therapy

18

As part of the discussion of therapy that is included in each chapter dealing with an infectious disease, the drugs of choice for treatment, alternative agents, and details of usage (dosage, administration, and duration of treatment) are specified. The doses are virtually always related to body weight because (1) antimicrobics and anthelmintics are drugs; and (2) in general, a large person needs more medicine than a small one. In this chapter, principles of rational selection and use of systemic antimicrobics and anthelmintics are related to several characteristics and properties of these remarkably effective therapeutic agents.

Classification

Of several bases advanced for classification of anti-infective drugs, the chemical structure (Table 18-1) is the most satisfactory because it is precisely known. Such classification facilitates the recognition of congeners—drugs with like structures and virtually identical activities, but with different pharmacodynamics and toxicity. Generally, one representative of a congeneric group can be identified as preferable for therapy and susceptibility testing *in vitro* (Chap. 12, Susceptibility Testing).

Classification according to mechanism of action is desirable, for it is more serviceable to the clinician. However, little is known of the mode of action of many useful drugs, and conversely, details of action are known for many compounds that are not applicable in therapy.

Sources and origins of antimicrobics have become less relevant to classification as more and more drugs have been discovered, and as increasing numbers have been altered after biosynthesis to obtain semisynthetic drugs with particular properties advantageous to therapy. Patterns of susceptibility are not dependable bases for classification because they vary from time to time and from place to place and depend greatly on the method of testing (Chap. 12, Susceptibility Testing). The kinds of infectious agents affected are of relatively little value to classification because the antiinfectives most often prescribed are, in fact, antibacterial agents.

Because the term *broad spectrum* is often misapplied, it requires clarification. It should be reserved for drugs that are therapeutically useful against more than one of the major groups of infectious agents (Chap. 1, Attributes of Infectious Agents). Thus, the penicillins and cephalosporins are active only against bacteria; no penicillin or cephalosporin possesses a broad spectrum. All of the tetracyclines and chloramphenicol are active against chlamydias, mycoplasmas, and rickettsias, as well as bacteria; the tetracyclines and chloramphenicol are broad-spectrum drugs.

Potential for inhibitory (static, *i.e.,* allowing no increase in the number of viable units of the inoculum within a specified, standard period of observation) and lethal (cidal, *i.e.,* producing a reduction in the number of viable units of the inoculum by at least 99.9% within a specified, standard period of observation) action also merits comment. Virtually any anti-infective agent suitable for systemic use can be shown by testing *in vitro* to inhibit the growth of the pathogen at a particular concentration—the minimal inhibitory concentration (MIC). In the same test system, a higher concentration of the drug often brings about the death of the infectious agent—the minimal lethal concentration (MLC). When the difference between the MIC and MLC is large, the drug is often regarded as primarily inhibitory or static in action; a close correspondence in MIC and MLC indicates a high potential for lethal effect. Also implied is a difference in the time required for a lethal effect; bacteria long held in a limbo of nonreplication by a bacteriostatic agent (*e.g.,* the tetracyclines) may eventually give up the host, whereas a truly bactericidal agent (*e.g.,* streptomycin) kills within 1 to 2 generation times. The relationship of the MIC to the MCL varies, not only with the drug but also with the kind of infec-

Table 18-1. Classification and Some Properties of Several Antimicrobics and Anthelimintics

Class	Agent(s)*	Spectrum	Mechanism(s) of Action	Concentration in Blood
Acridine dye	MEPACRINE	Broad—antiprotozoal anthelmintic	Intercalate, with DNA causing insertion of extra base during replication	50–60 μg/liter plasma
	SURAMIN	Broad—antiprotozoal, anthelmintic		150 mg/liter on day of dose (peak)
Acetanilide	DILOXANIDE FUROATE	Narrow—amebacide	Not known	?
Adamantine	AMANTADINE	Narrow—antiviral	Blocks penetration into host cell	200 μg/ml
Alkaloid	Dehydroemetine	Narrow—amebacide	Inhibit elongation of peptide chain by blocking tRNA	
	EMETINE	Narrow—amebacide		?
Aminocyclitol	AMINOGLYCOSIDE	Narrow—antibacterial	Interference with protein synthesis through ribosomal binding (30S subunit); surfactant	Variable with preparation, dose route of injection, 2–25 μg/ml Virtually unabsorbed from gut
	SPECTINOMYCIN	Narrow—antibacterial	Interference with protein synthesis through ribosomal binding (30S subunit)	About 100 μg/ml
Antimonial				
Trivalent	ANTIMONY POTASSIUM TARTRATE	Broad—antiprotozoal; anthelmintic	Inhibition of sulfhydryl enzymes; inhibition of phosphofructokinase	?
	ANTIMONY SODIUM DIMERCAPTOSUC-CINATE	Broad—antiprotozoal anthelmintic	Inhibition of sulfhydryl enzymes; inhibition of phosphofructokinase	?
Pentavelent	SODIUM STIBOGLUCONATE	Broad—antiprotozoal; anthelmintic	Inhibition of sulfhydryl enzymes; inhibition of phosphofructokinase	?
Arsenical				
Trivalent	MELARSOPROL	Narrow—antiprotozoal	Inhibition of sulfhydryl enzymes	0.3–0.6 μg/ml plasma
Pentavalent	TRYPARSAMIDE	Narrow—antiprotozoal	Inhibition of sulfhydryl enzymes	?
Bephenium	BEPHENIUM HYDROXYNAPHTHO-ATE	Narrow—anthelmintic	Paralyzes through depolarization	Low; very poorly absorbed
Biguanide	Chloroguanide	Narrow—antimalarial	Inhibition of reduction of folic acid	?
	Cycloguanil pamoate	Narrow—antimalarial	Inhibition of reduction of folic acid	?
Bithionol	BITHIONOL	Narrow—anthelmintic	Unknown	?
Chloramphenicol	CHLORAMPHENICOL	Broad—antibacterial antirickettsial, antimycoplasmal, antichlamydial	Inhibition of protein synthesis by binding to 50S ribosomal subunit, inhibiting peptide bond formation	10–12 μg/ml
Cyanine Dye	PYRVINIUM PAMOATE	Narrow—anthelmintic	Blocks uptake of glucose	Virtually unabsorbed from gut
	DITHIAZANINE IODIDE	Narrow—anthelmintic	Inhibition of both oxidative and anaerobic metabolism	Virtually unabsorbed from gut
Diamidine	Hydroxystilbamidine	Broad—antiprotozoal, antifungal	Inhibition of aerobic glycolysis	?
	PENTAMIDINE ISETHIONATE	Broad—antiprotozoal, antifungal	Inhibition of aerobic glycolysis	Around 0.2 μg/ml plasma

Table 18-1. (continued) *Classification and Some Properties of Several Antimicrobics and Anthelimintics*

Class	Agent(s)*	Spectrum	Mechanism(s) of Action	Concentration in Blood
Diaminopyrimidine	PYRIMETHAMINE	Broad—antibacterial, antiprotozoal	Inhibition of reduction of folic acid	?
	TRIMETHOPRIM	Broad—antibacterial, antiprotozoal	Inhibition of reduction of folic acid	1–3 μg/ml
Ethambutol	ETHAMBUTOL	Narrow—antitubercu-lous	Unknown	5–10 μg/ml
Griseofulvin	GRISEOFULVIN	Narrow—antifungal	Probably inhibition of nucleic acid synthesis	1–2 μg/ml
Hexylresorcinol	HEXYLRESORCINOL	Narrow—anthelmintic	Unknown	Low–poor absorption, rapid renal excretion
Imidazole				
Benzimidazole	THIABENDAZOLE	Narrow—anthelmintic	Inhibition of fumaric reductase	? (is absorbed)
	MEBENDAZOLE	Narrow—anthelmintic	Blocks uptake of glucose	? (poorly absorbed)
Nitroimidazole	METRONIDAZOLE	Broad—antiprotozoal, antibacterial	Unknown	10–20 μg/ml
Phenethylimidazole	Clotrimazole KETOCONAZOLE Miconzaole	Broad—antifungal, antibacterial	Inhibition of conversion of lanosterol to ergosterol	Topical 4–7 μg/ml 4–7 μg/ml
Isonicotinamide	Ethionamide	Narrow—antibuberculous	Unknown—possibly as for isoniazid	15–20 μg/ml
	ISONIAZID	Narrow—antituberculous	Inhibition of enzymes that require pyridoxal (or pyridoxamine) phosphate as cofactor (*e.g.*, transminases)	2–3 μg/ml
Lincomycin	CLINDAMYCIN Lincomycin	Narrow—antibacterial Narrow—antibacterial	Bind to 50S ribosomal subunit blocking initiation (clindamycin, lincomycin) and extension (erythromycin) of peptide chains	2–5 μg/ml
Macrolide	ERYTHROMYCIN	Broad—antibacterial, antimycoplasmal, antichlamydial		
	RIFAMPIN	Broad—antibacterial, antiviral (DNA)	Inhibition of DNA-dependent RNA polymerase.	10 μg/ml
	Triacetyloleandomycin	Narrow—antibacterial	As for erythromycin	3–5 μg/ml
Niridazole	NIRIDAZOLE	Narrow—anthelmintic	Augments glycogenolysis	?
Nitrofuran	NITROFURANTOIN	Narrow—antibacterial	Inhibition of initiation of formation of mRNA	Not detectable
	NIFURTIMOX	Narrow–antiprotozoal	Unknown	?
Novobiocin	Novobiocin	Narrow–antibacterial	Inhibits DNA gyrase	100–130 μg/ml
Organic Acid	HIPPURIC (methenamine)	Narrow–antibacterial	Unknown	?
	MANDELIC (methanamine)	Narrow—antibacterial	Unknown	?
	NALIDIXIC	Narrow—antibacterial	Inhibits DNA gyrase	10 μg/ml
Phenazine dye	CLOFAZIMINE	Narrow—antibacterial	Unknown	?
Piperazine	DIETHYLCARBAMAZINE CITRATE	Narrow—anthelmintic	Unknown	4–5 μg/ml
	PIPERAZINE	Narrow—anthelmintic	Paralyzes through hyperpolarization	?
Peptide	AZTHREONAM	Narrow—antibacterial	Interferes with cell wall synthesis	Variable with dose and route of administration: 20–150 μg/ml

Table 18-1. (continued) Classification and Some Properties of Several Antimicrobics and Anthelimintics

Class	Agent(s)*	Spectrum	Mechanism(s) of Action	Concentration in Blood
	Bacitracin	Narrow—antibacterial	Inhibition of cell wall synthesis	1–2units/ml
	Capreomycin	Narrow—antituberculous	Unknown	10–15 μg/ml
	CEPHALOSPORINS	Narrow—antibacterial	Inhibition of peptidases, activation of autolysins of cell wall	Variable with preparation, dose, route of administration, 5–200 μg/ml
	CLAVULANIC ACID	Narrow—antibacterial	Irreversible binding of β-lactamases	3–4 μg/ml
	Cycloserine	Broad—antichlamydial, antirickettsial, antibacterial	Inhibition of alanine racemase and *d*-alanyl-*d*-alanine synthetase	15–25 μg/ml
	Fosfomycin	Narrow—antibacterial	Inhibition of formation of UDP-*N*-acetyl muramic acid	10–40 μg/ml
	Penem	Narrow—antibacterial	Inhibition of cell wall synthesis	10–20 μg/ml
	PENICILLINS	Narrow—antibacterial	Inhibition of peptidases, activation of autolysins of cell wall	Variable with preparation, dose, route of administration, 2–200 μg/ml
	Polymyxins	Narrow—antibacterial	Surface active disruption of cell wall-membrane complex	2–8 μg/ml
	Saramycetin	Narrow—antifungal	Unknown	2–3 μg/ml serum
	Sulbactam	Narrow—antibacterial	Irreversible binding of β-lactamases	3–5 μg/ml
	N-FORMIMIDOYL-THIENAMYCIN	Narrow—antibacterial	Inhibition of cell wall synthesis	16–35 μg/ml
	VANCOMYCIN	Narrow—antibacterial	Inhibition of cell wall synthesis	25–40 μg/ml
	Viomycin	Narrow—antituberculous	Unknown	?
POLYENE Heptaene	AMPHOTERICIN B	Broad—antifungal, antiprotozoal	Interaction with sterols of cell membrane	0.5–2.0 μg/ml
	NYSTATIN	Narrow—antifungal	Interaction with sterols of cell membrane	Not absorbed from gut
Purine	ACYCLOVIR	Narrow—antiviral (DNA viruses)	Inhibition of viral DNA polymerase and DNA replication	<0.01–0.8 μg/ml (topical)
	ARA-A	Narrow—antiviral (DNA viruses)	Inhibition of viral DNA polymerase and DNA replication	3–6 μg/ml
Pyrazinamide	PYRAZINAMIDE	Narrow—antituberculous	Unknown	30–30 μg/ml
Pyrimidine	5-FLUROCYTOSINE	Narrow—antifungal	Competition with uracil (as 5-FU)	20–100 μg/ml
	5-IODO-2-DEOXYURIDINE	Narrow—antiviral (DNA)	Competition with thymidylic acid	?

Table 18-1. (continued) *Classification and Some Properties of Several Antimicrobics and Anthelimintics*

Class	Agent(s)*	Spectrum	Mechanism(s) of Action	Concentration in Blood
Quinoline				
4-Aminoquinoline	Amodiaquine	Narrow—antiprotozoal	Not known but appears to bind nucleoproteins	?
	CHLOROQUINE	Narrow—antiprotozoal	Inhibits nucleic acid synthesis by intercalating (base pairs) in DNA	Peak—150–250 μg/ml Low—20–40 μg/ml
8-Aminoquinoline	PRIMAQUINE	Narrow—antiprotozoal	Not known but appears to bind with nucleoproteins	?
	quinocide	Narrow—antiprotozoal	Not known but appears to bind with nucleoproteins	?
Isoquinoline	PRAZIQUANTEL	Narrow—anthelmintic	Not known	?
6-Methoxyquinoline	QUININE	Narrow–antimalarial	Possibly, interference with glucose metabolism	Around 7 mg/liter (average)
	quinidine	Narrow—antiprotozoal	May interfere with glucose metabolism	?
Oxyquinoline	DIODOHYDROXYQUIN	Narrow—antiprotozoal	Not known	Not absorbed
Salicylate	ρ-AMINOSALICYCLIC	Narrow—antituberculous	Replacement of ρ-aminobenzoic acid to yield a mock folic acid	5–7 mg/100 ml
	NICLOSAMIDE	Narrow—anthelmintic	Blocks conversion of ADP to ATP	Not absorbed from gut
Steroid	FUSIDIC ACID	Narrow—antibacterial	Unknown	25–35 μg/ml
Sulfonamide	SULFONAMIDES	Broad—antibacterial, antichlamydial, antiprotozoal	Competition with ρ-aminobenzoic acid	10–15 mg/100 ml
Sulfone	DAPSONE	Narrow—antimycobacterial	Probably competition with ρ-aminobenzoic acid	0.5 mg/100 ml
Tetrachlorethylene	TETRACHLORETHYLENE	Narrow–anthelmintic	Reversible paralysis	Absorbed to an unknown extent
Tetracycline	TETRACYCLINE	Broad—antibacterial, antimycoplasmal, antirickettsial, antichlamydial	Inhibition of protein synthesis by blocking tRNA in 30S ribosomal subunits	3–5 μg/ml
Thiosemicarbazone	METHISAZONE	Narrow—antiviral (DNA)	Inhibition of synthesis of protein through ribosomal disruption	0.3–3 μg/ml serum

*The agents of a group that are preferred for therapy are capitalized.

tious agent that is tested (*e.g.,* chloramphenicol is generally bacteriostatic but is bactericidal against *Haemophilus influenzae*) and the manner in which testing is carried out (*e.g.,* a single reading at 24 hours or multiple assays at timed intervals over 24–48 hours).

Because the determination of MICs and MLCs is strictly a laboratory exercise, it is reasonable to question the relevance of events observed in such a highly artificial situation to the treatment of infectious diseases in humans. Concentrations of antiinfectives that are potentially lethal to infectious agents are not always attained even in the blood of patients, let alone at the actual site of the infection. Moreover, both cellular and humoral defense mechanisms are ordinarily operative in the patient. There are, however, clinical situations that support the dictum, "Use an agent (or combination of agents) with potential for lethal activity in preference to a drug that is primarily inhibitory." For example, by susceptibility testing *in vitro,* it is usual to find that many antimicrobics are inhibitory to the bacterial causes of infective endocarditis. However, cure invariably requires the application of agents demonstrably lethal by *in vitro* testing (Chap. 134, Infective Endocarditis). It is similarly instructive to note that before the availability of penicillin, *Streptococcus pneumoniae* and group A *Streptococcus pyogenes* not uncommonly caused death in patients with florid, acute leukemias, an outcome virtually unheard of today.

Concentrations and Distribution

Measurements of the concentrations of antiinfective agents in the blood as guides to therapy can be questioned from the standpoint that the infectious process ordinarily is not actually intravascular. In fact, the concentration in the blood represents no more than the result of (1) absorption from the site of administration; (2) elimination—usually in the urine, sometimes in the bile or other secretions; (3) catabolism—primarily by the liver, but also by the kidneys and other organs with some drugs; and (4) passage into tissues and body fluids, with or without fixation by specific tissues or microorganisms. Notwithstanding these factors, it remains true that the blood is the one readily available tissue for assay, and in most instances there are no data specifying the concentrations of antiinfective drugs at the actual sites of infections. Because the blood is the transport medium that delivers the drug to the site of infection, the assumption is commonly made that concentrations of antimicrobics in the usual extravascular sites of infections are lower than those achieved in the blood. Whenever possible, therapy should provide maximal concentrations in the blood that are 4 to 5 times greater than the MIC of the infecting organism. A dash of empiric interpolation is often added, based on clinical experience and influenced by the severity of the illness or its location.

Infections of the central nervous system (CNS) were among the earliest noted to present special problems to the delivery of antiinfective agents. Bypassing barriers to penetration by the injection of drugs directly into the cerebrospinal fluid (CSF) has in some cases been superseded by resort to mass action, swamping of CNS barriers by huge doses; for example, of penicillins in bacterial meningitis. Other special compartments can also be affected in this way—the entry of penicillin and streptomycin into tracheobronchial secretions or into saliva. However, only a few antimicrobics are so nontoxic that a forcing, high-dosage approach can be used.

The penetration of drugs into various sites, organs, tissues, secretions, and compartments of the body is affected by factors other than the concentrations attained in the blood. Passage from the blood is favored by (1) small molecular size; (2) lack of electrical charge at pH 7.4; (3) solubility in lipids, and (4) ease of dissociation from plasma proteins. Although it is illuminating to consider these determinants of distributions, it must be realized that almost all studies of blood and tissue concentrations have been carried out in normal subjects. It is quite certain that the presence of infection can alter the pharmacodynamics of antiinfective agents—for example, the entry of drugs into the CSF in meningitis.

The relatively few antimicrobial agents that are small molecules (Table 18-2), appear to distribute throughout body water, regardless of charge or other properties.

The more nearly the pK_a of a drug matches the pH of the blood, the more significant nonionic diffusion becomes—for example, sulfonamides useful for systemic therapy (sulfadiazine, 6.5; sulfamethoxazole, 6.1). Most antimicrobics, however, are either weak acids with pK_a values much lower than pH 7.4 (penicillin V, 2.7; cephalexin, 4.5), or possess multiple ionizable groupings with differing pK_a values—for example, rifampin, 1.7 and 7.9. Molecular size lipid solubility and interaction with plasma proteins, then, are the critical determinants of distribution if there is no gradient in pH. Prostatic fluid is an example of the later situation because it is unique among nondigestive secretions in having a pH that is acid relative to the blood. Accordingly, there is actually concentration of drugs that are weak bases in prostatic fluid; for example, erythromycin and sulfanilamide (Chap. 49, Bacterial Prostatitis and Recurrent Urinary Tract Infections).

Solubility in lipids should facilitate passage through cell membranes. Such is the case experimentally, except for very small or very large molecules. If the

Table 18-2. *Molecular Weights of Various Antimicrobics**

Antimicrobic	Molecular Weight
Cycloserine	102.1
Ethionamide	166.2
Flucytosine	129.1
Fosfomycin	138.1
Isoniazid	137.1
Metronidazole	171.2
Pyrazinamide	123.1

*Relatively small molecular size is associated with distribution throughout body water.

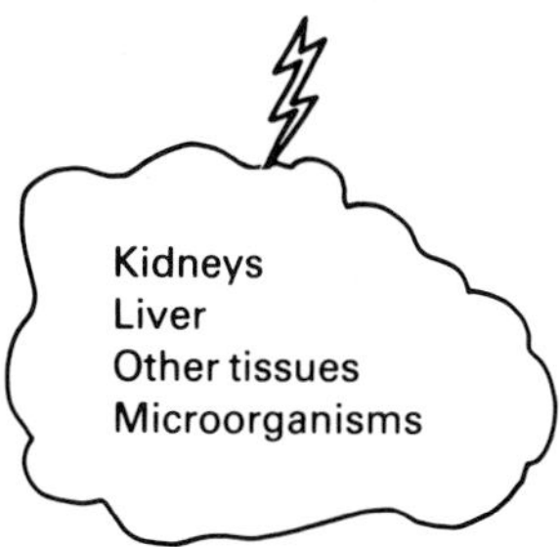

Fig. 18-1. In the blood, antimicrobics are reversibly associated with plasma proteins—principally albumin. As free drug is removed, dissociation of the albumin–antimicrobic complex occurs to maintain the proportion of free drug characteristic of that particular antimicrobic.

molecular radius is less than 1.5 nm, penetration is rapid, whereas molecules with radii greater than 3 nm are retarded in penetration despite solubility in lipids. Antimicrobics with molecular radii between 1.5 and 3 nm, such as the sulfonamides and chloramphenicol, may achieve wide distribution in part because of high lipid solubility.

Antiinfective agents, in common with virtually all drugs, are transported in the blood in association with plasma proteins, primarily albumin. Although it has become popular to measure the extent of "binding" of antiinfective agents to plasma proteins, the results may be specious because the values reported are usually static measurements made in an artificial environment *in vitro,* frequently at supratherapeutic concentrations. For example, the usual report gives only the percentage of the drug that is "bound" and is rarely complete in also providing the concentration of free drug at the equilibrium studied. It is certain that the *in vivo* situation is dynamic and composed of multiple, competitive systems. The association of antimicrobics with plasma albumin is reasonably thought of as an equilibrium reaction (Fig. 18-1). As free drug passes out of the blood, sufficient albumin–antimicrobic complex dissociates to satisfy the fractional requirement for free drug that is characteristic of the interaction of that particular antimicrobic and plasma proteins. The facts of urinary excretion and therapeutic efficacy of antimicrobics that are highly protein-bound according to *in vitro* measurements, for example, cloxacillin, is testimony to the appropriateness of this interpretation. Similarly, reversible binding may also occur with the proteins of various tissues and with nonprotein macromolecules. With susceptible microorganisms, binding appears to be irreversible.

Routes of Administration

Peroral

The convenience of peroral administration of antiinfective agents must be balanced against certain inherent disadvantages. *A drug is not absorbed if it is not ingested.* The fallibility of patients, particularly when directed to take medications by mouth as outpatients, has been documented in several studies and is confirmed by every physician's own experience.

Many agents are well absorbed in the normal subject but are erratically and poorly absorbed in the patient who is severly ill. Nausea, vomiting, diarrhea, and a variety of noninfectious causes of malabsorption may interfere with peroral therapy. Absorption of drugs such as penicillins is generally diminished when there is food in the upper digestive tract (Fig. 18-2). With several antimicrobics, moreover, peroral therapy is simply inefficient—through the formation of complexes (the tetracyclines plus Ca^{++} and Mg^{++}), enterohepatic cycling (nafcillan, ampicillin; Fig. 18-2), and unknown mechanisms (the aminocyclitol drugs).

Intramuscular

Antimicrobics such as amphotericin B, vancomycin, and erythromycin are so irritating that they should not be given intramuscularly. Several of the cephalosporins and some penicillins also may produce chemical myositis on intramuscular deposition—in addition to clinical manifestations, persistent elevation of the erythrocyte sedimentation rate (ESR) and serum lactic acid dehydrogenase may result. Intramuscular injection of all drugs, including antimicrobial agents,

Fig. 18-2. Only 15% to 20% of an oral dose of ampicillin attains to blood-borne distribution, whereas 50% to 80% of penicillin V is available for distribution. (Hoeprich PD: Cal Med 109:301–308, 1968)

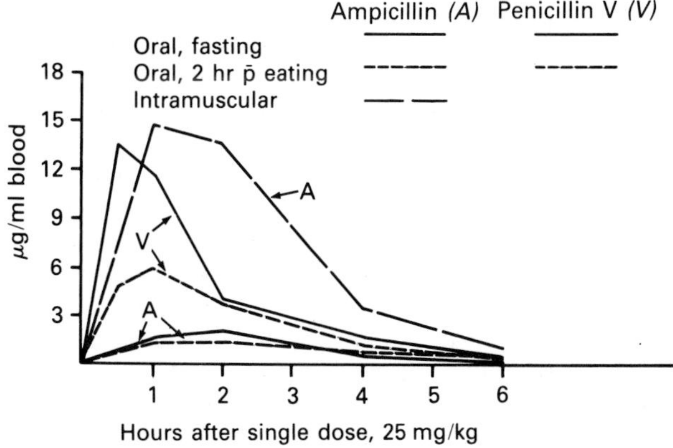

is contraindicated in patients who are in shock or who have a bleeding diathesis, and it should not be made into a paralyzed extremity or a region of fibrosis.

Intravenous

Not only is intravenous injection the humane route of parenteral administration with amphotericin B, vancomycin, erythromycin, salts of the polymyxins, and large doses of the penicillins and cephalosporins, but also it is the only effective route in the patient in shock, or safe route in the patient with a bleeding diathesis. This dictum should not be excepted even with agents customarily given by intramuscular injection (*e.g.,* the aminocyclitols). Any agent that can be injected intramuscularly can also be injected intravenously if the concentration is sufficiently low and the rate of injection is sufficiently slow.

Both continous and intermittent intravenous injection have been used with comparable success in therapy. Continuous injection results in a sustained concentration of the agent in the blood and offers less threat of chemical thrombophlebitis because the concentration of the drug in the solution for injection is generally lower than that used for intermittent injection. For example, cephalothin given by intermittent intravenous injection virtually always causes a florid thrombophlebitis, a complication that appears to be less frequent with continuous injection. Intermittent injection, however, provides higher concentrations of the drug in the blood for short periods; there is also less opportunity for either deterioration or contamination in the course of administration. The hazard of infection secondary to an indwelling intravenous catheter is directly proportional to the length of time that the catheter is left in place (Chap. 135, Septic Thrombophlebitis).

Intrathecal

As judged by simultaneous measurements of the blood and CSF, some antimicrobics penetrate the CNS barriers quite readily (Table 18-3). With other agents, for example, streptomycin and tetracycline, barriers to entry are sufficiently reduced by inflammation to enable successful treatment without direct intrathecal injection. Still other drugs are so safe that massive parenteral dosage can be undertaken and will assure penetration into the CSF/CNS even without inflammation (the penicillins but not the cephalosporins—except moxalactam and possibly cefotaxime and cefatriaxone; Fig. 18-3). However, if amphotericin B, the polymyxins, vancomycin, gentamicin, tobramycin, netilmicin, or amikacin must be used, there is no alternative to intrathecal administration.

In myelomeningitis, the convenience and safety of lumbar space injection has clinical support. However, the circulation of the CSF about the spinal cord in normally so sluggish that injection into the cistern is preferable if there is encephalomeningitis. If the direction of flow of the CSF is normal and there is infective ventriculitis, injection into a lateral ventricle would seem to be reasonable. The exact doses to be used are small, as is rational in view of the confined space and volume of CSF available for dilution. Thus, with amphotericin B, 0.5 mg per injection is the maximal dose (Chap. 41, Coccidioidomycosis). The usual adult doses are 5 mg to 10 mg with polymyxin B sulfate, gentamicin, tobramycin, and netilmicin (twice as much with amikacin), and 0.5 mg to 1.0 mg with vancomycin. Severe headache is often induced at the time of injection, and with continued intrathecal administration arachnoiditis and radiculitis may result. In addition, both amphotericin B and vancomycin are directly ototoxic.

Table 18-3. Concentraction of Various Antimicrobics in CSF*

Antimicrobic	CSF/Serum
Chloramphenicol	0.70–0.80
Ethambutol	0.25–0.50
Rifampin	≤0.5
Trimethoprim	≥0.5
Sulfonamides	
Sulfadoxine	≤0.3
Sulfamethoxazole	≥0.5
Sulfisoxazole	≤0.3

*In the absence of inflammation of the central nervous system and the leptomeninges, only certain antimicrobics will gain entry into the CSF.

Intraarticular

All antimicrobial agaents that have been examined enter the synovial fluid without restraint, although there is a time lag caused by equilibration with blood-borne drug (Fig. 18-4). Although periodic aspiration or the installation of flow-through devices may be considered useful in the treatment of infections of the joints (Chap. 151, Septic Arthritis), failure of penetration of antimicrobics is not a valid rationale.

Intraperitoneal and Intrapleural

Antimicrobics appear to enter serous fluids as readily as synovial fluids. That is, direct instillation into serous cavities is not necessary when systemic therapy is adequate. Overzealous intraperitoneal administration of polybasic antimicrobics (*e.g.,* aminocyclitols

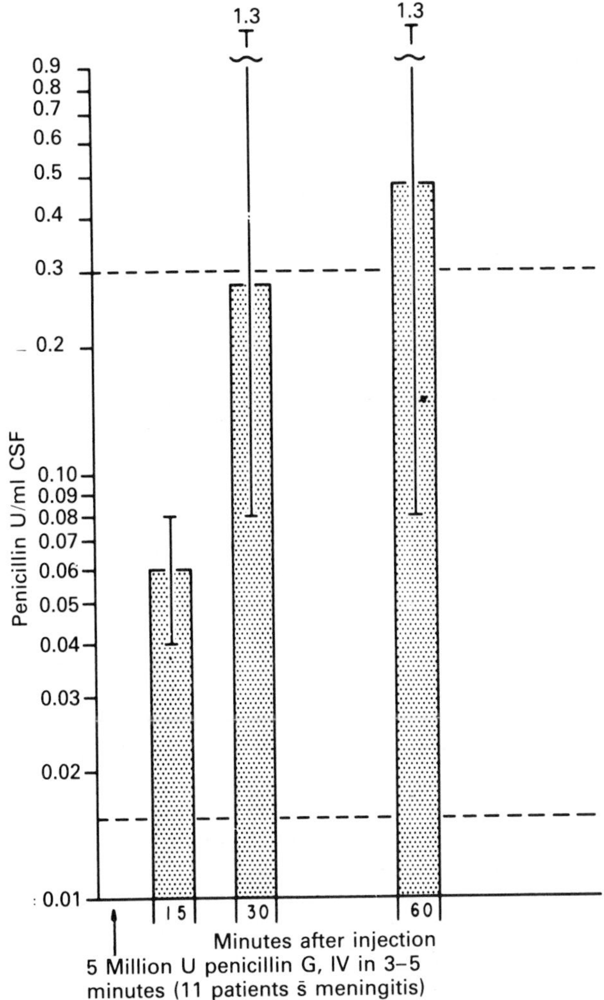

Fig. 18-3. In 11 patients without meningitis, the average concentration of penicillin G **(tops of bars)** in the cerebrospinal fluid after IV injection of 5 megaunits (3.15 g) exceeded the MIC for *Streptococcus pneumoniae* in 15 minutes **(lower dashed line)**, reaching an inhibitory concentration for *Neisseria meningitidis* in 30 minutes **(upper dashed line).** (After data of Bailey DJ: J Lab Clin Med 58:305–310, 1961)

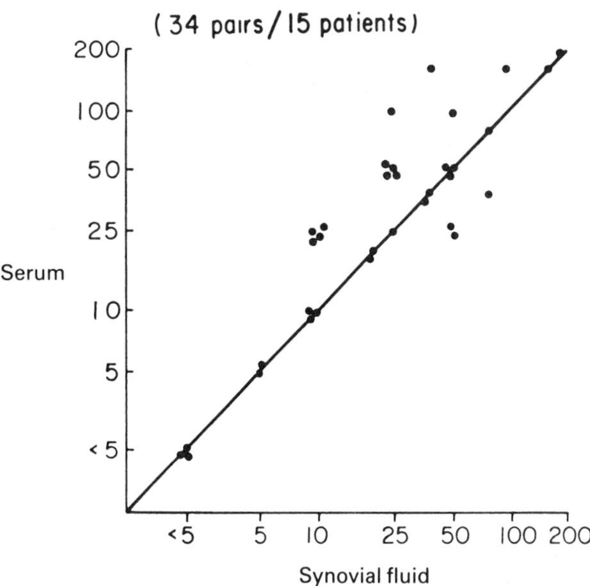

Fig. 18-4. The reciprocals of the bactericidal concentrations of antimicrobics in paired specimens of serum and synovial fluids cluster about a straight line corresponding to equality in concentrations. The specimens were obtained simultaneously from patients treated with penicillin G, nafcillin, cloxacillin, cephaloridine, tetracycline, erythromycin, and lincomycin. (Schmid FR, Parker RH: Arthritis Rheum 12:529–534, 1969)

and polymyxins) has resulted in acute neuromuscular blockade.

Inhalation

It is obvious that inhalation of air containing a finely dispersed antimicrobic will lead to a high concentration in the respiratory tract. It is less clear that successful treatment of an infection localized to the respiratory tract will result. Indeed, aerogenous administration of antimicrobics is of doubtful value. There are several reasons: (1) the site of deposition in the respiratory tract is primarily a function of particle size and is also influenced by respiratory dynamics; (2) the site of infection may be recondite to deposition of air-borne particles—as a result of the inaccessibility of exudate-filled bronchioles and alveoli and the convoluted anatomy of the upper respiratory tract; and (3) as particle size diminishes, the probability of the oxidative inactivation increases.

Irrigation

The introduction of antimicrobics as aqueous solutions or suspensions into hollow viscera, abscesses (soft or calcified tissues, through sinuses), or wounds should ensure high concentrations at the apparent sites of infections. Suppression of growth often results, but cure of the infection is generally not achieved. There is usually inadequate penetration into the interstices and recesses of the infected areas. Also, ease of access for irrigation implies ready access of bacteria, for example, colonization by *Pseudomonas aeruginosa* of a sinus tract leading to a chronic osteomyelitis caused by *Staphylococcus aureus*.

Adverse Reactions

Direct Toxicity

MISCELLANEOUS FACTORS

As the concentration of an antimicrobial agent increases, so also does the probability of a toxic effect. The range between therapeutic and toxic concentration is quite variable from one antimicrobial agent to another. It is maximal with the penicillins and minimal with amphotericin B. The occurrence of direct toxicity is influenced by several factors—age, genetic endowment, and hepatic and renal function.

Premature infants and neonates are particularly vulnerable to certain drugs as a consequence of immature (1) renal excretory capacity (aminocyclitols); (2) hepatic glucuronyl transferase activity (resulting in the grey syndrome of chloramphenicol and hyperbilirubinemia from novobiocin); (3) CNS barrier function (sulfonamide therapy in the mother leading to kernicterus in the fetus); and (4) osseous tissue (deposition of tetracyclines). In old age, the threshold for ototoxicity appears to be diminished; quite independently, the renal excretory capacity is often decreased as well.

If there is a deficiency of glucose-6-phosphate dehydrogenase (G-6-PD), antimicrobics such as sulfonamides, sulfones, nitrofurantoin, chloroquine, primaquine, and niridazole provoke hemolysis. Inactivation (acetylation) of isoniazid at an abnormally rapid rate appears to be a genetic trait that has little consequence in the treatment of tuberculosis (Chap. 34, Pulmonary Tuberculosis).

Hepatic metabolism (chloramphenicol, cephalothin, cefotaxime) and excretion (tetracycline, rifampin, several of the penicillins, certain cephalosporins, clindamycin, and amphotericin B) are often important in the handling of antimicrobial agents. Yet, accumulation of antimicrobics as a consequence of hepatic failure appears to be uncommon.

RENAL FUNCTION

Renal excretion of antimicrobial agents is so common that renal insufficiency is frequently a determinant of the toxicity of antimicrobics. The situation is complicated because several antimicrobics are directly nephrotoxic, and noninfectious renal diseases often set the stage for an infectious process.

In practice, the dose for a given patient should be reduced in quantity to match that patient's deficit in renal excretory capacity for the particular antimicrobic prescribed. Measurement of the disappearance of the antimicrobic from the blood as a function of time after administration of a dose is the obvious, direct, and proper approach to individually appropriate adjustment of dosage. Unfortunately, rapid, reliable, and inexpensive methods for assay of most antimicrobics are either not generally available or are yet to be devised. To be clinically valuable, results should be available to the clinician 4 to 6 hours after blood has been withdrawn from the patient. This is not possible with bioassay procedures, but is readily accomplished with chemical methods (the sulfonamides), immunofluorescence photometry (gentamicin, tobramycin, amikacin) and high-performance liquid chromatography (HPLC)—with flucytosine. Until these or other rapid methods are generally available, the dosage of many antimicrobics must continue to be adjusted empirically, that is, without the guidance of direct measurements of the drug. If an antimicrobic is eliminated primarily by the kidneys, conventional measurements of renal function should allow estimation of the reduction in dosage necessary to compensate for decreased renal function. Simply measuring the blood urea nitrogen or the creatinine may be deceptive. For example, both values are normal in patients whose creatinine clearances range from 30 to 130 ml/min/1.73 m^2. Rapid determination of the creatinine clearance is a readily available estimate of renal functional capacity—urine collection intervals as short as 4 hours will suffice. The necessary reduction in the maintenance dose (the initial or loading dose is the same as that given to patients with normal renal function) can then be estimated as a direct function of the creatinine clearance. The estimated maintenance dose must, of course, be modified as measurements of the low–high concentrations in the blood are carried out and as the status of the patient changes.

Such an approach maintains the usual or normal frequency of administration of the drug and compensates for diminished renal elimination by reducing the amount of drug given in each dose. Because a loading dose is given to start therapy, the time necessary to attain a steady state (ideally, low–high concentrations in the blood which bracket the desired therapeutic range) is shortened; generally, administration of one-third to one-half the daily dose is a sufficient loading dose. The attainment of such a steady state is a function solely of the half-life of the drug (it is independent of dose and frequency of administration); hence, regimens calling for reduced frequency of administration of usual or normal doses often subject patients to the double jeopardy of (1) potentially toxic concentrations in the period immediately following administration of a dose, and (2) subtherapeutic concentrations in the period prior to the next dose. A combination approach is often appropriate, that is, reduction of the dose and modest increase in the interval between doses, for it is probable that therapeutic concentrations of antimicrobics need not be constantly present.

SPECIFIC EFFECTS

Specific toxic effects are conveniently related to organ systems for discussion. Precise estimates of frequency of occurrence are not available, and in the presentation that follows rough estimates are given as three categories: common, occasional, and uncommon.

Nervous System

ENCEPHALOPATHY

common	melarsoprol
occasional	cycloserine, diethylcarbamazine, nalidixic acid, quinacrine
uncommon	amphotericin B, carbenicillin, chloramphenicol, isoniazid, methicillin, metronidazole, niridazole, penicillin G, piperazine, primaquine, sulfonamides, tetrachlorethylene

When the concentration of cycloserine exceeds 25 μg/ml serum, there may be progression of toxicity to seizures. If the premonitory evidences of toxicity—giddiness, confusion, and incoordination—are heeded with a reduction in dosage, seizures can be avoided.

The capacity of mechanisms that actively exclude penicillins from the CNS may be overwhelmed when there is extreme penicillinemia: concentrations of 400 units (250 μg) or more of penicillin G per milliliter of serum. Typically, massive dosage is augmented by some degree of renal failure to achieve such concentrations. Involuntary muscle tremors, confusion, and stupor generally occur before seizure activity. Although all of the penicillins appear to be capable of depolarizing neurons on direct application (penicillin G is one of the most active, and carbenicillin one of the least active), some are less likely to cause seizures on systemic administration than others. A critical factor may be excretory routes. Thus, penicillin G, penicillin V, and methicillin are excreted primarily by the kidneys; the isoxazolyl penicillins (oxacillin, cloxacillin, dicloxacillin, and flucloxacillin); nafcillin; ampicillin; amoxicillin; the acylureidopenicillins (mezlocillin, azlocillin, and piperacillin); ticarcillin; and carbenicillin—penicillins rarely associated with seizures—have quite significant egress through the liver, in addition to the kidneys.

VESTIBULAR DYSFUNCTION

common	streptomycin, viomycin
occasional	gentamicin, kanamycin, neomycin, paromomycin, tobramycin
uncommon	amikacin, capreomycin, netilmicin

It is clear that the vestibulotoxicity of one of the aminocylitol drugs is additive to that of another of the group. Accordingly, the total dose to which a person has been exposed should be recorded because approximately 75% of adults who have received 2 g streptomycin per day for 60 days or more sustain detectable vestibular dysfunction. Apparently, the cells of the cochlear nuclei are destroyed. Even though it is not certain that the injury caused by the vestibulotoxic peptide drugs is also cumulative, or is additive to damage inflicted by the aminocyclitols, error on the side of caution is recommended.

AUDITORY DYSFUNCTION

common	dihydrostreptomycin, neomycin, quinine, viomycin
occasional	kanamycin, paromomycin, quinidine, rifampin, vancomycin
uncommon	amikacin, amphotericin B, capreomycin, chloroquine, gentamicin, mepacrine, netilmicin, streptomycin, tobramycin

Neither dihydrostreptomycin nor neomycin should be used in parenteral therapy because of the high risk of ototoxicity. Viomycin has sometimes been necessary in the treatment of tuberculosis caused by strains of *Mycobacterium tuberculosis* resistant to safer agents—an application of diminishing importance.

With the ascendency of chloroquine-resistant *Plasmodium falciparum* as a cause of malaria, the use of quinine and quinidine has been revived. Concomitantly, there has been a resurgence of cinchonism, with a functional loss of hearing that is usually reversible.

In the United States, kanamycin is possibly the most widely used of the potentially ototoxic antimicrobics. Parenteral dosages of 15 mg/kg body wt/day given for 2 weeks have resulted in deafness. Insidious onset, weeks or even months after treatment, has been reported. The anatomic site of the lesion has not been precisely defined in humans, but it is probably identical for all the aminocyclitols. All appear to be additive in ototoxicity, and it is safer to assume that hearing loss caused by nonaminocyclitols is similarly additive.

Orally administered neomycin, kanamycin, and paromomycin may cause deafness if there is both (1) augmented enteric absorption—through inflammation or erosion of the mucosa of the gut or unnecessarily high dosage—and (2) poor renal function. Topical administration of large quantities of these drugs to extensive areas of denuded or burned skin might be similarly hazardous.

OPTIC DYSFUNCTION

common	quinine
occasional	chloroquine, ethambutol, quinidine, tryparsamide
uncommon	amodiaquine, chloramphenicol, ethionamide, isoniazid, quinacrine

Long-term administration of ethambutol, chloroquine, or quinacrine is required before optic neuritis appears, a complication seen also with chloramphenicol, ethionamide, and isoniazid. If the neuritis is recognized early and the causative agent is withdrawn, improvement usually results.

Although the visual disturbances of cinchonism are common, lasting damage from quinine or quinidine (*e.g.,* optic atrophy) is uncommon. Tryparsamide may also cause optic atrophy.

PERIPHERAL NEUROPATHIES

common	melarsoprol, suramin
occasional	cycloserine, emetine, ethionamide, isoniazid, nitrofurantoin, polymyxins
uncommon	aminocyclitols, amodiaquine, amphotericin B, chloramphenicol, ethambutol, vancomycin

Peripheral neuropathies are generally associated with high dose or long-term therapy. The effects are reversible on cessation of treatment.

NEUROMUSCULAR DYSFUNCTION

uncommon	aminocyclitols, polymyxins

Neuromuscular blockade is life-threatening when it takes the form of respiratory paralysis. Presumably the reaction involves the primary amino groupings of these antimicrobics. The effect is more marked in anesthetized persons, and there may be facilitation of blockade by curarelike drugs. The rapid absorption that may follow intraperitoneal application of these agents, as at abdominal laporotomy when gross fecal soiling of the peritoneal cavity is evident, may lead to the high concentrations required for significant blockade. In such instances, assisted respiration may be necessary temporarily until the concentration falls to nonblocking levels. Intravenously administered calcium gluconate may be of value.

INTRACRANIAL HYPERTENSION

uncommon	arsenicals, nalidixic acid, tetracyclines

Increased intracranial pressure that produces symptoms (headache, nausea, and vomiting) and signs (papilledema, bulging fontanelles, and cranial nerve palsies) may develop in the course of treatment. Termination of therapy is curative.

Hematopoietic System

LEUKOPENIA

common	5-iodo-2-deoxyuridine
occasional	adenine arabinoside (ara A), paraaminosalicylic acid, chloramphenicol, novobiocin, primaquine, pyrimethamine, sulfonamides, thiabendazole
uncommon	cephaloridine, cephalothin, clindamycin, griseofulvin, lincomycin, methicillin, metronidazole, nalidixic acid, ristocetin

If leukopenia is the result of direct toxicity, recovery will follow either reduction in dose or cessation of administration. However, leukopenia may warn of agranulocytosis, particularly with chloramphenicol, paraaminosalicylic acid, the sulfonamides, and novobiocin. Because agranulocytosis is apparently an adverse reaction of hypersensitivity, withdrawal of the inciting drug is obligatory.

THROMBOCYTOPENIA

common	5-iodo-2-deoxyuridine
occasional	adenine arabinoside, paraaminosalicylic acid, chloramphenicol, sulfonamides
uncommon	pyrimethamine, quinidine, quinine, rifampin

The depression in numbers of platelets may lead to the formation of petechiae and ease of bruising. Typically, the process is reversed with removal of the inciting drug.

ANEMIA

common	amphotericin B, primaquine
occasional	adenine arabinoside, chloramphenicol, certain cephalosporins, chloroquine, nitrofurantoin, pyrimethamine, sulfonamides, sulfones, suramin

uncommon paraaminosalicylic acid, isoniazid, niridazole, novobiocin, penicillins, trivalent antimonials

The anemias associated with administration of sulfonamides, sulfones, nitrofurantoin, chloroquine, primaquine, and niridazole are frequently the result of a deficiency in glucose-6-phosphate dehydrogenase in the erythrocytes. Immunohemolysis may also occur with the sulfonamides (as well as with quinine, penicillins, and paraaminosalicylic acid). The way(s) in which anemia results with novobiocin and the antimony compounds is not clear.

Systemic therapy with amphotericin B is virtually always associated with anemia. Although direct binding of amphotericin B to the cholesterol of the erythrocyte cell membrane occurs, the concentrations required for hemolysis *in vitro* far exceed those attained *in vivo*. Resolution of the anemia follows withdrawal of amphotericin B.

Pyrimethamine causes macrocytic anemia through the competitive inhibition of dihydrofolate reductase. Isoniazid, by competing with pyridoxine, may make clinically manifest a borderline or subclinical anemia of pyridoxine deficiency.

Because chloramphenicol causes a dose-related depression of bone marrow precursors, examination of the bone marrow and measurement of the serum iron (which is increased) are useful in predicting anemia. The serum iron-binding capacity should also be abnormal (decreased) but is so variable in patients with infections that it is of little value. Reduction of the dose or withdrawal of the drug is indicated.

Certain cephalosporins (*e.g.,* moxalactam, cefoperazone) may cause deficiency of vitamin K (possibly as a consequence of suppression of enteric bacterial flora), leading to hypoprothrombinemia and bleeding.

HEPATIC INJURY

common novobiocin
occasional paraaminosalicylic acid, cycloserine, erythromycin estolate, ethionamide, isoniazid, pyrazinamide, rifampin, sulfonamides, sulfones, tetrachlorethylene, tetracyclines, triacetyloleandomycin
uncommon amodiaquine, cephaloridine, cephalothin, ketoconazole, nalidixic acid, nitrofurantoin, penicillins, quinacrine, trivalent antimonials

Hepatic injury from systemically administered anti-infective agents varies greatly in severity. For example, transient elevation of the serum pyruvic-oxaloacetic transaminase is a trivial and unusual reaction to treatment with ampicillin, oxacillin, cloxacillin, cephalothin, and cephaloridine. On the other hand, the hepatocellular damage that may be caused by paraaminosalicylic acid, amodiaquine, ethionamide, isoniazid, ketoconazole, pyrazinamide, quinacrine, sulfonamides, sulfones, tetrachlorethylene, the tetracyclines, and the trivalent antimonials may be of grave significance because deaths have resulted.

Cholestatic jaundice may represent a hypersensitivity reaction. Although it is commonly engendered by treatment with novobiocin, and occasionally with erythromycin estolate, triacetyloleandomycin, and rifampin, it is an unusual complication of therapy with nalidixic acid and nitrofurantoin.

Renal Injury

common amphotericin B, bacitracin, melarsoprol
occasional aminocyclitols, capreomycin, cephaloridine, methicillin, polymyxins, sulfonamides, sulfones, suramin, tetracyclines, trivalent antimonials, vancomycin, viomycin
uncommon cephalothin, dithiazanine, ethambutol, griseofulvin, pentamidine isethionate

The nephrotoxicity of several antimicrobics is in a sense quite accidental. The concentrations of drugs such as the polymyxins, bacitracin, and the aminocyclitols reach levels toxic to the tubular epithelium simply as a consequence of resorption of water.

Although amphotericin B affects the renal tubules adversely (*e.g.,* hypokalemia, renal tubular acidosis), the glomeruli actually bear the brunt of the damage from this agent. Amphotericin B is cleared slowly, about 5 to 10 ml/min/1.73 m^2. The latter two observations may reflect the colloidal state of the drug as it is injected and probably exists in the blood and body fluids. Whatever the mechanisms, some degree of renal damage is virtually inevitable in the course of therapy with amphotericin B (Fig. 39-3). If renal function is normal at the outset and the dose of amphotericin B is moderate—not more than 0.75 mg/kg body wt every other day and no more than 2.0 g total—ordinarily there will be complete recovery of renal function. Although renal damage is also common with both bacitracin and melarsoprol, the injury with the latter drug is usually reversible.

Acute tubular necrosis in humans has resulted after the administration of cephaloridine, and the drug has been virtually replaced in therapy by safer congeners, for example, cefazolin.

Unusual but documented instances of nephropathy have been associated with tetracycline (deteriorated material), methicillin, cephalothin, ethambutol, viomycin, griseofulvin, and pentamidine isethionate.

Digestive Tract Dysfunction

common paraaminosalicylic acid, ampicillin, amphotericin B, bithionol, cephaloglycin, chloroquine, dithiazanine, ethionamide, 5-iodo-2-deoxyuridine, ketoconazole, lincomycin, mebendazole, melarsoprol, miconazole, nalidixic acid, nitorfurantoin, niridazole, novobiocin, paromomycin, pentamidine isethionate, quinacrine, quinine, tetracycline, thiabendazole, suramin

occasional amodiaquine, bephenium, cephalexin, cefoperazone, chloramphenicol, clindamycin, cycloserine, diiodohydroxyquin, emetine, erythromycin, griseofulvin, hexylresorcinol, isoniazid, methenamine hippurate or mandelate, metronidazole, niclosamide, nystatin, primaquine, pyrvinium pamoate, tetrachlorethylene, thiabendazole, triacetyloleandomycin, trivalent antimonials, tryparsamide

uncommon pyrimethamine, diloxanide furoate

Nausea and vomiting or diarrhea usually reflect irritation of the digestive tract by orally administered antiinfective agents. Derangement of the intestinal microbial balance has been implicated, especially with diarrhea, and is important with some antimicrobics (*e.g.,* clindamycin).

Some agents affect the gut adversely after parenteral administration: amphotericin B, clindamycin, melarsoprol, miconazole, pentamidine isethionate, tetracycline, suramin, emetine, trivalent antimonials, and tryparasamide. Of these, amphotericin B, clindamycin, and tetracycline may provoke adverse reaction after secretion into the gut. However, a central action is presumed to be important with most of the drugs that are injected.

Miscellaneous Dysfunctions

common

fever: amphotericin B, vancomycin

thrombophlebitis: amphotericin B, cefoxitin, cephalothin, erythromycin, vancomycin

cardiovascular abnormalities: antimonials, emetine, melarsoprol, pentamidine isethionate, quinidine, quinine

dizziness, headache: chloroquine, cycloserine, metronidazole, niridazole, quinacrine, thiabendazole, tetrachlorethylene

Hypersensitivity

OCCURRENCE

Virtually any drug, including the systemically administered antiinfectives, may engender hypersensitivity. Among the antiinfectives, the polymyxins almost never elicit hypersensitivity. At the other extreme, allergic reactions are very common with novobiocin. An approximate overall, relative ranking of the frequency of occurrence follows:

common bithionil, nalidixic acid, novobiocin, penicillins, sulfonamides, sulfones, suramin

occasional paraaminosalicylic acid, antiomonials, cephalosporins, diiodohydroxyquin, ethambutol, ethionamide, griseofulvin, isoniazid, lincomycin, methenamine hippurate or mandelate, metronidazole, miconazole, nitrofurantoin, nystatin, quinacrine, quinine, streptomycin, thiabendazole, tryparsamide, vancomycin, viomycin

uncommon amphotericin B, capreomycin, chloramphenicol, clindamycin, erythromycin, polymyxins, pyrazinamide, pyrvinium pamoate, rifampin, tetracyclines, triacetyloleandomycin

Generally, the statistical base for the assessment of hypersensitivity to a given drug is weak. The more severe the reactions, the more nearly accurate the reporting. Use is another factor. Although there is little question that the penicillins cause hypersensitivity in more people than almost any other drug, it is equally apparent that penicillins are among the most commonly prescribed drugs.

A true evaluation of the allergic potential of a drug must take into account not only the number of persons exposed but also the magnitude of the exposure of a particular person. With some antimicrobics, the probability of engendering hypersensitivity appears to be directly related to the dose, for example, with the sulfonamides and vancomycin.

The reported variation in the rate of occurrence of hypersensitivity reactions according to the route of administration of drugs is difficult to rationalize. For example, oral administration of penicillin G is said to cause hypersensitivity in about 0.3% of persons, whereas the various preparations for injection give rates of 0.4% to 5% (maximal with procaine penicillin, minimal with benzathine penicillin). Again, however, there are quantitative problems. The great bulk of the tons of penicillins that have been manufactured for systemic use has been given by injection—that is, the amount of penicillin per dose, the total amount given, and the number of persons exposed are all less with peroral application than with injection. There may also be problems with interpretation. For example, hypersensitivity to penicillins is said to be so common on intraconjunctival instillation that such use is contraindicated, but any drug placed in the conjunctival sac quickly attains high concentrations that may not be readily dissipated—the observed reactions may be evidence of physicochemical irritation.

MECHANISMS, PENICILLINS

In the blood, and presumably in other liquids and tissues of the body, virtually all antiinfective agents are protein-associated. If irreversibly bound to macromolecules, the drugs might act as haptenes. There is little evidence that such is the case. On the other hand, decomposition products arising during manufacture and storage and possibly in the patient after administration are often quite reactive and may form stable conjugates with proteins (possibly also with other macromolecules). Because the major adverse reactions to the penicillins are allergic, considerable effort has been expended in the study of hypersensitivity to penicillins. Although the following discussion draws primarily on work with penicillin G, it is generally accepted that the side chains that distinguish the various penicillins are of little consequence to hypersensitivity—that is, allergy to one is allergy to all.

Degradation of penicillin G proceeds at a finite rate, even in the solid, powdered state, to yield two primary products: benzylpenicillenic acid and benzylpenicilloic acid (Fig. 18-5). Both are much more reactive than penicillin G, forming stable, covalent bonds with proteins and possibly other macromolecules. Benzylpenicilloic acid reacts mainly with lysine groupings of proteins. The resulting conjugates are the antigenic substances most frequently identified in hypersensitivity to penicillins—the so-called major determinant.

TESTING, PENICILLINS

In view of the reactivity of benzylpenicilloic acid with lysine, it was reasonable to conjugate benzylpenicilloic acid with synthetic poly-*l*-lysine. Such benzyl penicilloyl-poly-*l*-lysine (PPL) preparations have been extensively evaluated as skin-testing reagents for the detection of allergy to penicillins. Although skin reactivity was common in patients who had recently experienced adverse reactions to a penicillin, persons who were nonreactive to PPL have developed adverse reactions, including anaphylaxis, when given penicillins, and rarely, adverse reactions have been precipitated by the skin test itself. In part, such drawbacks might be attributable to defects in some preparations of PPL, for example, a lack of definition of the size of the polymer, and failure of specification of the content of benzylpenicilloyl moieties.

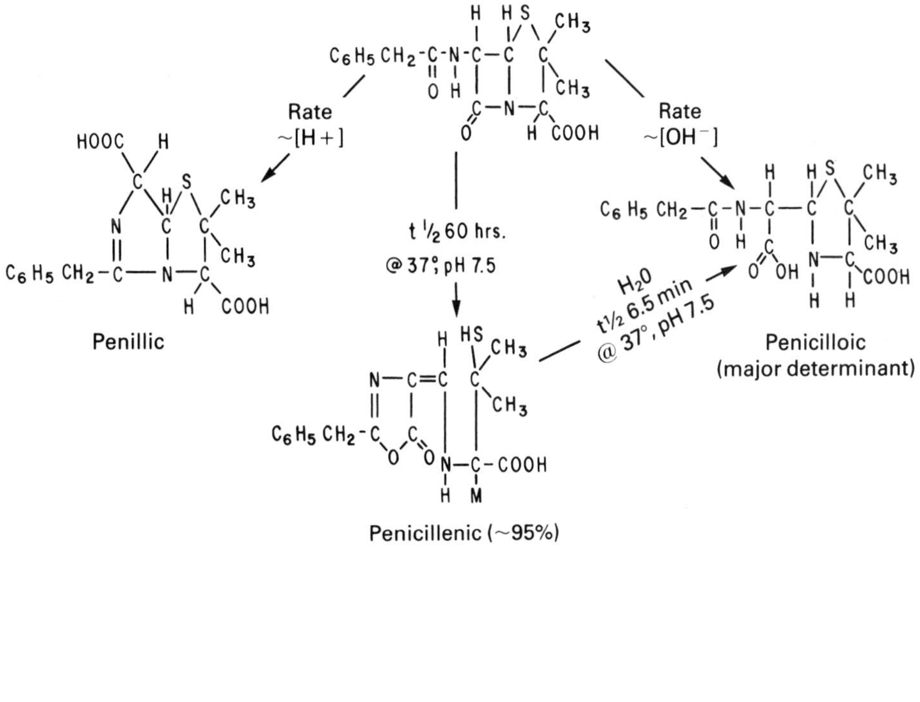

Rate ~[H+]

Rate ~[OH−]

$t_{1/2}$ 60 hrs. @ 37°, pH 7.5

H_2O $t_{1/2}$ 6.5 min @ 37°, pH 7.5

Penillic

Penicilloic (major determinant)

Penicillenic (~95%)

Fig. 18-5. The degradation of penicillin G proceeds at finite rates affected by variables encountered during manufacture, transport, storage, and use to yield compounds that are highly reactive with proteins, and possibly with other macromolecules. (Modified from Schwartz MA, Buckwalter FH: J Pharm Sci 51:1119–1128, 1962. Reproduced with permission of the copyright owner)

Expansion of the spectrum of testing, particularly to enable the detection of potential anaphylaxis, was sought through use of a mixture of other determinants of hypersensitivity to penicillins. Non-benzylpenicilloyl determinants have been lumped together as "minor determinants" and consist chiefly of penicillin G itself, benzylpenicillenoate, and benzylpenilloate. When a mixture of these three substances—minor determinant mixture (MDM)—is used in skin testing simultaneously with PPL, the results appear to be quite reliable. That is, persons who are nonreactive to both PPL and MDM do not develop anaphylactoid reactions if given penicillins; persons who react to both reagents should not be given a penicillin. Reaction to one of the test substances may not absolutely contraindicate penicillin therapy. PPL is available commercially; MDM preparations have not been marketed.

Outdated crystalline potassium penicillin G for therapy may be substituted for testing if diluted with sterile 0.9% NaCl solution for injection to contain 10,000 U (6.3 mg) per ml. Recently manufactured therapeutic material is less likely to contain sufficient benzylpenicillenoate and certainly will not contain sufficient benzylpenilloate to elicit skin reactivity to these minor determinants. The following regimen of testing is recommended for patients who give a history of adverse reaction to a penicillin. Supplies and equipment necessary to treatment of anaphylaxis should be kept at hand throughout testing (see p. 212).

1. Scratch test

   Using a sterile hypodermic needle, make two scratches about 3 cm apart on the volar surface of the forearm. The aim is to penetrate the epidermis without injuring the dermis. If blood is drawn, make a new scratch exerting less pressure. Apply 1 drop of MDM (or a 10,000 U/ml solution of outdated penicillin G) to the center of the proximal scratch (the distal scratch is a control for visual comparison).

   After 10–15 minutes, emergence of a wheal 3 mm or more in diameter (with or without erythema) or erythema 5 mm or more in diameter (with or without a wheal) constitutes a positive test. No further testing is necessary. Penicillins should be withheld and alternative drugs used.

2. Intradermal testing (carry out only if scratch test is negative or there is no history of adverse reaction to a penicillin)

   On the volar surface of the forearm (not used for scratch testing), inject 0.02 ml of 2.5×10^{-7}M PPL (a preparation certified to contain an average of 13 benzylpenicilloyl residues per molecule of polylysine—20 residues of lysine) and 0.02 ml MDM (10^{-2}M, each component). If MDM is not available, use 0.02 ml of the 10,000 U/ml solution of outdated penicillin G (200 U or 125.4 μg).

   After 10–15 minutes, a wheal 5 mm or more in diameter surrounded by erythema constitutes a positive test. If both reagents yield a positive reaction, no further testing is necessary. Penicillins should be withheld and alternative drugs used. If just one of the reagents yields a positive reaction and use of a penicillin is judged necessary, give a test dose.

3. Test dose

   With a blood pressure cuff secured about the thigh but uninflated, inject intramuscularly into the corresponding calf 10,000 U (6.3 mg) of penicillin G (*not* outdated material) or a corresponding amount of another penicillin to be used in therapy.

   If there is no adverse reaction (pruritus, urticaria, rhinitis, laryngeal edema, dyspnea hypotension, or shock) after 20 minutes, therapy can be undertaken without fear of provoking an *immediate* reaction.

Accelerated allergic reactions (onset 1–48 hours after beginning therapy) and *late allergic reactions* (onset 3–14 days after beginning therapy) may occur even though all skin tests are negative.

If the skin test is positive but alternatives to the penicillins are judged to be so inferior or are so toxic that a penicillin must be used, as in bacterial endocarditis, two courses are open: either rapid hyposensitization (desensitization) or suppression of the manifestations of allergic reactions.

HYPOSENSITIZATION

Rapid hyposensitization (desensitization is actually a misnomer because reduction in hypersensitivity sufficient to permit systemic therapy may only reduce cutaneous reactivity) has not been widely used. The risk of provoking serious allergic reactions (systemic reactions, laryngeal edema) is quite high. For example, of 45 patients from several reports, 10 experienced serious reactions, and there was one death. Not all were undergoing rapid hyposensitization—injection of a penicillin every 2–6 hours—a procedure more hazardous than a more leisurely regimen of 3 injections per week. Hyposensitization is an inpatient procedure requiring close surveillance as carefully graded doses, incremental from an intradermally administered quantity that does not elicit an adverse reaction, are injected. Progress through subcutaneous to intramuscular injections must precede therapy. For persistent effect, the treatment must be continued for months.

SUPPRESSION

In some patients, antihistamines suppress adverse reactions sufficiently to permit therapeutic use of penicillins. However, glucosteroids are more reliable. Although neither class of drugs prevents anaphylaxis or laryngeal edema with certainty, glucosteroids usually prevent other manifestations of hypersensitivity. A day of pretreatment—for example, dexamethasone, 0.25 mg/kg body wt, PO, as 3 equal portions, every 8 hours—should precede the administration of a test dose of the penicillin to be used in therapy. With all medications and equipment necessary for the treatment of anaphylaxis at hand (see p. 212), 5 to 10 mg (about 10,000 U of penicillin G) should be injected into a calf muscle (an uninflated blood pressure cuff should be in place on the corresponding thigh). If there is no reaction within 20 minutes, therapy may be started in full dosage. Reduction in the dose of glucosteroid is usually possible and must be guided by the clinical response of the patient.

Because the various penicillins should be considered as a group in terms of hypersensitivity, the structurally similar cephalosporins have been scrutinized carefully as possible cross-reactants. The gamut of hypersensitivity reactions, including anaphylactoid reactions, may be evoked by the cephalosporins, apparently independent of the allergic status of the patient with regard to the penicillins. Thus, humoral antibodies engendered by exposure to a penicillin react with penicillins, but not with cephalosporins, and vice versa. Although the frequency of allergic reactions to cephalosporins is higher in patients who have a history of allergic reaction to penicillins, such patients also respond with an identically high frequency to other drugs. That is, persons documented to have an allergic diathesis by displaying hypersensitivity to a penicillin clearly have the capacity to become allergic to the cephalosporins.

More pertinent to evoking hypersensitivity may be the chemical form of a given drug. Reference has been made previously to the apparent maximal frequency of occurence of hypersensitivity engendered by injection of procaine derivatives of penicillin G as contrasted with the benzathine derivative. Ampicillin provokes hypersensitivity distinctly more often than the other penicillins, particularly in children mistakenly given the drug in the treatment of a viral infection. Similarly, sulfathiazole has been associated with allergy much more often than other sulfonamides. Demethylchlortetracycline appears to cause photosensitivity more often than the other congeners of tetracycline. The estolate derivative of erythromycin provokes a cholestatic jaundice apparently not seen with other forms of erythromycin.

In the foregoing paragraphs the focus has quite appropriately been on the systemically administrable antiinfective agents. Drugs are, after all, manipulatable, and management of them is a primary responsibility of the physician. Yet, it is advisable to recall that persons vary greatly in their capacity to develop hypersensitivity. Although there is nothing the physician can do to alter permanently the so-called allergic diathesis, whenever drugs are prescribed there must be exercised a constant awareness, an alertness to the fact that such an inborn potential for hypersensitivity exists and may be expressed.

REACTIONS

The reaction of hypersensitivity may be no more than fever. Almost any kind of skin rash may result, with or without joint involvement. Nausea and vomiting, cholestatic hepatitis, and hemolysis may also occur. Reactions of this kind are not life-threatening. Usually, they can be controlled by stopping treatment with the inciting drug (substituting an alternative drug if antimicrobial therapy should be continued) and applying an antihistamine (*e.g.,* chlorpheniramine maleate, 4 mg, PO, 6- to 8-hourly for 3 to 5 days). In some patients, glucosteroids may be necessary—for example, dexamethasone, PO, as 3 equal doses, 8-hourly, each dose 0.25 mg/kg body wt on the first day, 0.15 mg/kg on the second day, and 0.05 mg/kg on the third and final day.

Nonanaphylactoid. Exfoliative dermatitis, agranulocytosis, and aplasia of the bone marrow are similar in the nonpredictability of occurrence, insidious onset, and primary dependence on self-repair after the inciting agent has been withdrawn. There are, of course, singular aspects of note:

1. Exfoliation of the skin is most commonly provoked by the sulfonamides (perhaps certain slowly excreted varieties are more often involved), tryparasamide, and the penicillins. The process may evolve despite prompt removal of the inciting drug. In such patients, and when the process is a serious erythema multiforme exudativum with predominant mucosal involvement, severe constitutional symptoms, and a high mortality (Stevens–Johnson syndrome), there is considerable doubt that antimicrobics or other drugs are in fact causative.

2. Agranulocytosis is classically brought on by sulfonamides. It is also seen as a hypersensitivity reaction to chloramphenicol, and it may occasionally follow the administration of pyrimethamine and streptomycin. Methicillin, penicillin, and tetracycline have uncommonly been associated with agranulocytosis. Ordinarily, the bone marrow recovers during the weeks after withdrawal of the provoking drug.
3. Aplasia of the bone marrow is more often secondary to chloramphenicol than to any other antimicrobic. The sulfonamides are next most frequently implicated; the tetracyclines and amphotericin B are quite rarely the cause of aplasia. Whatever the cause, the prognosis is extremely grave because at least half the patients die of the disease. No method is known that enables certain recognition of those rare persons who will develop aplasia in response to drugs. If there is a genetic susceptibility, as some claim, the drug should not be given to blood relatives of the patient with aplasia, particularly not to a twin. On the premise that in some cases the injury might be reversible and detectable by monitoring the peripheral blood (white blood cell count; differential, platelet, and reticulocyte count; hematocrit), examinations before treatment and at reasonable intervals thereafter may be valuable.

Anaphylactoid. Because angioneurotic edema is frequently part of an anaphylactoid reaction, the two reactions can be usefully considered together. The penicillins are incitants more often than are any other antimicrobics. However, it must be remembered that identical reactions may be caused by amphotericin B, the cephalosporins, the tetracyclines, the nitrofurans, novobiocin, paraaminosalicylic acid, the sulfonamides, streptomycin, and vancomycin. The reactions are dramatic, becoming manifest seconds to minutes after administration of the offending agent. The striking feature is hypotension that progresses rapidly to shock, followed by lethal cardiovascular collapse. Dyspnea, cyanosis, and coma are frequent, with or without convulsions. Treatment must be prompt and vigorous:

1. Administer epinephrine (aqueous, 1:1000), 0.5 ml–1.0 ml by IV injection (absorption after IM injection is not reliable if there is hypotension).
2. Insert an airway or a tracheostomy tube. Although there may be an element of bronchospasm (histamine-mediated, epinephrine- and antihistamine-responsive), dyspnea often reflects angioneurotic edema (kinin-provoked, poorly responsive to epinephrine and antihistamines).
3. Establish a means of continuous intravenous access. The salutary effect of the initial dose of epinephrine is short-lived, and additional doses may be needed.
4. Administer an antihistamine, *e.g.,* chlorpheniramine maleate, 10 mg IV.
5. Delay the absorption of the offending agent, *e.g.,* apply a tourniquet proximal to an IM injection site.
6. Administer a glucosteroid IV, particularly if prolonged absorption of the inciting agent is anticipated. For example, dexamethasone, 0.5 mg/kg body wt, may be infused IV over a period of 1–2 hours.
7. Observe the patient in hospital for at least 24 hours. Maintenance therapy with an antihistamine given PO (*e.g.,* chlorpheniramine maleate, 4 mg every 6 hours) is usually possible beginning 4–6 hours after intravenous dosage. Similarly, peroral administration of glucosteroids may be useful in a dosage sufficient to control symptoms as the depot of the inciting drug is absorbed.

Use of penicillinase has been suggested when the offending agent is a repository form of penicillin. However, penicillinase is a protein of bacterial origin that is antigenic and allergenic. Moreover, repository penicillins owe their persistence to insolubility; thus, penicillinase would have limited access to the penicillin. Finally, the end product of penicillinase activity is penicilloic acid, a major determinant of hypersensitivity to the penicillins. It is preferable to continue glucosteroid or antihistamine therapy in doses sufficient to control symptoms until penicillin breakdown products have been dissipated.

Ecologic Changes

The adverse ecologic impact of systemically administered antimicrobial agents is of two general kinds. First, there may be serious dislocation of the resident microbiota. Second, resistance to the therapeutic agent may be engendered in either the pathogen, elements of the resident microbiota, or both, or the infected site may be invaded by exogenous microorganisms also resistant to the antimicrobic.

RESIDENT MICROBIOTA

Ecologic vacuums are as thoroughly abhorred by nature as are physical vacuums. That is, some perturbation of the resident microbiota is virtually inevitable when an antimicrobic is applied systemically. This is the state of the art; as therapists we are still striving to meet Ehrlich's exhortation to "learn to aim, learn to aim with chemical substances." Efforts have focused on avoiding direct hits on the host and have been comparatively little concerned with hitting one specific pathogen while sparing other microorganisms.

The antibacterial agents that antagonize the synthesis of bacterial cell walls should provide the cleanest record of lack of adverse effect on the human. Indeed, the penicillins and cephalosporins are remarkably benign agents (not so other "cell-wall-active" antimicrobics). However, such agents are active not only against several kinds of pathogenic bacteria, but also against elements of the normal bacterial flora: most viridans group and microaerophilic *Streptococcus* spp., *Fusobacterium* spp., spirochetes, *Peptostreptococcus* spp., *Clostridium* spp., and some species of *Bacteroides.* With suppression of the growth of such normal inhabitants of the upper respiratory tract, as may occur during treatment of pneumococcal pneumonia with penicillin G, there is outgrowth of bacteria tolerant to penicillin in the concentrations attained in the upper respiratory tract. *Branhamella* spp. may become ascendant; other possibilities include *Staphylococcus aureus, Escherichia coli* or other gram-negative bacilli, and *Candida albicans.* The flora of the gut remains largely unaffected.

Broadly active antibacterial antimicrobics that attain high concentrations in the gut, particularly those that suppress the anaerobic flora of the colon, may allow proliferation of resistant bacteria capable of causing the syndrome of pseudomembranous colitis, for example, clindamycin and *Clostridium difficile.* With other drugs, the impact may become evident in several regions of the body.

For example, peroral administration of tetracycline will lead to profound changes in enteric, vulvovaginal, and skin flora. As the anerobic bacteria of the gut are suppressed, *Staphylococcus aureus* may become predominant and *Candida albicans* may also flourish. With inhibition of the normal vulvovaginal bacterial flora, candidal overgrowth may occur. Liberation of free fatty acids in the skin from lipolysis of sebum diminishes as *Propionobacterium acnes* is kept from growth; *Staphylococcus* spp. become predominant.

Hospitalized patients treated with antimicrobics run a greater risk of becoming colonized with bacteria that are resistant to several antimicrobial agents—varieties that abound in hospitals. Penicillin-resistant *Staphylococcus aureus* is classic (Fig. 100-3). A similar course of events can be cited for many other antibacterial agents.

There are comparatively few data regarding the ecologic impact of antiviral, antifungal, and antiprotozoal drugs. Perhaps this reflects the therapist's very poor aim with these agents because a major concern is avoidance of serious intoxication of the host. The antimicrobics active against chlamydias, rickettsias, and mycoplasmas are also effective against bacteria and spirochetes.

Resistance

In the course of therapy, the pathogen may develop resistance to the agent used in treatment. Peculiarities of both pathogen and drug appear to be involved. *Mycobacterium tuberculosis, Mycobacterium leprae, Staphylococcus aureus,* certain of the Enterobacteriaceae, *Neisseria* spp., *Candida* spp., *Cryptococcus neoformans Plasmodium* spp., and *Trypanosoma* spp. are notably resourceful in adapting to antimicrobics. It is difficult to rationalize this capability on the basis of infectious drug resistance, that is, acquisition of resistance to the very drug in use in the treatment of an infectious disease by mechanisms such as transformation (rare)—incorporation of genes loosed into the environment by resistant cells; transduction (occasional)—introduction of genes, piggyback on temperate phages; conjugation (common)—acquisition of cytoplasmic genes, called R factors, during cellular mating. Although R-factor-mediated resistance is quite rapidly acquired by gram-negative bacilli, the resistance usually includes several antimicrobics that are coded as a unit or group, for example, the simultaneous acquisition of resistance to the sulfonamides, chloramphenicol, tetracycline, kanamycin, neomycin, and streptomycin; of these drugs, the acquisition of massive resistance in a single step is common only with streptomycin when it is applied as the sole agent in therapy. With *Staphylococcus aureus,* infectious acquisition of resistance one drug at a time is the rule. However, with the possible exception of transduction; the operation of infectious processes has not been proved to occur with *M. tuberculosis, M. leprae,* fungi, or protozoa. Spontaneous gene mutations and the selective pressure favoring the outgrowth of resistant variants (either present in very small numbers before exposure to the drug, or by mutations after exposure) appear to be the important mechanisms.

Knowledge of mechanisms of action, albeit often incomplete, provides some insight into the rapid acquisition of resistance with a few drugs. Streptomycin and spectinomycin differ from other aminocyclitols in the speed, ease, and magnitude of the resistance that may develop (*e.g.,* with *E. coli* or *N. gonorrhoeae*). It may be pertinent to note that these two drugs stand out among the aminocyclitols as possessing the fewest amino groups. That is, they display the least surface active capability, and virtually depend on interaction with nucleic acids for antibacterial effect.

During treatment of infective endocarditis with high doses of 5-fluorocytosine, the causative *Candida parapsilosis* developed massive resistance through deletion of coding for cytosine deaminase (Fig. 18-6). Development of resistance to 5-fluorocytosine has also been reported with other *Candida* spp., *Cryptococcus neoformans,* and *Torulopsis glabrata,* but the exact mechanisms have not been detailed.

The antimalarials that most readily engender resistance are drugs that interfere with folic acid metabolism. Rapid emergence of profound resistance may occur in all species of *Plasmodium* that cause malaria.

From a practical standpoint, experience with tuberculosis, leprosy, other non-acid-fast bacteria, and malaria is quite supportive of a generalization: dapsone, erythromycin, ethionamide, flucytosine, fosfomycin, fusidic acid, isoniazid, lincomycin, nalidixic acid, novobiocin, proguanil, pyrazinamide, pyrimethamine, rifampin, streptomycin, or trimethoprim should not be used alone as a single agent in therapy. A second agent must always be given concomitantly. The second agent must also be effective against the pathogen under treatment and should be active by a different mechanism. There are exceptions—for example, erythromycin in diphtheria, isoniazid in the prophylaxis of tuberculosis, and dapsone in tuberculoid leprosy—but in the main, the generalization holds true.

Resistance may also develop in the host's resident microbiota. In the hospital, resistant strains are commonly acquired from outside the patient, as occurs with *Staphylococcus aureus* colonizing in the noses of inpatients (Fig. 100-3). Also, the selective pressure exerted on the patient's own resident microbiota as a

Fig. 18-6. Course of illness in a patient with infective endocarditis caused by *Candida parapsilosis* that mutated to resistance to 5-fluorocytosine during therapy. (Hoeprich PD, Ingraham JL, Kleker E, Winship MJ: J Infect Dis 130:112–118, 1974. © by The University of Chicago. All rights reserved.)

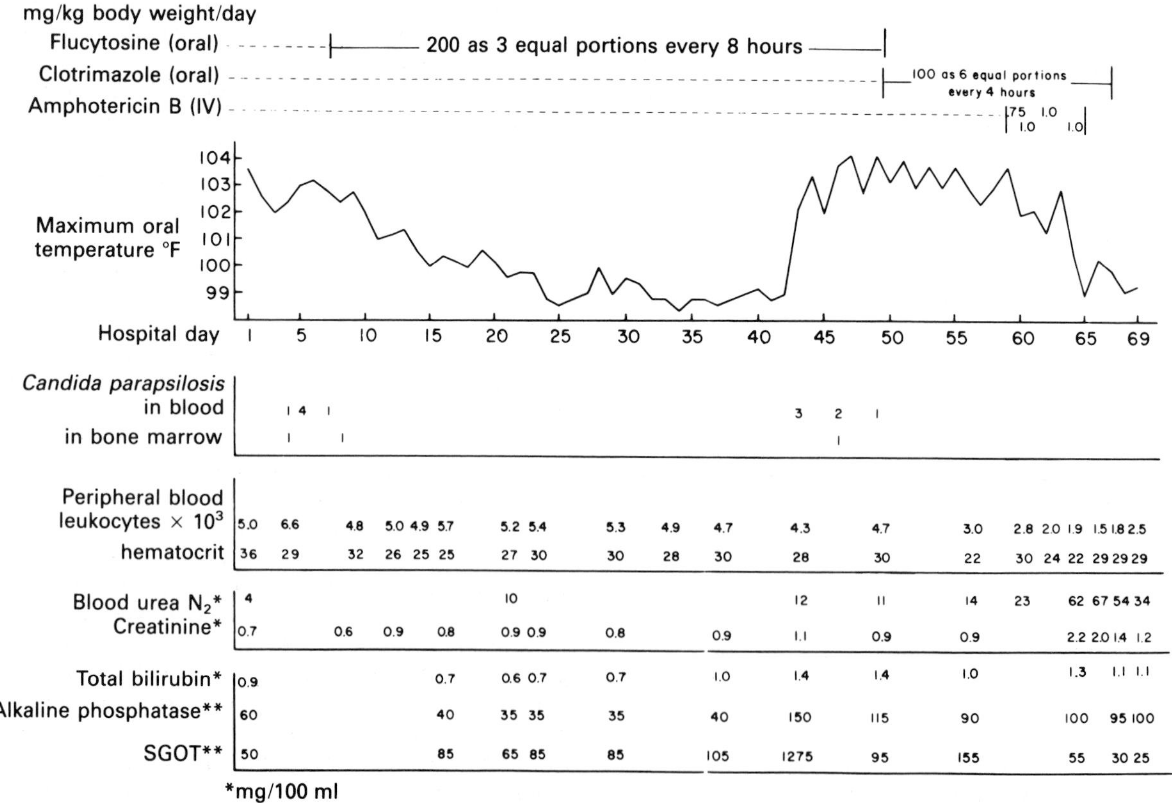

result of treatment favors the outgrowth of microorganisms that are resistant to the drug employed.

A third mechanism may be no more than a refinement of selective pressure. Despite systemic administration, many antimicrobics fail to attain effective concentrations in all areas of the body. The respiratory and digestive tracts are two areas served by secretions that exclude certain of the penicillins and cephalosporins and the aminocyclitols. Meager entry of these drugs would result in minimal selective pressure. Yet, the presence of subinhibitory concentrations might activate adaptive mechanisms eventuating in the development of resistance. Thus, long-term chemoprophylaxis of infection by *Streptococcus pyogenes*, using orally administered penicillin, is associated with the appearance of penicillin-resistant bacteria in the mouth—notably viridans streptococci and *Staphylococcus epidermidis*.

Choice Among Antiinfectives

Several groups of antiinfective agents consist of drugs that are similar in several properties such as chemical structure, kinds of organisms affected, and mechanisms of action. Substitution of one drug of a congeneric group for another of the same group does not constitute an actual change in chemotherapy. The bases for preference of particular agents vary somewhat according to clinical circumstances because pharmacodynamic differences and potential for adverse reactions are often quite marked.

Aminocyclitols

The aminocyclitols available for therapy include streptomycin, neomycin, kanamycin, paromomycin, spectinomycin (used only in the treatment of gonorrhea), gentamicin, tobramycin, amikacin (a semisynthetic derivative of kanamycin), and netilmicin (a semisynthetic derivative of sisomycin). Of these, neomycin and paromomycin should be restricted solely to peroral use and to topical application. Careful quantitative comparisons show that paromomycin is more effective in reducing the enteric microflora than neomycin. The difference may not be clinically significant. Moreover, paromomycin is considerably more expensive than neomycin.

The structural formulas of the systemically administrable aminocylitols are shown in Figure 18-7. With the exception of spectinomycin, these drugs are also aminoglycosides; that is, glycosidically linked aminosugars are substituents of the molecules either as streptidine (in streptomycin) or as deoxystreptamine (in kanamycin, gentamicin, tobramycin, amikacin, and netilmicin). However, aminoglycoside is too general a term because some macrolide and polyene antimicrobics are also aminoglycosides—erythromycin–desosamine (Fig. 18-10), and amphotericin B-mycosamine (Fig. 18-17)—whereas aminocyclitol is suitably specific.

The primary mechanism of antibacterial action is assumed to be the same for all aminocyclitols, although the information has been derived primarily with streptomycin. Irreversible binding of streptomycin to 30S subunits of ribosomes causes blockage of synthesis of essential proteins through failure of initiation of synthesis and misreading of mRNA. Apparently, the sites of ribosomal attachment are not necessarily identical for each drug, since there is not complete crossing of susceptibility resistance among the aminocyclitols. One-step, complete resistance to this mechanism may be acquired through mutations that lead to blocked or ineffective binding of drugs to ribosomes.

A secondary mechanism of antibacterial action is that of surface activity; it is important in direct proportion to cationicity as contributed by primary amino groupings. Thus, it is nonexistent with spectinomycin, of little importance with streptomycin, and contributory to the effectiveness of the other aminocyclitols. Such detergent capability is not readily accomodated by bacteria.

However, resistance may also be acquired through infection with plasmids encoding the synthesis of enzymes capable of inactivating the aminocyclitols. Key sites are inactivated by adenylation, phosphorylation, or acetylation.

Parenteral injection is necessary for systemic distribution. Entry into tracheobronchopulmonary secretions or exudates is known to be excellent for streptomycin and gentamicin. Some penetration into the CSF occurs when there is meningitis with streptomycin and possibly kanamycin; gentamicin, tobramycin, amikacin, and netilmicin enter poorly.

Streptomycin is the preferred aminocyclitol for the treatment of tuberculosis, although amikacin is also quite effective. Spectinomycin is the aminocyclitol of choice for the treatment of genitoanal gonorrheal disease. With other bacterial infections that require use of an aminocyclitol, either kanamycin, gentamicin, tobramycin, amikacin, or netilmicin may be used. Because kanamycin suffers from lack of activity against *Pseudomonas aeruginosa*, relatively high probability of causing hearing loss, and lesser antibacterial potency on both a mass and molar basis, it has been superceded by the other aminocyclitols.

Gentamicin, tobramycin, and netilmicin are interchangeable with regard to dosage and pharmaco-

Fig. 18-7. Structural formulas of six aminocyclitol antimicrobics. Commercial gentamicin consists of roughly equal parts of C_1, C_2, and C_{1a}.

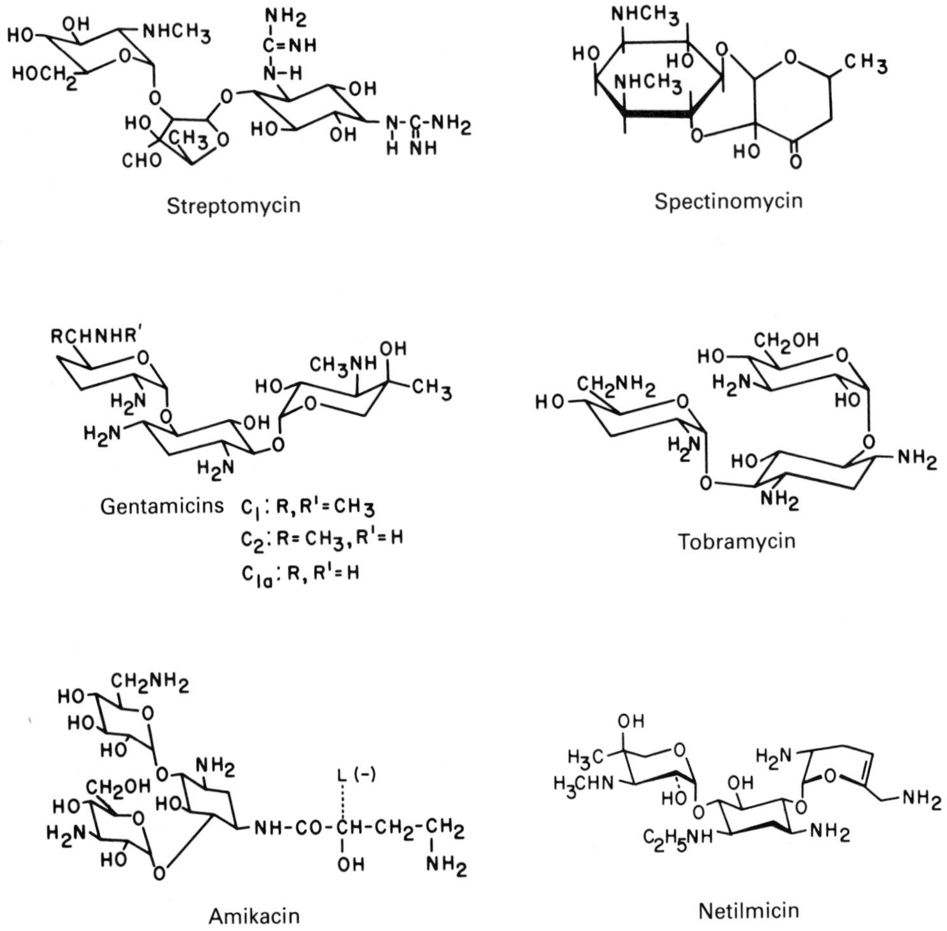

Streptomycin

Spectinomycin

Gentamicins C_1: R, R' = CH_3
C_2: R = CH_3, R' = H
C_{1a}: R, R' = H

Tobramycin

Amikacin

Netilmicin

dynamics: their potential for nephrotoxicity appears to decrease in the sequence as listed. Some clinical isolates that are resistant to one or two of these three drugs may be susceptible to the other(s), or to amikacin. Based on past experience, that of gradual development of resistance in the human-associated bacterial flora in hospitals—especially among the aerobic, gram-negative bacilli—there is a tendency to hold in reserve one of the newer aminocyclitols for use in situations of proved necessity.

Diaminopyrimidines

Apparently all forms of life depend on tetrahydrofolate (THF) for the synthesis of two-carbon fragments necessary to the formation of amino acids, pyrimidines, and purines for nucleic acid synthesis. Because the enzyme catalyzing the final reduction of dihydrofolate to THF differs in structure or configuration according to species of origin, it has been possible to synthesize a series of diaminopyrimidines that differ in their affinity for different dihydrofolate reductases (DHFRs). As is shown in Figure 18-8, 6-mercaptopurine has little selectivity, whereas trimethoprim is maximally active against bacterial DHFR, and pyrimethamine (and dihydrotriazine) against plasmodial DHFR. The other requirement for therapy, namely, a low affinity for DHFR of human origin, is met most successfully with the two diaminopyrimidines most often applied in antimicrobial therapy: trimethoprim and pyrimethamine (Fig. 18-9).

Trimethoprim virtually never causes clinically evident folate deficiency as it is used in therapy; however, it is excreted in the urine, and renal failure might result in accumulation to toxic concentrations. Suppression of the bone marrow by pyrimethamine is commonly observed when large doses are given or if therapy must be prolonged; again, renal failure increases the probability of toxicity unless the dose is reduced. Bone marrow function can be restored without loss of therapeutic efficacy by the administration of folinic acid, since bacteria and protozoa cannot utilize exogenous THF.

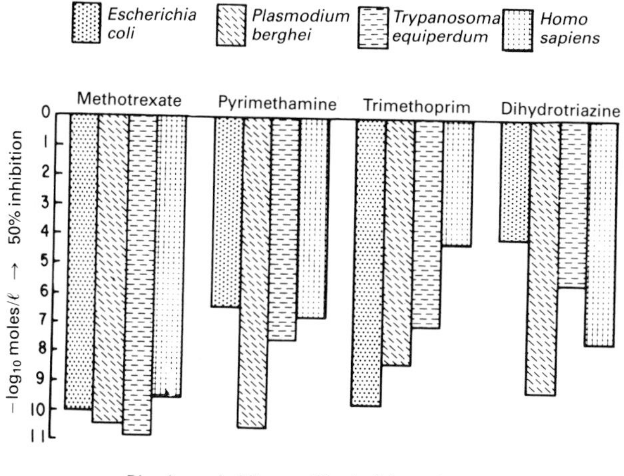

Fig. 18-8. Comparative affinities of four diaminopyrimidines for dihydrofolate reductases derived from three microorganisms and a human. (After Hitchings GH: Postgrad Med J 45 (Suppl): 7–10, 1969)

Neither trimethoprim nor pyrimethamine should be used as a single or sole agent in therapy because of (1) development of resistance (apparently through formation of DHFR isoenzymes), and (2) the potential for synergism in combination with a second, active drug. Both drugs are well absorbed from the gut and distribute generally in extravascular extracellular liquids; trimethoprim enters the CSF moderately well (Table 18-3).

Not only is trimethoprim active against many kinds of bacteria, but also its physicochemical characteristics facilitate collection in the prostatic fluid even without severe or acute inflammation. Moreover, it is active against *Pneumocystis carinii* and is currently the preferred agent (in combination with sulfamethoxazole) for the prevention and treatment of pneumocystosis (Chap. 45, Pneumocystosis).

Despite potential for toxicity, pyrimethamine is useful in the treatment of malaria (Chap. 145, Malaria) and toxoplasmosis (Chap. 129, Toxoplasmosis). It must always be used in combination with another effective antimicrobic—usually a sulfonamide.

Erythromycin–Clindamycin

Erythromycin (Fig. 18-10) has survived as the best of a group of macrolide congeners that included oleandomycin, carbomycin, and spiramycin. It is grouped with clindamycin (Fig. 18-11), a semisynthetic, nonmacrolide derived from lincomycin, because these drugs are used as alternatives to the penicillins. They also share the disadvantage of rapid, one-step, high-level development of resistance (not destructive of the drug) by *Staphylococcus aureus,* when used alone in therapy. Because group A β-hemolytic streptococci are sometimes resistant and gonococci are frequently resistant, erythromycin and clindamycin should not be relied on for treatment unless the infecting strain is proved susceptible by testing *in vitro.* Pneumococci are virtually always susceptible.

The antimicrobial activity of erythromycin extends beyond gram-positive cocci. It is the agent of choice for treatment of infections caused by *Legionella* spp. (Chap. 33, Legionnaires' Disease) and *Corynebacterium* spp., including *Corynebacterium diphtheriae* (Chap. 25, Diphtheria). When it is used as the sole therapeutic agent in treating corynebacterial infections, resistance has not developed during therapy. Also, on a mass or molar basis, erythromycin is particularly active as an inhibitor of *Listeria monocytogenes* (Chap. 51, Listeriosis). Erythromycin is truly a broad-spectrum antimicrobic, for it is clinically active against chlamydias (Chap. 55, Nongonococcal Urethritis, and Chap. 159, Trachoma) and *Mycoplasma pneumoniae* (Chap. 30, Nonbacterial Pneumonias). Because erythromycin base is poorly soluble in water, several derivatives have been prepared for therapy. Oral administration of a salt such as the stearate results in meager absorption—little changed from the free base. Esterification to yield the propionate or the ethylsuccinate makes for more efficient absorption from the gut. Either the lactobionate or the glucoheptonate salts are suitable for IV but not IM (pain, necrosis of tissue) injection. Marginally therapeutic concentrations may be attained in the

Fig. 18-9. Structural formulas of pyrimethamine and trimethoprim, two diaminopyrimidines useful in treatment of protozoal and bacterial infections.

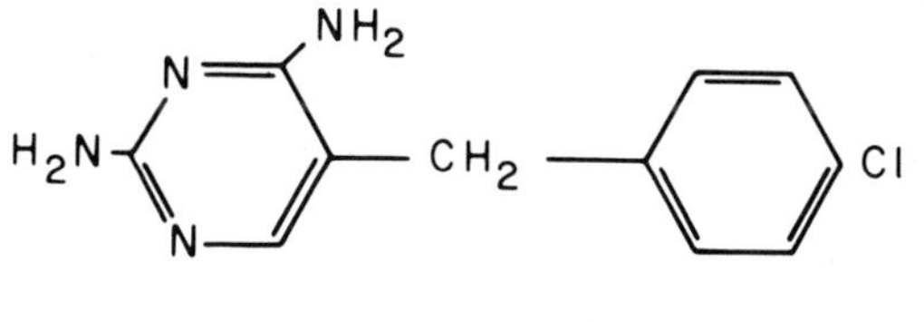

Pyrimethamine

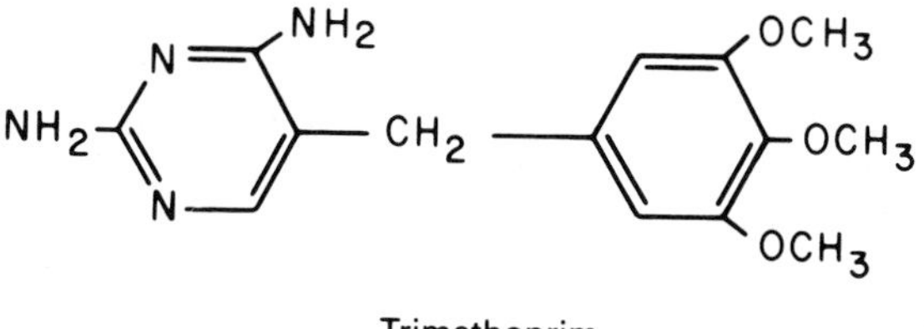

Trimethoprim

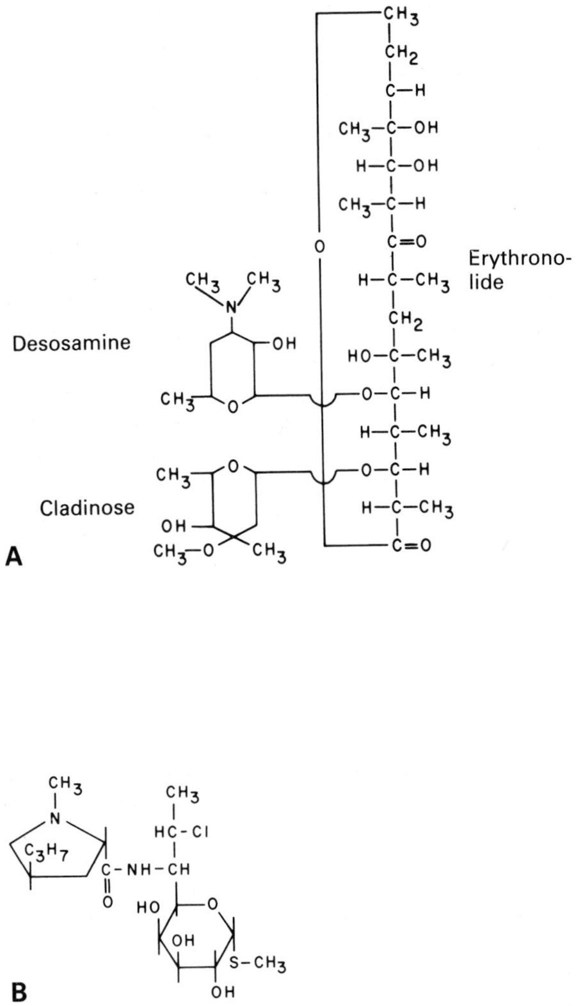

Fig. 18-10. Structural formulas of (*A*) the macrolide antimicrobic erythromycin and (*B*) the semisynthetic nonmacrolide clindamycin.

CSF when there is meningitis by IV injection of the drug. Catabolism is not extensive. As the primary route of excretion is the bile, there is no need to alter dosage because of renal failure. Increased frequency of defecation with passage of unformed feces is a common side-effect of peroral therapy. Hepatic dysfunction varying in severity from anorexia to jaundice with vomiting has been associated with ingestion, but not injection of the esterified forms.

Clindamycin (7-chloro-7-deoxylincomycin) has virtually replaced lincomycin because it is more active against bacteria, somewhat less likely to cause diarrhea, and better absorbed from the gut. Clindamycin, as the 2-phosphoric acid derivative, may also be given by IM or IV injection. There is little catabolism. Adjustment in dosage is not necessary when there is renal failure because hepatic excretion is the major egress for clindamycin. In the absence of meningitis, there is poor entry into the CSF. A special therapeutic niche was seemingly carved for clindamycin by the increased recognition of anaerobic bacteria as causes for infectious diseases. The drug is generally active against the nonsporulating, gram-negative anaerobic bacteria, notably *Bacteroides fragilis,* but is sometimes less than optimal against the anaerobic cocci and *Clostridium* spp. (see Table 32-4). Indeed, it is the resistance of toxinogenic *Clostridium difficile* to clindamycin that permits proliferation and elaboration of toxin(s) to cause enterocolitis. Clindamycin appears to have clinically useful activity against *Plasmodium* spp. and perhaps *Toxoplasma gondii.*

Imidazoles

BENZIMIDAZOLE

Two benzimidazole derivatives, thiabendazole and mebendazole, are clinically useful in treating enteric, nematodal infections (Chap. 68, Intestinal Nematodiasis). Both act to block energy generation but by different mechanisms: thiabendazole shuts off production of adenosine triphosphate (ATP) by blocking fumaric reductase; mebendazole prevents uptake of glucose. Although thiabendazole is absorbed, the adverse reactions associated with it (nausea, vomiting, and vertigo are common; skin rash, leukopenia, and hallucinations occasionally occur) are not life threatening because anaerobic glycolysis is not the primary energy-generating mechanism of humans (if the drug does, in fact, enter human cells). The lesser toxicity of mebendazole (occasional diarrhea and abdominal pain) may be related to poor absorption from the gut.

Mebendazole is preferable for treatment of the common enteric nematodal infections (trichuriasis, enterobiasis, ascariasis, hookworm) not only because of lesser toxicity and ease of treatment (uniform dose because of poor absorption), but also because it is highly active against *Trichuris trichiura* (whereas thiabendazole is not). With other intestinal nematodes, mebendazole is either the drug of first choice (hookworm), or at least as effective as thiabendazole or other drugs (enterobiasis and ascariasis).

Thiabendazole is preferred for the treatment of toxacariasis (Chap. 78, Visceral Larva Migrans), and it may be of some value in trichinosis (Chap. 150, Trichinosis), and possibly in echinococcosis. Infections caused by *Stronglyoides stercoralis* and *Capillaria phillipinensis* are also best treated with thiabendazole.

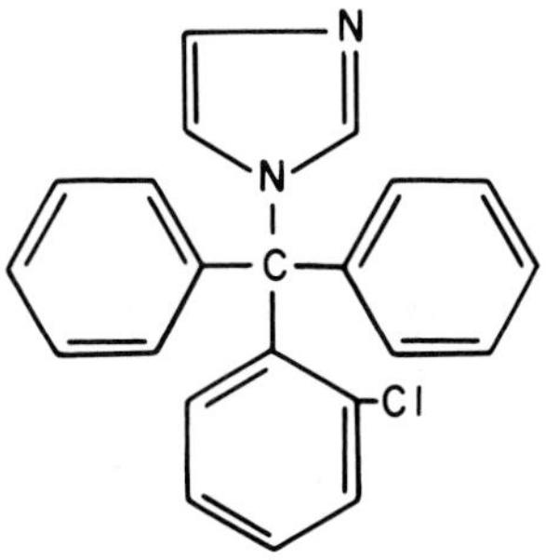

Fig. 18-11. Three phenethyimidazoles that have antifungal activity are in use in the United States. Only ketoconazole attains systemic distribution after peroral administration.

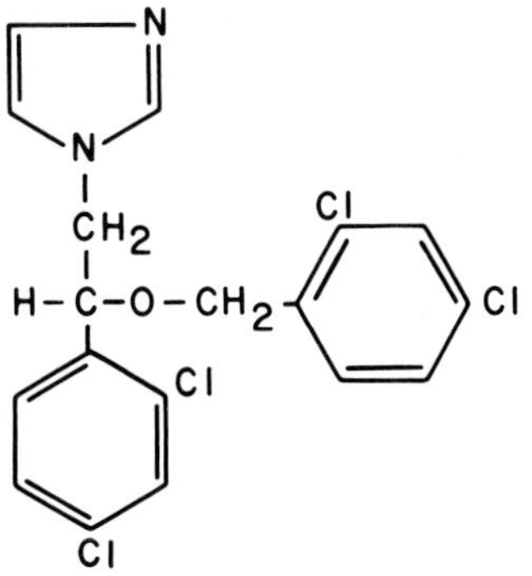

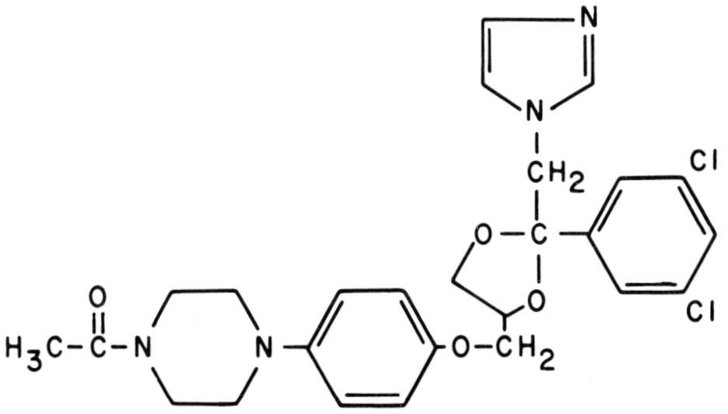

PHENETHYLIMIDAZOLE

Of the three phenethylimidazoles that are in use as antifungal agents in the United States (Fig. 18-11), clotrimazole and miconazole are virtually limited to topical application, as in treatment of candidal vaginitis (an application in which both are quite effective). Systemic use of miconazole by IV injection of a colloidal suspension has declined because of ineffectiveness, adverse reactions, and development of the perorally administrable ketoconazole.

Unlike predecessor antifungal imidazoles, ketoconazole is somewhat soluble in water, requiring normal gastric acidity for absorption after peroral administration. It is catabolized by the liver at a rate that is relatively constant,—that is, there is no induction of oxidative microsomes as occurs with clotrimazole. Neither the bile nor the urine contain antifungally active drug, but concentrations in the CSF after peroral administration may be 15% to 25% of the contemporaneous concentrations in the serum. Adverse reactions such as nausea and vomiting, lethargy, loss of libido, aspermia, and gynecomastia in males may be dose related. The nonenteric adverse effects may be related to suppression of synthesis of cortisol, as has been demonstrated in tissue culture systems, and of testosterone, as is implied by hypotestosteronemia in men under therapy. That is, the generally accepted mechanism of fungistasis by inhibition of conversion of lanosterol to ergosterol may, at appropriate concentrations, be paralleled in humans by interference with the endogenous synthesis of steroidal hormones. Other adverse reactions are infrequent: hypercholesterolemia, thrombocytopenia (which is reversible), and mild, usually transient, elevations of hepatic enzymes. However, severe toxic hepatitis has been reported, and may be lethal.

Ketoconazole appears to be the agent of choice for the treatment of chronic mucocutaneous candidosis (Chap. 39, Candidosis). It is effective in dermatomycoses, pityriasis versicolor, onychomycoses, paracoccidioidomycosis, and probably histoplasmosis. Usefulness in other systemic mycoses has not been proved by observation of sufficient numbers of patients for appropriate periods. Indeed, it is clear that long-term administration, possibly for life, will be necessary to sustain the spectacular successes achieved in chronic mucocutaneous candidosis. This points up the major therapeutic deficiency of ketoconazole, which is common to all of the antifungally active imidazoles thus far evaluated, namely, they are merely fungistatic at clinically practical concentrations (Fig. 18-12).

β-*Lactam Antimicrobics*

The β-lactam antimicrobics (penicillins, penems, carbapenems, monobactams, cephalosporins, oxycephams, and oxabetalactams) share many properties. They are among the least toxic of all therapeutic agents, having as their most serious drawback the occasional induction of hypersensitivity. The safety

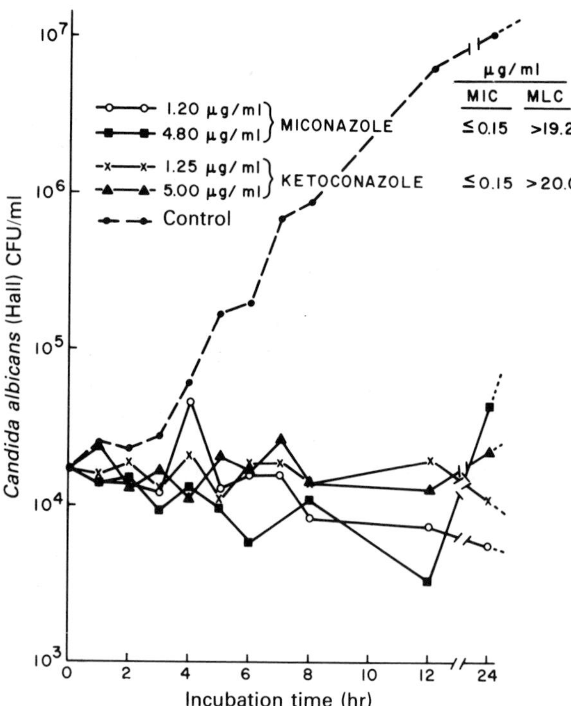

Fig. 18-12. Both miconazole and ketoconazole are fungistatic, effecting no decrease in viability of *Candida albicans.*

of these agents stems from their narrow—that is, solely antibacterial—activity. They affect enzymes concerned with the metabolism of the bacterial cell wall—sites that have no counterpart in eukaryotic cells. Different β-lactam antimicrobics produce different effects on a specific bacterial isolate; conversely, a particular β-lactam drug displays different effects on each of several different bacterial species. Inhibition of carboxypeptidases, endopeptidases, and particularly transpeptidases is undoubtedly important; failure of control or actual activation of autolysins is a feature of activity against some kinds of bacteria. The interactions are complex, and it is apparent that several mechanisms may lead to loss of viability or to lysis.

Essential to antibacterial activity is an intact β-lactam ring—a focus of structural fragility in these compounds. Prior to therapeutic use, physical degradation of the β-lactam ring can be minimized by storage at low temperature and neutral pH away from water and light, measures obviously inapplicable during and after administration to patients. However, the major threat to the β-lactam ring during therapy is enzymatic attack by β-lactamases elaborated by the infecting bacteria. Hydrolysis by β-lactamases results initially in penicilloic or cephalosporic acids from penicillins and cephalosporins, respectively; with most of the cephalosporins, there is virtually simultaneous expulsion of the substituent at C-3. Such destruction can be warded off by steric interference resulting from the introduction of bulky substituents at the 6-amino of the penicillins (*e.g.,* the napthamide of nafcillin) and the 7-α-methoxy substitution characteristic of the cephamycins. Clavulanate and sulbactam bind β-lactamases virtually irreversibly; possessed of only feeble antibacterial activity, their clinical usefulness arises from protection of β-lactamase-susceptibile compounds. In contrast, resistance to the β-lactamases is conferred on the penems, carbapenems, monobactams, and oxycephams by unique modifications such as substitution of carbon or oxygen for the sulfur in the ring fused to the β-lactam ring, or the fact that the free standing β-lactam ring is not strained. The result is diminished affinity for, or increased stability to, β-lactamases.

Beta-lactamases are elaborated only by bacteria. Moreover, it now appears that all bacteria are chromosomally constituted with β-lactamase capability. It may be expressed as copious production of β-lactamases loosed into the extracellular environment, as with some *Staphylococcus aureus* and certain *Bacillus* spp.; however, with some strains vigorous enzyme production may be inducible. With many gram-negative bacilli, β-lactamase activity may be barely detectable—only after bacteriolysis—that is, minimal elaboration of cell-membrane-bound enzyme. Thus, β-lactamases are detectable in bacteria that (1) have never been exposed to β-lactam antimicrobics and (2) remain susceptible to the β-lactam antimicrobics after decades of clinical use. It would appear, therefore, that chromosomally-mediated β-lactamases may have a normal function in the bacterial cell, perhaps in relation to cell wall metabolism.

Plasmids may encode β-lactamase synthesis, augmenting chromosomally determined production with β-lactamases that usually also differ qualitatively. Thus, β-lactamases vary in substrate preference—that is, they hydrolyze efficiently either penicillins or cephalosporins or utilize either kind of antimicrobic equally well. Other physicochemical differences are useful to characterizing β-lactamases: susceptibility to inhibition by cloxacillin and ρ-chloromercuirbenzoate (ρ-CMB), isoelectric focusing, antigenic specificity, molecular weight. From these several considerations, the classification of β-lactamases in the list on p. 221 was constructed.

There is another complexity. The advent of several

kinds of β-lactamase-resistant drugs has not resulted in antimicrobics that are active against all kinds of bacteria. This is curious because the very existence of a bacterial cell wall is testimony to peptidase activity—an activity obviously not blocked by the β-lactamase-resistant or β-lactamase-binding antimicrobics. Such resistance is apparently not mediated by β-lactamases and is often called intrinsic resistance; it appears to result from diminished binding of β-lactam antimicrobics by the proteins of the plasma membrane. Or, there could be diminished penetration of the drugs into the bacterial cells.

Tolerance of β-lactam antimicrobics is a different phenomenon. Inhibition of growth occurs at low concentrations; however, much higher concentrations are required to cause loss of viability. Again, β-lactamase activity does not appear to be implicated. It is possible that tolerance is achieved by the inaccessibility of β-lactam drugs to vital receptors. With some bacteria, there is failure of activation of autolysins (murien hydrolases).

A CLASSIFICATION OF β-LACTAMASES*

I. Enzymes active primarily against the cephalosporins, these are the usual chromosomally mediated β-lactamases of gram-negative bacteria (*Escherichia coli, Enterobacter* spp., *Citrobacter* spp., the indole-positive *Proteus* spp., *Serratia* spp., and *Pseudomonas* spp.). Enzyme production may be constitutive or inducible, and the relatively small quantities elaborated are cell membrane bound. They are inhibited by cloxacillin but not by ρ-chloromercuribenzoate.

II. Enzymes active primarily against the penicillins, these are the classic chromosomally mediated penicillinases. Often inducible, they are elaborated in large quantity and excreted into the environment by gram-positive bacteria (*e.g., Staphylococcus aureus, Bacillus licheniformis*). These enzymes are inhibited by cloxacillin, essentially inactive against all of the penicillinase-resistant penicillins and the cephalosporins, and unaffected by ρ-chloromercuribenzoate. Only a few strains of gram-negative bacteria have been shown to elaborate enzymes of this class.

III. Dual enzymes that are equally active against cephalosporins and penicillins, inhibited by cloxacillin but not by ρ-chloromercuribenzoate, these are the resistance-plasmid-mediated TEM β-lactamases. Augmentive of any background chromosomally mediated β-lactamases, the TEM enzymes are cell membrane bound and are produced in relatively small quantities; about 70% are of the TEM-1 variety and the remainder are TEM-2.

IV. Dual enzymes that are equally active against cephalosporins and penicillins, these chromosomally mediated, constitutive β-lactamases are not inhibited by cloxacillin (some actually hydrolyze cloxacillin) but are susceptible to ρ-chloromercuribenzoate. Typically, they are produced by *Klebisiella* spp., although rare strains of *Enterobacter cloacae* and *Escherichia coli* have been identified that are so endowed.

V. Enzymes that are primarily active against the penicillins, including cloxacillin and the other isoxazolyl penicillins, these heterogeneous, plasmid-mediated β-lactamases are also unaffected by ρ-chloromercuribenzoate. OXA-1, OXA-2, and OXA-3, the oxacillin hydrolyzing enzymes, and the *Pseudomonas*-specific enzymes (PSEs) are in this class.

*(After Richmond MH, Sykes RB: The β-lactamases of gram-negative bacteria and their possible physiological role. Adv Microbiol Physiol 9:31–88, 1973)

PENICILLINS (also referred to as *penams*). The 6-aminopenicillanic acid (6-APA) nucleus common to all penicillins arises from bicyclization of the dipeptide formed from *l*-valine and *l*-cysteine (Fig. 18-13). This condensation causes inversion of optical activity at C-3, a change that has been shown to be essential to antibacterial activity by the total synthesis of penicillin V. Since total synthesis of penicillins was commercially infeasible, and because modification of the molecule was practical only with regard to the substituent of the 6-amino grouping, the exploitation of biosynthesis of 6-APA on an industrial scale was essential to the production of penicillins not found in nature. Two methods were developed: harvesting 6-APA directly from fermentation beers (a special strain of *Penicillium chrysogenum* and special culture medium) and enzymatic (acylase) cleavage of a natural penicillin (*e.g.,* penicillin V). Seven penicillins of particular clinical interest are characterized by the structure of the substituent linked to the 6-amino in Figure 18-14. These penicillins are the fruits of intensive efforts seeking to satisfy three needs, namely, resistance to acid, resistance to β-lactamases, and alteration in antibacterial spectrum.

Resistance to Acid. Penicillin V (phenoxymethylpenicillin) is a natural penicillin much more resistant to degradation by acid than other natural penicillins.

Fig. 18-13. Biosynthetic origins of benzylpenicillin. (Hoeprich PD: Calif Med 109:301–303, 1968)

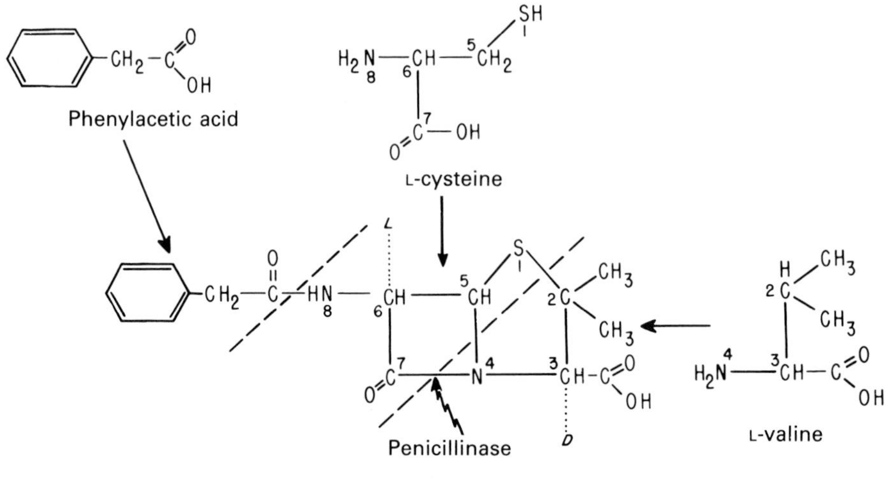

Phenylacetic acid

L-cysteine

L-valine

Penicillinase

Benzylpenicillin

The semisynthetic penicillins present a spectrum of resistance: (ampicillin = amoxicillin) ≫ (isoxazolyl penicillins [oxacillin, cloxacillin, dicloxacillin flucloxacillin] = nafcillin) ≫ (carbenicillin = ticarcillin and the acylureidopenicillins [piperacillin, mezlocillin, azlocillin]) ≫ methicillin. Because of lability with respect to acid, penicillin G, carbenicillin, ticarcillin, the acylureidopenicillins, and methicillin are unreliably, and generally poorly, absorbed after oral administration. Increasing the peroral dosage of these penicillins in no way alters their vulnerability to acid. Thus, the half-life of penicillin G at 37°C and pH 2.0 remains 3.5 minutes regardless of the number of units swallowed by the patient. The duration of exposure of a given dose to gastric acid is the critical determinant of survival to reach the alkaline safety of the duodenum where absorption takes place. This depends on the gastric emptying time—in turn a function of the amount and kind of food present in the stomach. Accepting as fact the vagaries of patients' compliance with instructions, it is reasonable to prescribe only acid-resistant penicillins for peroral therapy because they will be absorbed even in the presence of food. Yet, excellent resistance to acid does not ensure excellent absorption: oxacillin and nafcillin are erratically absorbed—for unknown reasons; ampicillin attains relatively low concentrations in the blood (Fig. 18-2—most likely because of enterohepatic cycling). Accordingly, for peroral therapy, the penicillins of choice are penicillin V; cloxacillin, dicloxacillin, or flucloxacillin; and amoxicillin.

Resistance to β-Lactamases. Penicillin G, penicillin V, ampicillin, amoxicillin, carbenicillin, ticarcillin, and the acylureidopenicillins are comparably susceptible to β-lactamases, whereas methicillin, the isoxazolyl penicillins, and nafcillin are resistant. There is one indication for the use of the penicillinase-resistant penicillins: infections caused by penicillinase-producing *Staphylococcus aureus.* If the infection is life-threatening, parenteral therapy, often with large doses, is necessary; nafcillin is the agent of choice for parenteral therapy. In virtually all respects, cloxacillin would be interchangeable with nafcillin if it were available in a form suitable for injection. Dicloxacillin is available for IM injection, a route of administration that is limiting when high-dosage therapy is necessary; for example, meningitis caused by *Staphylococcus aureus.* Flucloxacillin, also interchangeable with nafcillin, is not available for either parenteral or enteral use in the United States.

Oxacillin differs little from nafcillin in stability and activity against *Staphylococcus aureus.* However, oxacillin is less active against other gram-positive cocci—for example, *Streptococcus pneumoniae* and *Streptococcus pyogenes* (mistakes in diagnosis do occur)—and it is not as efficiently excreted by the liver. The latter characteristic of nafcillin may be a very important safety valve when high-dosage therapy must be used, as in patients with reduced renal function.

Methicillin was the first β-lactamase-resistant penicillin to come into clinical usage. However, it is now only of historical interest because it is the least stable, least potent, and most toxic of the penicillins. At pH 2.0 the half-life of methicillin is 2.3 minutes, whereas the other β-lactamase-resistant penicillins have half-lives of 160 minutes. The limitation of marked lability to acid requires prompt injection after the dry pow-

Generic Name (m.w.)*	Substituent at C-6	
	Chemical Name	Structure
Penicillin G (334.4 [372.5,K])	benzyl-	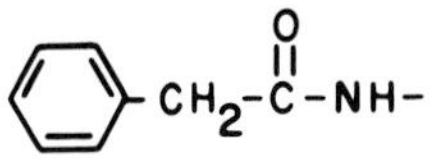 $C_6H_5-CH_2-C(=O)-NH-$
Penicillin V (350.4 [388.5,K])	phenoxymethyl	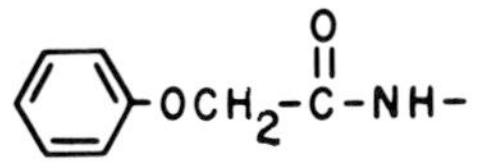 $C_6H_5-OCH_2-C(=O)-NH-$
Nafcillin (414.5 [436.5,Na])	6-(2-ethoxy-1)-napthamido-	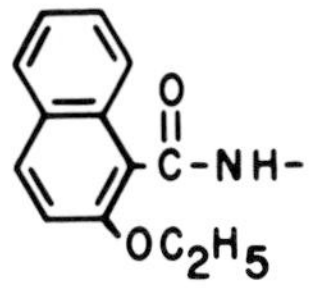 naphthyl ring with $-C(=O)-NH-$ and OC_2H_5
Dicloxacillin (470.3 [492.3,Na])	5-methyl-3-o-dichlorophenyl-4-isoxazolyl-	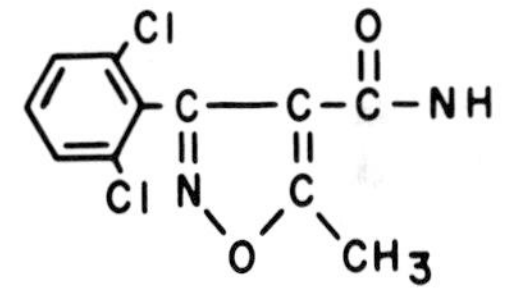 Cl, Cl-phenyl ring; C—C-C(=O)-NH; N, O, C, CH_3 (isoxazole ring)
Amoxicillin (365.4 [387.4,Na])	∝-amino-p-hydroxybenzyl-	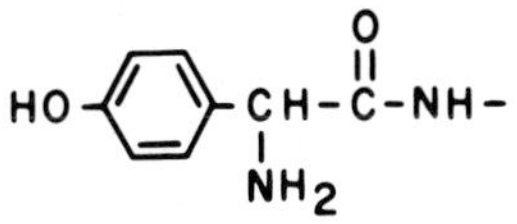 $HO-C_6H_4-CH(NH_2)-C(=O)-NH-$
Piperacillin (517.5 [539.5,Na])	3-dioxo-1-piperazinyl-carbonylamino-∝-phenylacetamido-	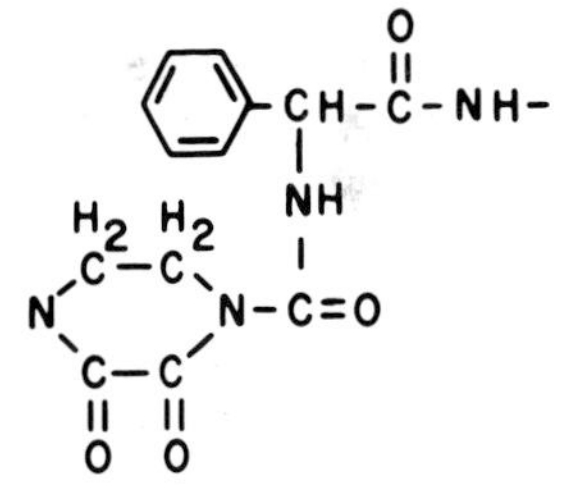 $C_6H_5-CH-C(=O)-NH-$; NH; N-C=O; ring: H_2C-CH_2, N, C(=O)-C(=O)
Mezlocillin (539.6 [561.6,Na])	3-methylsulfonyl-1-carbamoyl-carbonylamino-∝-phenylacetamido-	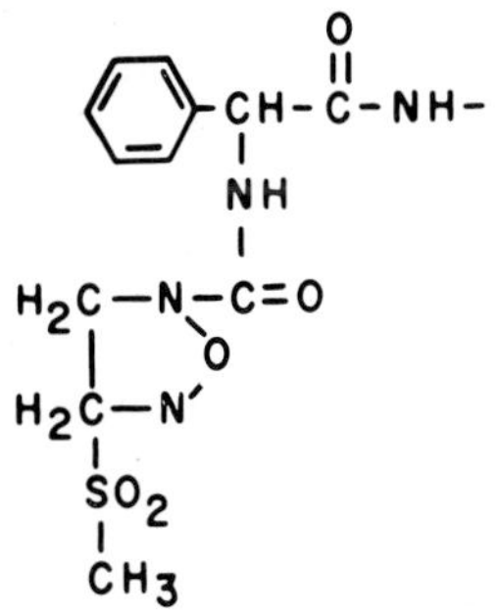 $C_6H_5-CH-C(=O)-NH-$; NH; $H_2C-N-C=O$, O, H_2C-N; SO_2; CH_3

*The first numbers = free acid; the second (in brackets) the salt.

Fig. 18-14. Seven penicillins of clinical interest and their characteristic substituents at C-6.

der is dissolved in one of the conventional, uniformly acidic solutions for injection. Because of low potency, at least twice as much methicillin is required for a therapeutic effect comparable to that exerted by any other β-lactamase-resistant penicillin—a requirement that may contribute to toxicity. The occurrence of direct toxicity to the CNS from penicillins depends in large part on a high gradient from the blood to the CNS; when the need for high dosage because of low potency is coupled with renal excretion as the sole exit for methicillin, the result is an unduly high probability of CNS toxicity. Possibly the same factors make for a frequency of occurrence of interstitial nephritis that is so striking in contrast with other penicillins that the term methicillin nephritis has come into use. The syndrome consists of hematuria with proteinuria, skin rash, and fever; mild to moderate renal insufficiency (although anuria has been reported); generally complete recovery after methicillin is withdrawn (although irreversible renal damage has been reported); and a characteristic histopathology (normal blood vessels and glomeruli, some tubular epithelial damage, prominent inflammation of the interstitium with granulocytes—many eosinophils—early, and mononuclear cells later). Toxic injury to the bone marrow manifested as agranulocytosis or aplasia has been reported almost exclusively with methicillin among the penicillins.

Only cloxacillin, dicloxacillin, and flucloxacillin, among the β-lactamase-resistant penicillins, are reliably absorbed from the gut. They may be used interchangeably.

Altered Antibacterial Spectrum. Ampicillin has significantly greater activity than penicillin G against *H. influenzae,* the enterococcal group of streptococci, *Salmonella typhi, Shigella* spp., and most strains of *E. coli* and *Proteus mirabilis.* Parenteral injection is necessary for reliable systemic therapy (Fig. 18-2) Diarrhea is common after peroral administration ($\geq$ 50% of patients when the daily dose is $\geq$ 2.0 g). Amoxacillin is identical with ampicillin in antibacterial effectiveness; because it is more efficiently absorbed from the gut, it is preferable to ampicillin when peroral therapy is sufficient.

Once unique among the penicillins in their antipseudomonal activity, carbenicillin and ticarcillin have been superceded by the acylureidopenicillins. Not only are the latter drugs at least as active against *Pseudomonas aeruginosa,* but also they carry less than one-half the load of sodium. Moreover, the acylureidopenicillins are more active against nonlactamase producing, pathogenic Enterobacteriaceae than are the other penicillins (comparable in this respect to the newer cephalosporins) and are at least as active against the enterococci as are ampicillin and amoxicillin (distinctly superior to the newer cephalosporins in this property). Penicillinase-producing *Staphylococcus aureus* is resistant to all of these penicillins.

Except in the CNS, the eyes, the upper respiratory tract, and the prostate, the penicillins enter all body liquids readily. Generally, mechanisms acting to exclude penicillins from these areas are less effective when there is inflammation, as in meningitis (this is not the case with prostatitis, however). Moreover, the penicillins are so well tolerated that sufficiently high concentrations can be safely attained in the blood to overcome the capacity for exclusion (again, except in the prostate).

Both glomerular filtration and tubular secretion are important to the renal excretion of the penicillins. The tubular secretory capacity can be diminished by the concurrent administration of probenecid. Penicillin G, penicillin V, and methicillin are excreted almost exclusively by the kidneys; when there is renal failure, or if the dose is excessive, these penicillins may attain toxic concentrations. Nafcillin, the isoxazolyl penicillins, ampicillin, amoxicillin, and the acylureidopenicillins are excreted sufficiently well by the liver to provide a safety valve against accumulation of these penicillins. Carbenicillin and ticarcillin are also excreted by the liver; in some patients, however, such large doses are necessary that hepatic excretion may also be inadequate in the face of hepatorenal failure.

If very high concentrations of penicillin G are attained in the blood (*e.g.,* $>$ 250 μg/ml of serum) sufficient penicillin may enter the CNS to cause intoxication. Muscular twitching, confusion, and grand mal seizures may result. The manifestations of toxicity disappear as the penicillin is eliminated. Hypersensitivity and the special problems of interstitial nephritis and bone marrow toxicity may also be related to very high concentrations of the penicillins.

β-LACTAMASE INHIBITORS

Two chemically different β-lactam compounds, which have intrinsically meager antibacterial activity, display such remarkably high affinity for β-lactamases that they protect β-lactamase-susceptible antimicrobics through irreversible binding of the enzymes. They are particularly active against penicillinases and penetrate bacterial cells to inactivate cell-bound enzyme. Potassium clavulanate and sulbactam (Fig. 18-15) are both absorbed from the gut and yield peak concentrations in the blood of 3 to 5 μg/ml. Clavulanate is more active than sulbactam and has

Generic Name (m.w.)*	Structure
Clavulanic Acid (199.2 [237.2,K])	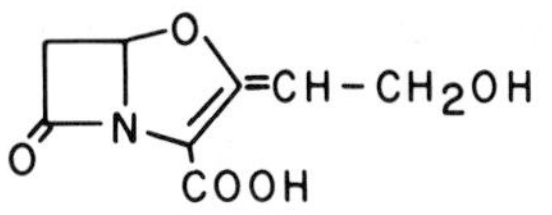
Sulbactam (347.4)	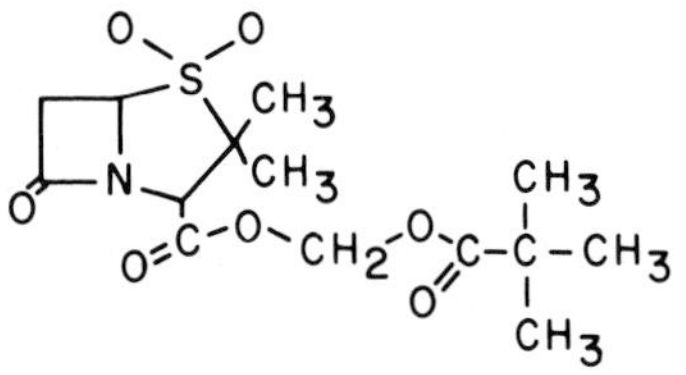
Sch 29482 (303.4 [347.3,di-Na])	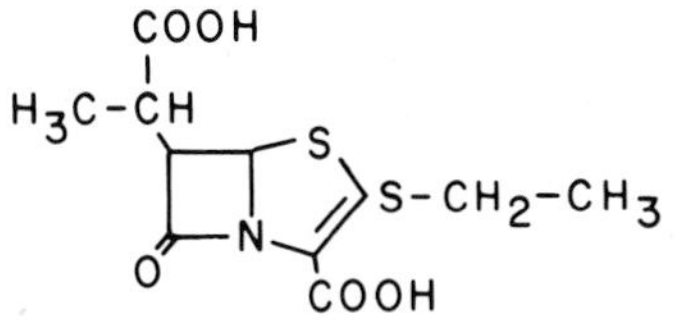
N-Formimidoyl-Thienamycin (299.4 [321.3, Na])	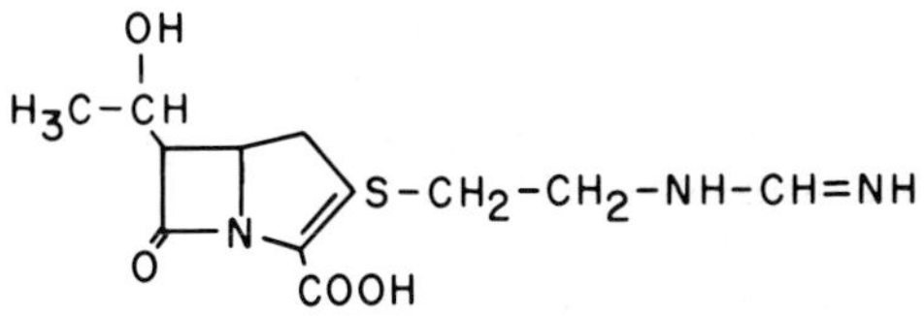
Azthreonam (435.4)	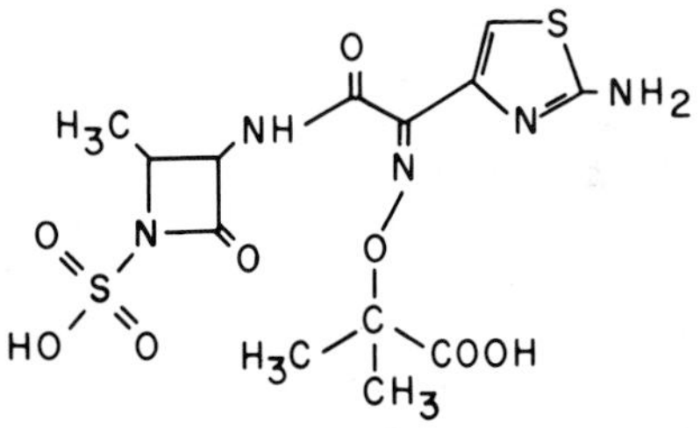

*The first number = free acid; the second (in brackets) the salt

Fig. 18-15. Structural formulas of some nonpenicillin, noncephalosporin β-lactam antimicrobics of clinical interest.

been used successfully in combination with amoxicillin in treating urinary tract infections caused by β-lactamase-producing bacteria. Additional studies may define other applications.

PENEMS

The penems (Sch 29482 in Fig. 18-15) are synthetic antimicrobics that differ chemically from the penicillins (penams) by (1) the presence of an unsaturated (double) bond between carbon atoms 2 and 3 of the five-membered thiazolidine ring of the penams (a change analogous to the unsaturation between carbon atoms 3 and 4 of the six-membered dihydrothiazine ring of the cephalosporins); and (2) lack of substituents at C-6 on the β-lactam ring. The penems are relatively lactamase-resistant, also binding tightly to some β-lactamases, and are active against many nonpseudomonal gram-negative bacilli, β-lactamase-producing gonococci, and gram-positive bacteria. They are stable molecules that are absorbed well from the gut, yielding peak concentrations in the blood of 20 to 30 μg/ml; they penetrate readily into special compartments such as the CSF and are rapidly excreted in the urine. The half-life in the blood after PO administration is 1 to 1.5 hours. Because only about 2% of the dose is present as antibacterially active drug in the urine, there appears to be brisk catabolism. The role of the penems in therapy remains to be defined.

CARBAPENEMS

Also analogues of the penicillins, the carbapenems also differ from the penems in having a carbon atom instead of a sulfur atom at the 1-position of the five-membered ring (Fig. 18-15). The thienamycins were the first carbapenems to be discovered. They are resistant to the β-lactamases and are active against many kinds of bacteria, including *Pseudomonas aeruginosa* and anaerobes. The initial problem of chemical instability was remedied by semisynthesis of the *N*-formimidoyl derivative. A second problem—rapid hydrolysis by human kidneys during excretion, reducing urinary recovery of the drug to 6% to 42% of the dose—appears to have been overcome by coadministration of an inhibitor of renal dehydropeptidase-1, which permits recovery of about 70% of the dose in the urine. *N*-Formimidoyl thienamycin must be given by parenteral injection; the peak concentration in the plasma is a function of the dose, for example, 16 and 35 μg/ml after IV injections of 250 mg and 500 mg doses, respectively. The half-life of *N*-formimidoyl thienamycin in the blood is about 1 hour; meningitis favors passage of it into the CSF. Clinical evaluations are in progress.

MONOBACTAMS

As the name implies, the monobactams do have the same four-membered β-lactam ring that is characteristic of the β-lactam antimicrobics. However, it is a β-lactam ring that stands alone—that is, it is not fused into a second five-membered ring (penicillins, penems, carbapenems) or six-membered ring (cephalosporins, oxycephams, oxabetalactams). Discovered as natural products of soil bacteria, the original monobactams had only modest activity; the evolution of the monobactams to potentially useful antimicrobics has proceeded by total chemical synthesis. Azthreonam is an α-oximino acyl derivative (Fig. 18-15) and is the first monobactam to come to clinical investigation. It is more stable to β-lactamases than the newer cephalosporins and is highly active against aerobic gram-negative bacteria, including the pathogenic genera of the Enterobacteriaceae, *Pseudomonas aeruginosa, H. influenzae,* and *N. gonorrhoeae.* Azthreonam is administered by parenteral injection of the arginine derivative. Peak concentrations in the blood reflect the dose: 20 to 150 μg/ml after 250 mg and 1000 mg, IV, respectively. The half-life in the blood is about 1.5 hours; dosage intervals of 6 hours are optimal if renal function is normal. About 60% to 80% of each dose of azthreonam is excreted in the urine by both glomerular filtration and tubular secretion. Entry into the CSF is facilitated by meningitis.

CEPHALOSPORINS, OXYCEPHAMS, AND OXABETALACTAMS

The 7-aminocephalosporanic acid nucleus common to the cephalosporins arises from bicyclization of the dipeptide formed from α, β-dehydro-γ-hydroxyvaline and L-cysteine (Fig. 18-16). Industrial production begins with cephalosporin C, a natural product with little antibacterial potency that is elaborated by *Cephalosporium acremonium.* Thus, the cephalosporins useful to therapy are semisynthetic antimicrobics derived through introduction of substituents at C-7 and at C-3. Over the years, there has been a chemical evolution that has resulted in compounds with desirable clinical properties properties in addition to remarkable antibacterial activity. The roster of the cephalosporinlike antimicrobics available for clinical use is long and seems always to be growing. Trimming the list to the 7 compounds depicted in Figure 18-17 may appear to be drastic but has rational bases.

The irritative capacity of cephalothin, cephapirin, and caphacetrile (severe pain on IM injection thrombophlibitis on IV injection); the susceptibility to catabolism by deacetylation of cephalothin, cephapirin, cephaloglycin, cephacetrile, and cefotaxime; and the potential for renal injury of cephaloridine and cephacetrile are undesirable properties. As a substitute for a penicillin in the treatment of infections caused by gram-positive cocci (except enterococci and "methicillin"-resistant *Staphylococcus aureus,* and any infection of the CNS), cefazolin is the cephalosporin of first choice because it is less irritating (IM injection is tolerated well), not catabolized, and not notably nephrotoxic. It is excreted primarily by the kidneys, therefore dosage should be reduced in patients with renal failure. If peroral treatment of the same infections is appropriate, cephalexin may be used; it is interchangeable with cephradine.

Resistance to degradation by β-lactamases was gained by cefoxitin, an oxycepham (cephamycin) drug, when a methoxy was added at C-7 (Fig. 18-16).

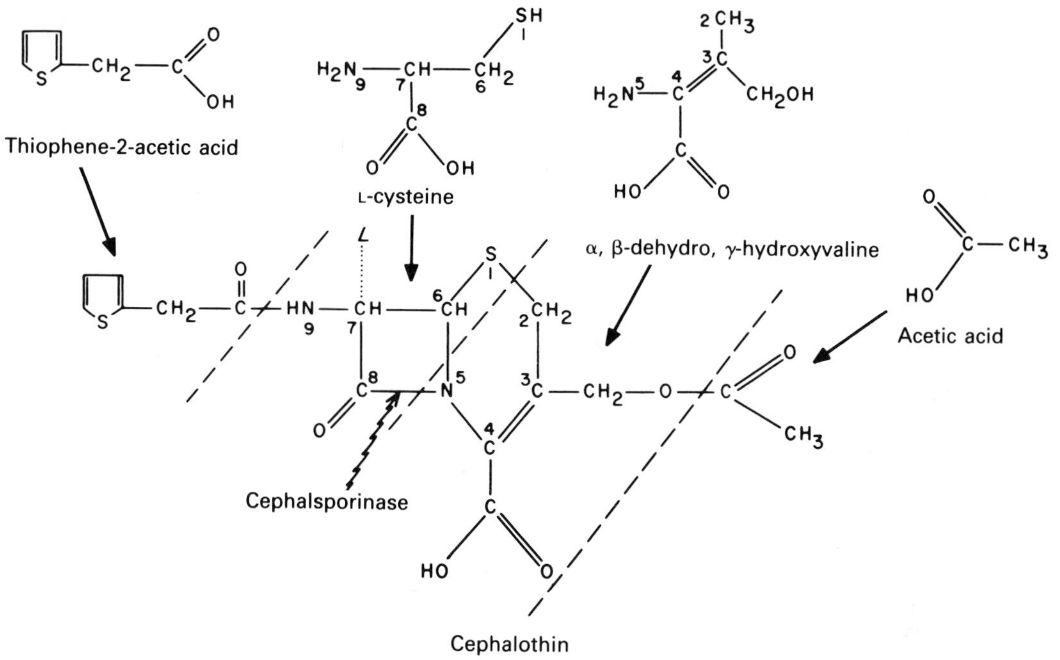

Fig. 18-16. Biosynthetic origins of 7-aminocephalosporanic acid (the two central panels) and the semisynthetic additions (the two external panels), which yield cephalothin.

There was also a gain in activity against enteric gram-negative bacilli, including the nonsporulating anaerobes, but with a concomitant decrease in potency against gram-positive cocci.

Moxalactam, an oxabetalactam, is also a variant of the cephalosporins (Fig. 18-16). Not only is there a methoxy at C-7 (as in cefoxitin), but also the sulfur of the six-membered ring is replaced by oxygen (*i.e.,* an oxazolidine ring is fused with the β-lactam ring instead of the usual thiazolidine ring). Furthermore, moxalactam is prepared by total chemical synthesis.

The theme of gain in activity against gram-negative bacilli with loss of activity against gram-positive cocci is repeated with the seven newer cephalosporins (and moxalactam), which are grouped according to the chemical structure of substituents in Table 18-4. These drugs are quite similar in possessing remarkable activity against most of the pathogenic Enterobacteriaceae, apparently useful activity against *Pseudomonas aeruginosa,* marked susceptibility to degradation by digestive enzymes (*i.e.,* they must be given by IM or IV injection), and high cost. Again, however, none appears to have potential usefulness against enterococci, and only one, moxalactam, has been shown to enter the CNS well enough to cure meningitis caused by enteric gram-negative bacilli.

Moxalactam has a half-life in the blood 2 to 2.5 hours; that is, injection every 8 or 12 hours is adequate. About 90% is excreted in the urine. Each gram carries along 3.5 mEq of sodium. Adverse effects include disulfiramlike reactions if ethanol is taken during therapy and hypoprothrombinemia, which is curable or preventable by injection vitamin K.

Cefoperazone (the half-life in the blood and dosage intervals are the same as those for moxalactam) is preferentially excreted by the liver—about 80% in the bile and 20% in the urine. The sodium load of each gram is 1.5 mEq. In addition to the adverse effects seen with moxalactam, cefoperazone has been associated with enterocolitis—possibly a consequence of the high biliary excretion.

Among the aminothiazyl cephalosporins, there is no basis for choice in antibacterial activity. In part because cefotaxime is catabolized (deacetylated), its half-life of 1 hour in the blood is the shortest of the newer cephalosporins; that is, dosage intervals of 6 hours, as are optimal for cefazolin and ceftizoxime, would appear to be necessary. Ceftriaxone, with a half-life of 8 to 9 hours in the blood, need be injected no more often than 12-hourly, partially offsetting the cost; moreover single-dose application appears to be sufficient for acute gonorrhea caused by penicillinase-producing *N. gonorrhoeae* and may be adequate in the chemoprophylaxis of postsurgical infections.

Generic Name (m.w.)*	Substituent at C-7		Substituent at C-3	
	Chemical Name	Structure	Chemical Name	Structure
Cefazolin (454.5 [476.5,Na])	2-(1H-tetrazol-1yl)acetamido-	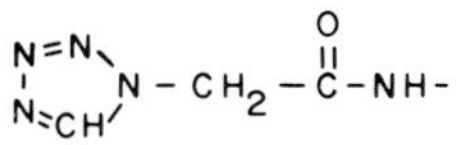 N=N, N=CH (tetrazole) N – CH_2 – C(=O) – NH–	(5-methyl-1,3,4-thiadiazol-2-yl) thiomethyl	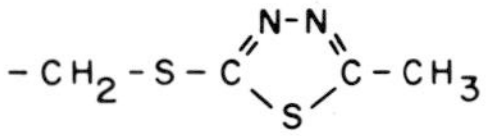 – CH_2 – S – C(N-N, S)C – CH_3
Cephalexin** (347.4 [365.4,Hy])	*D*-2-amino-2-phenyl-acetamido-	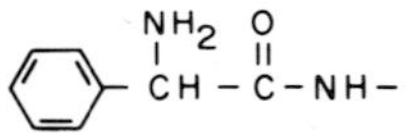 (phenyl)– CH(NH_2) – C(=O) – NH–	Methyl	– CH_3
Cefoxitin (427.5 [449.4,Na])	7-methoxy 2-(2-thienyl)acetamido-	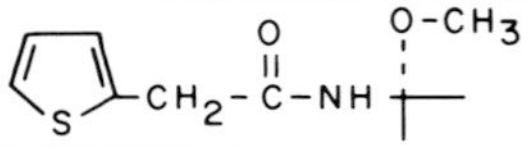 (thienyl)– CH_2 – C(=O) – NH – (O – CH_3)	Methylene carbamate ester	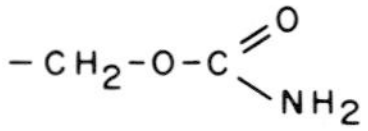 – CH_2 – O – C(=O) – NH_2
Moxalactam (518.5 [564.5,di-Na])	(carboxy [4-hydroxyphenyl] acetyl) amino-7-methoxy	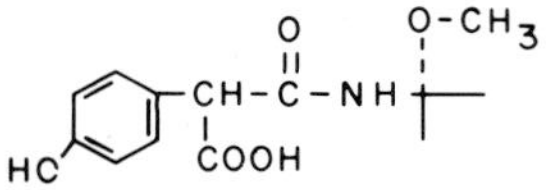 HO(phenyl)– CH(COOH) – C(=O) – NH – (O – CH_3)	(1-methyl-1H-tetrazol-5-yl) thiomethyl	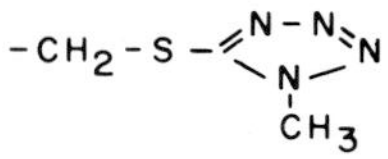 – CH_2 – S – (N – N = N, N – CH_3 tetrazole)
Cefoperazone (645.7 [667.7,Na])	α-(4-ethyl-2,3-dioxo-1-piperazinecarboxamido)-α-(4-hydroxyphenyl) acetamido-	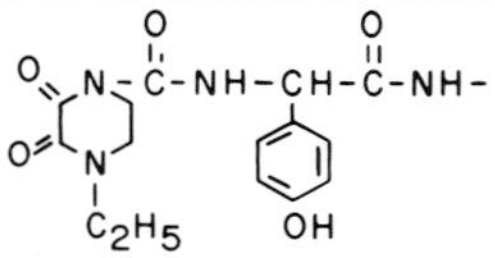 (2,3-dioxo-4-C_2H_5-piperazinyl)N – C(=O) – NH – CH(phenyl-OH) – C(=O) – NH–	(1-methyl-1H-tetrazol-5-yl) thiomethyl	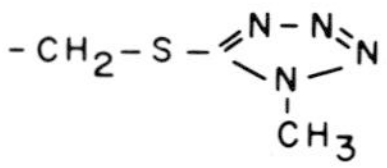 – CH_2 – S – (N – N = N, N – CH_3 tetrazole)
Ceftriaxone (552.5 [598.5,di-Na])	2-(2-amino-4-thiazolyl)-2-(methoxyimino)acetamido-	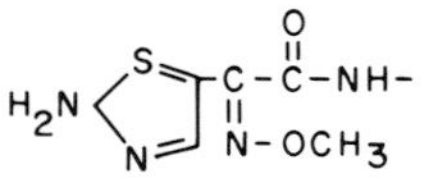 H_2N(thiazolyl: S, N)– C(=N – OCH_3) – C(=O) – NH–	(2,5-dihydro-6-hydroxy-2-methyl-5-oxo-as-triazin-3-yl)thio	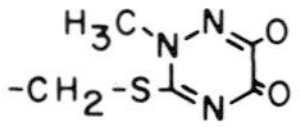 – CH_2 – S – (triazine ring: H_3C–N, N, O, O)
Cefsulodin (533.6 [554.5,Na])	β-(D-α-sulphophenyl-acetamido)-	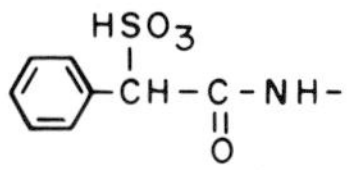 (phenyl)– CH(HSO_3) – C(=O) – NH–	Methylpyridinium amide	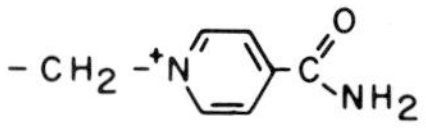 – CH_2 – ^{+}N(pyridinium)– C(=O) – NH_2

* The first figure-free acid; the second (in brackets) the sodium salt: Na or di-Na; or hydrate: Hy

** Zwitterionic

Fig. 18-17. Seven "cephalosporins" of clinical interest and their characteristic substituents at C-7 and C-3.

Table 18-4. *Grouping of nine Newer "Cephalosporins" by Chemical Structure*

Substituent at C-7	Substituent at C-3
Aminothiazyl	***Thiomethyltetrazol****
Cefotaxime	Moxalactam†
Ceftizoxime	Cefoperazone
Ceftazidime	***Methylpyridinium‡***
Ceftriaxone	Ceforanide
Cefmenoxime	Cefosulodin§

* Present also in cefazolin and cefamandole.

† Differing from the true cephalosporins in having an oxygen atom instead of a sulfur atom at position 1 in the 6-membered ring of the nucleus and a methoxy at C-7 (as in cefoxitin); moxalaction is produced by total chemical synthesis.

‡ Present also in cephaloridine.

§ Has in addition an amide substituent to the pyridine ring at C-4.

Each gram of ceftriaxone provides 3.3 mEq of sodium. Excretion is about evenly split between the bile and the urine.

Cefsulodin may offer an advantage in being less broadly antibacterial than the other new cephalosporins and more focused on *Pseudomonas aeruginosa.* With a half-life in the blood of 1.5 hours, injection every 6 hours appears to be appropriate. The obligatory sodium load is 3.0 mEq/g. Excretion is almost exclusively in the urine.

Polyenes

Elaboration of polyenes by soil-dwelling actinomycetes is quite common. However, only three polyenes are currently of clinical interest: nystatin, candicidin, and amphotericin B. Nystatin and candicidin are restricted to local use, as in irrigation, or to peroral administration because of potential for systemic toxicity. Amphotericin B has been used in the treatment of systemic fungal infections since 1957, and is one of the most toxic antimicrobics currently employed.

The biologic activity of the polyenes depends primarily on interaction with sterols. Thus, all life forms whose cell membranes are toughened or stabilized with sterols are, at least hypothetically, susceptible to the polyenes. In general, these are the eukaryotic cells. There is variation in the affinity of particular sterols for particular polyenes; that is, amphotericin B has a high affinity for ergosterol (the principal sterol of fungi), whereas candicidin interacts most strongly with cholesterol (the stabilizing sterol of mammalian cell membranes). A secondary site of action of the polyenes is the phospholipids of cell membranes.

Within minutes after exposure to a polyene, disorganization of the cell membrane is manifested by leakage of K^+ from the cell. As injury progresses, Mg^{++} escapes also, followed in turn by amino acids; protein synthesis stops and the cell dies.

Amphotericin B is of particular interest as the mainstay of the medical treatment of systemic fungal infections. As are other polyenes, amphotericin B is a macrolide antimicrobic (Fig. 18-18). It is elaborated by selected strains of *Streptomyces nodosus* grown under special conditions. The large ring, known also as the chromophore, consists of a rigid hydrophobic portion (because there are seven sequential unsaturated carbon–carbon bonds, amphotericin B is a heptaene) and a flexible hydrophilic portion (alcoholic–OHs). Of the two ionizable moieties, one is a carboxyl at C-16, near the hydrophobic–hydrophilic juncture of the ring, and the other is a primary amine that is a substituent of mycosamine, the characteristic six-carbon aminosugar glycosidically linked to the

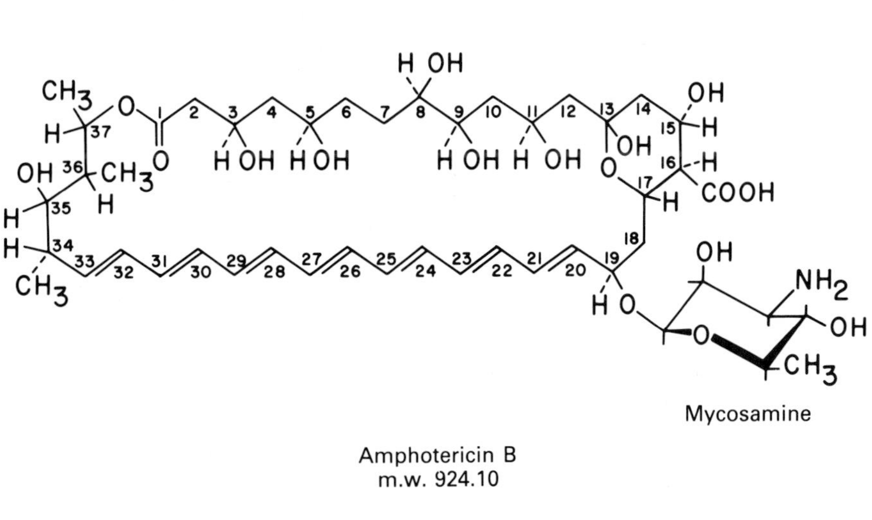

Mycosamine

Amphotericin B
m.w. 924.10

Fig. 18-18. Structural formula of amphotericin B, a heptaenic polyene antifungal antimicrobic applied in systemic therapy.

ring at C-19. The compound is aptly named for it is amphoteric, and is virtually insoluble in water at physiologic pH. The drug is used in therapy as an aqueous suspension that is stabilized with sodium deoxycholate. It is light sensitive and oxygen labile; it deteriorates rapidly in culture mediums, less rapidly in serum, still less rapidly in 0.9% NaCl or 5% glucose solutions and is stable for 1 week at 37°C in distilled water. There is no proof of catabolism in human or nonhuman mammalians.

For systemic therapy, an aqueous suspension of amphotericin B in 5% glucose solution must be injected IV or intrathecally: details of administration are given in Chap. 39, Candidosis, and Chap. 41, Coccidioidomycosis. There is virtually no penetration into the CSF and meager entry into the urine. The drug is excreted primarily in the bile, but at a slow rate—half-lifes of 17 hours in the serum and 275 hours in the whole body in rhesus monkeys.

The reversible adverse reactions engendered by amphotericin B include nausea, vomiting, abdominal pain, chills, fever, anorexia, thrombophlebitis, hypokalemia and hypomagnesemia, and rarely, neurotoxicity and hypotension. Irreversible nephrotoxicity is common and is the toxic reaction most feared. Bone marrow depression is a rare, but serious, consequence of treatment with amphotericin B. Subarachnoid injection of amphotericin B often causes arachnoiditis and radiculitis; diminished hearing may also result.

Sulfonamides

The ultimate combination of effectiveness and safety appeared to have been achieved in sulfadiazine. However, as additional sulfonamides were synthesized, special properties accrued that have in some instances proved to be desirable. All of the sulfonamides are quite stable compounds. Those that are absorbed are inactivated to a greater or lesser extent through obliteration of the ρ-amino group by hepatic conjugation with either acetate or glucuronate. Generally, the conjugate is preferentially excreted by the kidneys, although it may or may not be more soluble in the urine than the parent compound.

All of the sulfonamides inhibit competitively the synthesis of dihydropteroate (Fig. 18-22). Therefore, all of the sulfonamides are potentially capable of synergy with the 2,4-diaminopyrimidines. Thus, malaria and pneumocystosis have been treated successfully with sulfadiazine in combination with pyrimethamine. Sulfamethoxazole is generally paired with trimethoprime as a manufacturer's choice.

Native resistance to the sulfonamides appears to be the result of an isoenzymic dihydropteroate synthetase elaborated by the resistant bacteria. The isoenzyme has higher affinity for ρ-aminobenzoic acid than for the sulfonamides.

Adverse reactions are not uncommon with the sulfonamides. Hypersentivity; hepatotoxicity; bone marrow depression, especially of the granulocyte series; hemolytic anemia; thyroiditis; and confusion may occur. All are reduced in frequency of occurrence with the modern derivatives.

SYSTEMIC SULFONAMIDES

The six sulfonamides listed by chemical structure in Figure 18-19 may not include the ideal sulfonamide, but they do have properties ensuring current use. They are available in table form or as suspensions for peroral therapy. As sodium salts, several of the sulfonamides may be given by IM or IV injection.

All of the systemically administrable sulfonamides distribute widely in body water entering the aqueous humor, CSF, upper respiratory tract secretions, and, with derivatives having a basic pK, the prostrate. The concentrations attained in the blood are usually higher than in the extravascular fluids. Excretion is primarily in the urine. Of the drugs listed, sulfisoxazole is most rapidly excreted; indeed, it is relatively

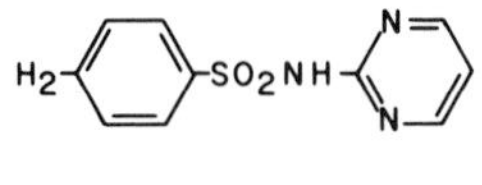

Sulfadiazine
m.w. 250.3

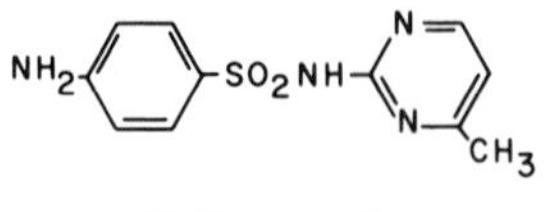

Sulfamerazine
m.w. 264.3

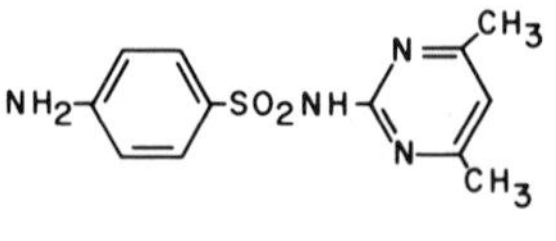

Sulfamethazine
m.w. 278.3

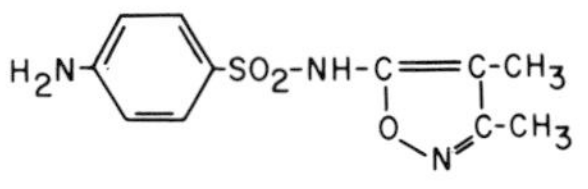

Sulfisoxazole
m.w. 267.3

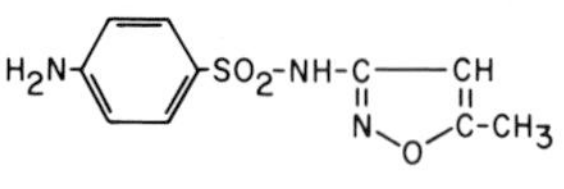

Sulfamethoxazole
m.w. 253.3

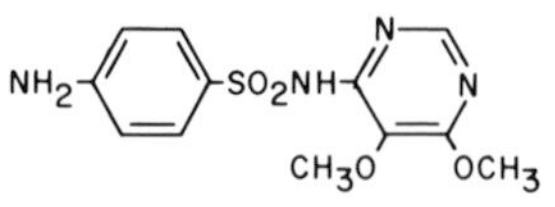

Sulfadoxine
m.w. 310.3

Fig. 18-19. Structural formulas of six sulfonamides. The three sulfapyrimidines in the top row are often prescribed as an equipart mixture.

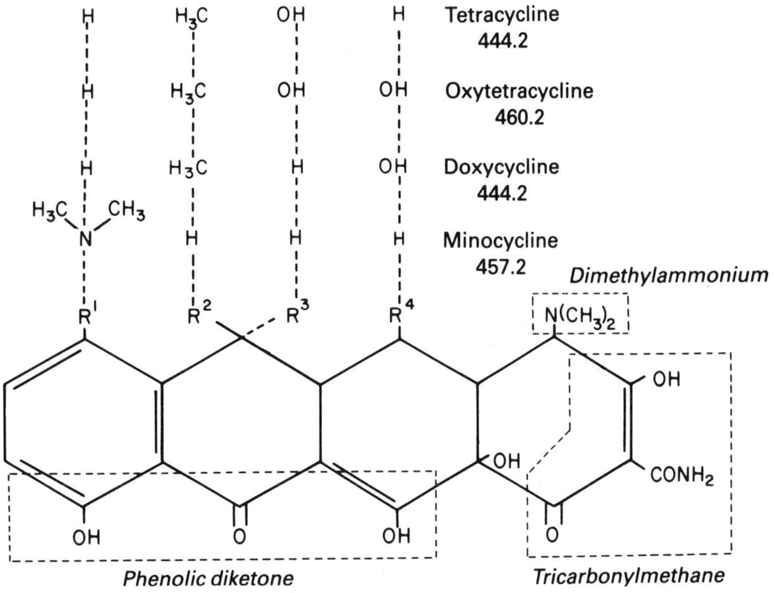

Fig. 18-20. Chemical variations of the tetracycline structure are possible at four sites with preservation of antimicrobial activity. Among these four congeners, lipophilicity is least with oxytetracycline and greatest with minocycline.

difficult to obtain therapeutic concentrations of this sulfonamide outside the urinary tract. The sulfapyrimidines are conveniently prescribed as triple sulfonamides (equal parts of sulfadiazine, sulfamerazine, and sulfamethazine). They, and sulfamethoxazole, are less rapidly excreted and 6-hourly dosage results in maintenance of therapeutic concentrations in the blood (10–15 mg/100 ml). Because the solubility of each component in the urine is independent of the others, the possibility of precipitation in the renal tubules is greatly reduced with the triple drug mixture.

Derivatives that persist in the blood and body fluids for long periods after absorption hold out the promise of convenience in dosages administered once a day (*e.g.*, sulfamethoxypyridazine) or once a week (*e.g.*, sulfadoxine). Unfortunately, adverse reactions may be more commonly engendered with such sulfonamides.

LOCAL SULFONAMIDES

Poorly absorbed sulfonamides are used to depress the microflora of the large bowel before surgery. There is little to choose between succinylsulfathiazole and phthalylsulfathiazole. Salicylazosulfapyridine has proved of value in the management of ulcerative colitis.

Mafenide has been used extensively with good effect in the form of a 10% cream for prophylaxis of burn wound infections. Disadvantages such as pain and acidosis may be circumvented by the substitution of silver sulfadiazine (Chap. 157, Infections Following Burns).

For use in the eye, collyria containing sulfacetamide and sulfisoxazole are equally useful.

Sulfathiazole and triple sulfonamides, as creams or tablets, are sometimes effective in treating vaginitis.

Tetracyclines

That variations were possible in the chemical structure of tetracycline with retention of antimicrobial activity was evident as soon as the structures of the first three congeners that were discovered (chlortetracycline, oxytetracycline, and tetracycline) were deciphered. Chemical changes were permissable at only four sites, labeled R^1 to R^4 in Figure 18-20. It was clear that the three microzones of ionization of the fermentation products were crucial to biologic activity—they could neither be altered chemically nor disturbed in physicochemical attributes without loss of activity. From this it follows that (1) the mechanism(s) of action and the spectrum of activity are virtually identical for all congeners and (2) variation in nonantimicrobic properties distinguishes the congeners. Four congeners, two from nature (oxytetracycline and tetracycline) and two semisynthetic (minocycline and doxycycline) offer a range in properties of possible clinical importance. As is evident from the structural formulas (Fig. 18-20), minocycline is the least polar and most lipophilic, whereas oxytetracycline is the most polar and least lipophilic.

With the exception of chlortetracycline, the tetracyclines are reasonably stable compounds, although decomposition—even in the dry powder form—occurs to a significant degree over the period of a year. Catabolism in humans is minor. About one-third to one-half of perorally administered oxytetracycline and tetracycline is absorbed, whereas absorption of both minocycline and doxycycline appears to be complete. Accordingly, parenteral dosage is identical to peroral dosage for minocycline and doxycline but should be reduced by about one-half if either oxytetracycline or tetracycline is injected.

Inhibition of protein synthesis by preventing the addition of amino acids is agreed on as the way in which the tetracyclines inhibit bacterial growth. Apparently, the tetracyclines attach to 30S ribosomal subunits and block the function of tRNA to mRNA. Perhaps nonbacterial microorganisms are affected in the same way as bacteria, although the avid chelating capability of the tetracyclines for divalent cations is also important.

Destruction or modification of the tetracyclines by resistant microorganisms has not been reported. Both gram-positive and gram-negative bacteria may be resistant.

Oxytetracycline is cleared most efficiently in the urine, and urinary excretion is also critical to the elimination of tetracycline and minocycline; these three drugs accumulate if renal dysfunction is not compensated by reduction in dosage. Doxycycline, on the other hand, does not depend on renal excretion for elimination and can be given in normal dosage to patients who are anephric. Although there is biliary excretion of the tetracyclines, reabsorption from the gut apparently does occur.

Oxytetracycline and tetracycline scarcely enter the CSF, the eye, or upper respiratory tract secretions. Doxycycline enters these liquids to a greater extent but still poorly, whereas minocycline penetrates relatively well. All of the tetracyclines appear to enter sebum and keratinizing cells, although excretion in perspiration may be more important to delivery of drug in the treatment of acne.

Because they are strong ligands for divalent cations, the tetracyclines are incorporated in calcifying tissues. If the permanant teeth are involved, the lesion is unsightly. More important is inhibition of formation of osteoid, for this leads to arrested bone growth and faulty dentition. Accordingly, tetracyclines should not be given to pregnant women or to children who are forming teeth and bones (the small doses prescribed for adolescent acne (*e.g.,* tetracycline, 250 mg/day) do not pose a hazard to calcifying tissues).

Acute hepatic necrosis has been precipitated by tetracyclines, a complication seen most often in women recently delivered and in shock. Decomposed tetracyclines, as might be encountered in outdated material, may poison renal function, causing glucosuria, amino aciduria, and loss of electrolytes. Hypersentivity to the tetracyclines is rare.

Except for urinary tract infections, doxycycline is the congener of choice for general use. It is easy to administer, relatively free of adverse effects such as gastrointestinal disturbances and candidal vaginitis, and is safe to use in patients with renal failure. Moreover, doxycyline has been shown to be of prophylactic value for traveler's diarrhea.

Oxytetracycline is preferable for treatment of urinary tract infections because of its high urinary clearance and stability.

Minocycline, because of superior entry into upper respiratory tract secretions, appears to have a special place in the chemoprophylaxis of meningococcal infections. Unfortunately, the frequent occurrence of headache and dizziness appears to have limited this application.

Vancomycin

Rendered obsolescent in the 1960s by the introduction of the penicillinase-resistant penicillins and the cephalosporins, vancomycin has had a renaissance principally because of the burgeoning importance of methicillin-resistant staphylococci and anaerobic bacteria as causes for disease. Vancomycin is a large glycopeptide (m.w. about 3300) of undeciphered structure that is lethal to susceptible, multiplying bacteria, principally through inhibition of cell wall synthesis by specific binding to the D-alanyl-D-alaine group on the side chain of certain cytoplasmic membrane-bound intermediates in peptidoglycan synthesis. Other mechanisms of action, as yet undefined, are implied by the lethal effect of vancomycin on protoplasts.

After IV injection, the half-life of vancomycin in the blood of patients with normal renal function is about 6 hours; thus, the administration of 30 mg/kg body wt/day, IV, as 2 or 3 equal portions, 12- or 8-hourly, yields concentrations around 10 ug/ml predose and 40 ug/ml postdose. There is virtually no catabolism and little biliary excretion; reduction of dosage in patients with renal failure is essential and is best guided by measurements of the concentrations in the blood.

Because it is irritating to the tissues at high concentrations, vancomycin should not be given by IM injection, and it causes thrombophlebitis on IV injection. Although it enters serous fluids, it does not normally penetrate into the CSF; with meningitis, entry into the CSF is facilitated but may not be adequate or reliable enough for treatment of meningitis. Absorption from the gut after peroral administration is meager, and the drug remains active even in the feces.

Vancomycin is bactericidal against *Staphylococcus aureus,* many coagulase-negative *Staphylococcus* spp., aerobic *Streptococcus* spp. (except enterococci), *Peptococcus* spp., *Peptostreptococcus* spp., nondiphtherial *Corynebacterium* spp., and *Clostridium* spp. (including *C. difficile*). The $Arg^{-}Hxy^{-}Ura^{-}$ strains of *N. gonorrhoeae* that typically cause gonococcemia are so susceptible to vancomycin that they are inhibited from growth on Thayer–Martin medium.

Treatment with vancomycin is indicated for infections caused by bacteria that are susceptible to it when the bacteria are resistant to the β-lactam antimicrobics and when patients cannot be treated with the preferred agents because of hypersensitivity. For enterococcal endocarditis, an aminocyclitol must always be given with vancomycin, a combination that may also be necessary for the successful treatment of corynebacterial (nondiphtheritic) endocarditis. It has been recommended for chemoprophylaxis of bacterial endocarditis in vulnerable patients who must undergo procedures likely to cause bacteremia with upper respiratory tract organisms and are allergic to the penicillins. Vancomycin is the preferred treatment for ileocolitis from *Staphylococcu aureus* and pseudomembranous colitis caused by *C. difficile* (0.5 g, PO, 6-hourly, for 3–5 days).

Although vancomycin frequently causes thrombophlebitis on IV injection and causes skin rashes in about 5% of patients, auditory toxicity is the major adverse effect. If the dose is adjusted to maintain the proper concentrations in the blood, the probability of nephrotoxicity is about that of netilmicin. Because auditory and renal toxic effects from vancomycin are additive to the same toxic effects of the aminocyclitols, combined therapy poses an increased hazard.

Combinations of Antimicrobics

In his zeal to aid the patient ill with an infectious disease, the physician may be tempted to argue that if one antimicrobial agent is good, two are better. There are circumstances where this is quite correct.

First, it is axiomatic that no combination can make something out of nothing. That is, each component must, by itself, be active against the microorganism that is the cause of the infection.

The second premise requires a different mechanism of action for each component of a combination. This must be observed with potentially toxic agents in particular so that the combination is not simply equivalent to a high dose of one of the components.

Two or more agents, each effective by a different mechanism, usually display activity that is quantitatively the sum of the respective individual activities. Such action is described as *additive*. Uncommonly, the effect may surpass addition; it is then termed *synergistic*. Also uncommonly, the effect may be less than summation, or *antagonistic*. A useful method of portrayal is the isobologram (Fig. 18-21). With precise regulation of cultures or experimental infections, as well as timing and dosage of antimicrobics, it is possible to assign combinations to one of these three categories. In practice, however, the several

Fig. 18-21. Assessment of the nature of the combined action of two antimicrobics is sharpened through calculation of the fractional inhibitory concentrations (FICs, per Elion GB, Singer S, Hitchings GH: J Biol Chem 208:477–488, 1954). When the plot of values falls along a line demarcated by the mean MIC of each antimicrobic exhibited alone (FIC = 1), the combination acts additively (curve ***ad***). Bowing toward the origin indicates synergism (curve ***sy***), whereas bowing outward, away from the origin, is consistent with antagonism (curve ***an***).

$$= \frac{\text{Geometric mean MIC in combination}}{\text{Geometric mean MIC singly}}$$

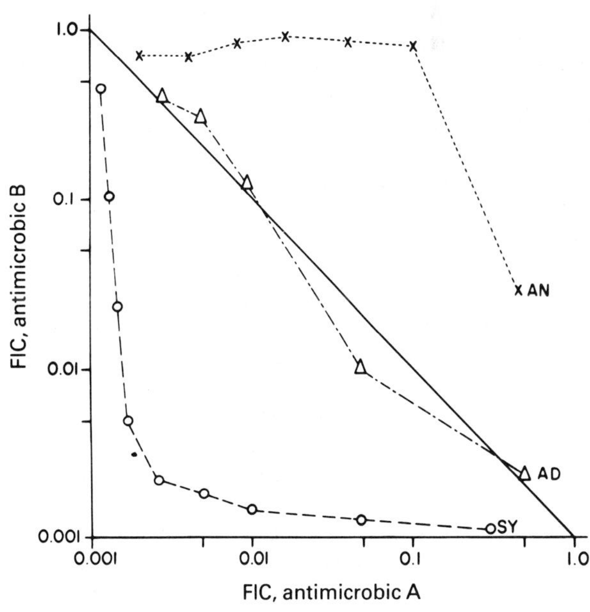

critical variables are not controlled, and the generalizations from the laboratory may not apply.

Proven Value

CELL-WALL-ACTIVE ANTIMICROBICS PLUS AMINOCYCLITOLS

All of the cell-wall-active antimicrobics (β-lactams, bacitracin, vancomycin, ristocetin, cycloserine, fosfomycin) may act synergistically with the aminocyclitols when tested *in vitro*. Clinical verification of this phenomenon is clear cut with penicillins plus aminocyclitols, and in most situations, a cephalosporin or one of the other cell-wall-active drugs may be used in place of a penicillin. However, as with a penicillin–aminocyclitol combination, the probability of efficacy of an alternative combination should be supported by testing *in vitro*.

Penicillins Plus Aminocyclitols. The combination of penicillin G plus streptocomycin is synergistic in effect on most strains of *Streptococcus* spp. The phenomenon is demonstrable in the test tube and verifiable in the patient; it is often crucial to the successful treatment of streptococcal endocarditis.

With enterococci, ampicillin, amoxicillin, and the acylureidopenicillins are clearly more active than penicillin G; the ampicillin–streptomycin combination is classic for the treatment of enterococcal endocarditis. However, with occasional isolates, streptomycin is ineffective; gentamicin, tobramycin, netilmicin, or amikacin may be active against such strains. Hence, in critical situations, before data from testing *in vitro* are available, it is reasonable to start treatment with a combination of ampicillin or one of the acylureidopenicillins plus one of the nonstreptomyin aminoglycosidic aminocyclitols.

The combination of nafcillin plus gentamicin is frequently synergistic against penicillinase-positive *Staphylococcus aureus.* In clinical situations requiring maximally bactericidal therapy (*e.g.,* staphylococcal endocarditis or extra-CNS infections in immunosuppressed patients), the combination has been used with good effect. By testing *in vitro,* either tobramycin, netilmicin, or amikacin may be used instead of gentamicin.

Carbenicillin, ticarcillin, and the acylureidopenicillins are synergistic by testing *in vitro* with the nonstreptomycin aminoglycosidic aminocyclitols against about one-half of the clinical isolates of *Pseudomonas aeruginosa* that are susceptible to the individual drugs. Although not proved of value by controlled clinical trial, use of such combinations can be defended on the grounds that the minimal gain, as additive effect, is helpful to any patient with diminished host defenses—as is implied by the existence of a serious pseudomonal infection.

ANTITUBERCULOUS THERAPY

The development of resistance in *Mycobacterium tuberculosis* occurs rapidly if antituberculous agents are applied singly in treatment. With administration of two or more agents, each individually effective by different mechanisms of action, resistance to any one agent of the combination develops quite slowly, if at all. The combinations commonly applied in tuberculotherapy are described in Chapter 34, Pulmonary Tuberculosis.

SULFONAMIDES PLUS DIAMINOPYRIMIDINES

The usefulness of the combination of a sulfonamide with a diaminopyrimidine (pyrimethamine, trimethoprim) rests on sequential competitive inhibition of a pathway that many microorganisms are obliged to follow (Fig. 18-22). Humans do not have the capacity to synthesize dihydropteroate, and sulfonamides have no adverse effect on humans in this connection. The affinity of pyrimethamine and trimethoprim for human dihydrofolate reductase is so much less than it is for the microbial enzyme, that the drugs are relatively safe.

Trimethoprim–sulfamenthoxazoe is not active against anaerobes. Because it is synergisitic against many of the Enterobacteriaceae, the combination is valuable in treatment of urinary tract infections. Because trimethoprim is one of the few antimicrobics that gains entry into the prostate, the combination is valuable in treatment of chronic bacterial prostatitis. Excellent entry into the respiratory tract may well be related to clinical usefulness in exacerbations of chronic bronchitis. Other bacterial infections that appear to be benefited by trimethoprim–sulfamethoxazole include typhoid fever, brucellosis, and gonorrhea. Trimethoprim–sulfamethoxazole is effective in the chemoprophylaxis of pneumocytosis and may also be the treatment of choice for this protozoal infection.

A combination of triple sulfonamides, or sulfadiazine alone, with pyrimethamine has proved to be synergistic against two kinds of protozoa: (1) Infections caused by *Toxoplasma gondii,* both experimental and in humans, respond to such treatment; (2) Acute clinical malaria, regardless of the species of *Plasmodium* or susceptibility to chloroquine or quinine, may also improve dramatically with such therapy; other sulfonamides—for example, sulfadoxine—are also effective.

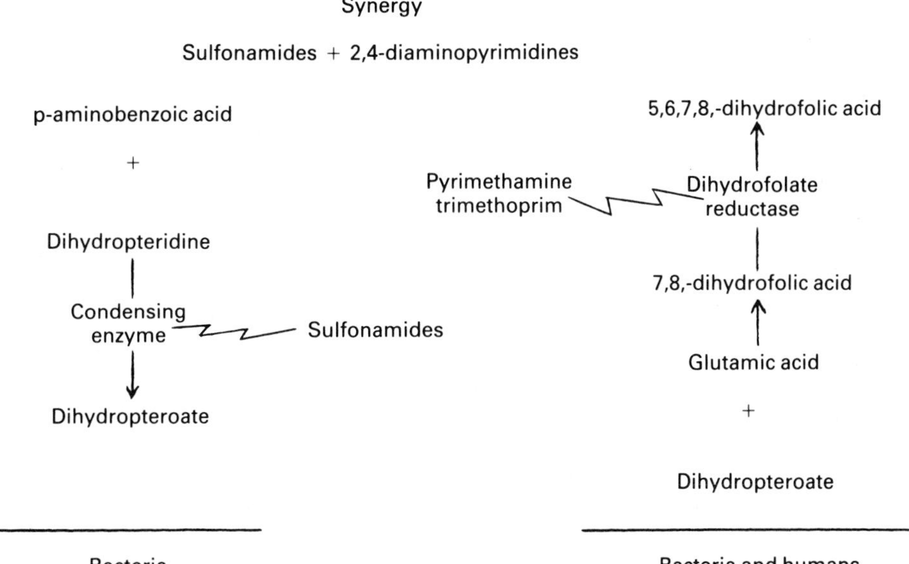

Fig. 18-22. The combination of a sulfonamide and a diaminopyrimidine offers potential for competitive inhibition at two sites in the pathway for synthesis of coenzymes essential to the synthesis of nucleic and amino acids. Humans are little affected by the combination because they cannot synthesize dihydropteroate, and human dihydrofolate reductase has particularly low affinity for trimethoprim—moderately low for pyrimethamine. (Hoeprich PD: Antimicrobial Agents and Chemotherapy, 1967. Ann Arbor, Mich, American Society for Microbiology, 1968, pp 697–704)

Unproven Value

MIXED AEROBE–ANAEROBE INFECTIONS

Infections that are caused by bacteria normally resident in the oropharynx, lower intestinal tract, and vagina almost always involve microaerophilic and facultatively anaerobic bacteria (generally lumped with obligately aerobic bacteria as "aerobes"), as well as obligately anaerobic bacteria. Accordingly, it seems reasonable to apply combinations of antimicrobics that should affect the potential pathogens of the region presumed to be the source of the infection. There is little doubt of the value of such therapy, although antimicrobics are adjuvant to surgical drainage and debridement. However, there are differences of opinion as to which agents should be coadministered, and proof is generally lacking that one regimen is superior to another.

Chloramphenicol should be active against most of the usual components of mixed aerobe–anaerobe bacterial infections. The advantages (capability of being administered by IM or IV injection and PO; efficient entry into the CSF and CNS; lack of nephrotoxicity and of need to adjust dosage in patients with renal failure as long as hepatic function is moderately well preserved) clearly outweighed the disadvantages (bacteriostaticity, except against *H. influenzae, Streptococcus pneumoniae,* and *N. meningitidis;* lack of activity against *Pseudomonas aeruginosa,* and poor activity against some of the Enterobacteriaceae and *Staphylococcus aureus;* potential for causing aplastic anemia—estimated at 1 case per 24,500 to 40,800 courses of treatment; dose-related bone marrow suppression in patients of all ages; and the grey baby syndrome) when there were no alternatives. But antimicrobics are now available that are safer and more effective against the aerobes (the β-lactams and the aminocyclitols). Also, there are alternatives for treatment of anaerobic infections: some of the penicillins and certain of the cephalosporins, clindamycin, and metronidazole.

Whenever possible, a β-lactam drug should be used, for example, in mixed infections caused by oropharyngeal flora. In other situations, either clindamycin or metronidazole is preferable to chloramphenicol because of bactericidal potential and lesser threat of toxicity. Although clindamycin can be given either by injection or perorally and is effective against most anaerobes (with the exception of some anaerobic cocci and *Clostridium* spp.—most notably, *C.*

difficile) and *Staphylococcus aureus,* it does not distribute widely, failing to penetrate into the CSF and CNS. Metronidazole may also be given parenterally, and perorally or per rectum; it is effective against most anaerobes (with the exception of *Actinomyces* spp., and some anaerobic cocci) and certain facultatively anaerobic bacteria when they are in an anaerobic environment, and it distributes into all body water, including the CSF and CNS. The major toxicity of clindamycin is provocation of pseudomembranous colitis; the most troublesome adverse reactions to metronidazole are nausea and vomiting and peripheral neuropathy.

From these considerations, a combination of an acylureidopenicillin–netilmicin–metronidazole might be appropriate for beginning treatment when a serious, life-threatening, mixed aerobe–anaerobe bacterial infection is thought to be caused by microorganisms drawn from lower intestinal or vaginal flora. The possible advantage over ticarcillin–gentamicin–clindamycin might be lesser toxicity with excellent activity against anaerobes, streptococci, Enterobacteriaceae and *P. aeruginosa,* but with somewhat poorer antistaphylococcal activity. As with any other initial regimen, modification may be necessary when information from smears and cultures becomes available.

PROPRIETARY COMBINATIONS

Several proprietary combinations made up of two antimicrobial agents have been advocated for the prevention or treatment of infections of unknown cause. The argument is advanced that the components of such mixtures provide activity against both gram-positive and gram-negative bacteria. In fact, mixtures such as penicillin–streptomycin, erythromycin–sulfonamides, and tetracycline–novobiocin have not been proved valuable. The fixed ratio of components frequently leads to inadequate dosage with one component—usually the antimicrobic most likely to cause an adverse reaction.

Combinations of tetracycline with nystatin or tetracycline with amphotericin B were available for peroral administration. Supposedly, the outgrowth of *Candida albicans* as a result of suppression of enteric bacterial flora by the tetracycline was prevented by the antifungal agent. If this did actually occur, no advantage to the patient from it was proved.

Bibliography

Books

ABRAHAM EP: Biosynthesis and Enzymatic Hydrolysis of Penicillins and Cephalosporins. Tokyo, University of Tokyo Press, 1974. 86 pp.

ANDERSON RJ, GAMBERTOGLIO JG, SCHRIER RW: Clinical Use of Drugs in Renal Failure, Springfield, Ill., Charles C Thomas, 1976. 251 pp.

CONTE JE JR, BARRIERE SL: Manual of Antibiotics and Infectious Diseases. Philadelphia, Lea & Febiger, 1981. 213 pp.

FRANKLIN TJ, SNOW GA: Biochemistry of Antimicrobial Action. 3rd ed. New York, Chapman & Hall, 1981. 217 pp.

GLASBY JS: Encyclopedia of Antibiotics. New York, John Wiley & Sons, 1976. 372 pp.

LASKIN AI, LECHEVALIER HA (eds): Handbook of Microbiology, Vol III, Microbial Products. Cleveland, CRC Press, 1973. 1143 pp.

LORIAN V ed: Antibiotics in Laboratory Medicine. Baltimore, Williams & Wilkings, 1980. 737 pp.

ROGERS HJ, PERKINS HR, WARD JB: Microbial Cell Walls and Membranes. London, Chapman & Hall, 1980. 564 pp.

TODD RG (ed): Extra Pharmacopoeia Martindale, 25th ed. London, Pharmaceutical Press, 1967

UMEZAWA H (ed-in-chief): Index of Antibiotics from Actinomycetes, Vol II. Tokyo, Japan Scientific Societies Press, 1978. 1466 pp.

Journals

ADKINSON NF JR, THOMPSON WL, MADDREY WC, LICHTENSTEIN LM: Routine use of penicillin skin testing on an inpatient service. N Engl J Med 285:22–24, 1971

BENNET WM, SINGER I, COGGINS CJ: A guide to drug therapy in renal failure. JAMA 230:1544–1553, 1974

BORDER WA, LEHMAN DH, EGAN ID, SASS HJ, GLODE JE, WILSON CB: Antitubular basement–membrane antibodies in methicillin associated interstitial nephritis. N Engl J Med 291:381–384, 1974

COOK FV, FARRAR WE: Vancomycin revisited. Ann Intern Med 88:813–818, 1978

COSTERTON JW, CHENG K–J: The role of the bacterial cell envelope in antibiotic resistance. J Antimicrob Chemother 1:363–377, 1975

DETTLI L, SPRING P, RYTER S: Multiple dose kinetics and drug dosage in patients with kidney disease. Acta Pharmacol Toxicol 29 (Suppl 3):211–224, 1971

DORNBUSCH K, HOLLANDER HO: Gentamicin resistance in gram-negative bacilli: Occurrence of modifying enzymes and their influence on susceptibility testing. Scand J Infect Dis 12:295–302, 1980

FEDER HM JR, OSIER C, MADERAZO EG: Chloramphenicol: A review of its use in clinical practice. Rev Infect Dis 3:479–491, 1981

FISHMAN RA: Blood–brain and CSF barriers to penicillin and related organic acids. Arch Neurol 15:113–124, 1966

GERACI JE: Vancomycin. Mayo Clin Proc 52:631–634, 1977

JACKSON D, PHILLIPS I (eds): From penicillin to piperacillin. J Antimicrob Chemother 9(Suppl B):1–101, 1982

KASS EH, EVANS DA (eds): Future prospects and past problems in antimicrobial therapy: The role of cefoxitin. Rev Infect Dis 1:2–239, 1979

LEVINE BB, REDMOND AP, FELLNER MJ, VOSS HE, LEVYTSKA V: Penicillin allergy and the heterogeneous immune responses of man to benzylpenicillin. J Clin Invest 45:1895–1906, 1966

MEYER RD: Amikacin. Ann Intern Med 95:328–332, 1981

NEU HC, WISE R (eds): Mezlocillin. J Antimicrob Chemother 9(Suppl A):1–299, 1982

NIGHTINGALE CH, GREENE DS, QUINTILIANI R: Pharmacokinetics and clinical use of cephalosporin antibiotics. J Pharm Sci 64:1899–1927, 1975

O'GRADY F: Antibiotics in renal failure. Br Bull Med 27:142–147, 1971

PEDERSEN–BJERGAARD J: Specific hyposensitization of patients with penicillin allergy. Acta Allerg 24:333–361, 1969

PEDERSEN–BJERGAARD J: The clinical diagnosis of penicillin allergy. Acta Allerg 25:98–130, 1970

PHILLIPS I, WISE R, NEU HC (eds): An oral penem antibiotic: Sch 29482. J Antimicrob Chemother 9(Suppl C):1–247, 1982

PISCOTTA AV: Drug-induced leukopenia and aplastic anemia. Clin Pharm Ther 12:13–43, 1971

SMITH CR, LIPSKY JJ, LASKIN OL, HELLMANN DB, MELLITS ED, LONGSTRETH J, LIETMAN PS: Double-blind comparison of the nephrotoxicity and auditory toxicity of gentamicin and tobramycin. N Engl J Med 302:1106–1109, 1980

SYKES RB: The classification and terminology of enzymes that hydrolyze β-lactam antibiotics. J Infect Dis 145:762–765, 1982

SYKES RB, MATTHEW M: The β-lactamses of gram-negative bacteria and their role in resistance to β-lactam antibiotics. J Antimicrob Chemother 2:115–157, 1976

SYKES RB, PHILLIPS I (eds): Azthreonam: A synthetic monobactam. J Antimicrob Chemother 8(Suppl E):1–148, 1981

TOMASZ A: Penicillin-binding proteins in bacteria. Ann Intern Med 96:502–504, 1982

TOMASZ A: The mechanism of the irreversible antimicrobial effects of penicillins: How the beta-lactam antibiotics kill and lyse bacteria. Ann Rev Microbiol 33:113–137, 1979

NEIL M. FLYNN
PAUL D. HOEPRICH

19 *Chemoprophylaxis of Infectious Diseases*

It is axiomatic in medicine that the best management for any disease is prevention, provided that the means are available and the cost:benefit or risk:benefit ratios are acceptable. This chapter deals with prevention of morbidity from infectious agents through the prophylactic and empiric use of antimicrobial drugs.

The basis for chemoprophylaxis is the belief that an antimicrobic that can bring about cure of an infectious disease also can prevent the development of that disease if it is given at or shortly after exposure to the causative agent. This implies that the time of exposure, the etiologic agent, and its susceptibility to the drug(s) to be used for prophylaxis are known. Failure to understand these concepts will lead to ineffective prophylaxis, overuse of antimicrobial agents, promotion of resistance in human-associated microorganisms, and waste of limited and costly medical resources. In some instances, the physician wishes to prevent disease from a single infectious agent (*e.g.*, the tubercle bacillus). In others, the aim is to prevent the growth of several possible pathogens (*e.g.*, staphylococci and streptococci in the prevention of surgical wound infection in total hip replacement). In general, the greater the number of species of organisms to be suppressed, the less effective and the more toxic the prophylactic regimen becomes. There is no ideal chemoprophylactic drug or combination of drugs that lacks toxicity and selectively inhibits only pathogens. Accordingly, specific situations are discussed in which the risk of toxicity is acceptably low and there is evidence of effectiveness in the prevention of morbidity.

Factors important in assessing the risk:benefit equation include the (1) likelihood that the patient will develop disease if chemoprophylaxis is not used; (2) severity of the disease to be prevented; (3) effectiveness of nonspecific host defenses; (4) efficacy of the drug in preventing the disease; (5) acceptability of the drug to the patient, physician, and community based on side-effects and toxicity of the drug; (6) duration of exposure to the infectious agent; (7) likelihood and consequences of promoting resistance to the drug(s) used; and (8) cost and availability of the prophylactic regimen.

New drugs and a better understanding of the factors that affect the development of disease following exposure to an infectious agent may permit expansion and refinement of the indications for chemoprophylaxis. Such an evolution over the past 5 years has led to inclusion of a discussion of empiric therapy in the compromised host and expansion of the discussion of the chemoprophylaxis of infections complicating surgical operations. These areas merit extended treatment because of the high mortality in patients with compromised host defenses and the expense in drugs, money, and time associated with chemoprophylaxis in surgery.

Effective Chemoprophylaxis

Prevention of Specific Infectious Diseases

INFLUENZA (Chap. 28, Influenza)
The introduction of influenza virus into a susceptible population may lead to disease in 10% to 20% of the exposed persons (up to 40% in certain closed populations). Both morbidity and mortality tend to be higher in the elderly and in compromised hosts, such as those with cardiorespiratory disease. Amantadine hydrochloride is approximately 75% effective in the prevention of disease from influenza A_2 when given in a dose of 100 mg, PO, 12-hourly, for 10–14 days following vaccination or for the duration of an outbreak in those who cannot be immunized (*e.g.*, be-

cause of allergy to components of the vaccine). Amantadine should be given to unvaccinated persons with chronic diseases at the time of an outbreak, to household contacts of a presumed case of influenza A, and to exposed hospital and nursing home patients and employees. Adverse effects include central nervous system (CNS) toxicity, orthostatic hypotension, urinary retention, and congestive heart failure—all potentially serious, particularly in the elderly and persons with renal dysfunction.

SMALLPOX (Chap. 92, Smallpox and Other Poxvirus Infections)
Although smallpox has been eradicated, the virus is stored in several laboratories. Moreover, there is a remote possibility of mutation of a nonvariola poxvirus to increased virulence for humans. Hence, it is prudent to note that methisazone was proved effective in preventing disease following exposure of unvaccinated persons to smallpox. Field trials of the drug were carried out in Madras, India among household contacts of persons clinically ill with smallpox. In trials using a single dose of 3 g or two doses of 3 g each, 12 hours apart, side-effects were minimal and the regimens were very effective. There were 5 cases and 2 deaths among 1199 contacts given the single dose, compared with 105 cases and 18 deaths among 2044 controls. The 2-dose regimen resulted in no cases among 610 treated contacts in contrast with 43 cases and 3 deaths in the 810 untreated controls. Administration of two doses of 3 g of methisazone, PO, 12 hours apart, prevents smallpox if given before the 7th day of incubation. Alastrim, or variola minor, may also be prevented using methisazone. The consequences of vaccinia virus infections may be modified by the drug, and its course may possibly be as well.

SCRUB TYPHUS (Chap. 99, Scrub Typhus)
Scrub typhus may be prevented from becoming clinically evident in persons exposed for short periods by the administration of chloramphenicol, 1 g, PO, every other day. However, clinical illness follows unless the treatment is continued for 1 month after exposure. Similar protection is afforded by the administration of a dosage of 3 g once a week during exposure and for 5 weeks after the last exposure. Although tetracycline has been effective in the treatment of disease, sufficient data are not available regarding its efficacy in prophylaxis. It may be that a long-acting tetracycline (*e.g.,* doxycycline) would be as effective for prophylaxis as chloramphenicol and would be potentially less toxic. Thus, if timed properly, chloramphenicol (and probably tetracycline) prevents classic clinical scrub typhus, but at the cost of delaying the development of immunity.

TUBERCULOSIS (Chap. 34, Pulmonary Tuberculosis)
The use of isoniazid (INH) alone is of value in the chemoprophylaxis of tuberculosis (1) following intimate or intense exposure to active tuberculosis; (2) during early, asymptomatic primary infection; and (3) when there is an apparently quiescent focus in a patient at risk of reactivation and spread. The risk of progressive tuberculous disease in these settings is influenced by the general health and adequacy of immune function of the patient. Gastrectomy, silicosis, prolonged immunosuppression, childhood, old age, malignancy, diabetes mellitus, malnutrition, and pregnancy increase the risk of disease in an infected person.

The need for chemoprophylaxis with isoniazid varies according to the likelihood of developing disease and is associated with the following groups, in descending order: (1) household contacts and other close associates (children in particular) of a person with active tuberculosis (the risk of overt disease during the first year after exposure is 2.5% overall and 5% among those with positive tuberculin skin tests at the time of initial examination); (2) recently infected persons as defined by skin test conversion within the prior 2 years and usually detected by annual or case contact skin testing (the risk of overt disease is 5% during the first year after infection); (3) persons with evidence of past tuberculous disease (positive skin test and nonprogressive granulomatous disease by chest radiography or a history of extrapulmonary tuberculous disease) who have never received adequate chemotherapy (the risk of overt reactivation of disease is 1%–4.5% per year); (4) other positive reactors (those with a positive skin test, no history of tuberculous disease, and a normal chest roentgenogram, who are not recent convertors and are not close contacts of an active case) who are less than 35 years of age, or who have one of the conditions other than pregancy that increase the likelihood of disease (the risk of reactivation disease is 0.1%–1% per year).

Once the decision has been made by the patient and the physician to undertake isoniazid chemoprophylaxis, certain screening procedures should be carried out. Active tuberculosis should be ruled out, since treatment of active disease should include two or more drugs. There should be no history of previous, adequate isoniazid therapy, toxicity from previous isoniazid therapy, heavy alcohol use (which may increase the risk of serious hepatotoxicity), acute or chronic liver disease, pregnancy, or concurrent medications that might interact with isoniazid to produce toxicity. Isoniazid may enhance the effects of diphenylhydantoin.

Isoniazid is given in a dosage of 300 mg/day, PO, for 12 months in adults, and 10 mg/kg body wt/day (not to exceed 300 mg/day), PO, for 12 months in children. Pyridoxine, 10 to 100 mg/day, should be given concomitantly to prevent neurotoxicity, particularly in patients with poor nutrition or with diabetes mellitus. Toxicity severe enough to require cessation of prophylaxis occurs in 10% to 20% of patients. The major toxicity is hepatic injury, which may be fatal if it is not detected early and if the drug is not stopped after the appearance of symptoms. Overall, chemical evidence of hepatic dysfunction in the form of abnormally high serum concentrations of transaminases occurs in 10% to 20% of persons taking isoniazid for 1 year. Generally, there is a spontaneous return to normal without interruption of treatment, and the patient has no symptoms of hepatitis. However, if there are symptoms of hepatitis, or the rise in serum transaminases on monthly testing exceeds threefold (monthly testing has been recommended for persons over age 35), isoniazid should be discontinued. The frequency of isoniazid hepatitis is age related. It is virtually absent in children, rare in persons aged 20 to 34, and has a 1.2% incidence in persons aged 35 to 49 years and a 2.3% incidence in persons 50 years of age and older. The risk of hepatitis ceases when treatment is stopped: follow-up has disclosed no delayed adverse effects 15 years postchemoprophylaxis.

The efficacy of isoniazid in the prevention of active tuberculosis has been proved in a series of well-controlled studies carried out under the aegis of the United States Public Health Service. Active disease does not occur during prophylaxis if it was not present at the time administration of isoniazid was begun, and the beneficial effect appears to extend for years after the completion of prophylaxis. Indeed, chemoprophylaxis with isoniazid may decrease the lifetime risk of developing active tuberculosis by as much as 80%.

MENINGOCOCCAL INFECTIONS
(Chap. 119, Bacterial Meningitis)

Meningococci must spread from person to person, for *Neisseria meningitidis* has no host other than the human. A clinical infection dramatically identifies a source for dissemination of *N. meningitidis* and enables recognition of a cohort of persons who have a greatly increased risk of developing meningococcal disease. The risk of disease among household or very close contacts of an index patient is 2 to 4 in 1000 in nonmilitary, nonepidemic settings, and 11 to 45 in 1000 during nonmilitary epidemics. These rates are 1 to 15 thousand times greater than the endemic rate of meningococcal disease.

Persons at highest risk include household contacts of an index patient; day care center contacts; medical personnel who resuscitated, intubated, or suctioned the patient before treatment was begun; and others who had contact with the patient's oral secretions. One-third of secondary cases become clinically manifest within 4 days of the diagnosis of the index case, indicating the need for rapid identification and prompt institution of prophylaxis of close contacts. That prophylaxis may not be carried out quickly enough is reflected in the finding that only 26% of eligible contacts in one study had received prophylaxis within 24 hours of admission of the index patient to the hospital.

The three drugs that have been demonstrated to be effective in eradicating the carrier state share the property of achieving high concentrations in tears and saliva. If the strain of *N. meningitidis* is known to be susceptible to sulfonamides, they are the drugs of choice. However, when the susceptibility is not known, as is usually the case, sulfonamides should not be relied upon because of the high frequency of resistant meningococci, even in nonepidemic, community-acquired disease (≥15%). When the infecting meningococci are susceptible to 0.1 mg sulfadiazine per 100 ml (1 μg/ml), the administration of 1 g twice daily to adults, 500 mg twice daily to children 1 to 12 years of age, and 500 mg daily for infants, for 2 to 3 days is effective in eradicating meningococcal carriage in 95% or more of those treated.

At the present time in the United States rifampin is the drug of choice for prophylaxis when the strain is resistant to sulfonamides or its susceptibility is unknown. Treatment for 2 days is recommended: 600 mg, PO, 12-hourly, for adults; 10 mg/kg of body wt/day, PO, as 2 equal portions, 12-hourly for children 1 month to 12 years of age; and 5 mg/kg of body wt/day, PO, as 2 equal portions 12-hourly for newborn infants. The effectiveness of such treatment is ≥ 85%. Some of the apparent failures may in fact represent recolonization from untreated carriers. Rifampin-resistant strains have emerged following prophylaxis among military personnel, but such strains have not persisted, and primary resistance is extremely rare.

Minocycline given in a dose of 2 mg/kg body wt/day, PO, as 2 equal portions, 12-hourly for 5 days is as effective as rifampin. Resistant strains have not been encountered. However, adverse vestibular reactions to minocycline have been reported in as many as 90% of recipients in the United States, as compared to 1% to 6% in Great Britain. Minocycline should not be given to young children or to pregnant women.

Meningococcal vaccines are of no value in preventing disease in close contacts because of the rapidity with which secondary cases occur. Immediate administration of a vaccine does not result in a protective antibody response for at least 10 to 14 days. Moreover, fewer than 20% of the meningococcal isolates associated with disease belong to groups A or C, for which vaccines are available.

Although meningococci are susceptible to penicillin, tetracycline, erythromycin, and other antimicrobics, none is effective in eliminating nasopharyngeal carriage. Meager entry into upper respiratory tract secretions appears to be the explanation.

The cooperation of the local health department should be sought in attempting to provide chemoprophylaxis for contacts of a patient with meningococcal disease. Assistance with rapid identification, notification, and treatment of contacts is generally forthcoming.

GONOCOCCAL INFECTIONS
(Chap. 56, Gonococcal Infections)
Chemoprophylaxis may be given following venereal exposure to gonorrhea and is routinely given to prevent neonatal ophthalmic gonococcal infection.

For several years after the introduction of penicillin for the treatment of gonorrhea, small doses of the drug given 3 to 4 hours after venereal exposure were effective in preventing disease. However, this is no longer the case, and lacking the evidence of controlled trials, it is probable that therapeutic doses of penicillin, tetracycline, or spectinomycin should be given for prophylaxis in this setting.

Asymptomatic carriage of gonococci at any site, whether in a male or female, should be treated with therapeutic doses of penicillin, tetracycline, or spectinomycin, and test-of-cure cultures should be taken following completion of therapy. Likewise, all sexual contacts of confirmed cases of gonorrhea should be treated and followed up with test-of-cure cultures.

Gonococcal ophthalmia neonatorum is a potentially serious infection that may result in impairment of vision as well as disseminated gonococcal disease. For this reason, and because unrecognized maternal gonococcal infection is not infrequent, 2 drops of 1% silver nitrate should be instilled in the conjunctival sac of each eye immediately after birth, and not removed by irrigation. It is effective and reasonably well tolerated, although a mild chemical conjunctivitis may occur in up to 20% of infants within the first 24 hours after birth.

SYPHILIS (Chap. 59, Syphilis)
Asymptomatic syphilis occurs in two settings: during the incubation period of primary syphilis and during the latent period after the primary and secondary lesions subside. During the 2- to 3-week period of incubation, the serologic tests for syphilis are generally negative. Thus, contact tracing of an infectious case may identify exposed persons who have neither clinical nor serologic evidence of infection. Such persons should be given preventive or epidemiologic treatment. To wait for seroconversion or the appearance of a primary chancre before treating is to risk loss of these contacts to follow-up, further spread of infection to subsequent sexual contacts, and fetal infection if the exposed person happens to be a pregnant woman. A single injection of benzathine penicillin G, 2.4 million units IM, provides effective treatment for such incubating syphilis. Alternatively, tetracycline hydrochloride or erythromycin, 15 mg/kg body wt/day, PO, as 4 equal portions, 6-hourly, for 15 days may be used in patients who are allergic to the penicillins (tetracycline and erythromycin must be avoided in pregnancy). Doxycycline (200 mg/day, PO, as 2 equal portions, 12-hourly, for 15 days) is at least as effective and may be better tolerated, though it is more expensive. Serologic testing should be carried out after therapy to detect seroconversion if it occurs, although further treatment is not necessary.

Before undertaking chemoprophylaxis in latent syphilis, the physician should determine whether neurosyphilis is present, both by clinical assessment and by examination of the CSF. If there is no evidence of neurosyphilis, benzathine penicillin G should be given in a dosage of 2.4 million units, IM, each week for 3 successive weeks. Tetracycline hydrochloride or erythromycin estolate (30 mg/kg body wt/day, PO, as 4 equal portions, 6-hourly, for 30 days), or doxycycline (200 mg/day, PO, as 2 equal portions, 12-hourly, for 30 days) may be substituted in patients who are allergic to the penicillins. Compliance with these regimens is often poor, a matter that should be considered carefully by the patient and physician before starting therapy.

If the CSF is abnormal, many authorities prefer to treat with aqueous procaine penicillin G, 600,000 units, IM, daily for 15 days, or to admit the patient to the hospital for aqueous crystalline penicillin G, 2 to 4 million units, IV, every 4 hours for 10 days. Patients who are allergic to the penicillins who have latent neurosyphilis may be treated with one of the alternative regimens given above, though proof of effectiveness by clinical trials is lacking. Follow-up examinations of the CSF should be performed to document improvement, especially in patients receiving an alternative therapy.

SHIGELLOSIS (Chap. 62, Shigellosis)
Epidemic shigellosis may occur in closed populations in which there is opportunity for fecal–oral spread of the organisms, for example, military camps or day-care centers. The epidemic may be aborted by treating the entire closed population with a subtherapeutic regimen of tetracycline, ampicillin, or trimethoprim–sulfamethoxazole, depending on the resistance pattern of the epidemic strain. Resistance to one or all of these drugs is increasing in frequency among *Shigella* spp.

MALARIA (Chap. 145, Malaria)
Prevention of malaria is feasible for travelers from developed countries who enter areas endemic for malaria. A number of compounds have been effective in the past, including mepacrine, proguanil, pyrimethamine, cycloguanil pamoate, and chloroquine. However, resistance to each of these compounds has been reported, most notably to chlorquine, the most useful of this group. Chloroquine-resistant *Plasmodium falciparum* has become a major problem in some parts of the world, including most of Southeast Asia, many areas of the South Pacific, central and northern South America, and East Africa. A complete description of the distribution of chloroquine resistance in *P. falciparum* is provided yearly in *Health Information for International Travel,* published by the United States Public Health Service Centers for Disease Control, Atlanta, GA. In areas where resistance to chloroquine is common, a combination of pyrimethamine and sulfadoxine (Fansidar), a long-acting sulfonamide, may be effective.

For chemoprophylaxis of malaria caused by *Plasmodium vivax* and chloroquine-susceptible *P. falciparum,* chloroquine phosphate should be given as a 500-mg dose, PO, weekly, beginning 2 weeks prior to exposure and continuing for 6 weeks after termination of exposure. Travelers with particularly high-risk exposure to *P. vivax* infection may also be given primaquine phosphate, 15 mg/day, for 14 days, following return from the malarious area or alternatively may be given a combination of chloroquine phosphate, 500 mg, plus primaquine phosphate, 79 mg, once a week during exposure and for 8 weeks after return from the endemic area. The physician should test the patient for G6PD deficiency before prescribing primaquine.

Travelers in areas where resistance to chloroquine is prevalent in *P. falciparum* should receive a single weekly dose of pyrimethamine, 50 mg, plus sulfadoxine, 1 g in addition to chloroquine, starting prior to exposure and continuing for 6 weeks after departure from the endemic region. Continuous prophylaxis with this combination is not recommended for periods exceeding 6 months.

Finally, it is important that travelers be counseled on techniques to prevent mosquito bites, and on the importance of seeking medical attention if unexplained fever or symptoms of malaria occur while in the endemic area or for several months after leaving it.

RHEUMATIC FEVER
(Chap. 24, Streptococcal Diseases)
Untreated infections caused by *Streptococcus pyogenes* of Lancefield's group A are followed by rheumatic fever in some 1% to 3% of previously well persons, after a latent period of several days to 6 weeks. Persons who have had rheumatic fever either have acquired, as a result of the infection, or persist in having innately, abnormal reactivity to group A streptococcal infections. Rheumatic fever develops in 40% to 50% of such persons if they have a streptococcal infection during the first year after the initial episode of rheumatic fever. As years pass without recurrences of rheumatic fever, hyper-reactivity wanes, but the probability of recurrence does not entirely disappear.

Not all streptococcal infection is clinically apparent. Inapparent infections may be detected only by serologic changes in the patient, that is, appearance of or increase in the titer of humoral antibodies specific for extracellular streptococcal enzymes. Such subclinical infections may be associated with activation of the rheumatic process. Thus, the patient and physician cannot rely on treatment of clinical streptococcal infection alone to prevent recurrences of rheumatic fever. Conversely, the simple carriage of group A. *S. pyogenes* (the presence of *S. pyogenes* by culture, but without serologic response) does not lead to rheumatic fever.

It is clear that if infection with group A *S. pyogenes* can be prevented, rheumatic fever recurrences can be reduced, although failure of prophylactic antimicrobics has been documented. The population at particular risk, the population in which streptococcal infection must be prevented, is identified primarily by the previous occurrence of rheumatic fever or equivalent disease. Thus, prophylaxis of infection by group A *S. pyogenes* must be continuous throughout life in all persons who have a well-documented history of rheumatic fever or chorea *and* who have definite evidence of rheumatic heart disease.

When rheumatic heart disease is not present, prophylaxis should also be given to persons who have had rheumatic fever or equivalent disease for several years after the episode. The necessary duration of chemoprophylaxis is less certain in this group. It should be prolonged if there is close contact with young children—a situation of high risk of reinfection with *S. pyogenes.* In addition to the risk of reinfection, other factors bear on the decision to forego lifelong prophylaxis following an episode of rheumatic fever, for example, the anticipated rate of recurrence of rheumatic fever following reinfection and the consequences of recurrence. Unfortunately, despite the best efforts of the physician, some patients elect to forego prophylaxis or simply fail to take the medication as prescribed. Careful explanation of the consequences of failure to take prophylaxis may improve compliance, and the physician should document such efforts in the patient's medical record.

Penicillin is the prophylactic agent of choice for the prevention of recurrences of rheumatic fever. Group A *S. pyogenes* is exquisitely susceptible to penicillin, and no resistant strains have been reported. Benzathine penicillin G injected intramuscularly at monthly intervals is the optimal regimen for patients not allergic to penicillin. It is effective, and compliance can easily be monitored. The monthly dose is 600,000 units for those under 25 kg in body weight, and 1.2 million units, equally divided in two injection sites, for those over 25 kg body weight. Two disadvantages—pain, sometimes severe and persistent for days or weeks after injection, and the potential for prolonged morbidity if hypersensitivity to penicillin develops—are outweighed by security in dosage and economy. Penicillin V, given PO in a dose of 125 mg twice daily for small children and 250 mg twice daily for children over 25 kg in body weight and for adults, is an effective alternative to benzathine penicillin; however, compliance is variable, and recurrence of rheumatic fever is therefore more likely. Penicillin V is most likely to be successful in young children with compulsive parents, and in patients who are taking other essential medications on a regular basis.

When hypersensitivity to penicillins precludes their use, alternatives include sulfonamides (triple and sulfonamides—equal parts of sulfadiazine, sulfamerazine, and sulfamethazine, 0.5 g per day for children less than 25 kg in weight and 1.0 g per day for those over 25 kg); erythromycin or clindamycin (250 mg twice daily for small children and 500 mg twice daily for larger children and adults); and possibly cephalexin or cephradine (125 mg twice daily for small children and 250 mg twice daily for large children and adults).

Even with continuous use of penicillin, prevention of infection by group A *S. pyogenes* may fail and rheumatic fever may recur. In one study, clinically overt pharyngitis was proved to be streptococcal by culture, serology, or both in 11 of 146 persons given benzathine penicillin by injection each month. An additional 13 asymptomatic patients developed serologic evidence of infection. Of these 24 patients, 2 developed rheumatic fever recurrences. None of the ten who failed to show an antibody response to group A streptococci isolated for their throat cultures had recurrences of rheumatic fever, suggesting mere colonization by the organism.

Many explanations for such prophylactic failures have been suggested. Failure to take peroral medication is probably a common cause, but cannot account for the failure of benzathine penicillin. Possibly, variation in the rate of absorption and excretion of the intramuscularly deposited penicillin results in periods when the concentrations of the drug are inadequate for protection from colonization and infection—a situation more likely to occur toward the end of the month.

In addition to postrheumatic fever prophylaxis, some physicians routinely treat siblings of children who have streptococcal pharyngitis (*e.g.,* pencillin V, 15 mg/kg body wt/day, PO, as 4 equal portions, 6-hourly, for 10 days). However, identification of carriers of group A streptococci by culture, and prophylaxis only for those positive on culture, is the preferred method of preventing infection in close contacts of a case of streptococcal pharyngitis. This approach avoids needless exposure to potentially sensitizing doses of penicillin.

Prophylaxis for the prevention of endocarditis in patients with rheumatic heart disease who must undergo a procedure that may produce bacteremia should not be confused with long-term prophylaxis to prevent recurrences of rheumatic fever.

Prevention of Infections at Particular Sites

RECURRENT URINARY TRACT INFECTION
(Chap. 48, Urethritis and Cystitis,
and Chap. 49, Bacterial Prostatitis
and Recurrent Urinary Tract Infections)

Some women experience repeated urinary tract infections (UTIs) at relatively frequent intervals. When the frequency of such infections exceeds two in any 12-month period, the physician should consider prophylaxis. Both trimethoprim-sulfamethoxazole, ½ tablet, and nitrofurantoin, 100 mg daily at bedtime, have been shown in 6-month trials of continuous prophylaxis to reduce recurrence of UTI, though the former regimen may be more effective. However, when prophylaxis is discontinued, the incidence of UTI returns to pretreatment levels—there appears to be no residual beneficial effect of prophylaxis, that is, prophylaxis would have to be administered for years for persistent good effect. Such prolonged chemoprophylaxis carries a theoretical risk of toxicity; however, the more frequent and troublesome the infections, the more justifiable long-term prophylaxis becomes.

A second approach to this problem has been to prescribe a single dose of an antimicrobic (nitrofurantoin, cephalexin, nalidixic acid, and penicillin G have all been used successfully) following sexual intercourse, in women whose infections seem temporally related to intercourse.

TRAVELERS' DIARRHEA (Chap. 60, Gastroenterocolitis Syndromes, and Chap. 61, Diarrheal Disease Caused by *Escherichia coli*)

Approximately 50% to 60% of persons from developed countries who travel to developing countries experience an episode of travelers' diarrhea (TD). The disease is often incapacitating in its severity. It is due most frequently to enterotoxinogenic strains of *Escherichia coli.* Not surprisingly, antimicrobics active against such strains appear to be effective in preventing TD, at least temporarily.

Doxycycline, taken PO in a dose of 100 mg/day, reduces the incidence of diarrhea to less than 10% for periods up to 3 weeks without serious side-effects. However, theoretical drawbacks to the routine use of doxycycline for prevention of TD include (1) augmenting the prevalence of tetracycline-resistant enterotoxinogenic *E. coli* (both properties appeared to be carried on the same plasmid); (2) increasing the transmission of R factors carrying resistance to the tetracyclines, other drugs, and toxinogenicity; (3) altering the intestinal flora, thus abrogating a protection from infection with salmonellas and shigellas (routinely tetracycline resistant); and (4) encouraging travelers to ignore basic preventive practices such as avoidance of contaminated food and water.

SURGICAL WOUND INFECTIONS

Since the advent of antibacterial agents, many surgeons have asserted that administration of antimicrobics to prevent complicating postoperative infections as effective. On the other hand, it has been argued that in many cases, such surgical chemoprophylaxis constituted overuse, or inappropriate use, of antimicrobial agents. As is often the case, proponents of each point of view were partially correct. Well-designed and well-executed clinical investigations have enabled recognition of the variables that influence the effectiveness of surgical prophylaxis. In many situations, the usefulness of chemoprophylaxis has been confirmed and quantitated. There is also ample evidence to establish that (1) there are many surgical operations in which chemoprophylaxis does not result in a measurable decrease in rates of infection and (2) short courses of antimicrobics (1 or 2 doses) are as effective as long courses of treatment. These findings provide strong support for the concepts of reserving antimicrobial agents for use in operations in which they have demonstrated effectiveness, and using the shortest course of prophylaxis documented to be effective. The principles basic to the rational use of antimicrobics in the prophylaxis of infections complicating surgical operations are given in the list below.

PRINCIPLES OF CHEMOPROPHYLAXIS OF INFECTIONS COMPLICATING SURGICAL OPERATIONS

Limit use of prophylaxis to procedures associated with relatively high rates of postoperative sepsis (>3-5%) (*e.g.*, colorectal surgery), or in which the consequences of infection are catastrophic (*e.g.*, cardiac valve replacement or total hip replacement).

Use antimicrobial agent(s) effective against the major anticipated contaminating bacterial species.

Use antimicrobics of the lowest possible toxicity and cost to the patient.

Avoid use of first-line therapeutic drugs.

Administer antimicrobics sufficiently in advance of an operation to permit absorption and distribution to the tissues, but not so far ahead of time that development of bacterial resistance is promoted.

Prolonged administration (24–48 hours) is not indicated in clean or clean-contaminated surgery.

Maintain serum and tissue concentrations of the antimicrobic(s) above the minimum inhibitory concentration of expected contaminating species throughout the procedure.

Monitor patient for side-effects of chemoprophylaxis.

If postoperative sepsis occurs, it will probably be caused by microorganisms resistant to the antimicrobial agent(s) used prophylactically.

There are three general influences on the incidence of surgical wound infection associated with various procedures. These are (1) the kind of surgical procedure, defined primarily by the degree of bacterial contamination that occurs at the surgical site; (2) the patient risk factors; and (3) the skill and routine practices of the surgeon.

Perhaps most influential in determining the expected surgical wound infection (SWI) rate for a given procedure is the degree of bacterial contamination of the operative site. A classification scheme useful in predicting the risk of SWI is presented in Table 19-1. The relatively wide range in the rates of postoperative infections is consistent with the interplay of many factors, including not only the number of bacteria contaminating the operative site, but also increasing age (the effect is measurable in persons more than 45 years old; duration of hospitalization prior to operation (this may reflect underlying disease or disability); duration of surgical procedures (the effect is measurable after 2 hours); the presence of infection at sites remote from the operative site at the time of surgical operation; glucosteroid therapy; morbid obesity; malnutrition; and probably diabetes mellitus. Local wound factors are also important: the competency of the blood supply to the injured tissues; the adequacy of postoperative drainage of loculated fluids; and presence of a foreign body in the operative site. The contributions of many of these factors to the risk of SWI have not been quantitated. As a result, it is often difficult to predict whether a patient with certain of these risk factors who must undergo a normally low-risk procedure is actually at sufficient risk of SWI to warrant chemoprophylaxis.

Possible overuse of antimicrobics in surgical chemoprophylaxis is of concern on 2 counts: the hazard posed to patients and communities (see list below) and the high cost of these agents ($10–$500 per course of prophylaxis—accounting for 25%–35% of all antimicrobics used in hospitals).

Specific recommendations for commonly performed surgical operations are outlined in Table 19-2. In general, cephalosporins are the most useful drugs for surgical prophylaxis. Cefazolin is preferred for routine chemoprophylaxis of clean and clean-contaminated procedures in which aerobic gram-positive cocci and common enteric gram-negative bacilli frequently cause postoperative wound infections. A relatively nontoxic drug, cefazolin may be given by IM injection (desirable for convenience and low cost); because it has a relatively long half-life in the blood, 6-hourly dosage is appropriate. Cefoxitin

Table 19-1. *Relationship of Classification of Surgical Procedures and Incidence of Postoperative Wound Infections*

Classification	% infected: OVERALL*	% infected: RANGE†
Class I (about 75% of surgical operations)		
Clean—The gastrointestinal, respiratory, and urinary tracts are not entered; no inflammation is encountered when normal tissues are incised; no breaks in aseptic technique occur; and there has been no preceding trauma.	2	1–5
Class II (about 15% of surgical operations)		
Clean-contaminated—A contaminated area is entered but there is no significant spillage. Cholecystectomy, incidental appendectomy, and hysterectomy are included in this category if no inflammation is present.	9	5–25
Class III (about 5% of surgical operations)		
Contaminated—Acute inflammation (without pus) is encountered or gross spillage from a hollow viscus occurs. Fresh traumatic wounds (<4 hours old and operations in which a major break in aseptic technique occurs are included.	18	15–50
Class IV (about 5% of surgical operations)		
Dirty—Pus spillage, or perforation of a viscus, and traumatic wounds untreated for >4 hours are included in this category.	42	40–60
Overall surgical wound infections	5	5–10

*Overall rates in patients who received various forms of chemoprophylaxis.
†Range of rates of infection without chemoprophylaxis.

HAZARDS OF CHEMOPROPHYLAXIS

- Direct toxicity of antimicrobics
- Alteration of the normal flora of the patient
- Promotion of resistance in the patient's own flora
- Surgical wound infection with resistant organisms
- Promotion of resistance in the nosocomial flora
- Failure of chemoprophylaxis
- Excessive cost

Table 19-2. *Summary of Bacteriology, Infection Rates, and Recommended Chemoprophylaxis of Surgical Wound Infection*

Surgical Operation	Reported SWI Rates	Infection Rates‡		Primary Pathogens	Recommended Prophylaxis	High Risk/Comments
		Placebo	Prophylaxis			
General						
Clean procedures (I)†						
Excisional breast biopsy	0.3–2.2			*Staphylococcus aureus,* group A *Streptococcus pyogenes*	Cephalosporin ‖	Rates <3–5%, particularly if infections are superficial and inconsequential, and do not warrant prophylaxis.
Modified radical mastectomy	4.3					
Vagotomy and pyloroplasty	6.0					
"Negative" laparotomy	5–7.8					
Inguinal hernia	0.5–1.9					
Splenectomy	0.7					
Thyroidectomy	1–2.2					
Nephrectomy (unilateral)	3.6					
Clean-contaminated (II)						
Biliary	1.2–27*	9.6 27*	1.2 4*	Enteric gram-negative bacilli, especially *Escherichia coli, Klebsiella* spp; *Staphylococcus aureus,* group D *Streptococcus* spp.	Cephalosporin ‖	Age >70, common duct stone, obstructive jaundice, acute cholecystitis.
Gastroduodenal	2–30*	25	10			Low gastric acidity, outlet obstruction, bleeding, low motility.
Elective colorectal	10–50*	10–25	5	Anaerobes, including *Bacteroides fragilis;* enteric gram-negative bacilli as above; *Staphylococcus aureus,* group D *Streptococcus* spp.	Oral 1 g neomycin plus 1 g enteric coated erythromycin at 1 P.M., 2 P.M., and 11 P.M., preoperatively Parenteral cefoxitin, 2 g, IV, just before anesthesia is induced, and every 4 hours for 12–24 hours; *or* tobramycin 1.7 mg/kg body weight plus clindamycin 600 mg, IV, just before anesthesia is induced	Abdominoperineal colon resection
Contaminated-dirty (III–IV)						
Abdominal trauma	40–70	?	7–15	Same as elective colorectal	Gentamicin plus clindamycin, IV, in full therapeutic dose for 5–10 days; stop if no perforation of bowel is found. Cefoxitin may be as effective	Empiric *treatment,* not true prophylaxis

Table 19-2. (continued) *Summary of Bacteriology, Infection Rates, and Recommended Chemoprophylaxis of Surgical Wound Infection*

Vascular						
Grafting Procedures (I)	0–12*	7 12*	1 3*	*Staphylococcus aureus,* enteric gram-negative bacilli	Cephalosporin‖ No prophylaxis for procedures restricted to brachiocephalic arteries	High-risk group includes abdominal aortic resection and femoral lower leg bypass. Prophylaxis may be continued 48–72 hours until vascular monitoring catheters are removed.
Obstetric–Gynecologic						
Clean-Contaminated (II) (numbers in parentheses indicate "febrile morbidity")§						
Vaginal hysterectomy	12–33* (15–70*)	25 (50)	2–8 (2–8)	Mixed aerobic–anaerobic infection, *Staphylococcus aureus, Streptococcus* spp. of Groups B, A, D	Cephalosporin#	Premenopausal women are at higher risk of infection following hysterectomy.
Abdominal hysterectomy	15* (50*)	15 (50)	4–8 (4–15)			
Cesarean section	3–25* (15–40*)	25 (40*)	10 (12–20*)			
Orthopedic						
Clean (I)						
Joint replacement	1–6*	2–6	1	*Staphylococcus aureus, Staphylococcus epidermis, Streptococcus pyogenes*	Cephalosporin‖	Prophylaxis may also decrease late (>6 months postoperative) site infections.
Total hip	1–6*	2–6	1			
Hip fracture	1–5*	1–5	1			
Miscellaneous, short duration, no foreign body inserted	1–5*	3–5	3		None	
Contaminated-Dirty (III–IV)	14	14	2	*Staphylococcus aureus,* group A *Streptococcus pyogenes,* aerobic gram-negative bacilli, *Clostridium* spp.	Cephalosporin‖	Empiric *treatment,* not true prophylaxis
Cardiovascular–thoracic						
Clean						
Valve replacement				*Staphylococcus aureus, Staphylococcus epidermis, Streptococcus* spp. gram-negative aerobic bacilli	Cephalosporin‖	Prophylaxis may be continued 48–72 hours until vascular monitoring catheters are removed.
Wound	1–4	?	1–4			
Endocartitis	?	?	≤1			
Coronary artery bypass graft	1–2	1–2	1–2	*Staphylococcus aureus, Staphylococcus epidermis,* group A *Streptococcus pyogenes*	Cephalosporin‖	Maintain inhibitory level throughout bypass.
Clean-contaminated (II)						
Pulmonary resection	17–50	17–50	17–19	*Staphylococcus aureus, Hemophilus influenzae*	Cephalosporin‖	One study shows benefit, another shows no benefit of cephalosporin prophylaxis.

Table 19-2. (continued) *Summary of Bacteriology, Infection Rates, and Recommended Chemoprophylaxis of Surgical Wound Infection*

Otorhinolaryngologic Clean-contaminated (II)	10–87	87	38	*Staphylococcus aureus*, *Streptococcus* spp., *Klebsiella* spp., anaerobic bacteria	Cephalosporin#	Investigational trial of cefoxitin vs. cefazolin is needed.
Ophthalmic Clean (I)†	—	—	—	*Staphylococcus aureus*, gram-negative aerobic bacilli	None, or an amino-cyclitol (*e.g.*, gentamicin) sub-conjunctivally	
Urologic (II–IV) Transurethral prostatectomy	50 (bacteriuria)			Gram-negative bacilli, group D *Streptococcus* spp.	Specific treatment of preoperative bacteriuria	Bacteriuria should be treated prior to prostatectomy

*Indicates presence of high risk group—see right hand column.
†Wound classification.
‡Data derived from controlled studies.
§Many gynecologists institute 3–5 days of empiric antimicrobial therapy in patients with "febrile morbidity."
‖Cefazolin, 1 g, IM or IV, every 6 hours beginning 30–60 minutes preoperatively and continuing throughout the procedure.
#Cefoxitin may have advantages over cefazolin in this procedure; dosage is 2 g, IV, every 4 hours, beginning 30–45 minutes prior to the procedure and continuing throughout.

may be preferable for chemoprophylaxis when anaerobic bacteria are likely to contribute to wound sepsis, as in gynecologic and large bowel surgery and in radical head and neck cancer surgery. Vancomycin is useful in patients allergic to the penicillins for chemoprophylaxis in clean surgery in which gram-positive aerobic cocci produce a majority of the SWI, for example, high-risk orthopedic procedures. Oral neomycin-erythromycin is effective in reducing SWI in elective colorectal surgery.

The use of antimicrobics in dirty (Class IV) surgery is in fact empiric therapy, not chemoprophylaxis. Consequently, antimicrobial agents of first choice against the pathogens most likely to cause infection should be administered in full therapeutic doses for periods appropriate to therapy, not prophylaxis.

In most instances, particularly elective clean surgery, a single dose of a cephalosporin such as cefazolin, 1 g, IV or IM, 30 to 45 minutes prior to surgery, has produced excellent results that are not improved upon by much longer periods of treatment. A second dose may be given 4 hours after the first if the procedure is prolonged. Perhaps only in cardiac valve replacement should treatment for 2 to 3 days be given routinely, since a foreign body has been implanted and intravascular pressure monitoring catheters are generally left in place for 24 to 72 hours postoperatively.

Periodic auditing of surgical prophylactic use of antimicrobic should be carried out by the hospital medical staff. The audit should answer the following questions: (1) has the surgeon chosen chemoprophylactic antimicrobics that are appropriate for the patient and the operation; (2) was the drug correctly prescribed, taking into account route of administration, dose, dosage interval, and duration of treatment; (3) did the patient receive the drug as ordered; (4) was an inhibitory concentration of the drug likely to be present in the patient's serum or operative site throughout the operation; and (5) could a less expensive or less toxic regimen have provided equal efficacy. Auditing teams should include members of the surgical staff as well as physicians, nurses, pharmacists, and administrators. The goal is improved use of antimicrobial agents to achieve maximum benefit at lowest cost with the least toxicity to the patient and minimal adverse effect on the hospital community.

Prevention of Infections in Compromised Hosts

Persons may become prone to infection as a result of breakdown in normal barriers to infection, diseases resulting in immune system dysfunction, or treatment of noninfectious diseases with immunosuppressive drugs. The variety of microorganisms that produce infection in such vulnerable persons is so great that chemoprophylaxis is infeasible—no antimicrobial agent or combination of agents is sufficiently effective or nontoxic to be used routinely. There are a few exceptions, for example, the prevention of burn wound sepsis and the prevention of some infections that occur in severely neutropenic patients.

BURN WOUND SEPSIS

Burn wounds render the patient susceptible to infection in direct proportion to the area of skin that has been destroyed. Despite advances in the care of burn wounds, they always become infected, usually repeatedly. General care of the patient is of primary importance in the success of treatment and in prevention and amelioration of infection. However, selective use of antimicrobial agents as adjunctive therapy is effective in reducing infectious complications. In the immediate postburn period, wound sepsis and septicemia are caused most frequently by either *Streptococcus pyogenes* or *Streptococcus pneumoniae.* Treatment with moderate doses of penicillin G prophylactically (2–5 million units per day in 4–6 equal doses) has markedly decreased early mortality from this cause. Later infections are most commonly caused by aerobic or facultative gram-negative bacilli, predominantly *Pseudomonas aeruginosa,* or by *Staphylococcus aureus.* These later infections may be reduced in frequency and severity by use of topical application of silver nitrate solutions, mafenide cream (10% paraaminoethylbenzene sulfonamide acetate), or 1% silver sulfadiazene ointment. Systemic chemoprophylaxis chosen on the basis of the predominant bacterial species in the eschar (usually an aminocyclitol, because the predominant bacteria are most often relatively resistant gram-negative bacilli) is useful. When the numbers of bacteria approach 10^4 to 10^5 per gram of eschar, septicemia is likely to occur; empiric antibacterial therapy and surgical intervention must be considered. In addition, empiric therapy for 3 to 5 days is frequently indicated because of systemic manifestations of sepsis.

Inconclusive Chemoprophylaxis

Prevention of Specific Diseases

In several infectious diseases, rigorous proof of prevention of infection by the administration of antimicrobial agents is generally lacking; yet, the physician often puts aside unease at lack of proof and gives antimicrobial agents. The choice of agent(s) and the manner of use (dosage form, route, frequency, duration of administration) depend on informed guesses about the microorganism(s) most likely to be encountered and on the evaluation of underlying diseases that contribute to vulnerability.

POSTSTREPTOCOCCAL GLOMERULONEPHRITIS
(Chap. 101, Streptococcal Skin Infections and Glomerulonephritis)

The occurrence of hemorrhagic glomerulonephritis (GN) as a complication of infection by certain strains of group A *S. pyogenes* is apparently predominantly a function of peculiarities of the parasite rather than of the host. In support of this view are the findings of (1) a clustering of cases among contacts of an index case, indicating communication of a nephritogenic strain of *S. pyogenes,* and (2) association with infection by particular strains of *S. pyogenes* (type 12, predominantly; also types 4, 25, 1, and others). Type-specific antistreptococcal immunity is also protective immunity, and if the immune response is not curtailed by effective antimicrobial therapy, type-specific protection may persist for decades. Acknowledging, in addition, that not all strains of a given type of group A *S. pyogenes* are nephritogenic, the futility of attempting to prevent recurrences of acute glomerulonephritis is apparent.

However, all persons with acute glomerulonephritis should be treated as though they have active streptococcal infection, for any source of continuing streptococcal antigenic stimulation must be eliminated. Benzathine penicillin G is the preferred agent and should be given by IM injection of 600,000 units in each of two sites (1.2 million units, total); for those under 25 kg in body weight, a total dose of 600,000 units is sufficient. If peroral therapy is preferred, penicillin V can be used: 15 mg/kg body wt/day, PO, as 4 equal portions, 6-hourly, for 10 days. Cephalexin or cephradine, and erythromycin are alternative agents for use in those with hypersensitivity to penicillins (same dosage as for penicillin V).

In the setting of epidemic glomerulonephritis, chemoprophylaxis should be given to all contacts of persons afflicted with acute GN, for example, members of the patient's family, and closed community groups such as the military, Indian tribes, and eleemosynary institutions. Benzathine penicillin G, injected as previously described, is again the preferred agent. Peroral penicillin V may also be used for 3 days; cephalexin, cephradine, or erythromycin may be prescribed for patients with hypersensitivity to the penicillins.

CLOSTRIDIAL INFECTIONS
(Chap. 126, Tetanus,
and Chap. 156, Gas Gangrene)

Gas gangrene and tetanus have their origin in contamination of wounds. Classically, gas gangrene complicates dirty, ragged wounds involving areas of deep muscle; tetanus may spring from superficial, trivial wounds. The primary preventive measure is adequate surgical debridement to rid the wound of all foreign materials and devitalized tissue. In itself, this is an impossible task, for small tags of nonviable tissue and tiny clots are always left in a wound carpeted with bacteria. Antibacterial chemoprophylaxis is a secondary measure and may be of value if thorough surgical debridement has been carried out.

Clostridium spp. contaminate wounds as spores. Spores *per se* are harmless and are not affected by systemically applied antimicrobial agents. Vegetative clostridia, the actual producers of exotoxins, are susceptible to penicillin G and to many other antimicrobics. Germination of clostridial spores requires a low redox potential, as is provided by dead tissue and the immediate environs of foreign bodies embedded in tissues. Thus, the very conditions favoring vegetative outgrowth of *Clostridium* spp. from spores are those in which absent or limited circulation of the blood also assures inadequate delivery of antimicrobial agents. Chemoprophylaxis is most effective if begun before anaerobic necrobiosis attains self-perpetuity, that is, within 1 to 2 hours of injury, or no later than the time when the patient is being prepared for surgical debridement.

Penicillin G is the agent of choice and must be given in large doses: 150 mg (240,000 units)/kg body wt/day, IV, (as 6 equal portions, 4-hourly, or by continuous IV infusion) for at least 4 days. Tetracycline, 10 mg/kg body wt/day, IV, as 4 equal portions, 6-hourly, may be a useful adjunct.

Prevention of Infections at Particular Sites

INFECTIVE ENDOCARDITIS
(Chap. 134, Infective Endocarditis)

Prevention of infective endocarditis (IE) is frustrated by lack of (1) identifiable bacteremia-producing procedures or events in at least 80% of patients and (2) any valvular or cardiac abnormalities that predispose to the development of IE in about 50% of patients. However, the consequences of IE are disastrous, and the cause–effect relationship between bacteremia-producing procedures and subsequent endocarditis is medical dogma. Hence, the prudent physician or dentist must at least *consider* administering theoretically effective chemoprophylaxis to any patient with a predisposing cardiac lesion who undergoes a procedure known to produce bacteremia. The following brief analysis of the components of procedure-related IE may assist the practitioner with decisions about chemoprophylaxis.

The first component is the nature of the patient's cardiac lesion. Most cases of IE that are apparently secondary to cardiac lesions occur in patients with rheumatic heart disease, congenital heart disease, prolapsing mitral valve with murmur, prosthetic valve, or previous IE. The risk of developing IE in cardiac lesions is apparently related to the degree of injury or alteration of the endocardium, turbulence of blood flow near the lesion, fibrin/platelet deposition, and other blood and tissue factors that retard or enhance bacterial adherence to the site. As a rule of thumb, persons at relatively high risk should be given prophylaxis more liberally than those with lower risk. For example, a patient with a prosthetic valve or previous IE should probably be given prophylaxis even for a relatively low-risk procedure such as colonoscopy or liver biopsy. If a procedure is known to produce bacteremia, chemoprophylaxis of patients at highest risk is the most prudent course.

The second component is the microorganisms involved in IE. Viridans streptococci and coagulase-positive staphylococci are the most frequent causative bacteria. Many viridans streptococci produce dextran, which promotes adherence to mucosal surfaces and, experimentally, to endocardial surfaces. *Staphylococcus aureus* also adheres well to tissue surfaces and induces fibrin/platelet deposition. In contrast, many of the organisms that cause endocarditis rarely (but commonly cause bacteremia), such as *E. coli,* not only adhere poorly to endothelium but also are killed by humoral antibodies and complement.

The third component of this problem is the procedure. Certain procedures are associated with a high incidence of bacteremia and have been empirically assigned the highest risk of causing IE. The relative risk of bacteremia for various procedures is given in Table 19-3. It is likely that risk from a given procedure is related to frequency of bacteremia, density of bacteremia (high numbers of bacteria per ml of blood) and the organism (streptococci *cf.* enteric bacilli). Procedures that only rarely cause bacteremia should not prompt prophylaxis except, perhaps, in extremely vulnerable patients.

The choice of the antimicrobic, or antimicrobics, used in chemoprophylaxis depends on the site of origin of the bacteremia, the pharmacokinetics of the drug(s), the allergic diathesis of the patient, and

Table 19-3. Percentage of Patients Developing Bacteremia Following Various Procedures

High Risk		Intermediate Risk		Low Risk	
Prostatectomy–infected urine		Prostatectomy–sterile urine		Sigmoidoscopy	2–10
Transurethral	58	Transurethral	11	Colonoscopy	3–6
Retropubic	82	Retropubic	13	IUD insertion	0
Esophageal dilation, unsterile dilator	100	Barium enema	11	Parturition	0.5
Tonsillectomy	28–38	Liver Biopsy	3–13	Esophageal dilation, sterile dilator	0
Dental extraction	18–85	Rigid bronchoscopy	15	Fiberoptic bronchoscopy	0
Peridontal surgery	21–28	Nasotracheal intubation	16	Orotracheal intubtion	0
Burn surgery	46	Nasotracheal suctioning, intensive care patients	16		
Surgery of infected areas	54				

(After Flynn NM, Lawrence RM: Antimicrobial prophylaxis. Med Clin North Am 63:1225–1244, 1979)

the severity of the predisposing cardiac lesion. The guidelines given in Table 134-9 may be modified as necessary to accommodate unusual circumstances.

The probability of compliance with a prescribed regimen is another variable that affects the decision to undertake chemoprophylaxis. While parenteral administration generally assures adequate concentrations of antimicrobics will be present in the blood when needed, peroral treatment is often more convenient and less painful, though less certain. If the risk of IE is high or the patient has a record of noncompliance, parenteral administration is necessary. If peroral treatment appears to be feasible, the patient must be forewarned of possible adverse effects such as the epigastric pain and nausea associated with erythromycin.

It is extremely important that patients with high-risk cardiac lesions be educated as to the need for prophylaxis whenever procedures likely to generate bacteremia are to be carried out, for example, dental manipulations. It must be the patient's responsibility to seek prophylaxis, but it is the physician's responsibility to make clear to the patient the lifelong need for prophylaxis.

CHRONIC OBSTRUCTIVE PULMONARY DISEASE

Encompassing singly or in combination chronic bronchitis, emphysema, and bronchiectasis, chronic obstructive pulmonary disease (COPD) is frequently complicated in the winter months by fever, malaise, and increase in quantity or purulence of sputum. Clinical demonstration of pneumonia is uncommon, but *S. pneumoniae* and *Haemophilus influenzae* are often ascendant in the sputum, and there may be a peripheral leukocytosis. Many studies, some controlled, appear to support the use of antimicrobics to prevent what appear to be bacterial infections complicating acute exacerbations of presumably viral causation. Several regimens are in use: tetracycline, 0.5 g every 12 hours, PO, for 10 to 14 days, and ampicillin, 250 mg to 500 mg 4 times a day for 10 to 14 days, among others. Such treatments provide no lasting benefits, although temporarily there may be a decrease in the quantity of sputum produced, the number of bacteria per unit volume, and the purulence. Ancillary features of management, such as postural drainage and the concomitant use of bronchodilator drugs and expectorant agents, may be of equal importance. Possibly the most useful prophylactic measure for patients with COPD is the administration of pneumococcal vaccine and annual influenza vaccination.

CEREBROSPINAL FLUID RHINORRHEA AND OTORRHEA

Trauma that results in the seepage of cerebrospinal fluid (CSF) is complicated by bacterial meningitis in 25% to 50% of cases, whereas overall only 6% of skull fractures are associated with infection. CSF rhinorrhea occurs in about 2% of patients with skull fractures, usually becoming evident within 2 days of the fracture and subsiding spontaneously within a week. This timing corresponds nicely with the timing of meningitis—more than half the cases occur within a week of fracture. *Streptococcus pneumoniae* clearly predominates as the causative bacteria, although staphylococci and various other streptococci are sometimes encountered.

Chemoprophylaxis, then, is indicated in patients who have sustained skull fractures and who have developed CSF rhinorrhea or otorrhea. When there is no indication for other agents, penicillin G, 600,000 units of the procaine derivative, by IM injection every 12 hours, should be given for 1 week or until leakage of CSF has ceased. Patients who develop signs of meningitis on this regimen should be considered infected with an organism resistant to penicillin until culture results are available.

Prevention of Infections in Compromised Hosts

CYSTIC FIBROSIS

There are nearly as many opinions on the use of prophylactic antimicrobics in patients with cystic fibrosis as there are centers for the treatment of the disease. On the other hand, there is agreement on the need for meticulous attention to supportive measures for preserving lung function, improving nutritional status, and treating exacerbations of infection when they occur. The tetracyclines, penicillinase-resistant penicillins, cephalosporins, trimethoprim-sulfamethoxazole, rifampin, and chloramphenicol have been prescribed blindly or with reference to the results of periodic cultures of expectorated sputum. A multicenter trial examining the effect of adding long-term prophylactic antimicrobics or placebo to the routine treatment of clinically apparent exacerbations of infection is needed to provide more information.

MALIGNANCY

Patients receiving chemotherapy for malignancies, particularly when they become severely granulocytopenic, are at high risk for serious infection with a wide variety of viral, bacterial, fungal, and protozoal organisms drawn primarily from the microbiota resident on or in the patients themselves. Bacterial infections are the most common, and much effort has been expended in devising preventive measures. Chemoprophylaxis alone or in combination with protected environments reduces infections and death from infection in large cancer treatment centers; however, remission rates and durations of survival may not be significantly improved. Various combinations of peroral and injected antimicrobics have been given, usually in large doses for weeks at a time. Adverse reactions to the drugs are common, and it is highly likely that such prolonged, high-dose administration selects for a resistant, in-hospital flora. There is some doubt whether such extensive use of antimicrobics is justified.

It is possible that trimethoprim-sulfamethoxazole given alone may reduce the incidence of clinical infections, but its usefulness for routine chemoprophylaxis remains to be defined. The combination is effective, however, in preventing pneumonia caused by *Pneumocystis carinii* in severely immunosuppressed patients. It should be given prophylactically if *P. carinii* is a frequent pathogen in a particular group of patients at a given institution. There appears to be considerable interinstitutional variation in the frequency of infection with this organism.

It is not surprising that attempts to protect severely immunocompromised patients from a wide variety of bacteria and fungi using antimicrobics prophylactically have met with only marginal success, and it is unlikely that the problems inherent in this endeavor will be overcome in the near future. The most effective management of severely compromised hosts with respect to infection remains meticulous attention to general preventive measures, careful observation, aggressive diagnostic intervention, and knowledgeable application of empiric and specific antimicrobial therapy.

POSTSPLENECTOMY

Surgical removal of the spleen predisposes the individual to increased risk of death from rapid, overwhelming infection with pneumococci, meningococci, or *H. influenzae.* The risk may be as high as 5% to 10% in young children splenectomized for congenital hemolytic anemia or Hodgkin's disease. It is slighter for adults and for persons who have had splenectomy following trauma. Up to one-half of patients whose splenectomy follows trauma apparently maintain splenic function either from accessory spleens or, more commonly, from implantation of splenic cells into the peritoneum with formation of nodules of functional splenic tissue. It is not clear whether the risk of overwhelming sepsis declines with time following splenectomy.

There is controversy as to the advisability and effectiveness of prolonged chemoprophylaxis with peroral penicillin in preventing septic death post-splenectomy. It may well be advisable in young children who have undergone elective or staging splenectomy. It should be considered for patients with posttrauma splenectomy for a period of 2 to 3 years following operation. Penicillin V, 7 to 10 mg/kg body wt/day, PO, as 2 equal portions, 12-hourly, is appropriate. However, pneumococci that are relatively resistant to penicillin may still pose a threat.

Pneumococcal vaccine should be administered to all patients who have undergone splenectomy and to patients who are being evaluated for splenectomy as soon as the procedure is considered. Giving the vaccine as early as possible prior to splenectomy may improve antibody response to it.

Ineffective Chemoprophylaxis

Clinicians frequently rationalize the use of antimicrobial agents for the prevention of infection simply because antimicrobics and the resources for administering them are available and because complicating infections are known to occur in a particular setting. The recognized guidelines for chemoprophylaxis are pushed aside by the psychological imperative to treat. Physicians should recognize their tendency to choose treatment or prophylaxis over nonintervention, even though risk of infectious disease is exceedingly small.

Examples of the ineffective use of prophylactic antimicrobics include prevention of bacterial pneumonia in patients with measles, influenza, poliomyelitis, the common cold, cardiac failure, respiratory failure with prolonged intubation, and urinary tract infections in patients with prolonged bladder catheterization by using irrigants containing antimicrobial agents. The law of diminishing returns is often operative—for example, it is not reasonable to administer 200 to 300 doses of a cephalosporin to 100 patients in order to prevent a single minor wound infection in a clean operative procedure that has an SWI rate of less than 1% when chemoprophylaxis is not given. It is costly and results in more morbidity from side-effects than it prevents by reducing wound infections.

Bibliography

Book

KEIGHLEY MRB, BURDON DW: Antimicrobial prophylaxis in surgery. Tunbridge Wells, England, Pittman Medical, 1979. 241 pp.

Journals

BAUER DJ, ST. VINCENT L, KEMPE CH, DOWNIE AW: Prophylactic treatment of smallpox contacts with *N*-methylisatin β-thiosemicarbasone (Compound 33T57, Marboran). Lancet 2:494–496, 1963

BEAM WE JR, NEWBERG NR, DEVINE LF, PIERCE WE, DAVIES JA: The effect of rifampin on the nasopharyngeal carriage of *Neisseria meningitidis* in a military population. J Infect Dis 124:39–46, 1971

BECKER GD, PARELL GJ: Cefazolin prophylaxis in head and neck cancer surgery. Ann Otolaryngol 88:183–186, 1979

BERGER SA, NAGAR H: Prophylactic antibodies in surgical procedures. Surg Gynecol Obstet 146:469–475, 1978

CARLSSON AS, LIDGREN L: Prophylactic antibiotics against early and late deep infections after total hip replacements. Acta Orthop Scand 48:405–410, 1977

CHETLIN SH, ELLIOTT DW: Preoperative antibiotics in biliary surgery. Arch Surg 107:319–332, 1973

CHODAK GW, PLAUT ME: Use of systemic antibiotics for prophylaxis in surgery. Arch Surg 112:326–334, 1977

CHODAK GW, PLAUT ME: Wound infections and systemic antibiotic prophylaxis in gynecologic surgery: A review. Obstet Gynecol 51:123–127, 1978

CONTE JE, COHEN SN: Antibiotic prophylaxis and cardiac surgery: A prospective double-blind comparison of single-dose versus multiple-dose regimens. Ann Intern Med 76:943–949, 1972

CROSSLEY K, GARDNER LC: Antimicrobial prophylaxis in surgical patients. JAMA 245:772–776, 1981

CRUSE PJE: Infection surveillance: Identifying the problems and the high-risk patient. South Med J 70:4–8, 1977

D'ANGELO LJ, SOKOL RJ: Short- vs long-course prophylactic antibiotic treatment in cesarean section patients. Obstet Gynecol 55:583–586, 1980

Editorial: Infections in leukaemia. Lancet 1:1294–1295, 1977

Editorial: Infective hazards of splenectomy. Lancet 1:1167–1172, 1976

EVERETT ED, HIRSCHMANN JV: Transient bacteremia and endocarditis prophylaxis: A review. Medicine 56:61–77, 1977

FEATHERS RS, LEWIS AAM: Prophylactic systemic antibiotics in colorectal surgery. Lancet 2:4–8, 1977

FEREBEE SH: Controlled chemoprophylaxis trials in tuberculosis: A general review. Adv Tuberc Res 17:28–106, 1969

FLYNN NM, LAWRENCE RM: Antimicrobial prophylaxis. Med Clin North Am 63:1225–1244, 1979

FUCHS GF: Criteria for prophylaxis in inactive tuberculosis. Arch Environ Health 10:937–941, 1965

FULLEN WD, HUNT J: Prophylactic antibiotics in penetrating wounds of the abdomen. J Trauma 12:282–289, 1972

GARROD LP, WATERWORTH PM: The risks of dental extraction during penicillin treatment. Br Heart J 24:39–46, 1962

GIBBONS RP, STARK RA: The prophylactic use—or misuse—of antibiotics in transurethral prostatectomy. J Urol 119:381–383, 1978

GIBBS RS, ST. CLAIR PJ: Bacteriologic effects of antibiotic prophylaxis in high-risk cesarean section. Obstet Gynecol 57:277–282, 1981

GOLDMAN DA, HOPKINS CC: Cephalothin prophylaxis in cardiac valve surgery: A prospective, double-blind comparison of two-day and six-day regimens. J Thorac Cardiovasc Surg 73:470–479, 1977

GOPAL V, BISNO AL: Fulminant pneumococcal infections in normal asplenic hosts. Arch Intern Med 137:1526–1530, 1977

GUTTLER RB, BEATY HN: Minocycline in the chemoprophylaxis of meningococcal disease. Antimicrob Agents Chemother 1:397–402, 1972

HASSELL TA, STUART KL: Rheumatic fever prophylaxis: A three year study. Br Med J 2:39–40, 1974

HEMLELL DL, CUNNINGHAM RG: Cefoxitin for prophylaxis in premenopausal women undergoing vaginal hysterectomy. Obstet Gynecol 56:629–634, 1980

HIRSCHMAN JV, INUI TS: Antimicrobial prophylaxis: A critique of recent trials. Rev Infect Dis 2:1–23, 1980

HUGHES WT, KUHN S, CHAUDHARY S, FELDMAN S, VARZOSA M, AUR

RJA, PRATT C, GEORGE SL: Successful chemoprophylaxis for *Pneumocystis carinii* pneumonitis. N Engl J Med 297:1419–1426, 1977

ITSKOVITZ J, FISHER M: The effect of a short-term course of antibiotic prophylaxis on patients undergoing total abdominal hysterectomy. Eur J Obstet Gynaecol Reprod Biol 11:101–107, 1980

JOHNSON EE, STOLLERMAN GH, GROSSMAN B: Rheumatic recurrences in patients not receiving continuous prophylaxis. JAMA 190:407–413, 1964

KAISER AB, CLAYSON KR: Antibiotic prophylaxis in vascular surgery. Ann Surg 188:283–289, 1978

KEIGHLEY MRB, ARABI Y: Comparison between systemic and oral antimicrobial prophylaxis in colorectal surgery. Lancet 1:894–897, 1979

KRAFT JK, STAMEY TA: The natural history of symptomatic recurrent bacteriuria in women. Medicine 56:55–59, 1977

LEDGER WJ, GEE C, LEWIS WP: Guidelines for antibiotic prophylaxis in gynecology. Am J Obstet Gynecol 121:1038–1045, 1975

MERSON MH: Doxycycline and the traveler. Gastroenterol 76:1485–1489, 1979

MOUNT RW, FEREBEE SH: Preventive effects of isoniazide in the treatment of primary tuberculosis in children. N Engl J Med 265:713–721, 1961

NICHOLS RL, BOIDO P, CONDON RE, GORBACH SL, NYHUS LM: Effect of preoperative neomycin–erythromycin intestinal preparation on the incidence of infectious complications following colon surgery. Ann Surg 178:453–462, 1973

PHELAN JP, PRUYN SC: Prophylactic antibiotics in cesarean section: A double-blind study of cefazolin. Am J Obstet Gynecol 133:474–478, 1979

POLK HC JR, LOPEZ–MAYOR JF: Postoperative wound infection: A prospective study of determinant factors and prevention. Surgery 66:97–103, 1969

Prevention of bacterial endocarditis in patients with valvular heart disease, prosthetic heart valves, and other abnormalities of the cardiovascular system. Med Lett Drugs Ther 23:92, 1981

Prevention of malaria in travelers. Morbid Mortal Week Rep Suppl 1982

Problems encountered with using Fansidar as prophylaxis for malaria Morbid Mortal Week Rep 31:232–234, 1982

REHU M, NILSSON CG: Risk factors for febrile morbidity associated with cesarean section. Obstet Gynecol 56:269–273, 1980

SMADEL JE: Influence of antibiotics on immunologic responses in scrub typhus. Am J Med 17:246–258, 1954

SPENCER WH III, THORNSBERRY C, MOODY MD, WENGER NK: Rheumatic fever chemoprophylaxis and penicillin-resistant gingival organisms. Ann Intern Med 73:683–687, 1970

STAMEY TA, CONDY M, MIHARA G: Prophylactic efficacy of nitrofurantoin macrocrystals and trimethoprim-sulfamethoxazole in urinary infections: Biologic effects on the vaginal and rectal flora. N Engl J Med 296:780–783, 1977

STONE HH, HOOPER CA: Antibiotic prophylaxis in gastric, biliary, and colonic surgery. Ann Surg 184:443–452, 1976

STRACHAN CJL, BLACK J: Prophylactic use of cefazolin against wound sepsis after cholycystectomy. Br Med J 1:1254–1256, 1977

Surg Clin North Am: Symposium on surgical infections and antibiotics. 55:1259–1474, 1975

TAGO Y, HORNICK RB, DAWKINS AT JR: Studies on induced influenza in man. I. Double-blind studies designed to assess prophylactic efficacy to amantadine hydrochloride against A_2/Rockville/1/65 strain. JAMA 203:1089–1094, 1968

TARANTA A, WOOD HF, FEINSTEIN AR, SIMPSON R, KLEINBERG E: Rheumatic fever in children and adolescents. A long-term epidemiologic study of subsequent prophylaxis, streptococcal infections, and clinical sequelae. IV. Relation of the rheumatic fever recurrence rate per streptococcal infection to the titers of streptococcal antibodies. Ann Intern Med (Suppl 5) 60:47–57, 1964

The Meningococcal Disease Surveillance Group: Meningococcal disease: Secondary attack rate and chemoprophylaxis in the United States, 1974. JAMA 235:261–265, 1976

TOMPKINS DG, BOXERBAUM B, LIEBMAN J: Long-term prognosis of rheumatic fever patients receiving regular intramuscular benzathine penicillin. Circulation 45:543–551, 1972

VOSTI KL: Recurrent urinary tract infections: Prevention by prophylactic antibiotics after sexual intercourse. JAMA 231:934–940, 1975

WINKELSTEIN JA: Splenectomy and infection. Arch Intern Med 137:1516–1517, 1977

WOOD HF, FEINSTEIN AF, TARANTA A, EPSTEIN JA, SIMPSON RR: Rheumatic fever in children and adolescents: A long-term epidemiologic study of subsequent prophylaxis, streptococcal infections, and clinical sequelae. III. Comparative effectiveness of three prophylaxis regimens in preventing streptococcal infections and rheumatic recurrences. Ann Intern Med (Suppl 5) 60:31–36, 1964

RUTH M. LAWRENCE
PAUL D. HOEPRICH

Immunoprophylaxis of Infectious Diseases

20

Very likely there was ancient observation of the special merit in surviving an infectious disease in terms of safety from future attacks on subsequent exposure to the same disease. However, the first definition of this phenomenon appears to have been the recognition in 1890 by Behring and Kitasato that acquired immunity to tetanus and to diphtheria resided in the blood plasma of animals that had been injected weeks before with sublethal doses of the respective toxins. The animals generated their own immunity—the acquisition of immunity was an *active* process.

As part of the proof that such protection was a property of the plasma, it was shown that animals fully susceptible to tetanus would acquire immunity if injected with plasma or serum from an immune animal. Such *passive* acquisition of immunity was soon put to use in the treatment of diptheria.

This early distinction between active and passive immunity also demonstrated the timing characteristics of acquired immunity. A period of several days or weeks is required before one exposure, or repeated exposures, to antigens result in active acquired immunity. On the other hand, if the dose of immune serum is adequate, passively acquired immunity is instantly effective.

There is another important difference. Not only does active immunity have the attractive connotation of self-help, but also it lasts longer than passively acquired immunity. Thus, immunity actively acquired in response to the injection of an antigen (*e.g.*, tetanal toxoid) is protective for several years without reinforcement. Passive antitetanus immunity acquired as homologous antibody (*e.g.*, antitetanal immunoglobulin of human origin) wanes in the weeks after injection, with a disappearance time corresponding to the normal catabolism of plasma proteins—that is, a half-life of 26 to 30 days. However, heterologous antibody (*e.g.*, tetanal antitoxin of equine origin), although prophylactic, is also antigenic in the human recipient. As a result, catabolism is especially rapid a week after administration (the half-life may be as short as 7 days) and serum sickness is frequently a complication.

Passive Immunoprophylaxis

Passive immunoprophylaxis should be possible with any infectious disease in which active immunization is possible. Although theoretically this is so, in fact, passive immunoprophylaxis and serotherapy have declined steadily in application. Several factors are important: (1) the morbid potential of injection of heterologous plasma proteins; (2) the development of agents for active immunization that are effective but not hazardous; (3) the discovery of specific antimicrobial drugs; and (4) the application on community, regional, and national bases of preventive measures such as sanitary engineering and vector control.

There are no reports of successful efforts at passive immunoprophylaxis of infections caused by fungi, rickettsias, chlamydias, or metazoan parasites. In Table 20-1, currently available passive immunoprophylaxis is listed by disease.

Antiviral

Gamma globulin (immune serum globulin, ISG), prepared from pooled human plasmas, is effective in preventing hepatitis A when administered within 1 to 2 weeks of exposure. It is recommended for close personal contacts of persons with hepatitis A and can also be employed for preexposure prophylaxis of travelers to areas of high risk.

The role of ISG in the prevention of hepatitis B has been more controversial. In some studies, standard ISG (with low or intermediate titers of antibody to hepatitis B virus) was thought to be less protective than hepatitis B immune globulin (HBIG) with high titers of antibody. When the two preparations were compared prospectively in a large cooperative study

Table 20-1. Passive Immunoprophylaxis

Disease	Antibody source and preparation	Dose and route of injection	Value	Adverse reactions
VIRUSES				
Hepatitis A (Chap. 70)	Human serum globulins	0.02–0.06 ml/kg body wt, IM	Definite	None
Hepatitis B (Chap. 71)	Human serum globulins	0.06 ml/kg body wt, IM	Definite	None
	Human hepatitis B immune globulin (HBIG)	0.06 mg/kg body wt, IM, repeat in 4 weeks	Definite	None
Mumps (Chap. 74)	Human hyperimmune serum globulins	5–10 ml, IM	Doubtful	Local pain, tenderness, induration
Measles (Chap. 86)	Human serum globulins	0.22 ml/kg body wt to prevent, IM; 0.04 ml/kg body wt to modify, IM	Definite	None
Rubella (Chap. 87)	Human serum globulins	20–50 ml, IM	Doubtful	Local pain, tenderness, induration
Smallpox and (Chap. 92)	Human hyperimmune serum globulins	0.3 ml/kg body wt, IM	Definite	None
Varicella (Chap. 93)	Human serum globulins	0.6 ml/kg body wt, IM	Slight	Local pain, tenderness, induration
	Human zoster serum globulins (ZIG), or Varicella–Zoster immune globulins (VZIG)	1.25–5.0 ml, IM	Definite	None
Poliomyelitis (Chap. 121)	Human serum globulins	0.35 ml/kg body wt, IM	Definite	None
Rabies (Chap. 124)	Horse serum, refined and concentrated	40 units/kg of body wt, part infiltrated in region of bite, the rest IM	Definite	Hypersensitivity; serum sickness
	Human immune serum globulins	20 units/kg of body wt	Definite	local pain, tenderness
BACTERIA				
Diphtheria (Chap. 25)	Horse serum, refined and concentrated	30,000–80,000 units, according to extent of membrane and degree of toxicity; IM and IV injection	Definite	Hypersensitivity; serum sickness
Pertussis (Chap. 29)	Human hyperimmune serum	20 ml IM	Unproved	Local pain, tenderness, induration
	Human hyperimmune serum globulins	2.5 ml IM	Unproved	None
Tetanus (Chap. 126)	Human immune serum globulins	250–500 units, IM	Definite	None
Botulism (Chap. 127)	Horse serum, refined and concentrated, trivalent (A, B, E)	Therapeutic 8–32 ml (about half IV/IM) depending on incubation period, severity, amount of incriminated food ingested. Per 8 ml: 7500 units A; 5500 units B; 8500 units E	Probable	Hypersensitivity; serum sickness
Gas Gangrene (Chap. 156)	Horse serum, refined and concentrated, pentavalent	26,000–104,000 units, IV	None	Hypersensitivity; serum sickness

of persons exposed by needlestick, there was no difference in protection against infection. However, disease occurred in 2% of the HBIG group and in 8% of the ISG group. As the administration of HBIG appeared to have induced passive–active immunity, it is recommended for prophylaxis in persons acutely exposed to blood or blood products positive for hepatitis B surface antigen and for babies born to mothers who are hepatitis B surface-antigen positive. HBIG may be protective for sexual contacts of persons with hepatitis B.

No attempt should be made to modify the course of mumps in children. In adults, however, it is possible, but not proved, that the probability of extrasalivary gland involvement, particularly orchitis, can be decreased by the injection of immunoglobulins of human origin during the incubation period (Chap. 74, Mumps).

In both measles (Chap. 86, Measles) and poliomyelitis (Chap. 121, Poliomyelitis), the situation is analogous to that in hepatitis A. There is a very high prevalence of these diseases; thus immunoglobulins obtained from pooled adult human plasmas always contain antibody. With measles, either modification or prevention can be accomplished if a suitable dose is given within 6 to 8 days of exposure (Table 20-1).

Lack of a predictable occurrence of antirubella antibody in lots of gamma globulin isolated from pooled human plasmas indicates that the effectiveness of immunoprophylaxis of rubella (Chap. 87, Rubella) is doubtful. Conflicting results were common in early trials, but as the dose of immunoglobulins was increased, suppression of the clinical mainifestations of rubella was the usual result. However, suppression is not necessarily prevention of infection. One-half of those given immunoglobulins who did not have clinical rubella nevertheless had the serologic responses characteristic of infection. Thus, protection of the fetus by passive immunoprophylaxis in the pregnant woman is still uncertain at best.

Immunoglobulins isolated from human plasma obtained 4 to 8 weeks after successful vaccination (vaccinia virus) are active against both smallpox and vaccinia viruses (Chap. 92, Smallpox and Other Poxvirus Infections). Significant protection against smallpox resulted when family contacts in India were given this material. Similarly, the spread of vaccinia was prevented in 25 children with eczema who either required vaccination or were exposed to recently vaccinated siblings, in 14 children in whom varicella became apparent after vaccination, and in 5 children who were burned after vaccination.

Pooled normal human serum immunoglobulins contain low titers of antibodies against varicella-zoster virus. As a consequence, tolerated doses cannot prevent disease, but may attenuate chickenpox if given within 3 days of exposure (Chap. 93, Varicella and Herpes Zoster). Because the disease is ordinarily benign, such passive immunomodification should be reserved for exposed persons under the age of 15 years who are vulnerable to serious consequences such as pneumonia and disseminated visceral disease. Vulnerable persons include those who have congenital or acquired immunodeficiencies, who have leukemia or lymphoma, and who require treatment with pharmacologic doses of glucosteroids, as well as infants born to mothers with varicella. Varicella-zoster immune globulin (VZIG), prepared from blood plasmas high in titer of complement-fixing varicella-zoster antibody, is much more effective than pooled normal human serum immunoglobulins; VZIG is actually preventive if given within 3 days of exposure. However, the supplies of VZIG are so limited that it is reserved for use in patients at risk of dire consequences as defined above.

From animal experiments, it is clear that passive immunoprophylaxis of rabies (Chap. 124, Rabies) requires the administration of the total dose of human rabies immune globulin within 24 hours of exposure. There appears to be no effect if treatment is delayed to 72 hours after exposure. Infiltration of the antiserum in and around the sites of bites is aimed at providing access of antibody to the extravascularly deposited virus. If injection of antiserum must be delayed beyond 24 hours (but less than 72 hours) from exposure, 2 to 3 times the usual recommended dose can be given. Multiple severe wounds around the face and neck are also indications for increasing the dosage of antiserum.

Antitoxic

Antitoxic immunity (diphtheria, tetanus, botulism), in affording specific neutralization of the most potent poisons that are known, is quite clear cut in its value to the patient. However, it must be borne in mind that clinical evidence of the diseases caused by bacterial exotoxins is at hand only after irreversible interaction between toxin molecules and host tissues has occurred. Passive acquisition of antitoxin, to be of greatest value, must be at the time of exposure, before there is overt disease.

In the case of diphtheria (Chap. 25, Diphtheria), there is some delay in the absorption of toxin from the membrane site of elaboration. Moreover, fixation by tissues of the host is not a rapid process. There is, then, some value to passive immunization when diphtheria is clinically apparent, although antitoxin is more effective the earlier in the disease that it is given (see Fig. 25-3).

With tetanus (Chap. 126, Tetanus), there is no

doubt about the prophylactic value of antitoxin given at, or very soon after, injury. Therapeutic administration of tetanal antitoxin when tetanus is overt is less firmly based, although there are both experimental and clinical data that support such use. There is less temporal leeway in passive immunoprophylaxis in tetanus than in diphtheria. For this reason, it is standard practice to give antitoxin in prophylaxis of tetanus to all persons with contaminated wounds who do not have a history of recently reinforced, active immunization. Adverse reactions are frequent with horse antitoxin; even the "refined and concentrated" preparations cause serum sickness in 15% to 30% of patients. Tetanal immunoglobulin of human origin is the preferred agent for passive immunization against tetanus. Because proteins of human origin are provided, the duration of immunity is greater than when heterologous proteins are delivered and there is no serum sickness.

The prophylactic value of botulinal antitoxin has been clearly demonstrated with experimental animals. From this, and from the clinical experience with other diseases caused by bacterial exotoxins, it is probable that immunoprophylaxis of botulism is possible. There is no proof, however, because exposure to botulism is virtually never suspected until the disease is overt. There is, however, proof of the utility of botulinal antitoxin in the treatment of botulism (Chap. 127, Botulism).

The prophylactic value of polyvalent gas gangrene antitoxin is unproved (Chap. 156, Gas Gangrene).

Antibacterial

It is probable that passive immunoprophylaxis of pertussis is achieved when antibody is given in the first week of incubation of the disease. The agent of choice is pertussis hyperimmune immunoglobulin of human origin (Chap. 29, Whooping Cough).

Passive serotherapy was used with good effect in pneumococcal pneumonia and in meningococcal meningitis. There is no certainty that antiserum is of any value in scarlet fever (antierythrogenic toxin) or in staphylococcal infections. Effective antimicrobial drugs have replaced these antiserums.

Active Immunoprophylaxis

Active immunoprophylaxis has been most clearly effective with bacterial exotoxins and viruses. At present, no useful immunizing preparations have been derived from fungi, chlamydias, protozoa, or metazoal parasites. Whole bacterial cells, mycoplasmas, rickettsias, and viruses vary from excellent to moderate effectiveness as immunogens. Substances presently available for active immunization are listed in Table 20-2. Some elaboration of this tabular material is appropriate.

Antiviral

Active immunization against viral infectious diseases has a long and successful history, beginning with Jenner's name-coining, epochal introduction of vaccinia virus inoculation in 1798. The introduction of hepatitis vaccine is the most recent development.

INFLUENZA

In persons who are not otherwise ill, influenza (Chap. 28, Influenza) is primarily a nuisance. However, in those with other diseases, particularly cardiopulmonary disease, metabolic disease (diabetes mellitus), age over 50 years, and pregnancy, (the increased mortality of pregnant women in the 1957–1958 pandemic was not seen before and has not occurred since), the stress of influenza may precipitate grave illness and death.

Two problems stand out with regard to active immunization against influenza. First, the extraordinary mutability of influenza viruses makes difficult the industrial production of an antigenically appropriate vaccine in advance of epidemic or pandemic influenza. Second, the immunity that results from the administration of the vaccine is effective for just one respiratory disease season, quite in contrast with the many years, even decades, of persistence of immunity earned by having had influenza.

Chemical (ether; tri-*n*-butyl phosphate) disruption of influenza viruses permits the discarding of antigenically unimportant components with preservation of the glycoprotein antigens (hemagglutinin and neuraminidase) important to immunogenicity. Such preparations are less likely to engender adverse reactions than are whole virus vaccines. Adjuvant mixtures secure more durable immunity, but are not well tolerated on injection. Side-effects are minimal with current vaccines. The Guillain–Barré syndrome (GBS) that followed immunization with swine influenza vaccine has not occurred with subsequent vaccines.

YELLOW FEVER

Attenuation of yellow fever virus by multiple tissue-culture passages yielded the 17D strain, which is grown in chick embryos for vaccine production. With the loss of hepatotropism, the 17D strain produces short-lived viremia and causes mild fever and malaise in some persons. The virus cannot grow in mosquitoes. Although immunity may last 15 years or more, vaccination at 10-year intervals is recommended. Yellow fever is controlled primarily through control of the vector (Chap. 73, Yellow Fever). Immunization is an adjunct, albeit an important one, for travelers in endemic areas and for those whose occupations involve exposure to the vectors of sylvatic yellow fever.

MUMPS

Mumps (Chap. 74, Mumps) generally runs a benign course in children, but meningitis or meningoencephalitis can occur. In adults, the frequency of complications such as overt meningoencephalitis, orchitis, and oophoritis, is higher than in children. Live, attenuated virus mumps vaccine (Jeryl–Lynn strain) causes antibody production in 95% of recipients and is recommended for all children at about 15 months of age. It is generally administered as combined measles–mumps–rubella (MMR) vaccine at age 15 months. Although the usual incubation period of 16 to 18 days (range: 2 to 3 weeks) theoretically gives time for active immunization, protection does not, in fact, result from postexposure inoculation of the attenuated, live-virus vaccine. The vaccine should not be given to pregnant women or to persons with compromised immunologic defenses.

MEASLES

The current live, attenuated measles virus vaccine (Schwarz and Attenuvax types) is extremely effective, producing immunity in 95% of patients immunized after the age of 15 months. It can be given alone or combined with rubella (MR) or (MMR). In the United States, proof of measles immunity is required for children entering kindergarten and first grade. Revaccination with live-virus vaccine is recommended for persons (now young adults) who previously received killed-virus vaccine. The risk of atypical measles in these persons exceeds the risk of a reaction (local pain, edema, fever) to the live-virus vaccine. Revaccination of persons who received live-virus vaccine or who had natural measles is not associated with an increase in vaccine reactions.

Live, attentuated measles virus vaccine should not be given to persons who are (1) pregnant; (2) ill with leukemias, lymphomas, or other general malignancies; (3) receiving immunosuppressive therapy (irradiation, alkylating agents, steroids, antimetabolites); (4) known to have tuberculosis or other severe febrile illnesses; (5) within 6 weeks of receipt of more than 0.025 ml human gamma globulin / kg body wt; or (6) hypersensitive to eggs, egg products, or feathers.

RUBELLA

Live rubella virus vaccine (RA 27/3) is recommended for all children over 1 year of age. It is given as a single subcutaneous injection. It is also recommended for susceptible adolescent and adult women to increase herd immunity and thereby decrease the risks of rubella-induced fetal injury. Because of the theoretical risk of the live vaccine virus to the fetus, RA 27/3 should not be given to pregnant women, and women should be advised not to become pregnant for 3 months following vaccination. Side-effects of rash, lymphadenopathy, arthralgias, or transient arthritis may occur and are more frequent in adult vaccinees. There is no evidence that use of the live rubella vaccine after exposure prevents the disease. The protection provided by the vaccine appears to be long-lived, and revaccination is not recommended.

SMALLPOX

Routine vaccination to prevent smallpox, that is, infection of a person with live vaccinia virus (a stable hybrid related to both smallpox and cowpox viruses) became obsolete with the achievement of global eradication of the disease in 1979. At this time smallpox vaccination is justified only for laboratory investigators working with vaccinia virus or other poxviruses.

Regardless of the vaccination experience of the person, unless some reaction occurs, vaccination must be considered a failure. The usual causes of failure are inactive virus, improper technique, or vaccination too early in infancy (virus neutralization by transplacentally acquired antibody). The typical evolution of primary vaccination and revaccination lesions is portrayed in Figure 92-4.

Complications of vaccination occur less often in children, particularly between 1 and 4 years of age, than in adults and are much less frequent in persons who were once vaccinated than in those never previously vaccinated. For example, in the United States, where childhood vaccination was nearly universal, postvaccinal encephalitis occurred in about 1 per 110,000 vaccinations. In young adults first vaccinated on entry into military training in the Netherlands, the incidence was 1 per 4000. The overall rate on revaccination was 1 per 50,000. While these data substantiate an increased hazard with increasing age at primary vaccination, it must be realized that different strains of vaccinia virus were used in the United States and Holland.

Postvaccinal encephalitis is an acute occurrence around the tenth day (range: 1–28 days) after vaccination. The clinical manifestations are in no way

Table 20-2. Active Immunoprophylaxis

Disease	Agent	Age Applicable	Dose				Adverse Reactions
			BASIC	BOOSTER	ROUTE	VALUE	
Viruses							
Influenza (Chap. 28)	Formalin-ethylene oxide inactivated multitypic, from chick embryos; either whole viruses or chemically split; epidemiologically current strains	>6 months	0.5 ml (700 CCA type A, 500 CCA type B) per month for two doses (half as much if <25 kg)	0.5 ml annually	Subcutaneous	75%–85%	Fever, malaise head and muscle aches, hypersensitivity to eggs and egg products
Hepatitis B (Chap. 71)	Formalin treated 22 nm HBsAg particles from plasma of human carriers	Any age	Two doses 1 month apart	One dose at 6 months	Intramuscular	>90%	Local pain, fever, fatigue
Yellow fever (Chap. 73)	Live, attenuated yellow fever virus from chick embryos	>6 months	0.5 ml	0.5 ml every 10 years if in endemic area	Subcutaneous	95%	Occasional, low-grade fever, malaise, headache, hypersensitivity to eggs and egg products
Mumps (Chap. 74)	Attenuated, live 5000 $TCID_{50}$/dose	>1 year	One dose	None	Subcutaneous	95%	Occasional mild induration
Measles (Chap. 86)	Live, attenuated virus from chick embryos 2000 $TCID_{50}$/dose	>12 months	0.5 ml	None	Subcutaneous	95%	Mild fever and rash in 15%
Rubella (Chap. 87)	Live attenuated virus from human diploid cells	>1 year to adulthood	One dose	None	Subcutaneous	>95%	Mild fever, anthralgia, arthritis, local induration
Variola (Chap. 92)	Live vaccinia virus, from calf lymph or chick embryos (10^3 pockforming units/ml)	>6 months	1 drop	1 drop every 3 years; annually if in endemic area	Multiple-pressure acupuncture	>90%	Fever, malaise, lymphadenopathy; local scarring
Poliomyelitis (Chap. 121)	Live, attenuated polio virus, types: **(1)** 800,000 $TCID_{50}$; **(2)** 100,000 $TCID_{50}$; **(3)** 500,000 $TCID_{50}$	>2 months	One dose, trivalent, at 8-week intervals for two doses, and a third dose 8–12 months later	One dose at 6 years of age after primary series or before travel to endemic area	Oral	>95%	None
	Inactivated polio vaccine grown in monkey cell cultures	Selected individuals	three doses 4–8 weeks apart, fourth dose 6–12 months later	One dose every 5 years	Subcutaneous	>95%	Local pain
Rabies (Chap. 124)	Rabies virus grown in human diploid cells inactivated with N-tributyl phosphate	Preexposure	Two 1-ml doses 1 week apart, third dose 2–3 weeks later	Every 2 years	Intramuscular	>90%	Local pain, erythema, myalgia, headaches, fever
		Postexposure	Five 1-ml doses days 0, 3, 7, 14, 28	One if no antibody response	Intramuscular	>90%	Local pain, erythema, myalgia headaches, fever

Table 20-2. (continued) Active Immunoprophylaxis

Disease	Agent	Age Applicable	Dose: BASIC	Dose: BOOSTER	Dose: ROUTE	Dose: VALUE	Adverse Reactions
Rickettsias							
Rocky Mtn. spotted (Chap. 96)	Formalin-killed ***Rickettsia rickettsii,*** from chick embryos	>6 months	0.5–1.0 ml every week for 3 doses	0.5–1.0 ml annually	Subcutaneous	Decreased severity	Hypersensitivity to eggs, chickens
Typhus (Chap. 98)	Formalin-killed ***Rickettsia prowazekii,*** from chick embryos	>6 months	0.2–1.0 ml every month for two doses	0.5–1.0 ml every 6–12 months	Subcutaneous	High	Hypersensitivity to eggs, chickens
Bacteria							
Diphtheria (Chap. 25)	Toxoid, 33 L_f/ml:	2 months to 5 years	0.5 ml each at 2, 4, 6 months	0.5 ml 1 year after basic and at age 4, or at entry into school	Intramuscular	>90%	Mild local pain, induration
Pertussis (Chap. 29)	Extracted *Bordetella pertussis,* phase 1, 8 units/ml					~85%	
Tetanus (Chap. 126)	Toxoid, 10 L_f/ml					~100%	
Tetanus	Toxoid, 10 L_f/ml	>6 years	0.5 ml each month for two doses	0.5 ml 1 year after basic and every 10 years thereafter	Intramuscular	~100%	Mild local pain, induration: rare allergic reactions
Diphtheria	Toxoid, 4 L_f/ml					> 90%	
Pneumococcal Pneumonia (Chap. 31)	Capsular polysaccharides, multitypic (1–4, 6, 8, 9, 12, 14, 19, 23, 25, 51, 56	≥50 years; underlying systemic disease	50 μg of each type	Unknown	Subcutaneous	High	Mild local pain, erythema
Tuberculosis (Chap. 34)	BCG, an attenuated, live strain of *Mycobacterium bovis*	Any	0.1–0.15 mg wet weight BCG (half dose for newborn)	None (full dose after 1 year if vaccinated as a newborn)	Subcutaneous or multiple percutaneous	~80%	Induration, ulceration, lymphadenitis; osteomyelitis; dissemination, death
Typhoid (Chap. 64)	Acetone-killed, *Salmonella typhi,* 10^9 ml	>2 years	0.25–0.5 ml every 4 weeks for two doses	0.25–0.5 ml on exposure, or triennially	Subcutaneous	70%–90%	Local induration, rare ulceration
Cholera (Chap. 65)	Phenol-killed *Vibrio cholerae* 8×10^9 ml	>6 months	0.25 ml (½–5 yr) 0.5 ml (>5 yr) every 4 weeks for two doses	0.5 ml subcutaneous or 0.2 ml intradermal if >5 yr, every 6 months if in endemic area	Subcutaneous, intradermal	40%–60%	Local inflammation, malaise, slight fever, headache
Anthrax (Chap. 104)	Cell free; alum-concentrated protein antigen	>6 months with high risk of exposure	0.5 ml every 2–3 weeks, for three doses	0.5 ml annually	Subcutaneous	95%	Local edema, induration
Meningococcal meningitis (Chap. 119)	Capsular polysaccharides, groups A and C, as mono- and di-valent preparations	>2 years	50 μg each A and C (repeat in 4–6 weeks if recipient 2–6 years)	Unknown	Subcutaneous	90%	Local erythema for 1–2 days
Tularemia (Chap. 139)	Live, attentuated *Francisella tularensis*	Usually >6 years	1 drop	3–5 years	Multiple pressure acupuncture	High	Local inflammation, with scarring
Plague (Chap. 140)	Formalin-killed *Yersinia pestis*	>6 months	0.5–1.0 ml initially; 0.2 ml 1 and 6 months later	0.2 ml every 6 months if in endemic area	Intramuscular	High	Local inflammation

uniquely different from encephalitis of other causation. There is headache, vomiting, drowsiness, and stupor that may progress to coma. Fever may be quite high, and a variety of central nervous system (CNS) disturbances may occur, including paralyses, convulsions, urinary retention, and meningeal irritation. Death follows in 30% to 40% of patients in Europe and in around 10% of patients in the United States. The pathogenesis of postvaccinal encephalitis is not clear. The isolation of vaccinia virus from brain tissue has been accomplished in some cases. In instances of successful isolation, there was no certainty that the vaccinia virus actually came from neural tissue and was not simply evidence of viremia at the time of death. The histologic findings of demyelination are identical with those seen in other diseases, such as allergic encephalomyelitis.

General vaccinia occurs spontaneously as a rare complication of primary vaccination. The widespread cutaneous lesions resolve without scarring in a course resembling that of an accelerated reaction. The requirement for viremia in the pathogenesis of general vaccinia is clear.

Eczema vaccinatum develops in a setting of prevaccination skin diseases such as eczema, intertrigo, and secondary syphilis. There is extensive tissue destruction, and the massed lesions are said to resemble confluent smallpox. The mortality is around 15%. The same clinical picture may occur when infection with herpes simplex virus (Chap. 91, Infections Caused by Herpes Simplex Viruses) complicates skin diseases. The name *Kaposi's varicelliform eruption* does not connote etiologic distinction. Autoinoculation of preexisting skin lesions may play a part in the development of this serious complication, although delivery of virus through the blood would suffice.

Primary vaccination should not be carried out in a pregnant woman unless actual exposure to smallpox is unavoidable; it may result in fatal vaccinia of the fetus. Fetal vaccinia has not been reported in a woman who was successfully vaccinated before pregnancy and was then revaccinated while pregnant. The residuum of some immunity from an earlier, primary vaccination apparently ensures against viremia with subsequent vaccinations.

Other contraindications to vaccination include immunodeficiency from any cause, and recent or current acute infectious diseases.

POLIOMYELITIS

Formalin inactivation of fully virulent polioviruses grown in tissue culture yielded a vaccine (Salk) that was at least 90% effective (Chap. 121, Poliomyelitis). Substitution of attenuated, live-virus strains (Sabin) for immunization was predicated not so much on gaining greater protection for the person as on the possibility of (1) engendering a persistent immunity, perhaps lifelong, without the necessity for multiple initial doses and periodic booster doses; (2) provoking enteric immunity—if attained in most of the population, wild polioviruses, with no place to hide, should die out; and (3) making immunization practical in any setting, in any country in the world. In persons completely without immunity, it is clear that both humoral and enteric immunity result from peroral immunization with live, attenuated polioviruses. Continued observation is needed to determine the duration of such immunity. It may be that with population-wide immunization there will now be so few opportunities for reaffirmation of immunity by contact with wild viruses that scheduled exposure to attenuated strains (*e.g.,* decennially) will be necessary.

Inactivated poliomyelitis vaccine, given by subcutaneous injection, is recommended for primary immunization of adults at increased risk of exposure (travelers to areas where poliomyelitis is endemic or epidemic, health care and laboratory workers, or persons in communities in which there is poliomyelitis).

RABIES

Rabies vaccine prepared in human diploid cells (HDCV) is safer and more effective than earlier vaccines prepared in duck embryos or neural tissues.

Preexposure vaccination is recommended for persons at high risk of exposure, such as veterinarians, animal handlers, mammalogists, certain laboratory workers, and persons venturing into countries where rabies is frequent. A primary series of three 1-ml intramuscular injections is given at 0, 1, and 3 weeks. Three weeks after the last dose of vaccine, serum should be tested for adequate antibody response. Booster doses of 1 ml should be given every 2 years to those with continued high risk.

Postexposure prophylaxis consists of use of the vaccine plus rabies immune globulin. Five 1-ml doses of vaccine are given, starting as soon as possible after exposure (day 0) and giving additional doses on days 3, 7, 14, and 28 after the first dose. A serum specimen should be obtained for rabies antibody testing on day 28 or 2 to 3 weeks later. If an adequate antibody titer is not detected, a booster dose of vaccine should be given and serum retested 2 to 3 weeks later.

HEPATITIS B

In November 1981, the United States Food and Drug Administration approved a vaccine for hepatitis B. The vaccine, inactivated 22-nm hepatitis B surface antigen particles obtained from the plasma of long-term carriers, produced high titers of antibody in 96% of high-risk persons given three doses and significantly reduced clinical and subclinical infections. At this time, the vaccine is indicated for health care workers, promiscuous male homosexuals and parenteral drug addicts. Because the vaccine is effective as soon as 10 weeks after administration, it is likely to be effective in postexposure prophylaxis.

Antirickettsial

Antirickettsial immunity can be actively induced with Rocky Mountain spotted fever (Chap. 96, Spotted Fevers) and with typhus (Chap. 98, Typhus Fevers) vaccines. Yolk sac cultures harvested from chick embryos infected with *Rickettsia rickettsii* and *R. prowazekii* are treated with formaldehyde. The use of these vaccines is sharply circumscribed by (1) the limited opportunity for contact of humans with infected vectors; (2) the limited duration of the protective immunity evoked by these vaccines—annual administration is recommended; and (3) the availability of effective chemotherapy. The efficacy of these preparations is not known, although typhus mortality appears to be lacking and morbidity is much reduced in vaccinated persons.

Antibacterial

DPT

The combination of diphtherial and tetanal toxoids with pertussis vaccine (DPT) is well established. Excellent antigens in themselves, both toxoids are potentiated in antigenic effectiveness by the presence of heat-killed *Bordetella pertussis.* Pertussis is particularly dangerous in infants (Chap. 29, Whooping Cough); once overt, the course of the disease is little influenced by antibacterial chemotherapy. Consequently, immunization should be undertaken at an early age. Reactions to the bordetellal whole-cell component of DPT generally become more severe as the person ages; moreover, pertussis is less severe after infancy. For these reasons, pertussis vaccine should not be given to persons over 5 years old.

Antitoxic immunity should be maintained in the adult because the hazard of diphtheria (Chap. 25, Diphtheria) and tetanus (Chap. 126, Tetanus) persists to an advanced age. Particularly with diphtheria, toxoid suitable for childhood immunization provokes untoward reactions in the adult. Somatic constituents of *Corynebacterium diphtheriae* may be to blame. Reduction in the content of both inert proteins and diphtherial toxoid results in a preparation safe for use in adults that is effective in provoking recall of antitoxic immunity. Unfortunately, diphtherial toxoid is not available by itself but is marketed solely in combination with tetanal toxoid. Although maintenance of antitoxic immunity to diphtheria requires the injection of toxoid at 4- to 6-year intervals, an interval of 10 years is more appropriate with tetanal toxoid.

Allergic reactions to tetanal toxoid are uncommon, generally occurring only after multiple injections. Because very small amounts of toxoid are sufficient to stimulate immunity, reduction in the concentration of the tetanal component of the tetanal-diphtherial toxoid mixture is indicated. In addition, after repeated injections of toxoid, most persons become truly hyperimmune to tetanus, displaying 100 to 1000 times the accepted minimal protective concentration of 0.01 IU of antitoxin per ml of serum. The intramuscular deposition of a highly concentrated mass of antigen, for example, 7.5 L_f (L_f = flocculating unit) of tetanal toxoid in 0.5 ml, the usual booster dose, can trigger Arthus-like or urticarial reactions in hyperimmune persons.

PNEUMOCOCCAL PNEUMONIA

The capsular polysaccharides typical of virulent *Streptococcus pneumoniae* were shown to be immunogenic and preventive of pneumococcal pneumonia in humans in 1945. Although some 83 types are known, and the humoral antibody response is type specific, active immunization is practical because (1) most pneumococcal disease in humans is caused by 20 types (1, 3–9, 11–20, 22, and 23); (2) immunizing doses (50 μg) of each of the 14 purified capsular polysaccharides can be given as a single, well-tolerated, subcutaneous injection; and (3) type specific immunity persists for years. Persons over 50 years of age and patients with underlying systemic diseases (*e.g.,* chronic obstructive pulmonary disease) should benefit most from immunization because they are at greatest risk of death from pneumococcal pneumonia.

The currently available vaccine contains polysaccharide from 14 bacterial types, which cause about 80% of the bacteremic pneumococcal disease in the United States. The vaccine's efficacy has been shown in healthy young men in an epidemic situation. Efficacy in high-risk groups has been more difficult to prove. Children under 2 years of age do not respond well to the antigens. Because the vaccine is relatively cheap and is well tolerated, its use is recommended for persons older than 2 years of age who have splenic dysfunction or asplenia and chronic illnesses that have an increased risk of pneumococcal disease, such as immunodeficiency states and lymphoreticular neoplasms. Such persons should be advised that the vaccine may not be completely effective. As yet, it is unproved that either the incidence or the severity of pneumococcal disease is reduced by pneumococcal vaccine, but it is a safe and cheap immunogen that should be offered to all persons 50 years of age or older.

BCG

The clinical occurrence of tuberculosis and its subsequent evolution is profoundly influenced by the state of the antituberculous immunity. There is no doubt that active immunization against tuberculosis is effective. The immunizing agent is a living culture descendent from an attenuated strain of *Mycobacterium bovis* derived by A. Calmette and C. Guérin by hundreds of passages on artificial culture mediums—who also contributed the name Bacille Calmette–Guérin (BCG). The original strain has undergone many, many additional subcultures; moreover, methods of vaccine production and preservation, and techniques for administration have changed so that BCG vaccination today is certainly different than in 1921, when it was first given to humans, and is probably different from the vaccine employed in the evaluative trails of the 1950s. Current vaccine must be capable of inducing reactivity to tuberculin in guinea pigs and must comply with standards of potency and safety. Adverse reactions are rare. However, as the following frequency data are drawn mostly from experience outside the United States, they may not pertain to BCG vaccines licensed in the United States: ulceration at the site of inoculation, regional lymphadenitis, 1 to 10 in 100,000; osteomyelitis, 0.1 to 5 in 100,000; dissemination and death (primarily immunoincompetent children), 0.008 to 0.1 in 100,000 vaccinations.

As with other measures of active immunization, BCG is of value only in persons who do not have tuberculosis and who do not react to tuberculin. In such persons, useful immunity is evoked—there is about an 80% reduction in clinical disease in vaccinated persons compared with nonvaccinated persons. Although effective, the value of BCG vaccination in a given population is influenced by the rate of occurrence of new, exogenous infections. Where this is high, the vaccine should be used—in children in areas of high prevalence of tuberculosis and in physicians, nurses, and paramedical personnel. BCG is best given by subcutaneous injection. Successful immunization leads to reactivity to tuberculin, which may wane during subsequent years.

CHOLERA

Cholera vaccine engenders definite protection against cholera for a few months after immunization. Presumably the good effect reflects elaboration of coproantibody (sIgA); there is also a serum antibody response. As the elimination of cholera from the western countries has shown, the essential factor in the control of cholera is the institution and practice of sanitation (Chap. 65, Cholera).

TYPHOID

Typhoid fever, like other salmonelloses (Chap. 64, Typhoid Fever; Chap. 63, Nontyphoidal Salmonelloses) is held in abeyance primarily by advances in sanitary engineering. Active induction of antibacterial immunity against *Salmonella* spp. is reserved for times of catastrophe, when disruption of normal water, food, and sewage processing is anticipated or has occurred. Considerable doubt has been expressed about the value of such vaccination. Large-scale, controlled field trials have substantiated the effectiveness of immunization against typhoid fever (particularly in children) with modern vaccines. There is no comparable evidence relating to nontyphoidal *Salmonella* spp.

ANTHRAX

Anthrax, as it occurs in the United States, is primarily an occupational disease of those handling cattle hides, wool, and goat hair (Chap. 104, Anthrax). The vaccine is prepared from a noncapsulated, nonproteolytic strain of *Bacillus anthracis* by alum concentration of "protective" antigen, a proteinlike component of anthrax toxin. Both laboratory and field-trial evidence of effectiveness has been obtained. The intimate relationship between protective antigen and anthrax toxin has stirred interest in immunotherapy with anthrax antiserum, particularly in the rapidly progressive pulmonary form of the disease.

MENINGOCOCCAL MENINGITIS

With the application of modern techniques, immunogenic, group-specific capsular polysaccharides have been prepared from group A (homopolymer of N-acetyl mannosamine phosphate) and group C (N-acetyl, O-acetyl neuraminic acid) *Neisseria meningitidis.* As a result of extensive trials both in military and nonmilitary populations, it is clear that group-specific protective immunity can be engendered safely by the subcutaneous injection of 50 μg doses of each of these antigens. The response is less marked in children under 6 years of age than in older children or adults, and it is inadequate for protection in children under 2 years of age. Although the decay of humoral antibody is also relatively rapid in the 2- to 6-year age group, there is a brisk response to a booster dose of antigen.

Comparable success has not been attained with group B (N-acetyl neuraminic acid) meningococci, currently the most frequent case for meningococcal meningitis in the United States. By microscopy, capsulation is minimal with group B isolates. They are also historically the most adaptable of the meningococci in terms of developing resistance to the sulfonamides.

At present, routine immunization of civilian populations against meningococcal disease is not recommended. The vaccine should be considered for close contacts of persons known to have group A or C disease because at least half of all secondary cases occur within 5 days after the primary case.

TULAREMIA

A live, attenuated strain of *Francisella tularensis* developed in Russia results in effective immunity in humans (Chap. 139, Tularemia). The necessity for stimulating such immunity is limited to those exposed in the course of work (rabbit-processing plants) or sport (rabbit hunters).

PLAGUE

Plague exists in a widely scattered sylvatic form in the United States and in endemic foci elsewhere in the world (Chap. 140, Plague). Vaccine immunoprophylaxis is of primary interest to those whose travels may involve exposure to the ectoparasite vectors of plague. A heat-killed preparation has been used, but requires biannual administration after basic immunization—a procedure that frequently produces local and systemic adverse reactions. For this reason, the apparently successful early trials in Vervet monkeys of an attenuated, perorally administered live vaccine are of great interest.

Bibliography

Journals

ARTENSTEIN MS, WINTER PE, GOLD R, SMITH CD: Immunoprophylaxis of meningococcal infection. Mil Med 139:91–95, 1974

AHONKAI VI, LANDESMAN SH, FIKRIG SM, SCHMALZER EA, BROWN AK, CHERUBIN CE, SCHIFFMAN G: Failure of pneumococcal vaccine in children with sickle cell disease. N Engl J Med 301:26–27, 1979

ARONSON JD, ARONSON CF, TAYLOR HC: A twenty-year appraisal of BCG vaccination in the control of tuberculosis. Arch Intern Med 101:881–893, 1958

AUSTRIAN R, DOUGLAS RM, SCHIFFMAN G, COETZEE AM, KORNHOF HJ, HAYDEN–SMITH S, REID DW: Prevention of pneumococcal pneumonia by vaccination. Trans Assoc Am Phys 89: in press, 1977

BARDENWERPER HW: Serum neuritis from tetanus antitoxin. JAMA 179:763–766, 1962

BEHRING E, KITASATO S: Ueber das Zustandekommen der Diphtherie-Immunität und der Tetanus-Immunität bei Thieren. Dtsch Med Wochenschr 16:113–114, 1890

BRACHMAN PS, GOLD H, PLOTKIN SA, FEKETY R, WERRIN M, INGRAHAM NR: Field evaluation of human anthrax vaccine. Am J Public Health 52:632–645, 1962

BREMAN JG, ARITA I: The confirmation and maintenance of smallpox eradication. N Engl J Med 303:1263–1273, 1980

BROOME CV, FACKLAM RR, FRASER DW: Pneumococcal disease after pneumococcal vaccination: An alternative method to estimate the efficacy of pneumococcal vaccine. N Engl J Med 303:549–552, 1980

CALMETTE A, GUÉRIN C: Vaccination des bovides contre la tuberculose et méthode nouvelle de prophylaxie de la tuberculose bovine. Ann Inst Past 38:371–398, 1924

EDSALL G, ALTMAN JS, GASPAR AJ: Combined tetanus–diphtheria immunization of adults: Use of small doses of diphtheria toxoid. Am J Public Health 44:1527–1545, 1945

EDSALL G, ELLIOTT MW, PEEBLES TC, LEVINE L, ELDRED MC: Excessive use of tetanus toxoid boosters. JAMA 202:17–19, 1967

ENDERS JF, KATZ SL, MILOVANOVIC MV, HOLLOWAY A: Studies on an attenuated measles-virus vaccine. I. Development and preparation of the vaccine: Techniques for assay of effects of vaccination. N Engl J Med 263:153–159, 1960

FIBIGER J: Om Serumbehandling af Difteri. Hospitalstidende 6:309–325, 1898

FINLAND M: Revival of antibacterial immunization: Meningococcal vaccines prove promising. J Infect Dis 121:448, 1970

GRAYSON JT, WATTEN RH: Epidemic rubella in Taiwan, 1957–1958. III. Gamma globulin in prevention of rubella. N Engl J Med 261:1145–1150, 1959

Guidelines for vaccine prophylaxis and other preventive measures: Diphtheria, tetanus and pertussis. Immunization practices advisory committee. Ann Intern Med 95:723–728, 1981

HOOFNAGEL JH, SEEF LB, BALES ZB, WRIGHT ED, ZIMMERMAN HJ, AND THE VETERANS ADMINISTRATION COOPERATIVE STUDY GROUP: Passive–active immunity from hepatitis B immune globulin: Reanalysis of a Veterans Administration cooperative study of needle-stick hepatitis. Ann Intern Med 91:813–818, 1979

JENNER E: An inquiry into the causes and effects of the variolae vacciniae, a disease discovered in some of the western counties of England, particularly Gloucestershire, and known by the name of cowpox. Printed and sold by S. Law, 1798

KABAT EA: Uses of hyperimmune human gamma globulin. N. Engl J Med 269:247–254, 1963

KATZ SL, KEMPE CH, BLACK FL, LEPOW ML, DRUGMAN S, HAGGERTY RJ, ENDERS JF: Studies on an attenuated measles-virus vaccine. VIII. General summary and evaluation of the results of vaccination. N Engl J Med 263:180–184, 1960

KEMPE CH, BERGE TO, ENGLAND B: Hyperimmune vaccinal gamma globulin: Source, evaluation and use in prophylaxis and therapy. Pediatrics 18:177–188, 1956

MADOFF MA, GLECKMAN RA: Immunizations: Where the money should be. J Infect Dis 133:230–232, 1976

MEASLES VACCINE EFFICACY: United States. Morbid Mortal Week Rep 29:470–472, 628, 1980, 1981

MEYER HM JR, PARKMAN PD, PANOS TC: Attenuated rubella virus. II. Production of an experimental live-virus vaccine and clinical trial. N Engl J Med 275:575–580, 1966

MONTO AS, BRANDT BL, ARTENSTEIN MS: Response of children to Neisseria meningitidis polysaccharide vaccines. J Infect Dis 127:394–400, 1973

MORTIMER ED JR: Pertussis immunization: Problems, perspectives, prospects. Hosp Pract 103–118, October, 1980

MULDER J, MASUREL N: Pre-epidemic antibody against 1957 strain of Asiatic influenza in serum of older people living in the Netherlands. Lancet 1:810–814, 1958

Oral poliomyelitis vaccine. Report of special advisory committee on dual poliomyelitis vaccines to the Surgeon General of the Public Health Service. JAMA 190:49–51, 1964

PARKMAN PD, MEYER HM JR, KIRSCHSTEIN RL, HOPPS HE: Attenuated rubella virus. I. Development and laboratory characterization. N Engl J Med 275:569–574, 1966

Recommendation of the Immunization Practices Advisory Committee: Immune globulins for protection against viral hepatitis. Ann Intern Med 96:193–197, 1982

Recommendation of the Immunization Practices Advisory Committee: Mumps vaccine. Morbid Mortal Week Rep 29:87–94, 1980

Recommendation of the Immunization Practices Advisory Committee: Pneumococcal polysaccharide vaccine. Ann Intern Med 96:203–205, 1982

Recommendation of the Immunization Practices Advisory Committee: Poliomyelitis prevention. Morbid Mortal Week Rep 31:22–34, 1982

Recommendation of the Immunization Practices Advisory Committee: Rubella prevention. Morbid Mortal Week Rep 30:37–47, 1981

Recommendation of the Immunization Practices Advisory Committee: Rabies prevention. Morbid Mortal Week Rep 29:265–280, 1980

Recommendation of the Public Health Service Advisory Committee on immunization practices: BCG vaccines. Morbid Mortal Week Rep 28:241, 1979

Recommendation of the Public Health Service Advisory Committee on immunization practices: Meningococcal polysaccharide vaccines. Ann Intern Med 89:949–950, 1978

SAPHRA I, WINTER JW: Clinical manifestations of salmonellosis in man: An evaluation of 7779 human infections identified at the New York salmonella center. N Engl J Med 256:1128–1134, 1957

SCHWARTZ JS: Pneumococcal vaccine: Clinical efficacy and effectiveness. Ann Intern Med 96:208–220, 1982

STUART–HARRIS C: The principles and practices of immunization. Practitioner 215:285–293, 1975

SZMUNESS W, STEVENS CE, HARLEY EJ, ZANG EA, OLESZKO WR, WILLIAMS DC, SADOVSKY R, MORRISON JM, KELLNER A: Hepatitis B vaccine: Demonstration of efficacy in a controlled clinical trial in a high-risk population in the United States. N Engl J Med 303:833–841, 1980

VARICELLA–ZOSTER IMMUNE GLOBULIN: United States. Morbid Mortal Week Rep 30:15–23, 1981

Section IV

Upper Respiratory Tract Infections

Indigenous Microbiota of the Upper Respiratory Tract

Species or Group	Nasal Passage	Nasopharynx	Oropharynx–Tonsil
Mycoplasmas			+
Bacteria			
Gram-positive cocci			
Staphylococcus epidermidis	**90***	++	**30–70**
Staphylococcus aureus	**20–80** **2–100†**	++	**35–45**
Anaerobic micrococci			+
Streptococcus mitis; undifferentiated α and γ streptococci	±	**24–99**	**100**
Streptococcus hominis (salivarius)		+	++
Enterococci or group D *Streptococcus* spp.			+‡
Streptococcus pyogenes (usually group A unless noted)	**0.1–5**	**0–9**	**8–66§**
Anaerobic *Streptococcus* spp.			+
Streptococcus pneumoniae	**0–17‖**	**0–50**	**7**
Gram-negative cocci			
Branhamella catarrhalis, Gemella haemolysans	**12**	**10–97**	**98**
Neisseria meningitidis		+	**0–15**
Veiilonella alkalescens		+	+
Gram-positive bacilli			
Lactobacillus spp.	**5–80**	+	**50–90**
Aerobic *Corynebacterium* spp.			
Propionibacterium acnes	+		
Mycobacterium spp.	±	±	±
Actinomyces israelii			+
Aerobic gram-negative bacilli			
Enterobacteriaceae		**21–23**	+
Escherichia coli		±	
Enterobacter spp.		±	±
Klebsiella spp.		±	+
Moraxella lacunata	+	±	
Acinetobacter calcoaceticus		±	
Haemophilus influenzae	**12**	**43–90**	**3–97**
Haemophilus parainfluenzae		**5**	**20–35**
Hemolytic *Haemophilus* spp.		+	**77**
Anaerobic gram-negative bacilli			
Bacteroides fragilis (5 subspecies)		+	+
Bacteroides melaninogenicus (3 subspecies)			+
Bacteroides oralis (2 subspecies)			+
Fusobacterium nucleatum			+
Fusobacterium necrophorum			+
Curved bacteria			
Selenomonas sputigena		+	
Campylobacter sputorum		+	
Treponema denticola			+
Treponema refringens			+
Fungi			
Candida albicans			**6–28**
non-albicans *Candida* spp.			±
Protozoa			
Entamoeba gingivalis			+
Trichomonas tenax			+

± to 0, rare; ±, irregular or uncertain (may be only pathologic); +, common; ++, prominent.

*Boldface values (*e.g.,* **30–60**) = range of incidence in percent, rounded, in different surveys.

†In infants and children; highest in hospital nursery infants.

‡In newborn.

§More common in school children.

‖More common in children.

CHIEN LIU

The Common Cold

21

The common cold is a self-limited clinical syndrome in which nasal catarrh is the predominant feature. Fever or other constitutional symptoms are absent. Complications are rare, but sinusitis, pharyngitis, and lower respiratory tract infections may follow. It is the most common infectious disease of man and is also the most costly, for it is the leading cause of absenteeism from school and work.

Etiology

A multitude of agents, mostly viruses, can cause the common cold syndrome. Conversely, a particular etiologic agent may reproduce a variety of different clinical syndromes depending on the population involved—for example, civilian versus military, and adult versus children. In children, particularly infants, the agents of the common cold of adults produce a much more severe disease that usually involves the lower respiratory tract. This is probably due to tissue susceptibility and the absence of immunity from lack of previous exposures.

More than 90% of upper respiratory infections are caused by nonbacterial agents, most of which are viruses. A list of such agents is shown in Table 21-1. Laboratory diagnosis is difficult. Even an excellent laboratory capable of applying the most sophisticated methods succeeds in identifying an etiologic agent in only about 60% of respiratory tract infections. The most important etiologic agents of the common cold in adults are the rhinoviruses, which are probably responsible for about 25% of colds.

Rhinoviruses

After many years of search, the first common cold virus was isolated in 1956. Subsequently, as investigators recovered many viruses from patients with colds, these agents were given different names such as ERC viruses, Salisbury agents, muriviruses, and coryzaviruses. At present, 113 immunologically distinct but biologically related rhinoviruses have been isolated.

All rhinoviruses are picornaviruses in that they contain RNA and are about 30 nm in diameter (Fig. 21-1). Rhinoviruses, unlike some picornaviruses, are inactivated at *p*H 3, which is probably why they do not parasitize the intestinal tract. They are not inactivated by ether, and they do not agglutinate red blood cells.

Some rhinoviruses are designated as M and H strains. The M strains can grow in monkey kidney cells as well as in human cells, whereas the H strains grow only in human cells. However, the pathogenicity of M and H strains for man is identical. Some rhinoviruses cannot be isolated in ordinary tissue cultures, growing only in organ cultures that provide differentiated, ciliated respiratory tract epithelium. Strains that grow in tissue cultures do so optimally at 33°C—at the temperature of the nasal mucosa of humans. Rhinoviruses are inactivated rapidly at 56°C, slowly at 4°C, and probably not at all at −70°C. Although drying in air inactivates rhinoviruses, they can be preserved by lyophilization. Antigenic variations have been found in strains of the same rhinovirus type isolated several years apart, suggesting that there is antigenic drift.

Coronaviruses

The first human coronavirus was isolated in 1965 from a boy with a common cold. Coronaviruses have a characteristic electron microscopic appearance with round or petal-shaped projections around the viral capsid resembling a solar corona. They are of medium size, varying from 80 nm to 160 nm in diameter. Their genetic material appears to be RNA, and they have essential lipid envelopes that are labile to ether or chloroform. More than 20 strains of coronaviruses have been obtained from humans, isolated chiefly from adults with upper respiratory in-

Table 21-1. *Nonbacterial Agents That Cause Upper Respiratory-Tract Infections of Man*

Agents	Human Serotypes	Nucleic Acid Types	Date of Discovery
Myxoviruses			
Influenza	A, B, C,	RNA	1933–1949
Parainfluenza	1, 2, 3, 4	RNA	1953
Respiratory Syncytial	1 (may be 2)	RNA	1956
Coronaviruses	1	RNA	1965
Picornaviruses			
Rhinoviruses	> 100 types	RNA	1960s
Coxsackie virus A	24 (perhaps only A_{21} causes respiratory illnesses)	RNA	1948
Coxsackie virus B	6 (perhaps only B_4, B_5 cause respiratory illnesses)	RNA	1948
Echoviruses	31 (perhaps only types 11, 20, 25 cause respiratory illnesses)	RNA	1950s
Adenoviruses	34 (types 1, 2, 3, 5, 7 14, 21 are responsible for respiratory illnesses)	DNA	1953
Chlamydia pittaci	1	DNA + RNA	1930
Mycoplasma pneumoniae	1	DNA + RNA	1944
Coxiella burnetti	1	DNA + RNA	1937

*Nonbacterial agents are responsible for more than 90% of the upper respiratory infections in man.

fections. Although coronaviruses may be isolated in human diploid fibroblast or human embryonic kidney tissue cultures, some strains can only be recovered in human embryonic tracheal organ cultures and cannot be adapted to grow in monolayer tissue cultures. Coronaviruses have also been isolated from nonhuman animals—for example, the avian infectious bronchitis virus (IBV) group, and the mouse hepatitis virus (MHV) group. There is some antigenic relationship between the human and murine strains, but no antigenic relationship has been detected between the avian strains and others. According to seroepidemiologic surveys, coronavirus infection is rare in children with lower respiratory tract illnesses. In adults, coronavirus infection occurred in 10% to 24% of patients with upper respiratory tract disease during a period when rhinovirus infection was uncommon but respiratory disease morbidity was high. The incidence and pattern seem to vary from year to year.

Coxsackieviruses and Echoviruses

Coxsackie- and echoviruses are picornaviruses that are also enteroviruses in that they are primarily inhabitants of the intestine. Coxsackieviruses consist of groups A and B, each of which is made up of serotypes. Echoviruses are not presently divided into groups, although several types are distinguished.

Aseptic meningitis and pleurodynia are the major clinical syndromes associated with these viruses. Occasionally, coxsackieviruses (group A, type 21; group B, types 4 and 5) and echoviruses (types 11, 20, 25) are associated with the common cold syndrome. Detailed descriptions of these agents are found in Chapter 149, Coxsackievirus and Echovirus Infections.

Myxoviruses

All three antigenic types of influenza virus classically cause influenza when they infect man. However, mild illness that simulates the common cold sometimes results from infection with influenza viruses. A detailed description of influenza is found in Chapter 28, Influenza.

Parainfluenza viruses consist of four antigenic types. In adults, these agents usually cause afebrile, common coldlike illnesses. However, in children, these agents can cause severe diseases, including

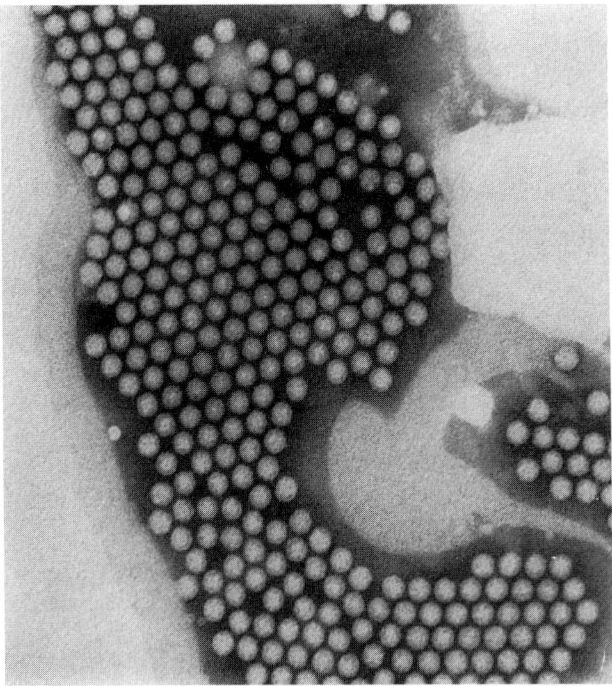

Fig. 21-1. Electron micrograph of purified rhinovirus type 14. (Original magnification × 125,000) (Courtesy of HD Mayor and S McGregor)

croup, bronchitis, and pneumonia. Parainfluenza viruses are described in detail in Chapter 26, Epiglottitis, Laryngitis, and Laryngotracheobronchitis.

Respiratory syncytial (RS) virus usually causes a mild common cold-like illness in adults. However, it is associated with severe lower respiratory tract disease in children, particularly in infants under 6 months. A description of RS virus is given in Chapter 23, Nonbacterial Pharyngitis.

Adenoviruses

Of the 34 serologically distinct adenoviruses isolated from humans, only a few are associated with respiratory illnesses, particularly in military recruits. A description of adenoviruses is given in Chapter 26, Epiglottitis, Laryngitis, and Laryngotracheobronchitis.

Mycoplasma pneumoniae

Not a virus but a pleuropneumonialike organism (PPLO), *Mycoplasma pneumoniae* causes respiratory tract illness that ranges in clinical form from the common cold to bronchopneumonia. A description of *M. pneumoniae* is presented in Chapter 30, Nonbacterial Pneumonias.

Coxiella burnetii and Psittacosis-Ornithosis Agents

One of the rickettsias, *Coxiella burnetii,* and the psittacosis-ornithosis agents of the genus *Chlamydia* do not cause the common cold syndrome but are responsible for more severe, systemic and lower respiratory tract infections. Descriptions of these agents are also given in Chapter 30, Nonbacterial Pneumonias.

Epidemiology

The common cold is world wide in distribution. It is spread by person-to-person contact, a fact that is of greater relevance to the increased frequency of occurrence of colds in the winter months than is the popular belief that cold weather of itself, or sharp changes in temperature, induce the common cold. Indeed, none of these beliefs was substantiated in volunteer experiments that involved exposure of subjects to cold. Neither humidity, wetness, nor atmospheric pollutants have been proved to activate latent respiratory viruses. Several waves of common colds are observed each year in the United States. Each wave is probably caused by different viruses.

Rhinoviruses are prominent among the identifiable causes—from 10% to 25% of adults and 5% to 10% of children with colds yield rhinoviruses on culture of nasal secretions. From 1% to 3% of adults without overt disease have rhinoviruses in their nasal secretions during the winter months; thus there appear to be human carriers of these viruses. Humans are the only natural host for rhinoviruses that have been identified.

Under natural conditions, transmission of colds may proceed from infected to susceptible persons by inhalation of infectious virus particles suspended in aerosols or droplets, by direct contact with infectious respiratory secretions on hands, fingers and environmental surfaces, or by a combination of both. With experimental rhinovirus infection, the virus appears to spread more efficiently by contaminated fingers and hands than by aerosols or droplets.

With the possible exception of chimpanzees, inoculation of rhinoviruses into experimental animals does not lead to common coldlike illnesses. However, agents closely related to human rhinoviruses have been isolated from cattle and horses with upper respiratory tract infections. Antibodies against equine rhinoviruses have been detected in stablemen who attended sick horses.

Pathogenesis and Pathology

Common cold viruses enter the respiratory tract by direct transfer, as on the fingers, or by inhalation of infected aerosols or droplets. The cells that line the nasal passages and pharynx appear to be most heavily infected because they support particularly active viral replication. Proliferation of viruses can often be demonstrated within 24 hours after inoculation of human volunteers. From biopsy specimens, inflammatory changes with hyperemia, edema, and leukocyte infiltration are seen. Desquamation of ciliated columnar epithelial cells reaches a peak on the second to the fifth day of a cold. Regeneration of epithelium soon follows, with new columnar cells reforming by approximately the fourteenth day following infection.

During the acute illness, nasal secretions rich in glycoproteins are produced in excessive quantities. Initially, this secretion is clear and mucoid, containing few bacteria. Later, after 1 to 2 days, as secondary bacterial infection is caused by the normal flora of the upper respiratory tract, the secretions become mucopurulent. When inflammatory changes become severe and marked swelling of the nasal mucosa is present, obstruction of the sinus ostia and the eustachian tube may lead to paranasal sinusitis and otitis media.

Manifestations

The incubation period of the common cold is usually 1 to 4 days. Initial symptoms consist of nasal stuffiness, sneezing, and mild headache. Feverishness and chilliness are also common. Rhinorrhea rapidly follows with increasing severity, and patients often use 10 to 20 or more paper handkerchiefs a day. There is usually a burning sensation and a scratchy feeling in the nasal passages. In moderate to severe cases, general malaise, lacrimation, sore throat, and headache are common. Anorexia and slight fever may be present. The patient often has a postnasal discharge, particularly on awakening and during the morning. Cough and substernal discomfort may be present when tracheobronchitis develops. These symptoms ordinarily run their course in about 5 to 7 days. In more severe cases, the course may be prolonged to 2 weeks.

Physical signs are usually confined to the nasopharynx. The nasal turbinates are boggy, swollen, and covered with secretions; they encroach on the nasal passages. There is mild hyperemia of the oropharynx; neither exudates nor membranes are present. Routine laboratory examinations, such as the hemogram and urinalysis, do not reveal abnormalities. However, in volunteers infected with rhinoviruses, a mild leukopenia, with a relative lymphocytosis, may occur during initial stages of the infection, shifting to a slight neutrophilic leukocytosis in later stages.

Complications are rare. A severe cold may spread to involve adjacent structures, giving rise to sinusitis, otitis media, and bronchitis.

Diagnosis

Establishment of a clinical diagnosis of the common cold depends primarily on the evaluation of the patient's symptoms—for example, the relative mildness of the infection, localization of the process to the nasopharynx, and an afebrile course. Clinically, there is no way of differentiating a cold caused by one etiologic agent from a cold caused by a different agent, although some strains of rhinoviruses sometimes cause more nasal secretions than others, and colds caused by influenza viruses tend to be more severe. However, the variation is so minor that it bears no predictive value. Allergic rhinitis is usually predictably seasonal, an annual recurrence, and is marked by the presence of eosinophiles in the nasal secretions. In young infants, infection caused by *Streptococcus pyogenes* may cause rhinorrhea simulating a chronic cold; a nasopharyngeal culture is diagnostic.

Etiologic diagnosis of the common cold depends on the isolation of viral agents and the documentation of a serologic response. Nasal washings or throat swabs obtained during the first 4 days of illness are the best materials for viral isolation. For rhinoviruses, the best tissue culture system is human embryonic kidney cells or human diploid fibroblast cultures, such as WI-38 cells. If possible, inoculation of specimens into tissue cultures should be performed immediately, without freezing the specimens. For influenza virus, embryonated hens' eggs are optimal for isolation. For parainfluenza viruses, monkey kidney cells may be used. Adenoviruses and respiratory syncytial virus can be isolated in susceptible, continuous human epithelial lines such as HeLa or Hep-2 cells. Picornaviruses other than the rhinoviruses can be isolated in monkey kidney cells. Isolation of *Mycoplasma pneumoniae* can be accomplished with PPLO medium containing yeast extract and fresh horse serum.

Complement fixation, hemagglutination inhibition, and neutralization tests against specific viral antigens comprise the range of useful serologic tests. Rhinovirus antibody can only be determined by neutralization tests. However, some patients infected with the H strains of rhinoviruses may not develop neutralizing antibodies, nullifying even this serologic procedure.

Prognosis

The prognosis of the common cold is extremely favorable; complete recovery within 1 week is the rule. Complications are generally related to extension of the infection to the lower respiratory tract, giving rise to bronchitis or to obstruction of the ostia of the paranasal sinuses, leading to sinusitis. Most commonly in children, obstruction of the eustachian tube may lead to otitis media (see Chap. 164, Infections of the Ear). A common cold may cause exacerbation of infection already complicating chronic respiratory tract disease such as chronic obstructive pulmonary disease in adults and cystic fibrosis with pulmonary involvement in children.

In naturally occurring common colds caused by M strains of rhinoviruses, homologous neutralizing serum antibodies develop in 90% or more of patients. In contrast, after colds caused by H strains of rhinoviruses, neutralizing antibodies are detectable in only about 37% of patients. M strain antibodies persist for months or years, whereas H strain antibodies fall off at a more rapid rate. Antibody responses of children do not appear to differ from those of adults.

Although rhinoviruses share minor antigenic determinants, there appears to be little cross reaction between them. In volunteer studies, the presence of rhinovirus antibody from an initial experimental infection with either M or H strains does confer protection against the rechallenge of homologous viruses, indicating that the preexisting neutralizing antibodies are protective.

The presence of serum antibodies for rhinoviruses, parainfluenza viruses, and respiratory syncytial virus and *M. pneumoniae* does not completely prevent reinfection or illness, but the clinical course may be milder. This incomplete protective effect of serum antibody, and the fact that there are so many different respiratory agents capable of causing the common cold syndrome, are the reasons that any one person may have several colds in a year. There is evidence that specific antibody is secreted in the upper respiratory tract (secretory IgA) following a naturally acquired common cold or as a response to vaccination. Neither the duration of production of secretory IgA, its persistence, nor its effectiveness in preventing infection is known with certainty.

Therapy

There is no specific treatment for the common cold. Supportive measures are aimed at reducing the discomfort of the patient during the acute stage of the illness. Bacterial complications of significance are infrequent. The routine use of antimicrobial agents either to treat a cold or to prevent secondary bacterial complications is condemned. Such practice leads to the selection of resistant bacterial strains, compounding the difficulty of management of bacterial complications if they arise. It will not otherwise alter the course of a common cold.

There is no accepted regimen for supportive therapy of the common cold. Bed rest or staying indoors, warm clothing, and the prevention of chilliness will add to the patient's comfort. Aspirin (600 mg for an adult, 10 m/kg body wt for children, give 3 to 4 times daily) alleviates the malaise and headache. Aqueous 0.25% to 0.5% phenylephrine hydrocholoride, given as nosedrops, may relieve nasal congestion. Oily nosedrop preparations should not be used, because aspiration into the lower respiratory tract may lead to a lipid pneumonia, particularly in the very young and the very old. A liberal intake of liquids, such as fruit juices, tea, or soft drinks, may be helpful. There is no proof of any curative value from the many proprietary remedies containing vitamins (including vitamin C), bioflavinoids, multiple analgesics, or antihistaminics in the treatment of the common cold. While the use of such remedies is of no benefit, the patient is exposed to agents with significant potential for engendering hypersensitivity. Throat lozenges without antimicrobics may help to relieve pharyngeal discomfort. If cough is nonproductive and is bothersome, a cough syrup such as elixir of terpin hydrate, with or without codeine, may be administered. In most cases, the acute symptoms usually last 1 to 2 days, and the patient is completely well in a week. If fever intervenes and symptoms persist, a careful physical examination must be carried out with particular attention given to auscultation of the lungs. A chest roentgenogram should be obtained because of the possibility of pneumonia.

Prevention

Virus excretion usually precedes the onset of symptoms of a cold. In addition, the common cold is really quite common. The net result is that prevention of the common cold by quarantine or by isolation of symptomatic patients is of no value. Patients should cover their noses during sneezing and should deposit used paper handkerchiefs soiled with nasal secretions and sputum in closed containers or in the toilet bowl. The rationales are courtesy and diminution of airborne dissemination of virus.

Although a formalinized vaccine prepared with a particular rhinovirus or another respiratory virus can be made and is effective, the large number of antigenically distinct viruses capable of causing the common cold syndrome militates against the production of a truly polyvalent vaccine. First, such a polyvalent vaccine would have to include more than 100 antigenically distinct components in a form that would not dilute one component to impotency. Second, for effectiveness, the human would have to respond equally with antibody formation specific for each of the simultaneously administered components. Third, the mixture would have to be devoid of either local or systemic toxicity. At present, no vaccines against common cold viruses are available. The commercial "cold vaccines" contain bacterial suspensions and provoke no protection against viral infections. Because the common cold is a benign disease that is a nuisance and personal inconvenience, the safety and effectiveness of a vaccine will have to be indubitable before it can be licensed for use.

Bibliography

Books

GWALTNEY JM JR: Rhinoviruses. In Mandell GL, Douglas RG Jr, Bennett JE (eds): Principles and Practice of Infectious Diseases. New York, John Wiley & Sons, 1979. pp. 1124–1134.

MONTO AS: Coronaviruses. In Evans AS (ed): Viral Infections of Humans: Epidemiology and Control. New York, Plenum, 1976. pp 127–141.

TYRELL DAJ: Common Colds and Related Diseases. Baltimore, Williams & Wilkins, 1965. 197 pp.

Journals

CHALMERS TC: Effects of ascorbic acid on the common cold: An evaluation of the evidence. Am J Med 58:532, 1975

DINGLE JH: The curious case of the common cold. J Immunol 81:91–97, 1958

DOUGLAS RD JR, CATE TR, GERONE PJ: Quantitative rhinovirus shedding patterns in volunteers. Am Rev Respir Dis 94:159–167, 1966

FOX JP, COONEY MK, HALL CE: The Seattle virus watch. V. Epidemiologic observations of rhinovirus infections, 1965–1969, in families with young children. Am J Epidemiol 101:122–143, 1975

HENDLEY JO, EDMONDSON WP JR, GWALTNEY JM JR: Relation between naturally acquired immunity and infectivity of two rhinoviruses in volunteers. J Infect Dis 125:243–248, 1972

HOWARD JC JR, KANTNER TR, LILIENFIELD LS, PRINCIOTTO JV, KRUM RE, CRUTCHER JE, BELMAN MA, DANZIG MR: Effectiveness of antihistamines in the symptomatic management of the common cold. JAMA 242:2414–2417, 1979

CHIEN LIU

Sinusitis

22

Sinusitis is an acute inflammatory affliction of one or more of the paranasal sinuses. Infection is virtually always a component of sinusitis, either from the outset or as the disease evolves.

Etiology

The paranasal sinuses are directly contiguous to, and communicate with, the upper respiratory tract. Accordingly, acute sinusitis most often follows rhinitis, which in itself is commonly of viral origin. Vasomotor rhinitis may also be antecedent to sinusitis. Deviation of the nasal septum, nasal polyps, tumors, and foreign bodies all set the stage for the development of acute sinusitis through the common mechanism of obstruction of the sinusal ostia. Less commonly, sinusitis may result from an abrupt change of pressure in the nasal passages, such as occurs in the rapid descent of an unpressurized airplane. Diving into a swimming pool may force infected water into the paranasal sinuses.

The most common bacterial agents responsible for acute sinusitis are *Streptococcus pneumoniae* and *Haemophilus influenzae.* These two pathogens were recovered in more than 50% of patients in whom specimens obtained from direct sinus puncture aspirates were cultured. Other organisms including anaerobes, *Staphylococcus aureus, Streptococcus pyogenes,* gram-negative bacilli, and respiratory viruses have also been recovered. Chronic sinusitis is commonly associated with anaerobic-bacteria, often as a combined infection with aerobes.

Infection of the maxillary sinuses may follow dental extractions or may result from the direct extension of infection from the infected roots of the upper teeth. The bacteria involved in such infections are often anaerobic streptococci or coliform bacilli.

Epidemiology

Sinusitis is common. Although there are no exact data regarding frequency of occurrence, the incidence of acute sinusitis closely parallels the incidence of acute infections of the upper respiratory tract—that is, acute sinusitis is common during cold weather, particularly in damp climates. Sinusitis associated with allergic rhinitis may show a seasonal increase in the frequency of occurrence coincident with an increase in atmospheric pollen.

Pathogenesis and Pathology

Obstruction of the paranasal sinusal ostia impedes drainage. Additionally, viral and bacterial infections impair the ciliary activity of the epithelial lining of the sinuses. The result is accumulation of mucous secretions. With bacterial multiplication in the sinus cavities the mucus is converted to mucopus. The pus also irritates the underlying mucosa causing further edema and aggravating the ostial obstruction.

Death of mucosal cells may result from viral multiplication, mechanical injury, or the inflammatory reaction of acute sinusitis. Some degree of sloughing of dead mucosal cells is part of the natural course of the disease. Ordinarily, regeneration is prompt, and the outcome is benign.

However, when acute sinusitis is not resolved but becomes chronic, the epithelial lining may be irreversibly damaged. This may lead to thickening of the mucosa and the development of polyps or mucoceles.

Manifestations

A sensation of pressure over a sinus heralds the development of acute sinusitis. Soon there follows local pain and tenderness; malaise and low-grade fever may also occur. In maxillary sinusitis, the pain is over the cheek and upper teeth. In frontal sinusitis, the pain is in the forehead above the eyebrow. In sphenoidal sinusitis, the patient may complain of headache in the suboccipital region. In anterior ethmoidal sinusitis, the headache is in the temporal area, and in posterior ethmoidal sinusitis it is over the distribution of the trigeminal nerve, particularly around the mastoid area. For patients suffering from acute frontal or maxillary sinusitis, the pain is typically absent in the early morning but appears 1 to 2 hours after arising. After increasing in intensity, it lasts 3 to 4 hours during the day. By late afternoon or evening, the pain becomes less severe again.

Physical examination may show no more than edematous and hyperemic nasal mucosa. If the ostia of the sinuses are not completely obstructed and the nasal turbinates have been shrunken by the application of a vasoconstrictor, mucopus may be seen around the ostial openings. The frontal, maxillary, and anterior ethmoidal sinuses drain through ostia located in the middle meatus; the ostia of the posterior ethmoidal and sphenoidal sinuses open into the superior meatus. Tenderness is best demonstrated by finger pressure over the sinus areas. Using transillumination, an involved maxillary or frontal sinus may appear opaque. Roentgenographically, diseased sinuses may be cloudy, at times with a fluid level.

In uncomplicated chronic sinusitis, purulent nasal discharge is the most constant finding. Usually, there is neither pain nor tenderness over sinus areas; recurrent headache is rarely caused by chronic sinusitis. Thickening of the sinus mucosa and a fluid level are usually seen in roentgenograms.

Diagnosis

A diagnosis of acute sinusitis can be made without radiographic examinations when there is a history of upper respiratory infection or allergic rhinitis, pain and tenderness over a sinus, and purulent discharge in the corresponding nasal meatus. In chronic sinusitis, a careful dental examination, transillumination, roentgenography, and antral puncture may be required to establish a diagnosis. When pain is persistent in a patient known to have a chronic sinus infection, the probability of an impending complication is high. Also, a previously unsuspected neoplasm should be looked for.

Prognosis

In properly treated cases of acute sinusitis, complications are rare and the prognosis is good. Spread of infection is signaled by chills and fever, general or persistent headaches, vomiting, convulsions, diplopia, edema and swelling of the forehead and eyelids, and signs of increased intracranical pressure. Periorbital abscess, cavernous sinus thrombosis, osteomyelitis of the skull, epidural or subdural abscess, brain abscess, and meningitis may result. Careful and meticulous diagnostic procedures are essential to application of appropriate medical and surgical therapy.

The frequent association of bronchiectasis and chronic sinusitis is remarkable, albeit unexplained. The concomitant occurrence of sinusitis, bronchiectasis, and situs invertus is known as the Kartagener's syndrome.

Therapy

Acute sinusitis should be treated medically. The pain may be quite severe, often requiring codeine or even morphine for alleviation. The application of moist heat over the affected sinus may also be helpful in relieving pain. A vasoconstrictor (aqueous 0.25% to 0.50% phenylephrine, or 2% ephedrine) should be applied as nose drops every 4 to 6 hours to promote drainage. The inhalation of warmed air that is saturated with water (not steam) is also quite useful. The position of the head must be appropriate to obtain drainage of the involved sinus.

For antimicrobial therapy, amoxicillin (25 mg/kg body wt/day, PO as 3 equal portions, 8-hourly) or ampicillin (30 to 40 mg/kg body wt/day, PO as 4 equal portions, 6-hourly) for 7 to 10 days may be given. Patients who are allergic to penicillins may be given 160 mg trimethoprim plus 800 mg sulfamethoxazole (8 mg trimethoprim/40 mg sulfamethoxazole/kg/day for children) PO twice daily. In rare cases, when the patient does not respond to the above regimens, a sinus puncture may be necessary to obtain specimens for culture to identify the etiologic organisms. A penicillinase-resistant penicillin is needed for the treatment of *Staphylococcus aureus*—for example, cloxacillin (30 mg/kg body wt/day, PO as 4 equal portions, 6-hourly). Other antimicrobics may sometimes be necessary, depending on the causative bacteria.

Surgical procedures should not be undertaken during acute sinusitis because of the hazard of spread of the infection. In subacute or chronic cases, when conservative treatment does not give a cure, irrigation of the affected sinus may be necessary. Antral puncture may be required in chronic maxillary sinusitis. Pus obtained from the puncture should be cultured and the offending microorganism(s) identified to enable the prescription of appropriate antimicrobial agents.

Prevention

There is no specific preventive of sinusitis. Proper treatment of rhinitis, whether allergic or infectious in origin, is important. Correction of nasal septal deviation and removal of polyps or foreign bodies will avoid obstruction of the sinusal ostia. If one must dive feet first into water, the nose should be held to avoid a sudden, forceful gush of infected water into the sinuses. Root abscesses of maxillary teeth require particular care in dental management to avoid secondary involvement of the maxillary sinuses.

Bibliography

Book

DEWEESE DD, SAUNDERS WH (eds): Acute and chronic sinusitis. In Textbook of Otolaryngology, 4th ed. St. Louis, C. V. Mosby, 1973. pp 240–255.

Journals

COURVILLE CB, ROSENVOLD LK: Intracranial complications of infections of nasal cavities and accessory sinuses. Survey of lesions observed in series of 15,000 autopsies. Arch Otolaryngol 27:692–731, 1938

FREDERICK J, BRAUDE AI: Anaerobic infection of the paranasal sinuses. N Engl J Med 290:135–137, 1974

HAMORY BH, SANDE MA, SYDNOR A JR, SEALE DL, GWALTNEY JM JR: Etiology and antimicrobial therapy of acute maxillary sinusitis. J Infect Dis 139:197–202, 1979

CHIEN LIU

23 Nonbacterial Pharyngitis

Nonbacterial pharyngitis is an inflammatory disease of the pharynx that is not caused by bacteria. It is the hallmark of a clinical syndrome that may result either from a process localized to the pharynx or from a systemic disease.

Etiology

Viral agents are commonly implicated in nonbacterial pharyngitis. Although it my be part of the clinical picture of a general illness such as infectious mononucleosis (see Chap. 137, Infectious Mononucleosis), nonbacterial pharyngitis is usually caused by one of the ubiquitous viruses responsible for the bulk of the respiratory infections. Although no single group of viruses is responsible for a major segment of these infections, some of the agents especially likely to be involved in nonbacterial pharyngitis merit individual consideration.

Adenoviruses

The first isolations of this group of viruses from human adenoid tissues grown in tissue culture were reported in 1953. At present, 35 antigenically distinct types have been isolated from humans. Of these, types 1, 2, 3, 4, 5, 7, 14, and 21 have been associated with epidemic or sporadic respiratory diseases in humans; type 8 appears to be the major etiologic agent of epidemic keratoconjunctivitis. Types 34 and 35 have been isolated from renal transplant recipients with interstitial pneumonia and fatal disseminated infections.

Morphologically, an adenovirus is arranged in an icosahedron 70 nm to 90 nm in diameter (Fig. 23-1). Its nucleic acid core is of the DNA type and is relatively stable to physical agents. Adenoviruses are not inactivated by ether or by exposure to acid (pH 1.5-2.5) for 30 minutes at room temperature. This acid-resistant characteristic may be associated with the survival and multiplication of adenoviruses in the gastrointestinal tract.

All adenoviruses, regardless of type, share a common, soluble, complement-fixing antigen. Individual types are distinguished by a specific antigen that is demonstrable by neutralization testing. Except for types 12 and 18, all adenoviruses that are pathogenic for humans agglutinate rhesus monkey or rat erythrocytes.

Adenoviruses are the major etiologic agents of acute respiratory disease (ARD) and pharyngitis. They cause bronchopneumonia only occasionally in civilians, but rather frequently in military recruits. Types 12 and 18, and certain strains of types 3, 7, and 21 are capable of producing sarcomas in the hamster cheek pouch and transforming normal tissue culture cells to malignant-appearing cells.

Herpes Simplex Viruses

The herpesviruses (Gr. *herpein,* to creep) consist of a number of DNA viruses found in both humans and animals (see Chap. 91, Infections Caused by Herpes Simplex Virus). They tend to produce latent infections. Herpes simplex virus is well known for its role in recurrent fever blisters. However, this virus may also cause ulcerted lesions in the pharynx and buccal mucosa and, occasionally, general fetal infections, including encephalitis (see Chap. 122, Viral Encephalitides).

Herpesviruses are 180 nm to 200 nm in size. They have icosahedral lipid-containing capsids and are inactivated by ether. The biosynthesis of herpesviral subunits begins in the host cell nucleus and is completed in the cytoplasm. The presence of eosinophilic, Cowdry type A, intranuclear inclusion bodies in infected cells is characteristic of herpesviral infections.

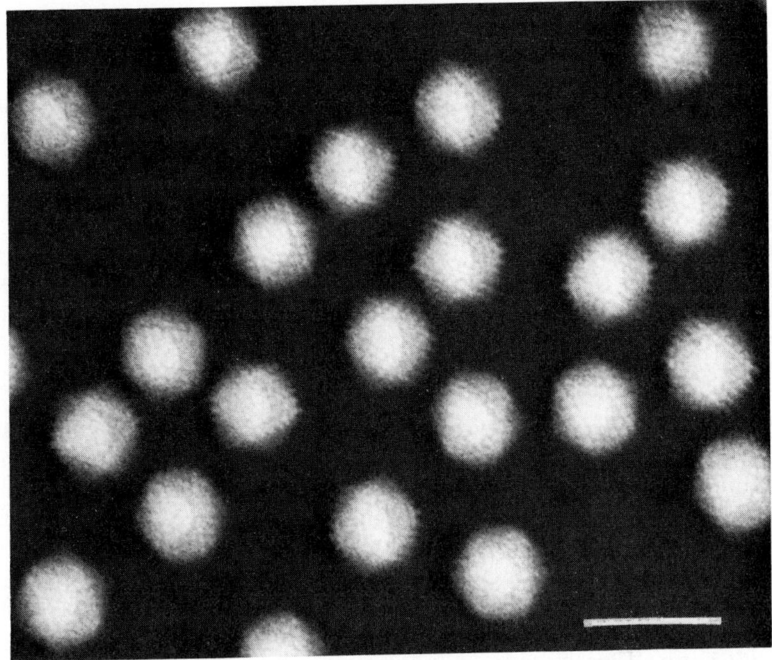

Fig. 23-1. Electronmicrograph of purified human adenovirus type 2. (Original magnification × 186,000). (Courtesy of HD Mayer and LE Jordan)

Coxsackieviruses

The name *Coxsackie* commemorates the New York town in which these agents were first isolated in 1948 from children with an acute, poliomyelitislike illness (see Chap. 149, Coxsackievirus and Echovirus Infections). Coxsachieviruses are now classified as picornaviruses. They can be distinguished from other picornaviruses by greater pathogenicity for suckling mice than for adult mice. In suckling mice, group A coxsackieviruses produce a diffuse myositis with acute inflammation and necrosis of the voluntary muscle fibers. Mice infected with group B coxsackieviruses exhibit focal degeneration of striated muscles and the interscapular fat pad; encephalomalacia is common, and hepatitis, pancreatitis, and myocarditis occasionally result.

Coxsackieviruses can produce a variety of clinical diseases, ranging from aseptic meningitis and myocarditis to upper respiratory tract infections. Among group A coxackieviruses, types 2, 4, 5, 6, 8, and 10 cause herpangina, a pharyngitis of children characterized by acute onset of fever, headache, sore throat, and dysphagia. The pathognomonic lesions are small vesicles or punched-out ulcers in and around the throat. Coxsackievirus, group A, type 10 is also associated with a summer febrile disease in children called acute lymphonodular pharyngitis. Coxsackievirus, group A, type 16 has been reported to cause hand-foot-and-mouth disease.

Mycoplasma hominis

Mycoplasma hominis type 1 has been reported to cause acute pharyngitis in volunteers. Its role in natural disease is not yet certain.

Epidemiology

The agents that cause pharyngitis are ubiquitous and are distributed throughout the world. Man is the principal reservoir. Most outbreaks and epidemics are due to intimate contact among crowded populations such as occur in military establishments and children's summer camps. However, the epidemiology of each group of viral agents is quite different and is discussed separately.

Adenoviruses

Primary infection with adenoviruses usually occurs early in life, producing an acute upper respiratory disease with pharyngitis, sometimes also with conjunctivitis. Rarely, a fatal pneumonia may occur. Outbreaks of adenoviral respiratory disease have occurred in children living together in institutions, boarding schools, and summer camps. Among college students and the civilian adult population, the incidence of adenoviral infections is low. However, in military recruits, adenoviruses of types 3, 4, 7, 14, and 21 frequently cause epidemics of undifferentiated febrile acute respiratory diseases (ARD) and primary atypical pneumonia. It has been estimated that, in the winter months, adenovirus infection rates approach 100% of susceptible military recruits during an 8-week period of basic training. Approximately 50% of these infections become clinically manifest as ARD.

Herpes Simplex Viruses

Herpesviruses are spread from person to person by direct contact and by the sharing of contaminated eating or drinking utensils. Oral secretions from persons with herpes stomatitis uniformly contain virus. Moreover, herpesvirus can be isolated from the saliva of apparently normal children (only occasionally) and adults (about 25%).

Initial infection of children usually occurs during the second year of life. The infection is clinically overt in about 15% of children as a herpetic gingivostomatitis—multiple vesicles on the buccal mucosa and oral mucocutaneous borders. By adulthood, approximately 80% of the population has been infected with herpes simplex viruses, judging from the relatively high titers of neutralizing or complement-fixing antibodies in serums. A substantial proportion of the infected population develops recurrent clinical disease, most often manifested as herpes labialis (fever blisters), keratitis, or ulcerated pharyngitis.

Coxsackieviruses

Worldwide in distribution, coxsackieviruses appear to have no reservoir other than man. They have been isolated from feces, pharyngeal swabbings, throat washings, and sewage. Because the lesions of herpangina are localized to the pharynx, aerosol and respiratory spread are possible. However, direct person-to-person contact is probably the most important means in the spread of coxsackieviruses.

In the United States, coxsackieviral diseases are encountered most frequently during July, August,and September. The frequency of virus excretion in feces and sewage is 3 to 6 times higher in the lower socioeconomic district of each city than it is in the middle-to upper middle-class districts. Virus isolation is more often successful from children than from adults. Close physical contact and crowding are conducive to outbreaks of herpangina caused by group A coxsackieviruses.

Pathogenesis and Pathology

On gaining access to the human host, respiroviruses multiply in the mucosal cells lining the nasopharynx and the oral cavity, giving rise to clinical symptoms of pharyngitis and stomatitis. The two DNA viruses of the group, adenovirus and herpes simplex virus, begin multiplication inside the nuclei of host cells, yielding intranuclear inclusion bodies. These same viruses also tend to persist in the host as latent agents. Adenoviruses can be isolated from adenoids and tonsils removed surgically from apparently healthy children. Herpesvirus frequently causes fever blisters when the host-parasite equilibrium is disturbed by environmental factors such as ultraviolet irradiation, fever, menstruation, nerve injury, and emotional upheaval.

The primary site of coxsackievirus multiplication is in the alimentary tract. Viruses can be isolated from the feces of infected persons as long as 47 days after acute infection. When the disease is herpangina, coxsackieviruses can be recovered from saliva, nasal secretions, the oropharynx, and stomach washings. Many investigators have been impressed by the high infectivity of herpangina, particularly within family and neighborhood groups. Group A coxsackieviruses have been isolated from 84% of patients with herpangina and 40% of their contacts. There is also strong evidence that strains of group A coxsackieviruses associated with herpangina may cause febrile illness without causing ulcerated lesions in the throat.

Manifestations

Fever, sore throat, and edema and hyperemia of the tonsils and pharyngeal walls mark the syndrome of nonbacterial pharyngitis. However, there are some differences in the diseases caused by each group of viruses that are helpful to clinical diagnosis.

Pharyngitis

Adenoviral pharyngitis occurs most commonly in young military recruits. The incubation period is estimated to be 5 to 7 days. Fever, chills, headache, anorexia, sore throat, hoarseness, and cough are present in about 75% of the patients. Physical examination may show a moderately red pharynx with lymphoid hyperplasia. Exudate may or may not be present on the tonsils and the posterior pharyngeal walls. Fever is usually present, ranging as high as 102°F, lasting about 3 to 4 days. If adenovirus type 3 is the etiologic agent, conjunctivitis usually accompanies the pharyngeal signs.

Acute pharyngitis caused by herpes simplex viruses and group A coxsackieviruses commonly occurs in children 1 to 7 years of age.

Gingivostomatitis

Primary herpetic gingivostomatitis occurs most often in children 1 to 4 years of age. The onset is usually abrupt. Constitutional symptoms may be severe, including fever of 103°F to 105°F, irritability, and anorexia. The throat is sore; the gums are swollen and bleed easily. Papulovesicular lesions 2 mm to 3 mm in diameter, each centered on a 4 mm to 6 mm erythematous base, are seen on the buccal mucosa, tongue, palate, and the oropharynx. These vesicular lesions rapidly change to punched-out ulcers. The disease is usually mild or moderately severe, with recovery in 5 to 7 days. In severe cases, fever persists and the child refuses oral intake because of the painful lesions. Dehydration and acidosis may develop, and clinical improvement may not be apparent until 10 to 14 days after onset.

Herpangina

Herpangina is primarily a disease of children 1 to 7 years old. The disease begins abruptly with a rise in temperature to 102°F to 103°F. Fever of 105°F does occur, and it may be accompanied by convulsions. Anorexia, dysphagia, and sore throat are common; vomiting, abdominal pain and diarrhea may also be present. On physical examination, the characteristic findings are grayish-white, papulovesicular lesions measuring 1 mm to 2 mm in diameter, located on the anterior pillars of the fauces and the tonsils, or along the free margin of the soft palate. These vesicles are occasionally seen on the posterior part of the buccal mucous membrane or the roof of the mouth. Within a day or two, the vesicles rupture and become punched-out ulcers. General and local symptoms last about 4 to 6 days; recovery is complete.

Diagnosis

Nonbacterial pharyngitis must be differentiated from streptococcal pharyngitis (see Chap. 24, Streptococcal Diseases) and diphtheria (see Chap. 25, Diphtheria)—much more serious diseases for which specific therapy is available. Exudate and hemorrhage over the tonsils and pharyngeal walls are common in streptococcal pharyngitis; however, exudates identical in appearance sometimes form in adenoviral pharyngitis. A throat culture for streptococcus is helpful in establishing the diagnosis. In diphtheria, a high index of suspicion is important. A moderate fever in a patient with a grayish-yellow to brownish pseudomembrane that leaves bleeding points on removal calls for smear and culture examinations for *Corynebacterium diphtheriae.*

Ulcerated lesions in the pharyngeal areas are typical of herpangina; herpetic lesions are more common in the buccal mucosa and gums. If conjunctivitis is present with pharyngitis, the infection is probably caused by adenovirus type 3. Tonsillopharyngitis is often the initial manifestation of infectious mononucleosis, preceding the appearance of atypical lymphocytes in the peripheral blood, general lymphadenopathy, and splenomegaly (see Chap. 137, Infectious Mononucleosis). The differentiation of infectious mononucleosis from other nonbacterial pharyngitides may be difficult.

Definitive etiologic diagnosis of nonbacterial pharyngitis requires either isolation of viral agents or documentation of a significant rise in specific serum antibodies during convalescence. These procedures are time consuming and expensive. They are valuable for the retrospective diagnosis of epidemics, but they contribute little practical diagnostic aid to the clinician who often deals with sporadic cases of pharyngitis and other respiratory illnesses.

Prognosis

Nonbacterial pharyngitis carries an excellent prognosis; complete recovery without complications is the rule. Occasionally, in severely ill young children, dehydration and acidosis may result from refusal of peroral intake because of painful, extensive lesions in the mouth and pharynx. If the pharyngitis is secondary to infectious mononucleosis, the complications are those of the primary disease—rupture of the spleen, neuropathy, thrombocytopenic purpura, and hemolytic anemia.

Homologous antibodies that develop following infections with specific agents can be demonstrated easily by serologic procedures such as complement fixation or neutralization tests. With adenoviruses, previous exposures appear to confer protection. Epidemics of ARD and pharyngitis are much less commonly seen among seasoned troops than among new military recruits. Herpes simplex virus persists as a latent virus in host cells even though there is demonstrable serum antibody from a primary infection. Recurrent herpesvirus disease appears to be the result of disturbance of the host–parasite equilibrium. Herpangina may recur because several types of coxsackieviruses can evoke this syndrome.

Therapy

There is no specific treatment for nonbacterial pharyngitis. Antimicrobial drugs do not affect the course of infection. Symptomatic treatment includes aspirin (10 mg/kg body wt for a child, 600 mg for an adult) and warm saline gargles. A diet liberal in fluids should be offered. Parenteral fluid replacement may be necessary in infants when acidosis and dehydration result from refusal of oral fluids.

Prevention

As in other respiratory infections, control measures attempting to limit virus spread by isolation of infected persons, installation of germicidal lamps, and use of disinfectant aerosols have little beneficial effect. No vaccine has been developed for immunization against herpangina because the disease is benign and because there are multiple serologic types of group A coxsackieviruses.

The search for an effective means of control of the herpesviruses has been unsuccessful. A killed herpesvirus vaccine was developed and proved to be either valueless or slightly beneficial. Inoculation with smallpox vaccine in an attempt to induce cross immunity to herpesvirus has been of equivocal value, and it is potentially dangerous in posing the threat of generalized vaccinia.

The loss of manpower in the military services from adenovirus-caused ARD and pharyngitis is significant. A trivalent killed vaccine containing types 3, 4, and 7 has been shown to be antigenic and brought about an 85% to 90% reduction of attack rate in military recruits. However, the vaccine was abandoned after the discovery of the oncogenic properties of some adenoviruses in nonhuman animals. A monovalent, attenuated, live type 4 adenovirus vaccine, when taken orally, results in viral multiplication in the alimentary tract with production of protective antibodies in recipients. Because adenoviral infection is of little medical significance in the civilian population, even in student dormitories, nonmilitary use of adenovirus vaccine for general immunization is not warranted at present.

Bibliography

Book

EVANS AS: Acute respiratory infections. In Top FH Sr, Wehrle PF (eds): Communicable and Infectious Diseases. St. Louis, C V Mosby,1972. pp 510–532.

Journals

BREESE BB, DISNEY FA: The accuracy of diagnosis of beta streptococcal infections on clinical grounds. J Pediatr 44:670–673, 1954

BUESCHER EL: Respiratory disease and the adenoviruses. Med Clin North Am 51:769–779, 1967

GLEZEN WP, CLYDE WA, SENIOR RJ, SHAEFFER CI, DENNY FW: Group A streptococci, mycoplasmas, and viruses associated with acute pharyngitis. JAMA 202:445–460, 1967

HAMRE D, CONNELLY AP JR, PROCKNOW JJ: Virologic studies of acute respiratory disease in young adults. IV. Virus isolation during four years of surveillance. Am J Epidemiol 83:238–249, 1966

MONTO AS, ULLMAN BM: Acute respiratory illness in an American community (the Tecumseh study). JAMA 227:164–169, 1974

PICKEN JJ, NIEWOEHNER DE, CHESTER EH: Prolonged effects of viral infections of the upper respiratory tract upon small airways. Am J Med 52:738–746, 1972

HUGH C. DILLON JR.
KENNETH L. VOSTI

Streptococcal Diseases (Groups A and B)

24

Diseases caused by *Streptococcus* spp. consist of lesions that either (1) contain live streptococci (most commonly in the respiratory tract, less frequently in the urogenital and integumentary systems, and occasionally as bacteremias with sundry metastatic involvements); or (2) are sterile and nonsuppurative (rheumatic fever and glomerulonephritis—delayed sequelae of infections caused by *Streptococcus pyogenes* of Lancefield's group A). Acute respiratory infections and rheumatic fever are considered in this chapter, along with infections caused by Group B *Streptococcus* spp.; pyoderma and acute glomerulonephritis are discussed in Chap. 101, Streptococcal Skin Infections and Glomerulonephritis.

Etiology

Streptococci are gram-positive, nonsporulating, generally nonmotile, spherical to ovoid bacteria 0.5 μm to 0.75 μm in diameter and occur in pairs or chains of variable length. On sheep blood agar, they grow as small, translucent to opaque, rarely pigmented colonies surrounded by unaffected culture medium (so-called γ-hemolysis), zones of greenish discoloration containing largely intact erythrocytes (α-hemolysis), or areas of complete destruction of red cells (β-hemolysis). Growth is generally optimal at 35°C to 37°C. Their metabolism is fermentative; they are cat-

Twenty-one species of *Streptococcus* have been differentiated by physiologic and immunologic characteristics. The scheme of classification developed by Lancefield is generally used (Table 24-1). It is based primarily on antigenic polysaccharide components of the cell wall that are group specific; however, the group-specific antigen of group D streptococci is lipoteichoic acid. It must be emphasized that not all Lancefield groups contain strains that are β-hemolytic and, more important, rare strains of group A streptococci may not be β-hemolytic.

Strains of the different serogroups may be recovered normally from several sites in humans and other animals. Pathogenicity for humans is not limited to a single group; however, strains of group A are most commonly associated with infections in humans and appear to be the only streptococci implicated in rheumatic fever. Group D streptococci frequently cause infective endocarditis (Chap. 134, Infective Endocarditis), and are occasionally implicated in infections of the urinary tract. Interest in group B streptococci has been renewed with the increased recognition of their role in bacteremia and meningitis of newborns. The range of diseases associated with non-group A streptococci is listed in Table 24-2.

Cellular Structure

Of the streptococci, *S. pyogenes* is the most important cause for disease, and there is an extensive body of information about it.

HYALURONIC ACID CAPSULE

The mucoid appearance of some strains of group A streptococci is related to the presence of hyaluronic acid capsules, which are most prominent in young cultures and in some epidemic strains. In certain group C strains that infect nonhuman animals, a hyaluronic acid capsule is also present and contributes to virulence by enhancing resistance to phagocytosis. Although a similar role has been proposed for the capsule of group A streptococci in infections of humans, M protein (see below) is the most important surface component associated with virulence.

SURFACE PROTEIN ANTIGENS

M proteins are the major surface protein antigens of the group A streptococci. They are type specific and enhance resistance to phagocytosis. More than 70 immunologically distinct M proteins have been identified, providing the principal means for serological classification of the group A streptococci. Lipotei-

Table 24-1. *Antigenic Groups of Streptococci, Habitat, and Pathogenicity*

Group	Species	Hemolysis	Host	Site	Recognized pathogenicity
A	*pyogenes*	Β, α, γ	Humans, cows, monkeys, rodents	Respiratory, skin, urogenital, feces	Humans—many clinical diseases Rodents—acute or chronic cervical adenitis and suppurative arthritis
B	*agalactiae*	β	Humans	Respiratory, urogenital	Humans—bacteremia, meningitis, suppurative arthritis
			Cattle	Milk and udder	Cattle—mastitis
C	*equisimilis*	β	Humans	Respiratory, urogenital	Humans—respiratory, bacteremia
	zooepidemicus		Horses		Horses—strangles, respiratory, others
	equi		Horses		Cattle—mastitis
	dysgalactiae		Cattle		
D	*faecalis*	α, γ, β	Humans	Intestine	Humans—urinary tract infection, bacteremia, endocarditis, abscesses
	faecium		Humans	Urogenital, respiratory	
	bovis		Cattle, humans		Cattle—endocarditis
	equinus		Horses		
	suis		Pigs		Pigs—bacteremia, meningitis, suppurative arthritis
E	Spp.	β	Humans Pigs	—	Humans—bacteremia Pigs—cervical adenitis, endocarditis
			Cattle		Cattle—mastitis
F	*anginosus*	β, α, γ	Humans	Respiratory, skin urogenital feces	Abscesses, sinusitis, meningitis
G	Spp.	β	Humans	Respiratory, urogenital, feces	Humans—pharyngitis, sinusitis, bacteremia
			Dogs		Dogs—adenitis, bacteremia
H	*sanguis*	α, β, γ	Humans	Respiratory, feces	Endocarditis, aphthous stomatitis (?)
J	Spp.	—	—	—	?
K	Spp.	γ, β	Humans	Respiratory, feces	Sinusitis, pulmonary, endocarditis
L	—	β	Humans, dogs, pigs	—	Miscellaneous infections
M	—	β, α	Humans, dogs	Respiratory, urogenital	Humans—endocarditis, abscesses
N	*lactis* *cremoris*	α, γ	Milk and milk products		Cattle—mastitis
O	—	α or β	Humans	Respiratory	Tonsilitis (?), pneumonia (?)
P	—		Pigs	—	Pneumonia, suppurative arthritis
Q	*avium*	α	Chickens, occasionally humans, dogs, pigs	Feces	?
R	—	γ	Pigs, humans	—	Pigs—septicemia Humans—bacteremia, meningitis
S	*suis*	α, γ	Pigs	—	Pigs—meningitis, bacteremia, suppurative arthritis
T	—		—	—	—

Table 24-2. *Diseases Associated With Non-Group A Streptococci**

DISEASE	Antigenic groups																				TOTALS
	B	C	D†	D‡	D§	E	F	G	H	J	K	L	M	N	O	P	Q	R	S	T	NG‖	
Bacteremia	20	6	36	95	29	1	6	12	25	0	6	2	0	0	1	0	0	0	0	0	30	269
Abscess	21	11	15	36	0	0	12	13	2	0	14	2	0	0	0	0	0	0	0	0	13	139
Arthritis	3	0	0	3	0	0	0	0	0	0	0	0	0	0	0	0	0	0	0	0	0	6
Endocarditis	13	2	3	87	42	0	0	2	4	0	2	0	0	0	0	0	0	0	0	0	17	172
Genital infection	3	1	0	1	0	0	1	1	0	0	0	0	0	0	0	0	0	0	0	0	1	8
Meningitis, brain abscess	8	0	1	4	0	0	3	0	3	0	3	0	0	0	0	0	0	0	0	0	0	22
Osteomyelitis	0	0	1	0	0	0	0	0	0	0	0	0	0	0	0	0	0	0	0	0	0	1
Upper resp. sinusitis, mastoiditis, otitis	3	0	2	2	0	1	2	0	0	0	4	1	0	0	0	0	0	0	0	0	2	17
Urinary tract infection	13	1	12	58	2	0	0	0	0	0	0	0	0	0	1	0	0	0	0	0	8	95
Totals	84	21	70	286	73	2	24	28	34	0	29	5	0	0	2	0	0	0	0	0	71	729

*Summarized from several published studies. The relative frequencies of occurrence of particulaı diseases with groups are approximations.
†Not differentiated.
‡Enterococcus.
§Nonenterococcus.
‖ Not groupable.

choic acid is the basic component of the hairlike fimbriae that protrude from the outer surface of the streptococcal cell wall. The M proteins appear to be associated with these fimbriae, and the complex promotes adherence of the streptococci to epithelial cells.

Other surface proteins are T, R, and serum opacity reaction (SOR). None of these is clearly implicated in virulence. However, T proteins are identified in a widely used serological typing system that is less specific than M typing, but is of epidemiological value. The T antigens of the lower numbered types correspond to M antigens of these same types. For example, M types 1, 3, 4, 6, and 12 commonly agglutinate with T antisera 1, 3, 4, 6, and 12. In contrast, many higher numbered M types share T agglutination antigens or complexes (Chap. 101, Streptococcal Skin Infections and Glomerulonephritis). SOR proteins are also antigenic. Not all group A strains produce SOR, but there is a general correspondence between M type and SOR antigen specificity.

Yet another surface component of group A streptococci has been shown to react with Fc portion of gamma globulin in a manner analogous to the protein A of *Staphylococcus aureus.* This streptococcal component, presumably also protein, is distinct from M antigen and is not type specific. It does not appear to be involved in resistance to phagocytosis.

GROUP-SPECIFIC CARBOHYDRATES

The group-specific antigen characteristic of group A streptococci is a multibranched polysaccharide consisting of *N*-acetyl-*d*-glucosamine and *l*-rhamnose. The immunodominant determinants are, typically, the terminal β-*N*-acetylglucosaminide residues. However, group A variants were developed by repeated passage in animals in which rhamnose was the determinant of immunologic specificity.

For group C streptococci, terminal α-*N*-acetylgalactosaminide residues are the important determinants of immunologic specificity. Pure group-specific carbohydrates are believed to be nontoxic. However, they are generally released from the cell wall in association with fragments of mucopeptide. Such mixed fragments produce a remittent nodular disease in experimental animals that is reminiscent of lesions observed in patients with rheumatic fever. Although antibodies to the group-specific carbohydrate are not protective, they remain elevated for longer periods in patients with rheumatic fever without carditis or acute glomerulonephritis. The implications of this observation to the pathogenesis of rheumatic carditis are not clear.

PEPTIDOGLYCAN (MUCOPEPTIDE)

Peptidoglycan, the rigid skeleton of the cell wall, is composed of repeating units of *N*-acetyl glucosamine and *N*-acetylmuramic acid (hexosamine polymers), cross-linked by complex peptide bridges. Streptococcal peptidoglycan is antigenic and is cross-reactive with similar material found in staphylococci. Peptidoglycan produces inflammatory responses in experimental animals, including dermal necrosis and carditis in rabbits. The role of peptidoglycan in the pathogenesis of streptococcal disease in humans is uncertain.

LIPOTEICHOIC ACID

The teichoic acid of group A streptococci consists of repeating units of polyglycerophosphate attached to lipids; it appears as fimbriae on the streptococcal cell surface, and promotes adherence to host cells. This mechanism is of importance in the initiation of streptococcal infections.

CYTOPLASMIC MEMBRANES

A thin, triple-layered cytoplasmic membrane lies within the cell wall of the group A streptococci. The cytoplasmic membrane is predominantly lipoprotein in structure and contains antigens distinct from cell wall antigens. The membrane forms the outer surface of streptococcal protoplasts or L forms. These altered form are osmotically fragile and are resistant to penicillin and other β-lactam antimicrobics.

STREPTOCOCCAL ANTIGENS CROSS-REACTIVE WITH TISSUE ANTIGENS

Numerous examples of cross-reactivity between streptococcal antigens and mammalian tissue have been described. Most studies have attempted to relate cross-reactions to the pathogenesis of rheumatic fever, chorea, or acute glomerulonephritis. Cell wall antigens, cytoplasmic membranes, and streptococcal hyaluronate have all been shown to cross-react with hear, skeletal muscle, glomerular basement membrane, and human brain tissue. Also, cross-reactive antibodies may promote cytotoxicity of sensitized lymphocytes. However, a definite role for the cross-reactive systems in the pathogenesis of streptococcal sequela has not yet been established.

Extracellular Products

Group A streptococci release into the extracellular environment substances that are mostly proteins, with toxic, enzymatic, or other biological activities. Certain other groups of β-hemolytic streptococci, notably groups C and G, produce similar substances, especially hemolysins and nucleases. Antibodies specific for the more commonly produced extracellular antigens often occur in association with infection and form the basis for several serological tests of clinical value. Though it seems reasonable that certain of these substances may contribute to the virulence of streptococci, a precise role in the pathogenesis of streptococcal disease in humans has been shown only for the erythrogenic toxin of scarlet fever. Several well-studied extracellular products are discussed in the following paragraphs.

DEOXYRIBONUCLEASE (DNase)

Groups A, B, C, and G streptococci elaborate DNases. Group A streptococci produce up to four antigenically distinct DNases, designated A, B, C, and D. DNase B is most common and is often produced in large amounts. Antibody directed against DNase B commonly developes during infection of either the skin of the throat. Anti-DNase B titers are strikingly elevated in patients with acute glomerulonephritis following skin infection (Chap. 101, Streptococcal Skin Infections and Glomerulonephritis). The anti-DNase B titer also remains elevated for a longer period than does anti-streptolysin O (ASO) and is therefore of value in the serological study of patients with acute rheumatic fever, including those with chorea.

EXOTOXINS

Group A streptococci may produce at least three immunologically distinct exotoxins (A, B, and C). Highly purified A toxin appears to be made up of protein complexed with hyaluronic acid.

Historically, the exotoxins were known for erythrogenic activity, as seen in the rash of scarlet fever. Other important biologic activities are now known to include the ability to stimulate fever, damage myocardial and liver tissue, blockade the reticuloendothelial system, suppress the early secondary immune response to injected sheep erythrocytes, promote lymphocyte-transforming activity, alter membrane permeability, and enhance susceptibility to the lethal shock of endotoxin. The immediate skin reaction caused by the intradermal injection of an erythrogenic exotoxin (Dick test) was originally thought to represent a toxic effect localized to the skin; however, it actually represents a reaction of acquired hypersensitivity to the toxin. The elaboration of the exotoxins has been shown to be an expression of lysogeny analogous to that involved in the production of diphtherial toxin (Ch. 25, Diphtheria).

HEMOLYSINS

Streptolysin O (Table 24-3) is the best known of the two major hemolysins produced by group A streptococci; it is the humoral response to this antigen that forms the basis for the ASO test so commonly employed for the serodiagnosis of streptococcal infection. Streptolysin S, the other hemolysin, is nonantigenic. However, unlike streptolysin O, which is oxygen labile, streptolysin S in stable under conditions of aerobic growth and is responsible for the clear zones of hemolysis seen around colonies of group A streptococci growing on the surface of blood agar. Hemolysis beneath the surface, that is, in the depths of the agar medium, and in cultures grown

Table 24-3. Properties of Hemolysins Elaborated by Streptococcus Pyogenes

	Streptolysin	
PROPERTY	O	S
Elaborated by	Most clinical isolates (also produced by strains of groups C and G)	Most clinical isolates (also produced by strains of all other groups); usually cell-bound but released by carrier molecules
Inactivated by	O_2, cholesterol, specific antibody, proteolytic enzymes	Heat, lecithin, lipoproteins, trypan blue, Congo red, proteolytic enzymes except trypsin
Active against	Erythrocytes, leukocytes, lysosomes, myocardial cells	Erythrocytes, leukocytes, lysosomes, platelets, bacterial protoplasts, Ehrlich tumor cells
Antigenic	+	−

under reduced oxygen tension, is likely a result of the actions of both hemolysins. A few strains of group A streptococci may produce only one or the other of the hemolysins, but it is the rare strain that produces neither. Although neither hemolysin has been shown to play a direct role in the development of streptococcal disease, it is apparent that both may exert toxic effects against a wide variety of mammalian cells. Streptolysin O may also transform lymphocytes and thus contribute to the cellular immune response in streptococcal infections; however, neither the mechanism of transformation nor its significance, especially with regard to pathogenesis of post-streptococcal sequela, is known.

The clinical significance of the ASO test is unequivocal. In untreated streptococcal respiratory infections, a rise in titer occurs within 2 to 5 weeks of onset. Persistence of an elevated titer depends in part upon the magnitude of the response. Patients with acute rheumatic fever commonly have higher antibody titers to streptolysin O, as well as to other extracellular streptococcal antigens, than patients with uncomplicated infection. Of particular interest, patients with pyoderma, including those who develop acute glomerulonephritis, mount a feeble ASO response; this is best explained by the probability that the hemolysin is antigenically inactivated by chloresterol and lipids at the primary site of infection in the skin.

HYALURONIDASE

Several groups of β-hemolytic streptococci produce hyaluronidase. Among group A strains, certain M types have been found to produce relatively large quantities of this enzyme and coincidentally lack a hyaluronic acid capsule. However, this inverse relationship is not uniform, and many strains of group A streptococci produce hyaluronidase that is antigenically specific for the group. Patients with either respiratory or skin infections, including those with either acute rheumatic fever or acute glomerulonephritis, frequently develop an immune response to this antigen.

STREPTOKINASE

Streptokinase is produced by β-hemolytic streptococci of groups A, C, and G. Two antigenically distinct streptokinases, designated SK-A and SK-B, have been identified among group A streptococci; a given strain produces one or the other form, and SK-A is more common. Streptokinase of group C origin (like that in commercial preparations of SK-SD) is closely related to SK-A, for example, the commercial preparation reacts with anti-SK-A antibody engendered in patients with group A streptococcal infections. Streptokinase appears to be an activator substance for the plasminogen-plasmin system. Periodically there have been attempts to use semipurified streptokinase as a fibrinolytic agent for clinical purposes, including efforts to lyse plural adhesions resulting from pulmonary infection, and clots in patients with coronary ar-

OTHER PRODUCTS

A number of other extracellular substances are elaborated by group A streptococci. Among them are a bacteriocin that appears capable of inhibiting various groups of β-hemolytic streptococci and certain other gram-positive bacteria; nicotinamide adenine dinucleotidase (NAD); amalyse; esterases; and proteinase. Production of these substances is variable. Certain of them, including NAD, are antigenic. However, antibody tests against them are not clinically useful.

Epidemiology

There are distinct differences in the epidemiology of streptococcal infections of the throat and of the skin. The latter subject is treated in detail in Chapter 101 (Streptococcal Skin Infections and Glomerulonephritis).

Humans are the natural hosts for group A streptococci. Certain domestic animals may become colonized as a result of close contact with infected humans, but seldom contribute to clinical infection. Respiratory strains of group A streptococci are commonly found in the nasopharynx, including tonsillar and other lymphoid tissues. Respiratory infections are spread among persons in close contact by way of large droplets of secretions from the respiratory tract. Streptococcal pharyngitis is most common in school-aged children, with a peak age incidence of around 10 to 12 years. Infected school children are the primary source of streptococcal respiratory infections that occur in family units.

Close contact indoors during the colder months undoubtedly makes for a higher incidence of streptococcal pharyngitis. However, it is not unusual to see a sharp rise in the incidence of disease when schools reopen in the later summer or early fall. Furthermore, it is now evident that streptococcal pharyngitis is a worldwide problem, occurring in tropical or subtropical as well as temperate and cold climates. Seasonal peaks of streptococcal respiratory infection are less evident in semitropical or tropical areas where temperatures are relatively constant. However, similar factors, such as the gathering together of children at school or other institutions, result in an increased incidence of disease at certain times of the year.

Certain populations, such as military recruits, are at increased risk for streptococcal pharyngitis. Factors include crowded or close living conditions as in barracks, as well as stress and climate. Common to the risk of disease in school children, military recruits, or others, is a relatively susceptible population, that is, one in which many or most persons lack immunity to the specific M types found in the community at a particular time.

Specific properties of group A streptococci that favor person-to-person transmission are incompletely understood. Production of M protein is involved because it is essential for attachment to epithelial cells, and all virulent strains have it. Also, a higher incidence of disease is associated with strains that cause scarlet fever and those that are highly mucoid.

In addition to direct person-to-person spread, streptococcal pharyngitis may also result from foodborne infection. This relatively unusual, epidemic form of streptococcal disease is particularly disabling, with a high ratio of disease to subclinical illness.

Strains of group A streptococci associated with acute respiratory infection may also be associated with infection at other sites or may cause disseminated disease. In cases of burn or wound infection, patients may be infected with strains carried in their own respiratory tract and may also become infected as a result of contact with others. Apparently, many classic cases of puerperal sepsis caused by group A streptococci occurred following acute respiratory tract infection in the mother.

Pathogenesis and Pathology

Attachment of group A streptococci to mucosal cells of the upper respiratory tract must occur before either colonization or disease can result. M proteins appear to be important because anti-M antibodies block attachment. The penetration of the mucosa, which causes clinical infection, may be related to diverse biologic activities associated with the many cellular and extracellular products of *S. pyogenes.*

Inoculation of the pharyngeal mucosa of volunteers with 2×10^7 group A streptococci is followed by a latent period of 36 to 72 hours when it is not possible to culture streptococci from the throat. As cultures become positive, rapidly increasing numbers of streptococci can be isolated; disease develops with sore throat, inflammation of the pharynx and tonsils (with or without exudates), fever, and leukocytosis. The severity of the clinical disease is variable for reasons that are not known precisely. However, the immunologic responsiveness of the host to the cellular or extracellular products of streptococci may be important because the severity of pharyngitis is definitely increased, and the occurrence of exudate is more frequent, in older, as compared with younger, children.

From the nasopharyngeal site, infection may be transferred to the skin, causing facial erysipelas or pyoderma. Extension to the adjacent paranasal sinuses, eustachian tube, and middle ear may be associated with obstruction which leads to the suppurative complications common prior to the development of antimicrobics. Futher direct extension may lead to mastoiditis, osteomyelitis, cavernous sinus thrombosis, or meningitis. Lymphogenous spread from the pharynx may result in cervical adenitis. Rarely, pneumonia may occur, usually secondary to a viral pneumonia (see Chap. 30, Nonbacterial Pneumonias);

massive serofibrinous empyema is a common, early complication. Bacteremia may arise from any of these foci of infection, resulting in purulent arthritis, osteomyelitis, meningitis, or other deep, septic processes.

Manifestations

Streptococcal diseases constitute a wide range of clinical syndromes. Manifestations are influenced by the variety of portals of entry, the potential for regional and distant spread of infection, and the age of the patient.

The clinical features of streptococcal respiratory infections are quite variable. In the infant or young child 3 to 4 years of age, respiratory infections may be manifested by (1) fever with acute cervical lymphadenitis (streptococci can be recovered from the affected lymph nodes), but little, if any, inflammation of the upper respiratory tract; and (2) a relatively nonspecific form of respiratory infection consisting of acute lymphadenitis, progressing to persistant enlargement of cervical lymph nodes, low-grade fever, and mild pharyngeal inflammation with purulent rhinorrhea. There are no contemporary epidemiological data on the frequency of these forms of infection. In general, acute exudative pharyngitis in the younger child is less likely to be streptococcal in etiology than is the similar syndrome in older children.

Acute exudative pharyngitis is the typical form of streptococcal respiratory infection seen beyond the first few years of life. In classic cases, the onset is so abrupt that the patient often recalls quite accurately when the illness began. There are fever, chills or chilly sensations, headache, an acutely sore throat with pain on swallowing, malaise, and not infrequently abdominal pain, nausea and vomiting. Examination of the pharynx reveals erythema; edema of lymphoid tissues, soft palate and uvula; and a filmy or purulent nonadherent exudate over the tonsils and posterior pharynx. Petechiae may develop on the soft palate and tonsillar pillars. The anterior cervical lymph nodes are acutely tender and may enlarge rapidly. In scarlet fever, there is a more pronounced hyperemia of the entire pharynx (enanthem) with petechial lesions and a strawberry tongue, and a fine, red skin rash that is most pronounced over the trunk and extremities. The rash usually develops within the first 48 hours of illness. Patients with scarlet fever often appear to be more acutely and severely ill than patients with acute pharyngitis. In dark-skinned patients, the rash may be difficult to discern, but when peeling begins, the rash becomes evident.

Not all patients have every classical feature of streptococcal pharyngitis. The clinical findings vary in relation to the duration of the illness. Early on, exudate may not be apparent and lymph node enlargement may not have occurred, although there may be tenderness beneath the angle of the jaw; typical features usually evolve within 48 hours of onset. Perhaps a third of the patients who experience acute streptococcal respiratory tract infection have either a mild or a subclinical infection. Such patients are of concern because the diagnosis is easily missed, and yet this form of streptococcal infection may be responsible for up to half the cases of acute rheumatic fever that now occur. Regardless of the clinical severity of the acute pharyngitis, a throat culture is required for diagnosis.

Group A streptococci are associated with other respiratory infectious syndromes, most of which are complications or extensions of pharyngeal infection. These include peritonsillar and retropharyngeal abscesses, acute sinusitis, acute otitis media, and pneumonia. Group A streptococci rank third, following *Streptococcus pneumoniae* and *Hemophilus influenzae,* as causes of acute otitis media in children. Historically, scarlet fever has been associated with a higher incidence of such suppurative complications. Streptococcal pneumonia occurs most often as a complication of influenza or other viral respiratory infections, including measles (Chap. 31, Bacterial Pneumonias).

Neonatal and puerperal infections caused by group A streptococci are discussed in conjunction with group B streptococcal disease.

Diagnosis

The isolation and characterization of *Streptococcus* spp. from appropriate cultures provides the only definitive means of establishing the diagnosis. Even a classic septic sore throat must be proved streptococcal by isolation of *S. pyogenes* because many of the manifestations of streptococcal infections can be associated with nonbacterial causes of acute pharyngitis (viruses, *Mycoplasma pneumoniae*—see Chap. 23, Nonbacterial Pharyngitis). Etiologic diagnosis is further complicated by the possibility that recovery of group A streptococci from pharyngeal cultures of symptomatic patients may reflect asymptomatic carriage in the presence of upper respiratory infections caused by other etiologic agents. Although an immunologic response (ASO or anti-DNase-B) should not result from carriage of streptococci, early treatment with penicillin can abort such an immune response.

That is, failure to demonstrate a serologic response may not exclude the possibility of streptococcal disease.

Streptococci are characterized initially by patterns of hemolysis when grown on nutrient agar plates containing 5% sheep red blood cells. Further characterization (Table 24-4) provides a presumptive diagnosis of serogroups. Definite, serologic classification can be obtained by the method described by Lancefield; this method employs hot hydrochloric acid extracts of whole cells and group-specific antisera in a precipitin test. The direct fluorescent antibody technique has been used in some laboratories to accelerate the identification of group A streptococci in throat swabs and spinal fluid (Chap. 9, Microscopic Examinations). Similarly, counterimmunoelectrophoresis has been used to provide rapid identification of solubilized group antigens in cerebrospinal or other body fluids (Chap. 14, Immunologic Diagnosis).

The initial isolation of hemolytic streptococci from mixed flora may be facilitated by the incorporation of neomycin sulfate (10 μg/ml) in blood agar plates to suppress the growth of *Staphylococcus* spp. or enteric bacteria, which may produce hemolysis. Various inexpensive commerical kits are available to the practicing physician for the diagnosis of suspected streptococcal infections. With a minimum of training, physicians can process and interpret throat cultures for streptococci with reasonable accuracy.

Measurements of antibodies to various of the extracellular products, for example ASO and DNase-B, are used to confirm past infections. It must be remembered that immunologic responsiveness may be reduced by age (under 4 years) and early effective treatment, and obscured by a high initial titer as a result of a past infection. However, a rise in titer is consistent with infection during the preceding 1 to 5 weeks. A high titer when first measured, for example ASO of 1:128 or greater, is compatible with either a recent infection or disease within the past 3 to 6 months. A hemagglutination test (Streptozyme) is available that appears to be more sensitive in detecting early antibody responses; unfortunately, little is known of the antigens involved because a concentrate of a crude culture filtrate is used to sensitize the red cells.

Prognosis

Prior to the availability of effective chemotherapy, the outcome of streptococcal infections was directly related to the extent of disease. Severe streptococcal pharyngitis generally subsided after 5 to 7 days unless it was accompanied by local suppurative complications, bacteremia, or metastatic foci in bones, joints, central nervous system, or other sites. The prepenicillin death rate of 1% to 3% was directly related to these complications. The use of antimicrobics has reduced sharply the occurrence of local suppurative complications, bacteremia, and metastatic septic complications.

The risk of developing late, nonsuppurative complications of streptococcal infection cannot be predicted with certainty for the individual patient. In part, this reflects an inability to assess the nephritogenicity or rheumatogenicity of the infecting strain; recognize host or environmental factors that may predispose to these diseases; and weigh the likelihood that early, effective therapy may reduce the risk of developing late sequelae. Despite these limitations, glomerulonephritis appears to follow infection with pharyngeal or skin strains of certain M types or T types of group A streptococci, whereas rheumatic fever may follow pharyngeal, but not skin, infections with any of the M types. In various studies, the likelihood of developing rheumatic fever has ranged from 0.5% to 3%.

Table 24-4. *Presumptive Identification of* Streptococcus *Spp.**

Group Identification	Hemolysis	Bacitracin susceptibility	Hippurate hydrolysis	Bile-esculin hydrolysis	Tolerance to 6.5% NaCl
Group A	β	+	−	−	−
Group B	β	−†	+	−	V‡
Non-group A, B, or D	β	−†	−	−	−†
Group D, enterococcus	β, α or None	−	V‡	+	+
Group D, nonenterococcus	α or None	−	−	+	−
Viridans, non-group D	α or None	V‡	−†	−	−

* Facklam RR. In Blair JE (ed): Manual of Clinical Microbiology, 2nd ed. Baltimore, Williams & Wilkins, 1974, pp 96–108
† An occasional exception
‡ Variable

Therapy

Penicillin continues to be the drug of choice for treating all forms of group A streptococcal disease. Strains resistant to penicillin have not been found, and group A streptococci are inhibited by concentrations of 0.02 to 0,005 μg/ml.

Effective treatment for upper respiratory infections can be attained with (1) one intramuscular (IM) injection of benzathine penicillin G (600,000 units in infants and children 8–10 years old and 900,000–1,200,000 units in older children and adults) or (2) a 10-day course of peroral (PO) potassium penicillin V (25–50 mg/kg body wt/day as four equal portions, 6-hourly), preferably taken on an empty stomach to ensure maximum absorption. Patients who are hypersensitive to penicillins may be treated with erythromycin (20 mg/kg body wt/day, PO, as four equal portions 6-hourly) or cephalexin/cephradine (25–50 mg/kg body wt/day, PO, as four equal portions 6-hourly) for 10 days. Sulfonamides are not recommended for the treatment of streptococcal infections because they neither eradicate streptococci nor prevent rheumatic fever. Although effective, clindamycin is not recommended because of the potential for causing enterocolitis. Tetracycline should not be used because 15% to 40% of group A streptococci are resistant to this agent.

Patients who have pharyngitis with unusual frequency, and patients with throat cultures persistently positive for streptococci after therapy, merit study to differentiate streptococcal disease from pharyngeal carriage of streptococci coincident with an unrelated respiratory illness. Serial antibody tests, such as that for ASO, should reveal a rising titer following repeated episodes of streptococcal disease. Clinical evaluation of each illness, in conjunction with quantitative streptococcal bacteriology, is also helpful. If the clinical manifestations are atypical or minimal, or if only a few streptococci are recovered from the throat, streptococcal carriage should be suspected rather than streptococcal disease. Occasionally, new infections may be distinguished from relapse or carriage only by detecting different M types in serial isolates submitted to a reference laboratory for serotyping.

Opinions differ as to the need for a throat culture after treatment if the patient is well 2 to 3 weeks after the onset of the acute illness. If cultures are positive after therapy, it is essential to determine whether the streptococci are group A, since carriage of group C or group G streptococci eliminates the need for further concern. Without recurrent disease, only rising titers of antibodies along with repeated isolations of group A streptococci from throat cultures should lead to additional antibacterial therapy. It is important to avoid the repeated administration of IM benzathine penicillin G to asymptomatic children who appear to be carriers.

Serious complications such as pneumonia, bacteremia, osteomyelitis, septic joint disease, puerperal sepsis, and meningitis are indications for parenteral treatment with larger doses of penicillin, for example 25 mg to 150 mg (40,000–235,000 units) /kg body wt/day, IV, as four or six equal portions, 6- or 4-hourly. In patients with hypersensitivity to penicillins, parenteral administration of a cephalosporanic acid derivative is the preferred form of treatment.

With the exception of group D enterococci, infections caused by other serogroups, including most isolates of group D nonenterococci, may be treated with the regimens of penicillin G used for group A streptococci. Group D enterococci are relatively resistant to penicillin G, with many strains having minimum inhibitory concentrations of 3 μg/ml or more. Because ampicillin is more active than penicillin G, it is preferred for the treatment of infections caused by group D enterococci; the dose and route of administration are related to the site of infection.

Prevention

There is no vaccine for the prevention of streptococcal infections. Chemoprophylaxis to prevent infections with group A streptococci is indicated in patients who have had rheumatic fever in order to prevent recurrences (see Rheumatic Fever). Tonsillectomy is not useful in the prevention of streptococcal infections or rheumatic fever.

Remaining Problems

The risks of chronic carriage of group A streptococci are poorly understood. This has important therapeutic implications, particularly if treatment is unnecessary and if chronic carriage is in some way related to the stimulation or maintenance of immunity. Little is known of the events facilitating the implantation of group A streptococci in the oropharynx and the initiation of infection. A better understanding of such events might lead to a better means of controlling infections and thus preventing sequelae.

Attempts to develop a vaccine are underway; however, numerous problems related to production, administration, and assessment of efficacy limit immediate availability. To be effective, highly immunogenic M proteins must be prepared free of toxic materials or antigens that cross-react with host tissues; mixtures of the most common M types are needed. Vaccine prevention of glomerulonephritis holds most promise because a limited number of M types is involved—particularly with pharyngeal infections where M 12 is the dominant type. However, prevention of streptococcal pyoderma will be more difficult because the strains involved possess M proteins that are only weakly immunogenic.

Rheumatic Fever

Pathogenesis

The relationship of infection with *S. pyogenes* of many different M types to the subsequent development of an initial or recurrent attack of rheumatic fever has been clearly established. Yet, the actual mechanism(s) by which streptococci provoke rheumatic fever and carditis is not known. Neither the occurrence of a rheumatogenic factor, limited to certain strains of group A streptococci nor the involvement of other infectious agents, such as viruses, has been convincingly implicated as important in the pathogenesis of this disease.

The onset of rheumatic fever occurs within a few days to 5 weeks (mean of 19 days) after a symptomatic streptococcal infection. This latent period does not appear to differ for primary or recurrent rheumatic fever. At the onset of disease, high levels of antibodies to many of the cell wall components and extracellular products of *S. pyogenes* are generally present. In addition, antibodies reactive with various components of heart tissue can be demonstrated in at least one half of the patients. The titers of the various antibodies appear to parallel the activity of the disease. Higher titers of antibody for group A carbohydrate appear to persist in patients with rheumatic carditis as compared with patients who have rheumatic fever without carditis. Such immunologic hyperreactivity to streptococcal antigens does not appear to represent an allergic diathesis because patients with rheumatic fever respond to nonstreptococcal antigens in a manner similar to those without rheumatic fever.

Some antigenic determinants are common to human cardiac tissues and streptococcal cell walls and membranes. Also γ-globulins are bound to myocardial tissues obtained from patients with rheumatic heart disease at necropsy or surgical operation. There is no reproducible experimental model of rheumatic carditis.

Several hypotheses constructed to explain the various clinical and experimental observations of rheumatic fever are listed in Table 24-5; none has been proved. A direct toxic effect from streptococcal cell wall components or extracellular products has some experimental support. However, the long latent period between infection and the clinical manifestations of rheumatic fever would be unusual for most toxic reactions. The suggestion that there is in fact no latent period because streptococci persist as L forms that continue to elaborate toxic factor(s) flounders for lack of demonstration of L forms and a suitably hyperosmolar environment in which L forms could persist.

The most intriguing of the postulated immunologic mechanisms holds that rheumatic fever may be mediated by host antibodies that were initially stimulated by streptococcal cell wall or membrane antigens. Because of the sharing of the antigenic determinants by streptococcal antigens and heart tissue, such antibodies can react not only with the streptococci but also with the heart. Although the host's shared antigens are normally covert, toxic injury by certain extracellular products of streptococci is postulated to result in exposure of the cardiac antigens to cross-reactive antibodies. Indirect support for this hypothesis is provided by the relationship of cross-reactive antibodies to the activity of disease (Fig. 24-1).

Alternatively, heart-reactive antibodies may be true autoantibodies that result secondarily from autoimmunization of the host with tissue antigens released as a result of toxic injury by the extracellular products of *S. pyogenes.* At this time, primary versus secondary antibody-mediated injury cannot be differentiated.

Although streptococcal antigen—antibody complexes provide the best candidate explanation of the pathogenesis of poststreptococcal glomerulonephritis, there is no convincing evidence to either confirm or exclude the operation of a similar mechanism in the development of rheumatic fever.

Hypotheses for the Pathogenesis of Rheumatic Fever and Glomerulonephritis

Toxic effect
Immunologic mechanism
Antigenic determinants shared by *Streptococcus pyogenes* and host tissues
Autoantibodies initiated by the release of host antigens by toxic injury
Streptococcal antigen–antibody complexes

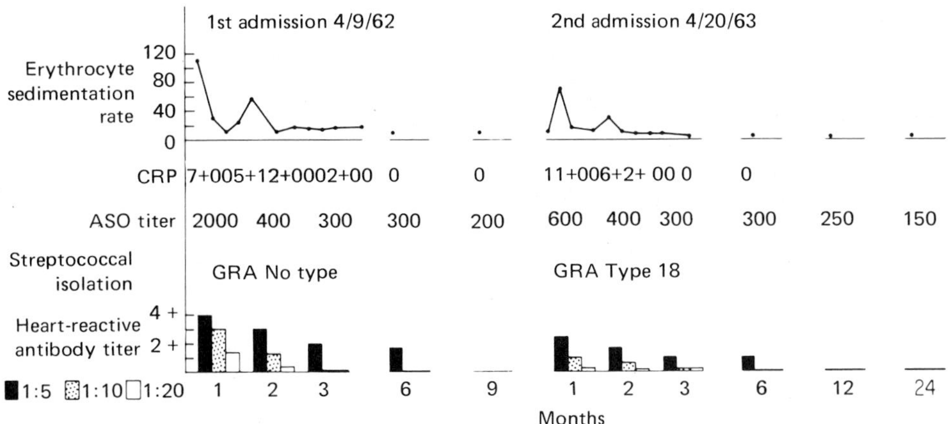

Fig. 24-1. Acute-phase reactants and heart-reactive antibody titers in a 7½-year-old boy during two episodes of acute rheumatic fever about 1 year apart. A soft, apical systolic murmur and a mild increase in cardiac size was noted with the attacks. Treatment with penicillin, prednisone, and salicylates was associated with recovery. There were no abnormalities on examination 3 years after the second attack. (Zabriskie JB: Advances in Immunology, Vol. 7, pp. 147–148 New York, Academic Press, 1967)

Manifestations

The clinical manifestations of rheumatic fever vary greatly and are determined by the sites involved, the severity of the attack, and the stage of the disease at which the patient is examined. In children over 6 years of age, rheumatic fever begins abruptly with onset of fever of 38°C to 40°C (101°F–104°F) and pain swelling of several joints such as the knees, ankles, elbows, or wrists. Several joints may be involved simultaneously, but characteristically the pain migrates from one joint to another. The pain is frequently more severe than seems to be warranted from the appearance of the joints.

Approximately 40% to 50% of children have evidence of myocarditis or valvulitis during the first attack of rheumatic fever. Recognition of carditis is particularly important because it is the only manifestation associated with significant sequelae. Murmurs almost always occur with carditis and typically reflect the presence of mitral regurgitation. A middiastolic murmur may be present that is not the murmur of mitral stenosis; the latter murmur, if it occurs, generally becomes apparent late in convalescence. The diastolic murmur of aortic insufficiency is found infrequently in children. Cardiac enlargement occurs in approximately 50% of patients with first attacks of rheumatic carditis and is accompanied by congestive heart failure (CHF) in around 5% to 10%. In less than 1% of these patients, severe, rapidly progressive carditis leads to death of the patient. Additional findings may include pericarditis, gallop rhythms, and other arrhythmias.

Subcutaneous nodules occure most commonly over the extensor surfaces of joints among children with severe carditis of several weeks' duration. Erythema marginatum—evanescent, macular, pink-to-reddish lesions with irregular central clearing—occurs in approximately 10% to 15% of children with rheumatic fever. Sydenham's chorea (spasmodic muscular movements and incoordination developing either during acute rheumatic fever or several months later) has become less common and recently has been reported in only 5% to 15% of patients. Epistaxis and abdominal pain occur as uncommon manifestations; the latter may be particularly perplexing, for it can mimic acute appendicitis.

Diagnosis

The diverse clinical manifestations and the nonspecific laboratory findings can make diagnosing acute rheumatic fever extremely difficult. In 1944, with the goal of providing uniformity and precision in diagnosis, T. Duckett Jones formulated a set of guidelines that became known as the Jones criteria. Last revised by the American Heart Association in 1965, the modified Jones criteria are given in Table 24-6.

Rheumatic fever frequently must be differentiated from other conditions manifested by fever and articular disease. Such conditions include rheumatoid arthritis, systemic lupus erythematosus (LE), Henoch–

Table 24-6. *Modified Jones Criteria for Diagnosis of Rheumatic Fever**

Major Manifestations	**Minor Manifestations**
Carditis	Fever
Murmurs	Arthralgia†
Prolonged apical systolic	Previous rheumatic fever or rheumatic heart disease
Apical middiastolic	
Basal diastolic	Increased erythrocyte sedimentation rate
Cardiomegaly	
Pericarditis	Positive C-reactive protein
Congestive failure	
Polyarthritis	Leukocytosis
Chorea	Prolonged PR interval‡
Erythema marginatum	
Subcutaneous nodules	

Evidence of antecedent streptococcal infection
Scarlet fever
Positive culture for group A streptococci
Increased anti-streptolysin O or other streptococcal antibody

* Two major, or one major and two minor, manifestations supported by evidence of an antecedent streptococcal infection indicates a high probability of rheumatic fever.

† Not a valid minor manifestation when polyarthritis is counted as a major manifestation.

‡ Not a valid minor manifestation when carditis is counted as a major manifestation.

Schönlein purpura, serum sickness, sickle cell hemoglobinopathies, postinfectious arthritis, septic arthritis, the early stages of leukemia, and infective bacterial endocarditis.

In children under 4 years of age, polyarthritis is most likely to be rheumatoid arthritis, particularly if there is involvement of the small joints of the hands, hectic fever, lymphadenopathy, and splenomegaly. Although tests for rheumatoid arthritis are frequently not helpful in children, persistence of joint symptoms in patients receiving adequate doses of salicylates should raise the possibility of rheumatoid arthritis.

The presence of a malar butterfly rash and a positive LE cell test support the diagnosis of disseminated lupus erythematosus. Petechiae that are prominent over the lower half of the body are consistent with Henoch–Schönlein's purpura; petechiae rarely occur in rheumatic fever. A serum sickness syndrome should be suspected in patients receiving penicillins or other drugs, particularly when arthralgia and fever are accompanied by angioneurotic edema and an urticarial rash or eosinophilia. Sickle cell hemoglobinopathies are best differentiated by appropriate laboratory tests; the coexistence of sickle cell disease and rheumatic fever is uncommon. The postinfectious arthritis of viral diseases, particularly rubella, should rarely be confused with rheumatic fever. A migratory polyarthritis is typical of gonorrheal joint disease (Chap. 56, Gonococcal Infections) and is a common manifestation of chronic meningococcemia (Chap. 151, Septic Arthritis). Other bacterial arthritides are usually monoarticular and may be related to infection at another site. Examination of a Gram-stained smear of synovial fluid and culture of the fluid should be helpful.

The early stages of leukemia may mimic rheumatic fever. Examination of smears of the peripheral blood and the bone marrow are required to establish the diagnosis of leukemia. The presence of scattered petechiae, splenomegaly, and the documentation of bacteremia should suggest the probability of infective endocarditis.

Therapy

Effective treatment of acute rheumatic fever includes administration of an antimicrobic to eradicate streptococcal infection and sufficient doses of an antiinflammatory agent to suppress the clinical manifestations of rheumatic fever.

The selection of an antiinflammatory agent is related to the extent of the clinical manifestations. Salicylates are the drugs of choice in patients with joint manifestations without carditis (*e.g.,* aspirin, 100 mg/kg body wt/day, PO, as four equal portions, 6-hourly, for at least 4 weeks). Carditis with cardiac enlargement or congestive failure should be treated initially with glucosteroids, (*e.g.,* prednisone, 2 mg/kg body wt/day, PO, as four equal portions, 6-hourly, for 2 to 4 weeks). The dose of prednisone should be decreased gradually during the final week; at the same time, salicylates should be given and continued for a week after the prednisone therapy is stopped to lessen the chance of relapse of carditis. Patients with carditis without cardiomegaly may be treated with salicylates, although some physicians prefer to treat all patients who have carditis with glucosteroids.

Ambulation is generally restricted during the acute stages of rheumatic fever with absolute bed rest continued until the clinical manifestations have disappeared. Activity should be more carefully controlled for a longer time in patients with carditis, particularly in the presence of cardiomegaly.

Prevention

Patients with rheumatic fever must be protected from streptococcal infections to minimize the risk of a recurrence of disease. The most effective antimicrobial regimen has been 1.2 million units of benzathine penicillin, given IM once per month. Sulfonamides (1 g/day PO) are nearly as effective. Unfortunately, failure to take oral agents regularly reduces their effectiveness. Patients must continue prophylaxis for at least 5 years after an episode of rheumatic fever because of the increased risk of recurrence during this period. The exact duration of prophylaxis beyond 5 years cannot be stated with certainty for all patients. Environmental and geographic factors known to be associated with an increased risk of developing rheumatic fever must be heeded.

Remaining Problems

The pathogenesis of rheumatic fever remains an enigma. Better understanding of the role of both the host and the parasite in the pathogenesis of this disease should prove valuable to its recognition as well as to possible prevention of the disease and its serious cardiac complications.

An additional perplexing problem is the lack of carefully defined guidelines for the duration of antimicrobial prophylaxis among patients who have had rheumatic fever.

Group B Streptococcal Infections

Etiology

Streptococcus agalactiae, or group B streptococci (GBS) resemble other β-hemolytic streptococci in their morphologic and cultural characteristics. They grow well in the enriched mediums suitable for the cultivation of group A streptococci. Such mediums, for example Todd–Hewitt broth and sheep blood agar, may be rendered usefully selective for GBS by the addition of nalidixic acid, polymyxin B, and crystal violet. In comparison with group A streptococci, the colonies of GBS on sheep blood agar are usually more mucoid, often larger, an off-white to pearl-gray color, and surrounded by smaller zones of hemolysis.

The CAMP test is a simple and reliable method for the presumptive identification of GBS. A positive test depends on augmentation of the action of the β-hemolysin of *Staphylococcus aureus* by a nonhemolytic polypeptide produced by GBS. The streptococcal isolate is streaked perpendicular to the indicator staphylococcal strain on blood agar; a positive test is signaled by a distinctive zone of enhanced hemolysis shaped like an arrowhead (with the base at the staphylococcal streak).

The group-specific antigen characteristic of GBS is found in the cell wall; it contains rhamnose (the major determinant), *N*-acetyl-glucosamine, and galactose. Serotyping (Lancefield) is based on carbohydrate (four type-specific, one shared—in a capsule-like structure) and protein antigens (Table 24-7). The major type-specific carbohydrate antigens contain galactose, glucose glucosamine, and sialic acid; the latter appears to be important in eliciting protective antibody. Type-specific antibodies in human serum protect chick embryos and appear to enhance opsonization of the homologous type when complement is present. The carbohydrate antigens of GBS elicit protective antibodies in rabbits.

Hippuricase and nucleases, which are antigenic, are produced by some strains. Neuraminidase (sialidase) is also produced by some strains, perhaps more often and in larger amounts by type III GBS; elaboration may correlate with virulence.

Some strains of GBS are lysogenic. A bacteriophage typing system has been developed and may afford increased sensitivity for epidemiologic studies, particularly when the spread of a single type requires study.

Epidemiology

Prior to serologic classification as group B streptococci, *S. agalactiae* were known to cause bovine mastitis. Infection of humans was first recognized in the 1930s by the isolation of GBS from the birth canal of parturient women who were usually asymptomatic or had mild postpartum fever. By the 1950s, it had become apparent that there was an association between maternal and fetal or neonatal infection. Over the ensuing decades, most epidemiologic studies to define reservoirs and carriage sites of GBS were carried out in pregnant women and their offspring.

Maternal carriage rates greater than 30% have been reported. Improved bacteriologic methods ac-

Table 24-7. *Type Antigens of Group B β-Hemolytic Streptococci*

Antigenic Determinants*	Types IA	IB	IC	II	III
Carbohydrate					
Specific	Ia	Ib	Ia	II	III
Nonspecific	Iabc	Iabc	Iabc	—	—
Proteins		Ibc	Ibc		

* Major type-specific antigens are the specific carbohydrate antigens Ia, Ib, II, and III. Some type II and III strains may have Ibc protein antigen and some type III strains have the R antigen, which is cross-reactive with that found in some group A streptococci.

count in part for such high rates, but there also appears to be a true increase in the prevalence of GBS. Increased prevalence of carriage is reflected in increased maternal and neonatal rates of disease, for example maternal infection rates of 2/1000 deliveries and neonatal sepsis rates of 5/1000 live births.

The highest incidence of disease occurs in the socioeconomically disadvantaged populace. Geographical and ethnic differences have also been reported. The highest rates of disease are reported from inner city urban populations, primarily in blacks, but not in Mexican-Americans in the same communities. During the past 10 to 12 years, as neonatal group B streptococcal disease has increased in the United States, it has declined in Great Britain and Western Europe.

The gut is the primary reservoir for GBS. Anorectal carriage rates are higher than vaginal or cervical carriage rates in pregnant women, and gut carriage precedes colonization of the birth canal. Anorectal carriage occurs in males as well as females, and anal cultures are more often positive than throat cultures in neonates and young infants who are colonized at or soon after birth. Thus, the epidemiology of group B streptococcal infection is much like that of gram-negative bacillary infections that are derived from the gut of the host. Moreover, GBS rank second to *Escherichia coli* as causes of bacteriuria in pregnancy.

Infection of the mother with GBS during pregnancy, as well as classic puerperal infection, appears to result from carriage strains. Bacteriuria is the most common infection during pregnancy; amnionitis and endometritis are generally recognized at parturition. There is a striking relationship between endometritis, abdominal delivery, and group B streptococcal bacteremia or sepsis in the parturient. Other kinds of bacteria are concomitantly involved in amnionitis and endometritis, although bacteremia with GBS clearly originates from endometritis.

Neonatal infections are arbitrarily but conveniently designated as early onset or late onset based on the interval from birth to disease. Approximately two thirds of early-onset group B streptococcal infections are recognized within the first 3 days of life; most are evident within 24 hours after birth. A maternal source of GBS is the rule in these cases. The fetus usually acquires GBS *in utero,* but may become infected intrapartum. Since the early form of neonatal group B streptococcal disease is seen most often in low birth weight, preterm, immature infants, GBS may be a cause of preterm delivery. Indeed, group B streptococcal infections acquired *in utero* may be a continuum from intrauterine fetal death—stillbirth—to early sepsis in the infant born live. All five major serotypes of GBS have been associated with early-onset disease.

Late-onset group B streptococcal infections of infants are less likely to be of maternal origin as the interval lengthens from birth to disease. Other sources include nonmaternal family contacts, the infant's own carriage flora (infrequently), and the environment (nosocomial infection). Following the peak of early-onset disease within the first 2 to 3 days of life, the rate of occurrence of group B streptococcal disease holds steady over the first 20 to 24 weeks of life. Previously healthy infants born at term of an uncomplicated pregnancy may be affected with septicemia, meningitis, cellulitis, pneumonia, and bone and joint infections. The late-onset infections also differ from early-onset disease in being caused most often by type III GBS or by type Ia.

Pathogenesis and Pathology

The pathogenesis of group B streptococcal infections is a matter of the interplay between the defenses of the host and the virulence of the bacteria that normally reside in the colon. The burden of pregnancy may predispose some women to vaginal and cervical colonization with GBS derived from their own fecal flora. If urinary-tract infection, amnionitis, or endometritis follow, infection of the preterm fetus is likely to occur. The risk of early neonatal infection is further increased by prolonged labor and premature rupture of the membranes.

The size of the inoculum is a determinant of the outcome, since the highest rates of disease occur in infants heavily contaminated with GBS at birth. The route of infection is also important; aspiration of amniotic fluid infected with GBS may lead to pneumonia with general sepsis following because the fetus and the immature infant have little ability to localize the infection. Thus, stillborn infants and infants born alive who then die in acute respiratory distress with pneumonia will have bacteria-laden lungs with little or no leukocyte response. Hyaline membranes may be present, and in other cases, there may be microscopic evidence of bronchopneumonia. Even when GBS are recovered from the cerebrospinal fluid (CSF) the histopathologic evidence of meningitis is scant to absent in cases of early onset neonatal sepsis, whereas the inflammatory response in late-onset cases may be typical of meningitis caused by other pyogenic bacteria.

Manifestations

Group B streptococci are associated with a wide spectrum of clinical diseases. Examples of diseases

Table 24-8. *Clinical Syndromes of Neonates and Infants That May Be Caused by Group B Streptococci*

Disease	Usual time of onset*
Acute undifferentiated septicemia	Early
Bone and joint infection	Late
Cellulitis	Late
Conjunctivitis	Early
Empyema with pneumonia	Late
Meningitis, purulent	Late
Otitis media, purulent	Late
Pneumonia	Early
Skin and soft tissue infection	Late
Septicemia	Late

* The time of onset of infections is an arbitrary basis for classification. The syndromes indicated here as early onset are often evident at or soon after birth. Those listed as late onset occur from a few days to a few months of age.

common to the neonate or young infant are given in Table 24-8. The two major clinical forms of infection are undifferentiated sepsis—the classic form of early-onset disease, and purulent meningitis or septicemia—predominantly delayed forms of disease.

The typical case of early infection is a low-birth-weight, immature infant with acute respiratory distress at, or soon after, birth. Apnea is an important early sign. There may also be hypothermia or instability of temperature; signs of cardiovascular collapse are ominous. Less often, there is insidious onset of infection early in the life of a newborn who has previously done well. When apnea and acute respiratory distress develop in an infant within 24 hours of delivery, infection with GBS should be suspected.

In the older neonate or infant, there may be systemic manifestations of infection such as fever, irritability, and change in feeding. Also, the typical focal signs of meningitis may be elicited. In general, the more mature the host, the more specific the signs and symptoms.

Other serious or life-threatening infections with GBS are probably consequences of bacteremia. These include skin and soft-tissue infection, cellulitis, bone and joint infection, and pneumonia, which may be complicated by empyema.

In adults, excluding pregnant women, GBS are most often associated with urinary-tract infections or infections in compromised hosts, for example patients with diabetes mellitus. Septicemia and infective endocarditis may occur. Pregnant women are not only at risk for urinary-tract infections, amnionitis, and endometritis, but also complicating bacteremias. Postpartum puerperal sepsis with GBS is a complication related to the route of delivery.

Diagnosis

In the newborn or neonate who may have sepsis, cultures of the blood, CSF, and urine must be obtained. Gastric aspirate cultures may be useful, especially when pneumonia is suspected. Cultures from the external ear canal, throat, umbilicus, and anus are of value for detecting the presence and extent of contamination or colonization with GBS; however, positive cultures from these sites do not confirm systemic disease. Positive cultures from the blood or CSF do establish the diagnosis of sepsis or meningitis. In cases of early-onset group B streptococcal infection, cultures should be obtained from the mother's birth canal, whether or not overt infection is evident, to document the source of GBS.

Tests to detect streptococcal antigens in blood, CSF, and urine have met with variable success. Countercurrent immunoelectrophoresis and latex-coated agglutination reactions may detect antigens, but a negative test does not exclude group B streptococcal disease. Other clinical and laboratory tests for documenting infection are nonspecific. The peripheral blood count tends to reflect the maturity of the host; the immature neonate is often neutropenic in the presence of overwhelming sepsis, whereas older infants with meningitis may have a pronounced leukocytosis. The clinical differentiation of penumonia caused by GBS from acute respiratory distress syndromes is not feasible, and it is essential to obtain cultures of the blood and from the lower respiratory tract. As is the case whenever there is serious illness in a neonate, it is important to review the history of the pregnancy and the condition of the parturient.

In adults other than women with puerperal infection, GBS are usually unsuspected as an etiologic agent until they are recovered from clinical specimens. The organism grows well on the conventional mediums employed in clinical laboratories for processing blood, CSF, and other specimens.

Prognosis

Among the factors that influence the outcome of infection with GBS in young infants, the degree of maturity and the extent of the infection are of particular importance. The mortality rates were in excess of 50% among young, immature neonates with septicemia, respiratory distress, and cardiovascular collapse. As the clinical patterns of group B streptococcal disease have been delineated and as the quality of supportive care has improved, the chances for survival have improved. However, mortality rates remain high in infants weighing less than 1500 g at birth. The mortality rate in septicemia or meningitis in the older neonate or young infant has generally been 20% to 30% in the past and is now probably lower. Factors that influence survival in meningitis include the presence or lack of seizures, and increased intracranial pressure early in the illness. Prompt therapy enhances the probability of survival and may reduce the risk of sequelae.

Therapy

The minimal inhibitory concentration of penicillin G for GBS is 0.06 μg per ml or less. Although ampicillin appears to be about as active *in vitro,* penicillin G is preferred for therapy. An aminocyclitol such as gentamicin is often prescribed initially, but once the diagnosis of group B streptococcal infections is established, it should not be continued. Synergism between penicillin and aminocyclitols has been demonstrated *in vitro,* but is not of proven clinical value. The penicillinase-resistant penicillins, the cephalosporins, and moxalactam are not active against GBS.

Penicillin G should be given in a dose of 200 mg (320,000 units) per kg of body weight per day, IV, as 6 equal portions, 4-hourly for newborns; beyond 1 week of age, the dose should be doubled. Treatment is continued for 10 to 14 days, but longer therapy may be needed in some patients with meningitis. Relapse or recurrent infection occasionally occurs, usually within a few weeks after the treatment was stopped, and is treated using the same regimen as employed initially.

Proper management of respiratory distress, shock, seizures, or other manifestatons of central nervous system infection is essential to assure an optimal outcome. The initial phase of treatment is best provided within an intensive care unit with full monitoring capability. Fresh blood, plasma, and plasma containing, type-specific antibody against GBS have all been used empirically and may be of benefit in the immature infant with fulminant sepsis.

Prevention

The possibilities of preventing neonatal group B streptococci disease include a reduction in obstetrical complications; antimicrobial prophylaxis for newborns; antimicrobial prophylaxis for women in labor or at parturition; and immunoprophylaxis. At the present time, neither of the approaches to prophylaxis with antimicrobics have proved to be of value.

Immunoprophylaxis has received considerable attention, especially for the prevention of infections caused by type III GBS. Although both mothers and infants who are infected with type III GBS are deficient in specific antibody, many who lack antibody escape the infection. However, there are limited data that indicate that type-specific antibody provides some protection, probably by enhancing the phagocytosis of the homologous type of GBS. Candidate vaccines prepared from purified carbohydrate antigens have been tested in a limited fashion and it is not known whether active immunization can elicit IgG that will provide the newborn with type-specific immunity.

Remaining Problems

The development of safe and effective methods for the prevention of both maternal and neonatal infections with GBS is a major challenge. A reduction in the obstetric complications and maternal morbidity that increase the risk of infection with GBS would be especially beneficial.

Bibliography

Books

BREESE BB, HALL C (eds): Beta Hemolytic Streptococcal Diseases. New York, John Wiley & Sons, 1978, 287 pp.

HAVERKORN MJ (ed): Streptococcal Disease and the Community. New York, American Elsevier, 1974, 356 pp.

MARKOWITZ M, GORDIS L: Rheumatic Fever, 2nd ed. Philadelphia, WB Saunders, 1972, 309 pp.

NAHAMIAS AJ, O'REILLY RF (eds): Immunology of Human Infection. New York, Plenum, 1981, 651 pp.

PARKER MT (ed): Pathogenic Streptococci. Surrey, England, Reedbooks Ltd, 1979, 291 pp.

Journals

GROUP A STREPTOCOCCI

Combined rheumatic fever study group: a comparison of short-term, intensive prednisone and acetylsalicylic acid therapy in treatment of rheumatic fever. N Engl J Med 272:63–70, 1965

DUMA RJ, WEINBERG AN, MEDREK TF, KUNZ LJ: Streptococcal infections: A bacteriologic and clinical study of streptococcal bacteremia. Medicine 48:87–127, 1969

GINSBURG I: Mechanisms of cell and tissue injury induced by group A streptococci: Relation to post-streptococcal sequelae. J Infect Dis 126:294–340, 419–456, 1972

GLEZEN WP, CLYDE WA, SENIOR RJ, SHEAFFER CI, DENNY FW: Group A streptococci, mycoplasmas and viruses associated with acute pharyngitis. JAMA 202:455–460, 1967

KRAUSE RM: Prevention of streptococcal sequelae by penicillin prophylaxis: A reassessment. J Infect Dis 131:592–601, 1975

POWERS GF, BOISVERT PL: Age as a factor in streptococcosis. J Pediatr 25:481–504, 1944

RAMMELKAMP CH JR: Epidemiology of streptococcal infections. Harvey Lect 51:113–142, 1955–1956

RANTZ LA, MARONEY M, DI CAPRIO JM: Hemolytic streptococcal infection in childhood. Pediatrics 12:498–515, 1953

SIEGEL AC, JOHNSON EE, STOLLERMAN GH: Controlled studies of streptococcal pharyngitis in a pediatric population. I. Factors related to the attach rate of rheumatic fever. N Engl J Med 265:559–566, 1961

STOLLERMAN GH: Factors determining the attach rate of rheumatic fever. JAMA 177:823–828, 1961

STOLLERMAN GH: The relative rheumatogenicity of strains of group A streptococi. Mod Concepts Cardiovasc Dis 44:35–40, 1975

ZABRISKI JB: Mimetic relationships between group A streptococci and mammalian tissues. Adv Immunol 7:147–188, 1967

GROUP B STREPTOCOCCI

ABLOW RC, DRISCOLL SG, EFFMAN EL: A comparison of early-onset group B streptococcal neonatal infection and the respiratory-distress syndrome of the newborn. N Engl J Med 294:65–70, 1976

ANTHONY BF, OKADA DM: The emergence of group B streptococci in infections of the newborn infant. Ann Rev Med 28:355–369, 1977

ANTHONY BF, OKADA DB, HOBEL CJ: Epidemiology of the group B streptococcus: Maternal and nosocomial sources of infant acquisition. J Pediatr 95:431–436, 1979

BAKER CJ: Summary of the workshop on perinatal infections due to group B streptococcus. From the National Institutes of Health. J Infect Dis 136:137–153, 1977

BAKER CJ, EDWARDS MS, KASPER DL: Immunogenicity of polysaccharides from type III, group B streptococcus. J Clin Invest 61:1107–1110, 1978

DILLON HC JR, GRAY E, PASS MA, GRAY BM: Anorectal and vaginal carriage of group B streptococci in pregnant women. J Infect Dis 145:794–799, 1982

FRANCIOSI RA, KNOSTMAN JD, ZIMMERMAN RA: Group B streptococcal neonatal and infant infections. J Pediatr 82:707–718, 1973

HOOD M, JANNEY A, DAMERON G: Beta hemolytic streptococcus group B associated with problems of the perinatal period. Am J Obstet Gynecol 82:809–818, 1961

LANCEFIELD RC, HARE R: The serological differentiaton of pathogenic and non-pathogenic strains of hemolytic streptococci from parturient women. J Exp Med 61:335–349, 1935

PASS MA, GRAY BM, KHARE S, DILLON HC JR: Prospective studies of group B streptococcal infection in infants. J Pediatr 95:437–443, 1979

PASS MA, GRAY BM, DILLION HC JR: Puerperal and perinatal infection with group B streptococci. Am J Obstet Gynecol 143:147–152, 1982

VOGEL LC, BOYER KM, GADZALA CA, GOTOFF SP: Prevalance of type-specific group B antibody in pregnant women. J Pediatr 96:1047–1051, 1980

WILKINSON HW: An analysis of group B streptococcal types associated with disease in human infants and adults. J Clin Microbiol 7:176–179, 1978

WOOD EG, DILLON HC JR: A prospective study of group B streptococal bacteriuria in pregnancy. Am J Obstet Gynecol 140:515–520, 1981

PAUL D. HOEPRICH

25 Diphtheria

Diphtheria is primarily a localized and generalized intoxication caused by diphtherial toxin, an extracellular protein metabolite elaborated by strains of *Corynebacterium diphtheriae* that are lysogenic for corynephages that carry the *tox*$^+$ structural gene in their genome. Classically, the diphtheritic lesion is located in the pharynx and consists of a tightly adherent, grayish pseudomembrane within which the bacilli multiply and produce diphtherial toxin.

The vanquishing of diphtheria became possible as a result of a series of discoveries beginning in 1883, when Klebs described the bacillus. In 1884, Loeffler proved that *C. diphtheriae* was the etiologic agent of diphtheria. To account for his inability to culture *C. diphtheriae* from sites other than the pharynx despite widespread disease, Loeffler postulated that there was dissemination of an extracellular poison. This theory was substantiated in 1888 when Roux and Yersin produced diphtheria in laboratory animals by the inoculation of cell-free filtrates of cultures of *C. diphtheriae.* Recognition of the key role of an exotoxin in diphtheria soon led to the discovery of the first successful antiserum by von Behring and Kitasato in 1890, and to the development of immunologic bioassay methods to titer antiserums by Ehrlich in the mid-1890s. These investigations, together with the development of active immunization (first with toxin neutralized with antitoxin [von Behring, 1913], and then toxoid [diphtherial toxin treated with 0.4% formaldehyde; Ramon, 1923]), are the bases for the near eradication of this once widespread, epidemic, and lethal disease.

Etiology

Corynebacterium diphtheriae is an irregularly staining, gram-positive, non-acid-fast, nonsporulating, preferentially aerobic, nonmotile, noncapsulated, pleomorphic bacillus that varies from 1 μm to 8 μm in length and from by 0.3 μm to 0.8 μm in diameter. The clubbed shape of bacilli grown in the laboratory is an artifact imposed by nutritionally inadequate culture mediums. Similarly, the metachromatic granules, or Babès–Ernst bodies, which are seen with methylene blue staining, represent an accumulation of long chain polymetaphosphates in a cell with retarded or already completed growth. The septa between attached or dividing microorganisms often appear as unstained transverse bands, giving diphtheria bacilli a barred appearance.

Corynebacterium diphtheriae can be cultured readily on mediums that contain tissue extracts. The usefulness of standard laboratory mediums stems either from nutritional inadequacy (Loeffler's coagulated serum-egg-glucose medium) or toxic ingredients (blood agar containing potassium tellurite) that retard the growth of contaminating microorganisms. Colonies of *C. diphtheriae* are grayish white on Loeffler's medium. Three colonial forms can be distinguished on tellurite-containing medium: mitis, gravis, and intermedius. The mitis colonies are smooth, convex, and black; the gravis colonies are semirough, flat, and gray to black; and the intermedius colonies are small and smooth with a black center. These three types also display differences in fermentation and hemolytic capabilities: mitis do not ferment starch or glycogen and are hemolytic; gravis ferment starch and glycogen but are not hemolytic; and intermedius do not ferment starch or glycogen and are not hemolytic. Because differences have not been detected in the exotoxins elaborated by these colonial types, and because toxinogenicity is now known to accord with infection by temperate bacteriophages, the previously postulated relationships of virulence and colonial form are no longer valid.

When parasitized by the specific, temperate bacteriophage β, carrying the *tox*$^+$ gene, *C. diphtheriae* elaborates diphtherial toxin, a protein that is released extracellularly and consists of a single polypeptide chain with two cystine bridges and a molecular weight of about 60,000. Strains of *C. diphtheriae* not so infected do not elaborate toxin. However, the production of toxin depends on genetic and nutritional factors. The Park–Williams strain (PW8) of *C. diphtheriae,* which is used to produce toxin commercially, devotes 5% of its protein synthetic capacity to the elaboration of toxin when nutrition is optimal, and at least 35% when there is a deficiency of iron ($Fe^{2+} \leq 0.2$ μg/ml). In descending order, Co^{2+}, Cu^{2+}, and Ni^{2+} also repress the synthesis of toxin without inhibiting bacterial growth; however, Fe^{2+} is by far the most effective repressant. The site of action of these four cations appears to be identical, although the mechanism of repression of synthesis of toxin remains to be determined. Toxin production may be enhanced by inducing lysogenized cells by ultraviolet irradiation.

The ability of a strain of *C. diphtheriae* to produce toxin can be demonstrated by testing it in the guinea pig or in agar. In the guinea pig test, the strain of *C. diptheriae* to be evaluated is injected intradermally into the shaved flank of the animal. Four hours later, antitoxin is injected intraperitoneally, and a second inoculation of the test strain is performed in the other shaved flank. If the isolate of *C. diphtheriae* is toxinogenic, only the initial site of inoculation will become necrotic. The agar gel diffusion test depends on the formation of a line of precipitation where optimal proportions of toxin–antitoxin are attained as they diffuse from a test strain of *C. diphtheriae* and from a centrally placed well, respectively. The gel diffusion technique is suited to rapid microbiologic diagnosis because toxin can be demonstrated in specimens obtained directly from the infected pharynx.

A diphtherialike disease, in the sense that it is a specific intoxication, can be caused by the one other species that elaborates diphtherial toxin—*Corynebacterium ulcerans.* Intermediate between gravis type *C. diphtheriae* and *Corynebacterium pseudotuberculosis* (also designated *Corynebacterium ovis*—primarily a pathogen of sheep and other nonhuman mammals), *C. ulcerans* is cultured most often from the nasopharynx of healthy persons; it has been isolated from the throats of patients with a diphtherialike disease. *Corynebacterium ulcerans* differs from gravis *C. diphtheriae* in some biochemical reactions, colonial morphology, antigenic structure, and by elaborating a second exotoxin that is akin to the toxin of *C. pseudotuberculosis.*

Pharyngitis, sometimes accompanied by a scarlatiniform rash, may occur as a consequence of infection with *Corynebacterium haemolyticum,* non-toxin-producing bacilli which are distinguished by an inability to grow on tellurite mediums, hemolysis on blood agar, and a lack of metachromatic granules.

Erythrasma is caused by *Corynebacterium minutissimum.* The disease and microorganism are considered in Chapter 102, Erythrasma and Trichomycosis Axillaris.

Other human-associated members of the genus *Corynebacterium* are usually saprophytes, capable of causing disease in humans only rarely and under quite special circumstances. *Corynebacterium hofmannii* normally inhabit the pharynx; *Corynebacterium xerosis,* the conjuctival sacs. In these loci, they are invariably nonpathogenic and on isolation from cultures of the throat or eye are reported as diphtheroids. They are readily distinguished from *C. diphtheriae* by morphology (often shorter, with inconspicuous granules and absence of clubbing), biochemical reactions, lack of hemolysis, and failure to elaborate an exotoxin. It is only in the compromised host that these microorganisms cause disease, most often an endocarditis engrafted on a prosthetic heart valve or a valve deformed by rheumatic fever. Susceptibility to antimicrobics should be determined for each isolate, although there is a high probability of activity with vancomycin, erythromycin, or penicillin G plus amikacin.

Propionibacterium acnes are usually anaerobic, but may be tolerant of 0_2, and were once classified as *Corynebacterium acnes.* Ordinarily, *P. acnes* are components of the resident microbiota of the skin. When there is hypersecretion of sebum, an increased production of free fatty acids through lipolysis by *P. acnes* contributes to the lesions of cutaneous acne. Although several antimicrobics are active against *P. acnes,* the tetracyclines are particularly useful because they penetrate sebaceous secretions and are secreted in the sweat.

Epidemiology

Diphtheria is worldwide in occurrence, typically striking in epidemic form. The incidence of the disease has declined sharply since the introduction of active immunization, and in many parts of the world, diphtheria has become rare. The disease is reportable in the United States, and fewer than 100 cases (0.03/100,000) now occur each year (Fig. 25-1). Most cases are reported from western states, with the incidence highest in South Dakota, New Mexico, Washington, Arizona, and Alaska. These are states with large populations of American Indians, who have attack rates of diphtheria 10 to 100 times higher than other races, but a lower mortality.

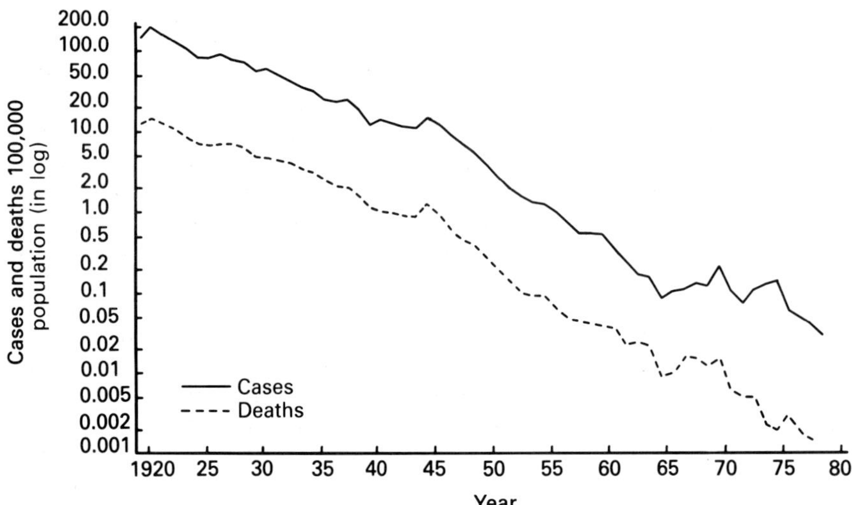

Fig. 25-1. Reported cases of diphtheria and death rates by year in the United States, 1920–1979. (Morbid Mortal Week Rep Ann Summary, 1979. DHEW Public Health Service, 1980)

Formerly, children 2 to 5 years in age were most commonly afflicted and suffered the highest mortality. Although children continue to have both high attack rates and high mortality, there has been a shift of diphtheria to older age groups. The case–fatality ratio of 7.5 in patients 50 years of age or older is comparable to that of children 10 years of age or younger (7.1). Overall, the ratio of fatalities to attack rate remained around 10% into the 1970s, when it fell to the present ratio of around 4% (Fig. 25-1), a change that may be related in part to the fact that cutaneous diphtheria now exceeds noncutaneous disease in the United States.

Humans are the only natural hosts for *C. diphtheriae.* The bacilli are transmitted from human to human during close contact by way of droplets of upper respiratory tract secretions. Spread is favored in the colder months of the year (crowding), although diphtheria now tends to occur at any time of the year in the United States. Those persons clinically ill with diphtheria generally have limited opportunity to spread the disease. Persons incubating the disease and convalescent or healthy carriers are much more important as disseminators of *C. diphtheriae.* Diphtheritic skin lesions, as may be seen in tropical areas and in alcoholic indigents in temperate regions, may serve as reservoirs and sources for dissemination. Fomites and dust have been implicated as vehicles of transmission, but they are probably of minimal importance.

Pathogenesis and Pathology

Diphtheria bacilli infrequently invade living tissue, commonly remaining localized to the mucosal surfaces of the upper respiratory tract. Ocular and genital mucous membranes are rarely involved. Burns or wounds are only occasionally the sites of localization. Cutaneous diphtheria has become more common than respiratory tract diphtheria in the United States.

The serious consequences of diphtherial infection are entirely the result of the production and dissemination of the toxin, an exceedingly active substance. Subcutaneous injection of 25 μg into a 250-g guinea pig is lethal in 4 to 5 days—the so-called standard minimal lethal dose. It has been estimated that about 100 ng/kg of body weight is lethal for humans.

Diphtherial toxin is lethal to susceptible eukaryotic cells through inhibition of the intracellular process of protein synthesis (*i.e.,* the toxin must get into the cell and then be activated). From studies using cell lysates and cell cultures, a probable sequence of events has emerged: (1) Intact diphtherial toxin attaches to the cell surface at specific binding sites that are receptive to a strongly cationic region on the COOH-terminal portion of the nontoxic B fragment (39,000 molecular weight) of the toxin; (2) after endocytosis, lysosomal processing releases the enzymatically active (*i.e.,* toxic) A fragment (21,145 molecular weight), which catalyzes the cleavage of nicotinamide adenine dinucleotide (NAD) and the transfer of its adenine diphosphate ribose (ADPR) moiety to polypeptidyl tRNA translocase (elongation factor-2 or EF-2); (3) the EF-2 is thereby rendered incapable of adding amino acids to a peptide chain, and protein synthesis stops.

Toxin adsorbed to cells, or toxin in extracellular fluids, can be neutralized by antitoxin and thus prevented from exerting a lethal effect. However, once toxin has penetrated into cells, it is beyond the reach of antitoxin, and the process of intoxication is irreversible. Intact nucleotides will block the attachment of diphtherial toxin to cell membrane receptors without detoxification or interference with reactivity to antitoxin.

In the host, the cytotoxic effect of diphtherial toxin is most marked initially in the vicinity of bacterial growth (*i.e.,* in the zone of highest concentration). A local inflammatory response results and is associated with a patchy, readily removed exudate. As patches coalesce during the 24 to 48 hours after onset, an adherent, tough membrane forms that characteristically transgresses anatomic boundaries—for example, not just the pharyngeal tonsil and tonsillar fossa are involved, but also the adjacent oropharynx. The color of the membrane varies from greenish gray to black, depending on the amount of blood it contains. Consisting primarily of fibrin, the membrane, as it is juxtaposed to living tissue, also contains necrotic epithelium, lymphocytes, polymorphonuclear leukocytes, some erythrocytes, and colonies of *C. diphtheriae* (Fig. 25-2). Stripping off a mature membrane leaves numerous bleeding points. Edema of the soft tissues subjacent to the membrane may be marked and is both a local reaction to the toxin and a consequence of secondary infection—classically by group A *Streptococcus pyogenes.* The combined encroachment on air space by the membrane and swelling, particularly in the limited confines of the juvenile larynx, results in respiratory embarrassment. When laryngeal diphtheria was common, death by suffocation occurred, and hence the synonyms *mobres suffocares* and *garrotillo.*

Although diphtheria bacilli rarely, if ever, extend beyond the membrane, some degree of invasiveness is an important component of pathogenicity. For example, a classic toxin-producing strain of *C. diphtheriae* such as PW8 is not invasive and is avirulent. The systemic effects which result from infection with a toxinogenic strain of *C. diphtheriae* that penetrates into, and proliferates within, mucous membranes are consequent on the absorption and the dissemination of the toxin. Although all human cells are susceptible to lethal injury by diphtherial toxin, lesions of the heart (myocarditis), kidneys (tubular necrosis), and nervous system (myelin degeneration) are clinically prominent.

Manifestations

The incubation period for diphtheria is less than 1 week—usually 2 to 4 days. Infection commonly begins within the pharynx, and the severity of symptoms depends on the extent of the pharyngitis. Some patients, especially those who have been immunized, have only minimal discomfort and often do not de-

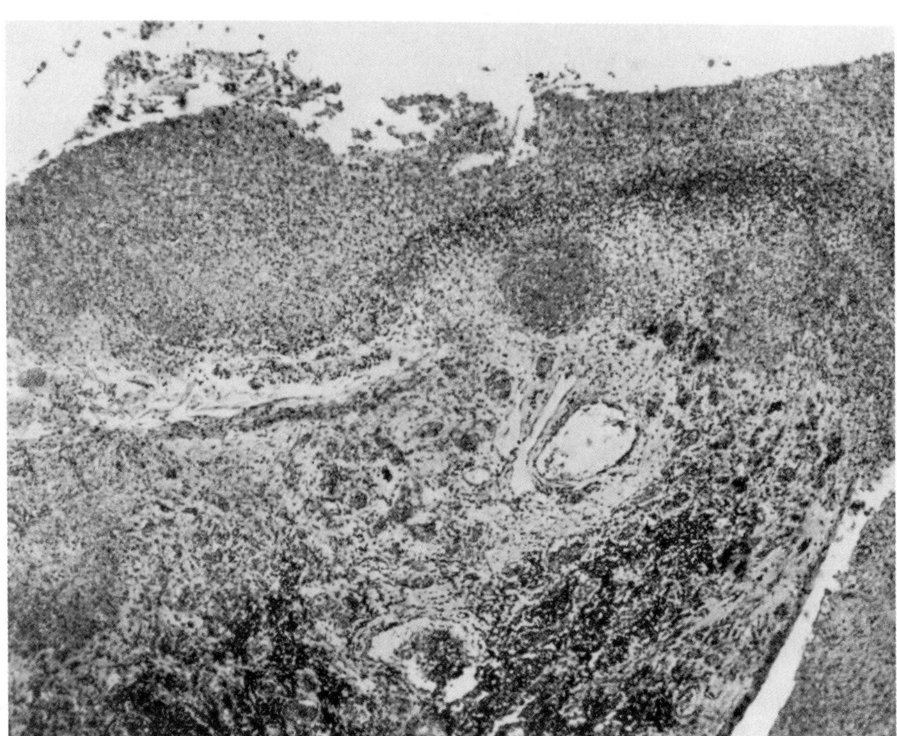

Fig. 25-2. Diphtheria involving a pharyngeal tonsil. The membrane–tissue junction is clearly marked by intense cellular infiltration. (Moore RA: A Textbook of Pathology. Philadelphia, WB Saunders, 1944)

velop diphtheritic membranes. In more severe infections, there is low-grade fever (rarely does fever exceed 39.5°C [103°F]), nonproductive cough, pharyngeal pain, membrane formation (Fig. 31-5*B1*), and cervical lymphadenopathy with soft tissue swelling. When the lymphadenopathy and swelling are extreme, the classic "bull neck" appearance results. In approximately 25% of patients nonspecific symptoms of headache, nausea, and vomiting are also present. A complicating streptococcal infection should be suspected if pharyngeal reddening is prominent and there is high fever.

Extension of the diphtheritic lesion to nasal and laryngeal regions indicates severe disease and a greater likelihood of complications or fatality. Patients with airway obstruction manifest varying degrees of tachypnea, infra- and suprasternal retractions, stridor, and cyanosis. Further extension of the diphtheritic membrane into the tracheobronchial airways increases the risk of suffocation. Occasionally, in younger patients, the primary site of infection is limited to the nasopharynx; a more benign form of the disease results—without general toxicity but with a serosanguineous nasal discharge.

Cutaneous diphtheria may occur in temperate as well as tropical regions in socioeconomically deprived persons with poor personal hygiene. Shallow ulcerations that are indolent and show little tendency to extend may involve infected seborrheic dermatitis, impetiginous, or other lesions. Although cutaneous infections often persist longer than respiratory infections, they usually do not cause systemic toxicity, and the postdiphtheritic complications of myocarditis or polyneuritis are rare.

Other less common sites of infection are the ear, conjunctiva, and genitalia.

Diagnosis

When diphtheria was prevalent or in epidemic situations, experienced personnel became highly skilled in recognizing *C. diphtheriae* in methylene blue or toluidine blue stained smears of throat swabbings. Present day competence requires the cultural isolation and biochemical identification of *C. diphtheriae* with laboratory proof of toxinogenicity for the microbiologic diagnosis of diphtheria. Rapid identification as *C. diphtheriae* is possible using immunofluorescence after isolation; however, toxinogenicity is not thereby established.

For culture, swabbings of lesions or preferably a bit of membrane removed from a lesion should be submitted promptly to the laboratory. *Corynebacterium diphtheriae* is relatively resistant to drying, but a nonnutritive, moist, reducing, transport medium prevents the overgrowth of competitors. Laboratory personnel must be informed of the possibility of diphtheria so that appropriate culture mediums (Loeffler's, tellurite) can be inoculated.

Other laboratory studies are of little aid in establishing the diagnosis. Examination of the blood shows a moderate leukocytosis. When neuritis is present, an increase in the concentration of protein in the cerebrospinal fluid can be expected. Less frequently, pleocytosis is observed.

The clinical diagnosis of diphtheria presents the most difficulty when the disease is mild. In these instances, the history of a sore throat with slight dysphagia and the presence of a nonmembranous pharyngeal exudate are likely to be attributed to viral or streptococcal infection, Vincent's angina, or infectious mononucleosis. The finding of a neurologic abnormality such as palatine paralysis or the presence of electrocardiographic abnormalities should alert the clinician to the possibility of diphtheria. More severe cases, with membrane formation (Fig. 31-5*B1*), myocarditis, or cranial nerve paralyses, are quite characteristic and permit clinical diagnosis. The development of peripheral neuritis is particularly perplexing in persons who have recovered from a primary nasal or pharyngeal lesion because cultural proof of diphtheria may not be possible.

Prognosis

In the late nineteenth century, before the use of serotherapy, the mortality from diphtheria was 30% to 50%; death was most frequent in children less than 4 years of age and was the result of suffocation. At present, the case fatality ratio is around 4% (Fig. 25-1), and there is no clear association of death with age.

The major complications resulting from the dissemination of diphtherial toxin are myocarditis and polyneuritis. Of the two, myocarditis is the more important because it is responsible for approximately half the mortality from diphtheria. Patients who have a toxin-induced amegakaryocytic thrombocytopenia as an early manifestation of diptheria are particularly likely to develop myocarditis, renal failure, and polyneutritis and die. The incidence of myocarditis has varied from 10% to 70%, depending on the patient population and the criteria used. Clinically significant cardiac abnormalities are present in approximately 20% of patients. These abnormalities appear 1 or more weeks after the onset of illness. The oropharyngeal lesion may be healing or may have healed at the time the myocarditis appears. In fact, it is common to have a deceptive period of well-being before the onset of cardiac dysfunction. Myocarditis may come on acutely or may develop insidiously, with diminishing intensity of heart tones, increasing dyspnea, and transient arrhythmias. Congestive heart failure may be an initial or late consequence of impaired cardiac function. The electrocardiogram may show T-wave changes, first-, second-, or third-degree heart block, bundle-branch block patterns, or other arrhythmias. Atrioventricular dissociation is a particularly ominous finding because it has been associated with a mortality rate of over 70%. Patients may have electrocardiographic abnormalities of serious portent even though appearing well, and therefore électrocardiograms should be obtained on a routine basis during the course of diphtheria.

When neurologic complications occur, they tend to appear relatively late in the course of diphtheria. It is not uncommon for paralysis to develop a month or more after the onset of infection. The incidence of neurologic complications is proportional to the severity of infection. Mild cases have a complication rate of 2%; severe infections, a rate as high as 75%. The cranial nerves are affected first. The most frequent symptoms are difficulty in swallowing and nasal regurgitation of liquids. The voice may also develop a nasal quality.

If the diphtheritic lesion is confined to one side of the palate, an ipsilateral palatal paralysis is a frequent and diagnostically valuable finding. Cranial nerve palsies involving the oculomotor, facial, and laryngeal nerves may also be present. Peripheral neuritis is manifest primarily as a motor defect. Dysfunction begins in proximal muscle groups and extends distally, and the severity of involvement varies from a mild weakness to paralysis. Tendon reflexes may be suppressed or absent. When sensory disturbances occur, paresthesias with a stocking-and-glove distribution are the usual form. Although the neuritis often persists for months, it is invariably a transient phenomenon; eventual return to normal function can be anticipated.

Recovery from diphtheria is followed by immunity, which is demonstrable a year after the illness in about 50% of the patients. Even though second attacks are rare, immunization with toxoid should be carried out.

Therapy

Diphtheria was the first disease in which specific antibody was proved to be of therapeutic value. Effectiveness in treatment relates to the vulnerability of the toxin to detoxification both before interaction with host cells, while still in body fluids, and when adsorbed to cell membranes prior to entrance into the cytosol. Antiserum treatment of humans with diphtheria was undertaken quite soon after the neutralizing power of specific humoral antibody was demonstrated in experimental animals. Actual proof of efficacy was delayed until 1898, when the results of a controlled trial of serum therapy were published: of 204 patients given antiserum, 5 died; of 201 not given antiserum, 14 died. In keeping with these toxin–host cell–antitoxin interactions, the earlier in diphtheria that antiserum is given, the more effective it is (Fig. 25-3).

The actual dosage of antitoxin is empirically geared to the probable quantity of toxin available, as implied by the extent of the membrane. In mild and moderately severe cases, 30,000 to 40,000 units are usually injected, intramuscularly. Patients with more severe disease should receive 40,000 to 80,000 units, with at least half (or all) the antitoxin given slowly, by intravenous infusion over a period of 60 min. Horse serum is still used in therapy because the presently available human serum immune globulin preparations do not contain sufficient antitoxin. Approximately 10% of patients will develop an allergic reaction. Nonspecific febrile reactions and serum sickness compose most of the adverse effects. Immediate reactions such as anaphylaxis are rare. Nevertheless, before antitoxin is administered the physician should (1) determine if an allergy to horse serum is known, (2) perform conjunctival and intracutaneous skin tests for hypersensitivity, and (3) have an appropriate amount of epinephrine at the bedside. If either the conjunctival or intracutaneous skin test is positive, desensitization with increasing doses of antiserum is recommended.

Neutralization of the toxin is essential and is clearly the most urgent task of therapy. The amount of antitoxin given is virtually always excessive in terms of the supply of toxin to be neutralized.

Antibacterial therapy is secondary to treatment with antitoxin, but it is necessary to (1) shut down the bacillary sources of supply of diphtherial toxin, (2) treat associated infections—for example, streptococcal, and (3) eliminate a known focus for the spread of diphtheria to other humans—a need that is critical to the control of diphtheria. If the isolation of *C. diphtheriae* from the throat or nose 3 months after the onset of diphtheria is taken to define a carrier, without chemotherapy some 1% to 15% of persons who recover from diphtheria become carriers. Decline in carriage follows an exponential curve, with

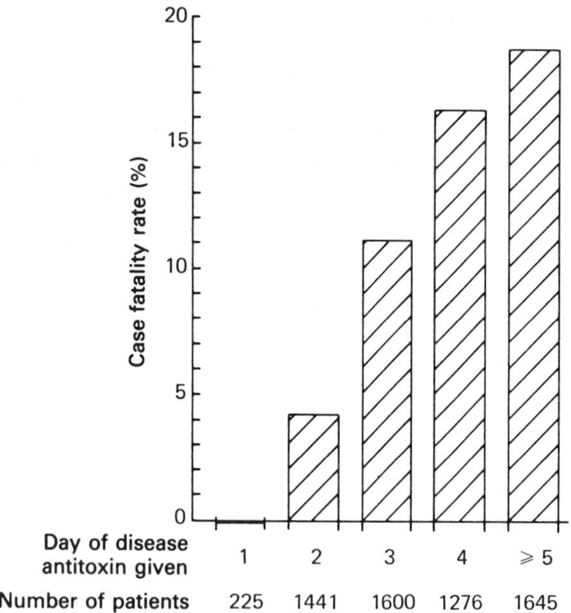

Fig. 25-3. Effectiveness of serotherapy in diphtheria. Antitoxin is most effective in preventing death when given within 4 days of the onset of diphtheria. With further delay, the antitoxin is apparently of little benefit. (Russell WT: Med Res Counc Spec Rep Ser 247;9–10, 1943)

the rate of decline significantly slower following nasal diphtheria (Fig. 25-4). Surgical removal of tonsils and adenoids has been of value in terminating the carrier state.

Corynebacterium diphtheriae is generally susceptible to benzylpenicillin. The usual dosage is 600,000 units of the procaine derivative every 12 hours by intramuscular injection for 2 weeks. Because *C. diphtheriae* is more susceptible to erythromycin than to penicillin G, and because erythromycin has been successful in eliminating the carrier state in persons not successfully treated with penicillin, erythromycin is recommended as primary therapy in a dose of 30 to 40 mg/kg body wt/day, for 2 weeks. If swallowing is difficult, the erythromycin must be given by intravenous injection (lactobionate or gluceptate preparations, as three equal portions, every 8 hours); thrombophlebitis may complicate the intravenous administration of erythromycin. Oral administration is preferable whenever feasible, although gastrointestinal disturbances sometimes occur.

One week after cessation of chemotherapy, cultures of the nasopharynx and oropharynx should be made to document the presence or absence of the carrier state. Uncommonly, a second course of therapy with erythromycin is necessary.

Patients with severe laryngeal obstruction require tracheostomy. Although of unproven value, glucosteroids have been advocated in such patients.

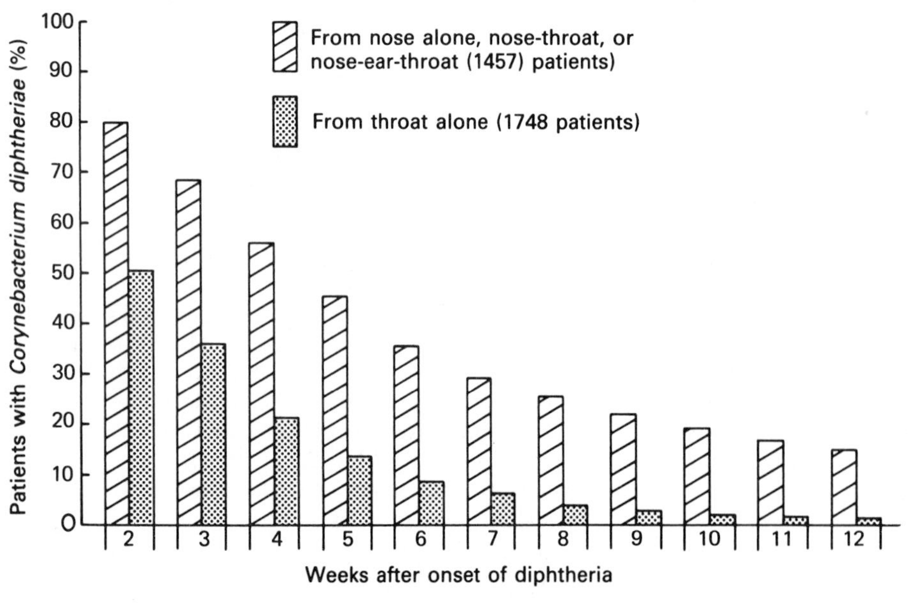

Fig. 25-4. Frequency of carriage of *Corynebacterium diphtheriae* in 3205 patients who recovered from diphtheria without specific therapy. True carriers, defined as persons yielding *C. diphtheriae* 3 months after onset of diphtheria, were more frequent in patients in whom there was nasal localization of the disease. (Thomas FH, Mann E, Marriner H: Metropol Asylum Board Ann Rep, 304–309, 1929)

Prevention

Immunity to diphtheria can be determined by the Schick test. A minute amount of diphtherial toxin (0.02 of a minimal lethal dose for a guinea pig) is injected intradermally (volar forearm). A local inflammatory reaction that reaches maximal intensity within 4 to 7 days, fading thereafter to yield a brownish discoloration with epidermal desquamation, indicates the absence of immunity (Schick-positive). The presence of circulating antitoxin (in the range of 0.02 units/ml of serum) blocks the response, indicating immunity (Schick-negative). Allergy to other antigens in the toxin preparations used in the Schick test may produce pseudoreactions distinguished by rapid resolution after attaining maximal intensity within 48 hours after inoculation and by the response to concomitant intradermal injection of heat-inactivated toxin in the opposite forearm. The test is most often used to determine the immune status of adults. It is generally presumed that preschool and young children who have not been given diphtherial toxoid are not immune.

Active immunization using toxoid (formalin-detoxified diphtherial toxin) prevents diphtheria. Preschool-aged immunization, as commonly practiced in the United States, is indubitably effective. However, the immunity engendered is not lifelong. When diphtheria was common, carrier rates were high, crowded dwelling was frequent, and almost everyone had contact with toxinogenic *C. diphtheriae* (*i.e.,* reinforcement of immunity was a phenomenon of nature). This is no longer true in industrialized countries. According to Schick test survey results and the clinical occurrence of epidemic diphtheria in American troops in Europe after World War II, from 20% to 75% of the adult population of the United States is largely without protective antitoxic immunity to diphtheria. For reinforcement of immunity in adults, a highly purified toxoid preparation must be used to avoid systemic effects attributable to anamnestic antibacterial immunity (as contrasted to the lacking antitoxic immunity). Such preparations are commercially available but only in combination with tetanal toxoid—an unfortunate situation because the ideal periodicity of booster inoculations to maintain immunity to diphtheria is 4 years, whereas it is 10 years with tetanal toxoid (see Chap. 126, Tetanus).

In the past, the Moloney test (intradermal injection of 0.1 ml of a 1:100 dilution of fluid diphtherial toxoid) was used to detect allergy to components of the toxoid (erythema-induration maximal in 24 hours). However, the test was not entirely reliable, and the highly purified toxoid is preferable.

Remaining Problems

Diphtheria is one of the best understood of all infectious diseases. Because adequate therapy and an excellent preventive are available, the remaining scientific problems are trivial. They are matters of improving the speed of diagnosis and reducing untoward drug reactions by replacement of horse antiserum with human antitoxin. Knowledge of diphtheria is sufficient to enable elimination of the disease, a task which is a social and political responsibility.

Bibliography

Books

WASHINGTON JA II: Bacteriology, clinical spectrum of disease, and therapeutic aspects on coryneform bacterial infection. In Remington JS and Swartz MN (eds); Current Clinical Topics in Infectious Diseases. New York, McGraw-Hill 1980. pp. 68–88.

WOOD WD JR: From Miasmas to Molecules. New York, Columbia University Press, 1961. 100 pp.

Journals

VON BEHRING E: Untersuchungen über das Zustandkommen der Diptherie-Immunität bei Thieren. Dtsch Med Wochenschr 16:1145–1148, 1890

COLLIER RJ: Diphtheria toxin: mode of action and structure. Bacteriol Rev 39:54–85, 1975

FIBIGER J: Om serumbehandlung af difteri. Hospitalstidende 6:237–325, 1898

GORE I: Myocardial changes in fatal diphtheria: A summary of observations in 221 cases. Am J Med Sci 215:257–266, 1948

MCCLOSKEY RV, ELLER JJ, GREEN M, MAVNEY CU, RICHARDS SEM: The 1970 epidemic of diphtheia in San Antonio. Ann Intern Med 75:495–502, 1971

MCCLOSKEY RV, GREEN MJ, ELLER J, SMILACK J: Treatment of diphtheria carriers: benzathine penicillin, erythromycin, and clindamycin. Ann Intern Med 81:788–791, 1974

NAIDITCH MJ, BOWER AG: Diphtheria: A study of 1433 cases observed during a ten-year period at the Los Angeles County Hospital. Am J Med 17:229–245, 1954

PAPPENHEIMER AM JR: Diphtheria toxin. Ann Rev Biochem 46: 69–94, 1977

PEDERSEN AHB, SPEARMAN J, TRONCA E, BADER M, HARNISCH J: Diphtheria on Skid Row, Seattle Wash., 1972–75. Public Health Rep 92:336–342, 1977

SCHEID W: Diphtherial paralysis. An analysis of 2,292 cases of diphtheria in adults, which included 174 cases of polyneuritis. J Nerv Ment Dis 116:1095–1101, 1952

Section V

Respiratory Airway Infections

Indigenous Microbiota of the Respiratory Airways

(None)

CHIEN LIU

Epiglottitis, Laryngitis, and Laryngotracheobronchitis

26

Epiglottitis, laryngitis, and laryngotracheobronchitis are acute inflammatory diseases of the upper airway. They are usually infectious diseases and are collectively designated as *croup*. Precise anatomic localization of site(s) of affliction in the airway may be difficult and is not really important because involvement of one structure generally connotes involvement of all, and the common hazard is obstruction of the airway. The latter danger is particularly great in the very young for their airways are relatively narrow.

Etiology

Bacteria and viruses, individually, and perhaps in combination, are the usual causes of epiglottitis, laryngitis, and laryngotracheobronchitis.

Haemophilus influenzae

Haemophilus influenzae is a minute (0.3 μm–0.4 μm by 1.5 μm long) pleomorphic, gram-negative bacillus that is nonacid-fast, nonmotile, nonsporulating, and usually capsulated in clinical specimens. After 24 hours of incubation at 37°C, the smooth, translucent colonies are less than 1 mm in diameter; if composed of capsulated strains, the colonies display a characteristic iridescence when viewed by obliquely incident light.

Haemophilus influenzae is aerobic and has no unique fermentive or other biochemical activities. It is further distinguished by requiring for growth an iron protoporphyrin compound (X factor) and some form of pyridine nucleotide (V factor). These requirements are conveniently met in culture mediums by the incorporation of peptic digest of blood—the culture medium of Fildes, or heat-disrupted erythrocytes—Levinthal's agar, and chocolate agar. The inclusion of nafcillin in a final concentration of 0.7 μg/ml renders these mediums usefully selective for *H. influenzae*.

Virulence appears to be associated with capsulation. On the basis of specific, capsular polysaccharides, six antigenic types have been distinguished—designated *types a* through *f*. Of these, type b accounts for almost all serious infections in humans. In clinical specimens, such as cerebrospinal fluid (CSF), etiologic diagnosis can be certified by the capsular swelling (quellung) reaction with a type-specific antiserum. Rapid detection of the type-specific capsular polysaccharide by counterimmunoelectrophoresis may prove to be diagnostically useful (see Chap. 14, Immunologic Diagnosis).

Genetically and immunologically, *H. influenzae* resembles *Streptococcus pneumoniae*. Indeed, some immunologic cross reaction between *H. influenzae* type b (HITB) and *S. pneumoniae* types 6, 15, 29, and 35 can be demonstrated.

In addition, cross reactions have been shown between HITB and some strains of *Escherichia coli*.

The usual disinfectants, drying, and ultraviolet light are quickly lethal to *H. influenzae*. Chloramphenicol, ampicillin, penicillin G, tetracycline, and the sulfonamides are usually active against influenza bacilli.

Since 1974, strains of ampicillin-resistant HITB have been isolated from CSF and blood in children under 5 years old with meningitis or bacteremia. Such ampicillin-resistant strains are not confined to a limited geographic region in the United States and have been isolated in Canada. The resistance is mediated by β-lactamase activity that is particularly efficient against the penicillins.

Corynebacterium diphtheriae

The pharynx and larynx are classic sites for the localization of diphtherial infection (see Chap. 25, Diphtheria).

Bordetella pertussis

Whooping cough is a special form of bronchitis that is caused by *B. pertussis* and is seen primarily in children (see Chap. 29, Whooping Cough).

Streptococcus pneumoniae

The major cause of bacterial pneumonia in adults and children (see Chap. 31, Bacterial Pneumonias), *S. pneumoniae* is also frequently recovered from the sputum of patients who have chronic bronchitis.

Parainfluenza Viruses

Generically, parainfluenza viruses are myxoviruses with binding sites for erythrocytes. Originally, because of this property, they were called hemadsorption (HA) viruses. Parainfluenza viruses are 150 nm to 250 nm in diameter, and they have an RNA core possessing helical symmetry that is enclosed in a projection-studded, ether-sensitive envelope. Infected tissue culture cells often form syncytiums with eosinophilic inclusion bodies indicating sites of intracytoplasmic multiplication.

Parainfluenza viruses have been isolated from humans, cattle, monkeys, and mice. The four types of parainfluenza viruses that parasitize man are designated *types 1, 2, 3, and 4*. These types appear to be antigenically homogenous. Unlike influenza viruses, which characteristically undergo antigenic alterations, the parainfluenza viruses have thus far been antigenically stable. They share related antigens but do not possess a common antigen. The clinical syndromes associated with parainfluenza viruses are as follows: Types 1, 3, and 4 are associated with the common cold and pharyngitis; types 1, 2, and 3 are associated with croup; types 1 and 3 are associated with bronchitis and bronchopneumonia.

Influenza Viruses

Influenza viruses typically cause lower respiratory tract infections, both in adults and children. Infection with influenza viruses is usually an epidemic phenomenon (see Chap. 28, Influenza).

Respiratory Syncytial Viruses

Although respiratory syncytial (RS) viruses can cause croup, they usually cause bronchiolitis or bronchopneumonia in infants. The properties of RS viruses are given in Chapter 27, Bronchitis and Bronchiolitis.

Epidemiology

Bacterial and viral agents of respiratory infections are ubiquitous and have a world-wide distribution. Animal reservoirs are not significant factors; person-to-person contact is the chief means of spread of respiratory diseases. Young children are more susceptible because they lack protective antibody. *Haemophilus influenzae* causes infection most commonly in the age group 6 to 24 months, with maximal frequency at 9 months; it rarely causes infection after 6 years of age. This age distribution of illness may relate in part to the nearly uniform presence of humoral antibodies that are bactericidal to *H. influenzae* in older children and adults.

Primary infection caused by type 3 parainfluenza virus seems to occur earlier in life than infections with types 1 and 2. By 2 years of age, most infants have acquired type 3 neutralizing antibody; the acquisition of type 1 and type 2 neutralizing antibody occurs at a slower rate. However, by 6 to 10 years of age, most children tested have antibodies against all types of parainfluenza viruses.

In a longitudinal study of pediatric patients in Chapel Hill, North Carolina, type 1 parainfluenza virus caused epidemics that began in the summer and extended into the fall and early winter. On the other hand, parainfluenza type 3 virus was isolated with regularity during almost the entire period of the study. Other studies have shown that type 1 and type 3 viruses are often endemic in large urban communities and can be recovered from children with respiratory illnesses during almost any month of the year. Type 2 parainfluenza virus infections tend to occur sporadically, usually in the fall and winter. Type 4 parainfluenza virus infections are usually mild and occur less frequently than the other three types.

Pathogenesis and Pathology

Haemophilus influenzae frequently resides in the upper respiratory tract without causing clinical illness. In children, carrier rates may be as high as 30%; of the encapsulated *H. influenzae* recovered from the throat, 80% are of the potentially pathogenic type b. It has been speculated that a viral upper respiratory tract infection may transform the carriage of *H. influenzae* into disease such as epiglottitis, otitis media, pneumonia, bacteremia, and meningitis. Acute epiglottitis caused by *H. influenzae* is notable for the severity of the inflammatory response, with gross swelling of the epiglottis that can lead to acute obstruction of the larynx. Bacteremia is usually present.

Because parainfluenza viruses rarely cause fatal diseases in humans, the pathologic changes of these infections have not been thoroughly investigated. Experimental infection of hamsters has been carried out with parainfluenza type 3 virus by intranasal inoculation. Viral multiplication in the nasal turbinates, trachea, and lungs reaches a peak 24 to 48 hours after infection. Viral antigens can be demonstrated by immunofluorescent staining in the cytoplasm of infected, ciliated, respiratory epithelial cells lining the nasal turbinates, the trachea, and the bronchi. Infectious virus and viral antigens persist in the respiratory epithelium for about 5 days and then disappear. However, during this entire period there are no appreciable histopathologic changes on examination of secretions of infected tissues stained with hematoxylin and eosin. Infection in humans probably starts in the upper respiratory tract and extends to the lower tract. Inflammation and edema of the larynx produce the croup syndrome. Involvement of the trachea and bronchi with an accumulation of inspissated mucus may result in further obstruction of the airway. When the bronchioles and pulmonary alveoli are involved, as may occur in severe infections with parainfluenza type 3 virus, bronchiolitis and bronchopneumonia may result.

Manifestations

Epiglottitis

An acute onset, with fever, sore throat, hoarseness, and a barking cough, is typical of epiglottitis. The disease may progress very rapidly, going from an apparently normal condition to one of toxicity, prostration, severe dyspnea, and cyanosis within hours. Retraction of the suprasternal notch and stridor are prominent with every breath. The throat is diffusely inflamed, and a beefy red, swollen, stiff epiglottis can be seen by direct laryngoscopy. Laboratory studies usually show a marked leukocytosis with increased polymorphonuclear cells. Acute epiglottitis is nearly always caused by HITB, and blood cultures are often positive for *H. influenzae*. The clinical course is fulminating, and the risk of a fatal outcome is high.

Laryngitis

Laryngitis typically begins as a common cold. The appearance of a barking cough, usually worse at night, and hoarseness is indicative of laryngitis. In mild laryngitis, constitutional signs such as fever and dyspnea are minimal or absent. In more severe cases, signs of subglottic obstruction appear. The patient has rapid and labored breathing. With each inspiration, there is stridor and retraction of the suprasternal notch and supraclavicular areas. Cyanosis of the lips and nail beds becomes evident. If the obstruction is not relieved, the patient becomes hypotonic owing to hypoxia. Physical examination may reveal only an infected pharynx, and auscultation shows only inspiratory stridor with decreased aeration of the lungs.

Laryngotracheobronchitis

Severe infection that extends downward from the larynx to include the trachea and the bronchial tree is termed laryngotracheobronchitis. It is almost exclusively a disease of children. Fever is higher, and restlessness and air hunger are more severe than with laryngitis. Substernal and intercostal retractions are added to suprasternal and supraclavicular retractions. There may also be nonsynchronous movements of the chest and abdomen during inspiration and expiration. Bronchitic inspiratory rales and expiratory wheezes are apparent on auscultation. Breath sounds vary, depending on the degree and area of obstruction by bronchial exudates. Localized areas of decreased to absent breath sounds, bronchophony, bronchial breathing, rhonchi, medium and fine moist rales may be heard on auscultation. Focal obstructive signs may change and disappear when bronchial exudates are cleared by coughing or by suction. If a main bronchus is completely obstructed, signs of massive atelectasis, with shift of the mediastinum to the affected side, may be present. On the other hand, partial obstruction of a bronchus may lead to compensatory emphysema resulting in mediastinal shift to the opposite side.

Diagnosis

The clinical diagnosis of croup is not difficult—the hoarseness, barking cough, inspiratory stridor, and retractions point to airway obstruction. Etiologic diagnosis must be instituted promptly; it may prove essential to therapy.

Acute spasmodic laryngitis may be difficult to differentiate from infectious laryngitis. However, spasmodic laryngitis usually occurs in 2- to 4-year-old children who are emotionally labile. It is generally less severe and is self limited, an attack lasting only a few hours.

Congenital laryngeal stridor usually occurs early in neonatal life without signs of respiratory infection. Most infants with this disorder do not have respiratory distress or cyanosis. Laryngeal spasm of the newborn due to tetany can be differentiated by documentation of hypocalcemia and demonstration of increased muscular excitability (*e.g.*, Chvostek's sign).

A foreign body in the larynx or in the trachea must be considered in children of crawling age and in toddlers. Direct laryngoscopy and bronchoscopy are indicated for diagnosis, as well as for removal of the foreign body causing the obstruction.

Retropharyngeal abscess may cause laryngeal obstruction. Usually there is no hoarseness. Digital palpation of the intrapharyngeal mass may reveal the fluctuation of the abscess.

Diphtheric laryngitis usually had a gradual onset, low-grade fever, and a less abrasive cough. The clinical course is usually that of progressive worsening; peripheral neuritis and myocardiopathy may develop.

Definitive etiologic diagnosis depends on laboratory procedures. Examination of smears and cultures of throat specimens may yield diphtheria or influenza bacilli. The blood culture is frequently positive for *H. influenzae* in patients with acute epiglottitis. Primary monkey kidney tissue cultures are best suited for isolation of parainfluenza viruses. Detection of viral growth may be accomplished by hemadsorption testing with guinea pig erythrocytes. Susceptible continuous culture cell lines such as HeLa or Hep-2 cells are useful for the cultivation of respiratory syncytial virus and adenoviruses. Chick embryos or primary tissue culture cells can be used for influenza virus isolation. Serologic tests such as neutralization, complement fixation, and hemagglutination inhibition may be used to measure the antibody rise during convalescence. These virologic procedures are timeconsuming and expensive. They are useful for epidemiologic studies rather than etiologic diagnosis of sporadic cases.

Prognosis

The outcome of laryngitis and laryngotracheobronchitis depends on the severity of the illness, the age of the patient, and the adequacy of treatment. In acute epiglottitis caused by *H. influenzae* and in diphtherial laryngitis, the morbidity and mortality rates are high. Bacteremia with *H. influenzae* may lead to meningitis, septic arthritis, or osteomyelitis. However, the prompt relief of airway obstruction by timely intubation or tracheostomy, and proper antimicrobial therapy, can save many lives and reduce complications.

Laryngotracheobronchitis may be complicated by the formation of a crusty, gummy exudate in the tracheobronchial tree as a consequence of inflammatory damage of the respiratory epithelium, inhalation of relatively dry air, and general dehydration. The crusted exudates often cause bronchiolar obstruction. Segmental atelectasis, obstructive mediastinal emphysema, and pneumothorax may further compromise the pulmonary function of a child who is already in great respiratory distress. If the obstruction is not relieved, bronchopneumonia, formation of pulmonary abscesses, and bronchiectasis may follow. The iatrogenic complications of laryngeal stenosis and perichondritis should be mentioned. These result from damage to the first tracheal ring or to the cricoid cartilage from a tracheostomy placed too high in the neck. Such complications are difficult to correct, even by competent otolaryngologists.

Therapy

The two basic principles of the treatment of infectious croup are maintenance of an adequate airway and control of the infection. Humidification of the inspired air helps prevent obstruction by preventing dryness of tracheobronchial secretions. A croup tent provided with a mechanical humidifier that supplies cold moist air (not steam) is quite effective. In the home, a portable humidifier with an aerosol spray of moist air is useful. If this is not available, the air of a closed bathroom can be saturated rapidly by turning on the hot water in the shower or tub. Oxygen therapy should be given as soon as respiratory distress is detected—for example, use of the accessory muscles for breathing, before cyanosis becomes apparent.

The patient should be kept quiet, and unnecessary examination and handling should be avoided. Fluid administration must be liberal to repair and to prevent dehydration.

Tracheostomy must be considered when the patient continues to show inspiratory retraction, restlessness, and increasing dyspnea despite adequate humidification and oxygen therapy. It should be done before the patient becomes exhausted from the struggle to breathe. Meticulous nursing care of the tracheostomy site and frequent aspirations to prevent plugging of the tube by bronchial secretions are essential.

Specific antimicrobial therapy should be given promptly if the disease is caused by *H. influenzae* or *Corynebacterium diphtheriae*. Ampicillin or chloramphenicol in dosages of 200 mg and 100 mg/kg body wt/day, respectively, should be given intravenously to patients with infection caused by *H. influenzae*. Diphtherial antitoxin should be administered as soon as the diagnosis of diphtheria is made (see Chap. 25, Diphtheria). Erythromycin (30–40 mg/kg body wt/day, perorally or intravenously) or penicillin G (25,000–50,000 units/kg body wt/day) should also be given.

Presently available antimicrobics do not affect the clinical course of viral croup. Supportive treatment is paramount. Glucosteroids, advocated in the hope of reducing inflammation and thereby mitigating airway obstruction, have not proved of value.

Prevention

Routine immunization of all infants against diphtheria, with regular, periodic boosters, is a preventive against diphtheria. No effective vaccines are commercially available for the prevention of infection by *H. influenzae* or the viral agents ordinarily the cause of croup. Experimental capsular polysaccharide (*H. influenzae* type b) and a parainfluenza virus vaccine are under development but are not yet ready for general use. Colonization by feeding with *E. coli* that cross reacts with HITB has been suggested as an alternate method for immunizing neonates.

Bibliography

Books

BALLENGER JJ: Acute inflammatory diseases of the larynx. In Diseases of the Nose, Throat and Ear, 11th ed. Philadelphia, Lea & Febiger, 1969. pp 336–347.

GLEZEN WP, LODA FA, DENNY FW: The parainfluenza viruses. In Evans AS (ed): Viral Infections of Humans: Epidemiology and Control. New York, Plenum, 1976. pp 337–364.

KRUGMAN S, KATZ SL: Acute respiratory infections. In Infectious Diseases of Children, 7th ed. St. Louis, CV Mosby, 1981. pp 260–298.

TURK DC, MAY JR: *Haemophilus Influenzae*: Its Clinical Importance. London, English Universities Press, 1967, 140 pp.

Journals

CHERRY JD: The treatment of croup: Continued controversy due to failure of recognition of historic, ecologic and clinical perspectives. J Pediatr 94:352–354, 1979

FADEN HS: Treatment of *Haemophilus influenzae* type B epiglottitis. Pediatrics 63:402–407, 1979

GLEZEN WP, DENNY FW: Epidemiology of acute lower respiratory disease in children. N Engl J Med 288:498–505, 1973

MCLEAN DM, BACH R, LAVKE RPB, MCNAUGHTON GA: Myxoviruses associated with acute laryngotracheobronchitis in Toronto, 1962–1963. Can Med Assoc J 89:1257–1259, 1963

MILLS JL, SPACKMAN TJ, BORNS P: The usefulness of lateral neck roentgenograms in laryngotracheobronchitis. Am J Dis Child 133:1140–1142, 1979

TAUSSIG LM, CASTRO O, BEAUDRY PH: Treatment of laryngotracheobronchitis (Croup). Am J Dis Child 129:790–793, 1975

CHIEN LIU

27 Bronchitis and Bronchiolitis

Bronchitis and bronchiolitis refer to inflammatory disease of the bronchial tree that does not extend to involve the pulmonary aveoli. Bronchitis and bronchiolitis are usually infectious in origin; the diagnosis is based primarily on clinical considerations. Acute bronchitis can occur in all age groups but is more commonly seen in the young and the old. Chronic bronchitis is usually an adult disease; bronchiolitis is typically a disease of infants.

Acute Bronchitis

Etiology

Acute bronchitis rarely exists as a solitary or primary illness, usually occurring together with inflammation of the trachea. The term *tracheobronchitis* is probably more accurate. An upper respiratory tract infection is the usual antecedent, with extension downward to the bronchi. However, acute bronchitis can be a part of specific infectious diseases such as measles, pertussis, scarlet fever, typhoid fever, and influenza. Throat or sputum cultures from patients with acute bronchitis often yield a variety of bacteria, including *Streptococcus pneumoniae, Haemophilus* spp., *Streptococcus* spp., and *Staphylococcus* spp. The etiologic significance of such culture results is difficult to assess because these bacteria are normally present in the upper respiratory tract. It is generally believed that *Mycoplasma pneumoniae* and the same respiratory viruses that cause upper respiratory tract infections are also etiologic agents for acute bronchitis.

Some persons are more prone than others to have respiratory tract infections associated with acute bronchitis. Predisposing factors play a role. In young children, such factors may be poor nutrition, allergy, and rickets; in the old, emphysema or chronic respiratory illness such as tuberculosis. Air pollution and rapid change of environmental temperature and humidity may also precipitate bronchitic episodes.

Epidemiology

The incidence of acute bronchitis follows the pattern of other acute respiratory tract infections—it is prevalent in the winter months. Cold, damp climates and irritatingly high concentrations of noxious gases, such as nitrogen oxides and sulfur dioxide, may precipitate outbreaks. The sharp increase in respiratory deaths in London during the 1962 smog was attributed to epidemic acute bronchitis in old persons and patients with chronic cardiopulmonary insufficiency.

Pathogenesis and Pathology

There has been little opportunity for the postmortem examination of patients who had acute bronchitis. From the meager data available, and from the study of experimental infections, it can be inferred that infection of the trachea and bronchi yields local inflammatory changes, increased bronchial secretions, and diminution of ciliary action. With fever and dehydration, the excessive bronchial secretions may become thick and tenacious, compounding the inefficiency of the impaired ciliary escalator. If cough is not provoked or is unsuccessful in bringing up secretions, obstruction of the bronchioles occurs. If secondary bacterial invasion occurs, the secretions (sputum) become mucopurulent. Microscopic examination of the bronchial walls may show infiltration with inflammatory cells, hyperemia, and distended mucous glands. Desquamation of the ciliated, columnar epithelial cells lining the trachea and bronchi is usually evident. The sloughed epithelial cells add to the viscosity of the mucopurulent bronchial secretions.

Manifestations

Symptoms of acute upper respiratory infections, such as malaise, headache, coryza, and sore throat, usually precede bronchitic symptoms by several hours or days. Cough soon develops; at first it is nonproductive, but later it yields mucopurulent sputum. There is usually some substernal discomfort, but true plueritic pain is quite uncommon. Dyspnea, cyanosis, and signs of airway obstruction are usually absent unless the patient has a preexisting pulmonary disorder such as asthma, chronic bronchitis, or emphysema. Fever, when present, is usually moderate, rarely exceeding 39°C (102°F).

Physical signs are absent to minimal early in the disease. The pharynx may be infected. Although rhonchi and coarse, moist rales may be heard bilaterally, there is usually no abnormality to percussion or ascultation. Roentgenograms of the lungs may reveal only some increase in bronchovascular markings. The blood leukocyte count is usually normal or may be slightly increased.

Diagnosis

The clinical diagnosis of acute bronchitis rarely presents much difficulty, except when cough is absent, as may occur in the very old. Differentiation of bronchitis from viral or mycoplasmal pneumonia may be impossible on clinical grounds because signs of consolidation are often lacking in these pneumonias. Roentgenographic examination of the lungs is usually necessary for their recognition.

Prognosis

In previously healthy persons, acute bronchitis is a self-limited disease—the prognosis is favorable. In the very young, the old, patients with chronic obstructive pulmonary disease, and in comatose patients, acute bronchitis may be unrelenting, leading to death. Obstruction of the bronchial tree by tenacious secretions may result in atelectasis and bronchiectasis. Pneumonia is a common complication that requires prompt and appropriate therapy.

Therapy

Supportive treatment should include bed rest and inhalation of warm, moist air. Aspirin (600 mg for an adult, 10 mg/kg body wt for a child) may be given every 4 hours to relieve malaise and fever. The distress of a nonproductive cough can be relieved by regular use of a preparation containing codeine of dihydrocodeinone. These and strong antitussives (*e.g.,* morphine or other opium derivatives) are contraindicated if the patient has sputum production. A sedative may be given at bedtime for sleep. In previously healthy individuals, the use of antimicrobial agents for treatment of acute bronchitis is rarely necessary However, in young children, in the elderly, and in patients with chronic pulmonary disease, if improvement does not occur within 3 to 5 days, procaine penicillin (600,000–1,200,000 units daily for an adult or 25,000–50,000 units/kg body wt/day for a child) may be used. If the sputum is purulent, a sputum smear and culture should be performed to look for gram-negative bacteria so that appropriate antimicrobics can be prescribed.

Prevention

Little can be done to prevent acute bronchitis, just as with most respiratory infections. With the exception of the killed influenza virus vaccines, respirovirus vaccines are not generally available. The commerically available respiratory vaccines that contain suspension of killed bacteria do not have documented beneficial effects.

Chronic Bronchitis

Chronic bronchitis is a nonspecific disease characterized by chronic and recurrent cough with expectoration. It is commonly, but not necessarily, associated with emphysema. Patients with chronic bronchitis may or may not have lower airway obstructions; by definition they do not have tuberculosis, bronchiectasis, pulmonary malignancy, cystic fibrosis, or primary cardiac disease.

Etiology

No single etiologic factor satisfactorily explains the incidence and prolonged nature of chronic bronchitis. Several factors appear to be contributory:

1. Cigarette smoking is clearly implicated, for there is a highly significant statistical difference in the incidence of chronic bronchitis in smokers and nonsmokers. There is also a graded relationship; both the prevalence of symptoms of chronic bronchitis and the death rate (Fig. 27-1) are directly related to the intensity of cigarette smoking.

Fig. 27-1. Standardized death rates for bronchitis and emphysema for men smoking cigarettes only. (From Doll R, Hill AB: Br Med J 1:1399–1410, 1964)

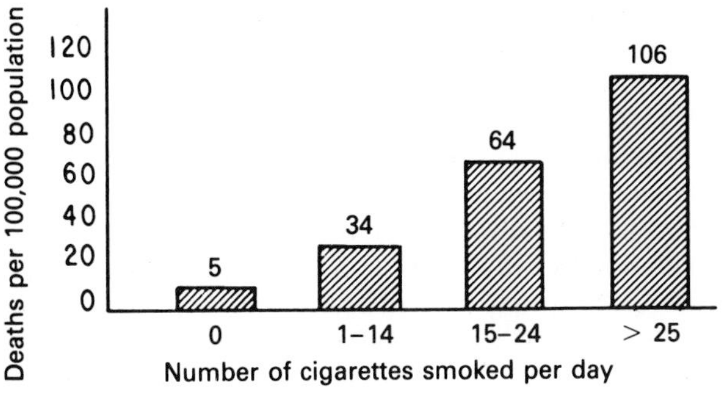

2. Air pollution with noxious gases such as ozone, oxides of nitrogen, and sulfur dioxide can cause exacerbation of symptoms and deaths in patients with chronic bronchitis. This effect was demonstrated by the London smogs of 1952 and 1962. However, the role of air pollution in the pathogenesis of chronic bronchitis is yet to be defined in man. Experimentally, rats exposed to 300 ppm to 400 ppm sulfur dioxide developed increased numbers of mucus-secreting globular cells in the bronchi, a finding of doubtful relevance to man exposed in smog to 1 ppm to 2 ppm sulfur dioxide.
3. Bacteria have been supposed to contribute to chronic bronchitis because (1) potentially pathogenic bacteria are frequently isolated from the purulent sputums dejected by patients with chronic bronchitis; (2) agglutinating antibodies for *H. influenzae* may occur more frequently in patients with chronic bronchitis than in normal controls; and (3) long-term suppression of the bacterial burden (decrease in both volume of sputum and number of bacteria per unit volume of sputum) with antimicrobics (*e.g.,* tetracycline) appears to contribute to well-being.
4. The etiologic role of viruses in chronic bronchitis is even less substantiated. Because many respiratory viruses can cause desquamation of the bronchial ciliated columnar epithelial cells, an acute viral infection may pave the way for bacterial invasion.

Epidemiology

Chronic bronchitis is a disease of older invidivuals. As many as 15% of the population may have chronic bronchitis. Cold and damp climates seem to favor the development of the disease. The possible contribution of cigarette smoking and air pollution has been commented on. Hereditary factors may also be involved because the incidence of chronic bronchitis appears to be higher in siblings than in the spouse of the patient with chronic bronchitis. The disease is also more prevalent in occupational groups exposed to pulmonary irritants (*e.g.,* miners).

Pathogenesis and Pathology

The normal secretory and ciliary functions of the bronchial mucosa are compromised by inhalation of pulmonary irritants such as cigarette smoke and noxious gases, and by repeated infections. Repetition of such insults over a period of years may lead to thickening of the mucosa and hypertrophy of the mucous glands, and in some patients, to diminution in the musculoelastic elements of the airways. Excessive mucus production and stasis of bronchial secretions provide a favorable environment for bacterial multiplication. Tenacious secretions in the bronchial tree may cause obstruction and emphysematous changes of the alveoli. Microscopic examination of the bronchial mucosa may show thickening, inflammatory changes with infiltrative cells, hypertrophy of the mucous glands, and an increase in the number of mucous-secreting cells. The ratio of the thickness of mucous glands to the thickness of the bronchial wall (gland–wall ratio) is greater in patients with chronic bronchitis than in normal persons (Fig. 27-2).

Manifestations

The symptoms of chronic bronchitis vary from the mildest form of smoker's cough to severe dyspnea, copious production of purulent sputum, recurrent infections, and severe physical disability. The first symptom is usually a chronic cough with the production of mucoid sputum. Patients with uncomplicated chronic bronchitis may have nothing more than cough and sputum production without progression to airway obstruction. In others, exertional dyspnea develops insidiously, and it is frequently aggravated by cold, dampness, exposure to dusty atmosphere, or minor upper respiratory infections. Once the exertional dyspnea develops, it progresses. The patient must limit his activity and finally give up working. Weight loss is evident. Commonly, disability is aggravated by episodes of superimposed acute bronchitis following upper respiratory infections. Wheezing is frequently associated with these acute exacerbations, but fever may or may not be present.

In early and uncomplicated chronic bronchitis, physical examination is usually unremarkable except for the presence of scattered rhonchi due to mucous secretions in the bronchial tree. However, patients with chronic bronchitis usually do not consult a physician until symptoms and signs of airway obstruction becomes bothersome. At this time, a variety of physical findings may be seen that are related to both chronic bronchitis and pulmonary emphysema: widening of intercostal spaces; an increase in the anteroposterior diameter of the thoracic cage; hyperresonance on percussion with obliteration of the area of cardiac dullness; low diaphragms with little mobility; fine to medium moist rales; and a prolonged expiratory phase, often with wheezing. Cyanosis is common and is associated with hypoxia and an erythrocytosis. Clubbing of the fingers may occur, but it is uncommon. Cardiac enlargement, hepatomegaly, and edema of the lower extremities may be present as a result of right heart failure.

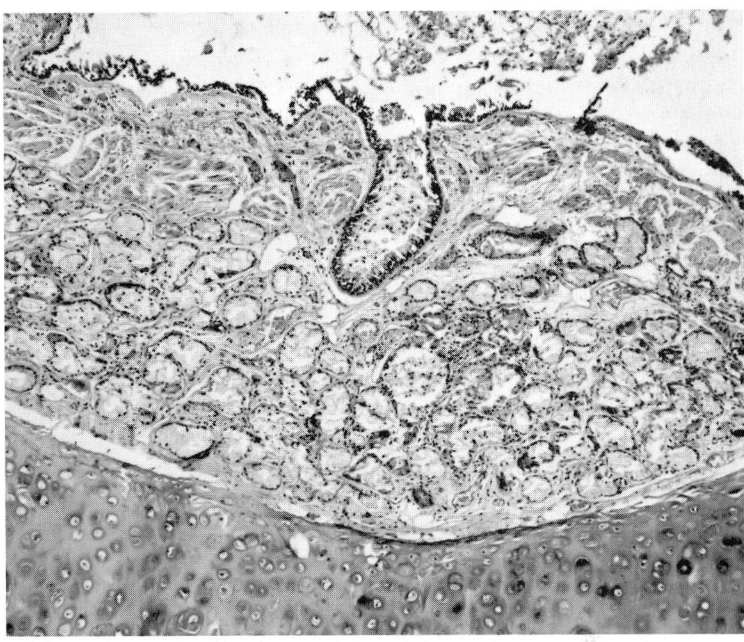

Fig. 27-2. Bronchus from a 78-year-old male with chronic bronchitis. Note the partial desquamation of ciliated columnar epithelium and the hypertrophy of mucous glands (the gland–wall ratio is 0.63 in this patient's bronchus; the normal ratio should be 0.14–0.36). (Original magnification × 55)

Diagnosis

A history of chronic cough productive of purulent sputum is highly suggestive of chronic bronchitis. Collection and inspection of the sputum are essential. The daily volume and the appearance of the sputum should be noted. Bacteriologic examinations by smears and cultures should be performed. Roentgenograms may show only increased bronchiovascular markings in chronic bronchitis. There may also be hyperaeration, widening of intercostal spaces, flattening of diaphragms, and a vertical position of the cardiac shadow when emphysema is present. Enlargement of the right ventricle may be seen when pulmonary hypertension is present. Pulmonary function studies usually reveal a decrease in the vital capacity and a prolongation of expiratory airflow. Measurement of arterial blood gas tensions is of great importance to diagnosis and in planning therapy.

Bronchial asthma, tuberculosis, bronchiectasis, cardiac failure, cystic fibrosis, and carcinoma of the lung must be considered in the differential diagnosis.

Prognosis

Some patients with chronic bronchitis manifested only by cough and sputum may remain stable for many years. Others may show progressive deterioration with each of a series of acute exacerbations leading to severe exertional dyspnea and serious disability. Emphysema and bronchiectasis are common complications. Erythrocytosis may occur in those patients with significant, persistent hypoxia. Pulmonary hypertension may lead to cor pulmonale, right ventricular hypertrophy, and finally cardiac failure.

Therapy

Most of the destructive changes of the respiratory tract associated with symptomatic chronic bronchitis and emphysema are irreversible. At best, treatment will delay further progression. The patient must stop smoking. He should avoid other irritating gases and dusts. Central heating and air-conditioning systems at home and at the place of employment will help reduce acute exacerbations by stabilizing the climate.

Administration of antimicrobial agents during acute attacks associated with the production of purulent sputum appears to shorten the course of acute exacerbations. Procaine penicillin G in a dose of 1.2 to 2.4 million units daily, by intramuscular injection; ampicillin (30–60 mg/kg body wt/day as four equal portions, every 6 hours, by month) or tetracycline (15 mg/kg body wt/day as four equal portions taken orally every 6 hours) may be prescribed. Such antimicrobial therapy should be given for 2 to 3 weeks. In selected patients with frequent exacerbations, prophylactic antimicrobial administration during the winter months or at the first signs of a "chest cold" may be useful. Either tetracycline (15–30 mg/kg body wt/day, PO as four equal portions, 6 hourly); ampicillin (30–60 mg/kg body wt/day, PO as four equal portions, 6 hourly); or one tablet of trimethoprim–sulfamethoxazole (80 mg plus 400 mg, PO, 12 hourly) appears to be effective. Patients with chronic pulmonary diseases should receive influenza virus vaccine and pneumococcal vaccine.

Bronchodilators are sometimes helpful for patients with airway obstruction. Theophylline, 2 to 4 mg/kg, can be taken orally every 6 hours. Terbutaline sulfate, 2.5 to 5.0 mg taken every 8 hours produces less cardiac stimulation than other sympathomimetics. Inhalation of aerolized 0.5% isoproteronol hydrochloride or 0.65 mg for each metered dose of metaproteronol sulfate is effective if the patient has been taught to use the nebulizer properly. Routine use of glucosteroids is not recommended.

Patients must be hospitalized when severe hypercapnia and hypoxia complicate acute exacerbations. The use of sedatives or narcotics must be avoided. Oxygen-enriched air is useful to correct hypoxia but must be carefully monitored to avoid ablation of the hypoxic drive to ventilation and further increase of carbon dioxide tension in the blood. Close clinical observation of the patients and frequent blood gas determinations are essential in guiding the course of therapy. Antimicrobial agents such as penicillin G and ampicillin should be administered if *S. pneumoniae* or *H. influenzae* are the cause of infection (procaine penicillin G, 600,000 units intramuscularly every 12 hours; ampicillin, 100–150 mg/kg body wt/day IV as four equal portions, 6 hourly for non-β-lactamase-producing strains of *H. influenzae*). If enteric gram-negative bacilli are contributory, either gentamicin, tobramycin, or netilmicin (3.0–6.0 mg/kg body wt/day, IM or IV as three equal portions 8 hourly) should be given.

Tracheostomy may be necessary in the patient who cannot mobilize tracheobronchial secretions. Mechanical aids to respiration may also be required; for example, intermittent positive-pressure breathing. Meticulous care of the tracheostomy, with aseptic precautions in cleansing and during suctioning, cannot be overemphasized.

Prevention

Among the multiple factors that contribute to chronic bronchitis, the elimination of cigarette smoking and the reduction of environmental air pollution constitute known, effective preventive measures. A concerted effort is required by the medical profession, public health agencies at all levels, civic leaders, and the population as a whole.

Bronchiolitis

Bronchiolitis is an acute, viral respiratory infection of young infants that is characterized by obstruction of the terminal branches of the bronchial tree. The infection is usually self-limited, with a favorable outcome; however, fatalities do occur.

Etiology

In the past, bacterial agents, including *H. influenzae,* have been implicated as causes of bronchiolitis. However, recent studies have shown that respiratory viruses such as influenza viruses (see Chap. 28, Influenza), adenoviruses (see Chap. 23, Nonbacterial Pharyngitis), rhinoviruses (see Chap. 21, The Common Cold), parainfluenza viruses (see Chap. 26, Epiglottitis, Laryngitis, and Laryngotracheobronchitis), and respiratory syncytial (RS) viruses are the actual causes of the disease. Among these agents, the type 3 parainfluenza virus and RS viruses are probably the most important.

First isolated in 1956 from a chimpanzee with a cold, RS virus was named chimpanzee coryza agent (CCA). In the following year, the same virus was isolated from human infants with lower respiratory tract illnesses. Because this virus induced the aggregation of tissue culture cells into large syncytial masses, the term *respiratory syncytial virus* was finally adopted. Respiratory syncytial viruses belong to the paramyxovirus group, even though they do not agglutinate erythrocytes. They are ether sensitive RNA viruses that measure about 90 nm to 130 nm in diameter. These viruses have not been adapted to grow in embryonated hens' eggs. There is a specific surface antigen detectable by neutralization and an internal soluble complement-fixing (CF) antigen present in the RS virus.

Respiratory syncytial virus is probably the most importnt respiratory pathogen of infants. During infancy and childhood, RS viruses are associated with 32% to 75% of pneumonias. In adults, RS viruses cause only a mild upper respiratory infection, simulating the common cold.

Epidemiology

The incidence of acute bronchiolitis in infants parallels epidemics or outbreaks of respiratory infections in older children and adults. It is more prevalent in the cold months during either late fall and early winter, or later winter and early spring. Neither nutritional status, sex, nor race affects the susceptibility of infants to bronchiolitis.

Primary infection with RS virus occurs early in life. Approximately 33% of infants develop neturalizing antibody to RS virus by 1 year of age and 80% to 90% by 4 years of age.

Pathogenesis and Pathology

Bronchiolitis probably results from the extension of an upper respiratory tract infection to the bronchioles by way of the trachea and bronchi. Even the parenchyma of the lung may be involved. Inflammation of the bronchiolar mucosa evokes exudate, leading to bronchiolar obstruction. This results in focal emphysema and atelectasis. In fatal cases, there is thickening of bronchial and bronchiolar walls, with exudate plugging the lumen. Microscopically, cellular infiltration with lymphocytes, plasma cells, and neutrophils is seen. In more severe cases, areas of atelectasis and emphysema are evident, as well as both interstitial and necrotizing pneumonitis.

Manifestations

The onset is usually insidious, following an upper respiratory infection with coryza and cough. An abrupt onset is unusual. Fever is moderate. As bronchiolar involvement progresses, dyspnea, cyanosis, and suprasternal, and intercostal retractions during inspiration become increasingly prominent. Fretfulness and irritability progress as bronchiolar obstruction increases; prostration with death from anoxia may result.

Physical findings may change quickly, but the signs of generalized obstructive emphysema are usually present. These include hyperresonance on percussion, expiratory wheezing, and medium and fine sibilant or musical rales. If bronchiolar obstruction is extensive, breath sounds may become inaudible.

Diagnosis

In an infant with generalized obstructive emphysema, the diagnosis of acute bronchiolitis is usually not difficult. Roentgenograms are of little help for the picture is that of hyperventilated lungs with depressed and flattened diaphragms; patchy consolidations may be seen if pneumonitis is present. Total and differential counts of blood leukocytes are usually normal. Specific bacterial pathogens are usually not isolated from nasopharyngeal cultures. With dehydration and hypoxia, abnormal serum electrolytes and blood gases are usually found.

Acute bronchiolitis may be difficult to differentiate from bronchial asthma. However, allergic asthma is rarely seen in infants under 18 months. A therapeutic trial of epinephrine or aminophylline may be helpful. Early pertussis, (see Chap. 29, Whooping Cough), cystic fibrosis, or the inhalation of irritant gases should also be considered.

Eitologic diagnosis depends on viral isolation and serologic tests. Nasopharyngeal secretions or swabs are the best sources for viral isolation. Parainfluenza viruses can be isolated in monkey kidney cells. For isolation of RS viruses, nasopharyngeal specimens should be inoculated directly, without freezing, into HeLa or Hep-2 cells. Complement fixation, neutralization, and hemagglutination-inhibition tests are used to demonstrate a rise in antibody titer during convalescence.

Prognosis

Most infants with bronchiolitis recover, although the clinical course may be stormy and alarming. The mortality rate is estimated to be about 1% to 2%, with higher rates in premature babies. Complications include pulmonary atelectasis, interstitial pneumonia, and cardiac failure. Permanent sequelae are rare.

Therapy

Provision of warm air that is saturated with water and contains 50% to 75% oxygen is the essential element of therapy. Bronchodilators such as epinephrine and aminophylline have not given consistently beneficial results; glucosteroids are of doubtful value. Yet, when there is progression of bronchiolitis in a severely ill infant, intravenous injection of 25 mg cortisol every 6 hours may be given. Presently available antimicrobial agents are ineffective in acute viral bronchiolitis. If pneumonitis associated with leukocytosis develops, a penicillinase-resistant penicillin should be applied—nafcillin in a dose of 150 to 200 mg/kg body wt/day intravenously. The proper replacement of electrolytes and fluids is important. Digitalis preparations should be given as soon as cardiac failure is detected.

Prevention

Experimental respirovirus vaccines, including those for parainfluenza and RS viruses, are under development. As yet, they have not shown great promise.

Bibliography

Books

CHANOCK RM, KIM HY, BRANDT C, PARROTT RH: Respiratory syncytial virus. In Evans AS (ed): Viral Infections of Humans: Epidemiology and Control. New York, Plenum, 1976. pp. 365–382.

REYNOLD HY: Chronic bronchitis and acute infectious exacerbations. In Mandell GL, Douglas RG Jr, Bennett JE (eds): Principles and Practice of Infectious Diseases. New York, John Wiley & Sons, 1979. pp. 484–489.

Journals

NELIGAN GA, STEINER H, GARDNER PG, MCQUILLIN J: Respiratory syncytial virus infection of the newborn. Br Med J 3:146–147, 1970

NIEWOREHUER DE, KLEINERMAN J, RICE DB: Pathologic changes in the peripheral airways of young cigarette smokers. N Engl J Med 291:775–758, 1974

REID L: Chronic bronchitis and emphysema. Adv Intern Med 12:256–294, 1964

ROBSON K: Acute bronchitis. Practitioner 181:681–685, 1958

ROSS CA, PINKERTON IW, ASSAAD FA: Pathogenesis of respiratory syncytial virus disease in infancy. Arch Dis Child 46:702–704, 1971

TAGER I, SPEIZER FE: Role of infection in chronic bronchitis. N Engl J Med 292:563–571, 1975

CHIEN LIU

Influenza

28

Influenza is an acute infectious disease characterized by the sudden onset of fever, malaise, headache, and myalgias. In uncomplicated cases, the disease is self limited, and affected individuals usually recover completely within a week.

Etiology

The etiologic agent is the influenza virus of the Orthomyxoviridae family. There are three antigenic types, designated *A*, *B* and *C*. Distinct subtypes are found in influenza A viruses and to a lesser extent in type B viruses. Influenza C does not appear to cause epidemics, and no subtypes are known.

Influenza viruses measure 80 nm to 120 nm in diameter (Fig. 28-1) and occur as spherical or filamentous forms with surface projections or spikes that correspond to the hemagglutinins (H) and neuraminidases (N), which determine the subtypes. There is a lipoprotein envelope. Inside, the single-strand ribonucleic acid RNA genome is a helix consisting of eight segments. Infectious virus is inactivated by heating at 56°C for a few minutes and by treatment with ether. Influenza viruses are pneumotropic agents with a selective affinity for tracheobronchial epithelial cells. Certain strains can be adapted to multiply in the mouse brain, and some strains produce a fatal hemorrhagic infection in chick embryos. On entry into susceptible cells, the influenza viral nucleoprotein rapidly becomes associated with the cell nucleus. A soluble antigen containing RNA is synthesized intranuclearly and diffuses from the nucleus to accumulate at the periphery of the cytoplasm. The assembly of viral components appears to take place at the cell surface, the site where infectious virus particles are released.

Influenza viruses were the first animal viruses found to be capable of agglutinating mammalian and fowl erythrocytes. Hemagglutination results when the virus interacts with the surface of erythrocytes. This phenomenon has been used extensively in the laboratory for studies of virus multiplication and for antibody titration.

Epidemiology

Epidemic influenza is cyclic in occurrence and is usually caused by type A or type B viruses. Type C influenza viruses rarely, if ever, give rise to epidemics; typically, they cause inapparent infections or small outbreaks in children. By 15 years of age, almost 100% of the population has developed antibody against influenza C viruses. Although not completely predictable, influenza A epidemics tend to have a cycle of 2 to 3 years, whereas influenza B epidemics usually occur 4 to 6 years apart. All pandemics of influenza have been caused by type A viruses. Since the latter part of the last century, at least three pandemics have been well documented: the first in 1889–1890, the second in 1918–1919, and the third in 1957. The 1918–1919 pandemic was devastating, accounting for the death of some 20 million people.

Epidemics of influenza usually occur in the cold months from late autumn to early spring. Within a community, the peak of a given epidemic is reached about 2 weeks after onset, and often the epidemic is over in a month. The attack rate may be as high as 40%, with the highest incidence in the 5- to 14-year age group. After the age of 40, the incidence decreases progressively. The overall case fatality rate in epidemics since the 1918–1919 pandemic has been low, perhaps in the neighborhood of 1%. At highest risk are the very young, the very old, the pregnant, and persons rendered vulnerable by underlying cardiopulmonary, metabolic, and renal diseases.

The influenza viruses that cause disease in humans

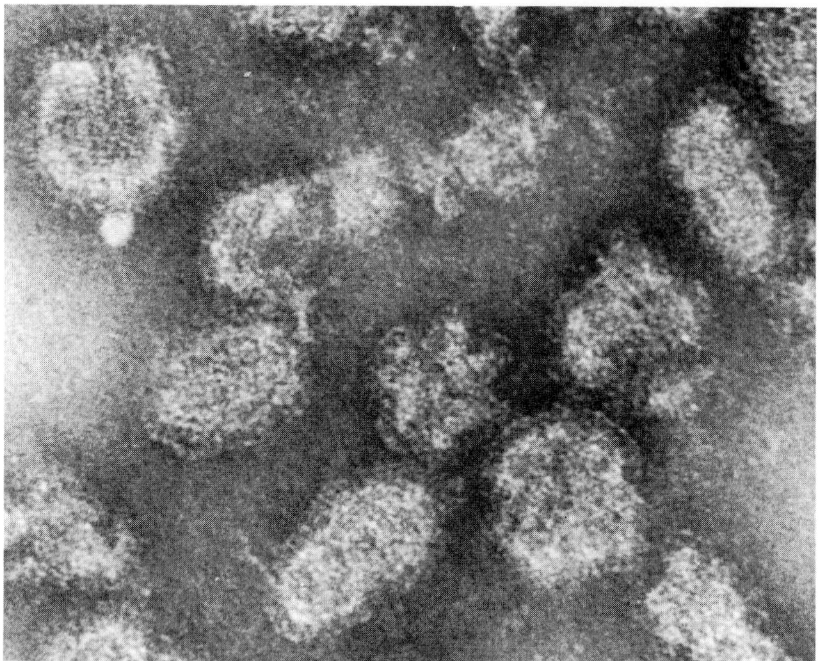

Fig. 28-1. Electron micrograph of Hong Kong influenza A virus. The internal nucleocapsid and outer envelope are apparent. (Original magnification × 155,000) (Courtesy of HD Mayor, Baylor College of Medicine)

appear to be peculiar to humans, although some strains isolated from swine and horses are antigenically related to human strains. It is not known where influenza viruses are harbored during interepidemic periods. Moreover, the mechanism of the transequatorial shift of occurrence of influenza, apparently in accord with the season, is not understood. The simultaneous eruption of influenza outbreaks in many areas distant from each other is also intriguing. Possibly, communities are seeded with virus through the occurrence of sporadic cases several weeks before an explosive outbreak.

The 1957 Asian influenza pandemic was studied most thoroughly by epidemiologists and virologists. The Asian virus (H2N2) apparently emerged in the central part of mainland China in 1956 or 1957. From there, it spread widely in China, then to Hong Kong and other parts of the world. The Asian virus was apparently brought to the United States by naval personnel arriving at Newport, Rhode Island, in early June of 1957 and perhaps also to San Diego, California, shortly thereafter. The first outbreak occurred on June 20, 1957, during a conference of high school girls at Davis, California. Several small outbreaks elsewhere in California soon followed. Apparently, the Asian virus was carried from the Davis conference to another meeting at Grinnell, Iowa, which was attended by some 1800 young people from 43 states and several foreign countries. Conferees returning home from the Grinnell conference seeded the Asian virus in many parts of the United States. After September, 1957, epidemics swept the country.

From serologic studies, there is evidence that the influenza A virus has a finite number of major antigenic mutations (Table 28-1). Recycling of these major antigenic components in a sequential manner may occur. The influenza viruses with Asian/57-like and Hong Kong 68-like hemagglutinins had occurred in the same sequence and caused epidemic influenza near the end of the 19th century. The A/Hong Kong/68 (H3N2) virus first appeared in 1968. These H3N2 viruses have undergone periodic antigenic drifts and have been responsible for most of the influenza epidemics for more than a decade. In 1976, the emergence of the "swine virus," A/New Jersey/76 ($H_{SW}N1$), at Fort Dix, New Jersey, generated a great deal of public and governmental concern over the possible resurgence of the 1918–1919 scourge. It was fortunate that this virus did not spread from the military base to the civilian population. In 1977, the A/USSR/77 (H1N1) virus reappeared after a lapse of two decades. During the period 1977–1981, influenza was caused by both H3N2 and H1N1 variants. Because most of the people born between 1947 and 1957 had contact with the H1N1 viruses, illnesses caused by A/USSR/77 and A/Brazil/78 were largely restricted to college and high school students and to younger children.

Table 28-1. Influenza Virus Types

Subtypes	Prevalence	Protypes
Type A		
H0,N1	1933–1943	A/PR/8/34
H1,N1	1947–1957	A/FM/1/47
H2,N2	1957–1968	A/Japan/305/57
H3,N2	1968–1972	A/Hong Kong/1/68
H3,N2	1973–1975	A/Port Chalmers/1/73
H3,N2	1975–1978	A/Victoria/3/75
Hswl,N1	1976	A/New Jersey/8/76
H3,N2	1977–1978	A/Texas/1/77
H1,N1	1977–1978	A/USSR/90/77
H1,N1	1978–1981	A/Bangkok/79
Type B		
	1936–1948	B/Lee/40
	1954–	B/GL/1739/54
	1959–	B/Md/1/59
	1962–	B/Taiwan/2/62
	1972–	B/Hong Kong/5/72
Type C		
	1947–	C/Taylor/1233/47
(No significant variants known)		1950 to present

Pathogenesis and Pathology

Influenza is transmitted by the inhalation of virus-containing droplets ejected from the respiratory tract of a person infected with influenza virus. In experimentally infected ferrets, the virus multiplies in the ciliated respiratory epithelium, particularly that lining the nasal turbinates. Desquamation of the ciliated epithelium coincides with the development of acute symptoms of fever and coryza. The regeneration and repair of respiratory epithelium passes through the stages of transitional, stratified squamous, and hyperplastic epithelium before the normal columnar ciliated cells are reestablished.

In uncomplicated influenza in man, essentially the same changes were observed throughout the tracheobronchial tree, by bronchoscopy with bronchial biopsy—namely, desquamation of ciliated epithelium, hyperplasia of transitional cells, edema, hyperemia, congestion, and increased secretions. During the 1957–1958 pandemic, 30 fatal cases of pneumonic influenza without bacterial complications were studied. Focal pneumonia with intraalveolar exudate, denuded alveolar walls, capillary thromboses, and necrosis were found. Because cells from foci of pneumonia stained with fluorescent antibody specific for A_2 virus, they may have been the sites of viral multiplication in the lungs. Bacterial infection complicating influenza is usually caused by *Staphylococcus aureus,* which penetrate to the tunica and form microabscesses.

Manifestations

After an incubation period of 1 to 3 days, influenza usually begins abruptly with fever ranging from 39°C to 40°C (102°F-104°F). Chilliness is common, and true rigors may precede or accompany the fever. Headache may be severe, and there may be retro-orbital pain. The conjunctivas are usually congested. There is often a sense of extreme prostration with myalgia that is particularly severe in the muscles of the back and limbs; patients voluntarily take to bed. Coryza is usually not a prominent symptom; indeed, dryness of the nasal passages and the pharynx is common. Cough that is only scantily productive is frequent and aggravates the substernal pain or discomfort that is complained of by many patients. During the acute stage of illness in uncomplicated cases, the physical signs consist of fever and injection of the conjunctivas and pharynx. There is no abnormality of the lungs, either by physical or radiographic examination. If there are no complications, the fever abates in 3 to 4 days, and recovery is complete within a week. However, in some patients, particularly older people, easy fatigability and lack of energy may persist for several weeks.

In some patients, notably infants, the symptoms may be mild and simulate a common cold or upper respiratory tract infection. However, in old people, in patients with underlying, chronic respiratory, cardiovascular, metabolic, and renal diseases, and in women in the last trimester of pregnancy, the course of influenza may worsen rapidly. Persistent fever, marked prostration, cough associated with rales, and pneumonia are poor prognostic signs. Although primary influenzal pneumonia may occur, pneumonia complicating influenza is usually a secondary bacterial infection caused by *S. aureus, Haemophilus influenzae, Streptococcus pneumoniae,* or *Streptococcus pyogenes.* Mental confusion and delirium, followed by coma, consistent with encephalitis. Development of a gallop rhythm and cardiovascular collapse may indicate myocarditis.

Diagnosis

The clinical diagnosis of sporadic cases of influenza may be impossible because the signs and symptoms are not pathognomonic. There is no clinical basis for differentiating influenza caused by types A, B, or C viruses. Whereas the typical common cold is an afebrile illness with profuse coryza, acute respiratory disease (ARD) caused by adenoviruses is difficult to differentiate from influenza. Conjunctivitis and pharyngitis are usually more severe in adenoviral ARD. In military populations, ARD primarily affects new recruits; influenza affects all personnel, seasoned and new. Streptococcal pharyngitis, as it occurs in older children and adults, is an exudative process with fever, leukocytosis, and tender, enlarged cervical lymph nodes.

Primary influenzal pneumonia is difficult to differentiate from other nonbacterial pneumonias. However, primary atypical pneumonia and other nonbacterial pneumonias usually have an insidious onset and are benign.

A complicating bacterial pneumonia is very serious. Although staphylococcal pneumonia rarely occurs in previously healthy persons (except for very young infants), *S. aureus* was the most common cause of bacterial pneumonia superimposed on influenza in recent epidemics. The course from onset to fatality may take only hours.

Definitive diagnosis of influenza depends on laboratory procedures: isolation of the virus from throat washings or sputum and the demonstration of a significant increase in antibody titer during convalescence. Isolation of the influenza virus is best accomplished by intraamniotic inoculation of chick embryos with specimens (throat washings, sputum) obtained during the first 3 days of illness. Primary mammalian tissue culture cells such as monkey kidney cells may also be used for viral isolation. Viral isolates can be identified serologically with type-specific antiserums.

Fig. 28-2. Nasal smears from patients with acute influenza infection, stained with antiinfluenza fluorescent conjugate. The white areas represent influenza viral antigen in infected cells. *(A)* Two infected ciliated columnar epithelial cells with antigen in cytoplasm and nuclei. *(B)* Three mononuclear cells with intracytoplasmic antigen. (Original magnification × 1600)

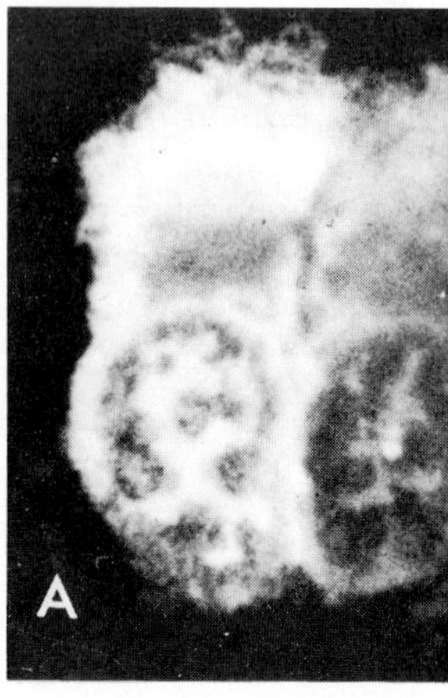

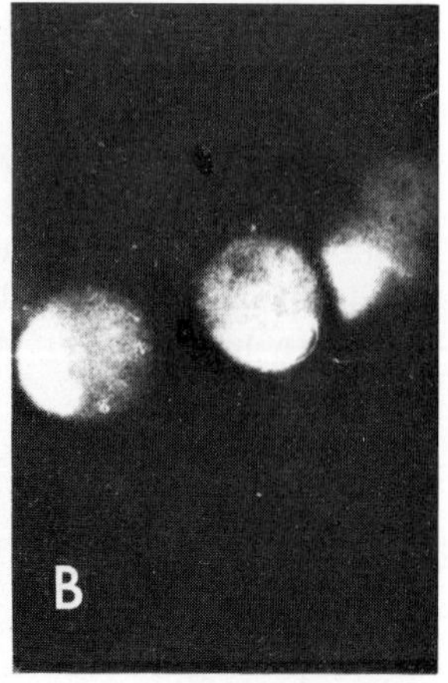

Serum antibody, detected either by hemagglutination-inhibition (HI), neutralization, or complement fixation tests, may rise as early as 8 to 9 days after the onset of illness. Maximal titers are usually not obtained until 2 to 3 weeks after infection. The diagnosis is satisfactorily established with the demonstration of a fourfold or greater rise in antibody titer, comparing serum obtained during the acute illness with serum obtained during convalescence.

Direct examination of exfoliated nasal epithelial cells after reaction with a fluorescent conjugate of antiinfluenza antiserum is a reliable and rapid method for diagnosis (Fig. 28-2). Best results are obtained when specimens are collected from febrile, acutely ill patients.

Prognosis

In uncomplicated cases, the prognosis of influenza is favorable. It is a self-limited disease resulting in complete recovery within a week, leaving no sequelae.

Complications are most common in patients with underlying, chronic cardiac or pulmonary diseases. That is, influenza epidemics are reflected in mortality rates that are higher than normal for the community when the aggregate of all respiratory tract illnesses are considered (see Fig. 31-2). Women who contract influenza late in pregnancy are also at a higher risk because elevation of the diaphragm compromises pulmonary function. Reye's syndrome—acute encephalopathy with fatty degeneration of the viscera—has been associated with influenza as well as other viral infections.

Patients who recover from influenza may contract the disease subsequently. Although active immunity is imparted by the natural disease, the protection is specific to the point of the subtypic variant of the influenza virus. Protection may wane with time, but there is evidence that it persists for many years.

Therapy

In uncomplicated influenza, treatment is symptomatic and supportive. Bedrest is essential and is almost always voluntarily undertaken because of the prostration. Antipyretics and analgesics, such as aspirin (300–600 mg every 4 hours) should be given to relieve fever, headache, and myalgia. If dry cough and substernal discomfort become bothersome, codeine (16–64 mg every 4–6 hours) may be given. A barbiturate such as secobarbital may be helpful for its sedative effect. Most patients are anorectic during the acute illness. Because of the fever, a liberal intake of fluids should be urged.

Antibacterial agents should not be given to patients with influenza in an attempt to prevent bacterial complications. The administration of antibacterial agents is not actually prophylactic and may be selective for *S. aureus* (when tetracycline is used). If bacterial infection is suspected, sputum smears and cultures of the sputum and blood should be obtained. Patients should then be treated with one of the penicillinase-resistant semisynthetic penicillins in full therapeutic dosages—for example, nafcillin, 150–200 mg/kg body wt/day, IV, as six equal portions, 4 hourly. If gram-negative bacilli predominate and the patient does not respond to the nafcillin, gentamicin or tobramycin (3–5 mg/kg body wt/day) should be given by IV or IM injection of three equal portions, 8 hourly. In addition, oxygen therapy with mechanical devices for positive pressure breathing may be helpful. Periodic blood gas determinations to monitor the adequacy of oxygen administration are necessary in the clinical management of such patients.

In controlled studies, amantadine hydrochloride was shown to shorten the clinical course of influenza A infections if given within 48 hours after onset of symptoms. However, in uncomplicated cases, influenza is a self-limited disease, and the routine use of amantadine is not recommended. In high-risk patients and in those with life-threatening primary influenza pneumonia or croup, amantadine may be considered for therapy, although effectiveness has not been documented by controlled studies. The dosage is 100 mg, PO, 12 hourly for adults and children over 9 years. For children less than 9 years of age, the dose is 4 to 8 mg per kg body wt/day, PO, as two equal portions (not to exceed 150 mg/day), 12 hourly.

Prevention

Quarantine is impractical in the control of influenza—the incubation period is too short, and modern man is highly mobile. Active immunization with vaccines remains the most effective means of prevention.

In the United States, the most current influenza viruses are grown in chick embryos and inactivated to make vaccine. For the 1980–1981 season, a trivalent vaccine formulation containing 7 μg of hemagglutinin of each antigen from A/Brazil/78 (H1N1), A/Bangkok/79 (H3N2), and B/Singapore/79 was available. Side effects and adverse reactions were few, consisting of local erythema and induration, fever, malaise, and myalgia lasting 1 to 2 days. The 1981–1982 vaccine is to contain the same three strains of influenza viruses as were in the 1980–1981 formulation but with 15 μg hemagglutinin per strain.

Guillain–Barré syndrome was associated with the 1976 swine influenza vaccination program at a rate of one case per 100,000 vaccinations. Although there was no such association in the 1978–1979 and 1979–1980 influenza seasons, any person who receives influenza vaccine should be made aware of the possible risk of Guillain–Barré and the risk of acquiring influenza and its complications.

The vaccine is injected subcutaneously or intramuscularly, according to the manufacturer's directions. Immunity is engendered in 65% to 70% of those vaccinated; the duration of protective immunity is about 3 to 6 months. The annual administration of vaccine is therefore necessary to assure protective immunity during the respiratory disease season. In the northern hemisphere, vaccinations should be completed before November. Hypersensitivity to eggs, chickens, and chicken products is the only contraindication to the administration of influenza virus vaccines. Influenza vaccines and the pneumococcal polysaccharide vaccines can be given to the patient during the same office visit.

Because uncomplicated influenza is a self-limited disease with low mortality, influenza vaccine has not been recommended as a routine primary vaccination procedure in the pediatric population, as have diphtheria–pertussis–tetanus (DPT), poliomyelitis, and measles vaccines. Debilitated patients, old persons, institutionalized persons, and patients with chronic pulmonary, cardiovascular, renal, or metabolic diseases should receive the vaccine. Pregnancy is not an indication for or against influenza vaccination. Health and public service personnel (policemen, firemen, and municipal government officials) have the next highest vaccination priority.

For chemoprophylaxis, amantadine hydrochloride has been approved by the Food and Drug Administration for all strains of influenza A viruses. It is not effective against influenza B viruses. Many studies have shown that amantadine is a preventative of approximately 70% of influenza caused by type A viruses. While immunization remains the preventative measure of choice, amantadine may be used to supplement a program of prophylaxis. When an influenza outbreak is detected in a given community, elderly persons and persons with chronic diseases who have not been vaccinated should be given the influenza vaccine together with amantadine, 100mg, PO, twice daily for 10 to 14 days until an antibody response has occurred. In persons who have hypersensitivity to eggs, amantadine may be given throughout the duration of the outbreak of influenza. During a severe outbreak, individuals who render essential public services should also be considered as possible candidates for amantadine chemoprophylaxis. About 7% of persons taking amantadine may develop central nervous system side effects consisting of insomnia, dizziness, and difficulty in mental concentration. These reactions disappear when the drug is discontinued. The decision to implement largescale use of amantadine must take into account the cost and side effects, as well as possible selection of amantadine-resistant viruses. In the laboratory, spontaneous development of resistance to amantadine by influenza A viruses has occurred in tissue cultures at a relatively high frequency.

Bibliography

Books

DAVENPORT FM: Influenza viruses. In Evans AS (ed): Viral Infections of Humans: Epidemiology and Control. New York, Plenum, 1976. pp 273–296.

KILBOURNE ED: Epidemiology of influenza. In Kilbourne ED (ed): Influenza Viruses and Influenza. New York, Academic Press, 1975. pp 483–538.

MULDER J, HERS JFP: Influenza. Netherlands, Wolters–Noordhoff, 1972, 300 pp

Journals

BOGART DB, LIU C, RUTH WE, KERBY GR, WILLIAMS CH: Rapid diagnosis of primary influenza pneumonia. Chest 68: 513–517, 1975

DELKER LL, MOSER RH, NELSON JD, RODSTEIN M, ROLLS K, SANFORD JP, SWARTZ MN: Amantadine: Does it have a role in the prevention and treatment of influenza? A National Institutes of Health consensus development conference. Ann Intern Med 92:256–258, 1980

DYKES AC, CHERRY JD, NOLAN CE: A clinical, epidemiologic, serologic and virologic study of influenza C virus infection. Arch Intern Med 140:1295–1298, 1980

GLEZEN WP, COUCH RB: Interpandemic influenza in the Houston area, 1974–76. N Engl J Med 298:587–592, 1978

LITTLE JW, HALL WJ, DOUGLAS RG JR, MUDHOLKAR GS, SPEERS DM, PATEL K: Airway hypersensitivity and peripheral airway dysfunction in influenza A infection. Am Rev Respir Dis 118:295–303, 1978

MEIKELJOHN G, EICKHOFF TC, GRAVES P: Antigenic drift and efficacy of influenza virus vaccines. 1976–1977. J Infect Dis 138:618–624, 1978

SWEET C, SMITH H: Pathogenicity of influenza virus. Microbiol Rev 44:303–330, 1980

DAVID H. SMITH

Whooping Cough

29

Whooping cough is an acute tracheobronchitis affecting only humans—particularly young infants. It is characterized by paroxysmal cough followed by inspiratory stridor. A highly contagious disease, whooping cough is usually caused by *Bordatella pertussis,* although the related *Bordatella parapertussis* and *Bordatella bronchisepticum* may be responsible for milder cases. Some patients with whooping cough are simultaneously infected with an adenovirus; however, *B. pertussis* plays the primary role in the disease. Respiratory disease lacking the classic clinical features of whooping cough may be caused by *B. pertussis,* especially in older children and adults.

Etiology

Bordatella pertussis is a small, ovoid, nonmotile, nonsporeforming, gram-negative bacillus that has fastidious requirements for growth. Replication is slow, even under optimal conditions, and is inhibited by many factors present in routine bacteriologic mediums (*e.g.,* toxic lipids). The blood and starch components of the commonly used Bordet–Gengou medium serve primarily as absorbents and can be satisfactorily replaced by other substances such as charcoal or an anion-exchange resin. The viability of *B. pertussis* is rapidly lost under environmental conditions.

Freshly isolated *B. pertussis* is in phase I, the virulent, morphologically uniform, encapsulated, and pilated form, which also produces several biologically active substances. These include lipopolysaccharide (endotoxin); a heat-labile dermonecrotoxin; a factor that sensitizes animals to histamine and serotonin; a hemagglutinin; and six serologically distinct agglutinogens (K antigens—at least two of which are present in each isolate). The pili appear to contain the lymphocytosis—promoting activity which is typical of *B. pertussis*. However, neither the capsular substance(s) nor the agglutinogens have been either isolated or characterized. With passage in the laboratory, a smooth to rough transition occurs, yielding phase IV cells that are pleomorphic, nonencapsulated, and avirulent. Only phase I *B. pertussis* bacilli are suitable for the preparation of vaccines.

Both *B. parapertussis* and *B. bronchisepticum* differ from *B. pertussis* by growing more rapidly on plain agar mediums and by seroreactivity. Moreover, *B. bronchosepticum* is enzootic in several species. Because *B. pertussis* shares certain physiologic properties with *Haemophilus influenzae,* some writers refer to pertussis bacilli as *Haemophilus pertussis,* although the genera are not closely related genetically.

Epidemiology

Whooping cough is distributed worldwide, with humans as both the natural host and the reservoir of *B. pertussis* (nonhuman primates and mice can be infected experimentally). Pertussis is one of the most contagious of infectious diseases, with 80% or more of exposed, susceptible persons developing disease. Asymptomatic infection does occur, and *B. pertussis* may colonize the upper respiratory tract. Although pertussis occurs endemically, epidemics may appear in susceptible populations. There is no consistent seasonal incidence, though overall, the summer and early fall are the periods of highest incidence. Pertussis afflicts infants primarily, with up to 50% of cases occurring in the first year of life; girls are more often affected than boys. Although adults were once thought to be resistant, recent studies have revealed endemic and clustered disease among adults. Disease among hospital personnel has been responsible for nosocomial outbreaks, and it is clear that adults are important, often asymptomatic, reservoirs of *B. pertussis*. Only about 3000 cases are reported annually in the United States, but most observers think this number is too low. Pertussis is a major health problem in developing countries, particularly in areas of poor nutrition and immunization. The recent decline in the rate of immunization against pertussis in the United Kingdom to 30% of children has been accompanied by an epidemic affecting as many persons as in prevaccine times.

Pathogenesis and Pathology

Inhaled in aerosols, pertussis bacilli attach to the respiratory epithelium by pili and multiply. Growth of *B. pertussis* inhibits the action of respiratory tract cilia, stimulates mucous secretion, and produces a necrotizing inflammation that results in patchy ulceration of the respiratory epithelium. It is presumed that the capsule of *B. pertussis* inhibits phagocytosis. The copious secretions and desquamated epithelial and inflammatory cells readily block the small tracheobronchial airways of infants, producing the characteristic symptoms and the frequent atelectasis. The infection occasionally spreads beyond the airways to become a primary pneumonia and may damage the bronchioles sufficiently to produce bronchiectasis. The cough may raise venous pressue high enough to rupture alveoli, producing transient interstitial or subcutaneous emphysema and hemorrhage. Whether the neurologic symptoms of pertussis result from a direct neurotoxic action of bacterial products or hypoxia or both remains undefined.

Adenoviruses are isolated from a small number of infants with whooping cough. However, *B. pertussis* plays the primary pathogenic role, and the virus may be activated from a latent phase by the disease.

The primary pathologic process is in the lower bronchi and upper bronchioles, taking the form of inflammation of the respiratory mucosa with congestion, infiltration by leukocytes (predominantly lymphocytes), epithelial necrosis and peribronchial lymphoid hyperplasia. Atrophy and necrosis of cells and hemorrhage may be found in the brain; necrosis and fatty infiltration may be found in the liver.

Manifestations

Following an incubation period of 10 to 14 days, rhinorrhea, mild fever, anorexia, and mild cough develop. This so-called catarrhal period cannot be distinguished from many other respiratory diseases, but it is during this period that the disease is most contagious. After approximately 1 to 2 weeks, the cough increases in frequency and intensity. A cascade of repeated coughs, during which no respiration occurs, is followed by a dramatic and audible, inspiratory gasp—the characteristic whoop of whooping cough.

The cough may be provoked by many stimuli, including nursing care, eating, drinking, and inhaled irritants. In its most severe form, the cough may occur at intervals of only a few minutes and interfere with respiration and oral intake of liquids and calories. Hypoxia is often more severe than is clinically appreciated. The cough may provoke hemoptysis, epistaxis, and conjunctival hemorrhage. Vomiting is commonly induced by the cough and swallowed mucous. Dehydration, electrolyte imbalance, and weight loss may be severe. Having no immunity and airways of small diameter, infants have more severe disease than older persons. Older children and adults do not whoop but usually have the symptoms of a common cold or a tracheobronchitis.

Diagnosis

The clinical diagnosis of pertussis is suggested by a history of contact, the classic symptoms of the paroxysmal phase of the disease, and a marked, absolute lymphocytosis. Thus, whooping cough is often not considered during the catarrhal stage and in older children and adults. Infants under 6 months of age may not exhibit a marked lymphocytosis; moreover, a relative lymphocytosis is common in infants with respiratory infections of various causes. The chest roentgenogram may reveal perihilar infiltrates, patchy atelectasis, or emphysema.

The diagnosis of whooping cough depends on the isolation of *B. pertussis* from respiratory secretions. Success in isolation is favored by immediate culture of a deep nasopharyngeal specimen on freshly prepared, selective medium. Cultures inoculated by having the patient cough into a Petri plate are seldom helpful. Because the characteristic, small, pearllike colonies cannot be appreciated for 4 to 6 days, inhibitors of the normal respiratory flora (*e.g.,* methicillin) must be added to the medium to prevent overgrowth of *B. pertussis*. The organism can be isolated in about 90% of cases during the catarrhal stage of the disease, but in no more than 50% during the paroxysmal stage.

Viable and nonviable *B. pertussis* can be found in nasopharyngeal smears using fluorescein-labeled antibody (*i.e.,* in specimens from culture-negative patients); however, false-positive tests may occur in as many as 30% to 40% of cases, and false-negative tests in around 10%. None of several serologic tests is accurate or sensitive enough for routine use.

Pertussis may be distinguished from viral, mycoplasmal and other bacterial causes of tracheobronchitis by a history of contact, the character and duration of symptoms, and the laboratory findings. The results of cultures are definitive.

Spasmodic coughing may also be associated with bronchiolitis; bacterial, mycoplasmal, and viral pneumonia; tuberculosis; cystic fibrosis; foreign bodies; and disease causing airway compression such as malignancy or chronic obstructive pulmonary disease. These diseases may be distinguished by their clinical and laboratory findings and by the course of the illness.

Prognosis

Improved general medical support, including management of fluid and electrolyte imbalance and respiratory dysfunction, has reduced the mortality rate of pertussis in developed countries to 1% or less. However, pertussis continues to produce mortality rates of up to 40% in developing countries, caused primarily by pulmonary complications and secondary infections. Patients who recover are usually well after approximately 6 weeks, but severe cough may be provoked in many convalescents by the inhalation of irritants, particularly tobacco smoke. Secondary bacterial pneumonia and otitis media are not uncommon; bronchiectasis is now a rare but severe complication, as are seizure disorders and cerebral dysfunction.

Persons who have been infected with *B. pertussis* are partially, but not completely, immune. Thus, older children, and particularly adults, may again contract whooping cough. Immunity is thought to be mediated by a combination of circulating and local respiratory antibody, but the antigenic specificity of protective antibody and the characteristics of that antibody remain incompletely defined. The question of whether the infant is at high risk owing to the absence of transplacental transfer of IgM antibody or low levels of IgG antibody in the mother is unresolved. The role of cellular immunity in pertussis has not been investigated.

Therapy

Erythromycin (50 mg/kg of body wt/day, PO, as four equal portions, 6-hourly) usually eliminates *B. pertussis* from the nasopharynx during the catarrhal stage, and thereby reduces communicability. However, such therapy does not alter the course of the disease once the paroxysmal phase has developed. Pertussis hyperimmune globulin is not effective.

Supportive care is critical and includes fluid and electrolyte therapy, adequate nutrition, oxygen, and careful, attentive nursing, especially for removal of secretions. The administration of glucosteroids worsened experimental murine pertussis, but reduced cough, vomiting, and duration of symptoms in a single, uncontrolled clinical study.

Prevention

Because the respiratory tract secretions are highly contagious, both contact and respiratory precautions should be applied to hospitalized patients to reduce the risk of infecting personnel and other patients. Several, but not all, studies have found that erythromycin may be preventive if administered promptly after exposure.

Immunization with the current vaccine (a partially purified extract of whole bacteria) markedly reduces the attack rate among susceptibles and decreases symptoms among those vaccinated persons who become infected. That is, the vaccine is not completely protective. It is currently recommended that 12 protective units of pertussis vaccine be administered as a component of DPT vaccine; starting at 2 months of age, three equal doses are given at 8-week intervals. A single dose of DPT should be given about 1 year after the completion of the primary series, and again on entry into kindergarten. The vaccine produces a relatively high rate of local reactions and fever, may be accompanied by extreme fussiness or screaming for several hours after vaccination, and is rarely associated with convulsions and neurologic complications. The efficacy of the vaccine far outweighs its toxic potential and the risk of the neurological complications of the disease. Children with a static central nervous system disease are at no increased risk of neurologic complications. Adverse reactions may be reduced and successful immunization attained by the administration of 12 protective units of vaccine in multiple smaller doses (0.05 ml–0.1 ml) given at intervals of 2 weeks. Convulsions, alteration of consciousness, shock, screaming, focal neurologic signs, and thrombocytopenic purpura following pertussis vaccination are contraindications to further doses. Because toxic reactions are more common in older persons, the vaccine is rarely given to those over 6 years of age. However, older persons with chronic pulmonary disease and hospital personnel who have been exposed may be candidates for an adsorbed pertussis vaccine (0.1 ml–0.25 ml).

Remaining Problems

Improved health care, nutrition, and housing, and the relative efficacy of the pertussis vaccine, have dramatically reduced the importance of pertussis as a health problem in the United States. As a result, pertussis has attracted limited investigative effort; yet many important questions remain. A better understanding of the epidemiology of pertussis is needed; unfortunately, most data were derived from studies of hospitalized or very ill patients. The frequency and contagiousness of asymptomatic carriers needs to be defined, as well as the true incidence of infection in the community, by age and severity of symptoms. The frequency and basis for the neurologic toxicity of the current vaccine should be defined by continuing studies. There is also a great need for a thorough biochemical definition of the bacterial factors involved in pathogenicity and elucidation of the details of the immune response of the host. This information is vital to the development of improved diagnostic capabilities and a new, more effective, less toxic vaccine. A controlled trial of chemoprophylaxis is critical to the rational management of family and hospital outbreaks.

Bibliography

Journals

BARAFT LJ, WILKINS J, WHERLE PF: The role of antibiotics, immunizations, and adenovirus in pertussis. Pediatrics 61:224–230, 1978

BASS JW, KLENK EL, KOTHEIMER JB, LINNEMANN CC, SMITH MHD: Antimicrobial treatment of pertussis. J Pediatr 75:768–781, 1969

KOPLAN JP, SCHOENBAUM SC, WEINSTEIN MC, FRASER DW: Pertussis vaccine—an analysis of benefits, risks and costs. N Engl J Med 301:906–911, 1979

LAMBERT HJ: Epidemiology of a small pertussis outbreak in Kent County, Michigan. Public Health Rep. 80:365–369, 1965

MUSE KE, COLLIER AM, BASEMAN JB: Scanning electron microscopic study of hamster tracheal organ cultures infected with *Bordatella pertussis*. J Infect Dis 136:768–777, 1977

NELSON JD: The changing epidemiology of pertussis in young infants: The role of adults as reservoirs of infection. Am J Dis Child 132:371–373, 1978

STROM J: Further experience of reactions, especially of a cerebral nature in conjunction with triple vaccination: A study based on vaccinations in Sweden 1959–1965. Br Med J 4:320–323, 1967

WHITAKER JA, DONALDSON P, NELSON JD: Diagnosis of pertussis by the fluorescent–antibody method. N Engl J Med 263:850–851, 1960

Whooping Cough Immunization Committee, Medical Research Council: Vaccination against whooping cough. Br Med J 1:994–1000, 1959

Section | *VI*

Parenchymal Respiratory Infections

Indigenous Microbiota of the Respiratory Parenchyma

(None)

CHIEN LIU

Nonbacterial Pneumonias

30

Nonbacterial pneumonias are a congeries of inflammatory diseases of the pulmonary parenchyma that have in common the lack of a bacterial etiology. Unlike bacterial pneumonias (see Chap. 31, Bacterial Pneumonias), they are less definite diseases—insidious in onset, mild or moderate in severity, producing minimal or evanescent signs. For the most part, nonbacterial pneumonias are infectious in origin; in this chapter, several of the more important infectious agents are considered.

Mycoplasmal Pneumonia

Pneumonia caused by *Mycoplasma pneumoniae* has often been called primary atypical pneumonia. It is an acute, self-limited illness of low mortality that evokes a variety of nonspecific manifestations.

Etiology

Primary atypical pneumonia is a clinical syndrome that may be caused by several agents. The most common etiologic agent, *M. pneumoniae,* is frequently associated with the development of cold hemagglutinins. *Mycoplasma pneumoniae* was originally thought to be a virus and was generally referred to as the Eaton agent in acknowledgement of M.D. Eaton's isolation of it in 1942. Visualization of the Eaton agent by immunofluorescence and the development of a specific etiologic test in 1957 by Liu further strengthened the etiologic relationship of this microorganism to primary atypical pneumonia. With successful cultivation in nonliving, agar culture medium in 1962, Chanock and coworkers established that the agent was a pleuropneumonialike microorganism (PPLO); the name *Mycoplasma pneumoniae* was then assigned.

Like other PPLOs, *M. pneumoniae* does not possess a rigid cell wall. The colonies grow into the agar, taking the form of spheres that vary from 10 μm to 100 μm in diameter (Fig. 30-1). They do not have the surrounding halo or fried-egg appearance often seen with colonies of other human-associated PPLOs, such as *M. salivarium* and *M. hominis.* The colonies consist of elementary bodies that can be distinguished by appropriate staining (Fig. 30-2). Individual *M. pneumoniae* measure 250 nm to 300 nm in diameter (Fig. 30-3). They are usually filamentous in broth cultures.

For growth, *M. pneumoniae* requires a sterol-containing medium fortified with horse serum and fresh yeast extract. It is facultatively microaerophilic and differs from other *Mycoplasma* spp. found in man by fermenting glucose and hemolyzing mammalian erythrocytes (human, equine, ovine, guinea pig).

Isolation of *M. pneumoniae* from clinical specimens to slow process requiring incubation of cultures for 2 to 3 weeks. Once adapted to artificial me-

Fig. 30-1. Colonies of *Mycoplasma pneumoniae* grown on PPLO agar. (Original magnification × 95)

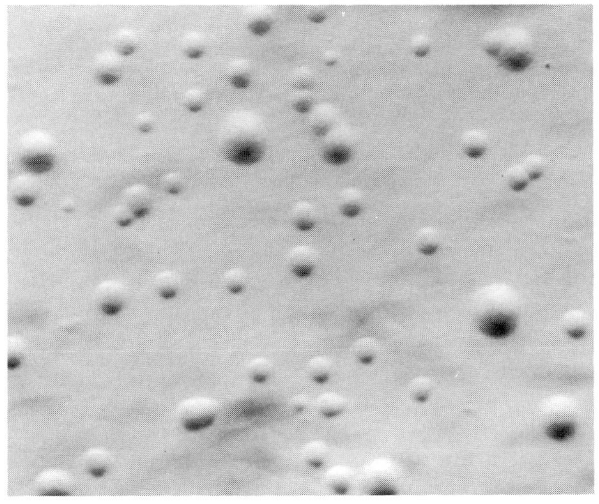

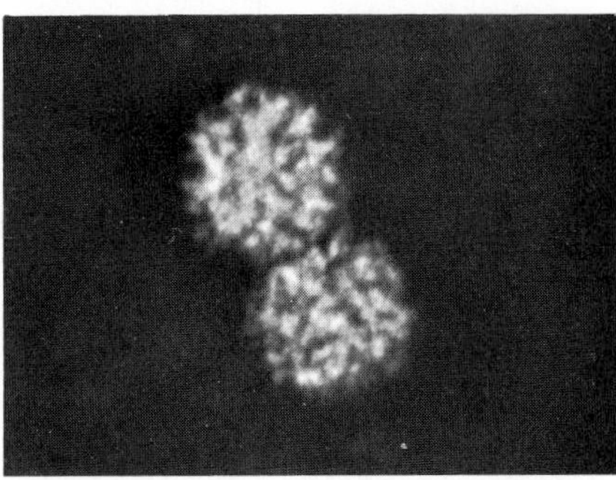

Fig. 30-2. Immunofluorescent staining of two colonies of *Mycoplasma pneumoniae.* The granular appearance represents elementary bodies. (Original magnification × 1200)

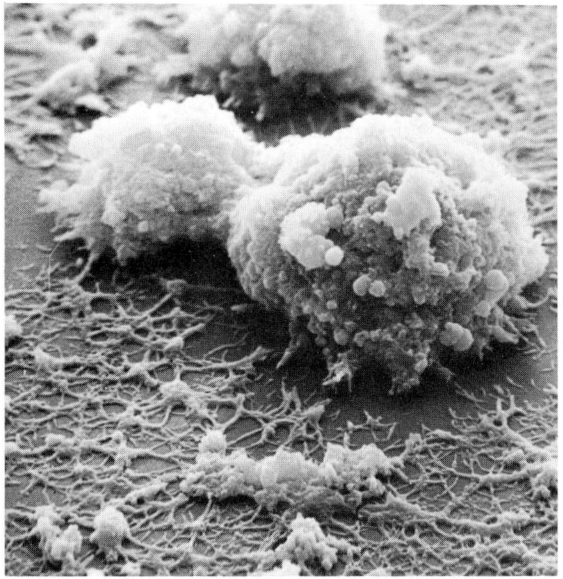

Fig. 30-3. Scanning electromicrograph of a 3-day-old culture of *Mycoplasma pneumoniae.* The microorganisms in the colonies are rounded in appearance, and there is a network of filamentous forms on the surface. (Original magnification × 2000) (Courtesy of G Biberfeld)

diums, maximal growth is attained in a few days. Because *M. pneumoniae* has no cell walls, like other PPLOs, it is completely resistant to inhibitors of bacterial cell wall synthesis (*e.g.,* penicillins). However, it is susceptible to antimicrobials that act at other sites (*e.g.,* the tetracyclines).

Epidemiology

The spectrum of respiratory infection caused by *M. pneumoniae* ranges from an inapparent infection to bronchopneumonia. Diseases involving other organ systems have also been associated with *M. pneumoniae.* These include cold agglutinin-positive hemolytic anemia, hepatitis, polyarthritis, pericarditis, myocarditis, erythema multiforme, cerebellar ataxia, peripheral and cranial neuropathy, and meningoencephalitis. Clinical disease occurs the year round, but the incidence rises during the winter. Mycoplasmal infection is usually endemic but is worldwide in distribution. Other than humans, no hosts have been identified.

Transmission involves the transfer of droplets of secretions from the respiratory tract of an infected person to a susceptible person. Spread is slow, and true epidemics are rare except in closed populations such as in the military or eleemosynary institutions. The average incubation period of natural mycoplasmal pneumonias is estimated to be 12 to 14 days; in volunteer experiments it was shown to be 8 to 10 days.

Although preschool children may be infected by *M. pneumoniae,* clinical illness usually does not occur in this age group. The ages of peak incidence of mycoplasmal pneumonia are 5 to 19 years (Fig. 30-4).

There are wide fluctuations in the frequency of mycoplasmal pneumonia, both with place and time, that do not correlate with population size, environment, or known stresses. For example, in 1961, in a study involving University of Wisconsin students, 25% of lower respiratory infections were caused by *M. pneumoniae.* In Marine recruits at Paris Island, South Carolina, 67% of nonbacterial pneumonias studied in 1959 had serologic evidence of *M. pneumoniae* infection; in 1963, only 7% of such patients were serologically positive for *M. pneumoniae.* In two other studies, the annual incidence of pneumonia caused by *M. pneumoniae* was 18 per 1000 persons in a military population, and 15 per 1000 persons in a civilian population.

However, it must be kept in mind that all persons infected with *M. pneumoniae* do not develop pneumonia. Overall, recognizable bronchopneumonia develops in 3% to 10% of infected persons.

Pathogenesis and Pathology

Mycoplasma pneumoniae grow extracellularly as filamentous forms that adhere to epithelial cells of the respiratory tract by specialized structures at one end of the microorganisms (Fig. 30-5). In view of their extracellular location, it is not surprising that isolation of *M. pneumoniae* from respiratory tract secretions or exudates is often possible as long as 3 to 4 weeks after the clinical onset of illness at a time when humoral antibody is present in the blood. The persist-

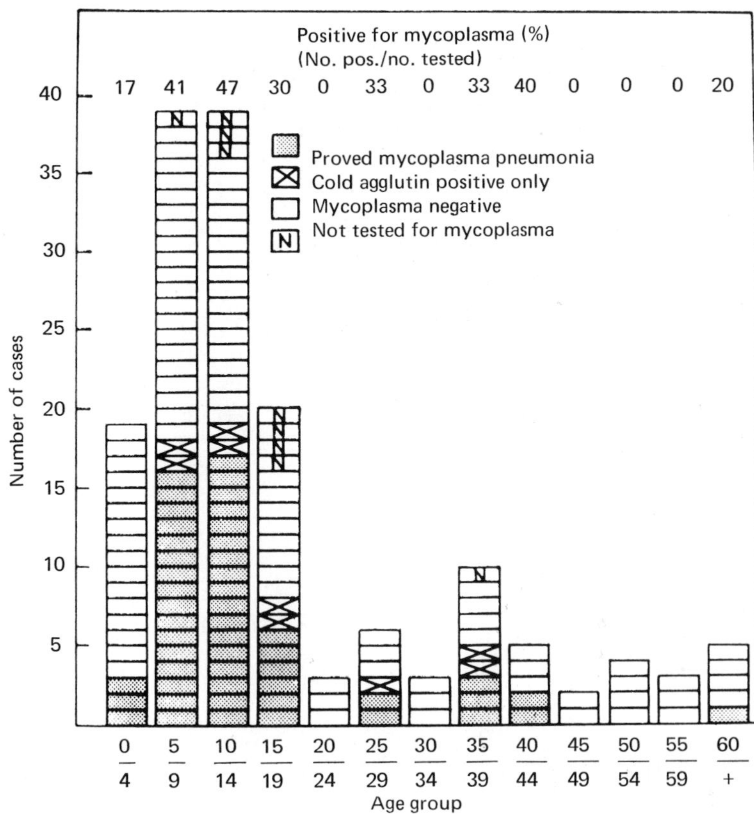

Fig. 30-4. Distribution according to age of patients with mycoplasmal pneumonia. (Copps SC, Allen BD, Sultmann S, Evans AS: JAMA 204:123–128, 1968. Copyright © 1968, American Medical Association)

ence of viable *M. pneumoniae* in sputum during and after the administration of antimicrobics that are effective by *in vitro* testing and by clinical assessment may reflect relatively poor penetration of these drugs into respiratory tract secretions.

Because the mortality of mycoplasmal pneumoniae is extremely low, reports on the pathology of this disease have been few. Parker and coworkers reported studies on fatal cases or primary atypical pneumonia seen at the Boston City Hospital in 1942 and 1943. On gross examination, the mucosa of the trachea and bronchi was hyperemic. The lungs were scattered on the pleural surface. The cut surfaces presented a characteristic miliary nodular appearance. Histologically, these nodules consisted of a mononuclear type of alveolar exudate, an interstitial infiltration composed predominantly of plasma cells, and swollen aveolar lining cells. The bronchiolar respiratory epithelium was intact, and bacteria were infrequently seen.

In 1955, using chick embryos, Liu isolated the Sil strain of *M. pneumoniae* from material preserved from the Boston City Hospital cases. By immunofluorescent staining, this Sil strain was antigenically identical with other strains of *M. pneumoniae* isolated from patients with primary atypical pneumonia.

Manifestations

The onset of mycoplasmal pneumonia is usually insidious. Fever and cough are almost invariably present. Chills, but not rigors, and malaise are seen in most patients. Sore throat, nasal congestion, and coryza are reported in about half the patients. In the early stage, the cough is usually nonproductive or yields small amounts of mucoid to mucopurulent sputum. As the disease evolves, increased production of sputum is common. Hemoptysis is rare.

On physical examination, the patient often has a flushed face but does not appear to be severely ill. The pharynx may or may not be injected, and cervical adenopathy is uncommon. Physical findings on examination of the lungs are usually not striking. Moist rales are commonly heard, but egophony and bronchial breathing are uncommon. The abnormalities are usually more extensive roentgenographically than would have been predicted from physical examination, with bronchopneumonia radiating from the hilar region toward the periphery of the lung, involv-

A
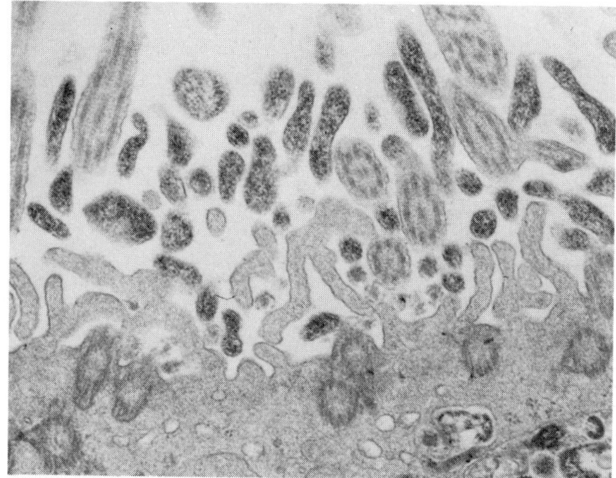

B
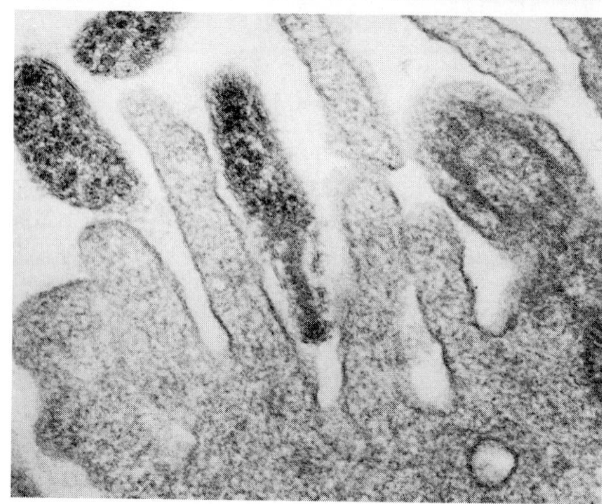

Fig. 30-5. Electron micrographs of clumps of respiratory tract epithelial cells expectorated by a man with pneumonia caused by *Mycoplasma pneumoniae. (A)* Lumenal border of ciliated epithelial cells heavily parasitized by *M. pneumoniae,* the round, oval, and elongate densely stained extracellular structures. (Uranyl acetate and lead citrate, original magnification × 26,500) *(B)* Higher magnification of specimen *A* showing extracellular location and attachment of *M. pneumoniae* to the epithelial cell membrane by specialized terminal organelles. (Uranyl acetate and lead citrate, original magnification about × 66,000) (Collier AM, Clyde WA, Jr: Am Rev Respir Dis 110:765–773, 1974)

ing one or more lobes. The lower lobes are involved more frequently than the upper lobes; lobar consolidations are rare. Small pleural effusions may be detected in 25% of patients with pneumonia when lateral decubitus chest roentgenograms are obtained.

The hemogram is usually normal, although occasionally a leukocytosis of 10,000/mm^3 to 20,000/mm^3 is seen. The cellular response in the sputum is typically mononuclear (Fig. 31-5*A*1). There are no characteristic abnormalities of renal or hepatic function. In about 50% of patients, a significant titer of cold agglutinins—that is, agglutinins for human blood group O cells that are active at 4°C—develops during the second to fourth week of illness, disappearing in 6 to 8 weeks. Agglutinins for streptococcus MG may also occur, with or without cold agglutinins. Biologic false positive reactions for syphilis sometimes appear.

The fever usually lasts about 8 to 10 days and gradually falls to normal by lysis. Cough and other symptoms begin to resolve as the fever declines. Roentgenographic clearance of pneumonic changes may take 2 to 3 weeks to return to normal.

The course of a patient documented to have mycoplasmal pneumonia is presented in Fig. 30-6.

Diagnosis

The clinical differentiation of mycoplasmal pneumonia from other nonbacterial pneumonias may be impossible, although the disease must be suspected if there has been a gradual onset of fever, malaise, and cough in a patient with roentgenographic evidence of pneumonia. The major entities that must be con-

Fig. 30-6. The course of mycoplasmal pneumonia in a 24-year-old male medical student who was hospitalized between the fifth and 11th days of illness. An accurate history was available from the first day of illness. No antimicrobial agents were given.

Day of illness	1 2 3 4 5 6 7 8 9 10 11 // 14 // 23 // 39
Temperature (°F)	98, 99, 100, 101, 102, 103
Anorexia	
Malaise	
Cough	
Rales	
Chest x-ray	
WBC×1000	6.6 6.5
Cold agglutinin	1/16 1/256
FA titer	1/10 ≥ 1/640

sidered in such patients include ornithosis, Q fever, and adenoviral infection. Bacterial infections, such as a mild pneumococcal pneumonia (see Chap. 31, Bacterial Pneumonias), tularemic pneumonia (see Chap. 139, Tularemia), legionella pneumonia (see Chap. 33, Legionnaires' Disease), nocardiosis (see Chap. 37, Nocardiosis), actinomycosis (see Chap. 38, Actinomycosis), and some cases of pulmonary tuberculosis (see Chap. 34, Pulmonary Tuberculosis), must be recognized. Primary pulmonary mycoses (see Chap. 40, Histoplasmosis, Chap. 41, Coccidioidomycosis, Chap. 42, Paracoccidioidomycosis, and Chap. 43, Blastomycosis), carcinoma of the lung, and even bronchiectasis should also be considered in the differential diagnosis. The diagnosis is usually arrived at by exclusion.

If a patient has a pneumonia and a positive cold agglutinin test (titer equal or greater than 1:32 in convalescent serum), the diagnosis of mycoplasmal pneumonia can be made with reasonable certainty. Cold agglutinins are evoked in other diseases *e.g.,* blood dyscrasias, liver diseases, and trypanosomiasis).

Definitive diagnosis requires the isolation of *M. pneumoniae* from sputum or throat specimens using a special culture medium. It is time consuming; *M. pneumoniae* may require 2 to 3 weeks to grow out on primary isolation. Specific serologic tests for the diagnosis of infections caused by *M. pneumoniae* include indirect immunofluorescent staining, complement fixation, and growth inhibition. Immunofluorescent staining of infected chick embryo lung sections is specific and sensitive, but the test is technically difficult and not available in most laboratories. Complement fixation (CF), although less sensitive, is the most practical test for diagnosis and antibody surveys. The correlation between the isolation of *M. pneumoniae,* CF reactivity, and the presence of cold agglutinins is shown in Fig. 30-7.

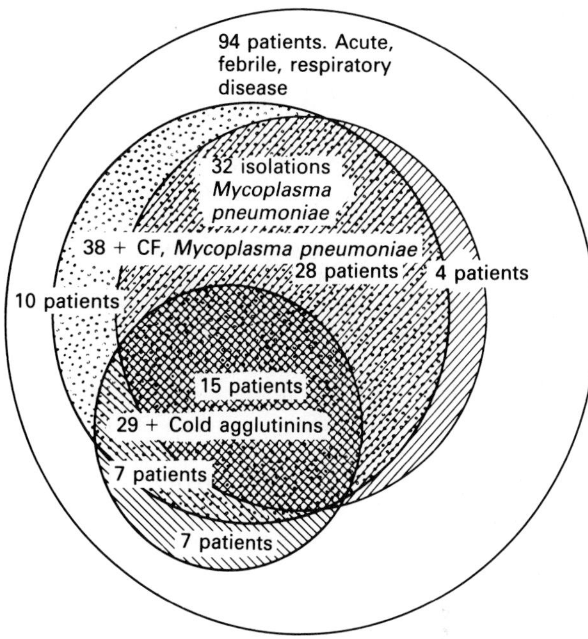

Fig. 30-7. Interrelationships between the isolation of *Mycoplasma pneumoniae,* CF reactivity, and cold agglutinins in 94 patients with acute, febrile respiratory disease. (After Grayston JT, Alexander ER, Kenney GE, Clarke ER, Fremont JC, MacColl WA: JAMA 191: 369–374, 1965)

Prognosis

Mycoplasmal pneumonia has a very favorable prognosis, even in untreated cases. Almost all patients recover completely without sequelae, and the mortality rate is less than 0.1%. Not only is the disease mild, but also those affected are usually previously healthy, young persons. Myringitis, reported in volunteers experimentally infected with *M. pneumoniae,* occurs rarely, if at all, in the natural disease. Some patients with high cold agglutinin IgM antibody against the I antigen of their erthrocytes may develop hemolytic anemia, paroxysmal cold hemoglobinuria, Raynaud's syndrome, peripheral gangrene, and diffuse intravascular coagulopathy.

Complications involving the central nervous system have been estimated to occur in 0.1% of all patients infected with *M. pneumoniae* and in 7% of those requiring hospitalization. Diverse neurologic involvements, including aseptic meningitis, meningoencephalitis, cerebral ataxia, Guillain–Barré syndrome, and transverse myelitis, have been described. The severity of the respiratory symptoms or the titer of cold agglutinins does not seem to correlate with the neurologic manifestations. Although recovery from neurologic syndromes usually occurs, it is generally slow and requires months for improvement; some patients may be left with permanent residual deficits. It has been thought that the neurologic syndromes are immunologically mediated. However, certain neurologic disorders may be related to direct central nervous system (CNS) infection with *M. pneumoniae.* Using special and sensitive microbiologic techniques, demonstration of viable *M. pneumoniae* in the cerebrospinal fluid and the buffy coat of the blood was reported in one patient with mycoplasmal pneumonitis complicated with neurologic dysfunction. In spite of search, no immune complexes were demonstrated in this patient.

Therapy

Many patients with mycoplasmal pneumonia recover spontaneously without specific treatment. For symptomatic therapy, codeine, 16 mg to 64 mg orally every 4 to 6 hours, may be given for the relief of headache and troublesome cough. Use of sponge baths with cold water or alcohol should be avoided in severely ill patients with high titers of cold agglutinins because a hemolytic crisis may be precipitated by suddenly lowering the temperature.

Tetracycline and its analogues and erythromycin are effective for the treatment of mycoplasmal pneumonia. Although *M. pneumoniae* is susceptible to clindamycin *in vitro,* it was not clinically effective. The dosage of tetracycline for adults is 15 mg to 30 mg/kg body wt/day given PO as four equal portions, 6-hourly; for children, the dosage is 25 mg/kg body wt/day given PO as four equal portions, 6-hourly. The dose of erythromycin for adults is 20 mg to 25 mg/kg body wt/day PO as three equal portions, 8-hourly; for children, the dosage is 35 mg to 50 mg/kg body wt/day PO as three equal portions, 8-hourly if less than 25 kg in weight (the same as for adults if over 25 kg in weight). Five to 7 days of treatment are generally sufficient.

The tetracyclines and erythromycin are about equally effective. In young children, the use of erythromycin instead of tetracyclines is prudent to avoid staining of the teeth. For adults, when the pneumonitis might be Q fever of psittacosis, tetracycline is the appropriate choice. However, if the patient is immunosuppressed or is the recipient of a transplanted kidney, legionellosis is a possibilty and erythromycin would be a logical choice.

Prevention

No specific prophylactic measures are available for the control of mycoplasmal infections. Isolating patients is seldom practical. A vaccine is under development and has been shown to have some protective value, but there is no immediate prospect for its general use.

Q Fever

Q fever is an acute, systemic rickettsial disease characterized by the sudden onset of malaise, fever, headache, chills, and pneumonitis. The disease is self limited and seldom causes death.

Etiology

Q fever is caused by *Coxiella burnetii.* This is a gram-variable rickettsia which follows an unusual developmental cycle in phagolysosomes of eukaryotic cells; it has been suggested that the morphogenesis of *C. burnetii* involves a process comparable to the formation of endospores. Two morphologic cell types predominate, large and small cell variants, and there is extreme pleomorphism, which may be related to the ability of *C. burnetii* to pass through filters which retain the other kinds of rickettsias.

By virtue of minimal metabolic activity at neutral or alkaline pH, *C. burnetii* is resistant to physical and chemical agents and persists viable for long periods (*e.g.,* prolonged desiccation in dust and excreta, survival for 36 to 42 months in water and milk). It remains viable after heating at 70°C for several minutes, and endures exposure to 0.5% formaldehyde for 48 hours and 0.4% phenol for several days. Multiplication follows inoculation of embryonated eggs, mice, guinea pigs, and hamsters. Antigenically, *C. burnetii* also differs from other rickettsias; for example, *C. burnetii* fails to evoke cross-reacting agglutinins for the *Proteus* strains used in the Weil-Felix reaction.

Epidemiology

Q fever was first recognized in Australia by Derrick in 1937. The infection is worldwide in distribution, except for northern Europe and the Scandinavian countries. It was first recognized in the United States in Montana and California. Subsequent studies have shown that it is prevalent in most states where cattle and sheep are raised. In nature, *C. burnetii* is maintained in wild animals through a tick vector. Domestic cattle and sheep are inoculated by infected ticks.

In contrast, humans acquire Q fever not by tick bite but by inhaling aerosolized particles containing infectious *C. burnetii.* The usual sources are the placental tissues, amniotic fluid, milk, and feces of infected cattle, sheep, and goats, all of which frequently have only mild or inapparent infections.

The incubation period in humans is 18 to 20 days. Although direct human-to-human transmission is theoretically possible, there is no documentation of this—that is, there is no known period of infectivity without the intervention of a nonhuman host.

Pathogenesis and Pathology

After being inhaled, *C. burnetii* multiplies in pulmonary tissues and other body organs. Rickettsemia is present and microorganisms are excreted in the urine. The pathology of the lung in Q fever is similar to that in viral or mycoplasmal pneumonias, with interstitial and peribronchiolar mononuclear infiltrations. Valvular vegetations are seen when endocarditis complicates Q fever.

Manifestations

The onset of Q fever is abrupt, with severe headache, chills, fever, myalgia, and malaise. Unlike other rickettsial infections, there is no rash. Pneumonitis is found in about 50% of cases. Hepatomegaly and splenomegaly are present. Laboratory findings are not diagnostic, and patients may have abnormal liver functions, with elevated transaminases and alkaline phosphatase, and a positive cephalin flocculation test. The clinical course is usually self-limited, with fever declining by lysis after 1 to 3 weeks. In a few patients, the fever may be prolonged for several weeks. Cardiac murmurs and embolic phenomena late in the course of the illness oblige the consideration of endocarditis. Although precise data on the incidence of this complication are not available, in approximately 2% of patients with apparently abacterial infective endocarditis, *C. burnetii* is the infecting microorganism.

Diagnosis

The clinical findings in Q fever are insufficient to enable a diagnosis to be made on these grounds alone. A history of direct or indirect contact with livestock is helpful to the physician. Early in the course of Q fever, the disease must be differentiated from brucellosis (see Chap. 138, Brucellosis), typhoid and paratyphoid fever (see Chap. 63, Nontyphoidal Salmonelloses, and Chap. 64, Typhoid Fever), infectious hepatitis (see Chap. 70, Hepatitis A, Chap. 71, Hepatitis B, Chap. 72, Non-A, Non-B Hepatitis), leptospirosis (see Chap. 76, Leptospirosis), and other rickettsial diseases (see Chap. 98, The Typhus Fevers). When pneumonitis is present, differentiation from other nonbacterial pneumonias of mycoplasmal, chlamydial, viral, and fungal origins should be undertaken.

The definitive diagnosis of Q fever rests on the isolation of *C. burnetii* from the blood, sputum, urine, or other clinical materials. However, *C. burnetii* is so contagious that isolation cannot be safely attempted in the usual clinical laboratory. When maximum precautions can be exercised, recovery of *C. burnetii* is best accomplished by the intraperitoneal inoculation of clinical specimens into guinea pigs. Inoculation into the yolk sac of chick embryos can also be used.

Serologic procedures are simpler and safer, and they are preferred in most diagnostic laboratories. Complement fixation (CF) or agglutination tests are most useful. A fourfold or greater rise of antibody during convalescence is diagnostic. The presence of significant CF antibody in the patient's serum against Phase I Q fever antigen—that is, *C. burnetii* newly isolated from mammals or ticks—indicates chronic infection and is particularly useful for diagnosis of Q fever endocarditis.

Prognosis

Q fever is a self-limited disease with a favorable prognosis; the mortality rate is less than 1%. Cardiovascular complications, including endocarditis, pleuropericarditis, and thrombophlebitis, are usually seen in chronic Q fever. Uveitis, optic neuritis, nephritis, hepatitis, meningitis, and congenital malformations have also been associated with infection caused by *C. burnetii*. Endocarditis complicating Q fever is uniformly fatal; it does not respond to therapy with antimicrobics. An attack of Q fever usually confers life-long immunity.

Therapy

Coxiella burnetii is susceptible to chloramphenicol and the tetracyclines according to *in vitro* tests. However, these agents do not appear to be as effective in the treatment of Q fever as they are in the other rickettsioses. The tetracyclines are generally preferred because of the potential of chloramphenicol for hematopoietic toxicity. The usual oral dosage of tetracycline for Q fever is 30 mg to 40 mg/kg body wt/day given PO as four equal portions, 6-hourly. Treatment is continued at least 5 days after defervescence.

Prevention

Vaccines made from formalin-killed *C. burnetii* (chick embryo cultures) engender protective antibody. However, owing to the high incidence of local reactions from vaccination, the vaccine should be used only in persons at high risk; for example, dairy and slaughterhouse workers, wool sorters, and tanners.

The flash method of pasteurizing milk—holding the temperature at 161°F for 15 seconds—reliably kills *C. burnetii,* unlike ordinary pasteurization by heating to 140°F for 30 minutes. Excreta, sputum, and clothing from infected persons should be autoclaved. The conduct of postmortem examinations and the handling of infected cadavers require the most stringent precautions to avoid infecting personnel. However, neither isolation nor quarantine measures are warranted in the care of patients.

Ornithosis (Psittacosis)

Ornithosis in humans is an acute infectious disease characterized by fever, malaise, myalgia, and pneumonitis. The disease varies in severity and may carry a significant mortality rate. When the agent *Chlamydia psittaci* is transmitted to humans from psittacine birds (parrots, parakeets, cockatoos, and budgerigars), the disease is often called psittacosis or parrot fever. Because other avian genera (pigeons, turkeys) are more common sources of infection in man in the United States, the more general term *ornithosis* is preferred.

Etiology

The genus *Chlamydia* is made up of two species: *psittaci* and *trachomatis*. In humans, *C. trachomatis* is mainly associated with occular and genitourinary infections of varying severity (see Chap. 159, Trachoma, and Chap. 55, Non-Gonococcal Urethritis). In many avian species and mammals, *C. psittaci* may produce various diseases including psittacosis, ornithosis, feline pneumonitis, arthritis, and bovine abortions.

Chlamydia psittaci is an intracellular parasite that is spherical, measuring 200 nm to 300 nm in diameter, and contains both DNA and RNA. Deficient in energy-yielding capabilities, *C. psittaci* depends on the host cell for energy-rich phosphate esters and other cofactors for growth and multiplication. *Chlamydia psittaci* multiplies by binary fission similar to bacteria. It is susceptible *in vitro* to penicillin, cycloserine, chloramphenicol, tetracycline, and erythromycin. Streptomycin and sulfonamides are not inhibitory.

Epidemiology

The ornithosis agent causes natural infections in turkeys, pigeons, ducks, chickens, pheasants, and other fowl as well as in parrots, parakeets, cockatoos, budgerigars, petrels, and finches. Although the avian disease may be fatal, infected birds more often show only minimal evidence of disease. The agent is found in the bood, tissues, and respiratory and cloacal discharges of sick birds. It is transmitted to humans through the inhalation of aerosolized particles—either droplets, droplet nuclei, or, because the agent withstands drying, dust.

Humans usually contract the disease as a result of contact with sick birds. Poultry workers, pet shop workers, and pigeon handlers are at high risk. Person-to-person transmission has been documented. Physicians, nurses, and other paramedical personnel caring for patients may contract the disease. Ornithosis contracted from turkeys, psittacine birds, or from an ill patient appears to be more severe than ornithosis acquired from other sources.

Pathogenesis and Pathology

Although the ornithosis agent gains entry into the human body through the respiratory tract, it rapidly disseminates through the blood to produce systemic disease involving the lungs and the reticuloendothelial system. During the first 2 weeks of illness, the agent can be isolated from the blood and sputum. In fatal cases, it can be recovered from the spleen.

Postmortem findings consist chiefly of lobular pneumonitis. There is inflammation with edema, exudate, and hemorrhage in the aveoli. Early in the disease, the exudates contain polymorphonuclear cells; in later stages, mononuclear cells and lymphocytes predominate both in the aveoli and in the interstitial areas. Vasculitis and thrombosis may also be present. The elementary bodies of the ornithosis agent may be seen in large monocytes and macrophages. In the liver, intralobular focal necrosis sometimes occurs, and swollen Kupffer's cells containing ornithosis elementary bodies may be found. Inflammatory changes, with or without intraphagocytic elementary bodies, have also been reported in other tissues such as the myocardium, pericardium, brain, meninges, and kidneys.

Manifestations

The incubation period is usually 7 to 14 days, but sometimes it may be longer. The onset may be sudden or insidious, with chills, fever, malaise, headaches, anorexia, sore throat, and photophobia. The initial temperature is 37.8°C to 38.9°C (100°F–102°F) and gradually rises to 39.4°C to 40.6°C (103°F or 105°F) during the first week of illness. Cough is generally prominent, with mucoid sputum that is occasionally blood streaked. Nausea and vomiting are frequent. In severe cases, mental confusion, delirium, or stupor may occur. Cyanosis and symptoms of anoxia may be present.

Physical findings include fever, tachypnea, and a relative bradycardia. Examination of the lungs may show fine, crepitant rales, but signs of true pulmonary consolidation by percussion and auscultation are not usually detectable. Chest roentgenograms frequently disclose interstitial pneumonitis that is more extensive than would be predicted by physical examination. Hepatosplenomegaly may be present. In rare cases, signs of pericarditis and myocarditis may be found.

Patients with mild illness usually recover in about 1 week. The clinical course in more severe infections may run for 3 weeks, with gradual defervescence and prolonged convalescence. The presence of severe dyspnea, tachypnea, cyanosis, tachycardia, jaundice, delirium, and stupor augurs a poor prognosis.

Diagnosis

The separation of ornithosis from other acute infectious diseases and nonbacterial pneumonias on purely clinical grounds may not be possible. Simple routine laboratory study of the blood and the urine is not very helpful in establishing the diagnosis. A clue is offered in a history of contact with sick birds or employment in poultry or pet shop businesses. When signs of pneumonia are present, differentiation from viral pneumonias, Q fever, mycoplasmal pneumonia, influenza (see Chap. 28, Influenza), Legionnaires' disease (see Chap. 33, Legionnaires' Disease), and pulmonary fungal infections should be undertaken.

The definitive diagnosis of ornithosis requires isolation of the agent or the demonstration of a significant rise in antibody specific for ornithosis. The ornithosis agent is present in the blood and sputum during the first 2 weeks of illness and can be isolated by inoculation of clinical specimens into mice (intraperitoneal) or into embryonated hens' eggs (yolk sac). The preferred procedure for primary isolation is inoculation of tissue cultures (McCoy cell line). Because the ornithosis agents are highly infectious, isolation should only be undertaken by experienced personnel working in well equipped laboratories. A fourfold rise of antibody is diagnostic, comparing acute with convalescent serum. The antibody is detected by complement fixation on reaction with a heat-stable group antigen prepared from infected chick embryos.

Therapy

Tetracycline is the drug of choice for the treatment of ornithosis; chloramphenicol is less effective. If peroral treatment is possible, 30 mg to 40 mg/kg body wt/day should be given in four equal portions, once every 6 hours. If parenteral therapy is necessary, 10 mg to 15 mg/kg body weight should be injected either intramuscularly or intravenously as four equal portions given every 6 hours. Prompt improvement of fever and other symptoms can often be detected 48 to 72 hours after treatment. Peroral therapy with tetracycline should be continued for 7 days after defervescence to ensure recovery and prevent relapses. Penicillin G in a dosage of 1 million units of an aqueous procaine preparation given by intramuscular (IM) injection every 8 hours may be used if the patient is intolerant to tetracycline. Supportive measures—such as oxygen therapy for cyanotic patients, and reduction of body temperature by sponging or cooling mattresses and blankets for hyperpyrexic patients—are also important.

Prognosis

Before the advent of antimicrobial therapy, ornithosis carried a case fatality rate of about 20%. With chemotherapy, the mortality rate is around 5%. Complications and sequelae are rare.

Prevention

The ecology and potential sources of infection for ornithosis are sufficiently well known to enable the institution of practical preventive programs. With the help of chemotherapy, parakeets in the United States have been bred, distributed, and sold that are free from ornithosis. However, the psittacine birds from abroad still are a potentially dangerous source of infection.

Chemotherapy with tetracyclines in commercial domestic flocks of turkeys and ducks has failed to eliminate ornithosis. The disease remains an occupational hazard among workers who may handle infected birds in the course of processing and marketing. Frequent inspections and careful supervision of flocks and procedures are required to minimize exposure. No effective vaccine is available.

Viral Pneumonias

A number of viral agents, including influenza viruses (see Chap. 28, Influenza), adenoviruses, variola (see Chap. 92, Smallpox and Other Poxvirus Infections), varicella (see Chap. 93, Varicella and Herpes Zoster), and measles viruses (see Chap. 86, Measles), can cause a primary bronchopneumonia both in children and adults. Parainfluenza viruses (see Chap. 26, Epiglottitis, Laryngitis, and Laryngotracheobronchitis) and respiratory syncytial viruses (see Chap. 27, Bronchitis and Bronchiolitis) are often responsible for pneumonia in infants and young children but rarely cause pneumonia in adults. Cytomegalovirus (see Chap. 75, Cytomegalovirus Infections) has become increasingly prominent as a cause of pneumonia in immunodeficient persons—for example, those given immunosuppressive therapy for organ transplantation or for malignant diseases. Viral pneumonias do not respond to treatment with presently available antimicrobics. The morbidity and mortality from viral pneumonias vary with the age and physical condition of the host at the time the infection is contracted, and the infecting viral agent. The pathologic changes of the lung are similar to those described in mycoplasmal, Q fever, or psittacosis infections. Etiologic diagnosis depends on laboratory examinations, although the presence of a primary disease, such as measles, chicken pox, or smallpox, preceding or concurrent with the development of the pneumonitis, may indicate the diagnosis.

Influenza Virus Pneumonia

Influenza is primarily a tracheobronchitis that is usually a self-limited disease (see Chap. 28, Influenza). Two kinds of pneumonia may intervene to change the course of influenza: bacterial *(Staphylococcus aureus, Streptococcus pneumoniae, Haemophilus influenzae)* pneumonias and primary influenza virus pneumonia. Influenza virus pneumonia usually affects persons who are old or who have an underlying noninfectious process such as a chronic pulmonary, cardiovascular, renal, or metabolic disease. Women in the last trimester of pregnancy are also hypervulnerable. Rheumatic heart disease with mitral stenosis appears to be particularly conducive to the development of influenza virus pneumonia. Pulmonary hypertension may be an important factor.

Within 24 to 48 hours after the onset of influenza, the patient develops a cough producing bloody sputum, marked cyanosis, and dyspnea. Fever is usually quite high. Substernal pain and discomfort are often present. Auscultation may reveal generalized expiratory wheezes and moist rales. Roentgenograms of the chest usually show diffuse bilateral bronchopneumonia radiating from the hilum. Routine laboratory studies, including leukocyte counts, sputum smears, and cultures, do not yield characteristic findings. The course is usually one of progression with unremittent fever, increasing pulmonary dysfunction, vascular collapse, and death a few days after the onset of illness. Antimicrobial and supportive therapeutic measures are usually without avail. There are no controlled studies to show that amantadine treatment for influenza virus pneumonia is beneficial. However, the use of amantadine should be considered because the disease often runs a fulminating course, and amantadine has been reported to reduce peripheral airway resistance in uncomplicated cases of influenza.

At postmortem examination there is a hemorrhagic pneumonitis. High concentrations of influenza virus are recoverable from the lungs. Examination of sections of quick-frozen lung by direct immunofluorescent staining for influenza virus antigen reveals specifically fluorescent macrophages and aveolar cells.

Adenovirus Pneumonia

Of the 35 known types of adenoviruses (see Chap. 23, Nonbacterial Pharyngitis), clinical respiratory diseases have been associated with types 1 through 7, 14, and 21. Pneumonia is relatively infrequent as the clinical expression of adenoviral infection.

Fatal pneumonias in infants have been associated with types 1, 2, 3, 7, and 7a adenoviruses. Necrotizing bronchitis and pneumonitis are the major findings at necropsy. Intranuclear inclusions are seen in infected cells, and adenoviruses may be recovered from the lung tissues.

The incidence of adenoviral infections in the adult civilian population is low. On the other hand, acute respiratory diseases (ARD) and atypical pneumonia caused by types 2, 4, and 7 adenoviruses are common in military recruits during basic training. Almost 100% of new military recruits develop infection with adenoviruses during the 8-week basic training period. Of these, only about 50% have overt illness, usually ARD. When adenoviral pneumonia occurs, its clinical course cannot be differentiated from that of mycoplasmal pneumonia. However, sore throat and injection of the pharynx are more common in adenoviral infections. Moreover, patients with adenoviral pneumonia do not develop either cold agglutinins or streptococcus MG agglutinins, antibodies that appear in about half the patients with mycoplasmal pneumonia.

There is no specific treatment for adenoviral pneumonia. The mortality is quite low, and patients generally recover completely, without sequelae.

The injection of a formalin-killed trivalent adenovirus vaccine (types 3, 4, and 7) resulted in a 70% reduction in the incidence of ARD in military recruits. However, the vaccine was withdrawn when it was discovered that it contained genetic material of the oncogenic (to hamsters) simian virus SV_{40}. Live attenuated type 4 adenovirus vaccine, given orally in enteric coated capsules, multiplies in the intestinal tract of man, evoking protective immunity. In field studies, the incidence of adenovirus type 4 infection in military recruits was reduced 95.5%. This vaccine is not commercially available.

Respiratory Syncytial Virus

Respiratory syncytial viruses (RSV) are the most important etiologic agents of respiratory tract infections in infants (see Chap. 27, Bronchitis and Bronchiolitis). The clinical syndromes vary from mild upper respiratory infections to severe bronchiolitis and bronchopneumonia. Apparently, the earlier in life that initial exposure to RSV occurs, the more severe the resulting infection. A reinfection occurring in older children and in adults in whom there is circulating antibody manifests itself as mild upper respiratory illnesses. However, severe lower respiratory tract infections and bronchopneumonia have occurred in elderly residents of nursing homes.

Respiratory syncytial viral pneumonia occurs most often in the winter. Over an 8-year period at the Children's Hospital in Washington, D.C., RSV was isolated in 9.5% of patients with pneumonia and in 29.6% of patients with bronchiolitis. Infants with pneumonia are usually listless, irritable, and tachypneic, and they show retraction of the intercostal muscles. Cough may or may not be present, and sputum production is slight. Auscultation may reveal minimal changes of breath sounds and some fine moist rales. Roentgenograms of the chest are helpful in diagnosis, often revealing patchy consolidation bilaterally. The leukocyte count is normal or slightly elevated. Bacteriologic throat culture is not contributory.

The clinical course varies with the severity of the infection, but most patients recover completely in 1 to 3 weeks. Treatment should be supportive and should include provision of cool, moist air and oxygen. Antimicrobics (*e.g.*, penicillin G) are not beneficial, but they are usually given because the differentiation of viral pneumonia from bacterial pneumonia is often impossible in this age group. When bronchial secretions are present and interfere with the exchange of air, tracheal suction is mandatory and may be aided by tracheostomy.

No practical prevention for RSV pneumonia is available. Experience with an experimental inactive RSV vaccine showed good antibody response, but did not confer protection. Moreover, infants who received this vaccine apparently developed a more extensive respiratory disease following natural RSV infection than did a nonvaccinated control group. In searching for a live attenuated RSV vaccine, a low-temperature-adapted laboratory strain of RSV was found to produce silent infection in infants and young children who had been infected with RSV previously. However, this vaccine produced mild lower respiratory tract disease in young infants who were seronegative to RSV. Another vaccine made from a temperature-sensitive RSV mutant was shown to be acceptably attenuated for young children, but it induced rhinitis followed by otitis media in young seronegative infants. The RSV recovered from some of the vaccines displayed altered genetic stability. These events were considered unacceptable for putting the RSV mutant vaccine into clinical use.

Measles (Rubeola) Pneumonia

Cough and signs of acute bronchitis are almost always present in measles (see Chap. 86, Measles). Although bacterial pneumonia is one of the serious complications of measles, primary measles pneumonia may occur in certain patients. Pathologically, the presence of giant cells with intranuclear and intracytoplasmic inclusion bodies is characteristic of measles pneumonia. Children with immunodeficient disorders or with malignant disease should not receive live attenuated measles vaccine. Giant cell pneumonia after receiving attenuated measles vaccine has been reported in such a hypervulnerable child.

Chickenpox (Varicella) Pneumonia

Chickenpox and the properties of the varicella-zoster virus are discussed in Chapter 93, Varicella and Herpes Zoster.

For reasons not known, 90% of primary varicella pneumonias occur in persons who are older than 19 years. One to 6 days after the onset of rash, the development of pneumonia is manifested by cough, dyspnea, tachypnea, chest pain, and hemoptysis. In 50% to 60% of patients, ausculation reveals rhonchi and wheezes. Chest roentgenograms generally reveal a pneumonia that is more extensive than would be predicted by the physical findings. Bilateral peribronchial nodular infiltrates radiate from the hilum to the periphery of the lungs. However, such radiographic findings are not specific and are found in other nonbacterial pneumonias, tuberculosis, sarcoidosis, and carcinomatosis. The leukocytes may be normal or slightly increased in number; the sputum yields normal flora on culture. The demonstration of intranuclear inclusions in epithelial cells shed in the sputum is useful in diagnosing varicella pneumonia.

The treatment of varicella pneumonia is supportive, including adequate hydration and oxygen therapy. In most cases, after the cutaneous lesions disappear, the pneumonic consolidation clears rapidly. In patients who are critically ill, glucosteroids may possibly have a life-saving effect by reducing pulmonary edema and lessening interstitial inflammation. When pneumonia complicates varicella, the mortality becomes 10% to 30% instead of the normal level of less than 1%. An increased severity of varicella pneumonia in pregnancy has been reported. Death in varicella pneumonia results from respiratory insufficiency.

At postmortem examination, the pulmonary lesions vary from focal necrosis to complete hemorrhagic consolidation. Vesicles may be seen on the pleural surfaces. Interstitial pneumonitis with intranuclear inclusions characteristic of varicella infection may be found in septal cells, giant cells, fibroblasts, capillary endothelium, and tracheobronchial mucosa. In severe cases, varicella lesions may even be found in the liver, pericardium, and endometrium.

There is no known preventive of varicella except avoiding contact with infected persons. Immunoglobulins separated from human hyperimmune varicella serum may be of value in prophylaxis and modification of the illness. Patients who have either congenital or acquired immunologic deficiencies should probably be given such hyperimmune immunoglobulin when exposed to varicella-zoster disease. No vaccine is available.

Cytomegalovirus Pneumonia

The use of immunosuppressive agents has been associated with an increased incidence of pneumonia caused by cytomegalovirus (CMV) (see Chap. 75, Cytomegalovirus Infections). Infections with CMV are also associated with natural immunologic deficiencies (*e.g.,* hypogammaglobulinemia) and chronic debilitating diseases.

CMV is a DNA virus that grows well in human fibroblast tissue cultures. Histologically, CMV-infected tissues show characteristic, enlarged cells that contain intranuclear and intracytoplasmic inclusion bodies. The intranuclear inclusion bodies are surrounded by a halo, stain reddish purple with hematoxylin and eosin, and measure about 9 nm in diameter (see Fig. 75-1). In generalized CMV infection, cells bearing such large inclusions are widely distributed and are particularly prominent in the salivary glands, kidney, liver, lung, and brain.

Clinically, pneumonia caused by CMV is impossible to differentiate from other nonbacterial pneumonias. The possibility of CMV pneumonia must be kept in mind in any patient whose immunologic capacity has been compromised congenitally, through disease, or as a consequence of therapy.

Definitive diagnosis requires material aspirated percutaneously from the involved lung or obtained by open lung biopsy. Microscopic examination and isolation in human fibroblast tissue cultures should be carried out.

There are neither specific treatments nor preventive measures for CMV infections. A CMV vaccine is under investigation which may be beneficial for use in high-risk patients.

Bibliography

Books

CLYDE WA JR: *Mycoplasma pneumoniae* infections in man. In Tully JG, Whitcomb RF (eds): The Mycoplasmas. Vol. 2. New York, Academic Press, 1979. pp 275–306.

LEEDOM JM: Q fever: An update. In Remington JS, Swartz MW (eds): Current Clinical Topics in Infectious Diseases. Vol. 1. New York, McGraw-Hill, 1980. pp 305–331.

Journals

ABDALLAH PS, MARK JBD, MERIGAN TC: Diagnosis of cytomegalovirus pneumonia in compromised hosts. Am J Med 61:326–332, 1976

BAYER AS, GALPIN JE, THEOFILOPOULOS AN, GUZE LB: Neurologic disease associated with *Mycoplasma pneumoniae* pneumonitis. Ann Intern Med 94:15–20, 1981

BOGART DB, LIU C, RUTH WE, KERBY GR, WILLIAMS CH: Rapid diagnosis of primary influenza pneumonia. Chest 68:513–517, 1975

CENTERS FOR DISEASE CONTROL: Respiratory syncytial virus—Missouri. Morbidity and Mortality Weekly Report 26:351, 1977

COLLIER AM, CLYDE WA JR: Appearance of *Mycoplasma pneumoniae* in lungs of experimentally infected hamsters and sputum from patients with natural disease. Am Rev Respir Dis 110:765–773, 1974

DERRICK EH: The course of infection with *Coxiella burnetii.* Med J Austral 1:1051–1057, 1973

DUDDING BA, WAGNER SC, ZELLER JA, GMELICH JT, FRENCH GR, TOP FH: Fatal pneumonia associated with adenovirus type 7 in three military trainees. N Engl J Med 286:1289–1292, 1972

GASSELL GH, COLE BC: Mycoplasmas as agents of human disease. N Engl J Med 304:80–89, 1981

GEORGE RB, ZISKIND MM, RASCH JR, MOGABGAB WJ: Mycoplasma and adenovirus pneumonias. Ann Intern Med 65:931–942, 1966

LEVINE DP, LERNER AM: The clinical spectrum of *Mycoplasma pneumoniae* infections. Med Clin North Am 62:961–978, 1978

MCCAUL TF, WILLIAMS JC: Developmental cycle of *Coxiella burnetii:* Structure and morphogenesis of vegetative and sporogenic differentiations. J Bacteriol 147:1063–1076, 1981

TRIEBWASSER JH, HARRIS RE, BRYANT RE, RHOADES ER: Varicella pneumonia in adults. Report of seven cases and a review of literature. Medicine 46:409–423, 1967

PAUL D. HOEPRICH

Bacterial Pneumonias

31

Over the past century, the physician's view of pneumonia—that is, inflammatory diseases of the lungs with alveolar involvement—has undergone several major changes. With the ascendency of pathology in the nineteenth century, emphasis was placed on anatomic localization (unilateral, bilateral, apical, basilar, central, lobar, bronchial, interstitial); histopathology (cellular response: acute, chronic, necrotizing, organizing; exudative response: fibrinous, hemorrhagic, suppurative); and pathogenesis (airborne, bloodborne). The burgeoning of bacteriology as a science at the turn of the century enabled etiologic diagnosis, a development that the advent of specific therapies has rendered absolutely essential. As the classic bacterial causes of pneumonia have come under increasingly successful attack, it has become apparent that the state of the host is of very great importance. In fact, whether the pneumonia is primary, or secondary to a preexisting, noncurable, defense-crippling, noninfectious disease now surpasses both extent and cause of the pneumonia as a determinant of outcome.

Etiology

Pneumococcus

Many kinds of bacteria may cause pneumonia in humans (see list below). However, *Streptococcus pneumoniae* are archetypal as causes of bacterial pneumonia and still account for about 90% of community-acquired cases in the United States. Pneumococci are nonmotile, nonsporulating, capsulated, gram-positive, ovoid bacteria that are 0.5 μm to 1.0 μm by 1.2 μm to 1.8 μm in size. In clinical specimens, a lancelike asymmetry of individual cocci may be apparent in mirror-image pairs—the classic diploids, with blunted contours juxtaposed—the two cells enveloped in a smoothly continuous capsule. Short chains also occur and are seen most commonly with serotype 3. Capsulation is generally demonstrable with clinical materials because only the smooth (*i.e.,* capsulated) form is virulent.

CAUSES OF BACTERIAL PNEUMONIAS

Streptococcus pneumoniae
Staphylococcus aureus
Streptococcus spp.
  Group A and Group B
Peptostreptococcus spp.
Peptococcus spp.
Neisseria meningitidis
Bacillus spp.
Legionella spp.
Haemophilus influenzae
Klebsiella spp.
Other Enterobacteriaceae
  Enterobacter spp.
  Escherichia coli
  Salmonella spp.
  Serratia spp.
Pseudomonas spp.
Francisella tularensis
Yersinia pestis
Bacteroides spp.
Fusobacterium spp.
Actinomyces spp.
Nocardia spp.
Mycobacterium spp.

The nutritional requirements of *Streptococcus pneumoniae* are complex and not precisely known. Glucose is the primary substrate for energy production. Not only must this nutrient be available for optimal growth, but also the culture medium must be well buffered to accommodate the organic acids generated by fermentation. Pneumococci are aerobic and facultatively anaerobic. Growth is favored by the presence of 5% to 10% ambient CO_2, a temperature of 37°C, and a pH of 7.4.

Colonies of virulent pneumococci growing on a nutritionally optimal blood agar medium for 12 to 18 hours are 0.5 mm to 1.0 mm in diameter, shiny, and smoothly convex. With continued incubation, the oldest, central part of the colony undergoes autolysis and collapses to give a crateriform appearance. Some strains, notably of serogroups 3 and 37, are more mucoid than others. All pneumococci, whether capsulated or not, cause greening on blood agar (alpha-hemolysis) that is, to the practiced eye, characteristically more intense than the similar change wrought by viridans *Streptococcus* spp. An oxygen-labile hemolysin (pneumolysin) is formed by some strains.

In addition to fermenting glucose and some other sugars, virtually all freshly isolated strains are quite unlike other *Streptococcus* spp. in being able to ferment inulin. The action of autolytic enzymes is uniquely accelerated by a number of surface-active compounds, such as bile salts, saponins, and commercial cationic laundry detergents, to provide a diagnostically useful laboratory test—the *bile* solubility test.

Some 83 types (according to the American typing system) of *Streptococcus pneumoniae* have been distinguished on the basis of capsular polysaccharides that are unique in being singular chemical expressions of genetic differences among the pneumococci, and specific immunogens. Capsular polysaccharides are relatively stable macromolecules. Several have been prepared in high purity and are generally acidic, often because they contain d-glucuronic acid residues or, less commonly, sialic acid (perhaps the basis for the cross-reactivity of type 14 polysaccharide with the A, B, O blood group isoantigens). Because capsulation is synonymous with virulence, specific identification can be made in clinical materials by demonstrating reaction with type-specific antibody. In the quellung reaction, a visibly detectable shift in refractive index renders the capsule distinct, with sharply defined borders, as a consequence of interaction between capsule and specific antibody. Capsules also become sticky and agglutination occurs. Polysaccharide that has dissociated from the capsule may be precipitated in the presence of an optimal quantity of specific antibody. In addition, type-specific anticapsular antibody is protective in experimental infections and has been therapeutically effective when applied in treatment. Dosage in such immunotherapy has been monitored by the intradermal injection of capsular polysaccharide corresponding to the serotype under treatment (Francis test). An immediate reaction signals the presence of specific humoral antibody in the patient.

Other antigenic components of *Streptococcus pneumoniae* are found in both capsulated and noncapsulated strains. There are species-specific somatic or C carbohydrate and nucleoprotein antigens, as well as type-specific M proteins. These antigens bear no relationship to virulence and do not engender protective immunity.

Capsulated *Streptococcus pneumoniae* are highly virulent, not only in humans, but also in many laboratory animals. Thus, as little as one viable unit of some strains of fully virulent (capsulated) pneumococcus will initiate a lethal infection on intraperitoneal injection into mice. Such virulence is extraordinary among bacteria that ordinarily inhabit or cause disease in the respiratory tract of humans, a fact that has been used to achieve isolation of *Streptococcus pneumoniae* by intraperitoneal injection of contaminated specimens, such as expectorated sputum, into mice.

Pneumococci are quite susceptible to physical agents such as heat (56°C for 20 minutes is lethal) and drying. They possess no outstanding resistance to the usual antiseptics and germicides. The susceptibility of *Streptococcus pneumoniae* to ethyl hydrocuprein chloride (Optochin) is so marked, so uniform, and in such contrast to viridans group and other *Streptococcus* spp. that disk testing with this compound has become routine for confirmation of identity in most clinical laboratories. Although many antimicrobics are active against *Streptococcus pneumoniae,* the aminocyclitols are notable exceptions, for example, gentamicin, 5 μg/ml final concentration, in blood agar aids in isolating pneumococci from contaminated specimens.

Exquisite susceptibility to penicillin G has been the rule with MICs typically $\leq$ 0.05 μg/ml ($\leq$ 0.08 U/ml). However, since 1966, rare clinical isolates with so-called intermediate resistance, MICs 0.1 to 1.0 μg/ml (0.2–1.6 U/ml) have been reported; disease caused by such strains will respond to treatment with penicillin G. Of greater concern was the appearance in 1977 of pneumococci with MICs of 2.0 to 10 μg/ml (3.1–15.6 U/ml) that caused serious disease that was refractory to treatment with penicillin G and other β-lactam antimicrobics. Some of these strains were also resistant to the tetracyclines, sulfonamides, erythromycin, lincomycin, clindamycin, and chloramphenicol. Rifampin, fusidic acid, vancomycin, novobiocin, and bacitracin were generally active. Resistant *Streptococcus pneumoniae* do not elaborate β-lactamases and do not carry R plasmids; except for an inducible enzyme that inactivates chloramphenicol, the bases for resistance are unknown.

Worldwide, 22 serotypes have been associated with resistance to penicillin G and other antimicrobics; high resistance has occurred, primarily with type 57, occasionally with type 6, and rarely with type 14 (American serotype nomenclature). Types 6 and 14 are components of the 14-valent capsular polysaccharide vaccine, whereas type 57 is not. It is probable that antibody engendered by the type 19 polysaccharide of the vaccine is not sufficiently cross-reactive to provide protection against type 57.

Other Bacteria

The frequency of occurrence of *Staphylococcus aureus* as a cause for bacterial pneumonia varies from 1% to 5%, depending primarily on the epidemicity of facilitating, nonbacterial respiratory infections. The characteristics of *Staphylococcus aureus* are reviewed in Chap. 100, Staphylococcal Skin Infections. In recent experience, over half the isolates from patients with influenza-associated staphylococcal pneumonia have been penicillinase-positive.

Klebsiella spp. (Chap. 48, Urethritis and Cystitis) also cause 1% to 5% of bacterial pneumonias. Multiantimicrobic resistance is common, with aminocyclitols and the newer cephalosporins among the most active and useful antimicrobics.

Many other kinds of bacteria are implicated as causes of pneumonias. *Haemophilus influenzae* (Chap. 26, Epiglottitis, Laryngitis, and Laryngotracheobronchitis) may be responsible for as many as 1% of cases, while *Legionella* spp. (Chap. 33, Legionnaires Disease) cause under 1% of cases. *Streptococcus pyogenes* (group A; Chap. 24, Streptococcal Diseases) rarely causes pneumonia at present. *Neisseria meningitidis* (Chap. 119, Acute Bacterial Meningitis), nonsporulating anaerobes (Chap. 32, Necrotizing Pneumonias and Lung Abscess), and bacteria of the family Enterobacteriaceae have been implicated, as have *Mycobacterium tuberculosis* (Chap. 34, Pulmonary Tuberculosis), *Nocardia* spp. (Chap. 37, Nocardiosis), *Francisella tularensis* (Chap. 139, Tularemia), and *Yersinia pestis* (Chap. 140, Plague). Clearly, the necessity for accurate bacteriologic diagnosis cannot be overemphasized.

Epidemiology

According to the National Health Interview Survey for 1979–1980, the estimated annual number of cases of pneumonia in the United States was 2,606,573. As a result, there were 45,910,907 days of restricted activity, and 28,039,272 days of bed disability. About 10% of admissions to acute medical hospital wards are due to pneumonia. Of the 15 leading causes of death, pneumonia (with influenza) ranks fifth, and it is first among infectious diseases. Death from pneumonia is most frequent among males, striking particularly at the extremes of age (Table 31-1). About half of all pneumonias, those producing serious morbidity and mortality, are bacterial pneumonias.

Table 31-1. *Death rates (per 100,000 population) from pneumonia for selected age groups, by sex, in the United States in 1978*

Sex	Under 1 yr	5–24			55–64 yr
		5–14 YR	15–24 YR	TOTALS	
Male	50.8	0.8	1.5	1.2	31.7
Female	42.6	0.8	1.0	0.9	14.7

Pneumococcus

Streptococcus pneumoniae, by far the most important cause of bacterial pneumonias, is a communicable commensal and parasite of humans. Pharyngitis is not caused by pneumococci; yet, *Streptococcus pneumoniae* must be regarded as an element of the normal flora because it may be isolated from the upper respiratory tracts of as many as 70% of normal persons. However, rates of carriage vary with the season (maximal October–April in the northern hemisphere), are higher in children than in adults, and increase with close cohabitation. The density of colonization has not been defined quantitatively.

Although noncapsulated *Streptococcus pneumoniae* is avirulent, there is type-specific variation in capacity to invade. With the exception of type 3 in adults and children, type 8 in adults, and types 6, 19, and 23 in children, the most commonly carried serotypes (3, 8, 9, 18, 19, 23 in adults; 3, 6, 19, 23 in children) do not correspond to the types most frequently responsible for pneumococcal disease (1, 3, 4, 7, 8, 12 in adults; 3, 6, 14, 18, 19, 23 in children). However, both carriage and disease serotypes vary with time and geographic area.

There is no racial predisposition to pneumococcal pneumonia. The disease occurs approximately three times more often in males than in females. Although the exact incidence is not known, it is estimated that 150,000 to 570,000 cases of pneumococcal pneumonia occur each year in the United States, giving an incidence of 68 to 260 cases per 100,000 population. The attack rate is highest in the 30- to 50-year age group; and occurrence appears to be favored by noninfectious diseases (splenic dysfunction, cirrhosis, multiple myeloma, hypogammaglobulinemia, nephrotic syndrome, alcoholism, congestive heart failure, and chronic obstructive pulmonary disease) and certain nonbacterial respiratory tract infections. Geography and climate influence the occurrence of pneumococcal pneumonia in that the disease is less frequent when it is warm and dry.

Other Bacteria

For the most part, the other relatively infrequent bacterial causes of pneumonia are also drawn either from a person's own flora or from that of other humans. There are epidemiologic peculiarities, however. *Staphylococcus aureus* afflicts infants and the aged most often. This age characteristic persists when influenza is epidemic but is expanded to include pregnant women, resulting in an overall increase in the frequency of staphylococcal pneumonia.

Children less than 5 years old, immunoincompetent persons, alcoholics, and elderly persons with chronic obstructive pulmonary disease are more likely than are others to contract pneumonia caused by *H. influenzae*. Klebsiellal pneumonia is primarily a disease of men 40 to 60 years old, and it occurs with increased frequency in alcoholics.

Pneumonia caused by various other Enterobacteriaceae and *Pseudomonas aeruginosa* has been attributed to the inoculation of the patient by means of contaminated respiratory-assistance apparatus; however, the need for mechanical ventilatory aids testifies to the underlying hypervulnerable state of the patient. The principal isolates of aspiration pneumonias contracted outside the hospital are the normal anaerobic flora of the upper respiratory tract, namely, anaerobic and microaerophilic streptococci, *Bacteroides melaninogenicus,* and *Fusobacterium nucleatum*; in hospitalized patients, aerobic bacteria (usually *Staphylococcus aureus* and enteric gram-negative bacilli) are commonly present, with or without anaerobes.

Pathogenesis and Pathology

Bacteria may reach the lungs through either the airways or the bloodstream. Aerogenous infection is the most common and also occurs with nonbacterial microorganisms. Whether an inhaled infectious particle actually reaches the alveoli or is halted en route is a problem in aerodynamic filtration. Particles varying from 5 μm to 10 μm in diameter will settle in the upper airways largely by inertial deposition consequent on turbulence and directional changes imposed on the air by the anatomy of the supralaryngeal respiratory tract. The particles are trapped in mucus on nasal, pharyngeal, or tracheobronchial surfaces and are swallowed (after delivery to the oropharynx from infralaryngeal deposition through the mucociliary stream). Smaller particles, down to 0.3 μm in diameter, may penetrate to the alveolar ducts and alveoli and be deposited, whereas still smaller particles tend to remain suspended in air and be exhaled. Bacteria-laden nuclei of droplets of respiratory tract secretions are of appropriate size to achieve alveolar deposition. Whether pneumonia results is determined primarily by the capacity of the cellular defenses of the host—especially the alveolar macrophages—versus the virulence of the bacteria.

The carriage of invasive bacteria in the upper respiratory tract as commensals is a matter of chance that appears not to be influenced by the administration of the capsular polysaccharide vaccines (pneumococcal, meningococcal, *Haemophilus influenzae* type b), although such vaccines are efficacious in preventing disease in certain populations. On the other hand, several factors may adversely affect the defenses of the host. For example, the physical stress of chilling appears to contribute to susceptibility to pneumonia. Defense mechanisms seem to be less effective in old age. Inadequate production of humoral antibodies, as may occur with asplenia, splenic dysfunctions, and diseases of the hematopoietic–lymphoreticular system favor the occurrence of pneumonias.

Many viral respiratory tract infections have a facilitating influence on the occurrence of bacterial pneumonias, a relationship well grounded in lore, for example from 50% to 80% of patients with pneumococcal pneumonias have had an upper respiratory infection in the preceding 1 to 2 weeks. Laboratory evidence firmly backs up the epidemiologic observation of the relationship of deaths from pneumonia to epidemicity of influenza (Fig. 31-1). In correlation with the present knowledge of pulmonary defense mechanisms, it is notable that viral infections of the respiratory tract (1) are not limited to the upper (supralaryngeal) tract; (2) compromise epithelial resources (diminished ciliary function, depression of alveolar macrophages), while augmenting bacterial adherence; and (3) cause hypersecretion and qualitative alterations in tracheobronchial surface liquids. Thus, endogenous formation of droplets is favored, the milieu for the proliferation of commensal bacteria is enriched, and at the same time, major pulmonary defense mechanisms are crippled.

Infection is favored whenever a bacterial inoculum is aspirated along with materials that cause injury to the respiratory tract. Foreign bodies, gastric contents (HCl, enzymes), and lipids (mineral oil) are prominent offenders. Noxious gases and vapors may predispose to pneumonias. For example, ozone impairs the bactericidal capacity of the lungs, and nitrogen diox-

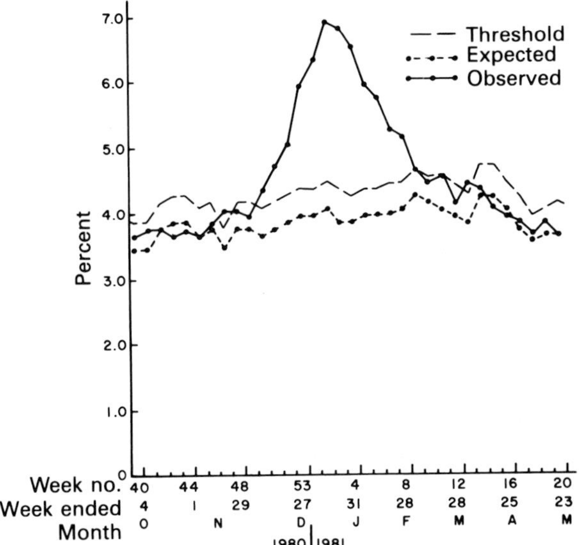

Fig. 31-1. Influence of epidemic influenza on the pneumonia-influenza death rate in 122 cities in the United States. (Morbid Mortal Week Rep Suppl Summary, 1980)

ide, as in silo-filler's disease, acutely compromises pulmonary defenses.

Alcoholics are vulnerable to pneumonias through aspiration and diminished function of pulmonary defenses as part of alcoholic stupor, impairments of leukocyte mobilization, and the effects of heavy cigarette smoking.

Bypassing the turbulence-producing, particle-trapping upper respiratory tract—as by tracheostomy and tracheal intubation—renders the patient susceptible to pneumonia. Repeated catheter suction of the tracheobronchial tree, the prolonged inhalation of dry air, and the irritant effect of devices indwelling in airways all predispose to the development of pneumonia.

Surgical operations, particularly those associated with general anesthesia, result in the interplay of several pathogenetic factors. Anesthetics compromise epithelial, cellular, and secretory pulmonary defenses. Cough and air exchange are depressed. Foreign bodies contaminated with upper respiratory tract flora are inserted into airways for variable periods.

Patients who require tracheostomy, tracheal intubation, or mechanical assistance to respiration already have underlying structural or functional disability that renders them vulnerable to pneumonia. Thousands of persons with advanced obstructive pulmonary disease, paresis or paralysis of the respiratory muscles, and coma or unconsciousness are in this category.

Lesser degrees of chronic obstructive pulmonary disease, pneumoconioses, congestive heart failure, and cystic fibrosis also predispose persons to bacterial pneumonias. Again, compromised function of both cellular and secretory defenses of the lung is implicated. In addition, it is probable that in some of these patients, immunologic reserves, both humoral and cellular, are limited or nonfunctional. Hypoxia may be a primary factor. Endogenous bacteria are commonly involved, and more than one kind may cause a pneumonia.

Actual obstruction of an airway leads to pneumonia in the lung distal to the obstruction. With foreign bodies, the inoculum is derived from the obstructing object. Yet even when the obstruction is endogenous (*e.g.,* bronchogenic carcinoma), the microorganisms that are isolated are normal upper respiratory tract flora. The isolation of more than one kind of bacterium is not uncommon in obstructive pneumonias.

Uremia and metabolic acidosis exemplify processes that impair pulmonary defenses without directly compromising ventilation or gas exchange.

Hematogenous inoculation of the lungs is infrequent in comparison with aerogenous pneumonia. Pulmonary trapping of infected emboli arising from a septic pelvic thrombophlebitis is classic. Heroin addicts develop pneumonia apparently as a consequence of induced bacteremia, often originating from right heart infective endocarditis. Similarly, infection localizes in the lungs as a consequence of bacteremia without embolization in plague.

The inflammatory response in pneumonias provokes exudation into the alveoli, displacing air. As one consequence, despite an augmented blood flow to zones of pneumonitis, gas exchange cannot occur and hypoxemia results. The severity of the hypoxemia is certainly related to the total volume of lung involved, and it may also depend on the cardiodynamic response. In about one-third of patients with acute pneumonias, there is depression of myocardial function rather than the hyperdynamic response that ought to occur in a febrile, hypoxemic patient. In such cardiodepressed patients, the arteriovenous oxygen difference is exaggerated.

The components of the exudate in acute bacterial pneumonia vary with the time course of the reaction and are reflected in grossly and microscopically evident changes in the lung. Study of experimental pneumococcal pneumonia has contributed greatly to our understanding of the course of events (Fig. 31-2):

1. In the outermost, leading edge of a pneumonic lesion, the pneumonia is in its earliest stages. Here, the bacteria proliferate virtually unhindered in a relatively acellular exudate that is akin

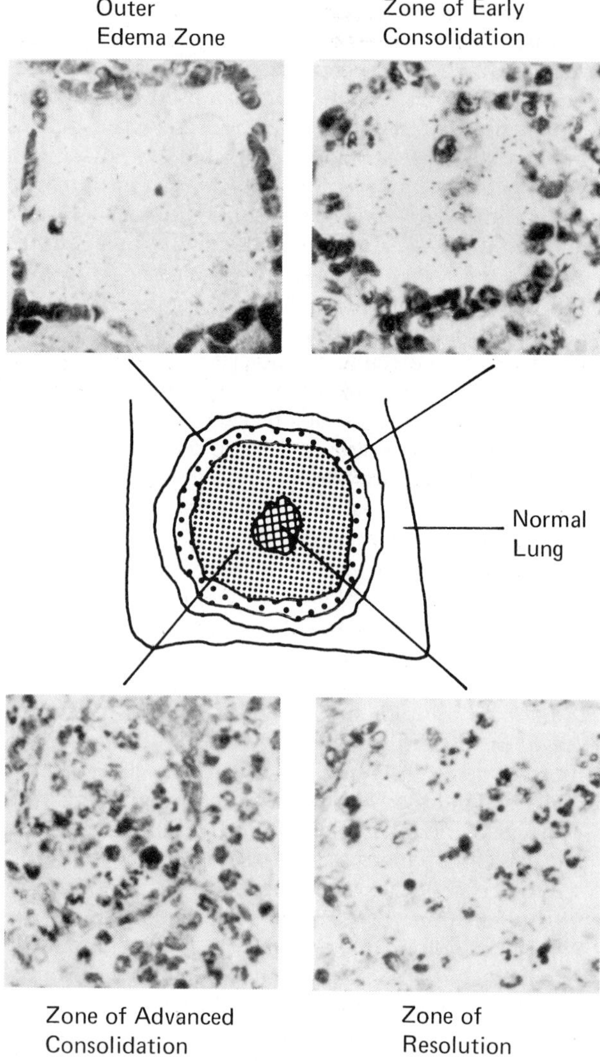

Fig. 31-2. Diagrammatic and photomicrographic representation of a pneumococcal pneumonic lesion. *Outer edema zone:* the leading edge of the lesion with exudate-filled alveoli laden with pneumococci; *Zone of early consolidation:* while bacterial density has decreased, neutrophils are now in evidence; *Zone of advanced consolidation:* pneumococci are no longer visible, and the neutrophilic cellular reaction is maximal; *Zone of resolution:* the neutrophils are gone and have been replaced with macrophages. (Wood WB Jr, Smith MR: J Exp Med 103: 487–498, 1956)

to blood plasma (outer edema zone, Fig. 31-2). If the exudate is poor in fibrinogen, or if the fibrinogen has not been converted to fibrin, the lung is flabby, and a light yellowish liquid oozes freely from the cut surface.

2. The zone of edema shades into a region in which bacterial growth has slowed as nutrients are exhausted, metabolites accumulate, and a neutrophilic cellular response occurs (zone of early consolidation, Fig. 31-2). The lung is usually firm, and the cut surface is dry, perhaps stubbly, if the formation of fibrin has advanced sufficiently. A gray color results from the fibrin (white) and leukocytes (buff).
3. In the next most central, yet older, part of the lesion (zone of advanced consolidation, Fig. 31-2), the bacterial population has declined as a combined effect of diminished replication and phagocytosis. The inflammatory response is maximal, resulting in myriads of polymorphonuclear leukocytes and erythrocytes. Hence, the cut surface of the firm lung is dry and reddish to an extent dependent on the number of erythrocytes.
4. At the center of the lesion, there are no bacteria or neutrophilic leukocytes; macrophages are present (zone of resolution, Fig. 31-2). If alveolar walls have not been destroyed (the usual outcome with *Streptococcus pneumoniae*), the lung is firm and resilient, whereas pulmonary necrosis (frequent with *Klebsiella* spp.) yields a soft, friable lung that is yellow in cut section.

Pneumonic infection spreads from one pulmonary segment to another by spillage of bacterial-laden exudate into a bronchiole and subsequent aspiration into previously uninvolved alveoli. As the lesion extends, pleural surfaces are involved, giving rise at first to an intrapleural collection of sterile exudate. If bacteria gain access to the effusion, the leukocyte response is greatly augmented and empyema results.

Depending on the location of the primary pneumonic lesion, involvement of the visceral pleura may, by direct spread, also involve the pericardium. The resultant pericardial effusion usually remains sterile but may become infected.

In the course of intrapulmonary spread, bacteria gain access to the lymphatics. If the regional nodes cannot cope with the bacteria delivered in the lymph, the bacteria pass on, causing bacteremia. Metastatic infections may result, for example, endocarditis, meningitis, and arthritis.

Characteristically, the tubules and air sacs of the pulmonary parenchyma are not irreversibly injured in a pneumococcal pneumonia. That is, with resolution of the exudate, the lung is restored to normal function. Very rarely with *Streptococcus pneumoniae,* but typically with other kinds of bacteria, there is destruction of pulmonary parenchyma. Necrosis with formation of abscesses occurs relatively early in the course of pneumonias caused by *Staphylococcus aureus, Klebsiella* spp., and nonsporulating anaerobes. In pseudomonal pneumonias, necrosis results from thromboses caused by the vasculitis typically engendered by *Psuedomonas aeruginosa.*

In some patients, even in pneumococcal pneumonia, fibroblasts and capillaries invade the fibrinous exudate to yield, by deposition of collagen, an organized nonfunctional zone. Organization may also occur with nonbacterial causes of pneumonia.

Manifestations

Classic pneumococcal pneumonia is primarily a disease of the adult male that strikes suddenly with a single, shaking chill, yielding fever that becomes sustained at 39°C to 41°C (102°F–106°F). Cough producing rusty (prune juice) colored, mucopurulent sputum, pleurisy, and signs of pulmonary consolidation complete the picture. Frequently, the patient can specify the exact hour of onset of the illness, so abrupt and dramatic was its beginning.

Repeated rigors are so atypical of pneumococcal pneumonia that other causes must be sought, especially *Staphylococcus aureus, Klebsiella* spp. nonsporulating anaerobes, and *Streptococcus pyogenes.* Shaking chills are generally lacking when *H. influenzae* is the causative agent.

Hectic fever is the rule in pneumonias caused by bacteria other than *Streptococcus pneumoniae* and *F. tularensis.* Although labial herpes is said to be typical of pneumococcal pneumonia, almost any severe infection, including nonbacterial pneumonias, may lead to this clinical expression of a dormant herpesvirus infection. Pleuritic pain is common to most bacterial pneumonias except those caused by *H. influenzae* and *F. tularensis.* About 75% of patients with pneumococcal pneumonia have pleurisy that is often quite severe—an excruciating, sharp pain that stabs with every breath. Flaring of the ali nasi at each inspiration is typical as the patient with pneumococcal pneumonia sits up and leans forward, attempting to achieve adequate air exchange while trying not to cough or breathe deeply.

In a particular patient, the gross appearance of sputum is not a reliable indicator of the etiologic agent. Rusty, bloody sputum is produced in pneumococcal, staphylococcal, klebsiellal, and streptococcal pneumonias. The sputum in klebsiellal pneumonia is often markedly viscous (like currant jelly), as it may be in any patient with pneumonia who is dehydrated. When *H. influenzae* cause pneumonia, the sputum may be "apple green" in color, an appearance that may reflect no more than purulence, and may also result from postexpectoration growth of *P. aeruginosa* or other microorganisms.

As exudate replaces air in the lung, or if there is pleurisy, the chest will lag both in timing and extent of excursion or will be splinted. The respirations will accordingly be shallow and grunting, although the patient may labor to breathe, employing accessory muscles. The hypoxemia that results may be manifest as a cyanosis of the lips and nail beds. Dullness to percussion, increased tactile fremitus, bronchial breath sounds, transmission of spoken and whispered voice, egophony—the gamut of signs of consolidation—all relate to replacement of parenchymal gas space with exudate.

Exudates also absorb x-rays more effectively than does air. The pulmonary opacifications evident in roentgenograms are a more sensitive means to detect pneumonias than is physical examination. Overall, certain radiographic patterns emerge associated with particular etiologic agents—associations that are usually deceptive when applied to a particular patient. Thus, a pneumonia involving all of an upper lobe, actually causing a downward bulging of the inferior margin of the lobe on posteroanterior projection, is said to characterize pneumonia caused by *Klebsiella* spp. The presence of multiple pneumatocoeles, several abscesses, and many areas of infiltration should bring to mind *Staphylococcus aureus* as the cause for the pneumonia. Small abscesses are said to be characteristic of pneumonia caused by *P. aeruginosa.*

A brisk leukocytosis, in the range of 15,000 to 30,000/mm^3, is usual in bacterial pneumonia. Polymorphonuclear leukocytes make up 70% to 90% of the leukocytes, about half of which are nonsegmented. If the pneumonia is overwhelming, the total number of leukocytes falls, toxic granulations become evident, and immature neutrophils appear.

Diagnosis

The clinical diagnosis of classic lobar pneumonia is readily accomplished on the basis of the manifestations. However, if the patient is seen quite early, at the onset of the illness, there may be only fever and pleuritic pain, perhaps associated with a nonproductive cough. Some 12 to 24 hours later, often only after parenteral hydration, signs of pneumonia are evident in physical and radiographic examinations. Atypical manifestations—lack of chills, moderate fever, dyspnea disproportionate to physical findings and radiographic changes, confusion, and lethargy—may be seen in alcoholics, the elderly, and patients with severe chronic obstructive pulmonary disease.

Although most bacterial pneumonias are caused by *Streptococcus pneumoniae,* the physician must always strive for the earliest possible identification of the responsible pathogen. Only in this way can optimal, specific therapy be assured. Microscopic examination of a gram-stained smear of sputum is of particular value in the rapid detection of pneumonias caused by gram-negative bacilli. Because gram-positive cocci predominate in the normal flora of the upper respiratory tract, the finding of gram-negative bacilli in a specimen of expectorated sputum from a patient with a pneumonia who has not received antimicrobics must be heeded.

The major pitfall is the inevitable contamination of sputum by upper respiratory tract secretions in the course of expectoration. For example, anaerobes indigenous to the mouth are always added to the specimen, rendering expectorated sputum uniformly unsuitable for anaerobic culture. For both smears and aerobic cultures, a choice portion of sputum must be selected—that is, a mucopurulent fleck. If bacterial pneumonia is the source of such a fleck, polymorphonuclear leukocytes should be abundant and epithelial cells should be lacking. Judgment of the gram reaction of bacteria in the smear should be made only in an area of the slide where the neutrophils are gram-negative.

Reducing the time between the collection of sputum and the inoculation of cultures is essential to minimizing the overgrowth of contaminating potential pathogens. Quantitative culture of the sputum has been recommended as an aid in identifying the actual cause of the pneumonia when a specimen yields more than one potential pathogen. *Streptococcus pneumoniae* is readily separated from contaminating oropharyngeal bacteria by intraperitoneal injection of sputum into mice.

Specimen contamination is best circumvented by obtaining material that can be certified as infralaryngeal in origin. Percutaneous transtracheal aspiration is readily accomplished at the bedside using a needle-polyethylene catheter set of the kind commercially available for intravenous infusion (Fig. 31-3). Specimens obtained in this way are valid for both anaero-

Fig. 31-3. Technique of transtracheal aspiration. The neck is hyperextended by placing a pillow under the shoulders. The skin over the cricothyroid membrane is cleansed (isopropanol) and anesthetized (lidocaine). Using a large, commercial, intravenous catheter set, a 14-gauge needle is inserted through the skin into the trachea. While pointed caudad, the polyethylene catheter is passed into the trachea; the steel is withdrawn leaving the catheter in place. Two to four ml of sterile, bacteriostat-free 0.9% NaCl solution is injected rapidly through the catheter. A paroxysm of coughing invariably results. Suction is immediately applied and tracheobronchopulmonary secretions/exudates are aspirated into the catheter/syringe. The catheter is withdrawn and pressure is applied over the puncture site.

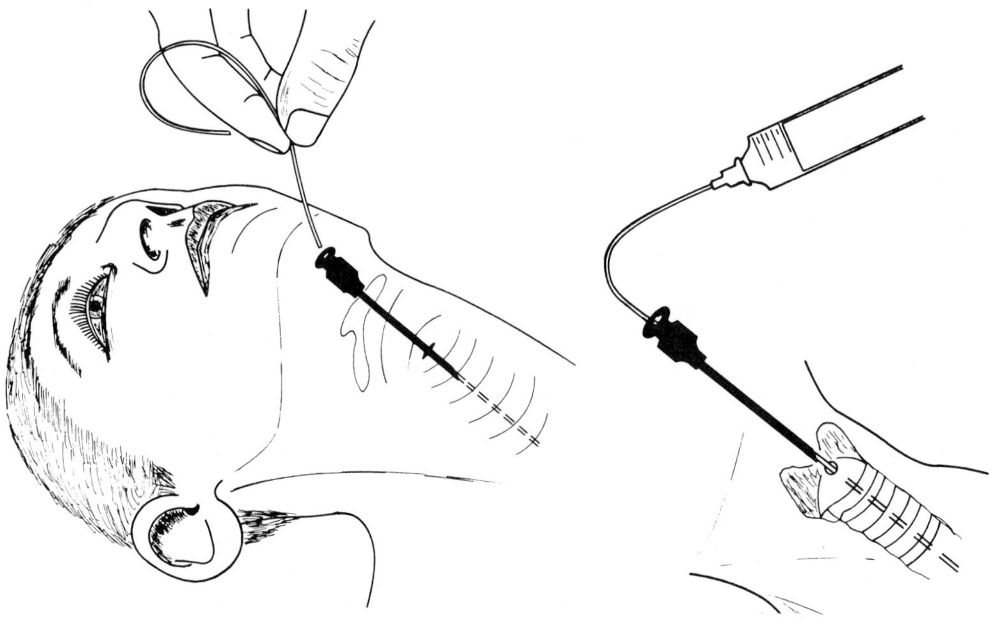

bic and aerobic cultures, and they are ideal for microscopic examination (Plate 31-1*A*). Moreover, the procedure often enables the collection of a specimen from patients with pneumonia who either cannot or will not produce sputum by expectoration. It is also of great value in patients who are hypervulnerable and in whom more than one kind of bacterium is cause for the pneumonia.

In every patient suspected of having a bacterial pneumonia, at least one blood culture should be obtained before antimicrobial therapy is given. Both aerobic and anaerobic culture mediums should be inoculated according to the technique described in Chapter 10, Clinical Specimens for Microbiologic Examinations. All pneumococci isolated from the blood or cerebrospinal fluid should be tested *in vitro* for susceptibility to penicillin G.

Tuberculous pneumonia represents a pulmonary and systemic tuberculin reaction set off by the endobronchial discharge of a tuberculous lesion (Chap. 34, Pulmonary Tuberculosis). Although pleurisy is common, the reaction is generally most severe in the perihilar regions. Chills and fever reflect the absorption and systemic distribution of tuberculin. It may be difficult to find tubercle bacilli by microscopic examination of the sputum, although cultures are usually positive. Leukocytosis is unusual. A history of tuberculosis and the chest film are valuable. However, the failure of conventional antimicrobial agents most often directs the diagnostic efforts toward tuberculosis.

Emphasis on a precise etiologic diagnosis of bacterial pneumonias presumes that differentiation from nonbacterial pneumonias has been accomplished. Infectious nonbacterial pneumonias are at least as frequent as bacterial pneumonias and are considered in detail in Chapter 30, Nonbacterial Pneumonias. The most consistent and useful clinical indicators of infectious nonbacterial pneumonias, as caused by *Mycoplasma pneumoniae* (5%–15% of pneumonias), viruses, *Chlamydia* spp. or *Coxiella burnetii,* include (1) an insidious onset of illness; (2) a history of similar illness in the family, occupational, or other social unit; (3) lack of true rigors and moderate fever; (4) headache as a major complaint with pleurisy virtually never mentioned; (5) scanty production of sputum, usually without grossly evident blood, (the exception is psittacosis), but with a predominance of mononuclear cells (Plate 31-1*A*), and a scattering of polymorphonuclear leukocytes, and cultures yielding only normal oropharangeal flora if expectorated, but no growth if obtained by transtracheal aspiration; (6) a total leukocyte count that is normal or slightly elevated, with a normal differential; (7) rales as the major sign with a radiographic picture of bronchopneumonia that is patchy and multilobar in distribution; and (8) except for pleural effusions, very few complications, with death rarely the outcome. Retrospectively, tissue culture and animal inoculation procedures, along with serologic tests, are of value in differentiation. Because specific antimicrobial therapy is of value in treating ornithoses, Q fever, and mycoplasmal pneumonia, the epidemiologic history is particularly important.

Pulmonary fungal infections have an insidious onset in normal persons. In patients with noninfectious predisposing illnesses (*e.g.,* Hodgkin's disease), the onset and course may be fulminant. Lack of a neutrophilic response, both in the sputum and in the peripheral blood, is usual in fungal pneumonias, but may also be found in bacterial pneumonias in patients with primary hematopoietic–lymphoreticular diseases, particularly after treatment with agents that suppress the bone marrow.

A variety of noninfectious processes may mimic bacterial pneumonias: congestive heart failure, pulmonary infarction, fractured ribs; inhalation of allergens, oils, fumes, toxins, or dusts; carcinoma (primary or metastatic); irradiation injury of the lung; drug-induced pulmonary disease; collagen-vascular disease of the lung; sarcoidosis (Chap. 168, Sarcoidosis); and uremia. Any of these processes in pure form is readily differentiable from classical lobar pneumonia. The difficulty lies in recognizing the addition of a bacterial pneumonia to one of these noninfectious pulmonary diseases. An abrupt worsening of the patient is highly significant and calls for immediate physical examination of the patient, chest radiography, gram-stained smear and culture of sputum (preferably, a specimen obtained by transtracheal aspiration), leukocyte and differential counts, and culture of the blood.

Prognosis

Pneumococcus

Formerly, without specific therapy, the die was cast in pneumococcal pneumonia 6 to 10 days after the illness had begun. The overall case–fatality rate was around 40%, earning for the pneumococcus the somewhat grandiloquent designation: "captain of the men of death." The 60% who recovered typically began improvement as abruptly as they became ill, with rapid defervescence and drenching diaphoresis—the crisis. When death was the outcome, circulatory collapse, with or without recognizable heart failure, culminated progression of the pulmonary involvement marked by dyspnea and cyanosis. With specific therapy, the overall case–fatality ratio is about 5%. Several factors influence the outcome significantly:

1. The age of the patient is quite important, as has long been recognized in another appellation for the pneumococcus: "the old man's friend." All other factors being equal, age alone is not associated with a deleterious effect until the fourth decade; thereafter, morbidity and mortality increase directly with increasing age, exceeding 25% despite the application of appropriate chemotherapy.
2. Any underlying disease that adversely affects pulmonary functions or interferes with either humoral or cellular defenses against infection contributes to a poor prognosis. The list is long; in addition to those already mentioned should be added: atherosclerotic cardiovascular disease, with or without congestive heart failure; diabetes mellitus; thyrotoxicosis; cirrhosis of the liver; anatomic and functional asplenia.
3. Several indicators of the severity of the pneumonia individually or collectively augur a poor prognosis: involvement of more than one lobe; toxic granulations of the neutrophils and relative leukopenia, for example, if the leukocyte count is $\leq 5{,}000/\text{mm}^3$ at the time treatment is begun, only about two-thirds of the patients will survive. Bacteremia indicates failure of confinement of the infection to the lungs; 25% of such patients die—especially if they are over 50 years in age.
4. The serotype of *Streptococcus pneumoniae* is important, with the poorest prognosis associated with type 3. During rapid growth *in vivo,* type 3 pneumococci are the least susceptible to phagocytosis of all serotypes, apparently as a consequence of a slime layer of polysaccharide that adheres to the capsule. Curiously, serotherapy was least effective with type 3—possibly because of the prodigous capacity of this serotype to synthesize capsular polysaccharide. Although pneumonia caused by type 2 is now rare in the United States, the virulence of this type remains inexplicably high.
5. Within the first 4 days of illness, delay in the application of specific therapy seriously diminishes the probability of cure. The decreasing prognostic import of delay thereafter may be related to the beginning of the specific antibody response.

Complications may be related to the same factors affecting the overall prognosis. Pleural effusion is detected in about 25% of patients with pneumococcal pneumonia. Typically, pleurisy diminishes, the percussion note changes to flatness from dullness, the trachea deviates away from the affected side, and there is shifting of a basilar radiodensity to a layer along the dependent chest wall in decubitus radiography. Fewer than 10% of patients with effusions go on to empyema. Development of empyema and delayed resolution are believed by many observers to be complications that are avoided by the early institution of specific therapy. Extension to involve the pericardium is quite uncommon and is signaled by the usual manifestations of pericarditis (Chap. 132, Pericarditis). Pulmonary abscess caused by *Streptococcus pneumoniae* is very rare.

Delayed resolution—persistence of infiltration by radiography 3 weeks after treatment was begun—appears to be related to delay in beginning therapy; it is most frequently seen in alcoholics. Because an underlying obstruction must be considered (*e.g.,* bronchogenic carcinoma), bronchoscopy is advocated when this complication becomes evident.

The metastatic infection of joints, heart valves, and meninges is quite uncommon in the treated patient. Occurrence of these infections depends on bacteremia, reflecting the interplay of severe disease, poor host response, and delayed therapy.

Paralytic ileus and jaundice are noninfectious consequences of pneumococcal infections. With prompt specific therapy, both occur quite infrequently.

Other Bacteria

With other bacterial causes of pneumonia, death may ensue quite rapidly through the final common pathway of cardiovascular collapse. Although many of the prognostic factors operative with pneumococcal pneumonia are probably also influential in nonpneumococcal bacterial pneumonias, documentation is not generally available.

STAPHYLOCOCCUS AUREUS

With *Staphylococcus aureus,* the patient has virtually always been rendered vulnerable by some clearly recognizable process. Thus, the hypersusceptibility of infants and their inability to localize staphylococci may be related to immunologic virginity with respect to *Staphylococcus aureus*—that is, they have neither cellular nor humoral antistaphylococcal capabilities.

The devastating potential of staphylococcal pneumonia complicating influenza (or other nonbacterial respiratory tract infection) is well known. Death may result after a clinical course as short as 12 hours. Despite the availability of the penicillinase-resistant penicillins and cephalosporins, the case–fatality rate in staphylococcal pneumonia ranges from 25% to 60%.

Pneumatoceles in children and abscesses in adults are the characteristic complications of staphylococcal pneumonia. There is no necrosis of tissue in children, and if recovery occurs, there is no residual pulmonary damage. In adults, however, there is destruction of pulmonary parenchyma; empyema is frequent and may communicate through a pulmonary abscess to form a pyopneumothorax.

KLEBSIELLA SPP.
Occasionally a primary infection, klebsiellal pneumonia is usually, like staphylococcal pneumonia, secondary to another process, such as alcoholism, old age, diabetes mellitus, congestive heart failure, chronic obstructive pulmonary disease, and influenza or other viral infections of the respiratory tract.

The case–fatality rate of 40% to 60% reflects the vulnerable state of those who contract klebsiellal pneumonia and the limitations of presently available antimicrobics. The disease may progress quite rapidly with an alert, apprehensive patient dying in shock within 24 hours of onset.

Necrosis of pulmonary tissue is quite common, with consequences in the form of cavities, bronchiectasis, and pulmonary fibrosis evident in about one-third of those who survive the infection.

Other

Necrotizing pneumonias with a virtually uniform production of abscesses are characteristic of pulmonary infections caused by nonsporulating anaerobes (Chap. 32, Necrotizing Pneumonias and Lung Abscess). The posterior segment of the right upper lobe is most frequently involved.

Accumulation of pleural fluid in large quantities very soon after the onset of pneumonia caused by group A *Streptococcus pyogenes* occurred in as many as 80% of patients before the availability of antimicrobics. Although this kind of pneumonia is now rare, infected pleural effusions appear to occur as frequently as in the past.

Therapy

General Therapy

Patients with bacterial pneumonias should be hospitalized. The measures necessary to etiologic diagnosis, sophisticated evaluation of pulmonary gas exchange, and surveillance of cardiopulmonary function are all best accomplished in the hospital. Bed rest is assured, and other supportive measures are expeditiously applied.

Parenteral rehydration is important, not only because the loss of water is augmented by fever and rapid breathing, but also because it is the most efficient means to decrease the viscosity of intrapulmonary exudate, enabling expectoration (*i.e.,* drainage). In pneumonia, drainage is perhaps even more important than in other infectious processes because the vital process of gas exchange is involved. Some patients may be too weak to mobilize sputum, particularly if it is tenacious and thick. Endotracheal intubation may occasionally be necessary to enable the removal of sputum by catheter suction.

The patient with hypoxemia should be given oxygen—a nasal catheter arrangement is usually adequate, but must be assessed by determinations of arterial blood gases. The patient with underlying chronic obstructive pulmonary disease whose major respiratory drive stems from hypoxemia may be a particular problem in management—his pO_2 should not be driven above 50 to 60 mm Hg. In the patient with an asthmatic component contributing to pneumonia, the administration of isoproterenol by aerosol–intermittent positive pressure may be beneficial.

The caloric requirements imposed by a bacterial pneumonia are severe, and parenteral nutrition may be necessary.

Pleuritic pain may be excruciating. Narcotic analgesics are contraindicated because they also suppress cough. Propoxyphene hydrochloride may be helpful and is neither antitussive nor antipyretic. Gratifying relief, albeit temporary, results from injection of an anesthetic agent (*e.g.,* lidocaine) subcostally to anesthetize the involved dermatomes.

Congestive heart failure and atrial fibrillation are indications for intravenous administration of a cardiac-active glycoside. If the patient is hypotensive, the central venous pressure (CVP) and output of urine should be monitored. Digitalization, restoration of the CVP with blood, and injection of dopamine should be applied, in that order, if shock develops. Rarely, norepinephrine may be necessary (see pp. 94–96).

The value of pharmacologic doses of glucosteroids is as unproved as is detriment from their use; 0.5 mg of dexamethasone/kg body wt/day (or the equivalent dose of another glucosteroid) intravenously may aid in supporting the blood pressure and should block hypersensitivity reactions to bacteria or drugs. The glucosteroid can be discontinued after 3 to 5 days without compromising the patient's adrenal function.

Specific Therapy

Antimicrobial therapy should not be withheld until the results of cultures and susceptibility tests become available. Substantial clues to etiology are provided by the history of the illness, physical findings, radiographic examinations, laboratory data, and epidemiologic information. From these data, the physician can derive the most probable cause for the pneumonia and undertake specific therapy.

Of all the factors influencing the physician's decision, the results of examination of gram-stained smears of sputum are the most important. It cannot be emphasized too strongly that the validity of such examinations is primarily a function of the validity of the specimens. If there is any doubt about the infralaryngeal origin of a specimen of expectorated sputum, if sputum cannot be obtained, or if aerobic bacteria are likely to be involved, transtracheal aspiration should be carried out. Among bacterial pneumonias, the possibilities that must not be missed are *Staphylococcus aureus* and gram-negative bacilli, particularly *Klebsiella* spp. In an authentic specimen of tracheobronchopulmonary exudate, clusters of round gram-positive cocci should be taken as indicative of *Staphylococcus aureus*. Large gram-negative bacilli should be regarded as klebsiellal until proved otherwise. Usually, the bacteria are ovoid gram-positive cocci in diploids or short chains–*Streptococcus pneumoniae*. That is, the initial therapy of a bacterial pneumonia is generally directed against the pneumococcus.

The antimicrobial therapy selected may require modification according to the clinical course of the patient and the results of culture and susceptibility studies. However, the physician sometimes needs to accommodate conflicting inputs. For example, improvement in a patient with a pneumonia caused by *Staphylococcus aureus* or *K. pneumoniae* is not the dramatic, overnight defervescence so often seen with pneumococcal pneumonia. Persistence in a course of therapy that is appropriate according to clinical experience and laboratory data may require courage. The other side of the coin is the knowledge that inappropriate therapy is, in fact, no therapy. Certainly, thorough reassessment is indicated in the patient who does not respond after 3 days of treatment.

Penicillin G is the agent of choice for the treatment of bacterial pneumonias caused by *Streptococcus pneumoniae* and *Staphylococcus aureus* that are penicillinase negative, *Streptococcus pyogenes, N. meningitidis,* and nonsporulating anaerobes (in combination with chloramphenicol—see Chap. 32, Necrotizing Pneumonias and Lung Abscess). The procaine derivative in aqueous suspension injected intramuscularly in a dose of 600,000 units (0.4 g) every 12 hours for 7 to 10 days is generally adequate for pneumococcal, streptococcal, and meningococcal pneumonias. If there is shock, empyema, or other serious complications, potassium penicillin G should be injected in a dose of 25 mg to 30 mg (40,000–50,000 units) kg/body wt/day, IV, as four equal portions, 6-hourly. In patients who are allergic to the penicillins, a cephalosporin should be used, for example cefazolin (15 mg/kg body wt/day, IV or IM, as three equal portions 8-hourly for 7–10 days) is generally adequate. If there are complications, the dose should be increased to 25 to 30 mg/kg body wt/day, IV, as four equal portions, 6-hourly.

Staphylococcus aureus should always be presumed to be penicillinase-positive when treatment is initiated. Nafcillin (or an isoxazolyl penicillin) should be given in a dose of 150 to 200 mg/kg body wt/day, IV, as six equal portions, 4-hourly. Patients who are allergic to the penicillins should receive cefazolin in a dose of 75 to 100 mg/kg body wt/day, IV, as four equal portions, 6-hourly. Should laboratory tests prove that the responsible strain of *Staphylococcus aureus* is penicillinase-negative, penicillin G should replace the nafcillin in a dose of 150 mg to 200 mg (240,000–320,000 units)/kg body wt/day, IV, as six equal portions, 4-hourly. Treatment should be continued for at least 1 week after defervescense in patients without complications. If there is empyema or lung abscess, 4 to 6 weeks' treatment is necessary. In addition, tube drainage of the pleural space is required for empyema; lobectomy or segmental resection may be necessary with abscesses.

Pneumonia caused by *H. influenzae* is best treated with ampicillin if the infecting strain is not β-lactamase-positive. A dose of 150 mg/kg body wt/day, IV, as four equal portions, 6-hourly, should be given for a period extending 7 days beyond defervescence. If the infecting strain does elaborate β-lactamase, or if the patient is allergic to the penicillins, chloramphenicol should be given in a dose of 50 to 75 mg/kg body wt/day, PO, as four equal portions, 6-hourly. If parenteral administration is required because of shock, coma, or other complications, chloramphenicol succinate should be substituted in a dose of 50 to 60 mg/kg body wt/day, IV, as four equal portions, 6-hourly. In premature infants and neonates under 1 week in age, the dose of chloramphenicol should not exceed 25 mg/kg body wt/day.

Heretofore, the essential component of regimens for the treatment of pneumonias caused by *Klebsiella* spp. has been either gentamicin or tobramycin (a loading dose of 2 mg/kg body wt, IV, followed by 5–6 mg/kg body wt/day, IV, as three equal portions, 8-hourly). The dose must be adjusted to compensate for the renal capacity to excrete the drug according to measurements of concentrations in the blood: 8 to 10 μg/ml at peak and 1 to 3 μg/ml at trough. Combination with a cephalosporin, most appropriately cefoxitin (150–200 mg/kg body wt/day, IV, as six equal portions, 4-hourly), was often advocated. However, single-agent therapy may prove to be adequate with one of the newer cephalosporins (moxalactam, or ceftriaxone) since these drugs are more active than either the penicillins (including the acylureido derivatives) or the previously available cephalosporins. Pneumonias caused by *Escherichia coli* are appropriately treated using the same regimens.

Infections caused by *Proteus mirabilis* may be treated with either penicillin G or ampicillin (200 mg/kg body wt/day, IV, as six equal portions, 4-hourly), or cefazolin (100 mg/kg body wt/day, IV, as four equal portions, 6-hourly). Pneumonias caused by other Enterobacteriaceae may require either the regimens described for klebsiellal infections or different agents, for example, amikacin (a loading dose of 10 mg/kg body wt, IV, followed by 25–30 mg/kg body wt/day, IV, as three equal portions, 8-hourly) plus one of the newer cephalosporins, chloramphenicol (dosage as for hemophilan pneumonia).

With *Pseudomonas aeruginosa* and the non-*mirabilis Proteus* spp., either gentamicin, tobramycin, netilmicin, or amikacin (dosages as above) plus one of the acylureidopenicillins (150 mg/kg body wt/day, IV, as four equal portions, 6-hourly) may be effective.

Prevention

Active immunization to prevent pneumococcal pneumonia has as its bases: (1) *Streptococcus pneumoniae* is the commonest cause of bacterial pneumonia; (2) the therapeutic efficacy of penicillin G cannot be improved upon; (3) type-specific capsular polysaccharides can be prepared in a high degree of purity; (4) purified capsular polysaccharides are immunogenic in humans and are also innocuous; and (5) relatively few types account for most of the fatalities from pneumococcal pneumonias. If bacteremia complicates pneumococcal pneumonia, the case–fatality rate may reach 17% overall and exceed 25% in patients over 50 years in age, despite treatment with penicillin G. Hence, serotype prevalence among isolates from the blood has particular relevance to active immunization. As is shown in Figure 31-4, a vac-

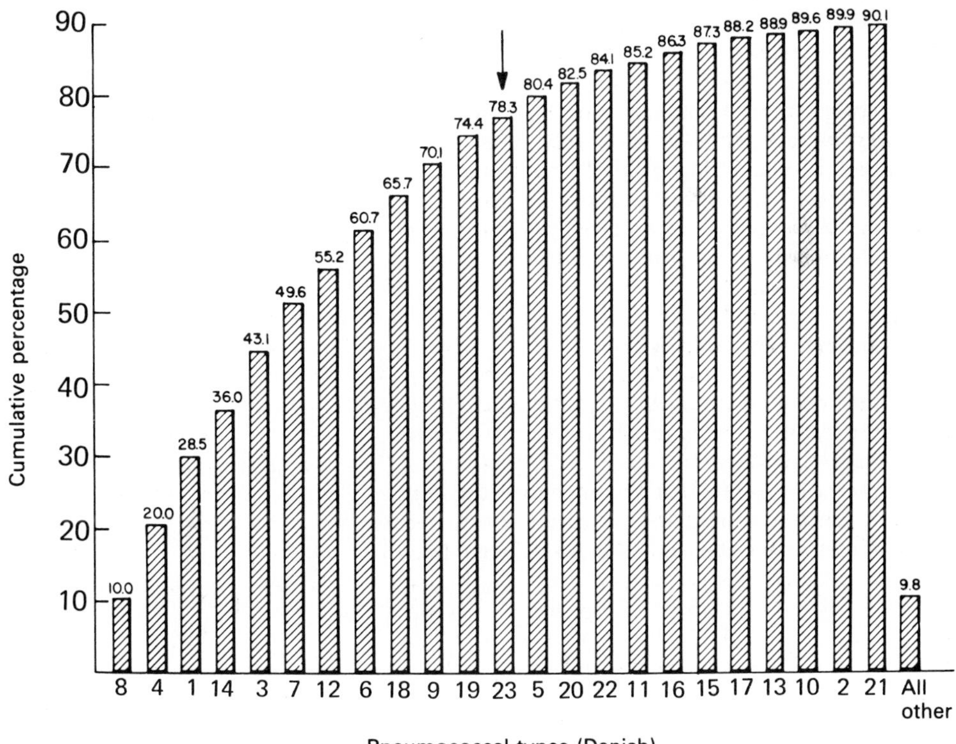

Fig. 31-4. Cumulative frequency of occurrence of serotypes of *Streptococcus pneumoniae* among 3644 isolations from the blood of patients with pneumococcal pneumonia during 1967–1975 in ten cities of the United States. (Austrian R, Douglas RM, Schiffman G, Coetzee AM, Koornhof HJ, Hayden–Smith S, Reid DW: Trans Assoc Am Phys 89:184–194, 1977)

cine containing 100 μg/ml of each of 14 serotypes (1, 2, 3, 4, 6A, 8, 9N, 12F, 14, 19F, 23F, 25, 7F, and 18C [Danish nomenclature]), enables active immunization against the serotypes that cause about 80% of bacteremic pneumococcal pneumonia. A single subcutaneous injection of 0.5 ml is generally well tolerated, with tenderness at the site of injection in about 40% of subjects, erythema in about 35%, and slight fever in about 3%. A humoral antibody response is engendered in 2 to 3 weeks. The efficacy of the vaccine in preventing pneumococcal disease in healthy young adults at high risk is 76% to 100%. Children under 2 years of age do not respond. Some 80% to 100% of adults over 45 years of age show a serologic response to the vaccine; however, a concomitant reduction in pneumococcal disease has not been proved. Patients who are immunodeficient may not develop antibodies. However, the vaccine is recommended for persons over 2 years in age who have splenic dysfunction or asplenia, and chronic illnesses including sickle cell anemia, multiple myeloma, cirrhosis, renal failure, alcoholism, diabetes mellitus, congestive heart failure, chronic pulmonary disease, and conditions associated with immunosuppression. The need for booster immunizations has not been established, but the interval will likely exceed 3 years.

At present, the group A and C meningococcal capsular polysaccharides, and the type b *H. influenzae* capsular polysaccharide are the only other specific preventive agents either proved immunogenic or under test; they are of numerically minimal importance to the prevention of bacterial pneumonias and are effective only in persons over 2 years in age.

Remaining Problems

The contribution of atmospheric pollutants to heightened vulnerability to bacterial pneumonias remains to be evaluated.

Antimicrobial agents that are safer than those previously available should be evaluated in the treatment of pneumonias caused by gram-negative bacilli.

Bibliography

Journals

AUSTRIAN R, DOUGLAS RM, SCHIFFMAN G, COETZEE AM, KOORNHOF HJ, HAYDEN–SMITH S, REID RDW: Prevention of pneumococcal pneumonia by vaccination. Trans Assoc Am Physicians 89:184–194, 1976

AUSTRIAN R, GOLD J: Pneumococcal bacteremia with special reference to bacteremic pneumococcal pneumonia. Ann Intern Med 60:759–776, 1964

BAYER AS, GUZE LB: *Staphylococcus aureus* bacteremic syndromes. Diagnostic and therapeutic update. DM 25:1–42, 1979

BROOME CV: Efficacy of pneumococcal polysaccharide vaccines. Rev Inf Dis 3(Suppl):82–88, 1981

DILWORTH JA, STEWART P, GWALTNEY JM JR, HENDLEY JO, SANDE MA: Methods to improve detection of pneumococci in respiratory secretions. J Clin Microbiol 2:453–455, 1975

GORBACH SL, BARTLETT JG: Anaerobic infections. N Engl J Med 290:1177–1184, 1237–1245, 1289–1294, 1974

GREEN GM: In defense of the lung. Am Rev Resp Dis 102:691–703, 1970

HERVA E, LUOTONEN J, TIMONEN M, SIBAKOV M, KARMA P, MAKELA PH: The effect of polyvalent pneumococcal polysaccharide vaccine on nasopharyngeal and nasal carriage of *Streptococcus pneumoniae*. Scand J Infect Dis 12:97–100, 1980

HIRSCHMANN JV, EVERETT ED: *Haemophilus influenzae* infection in adults. Reports of nine cases and review of the literature. Medicine 58:80–94, 1979

HOEPRICH PD: Etiologic diagnosis of lower respiratory tract infections. Calif Med 112:1–8, 1970

VAN METRE TE JR: Pneumococcal pneumonia treated with antibiotics. The prognostic significance of certain clinical findings. N Engl J Med 251:1048–1052, 1954

WOOD WB JR, SMITH MR: An experimental analysis of the curative action of penicillin in acute bacterial infections. I. The relationship of bacterial growth rates to the antimicrobial effect of penicillin. J Exp Med 103:487–498, 1956

SYDNEY M. FINEGOLD

Necrotizing Pneumonias and Lung Abscess

32

Necrotizing pneumonias are either acute or chronic suppurative processes; lung abscesses result from the localization and maturation of foci of necrotizing pneumonias. Neither is a distinct entity; both are clincopathologic conditions caused by many different agents that are not always easily differentiated.

Etiology

Anaerobes

Seventy percent to 90% of cases of necrotizing pneumonia and lung abscess involve anaerobic bacteria. In these conditions, anaerobic bacteria are found to the exclusion of other kinds of bacteria in one-half to two-thirds of cases. So-called nonspecific lung abscess is virtually always caused by anaerobes. Anaerobic bacteria are also quite important as causes of infection outside of pleuropulmonary areas (see Chap. 38, Actinomycosis; Chap. 53, Intrarenal and Perinephric Abscesses; Chap. 83, Appendicitis and Diverticulitis; Chap. 84, Pylephlebitis and Liver Abscess; Chap. 85, Subphrenic and Other Intraabdominal Abscesses; Chap. 125, Intracranial Suppuration; Chap. 126, Tetanus; Chap. 127, Botulism; Chap. 156, Gas Gangrene; Chap. 158, Infections Following Surgical Operations).

Modern specialized techniques necessary for the isolation and identification of anaerobic bacteria are now generally available in hospital diagnostic microbiology laboratories. Moreover, the taxonomic jungle which has impeded communication in this area has now been largely resolved.

The anaerobic bacteria which are most important as causes of disease in humans in all clinical situations including pulmonary infections are listed below. Of these, the anaerobes most often involved in necrotizing pneumonias and lung abscesses are the *Bacteroides melaninogenicus* group (Plate 32-1A), *Fusobacterium nucleatum* (Plate 32-1*E* and Fig. 32-1), various anaerobic cocci and streptococci (*Peptococcus* and *Peptostreptococcus,* Plate 32-1*A, B, C,* and *F*), and microaerophilic streptococci (Plate 32-1*B* and *G*). *Bacteroides fragilis* group strains (Fig. 32-2) and other β-lactamase-producing (penicillin-resistant) *Bacteroides* spp. are found in 15% of cases. *Fusobacterium necrophorum* (Plate 32-1*A* and Fig. 32-4), found frequently in the preantimicrobic era, is no longer encountered commonly. Spirochetes (*Treponema* spp.) are common and are often associated with *F. nucleatum* (so-called fusospirochetal disease), but their significance is doubtful. On the basis of experimental work, the *B. melaninogenicus* group may be key pathogens in this kind of mixed infection. The microaerophilic cocci are identical with species classified as aerobic (facultative) and officially belong in the genus *Streptococcus;* however, anaerobic techniques are often required for their isolation and characterization.

MAJOR ANAEROBES ENCOUNTERED CLINICALLY

Gram-negative bacilli

- *Bacteroides fragilis* group
- *Bacteroides melaninogenicus* group
- *Bacteroides ruminicola* ss. *brevis*
- *Bacteroides ureolyticus*
- *Bacteroides bivius*
- *Bacteroides disiens*
- *Fusobacterium nucleatum*
- *Fusobacterium necrophorum*
- *Fusobacterium naviforme*
- *Fusobacterium gonidiaformans*
- *Fusobacterium varium*
- *Fusobacterium mortiferum*

Gram-positive cocci

- *Peptococcus* (especially *P. magnus, P. asaccharolyticus, P. prevotii*)

Peptostreptococcus (especially *P. anaerobius, P. intermedius**, *P. micros*)
Microaerophilic cocci and streptococci

Gram-positive spore-forming bacilli
Clostridium perfringens
Clostridium ramosum
Clostridium septicum
Clostridium sporogenes
Clostridium sordellii
Clostridium difficile
Clostridium clostridiiforme
Clostridium innocuum

Gram-positive nonsporing bacilli
Actinomyces spp.
Arachnia spp.
Bifidobacterium eriksonii

**Peptostreptococcus intermedius* is actually microaerophilic and is properly placed in the genus *Streptococcus.*

Fig. 32-1. Microscopically, *Fusobacterium nucleatum* is long, thin, and crystallike with tapered ends. It stains pale pink by the gram method. (Finegold SM, Miller LG: The Anaerobic Bacteria. In Fredette V (ed): Proceedings Of An International Workshop, Oct. 1967. Laval-des-Rapides, P.Q., Canada, Institute of Microbiology and Hygiene, Montreal University)

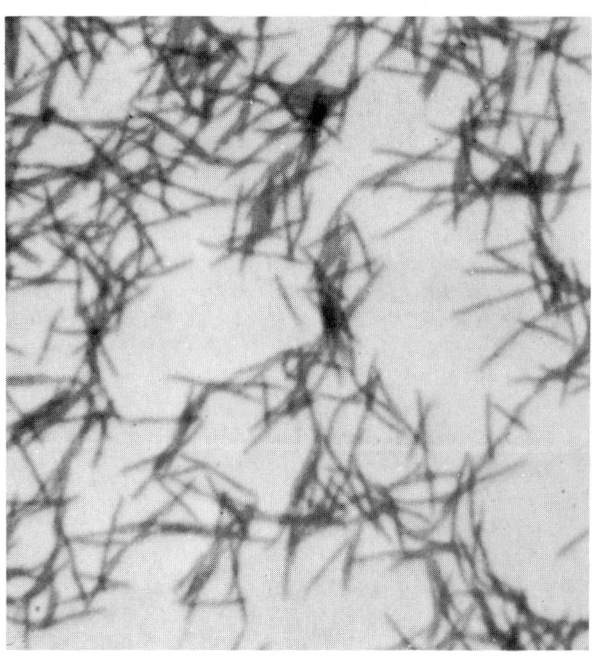

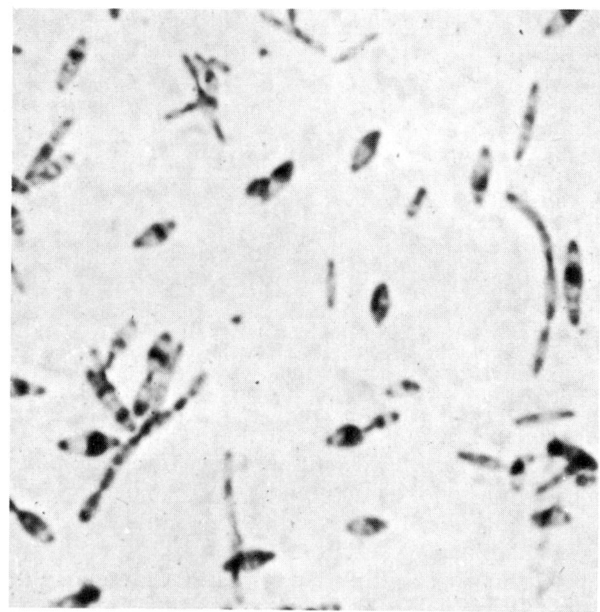

Fig. 32-2. Microscopic morphology of *Bacteroides fragilis*. Note the moderate degree of pleomorphism and the irregularity of staining. (Finegold SM, Miller LG: The Anaerobic Bacteria. In Fredette V (ed): Proceedings of an International Workshop, Oct. 1967. Laval-des-Rapides, P.Q., Canada, Institute of Microbiology and Hygiene, Montreal University)

Fig. 32-3. On microscopic examination, *Fusobacterium necrophorum* is highly pleomorphic. Note the long filaments with swellings and the large, free, round bodies. Irregularity of staining is also evident. (Finegold SM: Med Times 96:174–187, 1968)

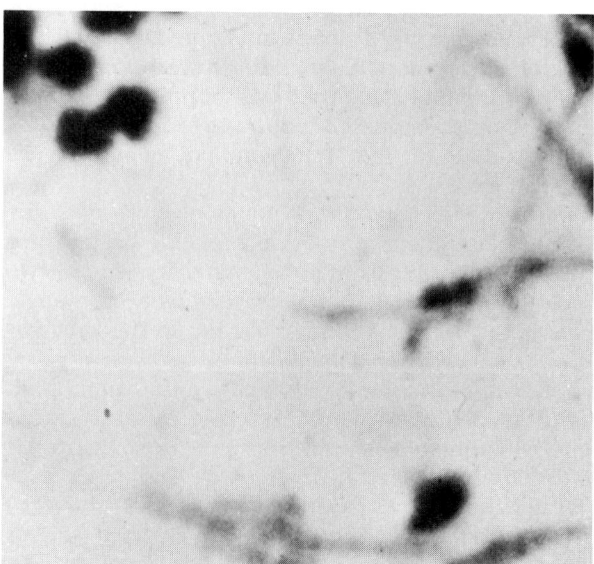

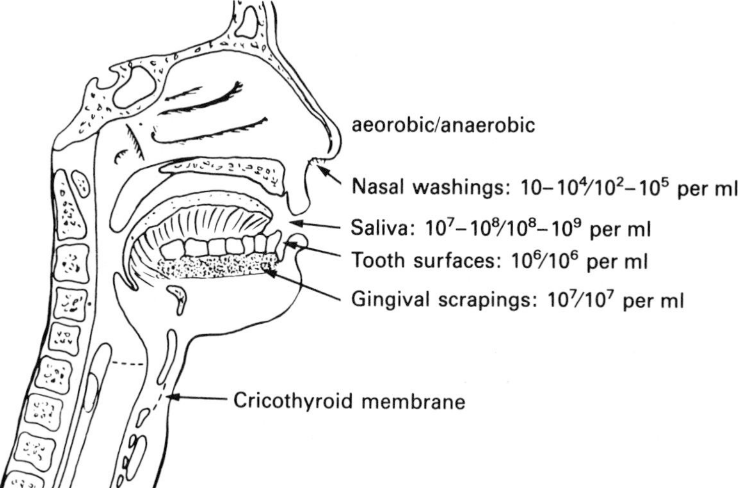

Fig. 32-4. Sagittal view of head and neck illustrating the high counts of anaerobic as well as aerobic bacteria that may be encountered as normal flora in various sites. Note that transtracheal aspiration through the cricothyroid membrane bypasses all sites of normal flora. (Hoeprich PD: Calif Med 112:1–8, 1970)

Because anaerobes are prevalent in the mouth and upper respiratory tract as normal flora (Table 32-1), expectorated sputum is unreliable for culture. Transtracheal aspiration (see Fig. 31-3) and transthoracic lung puncture are suitable techniques for bypassing normal oropharyngeal flora (Fig. 32-4). Specimens obtained with a rigid bronchoscope are not suitable. However, specimens collected through a flexible fiberoptic bronchoscope may prove to be useful if the following special precautions are observed: using a double lumen catheter containing a brush which is protected during insertion by a displaceable polyglycol plug; promptly placing specimens under anaerobic conditions immediately after collection; and employing quantitative anaerobic cultures. This remains to be established.

The unique morphology and staining characteristics of many anaerobes, given below, may enable the specific diagnosis to be predicted. *Actinomyces israelii* is an uncommon cause of necrotizing pneumonia (see Chap. 38, Actinomycosis).

BACTERIOLOGIC HINTS SUGGESTING POSSIBLE INFECTION WITH ANAEROBES

Gram stain of discharge (or subsequent culture growth) revealing (1) pale, irregularly staining, pleomorphic, slender gram-negative bacilli (*Bacteroides, Fusobacterium*), gram-negative rods with tapered ends (*Fusobacterium*); (2) large, broad, gram-positive bacilli, with or without spores (*Clostridium*); (3) thin, branching gram-positive bacilli (*Actinomyces, Eubacterium, Bifidobacterium*); or (4) tiny to small cocci or streptococci (anaerobic or microaerophilic cocci or streptococci) or cocci resembling staphylococci (*Peptococcus*).

No growth on routine culture—"sterile pus": growth in thioglycollate broth, or not.

Failure to grow, aerobically; organisms seen on Gram stain of original exudate.

Growth on mediums containing 100 μg/ml of kanamycin, neomycin, or paromomycin (or medium also containing 7.5 μg/ml of vancomycin, in the case of gram-negative anaerobic bacilli).

Production of much gas; foul odor in culture.

Growth in anaerobic zone of thioglycollate broth or of agar deeps.

Characteristic colonies on agar plates anaerobically.

Aerobes

The major aerobic causes of necrotizing pneumonia are *Staphylococcus aureus, Streptococcus pyogenes, Klebsiella pneumoniae,* and *Pseudomonas aeruginosa.* Although pneumococci only rarely cause lung abscess, type 3 is most commonly involved. Occasionally, other gram-negative bacilli, such as *Escherichia coli* and perhaps *Proteus* spp., may cause pulmonary necrosis. Uncommon but important causes of cavitating pneumonias are *Nocardia* spp. (see Chap. 37, Nocardiosis), *Legionella* spp. (see Chap. 33, Legionnaires Disease), *Pseudomonas pseudomallei* (see Chap. 141, Melioidosis), and *Entamoeba histolytica* (see Chap. 66, Amebiasis). Underlying tuberculosis must always be considered (see Chap. 34, Pul-

Table 32-1. *Incidence of Various Anaerobes as Normal Flora in the Human**

	Anaerobic Cocci	Anaerobic Gram-Negative Bacilli	Clostridia	Gram-Positive Nonsporulating Anaerobic Bacilli
Skin	++†			++ to+++
Upper respiratory tract‡	+++	++		+
Mouth	++++	+++	rare	++
Intestine	+++	++++	+++	+++
Genitourinary tract§	++	++	+	+ to ++

* After Rosebury T: Microorganisms Indigenous to Man. New York, McGraw-Hill, 1962.

† The ranking, + to ++++, reflects both consistency of occurrence and density of numbers.

‡ Includes nasal passages, nasopharynx, oropharynx, and tonsils.

§ Includes vagina, external genitalia, and urethra.

monary Tuberculosis). Cavitation may also occur in fungus infections (see Chap. 39, Candidosis; Chap. 40, Histoplasmosis; Chap. 41, Coccidioidomycosis; Chap. 42, Paracoccidioidomycosis; Chap. 43, Blastomycosis; Chap. 44, Aspergillosis).

Morphologic features that call to mind specific aerobes on direct smear include relatively large, round, gram-positive cocci separated from each other by half the diameter of a coccus (staphylococcus), lancet-shaped, gram-positive diplococci (pneumococcus), and gram-negative bacilli often showing bipolar staining with a trace of blue coloration (*Klebsiella* spp.). *Pseudomonas* spp. and other gram-negative bacilli may also show bipolar staining.

Epidemiology

Chronic lung abscess is uncommon at present, but acute necrotizing pneumonias are still seen frequently. The bacteria that cause these infectious diseases are elements of the normal flora and colonizers of the mouth and upper respiratory tract.

Pathogenesis and Pathology

Generally, there is no significant vascular involvement in either necrotizing pneumonia or lung abscess. However, pulmonary embolus (septic or bland) may be the initial event. Once underway, the infection itself may give rise to pulmonary arteritis, as in infection caused by *Pseudomonas* spp.

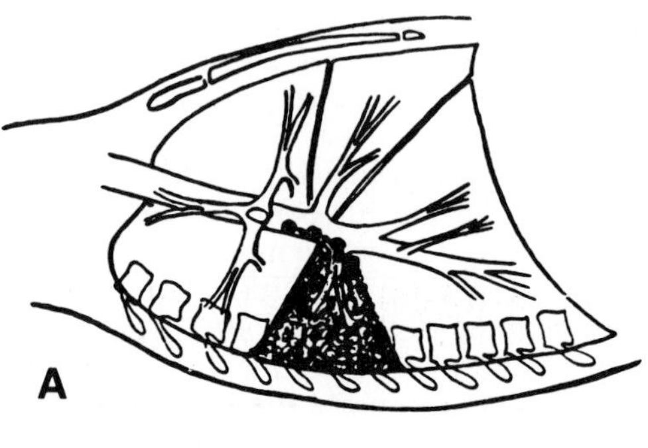

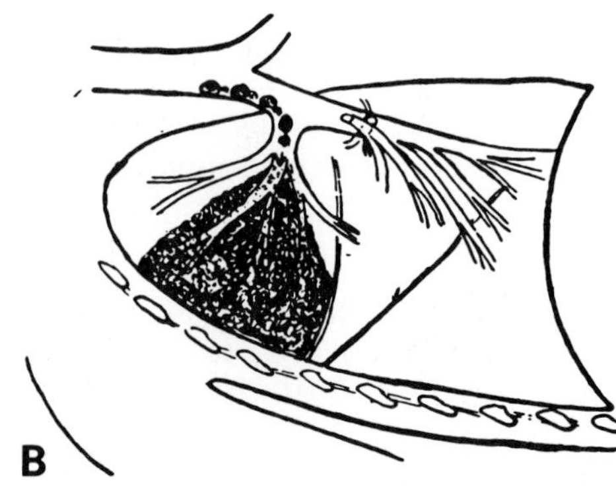

Fig. 32-5. Relationship between posture and localization of lung abscess. *(A)* With the patient on his back, the apical segment of the lower lobe is vulnerable. *(B)* With the patient on his side, the lateral and posterior portions of the upper lobe are affected. (Brock RC: Lung Abscess. Oxford, Blackwell Scientific Publications, 1952, p. 10)

The most common site of lung abscess is the posterior segment of the right upper lobe, with the same segment on the left less commonly affected. Next in frequency of involvement are the apical segments of both lower lobes. This distribution relates to the fact that inhalation or aspiration (bronchial embolism) is the primary incitant (Fig. 32-5). The inhaled material—saliva; nasal, oral, or nasopharyngeal secretions; blood; vomitus—is distributed according to gravity and the posture of the subject. Such inhalation of material occurs in many situations—for example, during sleep, deep narcosis and anesthesia, and after oral surgery. Normally, the inhaled matter is handled effectively by ciliary action, cough, and by alveolar macrophages. If the protective mechanisms are not effective, infection may result. Thick or particulate matter and foreign bodies are not easily removed and may produce bronchial obstruction and atelectasis. In aspiration pneumonia, gastric acid and enzymes are the primary offending agents.

Other important mechanisms leading to necrotizing pulmonary infection include the following: seeding as a result of bacteremia, with or without endocarditis; extension of infection by way of lymphatics and through the diaphragm (or defects in it); infection within or distal to a neoplastic obstruction of airway(s); and infection secondary to trauma to the chest. Gingivitis and periodontal disease are not infrequently the underlying problems. Other predisposing causes include alcoholic intoxication (Fig. 32-6), altered consciousness from any cause, factors tending to produce regurgitation, the postpartum or postabortal states, surgery (particularly oral surgery, tonsillectomy, and surgery on the bowel or genitourinary tract), pulmonary embolus (septic or not), and bronchogenic carcinoma.

The virulence of the infecting microorganism(s) and the size of the inoculum are the final factors that may determine the nature and extent of the necrotizing process.

During the early stages, the pathologic process of lung abscess is essentially that of an ordinary pneumonia. However, necrosis supervenes upon the inflammation. Later, the abscess cavity may be partially lined by regenerated epithelium, and local bronchiectasis and emphysema may develop.

Fig. 32-6. Posteroanterior *(A)* and lateral *(B)* chest films. Note lung abscess in the posterior portion of the right upper lobe. The bilateral multiple healed rib fractures are consistent with the history of chronic alcoholism. (Finegold SM: Med Times 96:174–187, 1968)

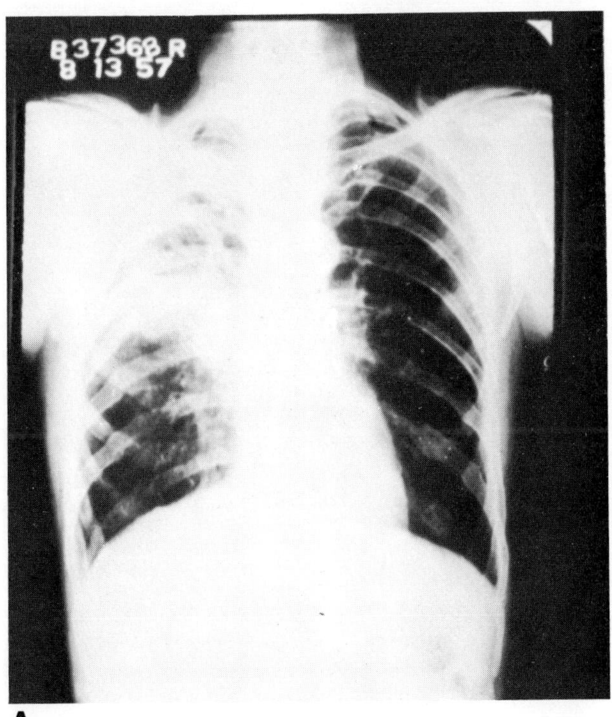

A

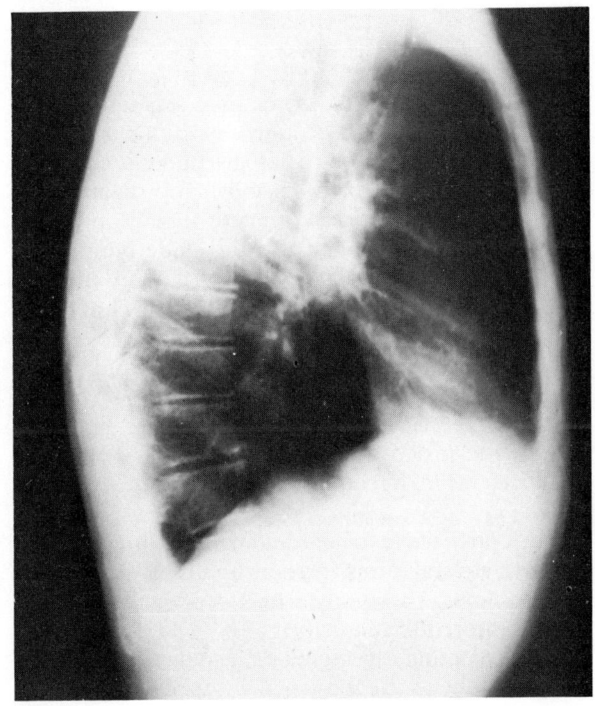

B

Manifestations

The usual picture is that of an acute pneumonic process, with fever, malaise, dry cough, and, frequently, pleuritic pain. Later, the cough becomes productive of copious amounts of purulent sputum that is usually foul smelling. The physical findings are those of a local pneumonia, with or without pleurisy; later, amphoric or cavernous breath sounds may be noted. Radiography occasionally reveals mediastinal lymphadenopathy in addition to the usual findings, making the differential diagnosis more difficult. Clubbing of the fingers occurs occasionally. Other findings, related to the pathogenetic factors, may be noted: diseased gums, absence of the gag reflex, and evidence of alcoholism. Leukocytosis and anemia are often present.

The onset is sometimes much more insidious than acute pneumonia. Weeks to months of malaise, low-grade fever, and cough, with significant weight loss and anemia, may precede consolidation. Neoplasia is a serious diagnostic consideration in such patients. Indeed, unless a definite abscess cavity is found, the diagnosis of necrotizing pneumonia without underlying cancer may first be made at the time of exploratory thoracotomy.

CLINICAL HINTS OF POSSIBLE INFECTION WITH ANAEROBES

Location of infection in proximity to a mucosal surface
Foul-smelling discharge
Necrotic tissue, gangrene
Infection producing gas in tissues or discharges
Infection associated with neoplastic or other processes producing tissue destruction
Infection related to the use of kanamycin, neomycin, or related agents (oral, parenteral, or topical)
Septic thrombophlebitis
Infection following human or other bites
Bacteroides melaninogenicus group strains may produce hematin in tissues, leading to black discoloration of exudate.
Lesions or discharges containing *Bacteroides melaninogenicus* group strains may fluoresce red under ultraviolet light.
Bacterial endocarditis with negative routine blood cultures
Presence of sulfur granules in discharges.

Diagnosis

Localization of a pneumonic process to a posterior upper lobe or superior lower lobe segment should suggest the possibility of lung abscess or aspiration pneumonia. Physical or radiologic findings of cavitation or an air-fluid level establish the diagnosis of lung abscess. However, complete definition of the process is important because the underlying problems vary widely in kind, prognosis, and therapy. Foul-smelling sputum is a very important clue to the diagnosis. Although anaerobic infections occur without a foul odor in about half of anaerobic pulmonary infections, the presence of such an odor is virtually unequivocal evidence that anaerobes are contributory to the process. Other clinical clues consistent with anaerobic infection in this setting are noted below.

The coexistence of carcinoma and lung abscess may take several forms and may be a difficult diagnostic problem. There may be secondary infection within a necrotic tumor (Fig. 32-7), infection distal to an obstructing carcinoma, or a spillover abscess in the same lobe as the tumor, in another lobe, or even in the other lung. Lung abscess in an edentulous person very often betokens bronchogenic carcinoma.

Fig. 32-7. Abscess, left upper lobe, within a carcinoma.

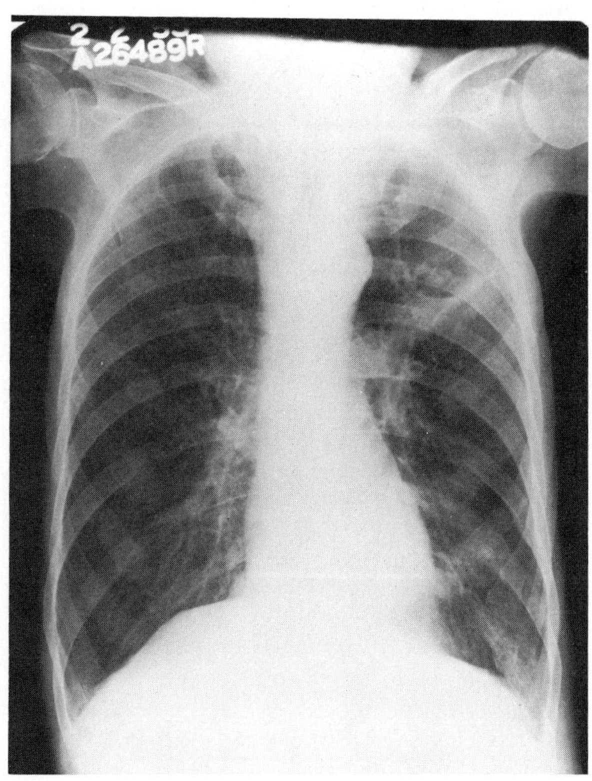

Differential diagnosis includes nonnecrotizing pneumonia, tuberculosis, carcinoma, infected lung cyst, bronchiectasis, and pyopneumothorax. It is important to keep in mind that rarefied areas may occasionally be seen in roentgenograms during the normal resolution of pneumonia.

Prognosis

The prognosis depends on the type of underlying or predisposing pathologic processes, if any, and, in the case of acute, severe necrotizing pneumonias, the speed with which appropriate therapy is instituted. Anaerobic lung abscess carries an overall mortality rate of 15% or less. The case fatality rate is significantly higher in acute pneumonias caused by *Staphylococcus aureus, Klebsiella* spp., *Pseudomonas* spp., and in anaerobic necrotizing pneumonias.

The most common complication is empyema, with or without bronchopleural fistula (also seen with high frequency). General infection occurs occasionally. The spillover of pus sometimes leads to the spread of infection and even, rarely, to asphyxiation. Other complications are now rare; these include brain or other distal abscesses, severe hemorrhage, and secondary amyloidosis. Superinfections caused by other bacteria or by fungi may occur in relation to antimicrobial therapy. In chronic lung abscess, there may be local bronchiectasis with subsequent recurrences of acute pneumonitis in the involved area. Loss of a variable amount of lung volume may occur.

Carcinoma is diagnosed relatively easily in patients with infection distal to the tumor. On the other hand, abscesses excavated in neoplasms present a serious paradox in that there will often be subjective and objective evidence of response to antibacterial therapy. It may be impossible to detect the neoplasm without thoracotomy. Such abscesses may achieve stability and even apparent cure with "residual fibrosis," only to reappear as inoperable carcinoma as long as 2 to 3 years later. Factors increasing the likelihood of a primary malignancy include the edentulous state, a history of cigarette smoking in the older age groups, the absence of precipitating causes for abscess (particularly aspiration), the location of an abscess in a nondependent bronchopulmonary segment, and the presence of hemoptysis or localized wheeze.

Therapy

Antimicrobial therapy is the keystone of treatment. Prolonged therapy is important to prevent relapse; the actual duration of treatment must be individualized, but periods of 2 to 4 months are often required.

Drugs effective against various anaerobes are listed in Table 32-2. Chloramphenicol is uniformly active. Tetracycline is less effective because many strains of the *B. fragilis* group and anaerobes of virtually all other kinds are now resistant. Doxycycline and minocycline are more active than tetracycline, but there are resistant strains in most anaerobic species. Penicillin G is more active than most of the other penicillins and the cephalosporins; penicillin and ampicillin are roughly comparable. Carbenicillin, ticarcillin, piperacillin, and mezlocillin, are active against 95% of strains of the *B. fragilis* group because very high concentrations may be safely attained in the blood. Cefoxitin, a β- lactamase-resistant cephamycin, is active against 90% to 95% of the *B. fragilis* group strains and against most other anaerobes except for about one-third of clostridia of species other than *C. perfringens.* Cefamandole has poor activity against the *B. fragilis* group. Other penicillins and cephalospirins are usually considerably less active. Clindamycin and metronidazole are very effective drugs.

The seriously ill patient with necrotizing pneumonia or lung abscess that may be caused by anaerobes should be treated with either clindamycin plus penicillin, metronidazole plus penicillin, or chloramphenicol without delay for bacteriologic diagnosis and susceptibility testing. In the adult, the succinate derivative of chloramphenicol should be given IV in a dose of 30 mg to 60 mg/kg body wt/day as four equal portions, 6-hourly. When the situation becomes less critical, peroral administration can be substituted—25 mg to 30 mg/kg body wt/day as four equal portions, 6-hourly. Penicillin G may be given if the *B. fragilis* group and other β-lactamase-producing anaerobes are known to be absent; it should be injected IV during the time of desperate illness in a dose of 150 mg to 200 mg (240,000 to 320,000 units)/kg body wt/day as six equal portions, 4-hourly.

The usual adult patient with lung abscess is not critically ill and generally responds quite satisfactorily to potassium penicillin G injected in a dose of 35 mg to 70 mg (55,000 U–110,000 U)/kg body wt/day as four equal portions, 6-hourly, even if *B. fragilis* is present as part of a mixed flora; when there has been good clinical response, the regimen can be changed to 1 million units of procaine penicillin G injected intramuscularly every 12 hours. If alternatives to penicillin G must be employed, clindamycin can be given intravenously or orally (15 mg–30 mg/kg body wt/day as four equal portions, 6-hourly, or metronidazole given IV or PO (30 mg/kg body wt/day as four

Table 32-2. *Susceptibility of Anaerobes to Some Antimicrobics*

Antimicrobial	Microaerophilic and Anaerobic Cocci	*Bacteroides*		*Fusobacterium*		*Eubacterium* spp. and *Actinomyces* spp.	*Clostridium*	
		FRAGILIS	OTHER SPP.	*VARIUM*	OTHER SPP.		*PERFRINGENS*	OTHER SPP.
Penicillin G	3 to 4+*	1+	2 to 3+	2+	2 to 3+	4+	4+†	3+
Chloramphenicol	3+	3+	3+	3+	3+	3+	3+‡	3+‡
Tetracycline	2+	1+ to 2+	3+	2+ to 3+	2+ to 3+	2+ to 3+	2+	2+
Erythromycin§	2+ to 3+	1+	2 to 3+	1+	1+	3+	1+ to 2+	3+
Cefoxitin	3+	2+ to 3+	2 to 3+	2+	3+	3+	3+	3+
Clindamycin	2+ to 3+	3+†	3+†	1 to 2+	2 to 3+	3+†	3+‡	2+ to 3+
Vancomycin§	3+	1+	1+	1+	1+	?3+	3+	3+
Metronidazole	2+	3+	3+	3+	3+	1+ to 2+	3+	3+

* Key: 4+, drug of choice; 3+, good activity; 2+, moderate activity; 1+, poor or inconsistent activity.
† Few strains resistant.
‡ Rare strains resistant.
§ Not listed by the Food and Drug Administration for use in anaerobic infections.

equal portions, 6-hourly) with erythromycin in the same dose if facultative streptococci are also present. If a tetracycline is used, doxycycline (2 mg–3 mg/kg body wt as a loading dose, followed by half as much every 12 hours—either by IV injection or PO) is recommended; the dosage of doxycycline need not be altered because of renal failure.

Vancomycin is generally reserved for the treatment of staphylococcal infections, but it is sometimes useful in gram-positive anaerobic infections. It must be given intravenously in a dose of 25 mg to 30 mg/kg body wt/day as two equal portions, 12-hourly (adults with normal renal function).

For staphylococcal infections, a penicillinase-resistant penicillin (*e.g.,* nafcillin) is preferable, although the cephalosporins or vancomycin may be used. Penicillin G is the drug of choice for group A streptococcal and pneumococcal infections, with cefazolin, erythromycin, and clindamycin as secondary, alternative agents.

Gentamicin, tobramycin, or netilmicin (4 mg–6 mg/kg body wt/day by IM or IV injection of three equal portions, 8-hourly) is effective in infections caused by *P. aeruginosa;* supplementation with carbenicillin (300 mg–500 mg/kg body wt/day by IV injection of six equal portions, 4-hourly), ticarcillin, piperacillin, or mezlocillin (200 mg–300 mg/kg body wt/day, IV, as 6 equal portions, 4-hourly). The most active agent is amikacin (15 mg/kg body wt/day by IM or IV injection of two equal portions, 12-hourly). Amikacin, gentamicin, tobramycin, or netilmicin (dosage as above) are preferred for infections caused by *Klebsiella* spp., depending on individual strain susceptibility. These drugs would also be suitable for treating pneumonia caused by *Escherichia coli.*

If *Proteus mirabilis* is the etiologic agent, penicillin G should be injected IV in a dose of 200 mg (320,000 U)/kg body wt/day as six equal portions, 4-hourly. With the other *Proteus* spp., either amikacin, gentamicin, tobramycin, metilmicin, or kanamycin is appropriate.

Postural drainage is an important component of therapy for lung abscess. Bronchoscopy may occasionally be helpful in effecting good drainage, permitting removal of foreign bodies, and enabling biopsy diagnosis of tumors. Tracheostomy and frequent suctioning may be required in selected patients.

Surgical resection is rarely required unless there is a coexisting malignancy. There is a hazard of uncontrollable spread before medical control can be achieved. Surgical drainage of a lung abscess through the chest wall is almost never indicated.

In the case of gross aspiration and pneumonia, immediate clearing of the airway by postural drainage and suctioning, preferably by bronchoscopy, is important. Some clinicians feel that if the pH of the aspirated contents is less than 2.5, or if this cannot be determined, the patient should receive at least 100 mg hydrocortisone by IV injection followed by 1 mg/kg body wt/ (either IV or PO) every 6 to 8 hours for 3 days to suppress the inflammation of the chemical pneumonitis. The value of this regimen is not established; indeed, it is quite questionable. Penicillin G should be administered intramuscularly in a dose of 1 megaunit every 6 hours for several days.

Prevention

Situations that facilitate the aspiration of liquids or solids into the tracheobronchial tree should be avoided—for example, if possible, general anesthesia should not be used for tonsillectomy, tooth extraction, and surgery on the paranasal sinuses. Nasogastric tube feedings should be administered with great care to avoid aspiration. The head of the bed should be elevated for patients with achalasia or similar problems. If aspiration does occur, the foreign material should be removed promptly.

Acute pneumonias and bacteremias should be treated promptly with appropriate drugs.

Remaining Problems

Definition of the bacterial etiology of necrotizing pneumonias is necessary. Such information requires careful anaerobic and aerobic cultures of specimens obtained by transtracheal aspiration.

Techniques for washing sputum free of mouth flora and for liquefying the sputum to permit even distribution of microorganisms may facilitate accurate bacteriologic diagnosis.

Bibliography

Books

BEERENS H, TAHON-CASTEL M: Infections Humaines à Bactéries Anaérobies Non Toxigènes. Bruxelles, Presses Academiques Européennes, 1965, 194 pp.

BROCK RC: Lung Abscess. Springfield, Charles C Thomas, 1952, 197 pp.

FINEGOLD SM: Anaerobic Bacteria in Human Disease. New York, Academic Press, 1977, 710 pp.

HOLDEMAN LV, CATO EP, MOORE WEC: Anaerobe Laboratory Manual, 4th ed. Blacksburg, Virginia Polytechnic Institute & State University, 1977, 152 pp.

PRÉVOT AR: Biologie des Maladies dues aux Anaerobies. Paris, Ernest Flammarion, 1955, 572 pp.

SUTTER VL, CITRON DM, FINEGOLD SM: Wadsworth Anaerobic Bacteriology Manual, 3rd edition, St. Louis, C.V. Mosby, 1980, 131 pp.

Journals

BARTLETT JG, FINEGOLD SM: Anaerobic infections of the lung and pleural space. Am Rev Respir Dis 110:56–77, 1974

BARTLETT JG, GORBACH SL, FINEGOLD SM: The bacteriology of aspiration pneumonia. Am J Med 56:202–207, 1974

BARTLETT JG, GORBACH SL, TALLY FP, FINEGOLD SM: Bacteriology and treatment of primary lung abscess. Am Rev Respir Dis 109:510–518, 1974

JORDAN GW, WONG GA, HOEPRICH PD: Bacteriology of the lower respiratory tract as determined by fiberoptic bronchoscopy and transtracheal aspiration. J Infect Dis 134:428–435, 1976

KIRBY BD, GEORGE WL, SUTTER VL, CITRON DM, FINEGOLD SM: Gram-negative anaerobic bacilli: Their role in infection and patterns of susceptibility to antimicrobial agents. I. Little-known *Bacteroides* species. Rev Infect Dis 2:914–951, 1980

RICHARD D. MEYER

33 Legionnaires' Disease and Related Infections

The appellation *Legionnaires' disease* derives from an outbreak of respiratory tract disease that afflicted war veterans attending a convention in Philadelphia in 1976. Subsequently, investigators at the Centers for Disease Control isolated and identified the causative bacterium, *Legionella pneumophila.* Serologic and bacteriologic methods were developed, which enabled retrospective diagnosis of sporadic cases dating from 1947, and major outbreaks since 1965 (Table 33-1). The manifestations of infection caused by *L. pneumophila* are protean and include asymptomatic seroconversion, nonspecific febrile illness, and fulminant pneumonia. Subsequently, microorganisms were isolated from patients with pneumonia which were not *L. pneumophila* but were atypical, or *Legionella* like, bacteria.

Etiology

Legionella pneumophila is weakly gram negative; that is, it retains the safranin counterstain so poorly that it is usually too pale to be seen in clinical specimens but will be visible in smears from cultures. It is not acid fast. The Dieterle silver impregnation stain and the Gimenez stain (see Chap. 9, Microscopic Examinations) are suitable.

Normally bacillary in shape (0.3 μm to 0.9 μm wide by 2 μm to 3 μm long) (Fig. 33-1*A*), *L. pneumophila* occasionally takes the form of elongated bacilli, and coiled or filamentous forms >50 μm long are seen in cultures or in tissues (Fig. 33-1). Spores are not formed. Polar and bipolar flagella have been demonstrated. Electron microscopy reveals the two triple unit membranes and cytoplasmic vacuoles typical of gram-negative bacilli (Fig. 33-1*B*).

Legionella pneumophila grows best at 35°C in an atmosphere of 2.5% to 5.0% CO_2; the optimal pH is 6.9 to 7.0. Cysteine and methionine are required, and growth will occur on enriched mediums including supplemented Mueller–Hinton agar medium. However, the best culture medium now available both for isolation and passage is buffered charcoal–yeast extract agar. The convex, circular, glistening grey colonies form in two sizes: >2 mm and <1 mm in diameter. The yolk sacs of embryonated hens' eggs and the peritoneal cavities of guinea pigs will also support growth.

The oxidase and catalase reactions are weakly positive. If 1-tyrosine and 1-phenylalanine are constituents of the culture medium, a brown, water-soluble melanin is produced. A β-lactamase is elaborated which is particularly active against the cephalosporins and is little affected by clavulinic acid. Large amounts of unusual branched chain fatty acids are cell constituents; these appear to be unique, and detection by gas chromatography is useful for identification. Base ratio analysis and DNA homology studies have shown that *Legionella* is a distinct genus. Based on antigenic differences, six serologic groups of *L. pneumophila* have been distinguished by immunofluorescence. Most of the isolates associated with disease belong to group I (prototype strains Knoxville and Philadelphia), with fewer isolates in group II (Togus), group III (Bloomington), group IV (Los Angeles), group V (Dallas), and group VI (Chicago). Some environmental isolates do not fit into recognized serogroups.

Legionellas other than *L. pneumophila* can be isolated primarily on charcoal–yeast extract agar and show similar biochemical reactions (Table 33-2). *Legionella micdadei* is, however, weakly acid fast with the Kinyoun stain. The colonies of *Legionella bozemanii* and *Legionella dumoffii* may show a blue fluorescence under ultraviolet light, but neither elaborates a β-lactamase. Some of these non-*pneumophila* legionellas can be differentiated by cellular fatty acid analyses, but DNA hydridization studies may be necessary.

Table 33-1. *Reported Clinical Infections Caused by* Legionella pneumophila

Type	Predominant Pattern*	Time	Place	Cases†
Pneumonic	Sporadic	1947–1979	United States	1005‡
	Epidemic	1965	Washington, D.C. Hospital	81
		1974	Philadelphia, PA, Hotel	20
		1976	Philadelphia, PA, Hotel	182§
		1977	Kingsport, TN, Hospital; area	33
		1978	Atlanta, GA, Golf course	8
		1978	Memphis, TN, Hospital	39
		1978	Dallas, TX, Convention	18
		1979	Eau Claire, WI, Hotel	12
		1979	Jamestown, NY, Factory	7
		1979	Västerås, Sweden, Shopping center	67
		1980	San Francisco, CA, Office building	8
	Hyperendemic	1973–1980	Benidorm, Spain, Hotel	≥20
		1976–1979	Norwalk, CN, Hospital	28
		1977–1979	Burlington, VT, Hospital and community	≥75
		1980	Burlington, VT, Hospital and community	~75
		1977–1981	Los Angeles, CA, Hospital	218
		1977–1979	Bloomington, IN, Hotel	39
		1977–1979	Columbus, OH, Hospital	25
		1978	New York, NY, Limited area	38
		1979–1980	Pittsburgh, PA, Hospital	25
Nonpneumonic	Epidemic	1968	Pontiac, MI, Building	144
		1973	James River, VT, Steam turbine condenser	10

* Centers for Disease Control epidemiologic classification used for cases from the United States (Cordes LG, Fraser DW: Legionellosis Med Clin North Am 64:395–416, 1980).

† Criteria for case definition vary.

‡ Additional cases reported in diverse areas worldwide.

§ 221 total cases.

Epidemiology

Legionella pneumophila appears to be widely distributed in soil and water. Survival in tap water for extended periods has been documented. Isolation of *L. pneumophila* has been accomplished from thermal effluents in association with blue green algae, fresh water lakes not known to be associated with disease, a number of cooling towers and evaporative condensers, and from shower water and tap water associated with outbreaks. Only in Pontiac, Michigan, and Memphis, Tennessee, were defective air-conditioning units directly related to outbreaks, although spatial and temporal relationships were found elsewhere.

Legionnaires' disease exists both as sporadic cases and outbreaks (see Table 33-1). Sporadic cases have occurred in all areas of the United States and have been reported from Australia, Canada, Great Britain, Israel, New Zealand, Scandinavia, and most of the countries of Western and Mediterranean Europe. In temperate areas of the northern hemisphere, the incidence is highest from June to October. The age span is 15 months to 84 years, but persons ≥ 50 years of age predominate. Males contract the disease more often than females. Other risk factors include smoking, alcohol abuse, immunosuppression, and chronic disease such as cardiopulmonary or renal disease. However, apparently healthy persons may contract severe disease, and asymptomatic persons may have had the disease. For example, the rates of indirect fluorescent antibody titers ≥ 1:128 vary, ranging from 1.3% nationwide, to 17% for groundskeepers in Los Angeles, to 22% for maintenance workers in New York City.

Legionella pneumophila may account for 1% to 4.1% of community-acquired pneumonias. Among fatalities from nosocomial pneumonias, 3.8% were caused by *L. pneumophila* and were sporadic infections occurring in geographically separate areas. The

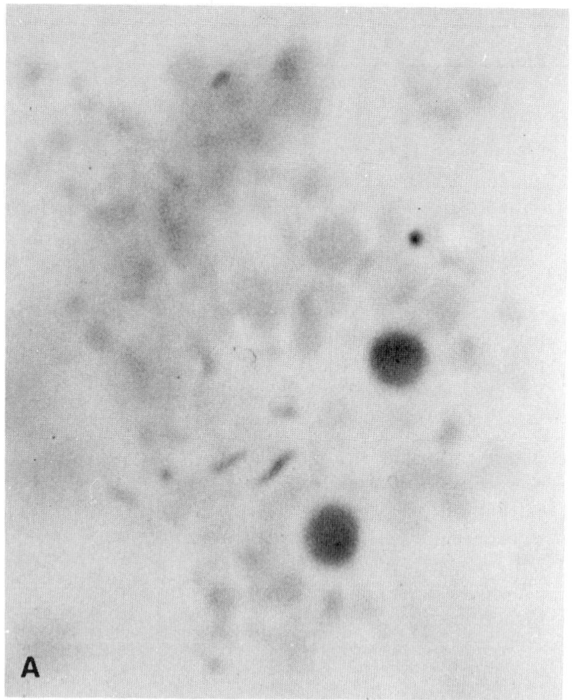

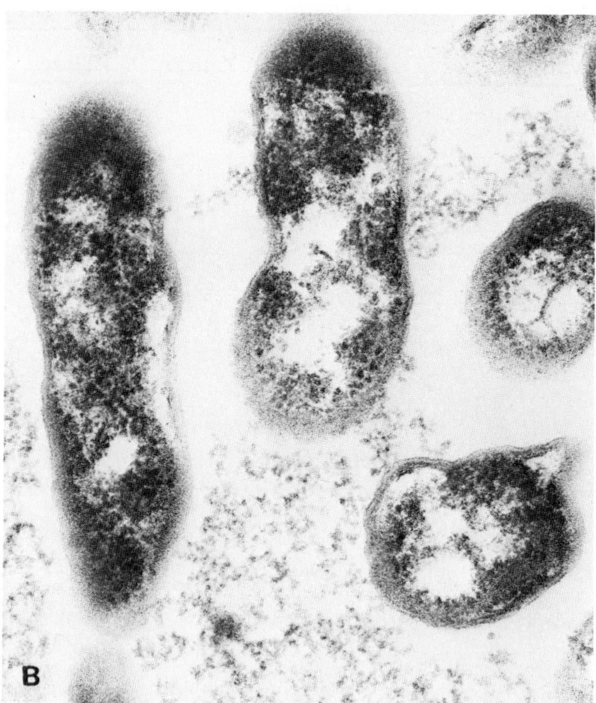

Fig. 33-1. *(A)* Gimenez stain of *Legionella pneumophila* from egg yolk sac culture. The usual bacillary form is shown along with elongated forms. (Original magnification × 1200) (Courtesy of Dr. Paul H. Edelstein) *(B)* Electron photomicrograph of *Legionella pneumophila* in human alveolar macrophage illustrating the two triple-layer membranes and vacuoles. (Original magnification × 59,800) (Courtesy of Drs. T. Stanley and F. Hernandez)

attack rate was 0.5% of admissions studied prospectively in one hospital.

The epidemiology of infections caused by non-*pneumophila Legionella* spp. is less clear. Patients with nonpneumonic disease in Pontiac and James River were younger, and nearly all of them were previously in good health.

Pathogenesis and Pathology

Legionnaires' disease appears to be acquired by inhalation of infected aerosols. Proliferation of *L. pneumophila* that has lodged in alveoli and terminal bronchioles leads to retrograde spread to larger bronchioles, and to the interstitium, pleuras, and lymphatics. Fever, rigors, and extrapulmonary manifestations could be the result of a toxin or toxins (not documented), or bacteremia (which has been documented). Endotoxin derived from *L. pneumophila* has relatively little activity in biological assays. Hemolysin, protease, and cytotoxic activities have been found, but they are of unproved pathogenetic significance.

Lobar consolidation and a fibrinous pleuritis are the major, common pathologic findings. Serous or serosanguinous pleural effusions are frequent. Although pulmonary nodules are found with *L. pneumophila* and the other *Legionella* spp., abscesses are uncommon. Histologic demonstration of *L. pneumophila* in hilar and other lymph nodes, the liver, spleen, kidneys, heart, or bone marrow has rarely been accomplished.

The intense inflammatory response in the alveoli consists of varying proportions of intact and lysed neutrophiles and macrophages bathed in proteinaceous exudate. The alveolar septa are generally spared; however, acute, diffuse alveolar damage and fibrosis have been seen after oxygen therapy. *Legionella pneumophila* survives inside pulmonary alveolar macrophages and is located mostly in phagolysosomes and also in the cytoplasm.

Routine tissue stains will not disclose *L. pneumophila,* although the Gimenez stain will reveal the ba-

Table 33-2. Summary of Reported Disease Caused by Legionella Pneumophila-like *Bacteria (Culture Positive)*

Proposed Name	Location and Name of Isolate	Date	Focus	Cases	Deaths	Comments
Legionella micdadei	Fort Bragg, NC * (Tatlock)	1943	Same	7		Isolate probably incidental to disease caused by leptospira
	* (Heba)	1959		1		? Sporadic (Pityriasis rosea)
	* Pittsburgh, PA	1978	University hospital	8	5	6 renal transplant recipients 2 others —steroid therapy
	* Charlottesville, VA	1978 –1979	Hospital	5	2	4 renal transplant recipients 1 lymphoma patient
Legionella bozemanii	* (WIGA)	1959	Key West, FL	1	1	Scuba diver; bronchopneumonia
	Decatur,GA * *(GA–PH)*	1978	Fresh water lake So. Carolina	1	1	Chronic lymphocytic leukemia
Legionella dumoffii	Houston, TX * *(TEX–KL)*	1979	?	1	1	Oat cell carcinoma of lung
Legionella longbeachae	California Georgia	1979	? Sporadic	4	1	4 steroid therapy

* Recovery of isolate

Additional serocoversion cases known. *Legionella gormani* (LS-13) and *L. jordanis* are environmental isolates (cases with seroconversion known).

cilli when applied to fresh or fixed lung tissue. If the Brown-Brenn tissue Gram stain is applied to tissue imprints, faintly staining *L. pneumophila* may be discerned, and *L. bozemanii* will be visible. Specific histologic diagnosis can be made using the direct fluorescent antibody test with polyvalent or monovalent antiserum directed against *L. pneumophila* or other *Legionella* spp.

Manifestations

Pneumonic Form

The clinical manifestations of Legionnaires' disease range from asymptomatic infection, to a mild febrile illness, to pneumonia, which is frequently severe and is the most commonly recognized form of disease. After an incubation period of 2 to 10 days, the disease begins with malaise, weakness, lethargy, anorexia, headache, and myalgia. Watery diarrhea occurs in about half of the patients, but abdominal pain is uncommon. Nausea and vomiting is not uncommon. Coryza and pharyngitis are unusual. A cough ensues; initially it is dry and becomes productive of nonpurulent or minimally purulent grayish secretions in about one-half of the patients. Hemoptysis is frequent. Rales may be heard before there is evidence of an infiltrate on radiographs. Pleuritic chest pain develops in about one-third of the patients, but physical evidence of pleural effusion is uncommon. Pulmonary consolidations may extend directly and may develop in apparently uninvolved lung as the disease progresses.

Almost all patients become febrile; the rise in temperature may be step wise and leads to an unremitting fever of $\geqslant$ 39°C. Shaking chills, which are recurrent, are observed in most of the patients. Severe sweats are noted in about one-fourth of the patients. Relative bradycardia is seen in two-thirds of the patients. The fever responds to specific antimicrobial therapy but not to antipyretics or to glucosteroids.

In about 25% of patients neuropsychiatric dysfunctions take the form of confusion, disorientation, obtundation, depression, emotional liability, insomnia, hallucinations, grand mal seizures, delerium, retrograde amnesia, and ataxia. Infrequently, there is tender hepatomegaly, jaundice, or gastrointestinal bleeding. Myositis or rhabdomyolysis is rare. Renal failure is usually related to hypotension or shock.

With *Legionella* spp. other than *L. pneumophila*, the clinical manifestations are similar, but the extrapulmonary manifestations are less prominent. Some patients with *L. micdadei* infections have had a more slowly progressing course and were afebrile when pulmonary infiltrates were seen on radiographs.

Nonpneumonic Form

The incubation period is shorter (usually ≤ 48 hr) followed by 2 to 5 days of malaise, chills, fever, headache and myalgia. Diarrhea and neurologic symptoms are infrequent. Although there may be symptoms of upper respiratory disease, cough, and even rales, radiographs of the chest have not shown infiltrates.

Diagnosis

At present, the most rapid method for specific diagnosis of pneumonia caused by *L. pneumophila* is direct immunofluorescent examination of expectorated sputum, transtracheal aspirates, pleural fluid, endotracheal tube aspirates, bronchoscopic washings, lung aspirates, or lung biopsies. The only known cross reactions occur with rare strains of *Pseudomonas fluorescens, Pseudomonas aeruginosa,* and *Bacteroides fragilis.*

Specimens suitable for immunofluorescence microscopy are also suitable for culture. However, growth may not be apparent for 3 to 10 days. Inoculation of the yolk sacs of embryonated hens' eggs and intraperitoneal injection of guinea pigs are additional methods for isolation that are available in certain reference centers. The non-*pneumophila Legionella* spp. can be isolated using similar methods.

Examinations of the blood and urine reveal abnormalities consistent with an acute infectious disease. The more severely ill the patient, the more pronounced the abnormalities. For example, leukocytosis, with or without immature forms, is common, whereas leukopenia, thrombocytopenia, and disseminated intravascular clotting are uncommon. Hematuria and hyaline, granular, or red blood cell casts occur uncommonly, but proteinuria is common; acute renal failure with myoglobinuria and nonoliguric renal failure is rare. Hyponatremia and abnormalities of liver function tests are common, whereas the concentrations of creatine phosphokinase and aldolase are only rarely abnormal.

The findings on radiographic examination of the chest are not specific. Thus, the lower lobes are commonly involved with a patchy alveolar infiltrate, which progresses to consolidation. As the disease evolves, it may become evident in ipsilateral or contralateral areas (Figs. 33-2, 33-3, 33-4, 33-5). Pleural effusions occur in about half the patients and may be found before infiltrates become evident. Nodular infiltrates and cavities are uncommon with *L. pneumophila* but are seen more often with other *Legionella* spp.

Specimens of serum for the indirect fluorescent antibody test should be obtained at the onset of illness and at least every other week for 6 to 8 weeks. Current criteria for serologic confirmation of the diagnosis are a fourfold rise in titer to ≥ 1:128, with compatible clinical disease. A convalescent titer ≥ 1:256 with compatible clinical disease is presumptive evidence. Cross reactions occur with plague, tularemia, leptospirosis, and rarely in association with *Bacteroides fragilis* bacteremia. About 65% of the patients become seropositive at 3 weeks, and an additional 25% by 6 weeks. That is, at least 10% of patients infected with *L. pneumophila* fail to show seroconversion even if all available antigens are tested.

Other causes for pneumonia must be differentiated from *L. pneumophila.* Recurrent rigors are more

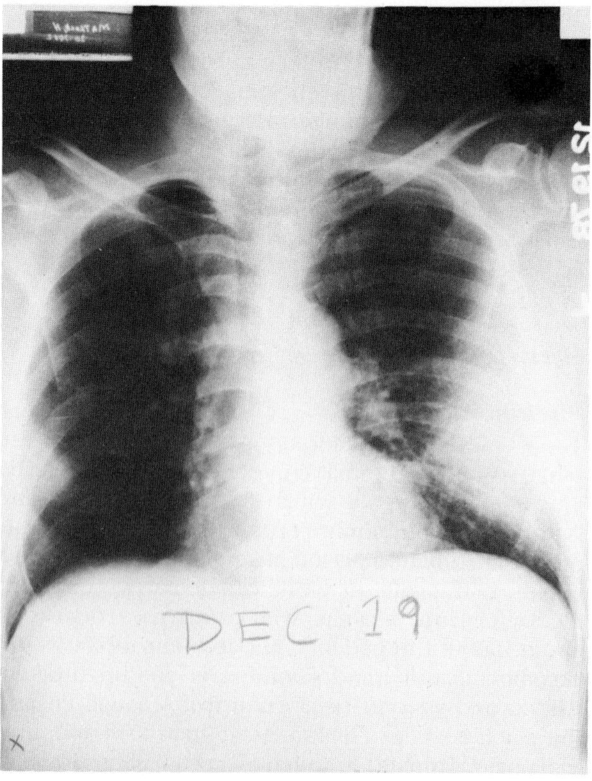

Fig. 33-2. Posterior–anterior chest radiograph with pleural based infiltrate in left lower lobe (superior segment). The patient had fever, shaking chills, pleuritic pain, and bloody sputum.

common with *L. pneumophila* than with uncomplicated pneumococcal pneumonia (see Chap. 31, Bacterial Pneumonias). *Mycoplasma pneumoniae* usually causes disease in a younger age group; the cough is hacking and more prominent (see Chap. 30, Nonbacterial Pneumonias). Pulmonary infiltrates in psittacosis are usually less prominent than with *Legionella* spp. The infiltrate in Q fever is usually diffuse and interstitial. Influenza, adenovirus infections, plague (see Chap. 140, Plague), and tularemia (see Chap. 139, Tularemia) are also manifest as pneumonias. Immunoincompetence should always alert the physician to the possibility of infection caused by *L. pneumophila* or other *Legionella* spp. Failure to isolate common bacterial pathogens or failure of response to therapy with multiple antimicrobial agents are the least specific aids to diagnosis of Legionnaires' disease.

Prognosis

The presence of underlying diseases and the specific therapy that is applied greatly influence the prognosis. Thus, the fatality rate will vary from < 10% in treated, nonimmunosuppressed patients to 80% in untreated immunosuppressed patients.

Some patients with severe clinical illness will improve spontaneously between the sixth and tenth day, and will recover after a long convalescence. Infiltrates may progress or clear slowly despite appropriate therapy and apparent clinical recovery. A decrease in the diffusing capacity of the lungs after therapy is uncommon. Convalescence may be marred by persistent malaise, weakness, easy fatigability, and, rarely, confusion, aphasia, ataxia, or retrograde amnesia. Second occurrences of infections with *L. pneumophila* are more likely reinfections than late relapses.

Therapy

The results of susceptibility tests *in vitro* do not correlate well with the clinical outcome of therapy. Erythromycin and rifampin are effective in experimental infections in guinea pigs induced with *L. pneumophila*. Clinically, the penicillins, cephalosporins, aminocyclitols, cefoxitin, and clindamycin are ineffective, whereas erythromycin is the most effective drug. A dosage of 30 to 60 mg/kg body weight/day should be given as four equal portions every 6 hours, either perorally or intravenously (seriously ill patients) for at least three weeks. Chloramphenicol is usually ineffective. The tetracyclines are probably somewhat effective but should not be used alone. Rifampin, 10 to 15 mg/kg body weight/day given perorally as two equal portions every 12 hours, can be used in combination with erythromycin or one of the tetracyclines; rifampin should not be used as a single agent. The treatment of disease caused by the non-*pneumophila Legionella* spp. is identical.

Prevention

Investigations to discover and interrupt the source of *Legionella* spp. may be effective. Hyperchlorination of cooling towers and potable water is under evaluation. No vaccine is currently available.

Fig. 33-3. Posterior–anterior chest radiograph showing clearing of a left lower lobe infiltrate and new right nodular pleural-based infiltrate. The latter was aspergillosis at postmortem examination. (Meyer RD et al: Ann Intern Med 93:240–243, 1980)

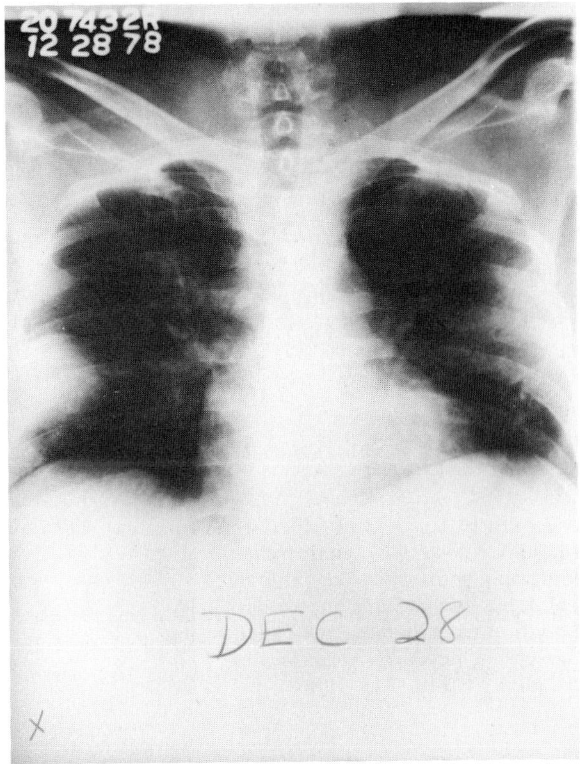

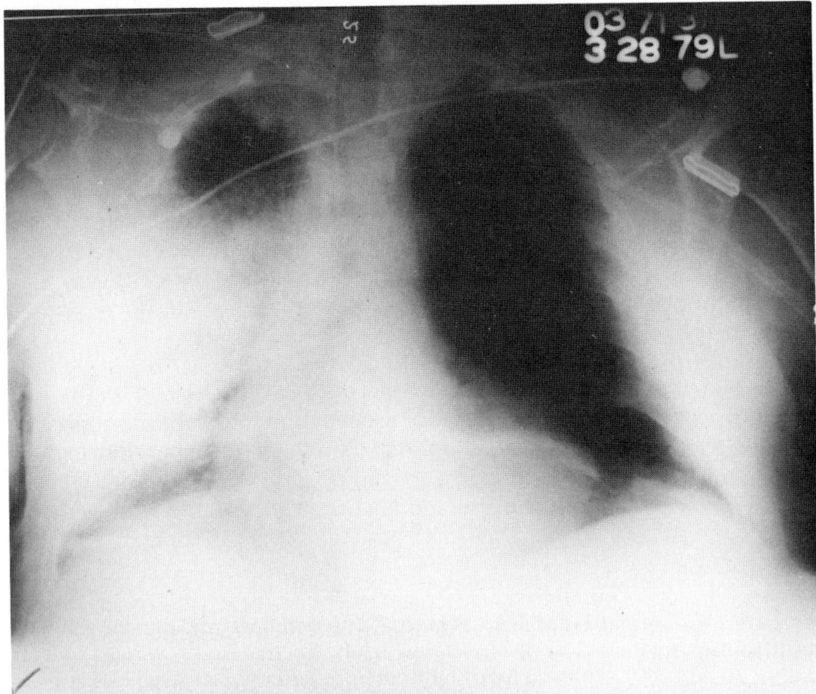

Fig. 33-4. Posterior–anterior chest radiograph demonstrating a dense right midlung field infiltrate extending to the pleura and involving all lobes on the right. The margins show alveolar infiltrates.

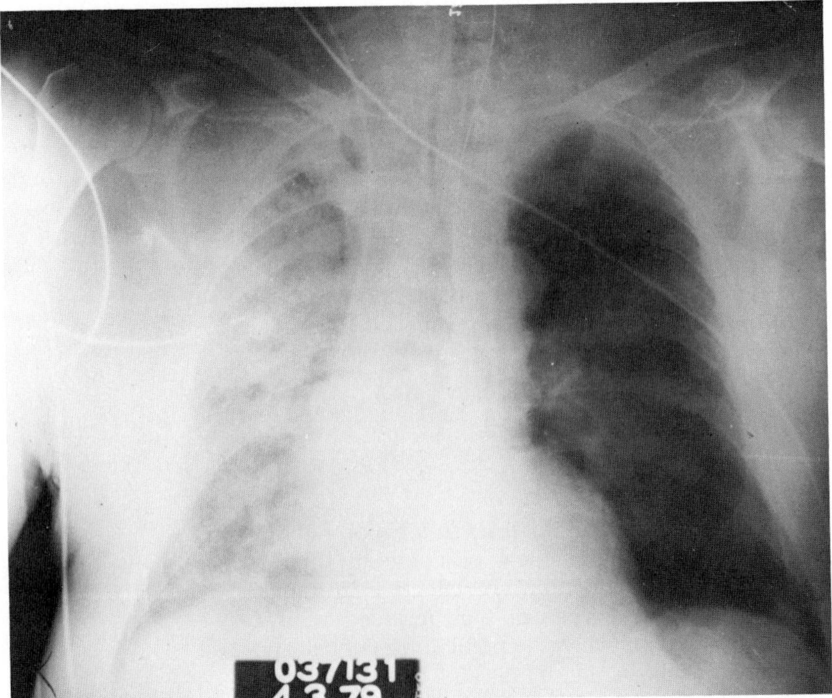

Fig. 33-5. Posterior–anterior chest radiograph with extensive infiltrate of all lobes of right lung after 6 days of erythromycin therapy. The patient recovered. (Meyer RD et al: Ann Intern Med 93: 240–243, 1980)

Remaining Problems

A better knowledge of the source and means of control of *Legionella* spp. in the environment is needed. More information is needed on the spectrum of the illness, the cross reactions in serologic tests, and the extent of infection as might be determined by prospective serosurveys.

Bibliography

Book

JONES GL, HEBERT GA (eds): Legionnaires' Disease: The Bacterium and Methodology. CDC Laboratory Manual. Atlanta, Centers for Disease Control, United States Public Health Service, Department of Health, Education, and Welfare, 1979, 173 pp.

Journals

BALOWS A: Legionella: "A rose is a rose. . ." Ann Intern Med 93:366–367, 1980

BALOWS A, FRASER DW (eds): International Symposium on Legionnaires' Disease. Ann Intern Med 90:489–736, 1979

CORDES LG, FRASER DW: Legionellosis. Med Clin North Am 64:395–416, 1980

EDELSTEIN PH, MEYER RD, FINEGOLD SM: Laboratory diagnosis of Legionnaires' disease. Am Rev Respir Dis 121:317–327, 1980

ENGLAND AC III, FRASER DW, PLIKAYTIS BD, TSAI TF, STORCH CV: Sporadic Legionellosis in the United States: The first thousand cases. Ann Intern Med 94: 164–170, 1981

FEELEY JC, GIBSON RJ, GORMAN GW, LANGFORD NC, RASHEED K, MACKEL BC, BAINE W: Charcoal–yeast extract agar: Primary isolation medium for *Legionella pneumophila.* J. Clin Microbiol 10:437–441, 1979

FRASER DW, TSAI TR, ORENSTEIN W, PARKIN WE, BEECHAM HJ, SHARRER RG, HARRIS J, MALLISON GF, MARTIN SM, MCDADE JE, SHEPARD CC, BRACHMAN PS, THE FIELD INVESTIGATION TEAM: Legionnaires' disease: Description of an epidemic of pneumonia. N Engl J Med 297:1189–1197, 1977

KIRBY BD, SNYDER KM, MEYER RD, FINEGOLD SM: Legionnaires' disease: Report of sixty-five nosocomially acquired cases and review of the literature. Medicine (Baltimore) 59:188–205, 1980

MEYER RD, EDELSTEIN PH, KIRBY BD, LOUIE MH, MULLIGAN ME, MORGENSTEIN AL, FINEGOLD SM: Legionnaires' disease: Unusual clinical and laboratory features. Ann Intern Med 93:240–243, 1980

TOBIN JOH, BEARE J, DUNILL MS, FISHER-HOCH S, FRENCH M, MITCHELL RG, MORRIS PJ, MUERS MF: Legionnaires' disease in a transplant unit: isolation of the causative agent from shower baths. Lancet 2:118–121, 1980

H. WILLIAM HARRIS
JOHN H. McCLEMENT

34 Pulmonary Tuberculosis

A disease that was probably tuberculosis was known as early as 1000 B.C. Hippocrates described the symptoms of a malady called *phthisis,* meaning to waste away, and recognized nodules (phymata) of the lung as a feature of the disease. Such nodules, termed *tubercula* in Latin, were called tubercles when they became recognized as a pathologic characteristic of disease. The term *tuberculosis* was first applied to the clinical and pathologic description of the disease in 1834. The causative microorganism, discovered by Koch in 1882, became known as the tubercle bacillus. By 1900, in addition to the human tubercle bacillus *(Mycobacterium tuberculosis),* two additional species of tubercle bacilli (*Mycobacterium bovis* and *Mycobacterium avium*) were recognized to cause disease in man, as well as infections in cattle and birds. Later, infections of rodents, fish, and reptiles caused by entirely separate mycobacterial species were accepted as additional examples of nonhuman tuberculosis.

Chronic pulmonary infections in man caused by still different mycobacterial species were recognized in the early 1950s. Collectively, these mycobacteria have been variously termed *atypical, anonymous,* or *unclassified* strains. The clinical and pathologic manifestations of infections with these microorganisms closely resemble those caused by *M. tuberculosis;* such infections can be distinguished from disease caused by *M. tuberculosis* only by isolating and identifying the mycobacterial species involved (see Chap. 36, Nontuberculous Mycobacterioses).

At present, tuberculosis is defined as an infectious disease caused by *M. tuberculosis* or *M. bovis*. Infections caused by other mycobacteria are designated *mycobacterial disease caused by (name of specific mycobacterial species)*.

Etiology

Microscopy

Mycobacterium tuberculosis is a nonmotile, noncapsulated bacillus varying from 1 μm to 4 μm long by 0.3 μm to 0.5 μm in diameter. Typically, the rods are straight or slightly bent, with parallel sides and curved ends. The bacilli are relatively resistant to staining with aniline dyes, requiring heat or the addition of surface-active agents to facilitate uptake of basic fuchsin; once stained, however, they are resistant to decolorization with alcoholic solutions of mineral acids (see Chap. 9, Microscopic Examinations). This remarkable property of acid-fastness results from lipoidal constituents in an intact cell structure; disrupted cells lose acid-fastness and become less resistant to aniline stains.

Cultures

With large inocula, *M. tuberculosis* will grow in completely synthetic mediums containing simple sources of nitrogen, carbohydrate, and minerals. Such mediums, however, are not suitable for primary isolation because clinical specimens may contain few bacterial cells. Two kinds of mediums are customarily used for culturing specimens: (1) a complex medium containing eggs or egg yolks and potato extract, such as the Löwenstein–Jensen medium or the American Trudeau Society medium; and (2) a semisynthetic medium containing oleic acid and albumin, such as the Middlebrook 7H-11 agar medium. The latter medium permits earlier detection of growth because it is transparent. In addition, it is superior for determining susceptibility to antimicrobials. Because some strains of mycobacteria grow better on one kind of medium than on another, it is worthwhile to culture on both an egg-potato medium and the 7H-11 medium.

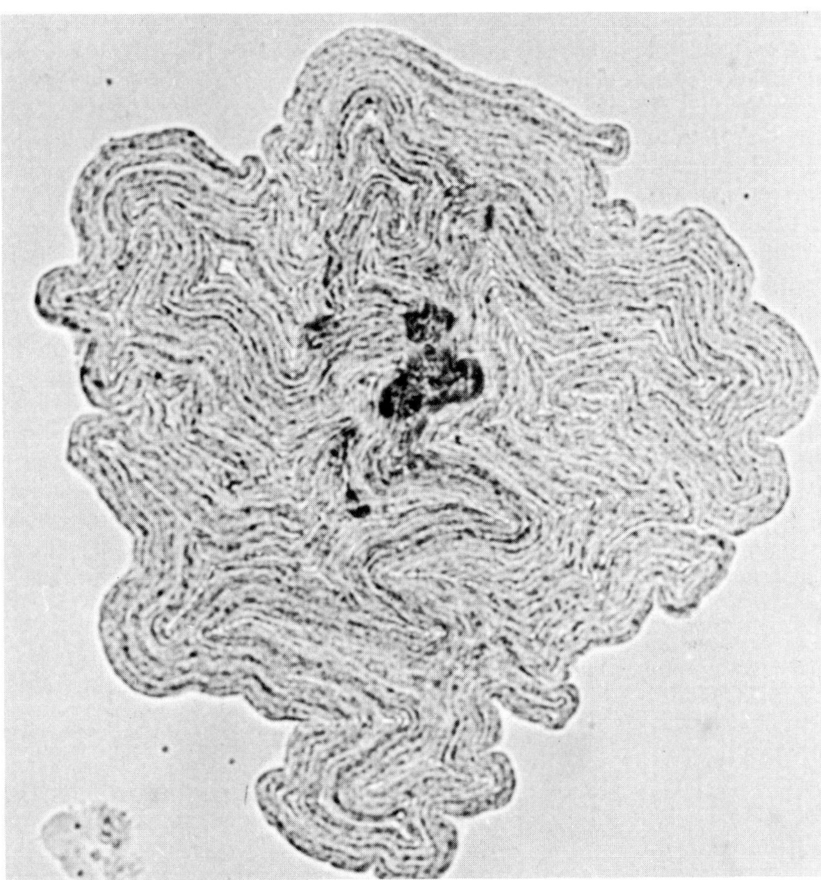

Fig. 34-1. Serpentine, cordlike growth is characteristic of virulent *Mycobacterium tuberculosis* and may result also with *Mycobacterium bovis.* (Original magnification approximately × 100) (Courtesy of Elliot Goldstein, M. D.)

Mycobacterium tuberculosis is an obligate aerobe. Optimum growth occurs in an atmosphere approximating alveolar air. In the laboratory, it is advantageous to enrich the ambient atmosphere with 5% to 10% carbon dioxide.

As compared with most bacteria, *M. tuberculosis* multiply slowly, dividing every 18 to 24 hours. Colonies are usually grossly visible within 3 to 4 weeks. The colonies are cream-colored, dry, and wrinkled with irregular edges. *Mycobacterium tuberculosis* is further distinguished from other mycobacterial species by its failure to develop yellow or orange pigment in the dark or after exposure to light, its ability to produce niacin, and by other characteristics.

Of particular practical importance is the tendency of *M. tuberculosis* to grow in a serpentine fashion, referred to as *cord formation* (Fig. 34-1). This characteristic pattern is caused by a distinct mycobacterial lipid, 6, 6'-dimycolytrehalose, called *cord factor.* The significance of cord formation is twofold: virulence is associated with its presence, and cords can be recognized within 2 weeks of incubation, enabling an early presumptive identification of *M. tuberculosis*. Other species of *Mycobacterium* may also form cords; however, in a clinical laboratory that deals with specimens from humans, at least 98% of isolates that form cords are *M. tuberculosis*.

Tubercle bacilli are relatively resistant to strong acids and alkalis, compared to most other bacteria. This property enables the use of 4% aqueous sodium hydroxide to digest particulate material and kill bacteria other than *Mycobacterium* spp. and fungi in sputum, gastric aspirates, and other grossly contaminated specimens. Such treatment, however, may kill a certain proportion of the mycobacterial cells. Accordingly, reduction in the concentration of NaOH, in combination with the potent, rapid-acting mucolytic agent, *N*-acetyl-*l*-cysteine, has become widely used for digestion/decontamination.

Chemical Composition

The chemical composition of tubercle bacilli varies somewhat, depending on the strain, age, and medium used for cultivation. Various complex, immunologically active polysaccharides and glycogen are present, as well as lipoproteins, nucleoproteins, nucleic acids, and several amino acids. Protein fractions have been studied extensively because a protein is used for the tuberculin reaction. Immunization of experimental animals with protein components stimulates various specific circulating antibodies but does not induce delayed hypersensitivity.

Tubercle bacilli contain large quantities of complex lipids, including waxes, fats, fatty acids, and alcohols. In experimental animals, the injection of certain lipid components may lead to the formation of tubercles and to caseation necrosis similar to that produced by injecting intact killed bacilli. The dose of lipids required, however, is greater than the amount present in a tubercle-provoking dose of intact bacilli.

Species Identification

Although most mycobacterial infections are caused by *M. tuberculosis,* specific bacteriologic diagnosis is essential because prognosis, treatment, and contagion vary according to species. In Table 34-1, the most common species that cause disease in humans are listed along with the saprophytic species commonly encountered in clinical specimens and some of the properties that enable their identification.

Of most importance are the rate of growth and pigment production when the microorganisms are cultivated in the dark and after exposure to light. Examination of cultures at weekly intervals enables the detection of *Mycobacterium fortuitum,* and other rapid growers that appear earlier than some mycobacteria. Scotochromogen colonies develop a yellow or orange color when cultivated in the dark *(e.g., Mycobacterium scrofulaceum)*. On the other hand, colonies of *Mycobacterium kansasii* are photochromogenic—nonpigmented when grown in the dark, becoming yellow when incubated after exposure to light.

Runyon's classification of atypical mycobacterial

Table 34-1. *Some Characteristics of a Few* Mycobacterium *Species*

			Colony		Growth					
			Pigment		Temperature, °C					
Runyon Group	***Mycobacterium* Species**	**Appearance**	IN DARK	PHOTO ACTIVATED	22–24	32–33	35–39	41–43	**Rate**	**Niacin Test**
Tuberculosis complex	*tuberculosis*	Rough	No	No	0	+	+	0	S	+
	bovis	Rough	No	No	0	+	+	0	S	0
I Photochromogen	*kansasii*	Usually rough	No	Yes	+	+	+	0	S	0
	marinum	Usually smooth	No	Yes	+	+	0	0	S	F
	simiae	Usually smooth	No	Yes			+	0	S	+
II Scotochromogen	*scrofulaceum*	Smooth	Yes	No	+	+	+	0	S	0
	szulgai	Smooth	Yes	No	+	+	+		S	0
	gordonae	Smooth	Yes	No	+	+	+	0	S	0
III Nonchromogen	*xenopi*	Smooth	Yes	No	0	F	+	+	S	0
	avium-intracellulare	Smooth	No	No	F	+	+	F	S	0
	ulcerans	Rough	No	No	M	+	0	0	S	0
	gastri	Smooth	No	No	+	+	+	M	S	0
	terrae complex	Smooth	No	No	+	+	+	M	S	0
IV Rapid Grower	*fortuitum* complex	Rough or smooth	No	No	+	+	+	M	R	0
	chelonei	Smooth	No	No	+	+	+	M	R	F

strains (see Chap. 36, Nontuberculous Mycobacterioses) included in group III organisms with smooth, nonpigmented or faintly yellow colonies which did not produce niacin. These were termed Battey bacilli. Subsequently, species were distinguished among group III strains; *Mycobacterium intracellulare* was shown to be the major species, occurring both as a cause for infection in humans and as a widely prevalent saprophyte in soil and water. It is closely related to *M. avium,* which it resembles in colony characteristics and biochemical reactions. However, the two species can be separated by serologic reactions and by the fact that *M. avium* is more pathogenic for chickens than *M. intracellulare*. In most clinical circumstances, it is not necessary to differentiate these two strains; rather, the isolate may be designated as *Mycobacterium* spp. of the *avium-intracellulare* complex. Other group III mycobacteria, such as *Mycobacterium gastri, Mycobacterium terrae, Mycobacterium triviale,* and others are largely saprophytic and must be distinguished from the *avium-intracellulare* complex.

Procedures

The niacin test is a useful method for screening cultures and for separating *M. tuberculosis* from other strains (Table 34-1). All niacin-negative isolates must be considered mycobacteria other than *M. tuberculosis* and must be subjected to more complete analysis. However, occasional isolates of other species, including *M. semiae, M. marinum,* and *M. chelonei,* may yield a positive niacin test; other cultural and biochemical characteristics must then be used to distinguish such isolates from *M. tuberculosis*. Loss of catalase activity at 68°C for 20 minutes, and a positive nitrate reduction test, provide confirming evidence for *M. tuberculosis*.

Except for *M. tuberculosis* and *M. bovis,* most

Catalase								
SEMI-QUANTITATIVE >45 MM	68°C FOR 20 MIN	Tween 80 Hydrolysis, 5 Days	Nitrate Reduction	Resistance to TCH at 10 μg/ml	Arylsulfatase Test, 3 days	Significance of Isolation from Clinical Specimens	*Mycobacterium* Species	Runyon Group
0	0	F	+	+	0	Always pathogenic	*tuberculosis*	Tuberculosis complex
0	0	0	0	0	0	Always pathogenic	*bovis*	
+	+	+	+	+	0	Usually pathogenic	*kansasii*	I
0	F	+	0	+	0	Usually pathogenic	*marinum*	Photochromogen
+	+	0	0	+		Pathogenic or nonpathogenic	*simiae*	
+	+	0	0	+	0	Pathogenic or nonpathogenic	*scrofulaceum*	II Scotochromogen
+	+	F	+		M	Usually pathogenic	*szulgai*	
+	+	+	0	+	0	Not pathogenic	*gordonae*	
0	+	0	0	+	M	Pathogenic or nonpathogenic	*xenopi*	III Nonchromogen
0	+	0	0	+	0	Usually pathogenic, may be nonpathogenic	*avium-intracellulare*	
+	+	0	0	+	0	Always pathogenic	*ulcerans*	
0	+	+	0	+	0	Not pathogenic	*gastri*	
+	+	+	+	+	0	Not pathogenic	*terrae* complex	
+	+	M	+	+	+	Usually nonpathogenic	*fortuitum* complex	IV Rapid Grower
+	+	0	0	+	+	Pathogenic or nonpathogenic	*chelonei*	

TCH = Thiophen-2-carboxylic acid hydrazide
S = Slow
F = Few (less than 50% of strains)
M = Most (more than 50% of strains)
R = Rapid

mycobacteria are relatively resistant to low concentrations of isoniazid, streptomycin, and various other antituberculous chemotherapeutic agents. If a resistant strain is isolated from a patient who has not previously received antituberculosis drugs, the infecting microorganism may not be *M. tuberculosis*. All such primary drug-resistant mycobacteria deserve careful study to distinguish nontuberculous mycobacteria from drug-resistant strains of *M. tuberculosis*.

Human strains that have become highly resistant to isoniazid display low or absent catalase activity, poor cord formation, and relative avirulence for guinea pigs.

Identification of mycobacterial species may require detailed analysis. Measurement of the ability of growing organisms to hydrolyze Tween-80 and tests for catalase activity are useful. *Mycobacterium kansasii* is more reactive than *M. intracellulare* in both tests. Cord formation and the ability to bind the dye neutral red are characteristic of human and bovine mammalian strains.

Most hospital microbiology laboratories can identify the mycobacterial species listed in Table 34-1 by use of these conventional cultural and biochemical tests. Because some isolates have characteristics of more than one species, more detailed diagnostic schemas may be necessary. A rare isolate may defy identification by the hospital laboratory; such organisms should be referred to a Mycobacteriology Reference Laboratory or to the Centers for Disease Control. In addition to the usual microbiological methods, serotyping, phagetyping, bacterial lipid analysis, and animal virulence tests may be applied in pursuit of species identification.

Epidemiology

Transmission

Aerosolized droplets of liquid containing tubercle bacilli are the primary means of transmission of tuberculosis. Dissemination of such droplets results if generation within the respiratory tract of a person with active ulcerative lesions of the lung is coupled with expulsion during talking, sneezing, laughing, singing, or coughing. The most important mechanism is coughing. Large airborne particles may settle out of the air to the floor or ground where the bacilli, although viable, remain relatively harmless. Droplet nuclei a few μm in diameter are produced by the rapid evaporation of water from aerosolized, small droplets. Containing only one or a few tubercle bacilli, these droplet nuclei may remain suspended in air for long periods. When air containing such droplet nuclei is inhaled by a previously uninfected person, the small particle is borne into the lung to the pulmonary alveoli, where the microorganisms become implanted and infection is initiated.

The risk of airborne transmission is influenced by many factors, such as the rate and the concentration of expelled organisms, the physical state of the airborne discharge, and the volume and the rate of exchange of the air in the physical space into which the bacilli are ejected. However, the most important risk factor is the length of time an individual shares a volume of air with an infectious case of tuberculosis. Thus, intimate, prolonged, or frequent contact, as in the home or work place, provides the greatest risk of transmission.

Transmission by contaminated fomites (clothes, books, personal articles) rarely, if ever, occurs. Tubercle bacilli are not easily suspended in air from objects, and most of them die rapidly from drying or sunlight. Dried secretions do not ordinarily become suspended in the air. Inhaled large particles are deposited in the upper respiratory passages, from which they are usually expelled. The tubercle bacilli that remain usually do not parasitize the upper respiratory tract, which is relatively resistant to tuberculous infection.

Persons with overt tuberculosis vary considerably in their efficiency as disseminaters-transmitters of tubercle bacilli. Extensive pulmonary lesions, the presence of cavities, and a heavy concentration of tubercle bacilli in pulmonary secretions increase the likelihood of generating infected droplet nuclei and of transmitting the disease to others. The factors of crowded living conditions and poor hygiene are very important, as attested by the striking decline in mortality that occurred even before the introduction of antituberculous chemotherapy (Fig. 34-2).

Tuberculosis acquired by ingestion of tubercle bacilli occurred before bovine tuberculosis was controlled and pasturization of milk was widely practiced. As contrasted to the airborne route of transmission, large inocula are required to initiate infection by the oral route. Discharges from extrapulmonary sources of tuberculosis (urine, abscess drainage) do not ordinarily become airborne and therefore provide little risk of transmission.

Accidental percutaneous or intraocular inoculation of tubercle bacilli may occur rarely in pathologists, microbiologists, and others. Venereal transmission from tuberculosis of the prostate is an extremely unusual mode of infection.

Natural History

Most infected persons remain entirely well and have no manifestations of tuberculous disease during their

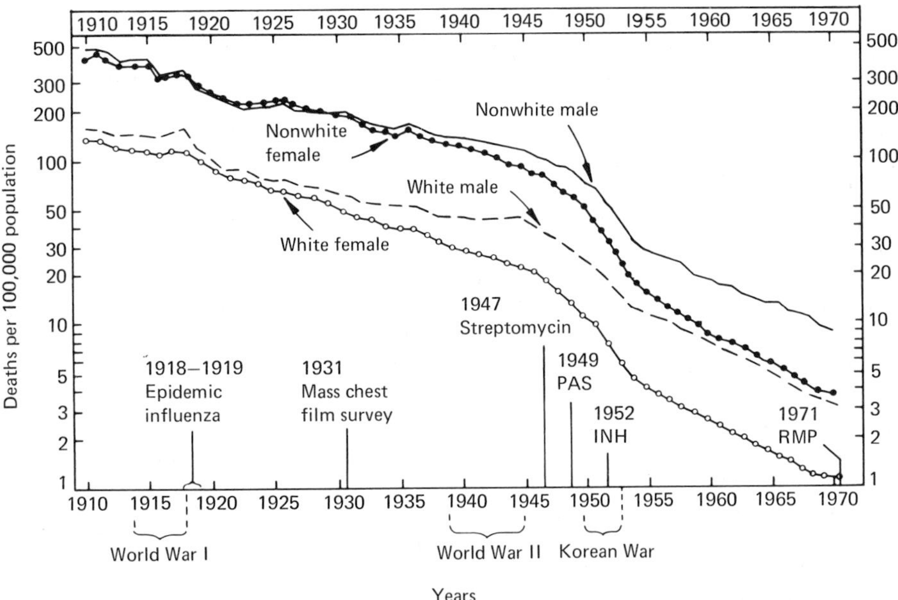

Fig. 34-2. Case fatality rate of tuberculosis in the United States. The most striking decline occurred before the introduction of effective antimicrobics: streptomycin in 1947, isoniazid (INH) in 1952, and rifampin (RMP) in 1971. (After Lowell AM: Tuberculosis. I. Morbidity and Mortality. Cambridge, Harvard University Press, 1969)

life span. Mycobacterial infection can be recognized in such persons by eliciting a reaction of delayed hypersensitivity through the intradermal injection of mycobacterial protein—the tuberculin skin test.

Progressive disease follows the initial infection promptly in some persons. When clinical or pathologic examinations provide evidence of an uninterrupted course, the term *progressive primary tuberculosis* is sometimes applied. Such early progression occurs most often in infants and young children and has been termed *the childhood type of tuberculosis*. However, progressive primary disease also occurs in certain adults who have a low level of native resistance to tuberculous infection as a consequence of genetic or constitutional factors. The common failing is an inability to halt the growth of the tubercle bacilli or to restrict or localize the site of infection in the tissues.

In other persons, the course of the disease is discontinuous. These persons usually remain free of clinical manifestations after the initial infection until years later, when overt, active, progressive tuberculous infection becomes evident. In most persons, the exacerbated infection is limited to the lungs, and it is the result of resurgent proliferation of tubercle bacilli residing in a long dormant, infected, caseous pulmonary focus. Such a course has been termed *reinfection tuberculosis*. In the past, it was widely believed that the late episode of active disease resulted from pulmonary invasion by newly inhaled, airborne tubercle bacilli from exogenous sources. The extent to which exogenous versus endogenous sources of tubercle bacilli account for reinfection tuberculosis has been the subject of controversy for many years. Present evidence supports the concept that in the United States most reinfection is in fact endogenous and is the result of reactivation of a preexisting tuberculous lesion. Late exacerbating tuberculosis occurs most often in older persons. Thus, at autopsy, late exacerbating disease was present in 71% of patients over 50 years in age, whereas progressive primary disease was present in 75% of those who died of tuberculosis between 16 and 30 years of age.

Identifying the Infected

The varied natural history of tuberculous infection necessitated the development of standard criteria for use in studies of prevalence. Three indices are widely used for this purpose. The *number of infected persons* in a given population is the sum of persons with positive tuberculin tests. The *new active case rate* refers to the number of persons discovered to have clinically apparent, overt tuberculous disease within a particular span of time. The *mortality rate* indicates the number of deaths directly due to tuberculosis occurring within a specific population and a specific interval of time.

In many parts of the world today, and in the United States early in this century, most individuals became infected with tubercle bacilli during childhood. Evidence for almost universal infection was obtained from early tuberculin surveys and from autopsy studies. For example, more than a thousand New York City residents who died suddenly and unexpectedly were autopsied by the Department of the City Medical Examiner at Bellevue Hospital between 1944 and 1947. There was evidence of previous tuberculous infection in 88% of those 60 years and older, and in 80% of those 40 to 59 years of age.

The tuberculin test is the basic tool used to identify infected persons (see Chap. 15, Skin Tests). Tuberculin hypersensitivity can be detected by a variety of methods that introduce tuberculoprotein into the tissues of the test subject. Among these, the intradermal, or Mantoux, test is the standard and offers the highest degree of consistency and reliability. Tuberculin was standardized in 1934 by Seibert, who developed purified protein derivatives of culture extracts of *M. tuberculosis*. A large quantity of this material, PPD-S, was prepared in 1940, and it still serves as the international standard for tuberculin of mammalian strains. In the past, three concentrations of PPD-S were used for testing: 0.00002 mg—first strength, or 1 tuberculin unit (TU); 0.0001 mg—intermediate strength, or 5 TU; and 0.005 mg—second strength, or 250 TU. Induration of 5 mm or more at the site of injection with any of these concentrations was considered positive and indicative of previous tuberculous infection. However, largely through epidemiologic studies, the influence of subclinical, nontuberculous mycobacterial infections on tuberculin reactivity was recognized, and more accurate, standardized criteria for the use of the tuberculin test were developed.

When diluted in a buffered diluent, tuberculoprotein is adsorbed in varying amounts by glass or plastic. Addition of a small amount of a detergent such as Tween-80, to the diluent will reduce adsorption.

The standard dose for tuberculin surveys and for diagnostic purposes is 0.0001 mg (5 TU, Test Units) of PPD-S. The test is read by measuring the transverse diameter of induration (not erythema) 48 to 72 hours after the intradermal injection.

Ideally, the tuberculin test would correlate perfectly (*i.e.,* infection with *M. tuberculosis* and a positive test, absence of infection and a negative test). Unfortunately, as was shown by extensive epidemiologic and other surveys, the correlations are not perfect, although they are very strong. At least 90% of persons who react to 5 TU of PPD-S with 10 mm, or more, of induration, have been infected by *M. tuberculosis* and have developed delayed hypersensitivity in response to the antigens of *M. tuberculosis*. Many persons develop 1 mm to 8 mm (and a few, 10 mm) reactions of induration as a result of cross-reactivity between PPD-S and the antigens of other, nontuberculous mycobacterial species to which they have become sensitized. Also, a skin test reaction of less than 10 mm of induration may have been augmented to 10 mm of induration in response to serial skin tests with PPD-S.

Other persons, some not ill but known to have been infected with tubercle bacilli, and some with clinical tuberculous disease, may respond to 5 TU of PPD-S with no induration or less than 10 mm of induration. Such hyporeactivity of the T-cell mediated immune response may result from overt immunosuppression accompanying diseases such as lymphoma and other malignancies, or may be caused by extensive pulmonary or miliary tuberculosis. Immunosuppressive drugs, viral infections, severe malnutrition and other systemic disorders may impair response to PPD-S. When tuberculous disease is suspected clinically and the tuberculin test is not reactive, the presence of anergy should be looked for by the application of other skin test antigens in a so-called anergy panel, as described in Chapter 15, Skin Tests.

Large-scale surveys, using protein derivatives of various nontuberculous mycobacterial strains, as well as PPD-S, were performed on white male recruits entering the United States Navy. These men ranged in age 17 to 21 years and came from all geographic sections of the United States. There was a much higher frequency of reaction to the other mycobacterial antigens than to PPD-S. Varying with the particular antigen used and with the geographic area of residence of the subjects, 10% to 40% showed evidence of previous infection with mycobacteria other than *M. tuberculosis*. Between 1958 and 1964, the overall reactor rate to PPD-S among more than 250,000 recruits was 4.1%.

The chances of an individual having been infected with tubercle bacilli, as evidenced by tuberculin reactivity, is markedly influenced by age, race, and socioeconomic status. In 1973 to 1974, more than 50,000 adult employees of the New York City Education Department were tested yielding reactor rates of 12.5% overall, 8.3% for whites and 23% to 25% for nonwhites. Among those with the highest socioeconomic status, 5.5% were reactors, as compared with 22.4% among those with the lowest socioeconomic status. Less than 6% of the employees between 20 to 29 years of age, but more than 18% of those over 50 years, were reactors.

The tuberculin reactor rate among children entering school has long been considered to be an indication of the level of tuberculous disease in the community. Although reactor rates among children also vary according to the population characteristics mentioned above, for most areas of the United States the rates are below 0.5%, and, in some rural and suburban areas, a tuberculin-positive seven-year-old is rarely found.

Continued efforts to detect and treat those with

Table 34-2. New Active Case Rates for Selected Countries, States and Cities

Year	Geographic Area	New Cases per 100,000 Population
1973	Australia	11.9
	Denmark	13.1
	United States	14.8
	Canada	16.1
	Yugoslavia	108.0
	Japan	118.4
	Korea	249.0
1979	United States	12.6
States	Nebraska	1.9
	Iowa	2.5
	New York	12.6
	Florida	18.4
	Hawaii	34.0
Cities	Wichita	8.8
	St. Louis	15.2
	New York	20.1
	Newark	51.5
	San Francisco	54.5

active disease and to intensify programs of prophylactic therapy have great potential for further reducing rates of infection. In rural Alaska in 1957, 75% of children entering school were tuberculin reactors; after intensive control measures were instituted, the number of reactors dropped to 3%.

Morbidity

The occurrence of overt tuberculous disease varies greatly with time and the characteristics of the particular population examined. Earlier in this century, the new active case rates in parts of the United States were around 500/100,000 population, and most of the new active cases were reported in infants, children, and young adults. This pattern persists today in areas of the world where the prevalence of tuberculosis remains high. Tuberculosis rates are greatest in densely populated, impoverished communities. Table 34-2 illustrates the enormous range of prevalence throughout different nations of the world and in various states and cities of the United States. In 1973, the new active case rate in Korea was more than 20 times higher than that in Australia. In 1979, the rate in the District of Columbia exceeded by more than 20 times that in Idaho. The incidence of new cases in the United States is related to counties in Fig. 34-3.

The risk of developing overt, progressive tuberculosis is influenced by age, sex, race, personal habits, coexisting disease, and socioeconomic circumstances. In the United States today, new active disease is found most often among older men. Although the disease occurs in all races and in all economic and social classes, tuberculosis is concentrated among the least affluent members of society. That is, circumstances that favor contact with persons who have active disease are the most important determinants of prevalence. Thus, in the large cities the incidence of tuberculosis is highest in the crowded, physically deteriorated sections. In rural areas, the disease occurs most often in squalid communities occupied by the poor. For example, in New York City in 1978, there were 1307 newly reported cases of tuberculous disease, for a case rate of 17.2 per 100,000 population. Whites made up 67% of the population and accounted for 22.6% of the new cases. Nonwhites and Puerto-Ricans represented 33% of the population and accounted for 54% of the new cases. Flushing, Queens, a residential area occupied principally by a white middle class, had a rate of 5.6 while Central Harlem, an economically depressed area occupied principally by blacks, had 52.2 new active cases per 100,000 population.

Mortality

Accurate vital statistics were not kept before the 19th century, but historically tuberculosis was a common cause of death from the Middle Ages to the turn of the 19th century. In London, phthisis was said to be responsible for 20% to 30% of all deaths during the 17th and 18th centuries. Between 1812 and 1880, the combined annual tuberculosis death rates for Boston, New York, and Philadelphia ranged from 300 to 400 per 100,000 population. Around 1880, a steady decline began, the rates averaging 245 in 1900, 119 in 1920, 69 in 1932, and 5.3 in 1970. A similar decline in mortality rates was noted as early as 1830 in Sweden; other countries noted improvement only within the past decade.

Table 34-3 illustrates the variation in tuberculosis mortality rates among different countries in 1973. In the United States, the rate was 202 per 100,000 in 1900, 4.1 in 1965, and 1.3 in 1978. However, these

Table 34-3. Death Rates from Tuberculosis for Selected Countries in 1973

Country	Deaths per 100,000 Population
Australia	1.0
United States	1.8
France	6.3
Japan	11.0
Chile	19.8
Hong Kong	27.7

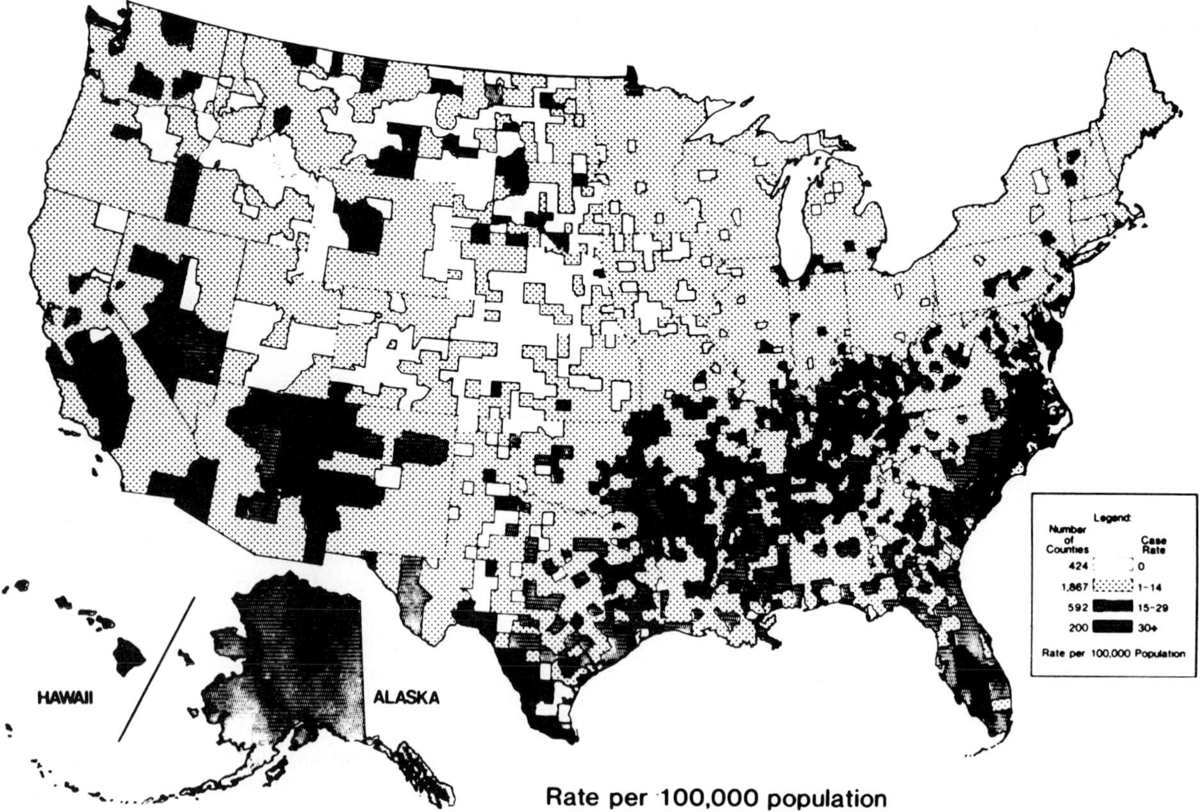

Fig. 34-3. Reported new cases of tuberculosis per 100,000 population by counties in the United States for the years 1976–1978.

rates vary markedly according to geographic area. In 1978, the tuberculosis death rate in Flushing, Queens, was 0.8 per 100,000 population, but in the same year, Central Harlem recorded a rate 20 times higher, at 16.3 per 100,000.

The decline in the mortality rate from tuberculosis is primarily the result of an overall reduction in the frequency of infection as a consequence of improved socioeconomic conditions. The influence of modern therapy is distinctly secondary, (see Fig. 34-2).

Pathogenesis and Pathology

Early Responses

Infected droplet nuclei inhaled by a previously uninfected person deposit randomly within the lungs. Tubercle bacilli lodging on the surface of an alveolus or an alveolar duct are phagocytized by alveolar macrophages; they multiply in spite of intracellular residence. The earliest local reaction is vasodilation of alveolar capillaries and moderate swelling of the cells lining the alveoli.

Inflammation and Spread

Soon thereafter, an inflammatory reaction occurs, and the alveoli fill with fibrin, desquamated alveolar macrophages, and a few polymorphonuclear leukocytes. The largely acellular early lesions consist principally of fibrinous exudate and contain relatively few tubercle bacilli. The less common lobular pneumonia is accompanied by dense accumulations of polymorphonuclear leukocytes and is associated with heavy concentrations of microorganisms. Such early tissue responses are not specific for the implantation of tubercle bacilli, but they may be evoked by other bacteria or irritating particulate material.

Before the emergence of delayed hypersensitivity and the histologic changes that typify cellular immunity, bacilli multiply within and outside of cells. The local inflammatory lesion may remain microscopic in size or in some cases may spread to involve a volume of lung tissue sufficient to become visible by chest radiography. Usually, bacilli escape from the local parenchymal focus and drain through lymphatic channels to the lymph nodes of the pulmonary hilum. From this site, they may reach the mediastinal lymph nodes. Inflammatory lesions also develop at the sites of implantation in the hilar and mediastinal lymph nodes. Tubercle bacilli may escape from the lymph nodes and then enter and traverse the thoracic duct to gain entry into the venous blood stream. *Mycobacterium tuberculosis* may also reach the pulmonary blood stream by direct extension of lesions in parenchymal foci into pulmonary veins. Blood-borne microorganisms become implanted throughout the body, and metastatic inflammatory foci develop in various organs, including the lungs.

TUBERCLE FORMATION

Both the evolution of lesions and the development of cellular immunity result in the replacement of the polymorphonuclear leukocytes of the early response by macrophages and lymphocytes. Bacilli are phagocytized, but continue to multiply; as they are expelled from disrupted cells, they are taken up by new macrophages entering the inflammatory lesion. Figure 34-4 illustrates the microscopic appearance of an early exudative lesion of the lung.

As macrophages become the predominant cellular

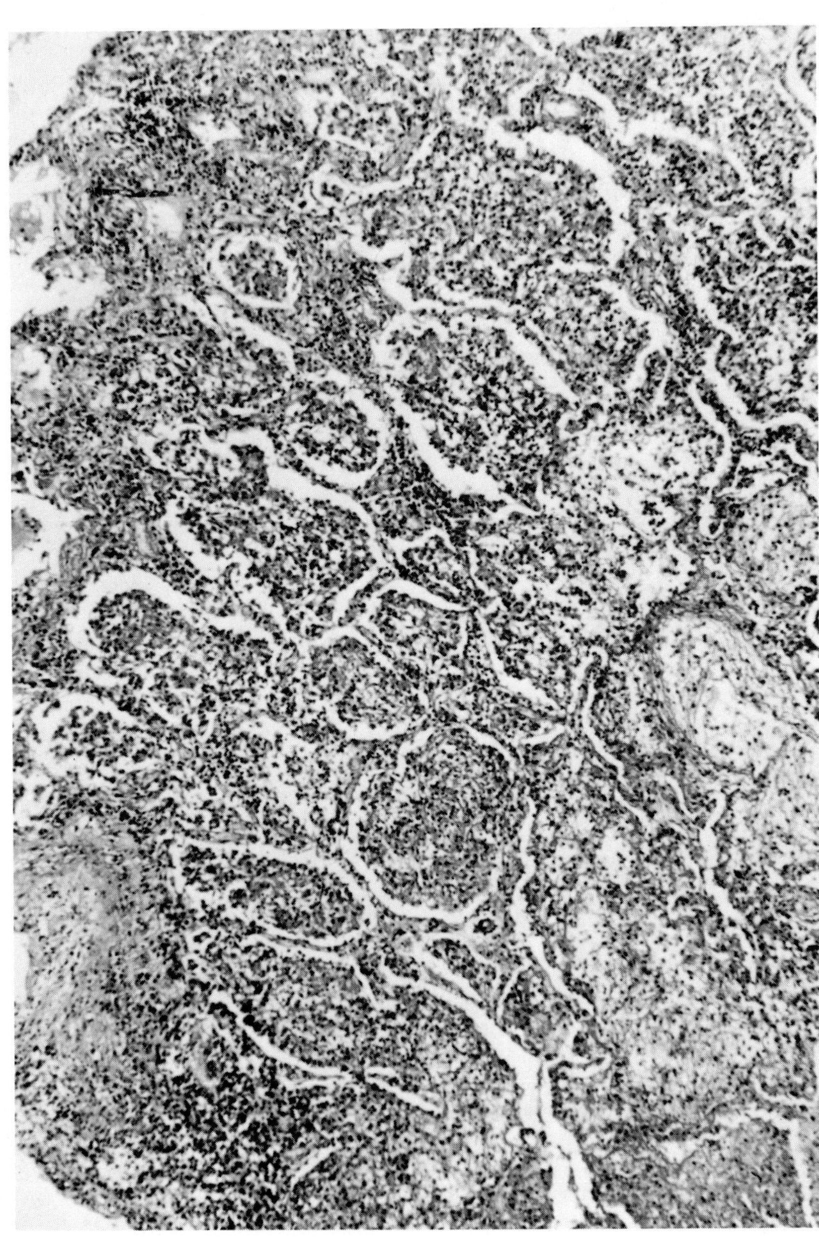

Fig. 34-4. Histologic structure of a small area of lubular pneumonia caused by *Mycobacterium tuberculosis.* (Original magnification approximately × 90)

component, the lesions evolve into productive tubercles composed of a central zone of Langhans' giant cells, a midzone of epithelioid cells, and a peripheral zone of lymphocytes interspersed among fibroblasts. Such lesions contain few tubercle bacilli, and those few are principally within epithelioid cells. The tubercle, a pathologic hallmark of tuberculosis, is the first characteristic feature to evolve in tuberculous infection. However, lesions with identical histologic appearance (lacking only mycobacteria) may be found in fungus infections, syphilis, sarcoidosis, and other diseases.

CASEATION

Caseation is a second characteristic feature of tuberculosis. At about the time hypersensitivity develops, approximately 6 weeks after initial implantation in humans, a portion of the inflammatory or productive lesion may undergo caseation necrosis. Caseation is characterized by the disintegration of host cells and tubercle bacilli to become a coagulated, homogenous, solid mass that may persist for many years. The term *caseum* was applied because the dry, crumbly appearance of the mass grossly resembles cheese.

The biochemical basis for caseation is not known. The tubercle bacillus has never been demonstrated to contain or elaborate toxins that injure host cells. Instead, the process appears to be intimately related to the local expression of the delayed hypersensitivity reaction—cell injury may be caused by toxic products released from sensitized lymphocytes influenced by mycobacterial antigen(s) (see Chap. 5, Immunopathology of Infectious Diseases).

Few intact acid-fast bacilli can be found on microscopic examination of caseum. However, because elastic fibers are particularly resistant to caseation necrosis, the ghost architecture of pulmonary lobules, vessels, and bronchi may be preserved by their elastic framework in the caseous mass. In Figure 34-5 the histologic appearance is shown.

Fig. 34-5. A lesion of pulmonary tuberculosis with central caseation surrounded by epitheloid cells. There is a Langhans' giant cell in the upper left. (Original magnification approximately × 700)

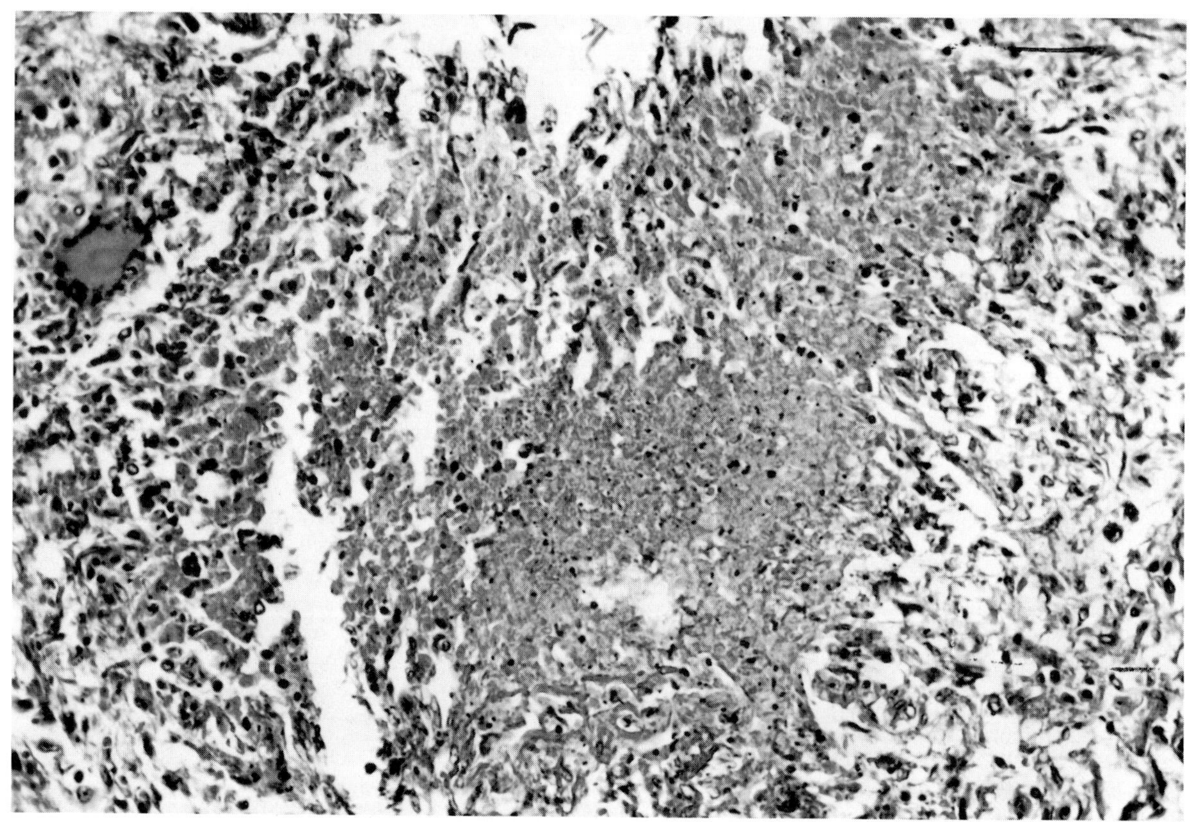

Evolution of Tuberculous Lesions

LOCALIZATION

The subsequent course of the early inflammatory, caseous primary lesion varies markedly in different persons. The ultimate consequences of primary infection are determined by the balance between the native resistance of the infected person and the extent to which tubercle bacilli can proliferate in host tissues. The property of virulence in *M. tuberculosis* varies from strain to strain, just as native resistance varies from person to person. Usually, the infection is interrupted, and the primary lesions heal spontaneously. The morphologic character of the healed lesions varies. Early exudative pulmonary lesions and noncaseous productive tubercles may resorb completely, leaving little or no residuum. Caseous material seldom, if ever, resorbs. Instead, the caseum heals by inspissation and hardening, and ultimately becomes encapsulated by dense collagenous tissue. The few tubercle bacilli that remain in caseum multiply slowly and are restricted by host defenses.

As years pass, calcium salts become deposited in the inspissated caseum of the primary pulmonary focus and the infected hilar or mediastinal lymph nodes. Such calcified primary lesions, the Ghon complex, may be apparent in chest roentgenograms or may be found years later at autopsy in the lungs of infected persons. Large caseous masses resulting from the primary infection may also become inspissated and encapsulated, leaving a residual tuberculoma. These may be quite large; they tend to be spherical, prominent, persistent abnormalities detectable by radiography.

If the primary infection is not localized, large numbers of tubercle bacilli may be disseminated throughout the pulmonary parenchyma, leading to extensive exudative and caseous lesions. One or more lobes may become the site of acute, caseous tuberculous pneumonia. In most cases, however, the host defenses are sufficient to confine the pulmonary lesions to a smaller volume of lung tissue, where they may heal, or slough and progress to a tuberculous cavity.

CONTIGUOUS SPREAD

Tubercle bacilli may enter the pleural space by extension from a subpleural parenchymal focus. Productive and caseous lesions develop at sites of implantation on the pleural membrane, and effusion into the pleural space may occur. The pericardial sac may also become infected by local extension from an adjacent parenchymal lesion or from tuberculous mediastinal lymph nodes.

LYMPHOHEMATOGENOUS SPREAD

Heavy and protracted bacillemia arising from lymphohematogenous dissemination may result in widespread metastatic miliary lesions throughout the body. These lesions are usually a few millimeters in size and typically are productive tubercles that may have caseous centers. Acute miliary lesions of the brain or meninges may be the source from which tubercle bacilli disseminate widely in the meninges, leading to tuberculous meningitis, one of the most serious complications of primary infection. Bacillemia is usually less marked, however, and only a few, scattered extrapulmonary foci result. In most instances, these heal; in some, the infection progresses at the metastatic focus, and an acute tuberculous abscess or an active caseous lesion evolves. Peripheral lymph nodes, bones, joints, and kidneys are common sites of such extrapulmonary lesions. Active disease may become manifest at these and other sites within a relatively brief interval—a few months after the initial infection. In other instances, the postprimary extrapulmonary focus remains quiescent for long periods, sometimes years, before bacilli begin to multiply, disseminate locally, and produce active lesions.

BRONCHIAL OBSTRUCTION

Other complications of primary tuberculous infection result from enlarged, infected lymph nodes in the pulmonary hilum. Lying in close proximity to major bronchi, such nodes may compress and obstruct a bronchus, resulting in an airless lobe or segment. Chronic pyogenic infection in the distal pulmonary parenchyma may result. When bronchial obstruction is irreversible, a contracted, nonventilated fibrotic lobe or segment results. The right middle lobe is most often involved in this fashion because of the distribution of lymph nodes surrounding the right middle lobe bronchus. Although the obstructed bronchus may become patent when tuberculous lymphadenitis subsides, irreversible bronchiectasis may have developed in the distal bronchi. Rarely, tuberculous hilar lymph nodes erode and rupture into the lumen of a bronchus. When this occurs, tubercle bacilli may drain from the infected node into the distal lung parenchyma, leading to tuberculous pneumonia at the latter site. Tuberculous mediastinal lymph nodes may adhere to the esophagus and heal spontaneously with considerable fibrous reaction, ultimately giving rise to an esophageal traction diverticulum.

CASEOUS LESIONS

The ultimate result of tuberculous infection of the lung is determined principally by the behavior of the caseous lesion. The most favorable reaction is inspissation, with hardening of the caseum and complete encapsulation by fibrous tissue. Softening and liquefaction of a caseonecrotic focus is less favorable because it may lead to chronic cavitary pulmonary tuberculosis. A portion of the caseous mass, usually its center, changes physically from a granular to a semisolid or creamy consistency and liquefies. Liquefaction proceeds radially from this focus. As yet, the basis for this alteration in the physical state of the caseum is not known, but regardless of the cause, liquefaction is accompanied by rapid proliferation of the mycobacterial population within the caseous mass.

Subsequently, if the liquid caseous lesion does not drain but remains encapsulated, the softened components may again inspissate, harden, and ultimately reorganize into a fibrous, encapsulated tuberculoma. Morphologic evidence of the ancient liquefaction of a solid caseous lesion may be found in the complete disruption and disarray of the elastic ghost architecture of the original lung framework.

More often, adjacent lung parenchyma is involved, and ultimately a bronchus is eroded, enabling the drainage of the bacilli-containing liquid contents of the lesion. Evacuation of the caseonecrotic focus initiates a new, deleterious chain of events.

CAVITATION

When air replaces the evacuated core of the lesion, an air-containing abscess, the so-called tuberculous cavity, results. As compared with the retarded growth of tubercle bacilli in the solid caseum, there is massive proliferation in the oxygen-rich, air-containing medium of the tissue-lined cavity. The inner walls of the cavity support extensive sheets of growing tubercle bacilli, often associated with heavy infiltration by polymorphonuclear leukocytes. Fig. 34-6 demonstrates the histologic appearance of a partially evacuated, liquefying caseous lesion. An early cavity is shown in Fig. 34-7. As tubercle bacilli extend into the lung parenchyma surrounding the cavity, caseation necrosis and liquefaction bring about sloughing into the cavitary chamber. Thus, the air-containing cavity may enlarge progressively. In some instances, an entire lobe may be destroyed and replaced by a giant, air-containing tuberculous cavity (Fig. 34-8). More often, however, expansion of the cavity is restricted by the wall of fibrous tissue that surrounds the lesion and offers resistance to microbial invasion and necrosis. Fig. 34-9 depicts the inner wall of such a chronic cavitary lesion.

Host defense mechanisms appear to have limited ability to suppress the growth of bacilli in the walls of established cavities; they rarely heal spontaneously, even in patients who demonstrate marked resistance to infection in previously undamaged lung tissue. Open cavities, encapsulated by fibrous walls, may persist for many years and may constantly drain microorganisms into the bronchial tree. Rarely, spontaneous healing of a tuberculous cavity occurs when the communicating bronchus becomes closed at the bronchocavitary junction. Without entry of air, the intracavity oxygen tension is reduced, bacterial growth is retarded, and necrosis is interrupted. The liquid contents may inspissate and ultimately harden, becoming solid caseum. Such an old, healed cavity may present the pathologic characteristics of a tuberculoma.

BRONCHOGENIC SPREAD

Another hazard inherent in the tuberculous cavity is that of transbronchial dissemination of the infection. Bacilli-laden exudate from the cavity drains into the bronchi, and may flow or become aspirated into previously uninfected lung tissue. Bacilli may implant at these new sites and the cycle of acute inflammation, caseation necrosis, liquefaction, and cavitation may occur here as well. Such new lesions may extend, coalesce, form large masses of caseum, and then cavitate. Some may resolve completely, and others may heal spontaneously by fibrous encapsulation of caseous nodules. Fig. 34-10 demonstrates the bronchogenic spread of infection as evidenced by serial chest films.

In view of the myriads of tubercle bacilli that reach the lumen of the bronchial tree during the course of chronic cavitary tuberculosis, it is remarkable that bronchogenic spread is usually limited, and that the infection does not often progress rapidly to involve all the lung parenchyma. Most microorganisms that are deposited in previously uninfected lobules succumb promptly to effective host defenses. The limitation of transbronchial spread is testimony to the efficiency of the basic immune mechanisms operating at the deposition sites of tubercle bacilli in the hypersensitive host. It is not known why these defense mechanisms fail in those instances of bronchogenic dissemination that result in new pulmonary lesions remote from the tuberculous cavity.

DIRECT EXTRAPULMONARY SPREAD

Sputum containing virulent tubercle bacilli is coughed from the major bronchi and trachea through the larynx and pharynx to the mouth. Although these structures are relatively resistant to local invasion, bacilli may become implanted, and tuberculous inflammation and ulceration may develop—especially in the larynx, and sometimes in the pharynx, buccal

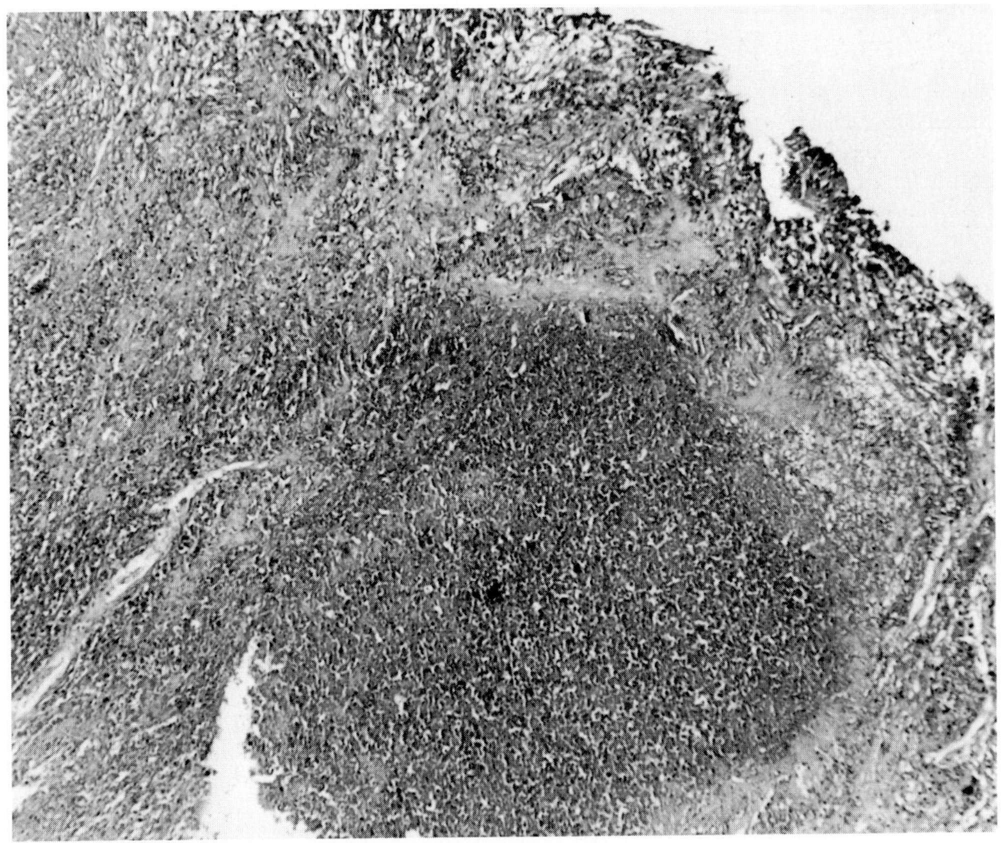

Fig. 34-6. A small caseous lesion in pulmonary tuberculosis with liquefaction at the lower border. (Original magnification approximately × 45)

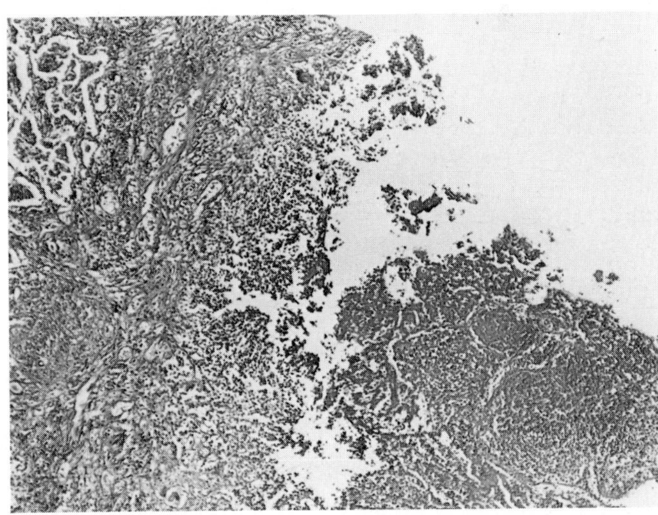

Fig. 34-7. The wall of a small tuberculous cavity is at the left. Liquefying caseous material extends from the wall into the lumen at the right. (Original magnification approximately × 45)

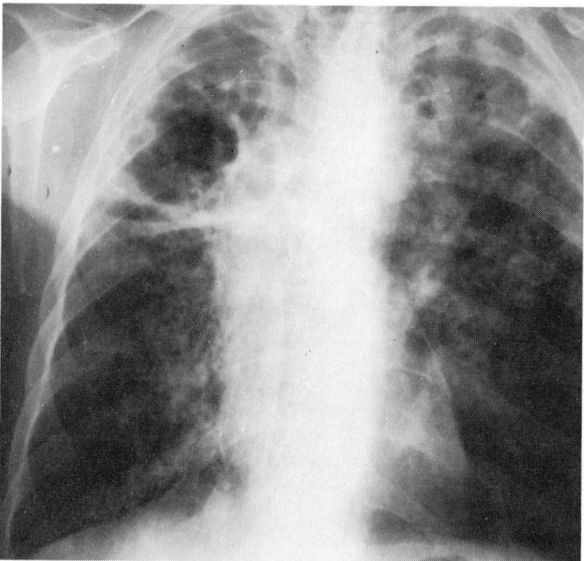

Fig. 34-8. Radiographic appearance of typical, far-advanced bilateral pulmonary tuberculosis. Note the extensive cavitation of both upper lobes and small, discrete soft infiltrates scattered throughout most of the remainder of the lung parenchyma.

Fig. 34-9. Wall of a chronic tuberculous cavity. Note the acute inflammatory reaction in the lower cavity border with organization and fibrosis of the outer (upper) border (Original magnification approximately × 320)

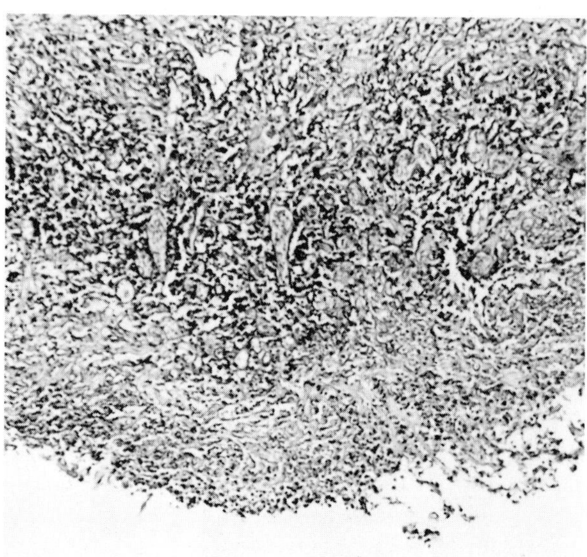

mucosa, tongue, or even the middle ear. Large numbers of microorganisms may be swallowed, thus invading the intestinal mucosa, leading to a proliferative inflammatory reaction and ulceration in the bowel, particularly in the mucosa of the ileum.

INFLUENCE OF AGE

Childhood Disease. The age of the patient greatly influences the clinical and pathologic manifestations of tuberculous disease. In infants and young children, the primary focus may be found in any portion of the lung parenchyma. Moreover, lymph node involvement is usual, lymphohematogenous dissemination is relatively common, and pulmonary cavities rarely occur. The pulmonary and lymph node lesions usually heal spontaneously. The most serious manifestations result from extrapulmonary foci established by blood-borne organisms.

Adult Disease. Typically, primary infection in teenagers and in adults differs considerably from that in young children. Lymph node involvement is not prominent, and massive lymphohematogenous dissemination occurs much less often. Progression of the infection is more apt to be the result of the development of a cavitary lesion in the lung, with subsequent pulmonary spread by the transbronchial route. A notable difference between the childhood and adult patterns of disease is the difference in the usual locations of the lesions in the lungs. In adults, as compared to young children, the lesions are most often found in the superior and posterior portions of the lung, particularly in the apical or posterior segments of the upper lobes. The occurrence of progressive infection in these areas is thought to be related to the favorable environment for the growth of tubercle bacilli provided by the higher tension of oxygen in these areas. It is not clear, however, why the same influence does not operate to favor the development of progressive primary disease in the upper lobes of children's lungs. It has been suggested that the lower level of native resistance in infants and young children makes possible the proliferation of tubercle bacilli in any portion of the lungs, including the lower lobes, despite a lower oxygen tension. Perhaps adults have a degree of native resistance sufficient to suppress the growth of tubercle bacilli in the less favorable parenchymal sites, but insufficient to prevent the multiplication and spread of bacilli that by chance become deposited in the apical or posterior segments of the upper lobes. The chest roentgenograms reproduced in Fig. 34-11 show a confluent tuberculous infiltrate and cavity in the posterior aspect of the left upper lobe. In this young adult tuberculosis developed within 1 year after tuberculin conversion.

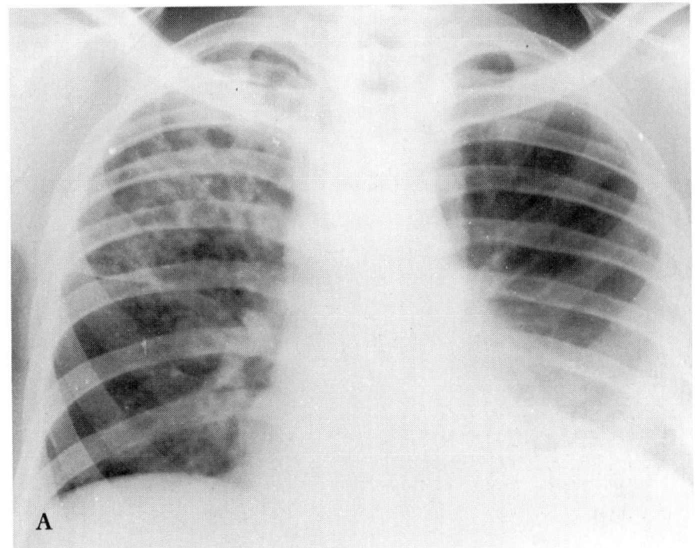

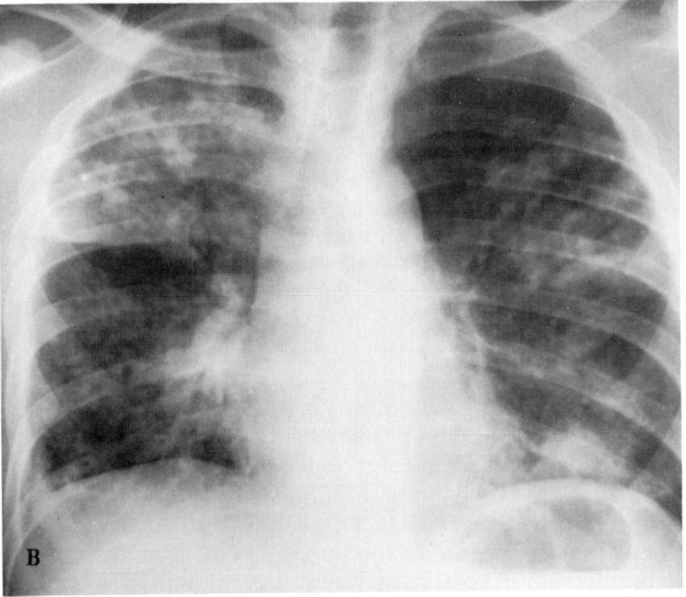

Fig. 34-10. *(A)* Radiographic appearance of local bronchogenic spread of tuberculosis in right upper lobe. Note the discrete and homogeneous lesions. There is also a homogeneous density with a roughly spherical air-containing cavity in its center at the first right anterior interspace and a left pleural effusion. *(B)* Radiographic appearance 5 months after the termination of 2 months of antituberculous chemotherapy. Although the left pleural effusion has disappeared, extensive new lesions have developed throughout the right lower lobe and the entire left lung.

LATE EXACERBATING TUBERCULOSIS

Late exacerbating tuberculosis develops principally in older individuals, usually many years after the primary infection and tuberculin conversion have occurred. Slowly progressive disease with chronic cavities and bronchogenic spread are characteristics of this form of tuberculosis. There is a marked predisposition for involvement of the upper and posterior portions of the upper lobes—also believed to be related to the higher oxygen tension at these sites. (Note: the major concentration of disease is in the upper lobes in the chest film shown in Fig. 34-8). It is not known why caseous lesions exacerbate after long periods of stability in some persons but remain entirely healed for life in others. In some cases, reactivation of tuberculosis appears to coincide with deterioration of the general health of the person due to another disease, such as chronic alcoholism, diabetes mellitus, or malignancy. Gastric resection and the administration of glucosteroids or other immunosuppressive drugs appear to increase the risk of reactivation. In other cases, no specific cause can be identified.

The source of the tubercle bacilli responsible for

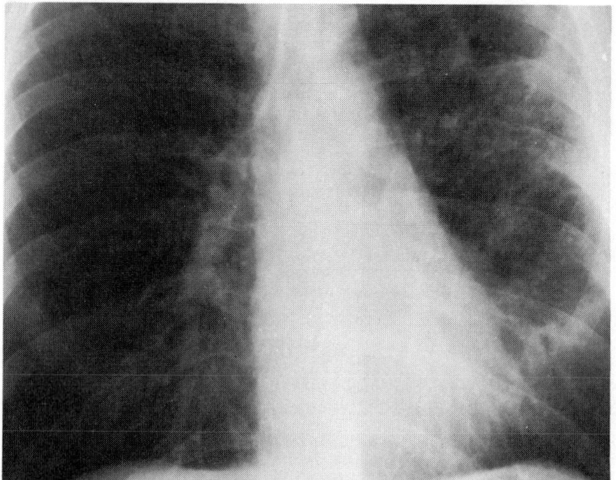

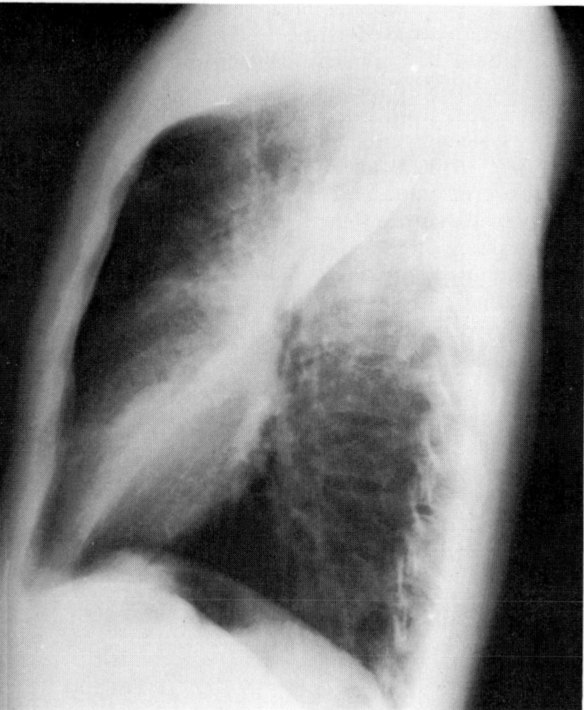

Fig. 34-11. Chest films (posteroanterior on left; left lateral on right) of a 24-year-old male obtained approximately 1 year after he was demonstrated to be tuberculin negative. A mild cough had been present for a few weeks. There is a large, thin-walled cavity and confluent disease in the posterior portion of the apical-posterior segment of the left upper lobe. In addition, bronchogenic dissemination to the anterior segment and lingular division of the left upper lobe has occurred.

late exacerbating tuberculosis is usually a caseous residuum of the original primary infection in the lung or caseous foci that have developed in the implantation sites of blood-borne bacilli during the early stages of primary infection. Exogenous sources may sometimes contribute to the development of recurrent infection in communities with large numbers of persons with communicable pulmonary tuberculosis. That is, a healthy, tuberculin-positive person may become reinfected by inhaling *M. tuberculosis* in droplet nuclei expelled by a person.

Host Defense Mechanisms

No protective value has been demonstrated with any of the several specific humoral antibodies that develop in the course of tuberculosis. It has long been recognized, however, that some kind of specific immune resistance to tuberculosis exists. Koch's phenomenon is illustrative: (1) Subcutaneous inoculation of a guinea pig with virulent *M. tuberculosis* yields no response for about 2 weeks, and then a nodule that ulcerates appears at the site of injection while a concomitant regional lymphadenitis may progress to caseation. (2) Several weeks later, a second subcutaneous inoculation of *M. tuberculosis* at a different site precipitates an acute inflammatory response followed in turn by necrosis, ulceration, and healing—with little reaction in the regional nodes. Koch also found that the intradermal injection of proteins of tubercle bacilli evoked a prompt inflammatory response in tuberculous guinea pigs but elicited no reaction in normal animals—the tuberculin test. Neither old tuberculin, such as used by Koch, nor PPD will induce hypersensitivity. Yet, either reagent will evoke the tuberculin reaction, which is specific for previous infection by mycobacteria.

HYPERSENSITIVITY

The hypersensitive state appears to depend on the presence of sensitized lymphocytes in the circulation (see Chap. 5, Immunopathology of Infectious Diseases). During the initial stages of infection, antigens released from tubercle bacilli in the lungs or lymph nodes become attached to monocytes or macrophages and, subsequently, are presented to helper T cells, which act as initiators for several aspects of the cell mediated immune reaction. One line of lymphocytes transforms and proliferates to establish a larger number of "memory" T cells. The exact mechanisms by which such cells provide tuberculin reactivity and cellular immunity are not entirely clear at this time. It is apparent, however, that macrophages are essential to the expression of both hypersensitivity and cellular immunity and are specifically involved as one consequence of effector substances (lymphokines) released as part of the interaction of sensitized lymphocytes and antigen(s) derived from tubercle bacilli. An example of such an effector substance is the migration inhibitory factor that causes macrophages to accumulate at the site of the lymphocyte–tuberculin reaction.

Another lymphokine, macrophage-activating factor, stimulates an increased concentration of hydrolytic enzymes within local macrophages and increases their ability to phagocytize and destroy tubercle bacilli. Also, a lymphocyte-transforming substance converts nonsensitive lymphocytes to tuberculin responsiveness by means of transformation and clonal proliferation.

TRANSFER FACTOR

The capacity to transfer specific delayed hypersensitivity from one person to another also resides in sensitized lymphocytes. Intact lymphocytes are not required, and in fact, a relatively low molecular weight, dialyzable, heatlabile, polypeptide or polynucleotide substance has been isolated from lymphocytes and designated transfer factor. Transfer factor is not immunogenic and differs also from the protein effector substances previously mentioned. Within hours to days after injection into normals, transfer factor engenders specific delayed hypersensitivity that persists for prolonged periods in man.

Precommitted, thymus-dependent lymphocytes become endowed with specific transfer factor on contact with antigen from the tubercle bacilli during the evolution of delayed sensitivity. Such antigen-stimulated cells proliferate and provide clones of sensitized cells that direct the activities of macrophages and other host defense mechanisms at the inflammatory site. After the initial infection has been curtailed and localized, progeny of such sensitized cells remain in the host. The future introduction of antigen, either by a tuberculin test or renewed proliferation of tubercle bacilli, leads to antigenic stimulation of a few of these cells, which in turn transform and proliferate. Under the influence of antigen, sensitized cells elaborate lymphokines and mediate the host cellular response.

Thus, the cell-mediated immune response to parasitism in tuberculosis essentially reenacts the cellular events that characterize the tuberculin reaction. In addition, the increased ability of macrophages to kill intracellular tubercle bacilli contributes significantly to control of the infection.

Manifestations

Symptoms and Signs

Most persons with active tuberculosis have no symptoms until the lesions are quite extensive. Delayed occurrence of symptoms applies both to progressive primary and late exacerbating forms of disease. As a result, persons with early disease of limited extent seldom seek medical attention, and often the diagnosis is not made until the disease has become far advanced. Among cases of advanced disease, the symptoms are not specific but may also be found in other kinds of chronic infection. Symptoms may be constitutional—the systemic effects of active infection—or local—the malfunction of an infected organ. The most common constitutional symptoms are malaise, easy fatigue, anorexia, weight loss, and fever. The temperature may rise as high as 39°C to 40°C (102°F–104°F) in the afternoon and evening, and defervescence, typically after midnight, is frequently accompanied by drenching night sweats. In tuberculosis, in contradistinction to most acute bacterial diseases, the patient is neither prostrated nor greatly discomforted by elevated body temperature and may not even be aware of fever. Some patients note chilly sensations, but shaking chills rarely occur.

Local manifestations of infection are quite variable. Pulmonary tuberculosis may cause little or no cough and sputum when the lesions are small, but patients with advanced cavitary disease are usually aware of chronic cough and expectoration. Typically, the sputum is mucopurulent, but with large, rapidly progressing cavities, frankly purulent sputum may occur. Hemoptysis is common, usually as bright red streaks of blood intermixed with sputum. Fortunately, massive, life-threatening pulmonary hemorrhage is rare. Shortness of breath follows extensive spread of infection throughout the lungs, or large pleural effusions. Tuberculous pleuritis is usually accompanied by pleuritic pain, and dyspnea if pleural effusion ensues.

Depending on the extent of disease, physical examination of persons with pulmonary tuberculosis may reveal no abnormalities or may disclose advanced parenchymal consolidation, pleural effusion, or fibrosis. Rales are often detected over the areas of diseased parenchyma, and they are usually accentuated by the posttussive maneuver. However, the physical signs do not provide a reliable basis for assessing the extent or activity of the disease.

Extrapulmonary Sites

Tuberculosis of extrapulmonary organs is discussed in Chapter 35, Extrapulmonary Tuberculosis.

Radiographic Findings

Usually, the diagnosis of pulmonary tuberculosis is suspected from an abnormal chest radiograph obtained because of symptoms or as part of a routine or screening health examination. In infants and young children, the abnormality is a nonspecific shadow suggesting parenchymal consolidation in any portion of the lung, accompanied by ipsilateral hilar lymphadenopathy. In some instances, only one or the other of these abnormalities is seen.

In adults, there are typically three characteristics of the lesions of pulmonary tuberculosis. First, the maximum concentration of the disease, particularly that due to confluent or cavitary lesions, is found in the apical or posterior segments of the upper lobes. Small, early lesions are usually confined to one of these segments, and in far-advanced disease, these are usually the most prominent sites of consolidation and destructive changes. Occasionally, the superior segments of the lower lobes are sites of maximal involvement. In adult tuberculosis, it is rare to find the major confluent lesions in the anterior portions.

Second, the major concentration of disease usually has the appearance of a homogenous, confluent infiltrate or a cavity. Homogenous shadows are produced by inflammatory or caseous changes in the lung parenchyma at the site of the original, or most active, tuberculous lesion. Such lesions vary in size from less than a centimeter in tiny, minimal lesions to the volume of one or more of the lung segments in advanced disease. The peripheral borders of such confluencies tend to be irregular and mottled because of nonhomogeneous consolidation of parenchymal lobules and the presence of productive tubercles surrounding the confluent lesion. In moderately advanced and far-advanced disease, cavities are usually apparent. A large, air-containing space may be the most prominent abnormality (see Fig. 34-11). In other instances, the cavitary space may be small, but surrounded by a thick, homogenous mass (see Fig. 34-10). Chest films obtained in the oblique and apical–lordotic positions or by body section roentgenography may be required to demonstrate and delineate a cavity. Solid, encapsulated tuberculomas seldom contain cavities, and they may be absent or undetectable in small lesions.

Third, roentgenographic evidence of bronchogenic dissemination is usually found. Fresh lesions from recent spreading will appear as multiple, discrete, soft, fluffy nodules scattered in the lung parenchyma adjacent to the confluent or cavitary lesion, or remote from this focus in another lobe or in the opposite lung. These lesions may occur in any portion of the lung, including anterior and inferior locations (see Figs. 34-10 and 34-11). Old, healed, or healing lesions from past bronchogenic spreads are sharply discrete and nodular, and they present smoother borders and a more rounded configuration than do recent lesions.

The diagnosis of tuberculosis cannot be established by roentgenography; many other diseases of the lungs result in identical or very similar radiographic characteristics. Nonetheless, chest films are a major component of the evidence required to formulate a meaningful differential diagnosis. In addition, analysis of the changes that occur in serial films provides a principal means for studying the natural history of the disease in a specific patient and for predicting the pathologic characterics of the lesions.

Diagnosis

The diagnosis of tuberculosis requires the isolation and identification of *M. tuberculosis* or, rarely, *M. bovis,* from tissue, body fluids, or inflammatory exudates. In pulmonary tuberculosis, a presumptive diagnosis is frequently based on the demonstration of characteristic acid-fast bacilli in smears of sputum (unconcentrated or concentrated) obtained either by spontaneous expectoration or induced by inhaled aerosols. Subsequent confirmation by culture is mandatory. Pulmonary secretions may also be obtained by aspiration of the trachea or bronchi by catheter or through a bronchoscope. In children and in adults in whom it is difficult to obtain sputum, a secondary method involves collecting gastric contents after the patient has fasted. The stomach may contain swallowed sputum, thus providing a specimen suitable for culture. Excepting those from infants and young children, gastric aspirates contain mycobacteria other than *M. tuberculosis* so frequently that examination of smears is not recommended. Tubercle bacilli may also be cultured from pleural fluid, ascitic fluid, cerebrospinal fluid, urine, and from pus drained or aspirated from abscesses. Tubercle bacilli may be grown from tissue removed by biopsy or surgical resection.

Tissue specimens that demonstrate the histopathologic characteristics of a tubercle or a caseated granuloma, and in which acid-fast bacilli are found, may be presumed to have resulted from mycobacterial infection. Identification of mycobacterial species, however, requires isolation of the microorganism in culture. Microscopic demonstration of characteristic acid-fast bacilli (see Chap. 9, Microscopic Examinations) in uncontaminated body fluids, such as pleural, ascitic, or cerebrospinal fluid, also enables a presumptive diagnosis of mycobacterial infection to be made. Repeated demonstrations of a heavy concentration of acid-fast bacilli in stained sputum specimens enables a preliminary, presumptive diagnosis of tuberculosis to be made, pending the results of cultures that should yield tubercle bacilli in this circumstance. Detection of a few acid-fast bacilli in a single sputum smear may denote a false positive result because of errors in the preparation or interpretation of the slide or to the presence of saprophytic acid-fast bacteria, or it may indicate the presence of tubercle bacilli. Unless confirmed by cultures, such an isolated demonstration of acid-fast microorganisms in the sputum should be interpreted as suggestive but not diagnostic. In adults, urine and gastric contents contain saprophytic acid-fast bacteria so often that stained smears have little value.

Some clinical situations require the use of circumstantial evidence rather than direct proof of active tuberculous infection. Children who have a positive tuberculin test must be assumed to have had recent infection because their age precludes long-standing, healed, or inactive disease. Similarly, a recent conversion to reactivity to tuberculin, regardless of age, must be presumed to indicate infection which occurred subsequent to an earlier, negative tuberculin test.

Whenever possible, the diagnosis of tuberculosis should be proved rather than assumed. There are, however, occasional circumstances in which serious, life-threatening manifestations require prompt treatment and do not permit delay for the bacteriologic confirmation of tuberculosis before therapy is initiated. In such cases, appropriate specimens should be collected promptly, examined immediately for acid-fast bacilli, and cultured. Therapy is then based on a presumed diagnosis pending the results of cultures.

Most cases of moderately advanced or far-advanced tuberculosis offer little diagnostic difficulty. Early disease and noncavitary pulmonary lesions provide a greater diagnostic challenge. Some acute, and many chronic, lung diseases may closely resemble tuberculosis. Upper lobe pneumonias caused by other bacteria, mycoplasmas, viruses, fungi, or the result of aspiration may be confused with tuberculous infections. Chronic fungus infection of the lung, especially histoplasmosis, may cause clinical and radiographic manifestations identical with those of tuberculosis. Lung cancer, chronic lung abscess, sarcoidosis, pneumoconiosis, and pulmonary manifestations of a variety of systemic disorders may also resemble tuberculosis.

Therapy

If a program of antituberculous chemotherapy is carefully designed and flawlessly executed, treatment is almost always successful. Conversely, selection of an inappropriate regimen by the physician or the patient's failure to adhere to a prescribed program may result in the failure of clinical response and the emergence of tubercle bacilli resistant to the antituberculous agents employed.

Soon after streptomycin (SM) became available in 1944, it was noted that some patients either failed to respond or relapsed promptly after initial improvement. Tubercle bacilli resistant to the action of streptomycin were usually isolated from such patients.

In 1950, after the introduction of paraaminosalicylic acid (PAS), it was possible to assess combined two-agent therapy. The emergence of SM-resistant mutants was markedly delayed when PAS was given concurrently with SM. Bacteriologic conversion, healing of active pulmonary foci, and ultimate cure occurred in most patients when these drugs were administered together.

Isoniazid (INH), introduced in 1952, was soon shown to be a remarkably effective and relatively nontoxic antituberculous drug. Regimens that combined INH with either PAS or SM, or the use of all three agents together, were superior to SM–PAS in clinical efficacy and in suppressing the emergence of drug-resistant bacilli.

Fundamental to rationalizing these observations was the demonstration of the presence of a few natively resistant cells in all large populations of *M. tuberculosis* newly isolated from untreated patients. With SM, the frequency is about one in 10^6 cells; with INH, one in 10^5 cells. Thus, in patients with lesions that contain myriads of actively multiplying tubercle bacilli, as in pulmonary cavities or other ulcerative lesions, use of a single antituberculous agent could be expected to result in the outgrowth of the small minority of natively resistant bacilli. Simultaneous exposure to two individually effective drugs suppresses the emergence of resistance, presumably as a consequence of the independent action of each drug on the small minority of cells resistant to the other.

Table 34-4. *Antituberculous Drugs*

Drugs	Route of Administration	Dose/Day MG/KG BODY WT	Dose/Day USUAL ADULT	Toxicity MANIFESTATIONS	Toxicity FREQUENCY	RELATIVE EFFICACY
Primary						
Isoniazid (INH)	Peroral	5–10, once daily	300 mg	Hepatic Neurologic	Uncommon	Highly effective
Rifampin (RMP)	Peroral	10, once daily	600 mg	Hepatic Hematologic	Uncommon	Highly effective
Secondary						
Ethambutol (EMB)	Peroral	15–25, once daily	800–1600 mg	Optic neuritis	Uncommon	Limited effectiveness, good secondary drug
Pyrazinamide (PZA)*	Peroral	20–30, once daily	1–3 g	Hepatic Hyperuricemia	Uncommon	Effective, useful as secondary drug, hepatitis may be severe
Streptomycin (SM)	Intramuscular	7–15, once daily	0.75–1.0 g	Eighth nerve Renal	Common	Highly effective
Tertiary						
Paraaminosalicylic acid (PAS)*	Peroral	200, 4 equal doses, 6-hourly	12–16 g	Gastrointestinal intolerance	Common	Limited effectiveness, poor patient tolerance
Ethionamide (ETA)*	Peroral	7–15, 4 equal doses 6-hourly	0.75–1 g	Gastrointestinal intolerance	Common	Moderately effective, poor patient tolerance
Cycloserine (CS)*	Peroral	10–15, 4 equal doses 6-hourly	0.75–1 g	Psychopathy Seizures	Common	Limited effectiveness, rarely indicated
Capreomycin (CM)*	Intramuscular	15, once daily	1 g	Eighth nerve	Common	Moderately effective
Kanamycin (KM)*	Intramuscular	15, once daily	0.5–1 g	Eighth nerve Renal	Common	Moderately effective

*Use generally restricted to retreatment.

In order to evaluate the efficacy of various combinations of antituberculous agents, systematic, controlled trials of chemotherapy were undertaken by cooperative, multicenter study groups in the United States, Great Britain, and Japan. The results of these studies form the major basis for current practices in the chemotherapy of tuberculosis. The antituberculous drugs currently available are listed in Table 34-4 (see also Table 18-1) along with conventional doses and major toxic manifestations. In a given patient, selection of the most appropriate regimen should be based on (1) the history of previous drug therapy, (2) the results of *in vitro* susceptibility tests, and (3) the relative risks of adverse reactions to the drugs. The prescribed regimen should not only provide maximum antimicrobial activity, but should also be convenient to administer, a factor of great importance to patient acceptance and adherence to the regimens of prolonged administration that are required.

Initial Therapy

Tuberculous infections of the lung can virtually always be controlled if the first attempt at therapy is implemented correctly. Since INH was introduced, a number of combined drug regimens have been used for this purpose. For the first 15 years, regimens composed of various combinations of INH, SM, and PAS were widely used. Overall, these were quite effective, the most efficacious being the triple regimen: INH, PAS, and SM, each given daily. Treatment was continued for 18 to 24 months in order to prevent posttherapy relapse. A large dose of PAS was required, 12 g to 14 g daily, and many patients suffered gastrointestinal distress, indigestion, nausea, and anorexia. Up to 50% of patients failed to take PAS as prescribed.

Ethambutol (EMB), a relatively weak, tuberculostatic agent, became available in 1968 and largely supplanted PAS as a companion drug to INH and SM. EMB is generally well tolerated and, except for the rare occurrence of optic neuritis, causes few adverse reactions. Combined with INH or SM, it is effective in preventing the emergence of drug-resistant mutants.

Rifampin (RMP) is the newest of the antituberculous antimicrobics. Used in Europe since the mid-1960s, RMP became generally available in the United States in 1971. It is highly effective against *M. tuberculosis* and is a very useful agent in the clinical management of tuberculosis.

The most effective and widely-used regimen today is INH, 300 mg, and RMP, 600 mg, both given in single daily dosages. Sputum conversion (*i.e.,* failure of growth of *M. tuberculosis* in cultures) occurs within 1 month in the majority of patients, and within 3 months in more than 95% of previously untreated cases with drug-susceptible organisms. This regimen causes a more rapid sputum conversion and has a higher level of bactericidal activity *in vivo* than does the combination of INH–SM–EMB. The addition of EMB to INH–RMP does not speed sputum conversion.

The major disadvantage of the INH–RMP is the occurrence of drug related hepatitis. As many as 20% to 30% of patients receiving INH–RMP will develop laboratory evidence of disturbed hepatic function on serial testing; most will have no symptoms, and liver function returns to normal in spite of continuing drug administration. Probably less than 5% of patients develop symptoms (anorexia, nausea, vomiting) jaundice, and progressive deterioration of liver function; in such patients, INH–RMP must be discontinued promptly. Depending upon the clinical circumstances and the severity of the reaction, another regimen should be substituted temporarily or permanently.

From the early trials of antituberculous chemotherapy, it was recognized that prolonged therapy was required and that the risk of relapse of tuberculosis after stopping therapy was greatly influenced by the duration of uninterrupted chemotherapy. A combined regimen of INH–SM–EMB in the initial phase, followed by INH–EMB, resulted in a higher rate of relapse after 12 months of therapy than after 18 to 24 months of treatment. Accordingly, the conventional duration of therapy recommended and attempted was 18 to 24 months. A number of important factors, however, have prompted organized efforts to reduce the total duration of treatment and the specific number of doses of medication required to achieve cure. The major unpredictable variable in the United States has been the level of patient compliance. The longer the course of treatment required, the greater the risk that the patient will terminate therapy prematurely. Also, in the United States and especially in developing countries, the cost of medication and services stimulated an interest in short-course chemotherapy. Clinical trails in Europe and in the United States showed that a regimen of INH–RMP daily for 12 months, or INH–RMP daily for 20 weeks followed by daily INH–EMB until the sputum has been free of viable *M. tuberculosis* for 1 year, were both highly effective and associated with a low posttreatment relapse rate. Thus, 12 months became the recommended duration of treatment with either of these regimens.

Clinical trials in Africa by the British Medical Research Council showed that a 6-month regimen of daily INH–RMP was effective and yielded an acceptably low rate of posttreatment relapse. In contrast, both in Europe and the United States, 6 months of daily INH–RMP were followed by excessive rates of posttreatment relapse. After review of the evidence, a committee of the American Thoracic Society and the Tuberculosis Control Division of the Centers for Disease Control recommended 9 months of INH–RMP as an acceptable alternative therapy for adults with previously untreated, drug-susceptible, uncomplicated pulmonary tuberculosis. In some circumstances, after 2 weeks to 2 months of daily therapy, treatment may be continued with twice-weekly supervised doses of INH (15 mg/kg) and RMP (600 mg). Patients with extrapulmonary tuberculosis, those who have received previous therapy for tuberculosis, and those following irregular or inconsistent regimens because of toxicity, should not be considered candidates for short-course chemotherapy.

Recent immigrants from areas with a high prevalence of INH-resistant organisms, such as Southeast Asia and South and Central America, should also be given EMB (15 mg/kg) along with INH–RMP until susceptibility tests are completed. Of organisms obtained from previously untreated cases in 1975 to 1977, the Centers for Disease Control reported 8.6% resistant to one or more drugs, and 4.4% resistant to INH. Fortunately, primary resistance to RMP is low at 0.3%.

Rapid reversal of infectiousness is achieved in approximately 95% of patients treated for the first time using properly selected regimens that are followed without interruption. Failure to respond or, more frequently, clinical and bacteriologic relapse after an initial temporary response is most often the result of inconsistent administration of drugs through default by the patient. The risk of haphazard drug intake and premature termination of therapy is the resurgent proliferation of tubercle bacilli, sometimes with emerging drug resistance, followed by bacteriologic and clinical relapse (see Fig. 34-10). Medical and psychosocial factors operate to impair therapy. Drug reactions are more frequent and hazardous in aged individuals and in those with coexisting diseases, particularly chronic disease of the gastrointestinal tract, liver, and kidneys. Ignorance, chronic alcoholism, drug addiction, and psychopathic personality traits blunt the patient's motivation for cure and frustrate cooperation through the need for immediate personal gratification. Accordingly, the physician must not only prescribe appropriate drugs, but must also utilize every possible resource to ensure the cooperation of the patient.

In the successfully treated patient, serial chest radiograms will document healing as bacterial growth is interrupted. Soft infiltrates may resolve, or may shrink and harden. Cavities usually shrink, and the air-containing space may be replaced by a homogenous density composed of encapsulated caseum and fibrous tissue. A large cavity may heal by complete sloughing of the inner wall to form a persistent, fibrous, cystlike structure, an open-healed cavity composed of fibrous tissue. It is sometimes lined with squamous epithelium and is often devoid of tuberculous residua such as tubercles, caseous tissue, or tubercle bacilli.

Retreatment

Posttreatment relapse is rare among persons who achieve a noninfectious state as a result of the primary regimen of therapy and who complete the entire course of treatment. The risk of late relapse increases as the initial regimen deviates from the ideal. The bacilli recovered from relapsed patients often retain full susceptibility to the antituberculous agents previously employed. In such patients, the primary regimen should be reinstituted. When partial or complete microbial resistance is found, however, a retreatment regimen should be used.

In patients who fail to respond to continuous or interrupted primary therapy, resistance to the agents employed can usually be demonstrated by testing *in vitro*. For this reason, retreatment regimens consist of two, sometimes three, agents that have not previously been given to the patient. If this is not possible, only those drugs used previously that are still active as shown by testing *in vitro* against contemporary isolates are rationally prescribed again. INH should always be included in the retreatment regimen if the infecting tubercle bacilli remain susceptible to it. On occasion, however, INH is also recommended when resistance can be demonstrated by testing *in vitro*. Apparently, the degree of resistance to INH may vary among the bacilli comprising a given mycobacterial population—that is, some of the microorganisms may remain susceptible to INH.

Regimens which include RMP have greatly improved the treatment of patients with disease caused by *M. tuberculosis* that are resistant to INH, SM, and other agents. Candidates for retreatment with INH-resistant organisms should be treated with RMP (600 mg per day perorally as a single dose) combined with SM and EMB, if the organism remains susceptible to these agents. Pyrazinamide (PZA) may also be used as a companion drug to RMP and SM. Of the two injectible antimicrobics which may be used if SM-resistant *M. tuberculosis* is present, capreomycin is preferable to kanamycin because there is less hazard of irreversible toxicity. Ethionamide, PAS, and cycloserine are rarely required—only when tubercle bacilli are shown by *in vitro* testing to be resistant to the more effective antimicrobics. These agents are not highly effective and may cause troublesome adverse reactions. New agents must never be introduced singly into an ongoing regimen that is clinically and bacteriologically ineffective because resistance to the added drug will result.

Because of the prior failure of treatment and the frequent necessity for the use of several antimicrobics with potential for toxic adverse effects, patients receiving retreatment therapy must be followed closely and carefully. Attention must be given to the clinical and bacteriologic response, with particular concern for the appearance of adverse reactions and changes from the original patterns of resistance to antimicrobics. When possible, an ongoing retreatment regimen should be modified by deletion of the most toxic agents. Although 18 to 24 months of continuous therapy is generally necessary, the total duration of treatment should be individualized.

Properly selected and carefully monitored retreatment regimens result in sputum conversion in over 90% of patients. Surgical excision of cavity-bearing lung tissue is rarely indicated. It may be required in a very few, selected patients who fail to respond to primary therapy and to multiple retreatment regimens.

Extrapulmonary tuberculosis may either dominate the clinical picture or may be the sole clinical manifestation of tuberculosis (see Chap. 35, Extrapulmonary Tuberculosis).

Glucosteriods

The chemotherapeutic effectiveness of antituberculous agents is unaffected by glucosteroids. On the other hand, pharmacologic doses of glucosteroids diminish the inflammatory and granulomatous changes in the tuberculous lesions and abolish systemic manifestations of illness such as fever, malaise, and anorexia. Although the latter effects are a comfort to the acutely ill patient, in terms of cure of tuberculosis, concurrent administration of glucosteroids generally offers no advantage. The exceptions are (1) overwhelming, life-threatening disease, (2) tuberculous meningitis with actual or impending subarachnoid block, and (3) hypersensitivity to one or more antituberculous agents judged to be essential to treatment. Prednisone, in a dosage of 0.5 mg/kg body wt/day, or equivalent dosage of another glucosteroid, has been given for periods of 1 to 3 months. Substantiation of efficacy by controlled clinical trial has not been accomplished.

Prevention

Socioeconomic Aspects

In the early 1900s, voluntary citizen groups and governmental agencies cooperated in the development of organized programs for tuberculosis control. These were directed principally at the detection of overt, communicable tuberculosis so that admission to sanitoriums and other institutions of treatment would interrupt air-borne transmission of infection to others. Case finding was based largely on campaigns of public education regarding the symptoms of the disease and its mode of transmission, as well as the use of mass surveys of the population by chest roentgenography. Such efforts probably contributed to the control of the disease during those decades when tuberculosis remained relatively common throughout all the United States and all segments of society. Even in retrospect, however, it is difficult to quantitate the specific contribution to prevention that resulted from such programs.

Beginning late in the 19th century and continuing to the present time, tuberculosis mortality and morbidity rates have declined markedly in most economically developed countries, particularly in Western Europe and the United States (see Fig. 34-2). The decline is generally attributed to improved standards of living and general health. Better housing, sanitation, and personal hygiene lessen the risk of airborne contagion, whereas better nutrition may increase an individual's native resistance. Periods of social and economic decline (*e.g.,* war and natural disasters) impair the general and community health, and they are associated with an increased incidence of tuberculosis.

Today, in some economically depressed countries of the world and in certain geographic sections of the United States the level of personal and community health continues to favor the occurrence and spread of tuberculous infection. Thus, a major potential for tuberculosis control in these communities remains inherent in improved standards of living.

Chemotherapy

Effective chemotherapy is accompanied by an almost immediate reduction in the number of tubercle bacilli expectorated by the patient. After 3 months of effective therapy, approximately 95% of patients no longer discharge culturable tubercle bacilli, and very few who complete 9 to 12 months of treatment ever again become disseminators of tubercle bacilli.

Epidemiologic studies have demonstrated the remarkable effectiveness of chemotherapy as a preventive of tuberculosis contagion. Contacts of sputum-positive patients have virtually no risk of becoming infected some 3 to 6 weeks after chemotherapy was initiated despite continuing personal association.

Case Finding

Case finding and early, effective treatment of the active case remain essential to the control of tuberculosis, regardless of the actual incidence of disease within the community. However, case finding techniques offer different levels of feasibility and success, depending on the prevalence of communicable tuberculosis within the population examined. Population surveys by chest roentgenography are valuable in communities with high prevalance, particularly in economically depressed countries. Mass surveys of selected populations by microscopic examination of sputum for acid-fast bacilli have even been used effectively for case finding purposes. Case detection must be followed by effective treatment, however, in order to serve preventively.

In the United States today, the incidence of active pulmonary tuberculosis has declined to a level that precludes mass chest radiographic surveys of unselected populations as a useful or economically feasible technique for case finding. However, routine chest films are productive as a case finding technique among groups in which new cases are most likely to be found, such as (1) patients with respiratory symptoms who consult physicians; (2) indigent patients admitted to municipal and similar hospitals; (3) contacts of newly diagnosed cases of tuberculosis; (4) homeless alcoholic men; (5) prisoners; (6) recent immigrants from countries with a known high incidence of tuberculosis; (7) persons with silicosis, diabetes, previous gastrectomy, and those receiving prolonged glucosteroid therapy; (8) residents of economically depressed sections of large cities and certain rural areas; (9) persons known to have recently become reactive to tuberculin; and (10) contacts of young children with positive tuberculin tests.

Chemoprophylaxis

The administration of INH for 1 year in a single daily dose of 300 mg for adults and 10 mg per kg body wt for children prevents active pulmonary tuberculosis. INH acts to diminish the myobacterial population of roentgenographically detectable, quiescent pulmonary lesions or of pulmonary foci which are radiologically inapparent. Extensive trials by the United States Public Health Service have demonstrated a significant reduction of morbidity in treated subjects; such protection persists for many years. Through chemoprophylaxis, the incidence of infectious tuberculosis is reduced, thus limiting the transmission of the disease. Chemoprophylaxis, then, not only reduces the risk of active disease in the treated individual, but also serves to prevent the spread of the disease to uninfected persons, thereby benefiting the community as well.

Because every tuberclin reactor is at some risk of developing active tuberculosis, all tuberculin-positive persons, theoretically, might be candidates for INH prophylaxis. Such a massive preventive program is impractical; it is also contravened by the inherent risk of hepatitis caused by INH. Mild hepatic dysfunction, manifested by transiently elevated concentations of glutamic-oxaloacetic transminase in the serum, occurs in 10% to 20% of persons taking the drug. Most patients have no symptoms, and serum enzyme levels return to normal even though the administration of INH is continued. In a few cases, liver damage progresses, as is evidenced by deterioration of liver function and the development of symptoms typical of hepatitis. In such cases, INH must be discontinued; liver function usually returns to normal without sequelae. The risk of symptomatic, severe hepatitis varies considerably with the age of the patient. It is rare under the age of 20, and ranges from 1.2% to 2.3% in persons between 35 and 50 years and older. In order to obtain the benefits of INH prophylaxis and yet minimize the risk of serious hepatitis due to INH, the following priorities have been recommended and widely accepted: (1) household members and other close associates of persons with recently diagnosed tuberculosis; (2) tuberculin reactors with chest roentgenograms demonstrating nonprogressive, "healed" or "quiescent" leisions; (3) persons whose tuberculin reaction has become positive within the past 2 years; (4) tuberculin reactors with conditions which increase the risk of developing tuberculous disease—such as prolonged glucosteroid therapy, immunosuppressive therapy, silicosis; (5) any positive tuberculin reactor under the age of 35 years and particularly children up to the age of 7.

When INH is prescribed, the patient should receive careful instruction as to the symptoms of toxicity and should be carefully followed during the year of drug administration.

Immunoprophylaxis

Bacillus Calmette–Guérin (BCG), a live attenuated strain of bovine tubercle bacilli, has been widely used as vaccine since 1921. Although efficacy has been proved in man, the degree of protection remains somewhat controversial. Some controlled clinical studies in the United States, England, and India have reported a 60% to 80% reduction in rates of infection in vaccinated persons, compared with unvaccinated controls. However, in other trials the level of protection ranged from 15% to 30%. Such discrepancies may have been due to a variation in the immunizing potency of the vaccines used and the degree to which the populations studied were protected by previous subclinical, nontuberculous mycobacterial infections.

Currently, BCG is used extensively in countries with a high prevalence of tuberculosis. Vaccination must be carried out in infancy or early childhood before natural infection takes place. In the United States, BCG has been restricted to persons who are heavily exposed to tubercle bacilli or who carry a high risk of clinical disease—for example, certain medical and nursing personnel, and American Indians. Some authorities recommend vaccination for tuberculin-negative Americans who are assigned to duty in highly endemic areas, particularly members of the armed forces and diplomatic corps.

A major disadvantage of BCG is the tuberculin reactivity that is induced temporarily, negating the diagnostic value of tuberculin tests as long as reactivity persists. A valid tuberculin test is essential to the selection of candidates for chemoprophylaxis, and it is widely believed that chemoprophylaxis offers the best prospect for the control and eventual eradication of the disease in the United States.

Remaining Problems

The ultimate goal is the elimination of tuberculous infection worldwide. Virtually all countries have made some progress toward this goal—to a degree that generally parallels their economic development. In the United States and certain other economically advanced countries, the incidence of tuberculosis has declined progressively for 50 to 75 years, whereas in some countries it has lessened only in the past decade. In the developed countries with relatively low rates of infection, the major remaining problems are those of program development; that is, finding ways to plan, organize, finance, and apply information, measures, and methods that are well known. These same programmatic problems also exist in underdeveloped areas of the world, but implementation is much more severely hampered by the twin ogres of greater needs and fewer resources. The core problem remains economic.

Methods to identify the infected would be greatly improved by the development of a highly specific antigen for skin tests, or lymphocyte stimulation tests, thereby eliminating the problem of cross reactions with other mycobacterial species. A specific immunologic or biochemical test to predict the total concentration of metabolically-active tubercle bacilli in the host would permit preventive therapy selected for those at greatest risk of subsequent disease.

New, more effective, and cheaper methods for prevention are badly needed—for example, an immunizing agent which is less expensive, easier to use, and more effective than BCG. New antimicrobics appropriate for prevention but free of adverse reactions would be an advance.

Active tuberculosis can now be treated successfully with the knowledge and means at hand. However, less than optimum therapy is used in areas of the world where the economy precludes use of the more expensive antimicrobics. Treatment would be simplified if new antimicrobics were developed which were inexpensive, well tolerated, easy to administer, and, particularly, which had a prompt bactericidal effect upon tubercle bacilli.

Bibliography

Books

BLAIR, JE, LENNETTE EH, TRUANT JP: Manual of Clinical Microbiology. Baltimore, Williams & Wilkins, 1970. 729 pp.

BURKE RM: An Historical Chronology of Tuberculosis, 2nd ed. Springfield, Charles C Thomas, 1955. 125 pp.

CANETTI G: The Tubercle Bacillus in the Pulmonary Lesion of Man. New York, Springer-Verlag, 1955. 125 pp.

Centers for Disease Control: Tuberculosis in the United States: 1978. Atlanta: Centers for Disease Control 1980, DHHS Publication No. (CDC) 80-8322. 63 pp.

EICKHOFF TC: The Current Status of BCG Immunization Against Tuberculosis. In Ann Rev Med 28:411–423, 1977. Palo Alto, Annual Reviews. 1977.

LINCOLN EM, SEWELL EM: Tuberculosis in Children. New York, McGraw-Hill, 1963. 61 pp.

LOWELL AM: Tuberculosis in the World: Centers for Disease Control: Atlanta, 1976. HEW Publication No. (CDC) 76-8317. 319 pp.

RICH AR: The Pathogenesis of Tuberculosis, 2nd ed. Springfield, Charles C Thomas, 1951. 1028 pp.

RILEY RL, O'GRADY F: Airborne Infection: Transmission and Control. New York, Macmillan, 1961. 180 pp.

Journals

American Thoracic Society: Standards for tuberculosis treatment in the 1970's: a statement by the *ad hoc* committee on quality care for tuberculosis. Am Rev Respir Dis 102:992–995, 1970

American Thoracic Society: Preventive therapy of tuberculous infection. Am Rev Respir Dis 110:371–374, 1974

American Thoracic Society: Treatment of Mycobacterial Disease. Am Rev Respir Dis 115:185–187, 1977

American Thoracic Society: Tuberculosis in the Foreign Born. Am Rev Respir Dis 116:561–564, 1977

American Thoracic Society: Guidelines for Short-Course Tuberculosis Chemotherapy. Am Rev Respir Dis 121:611–614, 1980

American Thoracic Society: Diagnostic Standards and Classification of Tuberculosis and Other Mycobacterial Diseases, 14th ed. Am Rev Respir Dis 123:343–358, 1981

COMSTOCK GW, EDWARDS PQ: The competing risks of tuberculosis and hepatitis for adult tuberculin reactors. Am Rev Respir Dis 111:573–577, 1975

COMSTOCK GW, BAUM C, SNIDER DE JR: Isoniazid prophylaxis among Alaskan Eskimos: A final report of the Bethel isoniazid studies. Am Rev Respir Dis 119:827–830, 1979

DUTT AK, JONES L, STEAD WW: Short-course chemotherapy for tuberculosis with largely twice-weekly isoniazid-rifampin. Chest 75:441–447, 1979

EDWARDS PQ, EDWARDS LB: Story of the tuberculin test. Am Rev Respir Dis (Suppl): 81:1–47, 1960

FOX W, MITCHISON DA: "State of the art". Short-course chemotherapy for pulmonary tuberculosis. Am Rev Respir Dis 111:325–353, 1975

GLASSROTH J, ROBINS AG, SNIDER DE JR: Tuberculosis in the 1980's. N Engl J Med 302:1441–1450, 1980

KHAN MA, KOVNAT DM, BACHUS B, WHITCOMB ME, BRODY JS, SNIDER GL: Clinical and roentgenographic spectrum of pulmonary tuberculosis in the adult. Am J Med 62:31–38, 1977

KOPANOFF DE, KILBURN JO, GLASSROTH JL, SNIDER DE, FARER LS, GOOD RC: A continuing survey of tuberculosis primary drug resistance in the United States: March 1975 to November 1977. Am Rev Respir Dis 118:835–842, 1978

KUBICA GP, GROSS WM, HAWKINS JE, SOMMERS HM, VESTAL AL, WAYNE LG: Laboratory services for mycobacterial diseases. Am Rev Respir Dis 112:773–787, 1975

LONG MW, SNIDER DE JR, FARER LS: U. S. Public Health Service cooperative trial of three rifampin-isoniazid regimens in treatment of pulmonary tuberculosis. Am Rev Respir Dis 119:879–894, 1979

MACKANESS GM: The immunology of anti-tuberculous immunity. Am Rev Respir Dis 97:337–344, 1968

MACKANESS GM: Resistance to intracellular infection. J Infect Dis 123:439–445, 1971

MCDERMOTT W: The John Barnwell lecture: Microbial drug resistance. Am Rev Respir Dis 102:857–876, 1970

MEDLAR EM: The behavior of pulmonary tuberculous lesions: A pathological study. Am Rev Pul Dis (Suppl) 71:1–241, 1955

MITCHELL JR: N.I.H. Conference: Isoniazid liver injury: Clinical spectrum, pathology, and probably pathogenesis. Ann Intern Med 84:181–192, 1976

MOULDING T: Chemoprophylaxis of tuberculosis: When is the benefit worth the risk and cost? Ann Intern Med 74:761–770, 1971

PALMER CE, EDWARDS LB: Identifying the tuberculous infected: The dual test technique. JAMA 205:167–169, 1968

RALEIGH JW: Rifampin in treatment of advanced pulmonary tuberculosis. Am Rev Respir Dis 105:397–409, 1972

REICHMAN LB, O'DAY R: Tuberculous infection in a large urban population. Am Rev Respir Dis 117:705–712, 1978

SALVIN SB, NETA R: A possible relationship between delayed hypersensitivity and cell-mediated immunity. Am Rev Respir Dis 111:373–375, 1975

SBARBARO JA, CATLIN BJ, ISEMAN M: Long-term effectiveness of intermittent therapy for tuberculosis: Final report of three Denver studies. Am Rev Respir Dis 121:172–174, 1980

STEAD WW: Pathogenesis of the sporadic case of tuberculosis. N Engl J Med 277:1008–1012, 1967

THOMPSON NJ, GLASSROTH JL, SNIDER DE JR, FARER LS: The booster phenomenon in serial tuberculin skin testing. Am Rev Respir Dis 119:587–597, 1979

VALL–SPINOSA A, LESTER W, MOULDING T, DAVIDSON PT, MCCLATCHY JK: Rifampin in the treatment of drug-resistant *Mycobacterium tuberculosis* infections. N Engl J Med 283:616–621, 1970

YOUMANS GP: Relationships between delayed hypersensitivity and immunity in tuberculosis. Am Rev Respir Dis 111:109–118, 1975

RUTH M. LAWRENCE

Extrapulmonary Tuberculosis

35

In the United States, tuberculosis is acquired almost exclusively by inhaling *Mycobacterium tuberculosis* (*i.e.,* all tuberculosis begins as pulmonary tuberculosis). Virtually any organ of the body may become secondarily infected as a result of intraluminal spread, direct extension, and lymphogenous-hematogenous dissemination. The resultant foci of extrapulmonary disease may remain quiescent for many years, cause an indolent infection localized to one or more organs, or produce a dramatic, rapidly progressive illness early in the course of massive dissemination.

The digestive tract may be an important primary site of infection in areas of the world where bovine tuberculosis is common. Other extrapulmonary sites may then be involved by extension or by lymphohematogenous dissemination from the gut.

Epidemiology

The number of new cases of pulmonary tuberculosis reported annually in the United States during the decade 1962–1972 declined steadily, although the number of cases of extrapulmonary tuberculosis reported annually during the same period remained stable (Fig. 35-1). This trend has continued; the reasons for the difference are not clear but may be related in part to differences in the populations most likely to develop pulmonary or extrapulmonary disease. In 1978, extrapulmonary disease accounted for 14.6% of all the cases of tuberculosis reported in the United States. Certain population groups accounted for a greater proportion of the extrapulmonary cases. For example, individuals under 45 years of age accounted for 47.8% of reported extrapulmonary cases and 36.0% of pulmonary cases; females accounted for 48.9% of extrapulmonary cases and 32.4% of pulmonary cases, and nonwhite individuals accounted for 48.9% of extrapulmonary cases and 32.4% of pulmonary cases.

The most common site of extrapulmonary tuberculosis is the lymphatic system, followed by the pleura and the genitourinary tract. Bone and joint, peritoneal, and meningeal tuberculosis are less common.

Pathogenesis and Pathology

Extrapulmonary tuberculosis generally results from extension or dissemination from a pulmonary infection. Acquisition from the gastrointestinal tract secondary to ingestion of infected foodstuffs is extremely rare, especially in the United States. Inoculation through the skin occurs occasionally and produces a cutaneous Ghon complex. When tubercle bacilli are deposited within the lung, a granulomatous reaction develops, which may resolve completely, fibrose and calcify, or go on to necrosis with erosion into the lymphatics or the blood stream. Hematogenous spread can occur at any time in the course of tuberculosis, but occult hematogenous spread typically occurs during the first 6 weeks of the primary infection and carries bacilli to extrapulmonary sites and other areas of the lung. Secondary lesions in the apices of the lungs are known as Simon foci and are important in reactivation tuberculosis.

If large numbers of tubercle bacilli reach the blood stream and disseminate widely, miliary tuberculosis results. This can occur either in primary infection or long after the primary infection from an extrapulmonary focus. The miliary tubercles are of fairly uniform size and age.

Bronchogenic spread of tuberculosis may occur if a tuberculous granuloma enlarges and penetrates into the lumen of the bronchus, or if infected hilar nodes rupture into the trachea or bronchi; when this occurs, coughing and ciliary action transport infected material up the respiratory tract so that it can be expectorated. However, aspiration of this infected ma-

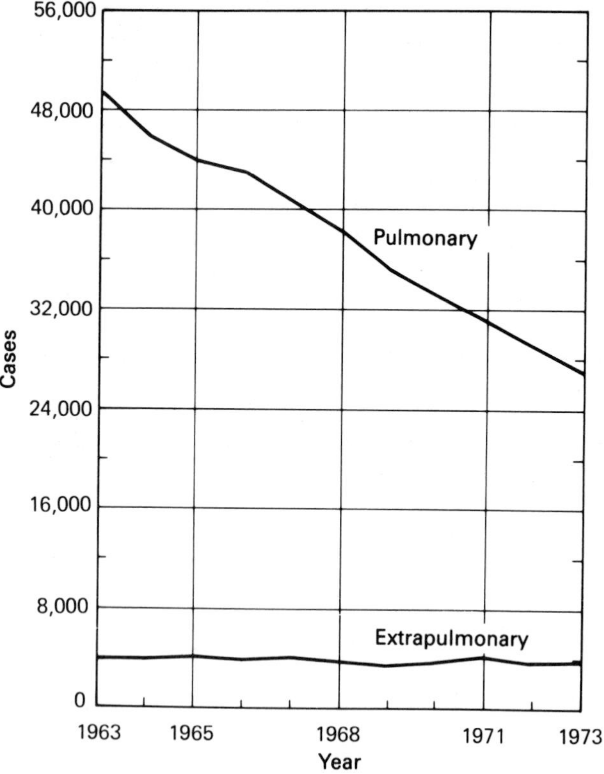

Fig. 35-1. Occurrence of pulmonary and extrapulmonary tuberculosis in the United States, 1963–1973. (After Reported Tuberculosis Data. DHEW Publications No. 75-8201, Atlanta, Center for Disease Control, 1972)

terial may lead to infection in other areas of the lung; also, secondary infection of the larynx, epiglottis, pharynx, or tongue may occur.

Direct extension to contiguous structures can result from necrotic foci in the lung or lymph nodes.

Manifestations

The manifestations of tuberculosis that has spread beyond the lungs are, of course, dependent on the organ or organ system involved. Because these infections may mimic other chronic infections or neoplasms, accurate diagnosis depends on obtaining proper specimens for smear and cultures. Although the liver and the spleen may contain many tubercles as a result of hematogenous dissemination, these organs rarely show progressive disease, perhaps because of the innate resistance of the reticuloendothelial system, or the low oxygen tension, or both. Miliary tuberculosis is usually an acute, rapidly progressive infection, but it may be an indolent process with low-grade fever, anemia, and debility. Any organ may be involved. Thus, all possible clinical manifestations cannot be described.

Tuberculosis of the Central Nervous System

Lymphohematogenous dissemination of tubercle bacilli to the brain and the meninges may result in a chronic meningitis or the manifestations of an intracranial neoplasm. Children who develop disseminated tuberculosis at the time of primary infection are at greater risk of developing meningitis than are adults who have disseminated disease. Commonly, there is active pulmonary tuberculosis in patients with tuberculous meningitis, but among the large numbers of adult patients reported in a Veterans' Administration–Armed Forces Study, 19% had no associated lesions that were detectable at the start of chemotherapy. The incidence of positive tuberculin tests varies greatly.

Clinically, there is an indolent meningitis with headache, stiff neck, vomiting, and occasionally cranial nerve deficits. The symptoms and signs are believed to be the result of a hypersensitivity reaction to tuberculoprotein released into the cerebrospinal fluid by rupture of a meningeal tuberculoma. As the infection involves vascular channels, causing an obliterative arteritis, infarction of the brain results. The cerebrospinal fluid is under increased pressure; there is an abnormal abundance of leukocytes, predominantly mononuclear, increased protein, and a reduction of the concentration of glucose to less than 40% of the concomitant blood glucose. The numbers of tubercle bacilli in the cerebrospinal fluid are small, and finding bacilli in direct smears is difficult. The fluid should be allowed to stand so that if a pellicle forms, tubercle bacilli will become enmeshed in it and be detectable after acid-fast staining.

Cultures may not show growth for several weeks; therefore, therapy should be started presumptively because the earlier therapy is initiated, the more successful the outcome. Survival has improved from 30% to 80% since isoniazid, a drug that enters the central nervous system freely, became available. Nevertheless, permanent neurologic sequelae may occur in as many as one-fourth of patients despite adequate treatment because the meningeal exudate collects at the base of the brain and entraps the major vessels of the circle of Willis and the cranial nerves. Hydrocephalus results when the foramina of exit of the fourth ventricle at the basal cistern are obstructed by this exudate. The resulting cerebral edema may lead to death from brain stem herniation. Administration of glucosteroids is associated with a reduction of cerebrospinal fluid pressure and normalization of cell counts, protein, and glucose; however, survival is not improved. The administration of glucosteroids is not recommended except in desperate situations to reduce cerebral edema. Antituberculous chemotherapy would be applied for 24 to 36 months as a combination of three drugs, always including isoniazid. Reduction of morbidity—quadriplegia, hemiparesis, optic atrophy, cranial nerve palsies, and chronic brain syndrome—appears to be dependent on early recognition of the disease and prompt application of therapy.

Cerebral tuberculomas large enough to mimic intracranial neoplasms are relatively uncommon in the United States but are still encountered in other areas of the world. The diagnosis is usually made at the time of surgery when an avascular, nodular mass is found. Meningitis may or may not be present.

Genitourinary Tuberculosis

Renal tuberculosis results from the hematogenous spread of tubercle bacilli. The cortex of the kidney is usually involved first; as the disease progresses to involve glomeruli, the bacilli are released into the urine and may then spread to the renal pelvis, ureters, and bladder, and to the prostrate, seminal vesicles, and epididymis in males. Urinary tract tuberculosis should be suspected whenever there is pyuria without bacteriuria, or unexplained hematuria or proteinuria. Diagnosis is dependent on the isolation of *M. tuberculosis* from the urine. Maximal yield is obtained by culturing at least three first voided early morning specimens. Smears of urine for acid-fast bacilli are not helpful because of the paucity of bacteria, and may be misleading if saprophytic *Mycobacterium smegmatis* is found.

Genitourinary symptoms may be minimal, and there is frequently evidence of tuberculosis in other organ systems. The roentgenographic signs of renal tuberculosis are varied, and lesions may remain stable for many years even without therapy. Intravenous urograms may show caliceal or renal pelvic dilation early in the course of the disease (Fig. 35-2). Later, multiple abscesses, parenchymal calcifications, or hydronephrosis of a kidney or ureter may be seen. Multiple urethral strictures may develop. Despite the structural abnormalities, surgical extirpation is rarely needed.

Tuberculosis of the female genital tract is usually secondary to hematogenous spread. Because ovaries, fallopian tubes, and endometrium are involved, the manifestations are those of a chronic, indolent pelvic inflammatory disease and sterility. Culture of endometrial curettings or biopsy specimens from involved sites will yield *M. tuberculosis.*

Gastrointestinal Tuberculosis

Gastrointestinal tuberculosis may result from ingestion of tubercle bacilli in infected foods and in spu-

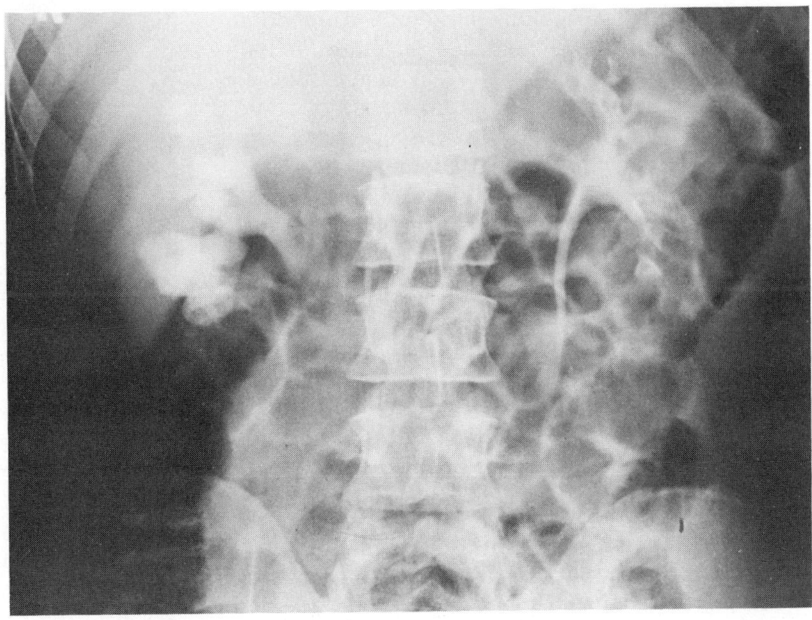

Fig. 35-2. Tuberculosis of the right kidney. Intravenous urogram shows a dilated and distorted caliceal system. (Courtesy of Dr. PES Palmer)

tum, or from hematogenous dissemination from another focus. With earlier and more effective therapy for pulmonary tuberculosis, the incidence of tuberculous enteritis has declined. The vague nature of the symptoms and signs may make the diagnosis difficult; confusion with intestinal neoplasm or Crohn's disease is frequent.

Anorexia, weight loss, and intermittent signs of partial small bowel obstruction are common. The ileocecal region is involved most commonly, but other parts of the intestinal tract may be affected. The following three forms are recognized: (1) ulcerative, (2) hypertrophic, and (3) mixed ulcerative–hypertrophic. Radiographically, the initial lesion appears as a polypoid defect in the intestinal submucosa, reflecting the formation of tubercle. Later, as caseous necrosis progresses, a circular ulceration is seen; this, in turn, progresses to fibrosis and narrowing. Hypertrophic changes in the wall of the bowel may occur and become clinically evident as an abdominal mass.

Abdominal symptoms in patients with pulmonary tuberculosis should cause the physician to suspect tuberculous enteritis. Surgical exploration may be necessary to relieve obstruction or to rule out neoplasm. If lesions are within reach of the endoscopist, diagnosis may be possible through microscopic and cultural examinations of biopsy specimens obtained from affected areas.

Tuberculous peritonitis may result from the direct spread of intestinal or pelvic tuberculosis. The presence of ascites and fever is an indication for diagnostic paracentesis; leukocytes, predominantly mononuclear cells, and a high concentration of protein are consistent with tuberculous peritonitis. An abdominal mass, consisting of thickened omentum and adherent bowel, is present in many patients. Tubercle bacilli may sometimes be found in smears of peritoneal fluid, but biopsy at peritoneoscopy or laparotomy is more likely to yield specimens that are diagnostic by histology or culture. With peritoneal infection, other serous membranes (pleura, pericardium) are frequently involved.

Tuberculous Pericarditis

Tuberculosis causes 7% to 10% of all cases of pericarditis (see Chap. 132, Pericarditis). Progression to chronic constrictive pericarditis may occur even with adequate antituberculous therapy. Death is usually the result of cardiac tamponade. Among patients studied between 1960 and 1966 in Brooklyn, New York, the addition of glucosteroids to regimens of antituberculous drugs improved survival. If the size of the heart remains increased, if the venous pressure remains elevated, or if cardiac failure is progressive, pericardiectomy should be performed.

Skeletal Tuberculosis

The spine and hip, in that order, are the most common sites of skeletal tuberculosis; the weight-bearing joints of the lower extremities follow next in frequency. Skeletal disease results from lymphogenous or hematogenous dissemination, commonly localizing on the mataphyseal side of the growing ends of long bones—apparently because of the high blood supply and oxygen content (Fig. 35-3). A monoarticular arthritis that is insidious in onset and is associated with roentgenographically evident destruction of the joint is quite probably tuberculous (Fig. 35-4). Smears of synovial fluid may be positive in about 25% of cases; the fluid must always be cultured. Biopsy of the synovium for histologic examination and culture boosts the diagnostic yield to nearly 100%.

Tuberculosis of the spine may cause back pain for several years before the diagnosis is established. The

Fig. 35-3. Tuberculous dactylitis in a child. Tuberculous osteomyelitis tends to localize on the metaphyseal side of the growing ends of bones. (Courtesy of Dr. PES Palmer)

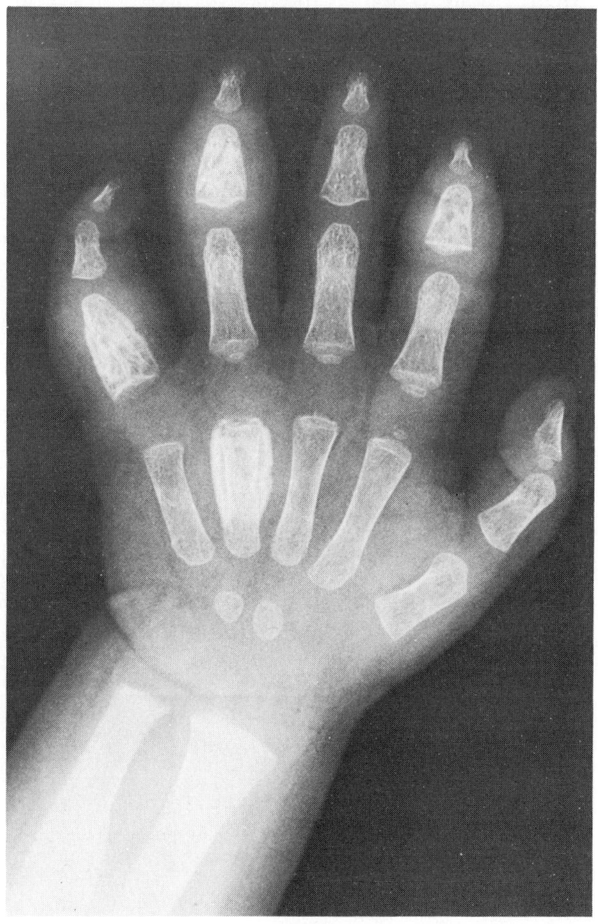

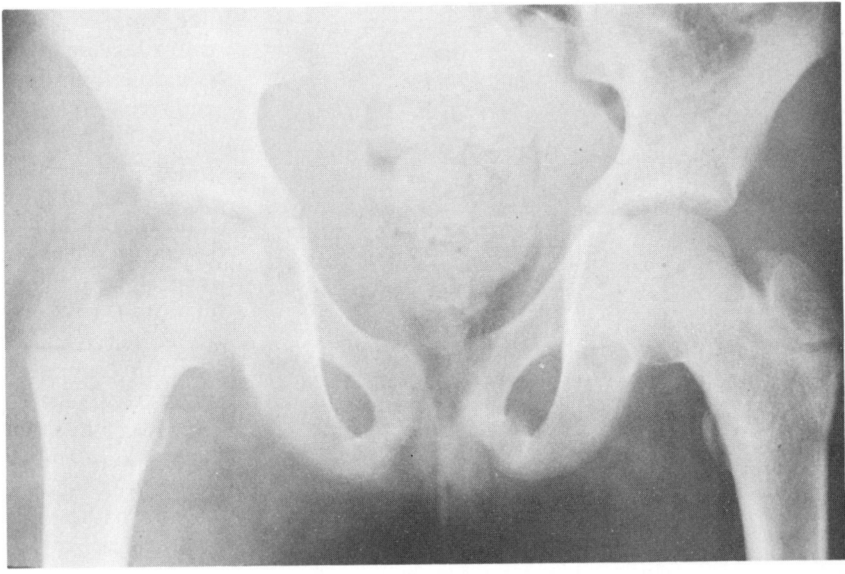

Fig. 35-4. Tuberculous arthritis of the right hip. Joint destruction is moderately advanced. (Courtesy of Dr. PES Palmer)

most common sites of involvement are the upper thoracic vertebrae in children and the lower thoracic and upper lumbar vertebrae in adults. Narrowing of the disk space is the first sign of infection; as the lesion progresses, there is destruction of the adjacent vertebral bodies. With collapse of vertebral bodies anteriorly, but with preservation of the posterior articulations, a gibbus forms—an abrupt angulation of the spine which is readily visible and palpable (Fig. 35-5). A contiguous paravertebral abscess is frequently present (Fig. 35-6). Diagnosis is accomplished by culture of pus aspirated from the abscess or of material obtained by biopsy of the bone.

Immobilization, once uniformly applied in the treatment of tuberculous spinal osteomyelitis, has not been shown to improve the results of antimicrobial treatment of tuberculosis of the thoracic spine. If destruction is extensive, or if necrotic bone or pus is present, surgical drainage or debridement is necessary. In all cases antituberculosis chemotherapy is the mainstay of treatment.

Lymphatic Tuberculosis

Scrofula, tuberculosis of the cervical lymph nodes, is usually accompanied by weight loss and fever, although painless swelling of the cervical nodes is the major finding. Excisional biopsy of a node for histologic examinaton and culture provides the diagnosis. Another common site for lymphatic tuberculosis is the intrathoracic lymphatic system (the hilar and paratracheal nodes). Systemic illness is common, and again the diagnosis is made by histologic and cultural examination of the nodes. Skin test reactivity to tuberculin is usual in lymphatic tuberculosis.

Fig. 35-5. Tuberculosis of the first lumbar vertebra. The characteristic anterior wedging with preservation of the posterior articulations is clearly shown in this lateral view. (Courtesy of Dr. PES Palmer)

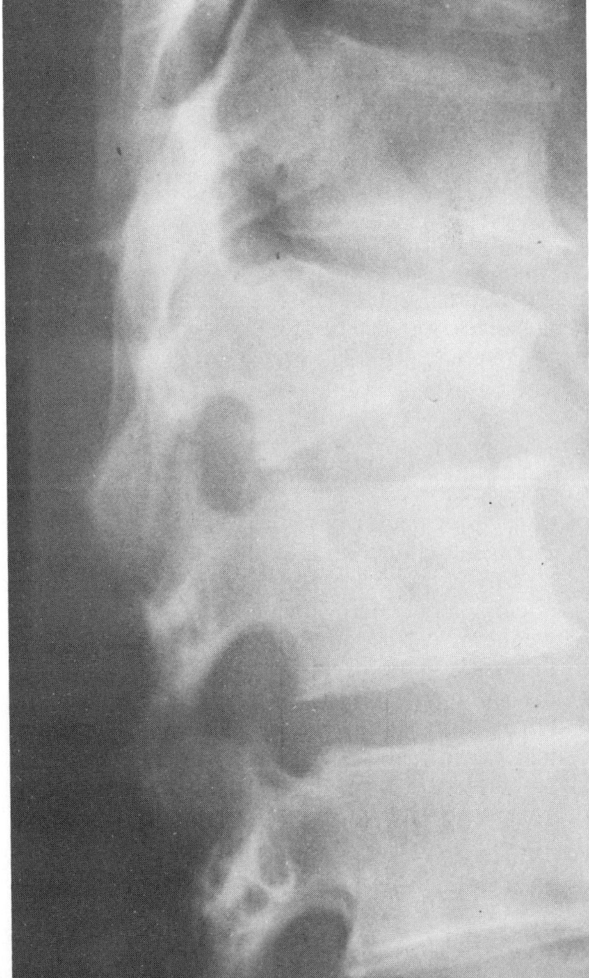

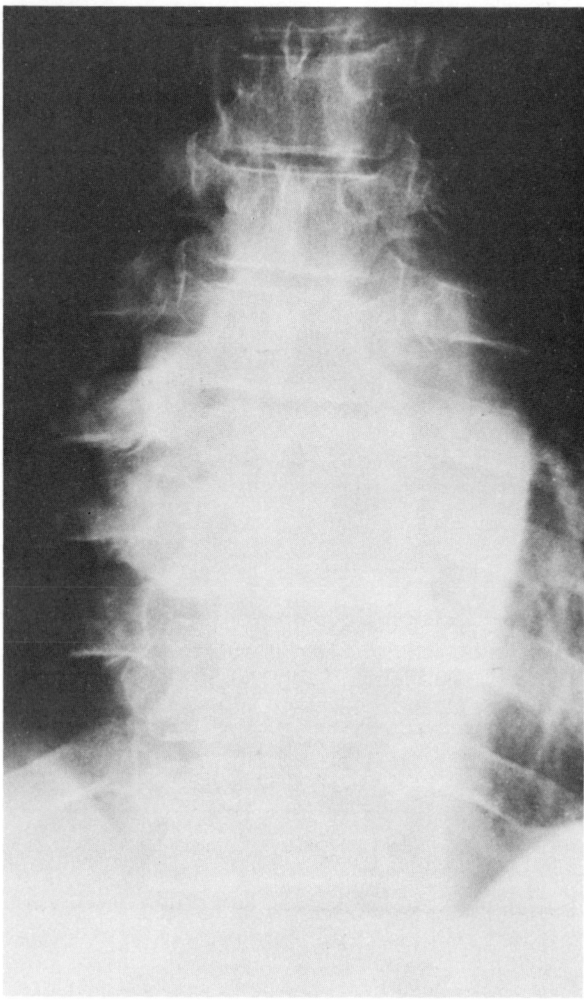

Fig. 35-6. Tuberculosis of the spine with collapse of the ninth thoracic vertebral body and a large paravertebral abscess. (Courtesy of Dr. PES Palmer)

Cutaneous Tuberculosis

Cutaneous tuberculosis may arise *de novo* as a result of direct inoculation or as a result of spread from other sites. It is uncommon in the United States and may easily be confused with other entities.

Inoculaton of an individual not previously infected with tuberculosis results in a local ulcer (analogous to the Ghon complex in the lung) followed by regional adenopathy. The process is usually contained, and there is gradual resolution of the ulcer; however, dissemination may occur. In an individual who has had tuberculosis, dermal inoculation produces a condition known as *tuberculosis verrucosa cutis:* wart-like papules that coalesce and eventually clear centrally, leaving a raised, irregular border. The process is indolent and may continue for years. Granulomas and rare acid-fast bacilli may be found in biopsy specimens; cultures are usually positive.

Tuberculosis of the skin that originates in other organs may take several forms. Lupus vulgaris—infiltrated, granulomatous lesions occurring most commonly on the face and neck—may arise by extension from adjacent lymphatics and occasionally from inoculation. Direct invasion of the skin from contiguous areas of active disease may cause scrofuloderma with necrotic, suppurating lesions. Occasionally, miliary tuberculosis may be manifest as numerous macules, papules, and vesicular skin lesions. A rare condition known as *tuberculosis cutis orificialis* occurs in seriously ill individuals when mucocutaneous areas are seeded with organisms from the respiratory or gastrointestinal tract, causing multiple irregular ulcerations.

Therapy

The principles of chemotherapy for tuberculosis that has extended beyond the lung are the same as those for pulmonary tuberculosis (see Chap. 34, Pulmonary Tuberculosis): Two or more drugs, each individually effective, must be given to reduce the chance of resistant organisms emerging; treatment must be prolonged—for 18 to 24 months. When the meninges or brain are involved, agents that reach effective concentrations in the central nervous system must be used. Of the primary drugs, only isoniazid diffuses readily into the cerebrospinal fluid. Cycloserine and ethionamide also attain therapeutic levels in cerebrospinal fluid, but they are secondary drugs. Meningeal inflammation may facilitate the entry of streptomycin and rifampin. Hence, three drugs are recommended for the treatment of tuberculous meningitis: isoniazid, 5 mg to 7 mg/kg body wt/day, perorally as a single dose; rifampin, 12 mg to 15 mg/kg body wt/day perorally as a single dose (or streptomycin, 15 mg to 17 mg/kg body wt/day, IM as a single injection); ethionamide, 7 mg to 15 mg/kg body wt/day, perorally as a single dose (alternatively, cycloserine may be given in a dose of 12 mg to 15 mg/kg body wt/day, perorally as three equal portions 8-hourly or ethambutol, 20 mg/kg body wt/day, perorally as a single dose). Treatment should be continuous for 24 to 36 months.

Because extrapulmonary tuberculosis is almost always the result of dissemination, widespread seeding should be assumed and a minimum of two antimicrobics should be given for at least 2 years. Isoniazid plus rifampin, given as above, provides a maximally active regimen.

Prevention

The best preventative of extrapulmonary tuberculosis is prevention of the primary pulmonary infection. Failing this, prompt identification of individuals with tuberculosis by periodic skin testing, and the application of isoniazid chemoprophylaxis to those who have become tuberculin positive will prevent extrapulmonary spread.

Remaining Problems

There is a need for improved, rapid diagnostic methods and for the development of drugs to which *M. tuberculosis* does not develop resistance. A means to control selectively the deleterious effects of hypersensitivity on the body's immune defenses would be a major advance.

Bibliography

Books

Diagnostic Standards and Classification of Tuberculosis. National Tuberculosis and Respiratory Disease Association, 1969, 94 pp.

JOHNSON JE III (ed): Rational Therapy and Control of Tuberculosis. Gainesville, University of Florida Press, 1970, 191 pp.

Journals

BORHANMANESH F, HIKMAT K, VAEZZADEH K, REZAI HR: Tuberculous peritonitis: Prospective study of 32 cases in Iran. Ann Intern Med 76:567–572, 1972

CHRISTENSEN WI: Genitourinary tuberculosis: Review of 102 cases. Medicine 53:377–390, 1974

DAVIDSON PT, HOROWITZ I: Skeletal tuberculosis: A review with patient presentations and discussion. Am J Med 48:77–84, 1970

FALK A: U. S. Veterans' Administration Armed Forces cooperative study on the chemotherapy of tuberculosis. XIII. Tuberculous meningitis in adults, with special reference to survival, neurologic residuals, and work status. Am Rev Respir Dis 91:823–831, 1965

FARER LS, LOWELL AM, MEADOR MP: Extrapulmonary tuberculosis in the United States. Am J Epidemiol 109:205–217, 1979

HAGEMAN JH, D'ESOPO ND, GLENN WWL: Tuberculosis of the pericardium: A long term analysis in 44 proved cases. N Engl J Med 270:327–332, 1964

LEPPER MH, SPIES HW: The present status of the treatment of tuberculosis of the central nervous system. Ann NY Acad Sci 106:106–123, 1963

O'TOOLE RD, THORNTON GF, MUKHERJEE MK, NATH RL: Dexamethasone in tuberculous meningitis: Relationship of cerebrospinal fluid effects to therapeutic efficiency. Ann Intern Med 70:39–48, 1969

ROONEY JJ, CROCCO JA, LYONS HA: Tuberculous pericarditis. Ann Intern Med 72:73–78, 1970

SHERMAN S, ROHWEDDER JJ, RAVIKRISHNAN KP, WEG JG: Tuberculous enteritis and peritonitis: Report of 36 general hospital cases. Arch Intern Med 140:506–508, 1980

SNIDER DE: Extrapulmonary tuberculosis in Oklahoma, 1965–1973. Am Rev Respir Dis 111:641–646, 1975

TABRESKY J, LINDSTROM RR, PETERS R, LACHMAN RS: Tuberculous enteritis: Review of a protean disease. Am J Gastroenterol 63:49–57, 1975

Tuberculosis in the United States, 1978. HHS No (CDC) 80-8322. Atlanta, Centers for Disease Control, 63 pp

H. WILLIAM HARRIS
JOHN H. McCLEMENT

36 Nontuberculous Mycobacterioses

Within 16 years after Koch's epic discovery of *Mycobacterium tuberculosis* in 1882, *Mycobacterium bovis* and *Mycobacterium avium* were recognized. Soon thereafter, other mycobacteria were discovered. Some were associated with disease in nonhuman mammals, fish, birds and reptiles, and others occurred as saprophytes.

After bacteriologic cultures became widely used in diagnosis, occasional patients with pulmonary or extrapulmonary "tuberculosis" yielded isolates that differed significantly from mammalian tubercle bacilli. In 1935, Pinner documented the isolation of bacilli he called *atypical mycobacteria* from cases of human disease. At first, such isolates were assumed to be saprophytic contaminants—fellow travelers in established cases of classic tuberculosis—because they lacked virulence for guinea pigs. By the early 1950s, cases were reported in which an atypical yellow bacillus was the sole isolate from diseased pulmonary tissue removed surgically and from widespread caseous lesions at autopsy. Concern about these bacteria was heightened after the introduction of antituberculous antimicrobics because the response was poor to absent.

In 1959, Runyon suggested a practical classification of atypical mycobacterial strains based on colonial morphology and pigmentation. Such classification was of great value to the subsequent study of the bacteriologic, epidemiologic, and clinical characteristics of nontuberculous mycobacterial infections. Runyon's classificaton separated nontuberculous mycobacteria into four groups, but lacked sufficient taxonomic standardization to permit species designation. Accordingly, all such nonspeciated strains became known, variously, as atypical, anonymous, or unclassified mycobacteria. Subsequently, intensive investigation of these mycobacteria using a number of biochemical, molecular and immunologic techniques resulted in species designation of all strains known to cause disease in humans and many saprophytic strains as well. Use of imprecise group designations is now both incorrect and outmoded; the correct phrasing is *mycobacterial disease caused by (name of specific mycobacterial species).*

Etiology

The tuberculosis complex consists of *M. tuberculosis* and *M. bovis.* As is noted in Table 34-1, *M. tuberculosis et bovis* are quite comparable microbiologically, except that *M. bovis* produces little or no niacin and differs in several other biochemical reactions.

The major species in Runyon's group I is *mycobacterium kansasii.* Although *M. kansasii* is like *M. tuberculosis* in slow growth of rough colonies, it is quite unlike *M. tuberculosis* in that colonies are photochromogenic (*i.e.,* nonpigmented) when cultivated in the dark, but distinctly yellow within 12 hours after young, growing colonies are exposed to light. In addition, *M. kansasii* does not produce niacin but does elaborate catalase. When isolated from clinical specimens, *M. kansasii* may be assumed to be responsible for infection.

The usual habitat of *Mycobacterium marinum* is warm water, either fresh or marine, in natural settings, swimming pools, or domestic fish tanks. Primary infections of the skin and subcutaneous tissue are usual; *M. marinum* does not cause pulmonary disease. *Mycobacterium marinum* is photochromogenic, shares other biochemical characteristics with *M. kansasii,* but grows poorly or not at all at 37°C. A few strains of *M. marinum* produce niacin.

Originally isolated from monkeys, *Mycobacterium simiae* has recently been recovered from a few cases of human pulmonary disease. Also photochromogenic, *M. simiae* differs from *M. kansasii* in a number of biochemical characteristics, susceptibility to antimicrobials, and vigorous production of niacin.

Scotochromogenic mycobacterial strains in Runyon's group II produce round, smooth, slowly growing colonies that are deeply pigmented with a yellow or orange color when cultivated either in the presence or absence of light. *Mycobacterium scrofulaceum* may, uncommonly, cause pulmonary infections in adults, but often infects cervical lymph nodes in children. In addition to its role in infection, *M. scrofulaceum* may exist as a saprophyte in water and soil.

Mycobacterium szulgai is a scotochromogenic species that has been isolated exclusively from humans, most often those with pulmonary infections. Biochemical characteristics, susceptibility to antituberculous drugs, and antigenic characteristics also set *M. szulgai* apart from other scotochromogens.

Mycobacterium gordonae and *Mycobacterium flavescens* are common ubiquitous, saprophytic, scotochromogenic bacteria that are not associated with disease in humans. They are distinguished by biochemical characteristics—particularly by ability to hydrolyze Tween-80

Mycobacterium intracellulare is the correct designation of the nonchromogenic mycobacteria formerly included in Runyon's group III and called Battey bacilli because they were particularly prevalent at the Battey State Hospital in Rome, Georgia. In most respects, *M. intracellulare* very closely resembles *M. avium*—except for serologic differences and the greater pathogenicity of *M. avium* for fowl. Indeed, Runyon and others have suggested that these species be linked as the *Mycobacterium avium–intracellulare* complex for clinical purposes. As listed in Table 34-1, the smooth, slowly growing colonies are nonpigmented and niacin negative. Bacteria of the *M. avium—intracellulare* complex cause pulmonary infections and (less often) disseminated disease in adults, and cervical adenitis in children (infrequent). They are readily isolated from soil and water and can be isolated sporadically from sputum or saliva produced by healthy persons or patients with lung disease unrelated to mycobacteria. Certain serotypes seem to be associated with disease in humans, and other serotypes occur principally in the environment.

Mycobacterium xenopi was first recovered from patients with pulmonary disease in England and has since been recognized in the United States as well. Although *M. xenopi* was classified in Runyon's group III, it's nonetheless, scotochromogenic and thermophilic (growing better at 45°C than at 37°C); it also produces aerial filaments.

Mycobacterium ulcerans causes ulceration of the skin and underlying tissue, but it has not been associated with pulmonary disease in humans. It grows only at temperatures below 37°C and is nonchromogenic and niacin negative.

Mycobacterium gastri and the *Mycobacterium terrae* complex are common saprophytes that can be differentiated from the potential pathogens of Runyon's group III by differences in biochemical reactions.

Mycobacterium fortuitum is a widely disseminated sapprophyte that very rarely causes disease in man. Rapid growth within 3 to 5 days is characteristic, yielding colonies that are noncorded, niacin-negative, and arysulfatase positive. Other mycobacteria formerly of Runyon's group IV are almost exclusively saprophytic: *Mycobacterium phlei, Mycobacterium smegmatis,* and *Mycobacterium vaccae.*

Epidemiology

Careful studies of contacts of patients infected with non-*tuberculosis* and non-*bovis Mycobacteriumn* spp. have failed to produce evidence of human-to-human transmission. The source of these mycobacteria appears to be nature; no vector has been identified.

Mycobacterium kansasii has been isolated from raw milk and from tap water. Sporadic cases have been reported from many areas of the United States—most often from the midwest (Illinois, Missouri, Nebraska) and the southwest (especially Texas). Men are infected about three times more often than women. Middle-aged and older white males who have chronic obstructive pulmonary disease are predisposed to this infection. The respiratory tract appears to be the portal of entry, but the source of infection is not known.

Mycobacterium marinum is world-wide in distribution and has been isolated from surfaces in contact with warm water—for example, artificial or natural pools, fish tanks, and aquarium. Infection is acquired by direct inoculation of the skin through abrasions.

Mycobacterium simiae was first isolated from monkeys in 1965. Subsequently, pulmonary infections caused in humans by *M. simiae* were identified. Extensive investigations of the mycobacterial species of water, soil, and other materials have failed to identify *M. simiae* (*i.e.,* the natural reservoir is unknown).

Mycobacterium scrofulaceum, gordonae, and *flavescens* can be isolated from water, foods, and soil; they may be found in the saliva, sputum, and gastric aspirates of persons without actual mycobacterial infections. Rarely, *M. scrofulaceum* may cause chronic cavitary pulmonary lesions closely resembling tuberculosis, especially in persons with silicosis and other chronic fibrotic pulmonary diseases. *Mycobacterium szulgai* has been recovered only from infections in humans.

The *M. avium–intracellulare* complex is worldwide in distribution, occurring in the soil. These species have been found as common saprophytes in house dust, raising the possibility that this is the source for infection of humans. Worldwide, a larger proportion of cases has been found in western Australia and Japan than elsewhere. In the United States, pulmonary infections caused by *M. avium—intracellulare* are concentrated in the Southeast, especially in Georgia and Florida. Reactivity to tuberculin derived from *M. intracellulare* was present in more than 65% of naval recruits from the southeastern and Gulf-bordering states. That is, subclinical, immunizing infection with *M. intracellulare* is prevalent in this region of the United States.

Mycobacterium ulcerans apparently also causes disease after direct inoculation into the skin. Although first described in Australia and reported from southeast Asia and Mexico, the infection is peculiarly endemic in inhabitants of the banks of the upper Nile River. Bacteria which resemble *M. ulcerans* have been isolated from certain grasses that occur in areas where the infection is common.

Bacteria of the *M. fortuitum* complex are truly ubiquitous. They have been isolated from soil, water, and nonhuman animals, and they have been recovered from sputum and gastric contents of normal persons.

Mycobacterium chelonei has been isolated from human sources, and was not found in soil or water in attempts to recover the organism from natural sources.

Pathogenesis and Pathology

The nontuberculous mycobacterial species do not produce progressive and fatal disease in the usual experimental animals, as do *M. tuberculosis* and *M. bovis*. *Mycobacterium marinum* and *M. ulcerans* will produce local skin ulcers in rats and mice. *Mycobacterium fortuitum* causes abscesses in the kidneys of mice, and some strains of *M. kansasii* are pathogenic for mice. However, the lack of a reliable animal model has handicapped investigations of transmission, pathogenesis, and the immunologic and histopathologic responses to infection with these species. Such information has been derived only from observations of disease in humans.

Three portals of entry are apparent by the diseases evoked: (1) inhalation to give pulmonary infection, (2) mucosal penetration in the oropharynx to give cervical adenitis, and (3) percutaneous inoculation to give dermal infections. The evolution of lesions has not been studied with the care applied to tuberculosis. However, the sensitivity of *M. marinum* and *M. ulcerans* to temperature is apparent in the limitation of infection to superficial lesions with a primarily acral distribution.

Pulmonary disease caused by *M. kansasii* or *M. avium–intracellulare* is identical in pathology with classic pulmonary tuberculosis. Tubercles, caseation, cavity formation, lesions secondary to bronchogenic spread, and healing by fibrosis are major pathologic features. However, pleural effusions, systemic dissemination, and extrapulmonary foci, except for cervical lymphadenitis in children, are uncommon in the nontuberculous mycobacterioses. Extensive and fatal dissemination by these nontuberculous species, including the least virulent strains such as *M. scrofulaceum* and *M. fortuitum,* has occurred in immunologically compromised persons.

Delayed hypersensitivity, immunologically distinguishable from that engendered by tubercle bacilli, results from infection with these nonmammalian mycobacteria. Individuals with pulmonary disease caused by *M. intracellulare* more consistently react to the tuberculin produced from this species than they do to PPD-S or other mycobacterial antigens. A similar but less impressive specificity of skin response has been shown for patients with *M. kansasii* pulmonary infections. Persons not infected by *M. tuberculosis* or *M. bovis* but infected with another mycobacterial strain demonstrate a larger area of cutaneous induration with the homologous skin test reagent than with PPD-S. However, in such subjects, PPD-S often evokes a cross reaction, yielding induration 8 mm or less in diameter. Such small reactions are especially common among residents of the southeastern United States, where a majority of the population reacts to tuberculin produced from *M. intracellulare* and, presumably, has had subclinical infection by this organism.

Manifestations

The diseases caused by *M. kansasii* are clinically and radiographically indistinguishable from classic tuberculosis. Examined collectively, the pulmonary lesions produced by *M. kansasii* appear to be more indolent and less often associated with pleural effusion or bronchogenic dissemination. However, on purely clinical grounds, infection caused by *M. kansasii* cannot be distinguished from that caused by *M. tuberculosis* in the individual patient. Cervical adenitis

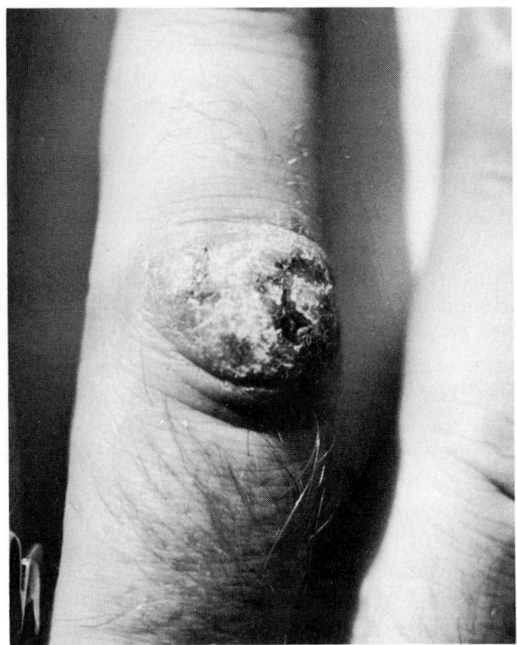

Fig. 36-1. A nodular, proliferating lesion on the knuckle of the middle finger of the right hand caused by *Mycobacterium marinum.* The patient cultivated tropical fish and recalled abrading his knuckle while cleaning a fish tank some 9 months earlier. The lesion resolved on treatment with isoniazid and cycloserine.

caused by *M. kansasii* has been reported rarely in children, and a very uncommon renal infection may occur. Other extrapulmonary manifestations are extremely rare.

Mycobacterium marinum produces chronic granulomatous nodules (Fig. 36-1) or ulcers involving the skin and subcutaneous tissue.

Mycobacterium scrofulaceum is a major cause of suppurative cervical adenitis in children; in countries with a relatively low incidence of tuberculosis, this species is more often the cause of cervical adenitis in childhood than is *M. tuberculosis.* A few instances of chronic pulmonary disease caused by *M. scrofulaceum* have been reported in adults. In a few cases, this organism appears to have been a primary pathogen, but in others, colonization of areas of preexisting lung damage seems more likely. The great majority of sputum isolates of scotochromogenic mycobacteria represent contamination from environmental sources rather than the presence of a pulmonary infection.

Chronic pulmonary disease caused by the *M. avium—intracellulare* complex is clinically and pathologically indistinguishable from that caused by *M. tuberculosis.* The incidence is highest among middle-aged and older white males, occurring most often in persons with chronic bronchitis and pulmonary emphysema. Extrapulmonary involvement is rare, but it has reportedly included cervical adenitis, osteomyelitis, renal abscess, and general dissemination. *Mycobacterium avium–intracellulare* also causes cervical adenitis in children, although less commonly than does *M. scrofulaceum.*

The pulmonary disease associated with *M. xenopi* is clinically and radiologically indistinguishable from tuberculosis or from other pulmonary mycobacterioses. *Mycobacterium ulcerans* causes extensive chronic granulomatous ulcerations of the skin and underlying tissue—termed Buruli ulcer in the endemic regions of Africa.

Rarely, *M. fortuitum* may cause cutaneous and ocular infections after inoculation through penetrating wounds or traumatized tissue. Pulmonary infection has been suspected because of repeated isolations of *M. fortuitum* from sputum produced by patients with pulmonary lesions that are consistent with mycobacteriosis in chest films. However, *M. fortuitum* is so often present as a contaminant that pulmonary infection is difficult to prove unless it is recovered directly from diseased lung tissue. A few instances of fatal infections have been reported, mostly in immunologically compromised patients.

Mycobacterium chelonei has been found as a rare cause for soft-tissue abscesses, chronic cavitary pulmonary disease, and infections of prosthetic heart valves, including porcine valve replacements.

Diagnosis

Nontuberculous mycobacterioses may be suspected on the basis of clinical characteristics suggesting tuberculosis, particularly in patients from areas recognized as endemic for such mycobacteria. The demonstration of acid-fast bacilli in patients who are nonreactive or minimally reactive (induration less than 8 mm in diameter) to 5 TU of PPD-S is also consistent with a diagnosis of nontuberculous infection. Actual diagnosis, however, requires the repeated isolation of nontuberculous mycobacteria from clinical specimens such as sputum. Culture from pus (aspirated directly from a lesion) or tissue specimens (biopsy or resected) are of greater significance. Single isolations from sputum or gastric contents probably reflect contamination. Renal infection is almost never caused by these mycobacterial species—isolation from the urine almost always reflects contamination of the specimen. The special requirements of temperature for the isolation of *M. marinum* and *M. ulcerans* can be accommodated if the clinical microbiology laboratory is told of the possibility of isolating these mycobacteria by the clinician.

Prognosis

A slow, indolent course, usually without dissemination from the initial focus of infection, appears to be characteristic of clinically manifest nontuberculous mycobacterioses. Most cases of nontuberculous mycobacterioses have been recognized since antimicrobials became available, and it is uncommon for the course of infection to be observed without the influence of antimicrobial therapy. Based on analysis of clinical manifestations before treatment is instituted and a few cases followed for many years without treatment, slowly progressive disease appears to be the most common course of lung infection caused by *M. kansasii* and the *M. avium–intracellulare* complex.

If appropriate drugs are prescribed and the regimen of therapy is adhered to by the patient, cure of *M. kansasii* mycobacterial infections should result. Because *M. avium–intracellulare* bacteria are relatively more resistant, bacteriologic conversion occurs in fewer patients. Surgical resection of diseased tissue may influence the prognosis favorably.

Cervical adenitis caused by *M. scrofulaceum* and *M. avium–intracellulare* responds poorly to antituberculous chemotherapy, undoubtedly because of the relative drug resistance of these species. Most are treated successfully, however, by surgical excision of the diseased nodes.

Therapy

Mycobacterium kansaii is usually inhibited by isoniazid (INH), rifampin (RMP), streptomycin (SM), paraaminosalicylic acid (PAS), and ethambutol (EMB), although the inhibitory concentrations are usually greater than those required for *M. tuberculosis.* Generally, the regimen should include INH (5 mg/kg body wt/day), EMB (20 mg/kg body wt/day), and RMP (10 mg/kg body wt/day). Streptomycin is often included until bacteriologic conversion has occurred and the pulmonary disease has stabilized. The combined chemotherapy regimen should be continued for at least 24 months. Clinical results are usually excellent among cases treated promptly with appropriate chemotherapy.

The rate of relapse is low, even among cases with persistent open-negative cavities. Depending on the results of drug susceptibility tests, other agents may also be used in patients who have received previous therapy and whose bacilli have become highly resistant to some of the primary drugs. Rifampin combined with the oral companion drugs to which the bacteria remain susceptible is usually an effective treatment regimen. Surgical resection is seldom required.

Most cases of *M. marinum* skin infections are self limited, although they may remain active for prolonged periods. The organism is usually resistant to the conventional antituberculous agents, but it may be susceptible to rifampin, cycloserine, ethambutol, and doxycycline. The infection has been controlled without surgical excision of the lesions by use of rifampin plus cycloserine, or by treatment with doxycycline.

Mycobacterium avium—intracellulare bacteria are either relatively or fully resistant to the available antimicrobial agents. Some isolates are partially inhibited by high concentrations of streptomycin and a few of the retreatment drugs. Chemotherapy regimens are usually composed of 4 to 6 agents selected on the basis of inhibition of growth *in vitro.* The initial regimen often consists of INH, RMP, EMB, ETA, and SM. Depending upon *in vitro* susceptibility, cycloserine may be added or substituted in the regimen. Adverse reactions are common, and close monitoring for drug toxicity is essential. Of investigative agents, clofazimine—used for many years in the treatment of leprosy (see Chap. 105, Leprosy)—is remarkably active *in vitro,* and has been applied with good clinical effect in limited trials.

In one center, 60% to 70% of patients become culture negative in 6 months after treatment with regimens consisting of 5 or 6 drugs. The probability of successful therapy is increased if it is possible to carry out surgical resection of the diseased lung parenchyma. In contrast to classic tuberculosis, surgical resection of lung tissue infected with nontuberculous mycobacteria can be undertaken with relatively low risk of morbidity and mortality, even though the sputum remains positive for mycobacteria. However, the results of chemotherapy appear to be highly unpredictable: (1) After 5 years of chemotherapy and observation of 45 patients with pulmonary infection caused by *M. intracellulare,* 20% died of active disease, about 10% relapsed, and the remainder had inactive or quiescent disease; (2) various combinations of 3 to 5 drugs given to 85 patients with pulmonary infections caused by *M. intracellulare–avium* brought initial sputum conversion in 68 (80%), with subsequent relapse in 16 (of these, seven responded to additional chemotherapy), but there was bacteriologic cure in 46% after 3 to 8 years; and (3) of 100 patients treated with a variety of regimens, less than half underwent bacteriologic conversion, but many remained clinically stable or improved despite persistently positive sputum cultures. It is not clear why the infection remains indolent in some patients but in others progresses relentlessly with enlarging cavities, extensive bronchogenic spread leading to new pulmonary lesions, and ultimate respiratory failure and death.

Mycobacterium xenopi is susceptible by *in vitro* testing to many antituberculous drugs. Clinical response to chemotherapy has been reported. Probably the regimen of choice is INH, RMP, and SM.

Mycobacterium szulgai is more susceptible to antituberculous drugs than are other scotochromogens. Chemotherapy may provide successful control of such infections. The combination of RMP, EMB, and, depending upon susceptibility tests, either ETA or SM, has been suggested.

Because presently available antimicrobics are seldom, if ever, effective against either *M. scrofulaceum* or *M. fortuitum,* surgical resection should be carried out whenever possible.

Prevention

No methods of immunization are available.

Remaining Problems

Worldwide, tuberculosis poses a much greater problem than the other mycobacterioses. Nonetheless, the nontuberculous mycobacteria also cause life-threatening and fatal disease. Drug treatment is less effective than in tuberculosis, especially with infections caused by *M. avium–intracellulare* and the other species with high degrees of resistance to antimicrobial drugs. More effective antimicrobics are needed to treat infections with predictable success.

Based on the high frequency of hypersensitivity, subclinical infection and sensitization to the nontuberculous mycobacteria has occurred in a large proportion of the world's population. How does sensitization to these ubiquitous mycobacterial strains influence immunity of humans to other intracellular parasites? Why does only a small fraction of the vast reservoir of infected humans develop clinical disease?

Bibliography

Book

CHAPMAN JS: The Atypical Mycobacteria and Human Mycobacteriosis. New York, Plenum, 1977, 200 pp

Journals

AWE RJ, GANGADHARAM PR, JENKINS DE: Clinical significance of *Mycobacterium fortuitum* infections in pulmonary disease. Am Rev Respir Dis 108:1230–1234, 1973

BATES JH: A study of pulmonary disease associated with mycobacteria other than *M. tuberculosis:* Clinical characteristics. Am Rev Respir Dis 96:1151–1157, 1967

BARKSDALE L, KIM KS: Mycobacterium. Bacteriol Rev 41:217–372, 1977

DUTT AK, STEAD WW: Long-term results of medical treatment in *Mycobacterium intracellulare* infection. Am J Med 67:449–453, 1979

HAND WL, SANFORD JP: *Mycobacterium fortuitum*—a human pathogen. Ann Intern Med 73:971–979, 1971

KRASNOW I, GROSS W: *Mycobacterium simiae* infection in the United States: A case report and discussion of the organism. Am Rev Respir Dis 111:357–360, 1975

KUBICA GP, GROSS WM, HAWKINS JE, SOMMERS HM, VESTAL AL, WAYNE LG: Laboratory services for mycobacterial diseases. Am Rev Respir Dis 112:773–787, 1975

LESTER W: Unclassified mycobacterial disease. Ann Rev Med 17:351–359, 1966

LINCOLN EM, GILBERT LA: Disease in children due to mycobacteria other than *Mycobacterium tuberculosis.* Am Rev Respir Dis 105:683–714, 1972

ROSENZWEIG DX: Pulmonary mycobacterial infections due to *Mycobacterium intracellulare–avium* complex. Chest 75:115–119, 1979

RUNYON EH: Whence mycobacteria and mycobacterioses. Ann Intern Med 75:467–468, 1971

RYNEARSON TK, SHRONTS JS, WOLINSKY E: Rifampin: In vitro effect on atypical mycobacteria. Am Rev Respir Dis 104:272–274, 1971

SCHAEFER WB: Incidence of serotypes of *M. avium* and atypical mycobacteria in human and animal diseases. Am Rev Respir Dis 97:18–23, 1968

WOLINSKY E: State of the art: Nontuberculous mycobacterial and associated diseases. Am Rev Respir Dis 119:107–159, 1979

YEAGER H, RALEIGH JW: Pulmonary disease due to *Mycobacterium intracellulare.* Am Rev Respir Dis. 108:547–552, 1973

PAUL D. HOEPRICH

Nocardiosis

37

Nocardiosis, infection with bacteria of the family Nocardiaceae, generally leads to disease, although tracheobronchial carriage may occasionally occur in patients with some form of chronic pulmonary disease. Clinical infections are either localized to the respiratory tract, disseminated to involve other organs as well (notably, the brain), or apparently primary subcutaneous processes, with or without vicinal lymphatic or osseous involvement. Tissue destruction with the formation of abscesses is characteristic of clinical infections. A chronic course spanning several months is usual, but in immunoincompetent patients, disease may be acute in onset and rapid in progression.

Etiology

Classification of the nocardias and certain other Actinomycetales has been and remains a challenge that continues to engross many investigators. New relationships have been disclosed as morphologic, physiologic, metabolic, antigenic, and chemoanalytic methods have been applied. The abbreviated classification of Table 37-1 is restricted to Actinomycetales currently recognized as medically important.

Nocardia spp. and *Actinomadura* spp., like *Actinomyces* spp., continue to be misrepresented as fungi. In fact, they are quite unlike fungi and are typically bacterial in having (1) stroma that are generally less than 1 μm in diameter; (2) cell walls consisting of peptidoglycans and containing neither chitin nor cellulose, (*i.e.,* they do not stain by the periodic acid-Schiff method) (see Chap. 9. Microscopic Examinations); (3) sterol-free cell membranes (*i.e.,* polyene antimicrobics such as amphotericin B are without effect); (4) susceptibility to antimicrobics devoid of antifungal activity (*e.g.,* sulfonamides); and (5) a prokaryotic arrangement of genetic materials (Fig. 37-1). Also, certain *Nocardia* spp. are parasitized by specific bacteriophages that will, in some instances, also accept certain *Mycobacterium* spp., as hosts.

Nocardias are aerobic, gram-positive, nonmotile, noncapsulated bacteria that may or may not grow as filaments. If filaments are formed, they may or may not be aerial; fragmentation into unequal bacillary (3 μm–4 μm long by 0.5 μm–1.0 μm in diameter) and coccoid (0.5 μm–1.0 μm in diameter) forms is characteristic (Fig. 37-2). Because the walls of the fragments are identical with the cell walls of the progenitor filaments, the fragments are not true spores. However, among certain nonpathogenic nocardias, coccoid cells called microcysts may form which can survive heating to 80°C.

Many strains of the pathogenic *Nocardia* spp. (*caviae, brasiliensis,* and *asteroides*) are acid fast, especially when mature colonies grown on glycerol-containing mediums are examined. Once basic fuchsin is taken up by such strains, it is not readily or completely removed by *aqueous* solutions of mineral acids (*e.g.,* 3% aqueous HCl, v/v). An acid–alcohol solution, as is used in the classic Ziehl–Neelsen staining procedure (see Chap. 9, Microscopic Examinations), is usually effective in decolorizing *Nocardia* spp., but not acid-alcohol-fast *Mycobacterium* spp. Similarly, the acid-fastness of *Nocardia* spp. (but not *Mycobacterium* spp.) is extractable with pyridine. Neither *Actinomadura, Actinomyces,* nor *Streptomyces* spp. is acid fast.

Table 37-1 is also a reminder of the close kinship the Nocardiaceae bear to the Mycobacteriaceae (absent or rare aerial hyphae, infrequent filamentation or branching), the Actinomycetaceae (branching filaments which fragment), and the Streptomycetaceae (nonfragmenting vegetative filaments, aerial hyphae bearing conidia). Generally, morphologic criteria enable separation of clinical isolates of Nocardiaceae from Mycobacteriaceae, and the morphologically similar pathogenic Actinomycetaceae are anaerobic to facultatively anaerobic. However, differentiation

Table 37-1. *Clinically Important Bacteria of the Order* Actinomycetales

Family	Genus	Species
Actinomycetaceae	*Actinomyces*	Several (see Chap. 38, Actinomycosis)
Mycobacteriaceae	*Mycobacterium*	Several (see Chap. 34, Pulmonary Tuberculosis, and Chap. 36, Nontuberculous Mycobacterioses)
Nocardiaceae	*Nocardia*	*caviae*
		brasiliensis
		asteroides
	*Actinomadura**	*madurae*
		pelletieri
		dassonvillei
Streptomycetaceae	*Streptomyces*	*somaliensis**

*Status *incertae sedis* (McClung NM: Family VI. Nocardiaceae Castellani and Chalmers 1919, 1040. In Buchanan RE, Gibbons NE (eds): Bergey's Manual of Determinative Bacteriology, 8th ed, pp 726–746. Baltimore, Williams & Wilkins, 1974)

of the Streptomycetaceae on morphologic grounds is often impossible; variations are especially frequent among clinical isolates, some of which are pathogenic *(e.g., Streptomyces somaliensis*—Africa, South America, Arabia, United States; *Streptomyces paraguayensis*—South America; *Streptomyces griseus*—United States).

Fortunately, there are the following differences in chemical constituents: (1) The Actinomycetales fall into four types according to major cell wall constituents; (2) the aerobic Actinomycetales display four patterns on whole cell sugar analyses; and (3) the mycolic acids of the Nocardiaceae differ from those of the Mycobacteriaceae and the Corynebacteriaceae. Thus, the cell walls of the Streptomycetaceae contain L-diaminopimelic acid, whereas the other Actinomycetales contain meso-diaminopimelic acid. On the basis of whole cell sugars, *N. asteroides, N. brasiliensis, N. caviae,* and *Mycobacterium* spp. contain arabinose and galactose (but no xylose or madurose [3-0-methyl-d-galactose]); *Actinomadura madurae* and *Actinomadura pelletieri* contain madurose (but no arabinose, galactose, or xylose), whereas *Actinomadura dassonvillei* does not; *Streptomyces* spp. do not display a characteristic pattern of sugars. The mycolic acids of *Mycobacterium* spp. contain 22 to 26 carbon atoms; *Nocardia* spp. (nocardomycolic acids), 12 to 18 carbon atoms; and *Corynebacterium* (corynomycolic acids), 14 to 18 carbon atoms. (The *Actinomadura* spp. and *Streptomyces* spp. do not contain mycolic acids.)

Several biochemical/metabolic tests are often used in the presumptive speciation of nocardial isolates (Table 37-2). The many cross reactions among *Nocardia* spp., *Actinomadura* spp., and *Streptomyces* spp. have limited serodiagnostic efforts.

The nutritional requirements of nocardias are not known, but it is clear that they are not fastidious. They will grow on mediums used for the culture of mycobacteria, on Sabouraud's glucose agar (*i.e.,* an acid *p*H is tolerated), and on blood agar. Although 5% to 10% ambient CO_2 is salutary and 37°C is the optimum temperature, growth is slow compared to that of enteric bacteria or pyogenic cocci. Colonies may not be apparent until 48 to 72 hours of incubation, a characteristic that may render isolation difficult because of the overgrowth of other bacteria in contaminated specimens. Selective culture mediums have not been developed. However, isolation from contaminated specimens may be facilitated by the so-called paraffin bait method, which takes advantage of the ability of *Nocardia* spp. to utilize paraffin as the sole source of carbon for growth.

When first visible, the colonies are usually white. Either they remain white, or they become yellowish tan, yellow, orange, pink, or red. The surface of the

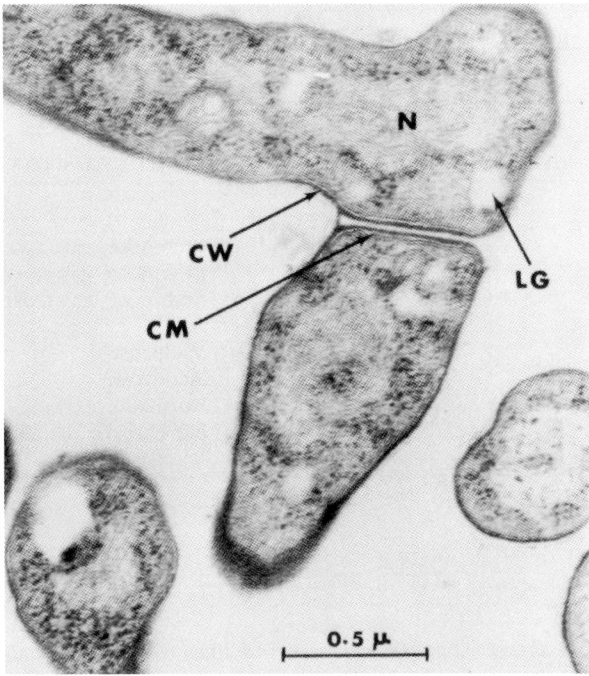

Fig. 37-1. An electron micrograph of *Nocardia asteroides*. The nuclear region *(N)* is prokaryotic. The cell wall *(CW)* and the cell membrane *(CM)* are distinct at branch points; a continuous sheath holds the cells together. A lipid granule *(LG)* is visible. (Farshtchi D, McClung NM: J Bacteriol 94:255–257, 1967)

colonies is powdery (aerial hyphae), wrinkled, and usually dry in appearance (*A. madurae* may be smooth and glistening). As stroma penetrate the agar, the oldest part of the colony may appear to sink as the culture ages. It becomes very difficult, even impossible, to pick up growth with a bacteriologic loop. An earthy odor is often quite pronounced.

Although a wide range of temperatures (6°C–50°C) is tolerated by nocardias, they possess no unique resistance to heat. Indeed, nocardias are as susceptible as other bacteria to physicochemical adversities such as ultraviolet light, drying, and disinfectants. Nocardias do not survive rigorous concentration procedures—for example, exposure to 4% NaOH as is used to process specimens for culturing *Mycobacterium tuberculosis*.

According to *in vitro* testing, nocardias are susceptible to many of the antimicrobial agents that are also active against other bacteria. Thus, inhibition may result with the aminocyclitols, the tetracyclines, chloramphenicol, rifampin, cycloserine, penicillins, cephalosporins, erythromycin, novobiocin, clindamycin, the sulfonamides, and trimethoprim. Demonstration of the activity of the sulfonamides, and trimethoprim *in vitro* requires the use of a culture medium that is free of p-aminobenzoic acid and thymine, respectively antagonists of sulfonamides and trimethoprim (see Fig. 18-22). It is important to note

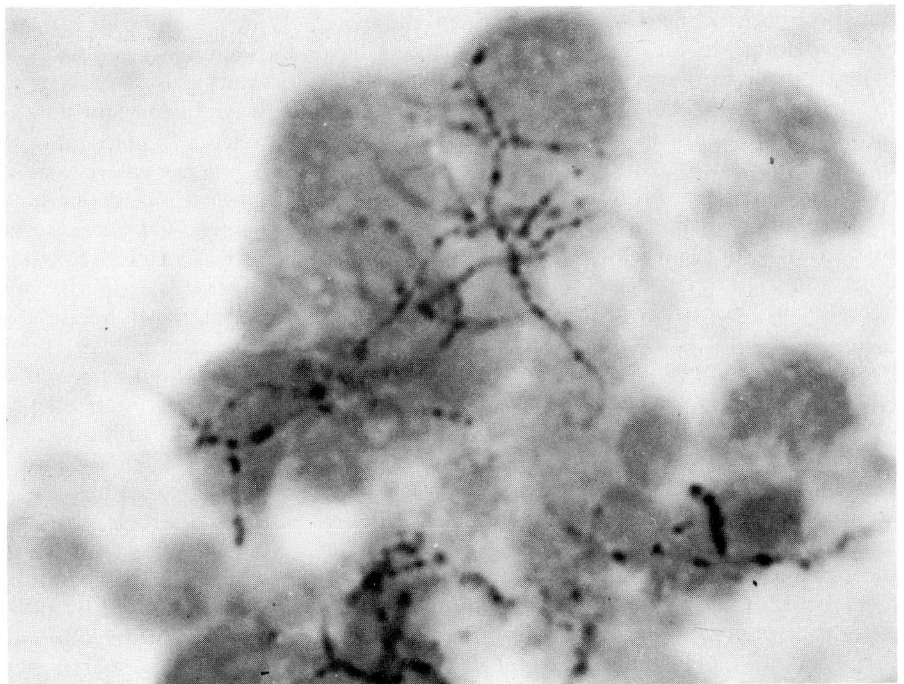

Fig. 37-2. Gram stain showing *Nocardia asteroides* in expectorated sputum from a patient with bronchopulmonary nocardiosis. Note the fragmentation of thin filaments into bacillary and coccoid forms. (Original magnification approximately × 1000)

Table 37-2. *Laboratory Test of Value in Presumptive Species Differentiation of* Nocardia, Actinomadura *(formerly* Nocardia*), and* Streptomyces*

	Decomposition of†					Cell Composition	
SPECIES	UREA	CASEIN	TYROSINE	XANTHINE	HYPOXANTHINE	DAP‡ ISOMER	WHOLE CELL SUGARS
Acid fast							
N. asteroides	+	−	−	−	−	Meso-	Arabinose, galactose
N. brasiliensis	+	+	+	−	+	Meso-	Arabinose, galactose
N. caviae	+	−	−	+	+	Meso-	Arabinose, galactose
Nonacid fast							
A. madurae	−	+	+	−	+	Meso-	Madurose
A. pelletieri	−	+	+	−	+	Meso-	Madurose
A. dassonvillei	−	+	+	+	+	Meso-	No madurose
S. somaliensis	−	+	+	−	−	L- (also glycine)	No characteristic sugars

*The reactions of *Streptomyces somaliensis* are indicated for comparison.
†+ corresponds to >85% positive; − to >85% negative.
‡Diaminopimelic acid in cell wall.

that the specifically antituberculous drugs (ethionamide, ethambutol, isoniazid, capreomycin, and pyrazinamide), and the antifungal antimicrobics, display little or no antinocardial activity.

Epidemiology

Since Nocard's report of isolation of the bacteria that now bear his name (in 1888, from cattle on the island of Guadeloupe in the West Indies), isolations have been reported from many countries. Just 2 years after the original report, humans were implicated as hosts for pathogenic nocardias by the isolation of *N. asteroids* from a patient with a brain abscess metastatic from chronic nocardial infection of the lungs and pleura. Other mammals have subsequently been proven to be hosts: nonhuman primates, goats, cats, dogs, guinea pigs, cetaceans, and marsupials. At least occasionally, nocardias are also pathogens of nonmammalian animals. Overall, however, nocardial infections do not appear to be common in humans; perhaps 1000 cases occur each year in the United States.

Nocardias are worldwide in occurrence, existing primarily in the soil as saprophytes, often in association with decaying organic matter. Humans and other animals apparently become infected accidentally, most often through inhalation. Traumatic inoculation through the skin (*e.g.,* puncture wounds of the bare feet) probably accounts for the association of *N. brasiliensis* and *Actinomadura* spp. with mycetomas (see Chap. 153, Mycetoma) in tropical and subtropical areas. There is no proof of man-to-man, animal-to-man, or animal-to-animal transmission.

In descending order of frequency in the United States (year to first isolation), nocardias potentially pathogenic for man are *N. asteroides* (1888), *N. brasiliensis* (1913), *N. caviae* (1924), *A. madurae* (1896), and *A. pelletieri* (1912). Isolation of these species from clinical materials (except gastric aspirates and occasionally from sputum) is of etiologic significance. In the United States, most clinical isolates are reported to be *N. asteroides.* However, caution is necessary because speciation has not always been vigorously pursued, and many strains labeled *N. asteroides* when isolated, prove to be *N. caviae* when examined in a reference laboratory. Despite the geographic implications of the species names, *N. brasiliensis* and *A. madurae* are encountered as causes for disease in the United States. *Nocardia brasiliensis* appears to be relatively more common in Mexico and South America, whereas *A. madurae* is predominant in Sudan and India, and *A. pelletieri* is found in Africa and South America.

Although persons of all ages may be infected, the third to the fifth decades are the ages of highest incidence. Males account for 3 to 4 times more cases than females, possibly reflecting occupational exposure. There is no discernible racial predisposition.

Nocardias, as many other infectious agents, flourish in patients with diminished host defenses, particularly as caused by neoplasia of the lymphoreticular system and by other diseases or therapies that depress cell-mediated immunity. Overall, about 70% of patients (United States) have evidence of immunoincompetence. Although depressed host resistance favors nocardial infection, it is not a prerequisite because approximately 25% of cases occur in persons without other discernible diseases.

Pathogenesis and Pathology

The respiratory tract is implicated as the usual portal of entry of *Nocardia* spp. because of the apparent primacy of pulmonary lesions. The course of untreated nocardiosis is usually chronic and must be reckoned in months. On the other hand, nocardiosis is generally more rapidly progressive than pulmonary tuberculosis.

Certain nocardial products may be important in pathogenesis: for example, nocobactins (complex lipid-soluble, iron-transporting substances) and nocardial cord factor. Moreover, some strains are able to survive and replicate inside phagocytes, a property which may relate to the chronicity of nocardiosis.

However, an acute, necrotizing, pneumonitic form of nocardiosis also occurs in which disease is evident for only a few weeks. It is quite often accompanied by dissemination and is seen most frequently in patients who have a generally debilitating, immunologically crippling, noninfectious disease.

Apparently, the initial lesion in the lung is a focus of pneumonitis that advances to tissue necrosis. The resultant abscesses may extend and coalesce with neighboring abscesses (Fig. 37-3). Typically, relatively little inflammatory response is engendered, there is little scarring, and the process does not become encapsulated (Fig. 37-4). There are several consequences. The sputum tends to be thick and purulent, and the nocardias may be seen in smears as loose aggregates of gram-positive, fragmenting filaments (Fig. 37-2); sulfur granules (see Chap. 38, Actinomycosis) are virtually never seen. True granulomas are quite uncommon but may occur most often in immunocompetent hosts infected with *N. brasiliensis,* the most virulent species in the setting of experimental infections. Often, however, neither the gross nor the microscopic findings are sufficiently distinctive to enable anatomic diagnosis of nocardiosis.

Direct extension from the lungs into the pleural cavity may go on to penetration of the chest wall, yielding sinuses that drain pus. Regional lymphadenitis may develop. Lymphohematogenous spread or bacteremia arising from the erosion of blood vessels gives rise to metastatic infection in approximately one-fifth of the patients. Spread by means of blood or lymph may occur from relatively small, inconspicuous pulmonary lesions. Brain abscesses result in almost every patient with disseminated disease (Fig. 37-5). However, involvement of virtually every organ has been reported: pericardium (~5%), bones (~3%), kidneys (~3%), and eye (~2%). In addition, lesions have been found in the spleen, heart, liver, peritoneum, adrenal glands, digestive tract, pancreas, thyroid, ear, bone marrow, pituitary, urinary bladder, and spinal cord.

Infections caused by *Actinomadura* spp. are generally consequent on percutaneous puncture inoculation. Typically, the disease is contained in the region of inoculation as a chronic, draining, low-grade infection.

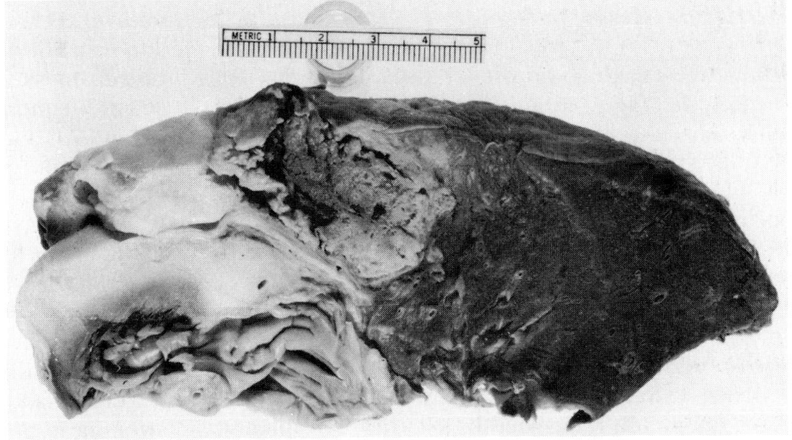

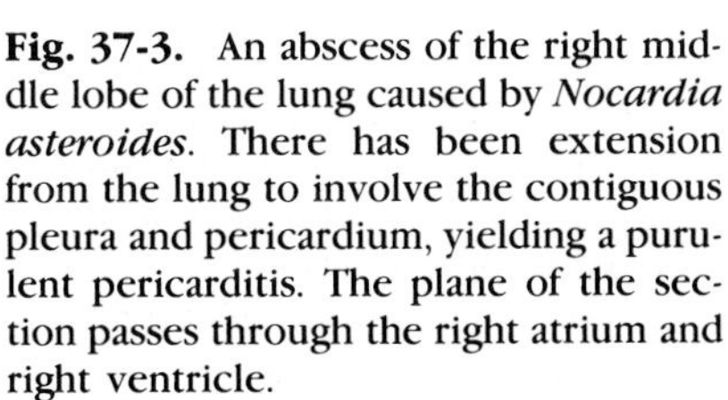

Fig. 37-3. An abscess of the right middle lobe of the lung caused by *Nocardia asteroides*. There has been extension from the lung to involve the contiguous pleura and pericardium, yielding a purulent pericarditis. The plane of the section passes through the right atrium and right ventricle.

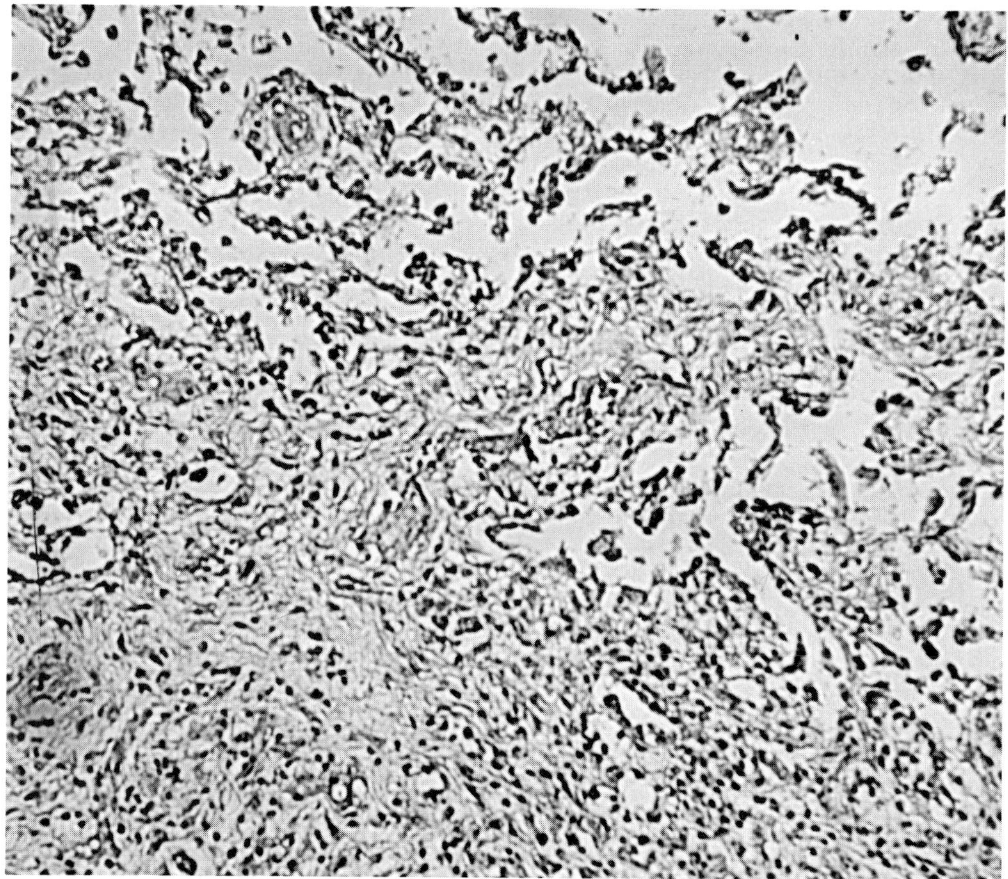

Fig. 37-4. The wall of a pulmonary microabscess caused by *Nocardia asteroides* (same specimen as shown in Fig. 37-3). Although the patient was ill for at least 3 months before death, there are no granulomas, the inflammatory response is only moderate, and encapsulation is incomplete. (Brown and Brenn modification of the Gram stain) (Original magnification approximately × 150)

Manifestations

Productive cough and fever are usual in pulmonary nocardiosis. The sputum is not malodorous, but it is thick, tenacious, purulent or mucopurulent, and may be tinged with blood. Although the temperature may be normal, fevers as high as 40.6°C (105°F) may occur, and they may be associated with chills. Other systemic reactions are also variable. Night sweats are not uncommon, and anorexia, malaise, and weight loss may occur. Leukocytosis may or may not be present; the anemia of chronic infection develops as the disease perists.

Direct extension from a pulmonary focus to involve the pleura is signaled by pleurisy. Intrapleural effusions frequently become infected, resulting in empyema. Metastasis to the brain results in diffuse abnormalities (difficulty in mentation, dizziness and unsteadiness, headache, nausea and vomiting, and seizures) and various focal neurologic abnormalities (of cranial and peripheral nerves).

Although pulmonary lesions are usually radiographically demonstrable, there are no etiologically diagnostic changes. There may be minimal shadows in the upper lobes that are quite consistent with early tuberculosis. Consolidated pneumonias occur, with or without demonstrable abscesses. If an abscess drains, cavitary disease will be apparent. Intrapleural liquid is readily detectable in chest films.

Actinomadural infections characteristically cause swelling in the area of involvement, with the formation of sinuses draining pus.

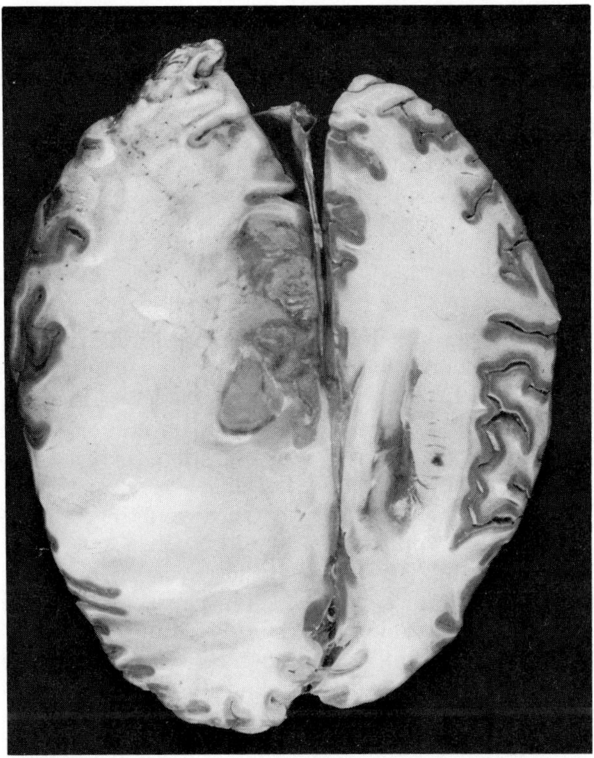

Fig. 37-5. An abscess of the left parietal lobe of the brain caused by *Nocardia asteroides*. (Weed LA, Andersen HA, Good CA Boggenstoss AH: N Engl J Med 253:1140, 1955)

Diagnosis

The lack of specificity of the manifestations of nocardiosis is reflected in the fact that about 40% of diagnoses are first made at autopsy. With any pneumonia that persists and is progressive despite conventional antimicrobial therapy, the possibility of nocardiosis should come to mind. The thought should lead to appropriate diagnostic activity, particularly in patients who also have leukemia, Hodgkin's disease, or other kinds of malignant neoplasms; iatrogenic immunosuppression, as in recipients of transplanted organs; dysproteinemias, disseminated lupus erythematosus, pemphigus vulgaris, diabetes mellitus, pulmonary alveolar proteinosis; and chronic obstructive pulmonary disease, asthma, or anthracosilicosis.

The diagnostic problem posed by the patient with nocardial infection of the brain may be especially vexing because the findings are so often nonspecific. Although scanning procedures may provide precise localization of lesions, the neurologic abnormalities may be either diffuse or focal, and the cerebrospinal fluid will show increased pressure, number of leukocytes, concentration of protein, and a slight to moderate decrease in the concentration of glucose. Because microorganisms are not found by smear or culture of the cerebrospinal fluid, a high degree of clinical acumen is necessary to insist on biopsy of the brain. Yet, biopsy is the one potentially definitive procedure in such desperately ill patients.

The isolation of nocardias from clinical specimens is essential to etiologic diagnosis. The clinical microbiology laboratory must be informed of the possibility of nocardiosis so that allowance can be made for the slow rate of growth, and the susceptibility to concentration procedures and selective additives to culture mediums. Etiologic diagnosis of pulmonary nocardiosis may result from culturing expectorated sputum. Although the paraffin bait method may be helpful with sputum (and other contaminated specimens), confusing overgrowth can be most readily avoided by obtaining a specimen for culture by transtracheal aspiration (see Chap. 31, Bacterial Pneumonias). In some patients, biopsy of intrathoracic lesions is necessary for diagnosis.

Similarly, sinus tracts may be colonized with bacteria which are unrelated to the underlying nocardial or actinomadural process. Biopsy of the seat of the infection may be necessary for etiologic diagnosis.

It is critically important that a portion of all biopsy specimens be cultured whenever there is even the slightest possibility of nocardial infection. Histopathologic diagnosis is not possible because the lesions of nocardiosis are not unique. In addition, neither *Nocardia* spp. nor *Actinomadura* spp. are visible in tissue sections stained either with hematoxylin and eosin, periodic acid-Schiff, or acid-fast methods. The Brown and Brenn modification of the Gram stain and the methenamine silver stain are often useful.

Despite a history of fitful investigative effort dating back to 1904, immunodiagnosis has not gained either wide acceptance or application in nocardiosis. Lack of specificity is the major problem. There is serologic cross reactivity between antigens from nocardial mycobacterial, corynebacterial, and rhodochrous complex bacteria (apparently nonpathogenic bacteria intermediate between nocardia and mycobacteria). Protein sensitins for skin testing of delayed hypersensitivity have been isolated from several *Nocardia* spp. and show promise in veterinary medicine; evaluation of such sensitins in humans is incomplete.

The primary problems in differentiation are the other causes for pulmonary infections. The usual bacterial pneumonias (see Chap. 31, Bacterial Pneumonias) have a more acute onset and course. Etiologic diagnosis is frequently accomplished by culturing sputum or transtracheal aspirate and blood. Tuberculosis (see Chap. 34, Pulmonary Tuberculosis) and fungal infections of the lungs (see Chap. 39, Candidosis; Chap. 40, Histoplasmosis; Chap. 41, Coccidioidomycosis; Chap. 43, Balstomycosis; Chap. 44, Aspergillosis; and Chap. 120, Cryptococcosis) may offer greater difficulty. Epidemiologic studies, cultures, and tuberculin and coccidioidin skin tests are useful measures. The nontuberculous acid-fast bacteria (see Chap. 36, Nontuberculous Mycobacterioses) and *Actinomyces israelii* (see Chap. 38, Actinomycosis) are surely recognized only by culture. Pneumoconioses (beryllium, silicon, and barium) are radiographically confusing. Biopsy investigation is quite valuable. Bronchogenic carcinoma of the lung sometimes leads to unilateral, suppurative, chronic pneumonia. Metastasis to the brain is frequent, and biopsy is often the most expeditious route to differentiation.

Prognosis

Before the advent of the sulfonamides, approximately three-fourths of patients proven to have nocardiosis died of the disease after a course that averaged 6 months from onset. Since sulfonamides have been included in most regimens of therapy, the overall case fatality rate is around 50%. The effectiveness of antimicrobial therapy may be reduced by the lapse in time from clinical onset of disease until therapy is applied—on the average, about 2 months. Dissemination, particularly as metastatic brain abscess, affects the prognosis adversely; the mortality may then exceed 70%. In the absence of an underlying disease, more than 90% of patients with nocardiosis restricted to the lungs should survive if treated with sulfonamides.

There is no documentation that protective immunity is acquired by patients who have recovered from nocardiosis.

Therapy

The utility of the sulfonamides in the treatment of nocardiosis, regardless of species, is well proved. Whatever sulfonamide is prescribed, the adequacy of the dosage regimen must be documented by measurement of the concentration in the blood. The dose for a given patient is the quantity that gives peak concentrations of 12 mg to 15 mg/100 ml. Triple sulfonamides in a dosage of 65 mg to 75 mg/kg body wt/day, PO, as four equal portions, 6-hourly, are quite satisfactory, whereas sulfisoxazole may be inadequate because it is excreted rapidly.

Several other antimicrobics are active against nocardias according to *in vitro* testing, notably the combination of trimethoprim–sulfamethoxazole. However, when the components are tested separately, not infrequently only the sulfamethoxazole appears to be active. It is possible that some of the reports of good clinical effect from the combination relate primarily to the sulfamethoxazole. For this reason, augmentation of trimethoprim–sulfamethoxazole by the coadministration of sufficient additional sulfamethoxazole or triple sulfonamides to attain therapeutically optimal concentrations of total sulfonamides appears to be desirable.

By testing *in vitro,* the penicillins and the cephalosporins may appear to be active against nocardias. However, they lack clinical effectiveness, probably because nocardias elaborate β-lactamases which are extracellular in about half the isolates and cell associated in the remainder. Although cefoxitin is active *in vitro,* there is no reported clinical experience using cefoxitin to treat nocardiosis.

Of the aminocyclitols, amikacin is often the most active by testing *in vitro*. Clinical experience is limited but may be corroborative. The poor penetration of the aminocyclitols into the central nervous system is a serious drawback to their use when there is intracerebral nocardiosis. Also, the necessity for long-term therapy is a demurrer to use of these potentially toxic agents.

Of the tetracyclines, minocycline appears to be most consistently active by testing *in vitro*. It is an observation of interest because minocycline enters the central nervous system efficiently and should pass into phagocytes to inhibit intracellular nocardias. The relatively small clinical experience using minocycline to treat nocardiosis that has been reported is favorable.

As nocardiosis is generally a chronic disease, a clinically effective regimen of chemotherapy must be applied for many months. There are no firm data regarding duration of therapy as might be derived from controlled clinical trials. Therefore, the clinical similarity of nocardiosis to tuberculosis and actinomycosis should be heeded, and treatment should be applied for 6 to 12 months.

Surgical drainage of abscesses and the excision of necrotic tissue must be carried out. General measures such as bed rest and adequate nourishment must also be provided.

Prevention

No preventive measures are known.

Remaining Problems

A selective medium that favors the outgrowth of nocardias would be of advantage in culturing contaminated specimens. Simpler, more generally applicable methods are needed for the laboratory identification of nocardias and for differentiating species within the genera. The utility of culture filtrate antigen to immunodiagnosis in humans should be assessed. Variation in susceptibility to antimicrobics according to species merits investigation.

Bibliography

Book

GOODFELLOW M, BROWNELL GH, SERRANO JA (EDS): The biology of the Nocardiae. New York, Academic Press, 1976, 517 pp.

Journals

BEAMAN BL, BURNSIDE J, EDWARDS B, CAUSEY W: Nocardial infections in the United States: 1972–1974. J Infect Dis 134:286–289, 1976

BERD D: Nocardia brasiliensis infection in the United States: A report of nine cases and a review of the literature. Am J Clin Pathol 60:254–258, 1973

CAUSEY WA: Nocardia caviae: A report of 13 new isolations with clinical correlation. Appl Microbiol 28:193–198, 1974

CURRY WA: Human nocardiosis: A clinical review with selected case reports. Arch Intern Med 140:818–826, 1980

EPPINGER H: Ueber eine neue, pathogene Cladothrix und eine durch sie hervorgerufene Pseudotuberculosis (cladothrichica). Wien Klin Wochenschr 3:321–328, 1890

GEISELER PJ, ANDERSEN BR: Results of therapy in systemic nocardiosis. Am J Med Sci 278:188–194, 1979

GOODFELLOW M, MINNIKIN DE: Nocardioform bacteria. Ann Rev Microbiol 31: 159–180, 1977

NOCARD ME: Note sur la maladie des boeufs de la Guadeloupe; Connue cous le nom de farcin. Ann Inst Pasteur (Paris) 2:293–302, 1888

ROSETT W, HODGES GR: Recent experiences with nocardial infections. Am J Med Sci 276:279–285, 1978

GEORGE GOLDSAND

38 Actinomycosis

Actinomycosis is a chronic granulomatous disease with a remarkable tendency to form external sinuses. It is an endogenous infection that develops when the anaerobic bacterium *Actinomyces israelii* invades tissues from its normal habitat in the tonsillar crypts and gingivodental crevices. Though most infections are caused by *A. israelii,* other, related normal oral commensals may also produce classic actinomycosis. Among these are the actinomycetes *A. naeslundii, A. viscosus* and *A. odontolyticus,* and a single species of the related genus, *Arachnia propionica.* The lesions of actinomycosis occur most commonly in the head and neck, lungs, pleura, ileocecal region, and uterus. Bone, pericardial, and anorectal lesions are less common, but virtually any tissue may be invaded; a disseminated, bacteremic form has been identified.

Etiology

Actinomyces israelii is a gram-positive, filamentous bacteria of the order *Actinomycetales.* One of the characteristic common features of infections with all members of this group is the production of a subacute form of granulomatous inflammation, such as occurs in nocardiosis (see Chap. 37, Nocardiosis) and tuberculosis (see Chap. 34, Pulmonary Tuberculosis).

Actinomyces spp., as *Nocardia* spp., have traditionally been misclassified as fungi; they are, in fact, bacteria. Several properties distinguish bacteria of the genus *Actinomyces* from fungi. Of greatest practical importance is a favorable response to treatment with penicillin or tetracycline, neither of which has any effect against fungi.

Colonies 1 mm to 2 mm in size appear after 3 to 7 days of anaerobic incubation on enriched mediums containing blood or brain–heart infusion. Growth is enhanced by the presence of CO_2.

On Gram stain, *Actinomyces* spp. are pleomorphic, gram-positive rods with forms varying from bacilli resembling diphtheroids to long, branching filaments. The same morphology may be observed in gram-stained smears of exudates or tissue sections. In addition, a unique morphologic form may develop *in vivo,* but not *in vitro:* the sulfur granule. If sufficient numbers of microorganisms are present and there is tissue inflammation, *Actinomyces* spp. will secrete a polysaccharide protein substance that cements filaments together to form yellow, macroscopic particles called *sulfur granules.* These are actually tiny colonies. When seen in tissue sections, the microscopic appearance of such colonies has given rise to the descriptive term *ray fungus.* Unfortunately the diagnosis of actinomycosis is often not made unless the typical sulfur granule or ray fungus is seen in exudates or sections of tissue. Careful anaerobic cultures are more useful in diagnosis, particularly in less severe infections in which sulfur granules are not

PROPERTIES OF BACTERIA OF THE GENUS ACTINOMYCES

There is no nuclear membrane; that is,they are prokaryotic (fungi have nuclear membranes; that is, are eukaryotic).
Cell walls contain basal mucopeptides and lack chitin (chitin is the principal structural macromolecule of fungal cell walls).
Filaments are 1 μm or less in diameter (fungal mycelia generally exceed 1 μm in diameter).
Filaments may segment into bacillary forms (fungal mycelia do not segment in the same way).
Reproduction is by fission, never by spores (fungi reproduce by spores or budding, not fission).
Growth is inhibited by penicillin, tetracycline, and other conventional antimicrobics but not by amphotericin B (fungi tolerate penicillin, tetracyline, and many other antimicrobics, but are inhibited by amphotericin B).

formed, or when tissues are not excised and viewed by the histologist. It is the branching properties of the *Actinomyces* spp. together with the fungus like appearance of the sulfur granule that has led to the erroneous inclusion of *Actinomyces* spp. with the legitimate fungi for so many years.

Antinomycosis was once thought to result from exogenous infection with *Actinomyces bovis,* a constitutent of the normal oral flora of cattle which is probably not capable of producing disease in humans. It is likely that infections of humans thought to be caused by *A. bovis* would have been found to be caused by *A. israelii* had there been more critical laboratory investigation. The differentiation of *A. bovis* depends on the ability of *A. israelii* to ferment xylose and its inability to hydrolyze starch.

Actinomyces viscosus differs from the other *Actinomyces* spp. in being catalase positive and growing under microaerophilic or aerobic conditions. Thus, a negative catalase reaction helps to distinguish all of the pathogenic, strictly anaerobic *Actinomyces* spp. from the other nonclostridial, anaerobic, gram-positive bacilli. *Arachnia propionica* is also anaerobic and is morphologically identical to *Actinomyces* spp.; however, it differs in serologic reactivity, contains diaminopimelic acid in its cell walls, and produces large amounts of propionic acid from glucose.

Epidemiology

Actinomycosis was first recognized in 1876, when Bollinger noted granules in the purulent discharge of a jaw lesion in a cow. Three years later, Ponfick found similar lesions in humans, and in 1885 Israel published the first detailed clinical description of the disease.

Actinomyces israelii appears to produce disease only in humans and has not been found outside the human body. It does not spread from human to human. *Actinomyces bovis* is responsible for granulomatous infections of the soft tissues surrounding the mouths of cattle and other ruminants, and it has a marked tendency to produce local osteomyelitic lesions of their jaws.

Pathogenesis and Pathology

The chief defense mechanism of the body against its endogenous anaerobic flora is the oxidation-reduction potential (Eh) of the tissues. At normal tissue Eh, anaerobes are unable to multiply at rates sufficient to produce tissue damage. Any factors that reduce the local Eh will enable such microorganisms to proliferate and invade surrounding tissues. In actinomycosis, the most frequent preceding event is dental extraction. The small foci of tissue necrosis and breaks in the mucous membrane that result from extractions are often sufficient to make the surrounding tissue susceptible to the proliferation of *Actinomyces* spp. or *A. propionica* resident in the gingivodental creases. Other factors that will lower the Eh of the tissues in the mouth include trauma, small foreign bodies, and previous chronic and recurrent infections with pyogenic aerobic and anaerobic bacteria. Recurrent viral or bacterial infections of the tonsils may enable the *Actinomyces* spp. within the tonsillar crypts to proliferate and spread through the pharyngeal tissues. The apparent increased occurrence of actinomycosis in people who habitually chew straw is probably a result of repetitive trauma to the gums and not, as was once believed, an exogenous infection with soil *Actinomyces* spp. transmitted by the straw. It is probable that infections occurring in thoracic and abdominal tissues begin with the aspiration or the escape of swallowed *Actinomyces* spp. through minute defects or breaks in the intestinal mucosa.

Once the microorganisms are able to proliferate and gain a foothold in the tissues, they eventually produce a subacute or chronic granulomatous inflammation that is followed by necrosis and fibrosis. Spread of the active lesion occurs primarily along the connective tissue planes toward the outside skin surfaces, with the eventual production of externally draining sinuses. Sparing of mucous membrane surfaces is characteristic of the disease.

Small sulfur granules can often be seen in the infected tissues and may be exuded from the external fistulas. Pus is usually scant, except in those rare instances when the course of the disease is very acute or if serous cavities such as the pleura or pericardium are involved.

Nodules of inflammation that are discrete or confluent constitute the usual reaction in actinomycosis. Colonies of *Actinomyces* spp. at the center of each nodule are surrounded by liquefaction necrosis and a polymorphonuclear leukocytic response; there is no caseation. Granulation tissue encloses the necrotic zone, and dense fibrous tissue, often with foci of calcification, is present peripherally.

Manifestations

Cervicofacial Actinomycosis (Lumpy Jaw)

The lesions begin as a painful, indurated swelling 1 to several weeks after dental extraction or trauma to the mouth. The mass, usually located at the angle of the

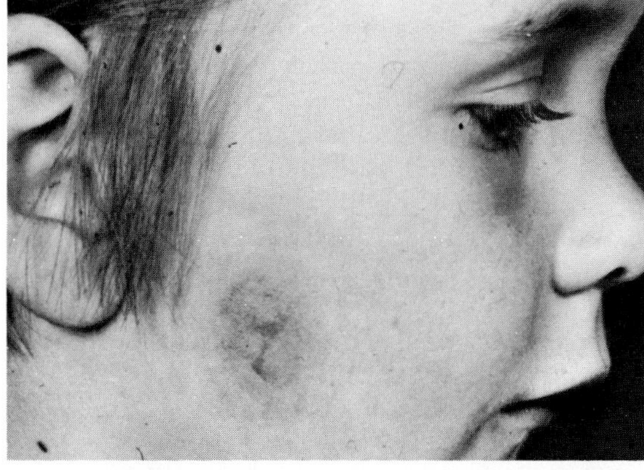

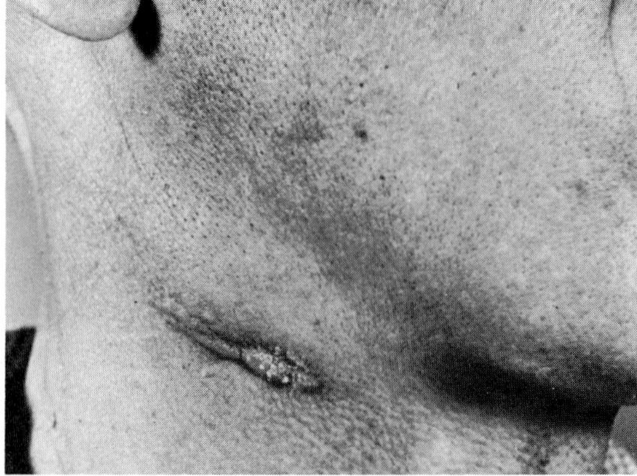

Fig. 38-1. External fistulas in cases of cervicofacial actinomycosis.

jaw, gradually increases in size and eventually forms fistulas that open onto the skin of the cheek or submandibular region (Fig. 38-1). Sulfur granules may be seen in the exudate. There is little tendency toward ulceration or lymphatic involvement. Less often, *Actinomyces* spp. spread to the mandible, causing periostitis or osteomyelitis. Direct extension into the orbit, lacrimal canaliculi, and paranasal sinuses has also been described.

Pulmonary Actinomycosis

Pulmonary actinomycosis develops when *Actinomyces* spp. from the mouth are aspirated into areas of the lung that have been rendered suitably anaerobic by atelectasis or infection with other kinds of microorganisms. A low-grade pneumonitis that tends to spread toward the pleura (Fig. 38-2) results. Prior to the pleural invasion, the only manifestation may be a nonproductive cough. As the lesion progresses, fever develops and the cough becomes productive, with occasional hemoptysis. The pleurae are eventually

Fig. 38-2. Pulmonary actinomycosis in a middle-aged male with cough and low-grade fever. *(A)* Before therapy. *(B)* After treatment with penicillin G.

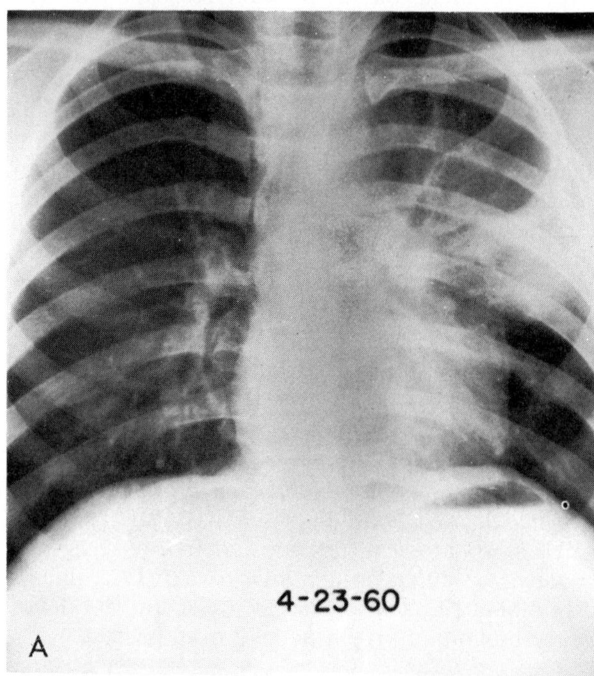

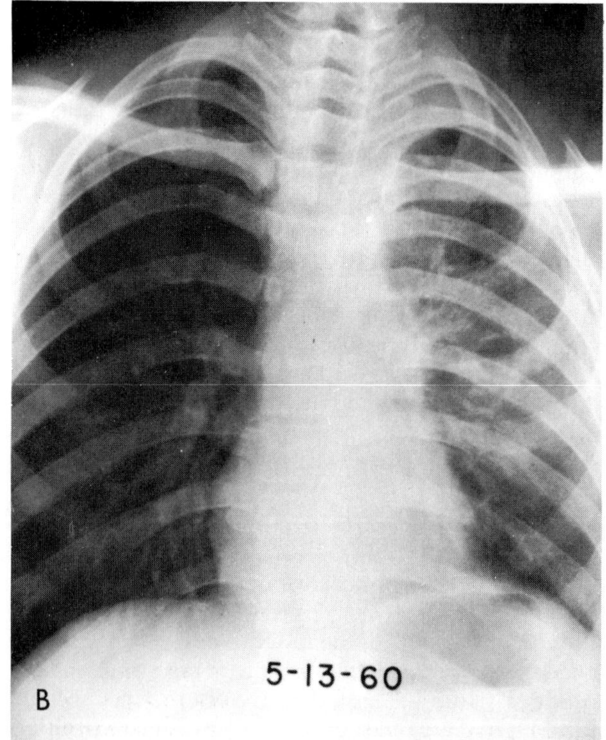

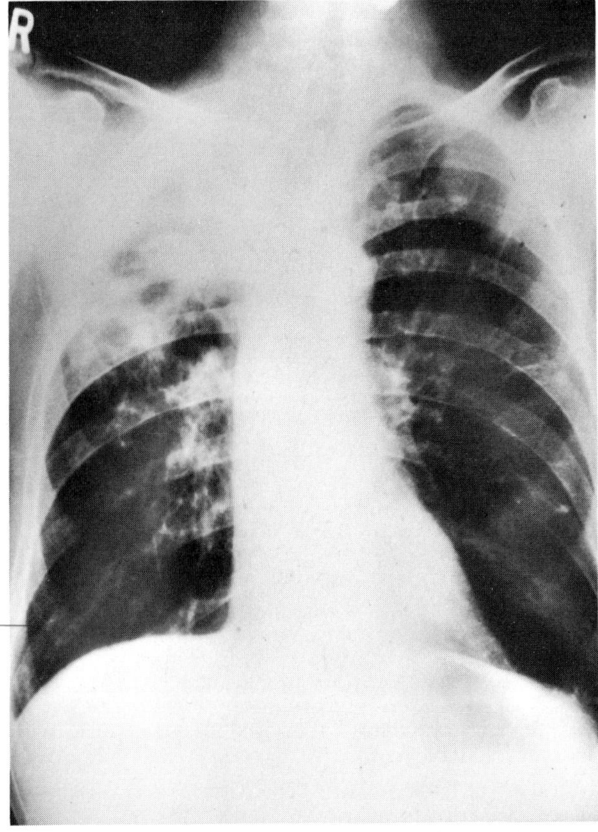

Fig. 38-3. Cavitary actinomycosis of right upper lobe in a 62-year-old male with a 1-1/2 year history of weight loss, cough, and sputum production.

invaded, resulting in empyema and the formation of a sinus through the chest wall. Lesions develop more often in the lower lobes but can occur anywhere in the lung. Cavitary disease resembling tuberculosis may also occur (Fig. 38-3).

A rare mediastinal form, characterized by empyema without obvious parenchymal disease, may also occur. The pathogenesis is not entirely clear, but the process may result from spread through the esophagus or from pleural exudation after a minimal lesion in the periphery of the lung. Sinuses that perforate the chest wall in the paravertebral area are frequent in this form of the disease. Periostitis of the ribs is a frequent radiographic sign.

Antinomycosis of the lung and pleura may be further complicated by direct extension into the pericardium, heart, or thoracic vertebrae, or through the diaphragm, producing subphrenic and hepatic abscesses. Pulmonary and thoracic lesions disseminate through the blood stream more frequently, carrying a relatively poorer prognosis than other forms of actinomycosis.

Gastrointestinal Actinomycosis

Gastrointestinal actinomycosis probably results when *Actinomyces* spp. are swallowed, escape through small defects in the bowel mucosa, and produce inflammatory masses in the adjacent connective tissues and mesentery. The lesions develop most commonly in the ileocecal region and less often in the anorectal or gastric areas. In many cases, there is a history of previous appendicitis. Where there is no such history, a subclinical form of appendicitis probably has occurred, rendering the tissue susceptible to infection with an anaerobe. Abdominal discomfort, fever, a palpable mass, and the development of an external sinus may be the presenting features. The disease is often recognized initially when drainage persists after surgery for an appendiceal abscess. Ileocecal actinomycosis may be mistaken clinically for tuberculosis, regional enteritis, cancer, or appendicitis. In patients with anorectal fistulas, sulfur granules should be sought in the exudate, and all drainage or excised tissue should be cultured anaerobically as well as aerobically. Gastrointestinal forms of actinomycosis may be complicated by direct spread to the kidneys or pelvic organs.

Female Pelvic Organs

Actinomycosis involving female pelvic organs was previously considered to be a relatively rare, chronic disorder characterized by lower abdominal and pelvic pain of several weeks to a month in duration. A pelvic mass was usually present, and the diagnosis was typically established at surgery for a suspected malignancy. Most cases probably developed by extension from the ileocecal region.

However, over the past decade, not only has the incidence increased but also the manifestations have shifted to those of pelvic inflammatory disease. Most cases appear to complicate intrauterine contraceptive devices (IUDs) that have been in place for months to years. Necrosis of endometrial tissue adjacent to the IUD provides an environment conducive to proliferation of anaerobic *Actinomyces* spp. that have probably been carried into the uterus from the vagina and perianal tissues.

Unusual Forms

BRAIN

Actinomycosis of the brain may result from bacteremia. In addition, *Actinomyces* spp. may be recovered together with anaerobic streptococci and *Bac-*

teroides spp. in pus from solitary brain abscesses arising from foci in the middle ear, sinuses, or lungs.

BONE

Actinomycosis of bone usually affects the mandible or vertebrae, producing periostitis or osteomyelitis. The long bones are seldom involved. Actinomycotic osteomyelitis of the mandible may remain confined to the bone and form a cystlike cavity, or it may extend to the surface, producing fistulas. Vertebral actinomycosis is usually a complication of throacic or abdominal disease. The bodies and transverse processes are attacked but not the intervertebral spaces. The slow progression of infection enables bone to be formed as fast as it is destroyed so that vertebral collapse is unusual. This process gives a sievelike appearance to the vertebral bodies on lateral radiography. The absence of vertebral collapse and the preservation of the intervertebral disk are helpful in distinguishing actinomycosis from spinal tuberculosis.

LIVER

The liver may be invaded from the bowel by way of the portal veins, by direct extension from another focus in the abdomen or thorax, or through the blood stream during bacteremia. The hepatic lesion is a suppurating granuloma that adheres to the abdominal wall or diaphragm before rupturing through it. The patient has an enlarged, tender liver and frequently complains of fever and chills.

Fig. 38-4. Pericardial effusion and pulmonary lesions in a male with disseminated actinomycosis.

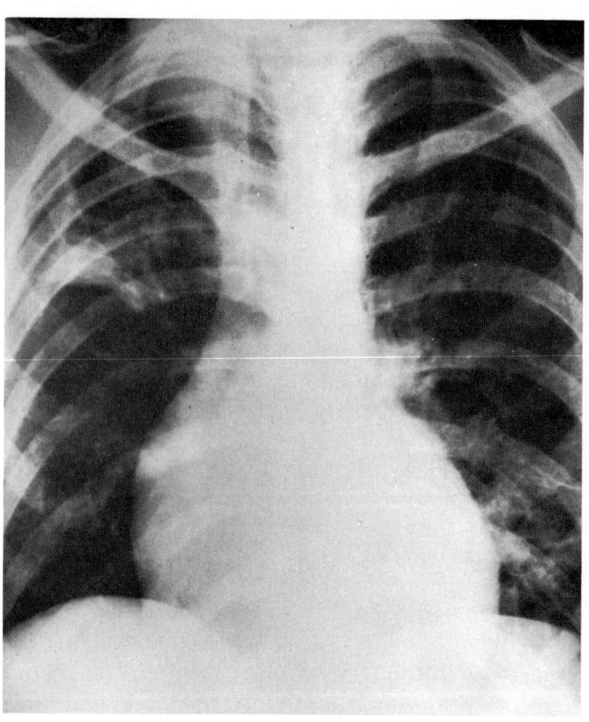

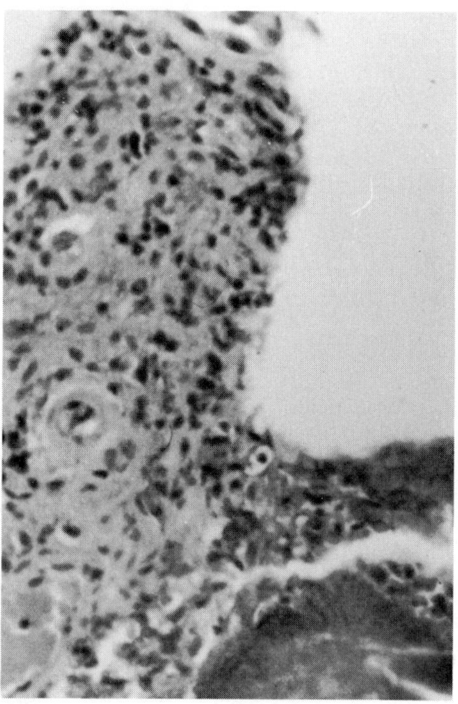

Fig. 38-5. Ray fungus in excised tissue of male with anorectal actinomycosis.

KIDNEY

Renal actinomycosis may result from the direct extension of lesions in the right iliac fossa or from bacteremia. Metastatic involvement usually takes the form of a circumscribed, chronic lesion that progresses slowly toward the renal capsule until it bursts through, producing a tender perinephric mass and flank pain.

ACTINOMYCOTIC SEPTICEMIA

Blood stream invasion usually begins from a focus in the lungs. Bacteremia may continue for months, producing low-grade fever, malaise, anorexia, weight loss, cough, and hemoptysis. Recurrent pleural and pericardial effusions (Fig. 38-4) are common, and painful red nodules may appear under the skin of the legs, arms, trunk, or scalp. These lesions become fluctuant as they enlarge and break down to form sinuses. Metastatic abscesses also occur in the liver, vertebrae, kidneys, and spleen.

Fig. 38-6. Appearance of *Actinomyces israelii* in Gram-stained smears of exudates. *(A)* Routine coughed sputum from patient in Figure 38-3. *(B)* Crushed sulfur granule from coughed sputum in the same patient. *(C)* From pleural fluid in a patient with empyema. *(D)* From pleural fluid. Note irregular staining, giving a beaded appearance.

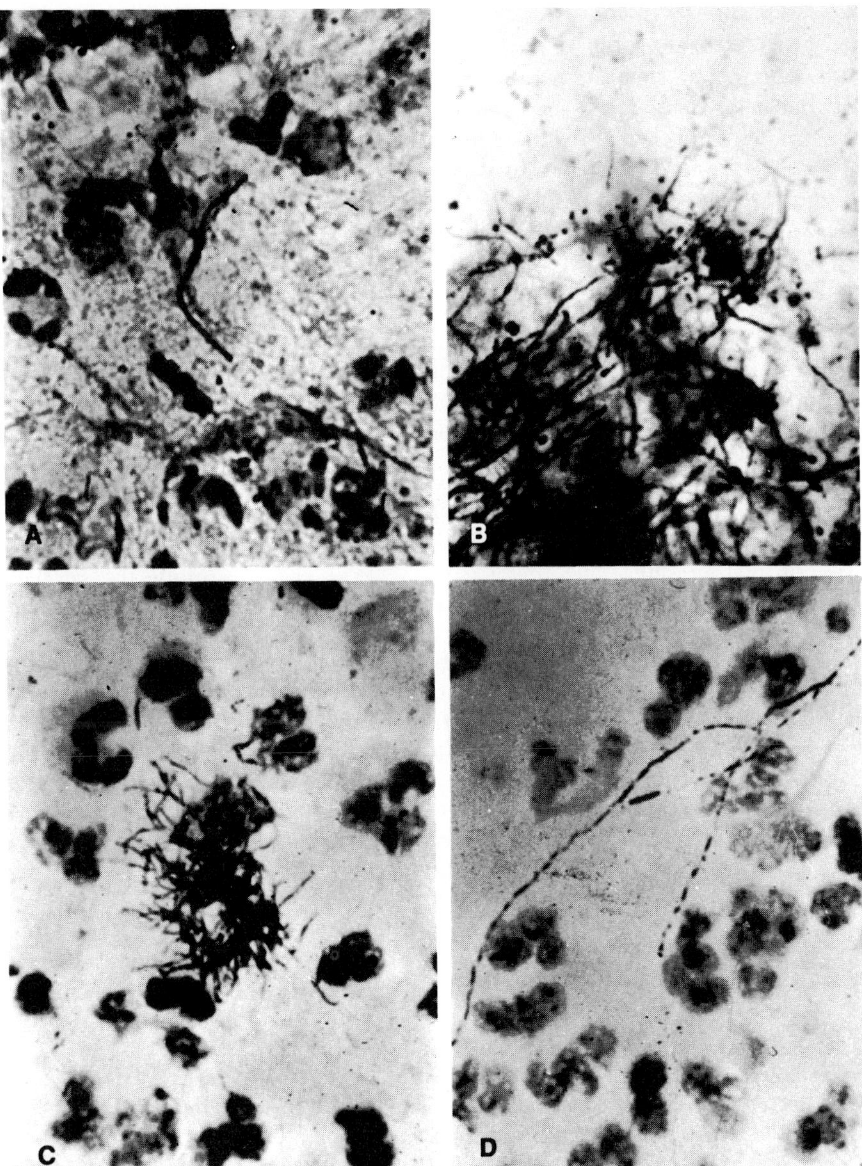

Diagnosis

The diagnosis of actinomycosis must be considered whenever typical sulfur granules are observed in exudates, when the typical ray fungus is seen in sections of excised tissues stained with hematoxylin and eosin (Fig. 38-5), and when gram-positive filaments are present in Gram stains of exudates or tissues. Such filaments measure 0.5 μm to 1 μm in diameter, and vary from pleomorphic, diphtheroid like bacilli to long, slender rods with definite branching. The rods may occasionally take up the Gram stain irregularly, producing a beaded appearance (Fig. 38-6). Thus, in Gram stains, *Actinomyces* spp. resemble *Lactobacillus* spp., diphtheroids, or *Listeria monocytogenes*. They must also be differentiated from *Nocardia* spp., particularly when isolated from an empyema or a sinus of the chest wall. This can often be done by demonstrating the acid-fast nonacid-alcohol-fast property of *Nocardia* spp. by decolorizing for only 1 min with aqueous 1% sulfuric acid solution rather than acid–alcohol solution as is done in the standard Ziehl–Neelsen technique (see Chap. 9, Microscopic Examinations, and Chap. 37, Nocardiosis).

The most important diagnostic procedure however, is recovery of the microorganism by culture. When actinomycosis is even remotely suspected, all exudates or excised tissues should be cultured promptly under anaerobic conditions. *It must be noted that any delay in culturing increases the probability of false-negative results because* Actinomyces *spp. may die on exposure to oxygen.* If present, sulfur granules are preferred for smear and culture because of a much higher rate of recovery. In females who may have uterine actinomycosis associated with an IUD, the diagnosis can be made by appropriate smear or culture of endometrial and endocervical biopsies, or by noting organisms of characteristic morphology in cytologic examination by the Papanicolaou method.

The exact and final identification of *Actinomyces* spp. depends on isolation in anaerobic cultures and identification by appropriate biochemical tests and gas chromatography.

Actinomyces spp. are seldom recovered from tissues in pure culture but often grow together with other anaerobes normally present in the mouth, such as *Peptostreptococcus* and *Bacteroides* spp. The typical granulomatous, spreading lesion of actinomycosis is seen when *A. israelii* is the predominant microorganism. Isolation of *Actinobacillus actinomycetemcomitans* and other small, poorly characterized gram-negative bacilli from conventional aerobic cultures may be a clue to the concomitant presence of the anaerobic *Actinomyces* spp.

Prognosis

The course of untreated actinomycosis is that of a very chronic, persistent infection with multiple draining sinuses. The prognosis is favorable with treatment, and complete recovery can be expected in more than 90% of cervicofacial and 80% of gastrointestinal cases. The prognosis is worse in the pulmonary form because bacteremic dissemination is more frequent and there is an increased risk of infection metastatic to vital organs.

Therapy

Penicillin is the preferred drug for treatment of patients with actinomycosis (Fig. 38-2*B*), although tetracyclines are also effective. Because *Actinomyces* spp. grow best in relatively avascular tissues, large doses of penicillin are necessary to ensure adequate tissue concentrations. Prolonged treatment is necessary to prevent recurrences.

Uncomplicated cases of cervicofacial actinomycosis should be treated initially with penicillin G (50 mg–75 mg [80,000 units–120,000 units]/kg body wt/day, IV, as four equal portions, 6-hourly) until the lesions have subsided. Patients with all other forms of actinomycosis should receive penicillin G in a dosage of 100 mg to 150 mg (160,000 units–240,000 units)/kg body wt/day, IV, as four equal portions, 6-hourly, for 4 to 6 weeks. Parenteral therapy should be followed by either penicillin V (25 mg–30 mg/kg body wt/day, PO, as four equal portions, 6-hourly) or tetracycline (15 mg–30 mg/kg body wt/ day, PO, as four equal portions, 6-hourly. Peroral therapy should be continued for periods varying from 6 to 8 weeks in mild, uncomplicated cases to up to 1 year in more severe, deep-seated infections. If neither the penicillins nor tetracycline can be tolerated, alternate drugs include the cephalosporins (same dosage as for the penicillins), clindamycin, erythromycin, or chloramphenicol (same dosage as for tetracycline). Definite abscesses or empyemas require surgical drainage. If large areas are involved, surgical excision may be a very helpful adjunct to antimicrobic therapy. Surgery alone is of little value in achieving complete eradication of the infection.

Prevention

The most important preventive of actinomycosis is the maintenance of a high standard of oral hygiene and an awareness of the increased risk of infection associated with insertion of an intrauterine device.

Remaining Problems

Actinomycosis must be recognized as an anaerobic bacterial infection and not one of the mycoses. Laboratory diagnosis of the disease should be made more frequently by the clinical bacteriology technologist than by the mycologist or pathologist. Delays in diagnosis can be minimized by an awareness that actinomycosis should be considered in the differential diagnosis of any inflammatory lesion of a subacute or chronic nature. The requirement for prolonged therapy, often as long as 1 year, must be recognized as comparable to the situation with infections caused by other microorganisms classified in the order Actinomycetales, (*e.g.,* those caused by *Mycobacterium* spp. and *Nocardia* spp.).

Bibliography

Books

COPE VZ: What the general practitioner ought to know about human actinomycosis. London, William Heinemann, 1952. 80 pp.

GEORG LK: The agents of human actinomycosis. In Balows A (ed): Anaerobic Bacteria: Role In Disease. Springfield, Ill, Charles C Thomas, 1974. pp 237–256.

Journals

BROCK DW, GEORG LK, BROWN JM, HICKLIN MD: Actinomycosis caused by *Arachnia proprionica:* Report of 11 cases. Am J Clin Pathol 59:66–77, 1973

BROWN JR: Human actinomycosis: A study of 181 subjects. Human Pathol 4:319–330, 1973

COLEMAN RM, GEORG LK: Comparative pathogenicity of *Actinomyces naeslundii* and *Actinomyces israeli.* Applied Microbiol 18:427–432, 1969

HAGER WD, DOUGLAS B, MAJMUDAR B, NAIB ZM, WILLIAMS OJ, RAMSAY C, THOMAS J: Pelvic colonization with Actinomyces in women using intrauterine contraceptive devices. Am J Obstet Gynecol 135:680–684, 1979

HARVEY JC, CANTRELL JR, FISHER AM: Actinomycosis: Its recognition and treatment. Ann Intern Med 46:868–885, 1957

HEINEMAN HS, BRAUDE AI: Anaerobic infection of the brain. Am J Med 35:682–697, 1963

HOLM P: Studies of the aetiology of human actinomycosis. 1. The "other microbes" of actinomycosis and their importance. Acta Pathol Microbiol Scand 27:736–751, 1950

LERNER PI: Susceptibility of pathogenic Actinomycetes to antimicrobial compounds. Antimicrob Agents Chemother 5:302–309, 1974

PEABODY JW JR, SEABURY JH: Actinomycosis and nocardiosis. Am J Med 28:99–115, 1975

SCHIFFER MA, ELGUEZABAL A, SULTANA M, ALLEN AC: Actinomycosis infections associated with intrauterine contraceptive devices. Obstet Gynecol 45:67–72, 1975

THADEPALLI H, RAO B: *Actinomyces viscosus* infections of the chest in humans. Am Rev Respir Dis 120:203–206, 1979

VARKEY B, LANDIS FB, TANG TT, ROSE HD: Thoracic actinomycosis: Dissemination to skin, subcutaneous tissue, and muscle. Arch Intern Med 134:689–693, 1974

PAUL D. HOEPRICH
MICHAEL G. RINALDI

39 Candidosis

Candidosis (or *candidiasis*) is fungal disease caused by *Candida* spp. Normally inhabitants of mucocutaneous body surfaces, species of *Candida* overgrow and invade tissues when permitted by alterations in the host.

Candidosis was once rare; it is now common because a patient population has burgeoned that (1) suffers from diseases that either involve the immune system primarily or require therapies that adversely affect immune competence; (2) is treated intensively with antibacterial agents; or (3) has been inoculated intravenously with *Candida* spp., thus bypassing normal defenses. Because candidal infections vary from asymptomatic to septicemic disseminated disease, it is often difficult to assess the role of a candidal isolate in a particular patient.

Etiology

Candida spp. are dimorphic fungi that grow as oval (about 2 × 8 μm), budding yeast cells–blastoconidia (buds) and as chains of connected, elongated cells—the pseudo or true hyphae. Of some 68 species, 9 have been associated with candidosis. The more virulent species, *C. albicans* var. *albicans, C. albicans* var. *stellatoidea,* and *C. tropicalis,* maintain their dimorphism when infecting tissues. The less virulent, but still pathogenic, species (*C. parapsilosis, C. guillermondii, C. krusei, C. pseudotropicalis, C. viswanathii, C. zeylanoides,* and *C. paratropicalis*) generally exist in tissues only in the yeast form.

The cell walls of *Candida* spp. are multilayered structures (Fig. 39-1) consisting mostly of polysaccharides, with some proteins and lipids. The main polysaccharides are mannans (mannan-protein complexes in the outer, electron-dense cell wall), and glucans (glucan-protein complexes in the inner, electron-transparent cell wall). Chitin is also present—mostly in bud scars and also in the glucan network. Mannan glycoprotein is antigenic and is responsible for the major humoral antibody response. There are physicochemical differences (*e.g.,* extent of branching, length of side chains, nature of bonding in the mannans of the different *Candida* species; yet, some degree of interspecies serologic cross-reactivity is usual. Within the species *C. albicans,* the two serotypes A and B reflect mannan-specific antigenic determinants.

The cell membranes of *Candida* spp. are morphologically unremarkable, but their lipid constituents are of interest. Sterol esters (mainly zymosterol), free sterols (mainly ergosterol), triglycerides, and phospholipids are present; the sterols are the primary interactive components necessary to the antifungal activity of the polyene antimicrobics.

Candida spp. grow readily at a pH of 3 to 8, a temperature of 20°C to 40°C, and with or without oxygen; they generate a characteristic yeasty odor. Soft, cream-colored colonies form on blood agar and Sabouraud's glucose agar; either pseudohyphae or true hypae are produced. Although most *Candida* spp. fail to form ascospores, ascomycetous teleomorphs have been discovered for some species, for example, *C. guillermondii* (teleomorph *Pichia guillermondii*), and *C. krusei* (teleomorph *Pichia kudriavzerii*). Presumptive identification of *C. albicans* var. *albicans* and *C. albicans* var. *stellatoidea* can be accomplished within 2 hours by demonstrating the formation of pseudogerm tubes (short filaments without constrictions at the point of origin from the yeast cell) on incubation at 37°C in human serum. This useful test is not only rapid, but also simple to carry out; it is valuable because fewer than 4% of strains of *C. albicans* var. *albicans* and *C. albicans* var. *stellatoidea* fail to produce pseudogerm tubes, structures that are formed but rarely by *C. tropicalis* and not at all by the other *Candida* spp.

Candida albicans var. *albicans* and *C. albicans* var. *stellatoidea* are also distinguished by profuse

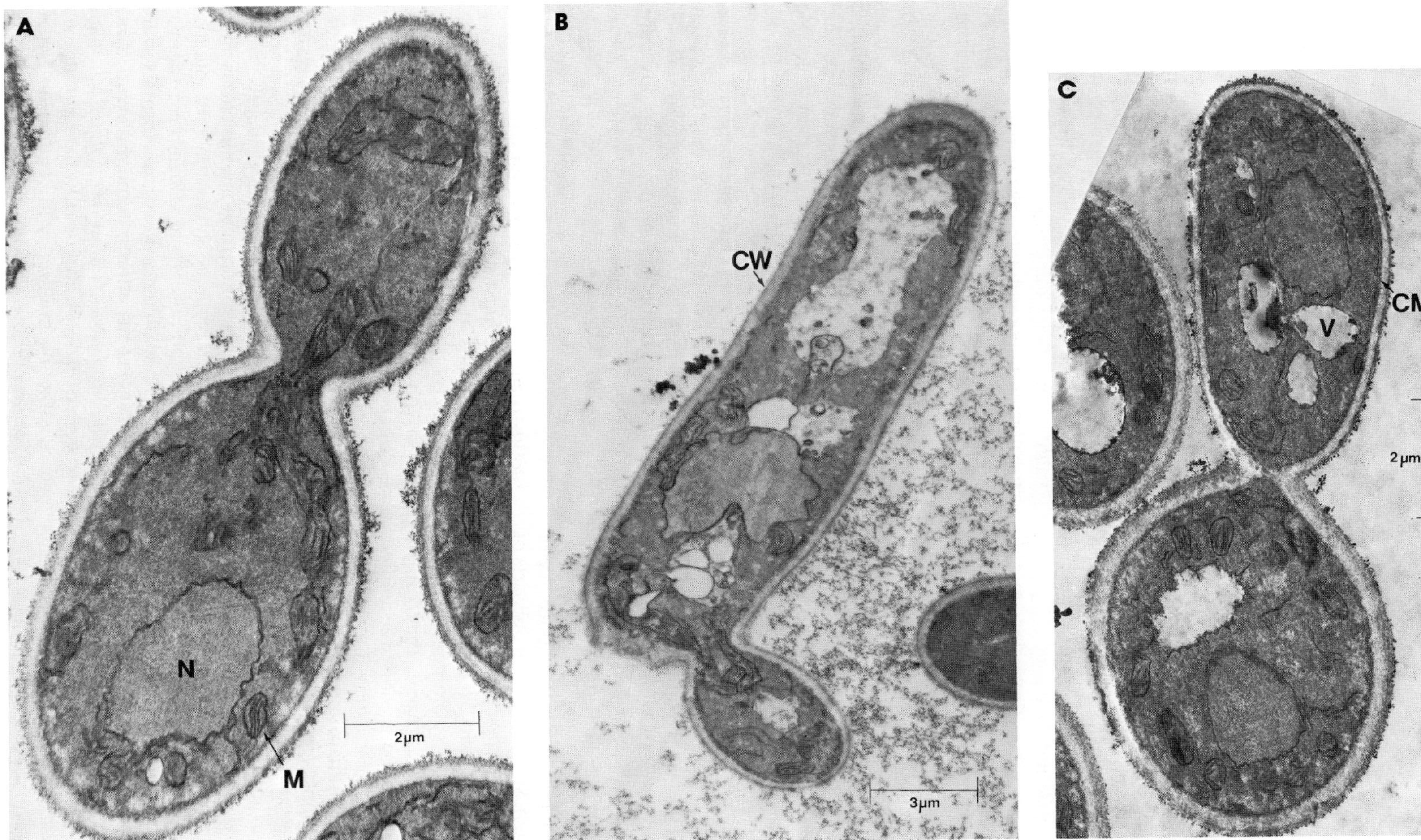

Fig. 39-1. Electron photomicrographs of three *Candida* species. N = nucleus; M = mitochondria; V = vacuole; CM = cell membrane; CW = cell wall. Fixed with permanganate. (Original magnification approximately × 7,000) (*A*) Mother and daughter blastoconidia of *C. albicans* in late logarithmic phase of growth. (*B*) Blastoconidia of *C. krusei* with young bud adjacent to bud scar. (*C*) Virtually completed bud cycle (septum forming between mother and daughter cells) in *C. parapsilosis*. (Odds FC: Candida and Candidosis, p. 18. Leicester, England, Leicester University Press, 1979)

production of chlamydoconidia in 3 to 4 days when cultured on corn meal agar. Occasionally, *C. tropicalis* exhibits meager production of chlamydoconidia that are often teardrop shaped.

All *Candida* spp. may be positively identified and differentiated in the course of 7 to 10 days by testing for fermentation and assimilation of glucose, maltose, sucrose, lactose, and galactose (Table 39-1). *Candida* spp. do not assimilate nitrogen from nitrates, and they are urease negative (except for *C. viswanathii* and *C. zeylanoides,* and occasional strains of *C. krusei*). Cycloheximide, as added to commercial culture mediums to render them selective, will inhibit *C. tropicalis, C. parapsilosis,* and *C. krusei.*

Virtually all isolates of the pathogenic *Candida* spp. are susceptible to the polyene antimicrobics and the antifungally active imidazole derivatives, whereas native resistance to griseofulvin is uniform and is not uncommon to flucytosine (10%–30% of clinical isolates of *C. albicans*). Antiseptics, such as quaternary ammonium compounds, chlorheximide, mercurials, iodine, and sodium hypochlorite, inhibit *Candida* spp.; topical anesthetics are inhibitory.

Epidemiology

Humans are the reservoir of *Candida* spp., and are the usual source of the inoculum leading to candidosis. That is, the epidemiology of candidosis reflects the normal status of *Candida* spp. as elements of the resident microbiota, the tenuous balance between colonization and infection, and the singular importance of *C. albicans* as a pathogen. Surveys from many parts of the world show that *Candida* spp., particularly *C. albicans,* are present in at least 50% of specimens of oropharyngeal and gastrointestinal contents as stable components of the microflora, that is, they can be isolated repeatedly when the same sites are sampled. The frequency of intraoral carriage is increased in patients with diabetes mellitus and is augmented by dental prostheses and smoking.

Candida albicans are also normal components of the vaginal microflora in at least 20% of nonpregnant and 30% of pregnant women. The skin is colonized less often—in about 2% of humans. Other *Candida* spp. are found on the same mucosal and skin surfaces; they are cultured less frequently than *C. albicans* from the oropharynx, gastrointestinal tract (where *C. tropicalis* is relatively common), and vagina, but more frequently from the skin.

Colonization with *C. albicans* commonly begins at birth when the fetus traverses the vaginal canal. This encounter often results in a self-limited, oral infection termed *thrush.* Such infections may be a source for the spread of *C. albicans* to other infants in the nursery. Although unproven, candidal colonization at later periods of life is believed to result from human-to-human transmission of the fungus. Animal-to-man transmission is also possible, since birds and mammals harbor the fungus. Because *Candida* spp. are seldom cultured from the air, or from soil not contaminated with feces, acquisition from the environment is unlikely.

The spectrum of candidosis includes skin infections; noninvasive overgrowth of the fungus on mucosa of the oropharynx, gastrointestinal tract, and vagina; superficial infections of these same mucous membranes; and systemic infections involving internal organs. Candidosis is usually caused by *C. albicans,* and occurs predominantly in patients who have diabetes mellitus, leukemia, lymphoma, or immunologic deficiency or who require treatment with antibacterial antimicrobics, glucosteroids, or immunosuppressive drugs. Regardless of the underlying cause or causes, most candidal infections remain superficial at the site of origin; invasion to gain access to the bloodstream and infect internal organs is exceptional.

Systemic infections may reflect spread of *Candida* spp. from the intestinal tract or may be consequent on the introduction of *Candida* spp. into the bloodstream through contaminated intravenous catheters, from the injection of unsterile materials by drug addicts and by physicians, from contamination of hyperalimentation solutions, and from contamination during cardiovascular surgery. These inadvertant bloodstream infections are often caused by species other than *C. albicans.* Such candidemias may result in endocarditis, the most important complication of self-induced or iatrogenic candidal infections, but may involve virtually any organ.

Urinary catheters may also lead to candidal colonization. Candiduria caused by *C. albicans* and *C. tropicalis* is common in hospitalized patients who have indwelling catheters and who are receiving antibacterial therapy.

Cutaneous infections occur primarily as diaper rashes in infants, intertriginous infections in obese and debilitated patients, and paronychial infections in housewives and others whose hands are traumatized by frequent washing. A very rare form of skin and oropharyngeal infection is termed *chronic mucocutaneous candidosis (CMC).* Typically, CMC begins in the first decade of life, usually before the age of 2 years, afflicting children with endocrine hypofunction, or severe immunologic deficiency, as is seen in DiGeorge's syndrome, Swiss-type agammaglobuline-

Table 39-1. *Laboratory Differentiation of Medically Important Species of* Candida, Torulopsis glabrata, *and* Rhodotorula rubra. *The Tests Are Arranged in a Sequence of Decreasing Value for Early Diagnosis, From Left to Right*

Fungus	Dimorphic In Tissues	Pseudogerm Tube (2 hr)*	Urease	Chlamydoconidia (4 Days)*	Fermentation/Assimilation (7–10 Days)*/(1 Day*)					Human Mycoses
					GLUCOSE	MALTOSE	SUCROSE	LACTOSE	GALACTOSE	
C. albicans var. *albicans*	+	+	−	+	F/A	F/A	v/A	−/−	F/A	All forms of candidosis
C. tropicalis	+	±	v	±**	F/A	F/A	−/A	F/−	F/A	Vaginitis; bronchopulmonary, systemic; onychomycosis; meningitis
C. albicans var. *stellatoidea*	+	+	−	+	F/A	F/A	−/−	−/−	−/A	Vaginitis
C. parapsilosis	±	−	−	−	F/A	−/A	−/A	−/−	v/A	Paronychia; endocarditis; otitis externa
C. guillermondii	±	−	−	−	F/A	−/A	−/A	F/−	F/A	Endocarditis; dermatitis; onychomycosis; meningitis
C. krusei	±	−	v	−	F/A	−/−	−/−	−/−	−/−	Endocarditis; vaginitis
C. pseudotropicalis	±	−	−	−	F/A	−/−	F/A	F/A	F/A	Vaginitis
*C. viswanathii****	−	−	+	−	F/A	F/A	−/A	−/−	F/A	Meningitis
C. zeylanoides	−	−	+	−	v/A	−/−	−/−	−/−	−/v	Onychomycosis
C. paratropicalis	?	−	−	−	F/A	F/A	−/v	−/−	F/A	Causative role not proved
T. glabrata	−	−	−	−	F/A	−/−	−/−	−/−	−/−	Urinary tract; vaginitis; systemic
T. candida	−	−	−	−	v/A	−/A	−/A	v/v	−/A	
R. rubra	−	−	+	−	−/A	−/A	−/A	−/−	−/A	
R. glutinis	−	−	+	−	−/A	−/A	−/A	−/v	−/A	Systemic; endocarditis
R. pilimanae	−	−	+	−	−/A	−/−	−/A	−/−	−/v	

*Usual incubation time for test on cornmeal agar (*C. albicans* is usually positive in 24–28 hours).
**Occasional strains produce teardrop-shaped chlamydoconidia.
***Incertus status.
F = fermentation; A = assimilation; v = variable; ± = uncommon.

mia, or thymus dysplasia. Deficiency of T cell mediated immunity is thought to be the critical defect, since humoral immunity is virtually always intact.

Pathogenesis and Pathology

Almost all cases of oropharyngeal, gastrointestinal, vaginal, systemic, and cutaneous candidosis are caused by *C. albicans,* although an increasing prevalence of *C. tropicalis* has been noted in immunocompromised patients. The virulence of *C. albicans* var. *albicans* has been related to its ability to grow in tissues as hyphal forms (Fig. 39-2*A*), which are apparently more resistant to the cellular defenses of the host than blastoconidia. Although *C. albicans* var. *stellatoidea* and *C. tropicalis* also may form pseudohyphae in tissues, in experimental studies, they are intermediate in virulence between *C. albicans* var. *albicans* and *C. parapsilosis* or *C. guillermondii,* species that do not convert to hyphae in the tissues (Fig. 39-2*B*). Thus, the association between dimorphism in tissues and virulence has support; however, it is not an absolute requirement because (1) blastoconidia and hyphae or pseudohyphae are almost always seen together in lesions; (2) conditions encountered *in vivo* favor filamentation—temperature >35°C, pH ≥7.0; and (3) species that are nondimorphic in tissues also cause disease.

Candida spp. have not been proved to produce toxin(s). However, hypersensitivity contributes to the pathogenesis of candidosis of the genital tract, skin, and respiratory tract.

Conditions that predispose to candidosis do so by (1) increasing the amount of nutrient available for fungal use (diabetes mellitus, treatment with glucosteroids, administration of antibacterial antimicrobics); and (2) depressing defense systems (leukemia, lymphoma, treatment with immunosuppressive drugs or glucosteroids). As a rule, overgrowth by

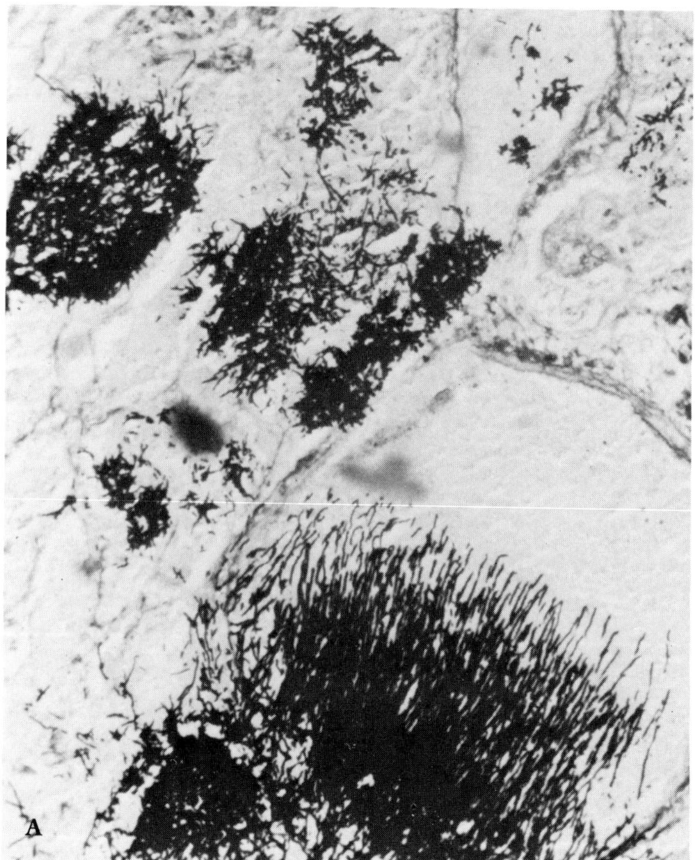

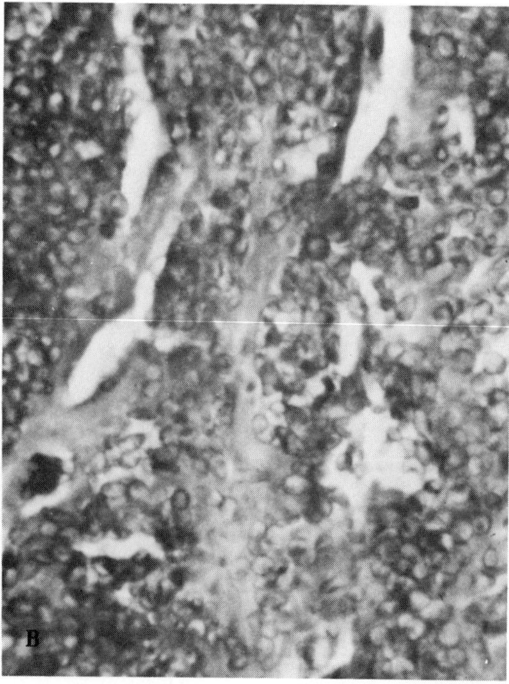

Fig. 39-2. Candidas in tissues. (*A*) Pneumonia caused by *Candida albicans*. Note predominance of pseudomycelia. (H&E, Original magnification approximately × 400) (*B*) Endocarditis caused by *C. parapsilosis*. The candidas are exclusively in the yeast phase. (Periodic acid-Schiff, original magnification approximately × 400)

Candida spp. that is conditioned by physiologic disturbances results in less serious illness than does overgrowth secondary to abnormalities of immune function.

The number of yeasts in oropharyngeal, gastrointestinal, and vaginal secretions is controlled primarily by the amount of available glucose. Increases in glucose concentration, as occur in diabetes mellitus and during treatment with glucosteroids, promote fungal growth without necessarily inducing tissue invasion. Treatment with certain antimicrobics, for example, the tetracyclines, also increases the amount of glucose available for fungal growth by reducing the number of bacteria capable of competing for glucose.

Normally, intact mucous membranes prevent proliferating *Candida* spp. from invading underlying tissues. Fungal penetration into submucosal tissues occurs in areas where the mucosa is damaged by trauma, tumors, instrumentation, or ulceration secondary to immunosuppressive therapy. Although the mechanisms responsible for preventing extension of candidal infections are not completely understood, polymorphonuclear leukocytes and tissue macrophages are quite active in killing fungi that invade submucosal tissues. The essential role of such phagocytic capability is clear from the lack of restraint of proliferation and dissemination of these fungi in patients whose cellular defenses are abrogated by lymphoreticular malignancies or immunosuppressive therapies.

Although all internal organs are susceptible to infection by blood-borne species of *Candida,* a descending order of involvement may be discerned using data pooled from several reports of postmortem examinations of patients who died with disseminated candidosis: digestive tract, kidneys, lungs, brain, heart, spleen, liver. In the living, it has been suggested that the high frequency of hematogenous infection of the kidneys might provide a diagnostically useful signal in candiduria; unfortunately, in disseminated candidal sepsis, candiduria is as infrequently documented as candidemia. Moreover, most patients with candiduria do not have upper-tract disease.

Cutaneous candidosis and candidal endocarditis are attributable to local abnormalities in the host. Unless a severe burn is present, infections of the skin occur in moist, intertriginous areas that are subjected to repeated trauma. Burn wounds that become colonized with *C. albicans* may serve as foci for fungal dissemination to internal organs, since the loss of the integrity of the skin provides access to the bloodstream. Although the skin lesions of chronic mucocutaneous candidosis frequently extend over large areas, dissemination to internal organs is rare.

Endocarditis occurs when blood-borne *Candida* spp. engraft on a normal, deformed, or prosthetic heart valve. These infections are not associated with general impairments of host defenses, and they are frequently caused by *Candida* spp. other than *C. albicans,* particularly *C. parapsilosis.*

Superficial mucosal lesions result in a mild inflammatory reaction, and a diffuse growth of pseudohyphae is evident on histologic examination. Deeper invasion by *Candida* spp. causes microabscesses with polymorphonuclear leukocytes as the predominant cell type. Granulomatous lesions may evolve if candidal infections persist. The blastoconidia and pseudohyphae of *C. albicans* can be identified in tissue sections stained with hematoxylin and eosin; however, they are better visualized by the Gridley stain or the Gomori methenamine silver stain (Chap. 9, Microscopic Examinations). The large vegetations observed in candidal endocarditis consist of eosinophilic debris, fibrin, and yeast cells (Fig. 39-2*B*); occasionally, pseudohyphae as well as blastoconidia are produced.

Manifestations

Superficial

Primary cutaneous candidosis is a superficial infection that is usually manifest about the nails and in intertriginous areas of the glabrous skin (axillae, groin, inframammary folds, intergluteal folds, interdigital spaces, glans penis, umbilicus) as erythematous macules with irregular edges that are scaly and sometimes covered by exudate. Candidal infection of the diaper area gives rise to an erythematous rash involving the genitocrural and intergluteal folds and the surrounding skin; scaling and papule formation is prominent at the periphery of the rash. Paronychial involvement causes tenderness, redness, and swelling that is sometimes associated with scaling, pus beneath the nail fold, and dark areas in the nail itself—indicating coexistent onychomycosis.

Superficial infections of oropharyngeal and vaginal membranes affect only the immediately subjacent mucosa. Oral candidosis causes numerous raised, discrete, or confluent cream-colored patches on the mucosal surfaces of the mouth, tongue, and pharynx. These lesions are usually asymptomatic, but may be painful; in infants, they may interfere with respiration. Scraping the candidal growth off reveals a hyperemic base.

The symptoms of vaginal candidosis are pruritus, dyspareunia, and a vaginal discharge. Candidal lesions of the vagina appear as raised gray or white patches surrounded by areas of erythema.

Chronic mucocutaneous candidosis usually begins with typical oral lesions, which then extend to involve the lips, the larynx, and rarely, the esophagus. Concomitant vaginal candidosis is typical. Onychial and paronychial lesions arise. In severe cases, the skin of the fingers, hands, shoulders, neck, face, ears, scalp, and groin may become desquammating, crusted, hyperkeratotic, and even granulomatous.

Deep

The manifestations of deep candidosis that is focalized in one organ or system are, perforce, related to that system. Thus, in serious candidal infection of the esophagus, dysphagia and retrosternal pain that increases with swallowing are the most important symptoms. Candidosis elsewhere in the digestive tract is not clinically evident.

Primary, nonhematogenous candidal infection of the lower respiratory tract is rare, even among debilitated patients. The suggestion that hypersensitivity to *Candida* spp. may be manifest as bronchial or pulmonary allergy has not received convincing support.

Lower urinary tract infection with *Candida* spp. or *Torulopsis* spp. that is provocative of urgency, frequency, nocturia, and hematuria is usually associated with >50,000 colony-forming units per ml of urine; in asymptomatic infections, the candiduria or torulopsuria is typically of lesser magnitude. Patients with candidal pyelonephritis may have fever, flank pain, nausea, vomiting, and sometimes, dysuria.

The clinical manifestations of candidal endocarditis are identical to those of bacterial endocarditis except for an increase in the frequency of occurrence of major emboli. Characteristically, candidal vegetations are bulky and friable; they fracture readily to yield large emboli that may occlude medium-sized arteries—a hallmark of candidal endocarditis.

Candidal endophthalmitis may or may not be associated with orbital or periorbital pain, blurred vision, and scotomas. On ophthalmoscopic examination (the indirect technique is preferable), the initial lesions are round, small, and white; surrounded by a margin of erythema; and located near a venule. They may resolve, or they may progress by simply enlarging—sometimes causing raylike processions into the vitreous or even causing retinal detachment. Intraocular candidosis is a sequel to candidemia.

Although *Candida* spp. infecting the central nervous system (CNS) are virtually always blood-borne, such a localization as the primary manifestation of candidosis is rare. The manifestations include headache, nuchal rigidity, papilledema, and focal neurologic abnormalities.

Candidosis of the bones and joints is a rare consequence of candidemia. The clinical manifestations are not unique.

Acute, hematogenous dissemination of *Candida* spp. (septicemic candidosis) may give rise to the same manifestations as are associated with acute, severe bacterial infections, namely, chills, high and spiking fevers, hypotension, and prostration. However, the concurrence of fever with an erythematous, maculopapular (lesions 3 mm–5 mm in diameter) skin rash on the trunk and extremities, and severe tenderness of the muscles in an immunosuppressed patient who has been, and continues to be, under intensive treatment with multiple antibacterial antimicrobics, is strongly suggestive of acute, hematogenous dissemination. Documentation of candidemia by culture of the blood is said to be successful in fewer than 50% of patients, with extremes of 20% to 80% possibly reflecting variation in technique. Focal growths of *Candida* spp. are usually evident in the oropharynges of such patients; there may also be symptoms of esophagitis, and infiltrates may be found in the lungs by radiography. Lesions consistent with candidal retinochoroiditis may be found in 5% to 50% of patients, but may not be detected until 1 to 6 weeks after the candidemia. Acute, hematogenous pyelonephritis may be rapidly destructive of renal tissue, leading to acute renal failure.

Diagnosis

Superficial

Because superficial candidosis involves regions of the body that may be visualized without special instruments, swabbings, scrappings, and biopsies are readily obtained for study using cultures and appropriately stained smears and sections. If invasion of tissues is documented, the causative role of the yeast fungi isolated in cultures is assured, whereas isolation alone leaves doubt as to the etiologic significance of candidas obtained in cultures.

Deep

Deep candidosis must always be suspected in immunosuppressed and immunoincompetent patients who are ill and have received antibacterial antimicrobics. Any localizing aid derived from signs and symptoms should be heeded in seeking a specific diagnosis. Thus, the manifestations of esophagitis should lead to contrast radiography; although the nodular defects and irregularities of the mucosa characteristic of ulcerative candidal esophagitis are not seen in every patient with the disease, the examination is often helpful. Moreover, the lesions may be seen on esophagoscopy when brushings can be obtained for smear and culture.

Expectorated sputum and tracheobronchial aspirates obtained perorally or through a bronchoscope are so readily contaminated with oropharyngeal *Candida* spp. that they are not useful for the diagnosis of lower respiratory tract candidosis. Either percutaneous transthoracic aspiration of a radiographically evident lesion or an open surgical biopsy of a pulmonary lesion will provide specimens that enable diagnosis of pulmonary candidosis.

Cystoscopy with biopsy of lesions suspected of being candidal may allow histologic demonstration of fungal invasion into the submucosa, a finding diagnostic of candidal cystitis. Candidal pyelonephritis, renal carbuncle, and perinephric abscess cannot be surely diagnosed without surgical exploration and biopsy or aspiration of pus.

The isolation of *Candida* spp. from several blood cultures taken from patients who do not have intravascular catheters but have clinical findings consistent with infective endocarditis is suggestive of candidal endocarditis. Detection of vegetations by echocardiography or the finding of *Candida* spp. in an embolus removed from an artery are strongly supportive findings.

Proof of the candidal etiology of an endophthalmitis is rarely possible, since retinochloroidal lesions are not amenable to biopsy. Vitrectomy is not useful, since the intravitreal extrusions appear to be sterile inflammatory exudate, and the aqueous humor is not ordinarily involved.

Smear and culture of the cerebrospinal fluid (CSF), and of aspirates or biopsies of intracerebral lesions detected by computed tomography (CT) is required for the diagnosis of candidosis of the CNS. Similarly, aspiration of synovial fluid and biopsy of bone lesions is necessary to the diagnosis of candidosis of the joints and bones.

Although septicemic candidosis may be suspected on clinical grounds, confirmation of the diagnosis must be sought by (1) culturing the blood—a procedure that is unsuccessful in 20% to 80% of the patients, and that may entail a delay of weeks if the *Candida* spp. is slowgrowing; (2) biopsy of skin lesions for examination by smear and culture—perhaps the speediest means to diagnosis; (3) aspiration or biopsy of lesions detected in any other organ; (4) culture of a specimen of bone marrow, since it is a safely and readily accessible component of the reticuloendothelial system; and (5) microscopic examination of Gram-stained smears prepared from the buffy coat of blood—an exercise fraught with the hazard of detection of yeastlike fungi present in reagents or on glassware. Culture of the urine has been advocated as an aid to the diagnosis of blood-borne dissemination. Unfortunately, candiduria is common in patients with diabetes mellitus and in hospitalized patients who have indwelling urinary catheters. Finding pseudohyphae in the urine is not proof of candidal invasion of the urinary tract. Also, *Candida* spp. may form fungus balls in the bladder; these are usually asymptomatic and can be demonstrated by cystoscopy or contrast cystography.

Immunodiagnosis

Failure to demonstrate *Candida* spp. in blood or tissues is all too common in patients suspected of having systemic or endocardial infection and in whom these forms of candidosis are eventually found at autopsy. Thus, there is an urgent need for improved diagnostic methods.

As a result of the intimate association of *Candida* spp. with humans, delayed hypersensitivity and humoral antibodies to these fungi are quite common. The intradermal injection of aqueous candidal extracts (*e.g.,* Oidiomycin) produces a zone of induration $\geqslant$10 mm in diameter after 48 hours in most normal persons. Such reactions may indicate remote or subclinical infections, but do not necessarily attest to recent or on-going infections. Lack of reaction may reflect anergy in patients with overwhelming candidosis, defective cellular immunity, or lack of contact with the fungus. Because cutaneous hypersensitivity to candidal antigens is present in most normal persons, skin testing is useful to determine whether a person is capable of a delayed hypersensitivity response. Lack, or transient suppression, of skin hypersensitivity has been correlated with the activity of candidal infection in patients with chronic mucocutaneous candidosis and lymphoma.

Serodiagnosis of systemic candidosis has been pursued vigorously for decades, but as yet there is no dependable method. Work aimed at diagnosis through detecting humoral antibodies has been hampered by the lack of standardized reagents, and failure of agreement about tests and methods. There is also the fact that many persons who are not ill carry antibodies to *Candida* species. Even so, the really crippling circumstance may be the limited or lacking capability to mount an antibody response that is characteristic of patients who develop systemic candidosis.

There may be more hope of serodiagnosis based on tests that seek to measure either antigenic components of these fungi, such as mannans or cytoplasmic proteins, or characteristic metabolic products such as D-arabinitol. As yet, there is no such test that is practical for routine use in the clinical laboratory. However, there is investigational application of the exquisite sensitivity of gas–liquid chromatography, mass spectrometry, and enzyme-linked immunosorbent assay.

Prognosis

The outcome of candidosis depends primarily on the correctability of the predisposing factor or factors that made the candidal disease possible. Most important is the state of the patient's immune capabilities. If these and other defenses are normal, removing unfavorable mechanical influences will make cure possible. If immune competence and other host defenses cannot be restored, the prospect for cure is dim.

Therapy

Prior to, or at least in concert with, antifungal chemotherapy, there must be correction of adverse mechanical conditions; control of diabetes mellitus; and cessation of administration or reduction in the dose of immunosuppressives, glucosteroids, and antibacterial agents.

The treatment of cutaneous candidosis is illustrative. The primary measures involve curtailing excessive exposure of the skin to water and detergents; halting maceration of the skin from intertrigo or tight, nonporous clothing; and protecting burn wounds from contamination. Antifungal agents are adjuvants that are applied in the form of creams or lotions containing nystatin or, preferably, one of the antfungal imidazole derivatives (clotrimazole, miconazole, econazole).

Ketoconazole is the treatment of choice for chronic mucocutaneous candidosis. The administration of 200 mg, PO, once a day secures improvement within 6 to 18 days and remission of the disease within 6 months. Because relapse occurs in most patients when treatment is stopped, the duration of therapy and the regimen appropriate for long-term suppression are under investigation.

Vaginal candidosis responds to the application of creams containing nystatin or, preferably, an antifungal imidazole (Chap. 50, Infections of the Female Genital Tract). However, cessation of treatment with systemic antimicrobics, particularly the tetracyclines, and control of diabetes mellitus is essential to avoid relapse or recurrence.

Holding suspensions of nystatin or amphotericin B in the mouth and gargling 4 to 6 times a day, or sucking on tablet or lozenge preparations of polyenes or imidazoles 3 to 4 times a day (held in the mouth or wedged in a pacifier and sucked until they disintegrate) aids in clearing oropharyngeal candidosis if predisposing diseases and therapies are also favorably manipulated. Ingestion of nystatin and other poorly absorbed antifungal antimicrobics has not been shown to be effective in the treatment of gastrointestinal candidosis, whereas systemically distributed drugs may be beneficial.

Candidosis associated with candidemia and involvement of internal organs warrants systemic therapy with antifungal antimicrobics. Some properties of four such drugs are listed in Table 39-2. As crippled host defenses so frequently predispose to systemic candidosis, merely inhibitory antimicrobics such as flucytosine and the imidazoles are less likely to be of value than is the fungicidal polyene amphotericin B.

Amphotericin B

Since 1955 when amphotericin B was first used in the systemic therapy of fungal infections, a lore has grown up surrounding its use that, in some respects, is not entirely rational. Three examples will suffice: (1) the IV injection of a dose by trickle over 6 to 8 hours does not really prevent adverse reactions and may in fact result in repeated chills, protracted nausea and vomiting, and thwarted peroral nutrition; (2) gradual increase in the daily dose from homeopathic to therapeutic over a period of 7 to 10 days may not secure the benison of tolerance to adverse reactions but does delay therapy unnecessarily; and (3) because the half-life of amphotericin B in humans is about 24 hours, daily administration is not necessary after loading the patient by giving daily doses for 3 days in beginning therapy. Additional commentary regarding the protocol given in the list below is appropriately related to the adverse reactions that are virtually obligatory when therapeutic doses of amphotericin B are injected intravenously.

Local irritation to peripheral veins is provocative of thrombophlebitis; it may be minimized by (1) adjusting the concentration of amphotericin B to less than 10 mg/dl and the pH to 6.0 to 6.5; and (2) adding heparin, 50 units/dl (glucosteroids should not be added, since they will inactivate the amphotericin B). The problem of thrombophlebitis is avoided altogether by using a Broviac or Hickman catheter. Because these catheters terminate in the superior vena cava, there is rapid mixing of the drug in a large volume of blood; thrombophlebitis does not occur, and higher concentrations may be used, that is, smaller volumes for infusion. Infection is prevented by insertion of the catheter by a surgeon in the operating theater and by scrupulous care of the external portion of the catheter, treating it always as a surgical wound.

Generally reversible systemic reactions may be diminished somewhat by regulation of the concentration, the rate of infusion, rapid mixing on injection, and continuing treatment, that is, some tolerance does develop. Such reactions include at least four categories. 1. Chills, fever, headache, nausea, and vomiting may sometimes be diminished by pretherapy and intratherapy medications; possibly, prochlorpromazine is more effective in combating nausea than other are medications. 2. Hypotension is uncommon, usually asymptomatic, and not often engendered after the first or second dose; typically, it responds promptly to raising the foot of the bed and administrating 0.9% NaCl solution IV. However, there are patients, fortunately quite rare, who develop such severe hypotension that they cannot be treated with amphotericin B. 3. Anorexia and malaise relate to other adverse reactions, but to some extent, they respond to the previously described maneuvers. 4. Anemia—a development in at least 75% of patients, sometimes with thrombocytopenia—results primarily from the direct suppression of erythropoiesis (and platelet formation) and also from renal failure. Hemolysis from direct interaction between erythrocytes and amphotericin B is unlikely to be contributory because much higher concentrations than are attained in therapy are necessary by testing *in vitro*. The hematocrit generally stabilizes at around 24% to 30%. Although transfusion may be temporarily beneficial, iron therapy is of no value—withdrawal of amphotericin B is critical to the correction of the anemia.

Nephropathy is virtually always produced by amphotericin B, but is variable in severity from patient to patient. It can be minimized only by limiting exposure of the kidneys to amphotericin B—see Figure 39-3. If renal function was normal at the outset of treatment and the total dose did not exceed 2 g (about 30 mg/kg in an adult), fewer than 15% of the patients will have detectable, not crippling, but permanent renal damage. When the total dose exceeds 5 g (about 75 mg/kg), approximately 80% of patients will have permanent, severe damage in the form of glomerular injury (decreased creatinine clearance, with or without azotemia) and prominent tubular injury as manifested by hypokalemia, hyposthenuria, and a diminished capacity to excrete acid. Histologic study of kidneys severely compromised or rendered nonfunctional by amphotericin B reveals necrosis and calcification of the renal tubules. In controlled trials, maneuvers such as alkalinizing the urine and giving mannitol were of no protective value.

Table 39-2. *Some Properties of Four Systemically Administrable Antifungal Antimicrobics*

Properties	**Amphotericin B**	**5-Fluorocytosine**	**Miconazole**	**Ketoconazole**
Route of administration (physical state)	Intravenous (suspension)	Peroral (dry solid)	Intravenous (suspension)	Peroral (dry solid)
Action	Interaction with sterols and phospholipids of cell membranes causing leakage	Enters pyrimidine anabolism to yield nonfunctional RNA; may also influence DNA synthesis	Antimetabolic	Antimetabolic
Effect	Fungistatic/fungicidal	Fungistatic	Fungistatic	Fungistatic
Toxicity	++++	±	+	+
Peak concentration in serum	2.5–3.5	80.0–100.0	3.5–5.5	3.5–6.0
Geometric mean MIC (*C. albicans*)	2.9	14.2	0.6	4.2
Distribution	Excluded from CSF, CNS, urine	In all body water	Excluded from CSF, urine	Limited entry into CSF; excluded from urine
Route of elimination	Bile	Urine	Catabolized	Catabolized
Effect of renal dysfunction	None	Accumulation	None	None
Development of resistance during therapy	Rare	Not uncommon	Very rare	Not reported

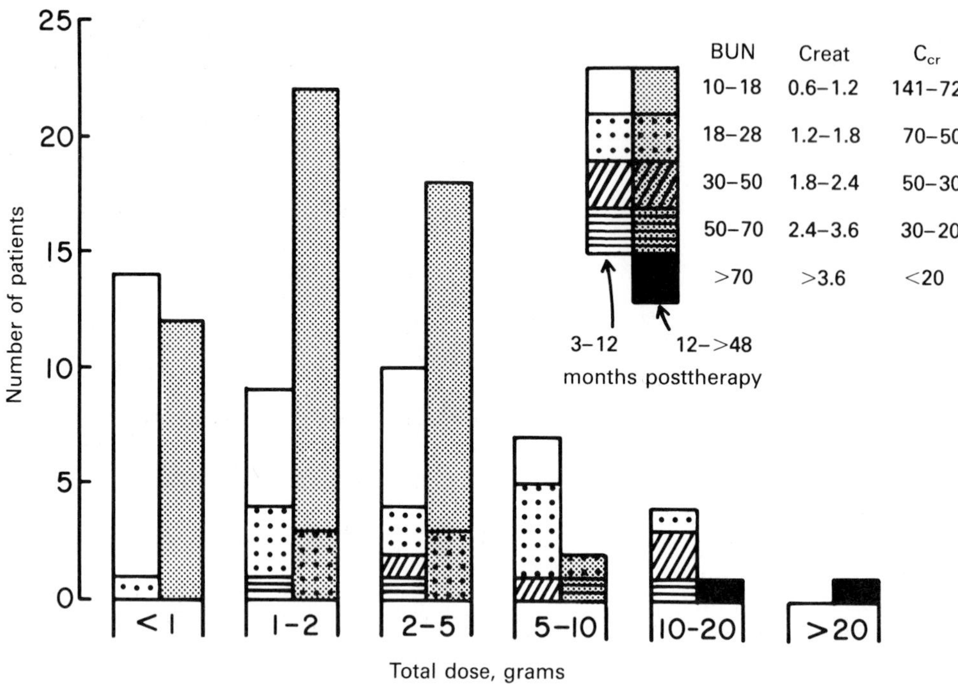

Fig. 39-3. Relationship of total dose of amphotericin B injected intravenously into patients with coccidioidomycosis, to renal function. Note the segregation of the duration of post-therapy follow-up into two periods. (After Winn WA: Coccidioidomycosis and amphotericin B. Med Clin North Am 47:1131–1148, 1963)

PROTOCOL FOR THE INTRAVENOUS ADMINISTRATION OF AMPHOTERICIN B

Pharmacy preparation

1. The desired dose is added to sufficient 5% glucose solution for IV injection to provide a final concentration of ≤10 mg/dl (peripheral vein—may be 15–20 mg/dl for infusion in a central vein).
2. Sufficient heparin solution is added to yield a final concentration of 50 U/dl.

Premedication—given 30 min before giving amphotericin B

1. Aspirin (or acetaminophen), 15–20 mg/kg body wt, PO (repeat dose every 3 hours for two additional doses)
2. One of the following (repeat dose once, 6 hours after initial dose)
   a. Prochlorpromazine, 0.3–0.6 mg/kg body wt, PO
   b. Trimethobenzamide, 3–4 mg/kg body wt, PO
   c. Diphenhydramine, 0.3–0.6 mg/kg body wt, PO

Injection

1. The patient should be supine in bed.
2. The temperature, pulse, and blood pressure must be recorded before starting treatment.
3. The infusion assembly should include a Y tube or similar arrangement (to provide access to both 5% glucose solution without additives and the dose of amphotericin B) and an infusion pump.
4. First day—0.25 mg/kg body wt
   a. Inject 5–10 mg over a period of 5 min, then switch to the 5% glucose solution without additives.
   b. Measure blood pressure at 5 min, 15 min, and 30 min.
      i. If there has been no fall in blood pressure, give the remainder of the dose of amphotericin B within 45 min.
      ii. If there has been a fall in blood pressure
         (A) Without symptoms

Elevate the foot of the bed, inject 0.9% NaCl solution (10 ml/kg body wt) over 30 min, and then give the remainder of the dose of amphotericin B within 45 min.

(B) With symptoms

Elevate the foot of the bed, inject 0.9% NaCl solution (10 ml/kg body wt) over 30 min, and give ephedrine, 0.3–0.6 mg/kg by IM injection.

If there is prompt restoration of the blood pressure and subsidence of symptoms, repeat the 5 mg–10 mg dose.

(1) If hypotension does not recur, give the remainder of the dose over 45 min.

(2) If hypotension recurs, put off therapy for 2–3 days before trying again.

5. Second day—0.50 mg/kg body wt
   a. If there was no hypotension with the first dose, inject the second dose over a period of 45 min (measure the blood pressure at 5 min, 15 min, 45 min, and 90 min).
   b. If there was transient hypotension with the first dose, again assess the effect of injection of 5 mg–10 mg, as with the first dose, before giving all of the second dose.
6. Third day—0.75 mg/kg body wt

   If there was no hypotension with the second dose, inject the third dose over a period of 45–60 min (measure the blood pressure at 5 min, 15 min, 45 min, and 90 min).
7. Fourth day—no amphotericin B
8. Fifth day—0.75 mg/kg body wt
9. Sixth day—no amphotericin B
10. Seventh day—0.75 mg/kg body wt
    a. Pretherapy, obtain blood (low, or trough specimen) for assay of the concentration of amphotericin B.
    b. Inject dose, noting exact duration of administration.
    c. Within 5 min posttherapy obtain blood (high, or peak specimen) for assay of the concentration of amphotericin B.
11. Continue alternate-day regimen of treatment, adjusting the dose to yield a peak concentration of 2.5—3.5 μg/ml serum (trough of 0.5–1.0 μg/ml).
12. When the appropriate dose is determined, continue therapy on alternate days for inpatients and thrice weekly (Monday, Wednesday, Friday) for outpatients.

Surveillance (in addition to clinical evaluations)

1. Before therapy
   a. Obtain pictures of lesions; radiographic, radionuclide, and ultrasound examinations; cultures; and serologic studies within 1 week before treatment.
   b. Determine creatinine clearance, urea nitrogen, creatinine, K^+, and Mg^{++} within 48 hours before treatment.
   c. Carry out urinalysis and complete blood count on the day treatment is started.
2. During therapy
   a. Weekly—perform studies of *1*b and c, above. If treatment goes smoothly, shift to biweekly to monthly observations after 4 weeks of therapy.
   b. Monthly—perform studies of *1*a, above, plus assays of peak/trough concentrations of amphotericin B in blood.
3. After therapy

   The studies of *1*a, b and c, above, should be repeated monthly for 3 months, then quarterly for 6 months, and finally semiannually for a period of years appropriate for the mycosis.

The duration and total dosage of systemic therapy with amphotericin B must be individually determined. The clinical course of the patient and the state of renal function are of major importance. Also of value are serial determinations of the (1) peak concentration of amphotericin B—it should be 2.5–3.5 μg/ml serum; and (2) peak candicidal titer of the patient's serum—it should be ⩾1:5.

Because endophthalmitis, intracerebral abscesses, pyolonephritis, and endocarditis may sometimes complicate candidemia, routine application of so-called low-dose, short-term treatment with amphotericin B has been suggested for all patients with candidemia. Such treatment—the intravenous injection of 0.25 mg/kg body wt/day for 7 to 10 days—has not been proven of value. Moreover, it is clear from the range in the susceptibility of clinical isolates of *C. albicans* that the concentrations of amphotericin B in the blood and tissues would often be subtherapeutic. To this must be added the poor penetration of amphotericin B into the CNS, the vitreous humor, the urine, and possibly, into vegetations. Details about the intrathecal administration of amphotericin B are given in Chap. 41, Coccidioidomycosis.

Flucytosine

Of available antifungal antimicrobics, only flucytosine (5-fluorocytosine) reliably penetrates into the CNS, the CSF, and the eye. Without renal failure, a dose of 200 mg/kg body wt/day, PO, as four equal portions 6-hourly, is usually well tolerated and yields peak concentrations in the serum (1 hour postdose) of 80 to 100 μg/ml, with contemporaneous concentrations in the CSF about two-thirds as great. To compensate for diminished renal excretory capacity, each 6-hourly dose should be reduced in direct proportion to the reduction of the creatinine clearance. Confirmation of the appropriateness of adjustment of dosage by assay of flucytosine in serums is desirable. Unfortunately, about 1% of serogroup A and about 85% of serogroup B isolates of *C. albicans* are natively resistant to flucytosine; also, *Candida* spp. and *Torulopsis glabrata* may develop resistance during therapy (see Fig. 18-7). Concomitant use of another effective antimicrobic might prevent clinical emergence of resistance. However, neither the polyenes nor the antifungal imidazoles, with the possible exception of ketoconazole, penetrate into either the CNS or the eye to attain therapeutic concentrations.

Since neither amphotericin B nor the imidazoles reliably achieve effective anticandidal concentrations in the urine, it is probable that they would be less useful in the treatment of candidal pyelonephritis than would flucytosine. The limitation of native resistance to flucytosine is detectable by susceptibility testing *in vitro.* Development of resistance to flucytosine during treatment of candidal pyelonephritis might be avoided by the concomitant administration of amphotericin B; this hypothesis has yet to be tested.

Imidazoles

Low concentrations of the antifungal imidazoles are generally inhibitory for *Candida* spp. However, they are not candidicidal at concentrations relevant to systemic therapy (Fig. 18-12).

Miconazole is not soluble in water, but can be injected IV as an aqueous suspension stabilized with polyethoxylated castor oil. Thrombophlebitis and irritation to tissues on extravascular deposition are relatively minor problems, as are giddiness, headache, anorexia, nausea, and vomiting. Hypersensitivity may occur, and may warrant cessation of therapy. Moreover, miconazole does not attain therapeutically significant concentrations in the urine or CSF. There is no proof that miconazole is effective in the treatment of systemic candidosis.

Ketoconazole is adequately absorbed after peroral administration, and in patients with fungal meningitis, attains concentrations in the CSF that are 15% to 25% of the concentrations in contemporaneous serums. Thus, in systemic candidosis that does not involve the urinary tract (ketoconazole does not enter the urine), ketoconazole should inhibit the infecting *Candida* spp. from growth. However, in immunoincompetent patients, fungistasis may not be enough. Prolonged suppressive treatment is costly and poses the problems of adverse effects: nausea and gastrointestinal distress (which are common), skin rashes, loss of libido and gynecomastia in males, and hepatitis. The place of ketoconazole in the treatment of systemic candidosis remains to be defined.

Combinations

It has been proposed that, if there is no barrier to the entry of amphotericin B to the site of infection, for example, in candidal pneumonia, a low dose of amphotericin B be combined with flucytosine. In this way, the development of resistance to flucytosine would be circumvented, the toxicity of amphotericin B would be avoided, and a therapeutic advantage would be gained by an additive or synergic effect from amphotericin B plus flucytosine. There are no data from controlled clinical trials that support this hypothesis. Such a combination might well be effective if the infecting strain is susceptible to flucytosine because the renal functional impairment engendered by amphotericin B would impede excretion of the flucytosine. However, when very high concentrations of flucytosine are attained in the body, adverse reactions (hepatic, bone marrow, gastrointestinal) are increasingly likely to occur.

In patients with normal host defenses, correction of mechanical predisposing factors may be all that is necessary for cure of candidosis—for example, the removal of an intravenous catheter that has been colonized by *Candida* spp. at its tip. Surgical excision or drainage of localized candidal lesions should be carried out in an effort to cure candidosis and to eliminate potential sources for dissemination; preoperative, intraoperative, and postoperative administration of amphotericin B is necessary. For example, cure of candidal endocarditis appears to depend primarily on surgical excision of the infected site; antifungal antimicrobics alone are rarely, if ever, curative, but may prevent postoperative recurrences.

Prevention

Since candidosis is usually endogenous in origin, prevention depends on preserving host defenses and disturbing the normally resident microbiota as little as possible. To these ends, restraint in application of blunderbuss therapies is desirable, for example, whole body exposure to x-irradiation, cytotoxic and antimitotic chemicals, broad-spectrum antibacterial antimicrobics, and radical surgery.

There would seem to be little hope from immunization in view of (1) the normally high prevalence of anticandidal immunity, and (2) the high frequency of immunoincompetence in patients with candidosis.

Remaining Problems

Improved methods are needed to (1) determine the clinical significance of *Candida* spp. isolated from clinical specimens; (2) diagnose candidal invasion of blood and tissues rapidly and accurately; and (3) treat candidosis. Advances in serodiagnosis may enable determination of the pathologic significance of candidal isolates. If there were confirmation of fingerprinting candidemia by unique, blood-borne compounds that are rapidly and specifically detectable, as by the newer chromatographic methods, powerful new diagnostic aids would become available.

Systemically administrable, nontoxic, fungicidal antimicrobics that are distributed in all body water are greatly needed.

Torulopsosis and Rhodotorulosis

Torulopsosis and rhodotorulosis are rare fungal infections that occur in patients who are debilitated or have catheters indwelling in blood vessels or in the urinary tract.

Torulopsis glabrata, (once called *Cryptococcus glabrata*) and *Torulopsis candida* bear a close kinship to *Candida* spp., and some mycologists favor abolition of the genus *Torulopsis* and transfer of its species into *Candida.* The causes of torulopsosis are small, ovoid yeasts (3.0 × 5.0 μm) that ferment glucose, trehalose, and occasionally lactose (*T. candida*) and have a unique pattern of carbon assimilation. Normally components of the oropharyngeal, gastrointestinal, genital, and skin microflora, *Torulopsis* spp. cause disease under the same conditions that predispose patients to candidal infections—hyperglycemia, impaired immune function, treatment with high doses of multiple antibacterial antimicrobics, pharmacologic doses of glucosteroids and other immunosuppressive agents, and contamination of the bloodstream or bladder by indwelling catheters. Systemic infections may be manifested by chills, high fevers, and hypotension; the clinical course may be fulminant. Infections of the bladder or kidney are usually secondary to an indwelling urinary catheter and are difficult to distinguish from the more common, benign colonization of the urine. Meningitis, endocarditis, and pulmonary infections are rarely caused by *Torulopsis* spp. Because these yeasts tend to be intracellular as well as extracellular, they may be seen within macrophages in specimens stained with methenamine silver. Torulopsemia secondary to a contaminated intravenous catheter usually remits after removal of the catheter. Systemic infections may be treated with amphotericin B or flucytosine; resistance to flucytosine may develop during therapy. Nystatin lavage has been used with apparent success to treat infections of the lower urinary tract. Amphotericin B and flucytosine may be valuable in the treatment of renal torulopsosis.

Rhodotorulosis is caused by *Rhodotorula* spp., principally *R. rubra* (there are over 30 synonyms) and sometimes *R. glutinis* and *R. pilimanae.* Both are environmental saprobes found occasionally as part of the microflora of sputum, feces, and skin. They grow readily on artificial mediums and form distinctive, coral red, mucoid colonies on Sabouraud's glucose agar. *Rhodotorula* spp. are relatively avirulent; in most reported infections, the fungi have entered the bloodstream from contaminated intravenous catheters or liquids for intravenous infusion. When bloodborne, *Rhodotorula* spp. cause nonspecific symptoms of fever and hypotension. In some instances, *Rhodotorula* spp. have caused serious, life-threatening infections. The diagnosis depends on culturing the fungi from the blood or infected tissues. Removal of the source of contamination is usually curative; treatment with amphotericin B is necessary only if infection persists.

Bibliography

Books

ODDS FC: Candida and Candidosis. Leicester, England, Leicester University Press, 1979. 382 pp.

RIPPON JW: Medical Mycology. The Pathogenic Fungi and the Pathogenic Actinomycetes. Philadelphia, WB Saunders, 1974. pp 175–204, 224–226, 226–227.

WINNER HI, HURLEY R (eds): Symposium on Candida Infections. Edinburgh, ES Livingstone, 1966. 249 pp.

Journals

ANDRIOLE VT, KRAVETZ HM, ROBERTS WC, UTZ JP: Candida endocarditis. Clinical and pathologic studies. Am J Med 32:251–285, 1962

DROUHET E, MERCIER–SOUCY L, MONTPLAISIR S: Sensibilité et résistance des levures pathogenes aux 5-fluropyrimidines. Ann Microbiol (Inst Pasteur) 126 B:25–39, 1975

EDWARDS JE JR, LEHRER RI, STIEHM ER, FISCHER TJ, YOUNG LS: Severe candidal infections: Clinical perspective, immune defense mechanisms, and current concepts of therapy. Ann Int Med 89:91–106, 1978

HENDERSON DK, EDWARDS TE JR, MONTGOMERIE JZ: Hematogenous candida endophthalmitis in patients receiving parenteral hyperalimentation fluids. J Infect Dis 143:655–661, 1981

HOEPRICH PD, HUSTON AC: Susceptibility of *Coccidioides immitis, Candida albicans,* and *Cryptococcus neoformans* to amphotericin B, flucytosine, and clotrimazole. J Infect Dis 132:133–141, 1975

JONES DB: Chemotherapy of experimental endogenous *Candida albicans* endophthalmitis. Trans Am Ophthalmol Soc 78:846–895, 1980

LOURIA DB, BLEVINS A, ARMSTRONG D, BURDICK R, LIEBERMAN P: Fungemia caused by "nonpathogenic" yeasts. Arch Intern Med 119:247–252, 1967

MECKSTROTH KL, REISS E, KELLER JW, KAUFMAN L: Detection of antibodies and antigenemia in leukemic patients with candidiasis by enzyme-linked immunosorbent assay. J Infect Dis 144:24–32, 1981

MEUNIER–CARPENTIER F, KIEHN TE, ARMSTRONG D: Fungemia in the compromised host: Changing patterns, antigenemia, high mortality. Am J Med 71:363–370, 1981

ODDS FC, MILNE LJR, GENTLES JC, BALL EH: The activity *in vitro* and *in vivo* of a new imidazole antifungal ketoconazole. J Antimicrob Chemother 6:97–104, 1980

PARKER JC JR, MCCLOSKEY JJ, LEE RS: The emergence of candidosis. The dominant postmortem cerebral mycosis. Am J Clin Path 70:31–36, 1978

PETERSEN EA, ALLING DW, KIRKPATRICK CH: Treatment of chronic mucocutaneous candiasis with ketoconazole. Ann Int Med 93:791–795, 1980

ROGERS TJ, BALISH E: Immunity to *Candida albicans.* Microbiol Rev 44:660–682, 1980

JOHN P. UTZ

Histoplasmosis

40

Histoplasmosis is a systemic fungal infection. *Histoplasma capsulatum,* the etiologic agent, is acquired by the respiratory route, and the primary focus of infection is in the lungs. Although a mild, self-limited course is the rule, a progressive, disseminated form is usually fatal.

Etiology

Histoplasma capsulatum (called *Emmonsiella capsulatum* in the perfect, sexual state) is a fungus that has two forms. In tissues, it is a yeast measuring approximately 3μm in diameter. On appropriate culture mediums (*e.g.,* Sabouraud's glucose agar), it grows as a white to brownish mold (mycelium), which microscopically is composed of filaments (hyphae) that bear both small spores (microconidia) measuring approximately 3μm in daimeter, and characteristic, diagnostic larger tuberculate spores (macroconidia) approximately 10 μm in diameter (Fig. 40-1).

African histoplasmosis is caused by *Histoplasma capsulatum* var. *duboisii* (perfect state, *Emmonsiella capsulatum* var. *duboisii*).

Histoplasma capsulatum are not known to elaborate either toxins, enzymes, or any other substances that play a role in producing disease.

Epidemiology

Histoplasmosis is worldwide in distribution and has been reported from more than 50 countries. However, studies using the histoplasmin skin test (see Diagnosis and Chap. 15, Skin Tests) have revealed an endemic area in the central United States, particularly in the Ohio River and Mississippi Riverr valleys but extending eastward into Virginia and Maryland, where as much as 85% of the population has been infected at some time with *H. capsulatum.* Characteristics of such areas include red yellow podzolic soil and special conditions of temperature, humidity, and wind.

Since the first isolation of the fungus from soil by Emmons in 1949, it has been shown that bird droppings, notably from chickens and starlings, and bat feces provide an optimal environment for the growth and persistence of *H. capsulatum.* It is not surprising, therefore, that a wide variety of domestic and wild animals have been infected. Except for sharing a common source, there is no apparent relationship between disease in animals and in humans. However, the prevalence of histoplasmin skin reactivity in children correlates with the number of nearby bird roosts. There have been several local outbreaks of histoplasmosis triggered by infected dust raised in vigorous cleanup or removal of accumulations of bird or chicken droppings, or by the demolition of an old, feces-laden coop. The largest reported outbreak occurred in Indianapolis, Indiana, from September, 1978 to August, 1979; an estimated 100,000 persons were infected, 15 of whom died of the disease.

Progressive disseminated and chronic cavitary forms of histoplasmosis occur most frequently in adult, middle-aged and older, men.

Pathogenesis and Pathology

Histoplasmosis is acquired by the inhalation and deposition of conidia of *H. capsulatum* in the periphery of the lungs. The alveolar macrophage is probably the first cell encountered by the microorganism. After initial phagocytosis, the fungus thereafter dwells inside the histocytes of the host, persisting in the yeast phase either in the lung or in the reticuloendothelial system. Such histiocytes are part of epithelioid cell granulomas, which commonly contain Langhans' giant cells. In older lesions, the central area may be-

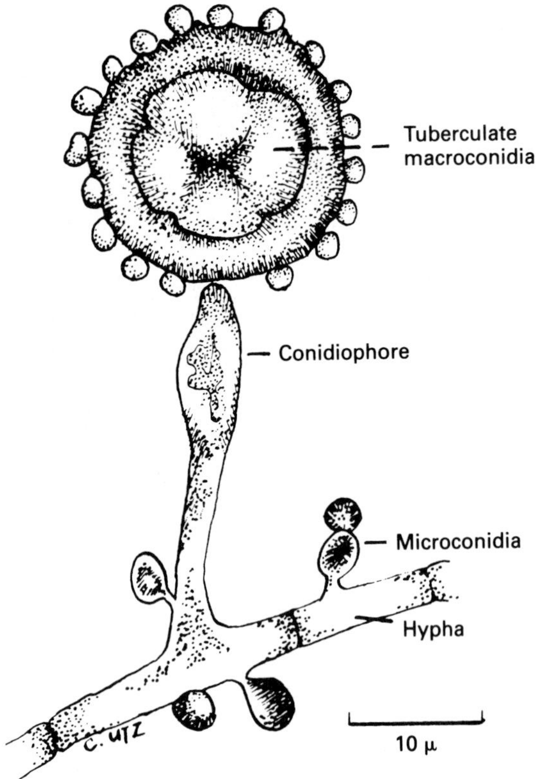

Fig. 40-1. Vegetative form of *Histoplasma capsulatum.*

come necrotic, and the outer edge of the granuloma more fibrotic. Central focal calcification in such lesions is a characteristic, but not pathognomonic, late finding.

Even in primary infections that run a benign course, dissemination from the lung probably occurs in most cases, because calcification later becomes evident in the spleen, liver, or adrenals. In fatal cases, larger numbers of microorganisms are present, and tissue destruction is more marked. Blood-borne *H. capsulatum* may cause platelet aggregation and release of sertonin, contributing to the thrombocytopenia and to the pathogenesis of progressive disseminated disease.

Histoplasmosis is apparently not an "opportunistic" infection (see Chap. 44, Aspergillosis).

Manifestations

It is convenient to consider histoplasmosis as having three forms in this country and one somewhat different form in Africa.

Primary Acute Disease

In endemic areas, primary contact with the fungus results either in no detectable illness or in a mild respiratory disease that is not distinguishable clinically from a severe cold or from influenza. Moreover, the commonest symptoms are nonspecific and general: fever, malaise, headache, myalgias, and anorexia. Symptoms referable to the respiratory tract include cough and chest pain.

Physical findings are remarkably scant—a few rales over the involved lung fields—but only rarely are there findings of consolidation or effusion. The chest film may show a local infiltrate and a vicinal lymphadenopathy that subsequently may become sites of scarring with calcification. In severe exposure, innumerable 2-mm to 5-mm pulmonary lesions may appear.

Progressive Disseminated Disease

Unlike coccidioidomycosis, progressive disseminated histoplasmosis does not occur in direct temporal evolution from acute primary disease. Moreover, it appears either in infants or, more commonly, in old men. There is hepatomegaly, splenomegaly, general lymphadenopathy, anorexia, weight loss, and fever. In some patients, involvement of a single organ or system predominates: endocarditis, meningitis, pericarditis, or Addison's disease. One particularly characteristic form is that of ulceration of the tongue, palate, epiglottis, larynx, or, somewhat less frequently, other gastrointestinal sites. Pain, hoarseness, and dysphagia are the usual symptoms from such lesions; bleeding is rare (Fig. 40-2).

Chronic Cavitary Disease

As a result of the classic studies of Palmer and Furcolow, chronic cavitary histoplasmosis was delineated and separated from chronic cavitary tuberculosis, which it mimics so closely. Presenting symptoms are usually productive cough, occasional hemoptysis, dyspnea, and eventually the other stigmata of chronic respiratory disease (weight loss, inanition, breathlessness, and cyanosis). The cavitary lesions of the upper lung fields are usually bilateral.

Acute cavitary disease has been induced experimentally in monkeys, and its natural counterpart in man has been suggested.

African Histoplasmosis

In 1952, Dubois and Vanbreuseghem reported on patients from Africa who had characteristic cutaneous lesions, lymphadenopathy, and bony and other visceral involvement caused by *Histoplasma capsulatum* var. *duboisii,* a fungus that is somewhat larger

Fig. 40-2. Large palatal ulcerative lesion caused by *Histoplasma capsulatum.* The arrow indicates the margin. The uvula has retracted to the left through scarring. The lesion was exquisitely painful and tender.

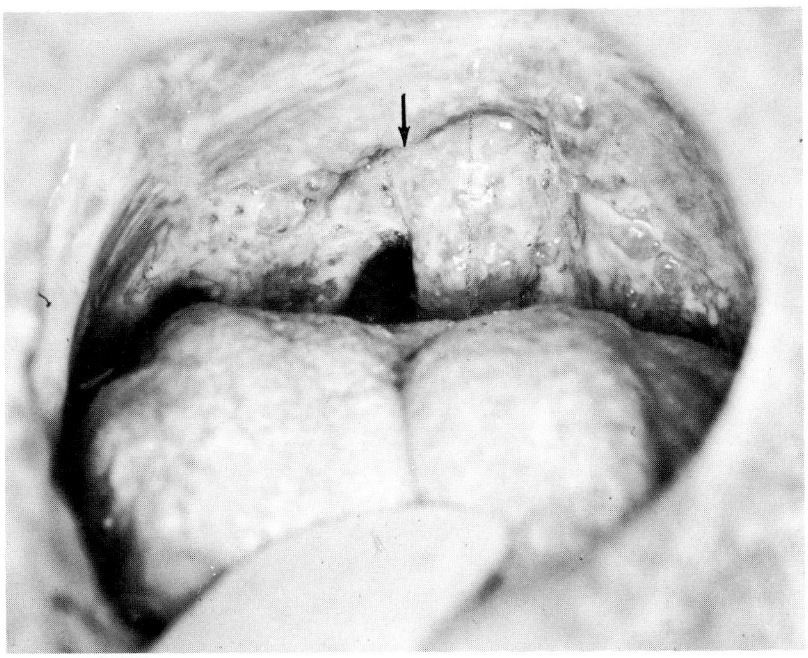

than *H. capsulatum.* The cutaneous lesions are most frequently nodules, papules, or ulcers. The bony lesions are usually at the site of subcutaneous or cutaneous disease, notably afflicting the skull and long bones. The lymph nodes are strikingly enlarged, with softening and liquefaction necrosis a frequent result. Remarkably, there are no pulmonary lesions.

Diagnosis

All forms of histoplasmosis are unequivocally diagnosed by the isolation and identification in culture of the causative fungus, *H. capsulatum.* In the acute primary form, the proper specimens for study are sputum (natural or induced), blood, and urine. In the progressive disseminated disease, they are bone marrow, lymph node, blood, and other specimens appropriate to the specific site of involvement (*e.g.,* cerebrospinal fluid, biopsy specimens of liver, and oral ulcerations). In the chronic cavitary form, the only specimen regularly helpful is sputum.

The experienced pathologist can make an etiologic diagnosis of histoplasmosis by finding characteristic forms in tissue sections stained by either Gomori's methenamine silver, periodic acid-Schiff, or the Gridley technique (Fig. 40-3). Fortunately, histologic diagnosis on surgical or postmortem specimens in the absence of clinical or cultural diagnosis is increasingly infrequent.

Although immunolgic methods are occasionally useful in suspected histoplasmosis, there has been far too much reliance on skin and serologic testing. The solid experimental methodology, the sucessful results, and the articulateness of some immunologists have led physicians away from classic methods of diagnosis to a degree that is decried by many immunologists. A positive histoplasmin skin test, like a positive tuberculin test, means past exposure to the antigen and not active disease. Furthermore, in acute illness in which the diagnosis is most desperately sought, the skin test has usually not yet become positive. Also, the high percentage of well persons in various areas of the country with a positive skin test further renders interpretation difficult. A positive reaction with complement fixation (or other) serologic methods, with a high or rising titer, is perhaps more helpful, but even here such results should only lead to more effort to culture the fungus, rather than acceptance of the serologic results as definitive.

Various forms of histoplasmosis are confused with tuberculosis, other fungal infections, or less frequently, bacterial diseases with a more chronic course. Special mention should be made of Hodgkin's disease and other lymphomas. Failure of histologic confirmation of the diagnosis of a lymphoma should

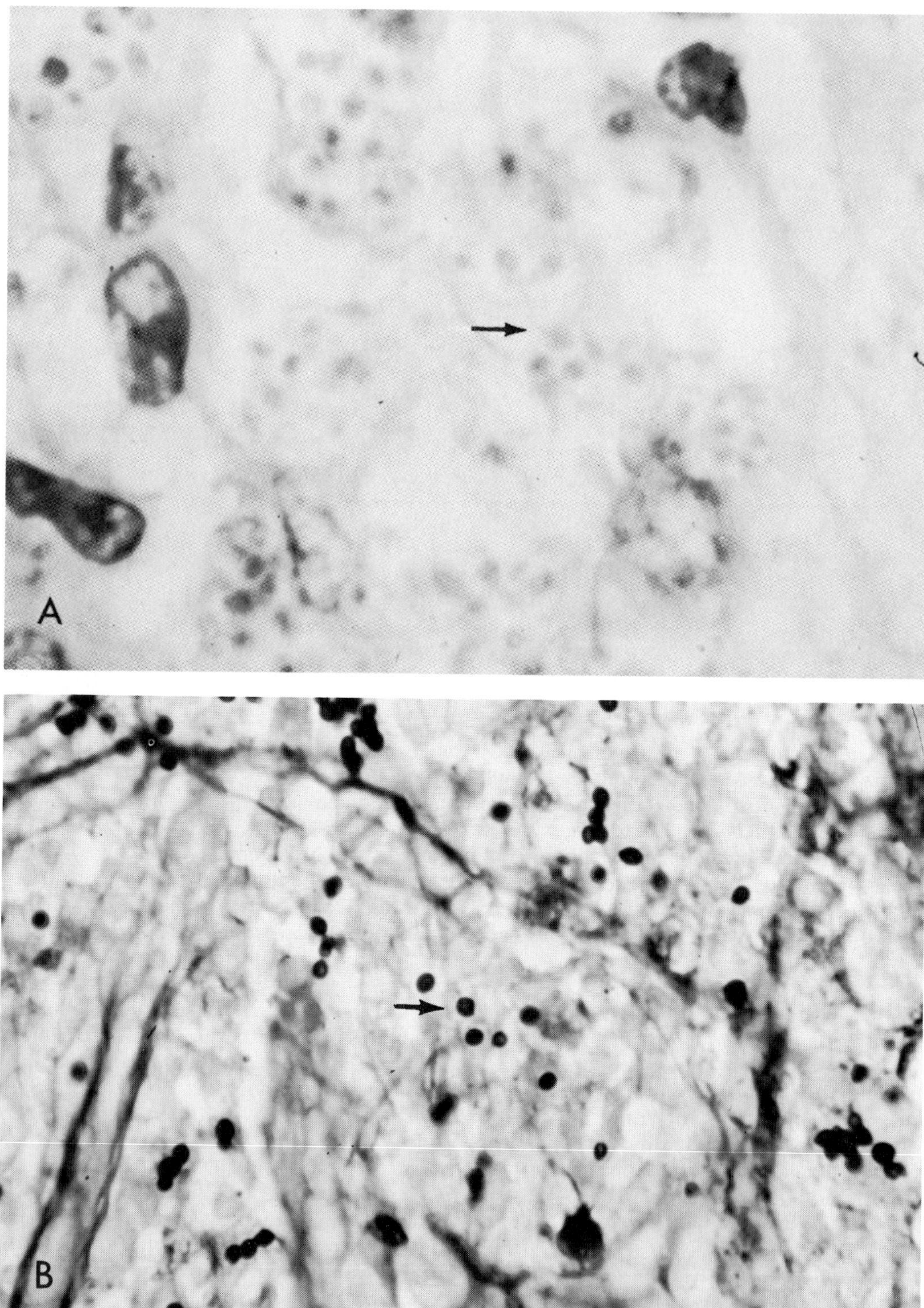

Fig. 40-3. Photomicrographs of tissue sections containing myriads of *Histoplasma capsulatum.* *(A)* Lymph node. Note contraction of cytoplasm (arrow), giving appearance of capsule, whereas none is truly present. Hematoxylin and eosin. *(B)* Laryngeal biopsy. "Capsules" are again apparent *(arrow)*. Note how the special staining renders the fungus readily visible. Gomori methenamine silver.

alert the physician to the possibility of progressive disseminated histoplasmosis. When histopathologic and cultural methods are applied to properly selected specimens, histoplasmosis can generally be distinguished conclusively.

Prognosis

It is apparent from skin testing that virtually the entire population of parts of the United States has been infected with *H. capsulatum,* developed no clinically distinctive illness, and is permanently immune to reinfection. However, in direct proportion to the intensity of exposure, primary acute disease can be serious and, indeed, fatal. In progressive disseminated disease, a fatal outcome occurs in at least 90% of patients. The chronic cavitary form is less often fatal, but progressive respiratory embarrassment is sufficient reason for attempting to control the infection. It is nevertheless a serious form of the disease; without chemotherapy approximately 20% of patients with chronic pulmonary histoplasmosis die within 1 year after diagnosis and 50% have succumbed within 5 years. Overall, of the major systemic fungal infections of man in the United States, histoplasmosis causes the largest number of deaths, according to the United States Public Health Service.

Primary acute disease rarely evolves into chronic cavitary or progressive disseminated histoplasmosis as a temporal continuum; indeed, chronic cavitary disease may be reinfection histoplasmosis. Therefore, therapy to prevent more severe disease is not justified.

Therapy

The treatment of histoplasmosis, like that of other systemic mycoses, can be divided into three parts for discussion. In actual practice, supportive care, surgery, and chemotherapy are intimately interrelated.

General Supportive Care

A patient with severe acute primary illness may have such extensive pulmonary involvement that oxygen therapy is required. In a patient with adrenal insufficiency, the administration of glucosteroids may be life saving (in conjunction with specific antifungal therapy). Patients with oral or laryngeal ulcerations often need parenteral feedings, and may in some cases benefit from a feeding gastrostomy.

Because prolonged hospitalization is necessary from chemotherapy, assistance by the social worker may avoid premature departure from the hospital. Occupational therapy and visiting teacher service can prevent boredom and subsequent failure in school.

Surgery

The dramatic effect of surgery in cases of histoplasmosis is epitomized in constrictive pericarditis. Probably the most frequently performed operation is resection of a solitary pulmonary nodule that is found postoperatively to be a histoplasmoma. Surgery must be considered almost as frequently in chronic cavitary disease, especially when chemotherapy has failed, or if there is hemoptysis. Additional indications for surgical intervention appear late in the course of histoplasmosis—middle lobe syndrome, mediastinal granuloma, broncholithiasis, and esophagotracheal fistula.

In meningitis, there is a profusion both of indications and of procedures for neurosurgery. In addition to diagnostic efforts the major therapeutic indication is for relief of increase intracranial pressure by some sort of shunting procedure. Such therapy may be life saving by itself and also helpful in the mechanical aspect of administering a chemotherapeutic agent (*e.g.,* via an Ommaya reservoir; see Chap. 41, Coccidioidomycosis).

Chemotherapy

Antifungal chemotherapy is probably the most important single mode of treatment. It is indicated in the more severely ill patients with acute primary disease. A case fatality rate in excess of 90% without chemotherapy clearly indicates the necessity for specific antifungal therapy in the progressive disseminated form, particularly because administration of amphotericin B in a total dose of 25 mg/kg body wt reduces the mortality to about 20%. The death rate in chronic cavitary disease is not nearly so high—50% by the end of the fifth year after diagnosis. However, if amphotericin B is given in a total dose of 35 mg/kg body wt, the mortality is significant reduced—to 28% by the end of the fifth year after diagnosis.

Opinion has been sharply divided on whether preoperative and postoperative chemotherapy is necessary; we favor such treatment. Chemotherapy is usually not necessary for the African form of the disease except in grave illnesses.

Amphotericin B is the best currently available chemotherapeutic agent, Details regarding administration of this agent are given in Chapter 39, Candidosis.

Neither the optimal dosage (bidaily or daily), the duration of therapy, nor the total amount of drug is firmly established for the treatment of histoplasmosis. One point of view holds that the optimal daily dosage is 1 mg/kg body wt/day (not to exceed 50 mg per infusion), with treatment continued until a total of 2.5 g has been given. With this dose, the concentration of amphotericin B in the serum is expected to be 10 times the minimal inhibitory concentration for most strains of *H. capsulatum.*

A second regimen consists of a 10-week course of therapy in which the daily dose of amphotericin B is defined as that quantity which yields a maximum concentration in the serum twice the mininal inhibitory concentration of the infecting strain of *H. capsulatum.* Both the daily dose and the total dose of drug are reduced from the first regimen. Because there is no detectable difference in success of therapy between these two regimens, the latter may be preferable, because the hazard to the patient from amphotericin B is less. It is important to minimize the amount of drug because of the striking toxicity associated with it (see Chap. 39, Candidosis).

Sulfonamides have a measurable effect in experimental histoplasmosis in laboratory animals, but they are generally less effective than amphotericin B. In a randomized study comparing amphotericin B alone with amphotericin B plus a sulfonamide, no benefit could be ascribed to the sulfonamide.

By testing *in vitro,* and from preliminary experience in humans, ketoconazole may be helpful.

Prevention

Efforts at producing vaccines have not yet been successful. Formaldehyde—233,000 gallons at a cost of $4000 applied to a 5-acre site—has been effective in clearing *H. capsulatum* from the ground, at least temporarily.

Remaining Problems

Some way to control birds to prevent the accumulation of bird excreta appears to be worthwhile. Better methods of decontaminating soil should be sought.

The complexity of the morphology of the fungus has made difficult the standardization and testing of vaccines; further work is necessary. Despite the excellent work on the immunology of histoplasmosis, why is it that neither circulating antibody nor cell-mediated (delayed cutaneous hypersensitivity) factors can be related to protection or immunity under experimental (or natural) conditions?

Ocular disease, notably uveitis, has been attributed on rather flimsy grounds to infection by *H. capsulatum.* Further diagnostic work is necessary, because histoplasmosis causes eye disease in birds and chickens.

Can any antimicrobic now in use be more unpleasant or more dangerous for the patient than amphotericin B? Work on any new agents must continue.

Bibliography

Book

VANBREUSEGHEM R, DEVROEY C, TAKASHIO M: Practical Guide to Medical and Veterinary Mycology, 2nd ed. New York, Masson, 1978. 270 pp.

Journals

AJELLO J: Comparative ecology of respiratory mycotic disease agents. Bacteriol Rev 32:6–24, 1970

CAMPBELL CC: Histoplasmosis outbreaks: Recommendations for mandatory treatment of known microfoci of *H. capsulatum* in soils. Chest 77:6–7, 1980

COX RA: Immunologic studies of patients with histoplasmosis. Am Rev Respir Dis 120:143–149, 1979

DRUTZ DJ, SPICKARD A, ROGERS DE, KOENIG MG: Treatment of disseminated mycotic infections. A new approach to amphotericin B therapy. Am J Med 45:405–418, 1968

EDWARDS LB, ACQUAVIVA FA, LIVESAY VT, PALMER DE: An atlas of sensitivity to tuberculin, PPD and histoplasmin in the United States. Am Rev Respir Dis 99:1–111, 1969

HERMANS P: Antifungal agents used for deep-seated mycotic infections. Mayo Clin Proc 52:687–693, 1977

REDDY P, GORLICK DF, BRASHER CA, LARSH H: Progressive disseminated histoplasmosis as seen in adults. Am J Med 48:629–636, 1970

SCHWARZ J, BAUM GL: The history of histoplasmosis, 1906 to 1957, N Engl J. Med 256:253–258, 1957

SWEET GH, CIMPRICH RS, COOK AC, SWEET DE: Antibodies in histoplasmosis detected by use of yeast and mycelial antigens in immunodiffusion and electroimmunodiffusion. Am Rev Respir Dis 120:441–449, 1979

WHEAT LJ, SLAMA TG, FITZEN HE, KOHLER RB, FRENCH MLV, BIESECKER JL: A large urban outbreak of histoplasmosis: Clinical features. Ann Intern Med 94:331–337, 1981

PAUL D. HOEPRICH

Coccidioidomycosis

41

Coccidioidomycosis refers to infection of human and nonhuman mammalians with the fungus *Coccidioides immitis,* a normally saprobic inhabitant of the soil in certain semiarid regions of the Americas. It is an environmental infection, since it is virtually always acquired through the accident of inhalation of air contaminated with coccidioidal arthroconidia; it is also a dead end for the fungus, since the infection is not communicable. The spectrum of infection in humans varies from inapparent to rapidly lethal with a high probability of there being no disease. Recovery from coccidioidomycosis confers permanent immunity.

Etiology

The genus *Coccidioides* contains but one species, *C. immitis,* which is normally a saprobe resident in the soil where it grows as mycelia composed of septate hyphae—the form displayed in the usual cultures in the laboratory. As mycelia age, perhaps also with the stimuli of drying and diminishing nutrients, certain hyphae form alternate arthroconidia, the *Malbranchea* state of *C. immitis* (Fig. 41-1*A*). About 2 μm × 5 μm in size, these thick-walled, barrellike, generally cylindrical structures are separated from one another by apparently empty cells. They are: (1) survival structures, since they resist drying; (2) units of dissemination — because they are very light, due to entrapped air, they become airborne by the slightest disturbance to be dispersed by air currents; and (3) the infectious elements of the fungus: inhalation of as few as ten may lead to pulmonary disease in rhesus monkeys.

After gaining access to a host, some arthroconidia survive phagocytosis and grow as globoid structures called spherules that are 20 μm to 100 μm in diameter (Fig. 41-1*B*). Internal nuclear divisions and cytoplasmic clevages result in the formation of as many as 10^5 endospores per spherule. The endospores (2 μm–3 μm in diameter) are released when the spherule ruptures (Fig. 41-1*C*) and form new spherules to continue the tissue cycle of *C. immitis* if they are neither dejected from, nor destroyed by, the host. Although coccidioidomycosis is not contagious, spherules/endospores yield mycelial growth when transferred to a suitable environment; they may remain viable for weeks in pus or blood.

Seven to ten days after inoculation of any morphologic form of *C. immitis* onto ordinary agar culture mediums, there is growth of cottony white colonies, which may become tan to brown as they age. This appearance is not characteristic. Moreover, there are neither unique growth requirements nor singular metabolic reactions that identify *C. immitis. To avoid infection of laboratory personnel* clinicians must always alert the laboratory to specimens that may contain *C. immitis,* and in clinical laboratories, all cultures even remotely suspected of containing *C. immitis* must be handled with the greatest care (class III precautions).

The relationships of the various morphologic forms, environments of development, and rates of growth are summarized in Figure 41-2.

Essential to the identification of *C. immitis* is the demonstration of the parasitic (spherule) form. This is accomplished most directly and quickly by microscopic examination of tissues and aspirates of closed space lesions (pus, exudates, and other body liquids) obtained from the host yielding the isolate (sputums and the contents of the digestive and urogenital tracts are not suitable for direct microscopic examination). At the cost of time, spherules may be demonstrated (1) with all strains in smears of peritoneal granulomas that form in mice 2 to 4 weeks after intraperitoneal (IP) inoculation, and (2) with some strains 3 to 6 weeks after inoculation of special culture mediums. A more rapid method of identification involves extraction of 7 to 10-day-old agar cultures and demonstration of specific coccidioidal antigens in the extracts by micro-immunodiffusion.

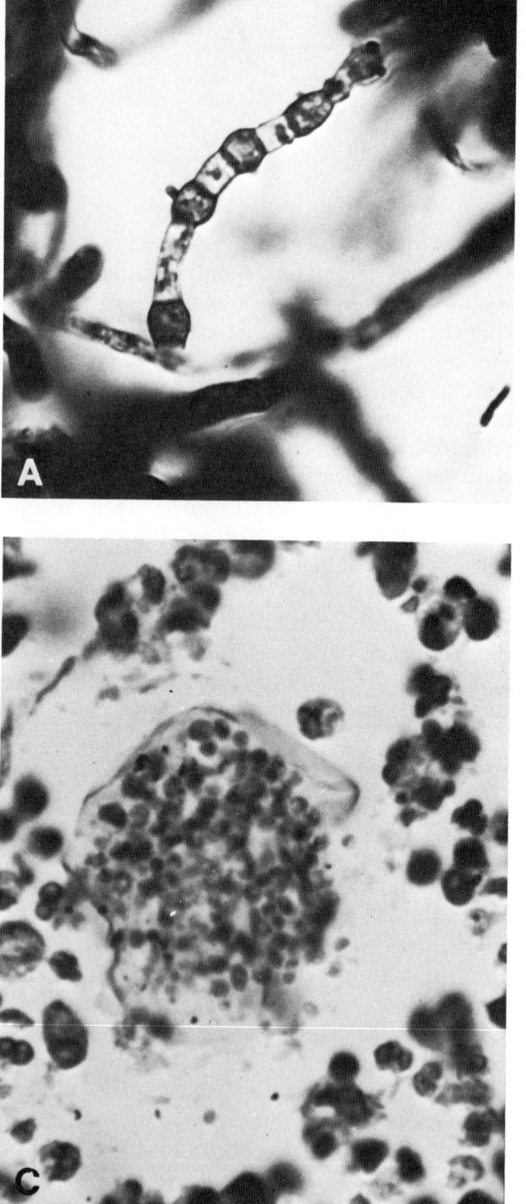

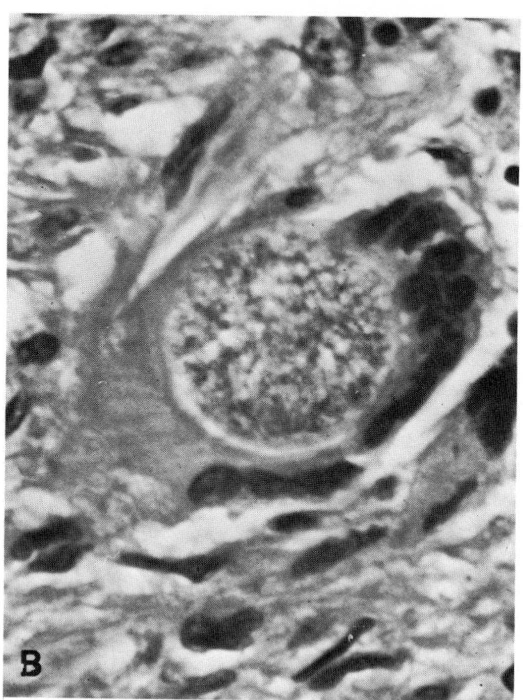

Fig. 41-1. Morphologic forms of *Coccidioides immitis.* (*A*) Hyphae showing the typical interposition of apparently empty cells between the heavy-walled arthroconidia. Lactophenol cotton blue. (Original magnification approximately × 150) (*B*) Spherule, showing endospores, inside Langhans giant cell. (H&E approximately × 450) (*C*) Mature spherule that has ruptured to release endospores. (H&E approximately × 450)

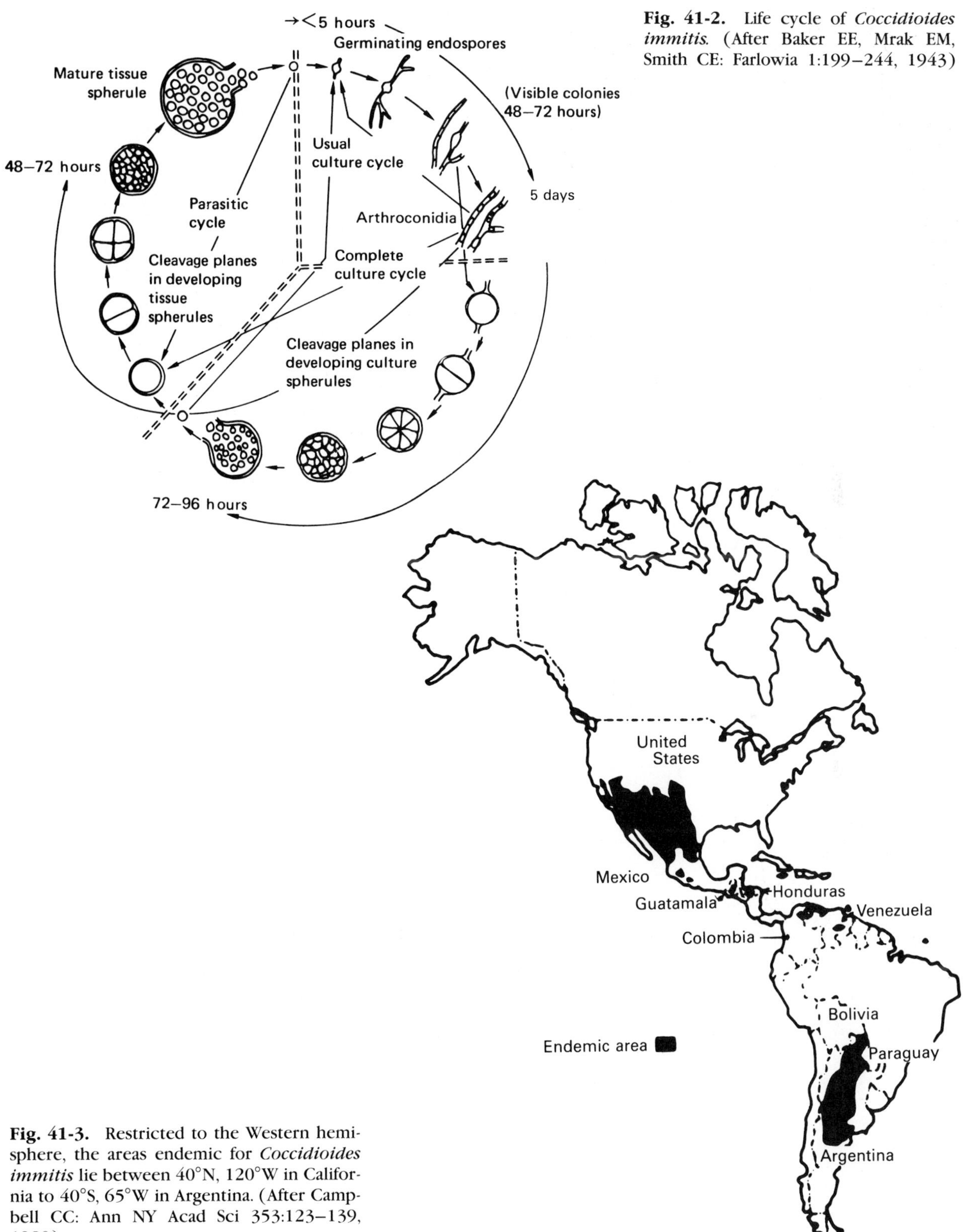

Fig. 41-2. Life cycle of *Coccidioides immitis.* (After Baker EE, Mrak EM, Smith CE: Farlowia 1:199–244, 1943)

Fig. 41-3. Restricted to the Western hemisphere, the areas endemic for *Coccidioides immitis* lie between 40°N, 120°W in California to 40°S, 65°W in Argentina. (After Campbell CC: Ann NY Acad Sci 353:123–139, 1980)

Although coccidioidal arthroconidia tolerate drying, they are susceptible to ultra-violet irradiation; they do not survive on the ground in direct sunlight. Heat, as in the steam autoclave, is lethal. Several chemical agents, such as elemental iodine (as a tincture or combined with surfactant) and glutaraldehyde, are effective in killing all forms of *C. immitis*. Several polyene and imidazole antimicrobics are inhibitory at clinically practical concentrations according to testing *in vitro,* whereas 5-fluorocytosine is without effect.

Epidemiology

Coccidioidomycosis is endemic in the Western Hemisphere from about 40°N 120°W in California to about 40°S 65°W in Argentina (Fig. 41-3). The endemic areas in the United States are in California (the San Joaquin, Sacramento, and adjacent valleys, and the southern counties); southern Arizona; New Mexico; Nevada and Utah; and southwestern Texas (Fig. 41-4). About 20% of the population of the United States resides in these states; moreover, these same states are favored by immigrants, and are commonly frequented by tourists. As a result, about 100,000 new cases occur each year. In the endemic areas, coccidioidomycosis is said to be as common as chickenpox. However, coccidioidomycosis may occur in areas far removed from endemic foci as a consequence of travel during incubation, and (rarely) the transport of arthroconidia on inanimate objects, for example, bailed cotton.

At least three major zones of endemicity have been delineated in Mexico by coccidioidin skin testing: a northern zone contiguous with the United States; regions in the Pacific littoral; and a central zone (Fig. 41-3). Curiously, at least two tropical areas are included in these endemic zones.

Coccidioidomycosis in humans has been recognized in Central America with cases reported in Guatemala, Honduras, and Nicaragua. Reactivity to coccidioidin has also been detected in natives of Panama and Costa Rica (Fig. 41-3).

In South America, the region most intensely endemic for coccidioidomycosis is in northwestern Venezuela. Cases have also been reported from Colombia, Paraguay, and Argentina (Fig. 41-3)—the source of the first description of the disease in a human in 1892.

A correspondence has been noted between major endemic areas of coccidioidomycosis and the bioclimatic lower sonoran life zone—arid or semiarid climates of low altitude, alkaline soil, hot summers, moderately wet winters and infrequent freezes. The conformity is not precise in the United States (Fig. 41-4) and appears to be excepted also in tropi-

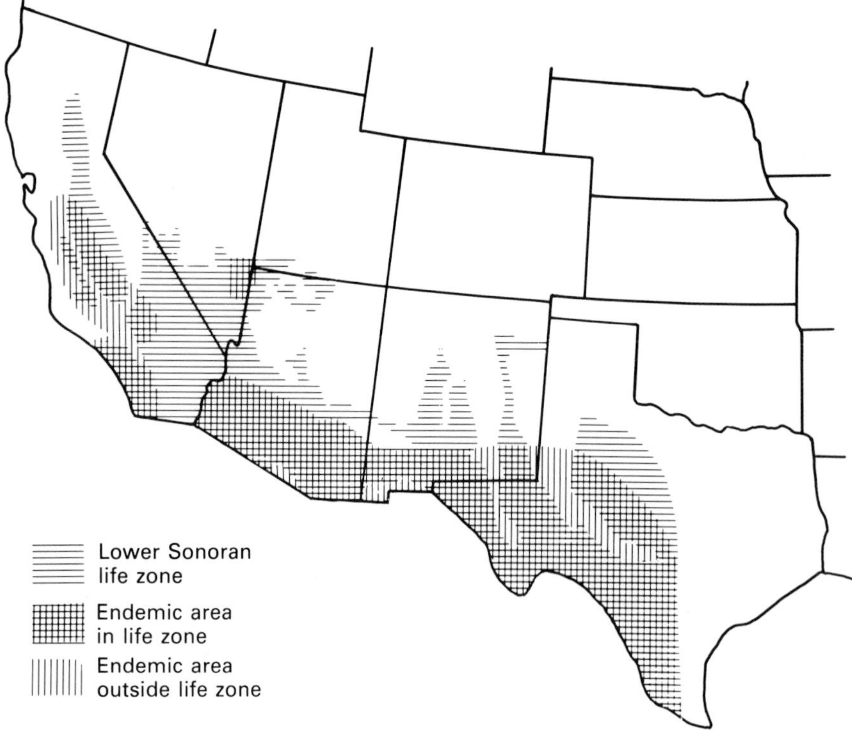

Fig. 41-4. The areas endemic for *Coccidioides immitis* in the United States extend beyond, but include, the lower sonoran life zone. (After Campbell CC: Ann NY Acad Sci 353:123–139, 1980)

cal areas of endemicity in Mexico. Moreover, *C. immitis* has been isolated from soils at relatively high altitudes (California, Arizona) and coexists with *Histoplasma capsulatum* in parts of Texas, Mexico, and Venezuela. It may be that the ecologic niche of *C. immitis* is defined primarily by conditions inimical to the growth of competitor saprobes in the soil. Thus, *C. immitis* grows well on conventional culture mediums and in a variety of soils from outside the lower sonoran life zone that were sterilized before inoculation, but fails to become established in cultivated (irrigated) soils in semiarid regions.

Except for rare instances of direct transcutaneous inoculation, human and nonhuman (domestic, feral, and captive) mammalians acquire coccidioidomycosis by inhalation of air contaminated with arthroconidia. That is, air currents are the vectors of *C. immitis*. It follows that the risk of infection is greatest when the soil is dry, for example, in the summer and autumn in California, and when arthroconidia are levitated by winds or disturbances as diverse as earth-moving machines and children playing.

The infectivity of coccidioidal arthroconidia under natural conditions was graphically illustrated on December 19 and 20, 1977 when a mammoth windstorm dispersed soil dust from an endemic region in the southern San Joaquin Valley of California northward over an area of about 87,000 square km. Of California's 58 counties, 15 experienced greater than tenfold increases in number of cases of coccidioidomycosis within the 22 weeks following the storm. In Sacramento County (area 2,797 square km; population 730,000) the attack rate was approximately 1 in 100, with a ratio of actual to reported cases calculated to be 50 to 1 (Fig. 41-5).

When the occurrence of coccidioidal infection is defined as reactivity to intradermal coccidioidin, 60% of infections are inapparent. There appears to be no predilection for either sex with regard to infection; however, the nonpregnant female is less likely to develop coccidioidal disease than the male, whereas the pregnant woman is at greater risk than the male.

Race also enters into the matter. Although much of the information is of limited statistical validity and does not always take into account factors such as intensity of exposure, nutritional status, habitation, and access to medical care, it appears that (1) dissemination (extrapulmonary disease) occurs five to ten times more often in blacks and Filipinos than in whites, whereas Asians and Mexicans may not be at substantially higher risk; (2) the risk of development of coccidioidal meningitis is about five times greater in blacks and ten times greater in Filipinos than in

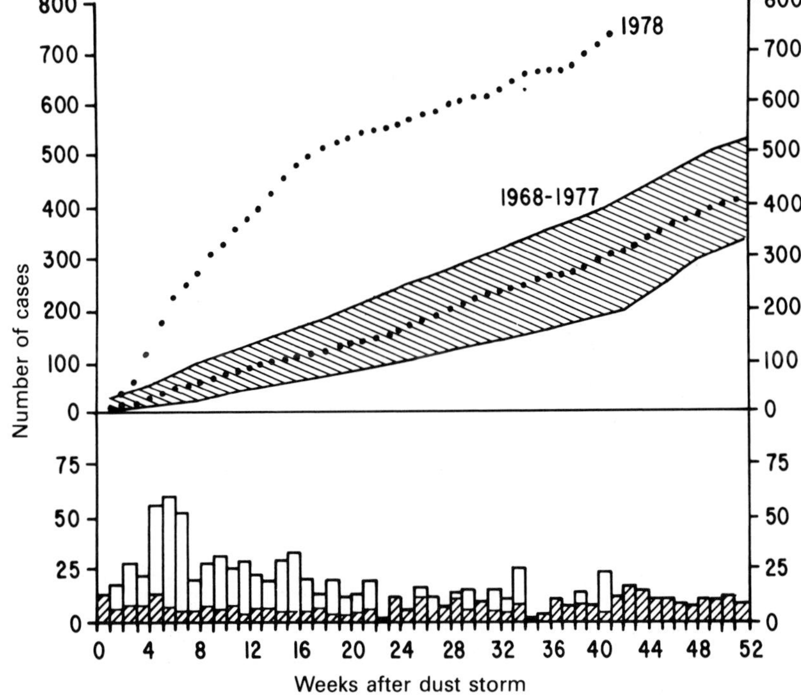

Fig. 41-5. Reported cases of coccidioidomycosis in California by week. The top curve reflects the cumulative cases in 1978 following windstorm dissemination of soil dust on December 19–20, 1977. The bottom curve gives the aggregate cumulative cases for the prior 10 years with the hatched area demarcating the range of values, and the dotted line the mean values. At the bottom, the numbers of cases reported each week is depicted as open bars for 1978 and hatched bars for the means of the prior 10 years. (After Flynn NM, Hoeprich PD, Kawachi MM, Lee KK, Lawrence RM, Goldstein E, Jordan GW, Kundargi RS, Wong GA: New Eng J Med 301:358–361, 1979)

whites; and (3) death from coccidioidomycosis occurs about five times more often in blacks than in whites, whereas Mexicans do not appear to be at higher risk.

Children are neither more susceptible nor more resistant to coccidioidomycosis than adults, either to acquisition of coccidioidomycosis or to dissemination. After puberty, the sex of the person becomes a determinant.

The massive dust storm in the Central Valley of California on December 19 and 20, 1977 delivered a relatively uniform suspension of coccidioidal arthroconidia to a known, large area over a finite period; probably all humans in the area who indulged in breathing inhaled arthroconidia. Yet, relatively few became ill with coccidioidal disease. This grand experiment of nature affirmed that there is a predisposition to coccidioidal disease in a small minority of persons in all races and both sexes, and that black males are at greater risk of dissemination and death than either black females, white males, or white females. The bases of this diathesis remain to be defined.

Pathogenesis and Pathology

By virtue of their size and buoyancy, inhaled arthroconidia deposit in the alveolar ducts and alveoli, as well as on the mucosal lining of the tracheobronchial tree. From observations in experimental animals, within the first 48 to 72 hours after infection, the surviving intrapulmonary arthroconidia metamorphose into spherule forms either intracellularly or extracellularly.

Initially, in human as well as nonhuman mammalians, the reaction is primarily pyogenic; with time, mononuclear cells and tissue macrophages become prominent, yielding either the typical mixed suppurative–granulomatous reaction (Fig. 41-6) or a frankly granulomatous process replete with epitheliod cells and giant cells that may contain spherules (Fig. 41-1*B*). Caseation necrosis occurs (Fig. 41-6), but calcification is uncommon. In short, the histopathology of coccidioidomycosis does not differ significantly from that of a number of other infectious and noninfectious diseases save for one unique feature, namely, the presence of spherules.

The lesions in the respiratory tract are primarily endobronchiolar, and are highly variable in extent and location; a patchy bronchopneumonia is the usual radiographic finding. Hilar lymphadenitis is common; extension to involve mediastinal, scalene, or supraclavicular nodes portends extrapulmonary dissemination, since it suggests failure of containment of the infectious agent within the pulmonary parenchyma and the nodes of the hilums. Sterile pleural effusions are common (Fig. 41-7).

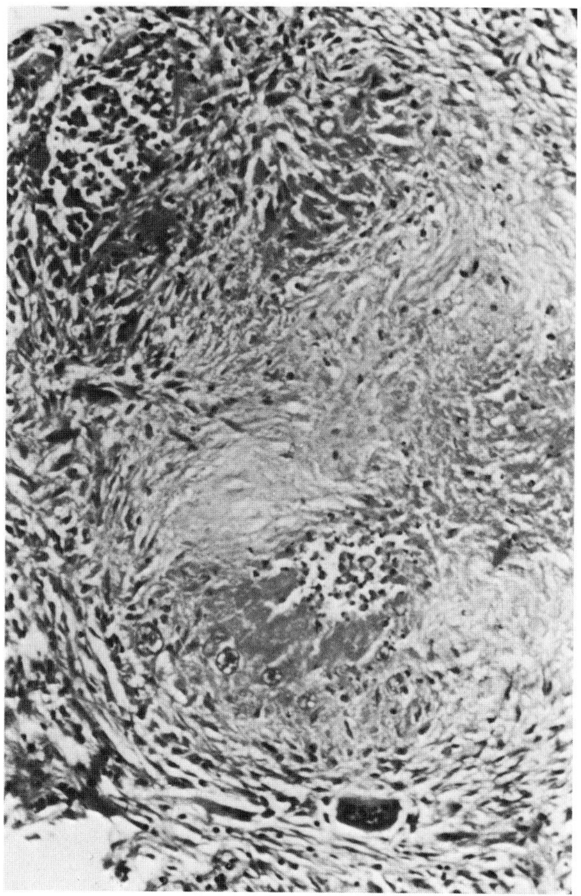

Fig. 41-6. Mixed pyogenic and granulomatous reaction in the lung. Caseation necrosis has occurred. H&E approximately × 100)

Complete healing without pulmonary residuals is the rule. However, acute coccidioidal pneumonia may be progressive and even lethal. Of all patients, 2% to 5% suffer necrosis of pulmonary tissue resulting in nodules (coccidioidal fungus balls) or abscesses; if such lesions excavate or drain, a coccidioidal cavity results (Fig. 41-7). Some newly formed cavities resolve quickly, but others persist. In chronic cavities, the spherules may not show endosporulation; hyphal elements are frequent, but arthroconidia have not been observed.

When endospores are released into the intercellular spaces, they may survive the influx of neutrophils engendered by such an event, escape engulfment by macrophages, and pass into the lymph to gain access

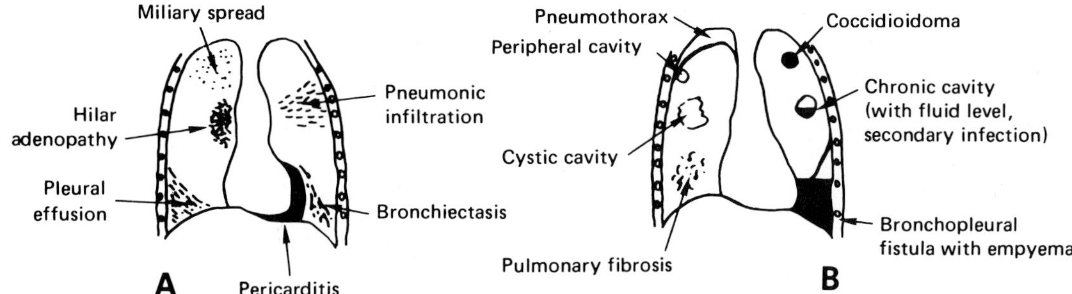

Fig. 41-7. The pulmonary manifestations of acute (*A*) and chronic (*B*) coccidioidomycosis. (Paulsen GA: Pulmonary surgery in coccidioidal infections. In Ajello L (ed): Coccidioidomycosis. Tucson, University of Arizona Press, 1967)

to the blood. The resultant hematogenous dissemination usually occurs during the early weeks of the pulmonary infection; however, dissemination may occasionally take place many years after the acute pulmonary process, usually from a chronic pulmonary focus. Although any tissue may be inoculated by blood-borne endospores, there is, overall, a descending order of frequency of sites in which proliferation is sufficient to yield disease: lungs, lymph nodes, spleen, skin and subcutaneous tissues, liver, kidneys, bones, meninges, adrenals, and myocardium. The mucous membranes of the digestive tract are virtually never involved. The reaction in disseminated lesions tends to be suppurative, yielding pus or exudate containing spherules.

Involvement of the meninges takes the form of a proliferative, granulomatous inflammation that is widespread but patchy in distribution, generally favoring the sulci. The reaction is most severe at the base of the brain. As a result, in some patients the normal flow of the cerebrospinal fluid (CSF) into the subarachnoid space is compromised by obstruction of the foramina of Luschka and Magendie or compression of the aqueduct of Sylvius; internal (noncommunicating) hydrocephalus follows, with dilation of the lateral ventricles. More commonly, the meningitis leads to interference with absorption of the CSF, causing external (communicating) hydrocephalus; diagnosis may be difficult, requiring assessment of the flow of the CSF, for example, by serial imaging after injection of colloidal ^{111}In into the lumbar subarachnoid space. Intracerebral coccidioidal lesions occur but rarely. Also rarely, arteritis may lead to foci of softening of the brain and spinal cord.

The development of humoral immunity begins with IgM (precipitins) and proceeds to IgG (complement-fixing antibodies) in a temporal sequence as diagrammed in Fig. 41-8. Circulating immunoglobu-

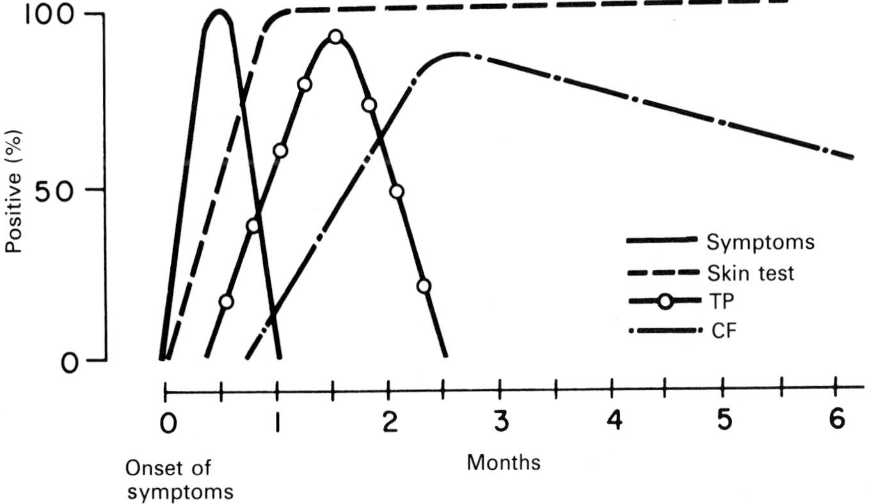

Fig. 41-8. Temporal relationships of skin test reactivity and humoral antibody response (TP = tube precipitin reactivity [primarily IgM]; CF = complement fixation [primarily IgG]) in acute symptomatic coccidioidomycosis. (Bayer AS: Chest 79: 575–583, 1981)

lins are not protective and apparently do not aid the host in overcoming the infection. However, detection and titration of IgG by complement fixation (CF) testing is of diagnostic and prognostic value.

The arousal of cell-mediated immunity—as may be detected by assessing reactivity to coccidioidin injected intradermally—appears to be critical to recovery from coccidioidal disease. Skin test reactivity to coccidioidin is typically lacking in patients with disseminated disease, whereas erythema nodosum (assumed to be a consequence of hypersensitivity to *C. immitis*) is alleged to signal a favorable outcome, an augury not always fulfilled.

Because the immune response of the host is a key determinant of the outcome of infection with *C. immitis,* it is helpful to conceive of coccidioidomycosis as a spectrum bounded by two poles. One pole is marked by a vigorous cell-mediated immune response (a predominance of granulomas in lesions with relatively few endosporulating spherules, inapparent or localized disease, reactivity—even hyperreactivity—to intradermal coccidioidin); low titers of IgG; and a high probability of self-cure. The other pole is marked by a poor cell-mediated response (a predominance of neutrophils in lesions with few granulomas and many endosporulating spherules, disseminated disease, poor to lacking reactivity to intradermal coccidioidin); high titers of IgG; and a low probability of self-cure. Fortunately, most persons who become infected with *C. immitis* mount a vigorous cell-mediated response and cure themselves; those whose response is marginal or inadequate require chemotherapy.

Manifestations

If coccidioidomycosis becomes evident as disease, it does so about 7 to 28 days after exposure (usually, 10–16 days). Typically, coccidioidal disease begins with cough, which is present in about 90% of patients and is usually nonproductive. Fever occurs in about 80% of patients, with chilliness, typically without rigors, but frequently with night sweats. Pleuritic chest pain, often substernal, is a complaint of about 70% of patients. Some patients may also note headache (75%), malaise (60%), sore throat (30%), myalgias (50%), and anorexia (10%). Eosinophilia, from 3% to 26%, is common 2 to 3 weeks into the illness. Single or multiple, rather hazy, segmental or lobar infiltrates are radiographically evident and are associated with regional paratracheal lymph node enlargements or pleural effusions in about 20% of patients.

These nonspecific manifestations of illness may be rendered indicative of coccidioidomycosis by the development of (1) toxic erythema—a fine, diffuse, macular, and sometimes urticarial rash on the trunk, extremities, and oral mucosa that occurs in about 10% of younger patients prior to attaining reactivity to intradermal coccidioidin; (2) erythema multiforme—commonly pruritic and located on the palms, lateral surfaces of the upper extremities, around the neck, and on the face and likely to appear at about the same time as skin test reactivity; (3) erythema nodosum—very tender and painful lesions symmetrically distributed on the shins and on the knees, lateral aspects of the thighs, and, uncommonly, on the arms and face, occurring with or without erythema multiforme in about 15% of patients (predominantly in whites) when the coccidioidin skin test is positive (with about five times greater frequency in females); and (4) arthralgias—tender joints with pain on motion, but without inflammation or large effusions in about 30% of patients with erythema nodosum. Such primary coccidioidal disease usually resolves without specific therapy in 2 to 8 weeks.

Persistent coccidioidal disease is conveniently thought of as either pulmonary or extrapulmonary (disseminated or metapulmonary). It is an operationally useful approach as long as the physician keeps always in mind the fallibility of any clinical categorization. Blood-borne spread from the respiratory tract early in the disease is probably a common occurrence, although it may never become apparent or may be recognized months or even years after the acute primary disease. Although the blood carries endospores to all tissues, there is variation from patient to patient not only in dose delivered to a given tissue, but also in defense capabilities (variation in the virulence of different strains of *C. immitis* for humans has not been documented). Hence, persistent coccidioidal disease is highly variable in manifestations, and unpredictable shifts in the course of the illness are common.

Persistent disease that is manifested primarily as involvement of the respiratory tract may take the form of (1) continued pneumonia—extensive infiltrates (sometimes appearing in previously uninvolved lung); productive cough (often with bloody sputum); chest pain; persistent fever; high titers of IgG with or without persisting IgM—with months-long morbidity, and even death although dissemination is not apparent; (2) progressive destructive pulmonary disease—continued fever; productive cough (with hemoptysis); chest pain, weight loss; and radiographically evident changes in the lungs (fibrosis, nodularity, cavities); and (3) late manifestations—

nodules (coccidioidal fungus balls); cavities inadvertantly discovered by chest film; and rarely, calcific changes—that are generally benign, although they may lead to pyopneumothorax, become secondarily infected, or give rise to pulmonary hemorrhage.

Dissemination is often marked by high fever, high titers of IgG, and lack of cutaneous reactivity to coccidioidin. Acute miliary dissemination is the most fulminant form. It may occur in as many as 3% of all patients with coccidioidal disease and is now recognized most frequently in immunocompromised patients. Virtually every organ of the body is involved, and death, 1 to 4 months after onset of symptoms, was the usual outcome prior to the availability of amphotericin B. It was once held that the central nervous system (CSN) was spared, an observation that may have been artifactual because of the speed with which the disease advanced; treatment with amphotericin B now secures survival long enough for meningitis to become manifest in about two-thirds of the patients.

In most patients with disseminated coccidioidomycosis, the evolution of the disease is slow and there is time for localization, classically as granulomas. Since there is little induration, pain, or tenderness, even necrosis with the formation of pus is not attended by inflammation. Clinically, single lesions are common in whites (men and nonpregnant women), the meninges being a frequent site, whereas multiple lesions are common in blacks, Filipinos, and pregnant women (regardless of race), the meninges being involved in some patients. However, occult localizations are common and include the lymph nodes (unless necrosis leads to vicinal formation of abscesses), spleen, liver, adrenals, kidneys, and prostate (isolation of *C. immitis* from urinary sediment and expressed prostatic secretions may lead to diagnosis).

Clinically apparent localizations of disseminated disease include the skin and subcutaneous tissues (virtually all patients), the bones and joints (10%–50%), and the meninges (30%–50%). The skin lesions are typically proliferating granulomas that often affect the nose. Subcutaneous abscesses may penetrate through the skin to yield indolent ulcers; sinus tracts may form that drain labyrinthine arborizations originating in viscera or osseous structures.

Lytic lesions involve more than one bone in 40% of the patients with osseous coccidioidal disease. In descending order, the bones afflicted are the vertebrae, tibias, skull, metatarsals, metacarpals, femurs, and ribs. Most lesions are asymptomatic and are detected by radiography or radioisotope (^{99}Tc or ^{67}Ga) scanning. Symptoms may arise either from breaching of the periosteum to yield an abscess, from a pathologic fracture, or from spread to involve a contiguous joint.

Joints, most often the knees and ankles, may also be primary sites of hematogenous seeding. Pain on motion, stiffness, and swelling are common complaints. The synovial fluid may yield *C. immitis,* but biopsy of the synovial membrane is more likely to yield the diagnosis by histopathology (villonodular synovitis) or culture.

Insidious in onset, coccidioidal meningitis is a chronic process that is the only clinically evident site of dissemination in about half of the patients. It usually begins within 3 months after the first clinical manifestations of coccidioidal disease, although intervals as long as 15 years have been recorded. Headache, severe and bilateral, is a prominent complaint of virtually all patients and is commonly associated with nausea and vomiting. Alterations of mental status suggestive of psychiatric illness (changed affect, disorientation, confusion, hallucination, lethargy); disturbances of vision (photophobia, anisocoria, diplopia, nystagmus); and focal neurologic signs (papilledema, hyperreflexia, cranial nerve palsies) are also present in almost all of the patients. Signs of meningeal irritation are not striking and are found in about half the patients. As the disease progresses, the manifestations of increased intracranial pressure come to dominate with constant headache, vomiting, and papilledema, and in many patients seizures, obtundation, stupor, and coma. Computed tomography (CT) and radionuclide scanning are useful in diagnosis and monitoring therapy.

Diagnosis

In endemic areas, the clinical findings alone may be highly suggestive of coccidioidomycosis. Yet, even in such settings, additional evidence is necesary for diagnosis. Often, the most readily accessible diagnostic finding is the demonstration of endosporulating spherules in specimens obtained by biopsy (*e.g.,* pulmonary nodules, lymph nodes, synovium, liver, kidney, prostate, thyroid, and other tissues) or aspiration (*e.g.,* exudates, pus, CSF). Lactophenol cotton blue, and hematoxylin and eosin stains will suffice, although some workers prefer methenamine silver (Chap. 9, Microscopic Examinations). Direct microscopic examination of sputum or specimens from the digestive and urogenital tracts is not recommended because of the frequent occurrence of spherulelike artifacts. Recovery of a cottony mould in cultures requires demonstration of conversion to endosporulating spherules preferably in an experimental animal or if this is not possible, by subculture in a special medium. Since cultures and animal inoculations are time-consuming and hazardous to laboratory personnel, investigation by skin and serologic testing should be pursued simultaneously.

Skin Testing

Coccidioidin consists mainly of nitrogen-containing polysaccharide products obtained by filtration of mycelial growth of strains of *C. immitis* in a synthetic, liquid culture medium. It is nonantigenic (except for the rare provocation of antibodies to yeast-phase *Histoplasma capsulatum*—Chap. 40, Histoplasmosis) and nonsensitizing, without clinical effect or impact on coccidioidal serology; usually specific (occasional cross-reactions in patients with histoplasmosis are prone to occur with 1:10 coccidioidin); and remarkably stable to heat (however, IgG reactivity is heat-labile). The usual test dose of 0.1 ml of 1:100 coccidioidin is injected intradermally on the volar forearm; a zone of induration ≥ 5 mm in diameter after 48 or 24 hours is a positive raction of delayed hypersensitivity. Some persons who fail to react to 1:100 coccidioidin give a positive test with the 1:10 dilution. At the other extreme, patients with erythema multiforme or erythema nodosum should first be tested with 1:10,000 coccidioidin; as long as there is no reaction, tenfold decremental dilutions proceeding to, and including, 1:1000 should be applied at 48-hour intervals (failure of reaction to 1:1000 coccidioidin excludes coccidioidomycosis as cause for the erythema). Virtually all patients with primary coccidioidomycosis give a positive reaction to 1:100 coccidioidin. On the other hand, patients who are moribund and those with disseminated disease are typically nonreactive to coccidioidin—as they frequently are to other skin test reagents. Also, about 10% of patients with chronic cavitary or nodular pulmonary disease fail to react to coccidioidin. Reactivity to coccidioidin is long-lived, though it may wane with time. Thus, a positive reaction is simply testimony that infection with *C. immitis* has occurred; the test is diagnostic of coccidioidal disease only if recent conversion from nonreactivity is documented.

Spherulin is the name given to a soluble fraction obtained by lysis of predominantly spherule growth of *C. immitis* harvested from a liquid culture medium. Although it was hoped that greater sensitivity in skin testing would be attained by using a product derived from a morphologic form akin to that predominant in lesions, careful comparison in patients has failed to disclose any advantage of spherulin over coccidiodin.

Serologic Testing

As the tube precipitin (TP) test (Fig. 41-8) detects IgM in serum, a positive result indicates recent infection with *C. immitis.* The test is almost always positive in patients with disease, but may not be positive in persons with asymptomatic coccidioidomycosis. In some patients undergoing dissemination, the TP test may become positive after having been negative. However, neither the intensity nor the duration of the IgM response is of prognostic import. The TP test is of no value with CSF.

Latex particles coated with coccidioidin have been used in a simple, rapid agglutination test—the LPA test—that may have utility in detecting serums with anticoccidioidal IgM. Since false-positive reactions do occur, positive serums should be tested by TP and complement-fixation (CF) methods. The LPA test is of no value with CSF.

Despite being cumbersome and intrinsically variable, the CF test remains the primary method for measuring anticoccidioidal IgG in the serum and other body liquids (synovial, serous, and cerebrospinal). Serums from persons with inapparent infection are unlikely to contain CF antibodies, whereas patients with coccidioidal disease usually develop CF reactivity following the TP response (Fig. 41-8). The titers of CF antibodies in synovial and serous fluids are generally one to two dilutions lower than in contemporaneous serums. The presence of CF antibodies in the CSF is diagnostic of coccidioidal meningitis except rarely, in a few patients with a parameningeal focus of infection.

Titration of CF antibodies by serial dilution of specimens is often of predictive value; in general, the higher the titer, the worse the disease. Moreover, some assessment of the course of the disease and the impact of therapy is possible through CF testing of specimens obtained at 3 to 4 week intervals, as long as sequential tests are carried out in the same laboratory with overlapping tests—the immediately prior specimen is tested along with the most recent specimen. In the serum (1) a rising titer that exceeds 1:16 or 1:32 may signal dissemination; (2) a falling titer is a favorable trend, although patients with no detectable lesions who are apparently well may carry titers ≤ 1:8 for many years; and (3) patients with chronic pulmonary residua or a single extrapulmonary lesion often have titers < 1:16. In the CSF (1) the titer of CF antibodies normally increases proceeding from the lateral ventricles to the lumbar sac if the flow is normal and there is no ventriculitis; and (2) the titer of CF antibodies should fall to nonreactivity (in all specimens from the lumbar sac) if remission obtains.

Of several other serologic tests under development and evaluation, immunodiffusion (IDCF) appears to be applicable in routine clinical laboratories as a substitute for the classic CF test, although titration may be more difficult.

Prognosis

The overview of the outcome in coccidioidomycosis diagrammed in Figure 41-9 is based on observations prior to the availability of amphotericin B. The disease was lethal in virtually all patients with meningitis and in at least half of those with nonmeningeal dissemination. Taking into account remote and contemporary observations, it appears that there is a greater risk of dissemination and death in blacks and in Filipinos; in pregnant women of any race; and in immunosuppressed patients of any race or sex.

Treatment with amphotericin B has increased the duration of survival in patients with coccidioidal meningitis to a mean of around 2.5 years; cure is usually elusive, but may have occurred when a patient has gone 8 to 10 years without a relapse. The mortality has been lowered and at least temporary benefit obtained in patients with the persistent pulmonary syndromes and those with nonmeningeal dissemination; in these situations, surgical treatment may be necessary in addition to amphotericin B.

Failures of treatment with amphotericin B are associated with underlying diseases and advanced coccidioidal disease when therapy is begun. The limitations of the drug are also important: acute and chronic toxicity restrict the amount per dose, the total dose, and the duration of treatment; the distribution is circumscribed; and some isolates of *C. immitis* are relatively resistant.

Because of the variable course of coccidoidal disease, valid judgment as to the efficacy of therapy requires observation for five or more years after treatment has been stopped.

Therapy

Nonspecific, supportive therapy is all that is needed in about 75% of the patients with coccidioidomycosis. Indeed, in the 60% of patients whose infection is inapparent, there is no opportunity for therapeutic intervention. The dilemma is posed by the need to determine as quickly as possible which of the 40% with clinically evident coccidioidal disease will contrive self-cure (about 15% of infected patients), and which are in danger of either persistent pulmo-

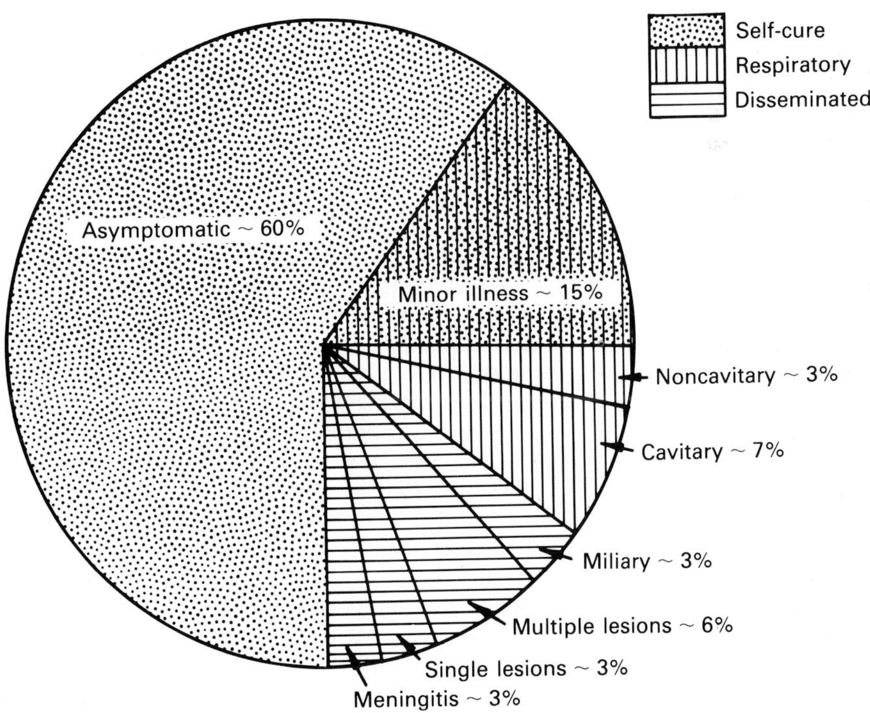

Fig. 41-9. An overview of the outcome of coccidioidomycosis in humans who did not receive specific chemotherapy.

nary disease (about 10%) or dissemination (about 15%). As yet, there is no means for positively identifying the vulnerable 25% of patients in the earliest stages of coccidioidal disease. If an effective, nontoxic, conveniently administrable antifungal antimicrobic were available, there would be no problem, since every patient with acute coccidioidal disease would be treated as soon as the diagnosis was reasonably certain. Unfortunately, no such anticoccidioidal antimicrobic is yet available. Accordingly, treatment is reserved for two categories of patients: (1) it is mandatory for all patients with any form of disseminated disease, persistent coccidioidal pneumonia with hypoxia, and chronic destructive coccidioidal pulmonary disease; and (2) it is strongly advised for patients with primary pulmonary coccidioidal disease who are at high risk of dissemination, namely, blacks and Filipinos; pregnant women of any race; and diabetics and immunosuppressed patients of any race and either sex.

Amphotericin B

Amphotericin B remains the most effective anticoccidioidal antimicrobic currently available for systemic therapy. Because of immediate and delayed or cumulative toxicities, only fungistatic concentrations are achieved in most regions of the body that are accessible to the drug, the duration of therapy is limited, and the requirement for intravenous (IV) administration makes treatment difficult (details about the IV administration of amphotericin B are given in Chap. 39, Candidosis).

The duration of IV therapy with amphotericin B is empirically determined by the limits of irreversible nephrotoxicity; patient tolerance to the misery of the therapy, and clinical and immunologic response. In general, a total dose of 30 mg/kg body weight delivered by IV injections of 0.75 to 1.0 mg/kg given every other day or thrice weekly will spread the treatment over 2 to 3 months without engendering renal damage that persists after therapy. Although a fourfold drop in the titer of CF antibodies has been held to indicate a favorable response, relapses may still occur. Greater assurance of adequacy of therapy is afforded by recession of the CF titer to $\leq 1:2$ and acquisition of reactivity to coccidioidin—goals rarely attained because of the toxicity of amphotericin B.

Because blood-borne amphotericin B does not attain therapeutic concentrations in the CNS, IV therapy must be supplemented by subarachnoid injection in the treatment of coccidioidal meningitis. This is topical therapy—a poor mode of antimicrobial therapy made even worse by the multiplicity of anatomically inaccessible recesses of the subarachnoid space, the difficulties and hazards of percutaneous entry into the region, and the toxicity of amphotericin B.

Four sites are used for injection: the lumbar space, the cisterna magna, the cervical space, and the lateral ventricles. Regardless of site, local pain, nerve damage, fibrosis, headache, nausea, and vomiting are consequences of the tissue injury caused by the amphotericin B itself and the deoxycholate with which it is complexed for therapeutic use. Lumbar injection is easiest but delivers medication into a limited volume for dilution in a region of normally sluggish flow of CSF, which is far removed from the basilar site of maximal meningitis. Arachnoiditis and injury to spinal nerve roots virtually always occurs and may lead to severe perineal pain, abnormal gait, pareses, paralyses, and impaired function of urinary and anal sphincters. It was hoped that intralumbar injection of amphotericin B suspended in 10% glucose solution followed by placing the patient's head down for 30 to 60 minutes (so-called hyperbaric therapy) might avoid, diminish, or delay complications while improving treatment by delivering the drug to the base of the brain. It is doubtful that therapeutic success is improved; arachnoiditis is not prevented, and subarachnoid blockage may occur.

Cisternal injection, like lateral cervical injection, has the attraction of delivery of the drug into a region vicinal to the site of maximal meningitis, although headache, nausea, and vomiting are not avoided. Both approaches suffer from the need for special and exquisite skill. Moreover, as therapy is continued, fibrosis occurs, rendering needle penetration ever more difficult, and the probability of hemorrhage and puncture of the brain or spinal cord ever greater—with increased potential for a fatal outcome.

Intraventricular injection into a lateral ventricle through an Ommaya or Rickham reservoir-catheter device is readily carried out. Although the drug is diluted in ventricular fluid, headache, nausea, vomiting, vertigo, tinnitus, and loss of hearing may result. Since coccidioidal ventriculitis is quite uncommon, a therapeutic effect depends on normal flow of the CSF for distribution of amphotericin B to the actual site(s) of meningitis. That this does occur is attested by suppression of the meningitis. Yet, it is possible that the device itself, since it is a foreign body, may be a haven for persistence of the fungus. Moreover, bacterial infection is not uncommon (about one episode per 2–3 patient years of use—almost always with *Staphylococcus epidermidis*), and generally requires removal of the device for cure; other complications include obstruction, hemorrhage, malposition, and neurologic sequelae.

Whatever method for intrathecal injection is used, at least 30 minutes beforehand the patient should be given codeine (30 mg–45 mg), perorally repeated after 4 hours), and either prochlorpromazine (5 mg–10 mg, perorally) or trimethobenzamide (200 mg–400 mg, perorally).

The amphotericin B should be dissolved in 5% (or 10%) glucose solution for injection. The final solution should contain 0.25 mg amphotericin B per ml. A volume of CSF at least equal to the volume to be injected should be withdrawn before dosage. The first dose should be 0.025 mg (0.10 ml); the dose is increased every 2 days as tolerated: 0.05 mg (0.20 ml), 0.10 mg (0.40 ml), 0.20 mg (0.8 ml), 0.30 mg (1.2 ml), 0.40 mg (1.6 ml), 0.50 mg (2.0 ml). The maximal dose that is tolerated, usually 0.25 mg–0.50 mg, is given 2 to 3 times weekly until there is disappearance of CF antibody and correction of other CSF abnormalities. Treatment should then be continued, consisting of 1 to 2 injections per week for at least an additional year. Periodic surveillance (every 4–6 months) is then necessary until 8 to 10 years have passed without relapse. If relapse does occur, the regimen of therapy is the same as that used for initial treatment.

Imidazoles

Several imidazole derivatives are inhibitory to *C. immitis* by testing *in vitro*. However, none are lethal, and none has proved capable of curing experimental coccidioidomycosis. Similarly, there was outright failure or only temporary beneficial effect in patients suffering from the forms of coccidioidal disease that require treatment when there was adequate follow-up after application of clotrimazole or miconazole. Ketoconazole, a perorally administrable imidazole derivative which attains concentrations in the CSF that are about 15% of contemporaneous serum concentrations, is under evaluation. However, the development of coccidioidal meningitis and the lack of resolution of persistent pulmonary infection during treatment with ketoconazole calls into question the efficacy of this compound in serious coccidioidal disease.

Immunoadjuvant

The application of transfer factor has not yielded convincing evidence of efficacy. Likewise, the administration of levamisole has not resulted in detectable improvement.

Surgical Measures

The administration of amphotericin B is facilitated by surgical placement of devices facilitating venous access (Broviac or Hickman catheters) and entry into the lateral ventricles (Ommaya or Hickman reservoirs-catheters). Hydrocephalus may require relief through surgical drainage of CSF by means of a ventriculoperitoneal or ventriculoatrial shunt.

When possible, purulent coccidioidal lesions should be drained by surgical incision, with debridement when appropriate. Pulmonary cavities should be resected when there is rapid expansion that threatens rupture into the pleural space, bronchopleural fistula, a fungus ball, or hemorrhage (recurrent or severe).

Prevention

Measures aimed at reducing exposure of humans to soil dust in areas endemic for *C. immitis* are useful, for example, planting grass, paving the ground, applying heavy oil.

A vaccine derived from cultured spherule–endospore phase *C. immitis* appeared to be effective in experimental animals and is under evaluation in humans.

Remaining Problems

Efforts at devising immunodiagnostic methods that are simple, inexpensive, and yet specific and sensitive should be continued. Perhaps the ELISA method (Chap. 14, Immunologic Diagnosis) will prove to be applicable.

The chemotherapy of coccidioidomycosis must be improved. A fungicidal antimicrobic that is less toxic than amphotericin B is desperately needed. Until such a drug becomes available, regimens of therapy using amphotericin B should be used that have a rational basis.

Bibliography

Books

AJELLO L (ed): Coccidioidomycosis. Tucson, University of Arizona Press, 1967. 434 pp.

AJELLO L (ed): Coccidioidomycosis: Current Clinical and Diagnostic Status. Miami, Symposia Specialists, 1977. 475 pp.

FIESE MJ: Coccidioidomycosis. Springfield, Ill, Charles C Thomas, 1958. 253 pp.

STEVENS DA (ed): Coccidioidomycosis. New York, Plenum Medical Book Co, 1980. 279 pp.

Journals

BAKER EE, MRAK EM, SMITH CE: The morphology, taxonomy, and distribution of Coccidioides immitis: Rixford and Gilchrist 1896. Farlowia 1:199–244, 1943

BOUZA E, DREYER JS, HEWITT WL, MEYER RD: Coccidioidal meningitis: An analysis of thirty-one cases and review of the literature. Medicine 60:139–172, 1981

CAMPBELL CC: (Philosophical) review of air currents as a continuing vector. Ann NY Acad Sci 353:123–129, 1980

DISALVO AF, SEKHON AS, LAND GA, FLEMING WH: Evaluation of the exoantigen test for identification of *Histoplasma* species and *Coccidioides immitis* cultures. J Clin Microbiol 11:238–241, 1981

DRUTZ DJ, CATANZARO A: Coccidioidomycosis. Am Rev Resp Dis 117:559–585, 727–771, 1978

FLYNN NM, HOEPRICH PD, KAWACHI MM, LEE KK, LAWRENCE RM, GOLDSTEIN E, JORDAN GW, KUNDARGI RS, WONG GA: An unusual outbreak of windborne coccidioidomycosis. N Eng J Med 301:358–361, 1979

FORBUS WD: Coccidioidomycosis: A study of 95 cases of the disseminated type with special reference to the pathogenesis of the disease. Mil Surg 99:653–719, 1946

GIFFORD J, CATANZARO A: A comparison of coccidioidin and spherulin skin testing in the diagnosis of coccidioidomycosis. Am Rev Resp Dis 124:440–444, 1981

HOEPRICH PD, HUSTON AC: Susceptibility of *Coccidicides immitus, Candida albicans,* and *Cryptococcus neoformans* to amphotericin B, flucytosine, and clotrimazole. J Infect Dis 132:133–141, 1975

KAFKA JA, CATANZARO A: Disseminated coccidioidomycosis in children. J Pediat 98:355–361, 1981

PUCKETT TF: Hyphae of *Coccidioides immitis* in tissues of the human host. Am Rev Tuberc 70:320–327, 1954

SMITH CE, BEARD RR, WHITING EG, ROSENBERGER HG: Varieties of coccidioidal infection in relation to the epidemiology and control of the diseases. Am J Public Health 36:1294–1402, 1946

SMITH CE, SAITO MT, SIMONS SA: Pattern of 39,500 serologic tests in coccidioidomycosis. JAMA 160:546–552, 1956

SWATEK FE: Ecology of *Coccidioides immitis*. Mycopathol Mycol Appl 40:3–12, 1970

WINN WA: Coccidioidomycosis and amphotericin B. Med Clin North Am 47:1131–1148, 1963

ALBERTO T. LONDERO

Paracoccidioidomycosis

42

Paracoccidioidomycosis (South American blastomycosis, Lutz–Splendore–Almeida's disease) is a systemic mycosis caused by *Paracoccidioides brasiliensis.* The disease was first described by Lutz in 1908 in a patient with oral lesions. Between 1909 and 1912, Splendore not only described the oropharyngeal and lymphatic lesions more fully, but also portrayed the morphology of the fungus. Between 1927 and 1930, Almeida clearly characterized the fungus and named it *P. brasiliensis.*

Typically, primary paracoccidioidomycosis occurs in young adults as a self-limited respiratory tract infection. Years later, reactivation may become manifest as progressive paracoccidioidomycosis of the lungs, with or without involvement of other organs.

Etiology

Paracoccidioides brasiliensis is dimorphic primarily as a function of temperature. In the soil and in cultures at room temperature, the growth is mycelial. The mycelia are composed of septate, branching, delicate hyphae bearing chlamydoconidia (15–20 μm in diameter); sessile conidialike projections (3–4 μm in diameter) may also appear. Under certain conditions of growth, aleurioconidia (3–10 μm) and arthroconidia may form (1–3 μm). Growth in cultures is very slow at room temperature, taking 2 to 4 weeks to form the typical white, tufted colonies, which become velvety and cracked as they age; brownish colonies sometimes form, which may be glabrous, or wrinkled to cerebriform in texture.

In tissues and in cultures at 35°C to 37°C, the growth is yeastlike. The individual elements are double-walled, oval to spherical, 1–40 μm in diameter, occurring singly or in chains of 3 or 4 cells bearing one or more buds. The buds have narrow necks and may be connected to the mother cells by cytoplasmic bridges (Figs. 42-1, 42-2). The variation in the size of buds (1 μm–>10 μm in diameter) is inversely related to the number borne on one parent cell (1–>100 buds, see Fig. 42-2*D*). Growth in cultures is more rapid at 35°C to 37°C; opaque, wrinkled, folded colonies appear in 6 to 8 days.

The variation in the size of the yeastlike cells and the multibud reproduction of these structures are diagnostic features when observed in potassium hydroxide (KOH) preparations (Fig. 42-1) or in methenamine silver-stained tissue sections (Fig. 42-2). There are no characteristic biochemical tests. However, the immunogenicity of *P. brasiliensis* is expressed in the development of skin test reactivity to paracoccidioidin, by the production of humoral antibodies detectable by precipitin reactions, and by complement fixation.

Epidemiology

Paracoccidioidomycosis is endemic in continental Latin American countries between latitudes 23°N and 34°S, with the exception of El Salvadore, Nicaragua, Guiana, Surinam, and Chile. The endemic regions are tropical or subtropical forests, where the temperature varies between 14°C and 28°C (average 23°C) and the annual rainfall varies from 800 to 2000 mm. Although the saprobic habitat and the ecologic associations of *P. brasiliensis* have not been fully elucidated, it is known that the intensity of endemicity varies from place to place within the endemic area.

Humans appear to be unique as hosts of *P. brasiliensis.* All races are susceptible, but non-natives of the endemic area appear to acquire more severe disease. The sexes are afflicted equally in the 10-to 29-year age group, which has the highest rate of infection. The progressive forms of the disease are rare in children (no sex preference) and occur most often in the 30-to 50- year age group, with more than 80% of the cases in men.

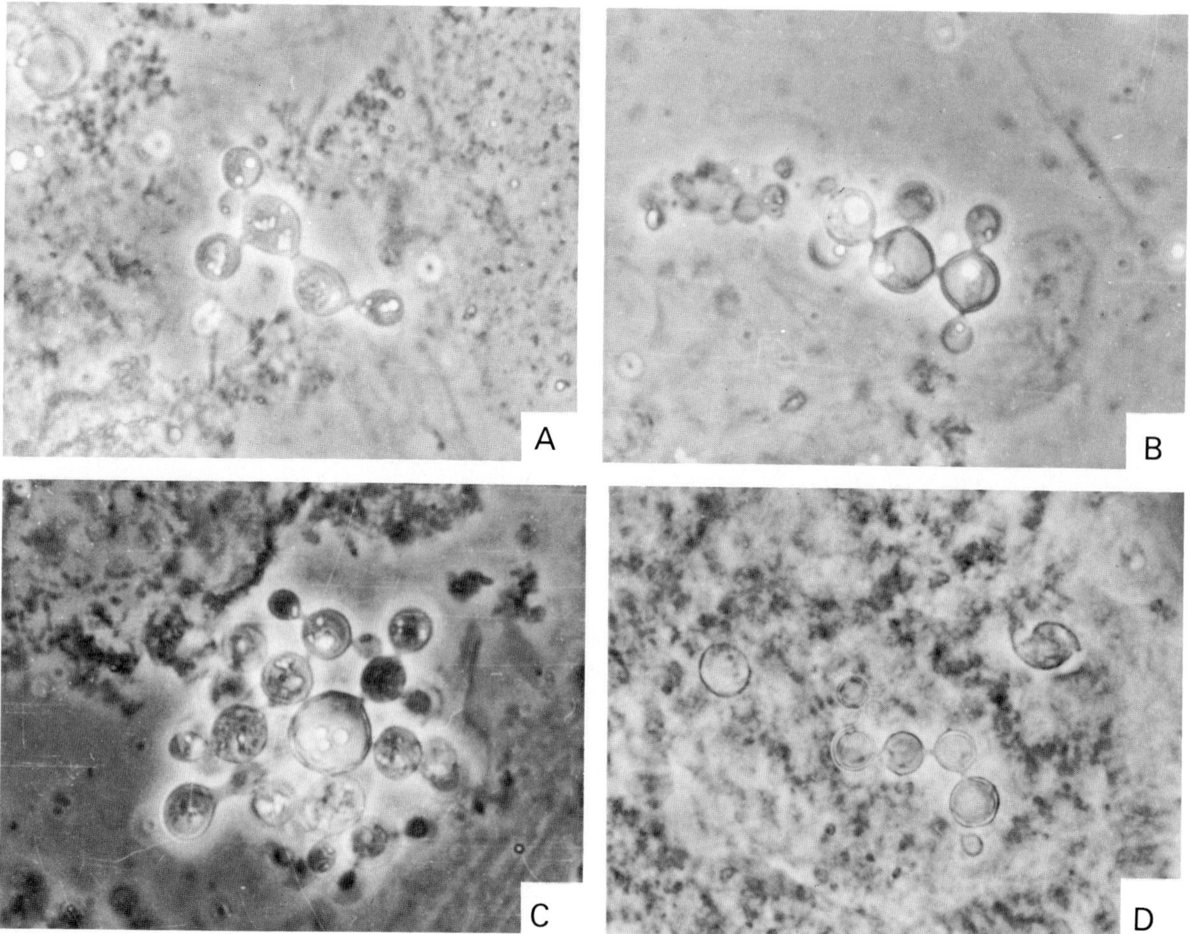

Fig. 42-1. Potassium hydroxide prepared slides with *Paracoccidioides brasiliensis* in *(A)* pus; *(B)* exudate; *(C)* sputum; and *(D)* crushed fragment from lung biopsy. (Original magnification × 400)

More than 6000 cases of progressive, disseminated paracoccidioidomycosis have been reported. However, these data are incomplete because patients with progressive pulmonary and regressive forms of the disease were overlooked or misdiagnosed. In addition, no data are available from vast regions within the endemic area—a point of importance because the disease occurs most frequently in people from rural areas who are in close contact with forests.

Although the respiratory tract is the portal of entry, there are no reports of epidemics. Human-to-human transmission has not been proved.

Pathogenesis and Pathology

Infection with *P. Brasiliensis* virtually always arises from inhalation of conidia. If intrapulmonary proliferation is not halted by the cellular defenders of the lung, a primary lymph node complex will result and hematogenous spread to other tissues and organs may take place. These events typically occur in the 10-to 29- year age group, and it is usual for the defenses of the host to bring about healing of the primary lesion—either through cure or conversion to latency. Years later, infected persons 30 to 50 years old who suffer an immune deficiency or imbalance may experience reactivation of latent lesions. The progressive disease of adults may result; mucocutaneous and lymphatic lesions are the most frequent manifestations of dissemination.

Direct intracutaneous inoculation of *P. brasiliensis* may produce a chancriform lesion, which appears to remain localized to the skin and regional lymph nodes.

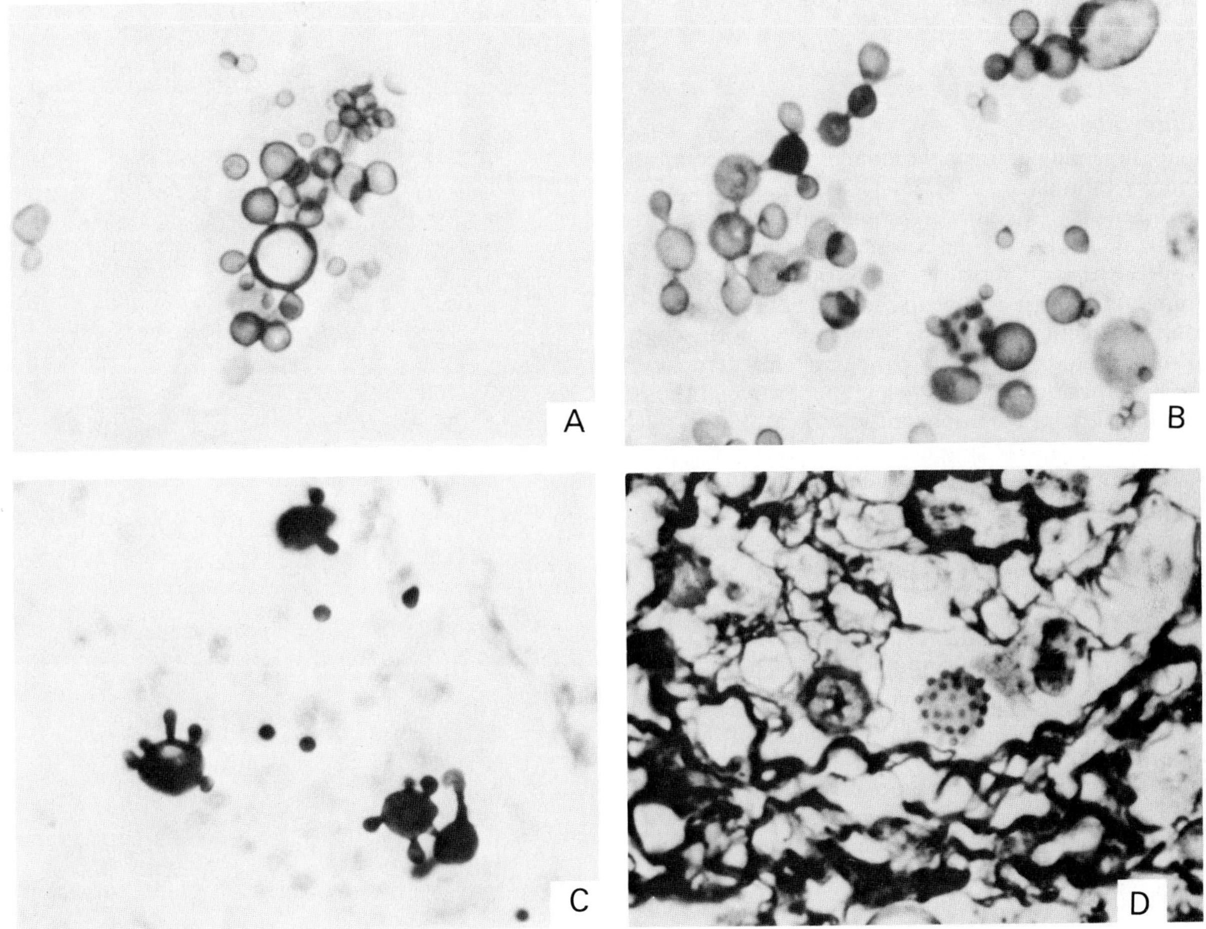

Fig. 42-2. *Paracoccidioides brasiliensis* in section obtained from lesions in the *(A)* epididymis; *(B)* skin; *(C)* lung; and *(D)* lymph node. Methenamine silver *(A, B, C)* and Laidlaw's stain *(D)* (Original magnification × 400)

The yeastlike forms of *P. brasiliensis* are abundant in lesions lying free or within giant cells. The reaction is typically granulomatous, with the formation of tubercles that may undergo caseation. At times, a pyogenic component to the reaction is evident in the formation of microabscesses. As lesions heal, fibrosis and hyalinization become dominant.

Manifestations

At least four clinical forms of paracoccidioidomycosis have been described: primary pulmonary, acute juvenile, progressive pulmonary, and disseminated.

Primary Pulmonary

The clinical and roentgenologic characteristics of primary pulmonary paracoccidioidomycosis have not been fully characterized. However, it is believed that the primary infection typically runs a subclinical course or, at most, evokes malaise, with or without cough or fever. A primary pulmonary lymph node complex may occur, which is similar to the primary lesion of tuberculosis (see Chap. 34, Pulmonary Tuberculosis) or histoplasmosis (see Chap. 40, Histoplasmosis) except that the enlargement of nodes is less marked and there is very little tendency for the lesions to calcify. Paracoccidioidomas have been reported. Metastatic foci may arise secondary to hematogenous distribution of the fungus. The lesions of primary pulmonary coccidioidomycosis usually heal but may become latent; however, the patient develops and retains cutaneous reactivity to paracoccidioidin.

Acute Juvenile

Acute juvenile paracoccidioidomycosis is a sequel to primary pulmonary infection. It is characterized by the following: (1) an acute course resembling septicemia, or an acute lymphoreticular malignancy; (2) general lymphadenopathy; and (3) occurrence in children over the age of 4 years, adolescents, and young adults. It occurs with equal frequency in both sexes. In addition to the hallmark of general enlargement of the lymph nodes, there is fever, anemia, weight loss, abdominal pain, vomiting, and diarrhea. Skin lesions are common, and enlargement of the liver and spleen may occur. Abscesses have been observed in bones, but pulmonary and oropharyngeal lesions are rare. The simultaneous involvement of many organs is usually seen in infantile paracoccidioidomycosis.

Progressive Pulmonary

Reactivation of quiescent lesions or (rarely) continuation of primary pulmonary disease results in the progressive pulmonary paracoccidioidomycosis seen in about one-third of patients less than 30 years of age. At first, the progressive lung lesions may be asymptomatic or, if symptoms are present, they are those of a nonspecific respiratory infection. Small apical infiltrations are roentgenographically visible (Fig. 42-3*A*). When these early lesions progress and extend through the lungs (Fig. 42-3*B*), symptoms worsen but continue to be nonspecific. The disease commonly runs a subacute or chronic course as a continuous or recurrent infection. Cough with expectoration is always present, and there may be hemoptysis; sooner or later, dyspnea appears. Fever, thoracic pain, anemia, and weight loss ensue. The physical signs are also nonspecific, and they vary with the localization and the extent of the lesions. In this stage of the disease, the roentgenographic picture is also nonspecific and may simulate many pulmonary conditions (Fig. 42-4).

As the disease advances, the roentgenograms reveal the typical bilateral nodular and infiltrative lesions distributed in the medial and lower fields of the lungs (Fig. 42-5). Cavitation is not uncommon. The course of this form of the disease is slow, and patients may show little change during 15 years of observation. However, metastatic lesions in other organs occur in about 7% of patients after months or years. Also, spontaneous cure of progressive pulmonary paracoccidioidomycosis has been reported.

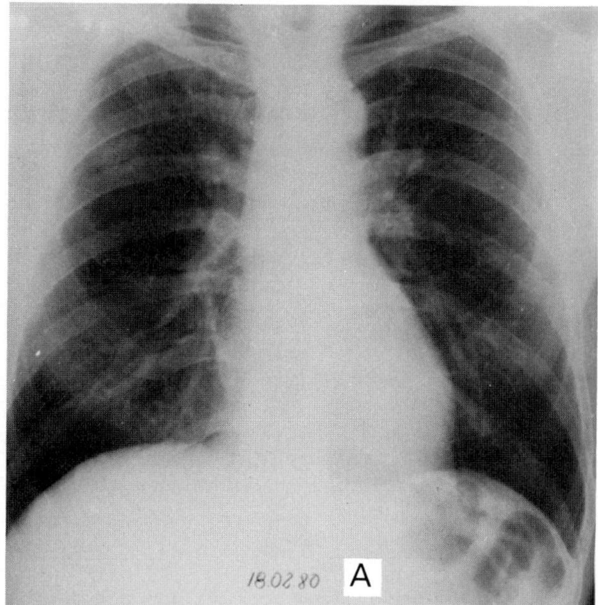

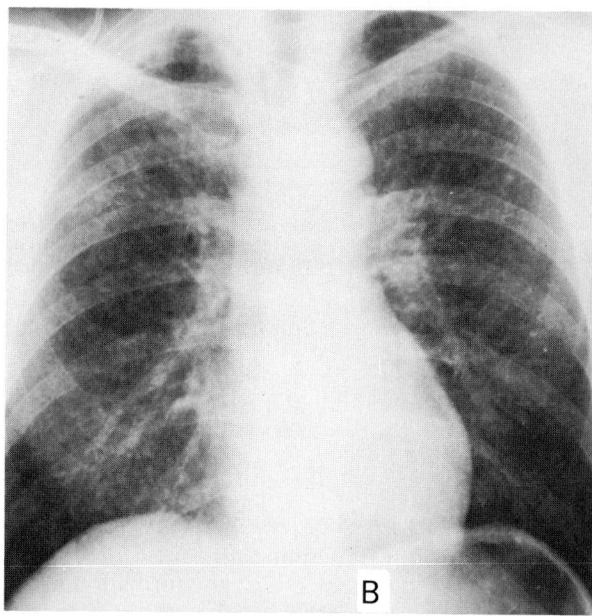

Fig. 42-3. Chest roentgenogram showing *(A)* an early lesion, as a small right apical infiltrate; and *(B)* the same patient at the time of diagnosis 6 months later when dissemination through both lungs was associated with glucosteroid therapy (Courtesy of Dr. L. C. Severo).

Disseminated

Disseminated paracoccidioidomycosis is present in about 70% of adult patients when their disease is diagnosed. Most patients have had previously over-

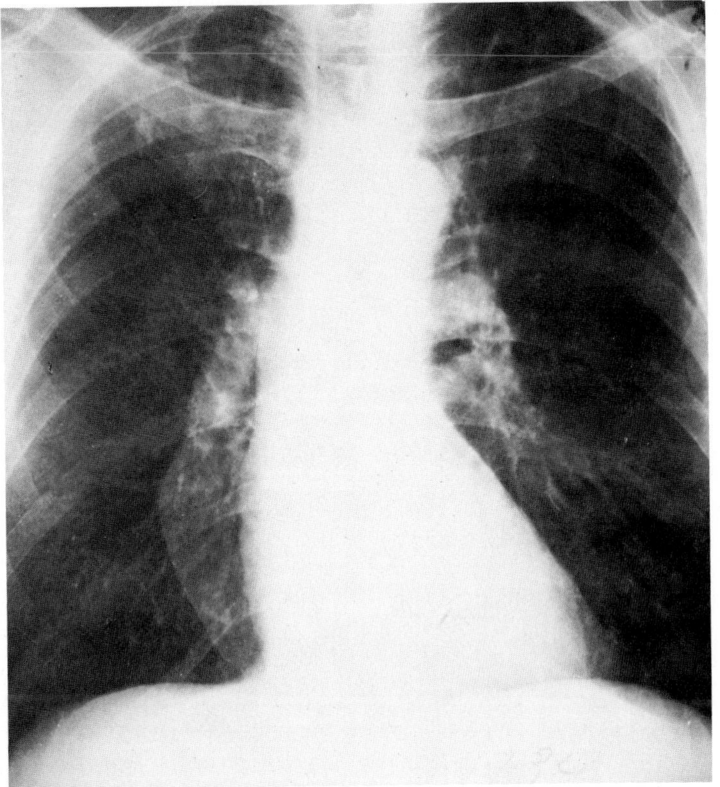

Fig. 42-4. Roentgenogram of chest of a patient with 2-year-long pulmonary infection. Note difuse interstitial infiltrations of both lungs, with confluence of the lesions in the right upper lobe.

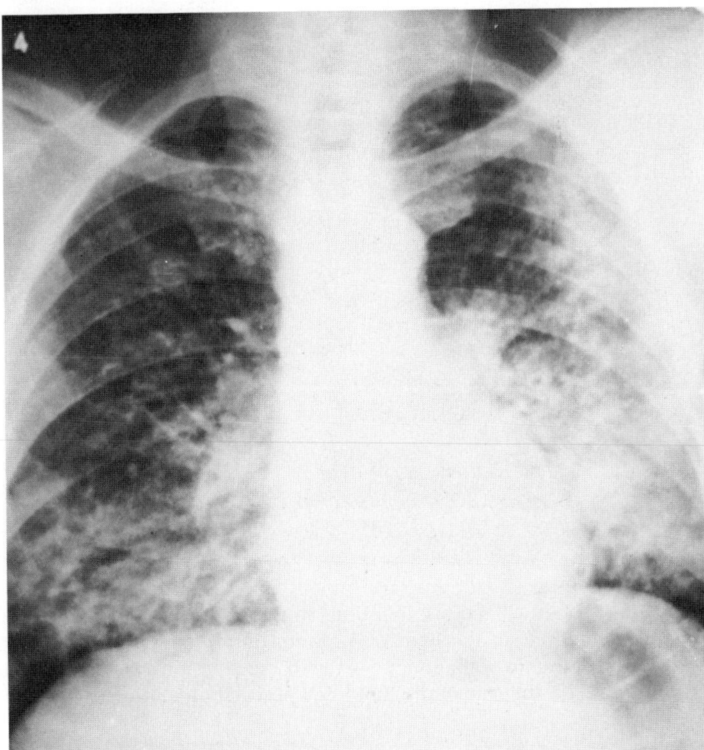

Fig. 42-5. In this roentgenogram of the chest, the distribution of lesions in the lower half of both lungs is consistent with a pulmonary mycosis. Note the heavy fibrosis, indicating an advanced stage.

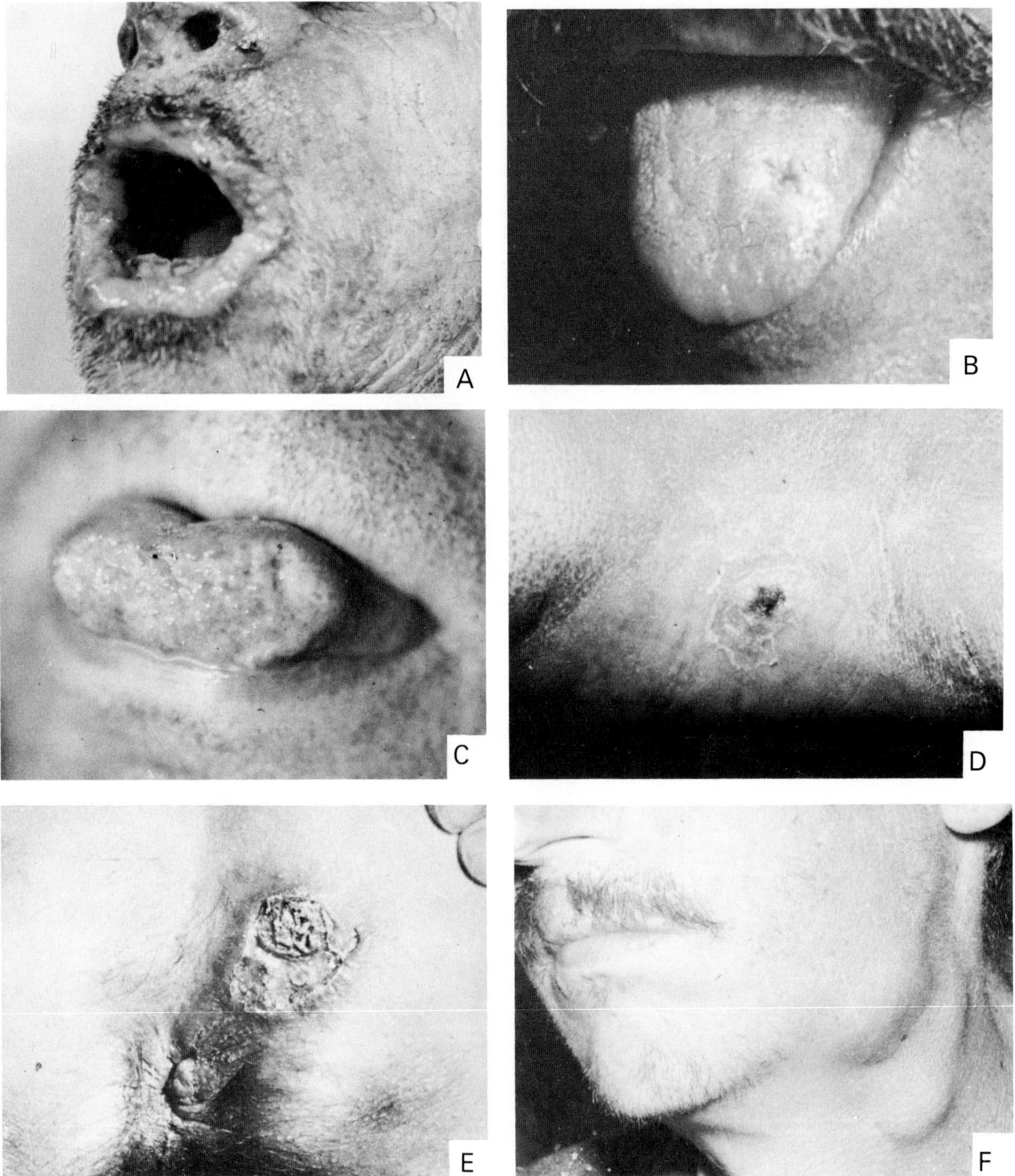

Fig. 42-6. The most accessible lesions in the disseminated form of paracoccidioidomycosis are *(A)* ulcerations of the lips (of 5-month duration); *(B)* early lesions of the tongue; *(C)* destruction of the tip of the tongue—an advanced lesion; *(D)* an ulcerated, crusted skin lesion (1-month old on the sole of the foot); *(E)* perianal ulceration; and *(F)* nonsuppurated lymphadenopathy.

looked pulmonary lesions that persisted as involvement elsewhere became evident. Dissemination is usually preceded by unexpected, rapid loss of weight. The oropharynx is the most frequently involved extrapulmonary site, with the lymph nodes and the skin next in frequency. The involvement of other organs is unpredictable, but virtually any organ or system is vulnerable. Accordingly, the manifestations of disseminated paracoccidioidomycosis are protean because they depend on which organ(s) is affected, the sequence of involvement, and the extent of lesions in particular organs.

The oropharyngeal lesions vary from a nonspecific, painful stomatitis or gingivitis to granulomatous or ulcerative, slowly spreading lesions of the lips (Fig. 42-6*A*), gums, palate, tongue (Fig. 42-6*B* and *C*), and pharynx. A granulomatous mulberrylike base with ulceration of large areas, occasionally with deep penetration, is consistent with paracoccidioidal disease. The larynx may be affected, and the vocal cords may be destroyed.

Ulcerated, crusted lesions of the skin usually reflect blood-borne dissemination of *P. brasiliensis* (Fig. 42-6*D*) but may result from extension of an oral lesion. The skin lesions may take on a wide variety of other forms and may be pleomorphic. Solitary, ulcerative, or granulomatous lesions of the penis and of the perineum have been reported.

Tender, cervical lymphadenopathy is frequent and may occur early in the course of disseminated paracoccidioidomycosis. The cervical nodes may become so large that Hodgkin's disease is mimicked. Massive visceral lymphadenopathy may simulate intraabdominal malignancy. In some patients, general lymphadenopathy is observed. The nodes sometime suppurate and drain pus that contains large numbers of yeastlike *P. brasiliensis*.

Adrenal gland involvement is very frequent and may lead to Addison's disease—in some patients, the only manifestation of the mycosis. The ileum and the colon are the most frequently involved regions of the gut. Ulcerative enteritis and colitis have been reported, but paracoccidioidal tumors of the gut are rare. Malabsorption syndrome has been related to paracoccidioidomycosis. Mild to severe hepatitis and cirrhosis of the liver have been reported; the spleen may also be affected. An intracranial hypertensive syndrome is more frequent than meningitis, but space-occupying lesions of the central nervous system have been also reported. The heart is rarely involved, but arteritis may be very severe, and thromboses of large blood vessels have been observed. Confined or diffuse osseous lesions may occur. The urinary tract is rarely involved. Involvement of the eye and endocrine glands is rare. A severe, septicemialike syndrome has been observed.

Paracoccidioidomycosis may complicate, or occur in association with, a wide variety of other infectious diseases. The manifestations are then quite unpredictable.

Diagnosis

The presence of oropharyngeal lesions typical of disseminated paracoccidioidomycosis enables clinical diagnosis in the endemic are. But with virtually any illness in the endemic area, paracoccidioidomycosis is among the diagnostic possibilities because the manifestations of this mycosis are protean. Thus, pulmonary paracoccidioidomycosis simulates tuberculosis and the other systemic mycoses. Mucocutaneous lesions must be differentiated from histoplasmosis, leishmaniasis, subcutaneous mycoses, neoplasms, yaws, syphilis, and tuberculosis. Lymphatic involvement simulates tuberculosis and lymphomas.

The laboratory diagnosis of paracoccidioidomycosis is based on the demonstration of the yeastlike forms of *P. brasiliensis* in clinical specimens: for example, exudate from ulcerative lesions (see Fig. 42-1*B*), pus from lymph nodes (see Fig. 42-1*A*) or abscesses, fragments of biopsied tissues (see Fig. 42-1*D*), sputum (see Fig. 42-1*C*), or feces. Bronchial washings or brushings, cerebrospinal fluid, and other body liquids should be centrifuged before examination; the sediment is then cleared of nonfungal elements by adding a drop of 10% KOH. If sputum is treated with 4% sodium hydroxide (NaOH), it will be cleared and liquefied so that centrifugation will provide sediment useful for microscopic examination. Sections cut from biopsy specimens should be stained with methenamine silver before examination (see Fig. 42-2).

Cultures should be planted on mediums selective for pathogenic fungi and incubated at 22°C. Heavily contaminated specimens (*e.g.,* sputum) should be inoculated intratesticularly in guinea pigs; the exudate or pus that forms may then be cultured. The identification of isolates as *P. brasiliensis* is based on conversion from the mycelial to the yeastlike form on incubation at 35°C.

Serodiagnosis depends on the availability of an adequate antigen for use in Yarzabal's modified immunodiffusion test—a practical and specific method. Immunoelectrophoresis and counterimmunoelectrophoresis are less time-consuming methods of equal reliability.

Prognosis

Without specific therapy, the progressive forms of paracoccidioidomycosis have a grave prognosis. The complement fixation test is a useful indicator of the activity of the disease.

Teeth may be lost, and parts of the tongue or vocal cords may be destroyed in advanced cases. However, the sequellae most often seen are consequent on therapeutic success: pulmonary fibrosis may cause right heart hypertrophy and failure; cicatricial constriction of the mouth may lead to microstomy; tracheal, glottic, or intestinal stenosis may occur.

Therapy

Sulfonamides (sulfadiazine, sulfamerzine, sulfamethoxypyridazine, sulfadimethoxine) are given in normal dosage for several months; when a clinical response is obtained, the dosage is reduced by one-half and continued for years or for life.

Amphotericin B is used as it is applied in histoplasmosis (see Chap. 40, Histoplasmosis). Alternating periods of therapy with sulfonamides and amphotericin B have been recommended.

Miconazole may be given both intravenously (200 mg/day) and perorally (3 g/day) for 1 month; peroral therapy (2 g–3 g/day) is then continued for 2 or more years. Ketoconazole is under evaluation (400 mg/day for 1–3 months; 200 mg/day for 1 or more years).

Prevention

There are no preventive measures of proved value.

Remaining Problems

The habitat and ecologic associations of *P. brasiliensis* should be elucidated.

Criteria of mycologic cure of paracoccidioidomycosis are not established. A cooperative study of therapy, with adequate follow-up research, is needed.

Bibliography

Journals

ALBORNOZ MB: Isolation of *Paracoccidioides brasiliensis* from rural soil in Venezuela. Sabouraudia 9:248–253, 1971

ANGULO-ORTEGA A: Calcifications in paracoccidioidomycosis. Are they the morphological manifestations of subclinical infection? In Paracoccidiodomycosis. PAHO Sci Pub No 254, pp. 129–133. Washington, DC: Pan Amer Hlth Organization, 1972

BRASS K: Observaciones sobre la anatomia patologica, patogenesis y evolucion de la paracoccidioidomicosis. Mycopathologia 37:119–138, 1969

LONDERO AT, RAMOS CD, LOPES JO: Progressive pulmonary paracoccidioidomycosis: A study of 34 cases observed in Rio Grande do Sul (Brazil). Mycopathologia 63:53–56, 1978

LONDERO AT, SEVERO LC: The gamut of progressive pulmonary paracoccidioidomycosis. Mycopathologia 75:65–74, 1981

PEDROSA PN: Paracoccidioidomicose. Inquerito intradermico com paracoccidioidina em zona rural do estado do Rio de Janeiro. Thesis, Faculdade Medicina Universidade Federale Rio de Janeiro, 1976

RESTREPO AM: Reapraisal of the microscopical appearance of the mycelial phase of *Paracoccidioides brasiliensis*. Sabouraudia 8: 141–144, 1970

RESTREPO AM, RESTREPO MI, DE RESTREPO F, ARISTIZABAL LH, MONCADA LH, VELEZ H: Immune responses in paracoccidioidomycosis. A controlled study of 16 patients before and after treatment. Sabouraudia 16:151–163, 1978

RESTREPO AM, ROBLEDO MV, GIRALDO R, HERNANDEZ H, SIERRA F, GUTIERREZ F, LONDONO F, LOPEZ R, CALLE G: The gamut of paracoccidioidomycosis. Am J Med 61:33–41, 1976

RESTREPO AM, ROBLEDO MV, OSPINA SC, RESTREPO MI, CORREA AL: Distribution of paracoccidioidin sensitivity in Colombia. Am J Trop Med Hyg 17:25–37, 1968

SEVERO LC, GEYER GR, LONDERO AT, PORTO NS, RIZZON CFC: The primary lymph node complex in paracoccidioidomycosis. Mycopathologia 67:115–118, 1979

YARZABAL LA, CABRAL NA, SANTIAGO AR: Evaluacion de una tecnica especifica de doble difusion en el diagnostico de la paracoccidioidomicosis. Acta Cient Venez 30:93–97, 1979

JOHN P. UTZ

Blastomycosis

43

Blastomycosis, a systemic infectious disease caused by the fungus *Blastomyces dermatitidis,* occurs predominantly in North America and has only recently been recognized in Africa. It is acquired by the respiratory route. From the primary focus in the lungs, there is occasionally hematogenous dissemination that can lead to a chronic, often fatal, course.

Etiology

Blastomyces dermatitidis (called *Ajellomyces dermatitidis* in the perfect, sexual state, with + and − mating types) is a fungus with two forms. In tissues, it is a yeast that measures approximately 10 μm in diameter, has a wall nearly 1 μm in thickness, and occasionally displays budding with a wide pore between parent and bud. On appropriate culture mediums (*e.g.,* Sabouraud's glucose agar), *B. dermatitidis* produces a mold (mycelium) of powdery consistency that is composed of microscopic filaments (hyphae) from which slender forms (conidiophores) project at right angles and bear conidia (spores) that are approximately 5 μm in diameter (Fig. 43-1).

Blastomyces dermatitidis is not known to elaborate toxins, enzymes, or other chemicals of pathogenic potential.

Epidemiology

Blastomycosis was for so long characterized as being limited to North America that it was frequently called North American blastomycosis. However, cases have been reported from the Middle East and widely scattered areas in Africa. Gilchrist reported the first case from Baltimore in 1898. Although the disease occurs most frequently in the southeastern United States, it is also seen in the Mississippi Valley. Recently a common source outbreak was described in Minnesota, where an acute, benign, self-limited illness occurred in 21 persons.

The saprophytic source in nature from which man and other animals acquire *B. dermatitidis* remains a mystery. Many attempts to isolate the fungus from soil in the vicinity of individual cases and in localities where there have been outbreaks have been essentially unsuccessful. Recent studies suggest that antibiotics or metabolites produced by other microorganisms lyse *B. dermatitidis* when unsterilized soil is baited with the fungus. Exposure to wood or lumber has been implicated epidemiologically, and the fungus has been cultured on woody plant material.

The disease occurs 6 to 10 times more frequently in males and is more common at ages 30 to 50 years.

The blastomycin for study of delayed cutaneous hypersensitivity is so unsatisfactory that its use has not enabled definition of the extent or frequency of the disease.

Pathogenesis and Pathology

Since the studies of Schwarz and Baum, it has been accepted that man acquires *B. dermatitidis* by way of the respiratory tract and that a primary but often subclinical focus of infection is established in the lung. From there, the fungus may disseminate hematogenously to various organs (*e.g.,* skin, bone, and internal genitalia). Spread by sexual intercourse has been described—from the infected epididymis, prostate, and testis to the endometrium, oviducts, and peritoneum.

Skin lesions are so frequent that is has been suspected that blastomycosis is acquired by accidental cutaneous implantation of the fungus. However, laboratory infections acquired by accidental implantation result in atypical skin lesions and lymphadenopathy (notably absent in natural infections), and are not followed by dissemination.

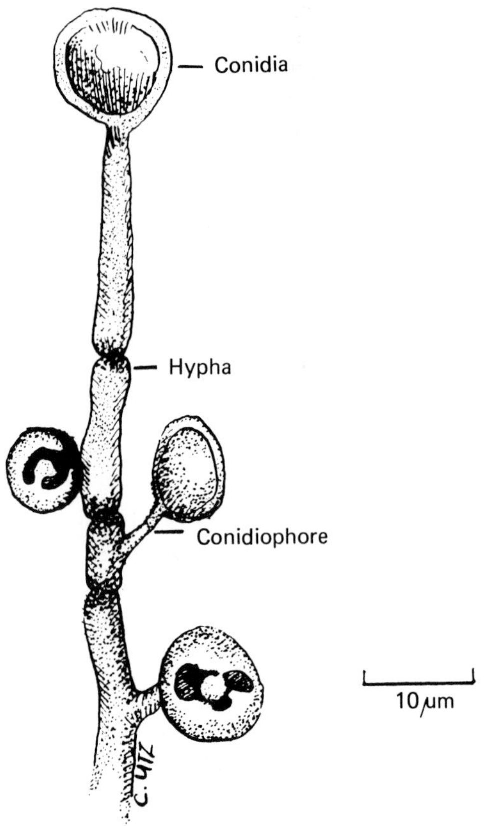

Fig. 43-1. Vegetative form of *Blastomyces dermatitidis.*

The tissue reaction to *B. dermatitidis* is variably suppuration and formation of granulomas. Abscesses occur frequently, ranging from microscopic to a size requiring surgical drainage. Polymorphonuclear leukocytes predominate in the pus. However, in areas surrounding or adjacent to abscesses, there are frequently epithelioid cell granulomas with Langhans' giant cells. Calcification occurs but is less frequent than in histoplasmosis or tuberculosis. With appropriate staining, *B. dermatitidis* can be seen both in pus and in granulomas.

Manifestations

Pulmonary Manifestations

Although not the most common manifestation of blastomycosis, pulmonary disease is still frequent, clinically important, and disabling. The onset is usually insidious, with cough that is commonly productive, pleural chest pain, and, occasionally, hemoptysis. Early in the course of the illness, general symptoms of fever, drenching night sweats, shaking chills, malaise, anorexia, and weight loss are present.

Examination of the chest may give disappointing results, but occasionally there are findings of consolidation. Radiographically, lesions vary from a small infiltrate to a dense, five-lobe consolidated pneumonia (Fig. 43-2); a characteristic finding is persistent or increasing infiltration in the face of antibacterial chemotherapy. Hilar lymphadenopathy occurs occasionally, and, despite the frequency of chest pain,

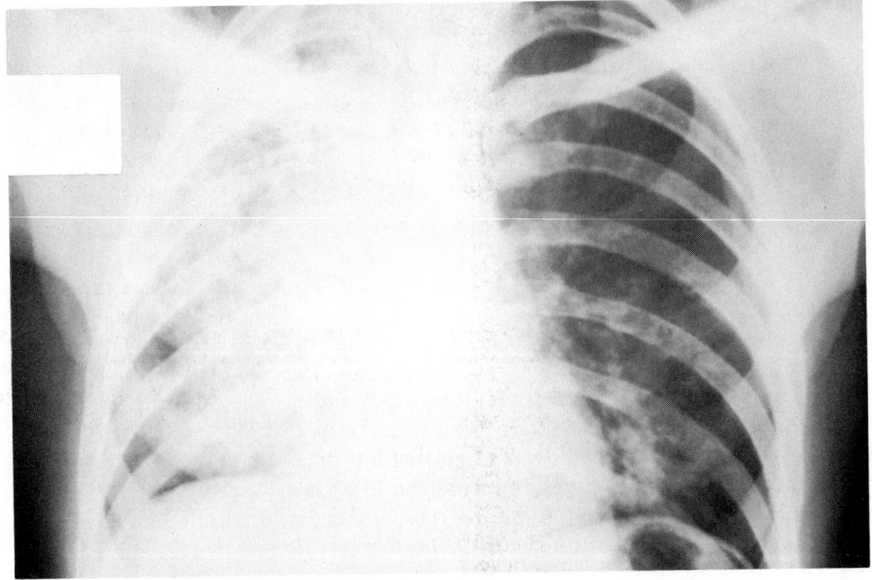

Fig. 43-2. Chest film of an adult male with diffuse blastomycosis of the right upper lung field and less severe involvement of the left lower lung field.

pleural effusions are rare. Cavitary disease occurs only occasionally, but it is important in terms of increased resistance to therapy and relapse after treatment. Solitary nodules, seen so frequently in histoplasmosis, coccidioidomycosis, and cryptococcosis, are rare in blastomycosis.

Cutaneous Manifestations

The characteristic skin lesions occur on the exposed parts of the body, notably the face and hands. They begin as small and nondistinctive macules or papules that gradually enlarge, becoming raised, verrucous, reddened, and, at various sites, alternately weeping and crusted. The outer border slants sharply, and the skin contiguous to it may be mildly erythematous (Fig. 43-3). The lesions are characteristically painless and nonitching. Extension may be more rapid in one area than in another so that the border is scalloped and the whole lesion becomes crescentlike. As the lesion progresses over several months, there may be central healing, leaving a thin, atrophic, depigmented scar, particularly noticeable in blacks. Less frequently, there may be multiple, peanut-sized, subcutaneous but raised abscesses, draining fistulas, and ulcers.

Fig. 43-3. Cutaneous blastomycosis of the face. The patient was unable to shave his beard at the lower margin. The lesion was raised and crusted, and it had a sharply slanting border, especially notable at the upper margin.

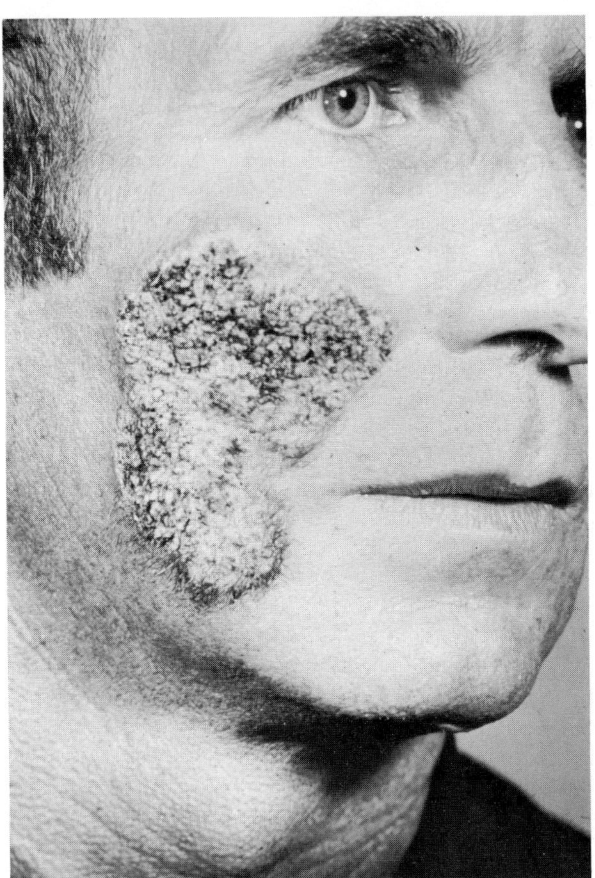

Genital Manifestations

Unlike most other fungi that cause systemic infections, *B. dermatitidis* characteristically infects the prostate, epididymis, and testis, while sparing the kidney. The onset is a painful swelling of the testis or the epididymis, or a vague, diffuse, deep, perineal pain. Occasionally, there is spontaneous drainage from the scrotum, but, more often, persistence as an indurated, thickened organ leads to surgical exploration and diagnosis. Pyuria and hematuria are frequent, but dysuria is uncommon.

Osseous Manifestations

Infections of bones occur frequently, and radiographic studies are indicated in all patients with blastomycosis. The thoracic, lumbar, and sacral segments of the spine are the most common sites of involvement. Next most commonly involved are the long bones of the lower extremities, then the pelvis and ribs. In children, skull lesions are common.

Bone lesions may sometimes be asymptomatic, but they are more commonly painful, with swelling of the covering soft tissues. As with other focal suppuration, there may be spontaneous drainage, and occasionally spinal involvement may be heralded by a fistula draiing below the inguinal ligament as a result of a psoas abscess.

Other Disseminated Forms

A number of other organs may be involved as a result of blood stream dissemination. Thus, there are reports of meningitis and cerebral abscesses, Addison's disease, pericarditis, endocarditis, and arthritis.

Diagnosis

The diagnosis of blastomycosis is established by the identification of *B. dermatitidis* in cultures. Physicians who have available the counsel of a mycologist can expect to obtain such a definitive laboratory diagnosis is more than 80% of patients. The specimen collected for culture must be appropriate to the lesion—scrapings from the skin and mucosal lesions, sputum, subcutaneous pus, or epididymal, testicular, and prostatic secretions. For reasons not well under-

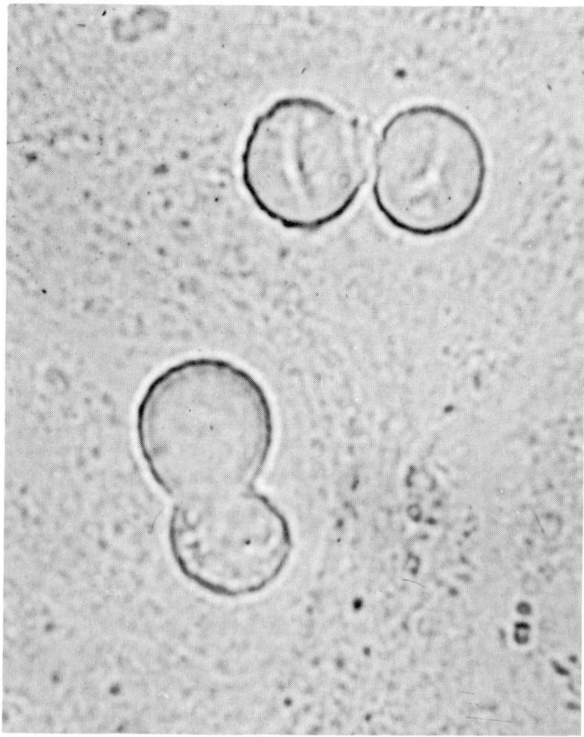

Fig. 43-4. Two budding cells of *Blastomyces dermatitidis* in sputum. Note the thick wall: inner, darker; outer, out of focal plane. Also, note the intervening bright (refractile) zone and the wide pore.

stood, the sputum of patients with pulmonary blastomycosis is rarely contaminated with *Candida* spp. or saprophytic yeasts that might make isolation of *B. dermatitidis* difficult.

Equally gratifying is microscopic examination of potassium-hydroxide-treated preparations of sputum, pus, or drainage from skin lesions. If spherical cells are found that have a diameter of 8 μm to 15 μm; thick walls with a refractile, double contour; no more than one bud per parent cell; and a granular internal structure, the fungus is almost certainly *B. dermatitidis* (Fig. 43-4). Immediacy of results coupled with a high degree of accuracy recommends such examinations.

Histopathologic diagnosis (Fig. 43-5) requires the use of three special stains (periodic acid Schiff, Gomori's methenamine silver, and Mayer's mucicarmine) to facilitate the recognition and differentiation of fungi. Thus, *Cryptococcus neoformans* (4 μm–7 μm in diameter) takes up the Mayer stain, whereas *B. dermatitidis* does not. *Blastomyces dermatitidis* is generally smaller than the sporangial form of *Coccidioides immitis* (20 μm–100 μm in diameter), and considerably larger than *Histoplasma capsulatum* (3 μm in diameter). *Histoplasma duboisii* is larger than *H. capsulatum* and rather closely resembles *B. dermatitidis* in size and morphology, but it lacks broad-based buds and is rarely encountered outside of Africa.

The blastomycin skin and serologic tests are of little use for diagnostic purposes. For example, in one large study, not one of 25 patients with culturally proved blastomycosis had a positive skin test, and fewer than 25% had a significant titer of complement-fixing antibodies.

Pulmonary blastomycosis is usually considered when the course is too prolonged for the usual bacterial pneumonia. On chest film, the infiltrate is generally more diffuse and linear than that seen in pulmonary carcinoma. In endemic areas, coccidioidomycosis and histoplasmosis are more common and must be distinguished from blastomycosis.

Cutaneous blastomycosis is often at first suspected of being a basal cell carcinoma, although the multiplicity of lesions in blastomycosis is unusual for cancer. Occasionally, the cutaneous–lymphatic form of sporotrichosis closely resembles blastomycosis, as may syphilid, tuberculid, other pyodermas, and the skin lesions of iodism. The other disseminated forms of blastomycosis closely mimic tuberculosis or other

Fig. 43-5. Periodic acid-Schiff stain showing, in an area of pyogenic inflammation, two cells of *Blastomyces dermatitidis (arrow)*, one of which is budding. The wall is preserved, but the cytoplasm has contracted in the process of fixation.

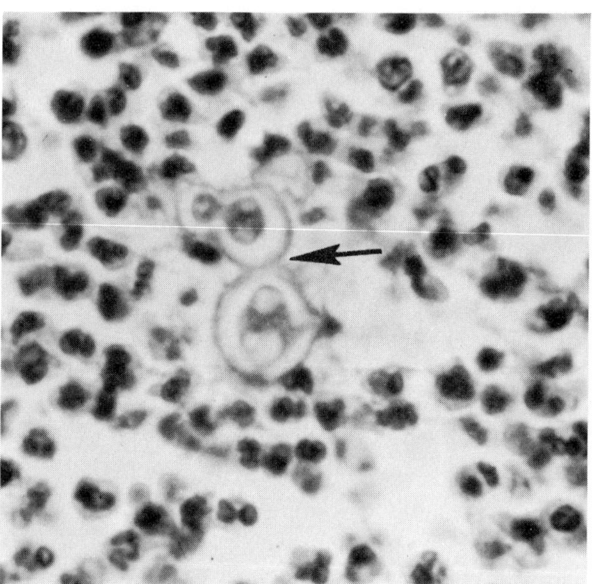

chronic bacterial diseases such as brucellosis. Confusion with salmonellal and staphylococcal infections of bones may also occur.

Prognosis

It has been widely held that blastomycosis is an inexorably fatal disease with a prolonged course marked by occasional, clear-cut remissions. This was not the case, however, in the recent outbreak in Minnesota, nor in an earlier study from Kentucky. Indeed, in one study, patients who refused treatment and left the hospital did better than those who were treated. However, these latter data must be viewed with caution, because the more seriously ill patients are more readily convinced that they should be treated. Despite some uncertainty, therapy is recommended for all patients with active disease.

The course of blastomycosis is generally characterized by slow progression, occasional spontaneous remission of lesions, and in some instances disappearance of pulmonary lesions without therapy. Progression from one form to another (*e.g.,* from pulmonary to cutaneous), or to another disseminated form, apparently does not occur.

The existence of an immune state has been much more difficult to establish in blastomycosis than in either histoplasmosis, coccidioidomycosis, or cryptococcosis. The lack of a satisfactory antigen for skin testing and the mystifying inability to find the fungus in man's environment have precluded authoritative assessment of immunity.

Therapy

General supportive measures and surgical treatment are as vital in blastomycosis as they are in the other systemic mycoses (see Chap. 40, Histoplasmosis, and Chap. 41, Coccidioidomycosis).

Of the major pathogenic fungi, *B. dermatitidis* is one of the most susceptible to antifungal agents by both *in vitro* and *in vivo* testing. Because many lesions remit spontaneously, therapeutic effectiveness has in the past been attributed to drugs that in fact had little or no activity. There are, however, several effective agents, judged on the basis of critical studies in humans and carefully controlled evaluations using experimental infections in laboratory animals.

Amphotericin B

It is important to note that success has been achieved with oral administration and with comparatively low doses of amphotericin B given intravenously (see Chap. 39, Candidosis). The total intravenous dose employed in the Veterans Administration Cooperative Study was 2 g. The alternative regimen—developed for histoplasmosis with smaller daily doses and a 10-week course of therapy—is more prolonged but better tolerated.

Hydroxystilbamidine Isethionate

Of the several aromatic diamidines effective in the treatment of blastomycosis, the preparation currently available is hydroxystilbamidine isethionate. It is administered intravenously in a dosage of 3 to 5 mg/kg body wt/day until a total of 8 g is given. Because some of the stilbamidines are sensitive to light, vials and bottles of solutions for infusion should be shielded during administration. The unfortunate side-effects of hypesthesia and anesthesia of the fifth cranial nerve seen with the parent compounds have rarely been encountered with the newer preparation. Because the drug is deposited in the liver (and skin), hepatic disease has been considered a relative contraindication to therapy.

The advocates of hydroxystilbamidine and committees on therapy agree the drug should be reserved for patients with nonprogressive, cutaneous disease.

Imidazoles

By testing *in vitro* and from preliminary experience in humans, ketoconazole may be helpful.

Prevention

Until more is known about the saprobic existence of *B. dermatitidis* in nature, it is difficult to envision successful efforts at the control of it in the environment. Neither circulating antibody nor cell-mediated (delayed cutaneous hypersensitivity) factors can be related to protection or immunity under either experimental or natural conditions. Despite this lack of association, there have been important studies with vaccines. Although some vaccines evoke increased resistance to subsequent challenge in laboratory animals, none is available at present for either investigative or general use in man.

Remaining Problems

Considering that blastomycosis is so common in the southeastern part of the United States, and that it is so clearly acquired by the respiratory route, it is both astonishing and humbling that the site of saprobic existence of *B. dermatitidis* is still completely unknown.

The occurrence of blastomycosis in the Southeast and the recent finding of cases in Africa led to the interesting speculation that the disease may have been introduced to the North American continent from Africa. If so, one might expect that the disease would be more frequent in blacks, whereas it is twice as common in whites. On the other hand, racial immunity could explain a lower frequency of occurrence in blacks.

The true frequency of blastomycosis of the internal genitalia should be ascertained with greater certainty. If some of the tissue resected at operations were set aside in the refrigerator for the 24 hours necessary to detect granulomas, the necessary cultural studies could then be done.

If *B. dermatitidis* is exquisitely susceptible to several antimicrobics, why do relapses occur so much more frequently than in other mycoses? Such poor responses may be associated with impaired immunity—a postulated but undefined defect.

Finally, development of an effective vaccine is as much needed for the prevention of blastomycosis as it is for prevention of other fungal infections.

Bibliography

Journals

BUSEY JF: Blastomycosis. I. A review of 198 collected cases from Veterans Administrations Hospitals. Am Rev Respir Dis 89:659–672, 1964

DENTON TF, DISALVO AF: Additional isolations of *Blastomyces dermatitidis* from natural sites. Am J Trop Med Hyg 18:697–700, 1979

DIXON DM, SHADOMY HJ, SHADOMY S: *In vitro* growth and sporulation of *Blastomyces dermatitidis* on woody plant material. Mycologia 69:1193–1195, 1977

KUTTEN ES, BEEMER AM, LEVIJ T, AJELLO L, KAPLAN W: Occurrence of *Blastomyces dermatitidis* in Israel: First autochthonous Middle Eastern case. Am J Trop Med Hyg 27:203–1205, 1978

MCDONOUGH ES, KUZMA JF: Epidemiologic studies on blastomycosis in the state of Wisconsin. Sabouraudia 18:173–183, 1980

RECHT LD, PHILIPS JR, ECKMAN MR, SAROSI GA: Self limited blastomycosis: A report of thirteen cases. Am Rev Respir Dis 120:1109–1112, 1979

SAROSI GA, ARMSTRONG D, BARBEE RA, BATES TH, CAMPBELL GD, GEORGE RB, GOLDSTEIN RA, SCHAFFNER W, STEVENS DA: Treatment of fungal diseases. Am Rev Respir Dis 120: 1343–1397, 1979

SAROSI GA, DAVIES SF: Blastomycosis. Am Rev Respir Dis 120:911–938, 1979

SAROSI GA, HAMMERMAN KJ, TOSH FE, KRONENBERG RS: Clinical features of acute pulmonary blastomycosis. N Engl J Med 290:540–543, 1974

WITORSCH P, UTZ JP: North American blastomycosis: A study of 40 patients. Medicine 47:169–200, 1968

JOHN P. UTZ

Aspergillosis

44

Aspergillosis is a term applied to a variety of conditions ranging from hypersensitivity with bronchospasm to an invasive, usually fatal, hematogenously disseminated disease—all associated with species of *Aspergillus,* notably *A. fumigatus* and *A. niger.*

Etiology

Aspergillus spp. are dimorphic fungi. In tissues they grow as filaments (hyphae) that are approximately 4 μm in diameter and characteristically branch abundantly in dichotomous fashion, typically at 45° angles (Fig. 44-1*A*).

During growth as a saprobe, a second, mycelial form arises. This form is distinguished by highly complex structures (conidiophores) that measure approximately 5 μm in diameter and reach a length of approximately 400 μm as they expand into dome-shaped vesicles approximately 20 μm in diameter. The upper half of each vesicle bears tubular structures (sterigmata) that produce conidia measuring approximately 3 μm in diameter (Fig. 44-1*B*). *Aspergillus fumigatus* is distinguished by the production of sterigmata that bend so that they are parallel, each supporting a columnar mass of greenish conidia. The conidia of *A. niger* are black, whereas those of *A. flavus* are reddish brown. The characteristic conidia are formed not only on appropriate culture mediums (*e.g.,* Sabouraud's glucose agar), but also during growth as nonpathogenic residents of the external auditory canal, in an ectatic bronchus, or in a pulmonary cavity.

Aspergillus spp. are the only fungi pathogenic for man that produce endotoxins. That elaborated by *A. fumigatus* does not appear to play an important role in disease in man. However, aflatoxin, the endotoxin produced by *A. flavus* growing on peanuts and other animal foods, is an important cause of abortion and death in sheep and cattle. It is also a remarkably potent carcinogen.

Epidemiology

Aspergillosis is worldwide in occurrence, but so many reports emanate from Europe (including Great Britain) that the disease appears to be relatively uncommon in the United States. Exposure to infected grains or to decaying vegetation on which the fungus grows was once thought to be important in acquisition of the disease by humans, according to early reports. Even today, fireproofing materials and outmoded ventilating systems, or proximity to solid sewage disposal residues, are important in exposure to *Aspergillus* spp.

A great number of *Aspergillus* spp. are natural saprobes and a few are pathogens for plants, insects, domestic animals, and birds, especially penguins. Because several species have been found in the oral and gastrointestinal tract of man, this fungus must be considered a commensal.

Saprophytic colonization of ectatic bronchi and pulmonary cavities, as well as actual invasion, almost always occurs in patients already compromised by diseases or conditions that reduce resistance to infection: leukemia and lymphoma (especially Hodgkin's disease), azotemia, sarcoidosis, alcoholism, glucosteroid therapy, ionizing irradiation, prolonged antibacterial therapy, indwelling urinary or intravenous catheters, immunosuppressive therapy, diabetes mellitus, leukopenia, the dysgammaglobulinemias, and impaired cell-mediated immunity. In this respect, aspergillosis strikingly resembles candidosis, cryptococcosis, and zygomycosis, standing in marked contrast to coccidioidomycosis, histoplasmosis, and blastomycosis. In aspergillosis and similar mycoses, the

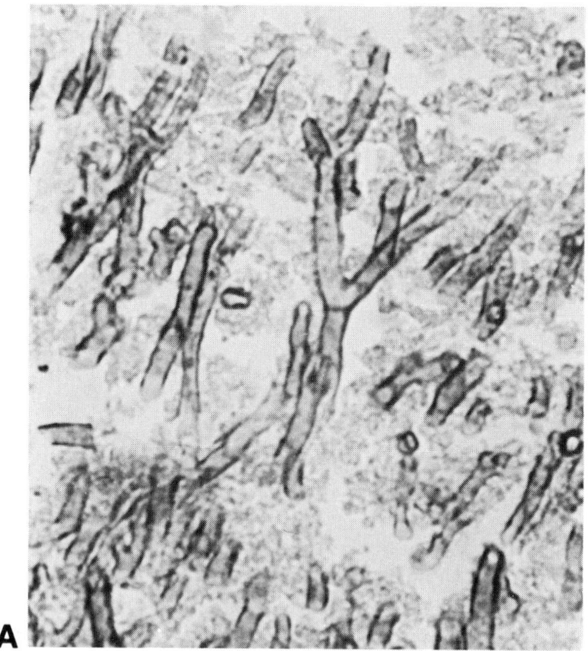

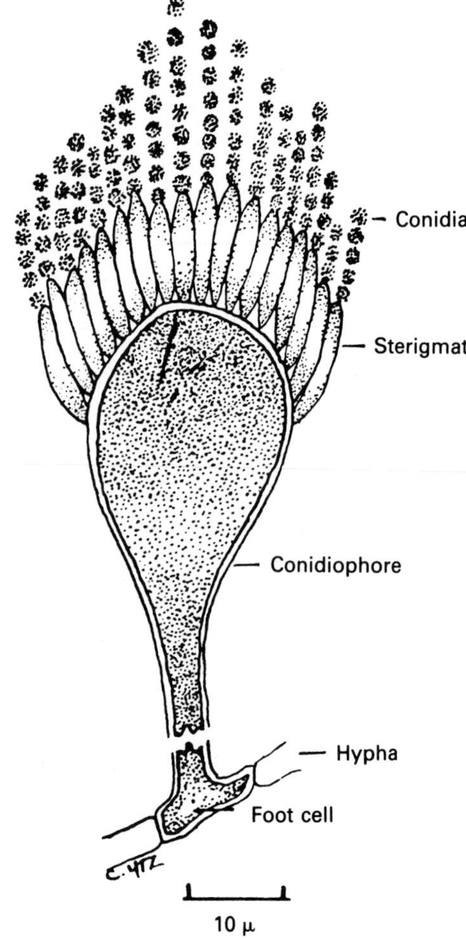

Fig. 44-1. *(A)* Photomicrograph of pulmonary tissue showing the profusion of a dichotomously branching fungus (*Aspergillus fumigatus* by culture) after periodic acid-Schiff staining. *(B)* Diagrammatic representation of the vegetative form of *Aspergillus fumigatus.*

pathogenicity of a common fungus is conditioned by a noninfectious disease that in some way compromises nonspecific or specific mechanisms of defense.

Pathogenesis and Pathology

It seems clear that aspergillosis is almost always acquired by the respiratory route, although there are rare instances in which the fungus may invade through the mucosa of the gut, producing severe or fatal disease. Involvement of the gastrointestinal tract is most often part of a general, disseminated process. Vaginitis has been ascribed to infection with *Aspergillus* spp. Kidney involvement is frequent in disseminated disease, but renal infection from the lower urinary tract must be at least as rare as bladder lesions caused by *Aspergillus* spp. The external ear is colonized directly. Empyema with *Aspergillus* spp. has been reported as a complication of therapeutic pneumothorax.

In two characteristic forms of aspergillosis—otitis externa and fungus ball—there is usually no invasion of tissues and rarely evidence of an inflammatory reaction.

Invasive pulmonary disease caused by *Aspergillus* spp. stands in marked contrast, in that hyphae penetrate the walls of bronchi and bronchioles, invading the pulmonary vasculature and inducing an acute, necrotizing, pyogenic pneumonitis. The bronchi and bronchioles are filled with pus, and sites of parenchymal involvement are marked by small white nodules of acute inflammation in response to invading hyphae.

When the fungus disseminates hematogenously from the lung, the metastatic lesions are characteristically also suppurative. Moreover, at both primary and secondary sites, hyphae may invade blood vessels, producing a thrombotic angiitis. Such invasion is less marked with *Aspergillus* spp. than with genera of Class Zygomycetes (see Chap. 128, Zygomycoses).

Manifestations

The term *aspergillosis* embraces, conveniently, a variety of conditions. Although *Aspergillus* spp. are involved, the manifestations vary according to the site of involvement and the kind of reaction from the host.

Otitis Externa

It is almost certainly an overstatement to represent a saphrobic colonization of debris in the ear canal as an otomycosis simply because *Aspergillus* spp. have been isolated from such detritus. The local application of antibacterial agents promotes such colonization, actual invasion of tissues almost never occurs, and colonization responds to nonspecific, nonantifungal therapy (*e.g.,* aluminum subacetate irrigations).

Allergy

The bases for implicating allergy to *Aspergillus* spp. in the genesis of manifestations of disease are as follows: (1) skin reactivity of the immediate type to skin test material derived from *Aspergillus* spp.; (2) the development of characteristic symptoms in some patients with asthma when exposed to this fungus; (3) the exacerbation of illness on exposure to *Aspergillus* spp. in many patients with chronic pulmonary disease, with the appearance of migratory infiltrates on the chest film, Curschmann's spirals and Charcot–Leyden crystals in the sputum, and a peripheral eosinophilia (perhaps a syndrome of reaction to mycelial plugging of a bronchus); and (4) elevated concentrations of IgE and the presence of precipitin (or other) antibodies in the serum.

Mycetoma

A striking manifestation of aspergillosis is the fungus ball, or pulmonary mycetoma. Radiographically, the typical fungus ball is a rounded opacification capped by a thin meniscus of air lying in an ectatic bronchus or old tuberculous cavity in an upper lobe (Fig. 44-2). Microscopically, the ball is composed of tangled hyphae, some inflammatory cells, fibrin, and amorphous debris. The fungus ball is generally asymptomatic, or the major manifestations are those of the underlying disease that caused the cavitation. However, hemoptysis may be the initial manifestation and, occasionally, the cause of death.

Endophthalmitis

Endophthalmitis is a dreadful infection characteristically arising 2 to 3 weeks after surgery or injury to the eye. In at least half the patients, an *Aspergillus* spp. is the cause. The earliest manifestations are clouding of vision, redness of the conjunctiva, and pain. Hypopyon then develops, and there is severe exudation into the anterior and posterior chambers (see Chap. 163, Intraocular Infections).

Disseminated Disease

Disseminated aspergillosis is an equally frightening disease that is usually acute and fatal. The brain and the kidney are involved in about two-thirds of the cases. Either as a result of the underlying disease or the infection, azotemia occurs rapidly. Hematuria is frequent, and there may be urinary tract obstruction.

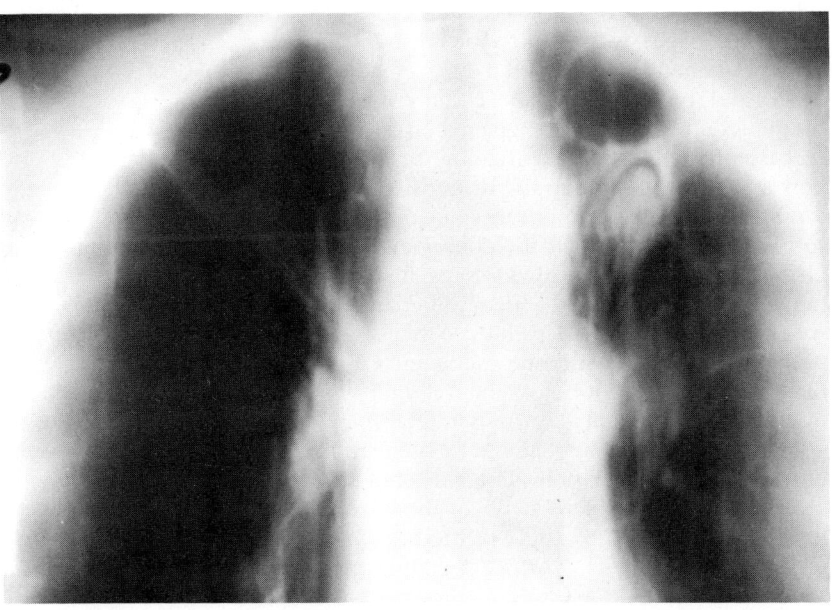

Fig. 44-2. Tomogram of the chest showing a lemon-shaped opacification (mycetoma or fungus ball) almost filling a cavity in the left upper lung field. Note the crescentic air space capping the mycetoma.

Central nervous system involvement is marked by headaches, seizures, and focal signs. More unusual presentations are hemiplegia and radicular pains. Endocarditis has been found, usually at autopsy, and may cause such characteristic findings as fever, heart murmur, peripheral emboli, splenomegaly, and cardiac failure. With osteomyelitic lesions there may be fever, bone pain and tenderness, soft tissue swelling, and fluctuance. Virtually any organ may be involved.

Diagnosis

The confirmation of a clinical impression of aspergillosis is fraught with extraordinary difficulty. Various species of *Aspergillus* are truly ubiquitous—present in the environment, including the clinical microbiology laboratory. Thom has colorfully called *Aspergillus* spp. "the weed of the culture room." Hence, the relationship of an isolate growing in a Petri dish or tube culture to a clinical specimen must always be questioned.

Many *Aspergillus* spp. are commensals of man and are frequently recovered from sputum, feces, urine, and conjunctival and vaginal swabs. Again, the relationship of such an isolate to any disease in the patient must be a matter for careful evaluation.

In at least one of the more classic and almost pathognomonic manifestations of aspergillosis—the fungus ball—it is frequently difficult to culture the fungus from sputum or bronchial washings. Similarly, in patients with endocarditis, it was not until 1968, and subsequently in only 1 of 40 cases by 1974, that the causative fungus was cultured from a specimen of blood obtained before death.

Skin and serologic tests have either not been available generally or have not given consistent results.

It is apparent from the foregoing that the present best means of confirming the diagnosis is the microscopic finding, in appropriately stained tissue, of microorganisms morphologically consistent with *Aspergillus* spp. that have invaded tissues. In addition, the fungus should be isolated and identified in cultures of specimens that originate from the actual site of infection—a so-called deep tissue specimen. Often, suitable specimens cannot be obtained if vital organs are involved, or if patients are desperately ill.

In fixed tissue, the hyphae can be seen readily with either the Gridley or periodic acid-Schiff stain. The smaller size, the septate hyphae, the dichotomous branching, and the 45° angle of the branches rather clearly distinguish *Aspergillus* spp. from the zygomycetes (see Fig. 44-1*A*). Only occasionally, when the fungus grows saprophytically, as in an ectatic bronchus or cavity, does a surgical specimen contain the diagnostic conidiophores.

When hyphal fragments and microconidia are found on direct microscopic examination of the sputum, it is certain that the fungus is present in the specimen. A culture medium rendered selective for fungi by the inclusion of antibacterial agents (*e.g.*, chloramphenicol or neomycin) is useful with contaminated specimens such as sputum. By incubating the specimen at 37°C to 40°C, or by including cycloheximide in the culture medium, fungal contaminants are usually inhibited. With deep tissue specimens, fewer precautions need to be taken against contaminants. With selective mediums incubated at 37°C to 40°C, characteristic conidiophores may be seen after 48 hours of incubation.

The activity of allergic or migratory pulmonary aspergillosis has been correlated with the presence of precipitins or other antibodies in the serum. Such tests are not generally available, and even when positive they are not convincing either microbiologically or academically regarding their relevance to the clinical state of the patient.

Otitis externa, the fungus ball, and endophthalmitis need to be distinguished only from identical lesions caused by other microorganisms. Asthmatic reactions and migratory infiltrations in the lung resemble asthma due to other allergens, Löffler's syndrome, or visceral larva migrans (see Chap. 78, Visceral Larva Migrans). Recurrent pulmonary emboli and pulmonary edema are more readily differentiated. Disseminated aspergillosis most closely resembles hematogenous candidosis or sepsis caused by gram-negative bacteria.

Prognosis

There is a striking variation in prognosis according to the form of disease, which in turn is conditioned primarily by the nature of the preexisting, underlying disease. Infections of the external ear canal, although irritating, are never serious and are usually self limited. Asthma due to *Aspergillus* spp., like asthma provoked by other allergens, can be severely disabling and even fatal. Because residence in ectatic bronchi or pulmonary cavities constitutes a saprobic existence of *Aspergillus* spp., disability and death are more often consequences of the underlying disease than colonization. The fungus ball is itself usually benign, although there have been instances of fatal hemoptysis. Endophthalmitis is a serious disease and usually leads to loss of the eye. The hematogenous, disseminated form is almost always fatal. There are only two known instances of recovery from endocarditis caused by *Aspergillus* spp.

Progression from one form of aspergillosis to another is not seen, and there is no urgency to treat milder forms of disease to forestall devolution.

It is obvious from the ubiquity of the fungus and the relative rarity of disease that *Aspergillus* spp. are low in virulence for man and that the normal human possesses strong natural defenses against them. These characteristics have not been further defined for either the parasite or the host. However, it is clear that the presence of precipitating or other antibodies cannot be correlated with either resistance to disease or the probability of subsequent infection.

Therapy

Specific antifungal chemotherapy is not necessary for the forms of aspergillosis in which the fungus is primarily a saprophyte. Thus, skin infections are best treated locally with nonantifungal preparations; for example, an astringent. Mild success in asthma has been ascribed to desensitization to the fungus. Surgical resection has been the usual treatment of fungus ball, although the local application of amphotericin B through a percutaneous endobronchial catheter has been reported to be effective. Systemic administration of amphotericin B is not indicated.

The high fatality rate is disseminated disease and the loss of vision from endophthalmitis are certainly indications for chemotherapy. However, two factors tend to nullify the utility of amphotericin B, the one antifungal agent available for systemic use: (1) The course of these forms of aspergillosis is usually so fulminant that there is not enough time to obtain an actual therapeutic effect, and (2) *Aspergillus* spp. are frequently resistant to amphotericin B, often requiring more than 50 μg/ml for inhibition. When invasive aspergillosis is chronic, amphotericin B may sometimes be beneficial. For details on the administration of amphotericin B, see Chapter 39, Candidosis. The course of therapy is usually shorter in aspergillosis—for example, in a patient with endophthalmitis who survives without enucleation, treatment beyond 2 to 3 weeks is unnecessary.

The rare success of treatment with flucytosine is testimony to the requirement for susceptibility testing *in vitro*. Resistance may be defined as lack of inhibition at or below 25 μg/ml.

Prevention

Although there have been sporadic attempts at preparing vaccines, none is currently available.

Patients allergic to *Aspergillus* spp. should avoid exposure to decaying vegetation and other sites where the fungus may abound.

The bronchial stump following lobectomy or pneumonectomy is apparently predisposed to infection by *Aspergillus* spp. by the use of silk sutures in closure. On the basis both of clinical and experimental studies in nonhuman animals, other materials (*e.g.*, absorbable sutures) are preferable.

Remaining Problems

It seems clear to workers on both sides of the Atlantic that there are real and mysterious differences in the frequency of the various forms of aspergillosis, the role of aspergillosis in pulmonary disease, and the usefulness of precipitin and other serologic tests in predicting resistance to the disease.

Fungal infections such as histoplasmosis and blastomycosis are common in discrete geographic areas of the United States; in those areas, why is aspergillosis peculiarly a problem of patients with compromised host defenses?

Can patients with clinically significant, preexisting pulmonary disease who develop a fungus ball be treated nonsurgically and yet effectively?

Would vaccines or effective and nontoxic chemotherapeutic agents be helpful in preventing aspergillosis in compromised patients?

The possible role of aflatoxin in human disease, either as a toxin or a carcinogen, needs exploration.

Why is it so difficult to culture *Aspergillus* spp. from the blood of patients with endocarditis (in 39 of 40 cases it was impossible)?

Bibliography

Journals

AISNER J, SCHIMPFF SC, BENNETT JE, YOUNG VM, WIERNICK PH: *Aspergillus* infections in cancer patients: Association with fire-proofing materials in a new hospital. JAMA 235:411–412, 1976

AISNER J, SCHIMPFF SC, WIERNICK PH: Treatment of invasive aspergillosis: Relation of early diagnosis and treatment to response. Ann Intern Med 86:539–543, 1977

CARBONE PP, SEYMOUR MS, SIDRANSKY H, FREI E: Secondary aspergillosis. Ann Intern Med 60:556–567, 1964

DOFT BH, CLARKSON LD, REBELL G, FORSTER RK: Endogenous *Aspergillus* endophthalmitis in drug abusers. Arch Ophthalmol 98:859–862, 1980

ENGLISH MP, HENDERSON AH: Significance and interpretation of laboratory tests in pulmonary aspergillosis. J Clin Pathol 20:832–834, 1967

FRASER DW, NORD JI, AJELLO L, PLIKAYTIS BD: Aspergillosis and other systemic mycoses: The growing problem. JAMA 242:1631–1635, 1979

LANDAU JW, NEWCOMER VD, SCHULZ J: Aspergillosis: Report of two instances in children associated with acute leukemia and review of the pertinent literature. Mycopathol Mycol Appl 20:177–224, 1963

REDDY PA, CHRISTIANSON CS, BRASHER CA, LARSH H, SUTARIA M: Comparison of treated and untreated pulmonary aspergilloma. Am Rev Respir Dis 101:928–934, 1970

LOWELL S. YOUNG

Pneumocystosis

45

Pneumocystis carinii is the commonest appellation applied to the putative protozoan cause of a diffuse pneumonitis that usually occurs in humans with congenital or acquired immunodeficiencies. The association between pneumonia in humans and cyst forms in the lungs was made during and after World War II, when Jirovec studied pneumonias in malnourished, premature infants cared for in orphanages. Years before, cyst and trophozoite forms morphologically similar to *P. carinii* were observed in the lungs of many nonhuman mammals, for example, in guinea pigs (Chagas, 1909) and rats (Carini, 1910). Clearly, a wide variety of pneumocystislike microorganisms exists, and the forms identified in tissues from humans should not be assumed to be the same as those found in other animals. Nonetheless, work with athymic mice and cortisone-treated rats has led to insights about the pathogenesis and treatment of pneumocystosis in humans. Such studies have been particularly valuable because *P. carinii* from humans has not been cultivated *in vitro* for extended passages in high titer.

Etiology

The taxonomic status of *P. carinii* and other pneumocystislike microorganisms is not fully resolved. They are protozoan on two counts: (1) Both light and electron micrographic examinations document the structural resemblance of the cyst and trophozoite forms to classic protozoa; and (2) both prevention and treatment of pneumocystosis are successful using antimicrobics that are active against classic protozoa. Although there are morphologic similarities between fungi and the cyst forms of *P. carinii,* antifungal antimicrobics are ineffective in the treatment of pneumocystosis in humans and nonhuman animals.

The primary evidence that pneumocysts are viable and pathogenic is the coincidence of the presence and fairly consistent morphology of pneumocysts in the alveoli of patients and nonhuman animals with pneumonitis and the reversal of such findings by appropriate treatment. The cyst form is a unicellular structure 4 μm to 6 μm in diameter, which contains up to eight oval bodies (intracystic bodies, sporozoites). Round cysts often contain structures shaped like opposing commas or parentheses that are probably thickened portions of the cyst wall.

In lung imprints and in bronchial washings, trophozoite forms may be identified with the Giemsa stain—the stain that is also best for the identification of intracystic bodies by light microscopy. Although the Giemsa stain can be applied relatively rapidly, it is limited because it also stains background alveolar material and cell fragments. Hence, the definitive method for the identification of cyst forms in lung tissues and respiratory secretions is the Gomori methenamine silver nitrate (GMS) stain (see Chap. 9, Microscopic Examinations). By this rather time-consuming method, pneumocysts have a thin, dark greyish or brown black capsule and may be perfectly round, disc shaped, or crescentic in form (Fig. 45-1). Cysts often occur in clusters lying within the intra-alveolar spaces rather than in the interstitium.

When there is need for rapid diagnosis, less definitive methods for detecting pneumocysts may be used. The Gram–Weigert stain, like the Giemsa stain, allows identification of both cysts and trophozoites, whereas the toluidine blue stain delineates the cyst form but not intracellular morphology. Nonetheless, the GMS stain should always be carried out for confirmation. Use of a positive and negative control is important because yeasts and erythrocytes might be mistaken for pneumocysts.

On the basis of electron microscopic studies, it is hypothesized that trophozoites are derived from intracystic bodies (sporozoites) that have escaped through the cyst wall. The trophozoites then evolve into larger forms, their walls thicken, and a precyst

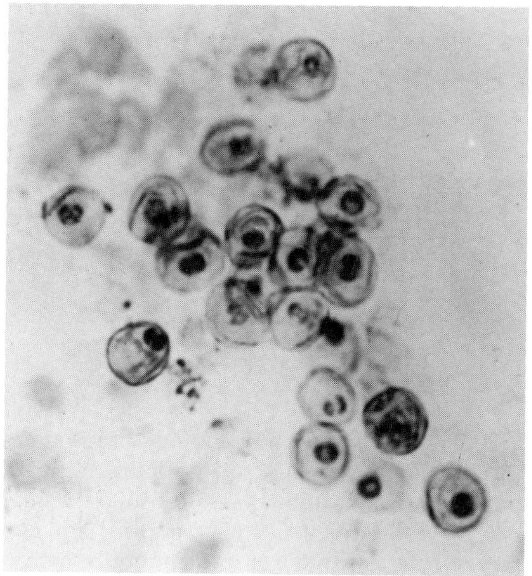

Fig. 45-1. Cysts of *Pneumocystis carinii,* shown in an impression smear of a lung biopsy. (Original magnification × 1000)

structure results. Final maturation of the precyst structure results in the formation of the classic cyst.

Epidemiology

Naturally occurring epizootics of pneumocystis infection have been documented in athymic (nude) mice. Airborne transmission and close contact have been implicated in experimental animals treated with cortisone. In humans, the observation of the epidemic occurrence of pneumocystosis in malnourished children in orphanages favors the concept of communicability. Moreover, there are reports of clusters of cases in normal populations among healthy family members and in institutions caring for immunosuppressed patients. On the other hand, there is serologic documentation of widespread acquisition of antipneumocystis antibody in early childhood. Thus, overt clinical disease occurring at a later age in patients given glucosteroid therapy or treated for neoplasms is thus logically conceived of as reactivation of latent infection. The attack rate in the United States is highest in children under 1 year of age, and most of these patients have some primary immunodeficiency. Lymphatic leukemia, Hodgkin's disease and nonHodgkin's lymphoma are the next most common underlying disorders. The most plausible unifying epidemiologic hypothesis is built on the following observations: (1) Low-grade or clinically inapparent infection is a common occurrence among young children and occasionally may be clinically manifest as pneumonitis even in children who are not immunosuppressed; (2) primary pneumocystosis that is clinically evident occurs primarily in children with congenital immunodeficiencies; (3) after childhood, most symptomatic pneumocystosis is associated with reactivation of latent infection; (4) clusters of institutional cases may result from reactivation of latent infection to an index case followed by person-to-person or airborne spread to immunosuppressed susceptibles; and (5) alternatively, if patients with similar underlying diseases are treated with identical chemotherapeutic protocols in a specific ward of a hospital, multiple cases of endogenous reinfection, triggered by therapy or disease, may yield clusters of pneumocystosis.

Pathogenesis and Pathology

According to studies *in vitro* using cysts harvested from nonhuman animals, humoral antibody enhances uptake and interiorization of cyst forms by alveolar macrophages. This is consistent with the findings *in vivo;* both experimental animals and humans with intact humoral antibody synthesizing mechanisms and mononuclear cell function are at relatively low risk of developing clinical pneumocystosis.

The great majority of patients with proven pneumocystosis have either congenital or acquired immunodeficiencies, or they are victims of protein-calorie malnutrition and crowding. Patients with congenital immunodeficiencies attributable to either T-lymphocyte deficits or impaired humoral antibody production (B-lymphocyte or plasma-cell abnormalities) are predisposed to pneumocystosis. Acquired immunodeficiencies stemming from impaired function of T lymphocytes are strongly associated with pneumocystosis: for example, malignancies (Hodgkin's disease, the histiocytic lymphomas, and the lymphatic leukemias) and treatment with glucosteroids, as given to patients with lymphoreticular malignancies and recipients of transplanted organs. Pneumocystosis continues to afflict malnourished infants, as in crowded refugee camps.

Confusion exists about the typical histologic pattern of pneumocystis pneumonia. The original descriptions often included the term *interstitial plasma cell pneumonia,* referring to pronounced infiltration of the interalveolar septa with plasma cells, as was seen in premature or malnourished children involved in nursery outbreaks of pneumocystosis. In contrast, infiltration with plasma cells is much less prominent in immunosuppressed patients cared for in medically sophisticated settings. The most striking finding in these patients is usually an intensely eosinophilic, foamy, or honeycombed material filling the alveoli. This material stains bright red with the paraaminosalicylic acid (PAS) stain and is composed primarily of inflammatory cells and degenerating pneumocysts. With the GMS stain, the cyst forms typically lie in the intraalveolar exudate. That is, the inflammatory process is primarily intraalveolar and not interstitial.

Pneumocystosis is almost always localized to the pulmonary tissues, and care must be taken to distinguish pneumocysts from similarly staining yeast forms in both pulmonary and extrapulmonary sites. Extrapulmonary pneumocystosis has been reported but appears to be exceedingly rare.

Manifestations

When pneumocystosis is epidemic in malnourished children, the onset of the disease is slow and insidious, and the manifestations are nonspecific. Restlessness, languor, and poor feeding are common. Fever is either low grade or absent. Tachypnea, perioral cyanosis, and cough may appear; dyspnea is common, but signs of pneumonia are usually absent.

In contrast, patients with an underlying immunodeficiency who contract pneumocystosis may have a fulminant course. Typically, many of these patients have prodromal agitation, fever, an increased rate of respiration, and episodes of cough and dyspnea for 1 to 2 weeks. Moreover, a reduction in the dose of immunosuppressant medication (*e.g.*, a glucosteroid) not uncommonly antedates the onset of pneumocystosis. As the disease progresses, dyspnea is observed in more than 90% of the patients; it is generally associated with marked hypoxia and tachypnea—findings typically more severe than would be expected by the relatively minimal radiographic findings. Cough is present in about 50% of the patients and is productive—with or without hemoptysis—in fewer than 10%. Fever is observed in about 67% of the patients.

The typical roentgenographic picture in pulmonary pneumocystosis is one of bilateral perihilar and basilar infiltrates that progress to diffuse alveolar consolidation in 3 to 7 days. Exceptions such as the following are common: (1) Some patients have not had abnormal chest roentgenograms within hours of dying of pneumocystosis; (2) although atypical, initial nodular lesions or lobar consolidations have been described; (3) pleural effusions are present in fewer than 5% of patients and probably relate to the underlying disease; and (4) the finding of a mediastinal mass does not argue against infection of the lungs caused by *P. carinii.* Thus, there is no radiologic finding that positively includes or excludes the diagnosis of pneumocystosis, but most of the patients have a bilateral pneumonitis.

Diagnosis

There is no set of clinical and laboratory data on which the diagnosis of pneumocystis infection can be reliably made. A large number of other infectious processes may be confused with pneumocystosis and, indeed, may be present simultaneously: cytomegaloviral pneumonia, nocardiosis, aspergillosis, zygomycosis, lymphangitic spread of a neoplasm, postirradiation changes, mycoplasmal pneumonitis, viral pneumonitis, and bacterial pneumonia caused by either gram-positive or gram-negative agents. The unequivocal diagnosis of pneumocystosis rests upon identification of cyst or trophozoite forms in bronchial secretions or in lung tissue. Securing authentic pulmonary specimens safely is the problem.

There are several diagnostic approaches, which vary not only in degree of invasiveness but also in probability of yielding definitive information. Open lung biopsy still remains the standard against which all other procedures must be judged. Examination of expectorated sputum, tracheal aspiration, transtracheal aspiration, fiber, bronchoscopic biopsy (forceps or brush), bronchoalveolar lavage, and percutaneous-transthoracic needle biopsy have all been used with varying success. The last-named procedure carries a substantial risk of pneumothorax and hemorrhage in adults but appears to be safer in young children. However, hemorrhage and pneumothorax are risks with all invasive procedures involving the removal of pulmonary tissue. Thrombocytopenia and intrinsic clotting abnormalities are relative contraindications that may be corrected by appropriate transfusion therapy. If specimens obtained by one of the tracheal aspiration methods or by bronchoscopy do not yield a diagnosis, open lung biopsy should be carried out.

Prompt staining of imprints of fresh lung and smears of infralaryngeal respiratory tract secretions may yield the diagnosis within a few hours. Fixed and stained tissues and secretions are valuable because they may reveal specific histologic patterns and aid in differentiating pulmonary inflammatory processes; however, such preparations may be available for days after collection. The detection of cysts and trophozoites in pulmonary secretions or lung tissue is sufficient basis for initiating antipneumocystis tratment in a patient with a pneumonitis.

Because safe, well-tolerated therapy for pneumocystis infection is available, it has been suggested that patients with diffuse interstitial pneumonia should be treated empirically, and only those who fail to respond should then be subjected to lung biopsy. However, as *P. carinii* does not account for more than one-third of diffuse interstitial pneumonitides, other diseases treatable with alternative medications might be missed. In patients with pulmonary infiltrates and a malignant neoplasm, the infiltrates are more likely to be neoplastic than pneumocystic. However, if the risk of an invasive diagnostic procedure is high, empiric therapy is justified. Because pneumocysts disappear from the lung after a few days of treatment, posttherapy biopsy may reveal only nonspecific inflammation; the clinician is then left to speculate about the cause of the pulmonary process and the need to continue or change antimicrobial therapy.

Humoral antibodies against *P. carinii* can be measured by indirect immunofluorescence. However, a diagnostic rise in titer would be a retrospective finding limited only to immunocompetent patients. The other side of the immunologic coin—the detection of blood-borne antigens derived from *P. carinii* by counterimmunoelectrophoresis—is experimental and needs further evaluation.

Prognosis

As the very occurrence of pneumocystosis indicates ominous malfunction of immune defenses, the prognosis is grave without specific antipneumocystis therapy. The case fatality rate in untreated, malnourished, or premature infants exceeds 50%, and approaches 100% in untreated, immunocompromised patients.

With specific therapy, most patients recover from pneumocystosis. However, the long-term outlook depends upon control of the underlying disease. If immunosuppression is not relieved, the rate of recurrence may be as high as 15%.

Particularly in younger patients, successful therapy will result in complete roentgenologic clearing of the lungs. In a minority of adults, postinfectious fibrosis with impaired diffusion capacity has been described. It is not clear whether this is a sequel to the infection or an effect of concomitant chemotherapy or irradiation.

Therapy

The first step in therapy should be diminution of immunosuppression as extensively as possible depending on the clinical circumstances. This follows from the observation of the following: (1) spontaneous recovery when immunosuppressive treatment with withdrawn or decreased (as in recipients of transplanted organs); and (2) failure rates of 20% to 40% with presently available antipneumocystis chemotherapy.

Success in the treatment of pneumocystosis has attended the use of pentamidine alone, the combination of trimethoprim–sulfamethoxazole (TMP–SMX), and pyrimethamine plus a sulfonamide. Pentamidine isethionate is an investigational, antiprotozoal, aromatic diamidine; it was the first antimicrobic shown to be effective in pneumocystosis, reducing mortality to less than 5% in malnourished and premature infants. The recommended dosage of 4 mg/kg of body weight/day is usually injected IM as a single dose (two sites should be used in patients over 50 kg in weight). If there is a bleeding diathesis, the drug may be injected IV—slowly, cautiously, and with continuous monitoring of the blood pressure. Depending on the response, the treatment is continued for 10 to 20 days. In addition to cardiovascular collapse, adverse reactions include hypoglycemia, tachycardia, facial flushing, erythema, nausea, vomiting, and pleuritis. Renal failure has been reported in almost 25% of the patients, and approximately 25% have other untoward reactions, including hepatotoxicity. Pain, sterile abscesses, and hematomas at sites of IM injections are not uncommon.

A 1:5 combination of TMP–SMX may be given either by PO or IV. The recommended PO dose for both children and adults is 20 mg of TMP (with 100 mg of SMX)/kg body wt/day as three equal portions, 8-hourly. Some patients may not be able to swallow tablets; moreover, the absorption of TMP–SMX from the gut may be so poor that PO therapy fails. In such patients, TMP–SMX can be injected IV in the same dosage that is used for PO therapy. Regulation of dosage by measurements of concentrations in the blood is especially important if there is renal dysfunction; the desired peak concentrations (specimens obtained either 1 hour after a PO dose or within 5 minutes after completion of IV injection of a dose) are TMP 5 μg to 6 μg/ml, and SMX 100 μg to 150 μg/ml. Clinical improvement may not be apparent for 4 to 7 days; if there is a good effect, therapy should be continued for an additional 1 to 2 weeks (*i.e.,* up to a total of 21 days). A history of a severe adverse reaction to a sulfonamide is a contraindication to the use of TMP–SMX. Nausea, vomiting, and skin rash are prominent among the relatively few adverse reactions to TMP–SMX. Bone marrow depression from the TMP is quite uncommon and may be overcome by administering folinic acid without nullifying the antipneumocystis efficacy of TMP.

Pentamidine and TMP–SMX appear to be equivalent in efficacy (*i.e.,* defervescence and clearing of pulmonary infiltrates result in 60% to 80% of patients. TMP–SMX is the treatment of first choice because it is less toxic than pentamidine. Yet, there are patients who will respond to pentamidine and not to TMP–SMX. Decision as to when to shift treatment is based on clinical assessment: If a patient remains stable but does not improve, therapy need not be changed until appropriate treatment (as verified by measurements of concentrations of TMP and SMX in the blood) has been given for 7 days; however, progressive impairment of oxygenation with a worsening of pulmonary involvement by serial roentgenograms during 4 days of appropriate treatment is indication for change. There is no evidence that addition of pentamidine to TMP–SMX is beneficial. One of the most important aspects of ongoing clinical evaluation of treatment must be due consideration of the possibility of concomitant pulmonary infection with another microorganism (*e.g,* cytomegalovirus; see Chap. 75, Cytomegalovirus Infection).

Although the combination of pyrimethamine plus sulfadiazine has been used successfully to treat proven pneumocystosis, there has been less experience with this regimen than with either pentamidine or TMP–SMX. Also, the toxic potential of pyrimethamine (bone marrow depression) is considerably greater than that of TMP (see Chap. 129, Toxoplasmosis). The usual dosage of pyrimethamine is 1 mg/kg body weight/day given PO as a single dose (all ages); the preferred sulfonamide is trisulfapyrimidines, 70 mg to 100 mg/kg body weight/day as four equal portions, 6-hourly, PO (the lower dose for adults, the higher for children).

Prevention

Trimethoprim–sulfamethoxazole in a dose of 4 mg to 8 mg of TMP/kg body weight/day as two equal portions, 12-hourly, PO (with 20 mg–40 mg SMX/kg body weight/day as two equal portions, 12-hourly, PO) has been remarkably effective in the prevention of pneumocystosis in children with lymphocytic leukemia. However, prophylactic use has not been rigorously assessed in other situations that predispose to pneumocystosis. Moreover, there is great variability in the incidence of pneumocystosis as a function of time and institution. Thus, routine chemoprophylaxis using TMP–SMX is not recommended unless there is a recognized problem with pneumocystosis. For example, recipients of bone marrow grafts frequently contract pneumocystosis, and so prophylaxis in such patients has been advocated. Because of the association of cytomegalovirus infection with pneumocystosis in recipients of renal homografts, it has been suggested that all such patients shown to be infected with cytomegalovirus be given TMP–SMX.

Remaining Problems

The present inability to grow *P. carinii in vitro* seriously hampers diagnosis. A noninvasive method for reliably diagnosing pneumocystosis is badly needed.

The impact of the widespread use of TMP–SMX in the treatment and prevention of bacterial infections on the effectiveness of this combination against *P. carinii* requires evaluation.

Bibliography

Books

ROBBINS JB, DEVITA VINCENT T JR, DUTZ W (eds): Symposium on *Pneumocystis carinii* infection. Bethesda, National Cancer Institute Monograph No. 43, 1976. 223 pp.

YOUNG LS (ed): *Pneumocystis carinii* Pneumonia: Pathogenesis, Diagnosis, and Treatment. New York, Marcel Dekker, 1981

Journals

BURKE BA, GOOD RA: *Pneumocystis carinii* infection. Medicine 52:23–51, 1973

DUTZ W: *Pneumocystis carinii* pneumonia. Pathol Annu 5:309–349, 1970

FRENKEL JK, GOOD JT, SCHULTZ JA: Latent pneumocystis infection of rats, relapse, and chemotherapy. Lab Invest 15: 1559–1577, 1966

GAJDUSEK DC: *Pneumocystis carinii*—etiologic agent of interstitial plasma cell pneumonia of premature and young infants. Pediatrics 19:543–565, 1957

HUGHES WT, FELDMAN S, CHAUDHARY SC, OSSI MJ, COX F, SANYAL SK: Comparison of pentamidine isethionate and trimethoprim–sulfamethoxazole in the treatment of *Pneumocystis carinii* pneumonia. J Pediatr 92:285–291, 1978

HUGHES WT, KUHN S, CHANDHARY S FELDMAN S, VERZOSA M, RHOMES JAA, PRATT C, GEORGE SL: Successful chemoprophylaxis for *Pneumocystis carinii* pneumonitis. N Engl J Med 297:1419–1426, 1977

HUGHES WT, PRICE RA, KIM HG, COBURN TP, GRIGSBY D, FELDMAN S: *Pneumocystis carinii* pneumonitis in children with malignancies. J. Pediatr 82:404–415, 1973

LAU WK, YOUNG LS: Trimethoprim–sulfamethoxazole treatment of *Pneumocystis carinii* pneumonia in adults. N Engl J Med 295:716–718, 1976

NORMAN L, KAGAN IG: Some observations on the serology of

Pneumocystis carinii infections in the United States. Infect Immun 8:317–321, 1973

WALZER PD, PERL DP, KROGSTAD DJ, RAWSON PG, SCHULTZ MG: *Pneumocystis carinii* pneumonia in the United States: Epidemiologic, diagnostic and clinical features. Ann Intern Med 80:83–93, 1974

WALZER PD, SCHULTZ MG, WESTERN KA, ROBBINS JB: *Pneumocystis carinii* pneumonia and primary immune deficiency disease of infancy and childhood. J Pediatr 82:416–422, 1973

WESTERN KA, PERERA DR, SCHULTZ MG: Pentamidine isethionate in the treatment of *Pneumocystis carinii* pneumonia. Ann Intern Med 73:695–702, 1970

WINSTON DJ, LAU WK, GALE RP, YOUNG LS: Trimethoprim–sulfamethoxazole for the treatment of *Pneumocystis carinii* pneumonia. Ann Intern Med 92:762–769, 1980.

PHILIP D. MARSDEN

Paragonimiasis

46

Paragonimiasis is a chronic pulmonary infection of humans caused by adult hermaphroditic flukes living in cystic spaces in the lungs.

Etiology

Measuring 0.8 cm to 1.6 cm in length by 0.4 cm to 0.8 cm in width, *Paragonimus westermani* is a reddish brown, plump, oval fluke that resembles a coffee bean. The flukes occur singly or in pairs in the lung parenchyma, where they feed on exudates secreted by the host. They live for 5 to 6 years, producing oval, yellowish brown, operculated ova (85 × 35 μm) that are coughed up in thick, blood-stained sputum. Under favorable conditions, the ova hatch, producing miracidia that invade specific snails, (*e.g.,* of the genus *Semisulcospira*). Subsequently, cercariae are produced by the snails; these encyst as metacercariae in the muscles and viscera of freshwater crabs and crayfish. Humans acquire the infection by eating these crustaceans raw or partly cooked. In the gut, larval flukes are released from the metacercariae, penetrate through the wall of the gut, and usually migrate from the peritoneal cavity through the diaphragm to the lung. Occasionally, they mature in the abdomen or brain.

Epidemiology

Paragonimus westermani is widely distributed in the Far East and is an important cause of human infection in China, Japan, Vietnam, Korea, Taiwan, the Philippines, and Thailand. Infection also occurs in parts of India and South America. In Africa, *Paragonimus africanus* is found in Nigeria, Cameróun, and Zaire. Two other species, *Paragonimus skrjabini* and *Paragonimus heterotrema,* are rarely pathogens in man. The natural nonhuman reservoirs of the disease include a wide range of animal hosts but are mainly feline.

Pathogenesis and Pathology

As the larval parasite tunnels into the periphery of the lung, an eosinophilic inflammatory reaction is produced. Later, the adult fluke occupies a cystic space demarcated by a fibrous tissue wall (Fig. 46-1). The cysts usually communicate with a bronchus and often become secondarily infected, with formation of abscesses. The death of the flukes is often followed by calcification. Ova may be aspirated back into the lungs, leading to an eosinophilic, inflammatory response and the formation of small granulomas.

The temporal and occipital lobes of the brain are occasionally sites of eosinophilic granulomas that contain flukes and rarely ova. Transverse myelitis has been reported. In the peritoneal cavity, flukes produce adhesions and abscesses. With ulceration of the intestine, ova will be passed in the feces. Adult flukes have been found in many other organs, including the intestine, spermatic cord, testis, scrotum, vagina, and muscles. Granulomas in the subcutaneous tissues of the thoracic and abdominal wall may also contain adult flukes.

Manifestations

Pulmonary paragonimiasis is associated with persistent hemoptysis, breathlessness on exertion, pleural pain, and recurrent pulmonary infections. Clubbing of the fingers is common, and persistent crepitations may be heard over affected lung segments. Lung abscess may be present. Pneumothorax, pleural effusion, and empyema are rare complications. Roentgen-

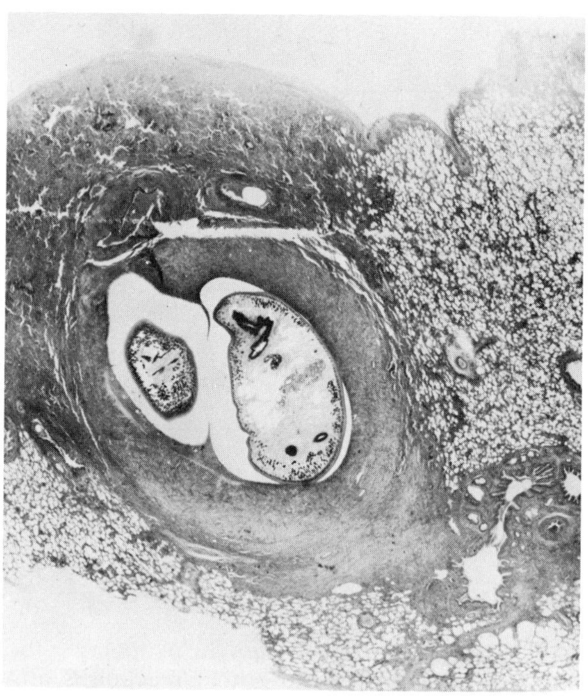

Fig. 46-1. Cross section of adult *Paragonimus westermani* encysted in lung. (Original magnification approximately × 20) (Ross JA, Kershaw WE, Kurowski AC: Br J Radiol 25:579–583, 1952)

ographic examination of the lungs will disclose infiltrates early in the disease. Later, dense nodular opacities and ring shadows indicate the sites of cysts. There are rarely more than 20 parasites in the lungs. Pleural adhesions and calcifications are late signs. Tuberculosis may coexist in some patients.

In one series, 25% of patients with pulmonary paragonimiasis also had cerebral symptoms. Cerebral paragonimiasis becomes clinically evident with signs of space-occupying lesions (Jacksonian epilepsy, paresis of varying degrees, and visual disturbances). The protein concentration in the cerebrospinal fluid is increased, and eosinophils are present. There may be intracerebral calcifications in radiograms of the skull.

Diagnosis

Demonstration of the ova of *P. westermani* in blood-stained sputum is diagnostic of paragonimiasis (Fig. 46-2) (see Chap. 11, Diagnostic Methods for Protozoa and Helminths). One-third of such patients also have ova in their feces either from sputum that has been swallowed or from a coincidental intestinal lesion. Precipitin tests (carried out either with crude or fractionated antigens), intradermal tests, and complement fixation tests all have been used for diagnosis. The complement fixation test is usually positive when living parasites are present, although there are cross reactions with other trematode infections.

Pulmonary paragonimiasis may resemble bronchiectasis, lung abscess, bronchial carcinoma, or most important of all, pulmonary tuberculosis. Cerebral paragonimiasis mimics other space-occupying lesions, including cysticercosis, hydatid cyst, and other helminthic lesions of the brain.

Fig. 46-2. Eggs of *Paragonimus westermani* in sputum. (Original magnification approximately × 200) (Courtesy of the Wellcome Museum of Medical Science, London)

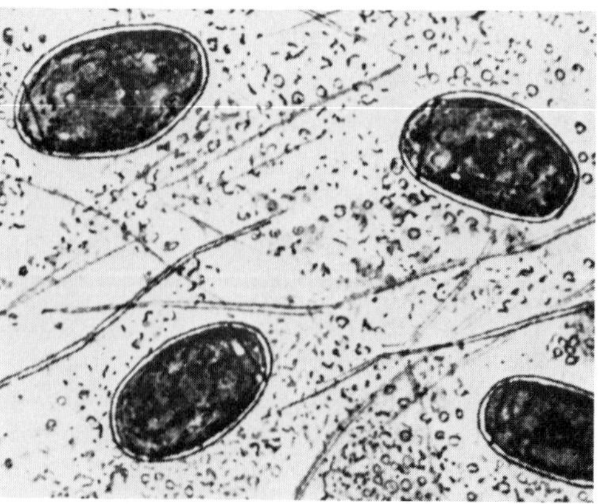

Prognosis

Fatalities are rare. The pulmonary lesions resolve spontaneously in 5 to 10 years. Some 2% of patients with lung paragonimiasis also have pulmonary tuberculosis. Cerebral involvement may be associated with persistent epilepsy.

Treatment

Bithionol (Actamer, Biton) is 2,2-thio,bis(4,6-dichlorophenol). It is given orally in a dosage of 30 mg/kg body wt on alternate days for 20 days. Skin reactions and gastrointestinal irritation are rarely severe enough to interrupt treatment. Results are better with bithionol than with either chloroquine or emetine, drugs used in the past. Granulomas containing adult flukes and ova may require surgical removal from the skin, testis, abdominal organs, or brain.

Prevention

It might be though a simple matter to dissuade people from eating raw, fresh salted, pickled, or imperfectly cooked crabs and crayfish, but such is not the case. Drunken crab, a favorite dish in the Far East, involves immersing live crabs in alcohol before consumption. In Korea and West Africa, fresh crab juice is used to treat measles. Such local customs, often involving esteemed gastronomic delicacies, are not easily relinquished.

Bibliography

Books

MIYAZADI I, HISHIMURA K: Cerebral paragonimiasis. In Hornabrook RW (ed): Topics in Tropical Neurology. Philadelphia, FA Davis, 1975. pp 109–132.

YOKOGAWA M: Paragonimus and paragonimiasis. In Dawes B (ed): Advances in Parasitology, Vol VIII. London, Academic Press, 1969. pp 375–387.

Journals

CHANG HT, WANG CW, YU CF, HSU CF, FANG JC: Paragonimiasis: A clinical study of 200 adult cases. Chin Med J 77: 3–9, 1958

SADUN EH, BUCK AA: Paragonimiasis in South Korea: Immunodiagnostic epidemiologic, clinical roentgenologic and therapeutic studies. Am J Trop Med Hyg 9:562–599, 1960

YOKOGAWA M, OKWA T, TSUJI M, IWASAKI M, SHIGEYASU M: Chemotherapy of paragonimiasis with bithionol. III. The follow-up studies for one year after treatment with bithionol. Jap J Parasitol 11:103–116, 1962

YOKOGAWA S, CORT WW, YOKOGAWA M: Paragonimus and paragonimiasis. Exp Parasitol 10:81–137, 139–205, 1960

Section | *VII*

Pleural Infections

Indigenous Microbiota of the Pleuras

(None)

SYDNEY M. FINEGOLD

Empyema

47

Empyema refers to the collection of a purulent, inflammatory exudate in the pleural cavity. It may be an acute or a chronic process. Acute empyema is invariably secondary to infection or disease elsewhere, most commonly a pulmonary infection.

Etiology

Staphylococcus aureus is the most common cause of thoracic empyema, accounting for about a third of the cases. Various gram-negative aerobic or facultatively anaerobic bacilli (particularly *Pseudomonas aeruginosa,* and also *Escherichia coli, Klebsiella* spp., and *Proteus* spp.) may cause thoracic empyema.

The same anaerobic bacteria commonly involved in necrotizing pneumonia and lung abscess may also cause empyema, usually as part of the same process. These bacteria (see Chap. 32, Necrotizing Pneumonias and Lung Abscess) are found in about 65% of cases of empyema that arise spontaneously (*i.e.,* nonpostoperative empyemas), and are the exclusive isolates in 50% of such cases. Various aerobic streptococci (including *Streptococcus pyogenes,* and viridans and enterococcal groups of streptococci), *Mycobacterium tuberculosis,* and fungi account for most of the rest of the cases. *Actinomyces israelii* and *Nocardia asteroides* are uncommon but important causes of empyema (see Chap. 37, Nocardiosis, and Chap. 38, Actinomycosis).

Epidemiology

Effective treatment of pneumonias with antimicrobial agents has reduced the frequency of empyema to less than 1%. However, the incidence is higher in necrotizing pneumonias. A significant cause of empyema today is infection after thoracic surgery.

Pathogenesis and Pathology

Acute empyema usually arises by extension from pneumonia or lung abscess. Extension from mediastinal lymph nodes or paravertebral asbcesses occurs primarily in granulomatous infections. Microorganisms may be introduced from the outside in relation to surgery or trauma. Empyema may also result from seeding during septicemia. Intraabdominal infection may extend into the pleural space directly or by way of the lymphatics or bloodstream. Rupture of the esophagus may lead to empyema.

The pathology may be divided into three phases, although the process is actually continuous. The exudative phase is the early response, with thin fluid and a low cell count. The fibrinopurulent stage is characterized by the accumulation of polymorphonuclear leukocytes and fibrin. This exudate tends to accumulate posteriorly and laterally and to become loculated. Finally, during the organizing phase, fibroblasts produce an inelastic membrane commonly referred to as "the peel."

Manifestations

Common findings are intermittent fever, sweating, chest pain, anemia, leukocytosis, and weight loss. The physical findings are those of pleural effusion; they may be limited to a small area or may be undetectable.

Diagnosis

Diagnosis is based on the demonstration of purulent pleural fluid. Lateral decubitus films and fluoroscopy may be helpful in localizing small empyemas, and ultrasound may distinguish between liquid and other roentgenographically similar substances. The following examinations of the pleural fluid should always be carried out: (1) volume; (2) color, consistency, and odor; (3) specific gravity; (4) pH; (5) total protein content; (6) red and white blood cell count and differential; (7) gram stain and acid-fast stain; (8) wet mount for fungi; (9) culture for aerobic and anaerobic bacteria, (10) tubercle bacilli, and fungi; and (11) cytology. The fluid may vary from moderately cloudy material with fibrinous webs to actual pus. Foul-smelling pus is a definite indication of the presence of anaerobic bacteria. Pus associated with infection caused by group A *S. pyogenes* is typically thin and turbid. The leukocyte count of empyema fluid is variable early in the illness, consisting almost exclusively of polymorphonuclear leukocytes. The presence of significant numbers of mononuclear cells indicates either sterile effusion or granulomatous infection. When the specific gravity is 1.018 or higher, the protein concentration above 3 g/100 ml, and the lactic dehydrogenase level above 550 units, the effusion is inflammatory in origin. With infectious empyemas, the pH is less than 7.20. Both infections and malignant neoplasms may give rise to inflammatory exudates. The microbiologic examination of empyema fluid is of the greatest significance and must always include microscopic examination of a Gram-stained smear. Clues to specific causes (see Chap. 9, Microscopic Examinations, and Chap. 32, Necrotizing Pneumonias and Lung Abscess) may be quickly obtained by this simple examination. Counterimmunoelectrophoresis, coagglutination, or latex-particle agglutination may be useful in detecting soluble polysaccharides of pneumococci or *Haemophilus* spp. Thick, purulent exudates that are sterile on culture may sometimes relate to previous antimicrobial therapy. Much more commonly, however, such empyema fluids yield anaerobic or other less common microorganisms on special culture.

A bronchopleural fistula may follow necrotizing pleuropulmonary infections and active tuberculosis, or it may reflect residual neoplasia at the point of surgical resection. A bronchopleural fistula is likely when an air–fluid level is seen in the absence of a previous thoracentesis. Radiopaque dye may be used to demonstrate the extent of an empyema space and the specific segment to which a bronchopleural fistula leads.

It is very important to define the underlying process that results in empyema. Blood cultures and other appropriate studies should be obtained to rule out distant sites of infection. Underlying causes of associated pulmonary parenchymal disease should be sought (see Chap. 32, Necrotizing Pneumonias and Lung Abscess).

Prognosis

Most forms of empyema respond well to therapy, although the course of illness is frequently prolonged. The major complications of empyema are metastatic infections, perforation through the chest wall or rarely into the lung itself, and chronic empyema. Failure to obliterate the pleural space during the course of management of acute empyema may lead to chronic empyema.

Therapy

The principles of treatment of empyema include the use of appropriate antimicrobics, the provision of adequate drainage, and the obliteration of dead space. The reader is referred to Chapter 32, Necrotizing Pneumonias and Lung Abscess, for a discussion of antimicrobial therapy for the microorganisms that may be involved in empyema and in lung abscess. Therapy should be prolonged, often for months.

In the early exudative phase of empyema, intermittent, closed drainage by repeated thoracenteses may provide adequate drainage. However, if the patient remains toxic or fluid reaccumulates rapidly, continuous closed drainage by intercostal catheter is required. Open drainage at this stage might result in collapse of the lung. During the fibrinopurulent phase, thoracenteses are unsatisfactory, and delay in instituting adequate drainage only allows further coagulation and loculation. Closed intercostal drainage with suction may be effective, but open drainage with rib resection is usually required. Drainage tubes should not be removed until the cavity is totally obliterated. Enzymatic debridement has been disappointing.

Decortication—that is, removal of the entire empyema sac—allows free expansion of the lung to obliterate dead space; this procedure is seldom required. More extreme procedures are rarely necessary; these include a modified thoracoplasty with resection of most of the extrapleural contents, or the creation of an Eloesser flap. At times, a muscle flap may be required to close a bronchopleural fistula.

Prevention

The prompt and effective treatment of pneumonia and other infections is a preventative of empyema.

This is particularly important in necrotizing pneumonias (see Chap. 32, Necrotizing Pneumonias and Lung Abscess) because of the frequency of empyema in this condition. Good surgical technique and careful asepsis in the operating room and elsewhere in the hospital minimize postoperative empyema. The prophylactic administration of antimicrobics is not indicated as a routine in thoracic surgery.

Remaining Problems

Improvement of our ability to prevent hospital-acquired infection of all types is very much needed.

Bibliography

Journals

BARTLETT JG, GORBACH SL, THADEPALLI H, FINEGOLD SM: Bacteriology of empyema. Lancet 1:338–340, 1974

FINILAND M, BARNES MW: Changing ecology of acute bacterial empyema: Occurrence and mortality at Boston City Hospital during 12 selected years from 1935 to 1972. J Infect Dis 137:274–291, 1978

GUILLEMOT L, LAHELLE J, RIST E: Recherches bactériologiques et expérimentales sur les pleurésies putrides. Arch Med Exp Anat Pathol 16:571–640, 1904

LUTZ A, GROOTEN O, BERGER MA: Considérations à propos des germes isolés dans 638 cas de pleurésies purulentes. Strasbourg Med 2:119–128, 1963

WEESE WC, SHINDLER ER, SMITH IM, RABINOVICH J: Empyema of the thorax then and now. Arch Intern Med 131:516–520, 1973

Section VIII

Infrarenal Genitourinary Tract Infections

Indigenous Microbiota of the Infrarenal Urinary Tract

Species or Group	Anterior Urethra
Mycoplasmas	±
Bacteria	
Gram-positive cocci	
Staphylococcus epidermidis	++
Staphylococcus aureus	±
Anaerobic micrococci	+
Streptococcus mitis; undifferentiated α and γ streptococci	±
Enterococci or group D *Streptococcus* spp.	**2–10***
Gram-negative cocci	
Branhamella catarrhalis	
Gemella haemolysans	+
Gram-positive bacilli	
Lactobacillus spp.	+
Aerobic *Corynebacterium* spp.	+
Mycobacterium spp.	±
Aerobic gram-negative bacilli	
Enterobacteriaceae	+
Escherichia coli	+
Enterobacter spp.	±
Klebsiella spp.	+
Proteus mirabilis, other *Proteus* spp., *Morganella morganii, Providencia* spp.	+
Pseudomonas aeruginosa	+
Alcaligenes faecalis	±
Moraxella lacunata	±
Haemophilus parainfluenzae	**5**
Corynebacterium vaginale	±
Fungi	
Candida albicans	±
non-albicans *Candida* spp.	±
Torulopsis glabrata	±
Protozoa	
Trichomonas vaginalis	+

± to 0, rare; ±, irregular or uncertain (may be only pathologic); +, common; ++, prominant.

*Boldface values (*e.g.,* **30–60**) = range of incidence in percentage, rounded, in different surveys.

ALLAN R. RONALD
PAUL D. HOEPRICH

Urethritis and Cystitis

48

The urethra and urinary bladder are the commonest sites of infection in the urinary tract. Infection may be limited to one or the other, but, because it frequently coexists, combined discussion is appropriate. Also, symptoms are often not specific to either site.

Urethrocystitis results in symptoms that range from a minor annoyance to a painful distressing illness. However, its major significance lies in the possibility of spread of infection upward to the kidneys.

Etiology

Many infectious agents have been implicated as causes for urethrocystitis. *Herpes simplex, Chlamydia trachomatis, Ureaplasma urealyticum,* and *Neisseria gonorrhoeae,* important causes of urethritis, are descirbed in Chapter 91 (Infections Caused by Herpes Simplex Viruses), Chapter 55 (Non-Gonococcal Urethritis), and Chapter 56 (Gonococcal Infections). Gram-negative bacilli of the family Enterobacteriaceae are responsible for almost 90% of all episodes of bacterial urethrocystitis. Anaerobic bacteria rarely cause urinary tract infections.

The Enterobacteriaceae are gram-negative bacilli 2 μm to 3 μm long by 0.6 μm in transverse diameter. They are aerobic and facultatively anaerobic, growing well on artificial culture mediums. All species ferment glucose. They are found in all animals and plants, often as nonpathogenic resident microbiota. A number of genera have been defined in the family as a result of common biochemical and antigenic properties.

Escherichia coli ferments lactose and are usually differentiated on the basis of biochemical tests that include the formation of indole, the production of acid from the glucose, and the inability to use citrate as the sole source of carbon. In addition, there is an antigenic mosaic provided by the following: group-specific, somatic, heat-stable, lipoprotein–polysaccharide O antigens (150 groups); type-specific, heat-labile, flagellar H antigens (50 types); envelope, or sheath, K antigens that are also heat labile (90 types). An isolate of *E. coli* from the urinary tract of a patient with acute urethrocystitis is almost always serologically identical with a strain of *E. coli* present in the feces of the same patient. Community-acquired *E. coli* is characteristically susceptible to a wide variety of antimicrobics (Table 48-1).

Klebsiella spp., *Enterobacter* spp., and *Serratia* spp. also usually ferment lactose but are generally the obverse of *E. coli* in other biochemical capabilities. They also differ from *Proteus* spp. and *Providencia* spp. in their relatively meager elaboration of urease and oxidative deaminases. The *Klebsiella* spp. are typically nonmotile and neither liquefy gelatin nor decarboxylate ornithine. They can be differentiated on the basis of 80 K (capsular) and 11 O (somatic) antigens. *Klebsiella* spp. are often susceptible *in vitro* to the cephalosporins. They are, however, resistant to ampicillin and more antimicrobics than is *E. coli* (Table 48-1).

Enterobacter spp. are motile and decarboxylate ornithine. Resistance to antimicrobial agents is more widespread than with *Klebsiella* spp. (Table 48-1).

Serratia spp. sometimes produce pigment (pink, red, magenta), although most pathogenic strains are nonpigmented when grown on ordinary culture mediums. The nonpigmented strains are differentiated on the basis of biochemical reactions (deoxyribonucleases and decarboxylases). *Serratia* spp. are almost always hospital acquired by patients with indwelling urethral catheters who are under treatment with antimicrobics.

Among the Enterobacteriaceae, *Proteus* spp., *Providencia* spp., and *Morganella* spp. have a remarkable ability to oxidatively deaminate aminoacids (*e.g.,* phenylalanine to phenylpyruvic acid). In addition, *Proteus* spp. and *Morganella* spp. rapidly split urea. Differentiation on the basis of unique antigenicity can

Table 48-1. *Disc Susceptibility of Common Gram-Negative Aerobic Bacilli**

		% Of Strains Susceptible										
	NO. OF STRAINS	AMPI-CILLIN	CEPHA-LOTHIN	CEFOX-ITIN	GENTA-MICIN	TETRA-CYCLINE	CHLORAM-PHENICOL	SULPHA-DIAZINE	NALIDIXIC ACID	NITRO-FURANTOIN	TRIMETHOPRIM–SULFAMETHOXAZOLE
Escherichia coli	2450	71	86	97	99	78	94	69	99	99	93
Klebsiella pneumoniae	445	14	97	97	99	92	95	72	99	70	90
Klebsiella oxytoca	247	4	84	96	99	98	94	86	98	88	97
Enterobacter spp.	276	16	14	26	99	88	96	94	99	86	96
Serratia spp.	78	4	24	64	99	11	91	4	99	8	94
Proteus											
mirabilis	537	81	93	99	99	<1	97	88	96	8	97
Indole positive†	85	24	20	92	97	56	99	65	99	24	90
Providencia spp.‡	105	45	65	86	68	65	60	12	85	8	15
Pseudomonas aerugiosa§	1362	<1	<1	<1	89						

* Based on consecutive isolates recovered at the University of Manitoba Health Sciencies Centre, January–June, 1981. Unpublished data from Gratton C, Ronald AR.

† Includes *Morganella morganii* and *Providencia rettgeri* as well as *Proteus vulgaris.*

‡ Does not include *Providencia rettgeri.*

§ 78% are susceptible to carbenicillin and ticarcillin.

now be carried out. Strains of *Proteus mirabilis* are relatively susceptible to penicillin G, ampicillin, the acylureidopenicillins, and many cephalosporins. *Proteus vulgaris, Providencia* spp., and *Morganella* spp. are resistant to many clinically useful antimicrobics with the exception of gentamicin–tobramycin–netilmicin–amikacin, carbenicillin–ticarcillin, the acylureidopenicillins, and the newer cephalosporins.

Pseudomonas aeruginosa, although not Enterobacteriaceae, are motile gram-negative bacilli that cause urethrocystitis—almost always secondary to urinary tract instrumentation. The production of water-soluble pigments (pyocyanin—bluish green, nonfluorescent; fluorescein—yellowish green, fluorescent) and the elaboration of indophenol oxidase are useful identifying characteristics. In addition, when there are high densities of *P. aeruginosa* either in culture mediums or in lesions, a characteristic sweet, fruity odor can be detected. Gentamicin–tobramycin–netilmicin–amikacin, carbenicillin–ticarcillin, and the acylureidopenicillins are active *in vitro,* displaying true synergism with about two-thirds of strains.

Among the gram-positive organisms, enterococcal *Streptococus* spp. (Lancefield Group D) and *Streptococcus aglactiae* (Lancefield Group B) each cause about 2% of episodes of urethrocystitis. *Staphylococcus aureus* is rarely isolated and usually is secondary to hematogenous renal infection. However, coagulase-negative *Staphylococcus* spp. are important urinary tract pathogens. *Staphylococcus saprophyticus* (formerly *Micrococcus* spp. subgroup 3), identified by its resistance to novobiocin, is the second most common cause of urethrocystitis in sexually active young females. *Staphylococcus epidermidis* is often a nosocomial pathogen in patients with indwelling urethral catheters.

Candida albicans and other *Candida* spp. may cause urinary infection without evidence of renal involvement—a situation most often encountered in patients with diabetes mellitus or indwelling urinary catheters. However, candiduria may be a clue to renal candidal infection resulting from bloodborne dissemination (see Chap. 39, Candidosis). Immunoincompetent patients and recipients of renal transplants appear to be vulnerable to candidal urinary tract infections. In the same clinical settings, *Torulopsis glabrata* is second in frequency to *Candida albicans.* Because of the high frequency of occurrence of *Candida* spp. and *T. glabrata* as normal residents of the mucous membranes in the vicinity of the external urethral meatus, documentation of funguria may require quantitative culture of urine obtained by suprapubic percutaneous aspiration (cystocentesis).

Viruria has been documented with many viruses, generally in association with viremia. Viruria in the absence of viremia probably represents viral replication in glomeruli or tubules or elsewhere in the urinary tract. Viral urinary tract infections may occur as acute illnesses (acute hemorrhagic cystitis in children caused by adenovirus type 11), during convalescence from viral infections that clinically did not involve the urinary tract (mumps, cytomegalovirus), and in persons in apparent good health (cytomegalovirus). Further, culture of renal tissue has yielded adenoviruses, cytomegaloviruses, coxsackieviruses, measles virus, and varicella virus in the absence of viruria. Although morphologic changes have been observed in the urinary tract with infections caused by cytomegalovirus (intranuclear inclusions in renal tubular cells; see Fig. 75-1*B*), measles (giant cells with inclusion bodies, characteristic of measles virus in Bowman's capsule, tubular epithelium, and ureteral and bladder mucosa), and adenovirus type 11 (acute hemorrhagic cystitis in children), functional changes (*e.g.,* reduced creatinine clearance) have been demonstrated only in association with mumps virus viruria.

Epidemiology

Because the infectious agents that cause urethrocystitis are drawn primarily from a person's own resident microbiota, the epidemiology of the disease should relate to factors within the person that make infection possible. In females, many factors have been suggested as precipitating events for infection, but most are poorly understood.

The incidence of the symptom complex referred to as dysuria syndrome has been delineated in population surveys of females. About one female in five experiences dysuria each year; approximately one-third of these symptomatic females will consult a physician for this complaint. In general practice, symptoms originating in the lower urinary tract will result in 6 physician visits per 100 patient years in females in their twenties. Most females experience an episode of urethrocystitis at some time during their life; about 5% of females have frequent episodes. The onset of urethrocystitis in females is often associated with initiation of an active sexual life.

Bacterial urinary tract infection in males occurs with prostatic hypertrophy and impairment of emptying of the urinary bladder. Instrumentation frequently antedates acquisition of bacteriuria.

The prevalence of bacteriuria in elderly people may be as high as 30%. Symptoms of urethrocystitis are common in this age group, but correlation between lower urinary tract symptoms and the presence of bacteriuria is poorly established.

Hospital-acquired urinary infections usually follow urethral instrumentation or continuous urethral catheter drainage. Infected urine is frequently a reservoir for cross infection with fomites and the hands of health care personnel acting as the vector between patients.

Pathogenesis and Pathology

The urethra has a normal flora consisting of diphtheroids, *Staphylococcus* spp., *Streptococcus* spp., and a variety of anaerobes. Colonization is heaviest in the distal urethra (Fig. 48-1). *Escherichia coli* and other enteric gram-negative bacilli are not normally present in large numbers in the human urethra or on the mucosal perineum. Females with a propensity to frequent urinary tract infections may be densely colonized for prolonged periods on the perineum. It is presumed that an altered biology, perhaps related to specific receptor sites on epithelial cells, permits perineal carriage of these potential pathogens. Although the male urethra is sometimes colonized with the same gram-negative bacilli present on the introitus of the sexual partner, there is no evidence to indicate that the male is a reservoir for infection in the female.

The urethra of the adult female is about 4 cm long, and its internal surface is punctuated by the orifices of numerous paraurethral glands. Bacteria resident in the urethra frequently gain access to the bladder. Although the role of sexual intercourse in the pathogenesis of urinary infection is undefined, almost certainly the minor urethral trauma and pressure that occur with intercourse can propel organisms into the bladder.

Fig. 48-1. Frequency of colonization of the urethra as a function of the distance inward from the external meatus. The single narrow column defined by a dotted outline refers to observations at the approximate midpoint of the female urethra; the columns marked by solid lines refer to studies in males. (After Helmholz HF: J Urol 64:158–166, 1950)

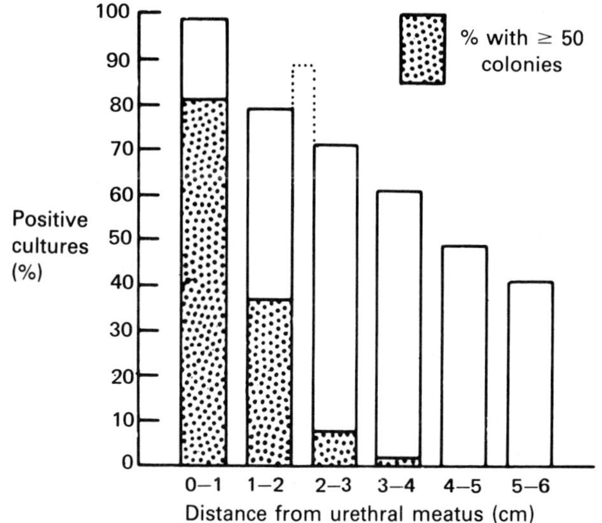

Voiding, with the flushing action of the outflow of urine, maintains the normal sterility of the bladder. Anatomic or physiologic abnormalities that lead to incomplete emptying of the urinary bladder facilitate bacterial infections. These abnormalities include congenital anomalies, urethral strictures, bladder diverticula, cystoceles, and prostatic enlargement.

Urine is a good culture medium *in vitro* for urinary pathogens. Although organisms grow less well in urine at a low *p*H (<5.5) and in hyperosmolar urine, manipulation of these parameters has not been shown to influence the acquisition of bacteriuria or to alter symptoms. Constipation, infrequent voiding, and incomplete emptying of the bladder may also influence urinary hydrodynamics and facilitate the persistence of microorganisms.

A poorly understood antibacterial mechanism intrinsic in the bladder mucosa is thought to prevent bacterial multiplication in the thin film of urine persisting on the bladder mucosa after complete voiding.

Both symptomatic and asymptomatic bacteriuria may spontaneously resolve without specific antibacterial treatment. Presumably, voiding and other host defenses clear the bacteria from the bladder. The role played by humoral and cell-mediated immunologic mechanisms is unknown.

Urinary symptoms appear to result from involvement of the mucous membranes lining the urethra and the bladder in a neutrophile-rich inflammatory response engendered by the infection. With severe inflammation, extravasation of blood may result, yielding a hemorrhagic cystitis. Organism or host factors that either lead to acute, symptomatic urethrocystitis or, permit asymptomatic bacteriuria for months or years are not understood.

Manifestations

The classic manifestations of lower urinary tract infection—dysuria (discomfort, pain, burning, stinging on urination), urgency, and frequency—are referable to inflammation of the urethra. Cystitis, on the other hand, produces suprapubic pain and tenderness. Ordinarily, there are no systemic manifestations as a result of urethrocystitis. Fever above 38°C (100.4°F) or true chills are indicative of renal or prostatic infection.

In some patients, the urine is grossly bloody. Excessive cloudiness of the urine may be noted when pyuria is dense. With some bacterial species, the urine may be malodorous.

On physical examination, the urethral orifice may be inflamed. The presence of pus at the urethral orifice is often caused by infection with *Neisseria gonorrhoeae* (see Chap. 56, Gonococcal Infections). There is ordinarily no local tenderness, although in some patients suprapubic palpation elicits tenderness referable to the inflamed bladder. In the female, it may be possible to demonstrate a urethrocele and stress-induced urinary incontinence. In the male, on rectal examination, prostatic enlargement may at times be evident. It should be emphasized that, in many men, hypertrophy of the prostate is not symmetric. The median lobe may undergo sufficient hypertrophy to interfere with urination, whereas the posterior lobe, by rectal examination, is normal in size.

Many females with the symptoms of urethrocystitis have a concomitant vaginal discharge, and irritation is noted as urine passes over the labia to cause the so-called external dysuria. In these patients, careful pelvic examination with appropriate investigation to diagnose infections such as trichomoniasis, candidosis, genital herpes, or other causes of vulvovaginitis is mandatory (see Chap. 50, Infections of the Female Genital Tract).

Diagnosis

Laboratory confirmation of bacteriuria is essential if the diagnosis of bacterial urethrocystitis is to be made with assurance. Clinical criteria cannot distinguish between bacterial urinary infections and symptom complexes without bacteriuria.

Bacterial contamination of the urine during micturition is unavoidable, and even collection of a specimen by urethral catheterization is no guarantee that the specimen will not be contaminated with microbiota resident in the urethra. Moreover, gram-negative bacillary contaminants may replicate rapidly in urine held at room temperature after collection. For these reasons, quantitative culture of urine was introduced to distinguish simple contamination of urine during collection from actual infection of the urinary tract on the premise that the greater the number of bacteria per unit volume of urine, the greater the probability of infection in the urinary tract. The term *true bacteriuria* is generally taken to mean there are at least 10^5 bacteria/ml of bladder urine. The connotation is that the probability of bacterial urinary tract infection is very high when there are more than 10^5 bacteria/ml (Fig. 48-2). However, it should never be assumed that the detection of fewer than 10^5 bacteria/ml excludes bacterial urinary tract infection. Indeed, detection of fewer than 10^5/ml in specimens collected without urethral contamination, as by

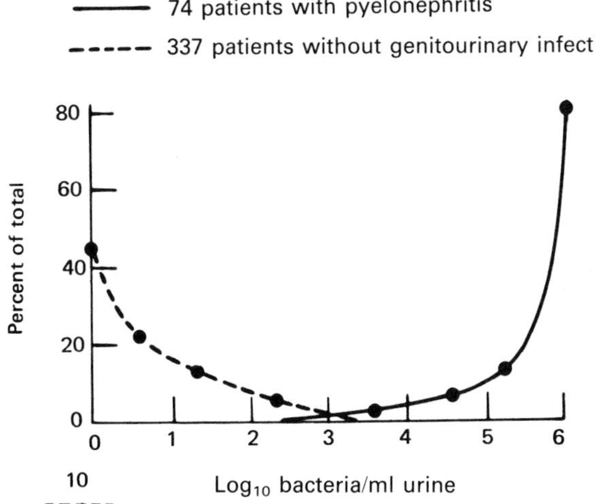

Fig. 48-2. Relationship bacteriuria in normals and patients with urinary tract infections clinically evident as acute pyelonephritis. (After Kass EH: Trans Assoc Am Phys 69:56–64, 1956)

cystocentesis, is diagnostic of "low count" urinary tract infection.

A specimen collected after the urethra has been flushed with the passage of about 100 ml of urine is referred to as a *clean-voided, midstream specimen.* When cultured promptly after collection or after refrigeration for no more than 6 hours, such a single specimen yields valid results at least 80% of the time. If two such specimens are collected at different times, the results of quantitative cultures are comparable in their validity to the result obtained with one specimen collected by urethral catherization.

Contamination of urine during the course of collection can be avoided entirely by suprapubic percutaneous aspiration of urine from the bladder—cystocentesis. This procedure can be carried out quite safely in patients who do not have a bleeding diathesis and who have a full bladder. The skin of the abdomen is cleansed with 70% ethanol at a point in the midline about one-third the distance from the symphysis pubis to the umbilicus; a 1½-inch 20-gauge needle affixed to a 20-ml syringe is passed through the skin into the bladder. Negative pressure is maintained on the syringe after insertion through the skin. Local anesthesia is unnecessary.

Numerous methods have been devised for the detection of bacteriuria. By far the simplest is mciroscopic examination performed immediately by the physician. A small drop or a bacteriologic loopful of freshly voided, uncentrifuged urine should be placed on a clean glass slide and allowed to extend as far as innate surface tension permits. When the urine has dried, it is fixed by gentle heating in a gas flame before Gram staining. One or more bacteria in each oil immersion filed correlate with more than 10^5 bacteria/ml of urine (see Fig. 52-4*A*). When 4 or 5 fields must be searched before bacteria are found, the count is probably lower, but in excess of 10^4 bacteria/ml. With experience, the correlation of smear examination with quantitative culture of the urine is in the neighborhood of 90%. In addition to being rapid and inexpensive, this procedure provides preliminary identification.

Quantitative loop culture of urine is precise and enables the direct categorization of bacteriuria into the three groupings of clinical interest: (1) equal to or greater than 10^5 per ml of urine; (2) 10^4 to 10^5 per ml of urine; and (3) fewer than 10^4 per ml of urine. It is quick and inexpensive in that two platinum loops, designed to pick up 10^{-3} and 10^{-2} ml of urine, respectively, are used to prepare half-plate streak cultures. The plates are inspected after overnight incubation, and the decision on the category of bacteriuria is readily made. The precision of colony counting to the last unit digit is unnecessary.

If the aim of the urine culture is simply to screen for infection—that is, the simple determination of the presence or absence of bacteriuria—a dip-inoculum culture is adequate. This technique makes use of an inexpensive, disposable plastic device that contains a small amount of culture medium. Inoculation is carried out simply by dipping the portion of the device bearing the culture medium into the urine specimen or by having the patient void over the agar surface. The inoculum that is deposited is a function of the surface area of the culture medium. By correlation with more precise techniques, interpretive factors have been derived that enable one to decide whether or not more than 10^5 bacteria/ml of urine were present.

Females with lower urinary tract symptoms whose urine fails to yield more than 10^5 bacteria/ml on culture have been considered to have an acute urethral syndrome or abacteriuric urethrocystitis. However, when urine is obtained from such females by cystocentesis, it frequently contains 10^4 to 10^5 bacteria/ml. That is, the typical symptoms of bacterial urethrocystitis may be provoked by low-count bacteriuria.

Urinary frequency, diuresis, and incomplete treatment may contribute to a reduced colony count in the presence of symptomatic infection. Some females with the acute urethral syndrome will have urethrocystitis caused by sexually transmitted pathogens, particularly *Chlamydia trachomatis* or *Neisseria gonorrhoeae.*

Radiologic and cystoscopic investigation of the urinary tract rarely provides information important to the management of lower urinary tract infection in females. Infection presumed to involve the kidneys or unexplained findings such as persisting hematuria warrant these procedures. Repeated studies are unnecessary.

Localization of the Site of Urinary Infection

In males, localization of infection to the prostate or urethra is important and should be carried out according to the instructions provided in Chapter 49 (Bacterial Prostatitis and Recurrent Urinary Tract Infections). In females, no clear guidelines have been established for the diagnosis of infection limited to the urethra.

Renal infection is common in patients without symptoms or signs referable to the kidneys (see Chap. 52, Pyelonephritis). From 15% to 30% of females with acute urethrocystitis and almost 50% of females with asymptomatic bacteriuria have organisms originating in one or both kidneys. Renal infection requires more intensive and prolonged therapy and more extensive investigation; it therefore puts the patient at greater risk of complications. As a result, the diagnosis of renal infection should be considered in all patients, even in the absence of symptoms referable to the kidneys.

Unfortunately a number of indirect methods, including examination of urinary sediment, renal function, intravenous urography, and enzyme excretion all are insufficiently sensitive or specific to be used to diagnose renal infection in an individual patient. Three techniques—bladder washout, detection of antibody coating the surface of bacteria in the urine, and the response to single-dose therapy—can predict the site of infection.

BLADDER WASHOUT TECHNIQUE

After voiding, a triple lumen number 18 retention catheter is aseptically inserted into the bladder, and the volume of residual urine is measured. A portion is submitted for quantitative and qualitative culture and complete urinalysis. One hundred ml of sterile 0.9% NaCl solution containing 10 mg gentamicin and 125,000 IU of streptokinase–streptodornase is instilled into the bladder. The catheter is clamped off for 45 minutes before the bladder is drained and then irrigated with 2 liters of sterile 0.9% NaCl solution; the final 5 ml of the washing is collected for quantitative culture. Five specimens of urine collected at successive 10-minute intervals are examined by quantitative culture. Localization of infection in the lower urinary tract is indicated by the presence of 10^4 or more bacteria/ml of urine residual in the bladder, no growth or fewer than 100 bacteria/ml in the post-washout specimens, and no increase in the number of bacteria/ml in successive specimens. Inoculation of the bladder urine from a renal site of infection is signaled by the presence of 100 or more bacteria/ml in the first post-washout specimen with a ten-fold or greater increase in the numbers of bacteria/ml from the first post-washout specimen with a tenfold or shed constantly or in great numbers from the kidneys in chronic pyelonephritis. Also, this method of study cannot be used to identify which kidney is involved if there is unilateral pyelonephritis. This procedure should be reserved for diagnosing renal infection in adult females in order to investigate the efficacy of therapeutic regimens.

ANTIBODY-COATED BACTERIA TEST

The antibody-coated bacteria test correlates well with renal localization by bladder washout in women. This test depends on the observation that bacteria originating in renal tissue are coated with antibody, whereas organisms that arise in the bladder do not have a coating of antibody. Presumably, the antibody is produced locally in the kidney in response to infection. The antibody is visualized by a fluorescence technique. The urine is centrifuged and the sediment is incubated with fluorescein-labeled antihuman globulin. If antibody is present on the bacterial surface, tagged antihuman globulin attaches to the antibody, and the organisms fluoresce under ultraviolet light. However, the technique is not adequately standardized and requires careful interpretation. Moreover, 1 to 2 weeks must pass after bacteria arrive in the kidneys before surface antibody is acquired. The antibody is directed against the lipopolysaccharide somatic antigen. In females, if urine is collected free of contamination, the test is specific for renal infection. However, false negatives are common and at least one-fourth of adult females with upper tract infection yield a negative antibody-coated bacteria test. In males, the test may be confused by antibody-coated bacteria shed into the urine from a bacterial prostatitis.

SINGLE-DOSE TREATMENT

Single-dose treatment was first put forward as a method to localize urinary infection in 1976. Following a single intramuscular injection of 500 mg of kanamycin, adult females with bladder infections were cured; most females with renal infections relapsed. That is, they recurred, usually within 48 hours with the same organism present before treatment.

The specificity of relapse as a means of localizing infection to the kidneys in patients without symptoms of pyelonephritis exceeded 90%. Females with infection confined to the bladder were cured, as were a proportion of those with uncomplicated, perhaps superficial renal infection. Localization of the site of infection by single-dose treatment depends upon the difference in the pathology at the two anatomic sites, the bladder mucosa and the renal medulla. Although a bladder infection is usually limited to the mucosa and is exposed to extremely high concentrations of antimicrobics, renal infection may be a deep, parenchymal process in the medulla, a region of the kidney to which antimicrobics have limited access. Following single-dose therapy, antibacterial activity in urine is adequate to cure a bladder infection but not sufficiently sustained to cure renal infections.

Subsequent studies have shown that single peroral doses of either amoxicillin, 3 g; sulfisoxazole, 2 g; or trimethoprim 320 mg/sulfamethoxazole 1600 mg, are all effective, alternative agents that will cure bladder infections and serve to identify renal infections in females. However, no studies have been carried out in males of any age or in pregnant patients.

Prognosis

Asymptomatic infection confined to the bladder is presumably of limited significance, except that it may ascend to involve the upper tract. However, asymptomatic infections should be treated in pregnant patients in order to prevent pyelonephritis and the premature delivery that may result. Also, bacteriuria should be suppressed with chemotherapy before instrumentation. Otherwise asymptomatic lower tract infection has not been proven to be of any consequence. For example, it is not known whether treatment of bacteriuria can prevent episodes of acute pyelonephritis or other syndromes of upper tract infection. During the course of 1 year of followup of women with asymptomatic bacteriuria, the bacteriuria disappeared spontaneously in one-third; one-third remained infected and asymptomatic; and one-third developed symptoms originating from either the upper or the lower tract.

Symptoms originating from inflammation of the lower urinary tract resolve quickly, perhaps aided by increased intake of fluids and frequent voiding. Relief of clinical symptoms does not correlate with eradication of bacteriuria, and almost all adult females with cystitis recover quickly with placebo treatment. Yet, one-half of the patients with untreated acute bacterial urethrocystitis remain bacteriuric at 1-month followup.

In both males and females, about 40% of infections recur within 1 year. The majority of recurrences in young females are symptomatic and tend to occur in clusters.

Therapy

Many antimicrobics are effective in the treatment of bacterial urethrocystitis. With normal renal function, the concentrations of antimicrobics in the urine exceed the minimum inhibitory concentration of most infecting bacteria. Nitrofurantoin; the well-absorbed, soluble sulfonamides such as sulfisoxazole and sulfamethoxazole; trimethoprim alone; ampicillin and amoxicillin; and nalidixic acid will cure over 90% of bladder infections when prescribed as conventional therapy for 7 to 14 days. However, such therapy is in fact gross overtreatment for urethrocystitis, and is inadequate for at least 50% of patients with pyelonephritis.

Single-dose therapy is appropriate for bacterial urethrocystitis. Whereas with conventional therapy, over 10% of patients experience adverse reactions which require medical attention, under 2% of females have significant side-effects following single-dose therapy. At least four regimens are effective when given as single-dose therapy—kanamycin, 500 mg by IM injection; amoxicillin, 3 g PO; sulfisoxazole, 2 g PO; and trimethoprim, 320 mg/sulfamethoxazole 1600 mg PO. Relapse is presumed to be caused by renal infection. Most often, relapses are asymptomatic; if symptomatic, the manifestations are less than or equal in severity to the initial illness.

Manipulation of either urinary *p*H or urinary specific gravity is not necessary to cure bladder infections. However, many patients do experience relief of symptoms with diuresis. Although urinary analgesics such as phenazopyridine may relieve dysuria, usually they are unnecessary. Antispasmodics are of unproven value. Antimicrobics with bactericidal activity have not been shown to be more effective than bacteriostatic agents.

Patients with remediable lesions such as a cystocele, bladder diverticula, or bladder calculi require surgery for cure of the infection. However, the vast majority of females with bladder infections have no underlying urologic disease. Operative procedures designed to correct supposed obstruction to urinary flow at the bladder neck or within the urethra have not been shown to prevent recurrences. Unfortunately, despite lack of evidence of efficacy, a variety of surgical procedures continue to be carried out.

Prevention

Both symptomatic and asymptomatic bladder infections often occur following urethral catheterization. With indwelling urethral catheters, the use of a closed drainage system is essential to reduce acquisition of bacteriuria to less than 5% per catheterized day for adult females. Infection control measures should require education and surveillance of catheter care.

Females with a propensity for frequent reinfections can be treated prophylactically with long-term low-dose antimicrobics. Such reinfections result from entry of bacteria from the perineal–fecal reservoir. A number of prospective studies have shown that the administration of any one of several antimicrobics at bedtime will prevent 90% to 95% of recurrences: nitrofurantoin, 50 mg; trimethoprim–sulfamethoxazole (40 mg/200 mg), every other day; and trimethoprim alone, 50 mg. Long-term continuous chemoprophylaxis with trimethoprim–sulfamethoxazole for periods as long as 2 years has been associated with few side effects and rare recurrences with resistant organisms. Prophylaxis should not be started until 2 weeks following therapy, after demonstrating that the urinary tract has been freed of infection. Perhaps other strategies to prevent infections such as antibacterial prophylaxis with sexual intercourse may be equally effective.

Remaining Problems

The epidemiology of urethrocystitis and its relationship to sexual intercourse requires further definition. Additional study of the pathogenesis of urethrocystitis is needed in order to devise more appropriate preventative strategies. Organism and host factors that lead to symptoms or that permit bacteria resident in the bladder to ascend to the kidneys are not understood. The significance of asymptomatic infection and the role of immunological responses remain enigmatic.

Bibliography

Books

KUNIN CM: Detection, Prevention and Management of Urinary Tract Infections. Philadelphia, Lea & Febiger, 1979. 381 pp.

STAMEY TA: Pathogenesis and Treatment of Urinary Tract Infections. Baltimore, Williams & Wilkins, 1980. 612 pp.

Journals

BOUTROS P, MOURTADA H, RONALD AR: Urinary infection localization. Am J Obstet Gynecol 112:379–381, 1972

FAIRLEY KF, BOND AG, BROWN RB, HABERSBERGER P: Simple test to determine the site of urinary tract infection. Lancet 1:427–428, 1967

FANG LST, TOLKOFF-RUBIN NE, RUBIN RH: Efficacy of single-dose and conventional amoxicillin therapy in urinary tract infection localized by the antibody-coated bacteria technic. N Engl J Med 298:413–416, 1978

FOWLER JE, PULASKI TE: Excretory urography, cystography, and cystoscopy in the evaluation of women with urinary-tract infection. N Engl J Med 304:462–465, 1981

HARDING GKM, BUCKWOLD FJ, MARRIE TJ, THOMPSON L, LIGHT RB, RONALD AR: Prophylaxis of recurrent urinary tract infection in female patients: Efficacy of low-dose, thrice-weekly therapy with trimethoprim–sulfamethoxazole. JAMA 242:1975–1977, 1979

HARDING GKM, MARRIE TJ, RONALD AR, HOBAN SA, MUIR P: Urinary tract localization in adult females: Comparison of bladder washout localization with antibody-coated bacteria in catheterized urine sediment and the patient's symptoms at the time of localization. JAMA 240:1147–1150, 1978

HOEPRICH PD: Culture of the urine. J Lab Clin Med 56:899–907, 1960

KRAFT JK, STAMEY TA: The natural history of symptomatic recurrent bacteriuria in women. Med 56:55–60, 1977

MABECK CE: Treatment of uncomplicated urinary tract infection in non-pregnant women. Postgrad Med J 48:69, 1972

RONALD AR, BOUTROS P, MOURTADA H: Bacteriuria localization and response to single-dose therapy in women. JAMA 235:1854–1856, 1976

RUBIN RH, FANG LST, JONES SR, MUNFORD RS, SLEPACK JM, VARGA PA, ONHEIBER L, HALL CL, TOLKOFF-RUBIN NE: Multicenter trial of single-dose amoxicillin of acute, uncomplicated urinary tract infection localized by the antibody-coated bacteria technique. JAMA 244:561–564, 1980

STAMEY TA, GOVAN DE, PALMER JM: The localization and treatment of urinary tract infections: The role of bactericidal urine levels as opposed to serum levels. Med 44:1–36, 1965

STAMM WE, WAGNER KF, AMSEL R, ALEXANDER ER, TURCK M, COUNTS GW, HOLMES KK: Causes of the acute urethral syndrome in women. N Engl J Med 303:409–415, 1980

THOMAS V, SHELEKOV A, FORLAND M: Antibody-coated bacteria in the urine and the site of urinary-tract infection. N Engl J Med 290:488–490, 1974

UTZ JP: Viruria in man: An update. Prog Med Virol 17:77–90, 1974

WATERS WE, ELWOOD PC, ASSCHER AW, ABERNETHY M: Clinical significance of dysuria in women. Br Med J 2:754–757, 1970

EDWIN M. MEARES, JR.

Bacterial Prostatitis and Recurrent Urinary Tract Infections

49

Prostatitis syndromes are common afflictions of men. Nonbacterial prostatitis, an inflammatory condition of uncertain cause, is the most common syndrome, but it is not associated with bacteriuria. Bacterial prostatitis, especially chronic bacterial prostatitis, is difficult to cure and is responsible for many relapsing urinary tract infections.

Etiology

Bacterial prostatitis is caused by strains of *Escherichia coli* associated with urinary tract infection in about 80% of the cases. The remainder are caused by *Klebsiella* spp., *Proteus* spp., *Pseudomonas* spp., *Enterobacter* spp., *Serratia marcescens,* and other gram-negative bacilli. Two or more kinds of gram-negative bacilli are present in about 10% of patients with bacterial prostatitis. Although various gram-positive bacteria (*e.g., Staphylococcus* spp.,) have been reported, only enterococci (*e.g., Streptococcus fecalis*) seem to be important prostatic pathogens, because other gram-positive bacteria seldom persist within the prostate and cause relapsing urinary tract infection. Likewise, obligate anaerobes are infrequent pathogens in bacterial prostatitis.

Despite careful searches by many investigators for causative agent, the cause of nonbacterial prostatitis remains obscure. Except in rare instances, a causative role for viruses, chlamydias, mycoplasmas, fungi, or protozoa has not been found in cases of nonbacterial prostatitis. Some patients whose symptoms mimic prostatitis have normal prostates but suffer from prostatodynia. That is, they yield normal prostatic expressates but they experience referred pain associated with tension myalgia of the pelvic floor or various kinds of voiding dysfunctions.

Epidemiology

Although prostatitis syndromes are commonly seen in clinical practice, accurate data regarding the incidence, particularly of bacterial prostatitis, are not available. Chronic bacterial prostatitis is uncommon, yet it is a major cause of persistent urinary tract infections in men.

Pathogenesis and Pathology

A key question, still largely unanswered, is how bacteria infect the prostate gland. Postulated routes of infection include the following: (1) ascending urethral infection; (2) reflux of infected urine into prostatic ducts; (3) invasion by rectal bacteria, either by direct extension or by lymphogenous spread; and (4) hematogenous infection. In certain instances bacterial prostatitis may be a sexually transmitted disease, caused by ascending infection following inoculation of the urethra by abnormal vaginal bacteria during intercourse. Although urethral instrumentation occasionally leads to bacterial prostatitis, most men with this disease give no history of such manipulation.

Acute bacterial prostatitis is characterized by marked inflammation of the prostate gland. Initially, the infection is usually focal, but often the entire gland becomes inflamed. Characteristically, numerous polymorphonuclear leukocytes, within and around the acini, are associated with intraductal desquamation, cellular debris, and varying degrees of tissue invasion by lymphocytes, plasma cells, and macrophages. Diffuse edema and hyperemia of the stroma are usually noted. Microabscesses may occur early in the course of the disease; large abscesses are late complications.

The histologic findings of chronic bacterial prostatitis are nonspecific. The inflammatory reaction is generally less marked and more focal than that seen in acute bacterial prostatitis. Varying degrees of infiltration by plasma cells and macrophages are prominent within and around the acini in association with focal areas of round cell invasion. Because these changes are noted frequently in patients who have no clinical or bacteriologic evidence of bacteriuria or prostatitis, they are not diagnostic of chronic bacterial prostatitis.

Manifestations

Acute bacterial prostatitis is a febrile illness, often accompanied by shaking chills, perineal pain, low back pain, dysuria, urinary frequency and urgency, and varying degrees of bladder outflow obstruction. On physical examination, the prostate is warm and exquisitely tender, diffusely enlarged, irregular, and indurated.

The clinical picture of chronic bacterial prostatitis is variable. Some patients have asymptomatic bacilluria, normal prostate glands according to rectal examination, normal excretory urograms, and no residual urine. Most patients, however, experience urgency and frequency of urination, with or without back pain, low-grade fever, and myalgia or arthralgia. Unless prostatic hypertrophy is also present, excretory urograms are usually normal, and residual urine is minimal to absent. Response to appropriate antimicrobial agents is usual, and these patients remain asymptomatic as long as the bladder urine is sterile. Symptoms recur when the prostatic bacteria reinfect the bladder urine. Other patients have chronic bacterial prostatitis in association with chronic pyelonephritis, with or without struvite or apatite urolithiasis.

Varying numbers of small prostatic calculi are common findings in men and are usually unrelated to prostatic infection. In an occasional patient, however, large numbers of *E. coli* have been recovered from deep within large prostatic calculi—that is, infected prostatic calculi can perpetuate prostatic infection and cause relapsing bacilluria.

The symptoms, physical findings, and microscopic appearance of the prostatic expressate (typically more that 10 leukocytes per high-power field, and numerous lipid-laden macrophages) are usually indistinguishable in chronic bacterial prostatitis and nonbacterial prostatitis. However, the patient with nonbacterial prostatitis typically has no history of documented urinary tract infection and does not yield bacteria from localization cultures of the lower urinary tract.

Diagnosis

Because the symptoms and physical findings are strikingly characteristic, acute bacterial prostatitis is usually recognized by the clinician. Although prostatic massage will produce purulent prostatic secretions yielding large numbers of bacteria on culture, bacteremia may result from manipulation of the acutely inflamed prostate gland—massage is contraindicated, unless appropriate antibacterial therapy has already been started. The etiologic agent can usually be identified by culture of the urine because cystitis is an early complication of acute bacterial prostatitis. Acute bacterial urethritis, acute pyelitis, and acute pyelonephritis are sometimes confused with acute prostatitis.

Chronic bacterial prostatitis cannot be accurately diagnosed by history, physical examination, radiographic studies, or cystoscopic examination. It is fallacious to base a diagnosis of chronic bacterial prostatitis on the number of leukocytes in the prostatic secretions. Culture of prostatic needle biopsy specimens is also ineffective for diagnosis: the infection is focal and needle biopsy specimens are random, small, easily contaminated, and difficult to quantify. Histologic examination of prostatic tissue is equally unreliable for diagnosis of chronic bacterial prostatitis, because diseases other than bacterial infection produce similar inflammatory changes.

The diagnosis of chronic bacterial prostatitis is validated when quantitative bacteriologic techniques clearly localize pathogenic bacteria to the prostate gland. Chronic bacterial prostatitis is characterized by the growth of small numbers of bacteria on a culture of prostatic fluid. Because bacteria resident in the urethra can contaminate prostatic fluid obtained by prostatic massage, culture of such fluid by itself is misleading. Diagnostic accuracy requires simultaneous quantitative culture of the urethra, midstream urine, and expressed prostatic secretions. Both the careful collection of segmemted specimens (Fig. 49-1) and the application of bacteriologic techniques capable of quantifying small numbers of bacteria are mandatory for the proper diagnosis of chronic bacterial prostatitis.

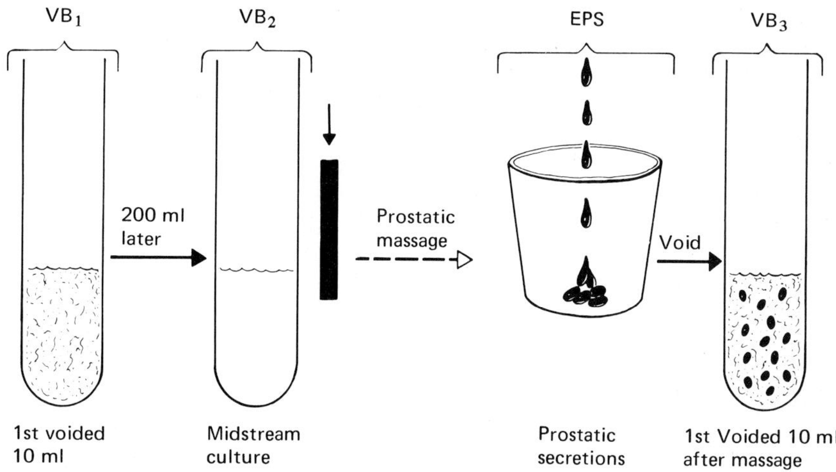

Fig. 49-1. To diagnose chronic bacterial prostatis, segmented specimens must be cultured immediately after collection. Bacteriologic methods capable of quantifying small numbers of bacteria must be used. If the bladder urine (*VB_2*) is sterile, bacterial urethritis is indicated by a much higher count (1 logarithm or greater) in the very first urine that is passed (*VB_1*) than is obtained from either prostatic fluid (*EPS*) or the last urine specimen (*VB_3*). With bacterial prostatis, the converse occurs. Because *VB_3* represents about a 1:100 dilution of prostatic fluid, the bacterial count off *EPS* in chronic bacterial prostatitis always exceeds that of *VB_3*. If the bladder urine (*VB_2*) is not sterile, 2—3 days of treatment with an antimicrobial agent that is active in the urine but not tissues (500 mg penicillin G by mouth every 6 hours; 100 mg nitrofurantoin by mouth every 6 hours) should precede the collection of segmented specimens. (Meares EM, Jr, Stamey TA: Invest Urol 5:494, 1968)

Prognosis

Acute bacterial prostatitis usually responds to appropriate antimicrobial therapy without sequelae. However, chronic bacterial prostatitis and relapsing urinary tract infections occasionally develop. Other complications include prostatic abscess, unilateral or bilateral epididymo-orchitis, seminal vesiculitis, pyelonephritis, and septicemia. Although chronic epididymitis can cause infertility, there is no proof that bacterial prostatitis causes impotence.

Chronic bacterial prostatitis, by contrast, is often a subtle disease, impossible to detect by physical or cystoscopic examination and extremely difficult to cure. Because chronic bacterial prostatitis causes recurrent bacteriuria, its complications include all the sequalae of chronic urinary tract infections.

Although antibody titers against prostatic pathogens are frequently elevated in the serum of patients

PROSTATIC FLUID ALTERATIONS IN BACTERIAL PROSTATITIS

Decreased compared to normal

- Specific gravity
- Prostatic antibacterial factor (PAF)
- Cation concentrations (zinc, magnesium, calcium)
- Citric acid concentration
- Spermine concentration
- Cholesterol concentration
- Enzyme concentrations (acid phosphatase, lysozyme)

Increased compared to normal

- pH value (alkalinity)
- Ratio of LDH isoenzyme 5 to LDH isoenzyme 1 (LDH-5/LDH-1 = >2)

Meares EM Jr: Kidney Internat. 20:122, 1982

who have acute or chronic bacterial prostatitis, little is known concerning the immunology of prostatitis.

Human prostatic fluid normally contains a potent inhibitor of gram-positive and gram-negative bacteria—the so-called prostatic antibacterial factor (PAF), a compound that contains zinc. Because men who have chronic bacterial prostatitis generally also have deficiency of both zinc and antibacterial activity in their prostatic fluid, it has been postulated that the normally present PAF may act as a natural defense mechanism against bacterial invasion. However, the prostatic fluid of men with chronic bacterial prostatitis is deficient in most of its normal constituents. That is, depression of both zinc content and antibacterial activity may be an effect rather than a cause of infection.

Therapy

Patients who have acute bacterial prostatitis often respond dramatically to therapy with antimicrobics that normally do not diffuse from plasma into prostatic fluid. Perhaps, as in acute meningitis, the intense, diffuse inflammatory reaction of acute bacterial prostatitis leads to the passage of antimicrobial agents from plasma into the prostatic acini. An appropriate antimicrobic, selected by *in vitro* susceptibility testing, should be given to the patient in doses that achieve bactericidal concentrations of the drug in the blood. General supportive measures, such as adequate hydration, analgesics, antipyretics, bed rest, and stool softeners, should also be used. Urethral instrumentation should be avoided. If acute urinary retention occurs, suprapubic needle aspiration of the bladder is safer and more comfortable for the patient than urethral catheterization. When prolonged bladder drainage is required, a suprapubic catheter (punch cystostomy) causes fewer complications than a urethral catheter.

Chronic bacterial prostatitis is unaccompanied by the active inflammation characteristic of acute bacterial prostatitis and presents a difficult challenge in therapy. The following three approaches are presently available: (1) to find a drug that will diffuse across the prostatic epithelium and kill the bacterial pathogen; (2) to remove the infected prostatic focus by surgical means; and (3) to use continuous, suppressive antimicrobial therapy to prevent reinfection of the bladder by the prostatic pathogen. The first alternative is the most appealing, but it is the most difficult to achieve.

Although total prostatectomy offers the most certain cure for patients who have chronic bacterial prostatitis, the morbidity of this procedure severely limits its usefulness. Transurethral prostatectomy is curative when all the infected prostatic tissue is removed; overall, about one-third of patients are cured by this operation. None of the two-thirds who are not cured is made worse; each simply resumes his previous pattern of recurrent bacteriuria with the same pathogen. Considering the uncertainty of cure by transurethral prostatectomy, most patients prefer continuous, suppressive antimicrobial therapy. These patients usually remain asymptomatic and maintain sterile bladder urine with only a single daily dose of an appropriate antibacterial agent. In all patients, despite prolonged drug therapy, the same pathogen is recovered in prostatic fluid cultures; cessation of drug therapy results in recurrence of bladder infection.

The failure to cure chronic bacterial prostatitis, even with prolonged treatment with apparently appropriate antimicrobics, may be related to failure of these drugs to penetrate into the prostatic fluid. Studies of the passage of antimicrobics into the prostatic fluid of dogs have documented free entry, indeed actual accumulation, of only the basic macrolides (rosamicin, erythromycin, and oleandomycin) and the antimicrobic bases trimethoprim and clindamycin. Rosamicin is an investigational drug which is not available currently for clinical use. Unfortunately, erythromycin, oleandomycin, and clindamycin are only useful against gram-positive bacteria. These studies demonstrate why chronic bacterial prostatitis is difficult to cure with antimicrobial agents: Most antimicrobics normally useful against gram-negative bacteria cross prostatic epithelium poorly, and therefore attain low-to-negligible concentrations in prostatic fluid.

The factors that determine the diffusion and concentration of drugs in the prostatic fluid are depicted in Figure 49-2. Although the principles of drug diffusion are probably the same for all epithelial membranes, the prostate gland is perhaps the only organ with secretory fluid that directly infects other major organs—the bladder and kidneys. To appreciate the therapeutic challenge of chronic bacterial prostatitis, one must understand the physiology of drug diffusion across prostatic epithelium.

Except for a few water-soluble compounds of small molecular size and specific spatial configurations, only unionized, lipid-soluble drugs that are not firmly bound to plasma proteins diffuse from the plasma across intact epithelial membranes. However, most antimicrobics dissociate to some extent, providing both unionized and ionized molecules in a ratio determined by the pK_a of the drug and the pH of the

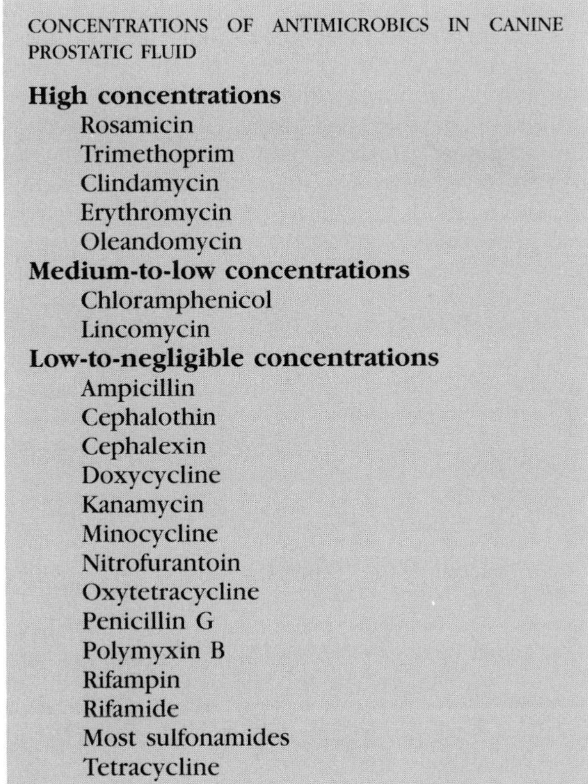

CONCENTRATIONS OF ANTIMICROBICS IN CANINE PROSTATIC FLUID

High concentrations
- Rosamicin
- Trimethoprim
- Clindamycin
- Erythromycin
- Oleandomycin

Medium-to-low concentrations
- Chloramphenicol
- Lincomycin

Low-to-negligible concentrations
- Ampicillin
- Cephalothin
- Cephalexin
- Doxycycline
- Kanamycin
- Minocycline
- Nitrofurantoin
- Oxytetracycline
- Penicillin G
- Polymyxin B
- Rifampin
- Rifamide
- Most sulfonamides
- Tetracycline

After Meares EM Jr: Kidney Internat 20:122, 1982

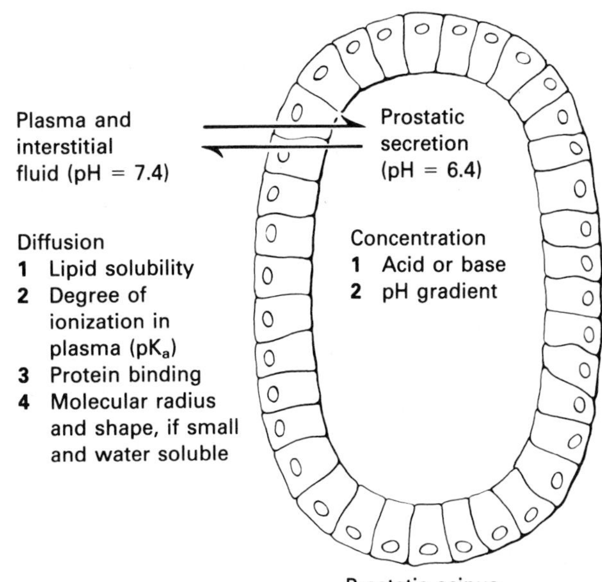

Fig. 49-2. Several factors determine the diffusibility of drugs into prostatic fluid. (Stamey TA, Meares EM, Jr, Winningham DG: J Urol 103:191, 1970)

milieu. In a stable system, the uncharged fraction of a lipid-soluble drug eventually equilibrates on each side of the membrane. In contrast, the charged fraction accumulates primarily on one side—a phenomenon called *ion trapping*.

In the normal prostate, the passage of drugs from the plasma (pH 7.4) into the prostatic fluid (pH 6.4) is strongly influenced by ion trapping. Acidic antimicrobial agents ionize to a greater extent in plasma than in prostatic fluid; therefore, ion trapping of antimicrobial acids occurs on the plasma side of the membrane, and the concentrations of such drugs in the plasma always exceed those in the prostatic fluid. Because prostatic fluid is more acid than plasma, antimicrobial bases ionize to a greater extent in prostatic fluid than in plasma. Accordingly, there is ion trapping of antimicrobial bases on the prostatic fluid side of the membrane; thus the concentrations of such drugs in the prostatic fluid can exceed the concentrations in the plasma.

Penicillins and cephalosporins are insoluble in lipids and are acids with low pKa values; therefore, these drugs do not accumulate in prostatic secretions. Many of the antimicrobial bases that are effective *in vitro* against gram-negative bacteria are not soluble in lipids (*e.g.*, the polymyxins). Despite being a lipid-soluble acid with a favorable pKa value, nalidixic acid is extensively (95%) bound to plasma proteins and is not freely diffusible. The basic macrolides are highly lipid soluble, dissociate as bases, and accumulate in prostatic fluid. Trimethoprim is a lipid-soluble base, has a pKa value of 7.3 (*i.e.*, about 50% is unionized in the plasma), and achieves concentrations in canine prostatic fluid that are 3 to 10 times higher than are simultaneously present in the plasma.

The prostatic secretions of men with chronic bacterial prostatitis typically are more alkaline than normal and may exceed the alkalinity of the plasma. Theoretically, this alteration of the pH relationship between the plasma and prostatic fluid should impede accumulation of trimethoprim in prostatic fluid and limit its concentration to that present in the plasma.

Nonetheless, trimethoprim–sulfamethoxazole (TMP–SMX) has given the best cure rates of chronic bacterial prostatitis attained by antimicrobic therapy.

Among patients who received full therapy (TMP 160 mg + SMX 800 mg twice daily) for 4 to 16 weeks, the rate of cure has been 32% to 71%—a significant improvement over short-term therapy. Furthermore, cures with TMP–SMX have been substantiated by serologic studies as well as by clinical observations.

Nonbacterial prostatitis is difficult to treat satisfactorily because it is a disease of unknown cause (or causes). There is as yet no documentation of chlamydial causation of nonbacterial prostatitis; however, if there is reason to suspect that either *Chlamydia trachomatis* or *Ureaplasma urealyticum* are involved, a trial of therapy with either minocycline (3 mg–4 mg/kg body wt/day, PO, as two equal portions, 12-hourly) or erythromycin (30 mg/kg body wt/day, PO, as four equal portions, 6-hourly) for 2 to 4 weeks is not unreasonable. Unless the clinical response is favorable, additional therapy with antimicrobics is unwarranted. Instead, treatment is best directed toward achieving symptomatic relief. Thus, flares of symptoms may respond to short courses of anticholinergics, antiinflammatory agents, and hot sitz baths. Although therapeutic prostatic massage is advocated by many, its benefits are questioned by others.

Prevention

Until the origin of bacterial prostatitis is clarified, effective preventive measures cannot be formulated. Without question, the physician who uses strict techniques of asepsis in regard to urethral instrumentation and in the management of urethral catheters minimizes iatrogenic infections.

Remaining problems

Because chronic bacterial prostatitis is a major cause of persistent urinary tract infection in men, it is important to (1) determine the portal of entry, especially the role of ascending infection during sexual intercourse, and develop methods for prevention of bacterial infections of the prostate; (2) explore the usefulness of trimethoprim alone in therapy; (3) search for other antimicrobics that will cross the prostatic epithelium and kill the infecting bacteria; (4) study the pathogenesis of prostatic calculi and their role in bacterial persistence; (5) clarify the role of PAF (zinc) in prostatic fluid and its role in preventing infections of the genitourinary tract; (6) elucidate further the nature of the secretory dysfunction of the prostate observed in prostatitis and its clinical sequalae; and (7) explore the immunology of prostatitis.

Nonbacterial prostatitis closely mimics chronic bacterial prostatitis in symptoms, but it is not caused by presently recognized bacterial pathogens. Exploration of nonbacterial causes is necessary; search for viruses, chlamydias, and mycoplasmas should continue. Because prostatic fluid normally inhibits the growth of various microorganisms, a reevaluation of present methods of culture and serodiagnosis may lead to greater success in the identification of pathogens.

Bibliography

Books

MEARES EM JR: Urinary tract infections in men. In Harrison JH, Gittes RF, Perlmutter AD, Stamey TA, Walsh PC (eds): Campbell's Urology, 4th ed. Philadelphia, WB Saunders, 1978. pp 509–537.

REEVES DS, ROWE RCG, SNELL ME, THOMAS ABW: Further studies on the secretion of antibiotics in the prostatic fluid of the dog. In Brumfitt W, Ascher AW (eds): Urinary Tract Infection. London, Oxford University Press, 1973. pp 197–205.

STAMEY TA: The Pathogenesis and Treatment of Urinary Tract Infections. Baltimore, Williams & Wilkins, 1980. 612 pp.

Journals

BLACKLOCK NJ, BEAVIS JP: The response of prostatic pH in inflammation. Br J Urol 46:537–542, 1974

FAIR WR, CORDONNIER JJ: The pH of prostatic fluid: A reappraisal and therapeutic implications. J Urol 120:695–698, 1978

FAIR WR, COUCH J, WEHNER N: Prostatic antibacterial factor: Identity and significance. Urology 7:169–177, 1976

MÅRDH P-A, COLLEEN S: Search for urogenital tract infections in patients with symptoms of prostatitis: Studies on aerobic and strictly anaerobic bacteria, mycoplasmas, fungi, trichomonads and viruses. Scand J Urol Nephrol 9:8–16, 1975

MÅRDH P-A, RIPA KT, COLLEEN S, TREHARNE JD, DAROUGAR S: Role of Chlamydia trachomatis in non-acute prostatitis. Br J Vener Dis 54:330–334, 1978

MEARES EM JR: Serum antibody titers in urethritis and chronic bacterial prostatitis. Urology 10:305–309, 1977

MEARES EM JR: Serum antibody titers in treatment with trimethoprim–sulfamethoxazole for chronic prostatitis. Urology 11:142–146, 1978

MEARES EM JR: Prostatitis syndromes: New perspectives about old woes. J Urol 123:141–147, 1980

MEARES EM JR: Prostatitis and related diseases. DM 26:1–40, 1980

MEARES EM JR: Prostatitis. Kidney Internat 20:117–126, 1982

MEARES EM JR, STAMEY TA: Bacteriologic localization patterns in bacterial prostatitis and urethritis. Invest Urol 5:492–518, 1968

STAMEY TA, BUSHBY SRM, BRAGONJE J: The concentration of trimethoprim in prostatic fluid: Nonionic diffusion or active transport? J Infect Dis (Suppl) 128:686–690, 1973

RUTH M. LAWRENCE

Infections of the Female Genital Tract

50

Infections of the female genital tract range from minor, but distressing, afflictions such as vulvovaginitis to major, life-threatening conditions such as pelvic cellulitis and septic thrombophlebitis. Microorganisms may reach pelvic structures from below—consequent to infection of the vulva and vagina, or from above—consequent to hematogenous dissemination. Of these two routes of infection, the former is more common. Because the vagina is normally colonized by a wide variety of microorganisms, listed below, culture results may be difficult to interpret unless cultures are collected properly. In addition, many pelvic infections are polymicrobial, compounding the difficulty of deciding which isolates are truly significant.

Many of the microorganisms which cause female genital tract infections are discussed in chapters dealing with veneral infections. Accordingly, only aspects of these diseases specific to women are discussed in this chapter.

BACTERIA AND FUNGI ISOLATED FROM THE VAGINAS IN 10 NORMAL WOMEN

Organism	No.
Nonpathogenic lactobacilli	8
Diphtheroids	2
Clostridium innoculum	1
Alcaligenes spp.	1
Gardnerella vaginalis	1
Gaffkya tetragena	1
Escherichia coli	2
Pseudomonas spp.	1
Enterococci	2
Eubacterium spp.	2
Lactobacillus catenaformi	2
Propionibacterium spp.	2
Bacteroides spp.	1
Fusobacterium spp.	1
Veillonella spp.	3
Candida albicans	1
Torulopsis glabrata	2

After Mead PB: J Reprod Med 13:135–141, 1974

Vulvovaginitis

Vulvovaginitis, inflammation of vulva and vagina, is one of the most common conditions for which women seek medical care and may be one of the most difficult gynecologic problems to treat satisfactorily. Vulvitis and vaginitis usually occur concomitantly, and the inflammatory process may involve the entire perineum and anal orifice as well.

Etiology

Infectious causes of vulvovaginitis are diverse and include viruses, chlamydias, mycoplasmas, bacteria, fungi, protozoa and metazoa (*i.e.,* almost any organism which can afflict the skin plus those whose growth is aided by the milieu of the lower genital tract). Local irritating factors—heat, perspiration, tight clothing, scented soaps, or medications—which predispose to maceration of the skin and inflammation, permit secondary infection by members of the resident microflora.

The motile protozoan, *Trichomonas vaginalis,* accounts for 15% to 20% of all cases of infectious vulvovaginitis and coexists with other microorganisms in another 10% to 20% of cases. It is usually 5 μm to 15μm in length, occasionally reaching 30 μm. Both its genital locus of infection and its morphology distinguish *T. vaginalis* from other trichomonads. *Trichomonas vaginalis* has four anterior flagella and a short undulating membrane which lacks a free posterior flagellum (Fig. 50-1). It grows optimally in a moist, acid environment at temperatures between 35°C and 37°C and *p*H between 5.5 and 5.8. It can be cultured in a casein hydrolysate serum me-

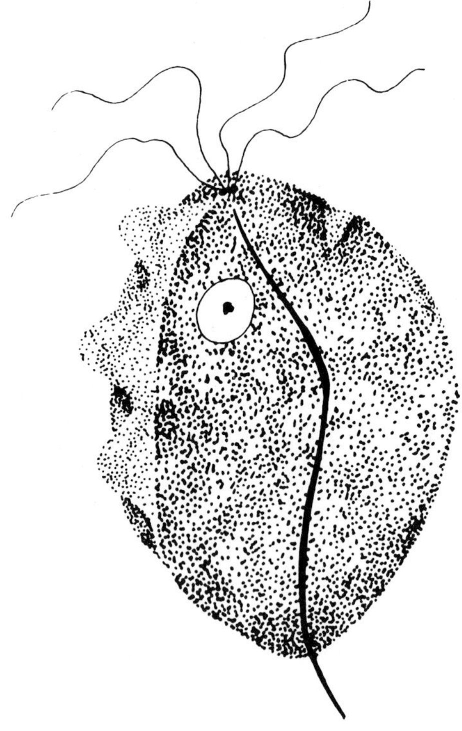

Fig. 50-1. *Trichomonas vaginalis.* (Beck JW, Barrett-Conner E: Medical Parasitology. St. Louis, CV Mosby, 1971)

dium, but in clinical practice it is usually identified by microscopic examination of wet mounts of vaginal secretions.

Small (1 μm–2 μm × 0.4 μm–0.6 μm), gram-negative, motile, pleomorphic coccobacilli, recently reclassified as *Gardnerella vaginalis* (formerly known as *Haemophilus vaginalis* or *Corynebacterium vaginale*) may be cultured from the vaginas of up to 90% of women with so-called nonspecific vaginitis and from the urethras of their sexual partners. The role of *G. vaginalis* in causing vaginitis has been debated, but it is probable that these bacteria are in part responsible for the symptoms. Increased numbers of anaerobic bacteria including *Bacteroides* spp. and *Peptococcus* spp. have been found in association with *G. vaginalis* in many women with nonspecific vaginitis. It is postulated that the anaerobic bacteria act in concert with *G. vaginalis* to produce nonspecific vaginitis. Small, translucent colonies are produced by *G. vaginalis* on chocolate agar; oxidase and catalase reactions are negative, and acid is produced from starch but not from mannitol. This last property distinguishes *G. vaginalis* from *Lactobacillus* spp., which are common normal inhabitants of the vagina. In clinical practice, *G. vaginalis* may be recognized on microscopy as masses of small, gram-negative coccobacilli covering vaginal epithelial cells (the so-called clue cell, Fig. 50-2).

Streptococcus spp. (see Chap. 24, Streptococcal

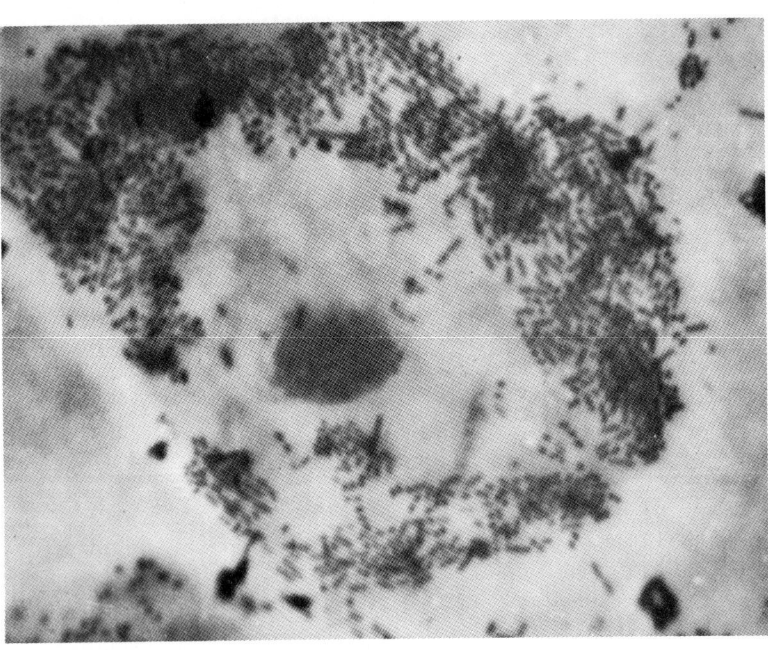

Fig. 50-2. Clue cell masses of gram-negative rods clustered about a vaginal epithelial cell—thought to be indicative of infection with *Gardnerella vaginalis.* (Marcuse PM: Diagnostic Pathology in Gynecology and Obstetrics. New York, Harper & Row, 1966)

Diseases), *Staphylococcus* spp. (see Chap. 100, Staphylococcal Skin Infections), enteric bacilli (see Chap. 48, Urethritis and Cystitis) and fusopirochetes (see Chap. 32, Necrotizing Pneumonias and Lung Abscesses) are other bacterial causes of vaginitis.

Fungal agents implicated frequently in vulvovaginitis include *Candida albicans* and other *Candida* spp. (see Chap. 39, Candidosis); *Entamoeba histolytica* (see Chap. 66, Amebiasis) may cause vulvitis; *Enterobius vermicularis* (see Chap. 68, Intestinal Nematodiasis) should be considered in children with vulvovaginitis. Ectoparasites such as *Sarcoptes scabiei* (see Chap. 116, Scabies) have been implicated in vulvovaginitis.

Epidemiology

Because of the multiplicity of causative agents, vulvovaginitis is worldwide in distribution and can occur at any age. Predisposing factors include poor personal hygiene; local irritation from trauma; reactions to chemicals used in perfumes, deodorants, contraceptive or douching medicaments; and lack of estrogen resulting in poorly stratified vaginal epithelium. The normal adult vagina is stimulated by estrogen and has a *p*H of 3.5 to 4.5 as a result of lactic acid production by *Lactobacillus* spp. When intravaginal secretions are increased (menstrual blood, exudate from cervical lesions), there may be a disruption of the normal flora with overgrowth of other bacteria. During pregnancy, progesterone levels are increased and the vaginal *p*H increases, permitting growth of many intravaginal pathogens. In patients with diabetes mellitus the increased glucose in vaginal secretions may contribute to a greater incidence of mycotic vaginitis. Women taking estrogen–progestin fertility control pills appear to have more yeast vaginal infections, but the reasons for this are not entirely clear. The selective pressure of some systemically administered antimicrobics, notably the tetracyclines and erythromycin, may favor candidal outgrowth and result in candidal vulvovaginitis.

Sexual practices are related to the incidence of vulvovaginitis because many agents are venereally transmitted. Women who are sexually active have a greater variety of agents cultured from vaginal secretions than women who are not active. The incidence of vaginitis also appears to be related to the number of different sexual partners.

Pathogenesis and Pathology

Proliferation of infecting microorganisms results in a roughened, congested vaginal mucosa which may show punctuate areas of hemorrhage. In most instances, involvement of the vaginal mucosa is associated with involvement of the vaginal vestibule, the labia, and occasionally the buttocks and thighs. The inflammatory response results in a vaginal discharge of varying degrees of purulence.

Herpetic infections of the vulva cause multiple, groups, ulcerating vesicles, especially of the labia minora. Localized abscesses may involve the labia or an obstructed Bartholin's gland as a result of secondary bacterial infection.

Manifestations

The cardinal manifestation of vulvovaginitis is increased vaginal discharge. This can usually be differentiated from physiologic leukorrhea (the clear mucoid discharge which may occur in the neonatal period, puberty and at the time of ovulation) by the concomitant presence of pruritus of the vagina and vulva. The time of onset of the discharge in relation to menses may be helpful. Trichomonal vaginitis is exacerbated with menses as the buffering effect of menstrual blood raises vaginal *p*H to 6.0–6.5, a range optimal for the growth of trichomonads. Candidal symptoms usually begin prior to menstruation, and symptoms in nonspecific vaginitis are not related to menstruation.

Classically, the discharge associated with *T. vaginalis* is copious, yellow green, frothy, and malodorous, while discharge caused by *Candida* spp. is scantier, thick and curdlike. The discharge in nonspecific vaginitis tends to be graywhite, frothy, and homogenous. A characteristic "fishy" odor of the discharge, which is intensified when KOH is added, is attributed to the production of amines by vaginal bacteria. Because mixed vaginal infections are so common, the nature of the discharge varies, and its character cannot be used as the sole diagnostic criterion. The vulva and perianal area are well supplied with sensitive receptors, so that sensations of pain, pruritus, stinging, and burning may be exquisitely intense. Dysuria and dyspareunia are common. Systemic signs of infection such as fever are usually absent.

Diagnosis

The diagnosis of vulvovaginitis, as based on history and physical findings, is usually not difficult. A general physical examination and a pelvic examination should be performed. The patient should not have douched or used intravaginal medications for at least 72 hours prior to examination. Inspection may reveal the labia and vaginal mucosa to be reddened and edematous. A sample of the vaginal secretions should be obtained by pipette for preparation of a wet smear and for culture. A small amount is placed on two glass slides and mixed with a drop of 0.9% NaCl solution. One drop of 10% KOH solution should be added to one slide to lyse epithelial cells and other vaginal debris. The two slides are examined microscopically for the presence of motile trichomonads (an oval organism moving jerkily across the field; Fig. 50-1), budding yeasts, or hyphae. A gram stain may demonstrate masses of *G. vaginalis* associated with epithelial cells (Fig. 50-2).

A Papanicolaou smear can aid in diagnosing trichomonal, fungal, and bacterial infections, in assessing hormonal status, and in detecting malignant lesions. Vesicular lesions should be unroofed and touch preparations on glass slides prepared for fluorescent antibody staining. Viral cultures can be performed if facilities are available. A bacterial culture for *Neisseria gonorrhoeae* should be performed on material obtained from the endocervix. Unless special procedures for the isolation of *G. vaginalis* are done, the results of other bacterial cultures are likely to be confusing. Discrete lesions of the vulva and vagina should be biopsied. In children, a scotch-tape swab of the perianal area may show pinworm *(Enterobius vermicularis)* eggs (see Chap. 68, Intestinal Nematodiasis, and Chap. 11, Diagnostic Methods for Protozoa and Helminths).

Prognosis

If a specific etiologic agent or contributing factor can be identified, therapy is usually successful. However, relapses are common and may require treatment. If pyogenic skin bacteria cause secondary invasion, severe local scarring resulting in vaginal stenosis may be the end result.

Therapy

Therapy for infectious vulvovaginitis includes antimicrobics aimed at the causative organism, local measures such as warm tub baths to help reduce edema and pain, careful attention to personal hygiene, and abstinence from sexual intercourse. Twice weekly douches with a solution of a tablespoon of white vinegar in a quart of warm water may be helpful.

Trichomonal vaginitis may be effectively treated with metronidazole. Cure rates of 95% have been reported with dosages of either 10 mg/kg body wt/day (about 750 mg), PO, as three equal portions, 8-hourly, for 7 days, or 30 mg/kg body wt (about 2 g) PO, as a single dosage. Systemic therapy is required to eradicate extravaginal infection and prevent relapse. Sex partners of women with trichomoniasis may also be treated with similar doses to prevent reinfection. *Trichomonas vaginalis* harbored in the male urethra usually disappears spontaneously within 3 to 4 weeks if venereal reinfection is avoided; hence, male sex partners who are not treated systemically may either abstain from coitus or use condoms for this period. Metronidazole should not be used in the first trimester of pregnancy. Symptomatic pregnant women may be treated with gentle vinegar douches. More definitive therapy late in pregnancy is important to prevent transmission of the organism to the newborn, and possibly to reduce the incidence of maternal postpartum fever and endometritis.

Metronidazole is effective against *G. vaginalis* and many anaerobic bacteria; it appears to be the most effective of several regimens in the treatment of nonspecific vaginitis when *G. vaginalis* is a component of the flora. A dose of 15 mg/kg body wt/day (about 1 g), PO, as two equal portions, 12-hourly, should be given for 7 days. Whether sex partners should be treated remains unknown.

Treatment of herpes simplex vulvovaginitis has been difficult. Applications of idoxuridine (2-deoxy-d-glucose) and trials of photodynamic inactivation have all failed to cause more rapid healing when tested in double-blind studies. A new antiviral compound, acyclovir, reduces viral shedding and pain in initial attacks. Local measures such as cool compresses and topical analgesics may provide relief.

Vaginitis caused by *Candida* spp. may be effectively treated with local application of antifungal agents. Insertion of one or two nystatin tablets (100,000 units of nystatin per tablet) high into the vagina once daily for 14 days or an applicator filled with miconazole nitrate 2% cream into the vagina once daily for 7 days is effective. It is recommended that therapy extend through one menstrual period. *Candidal vaginitis* may be more difficult to eradicate in women taking estrogen–progestin fertility control pills, and two courses of therapy may be needed. Systemic antibacterial therapy should be discontinued if possible. Male consorts of women with candidal vaginitis may acquire candidosis of the glans penis and prepuce; local treatment with nystatin cream is effective.

Gonococcal vaginitis demands systemic treatment with penicillin, tetracycline, or spectinomycin (see Chap. 56, Gonococcal Infections).

Local measures such as warm tub baths to which a mild solution of boric acid or colloids have been added, cool compresses, and avoidance of tight undergarments help to reduce inflammation and edema. In postmenopausal women with atrophic vaginitis (fewer epithelial layers of the vaginal mucosa and decreased vascularity), local estrogen cream applied daily helps to restore senescent tissues.

Vulvovaginitis is frequently overtreated with various douches or medications which can in themselves perpetuate symptoms. When this occurs, discontinuation of all medications and douching is necessary. Systemic analgesics or antihistamines may be required.

Prevention

Because most of the agents which cause infectious vulvovaginitis can be transmitted venereally, it is essential that women refer their sexual partners for appropriate therapy, if necessary. Good personal hygiene with careful cleansing of the perineum is vital for prevention of vaginitis, but the use of vaginal sprays or deodorants should be discouraged because these products can cause severe hypersensitivity vaginitis in many women.

Remaining Problems

The etiologic role of organisms such as mycoplasmas and chlamydias remains to be elucidated. The entity of nonspecific vaginitis needs further study to determine the exact role of the various microorganisms which may be isolated from the exudate.

Cervicitis, Endometritis, and Salpingo-Oophoritis

Cervicitis, endometritis, and salpingo-oophoritis usually imply the extension of infection from the lower parts of the female genital tract to higher structures. Extension may occur by way of the endometrium or by lymphatic or hematogenous dissemination.

Mycobacterium tuberculosis may be an exception, because the internal genitalia may be infected by direct extension from adjacent organs (see Chap. 35, Extrapulmonary Tuberculosis).

Etiology

Any of the bacteria found in the lower regions of the vagina can cause disease higher in the genital tract. The endocervix itself has a diverse microflora which includes many aerobic and anaerobic bacteria, mycoplasmas, chlamydias, and viruses. When mycobacteria and fungi are isolated from the cervix, it is usually an extension of disease from other organs.

The gonococcus *(Neisseria gonorrhoeae)* accounts for somewhat less than half of all cases of acute salpingo-oophoritis (pelvic inflammatory disease). The remainder are associated with a variety of aerobic and anaerobic bacteria, mycoplasmas, and chlamydias, with two or more microorganisms frequently present. These are listed below.

MICROORGANISMS CULTURED FROM THE PERITONEAL FLUID OF 54 PATIENTS WITH ACUTE PELVIC INFLAMMATORY DISEASE

Organism	Number
Anaerobes	
Bacteroides fragilis	14
Other *Bacteroides* spp.	5
Fusobacterium spp.	3
Peptostreptococcus spp.	16
Veillonella spp.	2
Clostridium ramosum	1
Propionibacterium acnes	1
Anaerobic lactobacillus	1
Aerobes	
Neisseria gonorrhoeae	7
Escherichia coli	3
Haemophilus influenzae, type B	3
Streptococcus pyogenes (group A)	1
α-hemolytic streptococci	12
Staphylococcus aureus	1
Staphylococcus epidermidis	6
Lactobacillus spp.	2
Gardnerella vaginalis	4
Diptheroids	8
Mycoplasma hominis	2
T mycoplasma	1
Chlamydia trachomatis	1

After Eschenbach DA, Buchanan TM, Pollock HM, Forsyth PS, Alexander ER, Lin J, Wang S, Wentworth BB, McCormack WM, Holmes KK: N Engl J Med 293:166–171, 1975

Chlamydia trachomatis has been implicated as a cause of salpingitis in other countries but has been reported relatively uncommonly in the United States.

Endometritis which results from septic abortion may be caused by *Clostridium* spp. (see Chap. 156, Gas Gangrene) and other anaerobic bacteria, as well as aerobic gram-negative bacteria.

Epidemiology

Because of the diverse nature of the infective organisms, cervicitis, endometritis, and salpingo-oophoritis may occur at any time in life. However, these infections are most common in sexually active women of childbearing age.

Factors which predispose to the development of pelvic inflammatory disease (PID) include the use of an intrauterine contraceptive device (IUD) (the risk appears 2 to 4 times greater for women with IUDs), multiple sex partners, and a previous episode of salpingitis. Gonococcal salpingitis occurs more frequently at the onset of menstruation than at other times in the menstrual cycle. This is attributed to the loss of the normal cervical mucus barrier with menses and to the increased numbers of bacteria present in the vagina at that time. The annual rate of diagnosis of salpingitis and PID in the United States is between 1000 and 1500 per 100,000 females discharged from hospitals, and it is estimated that 2500 to 3000 visits per 100,000 females in the adult population are made to a physician's office or clinic for treatment of PID. About 500,000 cases occur annually in the United States.

Septic abortion, formerly a major public health problem, has decreased dramatically because of the more widespread use of contraceptives and the availability of legal means for the termination of pregnancy. Nevertheless, infections occasionally occur even when abortions are carried out under the best of circumstances. Termination later in pregnancy is associated with increased risk of infection; hysterotomy and hysterectomy as modes of abortion have higher rates of infection than either uterine curettage or intraamniotic injection of hypertonic liquids.

In women beyond childbearing years, infections of the endometrium, tubes, and ovaries are usually secondary to a surgical procedure.

Pathogenesis and Pathology

The vagina and ectocervix are covered by stratified squamous epithelium, whereas the endocervix is covered by columnar epithelium arranged in an intricate system of tunnels, the so-called cervical glands. The transition between these two types of epithelium, the squamocolumnar junction, is usually located a few millimeters from the cervical os. Cervicitis implies diffuse inflammation at the squamocolumnar junction. With acute cervicitis polymorphonuclear and plasma cells infiltrate the subepithelial tissue; the mucosa becomes red and hypertrophic and may become desquamated. Occlusion of the glandlike structures leads to retention cysts (nabothian follicles). Chronic cervical infection may lead to fibroblastic hypertrophy, which results in stenosis of the cervical os. Granulomatous infections of the cervix produce typical granulomas with giant cells and epithelioid cells. The mature squamous epithelium of the vagina is relatively resistant to invasion by bacteria such as the gonococcus, which explains why the vaginal walls are not infected when the urethra and cervix are infected.

Organisms infecting the cervix can spread to involve the uterus and fallopian tubes by two routes. *Neisseria gonorrhoeae* spread from the cervix to the endometrium, causing a transient endometritis and extending to involve the endosalpinx. In contrast, other pyogenic bacteria such as the streptococcus reach the tubes by means of lymphatic spread. That is, the perisalpingeal areas and the wall of the tube are involved first, leaving the lumen of the tube free (Fig. 50-3). With acute endosalpingitis (Fig. 50-4) the submucosa is infiltrated with polymorphonuclear cells, and the lumen becomes filled with a purulent exudate, which may seep into the peritoneal cavity causing pelvic peritonitis. With chronic infection, the tubular lumen distends with retained secretions, all layers of the wall are infiltrated with inflammatory cells, and peritoneal adhesions are formed. The occluded, inflamed tube is termed a pyosalpinx; after resolution of the inflammatory process a hydrosalpinx results. If the fimbriated end of the tube adheres to the ovary, infected material from the tubular lumen has direct access to the ovary. A tuboovarian abscess may result, and there may be direct invasion of the ovarian cortex (*e.g.,* through a ruptured ovarian follicle).

Infection of the endometrium in the absence of pregnancy, an intrauterine device, or a septic abortion with retained products of conception, is usually self-limited. Retained, devitalized, necrotic tissue is an excellent culture medium which permits infection to spread from endometrium to myometrium and parametrium. Polymorphonuclear and plasma cells infiltrate the submucosa and fibroelastic tissues; new blood vessel growth occurs (Fig. 50-5). Multiple abscesses may result, and the inflammatory process may spread to involve blood vessels, leading to pelvic thrombophlebitis and pelvic cellulitis (Fig. 50-6).

Chronic endometritis (Fig. 50-7) may be associated with an earlier, severe acute infection, an intrauterine device, chronic pelvic inflammatory disease, or situations in which the cervical os is blocked by stricture or neoplasm.

Manifestations

Cervicitis may be asymptomatic or manifested by variable amounts of a vaginal discharge. Pelvic examination may show a zone of reddened mucosa in the area of the squamocolumnar junction. Such lesions should be evaluated by cytologic and colposcopic examinations to rule out neoplasia.

The patient with acute endometritis is usually postabortal or postpartum and experiences an abrupt rise in temperature within 24 hours of abortion or delivery. On examination, the uterus is large and tender; a foul-smelling discharge may be present (Fig. 50-8). Evidences of manipulation—vaginal lacerations, perforations, or foreign bodies—should be sought. Spread of the infection to pelvic veins may lead to septic emboli in the lungs with resultant dyspnea,

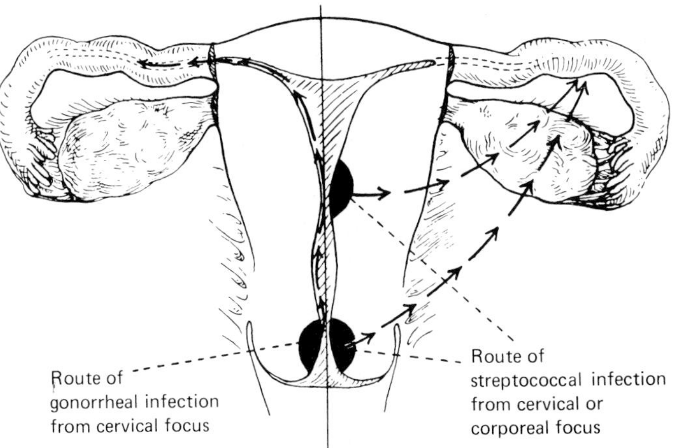

Fig. 50-3. Routes of spread of infectious agents to involve the oviducts. If untreated, both acute gonococcal and other pyogenic types of cervicitis may lead to salpingo-oophoritis—the former by way of the uterus (endometritis), the latter by lymphatic spread. (Novak ER, Woodruff JD: Novak's Gynecologic and Obstetric Pathology, 6th ed. Philadelphia, WB Saunders, 1967)

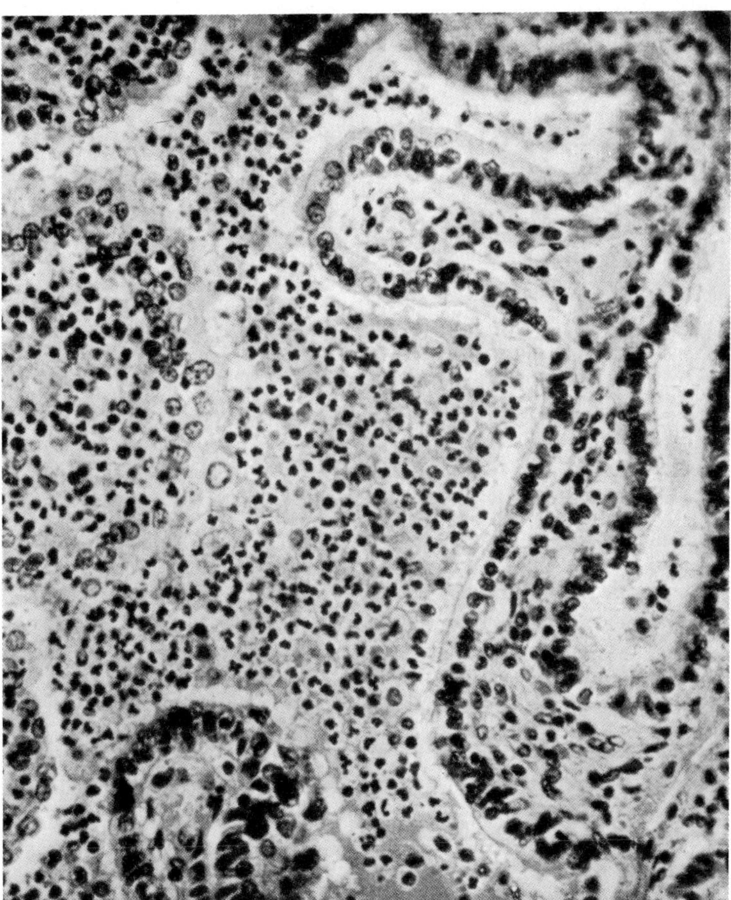

Fig. 50-4. Exudative, acute salpingitis. The acute exudative response almost invariably results in some damage to tubo-ovarian function. (Original magnification approximately × 100) (Novak ER, Woodruff JD: Novak's Gynecologic and Obstetric Pathology, 6th ed. Philadelphia, WB Saunders, 1967)

tachypnea, or pulmonary infiltrates. If signs of peritonitis are present, the possibility of uterine perforation or rupture of an abscess must be considered. Patients with severe endometritis may be critically ill with vascular collapse and evidence of disseminated intravascular coagulation.

Acute pelvic inflammatory disease causes fever, chills, malaise, and severe bilateral lower abdominal pain. The patient prefers to lie quietly with her legs flexed or walks bent forward from the waist in an attempt to reduce the pain. Both lower quadrants are tender to palpation. Pelvic examination may reveal a purulent discharge oozing from an inflamed cervical os. The size and consistency of the uterus are normal. Although the uterus itself is not tender, putting traction on the adnexal structures or pelvic peritoneum causes severe pain. The adnexal regions are very tender, and an adnexal or cul-de-sac mass may be palpable if the process is recurrent and chronic.

Rupture of a tuboovarian abscess causes severe pain referred to the site of involvement. Chills, fever, and signs of progressing peritonitis follow the onset of pain. Diarrhea may occur early but ceases as the peritonitis worsens. If large volumes of pus are released into the peritoneal cavity, infection may spread upward along the colonic gutters; subphrenic abscesses may form, causing pain in the shoulders as a result of irritation of the diaphragm.

Recurrent pelvic infections may lead to the development of an indolent form of pelvic cellulitis termed *ligneous cellulitis.* This is associated with nonspecific symptoms of malaise, fatigue, and pelvic discomfort with or without fever. On examination the pelvic floor has a hard, woody texture, which may be confused with cancer.

Diagnosis

Pelvic inflammatory disease must be differentiated from other acute lower abdominal processes such as acute appendicitis, rupture of an ovarian cyst, or a ruptured ectopic pregnancy. Right-sided unilateral symptoms and prominent gastrointestinal symptoms are suggestive of appendicitis. A history of irregular menses, a sudden drop in hemoglobin and hematocrit, and a positive pregnancy test should suggest a ruptured ectopic pregnancy.

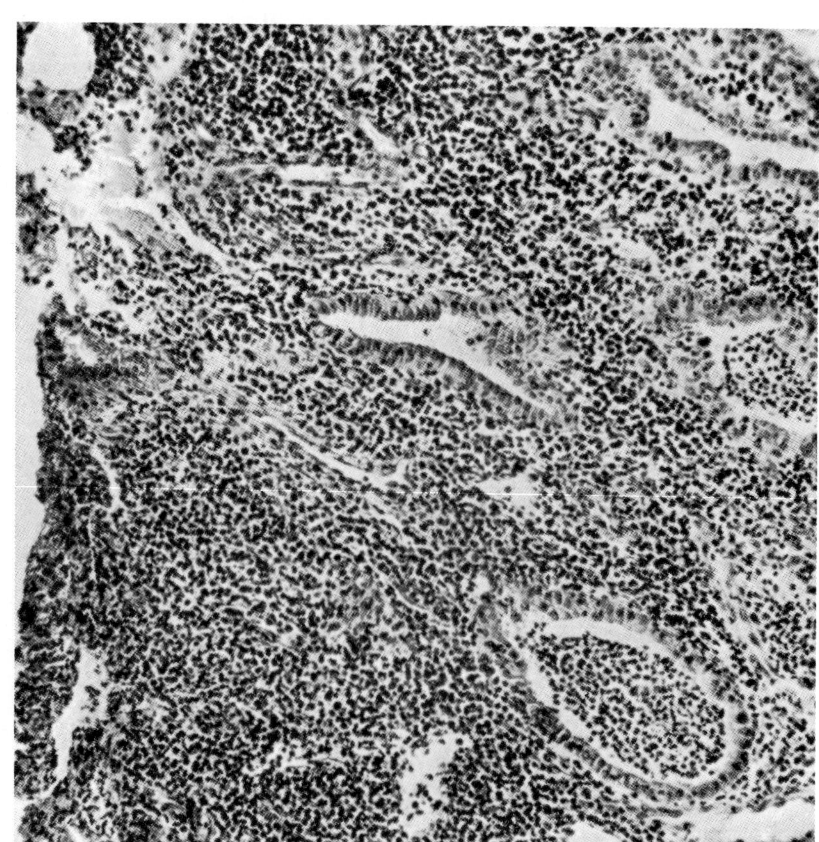

Fig. 50-5. Acute endometritis with marked leukocytic infiltration. Note exudate in the glands. (Original magnification approximately × 400) (Novak ER, Woodruff JD: Novak's Gynecologic and Obstetric Pathology, 6th ed. Philadelphia, WB Saunders, 1967)

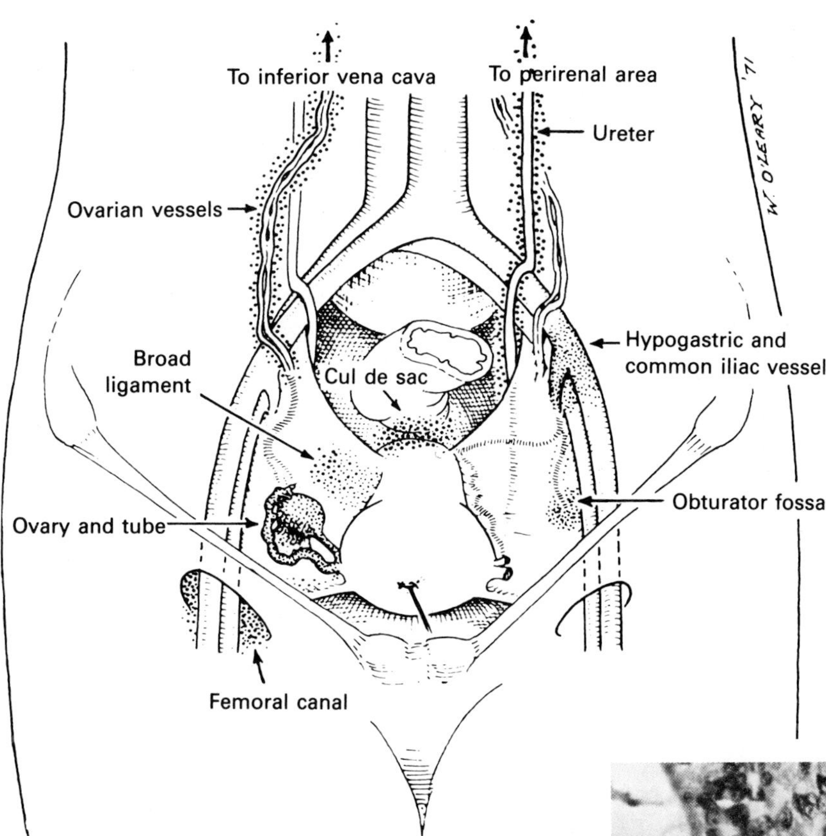

Fig. 50-6. Pathways by which acute uterine infections leading to pelvic cellulitis, thrombophlebitis, and peritonitis may spread. (Charles D, Klein JA: Postpartum Infection. In Charles D, Finland M (eds): Obstetric and Perinatal Infections. Philadelphia, Lea & Febiger, 1973)

Although an accurate bacteriologic diagnosis is desirable, the relative inaccessability of pelvic structures and the likelihood of external contamination of cultures obtained through the vagina have limited the information obtained. Procedures such as colposcopy, laparoscopy, or culdocentesis to obtain specimens for culture may increase diagnostic accuracy. Because cultures of peritoneal fluid may not always mirror infection in the fallopian tubes, cultures should be obtained from both sites. Material obtained for culture should be Gramstained and cultured aerobically and anaerobically. Blood cultures should be obtained but are frequently negative.

Diagnosis of septic abortion performed outside the hospital may be difficult because women who have undergone a criminal abortion frequently deny it. Clinical and laboratory findings may be nonspecific early in the course of a patient who has fever, rigors,

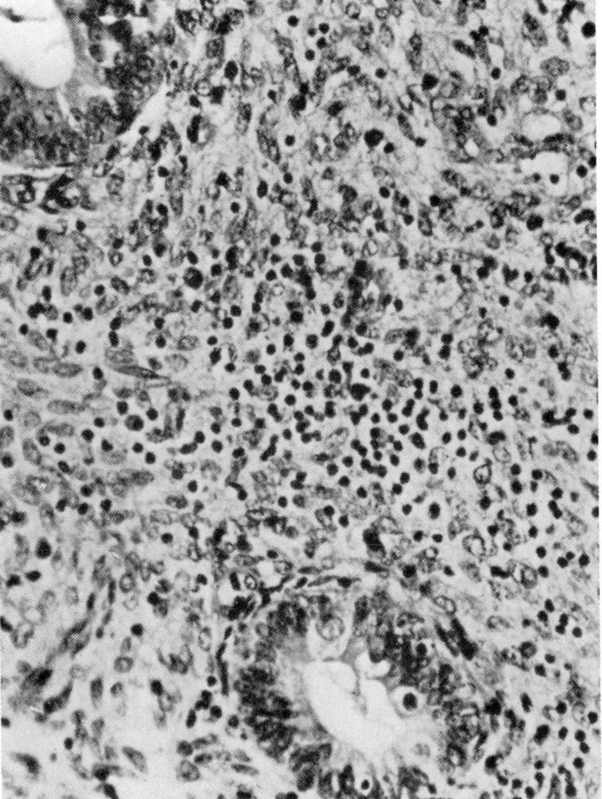

Fig. 50-7. Chronic endometritis is marked by round cell infiltration. (Original magnification approximately × 400) (Novak ER, Woodruff JD: Novak's Gynecologic and Obstetric Pathology, 6th ed. Philadelphia, WB Saunders, 1967)

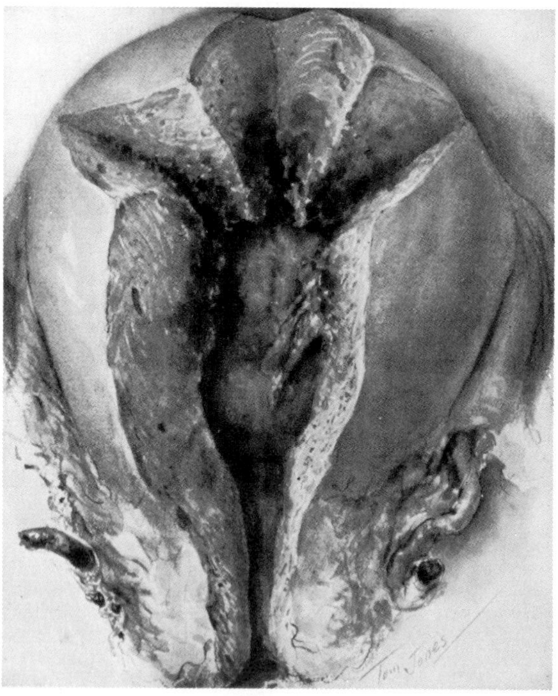

Fig. 50-8. Example of acute, postabortal infection in which the uterus is large and edematous. There is necrosis of the uterine wall at the site of placental attachment. There are remnants of retained placental tissue. Uterine veins are thrombosed bilaterally. (Novak ER, Woodruff JD: Novak's Gynecologic and Obstetric Pathology, 6th ed. Philadelphia, WB Saunders, 1967)

hypotension, and anuria. Pelvic examination may reveal a tender uterus or provide evidence that infection has spread far beyond the confines of the uterus. Placental fragments and purulent drainage from a patulous cervical os may be found; occasionally, the instrument used to induce the abortion is discovered. Roentgenographic examination of the abdomen is useful to determine the presence of intrauterine or extrauterine foreign bodies and gas. Free air or a foreign body in the peritoneal cavity indicates uterine perforation.

Tuboovarian abscess must be differentiated from recurrent pelvic inflammatory disease. Failure of the patient to respond to antimicrobial therapy and persistence of an adnexal mass are more in keeping with abscess than salpingitis.

Oophoritis without salpingitis is uncommon—viral infections, such as mumps, are occasionally implicated.

Prognosis

Acute pelvic inflammatory disease usually subsides with therapy. However, the patient may experience recurrences of pain with each menstrual period. When the infectious process becomes chronic or recurrent, fibrosis may cause structural changes, such as occlusion of the tubes, which may lead to sterility. Other complications include pelvic adhesions, hydro or pyosalpinx, tuboovarian abscess, chronic pelvic pain, and dyspareunia. Postabortal endometritis and rupture of a tuboovarian abscess may be fatal because of the widespread infectious process and complications of shock, disseminated intravascular coagulation, and renal failure.

Therapy

Medical therapy for pelvic infections is a matter of choosing an appropriate antimicrobic. This is made difficult by the problems of obtaining adequate material for culture and the diverse nature of the infecting microorganisms. Therapy cannot be directed against all possible etiologic agents; the clinician must choose antimicrobics on the bases of probabilities. The results of Gram stains of fluid from the peritoneal cavity of fallopian tube, as may be obtained by laparoscopy or culdocentesis, are helpful in selecting drugs prior to the availability of the results of cultures.

Women with mild symptoms may be treated as outpatients either with tetracycline (30 mg/kg body wt/day, PO, as four equal portions, 6-hourly, for 10 days) or with a penicillin. Aqueous procaine penicillin G, 4.8 million units as two equal portions injected IM using two sites, *or* ampicillin, 3.5 g PO *plus* 1.0 g probenecid PO, followed by ampicillin in a dose of 30 mg/kg body wt/day, PO, as four equal portions, 6-hourly, for 10 days. Tetracycline should not be given to pregnant patients.

The acutely ill patient with pelvic inflammatory disease should be hospitalized. Because *N. gonorrhoeae* is a frequent cause, penicillin G, 100 mg to 200 mg (120,000–360,000 units)/kg body wt/day should be injected IV as six equal portions, 4-hourly. After improvement (decrease in fever and pain), a total of 10 days of therapy may be attained using ampicillin in the dosage given above. An alternative regimen for nonpregnant patients is tetracycline injected IV in a dose of 15 mg/kg body wt/day as four equal portions, 6-hourly, to be followed after improvement by peroral treatment (dosage as for ampicillin) to complete a total of 10 days of therapy.

Severely, acutely ill patients should also receive an aminocyclitol (*e.g.*, gentamicin or tobramycin, 5 mg–6 mg/kg body wt/day, IV, as three equal portions, 8-hourly) plus clindamycin (20 mg–30 mg/kg body wt/day, IV, as four equal portions, 6-hourly), *or* chloramphenicol (50 mg/kg body wt/day, IV, as four equal portions, 6-hourly), *or* metronidazole (15 mg/kg body wt/ IV, as a loading dose followed by 30 mg/kg body wt/day, IV, as four equal portions, 6-hourly—maximum dose of 4 g/day). One of these regimens should be applied until the results of cultures become available to provide treatment for gram-negative enteric bacteria, enterococci, staphylococci, and anaerobes. Cefoxitin (100 mg/kg body wt/day, IV, as four equal portions, 6-hourly) is an alternative for use in patients who are allergic to penicillins; it is also active against many of the anaerobes.

A response may not be evident for 5 to 7 days, especially with nongonococcal infections. Surgical intervention may be required if the patient fails to respond to medical therapy, and it becomes mandatory when a tuboovarian abscess ruptures because the case fatality rate then approaches 90% with medical therapy alone. Rapid diagnosis of such an abscess is the keystone to a successful outcome; operation within 12 hours of rupture yields the best prognosis. Antimicrobics are adjunctive to surgical therapy; selection should be guided by the results of Gramstains of material obtained at surgery.

Pelvic thrombophlebitis is so frequently associated with infection caused by anaerobic cocci or *Bacteroides fragilis* that administration of penicillin G plus clindamycin is indicated. Anticoagulant therapy with heparin should also be given. If repeated pulmonary emboli occur despite adequate anticoagulation, ligation of the inferior vena cava and the ovarian vein may be necessary.

The treatment of septic, incomplete abortions is removal of necrotic tissue; this may be possible by uterine curettage, but in severe cases total hysterectomy may be required. The proper time for curettage is controversial; some clinicians favor early intervention, while others would delay if there is evidence of infection outside the confines of the uterus. Antimicrobial agents should be given prior to surgery because bacteremia may be caused by the operation. Anaerobic bacteria (*Clostridium* spp., *Bacteroides fragilis,* anaerobic cocci) play an important role in septic abortions, and therapy must be adequate to affect these pathogens. As in severe, acute pelvic inflammatory disease, penicillin G, an aminocyclitol, and clindamycin may be used in combination until the results of the cultures are available (dosages as given previously). Blood, urine, uterine drainage, and material aspirated from the cul-de-sac should be cultured aerobically and anaerobically. If curettage and antimicrobials fail—the patient becomes clinically worse with continued fever, increased hemolysis, or renal failure—laparotomy should be performed to assess the degree of pelvic damage, drain collections of pus, and excise necrotic tissue.

Postpartum endometritis, or puerperal fever, remains an important obstetric complication. Between 1964 and 1968 it was the leading cause of maternal death in Massachusetts. Many different kinds of bacteria can produce this disease, which characteristically begins with fever, profuse lochial flow, and an enlarged, tender uterus 3 to 4 days after delivery. β-hemolytic streptococci have historical significance as the causative agent of puerperal fever, but other aerobic bacteria and anaerobes are frequently present in mixed infections. Vaginal bacteria can be introduced into the endometrial cavity by examinations during labor; during delivery through the use of forceps; or by manual extraction of a breech presentation or of the placenta. When endometritis develops, retained tissue must be completely removed from the uterus and antimicrobial agents should be given. Penicillin G is the drug of choice: 150 mg to 200 mg (240,000 to 320,000 units)/kg body wt/day, IV, as six equal portions, 4-hourly; in severe cases an aminocyclitol and clindamycin should also be given (dosages as given previously).

Another common cause for fever in the puerperium is mastitis. *Staphylococcus aureus* is the most common cause of this condition. Treatment consists of cessation of nursing, drainage if an abscess forms, and administration of a penicillinase-resistant penicillin: cloxacillin or dicloxacillin (50 mg–60 mg/kg body wt/day, PO, as four equal portions, 6-hourly) or nafcillin (50 mg–60 mg/kg body wt/day, IV, as four equal portions, 6-hourly) for 7 to 10 days.

Prevention

Prevention of pelvic infections requires control of the venereal spread of disease by education and the use of condoms, through careful aseptic practices in instrumentation of the genital tract, and by careful attention to all details of delivery.

Postoperative Obstetric and Gynecologic infections

Because it is impossible to sterilize the vagina and cervix, areas which the gynecologic surgeon must frequently manipulate, infections following gynecologic surgery are a major problem. Vaginal cuff infections, pelvic cellulitis (extending from the cuff infection), pelvic thrombophlebitis, and ovarian abscess are infections which are commonly encountered. Pelvic infections following vaginal hysterectomy vary in frequency from 20% to 40%. Such infections tend to occur more commonly in younger women, perhaps because of the greater vascularity of the surgical field—predisposing to the formation of hematomas—and the richer bacterial vaginal flora of younger women.

Vaginal cuff infections usually begin with fever about 2 to 5 days postoperatively, with few other physical findings. If a vaginal cuff abscess forms, the collection may be palpable on pelvic examination, or a purulent discharge may be present in the vagina. Pelvic cellulitis is usually marked by fever, which begins 5 to 7 days after operation; it is associated with low abdominal pain and tenderness, ileus, or signs of peritoneal irritation. Ovarian abscesses which complicate pelvic surgery result from direct extension of infection from the vaginal cuff area to the ovary. Vaginal cuff abscesses, infected hematomas, and ovarian abscesses all require surgical drainage in addition to antimicrobics. The penicillin–aminocyclitol–clindamycin regimen (see Cervicitis, Endometritis, and Salpingo-Oophoritis) is applicable in severe postoperative gynecologic infections.

Because postoperative infections so commonly complicate gynecologic surgery, there have been several studies of chemoprophylaxis in vaginal hysterectomy. Brief courses using one of several antimicrobial agents have been shown to reduce rates of infection. As with any program of chemoprophylaxis, the drug employed must be relatively nontoxic, achieve therapeutic levels in the potentially contaminated area, and be effective against the most likely bacterial pathogens. It also seems evident that it is not necessary to obliterate all of the bacteria in a given area, because many successful regimens provide little activity against anaerobes. It may be sufficient to change the milieu only to the point that some bacterial growth is inhibited.

The use of antibacterial chemoprophylaxis certainly reduces the risk of postoperative infection in vaginal hysterectomy and is possibly effective in abdominal hysterectomy. Many regimens have made use of a cephalosporin for brief periods. A single dose of cefazolin (1.0 g IM or IV) on call to surgery appears to be as effective as multidose regimens of chemoprophylaxis in vaginal hysterectomy. With such a brief period of treatment, the potential for superinfection by drug-resistant bacteria is minimized and there is a low probability of adverse reaction to the antimicrobic.

Prophylactic antimicrobics appear to be beneficial in high-risk patients undergoing cesarean section. Women in the high risk category include those with onset of labor prior to surgery, those undergoing their first section, those who require internal fetal monitoring prior to cesarean section or who need general anesthesia, and those who present with obesity and other metabolic abnormalities such as diabetes mellitus. One effective regimen utilizes cefoxitin (2 g IV), started when the fetal cord is clamped, and repeated 4 and 8 hours later. This approach avoids potential complications from administration of the antimicrobic to the baby.

Chorioamnionitis

During pregnancy, the fetal membranes and the cervical mucus plug provide effective barriers to ascending infectious agents. Once the fetal membranes rupture, however, the potential for infection is great and increases as the length of time from rupture to delivery increases. Three-fourths of transabdominally obtained cultures of amniotic fluid contain bacteria when the membranes have been ruptured for 24 hours or longer. Bacteria growing in the amniotic fluid can infect the lungs of the fetus and result in overwhelming fetal infection. Another route of fetal infection involves penetration of the fetal circulation, which causes a venous vasculitis and septicemia. Maternal infection results from penetration of the maternal circulation, with resultant septicemia. The use of prophylactic antimicrobials in mothers with premature rupture of membranes does not reduce maternal or fetal morbidity.

When premature rupture occurs, 80% to 90% of women will go into labor within 24 hours. These patients should be hospitalized and examined vaginally using sterile technique to determine the fetal presentation, status of the cervix, and whether the umbilical cord has prolapsed. Immediate cesarean section should be done if the cord is prolapsed and the fetus is viable. Otherwise, the patient can be watched for 8 to 12 hours; if labor cannot be induced or does not occur spontaneously, cesarean section should be performed.

Once the diagnosis of chorioamnionitis is established by amniocentesis, antimicrobial therapy should be given. Gram-negative bacilli (especially *E. coli*) are the common causes of bacterial chorioamnionitis, along with anaerobes and *N. gonorrhoeae.* Effective therapy is the same as that recommended for acute endometritis and salpingo-oophoritis. Initial therapy should be guided by results of the gram stain of amniotic fluid.

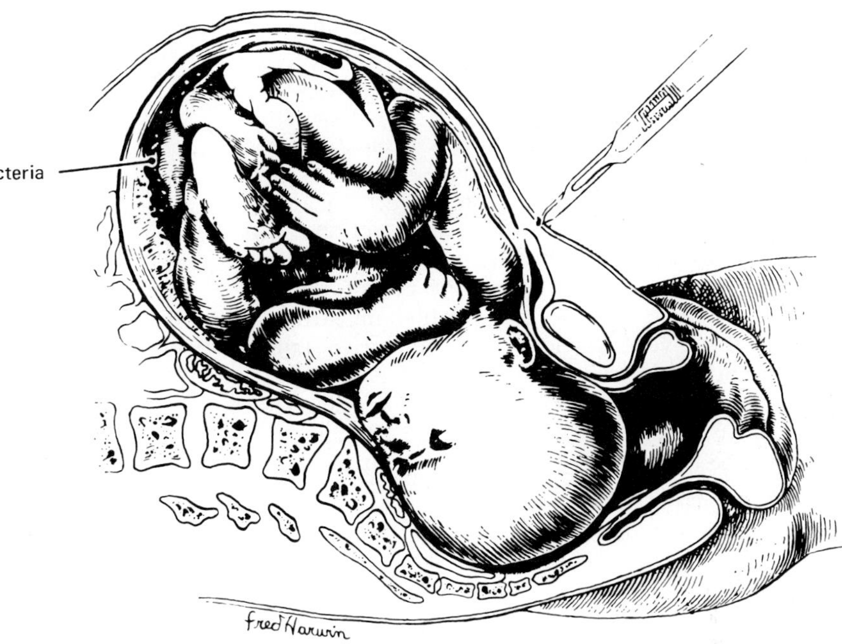

Fig. 50-9. When cesarean section is necessary in the face of chorioamnionitis, bacterial contamination of the surgical field is certain. Spread to the peritoneal cavity or to the surgical wound postoperatively is possible. (Ledger WJ: Clin Obstet Gynecol 12:160–282, 1969)

Other microorganisms, (*e.g.,* herpes simplex viruses, cytomegalovirus, and *Urea urealyticum*) have also been associated with chorioamnionitis; although the fetus may be severely damaged, there may be no signs of infection in the mother. Cesarean section in the presence of chorioamnionitis has inherent risks because the surgical wound is inevitably infected. Spread to other pelvic organs and the peritoneum is likely (Fig. 50-9). Cultures of the amniotic fluid, the placental surface, and the blood should be obtained at the time of surgery.

*Toxic Shock Syndrome**

Toxic shock syndrome (TSS) is an acute systemic illness which appears to be associated with infection or colonization by certain exotoxin-producing staphylococci. The majority of cases have occurred in menstruating women, especially those who use vaginal tampons. However, children, men, and women outside the reproductive age group have also been afflicted. Cardinal manifestations of TSS are fever, hypotension, multiple organ system dysfunction, a diffuse ("sunburnlike") erythematous rash typically seen on the trunk but less commonly involving the limbs and extremities as well, and a characteristic desquamation on the extremities during or after recovery. A prodrome of diarrhea, vomiting, and general, severe myalgias is common. Systemic involvement includes renal and hepatic insufficiency, pancreatitis, mild-to-moderate cardiac dysfunction, development of adult respiratory distress syndrome, and hematologic abnormalities including leukocytosis, thrombocytopenia, and prolongation of clotting parameters. *Staphylococcus aureus* has been isolated from vaginal exudates in women and from other focal infected sites in nonmenstruating patients. TSS can recur during subsequent menstrual cycles.

The pathogenesis of TSS is incompletely understood. Staphylococcal pyrogenic Exotoxin C, a protein of 22,000 MW that causes fever in rabbits and enhances the lethal effects of endotoxin, was produced by all TSS-associated isolates of *S. aureus* in preliminary studies. Whether this toxin is solely responsible for systemic manifestation of TSS, or whether it acts in concert with other toxins remains uncertain. Changes in the microflora and biochemical environment of the vagina during menses may predispose to overgrowth of the toxin-producing staphylococci. Further study is needed to elucidate the role of vaginal tampons in the pathogenesis of TSS; excoriation of the vaginal mucosa may facilitate absorption of exotoxin.

Treatment strategies in TSS depend on early recognition and appreciation of the potentially devastating systemic complications of prolonged hypotension, and should include vigorous fluid resuscitation with inotropic drug therapy if necessary and general sup-

* Discussion contributed by Sheila M. Nolan, M.D.

portive measures during the acute phase of the illness. Use of a β-lactamase-resistant antimicrobic (*e.g.*, nafcillin, 150 mg/kg body wt/day, IV) may attenuate or prevent recurrent episodes but does not appear to alter the course of the acute illness. Women who have had TSS should not use tampons.

Prevalence studies indicate that 5% to 15% of women harbor *S. aureus* in vaginal secretions. A small proportion of such isolates from normal women produce Exotoxin C, and the risk of TSS is very low—about 3 episodes per 100,000 menstruating women per year. Eradication of the carrier state may prevent TSS but may not be practical. The role of the immune response in modifying recurrent disease is under investigation. Development of an animal model of TSS is urgently needed to study further the pathogenetic mechanism in TSS.

Bibliography

Books

CHARLES DM, FINLAND M (EDS): Obstetric and Perinatal Infections. Philadelphia, Lea & Febiger, 1973. 652 pp.

MONIF GRG (ED): Infectious Diseases in Obstetrics and Gynecology. Hagerstown, Harper & Row, 1974. 470 pp.

NOVAK ER, WOODRUFF JF: Novak's Gynecologic and Obstetric Pathology, 8th ed. Philadelphia, WB Saunders, 1979. 795 pp.

Journals

CUNNINGHAM FC, HAUTH JC, STRONG JR, HERBERT WNP, GILSTRAP LC, WILSON RH, KAPPUS SS: Evaluation of tetracycline or penicillin and ampicillin for treatment of acute pelvic inflammatory disease. N Engl J Med 296:1380–1383, 1977

DAVIS JP, CHESNEY PJ, WAND PJ, LA VENTURE M AND THE INVESTIGATION AND LABORATORY TEAM: Toxic shock syndrome. Epidemiologic features, recurrence, risk factors, and prevention. N Engl J Med 303: 1429–1435, 1980

DIKERS JR: Single dose metronidazole for trichomonal vaginitis. N Engl J Med 293:23–24, 1975

ESCHENBACH DA: Epidemiology and diagnosis of acute pelvic inflammatory disease. Obstet Gynecol 55: 142S–152S, 1980

ESCHENBACH DA, BUCHANAN TM, POLLOCK HM, FORSYTH PS, ALEXANDER ER, LIN J. WANG S, WENTWORTH BB, MCCORMACK WM, HOLMES KK: Polymicrobial etiology of acute pelvic inflammatory disease. N Engl J Med 293:166–171, 1975

GALASK RP, OHM MJ: Abdominal hysterectomy. South Med J 70, Suppl 1:37–40, 1977

LETT WJ, ANSBACHER R, DAVIDSON BL, OTTERSON WN: Prophylactic antibiotics for women undergoing vaginal hysterectomy. J Reprod Med 19:51–54, 1977

MARDH PA, RIPA T, SVENSSON L, WESTROM L: *Chlamydia trachomatis* infection in patients with acute salpingitis. N Engl J Med 296:1377–1379, 1977

MEAD PB: Practical applications of antibiotics in prevention and treatment of pelvic infection. J Reprod Med 13:135–141, 1974

PHEIFER TA, FORSYTH PS, DURFEE MC, POLLOCK HM, HOLMES KK: Nonspecific vaginitis. Role of *Haemophilus vaginalis* and treatment with metronidazole. N Engl J Med 298:1429–1434, 1978

REIN MF, CHAPEL RA: Trichomoniasis, candidiasis and the minor venereal diseases. Clin Obstet Gynecol 18:73–88, 1975

SCHLIEVERT PM, SHANDS KN, DAN BB, SCHMID GP, NISHIMURA RD: Identification and Characterization of an Exotoxin from *Staphylococcus aureus* associated with toxic-shock syndrome. J Infect Dis 143:509–516, 1981

SHANDS KN, SCHMID GP, DAN BB, BLUM D, GUIDOTTI RJ, HARGRETT NT, ANDERSON RL, HILL DL, BROOME CV, BAND JD, FRASER DW: Toxic-shock syndrome in menstruating women: Its association with tampon use and *Staphylococcus aureus* and the clinical features in 52 cases. N Engl J Med 303:1436–1442, 1980

SPIEGEL CA, AMSEL R, ESCHENBACH D, SCHOENKNECHT F, HOLMES KK: Anaerobic bacteria in nonspecific vaginitis. N Engl J Med 303:601–607, 1980

SWEET RL, MILLS J, HADLEY KW, BLUMENSTOCK E, SCHACTER J, ROBBIE MO, DRAPER DL: Use of laparoscopy to determine the microbiologic etiology of acute salpingitis. Am J Obstet Gynecol 134:68–74, 1979

PAUL D. HOEPRICH

Listeriosis

51

Although uncommon, genital tract infection in the gravid female with perinatal infection of offspring is the most nearly unique of the many clinical varieties of disease caused by *Listeria monocytogenes*. Meningitis is the most frequent form of listeriosis in humans, but it is no more singular in manifestations than are the less common nonmeningitic infections of the central nervous system, primary listeremia, endocarditis, ocular infections, and rare incursions such as dermatitis, lymphadenitis, abscesses in various organs, pericarditis, peritonitis, and osteomyelitis.

Etiology

Operationally, the genus *Listeria* contains but one species, *monocytogenes*; the status of the nonpathogenic listerias, suggested as the species *denitrificans, grayi,* and *murrayi,* remains uncertain. The designation *monocytogenes* was applied because a monocytosis is characteristic of general listeriosis in rodents. In humans, ruminants, and other nonrodent mammals, a neutrophilic leukocytosis is the usual response.

The pathogenic, smooth colony form of *L. monocytogenes* consists of gram-positive, non-acid-fast, nonsporulating, facultatively anaerobic, motile (peritrichous flagellae) bacilli varying in size from 0.3 μm to 0.6 μm × 0.8 μm to 2.5 μm. A soluble hemolysin is elaborated, and several carbohydrates are fermented (acid, no gas), including glucose (acetoin formed), salicin, and, notably, esculin. As bile salts are not inhibitory, growth on conventional bile–esculin agar is useful to laboratory diagnosis. The isolation of listerias from contaminated specimens is aided by the use of the following: (1) culture mediums rendered selective by the addition of nalidixic acid with either trypaflavine or thallous acetate, and (2) cold enrichment (*i.e.,* holding specimens in broth at 4°C with periodic subculture for 2 weeks to 3 months, or even longer).

Listerias are catalase-positive but other common biochemical tests are not usefully distinctive. However, demonstration of motility (most pronounced at 20°C–25°C), ability to reduce tellurite and 2,3,5-triphenyltetrazolium chloride, and animal pathogenicity are generally adequate for differentiation of listerias from the other bacteria with which they are most often confused—namely, *Erysipelothrix* spp., *Corynebacterium* spp., and *Streptococcus* spp.

The most informative test for pathogenicity involves conjunctival inoculation in either rabbits, hamsters, or guinea pigs; in 3 to 5 days, keratoconjunctivitis develops, which is localized to the inoculated eye (Anton test). General listeriosis in the rabbit, induced by intravenous inoculation, is associated with a monocytosis 3 to 7 days after infection. Lethal infection follows 1 to 3 days after intraperitoneal injection of *L. monocytogenes* into mice; multiple hepatic abscesses, microscopic to pinhead in size, are characteristic.

Listeria spp. are serologically distinct and fall into seven major types on the basis of somatic and flagellar antigens. Typing serums are not generally available, but reference laboratories have been established that carry out typing (General Bacteriology Unit, Bacteriology Section, Centers for Disease Control, United States Public Health Service, Department of Health, Education, and Welfare, Atlanta, Georgia, 30333).

Epidemiology

Listeria monocytogenes is worldwide in distribution. It has been isolated from many kinds of nonhuman mammals and birds, ticks, crustaceans, stream water, mud, sewage, dirt, soil, and silage. It has been associated with either overt disease or a carrier state in humans, and it is possible that healthy human carriers are an important source of *L. monocytogenes* that infect humans. This possibility is supported by the finding (data from many countries) that 5% to 60% of asymptomatic adults are fecal carriers. However, some fecal isolates are nonhemolytic (*i.e.,* avirulent), and some are nontypable; of typable isolates, type 1 predominates, type 4 is next, and type 3 follows—a notable finding, since type 3 is uncommon as a cause for disease, whereas types 1a and 4b together account for more than 90% of listeriosis worldwide. The importance of nonhuman animals as sources of *L. monocytogenes* for infection of humans is further diminished by the following two additional observations: (1) most cases occur in city dwellers who have not had contact with nonhuman animals, and (2) the season of maximal frequency of disease is January to May in nonhuman animals, whereas it is July and August in humans (Northern Hemisphere).

Listeriosis is diagnosed with increased frequency in the United States and other countries. Diminished immune competence appears to play a predisposing role in about two-thirds of patients—most often from malignancies, iatrogenic immunosuppression (as in recipients of renal allografts), and hepatic disease (*e.g.,* cirrhosis). Listeriosis may occur as an occupational disease among veterinarians, abattoir workers, and poultry butchers through contact with infected liquids from nonhuman animals. In a very few instances, listeriosis in humans has followed ingestion of contaminated milk or inhalation of infected dust. Transfer of the infection from mother to offspring remains the only proved example of human-to-human transmission of listeriosis.

Overall, males are infected only slightly more often than females, but, in newborns, males clearly predominate. The age-related incidence is distinctly bimodal. Peak attack rates occur at ages less than 1 year and greater than 55 years.

Serotypes 1 (1b is about twice as frequent as 1a) and 4b occur with nearly identical frequency and together account for most disease; types 4d, 3b, 1, 4a, and 4 usually make up the remainder. *Listeria* spp. of type 2 have been isolated but rarely, and only from humans. Type 3 *L. monocytogenes* is quite uncommon in the United States, but may cause disease in both humans and nonhuman species.

Pathogenesis and Pathology

Although *L. monocytogenes* is ubiquitous, the way in which human and nonhuman animals become infected often remains obscure. Overall, meningeal localization is the most common clinical form of listeriosis, accounting for about 75% of all bacteriologically proved infections. The pathology of acute listerial meningitis does not differ from that of any other pyogenic meningitis. None of the other clinical forms of listeriosis gives rise to a unique pathology.

Whether an infection eventuates in disease is dependent on the interplay of at least three factors: (1) the state of the host, (2) the route of infection, and (3) the virulence of the infecting strain.

THE STATE OF THE HOST (AGE, IMMUNOCOMPETENCE)

Listerias are cytophilic parasites. It may follow that humoral immunity is of less importance in combating listeriosis than cell-mediated immunity. Indeed, the relatively high frequency of occurrence of listeriosis in patients with compromised cellular immunity (*e.g.,* patients with malignancies or other illnesses requiring treatment with drugs such as azathioprine or glucosteroids) is supportive of this construction.

THE ROUTE OF INFECTION

Prenatal (*i.e.,* transplacental) infection usually occurs during the third trimester and exposes the fetus to a blood-borne inoculum drawn from the infected placenta. The resultant widespread disease is quite reminiscent of the listeriosis that occurs in rodents—widely disseminated, small abscesses or granulomas, depending on the duration of the process. These fetal lesions vary in size from grossly visible to microscopic. They are always found in the liver (Fig. 51-1) and may also occur, in order of decreasing frequency, in the spleen, adrenal glands, lungs, pharynx, gastrointestinal tract, central nervous system, and skin. Because of the nature of the cellular response and the widespread involvement, the name *miliary granulomatosis* is often applied to this form of listeriosis. With gastrointestinal involvement, listerias are also present in the meconium, often in such great numbers that they can be seen on microscopic examination of a Gram-stained smear of meconium (distinctly abnormal, because normal meconium has too few bacteria to be seen microscopically) (Fig. 51-2).

Infection with *L. monocytogenes* that is contracted intrapartum is thought to result from contact with infected maternal secretions. The inoculum is smaller than with prepartum infection; if disease results, it is usually localized to the central nervous system and is manifest as meningitis.

THE VIRULENCE OF THE INFECTING STRAIN

In the laboratory, nonhemolytic strains are avirulent. Nontypable strains may also be avirulent because vir-

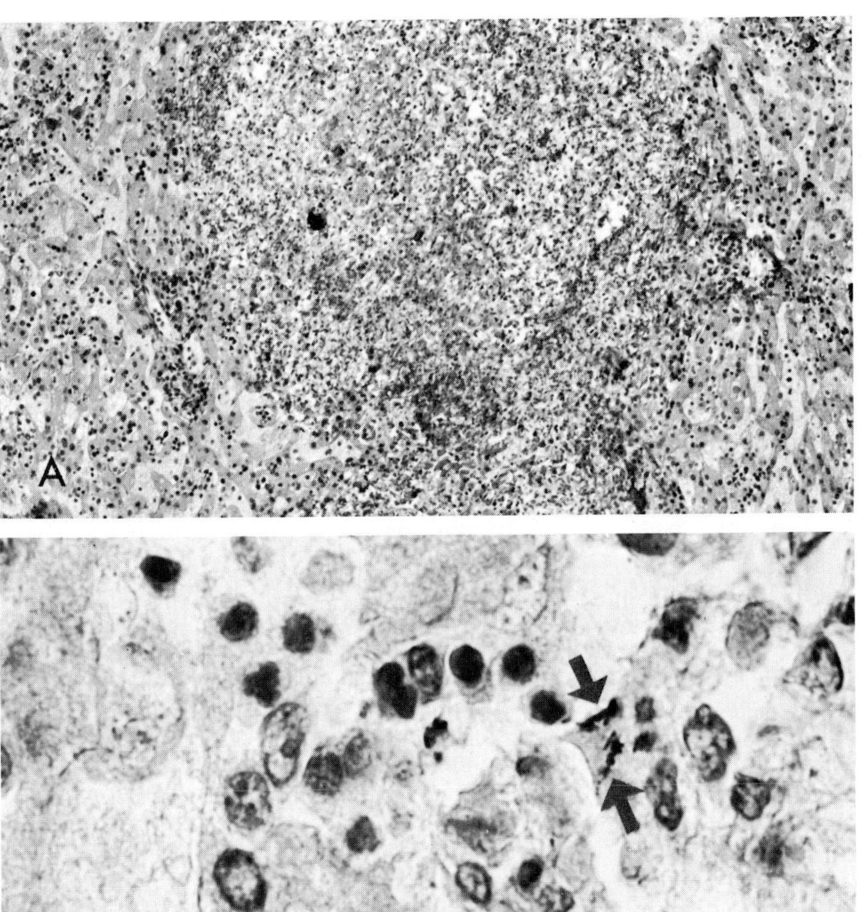

Fig. 51-1. Microabcess in the liver of a newborn who died of disseminated listeriosis. (*A*) Focal necrosis with intense inflammatory cell response (Hematoxylin and eosin, original magnification approximately × 100) (*B*) The listerias are predominantly intracellular (*arrows*) (Gram stain, original magnification approximately × 1600) (Courtesy of HPR Seeliger, Institut für Hygiene und Mikrobiologie, Universität Würzburg)

Fig. 51-2. Photomicrographs of Gram-stained smears of meconium. (*A*) Normal infant. (*B*) Newborn with listerial miliary granulomatosis. (Seeliger HPR: Listeriose. Leipzig, JA Barth, 1955)

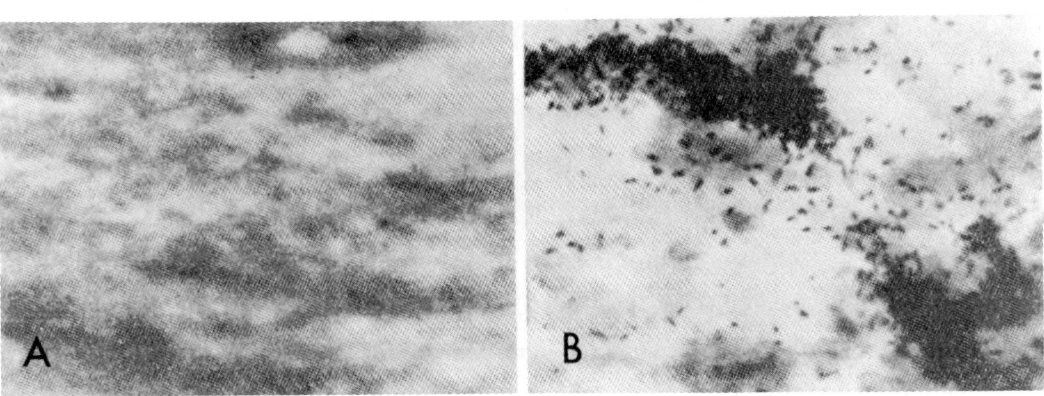

tually all isolates from patients with listerial disease are typable.

Manifestations

Listeriosis contracted prepartally results in abortion, premature delivery, stillbirth, or death within minutes to days following delivery. Active listeriosis of this kind may not cause fever. Cardiorespiratory distress, vomiting, and diarrhea are seen. Maculopapular skin lesions frequently involve the legs and trunk. Hepatosplenomegaly is frequent. Meningitis results in tense fontanelles, irritability, lethargy, convulsions, and coma. Curiously, there is usually no symptomatic illness in the mother. At most, a trivial, passing malaise, benign and self limited, may have occurred about a month before birth. Delivery is always before term when transplacental infection of the fetus with *L. monocytogenes* has occurred.

Listeriosis that occurs in infants under 1 month in age is referred to as *listeriosis of the newborn*. When infection occurs during the course of delivery, listeriosis of the newborn becomes clinically manifest 1 to 4 weeks postpartum. Meningitis, not different from any other bacterial meningitis, is the usual form of the disease.

Although listerial meningitis of newborns, children, and adults is not clinically differentiable from other bacterial meningitides, it is the commonest clinical form of listeriosis. Among patients with cancers, *L. monocytogenes* is one of the most common causes of meningitis. Yet, overall, fewer than 1% of all cases of bacterial meningitis are caused by *L. monocytogenes*.

Nonmeningitic listeriosis of the central nervous system implies either diffuse or focal involvement of the brain or spinal cord. The onset is nonspecific, with fever, nausea and vomiting, and headache. Listeremia is usually present, but the cerebrospinal fluid is normal. Localizing signs of neurologic dysfunction may come on abruptly, or the clinical picture may be that of an encephalitis. Brain scans (radionuclide or computed tomographic) may be helpful in diagnosis.

Primary listeremia, also known as *typhoidal listeriosis,* is characterized by high fever and severe, general illness without evidence of localized infection. Malignancies and immunosuppression are the commonest underlying conditions. However, cirrhosis, alcoholism, and pregnancy are not uncommon in patients who develop primary listeremia.

Infective endocarditis caused by *L. monocytogenes* has no clinically singular manifestations. Approximately one-half of the patients have cardiac lesions recognized as predisposing to bacterial endocarditis.

The ophthalmitis induced by conjunctival inoculation of listerias in the usual rabbit test for pathogenicity has its clinical counterpart in oculoglandular listeriosis. This rare form of listeriosis depends for its occurrence on the accident of inoculation into the eye.

Listerial dermatitis may afflict the skin of the arms of veterinarians who extract placentas manually from cows with genital tract listeriosis.

There is no reliable evidence that *L. monocytogenes* causes either habitual (repeated) abortion or infectious mononucleosis.

Diagnosis

The laboratory must be alerted to the possibility of isolation of *L. monocytogenes*. Confusion with diphtheroids or other bacteria can then be guarded against. Because enrichment procedures and selective culture mediums are not entirely satisfactory, isolation from contaminated clinical materials remains difficult.

Appropriate materials for culture vary with the clinical syndrome. In listeriosis of the newborn, some or all of the following would be appropriate: cervical and vaginal secretions and lochia from the mother; cord blood and the grossly abnormal parts of the placenta; and meconium, blood, cerebrospinal fluid, and exudate expressed from an incised skin papule from the newborn. Refrigeration of tissues appears to favor isolation, presumably by releasing *L. monocytogenes* from intracellular loci. Meningitis obviously requires culture of the cerebrospinal fluid and the blood. Blood cultures are essential to the diagnosis of listeremia, whether primary or secondary to endocarditis.

Serodiagnosis of listeriosis has been complicated by the frequency of occurrence of so-called natural antibodies. The term refers to agglutinins of listerias that are present in the sera of up to 90% of individuals of various species of vertebrates, including humans, although overt listeriosis has not occurred. On the other hand, in persons with bacteriologically proven listeriosis, agglutinins rise in titer, reaching a peak 2 to 4 weeks after onset of infection and falling off in the months following cure. This response is primarily IgM. Natural agglutinins are either IgG or IgM and may represent cross reactions with immunoglobulins engendered by *Staphylococcus aureus* or acquired in response to carriage of *L. monocytogenes.*

Prognosis

Without antimicrobial therapy, listerial meningitis has been fatal in more than 90% of patients. Although effective antimicrobics are available, death is not uncommon—possibly because diagnosis may be delayed. Encephalitis and brain abscesses may be acute complications of meningitis or may occur as primary localizations. Mental retardation and communicating hydrocephalus are late-appearing consequences that may be attributable to scarring. The other forms of listeriosis may yield to specific therapy, with the exception of infection of the newborn. If listeriosis is contracted transplacentally, death of the fetus virtually always results. Salvage of full- or near-term neonates infected during parturition is possible, but the death rate is still substantial, ranging to as high as 50% in many reports.

Humoral immunity, judged by titer of specific agglutinins, decreases with time after infection and may not have protective value. The participation of cell-mediated immune mechanisms appears to be essential.

Therapy

According to testing *in vitro,* many antimicrobics are active against listerias. On both a mass and a molar basis, rifampin is the most active agent (lowest MIC); erythromycin is next, followed by penicillin G, with ampicillin slightly less active. The aminocyclitols are also inhibitory; gentamicin and tobramycin are significantly more active than streptomycin. When capability for lethal activity is examined, there is a remarkable gap between MICs and MLCs with rifampin, erythromycin, penicillin G, ampicillin and streptomycin; in contrast, the MICs and MLCs of gentamicin and tobramycin are reasonably close. Further, combinations of penicillin G or ampicillin with gentamicin or tobramycin are often synergistic and listericidal.

From these considerations, maximally listericidal therapy should result from combined treatment with penicillin G (150–200 mg [240,000–320,000 units]/kg body wt/day, IV, as six equal portions, 4-hourly), and tobramycin (5–6 mg/kg body wt/day, IV, as three or four equal portions, 8- or 6-hourly). Ampicillin and gentamicin may be substituted but offer no advantage. This regimen is recommended for the treatment of listeriosis of the newborn (2 weeks), primary listeremia (4 weeks), listerial endocarditis (4–6 weeks), listeremia in pregnancy (with or without amnionitis; 2 weeks), and virtually any form of listeriosis outside the central nervous system in immunoincompetent patients (4–6 weeks).

For the treatment of meningitis, nonmeningitic infections of the central nervous system, and ocular infections, high-dosage therapy with penicillin G is the mainstay of treatment (200–300 mg [320,000–480,000 units] /kg body wt/day, IV, as six equal portions, 4-hourly). Treatment should be continued without alteration of dose or route of administration for at least 1 week after defervescence. Ampicillin may be substituted for penicillin G; however, the cephalosporins are not alternatives, since they penetrate into the central nervous system and the eye too poorly to be effective. Because tobramycin and gentamicin enter the central nervous system and the eye erratically and poorly, it is doubtful that the coadministration of either drug will be of value (local injection into the eye may be useful in the treatment of listerial endophthalmitis); streptomycin does not penetrate any better, and it suffers from lack of listericidal capability. Rifampin offers good penetration into the central nervous system, albeit without potential for listericidal action; by *in vitro* testing, it is at least additive to penicillin G, but the combination has not undergone clinical evaluation. Although chloramphenicol enters the central nervous system efficiently, relapses of listerial meningitis after treatment with this antimicrobic have been reported. Tetracycline penetrates into the central nervous system poorly, and failures of treatment with this agent have occurred; doxycycline should be more effective because it penetrates much better both into the central nervous system and into cells.

Listerial lymphadenitis and cutaneous listeriosis may be treated with erythromycin (25–30 mg/kg body wt/day, PO, as four equal portions, 6-hourly) or tetracycline (same dose as for erythromycin).

Supportive measures are critically important, particularly in listeriosis of the newborn. Patients with meningitis may also require respiratory assistance. Surgical drainage of listerial abscesses is as critical to cure as it is with any other abscess.

Prevention

Listeriosis of the newborn should be preventable by prompt, vigorous treatment (penicillin G plus tobramycin) of listeriosis in pregnant women. The problem lies in recognizing the disease, because maternal listeriosis is typically a minor, nuisance kind of ailment of infrequent occurrence.

Remaining Problems

Many aspects of the epidemiology of listeriosis remain obscure. If humans are infected with *L. monocytogenes* from carriers, which are more important, human or nonhuman carriers? Is the environmental reservoir of listerias of any consequence to listeriosis in humans? The rarity of type 2, and the infrequency of types 3, 5, 6, and 7 as infectious agents of listeriosis in humans in the United States is striking and unexplained.

Although the pathogenesis of transplacentally acquired listeriosis in the newborn seems clear, how and why is meningeal localization the most common development in listeriosis acquired in other situations?

In the laboratory, isolation from clinical materials is often difficult, although propagation after isolation is not. Improved methods for culture are needed. Serologic cross reactions with other infectious agents also require further definition.

Bibliography

Books

GRAY ML (ED): Second Symposium on Listeric Infection, August 29–31, 1962. Bozeman, Montana State College, 1962. 398 pp.

SEELIGER HR: Listeriosis. Basel, S Karger, 1961. 308 pp.

Journals

BOJSEN-MOLLER J: Human listeriosis: Diagnostic, epidemiological and clinical studies. Acta Pathol Microbiol Scand (B) (Suppl) 229:1–157, 1972

CHERUBIN CE, MARR JS, SIERRA MF, BECKER S: Listeria and gram-negative bacillary meningitis in New York City, 1972–1979. Am J Med 71:199–209, 1981

HALLIDAY HL, HIRATA T: Perinatal listeriosis—a review of twelve patients. Am J Obstet Gynecol 133:405–410, 1979

KAMPELMACHER EH, VAN NOORLE JANSEN LM: Listeriosis in humans and animals in the Netherlands (1958–1977). Zbl Bakt Hyg (Orig) 246:211–227, 1980

MOORE RM JR, ZEHMER RB: Listeriosis in the United States—1971. J Infect Dis 127:610–611, 1973

NIEMAN RE, LORBER B: Listeriosis in adults: A changing pattern. Report of eight cases and review of the literature, 1968–1978. Rev Infect Dis 2:207–227, 1980

RELIER JP: Listeriosis. J Antimicrob Chemother (Suppl) 5:51–57, 1979

SEELIGER HPR: New outlook on the epidemiology and epizoology of listeriosis. Acta Microbiol Acad Sci Hung 19:273–286, 1972

Section | *IX*

Renal Infections

Indigenous Microbiota of the Kidneys

(None)

GEORGE J. PAZIN
ABRAHAM I. BRAUDE

Pyelonephritis

52

Pyelonephritis is an inflammatory disease of microbial etiology that involves both the parenchyma and the pelvis of the kidney; it may lead to fatal bacteremia. It is an important illness in women of childbearing age and in the elderly. Although acute pyelonephritis produces renal scarring, the extent to which bacterial infection of the kidneys leads to chronic renal failure is uncertain.

Urinary tract infections are quite frequent among otherwise healthy women and are the most common nosocomial infections. Most such infections are not pyelonephritis but are afflictions of the lower (infrarenal) urinary tract (see Chap. 48, Urethritis and Cystitis, and Chap. 49, Bacterial Prostatitis and Recurrent Urinary Tract Infections). Yet, it is clear that pyelonephritis generally evolves from lower tract infection, contributes to the progression of chronic renal failure, aggravates other coexistent nephropathies, and jeopardizes the success of renal transplantation.

Etiology

Escherichia coli, the chief cause of pyelonephritis, is responsible for 90% of the first occurrences of urinary tract infections among out-patients. The distribution shown in Table 52-1 represents a cross section of hospitalized patients with urinary tract infections. Although *E. coli* remains the single most common cause of both in-hospital and recurrent urinary tract infections, the aggregate of other enteric bacilli accounts for more cases in these groups. *Escherichia coli* serogroups 01, 02, 04, 06, 018, and 075 are most frequent as causes of urinary infections and as components of the fecal flora of persons who do not have urinary infections (*i.e.,* there is no O group which is uniquely pathogenic for the kidney). However, serodifferentiation detailed to include flagellar H antigens, shell or slime layer K antigens, as well as somatic O antigens, has yet to be reported.

All species of *Proteus* have special significance inasmuch as they are uniquely potent producers of urease, an enzyme which decomposes urea to NH_3 and CO_2. The alkaline urine which results favors the precipitation of magnesium ammonium phosphate to form stones. Among the *Proteus* species, *P. mirabilis* is the most commonly encountered. *Klebsiella* spp. are also associated with the formation of urinary calculi; they are relatively poor producers of urease but elaborate extracellular polysaccharides, mucin, and slime that are suitable ligands for divalent cations.

Although enteric bacilli are microorganisms of relatively low virulence, they frequently cause urinary infections. In contrast, the *Salmonella* spp. and the *Brucella* spp. are virulent bacteria which are unusual causes of pyelonephritis. Although *Salmonella typhi* appears in the urine of 20% to 40% of patients during the second or third week of typhoid fever (see Chap. 64, Typhoid Fever), a focus of infection in the kidney is rarely established unless stones or obstruction are present. Renal brucellosis causes renal calcification, possibly through the urease activity of *Brucella* spp. (see Chap. 138, Brucellosis).

Gram-positive bacteria seldom cause pyelonephritis. Of the enteric gram-positive bacteria, only *Streptococcus faecalis* is responsible for a significant number of urinary tract infections. Staphylococcal bacteriuria may arise from renal abscesses of hematogenous origin and, in diabetics, it may be associated with papillary necrosis. Albeit uncommon, coagulase negative staphylococci do occasionally cause infection of the kidneys by means of retrograde spread from the bladder.

Anaerobes rarely cause pyelonephritis; they do so only in the presence of stones or tumors. *Actinomyces israelii* (see Chap. 38, Actinomycosis) is an exception and may infect normal kidneys.

Tuberculosis can cause extensive kidney destruc-

Table 52-1. *Etiology of Urinary Infections in 448 Hospitalized Patients*

Infectious Agent	% of Total
Escherichia coli	35.8
Proteus mirabilis	16.4
Enterobacter aerogenes	16.3
Klebsiella pneumoniae	10.1
Pseudomonas aeruginosa	5.8
Enterococci	4.0
Citrobacter spp.	3.3
Proteus spp., excluding *P. mirabilis*	3.0
Alcaligenes faecalis	2.2
Staphylococcus epidermidis	2.0
Staphylococcus aureus	1.1

tion (see Chap. 35, Extrapulmonary Tuberculosis) and should be suspected in patients with pyuria or hematuria and negative routine cultures. Spheroplasts and L forms have not been implicated as primary causes of kidney infections. However, they may be recovered from the urine of patients with pyelonlphritis and have been proposed as a cause of treatment failure because they can persist in a hypertonic environment and revert to the bacterial form after treatment. Although viruses, such as cytomegalovirus and mumps virus, may be recovered from the urine of a patient with the disease, they are not considered to be responsible for pyelonephritis. Similarly, adenovirus type 11 has been associated with hemorrhagic cystitis, but not pyelonephritis.

A variety of fungi may involve the kidney. The kidneys are a major target of *Candida* spp. (see Chap. 39, Candidosis) in candidemia and may occasionally be infected by candidas from the lower urinary tract. Either route of infection may result in ureteral obstruction by the fungus. *Aspergillus* spp. (see Chap. 44, Aspergillosis) may also obstruct the urinary tract, and cryptococci (see Chap. 120, Cryptococcosis) have a propensity to cause papillary necrosis.

Inability to recover bacteria from urine or renal tissue in chronic pyelonephritis does not preclude the possibility that bacteria played an important inciting role in the pathologic process. The demonstration of a common antigen of *Enterobacteriaceae* in sterile kidney tissue in chronic pyelonephritis is consistent with this concept.

Epidemiology

Although 10% to 20% of women are estimated to have a urinary tract infection at some time, the incidence of pyelonephritis in the general population is unknown. Surveillance programs generally indicate that 2% or more of hospitalized patients acquire a urinary tract infection, but again the frequency of renal involvement is undetermined. Hospitalized persons who come to autopsy may not be representative of the general population; moreover, the number of cases of pyelonephritis found at necropsy varies markedly with the diagnostic criteria applied. Older studies reported pyelonephritis in up to 30% of autopsies but used loose diagnostic criteria and probably included other diseases which mimic pyelonephritis histologically. More recent studies based on strict criteria and excluding cases with concomitant diseases such as diabetes or obstructive uropathy have reported less than 1% chronic pyelonephritis. The latter studies may underestimate the frequency of chronic renal infection because diabetes and obstruction predispose to kidney infection.

Much of our information on epidemiology is based upon surveys of different populations to detect bacteriuria (Table 52-2). Bacteriuria is generally defined as the presence of 10^5 or more bacteria per milliliter of urine in one or two voided, midstream specimens. It identifies patients who have a greater risk of symptomatic infections and some, but not all, who have asymptomatic renal infections.

Approximately 1% of infants have bacteriuria; the frequency is slightly greater among boys. Beyond infancy, bacteriuria is consistently more common in girls and women until the age of 50. Only about 1.5% of girls with asymptomatic bacteriuria will develop symptoms of urinary tract infections during each year of observation, and 25% of the group may show spontaneous clearing of the bacteriuria. Nevertheless, 15% to 20% of girls with asymptomatic bacteriuria will have pyuria, vesicoureteral reflux, or abnormal intravenous pyelograms (*i.e.,* are at risk of progressive renal damage).

Asymptomatic bacteriuria in young women is usually not associated with demonstrable urinary tract abnormalities. However, during pregnancy, bacteriuria is not only more frequent but is also more dangerous because acute, symptomatic cystitis or pyelonephritis occurs more often in bacteriuric (>20%) than nonbacteriuric pregnant women (1%–2%). Urinary infections during pregnancy are unlikely to clear spontaneously, tend to involve the kidneys, and are subject to a 60% recurrence rate.

Pyelonephritis is more common in adults with diabetes mellitus than in nondiabetics; bacteriuria is also more common, for it occurs in 18% of diabetic women and 5% of diabetic men. However, bacteriuria does not appear more often in diabetic girls;

Table 52-2. *Frequency of Occurrence and Possible Significance of Bacteriuria by Age Group*

Age group	Frequency of bacteriuria (%)	Possible significance
Infants		
Girls	1 (M > F)	Possibly related to the generally greater frequency of neonatal infections in males
Boys		
Childhood		
Girls	1–2	Radiologic abnormalities of renal collecting systems in 15%–20% of bacteriuric girls
Boys	< 0.1	Very uncommon in boys; require urologic evaluation
Young adult		
Women	2–5	Often associated with onset of sexual activity
Pregnant	6	Much greater risk of symptomatic infection in the third trimester or postpartum; greater likelihood of kidney involvement
Men	< 1	Infrequency in normal male implies prostatic infection, instrumentation, or obstructive uropathy if present
Older adult		
Women	5–15	Chronic bacteriuria and cystourethrocele major contributing factors; increases with parity and age
Men	5	Prostatic hypertrophy with obstruction or instrumentation major predisposing factors

hence, frequent hospitalizations, instrumentation, and urinary bladder dysfunction largely account for the apparent predisposition to urinary infections.

Pyelonephritis and bacteriuria are said to occur more often in hypertensive populations, and hypertension seems to be more common in patients with pyelonephritis than in the general population. However, the postulated causal relationship between pyelonephritis and hypertension is obscure—except, possibly, in the rare patient with hypertension and severe, unilateral pyelonephritis. Yet, acute pyelonephritis will aggravate existing hypertension and have an adverse effect on the course of the hypertension.

Obstruction or injury within the kidney, as from nephrocalcinosis, sickle cell anemia, or papillary necrosis, predisposes to pyelonephritis. Xanthomatous pyelonephritis is also an example of this phenomenon. This rare disease is often discovered only after infection with *P. mirabilis* or *E. coli*. Similarly, extrarenal obstruction enhances the susceptibility of the kidney to infection.

Instrumentation or catheterization of the lower urinary tract always involves a risk of infection. From 0.5% to 2% of patients will develop bacteriuria after one urethral catheterization. Indwelling urinary bladder catheters regularly result in bacteriuria after 3 days if connected to an open drainage system, whereas the urine may remain sterile for 10 days if a closed drainage system is used. Infection is frequent when a urethral catheter is left in place beyond 2 weeks despite closed drainage or irrigation of the bladder with solutions containing antibacterial substances.

Pathogenesis and Pathology

The usual route of infection of the renal pelvis and kidney is by way of the urethra, bladder, and ureters. Hematogenous infection of the kidneys occurs much less frequently, and lymphatic spread can be discounted.

The fact that women have a urethra that is short and close to the anus presumably accounts for their predisposition to urinary infections. Women who are particularly prone to urinary infections may be colonized more frequently with enteric bacteria in the area of the vaginal vestibule and urethral meatus. These bacteria can enter the urethra and bladder during sexual relations or urethral manipulation. Bacterial pili are involved in the adherence of bacteria to the urinary tract epithelium.

Bladder defenses against infection are both mechanical and chemical. Micturition eliminates many bacteria, and the remainder often die in the bladder, possibly because the mucosa has antibacterial capabilities or because urine with high concentrations of urea may inhibit bacterial growth. If micturition is disturbed by neurologic dysfunction or by mechanical obstruction, the urine retained in the bladder (residual urine) will contain bacteria that usually multiply rapidly. However, most women with recurrent urinary tract infections have no demonstrable abnormalities of the bladder or its function. That is, bladder emptying is but one process important to preventing infection.

Several conditions may promote movement of bacteria from the bladder up the ureters to the kidneys. Normally, the route is closed at the bladder by the vesicoureteral valves, but reflux may be produced by congenital defects, surgical trauma, or cystitis. The diminished vigor or loss of ureteral peristalsis in pregnancy makes it easier for bacteria to ascend to the kidney. Gram-negative bacteria and their endotoxins may also inhibit ureteral peristalsis.

Because men have a longer urethra, it is more difficult for bacteria to reach the bladder. The normal prostate may also help prevent infection by secreting low-molecular-weight antibacterial substances, a capacity that is usually lost in chronic prostatitis. The chronically infected prostate may be the chief source for recurrent urinary tract infections in men (see Chap. 49, Bacterial Prostatitis and Recurrent Urinary Tract Infections).

Acute hematogenous pyelonephritis occurs when patients with obstructed kidneys develop bacteremia. Even partial obstruction increases the susceptibility of the kidney to infection. In the absence of obstruction, the kidney is remarkably resistant to infection by most bacteria. However, coagulase-positive staphylococci and *Candida* spp. are capable of infecting unobstructed kidneys and are important causes of hematogenous pyelonephritis.

The renal medulla is particularly vulnerable to infection. It is an immunologic desert because its peculiar chemical environment inactivates all of the processes that normally destroy bacteria. Leukocytes, antibody, and complement may be exposed to 425 mM sodium, 850 mM urea, and *p*H below 5.5. During antidiuresis, the oncotic environment in the tip of a renal pyramid may reach 1300 mOsm/liter, or four times the osmotic pressure of plasma.

Such hypertonicity impairs exudation of leukocytes from blood vessels, phagocytosis, and stops the killing of gram-negative bacilli by complement and antibody. It is not surprising that *E. coli* and other components of the normal gram-negative intestinal flora can infect the kidney even though they are harmless elsewhere in the healthy body. Nor is it surprising that these bacteria are rapidly eliminated by inflammatory reactions in the medulla which diminish hypertonicity and restore effective resistance to infection. For this reason, most attacks of acute pyelonephritis terminate spontaneously, unless there is persistent obstruction.

Whether the kidney is infected by the ascending route or hematogenously, the inflammatory response usually begins with a purulent reaction in the interstitium of the medulla that extends to the cortex as an expanding wedge with its tip at the renal pelvis (Fig. 52-1). The lesions are patchy with normal areas interspersed between involved areas. Tubules, particularly in the proximal convoluted segments, are destroyed. Some tubular segments atrophy or become obstructed and distended with proteinaceous material as the process becomes chronic. In chronic pyelonephritis, such remnants of tubules resemble thyroid follicles and the pathologic picture is called thyroidization (Fig. 52-2*A*). Polymorphonuclear leukocytes in the tubular lumina become leukocyte casts. The glomeruli are usually spared. As the early neutrophilic reaction subsides, mononuclear cells, chiefly lymphocytes, come to predominate by 7 days after the onset of infection. If inflammation continues, it may lead to diffuse interstitial fibrosis,periglomerular fibrosis, and fibrosis at the fornices of the calyces (Fig. 52-2*B, C, D*). Eventually, the destroyed area is replaced by scars which have broad bases on the cortical surface (Fig. 52-3*A*). The overlying capsule often becomes thickened and tightly adherent. Contraction of parenchymal scars results in blunting of renal papillae and calyceal dilation which can be appreciated on excretory pyelography. The overall process may be strikingly unilateral, involve both kidneys in an uneven distribution, or result in extensive, bilateral renal parenchymal destruction with severely shrunken, deformed kidneys (Fig. 52-3*B*). Progression of acute pyelonephritis to scar formation has been well documented in children but has been difficult to prove in adults.

Although papillary necrosis may result in calyceal deformity, the combination of a dilated calyx with an overlying parenchymal scar (Fig. 52-3*C*) is considered unique to bacterial pyelonephritis. Chronic pyelonephritis cannot be diagnosed with certainty on needle biopsy because the requisite pelvicalyceal involvement cannot be discerned and there is a variety of other causes of chronic interstitial nephritis. A partial list of conditions that produce lesions resembling pyelonephritis includes ischemia, intra- or extrarenal obstruction, analgesic abuse, hereditary nephritis, Balkan nephritis, papillary necrosis, irradiation, and drug reactions from sulfonamides, methicillin, diphenylhydantoin, and phenindione.

Hematogenous infections of the kidneys by *Candida* spp. are distinctly different from bacterial pyelonephritis. The yeasts lodge in glomeruli and the pseudomycelia pentrate into the parenchyma and tubular lumina. Cryptococcal pyelonephritis appears to have a propensity for causing papillary necrosis.

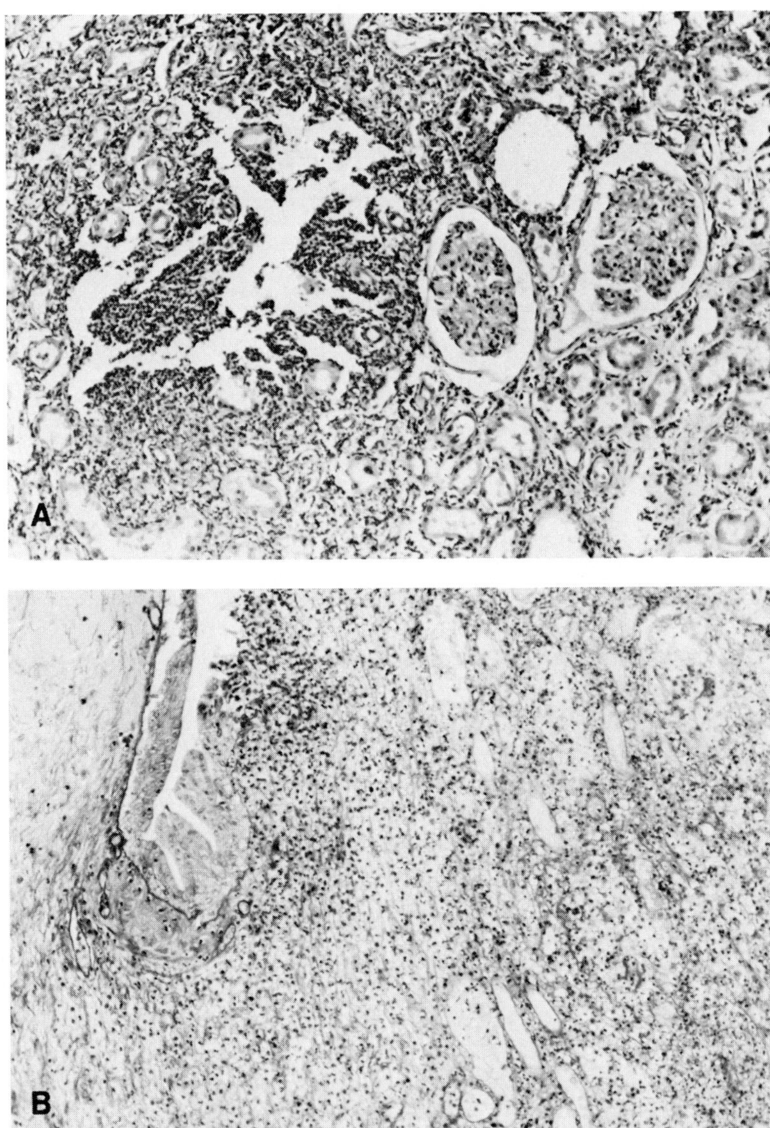

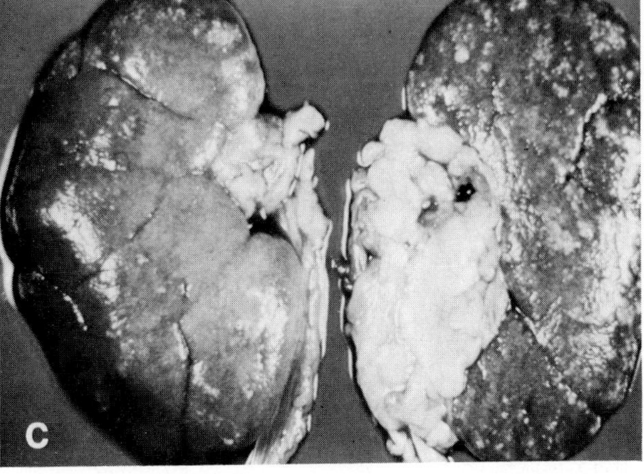

Fig. 52-1. (*A*) Histopathology of acute pyelonephritis in the corticomedullary region. The interstitium on the left side is infiltrated with many polymorphonuclear leukocytes, with a focal collection resulting in a microabscess. The tubules in the inflamed area are destroyed, whereas the glomeruli on the right are unaffected. (H&E × 350) (*B*) Histopathology of acute pyelonephritis in caliceal region. The reflection of transitional cell epithelium at the upper left margin represents the fornix of the calix. There is a diffuse infiltration of polymorphonuclear leukocytes throughout the renal papilla, which is most intense beneath the caliceal epithelium. (H&E × 350) (*C*) Gross appearance of acute pyelonephritis. Numerous small abcesses are on the surface of the kidneys.

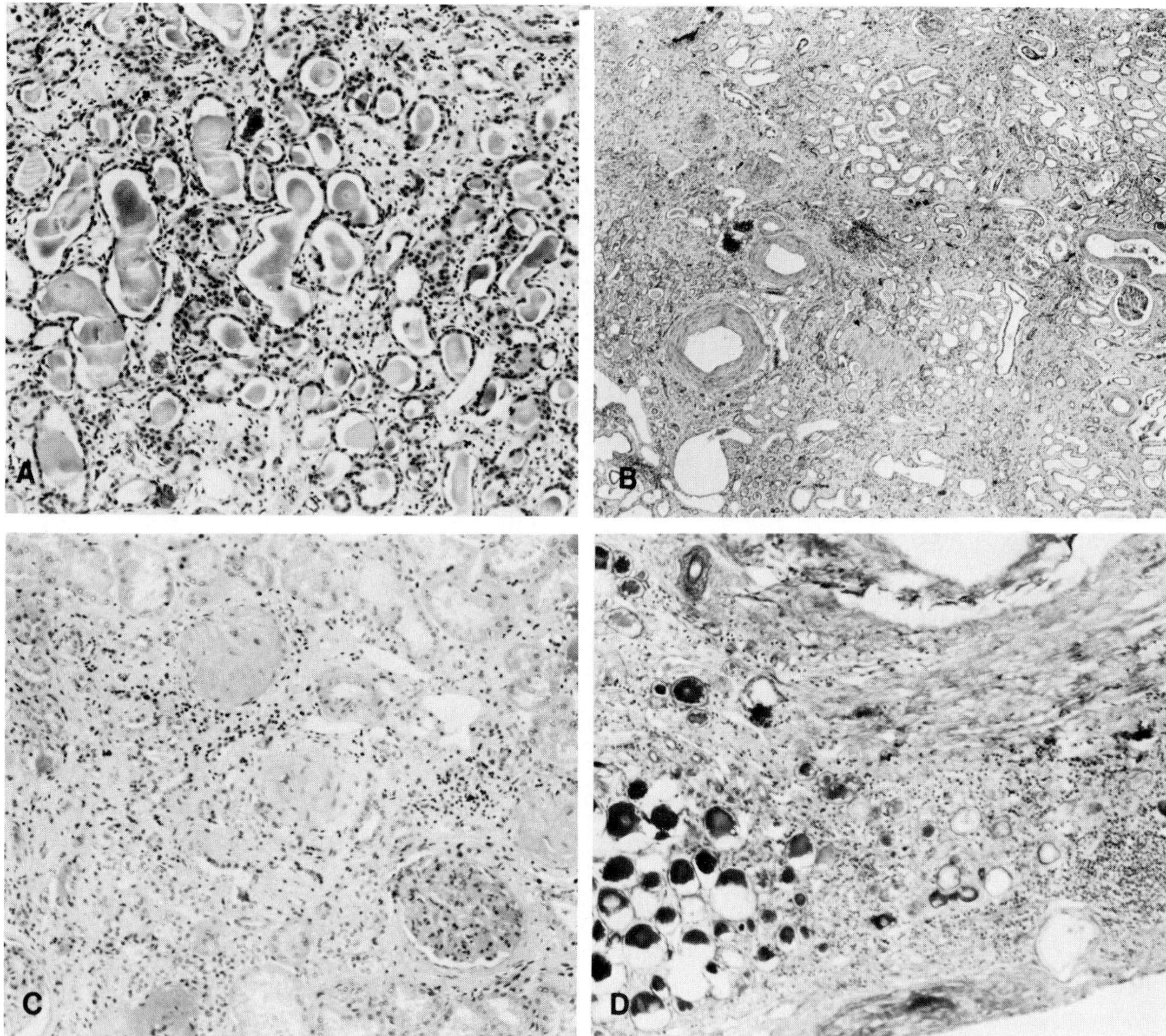

Fig. 52-2. Histopathology of chronic pyelonephritis. (*A*) The fibrous tissue is infiltrated with chronic inflammatory cells. Tubules are prominent with atrophic tubular cells and lumina distended with proteinaceous material (thyroidization). (H&E × 350) (*B*) There is diffuse interstitial fibrosis with focal collections of round cells. The glomeruli are relatively intact, but there is tubular atrophy. (H&E × 70) (*C*) In addition to chronic inflammatory cells and increased fibrous tissue, there is periglomerular fibrosis and solidification of two glomeruli. (H&E approximately × 350) (*D*) Beneath the scarred caliceal epithelium there is a focal collection of lymphocytes. (H&E × 350)

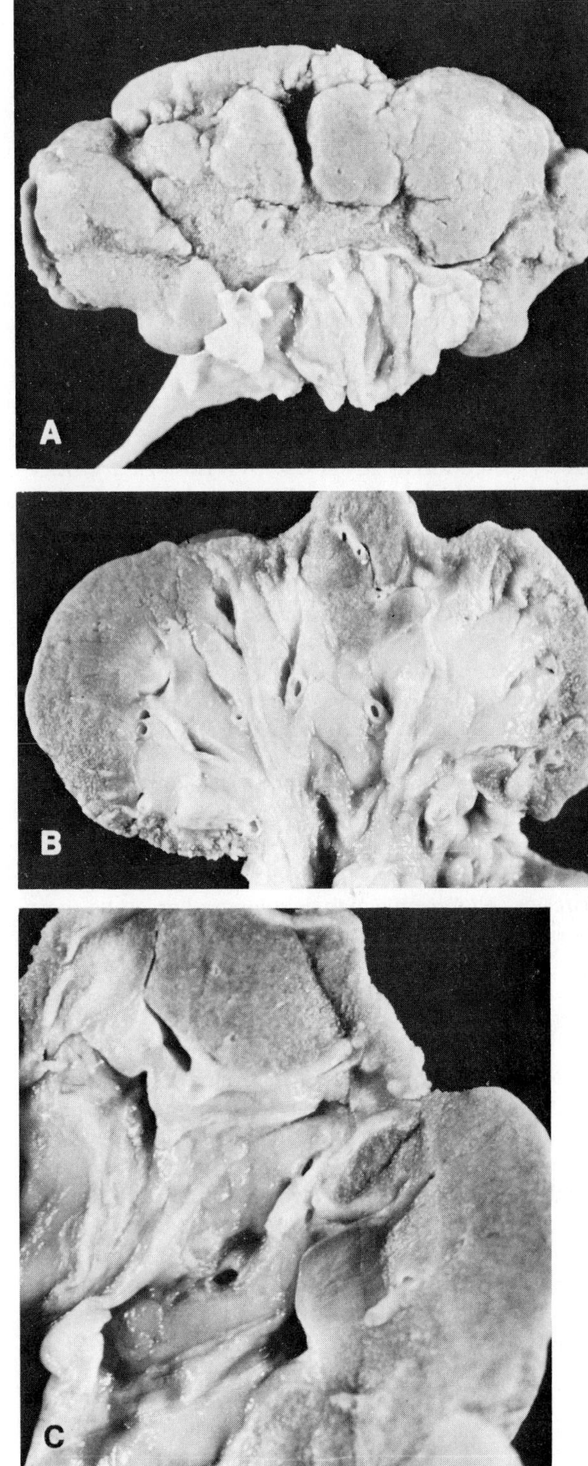

Fig. 52-3. Gross appearance of chronic pyelonephritis (*A*) Several broad-based scars mark the surface of this severely shrunken kidney. The kidney measured 8.5 cm, slightly more than half normal size. (*B*) Viewing the cut surface, scarred parenchyma is seen to overlie dilated, blunted calices at the upper pole. Note the cortical thickness in the relatively uninvolved lower pole. (*C*) View of cut surface showing a dilated, blunted calix with an overlying parenchymal scar.

When *Staphylococcus aureus* infects the kidney hematogenously, acute abscesses known as renal carbuncles often result.

Manifestations

The signs and symptoms of cystitis (*i.e.,* dysuria, urgent and frequent urination) often predominate in patients with acute pyelonephritis. Suprapubic tenderness is characteristic of cystitis, but does not exclude asymptomatic kidney infection. Loin pain or costovertebral angle tenderness, occurring with chills and fever, are typical of acute pyelonephritis but are not diagnostic because these same findings may occur in the absence of renal infection. Conversely, infection at any site within the urinary tract, including the kidneys, may be completely asymptomatic. Furthermore, dysuria, as well as urgent and frequent urination, may be present in the absence of infection.

Chronic pyelonephritis may be manifested as an acute infection, or as a low-grade fever with general malaise or weight loss. It may be asymptomatic. Pyuria and bacteriuria are the key findings. Proteinuria greater than 2 g in 24 hours is unusual, whereas a reduced ability to concentrate the urine is common (often reflected as nocturia and frequent urination—the patient can only produce dilute urine; therefore, a large volume is necessary to accomplish excretion).

If pyelonephritis is complicated by urinary obstruction, bacteremia may develop and produce shaking chills, toxicity, and hypotension or shock.

Diagnosis

Infection in the urinary tract is easier to prove than infection in any other organ/system save, perhaps, the skin. Properly collected, normal urine is free of bacteria or contains so few bacteria that infection is readily proved by microscopic examination and culture. Methods for collection and examination of urine for bacteria are detailed in Chapters 48, Urethritis and Cystitis, and 49, Bacterial Prostatitis and Recurrent Urinary Tract Infections. Usually, a single species of bacteria is recovered, but chronic or complicated pyelonephritis may yield mixtures. Generally, those species which number 10^5 or more bacteria/ml are considered to be actual agents of infection.

Neither clinical findings nor quantitation of cultures is sufficient to distinguish pyelonephritis from infection of the lower urinary tract. Leukocyte casts in the urine indicate renal parenchymal inflammation (*i.e.,* nephritis) (Plate 52-1). If bacteriuria is also present, it is highly probable that the leukocyte casts originated in pyelonephritis. However, leukocyte casts either are not recognized or are not regularly present in pyelonephritis. Definitive methods for localizing infections of the urinary tract which depend on cultures are discussed in Chapters 48, Urethritis and Cystitis, and 49, Bacterial Prostatitis and Recurrent Urinary Tract Infections.

High titers of serum antibody specific for the infecting bacteria, and a diminished concentrating ability are reliable indicators of renal infection. However, both may occur in a few patients with cystitis.

A sensitive, noninvasive method for distinguishing renal from bladder infections depends on the detection of antibody coating the causative bacteria. Bacteria are collected by centrifuging the urine. After washing, the sediment is stained with fluorescein-labeled antihuman globulin antiserum. Following incubation and washing, smears are prepared and examined by fluorescence microscopy. The presence of fluorescent bacteria is indicative of antibody coating and correlates well with a renal origin of the bacteria, whereas bacteria from the bladder are not antibody coated and do not emit fluorescence. False negative results may be found in some patients early in the course of renal infection. On the other hand, prostatic infections may yield bacteria that are coated with antibody in the absence of renal infection. Culture of sequentially collected specimens (see Chap. 49, Bacterial Prostatitis and Recurrent Urinary Tract Infections) makes it possible to differentiate prostatic from renal infections.

Patients with pyelonephritis must be evaluated carefully to determine if there is an underlying, predisposing condition which might be remedied by surgery. An excretory urogram should be obtained in all patients with urinary tract infections, with the possible exception of young women during their first infection. Flank pain consistent with renal colic is an indication for an emergency urogram because infection in an obstructed kidney requires prompt intervention by the urologist. A postvoiding plain film of the bladder will help detect urinary retention, and voiding cystograms are useful in children for diagnosis of vesicoureteral reflux. Most women with recurrent urinary tract infections do not have detectable abnormalities of the urinary tract (*i.e.,* one evaluation is sufficient).

Acute pyelonephritis and acute ureteral obstruction often present similar urographic findings. Gallium-67 has been used to localize urinary tract infections to the kidneys, but it may not differentiate infection from obstruction. Ultrasonic findings can be useful in making this distinction.

Prognosis

Asymptomatic bacteriuria disappears spontaneously within a year in 25% of patients. In the absence of mechanical or functional abnormalities of the urinary tract, treatment with antimicrobics easily cures bacteriuria and averts symptomatic infections. However, recurrences of bacteriuria are common.

The prognosis for recovery from an attack of cystitis or pyelonephritis is very good. Most patients respond to treatment, although they (almost always female) are subject to reinfections and very few progress to renal insufficiency.

The outlook for patients with acute pyelonephritis complicated by underlying renal disease or urologic abnormalities is considerably worse. The bacteria, whether *E. coli* or other gram-negative bacilli, are often resistant to antimicrobics, and thus treatment fails. Kidney stones preclude successful treatment unless they can be removed. Infections associated with intra- or extrarenal obstruction often become chronic and frequently lead to bacteremia—occasionally with a fatal outcome.

Chronic pyelonephritis occurs in patients who experience repeated episodes of urinary tract infection; these patients often demonstrate blunting of renal papillae, calyceal dilation, and parenchymal scarring on excretory urograms. Although pyelonephritis by itself does not often lead to renal failure, it contributes to progressive renal insufficiency in many instances. A sudden decline in renal function during an acute exacerbation of chronic pyelonephritis may not be restored with treatment, even when the infection is brought under control.

Therapy

The first step in the treatment of pyelonephritis is to relieve obstruction of the urinary tract. But even in the apparent absence of obstruction, no regimen of antimicrobial therapy can be depended upon to cure every patient with pyelonephritis. Moreover, improvement of clinical parameters such as fever, dysuria, or loin pain does not always indicate successful treatment. In fact, nearly one-third of patients who receive ineffective treatment experience clinical improvement. Therefore, bacteriologic assessment of response to therapy is every bit as important as the selection of antimicrobics.

Four categories of response are illustrated in Figure 52-4. They are defined by the results of bacteriologic examination of urine at intervals of 24–48 hours after starting treatment, and 7 days and 1 month or more after treatment was stopped. *Persistence* indicates that the quantity of bacteria has not decreased at 24–48 hours after starting drugs. Although nearly one-third of these patients will improve symptomatically, they are treatment failures because the bacteria are resistant to urinary concentrations of the antimicrobic. Another regimen must be selected according to the results of tests of susceptibility *in vitro.*

Relapse describes those instances in which the bacteria disappeared during therapy but reappeared after the drug was stopped. The significance of this kind of response depends upon the bacteria that are recovered after therapy. In patients with no obstructive lesions, the appearance of bacteria identical in kind and susceptibility to antimicrobics with the original isolate indicates that therapy was stopped too soon; a second, longer (*e.g.,* 6 weeks) course of therapy with the same drug is indicated. When permanent obstruction or other irremediable organic lesions are present, cure is often impossible; indefinitely prolonged administration of the drug may suppress the infection. If the infecting bacteria have become resistant, different antimicrobics are necessary. Occasionally, resistant bacteria originally present in small numbers will flourish, necessitating a change in drugs.

Reinfection or recurrence refers to reappearance of bacteriuria a month or more after treatment was stopped. If the same serogroup is found posttherapy as was present pretherapy, it is possible that reinfection occurred from a persisting colonic reservoir. Recovery of a different genus, species, serogroup or biotype always represents reinfection. Reinfections or recurrences warrant another course of antimicrobial therapy. In chronic pyelonephritis, treatment is followed by persistence in approximately 15%, relapse in 30%, reinfection in 20%, and cure for more than 6 months in about one-third of the patients. Successive courses of therapy with appropriate antimicrobics will cure more patients.

Data on which to base absolute guidelines for the selection of antimicrobics are not available because most studies have dealt with urinary tract infections in general and have not distinguished between pyelonephritis and infrarenal infections, such as cystitis and urethritis. This is quite important because (1) renal infections are more difficult to cure than infections of the bladder, as was reaffirmed by the demon-

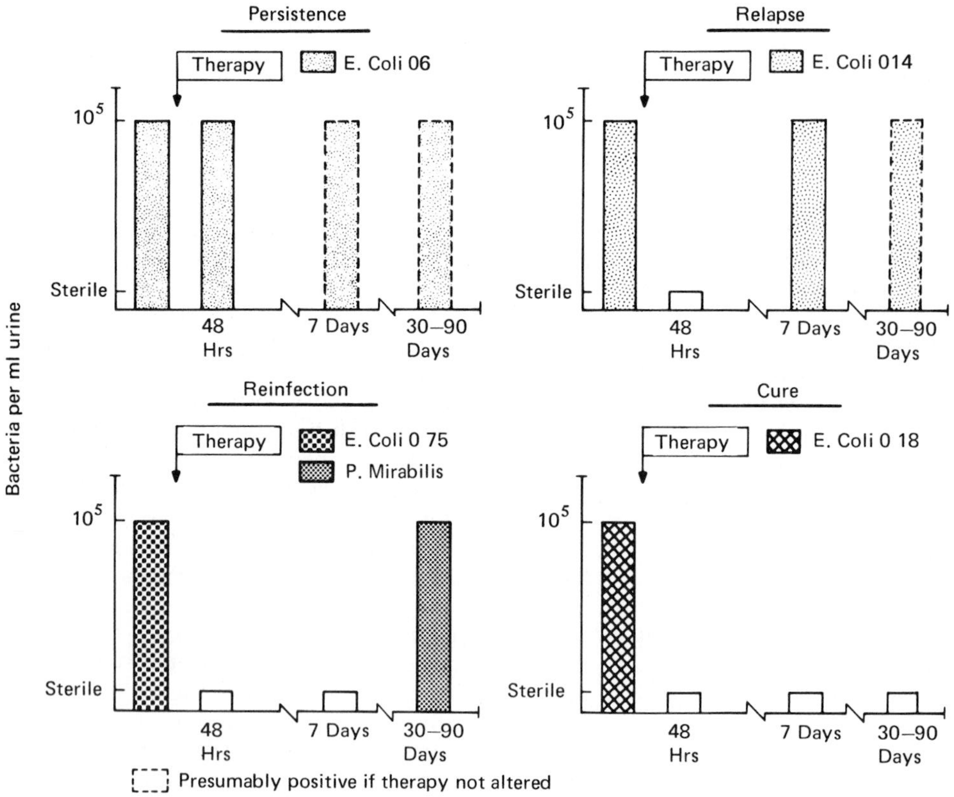

Fig. 52-4. Four general categories of response to antimicrobic therapy.

stration of cure of cystitis by single dose antimicrobial treatment, a regimen unsatisfactory for treating pyelonephritis (see Chap. 48, Urethritis and Cystitis); and (2) urethrocystitis is indubitably more common than pyelonephritis, although the actual proportion of cases varies from one study population to another. Thus, comparisons of drugs (bactericidal versus bacteriostatic; the value of effective concentrations in renal tissues alone, tissues and urine, or urine alone), schedules of administration, and duration of treatment remain largely invalid.

Despite these uncertainties, several observations are sufficiently well established to serve as guidelines. Although bacteriostatic, sulfonamides cure many urinary tract infections, including pyelonephritis. Nitrofurantoin or the tetracyclines, in doses that give negligible serum but high urinary concentrations, may be effective. Antimicrobics that are excreted by the kidneys will achieve high concentrations in the urine, but renal failure will impair excretion and may lead to dangerous accumulation. This is the reason that nitrofurantoin, for example, is contraindicated in renal failure.

Escherichia coli, the most common cause of pyelonephritis, is usually susceptible to most antimicrobials used to treat urinary tract infections. Orally administrable drugs, such as the sulfonamides, ampicillin, the tetracyclines, nitrofurantoin, or sulfamethoxazole–trimethoprim, are generally preferred. Ampicillin (or amoxicillin), penicillin, or cephalexin (or cephradine) are likely to be effective against *P. mirabilis. Klebsiella* spp. are generally resistant to ampicillin but may be susceptible to the cephalosporins. With cephalosporin-resistant *Klebsiella* spp., *Enterobacter* spp., *Serratia* spp., or *Pseudomonas* spp., gentamicin (or tobramycin) is generally useful. Carbenicillin (or ticarcillin) may also be effective against *Pseudomonas aeruginosa* and some *Enterobacter* spp. *Streptococcus faecalis* is usually susceptible to ampicillin and amoxicillin. Nalidixic acid is often active *in vitro,* but it has been disappointing because bacteria frequently develop resistance to it quite rapidly, and the drug is efficiently catabolized to an inactive form. Chloramphenicol is seldom used because the drug not only is capable of serious toxicity but also is excreted in the urine primarily as the inactive acetyl derivative. Details of antimicrobic regimens for pyelonephritis are given in Table 52-3.

Table 52-3. *Antimicrobic Regimens for the Treatment of Pyelonephritis in Adults*

Antimicrobic	Dosage	Bacteria	Comments
Ampicillin (amoxicillin)	15–30 mg/kg body wt/day perorally as 4 equal portions, 6-hourly, for 10–14 days	*Escherichia coli, Proteus mirabilis,* enterococci	May be given IV or IM during acute, septic phase. Because amoxicillin is quantitatively absorbed from the gut, it is preferable for peroral administration.
	250 mg perorally every 12 hours for 42 days or longer	*Escherichia coli, Proteus mirabilis,* enterococci	May be useful for relapse with susceptible bacteria or in chemoprophylaxis.
Cephalexin or Cephradine	15–30 mg/kg body wt/day perorally as 4 equal portions, 6-hourly, for 10–14 days	*Escherichia coli, Proteus mirabilis, Klebsiella* spp.	Cephalexin and cephradine are interchangeable. During acute, septic phase, an injectable cephalosporin may be given (*e.g.,* cefazolin).
Carbenicillin, ticacillin, piperacillin or mezlocillin	75–150 mg/kg body wt/day IV as 6 equal portions, 4-hourly, for 10–14 days	*Enterobacter* spp., *Pseudomonas aeruginosa, Proteus* spp., excluding *P. mirabilis*	Relatively low doses may be useful in urinary tract infections. Development of resistance is common. Indanyl derivative useful for peroral treatment.
Tetracyclines (oxytetracycline)	15–20 mg/kg body wt/day perorally as 4 equal portions, 6-hourly, for 10–14 days	*Escherichia coli*	Should not be used in pregnant women. Oxytetracycline has the highest urinary clearance of conventional tetracyclines.
Gentamicin, Tobramycin or Netilmycin	5–6 mg/kg body wt/day by IV or IM injection of 3 equal portions, 8-hourly, for 10 days	*Escherichia coli, Proteus* spp., *Klebsiella* spp., *Enterobacter* spp., *Serratia* spp., *Pseudomonas aeruginosa*	Gentamicin and tobramycin are interchangeable. Both must be reduced in dose when there is renal insufficiency (Fig. 17–5).
Kanamycin or Amikacin	15–20 mg/kg body wt/day by IV or IM injection of 3 equal portions, 8-hourly, for 10 days	*Escherichia coli; Proteus* spp., *Klebsiella* spp.,; *Enterobacter* spp.	Reduce dosage in patients with renal insufficiency.
Sulfonamides (sulfisoxazole)	4 g loading dose, then 30 mg/kg body wt/day perorally as 4 equal portions, 6-hourly, for 10–14 days	*Escherichia coli*	Should not be given during last 8 weeks of pregnancy
Trimethoprim, 80 mg *plus* Sulfamexthoxazole, 400 mg	2 tablets loading dose, then 1 tablet 12-hourly, for 10–14 days	*Escherichia coli*	Also useful in chronic bacterial prostatitis.
Nitrofurantoin	5–7 mg/kg body wt/day perorally as 4 equal portions, 6-hourly, for 10–14 days	*Escherichia coli*	Do not use if there is renal dysfunction or if bacteremia is suspected.

Although amphotericin B is sometimes effective in the treatment of fungal pyelonephritis, its utility is sharply limited by poor urinary excretion and nephrotoxicity. Flucytosine, on the other hand, is excreted by kidneys, and high concentrations are attained in the urine. Thus flucytosine may be useful in treating pyelonephritis caused by susceptible strains of *Candida* spp. and *Cryptococcus* spp.

A reduction of the intramedullary osmolality should result from inducing a water diuresis. Phagocytosis should be increased, and the formation of L forms of bacteria should be diminished. Although a water diuresis aggravated experimental pyelonephritis in mice, it prevented or cured the disease in rats. Assuming humans are rather more ratlike than mouselike, a liberal intake of liquids is recommended in the treatment of pyelonephritis in man.

Prevention

The dilation of the upper collecting system that normally occurs in pregnancy is associated with a marked susceptibility to pyelonephritis in pregnant women with bladder infections. Elimination of bacteriuria, by 8 to 10 days of treatment with sulfisoxazole (1 g perorally every 8 hours) or ampicillin (250 mg perorally every 6 hours), prevents pyelonephritis. If such treatment fails, the cause is almost never resistance to antimicrobics, because *E. coli,* which is susceptible to the sulfonamides and ampicillin, almost always cause the bacteriuria of pregnancy. Failure of cure or recurrence of bacteriuria warrants continuous chemoprophylaxis until term on the assumption that pyelonephritis was present.

There is a subgroup of women who appear to be prone to recurrent, symptomatic urinary tract infections. If more than three well-documented infections occur in a year, such women may benefit from taking an antimicrobic that is efficiently excreted into the urine after sexual relations or as a daily, low-dose medication (see Chap. 19, Chemoprophylaxis of Infectious Diseases).

Prostatic disease provides two situations that merit chemoprophylaxis: chronic bacterial prostatis and prostatectomy. The fact that it is difficult for most antimicrobials to enter into prostatic secretions accounts for the usual failure of antimicrobial therapy in chronic prostatitis. Because trimethoprim is an exception, entering the prostate freely (see Chap. 49, Bacterial Prostatitis and Recurrent Urinary Tract Infections), the regimen given in Table 52-3 will cure some cases of chronic bacterial prostatitis. Prostatis that is not cured may lead to recurrences of cystitis and possibly pyelonephritis. In such patients, continuous administration of ampicillin or oxytetracycline (250 mg perorally every 12 hours) will prevent recurrences of acute urinary tract infections but will not affect the underlying prostatic reservoir of infection. Following prostatectomy, the risks of lower tract infection and the possibility of pyelonephritis are decreased by the administration of gentamicin (80 mg) or kanamycin (500 mg) by intramuscular injection, once daily, for 2 days postoperatively.

Patients with indwelling urinary cathethers are prone to urinary infection, pyelonephritis, and even bacteremia. Either a sterile closed drainage system or a continuous antibacterial bladder rinse will decrease the morbidity and mortality from catheter-associated infections. For continuous bladder irrigation, buffered acetic acid solution (2.1% sodium acetate plus sufficient glacial acetic acid to lower the *p*H to 4.7) or 0.9% NaCl solution containing 20 mg polymyxin B and 40 mg neomycin/liter should be dripped continuously into the bladder through the inflow channel of the triple lumen catheter at a rate of 1 liter/day.

Remaining Problems

Testing for antibody-coated bacteria in the urine appears to aid localization of the site of infection within the urinary tract. Precise data regarding the frequency and significance of renal involvement in asymptomatic bacteriuria in various populations should be forthcoming. Valid studies of antimicrobial therapy, for example, investigation of the relative importance of the concentrations of drugs attained in the serum/tissues versus the urine or of bacteriostatic versus bactericidal agents, should be possible.

In relation to the pathogenesis of pyelonephritis, why are some women subject to recurrent urinary tract infections? If colonization of the vaginal vestibule and urethral meatus is a factor, why does it vary from woman to woman? The extent to which chronic pyelonephritis contributes to renal failure, the mechanisms by which bacteria may contribute to progressive renal insufficiency in the absence of overt infection, and the effect of antimicrobics in preventing or minimizing renal damage should be clarified.

Bibliography

Books

HEPTINSTAL, RH: Pathology of the Kidney. Boston, & Little, Brown & Co, 1974. 836 pp.

KASS EH (ED): Progress in Pyelonephritis. Philadelphia, FA Davis, 1965. 736 pp.

KAYE D (ED): Urinary Tract Infection and Its Management. St. Louis, CV Mosby, 1972. 200 pp.

KUNIN CM: Detection, Prevention and Management of Urinary Tract Infections. Philadelphia, Lea & Febiger, 1972. 230 pp.

NORDEN CW: Significance and management of bacteriuria of pregnancy. In Kaye E (ed): Urinary Tract Infection and Its Management. St. Louis, CV Mosby, 1972. pp 171–187.

QUINN EL, KASS EH (EDS): Biology of Pyelonephritis. Boston, Little, Brown & Co, 1960. 708 pp.

Journals

AOKI S, IMAMURA S, AOKI M, MCCABE WR: "Abacterial" and bacterial pyelonephritis. Immunofluorescent localization of bacterial antigen. N Engl J Med 281:1375–1382, 1969

BEESON PB: Factors in the pathogenesis of pyelonephritis. Yale J Biol Med 28:81–104, 1955

BRAUDE, AI: Current concepts in pyelonephritis. Medicine 52:257–264, 1973

HEPTINSTAL RH: The enigma of chronic pyelonephritis. J Infect Dis 120:104–107, 1969

KUNIN CM: A ten year study in school girls: Final report of bacteriologic, urologic and epidemiologic findings. J Infect Dis 122:382–392, 1970

KUNIN CM: New developments in the diagnosis and treatment of urinary tract infections. J Urol 113:585–594, 1975

PETERSDORF RC, TURK M: Some current concepts of urinary tract infections. DM, 1970

THOMAS V, SHELOKOV A, FORLAN M: Antibody coated bacteria in the urine and site of infection. N Engl J Med 290:588–590, 1974

MAURY E. MULLIGAN
JUDITH G. ROSE
SYDNEY M. FINEGOLD

Intrarenal and Perinephric Abscess 53

Intrarenal abscess (or renal carbuncle) is suppuration localized within the parenchyma of the kidney. Perinephric abscess is suppuration within the perirenal fascia, external to the capsule of the kidney (Fig. 53-1). The latter is reported much more frequently.

Etiology

Abscesses in or about the kidney may be hematogenous in origin or may result from direct extension of a preceding infection, either within the urinary tract or within a neighboring organ. Hematogenous infections are most frequently caused by *Staphylococcus aureus.* Enteric gram-negative bacilli, predominantly *Escherichia coli, Proteus* spp., and, less commonly, *Klebsiella* spp., *Enterobacter* spp., and *Pseudomonas* spp., are usually responsible for infections originating in the urinary tract. Occasionally, streptococci are implicated. Various anaerobic bacteria, including *Clostridium* spp., *Actinomyces* spp., the gram-negative anaerobic bacilli, and anaerobic cocci may cause perinephric abscess and may be the pathogens in patients with cultures reported to be sterile. *Mycobacterium tuberculosis* is an important occasional cause of perinephric abscess, as are fungi, most commonly *Candida* spp. The simultaneous presence of two or more kinds of microorganisms in pus from perinephric abscesses has been noted in some cases.

Epidemiology

Intrarenal and perinephric abscesses are currently reported to occur in 1 to 10 per 10,000 hospital admissions, affecting males and females with equal frequency. Intrarenal abscesses appear to be more common in younger individuals; perinephric abscesses occur mostly in older persons. The vast majority of abscesses are unilateral.

Diabetes mellitus is an important predisposing condition. Glucosteroid therapy is also said to facilitate the occurrence of perinephric abscess. Because intravenous drug abuse may lead to bacteremia, drug users are at an increased risk of hematogenous abscess. Preexisting renal disease is an important precursor to the formation of abscesses that follow primary urinary tract infections.

Pathogenesis and Pathology

Abscesses involving the kidney may arise through (1) hematogenous spread from a distant focus (2) ascending infection originating in the urinary tract or (3) direct extension from a preexisting infection involving an adjacent organ. Intrarenal abscess (renal carbuncle) is usually hematogenous in origin and generally occurs in the absence of underlying renal disease. Commonly caused by *S. aureus,* intrarenal abscess may follow a skin infection such as a furuncle, occur in a patient at risk for bacteremia (*e.g.,* persons who use drugs by IV injection), or be preceded by an unnoticed primary infection.

In contrast, perinephric abscess is usually preceded by either diffuse or focal intrarenal infection, although the hematogenous route of infection, still must be considered. Perhaps because of earlier detection and treatment of skin and other soft tissue infections, at present, the majority of patients with perinephric abscesses have underlying genitourinary tract abnormalities, and enteric gram-negative bacilli are the predominant etiologic agents. There is often obstruction to urinary outflow. Specific, underlying urinary tract problems or factors include renal or ureteral calculi, hydronephrosis, pyelonephritis, polycystic renal disease (with infected cysts), renal papillary necrosis, carcinoma, renal transplantation, tuberculosis, and trauma (including diagnostic instrumentation and renal biopsy or aspiration).

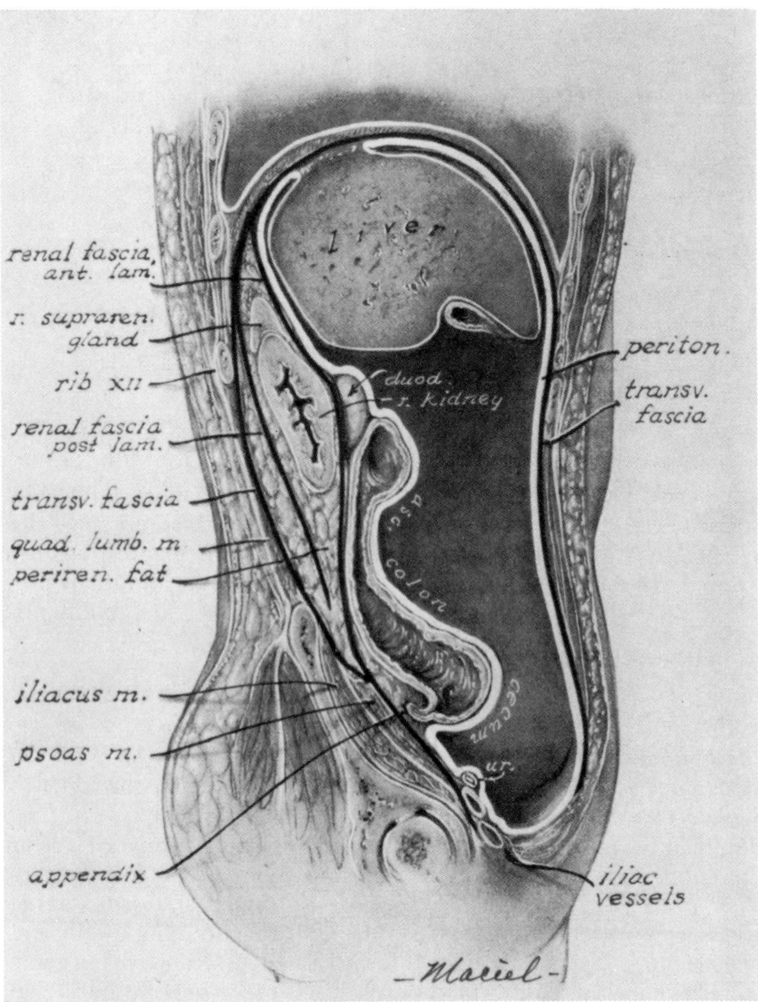

Fig. 53-1. Right sagittal section showing the retroperitoneal space. The anterior retroperitoneal space is limited by the peritoneum and the anterior layer of the renal fascia. The posterior space or perinephric space is further divided by the posterior layer of the renal fascia. (Altemeier WA, Alexander JW: Arch Surg 83:44–56, 1961)

Extension of infection from neighboring organs is an uncommon mechanism leading to perinephric abscess. Such infections include prostatic abscess; prostatitis; inflammatory lesions of the appendix, vertebra, rib, gallbladder, liver, pleura, and pelvic organs; and extension from primary pathologic processes in the colon (*e.g.*, carcinoma).

Manifestations

The patient with hematogenous intrarenal abscess typically has fever and chills. Costovertebral pain and tenderness usually suggest the localization to the kidney; however, there may be a lack of focal pain or, instead, symptoms suggesting an intraabdominal process. Coexistent infection at a distant site may be present, but often no primary source for the bacteremia is discovered.

In contrast, the onset of perinephric abscess is typically insidious. Patients are often sick for several weeks before they consult a physician. Fever, pain, and flank tenderness are the most common presenting features. Less common, but of diagnostic importance, is a palpable mass or bulging in the flank.

The fever is usually 39°C (102°F) or less, but occasionally very high fevers are noted; chills may occur. Although the location of the pain is variable, flank and costovertebral angle pain are the most common. Pain may also be located anteriorly in either the upper or lower quadrant, and less commonly may even be referred to the corresponding hip, thigh, or knee region, with minimal abdominal or back pain. The pain is often aggravated during extension of the corresponding thigh while walking, and it frequently is alleviated by flexion of the ipsilateral thigh while lying in bed, or by lying on the side opposite to that affected by the abscess. A mass is palpable in the renal area in somewhat less than half the patients. The abscess may point and then drain through the skin spontaneously. In the absence of a definite mass, there may be bulging of the flank or of distal sites such as the thigh or scrotum. Almost all patients have tenderness to palpation over the abscess. Nausea and vomiting, weight loss, psoas muscle spasm, and spasm of the paravertebral muscles leading to scoliosis with the concavity toward the abscess are other manifestations that are occasionally seen. Despite the frequency of underlying renal disease, dysuria is not always present. Hematuria or urinary retention occurs only occasionally.

Diagnosis

Distinction between intrarenal abscess and perinephric abscess is especially important because the treatment of the two diseases is usually different.

The laboratory findings associated with intrarenal abscess are variable. Leukocytosis is usual; azotemia is uncommon. If the abscess communicates with the collecting system of the kidney, urinalysis is likely to reveal pyuria, and a Gram stain of the urine will demonstrate the pathogen. However, if an abscess is localized to the renal parenchyma, especially the cortex, or if there is obstruction of the involved kidney, the urine sediment may be entirely normal. Occasionally, there is rupture of an abscess into the collecting system with the abrupt appearance of white blood cells and bacteria in the urine. Gross or microscopic hematuria may occur. The presence of gram-positive cocci in the urine, with or without white blood cells, may be the first evidence of hematogenous intrarenal abscess or of bacteremia without the actual formation of an abscess in the kidney. Cultures of urine and blood, although essential, may be negative.

In perinephric abscess, laboratory tests are usually indicative of a chronic illness. Although leukocytosis is the rule, even to the extent of a leukemoid picture, occasionally there is a normal white blood cell count or even leukopenia. Anemia is common. Urinalysis may reveal pyuria or proteinuria but is entirely normal in 25% to 35% of the patients. Azotemia may be present. Over half the patients will have more than 10^5 bacteria per ml of urine. As a rule, the bacteria isolated from cultures of the urine are the same as those present in the perinephric abscess itself. Positive blood cultures have been obtained in approximately 40% of the patients who have been evaluated.

Perinephric abscess is frequently a major diagnostic problem because of the insidious onset, variable symptoms, and variable physical and laboratory findings. Unfortunately, some cases are diagnosed only at autopsy. Most likely, failure to include the possibility of perinephric abscess in the differential diagnosis accounts for many of the diagnostic failures.

Roentgenographic examinations, including routine studies (plain abdominal films, chest films and intravenous pyelograms) and newer imaging modalities (gallium-67 imaging, ultrasonography, and computed tomography), are essential diagnostic aids in most cases. The chest roentgenogram may be normal or may show an elevated hemidiaphragm (with or without decreased diaphragmatic excursion), a pleural effusion, or a basilar infiltrate. Plain abdominal roentgenograms may demonstrate an abnormal psoas muscle outline, vertebral scoliosis, or obliteration of the renal outline by a soft tissue mass. Although an uncommon finding, the presence of gas bubbles in the area of the kidney is almost diagnostic of a gas-producing abscess.

Intravenous pyelography may be used to identify a perinephric or intrarenal abscess as well as to detect

Fig. 53-2. Perinephric abscess. The arrows point to calculi within a pyonephrotic kidney and gas shadows within the perirenal abscess.

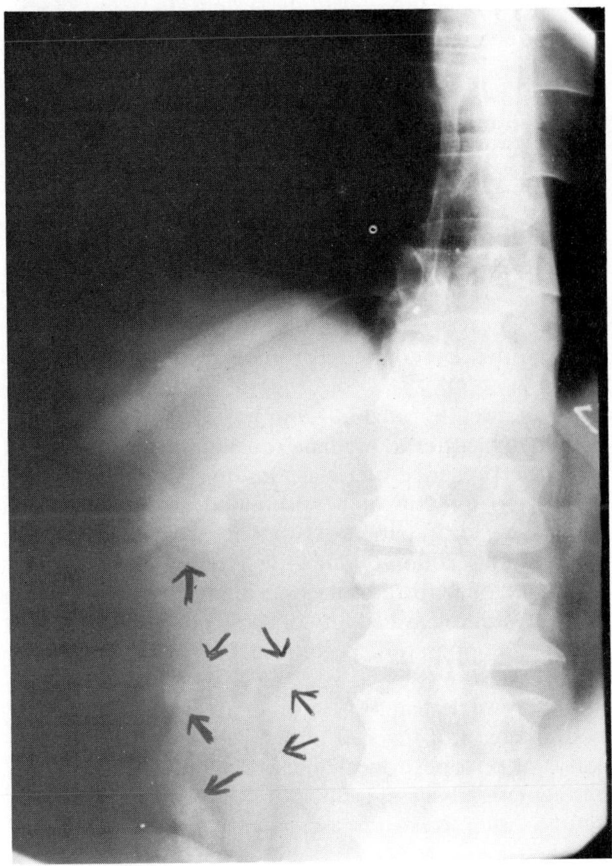

other coexisting renal pathology. The absence of respiratory motion of the kidney, pelvocaliectasis secondary to extrinsic pressure on the ureter by an abscess, displacement of the kidney or ureter, poor renal function, and calyceal abnormalities are important radiographic findings (Fig. 53-2). Extra-renal extravasation of contrast material is highly suggestive of an abscess. Fistula formation between the perirenal space and other structures, such as the colon, occasionally occurs. It is usually not necessary to perform retrograde pyelography.

Gray-scale B-mode and real-time ultrasound of the kidney are simple, rapid, noninvasive methods to evaluate further an abnormality suggested by intravenous pyelography. They may also serve as initial imaging procedures in patients for whom intravenous pyelography is unsuitable. Abscesses larger than 1.5 cm in diameter are easily visualized and appear as sonolucent mass lesions with irregular borders and some internal debris (Fig. 53-3). However, this pattern is nonspecific, and other renal pathology, such as hematoma, hydronephrosis, infected renal cyst, and neoplasm, may have a similar appearance. In addition, ultrasound may be useful to evaluate the extent of the abscess and to detect the presence of associated obstruction of the collecting system. In many cases, percutaneous needle aspiration under ultrasound guidance will assist in establishing the diagnosis and will provide an opportunity to obtain a reliable culture. Complications of the aspiration procedure are infrequent but include pneumothorax, hemorrhage and the introduction of microorganisms.

Of the imaging modalities, computed tomography provides the most precise anatomic information and permits detection of abscesses less than 2 cm in size (Fig. 53-4). It is especially useful if the ultrasound examination is negative or equivocal. Abscess aspiration guided by computed tomography is also possible.

Radionuclide renal imaging may be employed occasionally, either to evaluate renal function or to confirm the presence of a mass lesion. In patients with suspected infection but without localizing signs or symptoms, or in patients with a negative intravenous pyelogram, gallium-67 imaging may provide the first evidence of an intrarenal or perinephric abscess (Fig. 53-5). With the availability of these noninvasive techniques, angiography is unnecessary in most situations.

Differential diagnosis should include all the obscure causes of fever of undetermined origin, other kinds of retroperitoneal abscess, pneumonia, subdiaphragmatic abscess, gallbladder disease, and, importantly, other renal diseases, such as pyelonephritis, hydronephrosis, renal calculus, interstitial nephritis, xanthogranulomatous pyelonephritis, malakoplakia, and renal carcinoma. The most likely erroneous diagnoses are fever of undetermined origin and acute (uncomplicated) urinary infection.

Prognosis

Successful therapy of intrarenal abscess with antimicrobial agents alone has been reported; in most patients, symptomatic response occurs within one week, and no sequelae are noted.

Perinephric abscess is almost always fatal if not diagnosed promptly and treated properly. It is a surgical emergency. Even when the diagnosis of perinephric abscess is made and therapy is instituted, the mortality rate is commonly 25%. Factors that make for a poor prognosis include delay in diagnosis, the presence of an underlying disease (such as diabetes mellitus), bacteremia, azotemia, a significant leukocytosis, or an underlying urinary tract obstruction or infection. Sepsis is the immediate cause of death in almost all patients who die. Complications include rupture into the peritoneal cavity, pulmonary complications (particularly perinephrobronchial fistula), and spontaneous rupture to the outside. Extension or spontaneous rupture of the abscess into another site should be considered when there is any sudden change in the patient's clinical course. Persistent draining sinuses and incisional hernias are not infrequent postoperative complications.

Therapy

Because intrarenal abscess is usually hematogenous and caused by *S. aureus,* it often responds to antistaphylococcal antimicrobial therapy alone. If the history and physical findings are supplemented by finding only typical large, round, gram-positive cocci or no bacteria in a smear of the urine, antimicrobial therapy should be directed against *S. aureus.* Nafcillin (100 mg–150 mg/kg body wt/day, IV, as six equal portions, 4-hourly) or cefazolin (50 mg–75 mg/kg body wt/day, IM or IV, as four equal portions, 6-hourly) would be appropriate initial therapy for the patient with normal renal function. Radiologic and imaging techniques should be used to demonstrate that the abscess is localized to the renal parenchyma and to document the resolution of the infection. Modification of therapy may be required, based on the results of cultures of blood, urine, and, if available, pus aspirated from the abscess, as well as the clinical response.

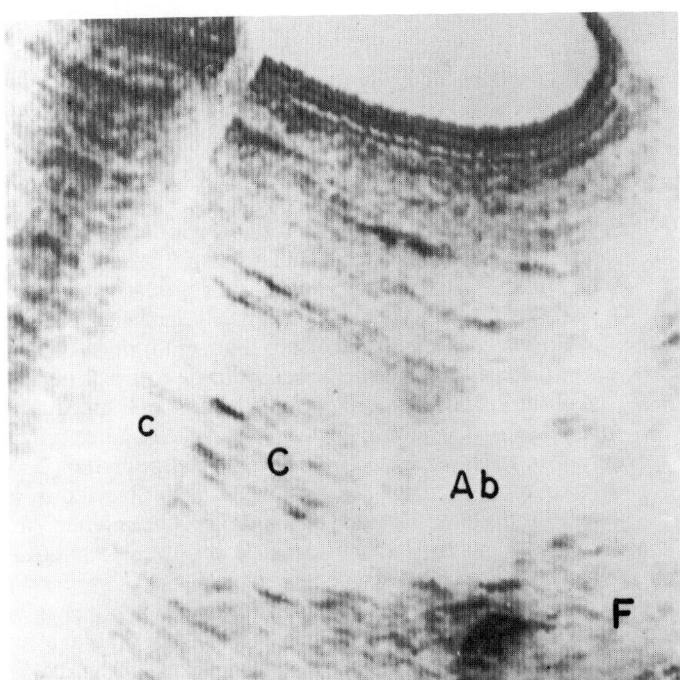

Fig. 53-3. Gray-scale ultrasound of the kidney demonstrating a lower pole intrarenal abscess. Longitudinal ultrasound of the kidney performed in the prone position revealed an echolucent mass in the lower pole. There was an irregular border to the mass. (*F* = feet; *Ab* = abscess; *C* = collecting system; *c* = renal cortex)

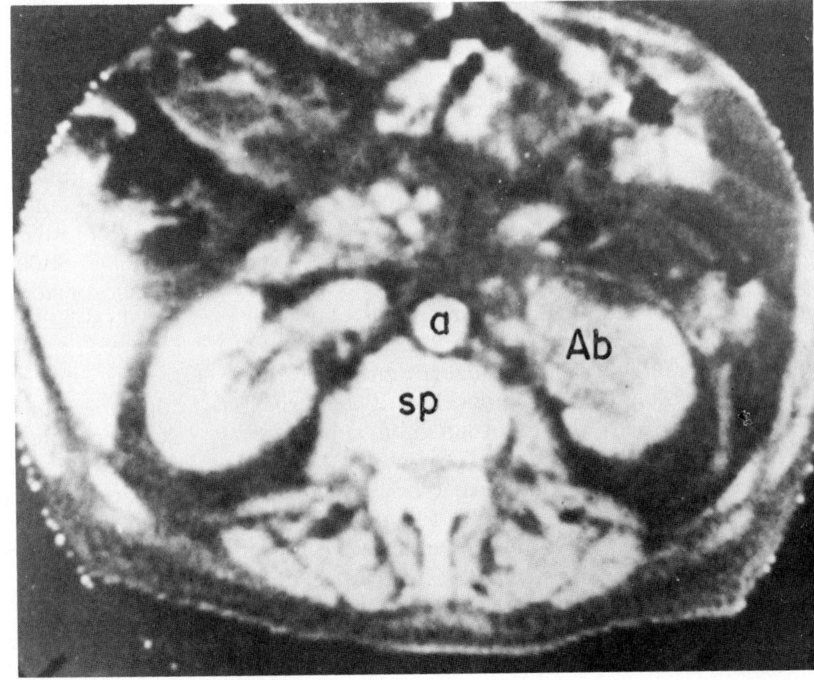

Fig. 53-4. Computed tomography (CT) of the abdomen demonstrating an intrarenal abscess with perinephric extension. Contrast-enhanced CT scan revealed a low-density left renal mass with extension into the perinephric space. (*Ab*=abscess; *sp*=spine; *a*= aorta)

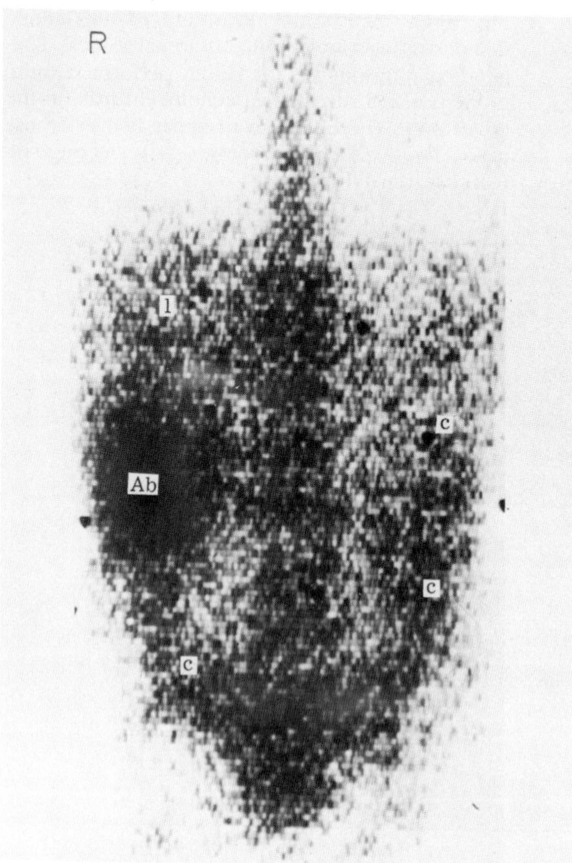

Fig. 53-5. Gallium-67 imaging study performed 24 hours after injection. The anterior image of the trunk demonstrated a large area of radionuclide in the right flank. (*Ab*=abscess; *L*=liver; *c*=colon)

In contrast, early, definitive surgical therapy for perinephric abscess is crucial; antimicrobial therapy serves as an adjunct. Incision and drainage is mandatory, even in the moribund patient in whom it may be performed under local anesthesia. Definitive surgery—for example, nephrectomy or removal of a stone from the kidney or the ureter—is commonly necessary; when possible, it should be performed at the time of initial drainage. Initial antimicrobial therapy should include an aminocyclitol if the urinary tract is the primary source of infection. Gentamicin or tobramycin (4 mg–6 mg/kg body wt/day, IM or IV, as three equal portions, 8-hourly (the dose must be adjusted to accommodate renal function) may be used. If the patient is seriously ill and there is reason to suspect bacterial resistance (*e.g.*, previous antimicrobial therapy or hospitalization), amikacin (15 mg/kg body wt/day, IM or IV, as two equal portions, 12-hourly, the dose adjusted for renal function) should be used. An additional antimicrobial agent may be needed as, for example, when *P. aeruginosa* is the cause of the infection: carbenicillin (300 mg–500 mg/kg body wt/day, IV, as six equal portions, 4-hourly, dose adjusted for renal function) or ticarcillin (200 mg–300 mg/kg body wt/day, IV, as six equal portions, 4-hourly, dose adjusted for renal function).

If the primary source of the infection appears to be outside the urinary tract (history of a recent skin infection: *S. aureus;* preceding gastrointestinal pathology: anaerobic bacteria), or if a Gram stain of the urine reveals bacteria other than gram-negative bacilli, additional antimicrobial therapy to treat the less common causes of perinephric abscess should be considered. Nafcillin or cefazolin (dosage as given above) may be added if *S. aureus* is suspected or documented. If anaerobic bacteria are involved, one of the following should be added: clindamycin (15 mg–30 mg/kg body wt/day, IM or IV, as four equal portions, 6-hourly), chloramphenicol (50 mg/kg body wt/day, IV, as four equal portions, 6-hourly), or metronidazole (IV injection of 15 mg/kg body wt as a loading dose, followed by 30 mg/kg body wt/day as four equal portions, 6-hourly). A combination of an aminocyclitol plus penicillin G (75 mg–100 mg [120,000 U–160,000 U] per kg body wt/day, IV, as six equal portions, 4-hourly) or ampicillin (same dose as for penicillin G) is the treatment of choice in enterococcal infections. Because cefoxitin (75 mg–100 mg/kg body wt/day, IV, as six equal portions, 4-hourly) is bactericidal for most aerobic and anaerobic bacteria, it may be used instead of combination therapy if resistant organisms (*e.g.,* virtually all strains of *Pseudomonas* spp. and most strains of *Enterobacter* spp.) are not implicated. The newer penicillins and cephalosporins presently under investigation may turn out to be valuable therapeutic agents. The results of cultures of urine, blood, and aspirates, and data from susceptibility testing, as well as the clinical response, should be used to determine the need to change or add antimicrobial agents. Renal function and, in some cases, hepatic function, and the concentrations of antimicrobics in the blood (peak and trough values) must be monitored to determine if adjustment of doses of antimicrobial agents is necessary. Specific therapy is necessary for abscesses caused by mycobacteria or fungi (see Chap. 34, Pulmonary Tuberculosis, and Chap. 39, Candidosis).

Prevention

Early recognition and treatment of soft tissue infections and of bacteremia from other sources may help to prevent intrarenal abscesses. Early, appropriate therapy of urinary tract disease is the major preventive of perinephric abscess. Of highest priority are the treatment of infection and the removal of calculi and other obstructions.

Remaining Problems

Despite major improvements in diagnostic technology, surgical therapy, and antimicrobial treatment, the mortality rate associated with perinephric abscess remains high. Failure to consider the diagnosis of perinephric abscess probably contributes substantially to this high mortality rate.

Bibliography

Journals

KAHN PC: Renal imaging with radionuclides, ultrasound, and computed tomography. (Semin Nucl Med 9:43–57, 1979

KLEIN DL, FILPI RG: Acute renal carbuncle. J Urol 118:912–915, 1977

MALGIERI JJ, KURSH ED, PERSKY L: The changing clinicopathological pattern of abscesses in or adjacent to the kidney. J Urol 118:230–232, 1977

RABINOWITZ JG, KINKHABWALA MN, ROBINSON T, SPYROPOULOS E, BECKER JA: Acute renal carbuncle: The reontgenographic clarification of a medical enigma. Am J Roentgenol Rad Nuclear Med 116:740–748, 1972

SALVATIERRA O JR, BUCKLEW WB, MORROW JW: Perinephric abscess: A report of 71 cases. J Urol 98:296–302, 1967

SCHIFF M, GLICKMAN M, WEISS RM, AHERN MJ, TOULOUKIAN RJ, LYTTON B, ANDRIOLE VT: Antibiotic treatment of renal carbuncle. Ann Intern Med 87:305–308, 1977

THORLEY JD, JONES SR, SANFORD JP: Perinephric abscess. Medicine 53(6):441–451, 1974

TRUESDALE BH, ROUS SN, NELSON RP: Perinephric abscess: A review of 26 cases. J Urol 118:910–911, 1977

Section X

Venereal Infections

Indigenous Microbiota of the Genital Tract

Species or Group	External Genitalia	Vagina
Mycoplasmas	+	+
Bacteria		
Gram-positive cocci		
Staphylococcus epidermidis	+	**3***
Staphylococcus aureus		**5–15**
Anaerobic micrococci		+
Streptococcus mitis; undifferentiated α and γ streptococci	+	**10–21** **47–50†**
Enterococci or group D *Streptococcus* spp.	+	**30–90**
Streptococcus pyogenes (usually group A unless noted)		**5–20‡**
Anaerobic *Streptococcus* spp.	+	**30–60**
Streptococcus pneumoniae		±
Gram-negative cocci		
Branhamella catarrhalis		+
Gemella haemolysans		
Veillonella alkalescens		+
Gram-positive bacilli		
Lactobacillus spp.		**50–75**
Aerobic *Corynebacterium* spp.	+	**45–75**
Mycobacterium spp.	+	
Clostridium perfringens		**0–10**
Other *Clostridium* spp.		**15–30**
Eubacterium limosum		**5**
Bifidobacterium bifidum		**10**
Actinomyces bifidus		**25–75**
Actinomyces israelii		±
Aerobic gram-negative bacilli		
Enterobacteriaceae		**15–40†**
	+	**3–10**
Bacteria (continued)		
Escherichia coli		+
Enterobacter spp.		**6†**
Proteus mirabilis, other *Proteus* spp.		+†
Morganella morganii		
Providencia spp.		
Moraxella lacunata	±	
Haemophilus parainfluenzae		+
Hemolytic *Haemophilus* spp.		+†
Corynebacterium vaginale		+
Anaerobic gram-negative bacilli		
Bacteroides fragilis (5 subspecies)	+	±
Bacteroides melaninogenicus (3 subspecies)	+	
Fusobacterium nucleatum	+	
Fusobacterium necrophorum		±
Curved bacteria		
Selenomonas sputigena	+	
Campylobacter sputorum		+
Treponema denticola	+	
Treponema refringens		
Fungi		
Candida albicans	+	**30–50**
non-albicans *Candida* spp.		**4–6§**
Torulopsis glabrata	+	+
Protozoa		
Trichomonas vaginalis		**10–25**

± to 0, rare; ±, irregular or uncertain (may be only pathologic); +, common; ++, prominent.

*Boldface values (*e.g.,* **30–60**) = range of incidence in percentage, rounded, in different surveys.

†Children.

‡Children; usually group B.

§*Candida stellatoidea,* principally.

PETER L. PERINE

Lymphogranuloma Venereum 54

Lymphogranuloma venereum (LGV) is a venereal disease caused by chlamydial microorganisms. It is also known as Durand-Nicholas-Favre disease, tropical or climatic bubo, poradenitis, lymphopathia venereum, and lymphogranuloma inguinale. Involving primarily the lymphatics and lymph nodes of the genital area and the lower urogenital tract, LGV is most commonly manifested by acute inguinal lymphadentitis (bubo), with or without genital ulceration. Late complications include urethral and rectal strictures, genital lymphedema, and rectovaginal fistulas.

Although Wallace described the disease in 1833, the account of Durand, Nicholas, and Favre in 1913 is regarded as definitive. The causative agent was not cultured until 1940, when Rake and associates grew it in the yolk sac of chick embryos.

Etiology

The characteristics common to all *Chlamydia* spp. are described in Chapter 1, Attributes of Infectious Agents. Two species are recognized, namely *C. trachomatis* and *C. psittaci.* The LGV chlamydias belong to *C. trachomatis,* along with the agents that cause trachoma, inclusion conjunctivitis, urethritis, and cervicitis. That is, subspecies of *C. trachomatis* can be biologically differentiated on the basis of the diseases that they cause in man, their only natural host. A more practical separation is based on characteristic surface antigens.

Twelve immunotypes, designated alphabetically A through K for trachoma, and three immunotypes, designated L_1, L_2, and L_3, are known for the LGV chlamydia. There are complicated immunologic interrelationships between LGV and some of the trachoma immunotypes. Although both trachoma agents and those causing LGV may be isolated from the genital tract of patients with LGV, the former are not responsible for the LGV syndrome.

The immunotype surface antigens of *C. trachomatis* are quite distinct from the group-specific, lipoprotein–carbohydrate antigen common to all *Chlamydia* spp. and demonstrable by the complement fixation test. On the other hand, the delayed hypersensitivity (skin test; blast transformation of lymphocytes *in vitro*) that is induced by infection with chlamydias is species-specific. The allergens used in the skin test are heat-stable proteins.

Epidemiology

Lymphogranuloma venereum occurs in most areas of the world but the greatest number of cases are concentrated in the tropical and subtropical nations of Africa and Asia. For example, between 200 and 400 cases are reported annually in the United States, whereas one clinic in Ethiopia treats more than 10,000 cases per year. However, most of the cases of LGV reported in the United States are diagnosed solely on clinical manifestations or on the basis of a positive complement fixation test that is not specific for LGV. In Western countries, LGV is usually found in homosexuals and prostitutes or in seamen, travelers, and military personnel returning from areas in which the disease is highly endemic.

Lymphogranuloma venereum is usually transmitted by sexual contact. The incidence of infection following exposure is not known, but it is lower than that of gonorrhea or chancroid. Nonvenereal transmission is rare, although it has been documented to result from direct contact with infected tissues, fomites, and laboratory accidents. The peak incidence of infection is in the second and third decades of life, which corresponds to the period of greatest sexual activity. For unknown reasons, clinically manifest infection is far more common in males than in females, the sex ratio often being as high as 6:1. In highly endemic areas, however, the ratio is more often less than 2:1, with infection in males predominant.

The incubation period is said to range from 5 to 21 days. Males are probably no longer infectious through sexual contact after the primary lesion heals, that is, approximately 3 weeks after LGV was acquired. The period of contagiousness in women is not known, but may be months in duration.

Pathogenesis and Pathology

The primary lesion of LGV is a small (2 mm–3 mm), painless, herpetiform vesicle or ulcer. It is found in only 10% to 30% of patients because it persists for only a few days, heals without scarring, and is inconspicious in terms of symptoms and location—on the posterior vaginal wall in women and the coronal sulcus in men. The histologic picture is that of a nonspecific granuloma consisting of an epidermal vesicle that usually extends into the dermis and produces a crater lined by epithelioid cells surrounded by a zone of mononuclear cells containing a few giant cells.

The mechanism(s) by which the chlamydias gain entry into the host is not known, but it is likely to involve entry through small abrasions in the epithelium or mucosa of the genital area and the urogenital tract. The chlamydias spread from the site of infection through the lymphatics to the regional nodes, and may then spread systemically. Rarely, the central nervous system is invaded, causing an acute meningoencephalitis—a complication that is unlikely to occur after the appearance of regional lymphadenopathy. The inguinal lymph nodes are affected primarily in men. Five to twenty-one days after infection and after the primary lesion has healed, the nodes swell, enlarging discretely but held together by periadenitis to form tender masses. In one-third of the cases, the lymphadenopathy is bilateral; less frequently, it is so extensive that the inguinal mass is cleaved by the inelastic inguinal ligament—the almost pathognomonic groove sign of LGV (Fig. 54-1). The histologic appearance depends upon the duration of the lymphadenopathy. Early lesions show central necrosis of the lymph node surrounded by epithelioid cells, scattered giant cells, and a zone of mononuclear cells. Later, there is matting of the nodes with the formation of multiple stellate abscesses that have a central, radiating area of necrosis surrounded by zones of histocytes and mononuclear cells. If untreated, the abscesses will coalesce to form caseous lesions that may erode through the tensely stretched, overlying skin to form sinus tracts. Thick, yellowish pus can be expressed from the sinus tracts, and drainage may continue for several weeks until healing eventually ensues, with formation of scars. In 20% to 25% of cases, the lymph nodes do not suppurate but slowly resolve over a period of weeks or months; less commonly, an indurated inguinal mass forms that persists for life.

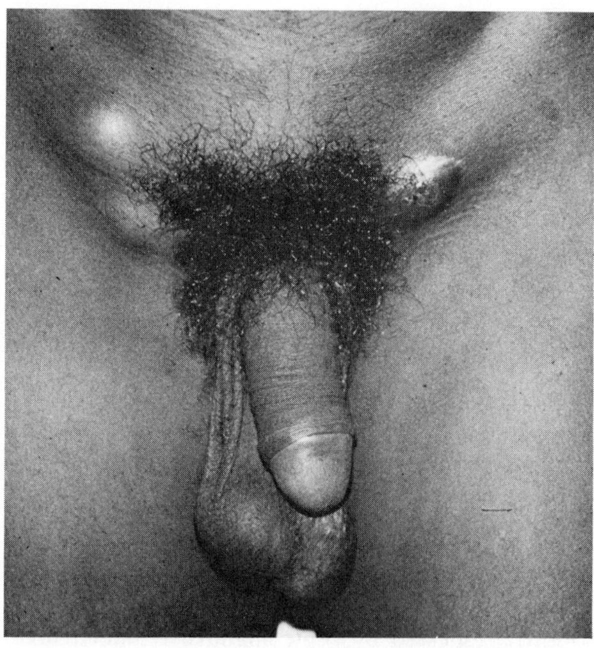

Fig. 54-1. Bilateral inguinal buboes, separated by the inelastic Poupart's ligament on the patient's right side, yielding the groove sign that is characteristic of lymphogranuloma venereum.

In women, the external and internal iliac lymphatics and the sacral lymphatics (*i.e.,* lymphatic drainage of the cervix, uterus, and rectum) are principally affected. Obstruction of the flow of lymph may result, leading to dilation and thrombosis of lymphatics, associated with hyperplasia and hypertrophy of the vulvar integument and subjacent connective tissue. The end-result of this process is lymphedema of the vulva and perineum. This may result in elephantiasis and ulcerations of the vulva (esthiomene) (Fig. 54-2), and pedunculated anal growths, lymphorrhoids, which clinically resemble hemorrhoids. If the urethra is involved in the ulceration, it may be shortened or destroyed, leading to proximal urethral perforations and urinary incontinence or difficulty in micturition.

Both men and women occasionally have a hemorrhagic proctitis or proctocolitis during the acute stages of LGV; the chlamydias can multiply in the epithelial cells of the intestinal tract. An identical proctocolitis may also be caused by non-LGV serotypes of *C. trachomatis* (types that commonly cause nongonoccal urethritis and cervicitis in heterosexual men and women) in homosexual men who practice anal intercourse. The process does not extend beyond the sigmoid colon and usually resolves completely. However, stricture of the rectum, found almost exclusively in women, follows after months or years. It is usually situated several centimeters above the anal orifice, and may be mistaken for rectal carcinoma. The lesion is cylindrical; ulceration of the mucosa is common, and there is marked fibrous thickening of the bowel wall with proliferation in the submucosa (Fig. 54-3).

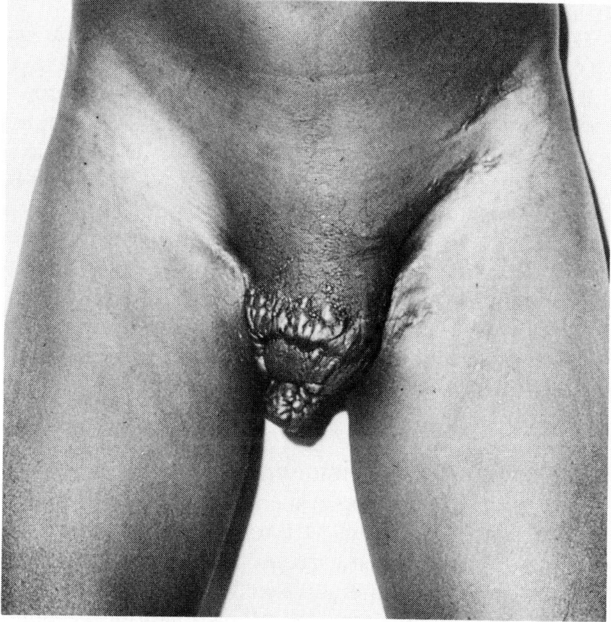

Fig. 54-2. Lymphedema of the vulva producing elephantiasis of the external genitalia (esthiomene). Note the scars in the left inguinal region due to rupture and healing of previous lymphogranuloma buboes.

Much of the pathophysiology of LGV is yet to be determined. Many clinical and pathologic manifestations of the infection resemble those of tuberculosis and other diseases in which cellular immune mechanisms play a significant role.

Manifestations

The manifestations of LGV are conventionally separated into the inguinal and the genitoanorectal syndromes. By far the most common, the former consists of the primary lesion, inguinal lymphadenopathy, and nonspecific systemic illness—fever, chills, headache, malaise, and weight loss, often with splenomegaly and hyperglobulinemia.

The genitoanorectal syndrome is seen in about 25% of patients; it occurs predominantly in women and homosexual men. The clinical hallmark is bloody, mucopurulent, rectal discharge. On proctoscopic examination, the rectal mucosa is inflamed, friable, and ulcerated. Without specific therapy, pararectal abscesses, rectal strictures, and rectovaginal fistulas may result. Despite the extensive inflammatory changes, the genitoanorectal syndrome is rarely associated with constitutional symptoms or with inguinal lymphadenopathy.

Acute meningitis, meningoencephalitis, pneumonia, and an exogenous keratoconjunctivitis with preauricular adenopathy and lymphedema of the eyelids

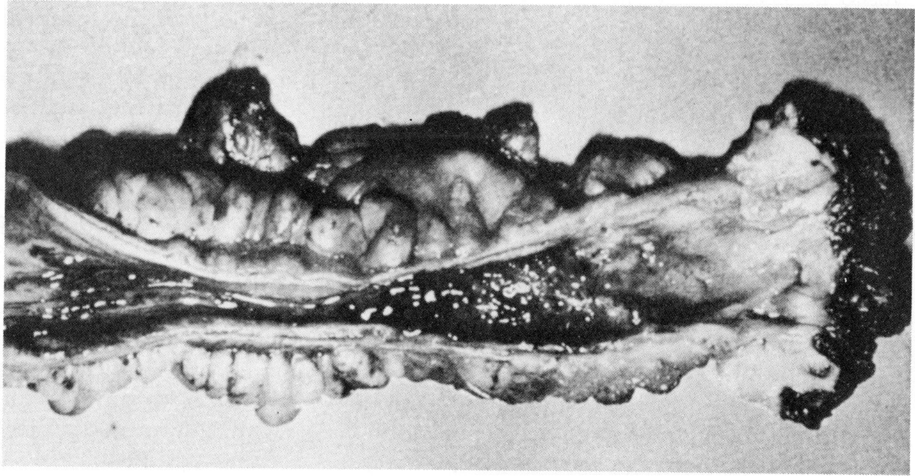

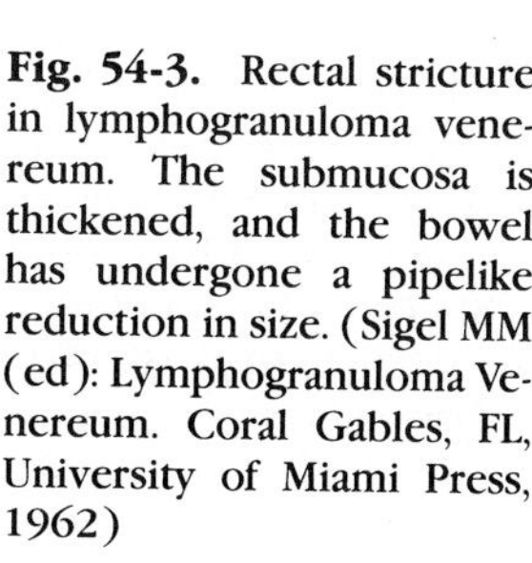

Fig. 54-3. Rectal stricture in lymphogranuloma venereum. The submucosa is thickened, and the bowel has undergone a pipelike reduction in size. (Sigel MM (ed): Lymphogranuloma Venereum. Coral Gables, FL, University of Miami Press, 1962)

(Parinaud's oculoglandular syndrome) are rare manifestations of LGV. An indolent polyarthritis with sterile joint fluid and a tendency to relapse is a rare, acute manifestation of LGV. Skin lesions, such as erythema multiforme, erythema nodosum, and scarlatiniform eruptions, may also occur in LGV—usually following surgical excision of lymph nodes, abscesses, or infected tissue.

Extragenital primary infections of LGV are rare. An ulcerating lesion may appear at the site of infection (*e.g.,* fingers, lips, tongue), but regional lymphadenitis is the usual cause of disease after extragenital inoculation.

Diagnosis

Although a number of diagnostic tests are available, the diagnosis of LGV can be proved only by isolating *C. trachomatis* from appropriate specimens and confirming the isolate as an LGV immunotype. Such laboratory diagnostic capabilities are not generally available, and the diagnosis of LGV is usually based primarily on clinical manifestations aided by other less specific tests and procedures.

Inguinal buboes are classic manifestations of LGV. However, there are other causes of inguinal swellings. The buboes of chancroid (see Chap. 57, Chancroid) are usually unilateral and not associated with general manifestations of illness. On the other hand, the lymphadenopathy of a malignant lymphoma and cat-scratch fever (Chap. 166, Cat-Scratch Fever) are part of a systemic illness.

The proctocolitis of the early genitoanorectal syndrome may be mistaken for idiopathic ulcerative colitis or amebic dysentery (Chap. 66, Amebiasis). Acute meningitis, meningoencephalitis, and polyarthritis caused by LGV usually cause diagnostic confusion. Smears, cultures, and serologic and skin tests are helpful to clinical differentiation.

Intradermal Skin Test (Frei Test)

Frei introduced a diagnostic skin test in 1925, using pus obtained from a bubo as antigen. A commercial skin test antigen prepared from LGV chlamydia grown in the yolk sacs of chick embryos was used for several decades, but its manufacture was discontinued in 1974. The test consisted of the intradermal injection of 0.1 ml of antigen into the flexor surface of the forearm; separately, 0.1 ml of normal yolk sac control material was also injected intradermally. The test was positive if a zone of erythema and induration 6 mm in diameter (or greater) developed 48 to 72 hours after injection at the site of inoculation of the antigen but not at the control site. The skin test became positive as early as 10 days after infection. Its sensitivity varied 36% to 95%. More important, the specificity of the Frei skin test for LGV was low because positive reactions occurred in other infections caused by *C. trachomatis.* The test was more likely to be positive the longer the infection had been untreated; once positive, the test remained so for life.

Complement Fixation Test

The heat-stable antigen used for complement fixation (CF) testing is group-specific for all *Chlamydia* spp. It is most commonly prepared from a psittacosis strain grown *in ovo* or in cell culture. The complement fixation test is usually positive in high titer (1:64 or higher) in more than 80% of cases. It is more sensitive than the skin test, particularly if there was a rise in titer between acute and convalescent serums. Unfortunately, an acute specimen is generally difficult to obtain, and antibodies cross-react broadly with other chlamydial antigens, including trachoma and psittacosis chlamydias. There is, however, no cross-reaction with syphilis, yaws, gonorrhea, or leprosy.

Microimmunofluorescence Test

The microimmunofluorescence (micro IF) test is more sensitive than the CF test. Trachoma and LGV immunotype antigens are used simultaneously and type-specific patterns of reaction are obtained. In LGV, very high titers of micro-IF antibodies and broad reaction to many trachoma–LGV strains are found, particularly to the LGV immunotypes.

Isolation of the Chlamydia of Lymphogranuloma Venereum

LGV chlamydia can be grown in cell cultures, in yolk sacs of chicken embryos, or in the brains of mice. Isolation of the agent from clinical material (blood, aspirated pus, cerebrospinal fluid, infected tissue) can be accomplished prior to treatment in 25% to 50% of patients. Cell culture (such as use of HeLa 229 cells) is simple to perform and is increasingly available in specialized venereal disease clinics.

Other Diagnostic Procedures

A trachoma–LGV-specific antigen extracted from LGV chlamydia grown in tissue culture has been used in counterimmunoelectrophoresis to detect antibodies in the serum. This experimental technique might prove to be useful in the diagnosis of LGV.

The histopathology of the lymph nodes involved with LGV is not diagnostic of the disease. A mild monocytic leukocytosis is common in LGV, as is mild elevation of the erythrocyte sedimentation rate. An increase in IgA, together with the occurrence of rheumatoid factor, has been reported in subacute and chronic LGV infections. Anticomplementary serum factors also occur. None of these abnormalities is specific for LGV.

Prognosis

Although LGV can cause disability and sometimes death, serious disease is the exception rather than the rule. For example, in areas of the world in which the disease is highly endemic, rectal stricture, the most serious complication, is rarely seen. Other factors, such as obstructed labor in childbirth, may contribute to complications such as rectovaginal fistulas. Secondary bacterial infections usually complicate rectovaginal fistulas, and concomitant infections are frequent (*e.g.,* gonorrhea and syphilis). These factors make it difficult to determine the contribution of LGV to the total disease process.

Late sequelae of the inguinal syndrome are seen in about 5% of cases. The most common lesions are fistular lesions of the urethra, penis, and scrotum in males, and ulcerative genital lesions in females. The most serious late sequelae of LGV are rectal strictures. In addition to tenesmus, pain, and constipation, there may be genital lymphedema, anal tags, or lymphorrhoids.

Therapy

Controlled trials of antimicrobic therapy in LGV are few and inconclusive. Treatment with tetracycline (25 mg–30 mg/kg body wt/day as 4 equal portions perorally every 6 hours) for 2 to 4 weeks or sulfonamides (*e.g.,* triple sulfonamides, 60 mg–75 mg/kg body wt/day as four equal portions perorally every 6 hours) for 2 weeks results in a prompt abatement of fever, decrease of pain in the involved lymph nodes, and an improved sense of well-being. Antimicrobial therapy may possibly prevent late sequelae such as rectal stricture and may ameliorate or prevent secondary bacterial infection of suppurated lymph nodes. Treatment does not seem to influence the resolution and healing of enlarged lymph nodes—usually 4 to 6 weeks. Keratoconjunctivitis should be treated with a tetracycline eye ointment applied twice daily for 14 days.

Fluctuant lymph nodes should be drained by aspiration with a syringe and 18-gauge needle. Aspiration is repeated as often as necessary to relieve pain and to prevent rupture. Open wounds should be covered with a nonadherent dressing moistened with an antiseptic solution, for example, benzalkonium chloride.

Rectovaginal fistulas, rectal strictures, and genital elephantiasis require surgical correction.

Prevention

Public health measures such as the identification and treatment of sexual contacts, the distribution of information about LGV, and education in personal hygiene have proven to be effective in reducing the number of cases of LGV in some areas of the world. There are no vaccines or other means of prophylaxis.

Remaining Problems

More information is required regarding the actual incidence of LGV, the frequency of infection following exposure, the incidence of subclinical infection, and the possibility of a carrier state. A more specific, readily available diagnostic test would be a distinct advantage, as would having information on the prognosis, particularly in terms of complications in both treated and untreated patients.

Bibliography

Books

HART G: Chancroid Granuloma Inguinale, Lymphogranuloma Venereum. Department of Health, Education, and Welfare Publication No. (CDC) 75-8302. Washington, DC, U. S. Government Printing Office, 1975

PERINE PL, ANDERSON AJ, KRAUSE DW: Diagnosis and treatment of lymphogranuloma venereum in Ethiopia. Curr Chemother Infect Dis, American Society for Microbiology, Washington, DC, 1980. pp 1280–1282.

SIGEL MM (ED): Lymphogranuloma Venereum. Coral Gables, FL , University of Miami Press, 1962. 197 pp.

Journals

HOLDER WR, DUNCAN WC: Lymphogranuloma venereum. Clin Obstet Gynecol 15:1004–1009, 1972

JAWETZ E: Chemotherapy of chlamydial infections. Pharmacol Chemother 7:253–282, 1969

KOTEEN H: Lymphogranuloma venereum. Medicine 24:1–69, 1945

SCHACHTER J: Chlamydial infections. N Engl J Med 298:428–435, 490–495, 540–549, 1978

WILLIAM R. BOWIE
KING K. HOLMES

55 Nongonococcal Urethritis

Nongonococcal urethritis (NGU) is urethritis in which urethral gonococcal infection cannot be demonstrated. Etiologically, it is a wastebasket diagnosis, but it is a clinical entity. It is usually restricted to men although the urethral syndrome in women (see Chap. 48, Urethritis and Cystitis) can be caused by *Chlamydia trachomatis,* one of the causes of NGU. Postgonococcal urethritis is indistinguishable from NGU and develops in 30% to 60% of men 2 to 3 weeks after curative treatment of gonorrhea with penicillin G or ampicillin.

During the 1800s, physicians began to suspect that venereally acquired urethritis was not a single nosologic entity. After Neisser's description of the gonococcus in 1879, culture of the gonococcus by Leistikow in 1882, and introduction of Gram's stain in 1884, it was possible to differentiate gonococcal and nongonococcal urethritis. However, it was the fact that urethritis could not always be cured by the sulfonamides and penicillin that called the attention of clinicians to NGU. It is a syndrome of growing clinical importance since it accounts for 30% to 90% of acute urethritis in males—the incidence varying with age group, population studied, and country surveyed.

Etiology

There is no evidence to support any of the nonvenereal causes of NGU put forward over the years and accumulated as an obscuring lore. Sexual transmission of an infectious agent is supported by (1) onset 2 to 3 weeks after coitus with a new partner, (2) outbreaks among sailors 2 to 3 weeks after shore leave, (3) an age distribution of incidence duplicating that of gonorrhea, and (4) success in therapy and prophylaxis with tetracyclines.

Although many saprophytic genital bacteria, various fungi, and protozoa have been implicated as possible causes of NGU in men, there is evidence that only two microorganisms, *Chlamydia trachomatis* and *Ureaplasma urealyticum,* commonly play an etiologic role.

Chlamydia trachomatis

The acceptance of *C. trachomatis* as a cause of NGU began with the demonstration of inclusion bodies in urethral discharge (men with NGU) and cervical secretions (mothers of infants with inclusion conjunctivitis). Isolation of the agent in yolk sac and tissue cultures, as well as demonstration of a humoral antibody response (immunofluorescence, IgM and IgG), closed the ring.

The biologic properties of the chlamydias and the bases for differentiating species and subspecies are discussed in Chapters 1, 54, and 159, Attributes of Infectious Agents, Lymphogranuloma Venereum, and Trachoma. As depicted in Table 55-1, immunotypes D through K (the genital strains) are of concern with regard to NGU, cervicitis, and inclusion conjunctivitis. Types D and E are the immunotypes most frequently isolated in NGU; types F and G are the next

Table 55-1. *Chlamydia Species That Cause Disease in Man*

Species	Disease	Immunotype
psittaci	Psittacosis	
trachomatis	Trachoma	A,B,Ba,C*
	Inclusion conjunctivitis	D,E,F,G,H,I,J,K
trachomatis (sexually transmitted)	NGU	D,E,F,H,H,I,J,K
	Cervicitis	D,E,F,H,K,I,J,K
	Lymphogranuloma venereum	L_1,$L_2$$L_{,3}$

* Immunotypes A, B, and C cause trachoma in most trachoma-endemic areas. Type Ba causes trachoma in American Indians. Other immunotypes can also cause trachoma in the populations of developed Western countries.

most common. These genital strains are also capable of causing sporadic, nonendemic trachoma, with onset either in childhood or after the patients have become sexually active.

In England and the United States, *C. trachomatis* has been isolated from the urethras of 30% to 60% of men with NGU, from 4% to 34% (usually about 20%) of men with gonorrhea, and from 0% to 5% of sexually active men with no urethritis. Among men experiencing their first episode of NGU and examined early after the onset of symptoms, 90% of those proved by culture to be infected by *C. trachomatis* had seroconversion of immunofluorescent antibody to *C. trachomatis* in paired sera; a transient rise of IgM antibody to *C trachomatis* was detectable in most patients.

Nearly all men simultaneously infected with *Neisseria gonorrhoeae* and *C trachomatis* who are treated with penicillin G or with gentamicin (also inactive against *C. trachomatis*) go on to develop postgonococcal urethritis. Such patients apparently acquire two venereal diseases simultaneously: one with a 2- to 7-day incubation period (gonorrhea) and one with a 2- to 3-week incubation period (chlamydial urethritis). The simultaneous acquisition of *C. trachomatis* in 20% to 30% of men with gonorrhea is not an unrealistic possibility because *C. trachomatis* have been recovered from the endocervix of 40% to 60% of women with gonorrhea. Chlamydial infection of the cervix is present in most female sex partners of men with chlamydia-positive NGU, but seldom in the sex partners of men with chlamydia-negative NGU.

Ureaplasma urealyticum

Of the two genital mycoplasmas of man, *Mycoplasma hominis* does not cause NGU, whereas *U. urealyticum* (T-strain mycoplasma) may be an etiologic agent. *Ureaplasma urealyticum* split urea and form tiny (=T) colonies on agar medium. Fourteen or more serotypes may be distinguished through metabolic inhibition or killing by type-specific antibody. In one study, the association of serotype 4 with symptomatic urethritis in men was significant. However, the etiologic significance of ureaplasmas in NGU is less well established than that of the chlamydias, because a humoral immune response to ureaplasmas is not usually demonstrable by available techniques in men with NGU, and because ureaplasmas are often recovered from men without urethritis.

The prevalence of urethral or cervicovaginal colonization with *U. urealyticum* is directly correlated with total number of sex partners. Among patients who attend venereal disease clinics, 50% to 80% carry urethral *U. urealyticum* regardless of diagnosis. Men with NGU often have an unusually high concentration of *U. urealyticum* in the urine first voided in the morning; persistence of ureaplasmas in the urine is associated with persistence or recurrence of NGU. There is a significantly higher rate of isolation and a higher concentration of *U. urealyticum* in men with chlamydia-negative NGU than in men with chlamydia-positive NGU.

The role of both *C. trachomatis* and *U. urealyticum* as separate causes of NGU is further supported by therapeutic studies. Sulfonamides and rifampin are active against *C. trachomatis* but not against *U. urealyticum,* and treatment with sulfonamides or rifampin produces a significantly higher rate of improvement in chlamydia-positive, ureaplasma-negative NGU than in chlamydia-negative ureaplasma-positive NGU.

Spectinomycin is active against *U. urealyticum* but has only slight activity against *C. trachomatis*; treatment with spectinomycin produces a significantly better response in chlamydia-negative, ureaplasma-positive NGU than in chlamydia-positive, ureaplasma-negative NGU. Furthermore, when spectinomycin failed to eradicate *U. urealyticum,* urethritis often persisted. Similarly, when tetracycline fails to eradicate *U. urealyticum* because of suboptimal dosage or resistance (approximately 10%), urethritis also frequently persists.

Intraurethral inoculation of *U. urealyticum* into two men and several nonhuman primates produced urethritis in both men and several of the primates.

Other Agents

Neither chlamydias nor ureaplasmas can be isolated from 20% to 30% of cases of NGU, and neither aerobic nor anaerobic bacteria have been implicated. However, bacterial prostatitis caused by coliform bacteria may produce a urethral discharge and be confused with NGU.

Candida albicans (see Chap. 39, Candidosis) and *Trichomonas vaginalis* (see Chap. 50, Infections of the Female Genital Tract) may rarely cause NGU. Type 2 herpes simplex virus (see Chap. 91, Infections Caused by Herpes Simplex Viruses) causes dysuria in about 30% of men with primary genital herpes-virus infection and sometimes also causes urethral discharge. Penile herpetic lesions are usually present and make the diagnosis obvious.

Epidemiology

The age distribution of males with NGU parallels that of men with gonorrhea, that is, most men are between ages 16 and 30 years. Among patients attending a venereal disease clinic because of urethritis, men with NGU differ from those with gonorrhea in that they (1) are more often white, (2) have attained a higher socioeconomic status (determined by educational attainment, occupation, and place of residence), (3) have had fewer sex partners and were older at the time of first sexual intercourse, and (4) are more likely to have had previous NGU but less likely to have had previous gonorrhea. There is no known genetic predisposition to NGU. The distribution of blood types and of histocompatibility antigens among NGU patients resembles that of the general population.

In England and Wales, the incidence of NGU has been increasing even more rapidly than that of gonorrhea in men, particularly in recent years (Fig. 55-1). The failure to control the incidence of NGU at a time when gonorrhea is coming under control may reflect failure to treat sexual contacts. In the United States, a further deplorable impediment to control is the failure of many public venereal disease clinics to provide treatment for sexually transmitted diseases other than gonorrhea and syphilis. Consequently, the prevalence of infection caused by *C. trachomatis* in the female is higher than that of gonorrhea.

Fig. 55-1. Comparative annual incidence of gonorrhea and NGU in men in England and Wales. (Courtesy Dr. Duncan Catterall, Middlesex Hospital, London)

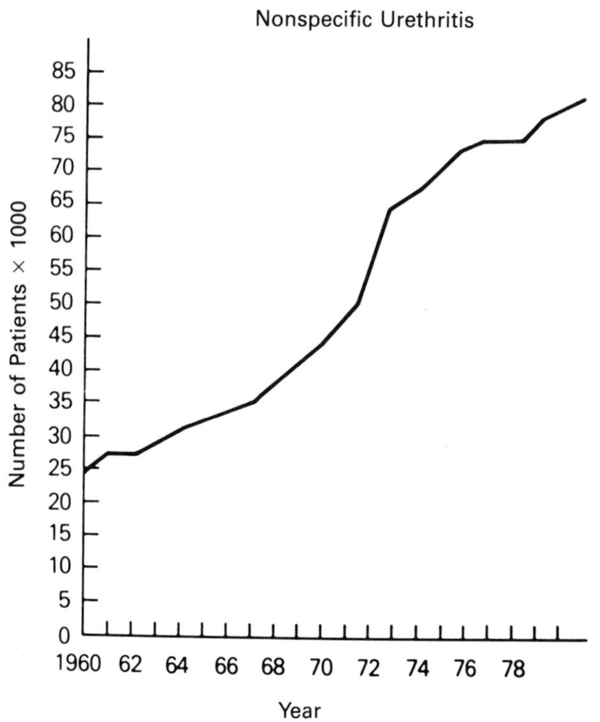

Chlamydia trachomatis is a cause of cervicitis, the acute urethral syndrome, and acute pelvic inflammatory disease in women. It may also cause the Fitz-Hugh–Curtis syndrome and late postpartum endometritis. Of near-term women, 2% to 13% are cervicovaginal carriers of *C. trachomatis* (about 10 times more frequent than *N. gonorrhoeae*), yielding infection in 60% to 70% of infants delivered vaginally despite ocular silver nitrate prophylaxis. Of the infected infants, 40% to 50% develop inclusion conjunctivitis, 10% to 20% develop a chronic, afebrile, interstitial pneumonitis, and the remainder have either asymptomatic carriage in the nasopharynx, rectum, or vagina, or develop serum antibody without an obvious focus of infection.

In some studies, *C. trachomatis* has been implicated in otitis media in infants, prepubertal vaginitis, bartholinitis and cervical dysplasia in adult women, culture-negative endocarditis, pneumonia in immunosuppressed or normal adults, and proctitis in homosexual men. It has been suggested that prematurity, stillbirth, and neonatal death may be related to antepartum maternal infection with *C. trachomatis.*

Pathogenesis and Pathology

Chlamydias produce infections that are characterized by prolonged latency, a unique intracellular growth cycle, and the development of incomplete host immunity. The elementary body appears to attach to susceptible cells by specific receptors. The mechanisms responsible for the penetration and persistence of *C. trachomatis* within cells, the epithelial cell damage, and the development of an inflammatory response are not well defined. Secretory and humoral antibodies form and there is some evidence of cell-mediated immunity. But the role of immune processes in pathogenesis or in resistance to infection is not understood, particularly in genital chlamydial infection.

The erosions down to the subepithelial connective tissue that characterize gonococcal urethritis do not occur with NGU. Without treatment, the urethra may eventually assume a cobblestone appearance reminiscent of trachomatous nodules.

Manifestations

Urethral infection by *C. trachomatis* and *U. urealyticum* may result in no urethritis, asymptomatic pyuria, or urethral exudate with or without dysuria. The majority of men who have infection of the urethra with *U.*

urealyticum do not have symptomatic urethritis, and most probably do not even have asymptomatic pyuria. A larger, though undefined, proportion of men who acquire *C. trachomatis* develop asymptomatic or symptomatic urethritis. For example, most men with acute urethritis who are infected with both *N. gonorrhoeae* and *C. trachomatis* develop postgonococcal urethritis if the gonorrhea is cured but the *C. trachomatis* is allowed to persist. It has been shown by prospective study of men that most of those who acquire gonococcal infection by sexual exposure also acquire acute urethritis.

The duration of the incubation period for NGU averages 2 to 3 weeks and may be as long as 5 weeks, whereas the incubation period for gonorrhea is usually 2 to 7 days. Dysuria occurs in most patients with gonorrhea and NGU, but is generally more severe with gonorrhea. Symptomatic patients with NGU generally have a white or mucoid urethral exudate containing fewer neutrophils than are found in gonococcal urethritis (Fig. 31-5*C*); the discharge is often noted only upon arising or after the urethra is stripped. Most men with gonorrhea have a more profuse urethral exudate that is yellow or green and contains large numbers of polymorphonuclear leukocytes. However, in an individual case, it is not possible to distinguish clinically the cause of urethritis.

Prognosis

Although not life-threatening, and generally not as productive of morbidity as gonorrhea, symptomatic NGU may be a persisting annoyance for months without antimicrobial therapy. It is probable that the disease is self-limited in most patients. However, epididymitis does occur in a small proportion of men with NGU, and *C. trachomatis* has been recovered from the urethra in nearly 50% of men under 35 years of age with acute epididymitis. The relationship of NGU to chronic nonbacterial prostatitis and to Reiter's syndrome is uncertain, although urethral cultures yield *C. trachomatis* in 30% to 70% of men with Reiter's syndrome; men whose histocompatibility antigens include HLA B27 appear to be at increased risk of developing Reiter's syndrome when they acquire NGU. However, one study showed that if HLA B27-positive men with NGU were treated with tetracycline before the onset of other manifestations, none went on to develop Reiter's syndrome. Infection with *C. trachomatis* or *U. urealyticum* does not appear to prevent reinfection, although very little research has been done on the effect of naturally occurring genital infection on possible development of partial type-specific immunity.

Diagnosis

The diagnosis of NGU is made by establishing the presence of urethritis, by excluding the presence of *N. gonorrhoeae,* and by excluding other conditions that may be confused with urethritis (Fig. 55-2). The presence of urethritis is established if a urethral discharge is demonstrable by milking the urethra from the base of the penis to the meatus, and the discharge when examined microscopically by Gram's stain contains more than four polymorphonuclear leukocytes per oil immersion field. For maximal sensitivity, specimens should be obtained before the first voiding of urine in the morning. If the patient has symptoms of urethritis but an increased number of polymorphonuclear leukocytes is not demonstrable in the urethral discharge, the first 10 ml of overnight urine and a midstream urine specimen should be collected separately and then centrifuged. All but 0.5 ml of supernatant urine is decanted from each specimen, the

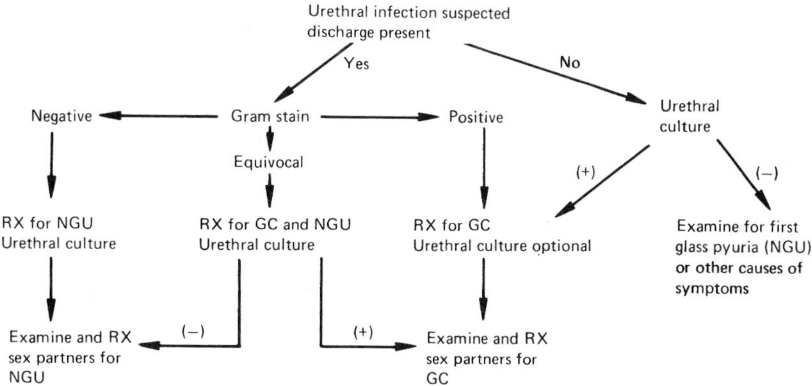

Fig. 55-2. Diagnosis and management of urethritis in males.

sediments are resuspended, and a drop of each sediment is examined under a coverslip. The presence of 15 or more polymorphonuclear leukocytes in two or more of five 400 × (high dry) fields in the first voided specimen, with fewer leukocytes in the midstream urine, indicates urethritis.

Urgency, hesitancy, perineal discomfort, or abnormal prostatic tenderness is consistent with prostatitis and should lead to quantitative culture and microscopic examination of urine and prostatic expressate. The urethra should be palpated for the presence of periurethral abscess or a foreign body inserted by the patient. The meatus should be spread and inspected for ulceration (*e.g.,* chancre) or condyloma acuminata. The clinician should also look for epididymitis and systemic manifestations of Reiter's syndrome or disseminated gonococcal infection.

Thus, a presumptive diagnosis of gonococcal or nongonococcal urethritis is made on the basis of a Gram-stained smear of urethral exudate. It can be interpreted while the patient is waiting, which permits rational selection of initial therapy. The smear is considered positive for gonorrhea (see Chap. 56, Gonococcal Infections) if typical gram-negative diplococci are seen within neutrophils, equivocal if only extracellular or atypical gram-negative diplococci are seen (Fig. 31-5*C*). A urethral culture for *N. gonorrhoeae* is necessary when the smear is equivocal. When the smear is negative, a culture is also desirable to exclude gonorrhea, particularly if the urethral exudate is scanty or absent. When the smear is positive, a culture is optional, but examination and treatment of the sex partner for gonorrhea should be initiated (see Chap. 56, Gonococcal Infections). If the Gram stain is negative or equivocal, treatment should be initiated for NGU.

Therapy

The optimal dose and duration of therapy for NGU and the value of treating the sex partners of men with NGU have not been clearly established. However, the initial regimen should consist of tetracycline hydrochloride, 30 mg/kg body wt/day, perorally, as four equal portions, 6-hourly for at least 7 days. Although tetracycline hydrochloride, 250 mg four times daily for 7 days, has been as effective as 500 mg four times daily for *C. trachomatis*-positive NGU, the higher dose regimen is required for treatment of gonorrhea and should be used for persons with an equivocal smear or undifferentiated urethritis. In two controlled trials, tetracycline was more effective than a placebo. After 7 days of therapy, nearly all patients with NGU are improved, although many still have a clear or mucoid urethral discharge that usually continues to resolve after therapy is discontinued. Those few patients who fail to show any improvement require evaluation for poor compliance, trichomoniasis, and other causes of urethritis, but many will have tetracycline-resistant *U. urealyticum.* If no other specific cause is found, a trial of erythromycin is appropriate (30 mg/kg body wt, perorally, as four equal portions, 6-hourly for 7 days). Continued failure to improve is an indication for urethroscopy in search of a urethral stricture, intraurethral ulceration, or condylomas. Occasionally, roentgenographic examination of the penis may reveal a foreign body that was not palpated or seen by urethroscopy.

Among patients given 1 week of therapy with tetracycline, 17% of chlamydia-positive cases and 47% of chlamydia-negative cases have an incomplete response or clinical recurrence of urethritis within the ensuing 6 weeks. Some recurrences are reinfections acquired from untreated sex partners, but many occur in men who deny being reexposed. Men with recurrences by 6 weeks after treatment rarely yield *C. trachomatis* and most do not have *U. urealyticum* by culture. Prolonging the initial course of treatment from 1 to 3 weeks did not improve results in one double-blind study. Use of newer congeners of tetracycline (*e.g.,* doxycyline or minocycline) does not appear to improve results. Treatment of the sex partner(s) of men with NGU is essential because a high percentage are known to be infected with chlamydias and/or ureaplasmas. Tetracycline (30 mg/kg body wt/day, perorally as four equal portions, 6-hourly for 7 days) is employed by many physicians, but erythromycin (15 mg/kg body wt/day, perorally as four equal portions, 6-hourly for 7 days) or sulfisoxazole (30 mg/kg body wt/day, perorally as four equal portions, 6-hourly for 10 days) is also effective for cervical infections caused by *C. trachomatis.*

There is no evidence that alcohol interferes with treatment, and it is probably sufficient to advise the patient to return only if symptoms fail to improve or to return 6 weeks after therapy. Management of recurrent NGU again requires exclusion of genital adnexal infection and gonorrhea. At this point, a more prolonged course of a tetracycline (*e.g.,* tetracycline, 15mg–17 mg/kg body wt/day, perorally, as four equal portions, 6-hourly for 30 days; doxycycline, 100 mg perorally every 12 hours for 30 days) is often effective.

Prevention

There is little doubt that the use of condoms during sexual intercourse will reduce the transmission of gonorrhea, chlamydias, and ureaplasmas. It is not known whether circumcision, washing, or voiding after intercourse influences transmission of these microorganisms. Controlled studies are in progress to determine whether prophylactic use of intravaginal spermicidal creams during intercourse will also reduce the transmission of venereal infections.

Chemoprophylaxis (a single dose of 200 mg minocycline taken 6–12 hours after intercourse) reduces the risk of acquiring NGU by 85% (compared with concomitant placebo-treated controls).

Vaccines for prevention of NGU are not in immediate prospect.

Remaining Problems

There are basic questions that must be answered concerning genital *C. trachomatis* infection. (1) Does natural infection produce species or type-specific immunity? (2) Is reinfection more or less severe than the initial infection? (3) Could a vaccine be developed that would reduce susceptibility to genital infection?

Further evidence that *U. urealyticum* causes urethritis should be sought through prospective cohort studies and improved serologic methods.

Bibliography

Books

BOWIE WR, ALEXANDER ER, WANG S–P, HOLMES KK: Etiology of NGU. In Holmes KK, Hobson DK (eds): Nongonococcal Urethritis and Related Oculogenital Infections. American Society for Microbiology, Washington, DC, 1977. pp 19–29.

Journals

BOWIE WR: Etiology and treatment of nongonococcal urethritis. Sex Transm Dis 5:27–33, 1978.

BOWIE WR, ALEXANDER ER, STIMSON JB, FLOYD JF, HOLMES KK. Therapy for nongonococcal urethritis: double-blind, randomized comparison of two doses and two durations of minocycline. Ann Intern Med 95:306–311, 1981

HOLMES KK, HANDSFIELD HH, WANG SP, WENTWORTH BB, TURCK M, ANDERSON JB, ALEXANDER ER: Etiology of nongonococcal urethritis. N Engl J Med 292:1199–1205, 1975

SCHACTER J: Chlamydial infections. N Engl J Med 298:423–435, 490–495, 540–549, 1978

SWARTZ SL, KRAUS SJ, HERRMANN KL, STARGEL MD, BROWN WJ, ALLEN SD: Diagnosis and etiology of nongonococcal urethritis. J Inf Dis 138:445–454, 1978

TAYLOR–ROBINSON D, MCCORMACK WM: The genital mycoplasmas. N Engl J Med 302:1003–1010, 1063–1067, 1980

KING K. HOLMES
STEPHEN A. MORSE

56 Gonococcal Infections

Gonorrhea is a sexually transmitted infection of columnar and transitional epithelium caused by *Neisseria gonorrhoeae*. The urethra, endocervix, anal canal, pharynx, and conjunctivae may be infected directly, and contiguous spread along mucosal surfaces may result in endometritis, salpingitis, peritonitis, and bartholinitis in the female, and periurethral abscess and epididymitis in the male. Systemic complications of gonococcemia include arthritis, tenosynovitis, dermatitis, endocarditis, and meningitis, as well as myopericarditis and hepatitis.

Etiology

Neisseria gonorrhoeae are nonmotile spherical or oval cocci usually found in pairs with flattened, adjacent sides (0.8 μm × 0.6 μm). They stain readily and are gram-negative. Formation of capsules has not been irrefutably demonstrated; spores are not produced.

Gonococci require both relatively high humidity and ambient CO_2 for growth. Narrow ranges of temperature (35°C–37°C) and pH (7.2–7.6) are optimal. In common with other neisserias, gonococci (as well as *Pseudomonas aeruginosa,* certain diphtheroids, Enterobacteriaceae, and some yeasts) elaborate cytochrome oxidase, the basis for the oxidase test, which is useful in laboratory diagnosis. Gonococci differ from other *Neisseria* spp. in their inability to utilize either maltose, sucrose, or lactose while metabolizing glucose. Since they are strict aerobes, they do not ferment glucose through the Embden–Meyerhof–Parnas pathway. The so-called fermentation reactions commonly employed to identify gonococci actually detect nonfermentive degradation of glucose through both the Entner–Duodoroff and pentose–phosphate pathways. Acetate accumulates, which drops the pH, changing the color of the phenol red indicator incorporated in the culture medium. Only glucose, pyruvate, and lactate can be used as energy sources by the gonococcus.

As growth requirements have been identified, nutritional peculiarities have been associated with groups of gonococcal strains. Such peculiarities are the bases for auxotyping—differentiation among gonococci according to stable, strain-specific requirements for amino acids, purines, pyrimidines, and vitamins. A synthetic, totally defined culture medium is necessary for auxotyping. Isolates from different geographic areas frequently differ in auxotype.

With appropriate reagents, specific immunofluorescence not only serves to distinguish gonococci from other species of *Neisseria,* but also permits serogrouping of the gonococcus. Such antigenic differences surely relate to unique structures in the cell envelope. As is shown schematically in Figure 56-1, the cell envelope of the gonococcus resembles that of other gram-negative bacteria, but with some important differences. One difference is that phospholipids are exposed on the outer surface, resulting in an outer membrane that is unusually permeable to hydrophobic molecules such as fatty acids and sterols. Mutation can alter the permeability of the outer membrane to hydrophobic molecules. A second difference is that the lipopolysaccharide (LPS) does not have the long repeating O- antigenic side chains characteristic of other gram-negative bacteria. Purified protein components and LPSs prepared from the outer membrane form the bases of additional systems for subtyping gonococci. In particular, by using selectively adsorbed antiserums and monoclonal antibodies specific for epitypes on the major outer membrane protein (protein I), it has been possible to distinguish three major serogroups, termed *WI, WII,* and *WIII.*

The cell envelope is traversed by pili—hairlike structures constituted primarily of protein that are about 0.07 μm in diameter and up to 2 μm long (Fig. 56-2). Pili appear to be important in the initial attachment of gonococci to epithelial cells. Gonococcal pili

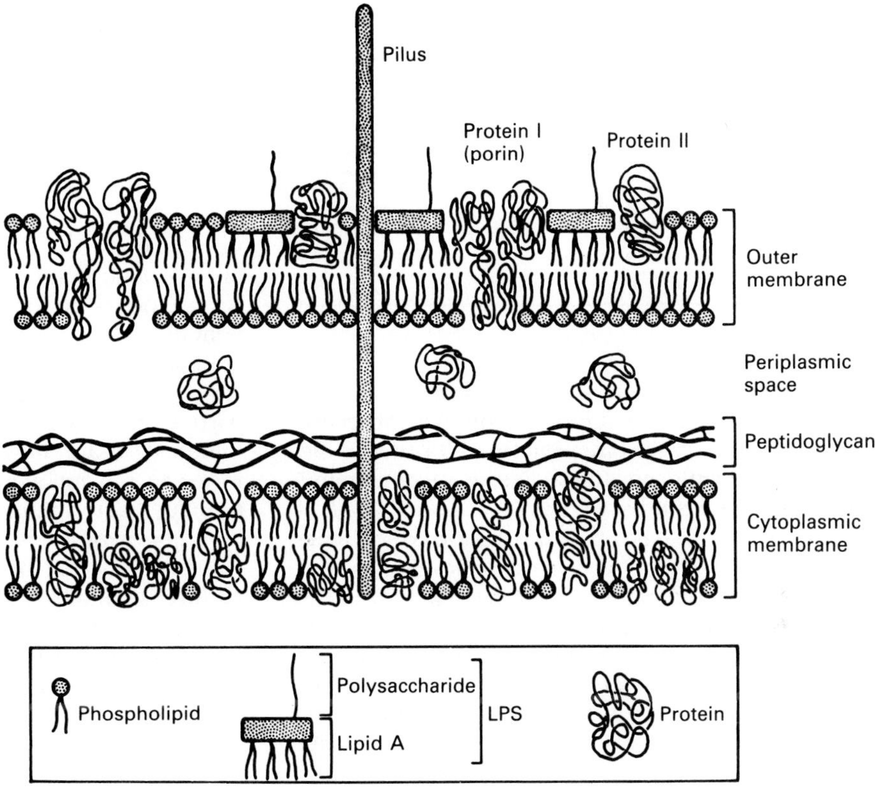

Fig. 56-1. Diagram of cell envelope of *Neisseria gonorrhoeae* Lipopolysaccharide, pilas, and other protein antigens in outer membrane are shown in relation to other components.

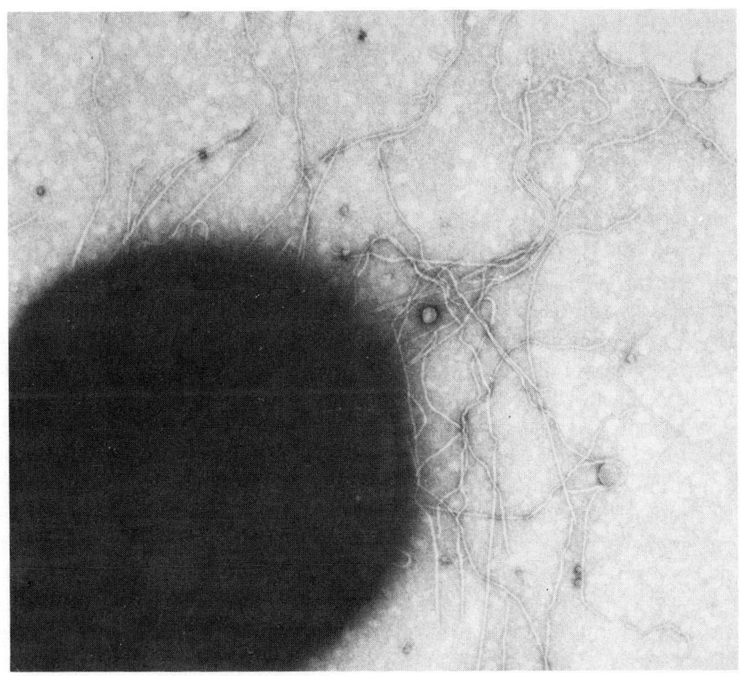

Fig. 56-2. Negative stain electron micrograph of T_2 (P^{++}) colonies of *Neisseria gonorrhoeae* showing pili projecting from the surface of an individual gonococcus. (Original magnification approximately 50,000) (Courtesy of Dr. John Swanson)

Table 56-1. *Characteristics of Colony Types of* Neisseria gonorrhoeae

Kellogg Type	Revised Typing Scheme	
	STATE OF PILIATION	COLONIAL OPACITY
T_1	P^+	O^+ or O^-
T_2	P^{++}	O^+ or O^-
T_3	P^-	O^+
T_4	P^-	O^-

exhibit antigenic heterogeneity. However, all antigenic types possess a common region that apparently recognizes a receptor on epithelial cell surfaces. Because pili are antigenic, their value as vaccine immunogens is under study.

Several morphologically distinct forms of colonies occur (Table 56-1). Fresh isolates develop colony forms that are conventionally termed T_1 (P^+) and T_2 (P^{++}) and are made up of piliated, fully virulent gonococci (experimental urethral inoculation of male humans or chimpanzees, IV injection of chick embryos). During repeated laboratory subculture, colony forms called T_3 and T_4 (P^-) appear; these lack pili and are less virulent. Gonococcal strains cannot be subtyped by colonial morphology because each strain gives rise to several colony forms.

Gonococcal colonies may also be classified on the basis of colonial opacity—an optical property that is independent of piliation but is related to the degree of aggregation among the gonococci comprising the colony. Gonococci from opaque colonies (O^+) have surface proteins (protein II) that are not present in isogenic gonococci from transparent (O^-) colonies. A family of proteins, separable by sodium dodecyl sulfate polyacrylamide gel electrophoresis, constitutes protein II species that are present in gonococci from O^+ colonies. These proteins are sensitive to protease and exhibit heat-modifiable behavior (*i.e.,* apparent increase in molecular weight with boiling). Protein IIs have been correlated with behavior of gonococci toward neutrophils *in vitro.* They may also mediate intercellular interactions between gonococci and surrounding cells.

The predominant protein in the gonococcal outer membrane is termed *protein I* (*POMP* or *MOMP*). The subunit molecular weight varies among strains (32,000–34,000). However, the same molecular weight subunit is present in all colonial variants of a single strain. This protein is not heat modifiable and exists in a trimeric form in the outer membrane. Protein I is thought to form hydrophilic channels through the outer membrane and thus functions as a porin. Hydrophilic molecules such as sugars and some antimicrobics penetrate outer membranes through porins. Gonococci may be divided into serogroups and serotypes based upon antigenic determinants on protein I.

Gonococci are fragile. Drying is lethal within 1 to 2 hours, a fact of vital importance to success in isolation from clinical specimens. Although inocula containing huge numbers of gonococci may survive for several hours on fomites, this probably has little epidemiologic significance. Moist heat at 55°C sterilizes cultures in less than 1 hour. Ultraviolet light and a variety of antiseptics kill gonococci. Silver salts are particularly active—1:4000 $AgNO_3$ is lethal in 2 minutes. Unsaturated fatty acids, such as those found in the cotton and wood used to prepare swabs and in ordinary bacteriologic grade agar inhibit many strains of *N. gonorrhoeae.* When starch, whole blood, or the insoluble fraction of yeast autolysates are added to culture mediums, they act as adsorbents, sequestering the inhibitors so that gonococci may grow.

The gonococcal chromosome has a molecular weight of 1.02×10^9 daltons. Plasmids of two sizes have been described in many gonococci. A small (2.4×10^6 daltons) plasmid of unknown function is present in 95% of the isolates from the United States. It is lacking in approximately 50% of Canadian isolates, particularly those with a Pro Cit Ura auxotype (a requirement for proline, citrulline and uracil). A large (24.5×10^6 daltons) plasmid is found in about 25% of strains and functions as a sex factor in conjugative transfer of plasmid DNA (including transfer of the β-lactamase plasmids).

The typical resistance of gonococci to antimicrobics is not associated with measurable destruction of drugs; that is, it is intrinsic in nature (Ch. 18, Antimicrobics and Anthelmintics for Systemic Therapy). There are regional differences in the magnitude of such intrinsic resistance. It is greatest in Southeast Asia and Africa where prophylactic or low-dose therapy is common; intermediate in the United States and Australia; and least in Scandinavia, the United Kingdom, and Western Europe. Increased resistance to penicillin G and tetracycline was noted in the United States during the 1960s when importation of resistant strains occurred during the Viet Nam war. From 1970 through 1975, no further increase in intrinsic resistance was detected. When gonococci collected from nine cities in the United States were tested *in vitro* at the Centers for Disease Control (CDC) in Atlanta, regional differences in susceptibility were found. For example, the proportion of isolates resistant to 0.25 μg penicillin G/ml—a level of resistance associated with failure of treatment in more than 5% of patients given 4.8 million U aqueous procaine penicillin G with probenecid—ranged from 7% in Des Moines to 27% in Denver.

In 1976, a new aspect of resistance to antimicrobics was recognized when strains were isolated in the United States and England that produced β-lactamases, conferring resistance to high concentrations of penicillin and to cephalothin and cefazolin. The β-lactamase producing strains of *N. gonorrhoeae* that first appeared in the United States probably originated in, and were imported from, the Philippines and contained a 4.4×10^6-dalton β-lactamase plasmid. Because most such "Asian" strains also contained the 24.5×10^6-dalton conjugative plasmid, it is not surprising that several different auxotypes and serogroups of gonococci have been found to contain the β-lactamase plasmid, probably reflecting conjugative transfer of this plasmid among gonococci.

In contrast, the first β-lactamase-producing strains of *N. gonorrhoeae* found in England contained a 3.2×10^6-dalton plasmid (a deletion variant of the 4.4×10^6-dalton plasmid), contained no 24.5×10^6-dalton plasmid, and were all of a single auxotype (Arg^-); all of these properties are characteristic of the β-lactamase-producing gonococci found subsequently in west Africa.

The simultaneous appearance of these β-lactamase plasmids in Africa and the Philippines is remarkable. Both plasmids (*i.e.*, the 3.2×10^6-dalton and the 4.4×10^6-dalton) contain the transposon TnA and share a high degree of homology with each other and with β-lactamase plasmids found in *Escherichia coli, Haemophilus influenzae, H. parainfluenzae,* and *H. ducreyi.*

Epidemiology

The only natural host for *N. gonorrhoeae* is the human. An estimated 2,000,000 cases of gonorrhea were treated in the United States during 1981. The annual age-specific incidence of reported gonorrhea tripled between 1963 and 1976, after which the reported incidence has fallen slightly each year. The rising incidence of gonorrhea and other sexually transmitted diseases in the West coincided with the introduction of orally administerable progestational contraceptives and intrauterine devices (IUDs) in the 1960s. These contributed to increased sexual freedom and to decreased use of condoms and spermicidal preparations, both of which offer protection against gonorrhea as well as providing contraception.

The highest incidence occurs between the ages of 20 and 24 years in men, and 18 and 24 years in women. In these age groups, the reported incidence is three times higher in the United States than in England and Wales. The relative incidence is probably even higher in the United States, where the reporting of gonorrhea is thought to be less complete than in England and Wales. Similarly, routine screening of endocervical cultures of gynecologic and obstetric patients documents an incidence of gonorrhea in women that is about ten times higher in the United States than in England and Wales. These remarkable differences in the rates of occurrence of gonorrhea point out the need for critical reexamination of the way in which patients with gonorrhea are managed by physicians in the United States.

The common failure of practicing physicians, hospitals, and some public clinics to trace and treat infected sex contacts probably contributes greatly to the high incidence of gonorrhea in the United States. Recent cutbacks of funding for contact tracing in public clinics will further exacerbate this problem. Physicians must remember that *gonorrhea is usually caught from a carrier who either has no symptoms or has ignored symptoms*. Thus, the primary goal of contact tracing is to identify source contacts—those who infected the index patient—because the source probably has no symptoms or has ignored symptoms, and may well reinfect the index patient. Both male and female source contacts must be identified and examined. A secondary goal is to identify contacts exposed to the index patient who may become infected. It is more important to trace exposed female contacts than exposed male contacts for these reasons:

1. Many males exposed to gonorrhea will not catch it. The risk of acquiring gonorrhea averages about 35% after a single exposure to an infected woman, but rises to about 75% with repeated exposure to the same woman. The risk of transmission from male to female is unknown, but may well be higher than the risk of female to male transmission.
2. Exposed male contacts who do become infected often develop symptoms and seek treatment. For example, over 95% of sailors (United States Navy) who acquired gonorrhea in the Philippines developed symptoms within 14 days after exposure. In contrast, women who acquire gonorrhea more often develop no symptoms or only nonspecific symptoms that do not bring them to treatment.
3. In a recent study, as many as 50% of exposed female contacts who became infected developed gonococcal pelvic inflammatory disease (PID),

Table 56-2. Guidelines for Contact Tracing of Gonorrhea

Index Case With Gonorrhea	Recommended Action for Contact Tracing
Man with acute urethritis	Examine all contacts* within 2 weeks prior to the onset of urethritis. Because two-thirds of the contacts have gonorrhea, and women are at risk for developing PID,† female contacts should be treated while initial culture results are pending—so called epidemiologic treatment.
Infected woman named as a contact by a man with gonococcal urethritis	Contact tracing is usually not productive. The original male source contact is often difficult to trace or identify, since the woman probably has chronic infection. Exposed male contacts will probably develop symptoms and seek treatment if they become clinically infected.
Symptomatic woman (*e.g.,* PID,† dysuria, new vaginal discharge, abnormal menses)	Examine all suspected male *source* contacts* within the previous 4 weeks. About one-half will have gonorrhea. If the man has no symptoms, perform an endourethral culture and treat him if the culture yields *Neisseria gonorrhoeae.*
Woman with nonsymptomatic gonorrhea (detected by routine endocervical culture (*e.g.,* during prenatal or family planning visit)	About one-third of the recent male sex partners have untreated gonorrhea. Therefore, examine any male sex partners within the previous 4 weeks.

*A note from the physician transmitted by a cooperative male patient to a female sex contact is often sufficient to bring her to examination. However, nonsymptomatic male contacts more often require direct discussion with the physician to convince them examination is necessary.

†Pelvic inflammatory disease caused by *Neisseria gonorrhoeae*

and ran a greater risk than males of developing disseminated infection. Early treatment during the incubation period prevents these complications.

The guidelines for contact tracing that follow from these considerations are summarized in Table 56-2.

Various properties of gonococci appear to be associated with a predisposition to destructive clinical manifestations. For example, isolates from patients with disseminated gonococcal infection are uniformly susceptible to low concentrations of penicillin G and tetracycline and resistant to normal human serum, and most are serogroup WI and auxotype $Arg^-Hyx^-Ura^-$. On the other hand, isolates from patients with PID are often relatively resistant to penicillin G and usually belong to other auxotypes. The $Arg^-Hyx^-Ura^-$ auxotype was not found prior to the 1950s but increased to account for 50% or more of all gonococcal isolates in certain areas of Scandinavia in the 1970s. This auxotype is associated with asymptomatic gonorrhea in men and is much less common in blacks than in whites. $Arg^-Hyx^-Ura^-$ strains are exceptionally uncommon among exclusively homosexual men, while gonococci possessing a gene for multiple drug resistance (*mtr*) are exceptionally common among homosexual men. Gonococci transmitted among homosexual men must be capable of surviving in the rectum in the presence of feces, which contain hydrophobic fatty acids and bile salts that are toxic for most gonococci. Thus, the antimicrobic-susceptible, $Arg^-Hyx^-Ura^-$ gonococci (which are markedly inhibited by hydrophobic compounds) may be poorly adapted for transmission among homosexuals, while the resistant *mtr* strains (which are unusually resistant to hydrophobic compounds) are best adapted for such transmission; both phenomena may account for the fact that rectal and throat infections with *N. gonorrhoeae* in homosexual men are particularly difficult to treat.

The incidence of acute gonococcal salpingitis, the major complication of gonorrhea in women, is estimated to be about a half million cases per year in the United States. An equal number of cases of nongonococcal PID occur each year, and many involve fallopian tubes previously damaged by gonococcal salpingitis.

A number of other properties of gonococci have changed dramatically during the past 30 years, illustrating the remarkable ability of this organism to adapt to new antimicrobics used for therapy and selective mediums. For example, no microorganism better illustrates the sequential emergence of increasing resistance to sulfonamides, penicillin G, and tetracycline as each of these agents became commonly used for treatment of gonorrhea. High-level gonococcal resistance to streptomycin also became common in areas of Europe where the drug was used for gonorrhea. The more recent occurrence of β-lactamase production provides a distinctive marker for analysis of the epidemiologic spread of gonococci. Beta-lactamase-positive strains now account for as many as 60% of all gonococcal isolates in certain areas of the Philippines, and these strains are increasingly common elsewhere in Asia. In the United States, the quarterly incidence of infections caused by β-lactamase producers remained fairly stable at a low level from 1976 through 1980, but took an alarming upswing in 1981 (Fig. 56-3). Microepidemics of such infections have now occurred in many areas of the United States where they have thus far been contained by (1) prompt screening of all isolates for penicillinase (2) active contact tracing and (3) increased use of drugs such as spectinomycin.

Paradoxically, an opposite trend has apparently occurred in a few cities in the emergence of vancomycin-*susceptible* strains of gonococci. Such strains, rarely seen before the introduction of the vancomycin-containing Thayer–Martin medium, may escape detection in cultures by virtue of their susceptibility to vancomycin.

Fig. 56-3. Increasing quarterly incidence of penicillinase-producing *Neisseria gonorrhoeae* in the United States. (Data reported to the Centers for Disease Control through the first quarter of 1982)

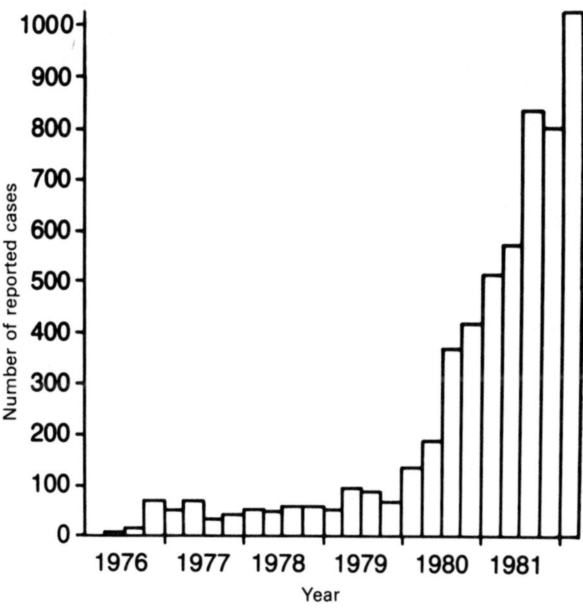

Pathogenesis and Pathology

Not everyone exposed to gonorrhea acquires the disease. It is uncertain whether this is due to variations in the size or virulence of the inoculum, to nonspecific resistance, or to specific immunity. It is still unknown whether naturally acquired gonorrhea confers any immunity to reinfection with the same or other strains of *N. gonorrhoeae.* However, in one small series of women followed prospectively after one episode of gonococcal salpingitis, reinfection with *N. gonorrhoeae* was significantly less likely to produce recurrent salpingitis if the reinfection was with a strain with the same principle outer membrane protein (protein I serotype) than if reinfection was with a new serotype. Thus, it appears that an episode of gonococcal salpingitis protects against recurrent salpingitis with the same serotype, but not against recurrent cervical infection with the same serotype or against recurrent salpingitis with a new serotype. The concentration of gonococci in vaginal irrigations from infected women averages 10^5 organisms per ml (range, 10^2–10^7), and the concentration is similar, though less well defined, in urethral exudates from men. Based on experimental urethral inoculation of male volunteers, it appears that approximately 10^3 organisms were required to establish an infection in 50% of the men (the ID_{50}). The microbial flora of the genital tract may contribute some resistance to gonorrhea, since various species, including *Candida albicans* and *Staphylococcus epidermidis,* and certain species and strains of lactobacillus produce compounds that inhibit gonococci *in vitro.* Progesterone inhibits the growth of *N. gonorrhoeae,* but only in concentrations exceeding those encountered *in vivo* in peripheral blood, even in pregnancy. The virulence of different gonococcal strains may be related to varying ability to remove iron from transferrin, or from lactoferrin, which is present in some mucosal sites. For example, $Arg^-Hyx^-Ura^-$ strains, which have an increased association with bacteremia, but a decreased association with salpingitis and a propensity for causing asymptomatic genital infection, remove iron readily from transferrin, but usually cannot remove iron from lactoferrin; in fact, such strains cannot grow on mediums containing lactoferrin as the sole source of iron. Nonpathogenic *Neisseria* spp. generally are not able to remove iron from transferrin or lactoferrin.

Attachment of gonococci to mucosal cells is mediated in part by pili, and rabbit antibody to pili reduces attachment of gonococci to mammalian cells. Nonpilus gonococcal surface antigens also may enhance attachment to mammalian cells. Secretory IgA

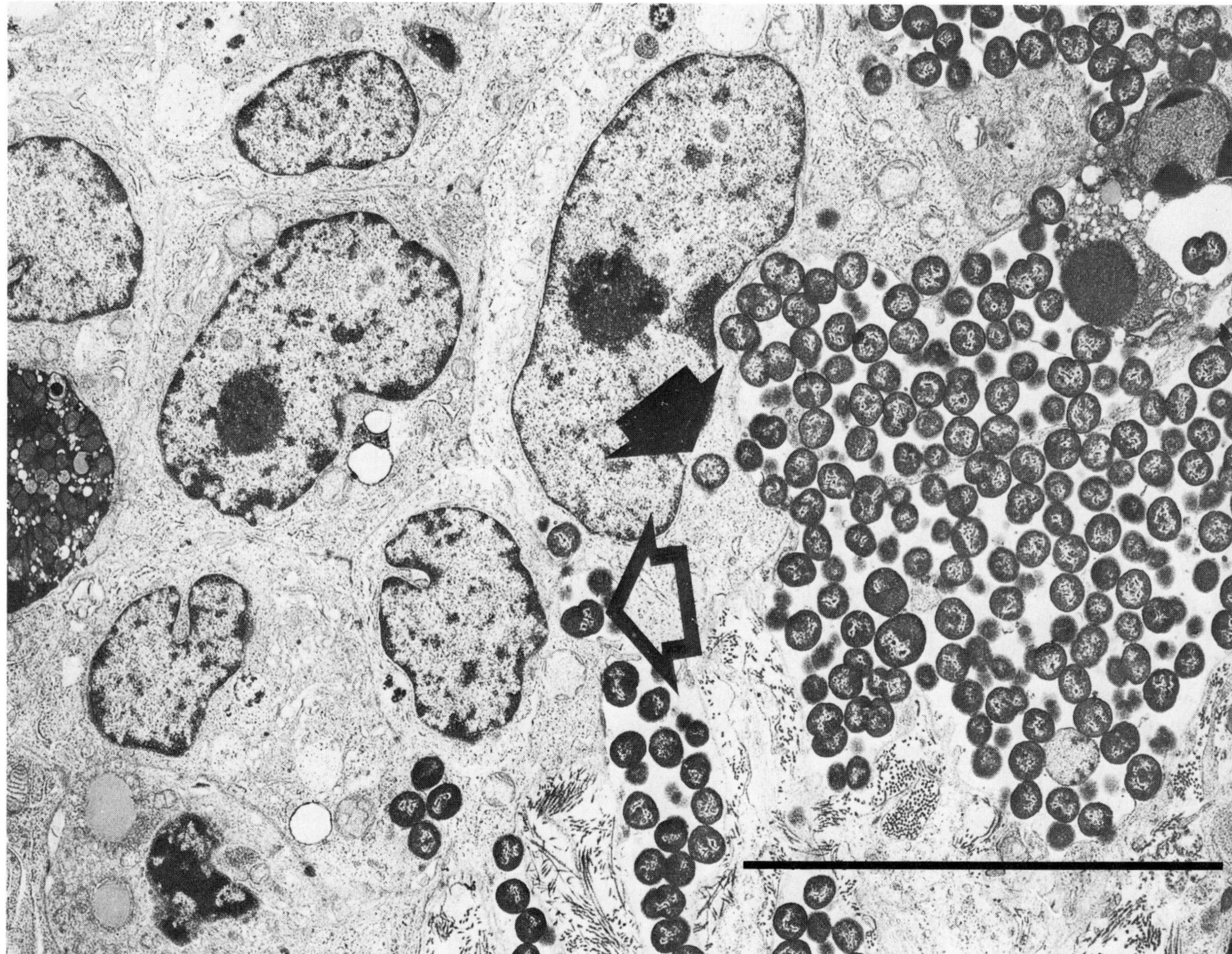

Fig. 56-4. Electron micrograph of late gonococcal invasion of a human fallopian tube organ culture *in vitro*. The bar represents 10 μm (Original magnification × 1600). Gonococci lie between the intercellular junctions (*hollow arrow*) and free within the cell cytoplasm (*black arrow*). Single gonococci were observed within membrane-bound cytoplasmic vacuoles as early as 3 hours after infection in this model system. (Courtesy of Drs. M. E. Ward and P. J. Watt)

antibody (sIgA) to *N. gonorrhoeae* appears in vaginal and urethral secretions in gonorrhea, but is shorter lived than serum antibody, usually disappearing soon after therapy. The role of sIgA has not been identified with any certainty, but it may inhibit gonococcal adherence to mucosal surfaces, or it may promote opsonization. In this regard, a gonococcal IgA_1 protease that inactivates sIgA by cleaving a specific peptide bond in the hinge region of the immunoglobulin molecule may be an important virulence factor.

Following attachment to columnar or transitional epithelium, histologic study of organs infected *in vivo* or in organ culture show that gonococci reach the subepithelial connective tissue either by penetrating the intercellular epithelial spaces or as a result of engulfment by and passage through epithelial cells (Fig. 56.4). Gonococci contain endotoxin (LPS), which produces mucosal damage in fallopian tube organ cultures, and brings about the release of enzymes (proteases, phospholipase, elastase) that may be important in pathogenesis. It is not yet known whether gonococci produce chemotaxin in the absence of serum antibody and complement, but a polymorphonuclear (PMN) leukocyte inflammatory response is apparent within 2 to 3 days after infection. With normal human serum plus complement, many gonococci stimulate formation of the chemotactic factor C5a, but $Arg^-Hyx^-Ura^-$ strains are less reactive than other strains in this respect. Piliated cells tend to remain extracellular, often in clumps, whereas nonpiliated cells are readily ingested and killed. Acquired IgA and IgG serum antibodies enhance the phagocytosis of gonococci by PMN leukocytes. Antibody specific for pilus antigen is known to be opsonic and to block attachment to epithelial cells.

It is interesting that adherent but noningested piliated cells nonetheless stimulate hexose monophosphate shunt activity and cyanide-independent oxygen consumption by PMN leukocytes.

Increased lymphocyte blastogenesis occurs when peripheral mononuclear cells from patients with recurrent gonorrhea are exposed to gonococcal antigens, but the role of cell-mediated immunity in gonorrhea is undefined.

Trypsinlike proteases present in cervical mucus may help to select for protease-resistant, transparent (O^-) colony phenotypes. Opaque (O^+) colony phenotypes (protease-sensitive) predominate in cultures taken during the middle portion of the menstrual cycle. Cervical proteases increase during the second half of the cycle, resulting in an increase in the O^- phenotype (protease-resistant). These O^- colony phenotypes can be isolated from tubal as well as endocervical cultures; O^+ colony phenotypes are isolated from endocervical cultures but not from tubal cultures.

Spread of gonococci from the endocervix to the urethra, anal canal, and Bartholin's duct probably occurs as a result of proliferation in the film of secretions covering the surfaces of these areas. Spread into the endometrial cavity and fallopian tubes is increased twofold to ninefold in women using IUDs and decreased about twofold in women using oral contraceptives. Menstruation facilitates spread to the upper genital tract, and 50% of women with gonococcal salpingitis experience onset of symptoms during the first week of the cycle. Gonococci attach to spermatozoa; conceivably, sperm could carry gonococci into the upper tract.

Menstruation also apparently facilitates bacteremic spread, perhaps by circumventing local mucosal and lymphoid barriers. Gonococci that cause bacteremia are usually resistant to complement-mediated killing by natural serum antibody. Exceptions have occurred in patients with a deficiency in one of the terminal components of the complement pathway. The bactericidal antibody appears to be IgM immunoglobulins directed against gonococcal LPS antigens. Theoretically, gonococci susceptible to this antibody might nonetheless produce bacteremia in newborns, since they lack gonococcidal antibody.

Skin pustules and septic arthritis are associated with gonococcal invasion of the skin and joints. Although gonococcemia is present in many patients with tenosynovitis and sterile synovial effusions, it is possible that circulating immune complexes alone can cause these manifestations. Gonococci isolated from synovial fluid appear less resistant to serum than gonococci isolated from blood. Resistance to natural serum IgM antibody is more common among gonococci of serogroup WI than among serogroups WII or WIII. Such resistance may be mediated by IgG antibody of uncertain specificity that blocks the bactericidal IgM antibody. On the other hand, persons convalescing from systemic gonococcal infection develop increased levels of bactericidal IgG antibody. Various mutations that alter surface protein and LPS antigens are associated with the resistance of gonococci to normal human serum. Variability between strains in their binding of the terminal C5–9 complex may also occur. Thus, susceptibility to gonococcemia appears to be determined by a complex interplay of host factors (*e.g.,* menstruation, anti-LPS IgM activity, blocking IgG activity, immune IgG activity, and complement deficiency) and of properties of the gonococcus (*e.g.,* auxotype, serotype, avidity for iron, and serum resistance).

Manifestations

The symptoms and signs of gonococcal infections depend on the site of inoculation, the age of the patient, the duration of the infection, and occurrence of local or systemic spread of the gonococci. These factors are influenced greatly by individual sex practices.

Gonococcal Infection in Men

In heterosexual men, gonococcal infection usually involves only the urethra, although pharyngeal gonococcal infection occurs in perhaps 5% of those exposed by cunnilingus. In homosexual men, gonococcal infection commonly involves the urethra, anal canal, and pharynx, with anorectal and pharyngeal infection often occurring concurrently.

The usual incubation period of gonococcal urethritis in men is 2 to 7 days, although longer intervals occur and some men never develop symptoms. A purulent urethral discharge is typical and is commonly associated with dysuria, frequency, and meatal erythema. Because most symptomatic men seek treatment, the disease is usually halted without further progression. However, those who develop no symptoms or minimal symptoms and those who ignore their symptoms not only serve as the main source of spread of infection to women, but also are at risk of developing local or systemic complications. Before antimicrobics became available, symptoms of urethritis persisted for an average of 8 weeks, and unilateral epididymitis occurred in 5% to 10% of untreated men. Epididymitis is now an uncommon complication, and gonococcal prostatitis rarely occurs. Most cases of nongonococcal epididymitis in young men are caused by *Chlamydia trachomatis,* and the specific etiology of most cases of prostatitis is not known. Other local complications of gonorrhea that are now unusual include inguinal lymphadenitis, edema of the penis from dorsal lymphangitis or thrombophlebitis, submucosal inflammatory infiltration of the urethral wall, paraurethral abscess or fistula, unilateral inflammation or abscess of Cowper's gland (palpable between the thumb and forefinger with the forefinger in the anal canal and the thumb positioned anteriorly on the perineum), abscess of Tyson's gland(s) that open on either side of the frenulum, and rarely, seminal vesiculitis.

Gonococcal Infection in Women

The most common site of infection in women is the cervix, followed in descending order by the urethra, anal canal, and pharynx. Urethral, rectal, and pharyngeal infection rarely lead to local complications, but salpingitis occurs in approximately 20% of women with cervical gonorrhea.

The primary site of inoculation of *N. gonorrhoeae* in women is thought to be the columnar epithelium of the endocervix. After a brief incubation period (less well defined than in males) any visible ectopic columnar epithelium exposed on the exocervix becomes dusky red and friable, with purulent exudate issuing from the os to cause vaginal discharge that is perceived by the patient as more copious and more yellow than normal. Compression of the cervix between the blades of a vaginal speculum may express otherwise inapparent cervical exudate. Contiguous spread of infected cervical secretions along the perineum to the anus and urethra presumably accounts for the occurrence of anorectal, urethral, and Bartholin's gland infections. Compression of the urethra against the pubic symphysis with the examining finger or speculum blade in the vagina expresses pus from the acutely infected urethral or Skene's glands. Acute gonococcal Bartholinitis is usually unilateral. The acutely infected duct is often surrounded by a red halo and exudes pus at the posterior third of the labium majus. Occlusion of the duct results in formation of a Bartholin's abscess. Chronic Bartholin's cysts are rarely caused by active gonococcal infection.

Upward spread of *N. gonorrhoeae* from the cervical os onto the endometrium causes endometritis that may be associated with abnormal menstrual bleeding and midline lower abdominal pain and tenderness. Extension to the fallopian tubes usually causes bilateral lower abdominal pain and adnexal tenderness, which is sometimes associated with fever, chills, and adnexal mass. Leukocytosis, and elevation of the erythrocyte sedimentation rate (ESR) may occur with either endometritis or salpingitis. The clinical diagnosis of salpingitis is made in about 20% of women with gonorrhea in the United States, but milder manifestations of endometritis or salpingitis may occur in a substantial proportion of the remaining 80%.

Further extension of infection into the pelvis may produce signs of pelvic peritonitis, accompanied by nausea and vomiting, and may lead to pelvic abscess. Bacteremia and suppurative pelvic thrombophlebitis are unusual in gonococcal PID. Treatment with antimicrobics before the development of pelvic peritonitis or adnexal mass restores normal tubal function and fertility in nearly all cases of gonococcal salpingitis. However, definitive studies in Sweden showed the average risk of sterility after PID (usually due to tubal occlusion) was 21% (13% were sterile after one infection, 35% after two infections, and 75% after three or more episodes of PID). Tubal occlusion was more common after nongonococcal PID than after gonococcal PID. Four percent of pregnancies that did occur after PID were ectopic; the relative importance of *N. gonorrhoeae* and *C. trachomatis* in this syndrome is under study. Spread of gonococci into the upper abdomen may cause perihepatitis (Fitz-Hugh–Curtis syndrome) manifested by right upper quandrant or bilateral upper abdomonal pain and tenderness and occasionally by a hepatic friction rub. Chronic abdominal pain persists in about 20% of patients after treatment for PID, presumably as a sequel of pelvic peritonitis.

The true rate of occurrence of symptoms and signs in women with gonorrhea is uncertain because the clinical manifestations of the disease vary with the clinical setting. Most women with gonorrhea who come to an emergency room or gynecology clinic complain of abnormal vaginal discharge (cervicitis), dysuria and frequency of urination (urethritis and Skenitis), abnormal menstrual bleeding (endometritis), anorectal discomfort, unilateral labial pain and swelling (acute Bartholinitis), or lower abdominal pain (salpingitis). For example, among indigent female emergency room patients, gonococci were isolated from 6% of women without genitourinary symptoms, whereas gonococci were isolated from 26% of women with abnormal vaginal discharge, 29% of women with urinary tract symptoms (including 61% of those who did not have coliform bacteriuria), 30% of women with abnormal menstrual bleeding, and 82% of women with acute PID or acute Bartholin's abscess. Although identical manifestations may be caused by *C. trachomatis,* any young woman with one of these five manifestations should undergo pelvic examination, and cultures appropriate for isolation of *N. gonorrhoeae* should be obtained. Failure to consider the diagnosis of gonorrhea may result in inappropriate therapy; for example, the topical vaginal preparations given for leukorrhea and antimicrobial regimens commonly used for urinary tract infections are ineffective for gonorrhea. Without therapy, cervicitis and endometritis may progress to salpingitis, and salpingitis to peritonitis, tubal occlusion, or superinfection; symptoms may subside spontaneously, leading to a chronic, asymptomatic carrier state and further spread of infection. Such carriers go undetected unless a routine screening culture for gonorrhea is obtained or the patient is named as a sex contact by a man with acute urethritis. In venereal disease, prenatal, or family planning clinics where screening cultures are performed, women with nonsymptomatic gonorrhea predominate. The average duration of the carrier state is not certain, but it may exceed a year.

Anorectal Infection

Anorectal gonococcal infection occurs in homosexual men, in women, and in the neonate. Symptoms include rectal pain, tenesmus, constipation, mucopurulent rectal discharge, and rectal bleeding. By anoscopic examination, a mucopurulent exudate covers an erythematous, somewhat friable rectal mucus membrane. Involvement is patchy; it is limited to the distal 5 cm to 10 cm of the rectum and is maximal just above the pectinate line in the area of the columns of Margani and the perianal glands. Anorectal infection may be completely asymptomatic, although anoscopy may show exudate or PMN leukocytes may be found in gram-stained smears of material obtained by swabbing the rectal mucosal surface.

Pharyngeal Infection

Pharyngeal infections are more common in women and in homosexual men, because fellatio is much more likely than cunnilingus to result in pharyngeal infection. In addition, pharyngeal infections occur more often in whites than in blacks, because whites currently engage in oral sex more often than blacks.

Nasopharyngeal or tonsillar swabs are equally likely to yield *N. gonorrhoeae* on culture. Because gonorrhea is seldom transmitted from the pharynx to a sex partner, pharyngeal infection is important mainly as a cause of sore throat or as a focal source of gonococcemia.

Disseminated Infection

Disseminated gonococcal infection has been detected in about 1% of men and 3% of women with gonorrhea in Seattle and in Sweden, but the frequency of this complication may vary regionally. The majority of men and women with gonococcemia do not have symptoms of urogenital, anorectal, or pharyngeal infection. Gonococcemia may occur soon after acquisition of a new infection, but the average interval from the last sexual exposure until the onset of symptoms is significantly longer than for uncomplicated genital infection. Fifty percent of women with disseminated gonococcal infection develop symptoms of gonococcemia during or just after menstruation. Gonococcemia does occur somewhat more commonly in women than in men. Factors that may be contributory include menstruation *per se,* a higher frequency of pharyngeal infection in women than in men, and relatively prompt institution of therapy in men as compared with women.

Onset of gonococcemia is characterized by fever; polyarthralgias; and papular, petechial, pustular, hemorrhagic, or necrotic skin lesions (Fig. 56-5). Approximately 3 to 20 such lesions appear, usually on the distal extremities. Gonococci are demonstrable by immunofluorescent staining in about two-thirds of gonococcal skin lesions, but this technique is seldom employed diagnostically. The initial joint involvement is characteristically limited to tenosynovitis involving several joints asymmetrically. Circulating immune complexes have been demonstrated in patients with tenosynovitis, but serum hemolytic complement activity is not significantly depressed and glomerulitis is uncommon, except in the presence of gonococcal endocarditis. The extensor tendons of the wrists, fingers, knees, and ankles are most often involved. Without treatment the systemic manifestations of bacteremia may subside spontaneously within a week. It is possible that many such cases go undiagnosed and that the actual frequency of occurrence of gonococcemia exceeds current estimates.

Alternatively, septic arthritis may ensue, sometimes without prior symptoms of bacteremia. Pain and swelling then increase in one or two joints, with accumulation of purulent synovial fluid, leading to progressive destruction of the joint if treatment is

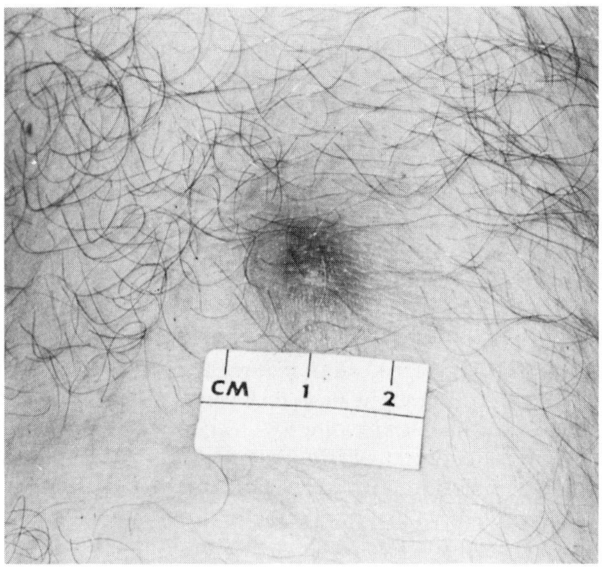

Fig. 56-5. Hemorrhagic pustule on the forearm of a patient with disseminated gonococcal infection.

delayed. Gonococcal arthritis is now the most common kind of septic arthritis among persons in the 16- to 50-year-old age group; about 60% of cases occur in women. A continuum exists from the manifestations of bacteremia (polyarthralgias, new skin lesions) to septic arthritis, but the probability of recovery of gonococci from the blood decreases with increasing duration of illness, whereas the likelihood of recovery from synovial fluid increases. Gonococci are infrequently recovered from early effusions containing less than 20,000 leukocytes per mm^3, but are usually recovered from effusions containing more than 80,000 leukocytes per mm^3. In a given patient, gonococci are seldom recovered from blood and synovial fluid simultaneously.

Other common manifestations of disseminated gonococcal infection include myopericarditis and toxic hepatitis. Endocarditis and meningitis are rare but serious complications.

Neonatal Infections

Infections of the newborn may involve the conjunctivas, pharynx, respiratory tract, or anal canal. The risk of neonatal infection increases with prolonged rupture of membranes.

Conjunctival infection is usually bilateral. Two to three days postpartum, a purulent discharge exudes from between the eyelids, which are edematous and erythematous (Fig. 56-6). It is a medical emergency, since blindness may result (corneal ulceration may lead to perforation and extrusion of the lens; scarring may opacify the cornea). The same disease, bearing the same prognosis, occurs quite rarely in adults as a consequence of autoinoculation. Asymptomatic or minimally symptomatic conjunctival infection has been well documented in infants and adults. Routine prophylaxis with 1% silver nitrate eyedrops has greatly reduced the frequency of occurrence of gonococcal opthalmia neonatorum; inclusion conjuncti-

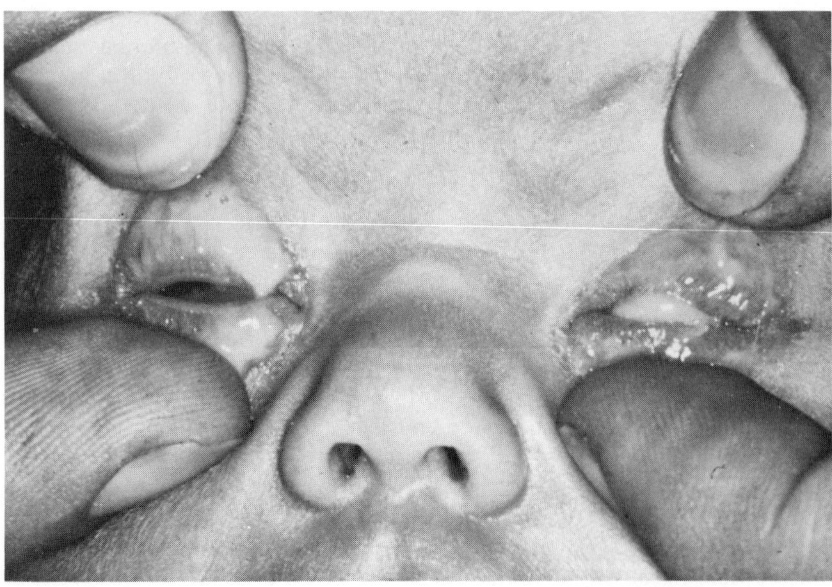

Fig. 56-6. Bilateral gonococcal ophthalmia neonatorum.

vitis caused by *C. trachomatis* is far more common in neonates in most countries.

The most common manifestation of gonorrhea in the newborn is the gonococcal amniotic infection syndrome, consisting of chorioamnionitis and nonspecific signs of sepsis in the newborn, together with the presence of *N. gonorrhoeae* in the orogastric aspirates of affected neonates.

Other Prepubertal Infections

During the first year of life, infection of the infant usually results from accidental contamination of the eye or vagina by an adult. Between 1 year and puberty, gonorrhea is usually manifest as a vulvovaginitis in girls who have been molested by another household member; medicolegal considerations necessitate a complete bacteriologic diagnosis. Dysuria and vulvar pain are typical symptoms, and there may be perianal soreness and discomfort on defecation. The vulva is erythematous and edematous; a yellowish green discharge may issue from the vaginal and urethral orifices. The perianal area may also be erythematous, and occasionally a purulent anal discharge appears in children who develop anorectal gonorrhea as a result of sexual abuse.

Diagnosis

Clinical Aspects

Gonococcal infection produces several common clinical syndromes that have multiple etiologies or that mimic other conditions. The diagnosis of urethritis is discussed in Chapter 55, Nongonococcal Urethritis, and Chapter 48, Urethritis and Cystitis.

Clinical and laboratory aspects of the diagnosis of vaginitis and cervicitis are discussed in Chapter 50, Infections of the Female Genital Tract. The simplest maneuver to establish the clinical diagnosis of cervicitis is to demonstrate pus mixed with mucus emanating from the cervical os. A swab inserted in the os and withdrawn shows a yellow or green color indicative of mucopus. Cervicitis may be caused by *C. trachomatis, N. gonorrhoeae,* or herpes simplex virus (HSV). In developed countries, *C. trachomatis* is the most common cause of cervicitis. Edema of the area of ectopic epithelium with a follicular appearance (not to be confused with Nabothian cysts) suggests a chlamydial infection. Herpetic cervicitis is usually associated with vesiculoulcerative cervical and labial lesions. Also, so-called cervicitis with clear cervical mucus may represent cervical ectopy—an outward migration of the squamocolumnar junction of the cervix, as occurs commonly during adolescence or pregnancy or with use of oral contraceptives. *Trichomonas vaginalis* and some yeasts may cause cervicitis associated with vaginitis—unlike cervical infections caused by gonococci, chlamydia, or HSV.

Gonococci can be demonstrated by gram-stain of the exudate in about half of women with gonococcal cervicitis if the exocervix is first thoroughly wiped clean before the exudate is expressed. *Trichomonas vaginalis* should always be excluded by wet mount examination, and *N. gonorrhoeae* should be looked for by endocervical culture in any woman with an abnormal vaginal discharge. Similarly, *C. trachomatis* and HSV are best detected by culture (Chap. 30, Nonbacterial Pneumonias, and Chap. 91, Infections Caused by Herpes Simplex Viruses).

Clinical diagnosis PID is imprecise, and this diagnosis must always be considered in young women with low abdominal pain and tenderness (Chap. 50, Infections of the Female Genital Tract). On pelvic examination, tenderness is maximal in the adnexal areas in salpingitis (it is usually bilateral and in the midline in endometritis) and is brought on by moving the cervix. The recent onset of an abnormal vaginal discharge or abnormal menstrual bleeding in a patient with abdominal pain is characteristic of PID. Also, the risk of salpingitis is increased fourfold to ninefold in women wearing an IUD. Although the risk is maximal during the first 2 months after insertion, it persists at least for the first 2 years. According to laparoscopic results, fewer than two-thirds of women with clinically suspected salpingitis actually have visible tubal inflammation. About 12% have an unsuspected problem, for example, a surgical emergency such as appendicitis or ectopic pregnancy, whereas many of the remainder may be presumed to have endometritis or cervicitis.

The presence of abnormal menstrual bleeding or mucopurulent cervicitis, a history of PID, use of an IUD, or exposure to gonococcal or nongonococcal urethritis all provide evidence for salpingitis or endometritis as opposed to other surgical problems. Onset with menses, dysuria, or proctitis favor gonococcal PID. Fever, leukocytosis, or elevation of the ESR favors salpingitis as opposed to normal laparoscopic findings.

Etiologic diagnosis of salpingitis and pelvic peritonitis is quite difficult because mixed infections are common and laparoscopy is required to obtain appropriate cultures. Endocervical cultures for *N. gonorrhoeae* and *C. trachomatis* are a minimum requirement, and laparoscopy to inspect and take cultures from the fallopian tubes and pelvic peritoneum should be taken whenever pain is unilateral, when the initial diagnosis is in doubt, or when early response to treatment is unsatisfactory. Optimal treatment regimens for PID should provide coverage for these two common pathogens.

Gonococcal perihepatitis may mimic acute cholecystitis, and transient nonvisualization of the gall bladder and mild liver function abnormalities may be demonstrated. The presence of fibrinous adhesions between Glisson's capsule and the abdominal peritoneum (*i.e.,* perihepatitis) should be distinguished from the hepatitis that occurs during gonococcemia. Perihepatitis may also complicate chlamydial PID.

The gonococcal arthritis–dermatitis syndrome must be differentiated from Reiter's syndrome in particular, and from other septic arthritides (Chap. 151, Septic Arthritis), acute rheumatoid arthritis, and systemic lupus erythematosus; meningococcemia and infection with *Yersinia enterocolitica* are less common causes of acute polyarthritis. Demonstration of *N. gonorrhoeae* by culture or specific immunofluorescent antibody stain in synovial fluid, blood, cerebrospinal fluid (CSF), or skin lesions is diagnostic of acute gonococcal arthritis. Failing this, the diagnosis of gonococcal arthritis is virtually certain if (1) *N. gonorrhoeae* is recovered from the urethra, cervix, pharynx, anal canal, or conjunctiva, or from the patient's sex partner; (2) pustular, hemorrhagic, or necrotic skin lesions are distributed on the extremities; and (3) a therapeutic trial of antimicrobial therapy produces subjective improvement and normal temperature within 48 hours and loss of all objective signs of arthritis within 2 weeks (except for patients with highly purulent synovial fluid). Even if only two of these three criteria are met, the diagnosis of gonococcal arthritis remains probable, particularly if other diagnoses are excluded. Conjunctivitis occurs rarely in gonococcal arthritis, and Reiter's syndrome is more likely in men with acute arthritis and conjunctivitis than in others. Haplotype B 27 histocompatibility is associated with Reiter's syndrome but not with gonococcal arthritis. Gonococcal arthritis may occur in women with active lupus erythematosus; indeed, hypocomplementemia may predispose to gonococcemia.

Laboratory Aspects

The gram stain of urethral or endocervical exudate is considered diagnostic for gonorrhea when typical gram-negative diplococci are seen within leukocytes, it is equivocal if only extracellular gram-negative diplococci are seen, and it is negative if no gram-negative diplococci are seen (Fig. 31-5*C*).

When these criteria are employed by experienced microbiologists, the sensitivity and specificity of the gram stain of the urethral exudate approach 100%. The specificity of gram stain examination of purulent cervical exudate obtained after the cervix is wiped clean to remove vaginal secretions also is high, but the sensitivity is only 60% or less. Modified Thayer–Martin (MTM) medium, Martin–Lewis (ML) medium and, modified New York City (MNYC) medium contains antimicrobics that suppress contaminants. They are most useful for isolating *N. gonorrhoeae* from the endocervix, anal canal, and pharynx, areas normally colonized by a mixed bacterial flora. The addition of 3 μg trimethoprim/ml inhibits swarming *Proteus* spp. and is especially desirable for anorectal cultures. Some strains of gonococci are inhibited by vancomycin if it is present at concentrations >3 μg/ml. Because some commercial culture mediums contain 4 μg of vancomycin per ml and $Arg^-Hyx^-Ura^-$ auxotypes (DGI strains) are particularly susceptible to vancomycin, there may be failure of confirmation of disseminated infection by culture of the blood, joint fluid, or skin lesions. As alternatives, both selective and nonselective mediums should be used, and lincomycin may be used in place of vancomycin in the MNYC medium.

Swabs free of cotton and wood should be transported from hospital wards or clinics to the microbiology laboratory in a nonnutrient, reducing medium containing activated charcoal to adsorb any inhibitors that may be present. If transportation requires more than a few hours, it is preferable to inoculate growth medium and incubate at ambient temperature in a candle jar or in a sealed bag with a CO_2 generating system.

Carbon dioxide is an absolute requirement for some strains of gonococci, and it enhances the growth of all strains, particularly when freshly isolated. Carbon dioxide decreases the lag phase of growth and decreases the number of gonococci needed to initiate growth. It is usually supplied in the gaseous form (3%–8%) but can be replaced by the addition of sodium bicarbonate to the growth medium.

Cultures should be incubated under CO_2 at 36°C for 24 to 48 hours, in an environment of at least 70% humidity. Cells from typical colonies are presumptively identified as gonococci by oxidase reaction and gram stain. Such isolates may be confirmed as *N. gonorrhoeae* by degradation of sugars or by simple immunologic tests (*e.g.,* those that employ staphylococcal coagglutination or fluorescence). These confirmatory tests are especially important for isolates from the pharynx and anal canal in order to differentiate gonococci from meningococci and for cervical cultures from populations of women who have a low prevalence of gonorrhea.

In men with incubating or chronic asymptomatic urethral infection without exudate, or as a test of cure following treatment, a very thin swab or wire bacteriologic loop should be inserted 2 cm into the anterior urethra and used to inoculate MTM medium. Cultures of the pharynx and anal canal should be obtained from all homosexual men suspected of having gonorrhea.

The most efficient test for gonorrhea in women is the endocervical culture; it is positive on a single examination in approximately 80% to 90% of those with gonorrhea. In areas where β-lactamase-producing strains of *N. gonorrhoeae* are encountered, cultures should not be replaced by gram stain or antigen detection tests, and all gonococcal isolates should be tested for production of β-lactamase to ensure proper treatment and prompt epidemiologic follow-up of contacts to prevent spread of such strains. The diagnostic yield may be increased by (1) obtaining a second endocervical culture with a second swab and streaking it on an enriched chocolate agar medium without antimicrobics; (2) simultaneously culturing the urethra, anal canal, and pharynx; and (3) having the patient return for a second examination if the initial cultures are negative.

Many gonococcal isolates are inhibited by the sodium polyanethol sulfonate present in standard liquid blood culture mediums. The inhibitory effect can be reversed by the addition of 1% gelatin (final concentration) to the medium, making it suitable for culturing blood and synovial fluid. In pus from skin lesions, *N. gonorrhoeae* is more often demonstrable by immunofluorescent staining than by culture.

A number of alternatives have been developed for the diagnosis of gonorrhea. Antisera to *N. gonorrhoeae*, prepared as monoclonal antibodies or as polyclonal antiserums cross-adsorbed to increase specificity, may be used to detect gonococci in exudates by enzyme linked immunoassay or by direct immunofluorescence. Although gram stain and culture are relatively simple and inexpensive, newer diagnostic tests for gonococcal antigens may find a role in testing specimens shipped over long distances.

Detection of gonococcal cytochrome oxidase in exudates and detection of antibody to *N. gonorrhoeae* in single-serum specimens are so nonspecific that they cannot be recommended. However, detection of an increase in antibody titer in paired serums against highly purified gonococcal antigens has been useful as a research procedure.

Prognosis

Untreated gonorrheal urethritis is probably self-limiting in most patients, and spontaneous recovery without sequelae or complications is probably the rule. However, in both sexes there may be spread to contiguous parts of the genitourinary tract and bacteremic distribution to other organ systems. With proper antimicrobial therapy, prompt cure should always result. Recurrent infection is common.

Urethral stricture is now very uncommon. Occurrence of stricture before specific antimicrobics became available may have been in part consequent on the use of caustic urethral irrigants. As a stricture develops, there is progressive difficulty in micturition, narrowing of the urinary stream, delay in emptying the bladder, and eventually, retention of urine.

Epididymitis causes unilateral thickening and tenderness of the spermatic cord. Painful orchitis and secondary hydrocele may also occur.

Gonococcal prostatitis has been described in the past, but is now rarely, if ever, seen.

In women, gonococcal cervicitis may progress to acute endometritis, salpingitis, peritonitis, and perihepatitis. Subsequent sequellae included ectopic pregnancy, sterility due to tubal occlusion, or chronic abdominal pain from pelvic adhesions.

Gonorrhea has been associated with septic abortion during early pregnancy and with premature delivery, chorioamnionitis, and the amniotic fluid infection syndrome later in pregnancy.

Therapy

For the past decade, the preferred drugs for the treatment of gonococcal infection have been penicillin G, ampicillin or amoxicillin, tetracycline, and spectinomycin. Certain of the newer cephalosporins are highly effective, though more expensive, alternatives. The regimens recommended in Table 56-3 have been adapted from the Centers for Disease Control recommendations for treatment of gonorrhea. The recommended dose of aqueous procaine penicillin G plus probenecid cures incubating syphilis and was found to be 97% effective for gonorrhea in a national cooperative study (1972–1974). With parenteral penicillin G, the risk of anaphylaxis in patients who deny previous penicillin allergy is 0.04%. With the currently recommended dosage, the risk of adverse reaction to the procaine is probably between 0.1 and 1.0%. The usual reactions of acute disorientation and psychosis beginning within a few seconds after the

Table 56-3. Recommended Treatment for Gonococcal Infections

	Treatment of Choice*	Advantages/Disadvantages
Uncomplicated infections in adult heterosexual men and women	Amoxicillin, 3 g with 1 g probenecid, PO, *plus* Doxycycline hyclate, 100 mg twice a day, PO, for 7 days (ampicillin, 3.5 g may be substituted for amoxicillin; and tetracycline HCl, 500 mg 4 times a day for 7 days, may be substituted for doxycycline)	Effective against *Neisseria gonorrhoeae* and *Chlamydia trachomatis*
	Tetracycline or doxycycline alone, as above	Requires compliance with multiple doses Less effective for *N. gonorrhoeae* Ineffective for anorectal gonococcal infection in men
	Ampicillin or amoxicillin alone, with probenecid, in single dosage, as above	Ineffective for *C. trachomatis* Ineffective for anorectal and pharyngeal gonococcal infections
	Aqueous procaine penicillin G, 4.8 million units, IM, at 2 sites, with 1 g of probenecid, PO	Painful Procaine reaction Anaphylaxis Ineffective against *C. trachomatis*
Special considerations		
Gonorrhea in homosexually active men	Aqueous procaine penicillin G, as above	
Penicillinase-producing *N. gonorrhoeae* infection (PPNG)	Spectinomycin, 2 g, IM, *or* Cefotaxime, 1 g, IM, without probenecid *or* Cefoxitin 2 g, IM, plus 1 g of probenecid, PO	None of these regimens effective for pharyngeal gonorrhea None of these regimens effective for *C. trachomatis* (therefore, consider adding tetracycline or doxycycline, as described above)
Pharyngeal PPNG infection	A single daily dose of 9 tablets of trimethoprim/sulfamethoxazole, 80 mg (400 mg) for 5 days	CNS side-effects, such as dizziness
Gonorrhea treatment failure	Spectinomycin 2 g, IM	No cross-resistance with other antimicrobials
Gonorrhea in pregnancy	Aqueous procaine penicillin G, as above	
Disseminated gonococcal infection	Aqueous crystalline penicillin G, 10 million units, IV, per day until improvement occurs, followed by amoxicillin, 500 mg or ampicillin 500 mg, PO, 4 times a day, for at least 7 days *or* Amoxicillin, 3 g, or ampicillin 3.5 g, PO, each with 1 g probenecid, PO, followed by amoxicillin 500 mg or ampicillin 500 mg, PO, 4 times a day for at least 7 days	Alternatives PPNG infection: Cefoxitin, 1 g, or cefotaxime 500 mg, given 4 times a day IV for at least 7 days. Penicillin allergy Cefoxitin or cefotaxime, as above *or* Tetracycline HCl 500 mg, PO, 4 times a day for at least 7 days. Should *not* be used for complicated gonococcal infection in pregnant women.
Gonococcal Salpingitis		
Inpatient	Cefoxitin 2 g, IV, 4 times a day, plus doxycycline 100 mg, IV, twice a day; continue drugs, IV, for at least 4	

	days and at least 48 hours after defervescence. Continue doxycycline 100 mg twice a day, PO, at home to complete 10–14 days total therapy	
	Gentamicin or tobramycin 2 mg/kg body wt, IV, followed by 1.5 mg/kg body wt, IV, 3 times a day in patients with normal renal function, plus clindamycin 600 mg, IV, 4 times a day. Continue drugs IV for at least 4 days and 48 hours after defervescence. Continue clindamycin at home, 450 mg, 4 times a day, PO, to complete 10–14 days therapy	May not be optimal against *C. trachomatis*
	Doxycycline 100 mg, IV, twice a day, plus metronidazole 1 g, IV, twice a day. Continue both drugs IV for at least 4 days and at least 48 hours after defervescence. Continue both drugs at home in same dosage, PO, to complete 10–14 days total therapy	Not optimal against *N. gonorrhoeae* and some facultative gram-negative rods
Outpatient	Cefoxitin 2 g, IM, with probenecid 1 g, PO, plus doxycycline 100 mg, PO, twice daily for 10–14 days	Probably not optimal for some anaerobic and facultative gram negative rods Compliance required
Sexually transmitted epididymoorchitis		
With gonococcal urethritis	Cefoxitin 2 g or aqueous procaine penicillin G, 4.8 million units, IM, with 1 g probenecid, PO, plus doxycycline 100 mg twice a day, PO, for at least 10 days	
With nongonococcal urethritis	Doxycycline 100 mg twice daily, PO, for 10–14 days	

****Children who weigh greater than or equal to 100 pounds (45 kg)***	Should receive adult doses
Children who weigh less than 100 pounds should be treated as follows:	
For uncomplicated gonococcal infection	Amoxicillin 50 mg/kg body wt, PO, at one visit with probenecid 25 mg/kg body wt (maximum 1 g) *or* Aqueous procaine penicillin G, 100,000 units/kg body wt, IM, plus probenecid, PO, 25 mg/kg body wt
For peritonitis, arthritis, conjunctivitis	Aqueous crystalline penicillin G, 300,000 units/day, IV, as 3 equal portions, 8-hourly, for 10 days

first or second injection, must be differentiated from vasovagal and anaphylactic reactions and from the very rare but life-threatening syndrome of cyanosis and cardiac arrhythmia thought to result from the intravenous injection of procaine penicillin. The latter reaction can be prevented by pulling back on the syringe plunger to be sure the needle is not lying in a vein before injecting the procaine penicillin. In the national cooperative study, reactions to procaine occurred more commonly with use of presuspended procaine penicillin than with procaine penicillin that was suspended just before injection. Ampicillin, 3.5 g (or amoxacillin, 3.0 g) can be given orally with probenecid with nearly equal efficacy, greater patient acceptability, and greater cost. Tetracycline must be given as a multiple-dose, 7-day regimen because single dose therapy with tetracycline is not reliable. However, in compliant patients, tetracycline has the significant advantage of eradicating coexisting *C. trachomatis* infection, which is present in about 20%

of men and 30% to 40% of women with gonorrhea. Such concurrent chlamydial infections may cause postgonococcal urethritis in men and postgonococcal cervicitis and salpingitis in women treated for gonorrhea with penicillin, ampicillin, amoxicillin, or spectinomycin. Since gonocococci that are resistant to penicillin, ampicillin, or tetracycline show no cross-resistance to spectinomycin, a single 2-g dose of intramuscular spectinomycin is adequate for gonorrhea in both sexes and is recommended for treatment failures. Spectinomycin and ampicillin–probenecid are much less effective than procaine penicillin or tetracycline for pharyngeal gonococcal infection, particularly in men.

Either spectinomycin or tetracycline may be given to patients who are allergic to the penicillins.

The increasing clinical occurrence of β-lactamase-producing gonococci may lead to changes in the recommended therapy for gonococcal infection in regions where such strains are prevalent. Spectinomycin and certain cephalosporins (*e.g.,* cefotaxime, cefoxitin) are highly effective for treatment of infections caused by β-lactamase-producing strains of *N. gonorrhoeae.*

It is now more important than ever to obtain a test of cure from patients treated with penicillin G or ampicillin. Patients who are not cured should be treated with spectinomycin. Tetracycline should not be used for treatment failures because gonococci which are relatively resistant to the penicillins are usually also resistant to the tetracyclines. Genetic loci (variously termed *mtr, pen B,* and *pen A*) that code for low-level multiple drug resistance appear to be involved—perhaps through altered permeability of the cell envelope. In addition, gonococci that produce β-lactamases are moderately resistant to tetracycline, having arisen in areas where gonococci were already moderately resistant to tetracycline.

Gonococcal infection in homosexual men, particularly rectal gonorrhea, frequently does not respond to the single-dose oral ampicillin–probenecid regimen or a 5-day regimen of tetracycline. That is, gonococci isolated from homosexual men tend to be more resistant to penicillin, ampicillin, and tetracycline than are isolates from heterosexuals. This increased resistance is attributable to certain genetic loci (*e.g., mtr*) that also confer resistance to the inhbitory hydrophobic compounds normally present in feces (*e.g.,* bile salts, fatty acids). Rectal gonorrheal infection in homosexual men should be treated with procaine penicillin G and probenecid, or with spectinomycin.

Postgonococcal urethritis (PGU) appears 2 to 3 weeks after therapy in up to 50% of men treated for gonorrhea with penicillin or ampicillin. Many cases of PGU appear to be caused by *C. trachomatis,* and others may be caused by *Ureaplasma urealyticum.* Either or both of these agents could be acquired at the same time as *N. gonorrhoeae* with the infection(s) incubating during the time of acute gonococcal urethritis. PGU should be treated with tetracycline as described in Chapter 55 (Nongonococcal Urethritis).

All patients diagnosed as having gonorrhea should have a serologic test for syphilis. A follow-up test is unnecessary in patients treated with a recommended regimen of procaine penicillin G, since this regimen cures incubating syphilis. However, if an alternative regimen of therapy has been employed, wherever syphilis is endemic, and in all homosexual men, additional serologic tests for syphilis are recomended 6 weeks and 3 months after treatment of gonorrhea.

Cultures from appropriate sites should be obtained 7 to 14 days after completion of therapy as a test of cure of gonorrhea. Additional follow-up cultures 6 weeks after therapy are advisable in women because about 15% of women who have a negative culture 7 to 14 days after treatment are again positive 6 weeks later, probably because of reinfection in most cases. Similarly, as many as 30% of women treated and apparently cured of gonorrhea during the first trimester of pregnancy become culture-positive before delivery. Thus, repeat cultures are advisable late in pregnancy for women treated for gonorrhea earlier in pregnancy.

Hospitalization is recommended for women suspected of having salpingitis to permit parenteral therapy with antimicrobial combinations active not only against *N. gonorrhoeae,* but also against *C. trachomatis,* facultative gram-negative rods, and vaginal anaerobic organisms, and to permit evaluation of the diagnosis and early response to therapy. Combinations of antimicrobics are necessary because mixed infections are common and because the causes of tubal infections are unknown at the time treatment is started. Hospitalization may not be practical in all cases of suspected salpingitis, but it is essential when (1) the diagnosis is uncertain and surgical emergencies must be excluded (especially if pain and pelvic tenderness are unilateral), (2) a pelvic abscess is suspected (3) the patient is pregnant or cannot follow an outpatient regimen or take peroral medication because of nausea and vomiting, or (4) there is no favorable response to outpatient therapy. Outpatient peroral treatment with either ampicillin, amoxicillin, or tetracycline alone is often ineffective, possibly because of poor compliance, infection with a β-lactamase producing strain of *N. gonorrhoeae,* or a mixed infection. The single-dose, procaine penicillin G-probenecid regimen recommended for uncomplicated gonorrhea is inaequate even for gonococcal PID, and there is no consensus on the optimal therapy. Antimicrobial combination regimens that deserve further evaluation in salpingitis include doxycycline plus metronidazole, tobramycin plus clindamycin, and doxycycline plus one of the newer cephalosporins such as moxalactam. The duration of therapy should not be less than 10 days, and dosages appropriate for intrabdominal infection should be used.

Gonococcal arthritis can be treated satisfactorily with several regimens. Five separate studies in different cities in the United States are in agreement that gonococci recovered from patients with gonococcal arthritis are significantly more susceptible to penicillin or tetracycline than are isolates from patients with uncomplicated gonorrhea. However, because of the threat of endocarditis, meningitis, and joint sepsis, all patients with disseminated infection should be hospitalized for initial treatment.

Failure to improve with treatment according to the regimens given in Table 56-3 casts serious doubt on the diagnosis of disseminated gonococcal infection. If the synovial fluid is highly purulent and viscous, serial aspirations or closed irrigation of the joint with sterile 0.9% NaCl solution may help to reduce inflammation. Open surgical drainage is virtually never required for gonococcal arthritis. Immobilization of the joint may reduce discomfort and may be useful during initial ambulation in patients with persistent effusions of the knee or ankle. Antimicrobics need not be injected directly into the joint space (Fig. 18-4).

The alternative regimen listed in Table 56-3 for pregnant women who are allergic to penicillin has a possible or potential disadvantage. Spectinomycin may, theoretically, cause otovestibular damage to the fetus. Erythromycin is no longer recommended as an alternative, because of an unacceptably high rate of failure with this antimicrobic.

Gonococcal conjunctivitis in the adult or newborn should be managed as a medical emergency by irrigation of the conjunctivas with saline solution, together with intravenously administered penicillin G.

Prevention

Theoretically, gonorrhea should be totally eradicable. There is no host other than the human, and there is no intermediary for transmission of the disease from one person to another. *Neisseria gonorrhoeae* is generally quite susceptible to penicillins—extraordinarily benign drugs. The persistence of gonorrheal disease is a socioeconomic problem. In older age groups, fear of gonorrhea has diminished because the ease of cure is well known; in younger age groups, there seems to be a lack of awareness of the existence of the disease.

Increased education about all aspects of gonorrhea is important. In order to eradicate as many reservoirs as possible, contacts must be located, interviewed, and treated.

At present, there is no vaccine. However, candidate vaccines consisting of pilus protein or protein I are under evaluation. Systemic antimicrobial chemoprophylaxis, although individually effective, has not been of value on a large scale. The use of intravaginal spermacides, as directed for contraception, may reduce the risk of acquiring gonorrhea in women. The condom is also effective in preventing the transmission of gonorrhea.

Chemoprophylaxis is effective in preventing neonatal gonococcal conjunctivitis. When required by law or indicated by local epidemiologic considerations, opthalmic ointment containing tetracycline or erythromycin or a 1% silver nitrate solution is an effective and acceptable regimen for prophylaxis of neonatal gonococcal conjunctivitis.

Remaining Problems

Gonorrhea is still a major problem. Experience has shown that the availability of effective antigonococcal agents is not sufficient to eradicate the disease. Behavioral research must be directed toward developing attitudes of personal responsibility in sexual behavior and illness. Clinical training of health care professionals in sexually transmitted diseases must be upgraded from the limited, didactic training now provided in this subspeciality in the United States and elsewhere.

Further information about mechanisms of gonococcal pathogenesis and the fundamental nature of acquired immunity to gonorrhea is needed.

The emergence of β-lactamase-producing gonococci may pose a major problem for therapy of gonococcal infection—particularly in underdeveloped countries. At present, spectinomycin remains effective, and the newer cephalosporins such as moxalactam, cefotaxime, and cefoxitin offer additional alternatives for single-dose treatment of infections caused by gonococci that are either susceptible or resistant to penicillin G.

Bibliography

Journals

BISWAS G, COMER S, SPARLING PF: Chromosomal location of antibiotic resistance genes in *Neisseria gonorrhoeae*. J. Bacteriol 125:1207–1210, 1976

BUCHANAN TM, SWANSON J, HOLMES KK, KRAUS SJ, GOTSCHLICH EC: Quantitative determination of antibody to gonococcal pili: Changes in antibody levels with gonococcal infection. J Clin Invest 52:2896–2909, 1973

CURRAN JW, RENDTORFF RC, CHANDLER RW, WISER WL, ROBINSON H: Female gonorrhea. Its relation to abnormal uterine bleeding, urinary tract symptoms, and cervicitis. Obstet Gynecol 45:195–198, 1975

DILWORTH JA, HENDLEY JO, MANDELL GL: Attachment and ingestion of gonococci by human neutrophiles. Infect Immunity 11:512–516, 1976

ESCHENBACH DA, BUCHANAN TM, POLLOCK HM, FORSYTH PS, ALEXANDER ER, LIN J, WANG S, WENTWORTH BB, MCCORMACK WM, HOLMES KK: Polymicrobial etiology of acute pelvic inflammatory disease. N Engl J Med 293:166–171, 1975

HANDSFIELD HH, LIPMAN TO, HARNISCH JP, TRONCA E, HOLMES KK: Asymptomatic gonorrhea in men: Diagnosis, natural course, prevalence and significance. N Engl J Med 290:117–123, 1974

HANDSFIELD HH, SANDSTRÖM EG, KNAPP JS, PERINE PL, WHITTINGTON WL, SAYER DE, HOLMES KK: Epidemiology of penicillinase-producing *Neisseria gonorrhoeae* infections: Analysis by auxotyping and serogrouping. N Engl J Med 306:950–954, 1982

HARKNESS AH: The pathology of gonorrhea. Br J Vener Dis 24:137–147, 1948

HOLMES KK, BEATY HN, COUNT GW: Disseminated gonococcal infection. Ann Intern Med 74:979–993, 1971

HOOPER RR, REYNOLDS GH, JONES OG, ZIADI A, WIESNER PJ, LATIMER KP, LESTER A, CAMPBELL AF, HARRISON WO, KARNEY WW, HOLMES KK: Cohort study of venereal disease. I. The risk of gonorrhea transmission from infected women to men. Am J Epidemiol 108:134–144, 1978

KAUFMAN RE, JOHNSON RE, JAFFE HW, THRONSBERRY C, REYNOLDS GH, WIESNER PJ, Cooperative Study Group: National gonorrhea therapy monitoring: Treatment results. N Engl J Med 294:1–4, 1976

MORSE SA: The biology of the gonococcus. CRC Crit Rev Microbiol 7:93–189, 1978

ST. JOHN RK, NEW HC, THOMPSON SE: Gonorrhea therapy 1979: Position papers for the current USPHS Recommendations. Sex Trans Dis 6 (Suppl):87–194, 1979

RUDOLPH H. KAMPMEIER

57 Chancroid

Chancroid (soft chancre, ulcus molle) is classified as one of the lesser venereal diseases because it occurs relatively infrequently and causes local lesions but no serious, distant, systemic manifestations.

The differentiation or identification of genital ulcers has been confused over the centuries. Physicians of ancient Greece and Rome wrote of dry and moist ulcers of the genitalia. The first clear-cut differentiation began with Ricord's classification in 1838 of a simple chancre as contrasted to an indurated chancre; he reserved treatment by mercury for the latter. In 1852, Bassereau observed that the indurated chancre transmitted only a genital ulcer of the same type. Shortly thereafter, others determined that the indurated chancre was not inoculable on the patient himself. Experiments as early as 1850 had shown that if a patient was inoculated elsewhere on the body with material from a simple chancre (chancroid), a sore developed within 2 to 3 days of inoculation.

The credit for describing the causative microorganism, *Haemophilus ducreyi,* belongs to the Italian, Ducrey, who published his observations in 1889. Nicolle reported successful transmission of the disease to monkeys in 1893.

Etiology

Haemophilus ducreyi are short bacilli (1 μm–1.5 μm × 0.6 μm) that are nonmotile, non-acid-fast, and generally gram-negative. Staining characteristics are variable, as is the length of the chains typically found in smears of exudates (Fig. 57-1).

In a recent endemic of chancroidal ulcers in West Berlin, confirmed by direct smears and culture, biopsies were taken from the edges of the ulcers for study by electron microscopy. Additionally, serum medium cultures were injected into the spleens and livers of mice for a similar study of the organism in tissues. Grouped in interstitial spaces of the biopsy specimen, the *H. ducreyi* were 1.25 μm to 1.40 μm in length and 0.55 μm to 0.60 μm in breadth. The cell wall–membrane complex was a trilaminar structure made up of two electron-dense layers separated by a translucent layer; the cytoplasm was rich in ribosomes. In the vascular spaces of the mouse liver and spleen, the bacilli were larger—up to 3.8 μm long—but had identical fine structure.

Culture mediums containing blood or serum are necessary for the isolation of *H. ducreyi*. Contaminating microorganisms are inhibitory; unfortunately, attempts at selective suppression of contaminants by adding bacteriostatic agents to culture mediums have generally resulted in the death of *H. ducreyi*. However, a recent report describes a selective medium of chocolate agar containing vancomycin as being effective in suppressing contaminants and increasing the number of colonies of *H. ducreyi*.

Positive cultures may be obtained in about 75% of cases. There is a male–female disparity in success (92% compared with 68%), which is likely related to the heavier bacterial contamination of specimens obtained from women. A technique of using the patient's own inactivated blood as a culture medium may result in identification of *H. ducreyi* within 48 hours in most cases.

Epidemiology

Chancroid occurs much more frequently in the underdeveloped countries (Africa, West Indies, Southeast Asia) than in the Western countries. In the United States, it is encountered more often in the southeastern states, and in past years was 10 times more prevalent among blacks than among whites. As reported by the Center for Disease Control, the frequency has declined in this country from a high of 9039 (6.4 per 100,000 population) in 1947 to 1064 (0.5 per 100,000) in 1974. In the venereal disease

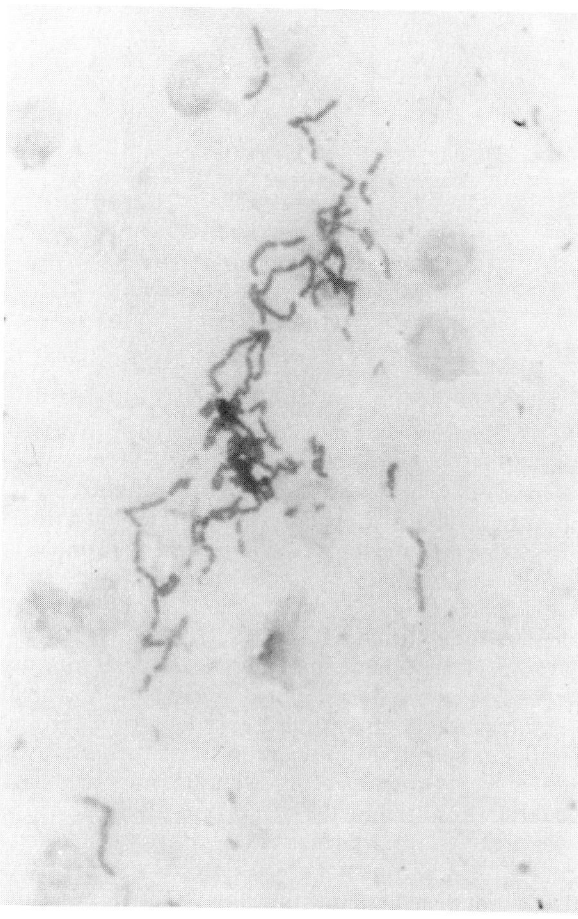

Fig. 57-1. Smear of exudate from a chancroidal ulcer showing *Haemophilus ducreyi* in pairs and short chains of several bacilli. Some show bipolar staining. (Courtesy of Norfolk Department of Public Health, Norfolk, VA; Grams stain, approximately × 700)

clinics of England and Wales, only 64 cases of chancroid were reported in 1967, and these were apparently imported mainly by seamen. Of historical interest and by contrast, these statistics represent a marked decline from a century and more ago; in two reports from France (cited by Lancereaux in 1868) Puche found that among 10,000 chancres, 1955 were indurated lesions (syphilitic, presumably) and 8045 were soft chancres; Fournier observed that among 341 chancres, 126 were of the indurated type and 215 were soft lesions.

The first epidemic of chancroid to be documented by modern technologic methods occurred in 1977 on the west coast of Greenland. Chancroid was apparently introduced in January of 1977; the epidemic mounted rapidly and came under control by early 1978. Among an adult population of 32,500, a total of 975 cases were reported: 401 from Godthaab, Greenland's main city, and 574 from 10 of the 15 district clinics on the west coast.

A detailed study of 186 cases was made in Godthaab during the first 6 months of 1977. The male patients were both Eskimoan and Danish, but the female patients were solely Eskimoan; the sex ratio (M:F) was 1.6:1. In the 3-month period before infection, half of both the male and female patients had had three or more different sexual partners. In the preceding year, 50% of the patients had been registered in the clinic because of gonorrhea—the majority of them had registered several times; syphilis had been diagnosed in 5% of male and 12% of female patients within that period. The mean incubation period of chancroid was 4 days for men and 13 days for women. It was suggested that a longer incubation period for women paralleled a longer period of communicability in women.

Almost 300 probable cases of chancroid were identified from May 1, 1981 to January 31, 1982 in Orange County, California. The great majority of the infections occurred in males 18 to 24 years of age who were recent immigrants from Mexico and lived in crowded quarters in the Santa Ana area; the contacts were prostitutes who solicited by knocking on doors. Careful differential laboratory studies, as well as the clinical characteristics of the disease, established the diagnosis of chancroid. In spite of the known difficulties attending the isolation of *H. ducreyi,* the organism was identified in cultures from 59 patients between December 1981 and January 1982.

Transmission of *H. ducreyi* by other than sexual contact must be exceedingly rare. It clearly is a disease accompanying sexual promiscuity and, most probably, uncleanliness. It would seem probable that rising levels of personal cleanliness account for the sharp decline in the prevalence of this infection in the Western nations, for promiscuity certainly has not fallen off.

Although easily identified in the male, the chancroidal ulcer is less obvious in the female. Either no lesion may be identified on the genitalia of the female, or there may be a nondescript, superficial ulcer or erosion. More often than not, there is no evidence of disease in female contacts of infected males. Since the disease has an incubation period of only several days, either the lesions are so small that they are missed, or there are carriers of *H. ducreyi*. Nevertheless, in the Greenland epidemic it was found that symptom-free females did seem to be an important reservoir of infection, although a few women without symptoms who were contacts had lesions on the portio or in the vagina.

Infection does not produce immunity. Reinfection is not uncommon in promiscuous men. Autoinoculation will produce a lesion.

Pathogenesis and Pathology

The portal of entry for the Ducrey bacillus is presumably a minute break in skin or mucosa which permits inoculation. The initial lesion is a vesicle or papule which quickly becomes an ulcer; there is sloughing of the epidermis. The base of the ulcer consists of a dense inflammatory exudate of polymorphonuclear phagocytes and round cells. In the depths of the corium, edema and perivascular accumulation of lymphocytes and plasma cells occur. Regional adenitis is characteristic, progressing to central suppuration in 50% of cases.

Manifestations

The characteristics of the soft chancre are more easily identified and described in the male. Some 3 to 5 days after sexual exposure, the initial evidence of infection is either a vesicle or papule that quickly progresses to pustulation and ulceration. Rather characteristically, the lesion is solitary and is located at the frenulum of the prepuce, but may appear on the shaft or the glans of the penis. Frequently, a number of ulcers appear on the edge of the foreskin. Not uncommonly, the ulcer enlarges progressively and by autoinoculation produces multiple ulcers elsewhere on the penis, scrotum, perineum, or thigh (Fig. 57-2). In the female, there are usually multiple lesions about the clitoris, on the labia, or at the vaginal introitus or fourchette by the time a physician is consulted.

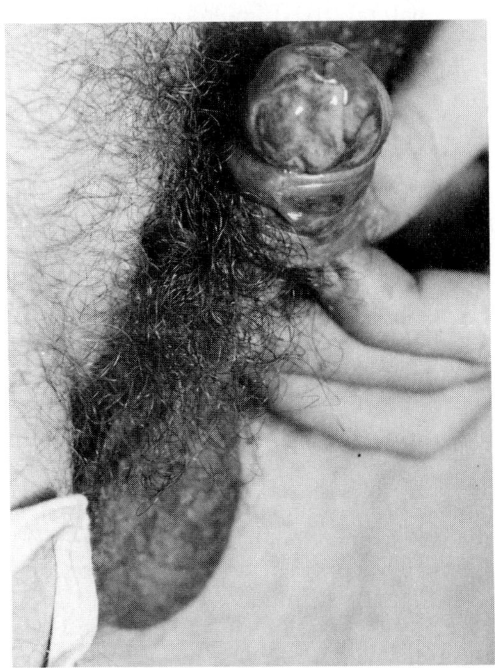

Fig. 57-2. Characteristic, destructive chancroidal ulcer at the frenulum with a second preputial ulcer. (Kampmeier RH: Physical Examination in Health and Disease. Philadelphia, FA Davis, 1970)

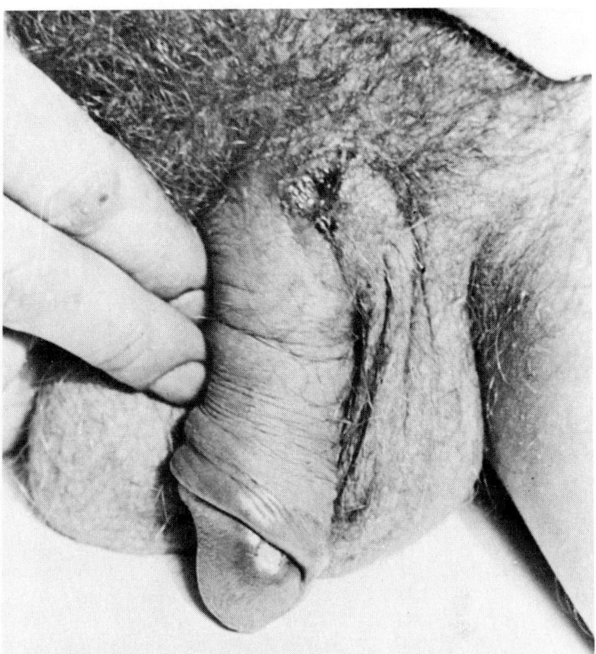

Fig. 57-3. Typical soft chancre (darkfield negative) on the glans accompanied by a typical darkfield positive hard chancre at the root of the penis (seronegative). Presumably, these chancres were acquired upon exposure without and with a condom, respectively, based upon epidemiologic information. (Kampmeier RH: Essentials of Syphilology. Philadelphia, JB Lippincott, 1944)

The typical uncomplicated soft chancre is a true ulcer with a red, overhanging edge and a base that is covered by a dirty, grayish white exudate. When irritated, as in the collection of exudate for a darkfield examination, the lesion bleeds readily (Fig. 57-3). The ulcer is painful and is so tender that contact with clothing may be uncomfortable and may even cause bleeding. Actually diagnostic, and in glaring contrast to the syphilitic chancre, the patient not uncommonly comes into the clinic or office with his penis wrapped in gauze or absorbent cotton. Urine flowing

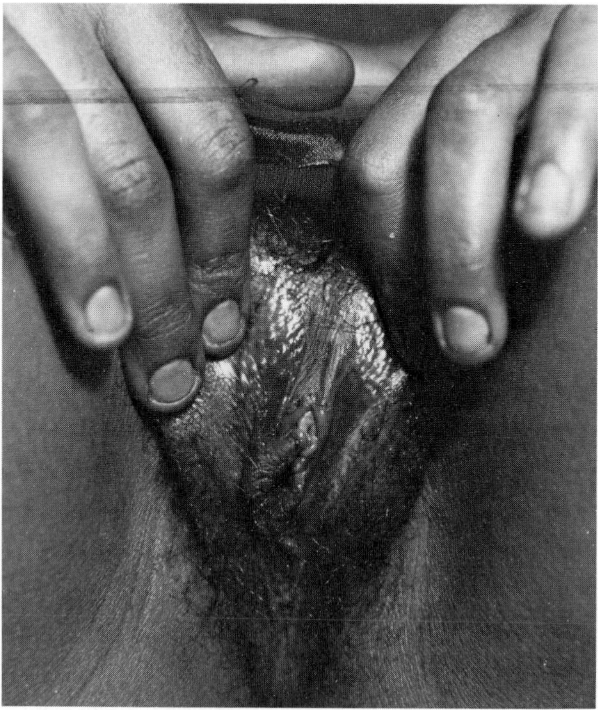

Fig. 57-4. Tender ulcer at the junction of the labia minora with sharply defined, red borders. It measured 1.0 × 0.5 cm. The exudate was darkfield negative and contained a variety of cocci and bacilli. The urethral meatus was inflamed and friable, probably accounting for the complaints of stinging and burning on urination, as well as frequent urination. The skin test (dmelcos) was positive.

over the ulcer may cause a burning sensation, often the chief complaint of infected women (Fig. 57-4). The chancroidal ulcer lacks induration, hence the terms soft chancre and ulcus molle.

The bubo of chancroid usually develops within a week, may resolve spontaneously, or in 50% of cases go on to suppuration. Drainage may be spontaneous, through incision (commonly in the past by the patient wielding his razor), or by needle aspiration by the attending physician. Healing is usually fairly rapid and results in a single, nonadherent scar. Of the 186 patients studied in the Greenland epidemic, 29% had inguinal lymphadenopathy which became fluctuant in one-fourth of cases.

Extragenital chancroidal ulcers have been reported, but must be rare.

Diagnosis

The first rule of diagnosis of genitoinfectious diseases applies also to chancroid, namely: every genital lesion, of whatever character, must be suspected of being syphilitic. Thus, every genital ulcer must be examined by darkfield microscopy (Chap. 9, Microscopic Examinations) and serologic testing (Chap. 59, Syphilis).

Clinically, the reverse of the soft chancre, the syphilitic chancre has a firm, infiltrated, clean base with little exudate. Typically, it is painless, relatively nontender, and bleeds scantily when a curette or scalpel is used to obtain exudate for darkfield examination.

Chancroidal ulcers may be multiple. Thus, at first, they may imitate the superficial and coalescing lesions of herpes genitalis (Chap. 91, Infections Caused by Herpes Simplex Virus). However, untreated, the lesions caused by *H. ducreyi* are more likely to be progressive and show deeper invasion of tissues.

The vesicle or papule that signals the site of entry of the infectious agent of lymphogranuloma venereum (Chap. 54, Lymphogranuloma Venereum) usually offers no diagnostic problem because it is so short-lived. The clinical differentiation of chancroid from early granuloma inguinale (Chap. 58, Granuloma Inguinale) should rarely pose any difficulty. The character of the ulcer, the presence of papules, and the demonstration of Donovan bodies will establish the diagnosis.

The lymphadenopathy accompanying chancroid is much more tender than the sentinal node of primary syphilis; the latter never breaks down unless complicated by other infection. The unilocular suppuration of the chancroidal bubo should not be confused with the typically bilateral, fixed, multilocular, suppurative lymphadenopathy of lymphogranuloma venereum. Retrospectively, the scar is diagnostic even decades later.

All authorities recommend specific diagnosis of chancroidal infection by demonstration of *H. ducreyi* in smears of scrapings from under the edge of the ulcer (Fig. 57-1) or by culture from the ulcer or bubo; most also warn that such identification is no simple matter. It is implied, or frankly admitted, that the clinical diagnosis and therapeutic results are more reliable than attempts at isolating the microorganisms. In fact, it is probable that examination of smears from ulcers will be useful in no more than 30% of cases. Cultures are even less likely to be of diagnostic value, principally because of inexperience in clinical laboratories.

Smears and culture examinations of pus aspirated from an intact bubo are much more likely to yield valid information. Accordingly, the diagnosis may be made upon any one of the following criteria: (1) culture of *H. ducreyi;* (2) finding *H. ducreyi* as the sole microorganism in the aspirate of a bubo; (3) smears showing bacteria resembling *H. ducreyi* in chains or clumps, provided these are not scattered among other microorganisms; and (4) a clinical appearance typical of a chancroidal ulcer, *i.e.,* a ragged, serpiginous ulceration of the coronal sulcus that is severely erosive and is associated with the classic unilateral bubo. Success in specific diagnosis by culture is usually the result of obtaining pus from an unbroken bubo.

Histologic examination of a biopsy may be specific, but it is not feasible in the private office or public health clinic. Inoculation of infectious material at another site in the patient's skin has been used for diagnostic certainty upon occasion. A vaccine (now unobtainable) was used in a diagnostic skin test (dmelcos test) in years past, but was of uncertain value and is obsolete.

Finally, the physician must always be alert to the possibility of two concomitant diseases, especially of more than one genitoinfectious disease in promiscuous persons, most important to the possibility of syphilis (Fig. 57-3).

Prognosis

Chancroidal ulcers may heal quickly and apparently spontaneously, if soap and water are given no credit. However, the ulcers often leave deep scars. The penis may be deformed, especially if the preputial frenulum was involved (Fig. 57-2). Phimosis and paraphimosis are not uncommon results.

Secondary infection of the soft chancre by other pathogens, especially by the fusospirochetal bacteria, may lead to a rapidly destructive, phagedenic ulcer with much loss of tissue; healing may leave a grotesque deformity of the penis. Systemic manifestations of uncomplicated infection with *H. ducreyi* do not occur.

Therapy

Local treatment should be delayed until darkfield examination has been carried out one or more times. Early and small lesions may respond to cleansing with soap and water and the application of hot packs. In women, healing may be rapid with use of soap and water and hot sitz baths.

In 1938, sulfanilamide was shown to be effective in the treatment of chancroidal infection. The sulfonamides have remained the drugs of choice. Sulfadiazine proved to be satisfactory in the Greenland epidemic, the lesion usually healing within a week of beginning a 2-week course of treatment. A sulfadiazine-streptomycin combination along with needle aspiration was used in those having fluctuant buboes. Sulfisoxazole is most commonly used in a peroral dose of 1 g taken four times daily for 2 weeks. The lesions usually heal within this time.

In patients who are allergic to the sulfonamides, tetracycline (30 mg/kg body wt/day, PO as four equal portions, 6-hourly, for 2 weeks) is an alternate choice, but it is less effective than sulfisoxazole. A combination of these two drugs has been recommended on the basis of experience in Vietnam. Chancroid resistant to the combination of sulfisoxazole and tetracycline may respond to (1) scrubbing the lesions four times daily with providone iodine, (2) needle aspiration of closed buboes or, if draining, scrubbing the abscess cavities with providone iodine; and (3) kanamycin (15 mg–17 mg/kg body wt/day, IM as two equal portions, 12-hourly for 7–14 days). Needle aspiration of buboes, if seen early, is indicated; dorsal slit of the prepuce is ill-advised because of probable autoinoculation of the incision.

In a prospective study of the use of doxycycline in a single dose of 300 mg PO compared with a week of sulfisoxazole (1 g PO 4 times daily), the response was inadequate in 6 of 19 (32%) patients receiving sulfisoxazole and in 8 of 30 (27%) receiving doxycycline. Four of the eight failures with doxycycline occurred in patients who vomited within 2 hours of taking the medication; however, compliance was better with doxycycline.

The susceptibility of *H. ducreyi* may vary from one outbreak to another. Thus, some isolates from the 1981–1982 epidemic in California were resistant to tetracycline and sulfamethoxazole but susceptible to erythromycin and trimethoprim–sulfamethoxazole by testing *in vitro.* Accordingly, the treatment prescribed was (1) for early penile or vaginal lesions without enlarged lymph nodes, trimethoprim 160 mg plus sulfamethoxazole 800 mg, PO, 12-hourly, for at least 10 days or until the lesions cleared and (2) for long-standing lesions with enlarged lymph nodes, erythromycin, 30 mg/kg body wt/day, PO, as 4 equal portions, 6-hourly, for at least 10 days or until the lesions healed.

Prevention

Personal cleanliness reduces the incidence of chancroidal infection. (The circumcised penis is less likely to become infected.) A condom is the best preventive measure. Chemoprophylaxis is unwarranted in the Western countries because of the rarity of the disease.

Bibliography

Books

KAMPMEIER RH: Essentials of Syphilology. Philadelphia, JB Lippincott, 1944. 131 pp.

KING A, NICOL C: Venereal Diseases, 3rd ed. London, Bailliere Tindall, 1975. 369 pp.

LANCEREAUX E: A Treatise on Syphilis: Historical and Practical, Vol I. London, New Sydenham Society, 1868. 99 pp.

Journals

BEESON PB, HEYMAN A: Studies on chancroid. II. Efficiency of the cultural method and diagnosis. Am J Syph 29:663–640, 1945

BORCHARDT KA, HAKE AW: Simplified laboratory technique for diagnosis of chancroid. Arch Dermatol 102:188–192, 1970

HAMMOND GW, SLUTCHUK M, CHANG JL, WILT JC, RONALD AR: Comparison of specimen collection and laboratory techniques for isolation of *H. ducreyi*. J Clin Microbiol 7:39–43, 1978

HAMMOND GW, SLUTCHUK M, LIAN JC, WILT JC, RONALD AR: The treatment of chancroid: Comparison of one week of sulfisoxazole with a single dose doxycycline. J Antimicrob Chemother 5:261–265, 1979

HART G: Chancroid, donovanosis, lymphogranuloma venereum. DHEW publication No. 75-8302, pp 1–10. Atlanta, Center for Disease Control, 1968

KERBER RE, ROWE CE, GILBERT KR: Treatment of chancroid. A comparison of tetracycline and sulfisoxazole. Arch Dermatol 100:604–607, 1969

LYKKE-OLESEN L, PEDERSEN TG, LARSEN L, GAARSLEY K: Epidemic of chancroid in Greenland, 1977–78. Lancet 1:654–655, 1979

MARMAR JL: The management of resistant chancroid in Vietnam. J Urol 107:807–808, 1972

MARSCH WC, HAAS N, STUTTGEN G: Ultrastructural detection of *H. ducreyi* in biopsies of chancroid. Arch Dermatol Res 263:153–157, 1978

NICOL CS: Venereal disease in women. II. Br Med J 2:383–384, 1971

PRENDERGAST T: An outbreak of chancroid in Orange County. California Morbidity No. 5, February 12, 1982

VD fact sheet, 1974. DHEW publication No. 75-8195, p 9. Atlanta, Center for Disease Control, 1975

RUDOLPH H. KAMPMEIER

Granuloma Inguinale

58

Granuloma inguinale is a chronic, indolent ulcerogranulomatous disease of the skin and mucous membranes. It is known as one the lesser venereal diseases because of its rarity in temperate climates and its low degree of contagiousness.

Granuloma inguinale was probably one of the variants of genital lesions described by writers in ancient and medieval medicine, and eventually, it was recognized as an entity by those interested in tropical medicine. McLeod, in 1882, described the disease from India as serpiginous ulceration. Additional descriptive terms in succeeding years included lupoid ulceration, granuloma of the pudenda, granuloma contagiosa, and granuloma venereum. In 1905, Donovan, a British army officer stationed in Madras, India, described the intracellular bodies which thereafter carried his name.

Etiology

The infectious agent was at first classified as *Donovania granulomatis* but is currently known as *Calymmatobacterium granulomatis.* They are nonmotile, rather plump, gram-negative bacilli (1 μm–2 μm long × 0.6 μm–0.8 μm wide) that often show bipolar staining. They stain also by Wright's, Giemsa's and silver methods. Both intracellular and extracellular forms are present in smears of scrapings of ulcers or in biopsy materials. When intracellular, they are generally unencapsulated and are found mainly in vacuoles of large mononuclear cells as well as in polymorphonuclear cells (Fig. 58-1).

Capsulation appears to be related to maturation. The extracellular bacilli are capsulated; when intracellular, replication yields unencapsulated bacilli within intracytoplasmic vacuoles. Encapsulation occurs as the bacilli mature, and the infective encapsulated, mature *C. granulomatis* are released when the host cell ruptures. By electron microcscopy, both extracellular and intracellular forms have capsules and their ultrastructure is characteristic of gram-negative bacilli.

Although Donovan bodies were quickly accepted as the causative agent of granuloma inguinale, early attempts at culture failed. Forty years passed before Anderson and co-workers succeeded in isolating what was probably *C. granulomatis* by yolk sac inoculation of chick embryos with exudate from active lesions of granuloma inguinale. The isolates (1) had the morphologic characteristics of the Donovan body in both encapsulated and unencapsulated forms; (2) would not grow in the available nonliving culture mediums but were carried through 25 successive yolk sac passages over a 3-month period; and (3) were not pathogenic for several kinds of laboratory animals. Washed bacteria provoked a skin reaction in six patients with granuloma inguinale; a so-called capsular substance reacted with serums from patients with the disease, yielding precipitin reactions in 18 of 19 and complement fixation in 12 of 15 specimens.

Epidemiology

Granuloma inguinale is most prevalent in India, Guiana, Brazil, the West Indies, the islands of the South Pacific, Northern Australia, the West Coast of Africa, and the southern part of China. The higher incidence of the infection in women in these areas may be related to polyandry as practiced among some native populations. The disease occurs during the years of greatest sexual activity, ages 14 to 50 years.

In the United States granuloma inguinale has been most prevalent in the southeastern states, with the disease almost confined to blacks. In 1941, 639 cases were reported nationwide, a rate of 0.4 per 100,000 population; a maximum of 2611 cases was reported

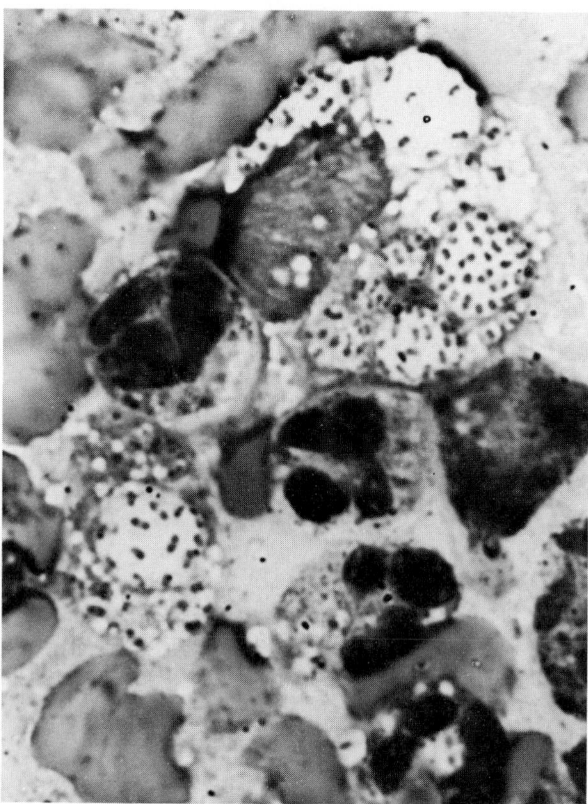

Fig. 58-1. Smear from the border of an ulcer of granuloma inguinale. The Donovan bodies are bipolar-staining, encapsulated bacilli lying mainly within vacuoles in macrophages. (Wright's stain, original magnification × 1400)

in 1949, *i.e.,* a rate of 1.8 per 100,000. There followed a gradual but progressive decline to 51 cases in 1974, with a rate 0.02 per 100,000 population.

The rariety of the disease in England, in spite of immigration from underdeveloped countries of the Commonwealth, is shown by reports of 11 cases in women in 1968 and only 3 in 1969. Quite in contrast, the incidence was 23.5% in male patients attending an urban clinic in New Guinea in 1972.

Sexual transmission of the disease is affirmed by (1) the fact that the initial lesions usually appear on the genitalia or adjacent regions, (2) the relationship of the first lesion to an incubation period (9–50 days as determined by inoculation of volunteers) following coitus, (3) the occurrence of lesions inside the vagina and on the cervix, and (4) apparent lymphogenous spread to pelvic structures following abortion or delivery.

On the other hand, the apparent low level of contagiousness has raised doubts of the sexual transmission of granuloma inguinale. The sexual partners of women with chronic granuloma inguinale often do not contract the disease in spite of continued, unprotected sexual exposure for months or years. However, there are reports of infection in 12% to 52% of the marital or steady sexual partners of these women. Of 87 cases studied recently in the Port Moresby Hospital, few were women; three denied any sexual contact, a fourth was a wife of a healthy man, and the others denied casual sexual contacts. Most of the males admitted having coitus with prostitutes. Also, investigations among male homosexuals point to transmission of granuloma inguinale by anal intercourse. In this connection, it has been speculated that *C. granulomatis* is an intestinal inhabitant that leads to granuloma inguinale through autoinoculation, or sexually through vaginal intercourse if the vagina is contaminated by enteric bacteria, or through rectal intercourse, both heterosexual and homosexual. It is reasonable to expect, however, that *C. granulomatis,* as bacteria of low pathogenicity which grow only in living tissues, will require direct inoculation through a break in the skin or mucosa to cause infection.

Occasionally, granuloma inguinale is encountered in the mouth and throat, and rarely elsewhere upon the body. On the basis of a few well-studied cases, it appears that both orogenital sexual contact and autoinoculation by contaminated fingers may lead to oral donovanosis.

Pathogenesis and Pathology

One or more indurated papules appear at the portal of entry of *C. granulomatis.* The papules progress to irregular-shaped ulcers which are usually nontender, 1 cm to 4 cm in diameter, marginated with thickened edges, and marked by a base of beefy red, granulation tissue which is usually exuberant. Tissue from the base of the ulcer is infiltrated by round cells and histiocytes. The hallmark of the lesion is the presence in smears (not in tissue sections) of mononuclear cells, 25 μm to 90 μm in size, which contain intracytoplasmic vacuoles packed with Donovan bodies. The marginal epithelial proliferation of long-standing ulcers may be the site of malignant transformation. Healing through deposition of fibrous tissue produces atrophic, but supple, depigmented scars.

Hematogenous spread with metastatic involvement in bones, joints, and liver occurs occasionally—most often in pregnant women. Subcutaneous spread by way of the lymphatics may result in indurated swellings or abscesses of the groin called pseudobuboes.

Manifestations

The genitalia are involved in 90% of cases and represent the clinical limit of the disease in 80% of patients. The less common areas of invasion are anal and inguinal. In men, papules appear most often on the glans or prepuce; in women, on the labia.

Initially, papules are flat or rounded on top; they ulcerate slowly. The ulcers are usually irregular lesions 1 cm to 4 cm in diameter with a rolled border, a beefy red, so-called cobblestone base, and scattered granulomatous masses. The ulcer is rarely without granulomatous tissue. Older portions of the ulcer may show the characteristic depigmented scarring at the same time that additional papules demarcate an active border; by confluence, the new papules produce a chronically extending ulcer (Figs. 58-2 and 58-3). Ulceration may be extensive; rarely, it may proceed so far as to involve the abdominal skin almost to the costal margins. Autoinoculation may occur between granulomas and apposed skin (kissing lesions) as in the groin, on the scrotum, thigh, or intergluteal areas. Pseudobuboes represent subcutaneous granulomas that extend into the inguinal regions (Fig. 58-4). Swelling of the vulva (elephantiasis) may appear during the period of active ulceration (Fig. 58-5), although there is no evidence of blockage of the lymphatics.

Fig. 58-2. Scar of healed granuloma inguinale bordering on active, progressing ulceration. Smears of exudate from the ulcer were positive for Donovan bodies, although administration of potassium antimony tartrate had resulted in healing on several occasions. Permanent healing followed treatment with streptomycin.

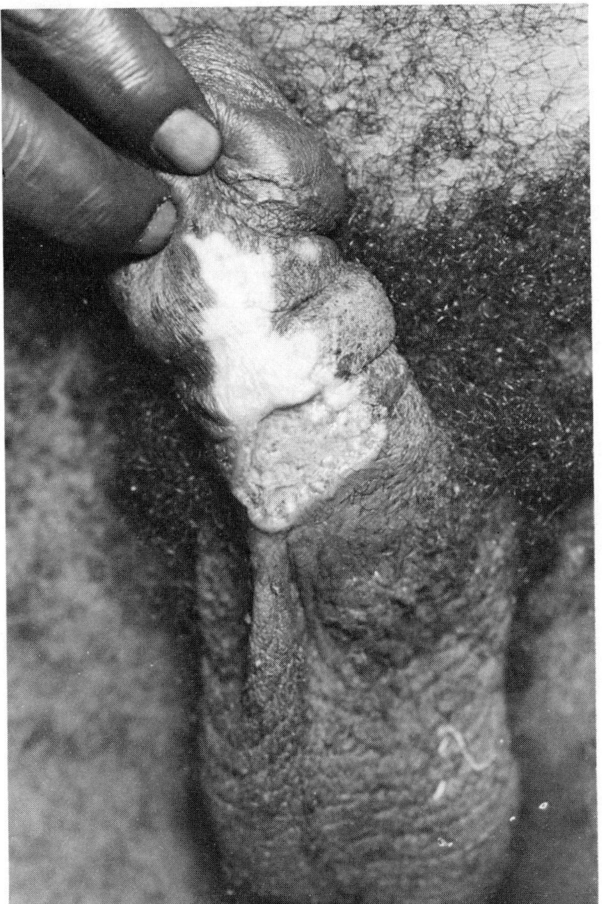

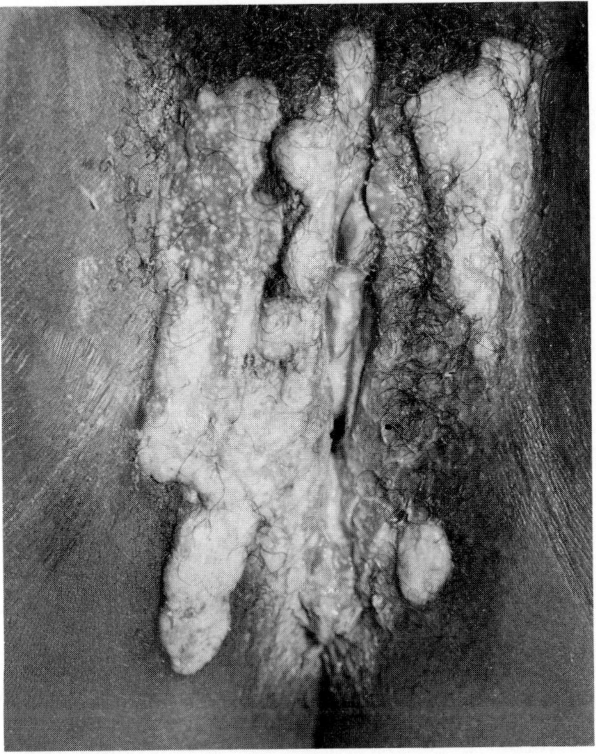

Fig. 58-3. Hypertrophic, granulomatous lesions of labia, groin, and perianal area which were smear-positive for Donovan bodies. The lesions had improved after treatment with stibophen 8 months previously. Improvement–relapse cycles followed addition of antimony therapy. (Kampmeier RH: Physical Examination in Health and Disease. Philadelphia, FA Davis, 1970)

The granulomatous tissue seems to be painless and the ulcer relatively so. Yet, manipulation with a curette or scalpel to obtain scrapings for microscopic study causes pain and bleeding.

Systemic manifestations rarely are a part of the clinical picture. Nevertheless, deaths have been re-

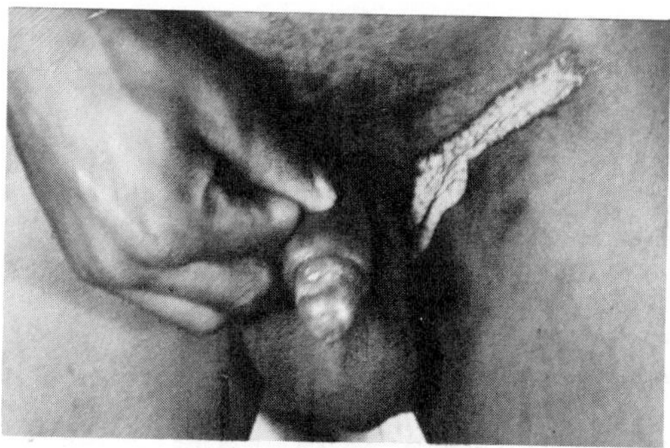

Fig. 58-4. A 29-year-old man had a 2-month history of an ulcer on the glans and in the groin, the latter spreading downward. Donovan bodies were demonstrated in the weeping, reddish granulations of the inguinal process. Treatment with oxytetracycline resulted in prompt improvement.

ported from invasion of parametrial structures following abortion or delivery. Metastatic lesions have been described as involving bones, joints, and viscera.

Diagnosis

The clinical characteristics generally are sufficient to suggest the probable diagnosis to the experienced clinician; scrapings or biopsy of the ulcer are necessary to enable microscopic examination for the diagnostic Donovan bodies. Material should be gathered by scraping or curetting rather deeply beneath an actively extending border of the ulcer. If scrapings are nonproductive, Donovan bodies are usually found in tissue (obtained by biopsy across the border of the ulcer and crushed for making a smear). Even if the diagnostic cellular inclusions are not found, the clinical findings are commonly so suggestive that treatment is indicated; resolution of the lesions verifies the clinical diagnosis.

In a research setting, complement fixation testing using an antigen derived from *C. granulomatis* appeared to be superior in sensitivity to a klebsiellal antigen.

The differential diagnosis conceivably may include several diseases presenting as genital lesions. A solitary papule might possibly be confused with the primary sore or hard chancre of syphilis. Also, a solitary papule, or several papules, may be mistaken for condyloma latum of secondary syphilis. An adequate darkfield examination should settle the matter with rare exceptions, provided neither penicillin nor tetracycline therapy antedated the examination. If there is uncertainty in regard to the darkfield examination, the screening VDRL test is helpful in the later days of a chancre and is decisive with regard to the secondary stage of syphilis. However, a positive serologic test may be evidence of latent syphilis in a patient developing granuloma inguinale.

A chronic ulcer is frequently associated with a thickened, rolled border, and a carcinoma may be suspected. Because malignancy may arise in any chronic ulcer of the skin or mucous membrane, as from granuloma inguinale or an ulceronodular lesion of later syphilis, biopsy should be performed. Granuloma inguinale may be premalignant, as evidenced by the frequency of carcinoma of the penis or vulva among young Jamaicans with a history of prior lesions characteristic of granuloma inguinale, although the lesions had healed with antimicrobial therapy.

The granulomatous characteristic of granuloma inguinale, whether as a papule or an ulcer, actually precludes confusion with chancroid, herpes genitalis, or the initial lesion of lymphogranuloma venereum. However, again, mixed infections can and do occur (Fig. 58-6).

The pink, tough cauliflowerlike excresence of condyloma acuminatum is easily recognized and is very unlikely to be confused with the manifestations of granuloma inguinale (Fig. 58-7).

Fig. 58-5. Nine months after cure of apparent syphilis by injection of penicillin, a vulval ulcer developed and was followed by swelling of the labia. The ulcer encircled the introitus at the time this picture was taken and involved the clitoris and labia minora; the posterior border is visible at the posterior fourchette. Smears were positive for Donovan bodies. Response to streptomycin was prompt.

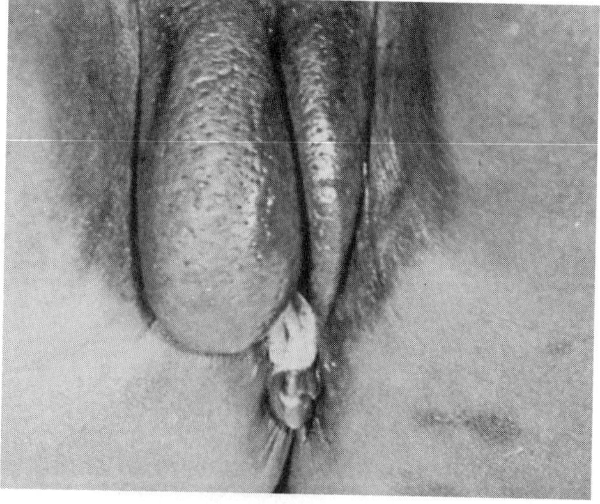

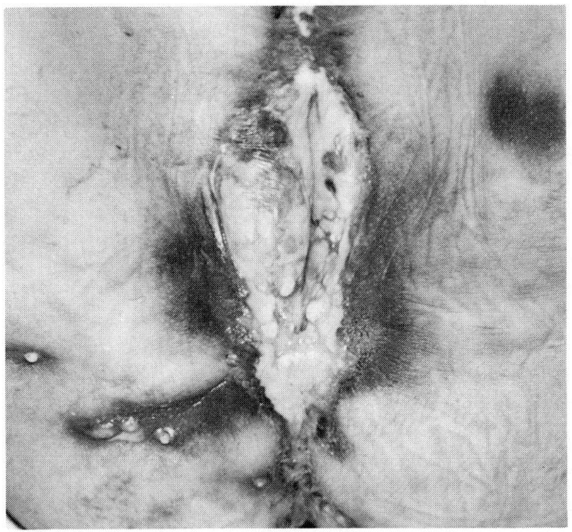

Fig. 58-6. Vulval disease, slowly progressive for 5 years. There was dual etiologies: (1) granuloma inguinale manifest as vulval ulcerations with islands of granulation tissue (smears were Donovan body positive) and (2) lymphogranuloma venereum which caused sinuses exuding pus on the buttocks and rectal stricture (Frei test positive). Treatment with streptomycin and sulfonamides were curative, but colostomy was later necessary.

Prognosis

With early diagnosis and prompt, adequate treatment, cure should result. Recrudescences may appear even after several years have passed despite apparently adequate therapy.

The possibility of malignant change in the margin of a chronic ulcer must be kept in mind.

Cicatrix following healing may lead to narrowing of urethra, vagina, or anus, interfering with function.

Therapy

Streptomycin, chloramphenicol, erythromycin, tetracycline, chloretetracycline, oxytetracycline, and gentamicin are effective in treatment of patients with granuloma inguinale. Tetracycline is recommended in a dose of 25 mg to 30 mg/kg body wt/day, PO as four equal portions, 6-hourly, for 10 to 20 days. Other regimens include streptomycin (15 mg–30 mg/kg body wt/day, IM, as two equal portions, 12-hourly, for 5 days); gentamicin (1 mg–2 mg/kg body wt/day, IM, as two equal portions, 12-hourly, for 10–20 days); or chloramphenicol (15 mg–20 mg/kg body wt/day, PO, as three equal portions, 8-hourly, for 10–20 days). Response to treatment will be apparent by the end of a week.

Recrudescence after healing may occur, but generally respond to a repetition of the previous treatment regimen. However, streptomycin was ineffective in patients treated in the Port Moresby Hospital; hence, the possibility of resistance to antimicrobics by *C. granulomatis* must be kept in mind. From limited experience, trimethroprim-sulfamethoxazole (160 mg–800 mg, PO, 12-hourly for 10 days) appears to be an alternative if the response to streptomycin or tetracycline is unsatisfactory.

Prevention

Because of the low level of infectiousness of *C. granulomatis,* cleanliness should be the best prophylaxis. The rariety of granuloma inguinale in the Western countries bears out this supposition.

Attitude is a major hurdle in control. The disease has been present for 2 to 6 months in the majority of patients before they seek help. Earlier treatment

Fig. 58-7. One year following cure of secondary syphilis by injection of penicillin, four circular, fleshy, granulomatous lesions (all Donovan body positive) appeared among cauliflowerlike condylomata acuminata. Healing of the granuloma inguinale was prompt following treatment with streptomycin.

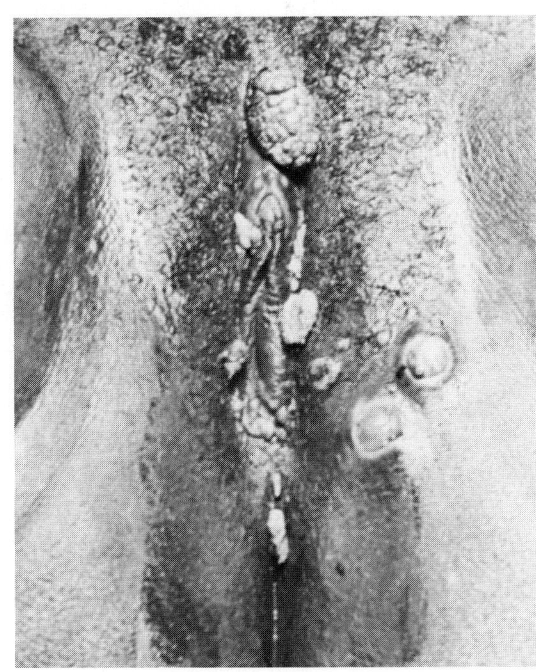

would not only reduce spread, but would almost certainly eliminate the probability of extensive scaring and possible chronic disability.

Bibliography

Books

KAMPMEIER RH: Essentials of Syphilology. Philadelphia, JB Lippincott, 1944. 131 pp.

MANSON-BAHR SIR PH (ed): Manson's Tropical Diseases; A Manual of the Diseases of Warm Climates, 14th ed, London, Cassell & Co, 1954. 1144 pp.

Journals

ANDERSON K: The cultivation from granuloma inguinale of a microorganism having the characteristics of donovan bodies in the yolk sac of chick embryos. Science 97:560–561, 1943

ANDERSON K, DE MONBREUN WA, GOODPASTURE EW: An experimental investigation of the etiology and immunology of granuloma inguinale. Am J Syph 29:165–173, 1945

D'AUNOY R, VON HAAM E: Granuloma inguinale. Am J Trop Med Hyg 17:747–763, 1937

GARG BR, LAL S, BEDI BMS, RATNAM DV, NAIK DN: Donovanosis (granuloma inguinale) of the oral cavity. Br J Vener Dis 51:136–137, 1975

GARG BR, LAL S, SIVAMANI S: Efficacy of co-trimoxazole: A preliminary report in donovanosis. Br Vener Dis J 54:348–349, 1978

GOLDBERG J: Studies in granuloma inguinale. VII. Some epidemiological considerations of the diseases. Br. J Vener Dis 40:140–145, 1964

HART G: Chancroid, donovanosis, lymphogranuloma venereum. DHEW publication No. 75–8302. pp 13–23. Atlanta, Center for Disease Control, 1968

HART G: Psychological and social aspects of venereal disease in Papua New Guinea. Br J Vener Dis 50:453–458, 1974

MADDOCKS I, ANDERS EM, DENNIS E: Donovanosis in Papua New Guinea. Br J Vener Dis 52:190–196, 1976

NICOL CS: Other sexually transmitted diseases. Br Med J 2:488–449, 1971

RAO MS, KAMESWARI VR, RAMULU C, REDDY CRRM: Oral lesions of granuloma inguinale. J Oral Surg 34:1112–1114, 1976

STEWART DB: The gynecologic lesions of lymphogranuloma venereum and granuloma inguinale. Med Clin North Am 43:773–786, 1964

VD fact sheet 1974. DHEW publication No. 75–8195, 33 pp. Atlanta, Center for Disease Control, 1974

ANDREW H. RUDOLPH

Syphilis

59

Syphilis is an infectious disease caused by *Treponema pallidum.* Although the disease is a continuum, for ease of discussion, untreated acquired syphilis is divided into the following stages: (1) an incubation period of approximately 3 weeks, followed by a primary stage manifested by a chancre; (2) a secondary stage manifested by widespread cutaneous and systemic manifestations; (3) a latent stage detected only by the presence of a reactive serologic test; and (4) a late stage which occurs in approximately one-third of infected, untreated persons and is characterized by serious complications that may lead to debilitation and death. Infectious syphilis includes the primary, secondary, and early latent stages of acquired syphilis; the late latent and late stages are considered noninfectious. Congenital (prenatal) syphilis is contracted *in utero* and is classified as early and late congenital syphilis.

Etiology

The etiologic agent of syphilis *T. pallidum,* is a thin, delicate spiral bacterium 6 μm to 15 μm long by about 0.25 μm in diameter (a dimension less than the resolving power of the ordinary light microscope). Six to fourteen rigid, tightly wound, regular spirals occur approximately 1μm apart and have a depth of 0.5 μm to 1 μm. The spirochete is actively motile with a characteristic slow, forward and backward movement (translation) along the long axis, a corkscrewlike rotation about the long axis, and a slight undulation at the middle of the organism. This characteristic motility of *T. pallidum,* together with its morphologic features, aids in its identification by darkfield microscopy.

By electron microscopic examination (Fig 59-1), *T. pallidum* exhibit a protoplasmic cylinder enclosed by a multilayered covering, which in turn is covered by a loose-fitting, 3-layered outer envelope. Axial filaments lie between the external cell envelope and the protoplasmic cylinder. Fibrils, nuclear vacuoles, mesosomes, and ribosomes have also been described.

Although nonpathogenic treponemes, such as the Reiter strain, have been grown and maintained in artificial mediums, *T. pallidum* has not been successfully cultivated *in vitro.* However, the organism has been successfully grown in chambers implanted in various host animals. Traditionally, *T. pallidum* has been considered anaerobic, requiring moisture and tissue for survival. However, virulent *T. pallidum* have recently been shown to consume oxygen at a rate similar to that of known aerobic spirochetes, and oxygen may therefore be needed for growth and reproduction. Thus, *T. pallidum* may be a microaerophilic bacterium, and the use of a modified tissue culture system may someday allow the growth of the spirochete *in vitro.*

Treponema pallidum are readily destroyed by a variety of physical and chemical agents including heat, drying, and mild disinfectants such as soap and water. Bismuth, trivalent arsenicals, and mercurial compounds rapidly immobilize the organism. Penicillin is spirocheticidal.

Epidemiology

Although *T. pallidum* have been maintained in other animal hosts by inoculation, humans are believed to be the only natural hosts. Survival of *T. pallidum* outside the body is brief, and transmission by fomites is extremely rare; therefore, infection virtually requires direct contact with infectious lesions. Congential syphilis, wherein infection is transmitted from mother to her fetus *in utero,* is an exception. Syphilitic infection has also been recorded after accidental inoculation or following transfusion of blood from a syphilitic donor.

Syphilis is most common during the sexually active

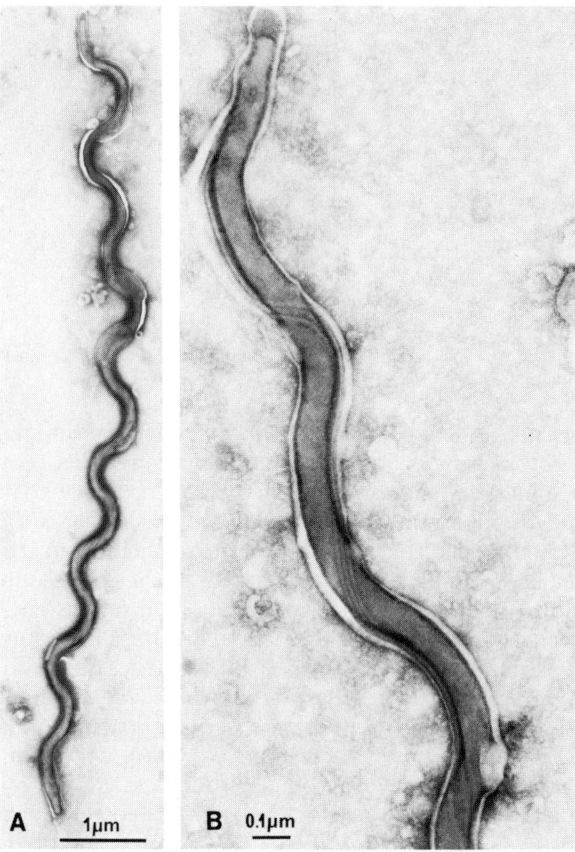

Fig. 59-1. Electron photomicrographs of *Treponema cuniculi* negatively stained with ammonium molybdate 1%. The cause of venereal spirochetosis in rabbits, *T. cuniculi* cannot be distinguished from *Treponema pallidum* serologically or morphologically. (*A*) The delicate flagella can be seen to wind around the regularly wavy body below the tip of the spirochete. (Original magnification approximately × 12,000) (*B*) Below the tip, the cell wall, cytoplasmic membrane, and flagella are clearly shown. (Original magnification approximately × 50,000) (Hovind–Hougen K, Birch–Anderson A, Jensen HJS: Acta Pathol Microbiol Scand [B] 81:15–26, 1973)

years; most new cases occur between 15 and 39 years of age. The highest rate of infection in both men and women occurs between the ages of 20 and 24; the second highest occurs between 25 and 29.

Pathogenesis and Pathology

Treponema pallidum enter the body through minute abrasions of the epithelium, by penetrating intact mucous membranes, or possibly through unbroken skin by way of hair follicles. In rabbits, spirochetes reach the lymphatic system within 30 minutes of dermal penetration and hematogenous spread follows. This is also assumed to be the case in humans. The length of the incubation period and the appearance of the primary lesions have been shown to be dependent upon the number of treponemes inoculated. The immunologic response of the host is undoubtedly another factor. In congenital syphillis, fetal infection is blood borne, through the placenta.

The most prominent histologic features of the response of humans to the presence of *T. pallidum* are vascular changes characterized by an endarteritis and a periarteritis. The endarteritis takes the form of dilation of arterioles and arteriolar capillaries with swelling and proliferation of the endothelial cells, which decreases the caliber of the lumen of the vessel. Proliferation of the adventitial cells and cuffing of the vessels by an inflammatory infiltrate consisting of monocytes, plasma cells, and lymphocytes are features of the periarteritis. With healing, fibroblastic proliferation leads to fibrosis and the formation of a scar. Syphilis may also produce a granulomatous infiltrate, tuberculoid in nature, with caseation necrosis.

Natural immunity to syphilis does not occur in humans. However, after infection with *T. pallidum*, an immune response occurs that is both humoral and cell-mediated. Exactly which immunologic mechanisms influence the course of the disease is still incompletely understood. Most likely, both humoral and cell-mediated immunity have a protective function in syphilis and both are probably responsible for the pathogenesis of the disease (Chap. 5, Immunopathology of Infectious Diseases).

Manifestations

Primary Syphilis

The prinicipal lesion of primary syphilis is the chancre that usually develops at the site of treponemal inoculation after an incubation period of 10 to 90 days (average 21 days) following infection. The typical chancre begins as a papule that passes through a series of evolutional stages. Superficial erosion occurs; scanty serous exudate may be observed and may result in the formation of a thin, grayish, slightly hemorrhagic crust. The base of the chancre is usually smooth, and the borders are raised, firm, and indurated. Chancres are painless if free of secondary infection. Traditionally, the chancre is described as a single lesion (Fig. 59-2), but multiple lesions are not unusual (Fig. 59-3). Also, the appearance of a chancre is often more atypical than typical, and until proven

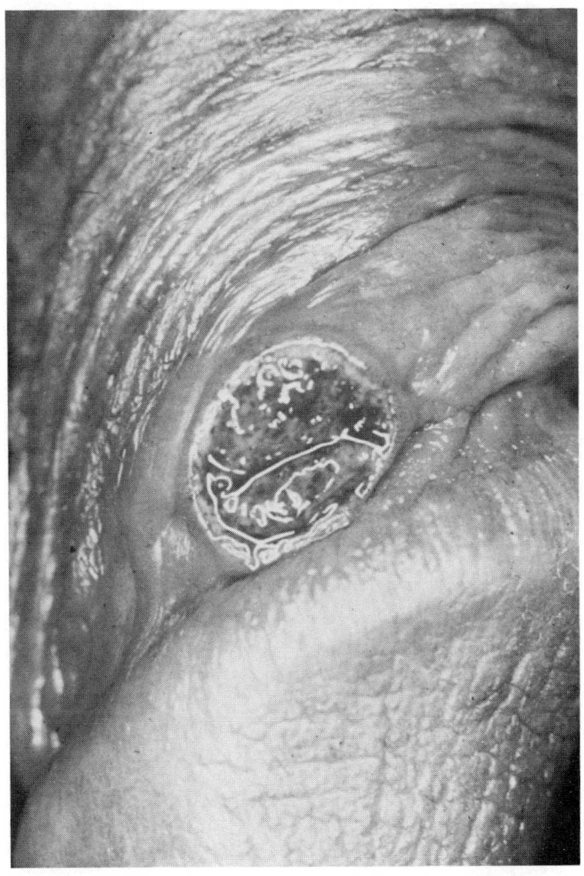

Fig. 59-2. Chancre of primary syphilis. (Courtesy of W Christopher Duncan, MD)

otherwise *every* genital lesion should be considered syphilitic. In women, genital chancres may be less commonly observed because they are frequently located on the cervix and cause no pain. Often, only careful examination with a speculum reveals their presence.

Regional lymphadenopathy (Fig. 59-4) usually accompanies primary syphilis. The inguinal adenitis is characterized by firm, movable, discrete, nonsuppurative, painless nodes without noticeable change of the overlying skin. Lymphadenopathy may be unilateral or bilateral, and in the case of a cervical or rectal chancre, may not be palpable.

Primary lesions may occur in areas other than the genitalia, and a high index of suspicion must be maintained if a diagnosis of syphilis is to be made. Extragenital chancres may occur on any portion of the body, but most frequently occur about the anus, within the rectum, on the lips, tongue, tonsils, eyelids, breasts, and fingers. They may be more painful

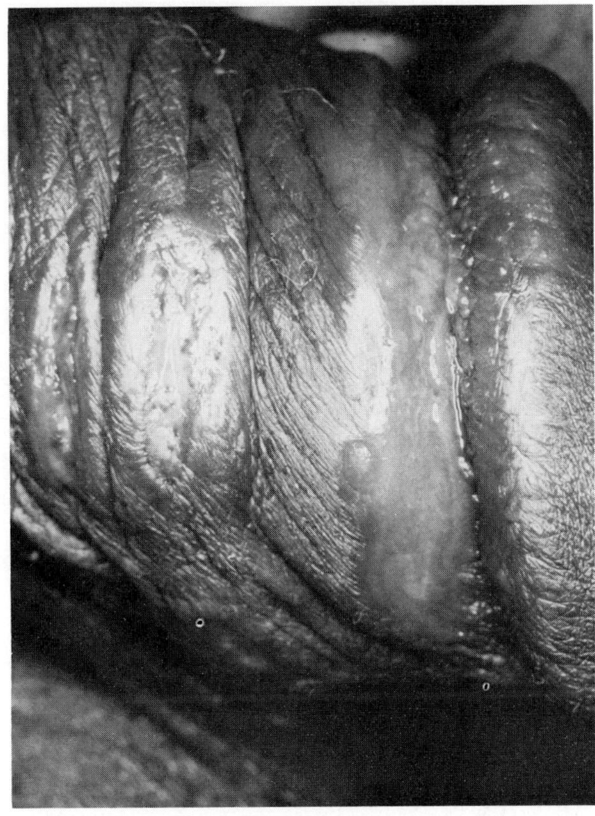

Fig. 59-3. Multiple primary chancres of syphilis. (Courtesy of W Christopher Duncan, MD)

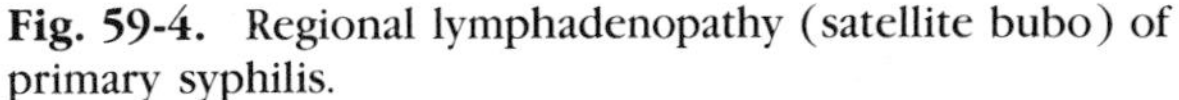

Fig. 59-4. Regional lymphadenopathy (satellite bubo) of primary syphilis.

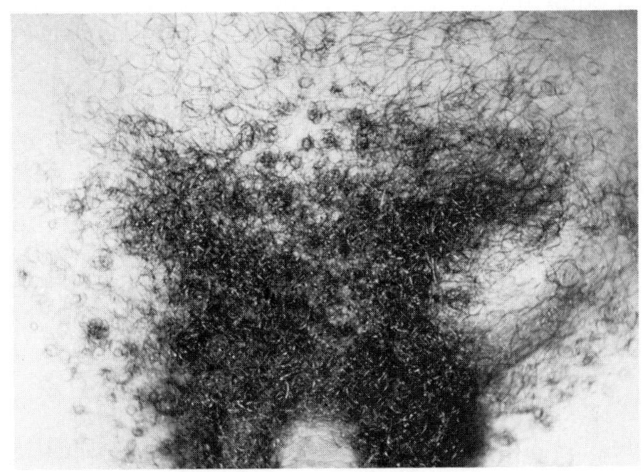

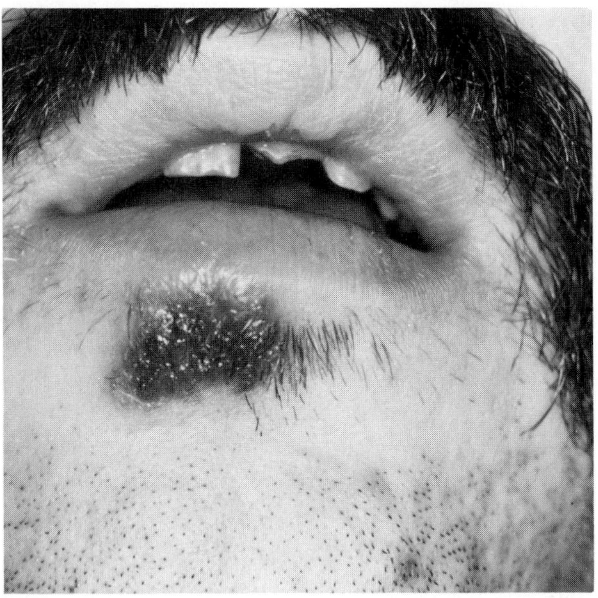

Fig. 59-5. Extragenital chancre with appearance of an ecthyma. (Courtesy of W Christopher Duncan, MD)

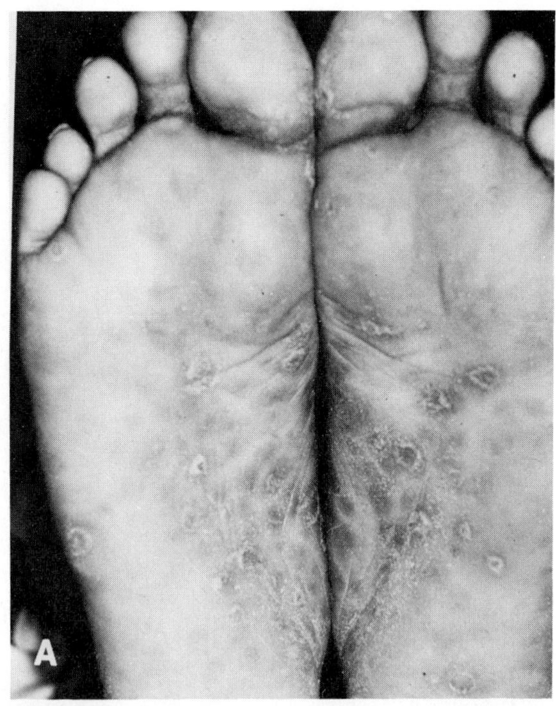

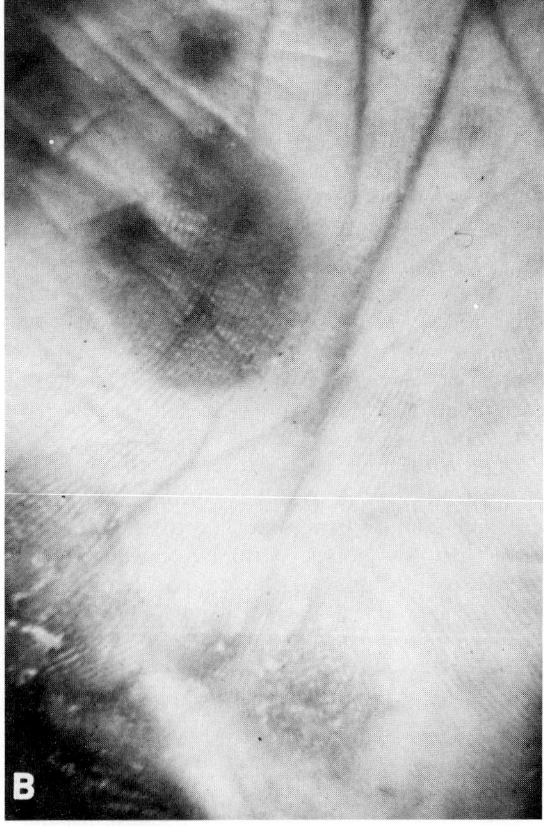

and may follow a more chronic course than genital chancres. At times they may assume an ecthymatous appearance (Fig 59-5) without the definite circumscribed buttonlike induration found in lesions of looser and thinner tissues.

As the primary stage progresses, healing gradually occurs. The epidermis regenerates over the erosion, and eventually the induration subsides leaving a thin atrophic scar. The chancre remains a visible manifestation of primary syphilis for only a short time, healing without treatment, usually within 3 to 6 weeks. Although the chancre of primary syphilis is usually gone before the onset of secondary syphilis, it may be present when secondary lesions appear.

Secondary Syphilis

Typically, the manifestations of secondary syphilis are noted about 6 to 8 weeks after the appearance of the primary chancre. The signs and symptoms are protean and may affect nearly any organ of the body; atypical presentations are not uncommon. Secondary syphilis is usually suspected on the basis of skin and mucous membrane lesions.

Fig. 59-6. Lesions of secondary syphilis. (*A*) Plantar lesions. (Courtesy of W Christopher Duncan, MD) (*B*) Palmar lesions.

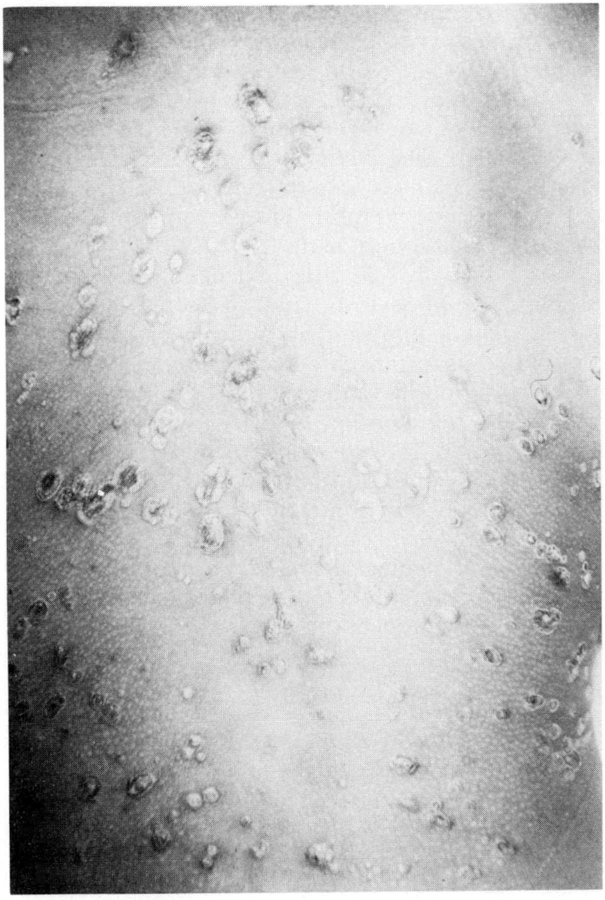

Fig. 59-7. Papulosquamous (psoriasiform) lesions of secondary syphilis.

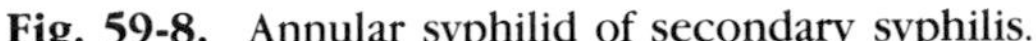

Fig. 59-8. Annular syphilid of secondary syphilis.

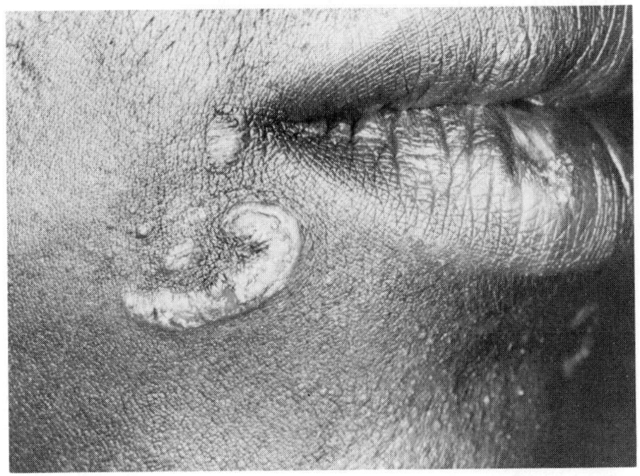

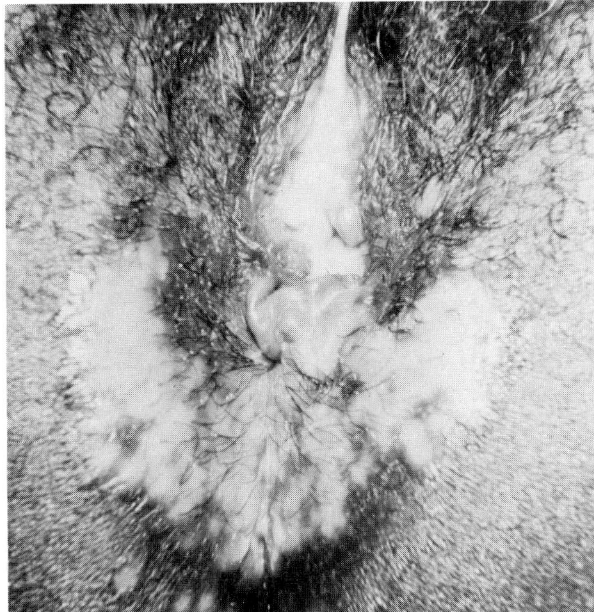

Fig. 59-9. Condyloma latum of secondary syphilis.

The cutaneous manifestations include macular, papular, papulosquamous, pustular, and follicular or nodular lesions; vesiculobullous lesions, as seen in early congenital syphilis, do not occur in adults. The lesions are often the same size, well demarcated, generalized, and symmetric. They often appear as discrete erythematous macules on the thorax or as reddish brown hyperpigmented lesions on the palms and soles (Fig. 59-6). Papular lesions may be present, and if scaling develops, papulosquamous (Fig 59-7) or even psoriasiform secondary syphilis results. Ringed or arciform lesions (Fig. 59-8), so-called annular syphilids, may occur, especially on the face of dark-skinned persons. In moist, intertriginous areas, lesions of secondary syphilis may take the form of large, pale, flat-topped papules that coalesce to form small plaques called condylomata (Fig. 59-9). These lesions are highly infectious. Because they are usually darkfield positive, they are also useful in making an absolute diagnosis of secondary syphilis.

Mucous membrane lesions (mucous patches) that may be present in secondary syphilis may occur alone or coincidentally with other cutaneous lesions. They appear as painless, dull, erythematous patches or as grayish white erosions (Fig. 59-10*A* & *B*). Any mucous membranes may be involved including the lips, oral mucosa, tongue, palate, throat, glans penis,

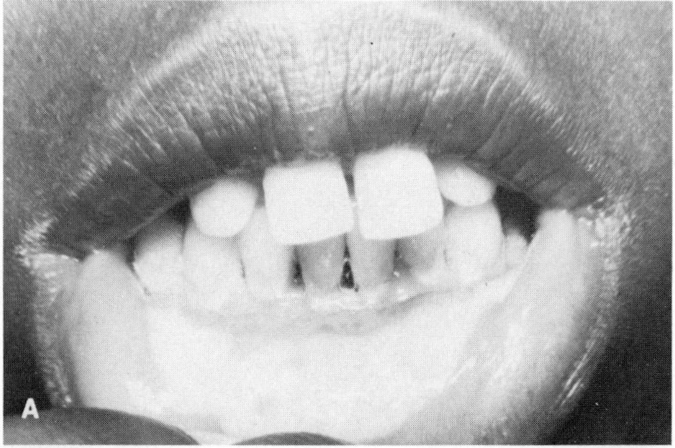

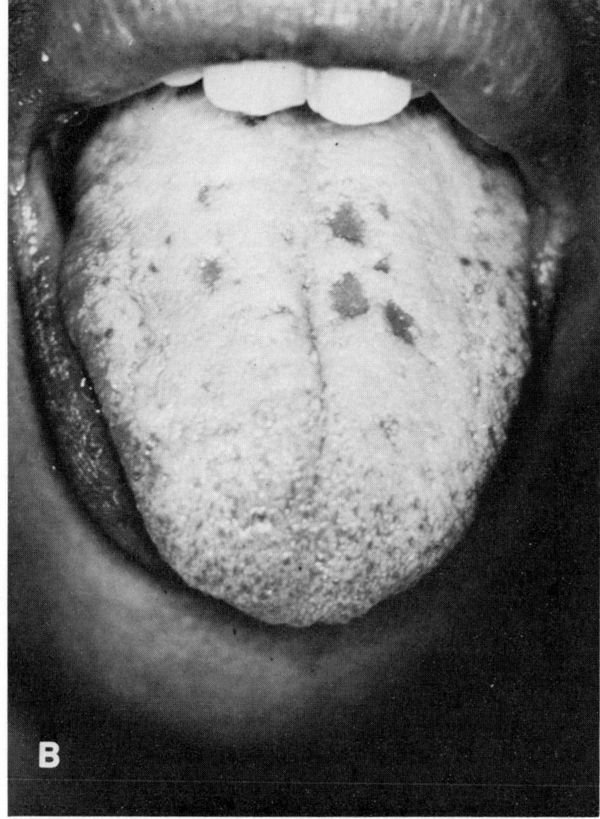

Fig. 59-10. Mucous membrane lesions of secondary syphilis. (*A*) Mucous patch of lower lip. (*B*) Mucous patches of tongue. (Courtesy of W Christopher Duncan, MD)

foreskin, vulva, vagina, and cervix. The lesions are highly infectious and are a valuable diagnostic sign.

Alopecia may also appear in secondary syphilis and most commonly occurs as random patches over the scalp. Occasionally, hair may be lost from the beard or the outer half of the eyebrows. The alopecia is temporary; regrowth occurs when the secondary stage passes, whether or not treatment has been received.

Malaise, anorexia, headache, sore throat, arthralgias, and low-grade fever commonly occur in secondary syphilis. Some weight loss may occur. General lymphadenopathy is present in most cases of secondary syphilis; the lymph nodes are large, nontender, discrete, and rubbery hard.

There may also be anemia, leukocytosis with an absolute lymphocytosis, and an increased erthrocyte sedimentation rate. Syphilitic hepatitis may be present, causing an elevated alkaline phosphatase; jaundice is unusual, and liver biopsy reveals a periocholangitis. A nephropathy, possibly the result of immune-complex deposition, may be associated with secondary syphilis. A low-grade, transitory proteinuria is common; however, a mild nephrotic syndrome or a hemorrhagic nephritis may also occur. Signs and symptoms of meningeal irritation may occur, but actual acute meningitis is rare. Syphilitic iritis and periostitis occur infrequently.

Latent Syphilis

By definition, latent syphilis is that stage of syphilis in which there is a reactive serologic test for syphilis in the absence of any clinical signs or symptoms of the disease. There may or may not be an history consistent with either infection or treatment. The cerebrospinal fluid must be normal, eliminating the possibility of asymptomatic neurosyphilis. Congential syphilis should also be ruled out. In addition, the possibility of a biologic false-positive reaction must be considered: the serologic test should be reactive when repeated with several serums; a specific treponemal test such as the Fluorescent Treponemal Antibody–Absorption (FTA–ABS) should be reactive; and diseases known to produce a false-positive reaction should be absent.

Latent syphilis begins with the passing of secondary syphilis and persists until the manifestations of late syphilis develop. It is arbitrarily divided into two periods: (1) early latency, infection of less than 4 years' duration; and (2) late latency, infection of more than 4 years' duration. During early latency, approximately 25% of untreated patients have one or more relapses in the form of infectious mucocutaneous lesions typical of secondary syphilis. Because of this potential for communicability, early latency is included in infectious syphilis. Approximately 1 year following infection, immunologic changes apparently begin to take place within the body and relapses are less common; after 4 years, relapses do not occur.

Late latent syphilis is considered noninfectious except in the case of a pregnant woman who may transmit the disease to her fetus or, rarely, in the case of an infected person who donates blood for transfusion. Late latent syphilis continues throughout life except in those patients who progress to the late symptomatic stages of syphilis.

Late Syphilis

Late syphilis, also called tertiary syphilis, is the destructive stage of the disease. It is noninfectious and can be considered a complication of untreated early infectious syphilis. Any organ of the body may be involved. In untreated or inadequately treated patients, the signs and symptoms of late syphilis usually do not occur until years after the initial infection. Late syphilis includes late benign (gummatous) syphilis, cardiovascular syphilis, and neurosyphilis. Although serologic tests are usually reactive, late syphilis can be present in spite of a nonreactive serologic test for syphilis.

LATE BENIGN SYPHILIS

The gumma is the typical granulomatous lesion of syphilis. It is the characteristic lesion of late benign syphilis and develops in approximately 15% of untreated syphilitics 1 to 10 years after initial infection. Gummas are found mainly in the skin and bones, but visceral lesions involving the liver, cardiovascular system, and central nervous system may occur. If a gumma occurs in a vital organ such as the brain, the term late benign syphilis may be a misnomer.

The cutaneous manifestations of late benign syphilis may appear as superficial nodules or as deep granulomatous lesions that break down to form punched-out ulcers. Gummas of the skin (Fig. 59-11) are usually solitary indolent lesions, asymmetrically distributed, with sharply marginated serpiginous or polycyclic borders. They are indurated on palpation, are locally destructive, heal incompletely (centrally or on one side), and leave atrophic, noncontractile scars that are often surrounded by hyperpigmented borders. Gummatous lesions respond quickly and dramatically to antimicrobial therapy.

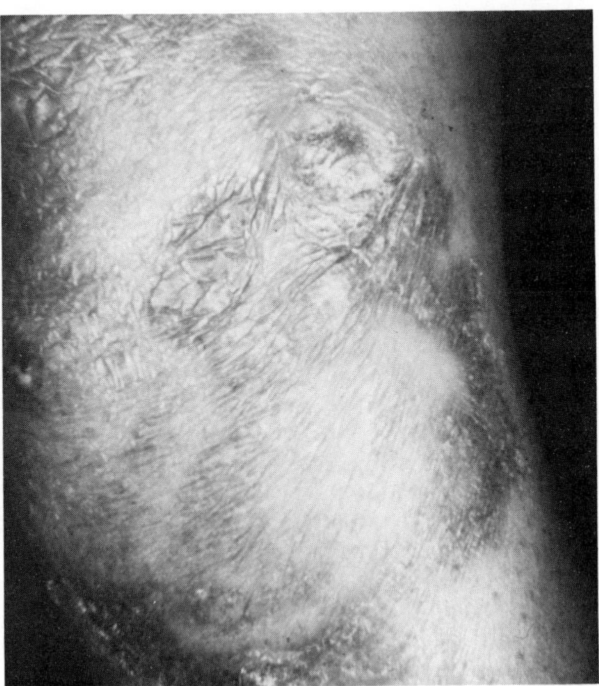

Fig. 59-11. Cutaneous gumma of late syphilis.

CARDIOVASCULAR SYPHILIS

Clinical manifestations of syphilitic involvement of the cardiovascular system develop in approximately 10% of late untreated syphilitics; they usually do not appear for 10 or more years after initial infection. Men are more frequently affected than women, and the incidence is higher in black than in white patients.

The basic lesion is an aortitis. It occurs predominantly and possibly only in acquired syphilis. Syphilitic aortitis consists of medial necrosis secondary to an obliterative endarteritis of the vasa vasorum. The elastic tissue is destroyed and replaced by fibrous tissue. The ascending and transverse segments of the aortic arch are most commonly involved. The process may be an asymptomatic (uncomplicated) aortitis detected radiographically as a linear calcification of the ascending aorta, or it may be found only at autopsy. The complications of syphilitic aortitis in order of frequency are aortic regurgitation, aneurysm, and obstruction of the coronary ostia. In syphilitic aortitis, the ring of the aortic valve and the valve cusps are frequently involved with widening of the commissures and thickening of the valve leaflets. Weakness of the valve ring and distortion of the cusps produce the incompetence of the aortic valve which results in regurgitation. If the aortic wall is also weakened by the destructive process, dilation may occur and may lead to formation of saccular and, less commonly, fusiform aneurysms. The thoracic aorta arch is most commonly involved, but the abdominal aorta above the renal artery may also be afflicted. Aneurysms of the ascending arch are associated with a higher incidence of aortic regurgitation than those located elsewhere.

Neurosyphilis

Symptomatic neurosyphilis develops in approximately 8% of cases of untreated syphilis. It is seen more frequently in white than in black patients and in men than in women. Although invasion of the central nervous system occurs during the early stages of syphilis, symptoms generally do not appear until 5 to 35 years after infection. Early involvement of the central nervous system is usually asymptomatic, but occasionally a person may develop an acute syphilitic meningitis 2 to 5 years after the primary infection. This form of meningitis resembles other acute meninigitides; it is rare and usually occurs in young men.

Because nonreactive nontreponemal tests (see Nontreponemal Tests) occur in approximately one-third of patients with neurosyphilis, a treponemal test should be included in the evaluation of patients suspected of having neurosyphilis. However, even treponemal tests may be nonreactive in the presence of clinical neurosyphilis.

Neurosyphilis is usually catagorized as asymptomatic, meningovascular, or parenchymatous. However, clear-cut classic forms of the disease are increasingly uncommon, and atypical or mixed manifestations are often seen.

In asymptomatic neurosyphilis, there are no signs or symptoms of central nervous system involvement; the abnormalities are present in the cerebrospinal fluid (CSF). A reactive serologic test is usually the first indication of syphilis, and often asymptomatic neurosyphilis is discovered only when the CSF is examined during a diagnostic work-up of a patient with possible latent syphilis. Untreated, asymptomatic neurosyphilis may resolve spontaneously, persist as such, or progress to symptomatic neurosyphilis. If treatment is instituted in the asymptomatic stage, progression to symptomatic neurosyphilis is usually prevented. Because asymptomatic neurosyphilis may coexist with other stages of late syphilis, the CSF should be examined in the evaluation of all patients with late complications.

The major clinical categories of symptomatic neurosyphilis include meningovascular and parenchymatous syphilis, although many patients have mixed features of both or incomplete syndromes. Meningovascular syphilis includes meningitis and central nervous system damage resulting from cerebrovascular occlusion, infarction, and encephalomalacia. The CSF is abnormal and the serologic tests are usually reactive.

The parenchymatous form of neurosyphilis includes syphilitic paresis and tabes dorsalis. Signs and symptoms of general paresis are extremely variable and reflect widespread damage. Personality changes and focal neurologic signs are often present. The CSF is usually abnormal and serologic tests are reactive.

Signs and symptoms of posterior column degeneration are the prime features of tabes dorsalis. The CSF findings are normal in approximately 10% of patients with tabes dorsalis. Nontreponemal serologic tests may also be nonreactive, whereas the treponemal tests are positive. Features of both paresis and tabes dorsalis may coexist in the same patient. Syphilitic optic atrophy is most often associated with tabes dorsalis but should be suspected in every patient with neurosyphilis. The Argyll Robertson pupil—small and irregular, reacting normally to convergence, but failing to react to light—is seen with both tabes dorsalis and general paresis.

Prenatal (Congenital) Syphilis

A pregnant woman with acquired syphilis can transmit the infection to her fetus. This form of syphilis is the result of prenatal infection rather than an inherited tendency, and the term prenatal, rather than congenital, is more accurate, although usage has made the latter term acceptable. The changes recognized as prenatal syphilis rarely occur before the 16th week of gestation. It has been suggested that the Langhans' layer of the chorion, which begins to atrophy at the 16th week of placental development, functions as an effective barrier to the passage of *T. pallidum.* However, fetal infection may actually take place earlier, before the fetus has begun to mature immunologically, with tissue changes recognized as prenatal syphilis delayed until approximately the fifth month of development when the fetus is capable of mounting an immune response.

In untreated prenatal syphilis, 25% of fetuses infected *in utero* die before birth, another 25% to 30% die shortly after birth, and among those who survive infancy, 40% develop late symptomatic syphilis.

The clinical manifestations of prenatal syphilis may be arbitrarily divided into lesions of early prenatal syphilis occurring before age 2 and those of late prenatal syphilis occurring after age 2. The earlier the onset of signs and symptoms of prenatal syphilis, the poorer the prognosis; active disease at birth is associated with a high neonatal death rate. More often, however, the infant is apparently healthy at birth and does not develop signs or symptoms of infection until the third week of life.

EARLY PRENATAL SYPHILIS

A large variety of cutaneous lesions may occur in early prenatal syphilis. There may be vesicular and bullous eruptions which frequently involve the palms and soles, although these vesiculobullous lesions are more commonly seen at birth. Later, the cutaneous lesions are more frequently maculopapular and resemble those of secondary syphilis; they are distributed about the face and mouth, the genital regions, and the palms and soles. Potentially infectious condylomatous lesions occur in the anogenital region. Mucous patches may involve the oral, pharyngeal, and nasal mucous membranes. Nasal obstruction with a mucoid, occasionally hemorrhagic, discharge (snuffles) is almost diagnostic. The discharge should be regarded as infectious, for it contains large numbers of treponemes. Osteitis of the nasal bones may follow snuffles and lead to the saddle-nose deformity. Laryngitis may produce a rather characteristic weak, forced cry. Periostitis and osteochondritis of the long bones are almost always radiographically evident after the first month of life, even in infants without signs of bone involvement. Hepatosplenomegaly and ascites are not unusual. Renal disease, thought to be secondary to immune-complex deposition, may be manifest as both an acute nephritis and a nephrotic syndrome.

LATE PRENATAL SYPHILIS

Late prenatal syphilis is manifested only be a reactive serologic test in 60% of the cases. Stigmas resulting from healed early or late lesions may also be present. Those most suggestive of prenatal syphilis are screwdriver-shaped central incisors with notching of the occlusal surfaces (Hutchinson's incisors); first molars with supernumerary, defective cusps (mulberry or Moon's molars); and interstitial keratitis. Other signs of prenatal syphilis include unilateral thickening of the inner third of the clavicle (Higouménakis' sign), saber shins, scaphoid scapulae, frontal bossing, short maxillae, nasal septal perforation, saddle nose, and rhagades. Eighth nerve deafness and hydrarthrosis, usually of the knees but also involving other large joints (Clutton's joints), may occur. Neurosyphilis, as seen in acquired syphilis, is also a potential complication.

Diagnosis

Primary Syphilis

A positive darkfield examination is the only means of making an absolute diagnosis of primary syphilis. If the initial darkfield examination is negative, syphilis is not excluded. The lesion should be examined by darkfield microscopy on 2 successive days and serologic tests should be obtained. During this time, the patient may apply compresses wet with 0.9% NaCl solution to the area. If secondary infection appears to be present, sulfonamides may be given, but antimicrobics that might affect *T. pallidum* must be avoided.

A presumptive diagnosis of primary syphilis can be made in those patients with darkfield-negative lesions if they have characteristic lymphadenopathy, have a reactive serologic test, and have been exposed to an infected person within 3 months. However, the diagnosis will become more tenable if the serologic test rises in titer. Because nontreponemal tests (see Nontreponemal Tests) for syphilis may remain nonreactive for a week or more after the appearance of a chancre, an initially nonreactive test does not exclude the diagnosis of primary syphilis. If the initial serologic examination is nonreactive, serologic examination should be repeated at weekly intervals for 4 weeks and then monthly for 2 months. The FTA–ABS test is more sensitive in primary syphilis than the veneral disease research laboratory test (VDRL), and it may be a useful diagnostic aid if the VDRL is negative.)

When a presumptive diagnosis of primary syphilis is made, other diseases of the genitalia must be considered in the differential diagnosis. These include trauma, herpes simplex (Chap. 91, Infections Caused by Herpes Simplex Viruses), chancroid (Chap. 57, Chancroid), granuloma inguinale (Chap. 58, Granuloma Inguinale), lymphogranuloma venereum (Chap. 54, Lymphogranuloma Venereum), drug eruptions, lichen planus, psoriasis, Reiter's syndrome (Chap. 55, Nongonococcal Urethritis), superficial (Chap. 107, Superficial Fungus Infections of the Skin) and deep mycotic infections (Chap. 39-44, Candidosis, Histoplasmosis, Coccidioidomycosis, Paracoccidioidomycosis, Blastomycosis, Aspergillosis), and carcinoma. These usually can be differentiated from syphilis by a negative darkfield examination and a nonreactive serologic test. However, it is important to remember that these diseases may also coexist with primary syphilis. Trauma to the genital area is not uncommon, but a corroborating history is often lacking.

The lesions of lichen planus are typically multiple, polygonal flat-topped violaceous papules. They are often pruritic. Biopsy usually shows a characteristic histologic picture.

Psoriasis is a papulosquamous disease characterized by well-demarcated scaling plaques on an erythematous base. Lesions commonly involve the scalp, elbows, knees, and sacrum. The nails may also be characteristically involved. Psoriasis may involve the glans penis as an erythematous macular or papular eruption without scaling. The presence of typical, psoriatic lesions elsewhere aids in the diagnosis.

Drug eruptions, especially a fixed drug eruption,

may involve the genital area. A careful history is mandatory.

Genital carcinoma is not usually confused with a primary chancre; biopsy is mandatory and diagnostic.

Secondary Syphilis

The signs and symptoms of secondary syphilis are variable, and a high index of suspicion on the part of the examining physician is required for a correct diagnosis. Because of the many kinds of cutaneous lesions and various systemic manifestations, secondary syphilis can mimic many diseases. For an absolute diagnosis, a darkfield examination should be performed on exudate from a moist, cutaneous, nonoral lesion. A presumptive diagnosis of secondary syphilis can be established if characteristic cutaneous and mucous membrane lesions are present and serologic tests are reactive.

The cutaneous eruption of secondary syphilis must be differentiated from pityriasis rosea, drug eruptions, acute exanthems, psoriasis, lichen planus, mycotic infections, and scabies (see Chap. 116, Scabies). Fortunately, serologic tests for syphilis are invariably reactive during the secondary stage, whereas they are nonreactive in the other conditions mentioned.

Pityriasis rosea is characterized by oval, papulosquamous lesions occurring along the lines of skin cleavage. The distal extremities, palms and soles, and mucous membranes are usually spared. Often the generalized eruption is preceded by a single lesion, the herald patch.

Prenatal Syphilis

The absolute diagnosis of early prenatal syphilis is dependent upon a positive darkfield examination of specimens from the umbilical vein or moist lesions of the skin and mucous membranes. Clinical manifestations, placental changes, and radiographic studies may be helpful. As in secondary syphilis, nontreponemal tests are reactive but do not give absolute evidence of infection. Reactive serologic tests in the newborn may reflect passive transfer of reaginic and IgG treponemal antibodies from the mother and not active disease in the infant. Repeated, careful clinical assessment and repeated serial quantitative VDRL testing of the newborn are mandatory. A significant rise in the VDRL titer justifies a diagnosis of syphilis, and treatment should be instituted. Decreasing quantitative titers call for further observation. A reactive nontreponemal test in the newborn from passive transfer of antibody should become nonreactive by the end of the third month; a persistent positive reaction strongly indicates active infection.

Early prenatal syphilis must be differentiated from other *in utero* infection such as rubella (Chap. 87, Rubella), cytomegalovirus infection (Chap. 75, Cytomegalovirus Infections), and toxoplasmosis (Chap. 129, Toxoplasmosis). The bullous eruption of early congenital syphilis may resemble bullous impetigo or infantile scabies. Lesions involving the buttocks or genital area may resemble a diaper dermatitis.

Darkfield Examination

The only specific and immediate means of diagnosing syphilis is by positive identification of *T. pallidum* on darkfield examination of specimens from an infected person. Darkfield examination is most productive during primary, secondary, infectious relapsing, and early congenital syphilis because moist lesions, *e.g.,* chancres, condylomata, or mucous patches, are present and contain large numbers of treponemes. Oral lesions are diagnostic problems; it is difficult, if not impossible, to differentiate *T. microdentium,* a saprophytic spirochete of the mouth, from *T. pallidum* by darkfield examination.

An accurate diagnosis on darkfield examination requires familiarity with the morphology and motility characteristic of *T. pallidum* and other spirochetes, as well as with the many problems that arise in the performance and interpretation of a darkfield examination (Chap. 9, Microscopic Examinations). Because most physicians lack the training, experience, and equipment necessary for darkfield microscopy, many local health departments provide darkfield examination as a service.

Fluorescent Antibody Methods

Both direct and indirect fluorescent antibody methods have been used to detect the presence of *T. pallidum* in tissue, ocular fluid, cerebrospinal fluid, tracheobronchial secretions, and exudates from lesions. Proper controls of the technique and reagents are mandatory if meaningful results are to be obtained.

The direct fluorescent antibody darkfield is an immunofluorescent staining technique using specific, fluorescein-labeled antibodies to identify *T. pallidum* in exudates from tissues. Because motility need not be maintained, specimens may be sent to a central laboratory. However, the specificity, sensitivity, and practicality of this procedure need to be further defined before it can be fully utilized.

Serologic Tests for Syphilis

Both nontreponemal and treponemal tests are used in the serologic diagnosis of syphilis. These tests differ in the antigens that are used, and in the kinds of antibodies that are measured.

NONTREPONEMAL TESTS

Nontreponemal tests measure reaginic antibody (primarily IgG and IgM—not IgE), which is detected by a highly purified cardiolipin–lecithin antigen. Although nontreponemal tests are relatively specific, they are not absolute for syphilis, and false-positive reactions may occur. They are also reactive in other treponemal diseases such as yaws, endemic syphilis, and pinta (Chap. 106, Nonsyphilitic Treponematoses). However, for screening or epidemiologic purposes in the United States or in the presence of clinical or historical evidence of syphilis, they are adequate.

Many nontreponemal tests have been developed over the years, and tests such as the Wassermann, Eagle, Hinton, Kahn, and Kline are now of historical importance only. Nontreponemal tests now in common use in the United States include the veneral disease research laboratory (VDRL) slide test, the rapid reagin (RPR) circle card test and the automated reagin test (ART). These tests can be carried out both as qualitative and quantitative procedures. When used as qualitative tests, they compare favorably in terms of their sensitivity and specificity. However, the quantitative titers obtained with the VDRL, RPR circle card test, and the ART cannot be interchanged or directly equated to each other. Thus, when these tests are performed on the same serums, the titer obtained with each may not be on the same. Moreover, change in the titer with the RPR circle card test or the ART has not been correlated with treatment, relapse, or reinfection. In some patients, therefore, it may be advisable to obtain a quantitative VDRL slide test simultaneously with the quantitative RPR circle card test or the quantitative ART.

Since the qualitative nontreponemal tests simply determine the presence or absence of antibody, any degree of reactivity is an indication for performing a quantitative test. Quantitation is carried out by diluting the serum in geometric progression and testing until an endpoint of reactivity is reached. Quantitative reactions are reported in terms of the highest dilution (dils) at which the specimen is reactive. Quantitative tests are much more informative than qualitative tests alone, for they establish a baseline of reactivity from which change can be measured. A recent infection can be evaluated by demonstrating a rise in titer, a feature that is also valuable in detecting reinfection or relapse in patients with a persistently reactive (serofast) test for syphilis. Quantitative nontreponemal tests are also the best serologic tests for assessing the results of treatment, especially in syphilis of less than 2 years' duration. Serial quantitative testing is also an important means of evaluating newborns suspected of having prenatal (congenital) syphilis.

Figure 59-12 depicts the quantitative serologic response of the various stages of untreated syphilis as

Fig. 59-12. Time course of reaginic antibody in untreated syphilis. Thirty years after the infection, about 50% of reagin tests are nonreactive. (Public Health Service Publication No. 743, July, 1961)

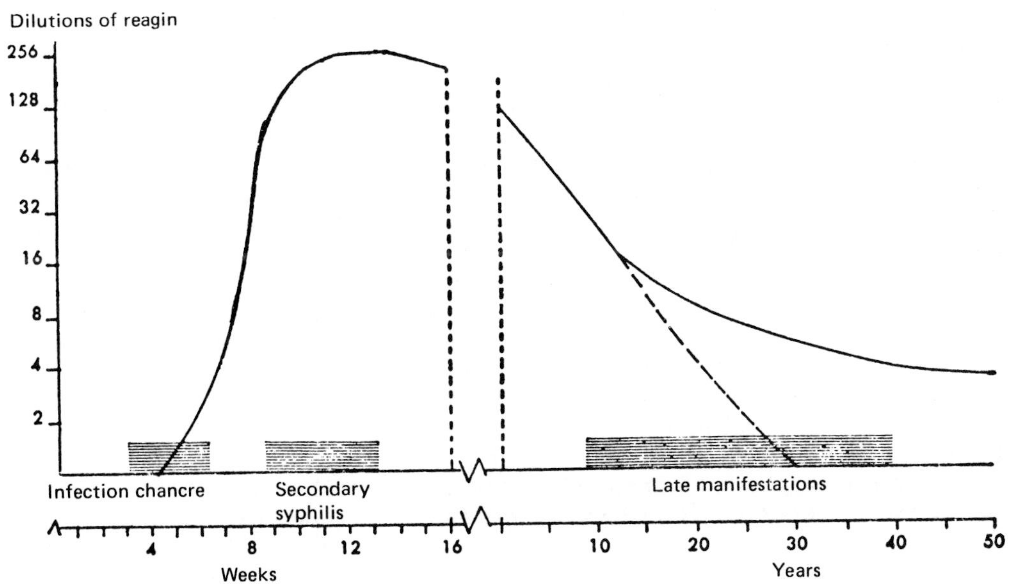

measured by titers in the VDRL test. The VDRL test usually becomes reactive 1 to 3 weeks after the chancre appears. The titer then increases during the secondary stage and begins to fall during the latent stage. Even without treatment, the VDRL may be reactive in only a low titer or may even be nonreactive in the late stages of syphilis.

Occasionally serums containing large amounts of reaginic antibody demonstrate a prozone (zonal) reaction in nontreponemal serologic tests. A strongly reactive serum may show a weakly reactive, atypical, or, on rare occasions, a nonreactive result when undiluted. The inhibitory effect of the excess antibody can be overcome by diluting the serum containing the antibody. Therefore, dilution testing should be performed on all serums showing any degree of reactivity when undiluted and on specimens which might be expected to show this phenomenon, as in secondary syphilis (approximately 1% of patients), even when the initial testing is completely nonreactive. Because many laboratories do not routinely perform quantitative VDRL tests unless the undiluted serum is reactive, the physician should alert the laboratory to those specimens which might be expected to exhibit a prozone phenomenon.

TREPONEMAL TESTS

Treponemal tests employ *T. pallidum* as the antigen and detect specific antitreponenal antibodies that are usually related only to treponemal infections, such as syphilis, yaws, endemic syphilis, and pinta (Chap. 106, Nonsyphilitic Treponematoses). Because of their greater specificity, they are primarily employed as verification procedures. Unfortunately, treponemal tests are also technically more difficult and more costly to perform than nontreponemal tests.

The *Treponema pallidum* Immobilization (TPI) test was the first acceptable treponemal verification test. Although it is highly specific, the test is expensive, difficult to standardize, and cumbersome to perform. It is not as sensitive as the fluorescent antibody method, and its use is now limited to special cases.

Indirect fluorescent antibody tests employing *T. pallidum* as the antigen have progressed through many stages of development and refinement. The manual fluorescent treponemal antibody–absorption (FTA–ABS) test has evolved as the standard treponemal test in use today. In the United States, the manual FTA–ABS test has replaced the TPI, as well as treponemal test based on complement fixation such as the Reiter protein complement fixation (RPCF) test and one-fifth volume Kolmer test with Reiter protein antigen (KRP).

The FTA–ABS test is reported as nonreactive, borderline, or reactive. Borderline tests should always be repeated and are not indicative of the presence or lack of syphilis. The FTA–ABS test has also been partially automated, becoming the automated fluorescent treponemal antibody (AFTA) test, but this modification is less specific and less sensitive than the manual test.

In the routine FTA–ABS test, the conjugate used in fluorescein-labeled antihuman globulin. A modification using monospecific fluorescein-labeled antihuman IgM conjugate has been adapted to the diagnosis of congenital syphilis. Unlike the IgG antibody detected by the VDRL and conventional FTA–ABS test, IgM antibody normally cannot cross the placenta. The presence of fetal IgM antitreponemal antibody detected by the FTA–ABS–IgM test would therefore indicate active syphilitic infection of the newborn. Because false-positive reactions occur in less than 10% of cases, this test was thought to be a useful confirmatory procedure to differentiate passive transfer of maternal antibody from active infection. However, in late onset congenital syphilis, the FTA–ABS–IgM test may be falsely negative in over 35% of cases, a degree of insensitivity that limits its usefulness as a screening procedure. Moreover, the specificity of the FTA–ABS–IgM test for neonatal congenital syphilis has been questioned. It has been suggested that newborns may produce IgM antibodies in response to passively transferred maternal IgG antibodies rather than in response to the infectious agent. Thus, the antibodies detected by the FTA–ABS–IgM test for congenital syphilis may be those produced in response to passively transferred maternal IgG syphilitic antibodies rather than in response to an active infection with *T. pallidum* in the newborn. Therefore, at this time, the FTA–ABS–IgM test for prenatal syphilis cannot replace repeated careful clinical assessment combined with serial quantitative nontreponemal tests, such as the VDRL, in the evaluation of the newborn with possible congenital syphilis.

The development of simpler, less costly, more specific tests for the serologic diagnosis of syphilis has continued with the adaptation of hemagglutination procedures to treponemal tests. The first reliable application of hemagglutination techniques to the serologic diagnosis of syphilis was reported in 1965. The antigen was formalinized, tanned sheep erythrocytes sensitized with material from *T. pallidum* (Nichols strain); antitreponemal antibody was indicated by macrohemagglutination. Subsequent modifications have included the *Treponema pallidum* Hemagglutination Assay or TPHA test, and an automated, qualitative microhemagglutination assay for *T. pallidum* antibodies, the AMHA–TP test. The latter procedure can also be performed equally well as a manual, qualitative or quantitative procedure, the MHA–TP test.

Hemagglutination tests for antibodies to *T. pallidum* are less expensive, easier to perform and easier to read than other treponemal tests. The MHA–TP test is now accepted as a reliable confirmatory treponemal test for syphilis and in some laboratories has replaced the FTA–ABS test as the routine treponemal confirmatory test. The MHA–TP test is less sensitive than the FTA–ABS test during the primary stage of syphilis but in the secondary, latent, and late stages the MHA–TP test compares favorably with the FTA–ABS test.

The comparative sensitivities of nontreponemal and treponemal tests in the various stages of untreated syphilis are summarized in Table 59-1. The FTA–ABS test is the most sensitive serologic test in primary syphilis. Because the VDRL test may be nonreactive in approximately 25% of patients with early primary syphilis, the FTA–ABS test may be helpful in the diagnosis of primary syphilis in selected instances. Similarly, because the VDRL test may be nonreactive in approximately 30% of patients with latent and late syphilis, the FTA–ABS test or MHA–TP test should be performed if the VDRL test is nonreactive and syphilis in these stages is suspected. Although the FTA–ABS test are especially useful in diagnosing syphilis, they are not useful for post-treatment follow-up. Quantitation of the FTA–ABS test is not practical and a titer cannot be followed. Moreover, the FTA–ABS test is positive in more than 80% of patients adequately treated for early syphilis as long as 2 years after treatment.

Since the MHA–TP test can be quantitated, obtaining titers does not seem to be advantageous because:

Table 59-1. ***Comparative Sensitivity of Nontreponemal and Treponemal Tests in Untreated Syphilis***

	Approximate % of Serums Expected to Give Reactive Test Results		
	NONTREPONEMAL	TREPONEMAL	
Stage of Syphilis	VDRL SLIDE, RPR CIRCLE CARD, ART	MHA-TP	FTA-ABS
Primary	76	65	90
Secondary	100	100	100
Latent	72	97	97
Late (tertiary)	70	95	95

(1) no relationship has been demonstrated between the titer and either the clinical stage or evolution of the disease; (2) titers obtained in untreated and treated patients overlap and are of little use in measuring response to therapy; and (3) the MHA–TP titers cannot be correlated with the titers of a quantitative nontreponemal test such as the quantitative VDRL. Futhermore, like the FTA–ABS test, the MHA–TP test shows little tendency for seroreversal after adequate therapy. Thus, the MHA–TP test would not be useful in evaluating response to therapy and cannot replace serial quantitative nontreponemal tests.

The FTA–ABS test or MHA–TP test should be used only to evaluate the serologic status of a patient. Once the diagnosis of either past or present syphilitic infection is made, the treponal tests are of little help and the physician must rely on clinical evaluation of the patient in conjunction with the information supplied by the quantitative nontreponemal tests.

FALSE-POSITIVE REACTIONS

False-positive reactions to nontreponemal tests are a major drawback. The titer of false-positive reactions is usually low but on rare occasions it is high; therefore, the level of the titer cannot be used to differentiate between a false-positive reaction and syphilis. Moreover, the antibodies responsible for false-positive reactions can cross the placenta and cause a false-positive test for syphilis in the newborn. The incidence of false-positive reactions depends upon the test employed and the population studied. Long lists of diseases linked with false-positive nontreponemal tests have been published. However, the present-day incidence of false-positive reactions probably much reduced as a result of the general use of newer, purified cardiolipin–lecithin–cholesterol antigens. In the older studies, very few patients were evaluated with the more specific treponemal tests, and many could have had both syphilis and a nonsyphilitic disease. Critical reexamination using the newer tests has been done with only a few diseases and it is difficult to compile a meaningful list of diseases or agents known to cause false-positive nontreponemal serologic tests for syphilis.

False-positive reactions occurring with the nontreponemal tests can be divided into two groups: (1) acute false-positive reactions of less than 6 months' duration and (2) chronic false-positive reactions which persist for more than 6 months. Acute false-positive nontreponemal reactions have been associated with hepatitis, infectious mononucleosis, viral pneumonia, chickenpox, measles, other viral infections, malaria, immunizations, pregnancy, and laboratory or technical error. Chronic false-positive reactions are narcotic addiction, aging, leprosy, and malignancy.

False-positive nontreponemal tests have also been obtained in apparently healthy persons. Patients who exhibit a false-positive reaction must be evaluated thoroughly to make certain they have no serious illness and should be followed closely for several years. The facile acceptance of a positive serologic test as a false-positive because the patient has a disease commonly associated with a false-positive reaction is dangerous because syphilis itself may be overlooked. Syphilis can coexist with many diseases. Only those patients without clinical, historical, or epidemiologic evidence of syphilis who have repeatedly reactive nontreponemal tests and a nonreactive FTA–ABS test on at least two separate occasions should be considered as having a false-positive reaction. If the FTA–ABS is reactive, a presumptive diagnosis of syphilis should be made. The patient with systemic lupus erythematosus may be an exception; in addition to a chronic false-positive nontreponemal test for syphilis, such a patient may have a false positive FTA–ABS test as well.

Though rare (less than 1%), false-positive FTA–ABS tests do occur—primarily in conditions associated with increased or abnormal immunoglobulins such as the autoimmune or connective-tissue diseases. Patients with systemic lupus erythematosus (SLE) can give false-positive FTA–ABS tests that exhibit an atypical, beading fluorescence pattern. Although the beading pattern was initially reported with lupus erythematosus, it can occur with other diseases. Borderline FTA–ABS reactions also occur in a significant number of patients with SLE; that is, a borderline FTA–ABS result is not conclusive evidence of syphilis and should not be interpreted as either reactive or nonreactive. Also, a small number of patients with SLE give a reactive FTA–ABS with the typical homogeneous pattern of fluorescence, indistinguishable from that normally seen in syphilis. False-positive, borderline, or atypical fluorescence has also been reported in drug-induced lupus erythematosus, drug addiction, smallpox vaccination, and pregnancy.

Presumably false-positive FTA–ABS tests must be viewed with caution. Syphilis is a relatively common disease, and a reactive FTA–ABS test might be the only evidence of it. Although the results of any laboratory test must be considered in light of the clinical evidence, a reactive FTA–ABS test must be considered indicative of syphilis until proven otherwise.

In general, the specificity of the MHA–TP test is probably equal to that of the FTA–ABS test and the rate of false-positive results is probably less than 1% of the normal population. False-positive or inconclusive hemagglutination tests have been reported in drug addicts and in patients with infectious mononucleosis, collagen disease, leprosy, and miscellaneous conditions associated with increased or abnormal immunoglobulins.

Cerebrospinal Fluid Examination

Three major determinations are necessary for the proper evaluation of the cerebrospinal fluid (CSF): (1) a cell count, (2) a total protein measurement, and (3) a VDRL slide test. More than 5 mononuclear cells/mm^3, a total protein in excess of 40 mg/100 ml, and a reactive VDRL are indicative of active central nervous system syphilis. The CSF cell count is the most reliable indicator of activity and of therapeutic response.

The sensitivity of the CSF–VDRL has been questioned and in an attempt to develop a more sensitive procedure, testing for treponemal antibodies in the CSF has been advocated. As in serologic tests for syphilis in blood, treponemal CSF tests are, in general, more sensitive than nontreponemal CSF tests. However, the clinical significance of the greater sensitivity offered by treponemal tests in CSF remains to be determined. At present, tests for treponemal antibodies on CSF should not be used to diagnose neurosyphilis without other supporting clinical and laboratory data.

Prognosis

The natural course of untreated, acquired syphilis and the response to nontreponemal serologic tests is depicted in a simplified manner in Figure 59-13. Approximately 25% of untreated patients experience one or more relapses with the development of infectious mucocutaneous lesions during the first 4 years of illness. At a later time, approximately one-third of untreated patients will develop manifestations of late syphilis; of these, approximately 15% develop late benign lesions, 10% cardiovascular lesions, and 8% central nervous system lesions. In addition, some patients develop lesions of one or more systems. The remaining two-thirds of the total number of untreated, infected persons do not develop clinically evident lesions, although in a number of these patients there is evidence of syphilis at autopsy. Many of these patients have nonreactive nontreponemal tests, but the occurence of an actual spontaneous cure, as evidenced by nonreactive treponemal tests, is doubtful. Also spontaneous seroreversal is not necessarily synonymous with spontaneous cure, and occasionally a patient may have active late syphilis but a nonreactive nontreponemal serologic test.

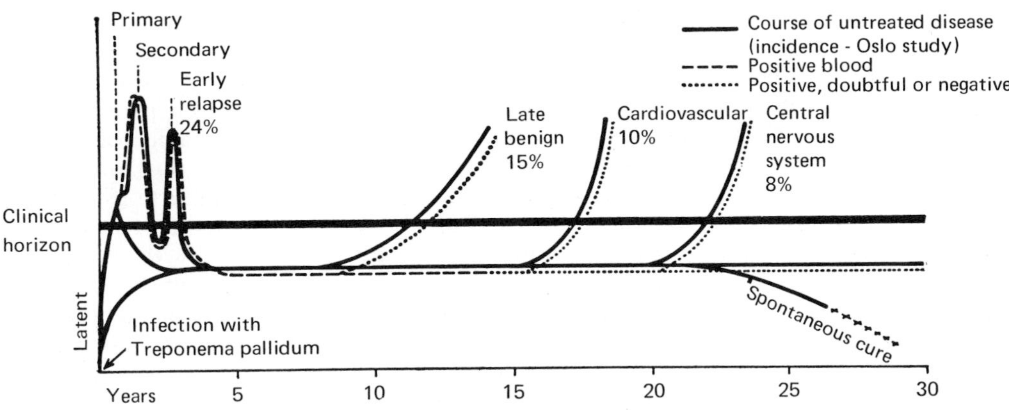

The clinical course of treated syphilis is dependent upon the length of time that the infection was present before treatment was initiated. Adequate treatment before the appearance of the chancre (as with epidemiologic treatment) will completely abort the disease before lesions are detectable. Adequate treatment and follow-up of primary, secondary, or early latent syphilis prevents crippling complications and death. However, many destructive lesions of late syphilis, such as aortic insufficiency, saccular aneurysms of the thoracic aorta, or the posterior column degeneration of tabes, dorsalis, and unresponsive to antimicrobial therapy.

Therapy

Acquried Syphilis

Parenteral penicillin is the treatment of choice for all stages of acquired syphilis. Benzathine penicillin G, penicillin aluminum monostearate (PAM), or aqueous procaine penicillin G are all effective. The schedules in the list below represent minimal therapy for various stages of syphilis. In most instances, benzathine penicillin G is preferred because adequate treatment can be given with a limited number of injections and, in the case of infectious syphilis, administered under direct supervision at the initial visit.

TREATMENT SCHEDULES FOR ACQUIRED SYPHILIS

Early Syphilis* and Contacts

Benzathine penicillin G: 2.4 million units total (1.2 million units in each buttock) by intramuscular injection

Aqueous procaine penicillin G: 4.8 million units total, given as 600,000 units by intramuscular injection daily for 8 days

Procaine penicillin G in oil with 2% aluminum monostearate (PAM)‡: 4.8 million units total usually given 2.4 million units (1.2 million units in each buttock) at the first visit and 1.2 million units at each of 2 subsequent injections 3 days apart

Late Syphilis†

Benzathine penicillin G: 7.2 million units total; 2.4 million units by intramuscular injection weekly for 3 successive weeks

Aqueous procaine penicillin G: 9.0 million units total; 600,000 units by intramuscular injection daily for 15 days

Alternatives for patients in whom penicillin is contraindicated

Early Syphilis* and Contacts

Tetracycline hydrochloride: 500 mg perorally 4 times a day for 15 days

Erythromycin (stearate, ethylsuccinate or base: as for tetracycline)

Late Syphilis†

Tetracycline hydrochloride: 500 mg perorally 4 times a day for 30 days

Erythromycin (stearate, ethylsuccinate, or base: as for tetracycline)

*Primary, secondary, and latent syphilis of less than 1 year's duration

†Includes latent syphilis of indeterminate or greater than 1 year's duration and late benign syphilis, cardiovascular syphilis, and asymptomatic and symptomatic neurosyphilis

‡PAM is not available in the United States

In general, the treatment of syphilis of more than one year's duration with either a total of 7.2 million units of benzathine penicillin G or 9 million units of aqueous procaine penicillin G is adequate. More penicillin provides no additional benefit. A possible exception is the patient with active symptomatic neurosyphilis. Because benzathine penicillin G and aqueous procaine penicillin G may not yield adequate concentrations in the cerebrospinal fluid when given intramuscularly, other forms of penicillin and routes of administration may be required. Thus, in those patients with active, symptomatic neurosyphilis or with neurosyphilis who do not respond to initial therapy, hospitalization may be necessary, at which time treatment may be given with 100 mg to 200 mg (160,000–320,000 units) /kg body wt/day, IV, as six equal portions, 4-hourly, for 10 days.

Although the clinical response to the treatment of early syphilis with chloramphenicol, erythromycin, doxycycline, or cephaloridine has been satisfactory, long-term follow-up of patients treated with these antimicrobics is not available. They are best reserved for special circumstances.

The treatment of a pregnant woman with syphilis is related to the stage of her syphilis; additional treatment is not necessary simply because the woman is pregnant. Erythromycin and not tetracycline should be used for the treatment of a pregnant woman who is allergic to penicillin. When erythromycin is used (30 mg/kg body wt/day, PO, as four equal portions, 6-hourly, for 30 days), especially careful follow-up is mandatory for both the mother and child.

The proper management of a patient with infectious syphilis does not end with the treatment of that patient alone. For every person with infectious syphilis, there is at least one other person with active syphilis. All contacts of the patient, from the beginning of the incubation period to the time of treatment, must be located, examined, and treated. Assistance in tracing contacts may be obtained from many local and state health agencies.

If a contact exhibits no manifestations of syphilis when first examined, the question often arises whether to treat purely on an epidemiologic basis or to follow the contact by reexamination at periodic intervals until a definite diagnosis is established or rejected. Experience has shown that waiting for signs and symptoms to develop or attempting to follow contacts is almost impossible. Approximately one-third of apparently uninfected contacts of a patient with infectious syphilis have syphilis in the incubation stage within 1 month of initial examination; if untreated, they develop infectious lesions. Even if not lost to follow-up, these persons develop infectious lesions between examinations and contribute to the spread of syphilis. This is especially true for promiscuous persons who will have many contacts before syphilis becomes apparent.

One of the major concerns with epidemiologic treatment is the possibility of allergic reactions to penicillin. Such reactions do occur, but are quite uncommon in patients treated in venereal disease clinics: approximately 0.06% of patients overall, with anaphylactoid reactions in about 0.04%.

Preventive or epidemiologic treatment is most easily accomplished with benzathine penicillin G, 2.4 million units administered intramuscularly as a single dose.

Prenatal Syphilis

Adequate treatment of the syphilitic mother before the 16th week of pregnancy prevents prenatal syphilis. Adequate treatment of the mother after the 16th week of pregnancy also treats the fetus *in utero* if fetal infection has occurred. Although treated, the infant may be marked by some of the stigmas of congenital syphilis, especially if therapy was not given until late in pregnancy.

Treatment of the infant with prenatal syphilis is divided into two treatment schedules, depending upon whether the cerebrospinal fluid findings are normal or abnormal (see Table 59-2). Antimicrobics other than penicillin should not be used in the treatment of infants with prenatal syphilis. Although the dose of either benzathine penicillin G or aqueous procaine penicillin G is the same for both neonatal and early postneonatal children, larger children need not receive more penicillin than is recommended for adults with syphilis of more than 1 year's duration.

Older children with congenital syphilis who are allergic to penicillin may be treated with erythromy-

Table 59-2. *Treatment Schedules for Congenital Syphilis*

Infants With Normal CSF	Infants With Abnormal CSF
Benzathine penicillin G—one injection of 50,000 units/kg body wt, IM	Aqueous crystalline penicillin G—50,000 units/kg body wt/day, IM or IV, as two equal portions, 12-hourly, for a minimum of 10 days or Aqueous procaine penicillin G— 50,000 units/kg body wt/day, IM, for a minimum of 10 days

cin or tetracycline. The total dose should be individualized depending upon the age and size of the child but should not exceed that used in adult syphilis of more than 1 year's duration. Tetracycline should not be given to children under 8 years of age because of the possible staining of the teeth and toxicity to bone. Children treated with tetracycline or erythromycin should be followed closely since the treatment of prenatal syphilis with these antimicrobics has not been adequately studied.

Post-treatment Follow-Up

ACQUIRED SYPHILIS

Post-treatment follow-up is essential in the management of the patient with acquired syphilis. Although penicillin is highly effective, treatment failures may occur and retreatment may be required. After treatment with any of the alternative antimicrobics, follow-up is particularly important to make certain that the treatment was adequate.

A quantitative nontreponemal test and not the FTA–ABS or MHA–TP test should be used to document the adequacy of treatment. Patients treated for primary and secondary syphilis should be followed with a quantitative VDRL at 3, 6, and 12 months. The treated latent and late syphilitic patients should be followed an additional 12 months at 6-month intervals.

The effect of treatment on the serologic titer of nontreponemal tests varies according to the stage and duration of disease at the time of treatment; not all adequately treated patients revert to seronegativity. Adequately treated seropositive primary syphilis should be followed by a progressive decline in titer; nearly all patients should exhibit a nonreactive VDRL within one year after treatment. Nearly all patients with adequately treated secondary syphilis should revert to a nonreactive VDRL within 2 years after treatment.

The response of the post-treatment titer in latent syphilis is unpredictable. In late latent or late syphilis, adequate treatment may sometimes result in a decrease or stabilization of the titer. If syphilis has gone untreated for more than 2 years, no amount of antimicrobial therapy will revert the serology to a nonreactive state; such patients are serofast for life.

All patients with neurosyphilis should be carefully followed at 6-month intervals for at least 3 years with clinical evaluations, full examinations of the CSF, and serological testing. A pregnant woman who has been treated for syphilis should have a quantitative nontreponemal serologic test at monthly intervals for the remainder of her pregnancy. Therapy of any stage of syphilis is considered a failure if any of the following occur: (1) the signs and symptoms of syphilis persist or return; (2) there is a 4-fold increase in the titer of the nontreponemal test, (3) a 4-fold decrease from an initially high-titer nontreponemal test does not occur within one year.

When treating patients with early syphilis, the possibility of reinfection should always be considered. Distinction between treatment failure and reinfection is often possible. A CSF examination should be performed before retreatment unless reinfection and a diagnosis of early syphilis can be established. If retreatment is required, the schedules recommended for syphilis of more than 1 year's duration should be followed. It should be kept in mind that some patients remain serofast despite adequate treatment and therefore usually only one retreatment course is indicated.

PRENATAL SYPHILIS

As in acquired syphilis, post-treatment follow-up is mandatory for the proper management of prenatal syphilis. A quantitative VDRL test should be obtained before treatment to establish a baseline titer. Serial quantitative VDRL tests should then be made to document a decrease in titer. In children treated for early congenital syphilis, these tests should be performed at monthly intervals for 6 months and then every third month for 1 year. Older children should be followed for an additional year at 6-month intervals. In general, early congenital syphilitic lesions heal rapidly, and the serologic titer usually reverts to a nonreactive state. In children 2 years or older when first treated, the titers may decrease very slowly; some patients may never revert to a nonreactive state, becoming serofast as occurs in acquired syphilis.

Persistent Treponemal Forms

The persistence of treponemes in aqueous humor, cerebrospinal fluid, lymph nodes, brain, arteries, and other tissues has been reported following treatment both with recommended and even larger doses of penicillin. Clinical findings suggestive of late syphilis were present in some cases although both nontreponemal and treponemal tests were negative. In a few cases, the virulence of these persistent treponemes has been documented by injecting them into rabbits in which they produced syphilitic lesions. Such findings may explain the persistence of antitreponemal antibody as measured by treponemal tests, but they do not provide a basis for altering the recommended treatment schedules for latent or late syphilis.

Jarisch–Herxheimer Reaction

The Jarisch–Herxheimer reaction may occur following treatment of any stage of syphilis, and patients should be warned to expect it. The patient with early infectious syphilis, especially secondary syphilis, is most likely to experience a reaction. Within hours after treatment is begun, the patient may experience transient fever and symptoms of malaise, chills, headache, and myalgia. An intensification of existing syphilitic lesions or exacerbation of old ones may occur. Cutaneous lesions of developing secondary syphilis first may be seen at this time. A transient neutrophilic leukocytosis occurs at the height of the reaction. In patients with syphilitic hepatitis, liver function tests may become markedly elevated. The reaction subsides within 24 hours, and its occurrence is not an indication for stopping treatment. Most reactions can be adequately managed by bed rest and aspirin.

Prevention

A vaccine against syphilis is still remote. Local prophylactic methods, such as thorough cleansing of the genitalia and adjacent areas with soap and water or the application of various chemicals, have limited effectiveness. Mechanical prophylaxis with condoms can be highly effective if properly used.

At present, the major means of preventing syphilis is through control programs that include such activities as syphilis epidemiology and serologic screening. Syphilis epidemiology is directed toward preventing the spread of infection by treating the contacts of infected persons, even though the contacts may have no manifestations of syphilis on initial examination. If the epidemiologic process is to work, however, all cases of infectious syphilis must be reported to state and local public health authorities. Thus, active involvement of the physician in private practice is needed; private physicians treat 80% of infectious syphilis but report only 20% of their cases to health departments.

Over 40% of primary cases, 50% of secondary cases, and 80% of early latent cases are detected because of either routine serologic testing or epidemiologic efforts. The latter consist of (1) interviewing and reinterviewing every reported case of early syphilis to identify sexual contacts (2) intensive effort by field workers to locate and offer medical examinations within a minimal period so that further spread of the disease is reduced, (3) counseling and blood testing of social-sexual peers who are possibly involved sexually in an infectious chain (cluster procedure), and (4) treatment of all sexual contacts of persons with infectious syphilis.

Finally, prenatal syphilis can be prevented through adequate prenatal care. Minimally, a serologic test for syphilis should be obtained during the first and third trimesters of pregnancy.

Remaining Problems

There are many problems still to be solved: more sensitive, specific, and inexpensive serologic screening tests for the early identification of syphilis need to be devised; the immunologic response to infection with *T. pallidum* should be defined; an effective vaccine remains to be developed. To accomplish these goals, large numbers of uncontaminated treponemes are needed; thus, the *in vitro* cultivation of *T. pallidum* is an urgent matter. At present, *T. palladium* must be extracted from the tissues of animals, so only small quantities of treponemes, which are invariably contaminated by tissue components from the donor animal, are available. Safe and effective topical or systemic prophylactic agents for syphilis are also needed. The role of persistent treponemal forms and their relationship to the production of disease, serologic reactivity, and therapeutic efficacy remain to be elucidated. Finally, problems remain in venereal disease education both at the public and professional levels. Research into the best means of distributing venereal disease information and the best ways to motivate persons to seek medical help is needed. Also, the problem of providing adequate training at both the undergraduate and postgraduate levels in clinical, epidemiologic, and social aspects of syphilis remains to be solved.

Bibliography

Journals

BIRRY A, KASATIYA S: Evaluation of microhemagglutination assay to determine treponemal antibodies in CSF. Br J Vener Dis 55:239–244, 1979

BREASETTE M: The laboratory diagnosis of congenital syphilis: A review. Am J Med Technol 45:645–646, 1979

CAMPISI D, WHITCOMB C: Liver disease in early syphilis. Arch Intern Med 139:365–366, 1979

DANIELS KC, FERNEYHOUGH HS: Specific direct fluorescent antibody detection of *Treponema pallidum.* Health Lab Sci 14:164–171, 1977

DANS, PR, JUDSON FN, LARSEN SA, LANTZ MA: The FTA–ABS test: A diagnostic help or hindrance? South Med J 70:312–315, 1977

FITZGERALD T: Editorial: The future of tissue culture methods for growth of *Treponema pallidum* in vitro. Sex Transm Dis 7:97–99, 1980

FIUMARA NJ: Serologic responses to treatment of 128 patients with late latent syphilis. Sex Transm Dis 6:243—246, 1979

FIUMARA NJ: Treatment of seropositive primary syphilis: An evaluation of 196 patients. Sex Transm Dis 4:92—95, 1977

FIUMARA NJ: Treatment of secondary syphilis: An evaluation of 204 patients. Sex Transm Dis 4:96–99, 1977

FIUMARA NJ, LESSELL S: Manifestations of late congenital syphilis. An analysis of 271 patients. Arch Dermatol 102:78–83, 1970

GRAVES S, BILLINGTON T: Optimum concentration of dissolved oxygen for the survival of virulent *Treponema pallidum* under conditions of low oxidation-reduction potential. J Vener Dis 55:387–393, 1979

JAFFE HW, LARSEN SA, PETERS M, JOVE DF, LOPEZ B, SCHROETER AL: Tests for treponemal antibody in CSF. Arch Intern Med 138: 252–255, 1978

THE JARISCH–HERXHEIMER REACTION. Lancet 1:340–341, 1977

KAUFMAN RE, OLANSKY DC, WIESNER PJ: The FTA–ABS (IgM) test for neonatal congenital syphilis: A critical review. J Am Vener Dis :79–84, 1974

LEE TJ, SPARLING PF: Syphilis: An Algorithm. JAMA 242:1187–1189, 1979

MACKEY DM, PRICE EV, KNOX JM, SCOTTI A: Specificity of the FTA–ABS test for syphilis: An evaluation. JAMA 207:1683–1685, 1969

MCGEENEY T, YOUNT F, HINTORN DR, LIU C: Utility of the FTA–ABS test of cerebrospinal fluid in the diagnosis of neurosyphilis. Sex Transm Dis 6:195–198, 1979

METZGER M: THEME 2: recent advances in the immunology of syphilis: Role of humoral versus cellular mechanisms of resistance in the pathogenesis of syphilis. Br J Vener Dis 55:94–98, 1979

MORRISON GD, EGGLESTONE SI, NORTHWOOD JL: Cultivation of *Treponema pallidum* in subcutaneous chambers implanted in golden hamster. Br J Vener Dis 55:320–324, 1979

RUDOLPH AH: Antibiotic treatment of venereal diseases: Update 1979. Internat Soc Trop Dermat Inc 18:797–804, 1979

RUDOLPH AH: The microhemagglutination assay for *Treponema pallidum* antibodies (MHA–TP test): Where does it fit? J Am Vener Dis 3:3–9, 1976

RUDOLPH AH: Serological diagnosis of syphilis: An update. South Med J 69:1196–1198, 1976

RUDOLPH AH, PRICE EV: Penicillin reactions among patients in venereal disease clinics: A national survey. JAMA 223:499–501, 1973

SCHROETER AL, LUCAS JB, PRICE EV, FALCONE VH: Treatment for early syphilis and reactivity of serological tests. JAMA 221:471–476, 1972

SOBEL HJ, WOLF EH: Liver involvement in early syphilis. Arch Pathol 93:565–568, 1972

STERZEL RB, KRAUSE PH, SOBEL HJ, KUHN K: Acute syphilitic nephrosis: A transient glomerular immunopathy. Clin Nephrol 2:164–168, 1974

SYPHILIS: CDC Recommended Treatment Schedule, 1976

WILLCOX RR: Recent advances in venereology. I. Syphilis. Br J Clin Pract 27:115–120, 1973

Section | *XI*

Infections of the Digestive Tract

Species or Group	Mouth			Lower Intestine		
	PREDENTULOUS	SALIVA-TOOTH SURFACES	GINGIVAL CREVICE	UPPER LEVELS	FECES	
					INFANT	ADULT
Mycoplasmas		+				+
Bacteria						
Gram-positive cocci						
Staphylococcus epidermidis	+	**75–100*** 1–4/ml			**31–59†**	+ 2–4/g
Staphylococcus aureus		+ 16–35		+	**10–93‖**	**30–50‡**
Anaerobic micrococci		+		+		
Streptococcus mitis; undifferentiated α and γ streptococci	++	**100** 6–8/ml	**100** 6/mg	+	**14–32**	+
Streptococcus hominis (salivarius)	**100**	**100** 7/ml	++	+	**0–6**	+
Enterococci or group D *Streptococcus* spp.	+	**4–22**[a]		+	**87** 6–9/g	**100** 3–8/g
Streptococcus pyogenes (usually group A unless noted)		**12–68**[b] 3–6/ml[b]			**0.7–19**[c]	**16**[d]
Anaerobic *Streptococcus* spp.	+	++	++ 6/mg			+
Streptococcus pneumoniae	+	**26**				
Gram-negative cocci						
Branhamella catarrhalis *Gemella haemolysans*		**95–100** 5–7/ml	+			
Veillonella alkalescens	+	**100** 6–8/ml	+			
Gram-positive bacilli						
Lactobacillus spp.	+	**95**[e] 0–6/ml		+		**20–60**[e] –7/g
Aerobic *Corynebacterium* spp.		**59**			**10–21**	**6**
Propionibacterium acnes	±					
Mycobacterium spp.						+
Clostridium perfringens		±		++	**13–19**	**25–35**
Clostridium tetani						**1–35**
Other *Clostridium* spp.						**5–25**
Eubacterium limosum						**30–70**
Bifidobacterium bifidum						**30–70**
Actinomyces bifidus	+	+			**15–60**[f] **90**[g] 7–11/g[g]	
Actinomyces israelii		+	+			
Leptotrichia buccalis		++ 0–3/ml	++			
Aerobic gram-negative bacilli						
Enterobacteriaceae	+	**65** 0–3/ml			**86–100** 7–9/g	**100** 5–8/g
Escherichia coli		**4.2**		++	**67–99**	**100**
Enterobacter spp.		**31**			**28–52**	**40–80**
Klebsiella spp.		**52**		++	**19–48**	**40–80**
Proteus mirabilis, other *Proteus* spp., *Morganella morganii* *Providencia* spp.	+				**48**	**5–55** –6/g
Pseudomonas aeruginosa					+	*3–11*
Alcaligenes faecalis		±			**0–2.1**	+

Species or Group	Mouth			Lower Intestine		
					FECES	
	PREDENTULOUS	SALIVA-TOOTH SURFACES	GINGIVAL CREVICE	UPPER LEVELS	INFANT	ADULT
***Bacteria** (cont.)*						
Haemophilus influenzae		**25–100**				
Haemophilus parainfluenzae		**25**				±
Hemolytic *Haemophilus* spp.		+				
Anaerobic gram-negative bacilli						
Bacteroides fragilis (5 subspecies)		+	+	+		**100** 7–10/g
Bacteroides melaninogenicus (3 subspecies)		+	+ 6/mg			**100**
Bacteroides oralis (2 subspecies)		+	+			**100**
Fusobacterium nucleatum	+	**15–90** 3–5/ml	+ 4/mg			**100**
Fusobacterium necrophorum			+			**100**
Curved bacteria						
Selenomonas sputigena	±	+	+			+?
Campylobacter sputorum	±	+	+			
Treponema denticola			**60–88**	+	**18**[h]	**28**
Treponema refringens		+	6/mg			
Fungi						
Candida albicans		**5–50** 0–5/ml	**15–40**		+	**1–3** 0–4/g
non-albicans *Candida* spp.		**1–4**				**1–12**
Torulopsis glabrata		+				+
Protozoa						
Entamoeba gingivalis			**0–72.6**			
Entamoeba coli						**8.0–32.1**[i]
Endolimax nana						**9.3–16.0**
Dientamoeba fragilis						**0.2–5.9**
Iodamoeba buetschlii						**1.4–5.0**
Trichomonas tenax			**4.0–33.8**			
Trichomonas hominis						**0.3–4.1**
Giardia lamblia						**2.9–14.7** **17.6**[#]
Chilomastix mesnili						**0.4–6.1**
Enteromonas hominis						**0.1–3.2**
Retortamonas intestinalis						**0.1–1.3**

± to 0, rare; ±, irregular or uncertain (may be only pathologic); +, common; ++, prominent.
* Boldface values (*e.g.,* **30–60**) = range of incidence in percentage, rounded, in different surveys.
† Predominant first day; decreasing during first month.
‡ Associated with nasal carriage.
§ Percentage of strains isolated.
|| In infants and children; highest in hospital nursery infants.
Children.
a More common below age 20.
b Associated with presence in throat.
c "Hemolytic": Lancefield group not given.
d Groups B, C, F, and G; no A.
e Especially in dental caries.
f Bottlefed infants.
g Breastfed infants.
h After the second week.
i Values in this column are for North America and western Europe.

RICHARD B. HORNICK

Gastroenterocolitis Syndromes

60

Exposed to every variety of infectious agent, the digestive tract is also beset with ingested toxic materials (Table 60-1). Some are preformed in food by microbial action; others are contained in medications, chemical products for industrial and domestic applications, poisonous plants and animals, and irritant and toxic food and drink. Even allergies and emotional stresses affect the gut. Acute illnesses caused by these agents may be clinically homogeneous—the gastroenterocolitis syndromes characterized by abdominal distress and diarrhea, often with nausea and vomiting. Although one region may be the particular focus of disease, the gut is continuous and disease of one portion is reflected to a greater or lesser extent throughout the digestive tract.

Gastroenteritis Syndrome

Gastroenteritides are usually self-limited and may be caused by a variety of infectious and toxic agents. The vast majority of outbreaks of microbial origin in which a specific cause is identified are caused by bacteria. Two general varieties are recognized: intoxications caused by the ingestion of preformed toxins produced by microorganisms growing in contaminated foods, and true infections, requiring the ingestion and proliferation of microorganisms to produce illness.

Preformed Toxins

STAPHYLOCOCCAL FOOD POISONING

Staphylococcal food poisoning results from the ingestion of an enterotoxin preformed by toxinogenic *Staphylococcus aureus* growing in contaminated food. It is a common cause of bacterial food poisoning in the United States (see Table 60-1). However, because the illness is of short duration and complete recovery occurs in most cases, it is usually not recognized unless many people are involved.

Etiology. Staphylococcal enterotoxin is an exotoxin elaborated by only a few strains of *S. aureus,* often of phage groups III and IV and particularly of phage types 6/47 and 42D. Despite the frequency of phage groups III and IV in enterotoxin-producing strains, most isolates of these phage groups do not produce enterotoxin. Coagulase-negative staphylococci rarely produce enterotoxin. The cultural and biochemical characteristics of enterotoxinogenic staphylococci do not differ in any significant way from other strains of *S. aureus,* except that nearly all produce penicillinase, even those isolated before 1941. Although the biologic activity of enterotoxin can be assessed in human and nonhuman primates and in kittens, serologic methods are preferable. At least five antigenically distinct types of enterotoxin have been identified, and it is probable that there are others. Types A and B are the most common; both have been purified, as has type C. The toxins are water-soluble, low molecular weight proteins that can produce illness in man even after being boiled for 30 minutes or refrigerated for many months.

Epidemiology. Humans are the most important sources of enterotoxin-producing staphylococci, and in outbreaks of staphylococcal food poisoning it is usually possible to isolate identical staphylococci from the suspected food and from the hands of a person involved in its preparation. Often only minor skin lesions are present; occasionally, nasal carriers are implicated. Outbreaks apparently have originated in fresh cow's or goat's milk; animals need not have clinical mastitis to excrete *S. aureus* from the udder. Staphylococcal food poisoning has followed the consumption of a wide variety of foods that have in common only the capacity to support the vigorous growth of *S. aureus.* Foods previously sterilized by cooking apparently support the growth of staphylococci better than uncooked foods. Custard-filled bakery goods, canned foods, and processed meats are most commonly responsible for infections. Cheese,

Table 60-1. *Confirmed Food-borne Disease Outbreaks, Cases, and Deaths by Etiology in the United States in 1979*

Etiology	Outbreaks		Cases		Deaths
	NUMBER	%	NUMBER	%	NUMBER
VIRAL					
Hepatitis (non-B)	5	(2.9)	74	(1.0)	–
Other Viral	1	(0.6)	155	(2.1)	–
Subtotal	6	(3.5)	229	(3.1)	0
BACTERIAL					
Brucella spp.	2	(1.2)	18	(0.2)	–
Clostridium botulinum	7	(4.0)	9	(0.1)	–
Clostridium perfringens	20	(11.6)	1110	(15.0)	5
Enterobacter cloacae	1	(0.6)	37	(0.5)	–
Salmonella spp.	44	(25.6)	2794	(37.9)	–
Shigella spp.	7	(4.0)	356	(4.8)	1
Staphylococcus aureus	34	(19.8)	2391	(32.4)	–
Streptococcus spp. Group G	1	(0.6)	73	(1.0)	–
Vibrio cholerae (non-01)	1	(0.6)	5	(0.1)	–
Vibrio parahaemolyticus	2	(1.2)	14	(0.2)	–
Subtotal	119	(69.2)	6806	(92.3)	6
METAZOAL					
Trichinella spiralis	11	(6.4)	93	(1.3)	–
CHEMICAL					
Heavy metals	1	(0.6)	18	(0.2)	–
Ciguatoxin	18	(10.4)	85	(1.2)	–
Scombrotoxin	12	(6.9)	132	(1.8)	–
Mushroom poisoning	1	(0.6)	2	(0.03)	–
Other chemical	4	(2.3)	13	(0.2)	–
Subtotal	36	(20.9)	250	(3.4)	0
	172	(100.0)	7378	(100.0)	6

Centers for Disease Control, Foodborne Disease Surveillance, Annual Summary, 1979

dried beef, sausage, ham, tongue, potato salad, meat pies, ice cream, and a variety of frozen foods have also been implicated. Foods containing sufficient enterotoxin to produce violent illness are usually normal in appearance, odor, and taste.

Pathogenesis and Pathology. Enterotoxins apparently have no local effect on the digestive tract. They must be absorbed to reach the central nervous system, presumably by way of the blood. There are no characteristic gross or microscopic pathologic changes in the digestive tract or the central nervous system. The disease can be reproduced by the parenteral injection of enterotoxins.

Manifestations. The symptoms of staphylococcal food poisoning appear 1 to 6 hours after ingesting food containing enterotoxin. The incubation period and the severity of symptoms are influenced by the amount of enterotoxin ingested. In addition, there is considerable variation in the susceptibility of persons, but the factors responsible have not been well defined. The first symptom is usually increased salivation, followed by nausea, vomiting, abdominal cramps, and diarrhea. Headache, sweating, chills, and muscular cramps are occasionally seen, but fever is not present unless there are complications. In severe cases, blood and mucus may be present in the vomitus and feces, and severe prostration, even shock, may occur.

Diagnosis. An acute gastrointestinal illness in a group of persons 1 to 6 hours after eating the same meal is strongly suggestive of staphylococcal food poisoning. Of those who ingest contaminated food, only a few will escape clinical illness. The rapidity of onset and lack of neurologic symptoms aid in distinguishing the illness from botulism. Isolated cases of severe staphylococcal food poisoning may occasionally be confused with acute abdominal crises such as acute cholecystitis, perforated peptic ulcer, severe gastritis, or appendicitis.

Potentially contaminated food should be examined by Gram-stained smear (an abundance of gram-positive cocci), culture (luxuriant growth of *S. aureus*), and testing for enterotoxin. The latter is particularly important because staphylococci may have been rendered nonviable by heat. Serologic assays employing gel diffusion, fluorescent antibody, and passive hemagglutination—inhibition techniques have recently been developed as tests for the presence of enterotoxin. However, none of these methods is either a routine or readily available test. The older methods of testing food for enterotoxin in volunteers, nonhuman primates, or kittens are often the only methods available. A less satisfactory course involves growing *S. aureus* isolated from foods in cultures, followed by the assay of whole cultures or filtrates, either serologically, or by enteral or parenteral administration to rhesus monkeys or kittens.

Therapy. In severe cases, particularly in the young or debilitated, dehydration can be severe, and the IV injection of solutions containing potassium and sodium chloride are necessary. Because neither antimicrobial nor serum therapy has been shown to be of value, neither is indicated.

Prognosis. In most patients, the symptoms subside within 8 hours, and recovery is complete in 1 to 3 days. Rarely, shock and death result from severe dehydration in infants and debilitated persons.

Prevention. Staphylococcal food poisoning depends on three factors: (1) the food must be contaminated with an enterotoxin-producing strain of *S. aureus,* (2) it must be nutritionally adequate for the growth of *S. aureus* and for the production of enterotoxin, and (3) it must remain at or above room temperature for several hours. Because enterotoxin is not formed in significant quantities at temperatures below 6.7°C, the best preventive measure is refrigeration of all perishable foods. Furthermore, food distributed in bulk lots must be handled so that refrigeration temperatures are rapidly attained throughout the food. In addition, workers should be excluded from handling food products when they have active staphylococcal lesions. Reheated foods should not be allowed to stand for long periods before being served.

BOTULISM

Botulism is discussed separately in Chapter 127, Botulism.

Actual Infections

VIRUSES

The exact incidence of virus-caused gastroenteritis is unknown. Overall, the highest attack rates of diarrheal diseases occur in infants and children under the age of 5 years. Although it is suspected that much of this illness is caused by viral agents, in children as in adults, failure of isolation of enteric bacterial pathogens from the feces is not in itself sufficient to affix the label of viral gastroenteritis or viral diarrhea. For example, enterotoxins produced by coliform bacteria but not readily detected by current methods may be implicated. Or, bacteria that require special conditions for isolation may be missed or not identified.

In some cases, the association of gastroenteritis with viruses may reflect no more than coincidence. Thus, adenoviruses detected by electron microscopy in the feces of infants and young children with nosocomial enteritis were not recovered in cell cultures of the same specimens. Possibly, the adenoviruses found by electron microscopy actually came from the respiratory tract, were swallowed, and inactivated in the stomach.

Reoviruslike Agent. The reoviruslike agent (HRVLA), also called rotavirus, duovirus, orbiviruslike, and infantile gastroenteritis virus, is about 70 nm in diameter and occurs worldwide, causing about 50% of the enteritis in hospitalized children. Hospital outbreaks have occurred among pediatric patients, and adults in contact with sick children may develop subclinical infections. Fecal–oral transmission is important. The incubation period is about 48 hours. The peak incidence is in the winter months.

In specimens obtained by duodenal biopsy, there may be mild to severe alterations of the mucosal architecture with shortening of villi and hyperplasia of crypts. Mononuclear cells and polymorphonuclear leukocytes infiltrate the lamina propria, and the surface cells contain vacuoles and appear to be cuboidal. By electron microscopy, HRVLA particles may be demonstrated in epithelial cells. Infants with these changes may have malabsorption of d-xylose.

The clinical manifestations of disease caused by HRVLA are not distinctive. Nausea and vomiting may precede diarrhea. Dehydration is common, and fever is present in about 75% of patients. Erythema of the pharyngeal mucosa and the tympanic membrane has been described. The disease may last 5 to 8 days.

Sophisticated serodiagnostic methods have been developed but are not readily available. However, a complement fixation test employing virus of nonhuman origin but similar to HRVLA may become widely used. Immunity usually develops by the time a person is 4 to 5 years of age; the basis for this acquired resistance is not known.

Parvoviruslike Agents. Parvoviruslike agents (PLA) are about 27 nm in diameter. Three groups are distinguished by place names of recognized outbreaks of disease in the United States: Norwalk, Hawaii, and Montgomery County, Maryland.

The disease, consisting of nausea, vomiting, and diarrhea (in various combinations) afflicted about 50% of the children of elementary schools. The incubation period was about 48 hours. The virus was disseminated by fecal–oral transmission or by contaminated water supplies—a route causing widespread epidemics. The so-called winter vomiting disease or viral diarrhea may be caused by PLA.

The enteric histopathology of PLA infections is identical with that of HRVLA except that viral particles in epithelial cells are unable to be detected by electron microscopy. Volunteers infected with PLA have malabsorption of fat and glucose.

As immune electron microscopy is the only diagnostic laboratory test currently available, proof of PLA causation of enteritis is possible only in certain research laboratories.

Prior illness does not guarantee resistance to reinfection; perhaps this is a reflection of lack of antibody synthesis in the gut.

BACTERIA

Clostridium perfringens. *Clostridium perfringens* is a major cause of food poisoning. In 1973, *C perfringens* accounted for about 3% of the reported food-borne disease outbreaks in the United States (Tables 60-1).

The disease is associated with the ingestion of strains of *C. perfringens* of type A that are capable of forming heat-resistant spores. These strains are widespread in nature, and they have been isolated from a high proportion of samples of raw meat, animal feces, and occasionally from the feces of healthy persons. Outbreaks of clostridial food poisoning are usually associated with products such as gravy that provide an anaerobic environment. The meat is cooked at a temperature that enables the spores to survive; it is then allowed to stand at temperatures that encourage germination and growth. Although the disease has been produced experimentally in humans and lambs after the ingestion of vegetative *C. perfringens,* but not after the ingestion of supernatant fluid from cultures, it is probable that actual food poisoning is caused as much by preformed toxin as by actual replication of *C. perfringens* in the gut.

Symptoms usually appear within 10 to 24 hours after ingestion of the contaminated food (range 8–24 hours). Crampy abdominal pain and diarrhea are the major symptoms; nausea and vomiting are rare. Fever, headache, and other signs or symptoms of infection are seldom prominent. The illness is of short duration, usually subsiding in less than 24 hours. The diagnosis is established by finding large numbers of *C. perfringens* in anaerobic cultures of the incriminated food. It is often possible to isolate the same bacterium from the feces of affected persons. Treatment is symptomatic, and no specific therapy is indicated.

A rare type of clostridial food poisoning termed enteritis necroticans occurs after the ingestion of foods heavily contaminated with type F strains of *C. perfringens.* This illness is characterized by an acute onset of severe abdominal pain, vomiting, diarrhea, prostration and shock; it may be rapidly fatal. Postmortem examination reveals a diffuse, necrotizing enteritis of the jejunum, ileum, and colon.

Food poisoning from *C. perfringens* is best prevented by avoiding long periods of warming or cooling of foods that have already been cooked. If foods are to stand for more than 10 hours before being served, they should be stored at temperatures above 60°C or below 5°C.

Vibrio parahaemolyticus. *Vibrio parahaemolyticus* bacilli are gram-negative, facultative anaerobes that can be cultured readily on ordinary mediums if 1% to 3% sodium chloride is added. These enteropathogenic, halophilic bacteria were first isolated in an outbreak of food poisoning in Japan in 1951, and now as many as 70% of cases of bacterial gastroenteritis in Japan are caused by these bacteria. Outbreaks have also been documented in the United States.

These vibrios have been found in the coastal sea waters of the United States, Japan, and other Pacific nations. The causative foodstuff in vibrio food poisoning is associated directly or indirectly with sea fish or sea water. Raw fish is the most important vehicle in Japan, whereas cooked seafood is the usual source in the United States. Vibrio gastroenteritis occurs only during the warmer months of the year, when there are large numbers of vibrios present in the coastal sea waters and when bacterial multiplication in unrefrigerated food is favored.

Vibrio parahaemolyticus appears to be pathogenic only for man. The vibrios are not found in the feces of asymptomatic persons. From epidemiologic and clinical studies, it has been found that the gastroenteritis produced by the vibrios is infectious rather than toxic in origin. Only vibrios that are hemolytic *in vitro* are enteropathogenic for man. The diagnosis is established by isolating *V. parahaemolyticus* from the feces or vomitus of patients.

Symptoms usually appear 12 hours after the ingestion of contaminated food, but the incubation period can range from 2 to 48 hours. The most prominent symptoms are abdominal pain, diarrhea, nausea, and vomiting. Mild fever, chills, and headache are often present. The symptoms may be clinically indistinguishable from gastroenteritis caused by *Salmonella* spp. or *Shigella* spp.

Recovery is usually complete within 2 to 5 days. The fatality rate is very low, and most deaths occur in old, debilitated patients.

Bacillus cereus. *Bacillus cereus* is a spore-forming, gram-positive, aerobic bacillus incriminated in several outbreaks of food poisoning. Illness has been produced in a volunteer after the ingestion of large numbers of viable *B. cereus* but not after the ingestion of culture filtrates. The incubation period is about 10 hours. The symptoms include abdominal pain, profuse watery diarrhea, rectal tenesmus, and nausea. Fever and vomiting are quite uncommon. The duration of the illness is about 12 hours, and no specific therapy is indicated.

Miscellaneous Microorganisms. Several microorganisms have been implicated as etiologic agents in outbreaks of food poisoning. In most cases, the isolation of large numbers of a specific microorganism from food suspected of contamination has been the basis for the implication. When the isolate is part of the normal fecal flora, it is extremely difficult to prove a causative role. It is on such grounds that food-borne outbreaks have been attributed to enterococci, *Proteus* spp., *Klebsiella* spp., *Providencia* spp., *Citrobacter* spp., *Actinomyces* spp., *Pseudomonas* spp., and *Enterobacter* spp.

Enterocolitis Syndrome

The enterocolitis syndrome is characterized by diarrhea, inflammation, ulcerations, and even pseudomembrane formation, primarily in the large bowel and in some patients also in the lower small bowel. Several etiologic agents and predisposing factors are now recognized, although some aspects of this syndrome are still not well understood.

Salmonellosis, Shigellosis, and Cholera

Salmonella spp. (Chap. 63 and 64, Nontyphoidal Salmonelloses and Typhoid Fever), *Shigella* spp. (Chap. 62, Shigellosis), and *Vibrio cholerae* (Chap. 65, Cholera) are important causes of the enterocolitis syndrome. The incubation periods may be as long as 48 hours, and fever is typical. Diarrhea is often prominent.

Escherichia coli

Enterocolitis caused by *Escherichia coli* is discussed in Chapter 61, Diarrheal Disease Caused by *Escherichia coli.*

Campylobacteriosis

Campylobacter fetus, subspecies *jejuni,* was formerly called *Vibrio fetus.* These curved, bent bacilli are not true vibrios, although they do cause enterocolitis. The reservoir appears to be nonhuman animals, both domestic and wild. Humans become infected through contaminated food, water, and raw milk. The epidemiology of campylobacteriosis is not completely worked out, but human-to-human transmission is probably not essential to maintenance of the *Campylobacter* spp., although from 5% to 10% of humans may shed campylobacters in their feces as long as one year after the acute disease.

The heat-stable enterotoxin elaborated by *C. fetus* ss. *jejuni* is similar in its activity to the heat-stable enterotoxin of *E. coli.* This enterotoxin appears to be responsible for the diarrhea.

Watery diarrhea is the most common manifestation of campylobacteriosis. Indeed, in children worldwide, *C. fetus* ss. *jejuni* are the most common cause of the diarrheas previously labeled nonspecific (up to 30%). In these children, the infection is probably confined to the proximal small bowel, and the enterotoxin induces the diarrhea. Because *C. fetus* ss. *jejuni* penetrates the epithelial barrier, the resulting inflammatory response may provide the mediator(s) that stimulate or enhance the production and transfer of liquid into the lumen of the gut to cause diarrhea.

Involvement of the colon results in a friable, edematous mucosa that may become ulcerated. The gross appearance, as seen through an endoscope, may in some patients be suggestive of ulcerative colitis. Colitis represents the severest form of enteric campylobacteriosis. Rarely, bacteremia, hepatitis, and pneumonitis may complicate the enterocolitis caused by *C. fetus* ss. *jejuni* (in marked contrast, *C. fetus,* subspecies *intestinalis* does not cause diarrhea in humans, but causes disseminated disease).

The diagnosis of campylobacteriosis depends on

the isolation of *C. fetus* ss. *jejuni* from feces or blood. Because they are slow-growing and fastidious bacteria, a selective medium should be inoculated as a routine in the work-up of any patient with enterocolitis. Brucella agar containing 10% sheep blood is satisfactory when fortified with vancomycin (10 μg/ml), polymyxin B (2.5 IU/ml), trimethoprim (5 μg/ml), and cephalothin (15 μg/ml).

Erythromycin is uniquely active against *C. fetus* ss. *jejuni.* Treatment with this drug (30 mg/kg body wt/day, PO, as four equal portions, 6-hourly, for 1 week beyond defervescence) promptly diminish the symptoms and shortens the period of diarrhea. Supportive management with replacement of fluids and electrolytes by IV injection is sometimes necessary, especially in the very young and the very old. The mortality rate is generally low in patients at the extremes of age and at the greatest risk of death.

Yersiniosis

Yersinia enterocolitica may occasionally cause an enterocolitis that can be confused with acute appendicitis because of abdominal pain, fever, diarrhea, vomiting, and leukocytosis. Histologically, there is necrosis of intestinal epithelium resulting in the formation of ulcers. Failure to isolate *Y. enterocolitica* may reflect failure to distinguish it from other enteric bacteria Although *Y. enterocolitica* may ferment sucrose, colonies on eosin—methylene blue or MacConkey mediums may appear to be nonfermentive. In addition to enterocolitis, *Y. enterocolitica* may cause mesenteric adenitis, ileitis, or acute appendicitis. In some studies, dogs were shown to be the source of the organism. Clinicians should be aware of *Y. enterocolitica* and should alert the clinical microbiology laboratory to the possibility of the infection so that appropriate methods for isolation can be applied. The mortality rate from this infection has not been defined, but *Y. enterocolitica* infections are generally severe. Previously healthy persons may rapidly develop life-threatening disease.

Antimicrobic-Associated Syndromes

Clarification of the pathogenesis of some of the enterocolitis syndromes that may develop following the administration of antimicrobics has provided a rational basis for treatment, and an extension of knowledge of the role of enterotoxins in causing diarrhea.

ETIOLOGY

Formerly, it was taught that staphylococci were common causes of enterocolitis. However, in recent years, this organism has rarely been implicated, and indeed, the evidence supporting a staphylococcal etiology is inconclusive. The major cause of antimicrobic-associated colitis now appears to be strains of enterotoxin-producing *Clostridium difficile.* Perhaps some other components of the anaerobic flora of the colon are involved in some cases.

EPIDEMIOLOGY

Clostridum difficile are anaerobic, gram-positive bacilli that are normal components of the fecal flora in 2% to 8% of humans. They are resistant to most antimicrobics and may grow to huge numbers (10^4–10^6 colony forming units/gram of feces) when antimicrobics inhibit bacterial competitors. In hamsters, homogenates of cecal contents (consisting primarily of anaerobes) suppress the growth of *C. difficile* and prevent the development of antimicrobic-induced colitis. Moreover, *C. difficile* can be cultured from the diarrheal feces of 95% of patients with antimicrobic-associated pseudomembranous colitis (PMC).

Although virtually all antimicrobics have been implicated in the development of PMC, clindamycin and ampicillin have been associated with PMC most frequently. Both perorally and parenterally administered antimicrobics can produce the disease. The dose and duration of the antimicrobial therapy have not been regularly correlated with the development of PMC.

The risk of developing antimicrobic-associated enterocolitis appears to increase with increasing age.

PATHOGENESIS AND PATHOLOGY

Enterotoxin-producing strains of *C. difficile* cause a lethal typhilitis when experimental animals are also given clindamycin. Intracecal injections of either whole broth cultures or cell-free filtrates of such cultures reproduce the disease. The enterotoxin is cytopathic in tissue cultures and stimulates the adenylate cyclase system, augmenting the secretory activity of epithelial cells.

Pseudomembranous enterocolitis varies in extent from discrete to confluent, with the latter a life-threatening consequence of the administration of antimicrobics. Regardless of extent, the pseudomembrane consists primarily of inflammatory cells plus fibrin, and is adherent to the denuded surface of the distal colon. The intervening mucosa is marked by hemorrhagic inflammation.

In three other forms of antimicrobic-associated diarrhea, pseudomembranes are not identifiable by endoscopy with biopsies. The mildest and most common form is diarrhea with normal colonic mucosa.

Frequently, the diarrhea ensues after the antimicrobic (usually clindamycin) has been stopped. In only about 20% of these patients, the enterotoxin of *C. difficile* will be detected in the feces. This may explain why there is no evidence of inflammation of the colonic mucosa. The cause(s) of the diarrhea in the other 80% of the patients is unknown.

A second group of patients has a nonspecific colitis with erythema, edema, and mild congestion, as observed by inspection and histology. A third group develops ulcerative proctitis or colitis with a friable, granular, or hemorrhagic mucosa seen at endoscopy, and a round cell infiltration in the lamina propria with extravasation of erythrocytes by histopathology.

MANIFESTATIONS

Moderate to severe diarrhea occurs in all patients with antimicrobic-associated enterocolitis. The onset is often sudden, beginning 2 days to several weeks after the start of antimicrobial therapy.

The manifestations of developing PMC are not distinctive. Diarrhea is common and consists of small volumes of watery feces, usually devoid of visible blood or mucous. Abdominal cramps and abdominal tenderness, fever, and leukocytosis are common findings.

DIAGNOSIS

The onset of diarrhea in any patient receiving antimicrobics, particularly clindamycin, lincomycin, or ampicillin, should raise the possibility of a causative association with the therapy. Sigmoidoscopy early in the disease may reveal minimal evidence of colitis or perhaps a single, small pseudomembranous plaque will be seen. In addition to culturing the feces for aerobic enteric pathogens, isolation of *C. difficile* may be attempted. A specimen of feces should be tested for the presence of the enterotoxin of *C. difficile.*

PROGNOSIS

Many patients improve promptly when the antimicrobic is discontinued; these patients usually have little or no evidence of colitis. In others, the diarrhea may persist for 2 to 8 weeks. Such patients invariably have readily demonstrable pseudomembranes, and may be debilitated by dehydration, electrolyte imbalance, and hypoalbuminemia; death may result.

Toxic megacolon is a rare, but serious, complication that has developed in a few patients, especially those who have received antiperistaltic drugs. Fatality rates vary widely, and may be as high as 20% to 30% in patients with serious disease.

THERAPY

In most patients, aside from stopping the antimicrobial therapy, nothing more need be done. This is the case even when the diarrhea persists for 10 to 14 days without systemic manifestations because as it is a period of slow restoration of a normal bowel flora, and healing of the mucosa. Similarly, if several small pseudomembranes are found by endoscopy, conservative management should be continued if the patient is doing well. The general supportive measures appropriate in all forms of diarrheal disease are useful—fluid replacement and correction of electrolyte abnormalities are essential. Hypoalbuminemia may develop in patients with severe colitis. Antiperistaltic or narcotic drugs must not be used because they may prolong and worsen the disease, leading to the development of toxic megacolon.

In patients with severe manifestations of colitis caused by *C. difficile,* that is, demonstration of both the organism and its toxin in the feces, specific therapy should be used. Vancomycin given PO is the preferred treatment. Either of two regimens (7.5 or 30 mg/kg body wt/day, PO, as 4 equal portions, 6-hourly, for one week) will relieve symptoms and diarrhea over a period of days. Although the lower dose is less costly, relapses may be more frequent. Overall, relapses occur in 10% to 12% of patients, apparently not as a consequence of the development of resistance. Rather, there is persistence of spores of *C. difficile* that germinate after the vancomycin has been excreted.

Cholestyramine benefits as many as 75% of patients, apparently by binding the toxin produced by *C. difficile.* Some clinicians prefer to treat first with cholestyramine (200–250 mg/kg body wt/day, PO, as 3 or 4 equal portions, 8- or 6-hourly). If there is no improvement within 3 to 5 days, vancomycin is then prescribed.

PREVENTION

Patients must be informed that diarrhea may develop when an antimicrobic is taken. If changes occur, for example, increased frequency of defecation or the passage of loose or unformed feces, the antimicrobic should be stopped.

Unknown

Necrotizing enterocolitis, a serious idiopathic disease of the newborn, occurs primarily in infants weighing less than 1500 g. It is characterized by gastric retention, the vomiting of bile, abdominal distention, and blood-streaked diarrhea. The most frequently involved site is the terminal ileum, followed by the ascending and transverse colon. Pathologically, there is fibrinoid necrosis of the bowel with ulceration and pseudomembrane formation; perforation is a frequent complication. Pneumatosis (intramural gas) of the intestinal wall is common, and it is often a premonitory sign of perforation. Therapy is mainly supporative, although gastric suction and antimicrobics are frequently used. The condition is not necessarily fatal if intestinal perforation is recognized early and repaired promptly.

Enterocolitis of unknown origin was recognized before the advent of antimicrobics. Occasionally, even at present there are patients with enterocolitis who have not received antimicrobial agents. Many of these patients develop pseudomembranous enterocolitis after surgery, and in some patients shock occurring at the time of surgery has been proposed as the cause. Abdominal operations, particularly gastric resections, are the most frequent predisposing procedures. The mortality rate is high, although there are isolated reports of the resection of necrotic, perforated bowel resulting in survival. The possible role of *C. difficile* or other anaerobes in this process remains to be explored.

Bibliography

Books

DACK GM: Food Poisoning, 3rd ed. Chicago, University of Chicago Press, 1956. 251 pp.

RIEMANN H (ED): Food-Borne Infections and Intoxications. New York, Academic Press, 1969. 698 pp.

RYSER RJ, HORNICK RB: A review of "new" bacterial strains causing diarrhea. In Remington JS, Swartz MN (eds): Current Clinical Topics in Infectious Diseases. New York, McGraw-Hill, 1981. pp 184–210.

STROEBELL FW, CRAMBLETT HG: Enteropathogenic *Escherichia coli* gastroenteritis. In Current Pediatric Therapy, 3rd ed, Philadelphia, WB Saunders, 1968. pp 719–722.

Journals

Acute gastroenteritis among four groups to the orient. Morbid Mortal Week Rep 18:301–303, 1969

BARTLETT JG, CHANG TW, GURWITH M, GORBACH SL, ONDERDONK AB: Antibiotic-associated pseudomembranous colitis due to toxin-producing clostridia. N Engl J Med 298:531–534, 1978

BARTLETT JG, MOON N, CHANG TW, TAYLOR N, ONDERDONK AB: The role of *Clostridium difficile* in antibiotic-associated pseudomembranous colitis. Gastroenterology 75:778–782, 1978

BARTLETT JG: Antibiotic-associated colitis. Clin Gastroenterol 8:783–801, 1979

BOKKENHEUSER VD, RICHARDSON NJ, BRYNAR JH, ROUX DJ, SCHUTTE AB. KOORNHOF HJ, FREIMAN I, HARTMAN E: Detection of enteric campylobacteriosis in children. J Clin Microbiol 9:227–232, 1979

EDITORIAL: Necrotizing enterocolitis in premature infants. Br Med J 2:1089–1090, 1966

GEORGE WL, SUTTER VL, FINEGOLD SM: Antimicrobial agent-induced diarrhea—a bacterial disease. J Infect Dis 135:822–828, 1977

HELSTAD AG, MANDEL AD, EVANS AS: Thermostable Clostridium perfringens as cause of food poisoning outbreak. Public Health Rep 82:157–161, 1967

KEIGHLEY MRB, BURDON DW, ARABI Y, ALEXANDER–WILLIAMS J, THOMPSON H, YOUNGS D, JOHNSON M, BENTLEY S, GEORGE RH, MOGG GAG: Randomized controlled trial of vancomycin for pseudomembranous colitis and postoperative diarrhea. Br Med J 2:1667–1669, 1978

MEYER KF: Food poisoning. N Engl J Med 249:765–773, 804–812, 843–852, 1953

RABSON AR, HALLETT AF, KOORNHOF HJ: Generalized Yersinia enterocolitica infection. J Infect Dis 131:447–451, 1975

RENWICK SB, MCGOVERN VJ, SPENCE J: Necrotizing enterocolitis: a report of six cases. Med J Aust 2:413–417, 1966

ROLAND FP: Leg gangrene and endotoxin shock due to Vibrio parahemolyticus: An infection acquired in New England coastal waters. N Engl J Med 282:1306, 1970

TANNER NC, HARDY KJ: Acute necrotizing enterocolitis: survival following perforation and resection in two postoperative patients. Br J Surg 55:379–381, 1968

CHARLES C. J. CARPENTER

Diarrheal Disease Caused by Escherichia Coli

61

Escherichia coli may cause at least three diarrheal syndromes. Most frequently, noninvasive, enterotoxin-producing bacilli cause diarrhea that ranges in severity from mild disease to (rarely) fulminant and potentially fatal, choleralike illness. Less frequently, invasive *E. coli* penetrate the large bowel mucosa and cause a shigellalike dysentery. Least often, *E. coli* that neither produce an identifiable enterotoxin nor invade the gut mucosa can produce a short-lived diarrheal illness that poses a major problem only in infants and very small children. Generally, diarrheas caused by *E. coli* are mild, self-limited illnesses in adults, but are often life-threatening in small children. In extreme cases, both the choleralike and the dysenterylike syndromes may be fatal in the absence of appropriate therapy.

Etiology

The characteristics of *E. coli* are given in Chapter 48, Urethritis and Cystitis. There are no histologic, colonial, or cultural peculiarities to distinguish those *E. coli* that cause diarrheal disease from those that do not. Therefore, neither a gram-stained smear nor a culture of feces can be used to identify *E. coli* that are diarrhea-causing pathogens.

Epidemiology

Many years ago, the so-called enteropathogenic *E. coli* (EPEC) were incriminated in limited outbreaks of infantile diarrheal disease, especially in nurseries. However, it was not until the late 1960s that enterotoxigenic *E. coli* (ETEC) were recognized as etiologic agents of diarrheal disease in humans when they were shown to be responsible for severe choleralike disease in adults in Calcutta. ETEC have subsequently been shown to be worldwide in distribution. In most of the developing countries, they have been incriminated as the most common cause of acute diarrhea in small children, and they have clearly been identified as the most common etiologic agent in traveler's diarrhea, as well as of common source (food or water) outbreaks in the developed nations.

At present, serotyping of ETEC strains is most valuable as an epidemiologic tool for identifying transmission of organisms. Serotyping may eventually be more useful as a diagnostic test, when pools of appropriate antiserums become available.

Invasive *E. coli* have been clearly related to diarrheal disease in humans in Southeast Asia, Eastern Europe, South America, and in limited food-borne outbreaks in the United States. The epidemiology of invasive *E. coli* has not been systematically investigated.

The fact that diarrheal disease can also be produced by nonenterotoxin-producing noninvasive *E. coli* has only recently been recognized, and neither the extent nor the epidemiology of this illness has been clarified.

Pathogenesis and Pathology

Diarrheal disease caused by *E. coli* generally results from either the production of enterotoxin or direct invasion of the gut wall, and the pathology differs accordingly. The pathophysiologic events in the illness caused by nonenterotoxin-producing, noninvasive *E. coli* have not yet been clarified, although infection with such strains clearly causes alterations in the brush border of the small bowel epithelial cells.

Enterotoxigenic Escherichia coli *(ETEC)*

Diarrheal disease caused by *E. coli* is far more variable than that caused by cholera, because of the multiple pathogenetic mechanisms which may be involved. As with cholera, a true secretory diarrhea is caused by enterotoxigenic ETEC, and at least two distinct toxins, a heat-labile toxin (LT) and a heat-stable toxin (ST), may be produced by *E. coli* that have colonized the small bowel. Unlike cholera, in which the ability to produce enterotoxin is chromosomally mediated and a single toxin is produced by all pathogenic strains, the ability of *E. coli* to produce enterotoxins is plasmid-mediated, and specific plasmids code for the production of LT and ST. Genes for either or both of these toxins may be on a single plasmid.

The *E. coli* LT has a molecular weight of approximately 83,000 daltons, and is structurally similar to, but not identical with, the cholera toxin. As in the case with cholera enterotoxin, the primary binding site for the *E. coli* LT is the GM-1 monosialoganglioside. Having bound to the gut mucosal cell, the *E. coli* LT also stimulates adenylate cyclase by means of ADP ribosylation with kinetics similar to those of cholera toxin, causing delayed secretion of isotonic fluid, which persists for many hours after binding the toxin. Like the cholera enterotoxin, the *E. coli* LT also has binding and activating moieties. The binding subunits are antigenically similar to, but not identical with, those of the cholera toxin. The activating, or A1 subunit, of the *E. coli* LT is also similar to, but not identical with, the A1 subunit of the cholera enterotoxin. Although the LT may be produced by a large number of *E. coli* serotypes, an identical LT molecule appears to be produced by all such strains.

The *E. coli* ST is quite different from the LT because it exhibits a rapid onset of action, does not bind to gangliosides of the mucosal cell membrane, and is of low molecular weight, that is, less than 2000 daltons. It is not antigenic in its natural state. The ST appears to act by stimulation of guanylate cyclase with resultant cyclic GMP accumulation in mucosal cells. The kinetics of ST action are strikingly different from LT, because it causes an almost immediate increase in the secretion of gut fluid, an effect that disappears rapidly when ST is washed out of the gut lumen. The increase in intracellular guanylate cyclase causes chloride secretion by gut mucosal epithelial cells in a manner similar to that seen with the cholera enterotoxin, but the ST does *not* alter neutral sodium chloride absorption by the brush border cotransport route. Although the binding properties have not yet been established, the binding appears to be specific for small bowel mucosal cells. Unlike the cholera enterotoxin and *E. coli* LT, the *E. coli* ST does not exhibit its characteristic effect of cyclase activation on nonintestinal tissues. Despite the different kinetics, the major physiologic effect of ST is also to increase net movement of isotonic fluid from blood to gut, resulting in a watery diarrhea that may be indistinguishable from cholera.

An *E. coli* strain may produce LT, ST, or both enterotoxins, depending upon the plasmids which it carries. The enterotoxin types may vary with the geographic location and serotype. In certain geographic areas, diarrheal disease is more commonly produced by *E. coli* that produce both ST and LT; in other regions, *E. coli* that produce ST alone predominate. The plasmids carrying the genetic material controlling enterotoxin production have been well characterized. These are for the most part transferable plasmids (like R factors) and can be transferred among strains through bacterial conjugation. The plasmid DNA sequences controlling enterotoxin production have been studied extensively by recombinant DNA technology. The LT and ST genes have been cloned; the ST gene has been shown to be a transposon (a DNA replicon that can insert itself into the chromosome as well as on different areas of the plasmid). Furthermore, DNA responsible for the production of only the A or the B subunits can be placed on separate plasmids, an observation that may be useful eventually in vaccine production.

Enterotoxinogenic *E. coli* also produce colonization factors that allow them to adhere to the small bowel mucosa. Some of these factors have been identified as fimbria or pili (hairlike projections of protein material extending from the cell surface) and designated as colonization factor antigens (CFA-I and CFA-II) (Fig. 61-1). These occur, however, only on certain ETEC, and are related to the serotype of the organism; it is suspected that other colonization factors will be found to account for the remainder of the strains. Colonization factors are also plasmid-mediated, and indeed a single plasmid may carry genes for both enterotoxin and CFA production.

Certain serotypes of *E. coli* seem to be especially adept at carrying one or more of these transmissible plasmids; moreover, it seems that there must be a combination of O, K, and H antigens, and often a certain characteristic fermentation pattern, or biotype, in order for the enterotoxin plasmid to be harbored successfully. Some serotypes more often produce both LT and ST, such as 06:K15:H16, and others produce ST only, such as 0128:H (antigens variable). Likewise, some serotypes carry CFA-I, *e.g.,* 078:H11, and others CFA-II, *e.g.,* 06:K15:H16. A summary of some characteristic associations is given in Table 61-1. Some enterotoxigenic serotypes are found worldwide, whereas others are more localized in distribution. In fact, each geographic area studied appears to have a characteristic spectrum of typical ETEC sero-

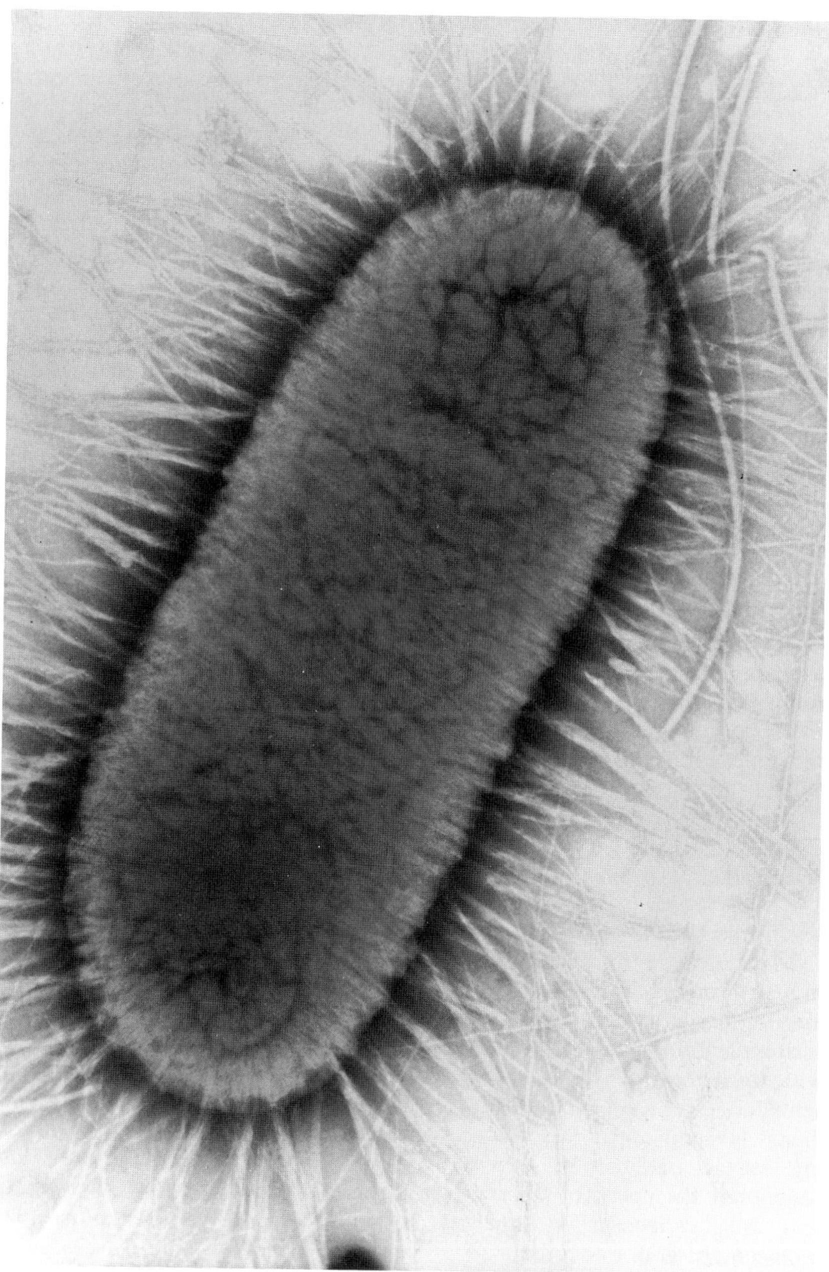

Fig. 61-1. Isolate of enterotoxigenic *Escherichia coli* demonstrating pili; the hairlike projections are designated colonization factor antigens (CFA). The CFA appear to be critical virulence factors in causing adherence of the *E. coli* to the small bowel mucosa. (Evans DG, Evans DJ, DuPont HL: J Infect Dis 136: S118–123, 1977)

types. The ETEC serotypes, with a few exceptions, are different from the enteropathogenic serotypes of *E. coli* (EPEC) described in the past as the cause of nursery outbreaks of diarrhea.

Invasive Escherichia coli

Certain strains of *E. coli* are closely related taxonomically to *Shigella* species and may produce invasive diarrhea that is clinically similar to shigellosis (Chap. 62, Shigellosis). These strains appear to belong to a limited number of serotypes, generally different from ETEC. Invasive *E. coli* are recognized as rare causes of acute diarrheal disease in Southeast Asia and North America, but are somewhat more frequently implicated in clinical illness in Eastern Europe. Thus far, no clinical isolates of invasive *E. coli* have been found to produce enterotoxin.

Table 61-1. *Recognized Associations Among Serotype, Enterotoxin Production, and Colonization Factors*

Serotype	Enterotoxin Production	Colonization Factors
078:HII	LT and ST	CFA I
078:H12	LT and ST	CFA I
06:K15:H16	LT and ST	CFA II
08:K40:H9	LT and ST	CFA II
0128:H (variable)	ST	CFA I variable
027:H (variable)	ST	CFA negative

Nonenterotoxin-Producing Noninvasive Escherichia coli

It is clear that some factors in addition to the ST and LT may play a pathogenic role in diarrheal illnesses caused by ETEC; for example, malaise, abdominal pain, and myalgias cannot be attributed to either of these two enterotoxins. Moreover, diarrheal disease may be associated with *E. coli* that neither invade nor produce enterotoxin, either *in vitro* or in animal models. Although such strains do colonize the small bowel heavily and cause demonstrable damage to the intestinal microvilli, the mechanism(s) by which diarrheal disease is produced remain unclear.

Manifestations

Severe diarrheal disease caused by ETEC is generally characterized by the abrupt onset of watery diarrhea. In severe cases, the clinical picture is identical with that of cholera (Chap. 65, Cholera) except that cramping abdominal pain is more commonly present with the *E. coli* diarrheas. However, even in the absence of antimicrobial therapy, the duration of the illness is significantly less than cholera, seldom lasting more than 24 hours after initiation of fluid replacement therapy. The mortality rate may be appreciable, especially in small children, if fluid replacement is not adequate.

There is no reliable clinical means for distinguishing clinical illnesses caused by ST or LT alone from those caused by *E. coli* which produce both ST and LT. Although the mean fecal volume is less in patients with *E. coli* that produce ST alone, neither the presenting features nor the responses to treatment are different from those in the illness caused by *E. coli* that produce both LT and ST.

The disease caused by the invasive *E. coli* may be clinically indistinguishable from that produced by *Shigella* spp. (Chap. 62, Shigellosis); there is an abrupt onset of fever, frequently with chills, followed initially by watery diarrhea and then dysentery. The disease is generally self-limited.

The nonenterotoxin-producing, noninvasive *E. coli* have thus far been incriminated only in relatively mild diarrheal illness in infants and small children. The full spectrum of illness related to these enteropathogens has not yet been defined.

Diagnosis

On primary isolation, the colonies of ETEC look the same as all other *E. coli.* The ability to make enterotoxin can be demonstrated by randomly picking approximately 5 to 10 typical colonies, and placing them in a medium in which enterotoxin production can be demonstrated. For LT, a tissue culture system, such as the mouse Y1 adrenal cell, or the Chinese hamster ovary cells, is inoculated. These cells respond morphologically to stimulation of their adenylate cyclase systems by the LT. A newer method, which will probably largely replace the tissue culture assays, involves the use of an ELISA (enzyme-linked immunosorbent assay, see Chap. 14, Immunologic Diagnosis) method in which either GM_1 ganglioside or specific antibody is used to bind the LT as the initial step in the assay.

For ST, the infant mouse is still the most useful assay. Once methods for producing an antiserum to ST are successful, an immunologic test, perhaps using ELISA, should replace this cumbersome test. Once ETEC are recognized, they can be further characterized according to serotype, ability to produce colonization factor, and susceptibility to antimicrobics.

Invasive *E. coli* can be identified by the Sereney test, in which the rabbit or guinea pig conjunctival sac is inoculated with *E. coli* isolated from a patient with a shigellosislike illness. Invasive strains of *E. coli* cause grossly detectable keratoconjunctivitis within 1 to 7 days.

An adequate laboratory means of identifying nonenterotoxigenic, noninvasive *E. coli* has not yet been developed. To date, this diagnosis has been made only by the isolation of *E. coli* from the upper small bowel of small children with an acute diarrheal illness.

Prognosis

With adequate therapy, the mortality in disease caused by enterotoxin-producing *E. coli* approaches zero. Without adequate fluid and electrolyte therapy, the mortality is directly proportional to the volume of fluid loss caused by the enterotoxin and may be quite high in small children. The mortality rate in diseases caused by invasive *E. coli* is low, but precise figures are not available. Adequate data are not available to determine the mortality rate in the illness caused by nonenterotoxigenic, noninvasive *E. coli.*

Therapy

Replacement of fluid and electrolytes lost in the feces by either IV or PO administration is the mainstay of therapy. Because most ETEC diarrhea is mild to moderate, PO therapy alone is almost always adequate. Packets of dry solids to be dissolved in tap water for PO administration—as used in the rest of the world—are not yet commercially available in the United States. Liquids such as juices containing some sugar and salt are probably adequate for most adults in the developed world because the disease is relatively mild in these persons.

ETEC in many parts of the world are unusually susceptible to antimicrobics, possibly because some plasmids are mutually incompatible; that is, they cannot be harbored simultaneously within a bacterium. Thus, *E. coli* that contain an enterotoxin plasmid cannot also carry a similar R factor plasmid. Antimicrobial therapy is not routine although in a controlled trial in Bangladesh, treatment with tetracycline caused a statistically significant, but clinically modest, reduction in the duration of diarrhea. Prophylaxis with doxycycline (100 mg/day, PO) has been shown to be highly effective in preventing diarrhea caused by *E. coli* in travelers to Kenya, Morocco, and Mexico, and should be offered to elderly travelers to the developing areas of the world. Bismuth subsalicylate may provide symptomatic relief (less severe abdominal cramps, less frequent stools) to persons with diarrhea caused by enterotoxigenic *E. coli;* the mechanism of action of bismuth subsalicylate is not known.

With both invasive *E. coli* and with nonenterotoxigenic, noninvasive *E. coli,* the principles of fluid repletion therapy are identical with those for ETEC. The role of antimicrobial agents, if any, in illnesses caused by these enteropathogens has not been established.

Prevention

Both the heat-labile enterotoxin and the colonization factor antigens (CFA) are immunogenic. Although immunization against either the heat-labile enterotoxin or specific CFAs confers partial protection in experimental animals, no vaccine is currently available for use in humans. Immunologic control may eventually be possible through the use of live *E. coli* containing appropriate nontoxic virulence antigens that have been developed through recombinant DNA technology.

Although prophylaxis with doxycycline is very effective in preventing traveler's diarrhea caused by *E. coli* in North American visitors to tropical areas, its use should probably be restricted to old persons and patients with underlying chronic illnesses. The indiscriminate use of prophylactic antimicrobials might result in a far greater worldwide prevalence of antimicrobic-resistant *E. coli.*

A relatively large dose of *E. coli* appears to be essential to produce enteric infection in humans. Accordingly, in areas in which *E. coli* diarrhea is prevalent, a high degree of protection can be afforded by careful hygiene, sterilization of drinking water, and avoidance of uncooked food.

Remaining Problems

A major need is a clear-cut definition of the epidemiology of diarrheal illnesses caused by *E. coli.* Because standard cultures of feces do not identify pathogenic *E. coli,* the prevalence of *E. coli* as a cause of diarrhea has thus far been determined only in a few geographic areas.

Why do ETEC cause severe, choleralike diarrheal disease in adults in Southeast Asia but not in other parts of the world?

Likewise, the apparently limited geographic distribution of disease caused by invasive *E. coli* is unexplained.

Finally, vaccines effective against ETEC are needed for use in areas in which diarrheal disease is endemic. Major efforts are currently directed both toward utilizing recombinant DNA technology to develp a nontoxic live oral vaccine and toward developing a multivalent parenteral vaccine directed against the more prevalent CFAs of *E. coli.*

Bibliography

Journals

CLEMENTS JD, FINKELSTEIN RA: Isolation and characterization of homogenous heat-labile enterotoxins with high specific activity from *Escherichia coli* cultures. Infect Immun 24:760–769, 1979

DUPONT HL, SULLIVAN P, PICKERING LK, HAYNES G, ACKERMAN PB: Symptomatic treatment of diarrhea with bismuth subsalicylate among students attending a Mexican university. Gastroenterology 73:715–718, 1977

EVANS DG, EVANS DJ, DUPONT HL: Virulence factors of enterotoxigenic *Escherichia coli.* J Infect Dis 136:S118–123, 1977

FIELD M, GRAF HL, LAIRD WJ, SMITH PL: Heat-stable enterotoxin of *Escherichia coli: in vitro* effects on guanylate cyclase activity, cyclic GMP concentration, and ion transport in the small intestine. Proc Natl Acad Sci USA 75:2800–2804, 1978

GORBACH SL, KEAN BH, EVANS, DG, EVANS, DJ, BESSUDO D: Traveler's diarrhea and toxigenic *Escherichia coli.* N Engl J Med 292:933–936, 1975

GUERRANT RL, MOORE RA, KIRCHENFIELD PM, SANDE MA: Role of enterotoxigenic and invasive bacteria in acute diarrhea of childhood. N Engl J Med 293:567–573, 1975

GYLES CSM, FALKOW S: The enterotoxin plasmids of *Escherichia coli.* J Infect Dis 130:40–49, 1974

MERSON M, ORSKOV F, ORSKOV I, SACK RB, HUQ I, KOSTER FT: Relationship between enterotoxin production and serotype in enterotoxigenic *Escherichia coli.* Infect Immun 23:325–329, 1979

MERSON ML, SACK RB, ISLAM S, SAKLAYEN G, HUDA N, HUQ I, ZULICH AW, YOLKEN YH, KAPIKIAN AZ: Disease due to enterotoxigenic *E. coli* in Bangladeshi adults: Clinical aspects and a controlled trail of tetracycline. J Infect Dis 141:702–711, 1980

SACK RB, GORBACH SL, BANWELL JG, JACOBS B, MITRA RC: Enterotoxigenc *E. coli* isolated from patients with severe cholera-like disease. J Infect Dis 123:378–385, 1971

SACK RB: Enterotoxigenic *Escherichia coli:* Identification and characterization. J Infect Dis 142:990–998, 1980

SACK DA, KAMINSKY DC, SACK RB, ITOTIA JN, ARTHUR RR, KAPIKIAN AZ, ORSKOV F, ORSKOV I: Prophylactic doxycycline for traveler's diarrhea. N Engl J Med 298:758–763, 1978

ULSHEN MH, ROLLO JL: Pathogenesis of *Escherichia coli* gastroenteritis: another mechanism. N Engl J Med 302:99–101, 1980

RICHARD B. HORNICK

Shigellosis

62

The term shigellosis refers to an acute inflammatory reaction of the intestinal tract caused by bacteria of the genus *Shigella.* This infection is most commonly manifested by a clinically nonspecific diarrhea that may extend and cause bacillary dysentery. Dysentery implies that the colon is primarily involved since there is the passage of small volumes of feces consisting of blood and mucus. Spread of *Shigella* spp. beyond the intestinal tract to cause disease in other organs is extremely rare.

Etiology

Shiga, in 1897, established as the cause of bacillary dysentery the bacteria that bear his name. *Shigella* spp. are nonmotile, short, gram-negative bacilli that ferment lactose very slowly or not at all. Four major serologic groups, A through D, have been delineated according to specific cell wall antigens. Approximately 50 serotypes make up the four groups. Serotypes are indicated by Arabic numbers placed after the serogroup designation.

Group A consists of *S. dysenteriae (S. shigae),* a species not encountered in the United States except for rare instances of imported disease. Inability to ferment mannitol is characteristic.

Group B includes *S. flexneri,* a species commonly isolated in the United States. Serogroup B shigellae may or may not ferment mannitol.

Group C strains are biochemically indistinguishable from group B isolates, but they are serologically unique and are rarely isolated in the United States. The classic serotype of group C is *S. boydii.*

Shigella sonnei, the single serotype in group D, is the most common cause of shigellosis in the United States. While serologically homogenous, strain differentiation in *S. sonnei* has been obtained with xylose fermentation (two strains) and by the ability to produce colicines. Sixteen colicine types of *S. sonnei* have been identified.

Epidemiology

Shigellas have a worldwide distribution. In the United States, the incidence of shigellosis, as reported to the Centers for Disease Control, was 9.15/100,000, as contrasted with 15.06/100,000 for nontyphoidal salmonellosis. Since the 1960s, *S. sonnei* has been more common than *S. flexneri* except in American Indians, who are more commonly infected with the latter species.

Group A and C strains represent less than 2% of the isolations in the United States. However, in the Orient and Central America *S. dysenteriae* is commonly responsible for severe cases of dysentery. Epidemic infection with *S. dysenteriae* in Central America spread into Mexico in 1969–1972. Early in the epidemic, the mortality rate reached 32% because of the severity of the disease, mistakes in diagnosis, and inappropriate antimicrobic therapy—the *S. dysenteriae* were resistant to multiple drugs. A few isolated cases of disease caused by *S. dysenteriae* occurred in tourists returning to the United States; no secondary spread occurred.

Shigella, unlike nontyphoidal salmonellas, have no natural intermediate host. Because they reside in the intestinal tract of man, shigellosis is primarily a disease of direct anal–oral transmission. A few well-documented waterborne or foodborne outbreaks have been reported (25 from 1964–1968). Experimentally, shigellas can survive in various foods. Under optimal conditions of temperature, without severe acidity, shigellas may be recovered after 30 days from milk, eggs, cheese, and shrimp. They can also persist for as long as 3 days in seawater. Formerly, it was believed that the endemicity of shigellosis in many countries was directly related to inadequate sanitation facilities. However, in technically advanced countries such as Great Britain, the incidence of shigella infections has actually increased in recent years, despite modern environmental hygiene.

Several fundamental characteristics of shigellas are important in considering why shigellosis persists despite modern plumbing. Shigellas are present in large numbers around the bases of toilets used by infected persons. Moreover, they readily pass through toilet paper onto the fingers, and they can be recovered in cultures taken as long as 3 hours after contamination. In healthy, male volunteers, shigellosis followed the ingestion of as few as 2000 *S. flexneri* 2a. No other enteric bacterial pathogen (including *Salmonella* spp. and *Vibrio cholerae*) is so efficient in causing overt disease in man. The high infectivity of shigellas also accounts for the frequency of laboratory acquired infections. Apparently, lapses in personal hygiene enable the person-to-person spread and persistence of shigellosis.

Epidemics of bacillary dysentery have been attributed to houseflies. In tropical regions, the peak incidence of shigellosis correlates with the peak of fly infestation. Several studies have demonstrated the passive passage of *Shigella* spp. through the gut of the fly without either increasing in numbers or engendering illness in the fly. The actual importance of flies as vectors relates to the physical transport of infected feces on the legs of flies. In England, flies are not important carriers because the highest incidence of infection occurs in the winter months. Similarly, flies appear to be of little significance in the transmission of shigellas in the United States. Although there is usually an increased incidence of shigellosis in the late summer, seasonality is not as marked as it is with salmonellosis (Chap. 63, Nontyphoidal Salmonelloses).

Closed population groups with substandard environmental sanitation are at highest risk of epidemic shigellosis. Prisoner-of-war camps, homes for retarded or mentally defective children, and Indian reservations have high carrier rates and frequent outbreaks of bacillary dysentery. The term "asylum dysentery" was in use before the discovery of Shiga's bacillus. Shortly after 1900, the role of *Shigella* spp. in causing most cases of asylum dysentery was documented. However, 80 years later, despite knowledge of the mode of spread of shigellas and the availability of effective treatment, institutional epidemics still pose a significant problem.

The highest incidence of shigellosis is in children between the ages of 1 and 4 years. During the first year of life, infection occurs less frequently. About 30% of all reported cases occur in adults in the United States. Over the past decade, the number of reported cases has varied from 16,052 (1977) to 22,642 (1973) (Fig. 62-1). It is unlikely that any significant improvement will occur unless an effective vaccine is found or an effective means for interrupting anal–oral transmission is developed.

Pathogenesis and Pathology

Shigella spp. must penetrate the cells of the epithelial lining of the large intestine to induce dysentery. Following intracellular penetration, multiplication occurs in the submucosa or lamina propria. However, the greatest concentration of bacteria is found near

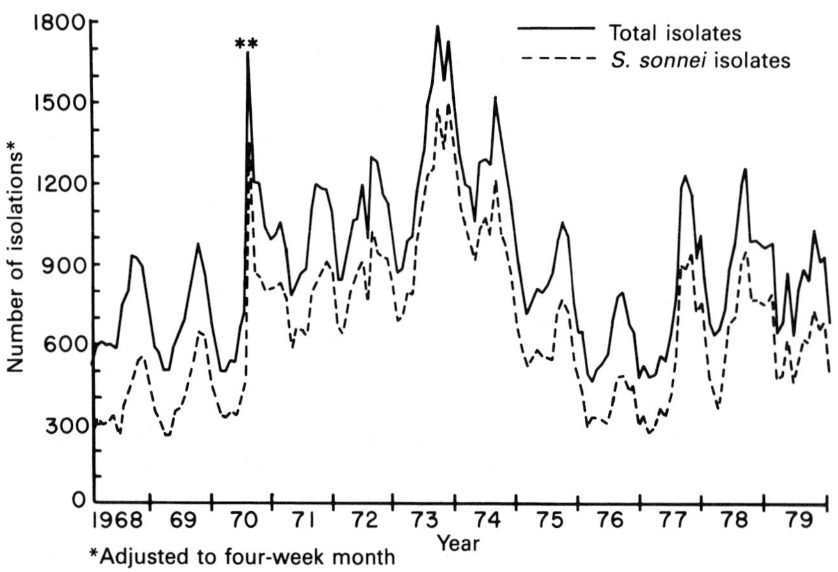

Fig. 62-1. Isolations of *Shigella* spp. by month from humans in the United States, 1968–1979. (Morbid Mortal Ann Suppl, 1979) No reports were received from California or the Virgin Islands after 1969.

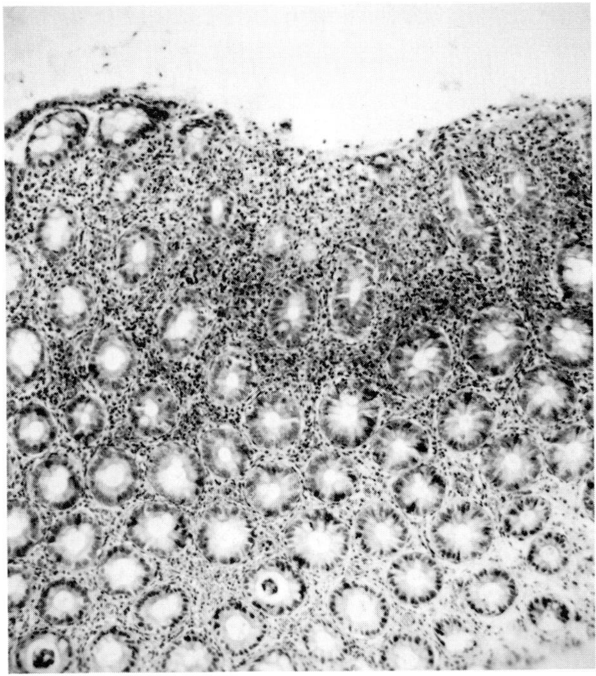

Fig. 62-2. Microabscesses in a rectal biopsy specimen obtained from a volunteer infected with *Shigella flexneri.* The site of biopsy was grossly hyperemic. (Original magnification approximately × 105).

the luminal surface. The areas of most intense inflammation usually correspond with those of heaviest bacterial invasion. Distortion of crypts occurs as clumps of cells are sloughed. This causes blockage. The accumulation of inflammatory cells behind the obstruction leads to the formation of microabscesses (Fig. 62-2). Through spread and coalescence, larger abscesses form. Long segments of affected colon or sigmoid may be covered by fibrinous exudate containing huge numbers of neutrophils. Bleeding occurs from superficial ulcerations that are about 5 mm in diameter. Perforation is not a complication because of the superficial localization of the infection. Invasion of the bloodstream is uncommon, occurring in 3% to 6% of patients—principally immunosuppressed and neonatal patients. The acute colitis leads to fever, abdominal pain, and the production of bloody, mucus-containing, diarrheal feces. Spontaneous recovery 2 to 7 days after onset is the rule. There is no evidence that shigellosis leads to chronic ulcerative colitis.

Many patients infected with shigellas do not develop dysentery but only have a watery diarrhea of short duration—as is also common prior to the onset of dysentery. The mechanisms involved are unknown but may include an enterotoxin with biologic activity similar to that of *Vibro cholerae* and *Escherichia coli.* An exotoxin is produced by *S. dysenteriae* and is perhaps associated with neurotoxicity (convulsions in children) as well as enterotoxicity. The enterotoxic activity of the exotoxin appears to be neutralized *in vitro* by antibodies which develop in patients infected with *S. sonnei* or *flexneri* 2b; that is, non-*dysenteriae* species of *Shigella* may elaborate an enterotoxin. However, enterotoxin causation of shigellosis by such species has not been proved. Volunteers infected with nonpenetrating mutants of *S. dysenteriae* did not develop diarrhea; apparently, this enterotoxin does not operate as those released by *V. cholerae* (Chap. 65, Cholera) and *E. coli* (Chap. 61, Diarrheal Disease Caused by *Escherichia coli*).

The inflammatory response induced by shigellas in the intestine may (1) release substances that stimulate the secretory mechanisms of the gut or (2) interfere with the normal absorptive capacity of the colon. Both of these abnormalities could result in excessive fluid in the terminal colon and hence diarrhea. Prostaglandins (PG) have been found in the polymorphonuclear leukocytes which make up the bulk of the cellular inflammatory response, and possibly PG stimulates the secretion of liquid. Evidence for this was obtained in rabbits infected with shigellas. Indomethacin, a potent inhibitor of PG, when given prior to and during infection, significantly inhibited fluid production without preventing the usual histologic manifestations of shigellosis. This attractive hypothesis may not be correct. Intestinal tissue may be stimulated *in vitro* by aspirin (and presumably by indomethacin) to absorb fluid and electrolyte, although the underlying infectious process results in loss of fluid. The algebraic sum of these two opposing forces results in a lessening of the secretory loss.

Before *Shigella* spp. can initiate the sequence of changes just described, they must traverse the proximal digestive tract. Although gastric acid destroys many shigellas, they have been isolated from the gastric juices of volunteers as long as 4 hours after ingestion. Sodium bicarbonate given before the administration of shigellas to volunteers increased the survival of shigellas and enhanced the incidence of infection.

Multiplication of shigellas does occur in the small intestine. Such growth appears to facilitate a temporary colonization of the small bowel with fecal flora. Whether this alteration in bacterial flora is related to the prolongation of diarrhea after the early phase of shigellosis is not known at present.

The multiplication of shigellas in the large bowel is associated with a diminution in some elements of the normal flora, particularly *Escherichia coli.* Metabolic competition may be responsible, and as the shigellas flourish, colicine production may maintain and aggravate the floral perturbation. As one consequence, the production of short-chain fatty acids is curtailed. Significant decreases in these acids can be demonstrated as long as shigellas are found in large numbers. As shigellas wane in numbers, fatty acids are replenished in the bowel. Fatty acids, presumably by maintaining an inhibitory acid environment, appear to protect against certain pathogens; for example, *Salmonella* spp. in mice. A similar correlation may exist in humans.

Manifestations

Humans are very susceptible to infection with *Shigella* spp. As few as 200 bacilli cause overt disease in 25% of healthy volunteers. Increasing the dose to 100,000 *S. flexneri* causes infection in more than 75%. The incubation period ranges from 36 to 72 hours. Initial symptoms are nonspecific; fever and cramping abdominal pain are prominent. Diarrhea usually appears after 48 hours, with dysentery supervening about 2 days later. Many persons do not present the classic picture just described. Fever may be absent, and diarrhea may continue without the appearance of blood and mucus. In such cases the diagnosis can be made only by the isolation of *Shigella* spp. from the feces. Abdominal tenderness is usually general, and the abdominal wall is not rigid. Sigmoidoscopy reveals intense hyperemia, multiple, small bleeding sites, loss of transverse mucosal folds, and thick, purulent mucous secretions. In patients with these findings, tenesmus is present, and the feces are bloody, mucoid, and of small volume.

Fluid and electrolyte loss may be quite significant, particularly in pediatric and geriatric populations. Infection with *S. dysenteriae* is occasionally associated with a peripheral neuritis. In children with shigellosis, convulsions are not unusual. Septicemia caused by *E. coli* has been initiated by shigellal infections.

Diagnosis

Shigellosis should be suspected in any patient with fever and diarrheal disease. The presence of blood and mucus in the feces of patients with diarrheal disease of acute onset strongly suggests shigellosis. However, the isolation of *Shigella* spp. from the feces is essential to definitive diagnosis.

Bacillary dysentery has a more acute onset than amebic colitis, and it is ordinarily a self-limited disease. Microscopic examination of freshly passed feces or a specimen swabbed from an ulcer at sigmoidoscopy will aid in differentiation. Clumps of neutrophils, macrophages, and erythrocytes are quite typical of shigellosis (Fig. 62-3), but they are not seen in diarrheas caused by enterotoxins (Chaps. 61, 65, 100: Diarrheal Disease Caused by *Escherichia coli*, Cholera, and Staphylococcal Skin Infections) or *Salmonella* spp. (Chaps. 63, 64: Nontyphoidal Salmonelloses and Typhoid Fever); trophozoites are consistent with amebic colitis (Chap. 66, Amebiasis). The appearance of the colon on sigmoidoscopic examination is helpful. Diffuse involvement of the mucosa with multiple shallow ulcers 3 mm—7 mm in diameter is typical in shigellosis; ulcers with undermined edges leaving islands of apparently uninvolved mucosa are classic in amebiasis.

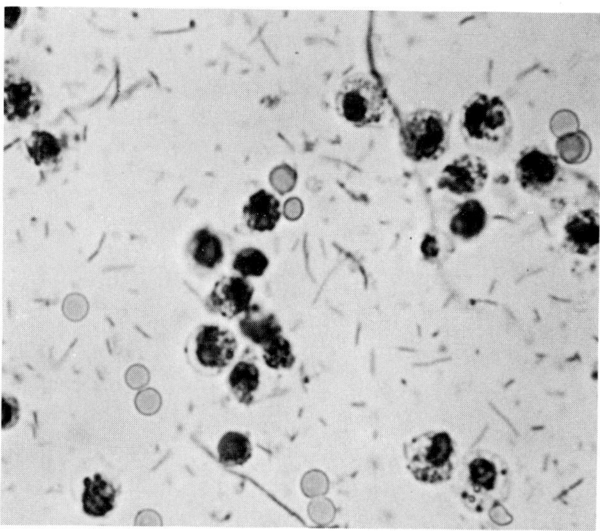

Fig. 62-3. Smear of feces from a patient with shigellosis. Note polymorphonuclear leukocytes, singly and in clumps, and many erythrocytes. (Methylene blue, original magnification approximately × 1000)

Other causes of diarrhea, such as *Salmonella* spp., staphylococcal enterotoxin, and viral agents, do not usually cause actual dysentery. Fever is a prominent feature of shigellosis and is typical in salmonellosis; it is low-grade or absent in viral enteritis and staphylococcal food poisoning. Nausea and vomiting, though sometimes present in *S. sonnei* infections, are much more common in viral infections and staphylococcal food poisoning.

The yield of *Shigella* spp. on culture of feces is critically dependent on minimizing the time from collection to inoculation (apparently, the continued growth of other microorganisms gives rise to acids that inactivate shigellae); and the selection of a choice portion of a specimen for culture (blood-tinged flecks of mucus are ideal).

Direct immunofluorescence, using type-specific, labeled antiserums, has been used to demonstrate shigellae in fresh feces. Unfortunately, polyvalent conjugated antiserums are not readily available, In an epidemic caused by a single known serologic type, immunofluoresence will give the most rapid and precise information on the extent of the epidemic.

Success in the serologic diagnosis of shigellosis is directly related to the severity of the disease. Patients with dysentery and fever generally have a demonstrable rise in hemagglutinating antibodies; a smaller number also develop agglutinating antibodies. Minor forms of the infection (*e.g.,* diarrhea) may lack serologic confirmation.

Prognosis

In previously healthy adults, shigellosis is a self-limited infection with fever that lasts about 3 days and dysentery that subsides within 1 week. Dehydration and electrolyte imbalance may become so severe in children that profound shock may result. It is in such patients that fatalities occur; the mortality of shigellosis in children in the United States is less than 1%.

Shigella spp. can be isolated for as long as a month after subsidence of bacillary dysentery in many untreated patients. Persistence beyond 3 months in otherwise healthy adults is unusual. Prolonged carrier states were demonstrated in malnourished Guatemalan children. Among these same children, those with more than 10^4 to 10^8 shigellas/g of feces were likely to develop repeated attacks of bacillary dysentery.

Asylum dysentery has been associated with an increased mortality (1%–25%) and morbidity, a relatively poor prognosis probably consequent to the general ill health of many patients with shigellosis. Also, in these circumstances, the carrier state tends to be chronic, probably reflecting repeated infections.

The mortality from shigellosis is less than 1% in the United States. In Central America, death is the outcome in 3% to 8% of children infected with *S. dysenteriae.* Malnutrition is the primary adverse factor in such a negative prognosis.

Complications following shigellosis are rare, even when specific therapy is omitted. Beyond the dire, immediate complications of dehydration—electrolyte imbalance and shock—a few patients develop a conjunctivitis if the disease persists for a week or more. In such patients, iritis occasionally occurs. Perforation of the colon following sigmoidoscopy has been reported. Thus, particular care must be exercised in performing this procedure in patients with shigellosis. Rectal prolapse has been a distressing problem in adults with unrelenting diarrhea. Fortunately, it is uncommon. Arthritis is an unusual, late complication that tends to occur in patients with chronic, untreated disease caused by *S. dysenteriae.* Usually, a large weight-bearing joint is involved, and the fluid aspirated from the joint is sterile.

Shigellal infections have been related to the initiation of chronic diseases. Ulcerative colitis and Reiter's syndrome are most often implicated. There is no evidence that ulcerative colitis is a sequel to shigellosis. However, there may be a relationship between *Shigella dysenteriae* and Reiter's syndrome. The association is clearest in persons who have HL-A B27; about 16% of HL-A B27 positive patients in an epidemic of dysentery developed Reiter's syndrome that persisted for at least 13 years.

Immunity following shigellosis is thought to be species-specific. Poorly nourished persons who are frequently exposed to large inocula may have multiple episodes of dysentery caused by a single species. In prisoner-of-war camps, second attacks of shigellosis a year or more after the first episode were frequent and were caused by the same *Shigella* sp. When volunteers were rechallenged with the same strain of shigella 10 weeks after an initial episode of experimental shigellosis, the attack rate was decreased, and fever, diarrhea, and dysentery were all less severe. It is evident that homologous immunity following shigellosis is incomplete. There is no evidence of heterologous immunity; that is, infection by multiple serotypes is possible.

Therapy

Because shigellosis is usually a self-limited infection, the need for antimicrobial therapy has been questioned. However, the effectiveness of antimicrobial agents and the threat posed to children by severe loss of fluids and electrolytes are persuasive arguments for treatment. Sulfonamides, formerly the drugs of choice, are no longer reliably effective. The worldwide spread of resistance mediated by resistance transfer factor (RTF) has been responsible for this change. Resistance of shigella strains to other antimicrobics, for example, tetracycline and ampicillin, has increased nonuniformly within species of *Shigella.* In most areas, *S. dysenteriae* and *S. sonnei* have become resistant to ampicillin and tetracycline;

such strains are susceptible to trimethoprim-sulfamethoxazole, nalidixic or oxolinic acid. *Shigella flexneri* are usually susceptible to ampicillin and patients respond to 50 mg to 60 mg/kg body wt/day, PO, as four equal portions, 6-hourly, for 3 to 5 days. Nonabsorbable oral antimicrobics are less effective in the control of shigellosis and their use is not advocated. In areas in which strains are not susceptible to tetracycline, for example, Yugoslavia, administration of 2.5 g of tetracycline as a single dose (0.5 g PO every 30 min × 5) has nevertheless given excellent results. Effective antimicrobics quickly eliminate shigellas from the feces, a practical public health measure. Fever and diarrhea usually abate within 12 to 18 hours after effective therapy is initiated.

Fluid and electrolyte replacement is the most prompt method of restoring the patient's sense of well-being. Infusions adequate to maintain a urinary output of 40 ml to 50 ml/hr should be administered. Rarely is blood loss sufficient to warrant transfusion.

Antidiarrheal drugs that act to inhibit intestinal peristalisis are contraindicated in patients with shigellosis. These drugs prolong fever, diarrhea, and excretion of shigellas in the feces. Their use should be strictly limited to relieving severe abdominal cramps (atropinelike drugs). Actual or threatened rectal prolapse and severe abdominal cramps are indications for the administration of paregoric or morphine.

Prevention

Proper sanitation and adequate sewage disposal are the most important means of prevention. In closed population groups, the detection of carriers and treatment of the disease will interrupt an epidemic.

Killed vaccines and the prophylactic administration of antimicrobics have failed to control the spread of epidemics. Orally administered vaccines containing attenuated strains show promise and are currently under investigation. The availability of an effective vaccine would find ready application in various closed population groups, such as asylums, reservations, and military camps, and perhaps for visitors to endemic areas of the world.

Remaining Problems

The exact mechanism of immunity in shigellosis remains to be deciphered. Local or coproantibodies may be important. The best means to stimulate the lifelong production of protective quantities of coproantibodies is yet to be discovered. The enzymes that facilitate the penetration of shigellae into mucosal cells and ultimate mechanisms that initiate diarrhea are questions pertinent to other diarrheal diseases.

Bibliography

Book

DUPONT HL., HORNICK RB: Diarrheal Diseases. Disease-a-Month. Chicago, Year book Medical Publishers, 1969. 40 pp.

Journals

CONNOR EB: Shigellosis in the adult. JAMA 198:717–720, 1966

DUPONT HL, HORNICK RB, DAWKINS AT, SNYDER MJ, FORMAL SB: The response of man to virulent *Shigella flexneri* 2a. J Infect Dis 119:296–299, 1969

HALTALIN KC, NELSON JD: Coliform septicemia complicating shigellosis in children. JAMA 192:441–443, 1965

HALTALIN KC, NELSON JD, KUSMIESZ HT, HINTON LV: Optimal dosage of ampicillin for shigellosis. J Pediatr 74:626–631, 1969

KEUSCH GT: Shigella infections. Clin Gastroenterol 8:645–662, 1979

TAYLOR BC, NAKAMURA M: Survival of shigellae in food. J Hyg (Camb) 62:303–311, 1964

RICHARD B. HORNICK

Nontyphoidal Salmonellosis

63

Salmonellosis refers to infections caused by bacteria of the genus *Salmonella.* The term does not differentiate between asymptomatic and symptomatic infections such as acute enterocolitis, bacteremia, localized infection, typhoid, or paratyphoid fever. Typhoid fever is discussed separately in Chapter 64.

Nontyphoidal salmonellosis is common and therefore ranks among the most important infectious diseases in the United States today. *Salmonella* spp. are transmitted either from animal to human or from human to human, causing infections that are usually brief, self-limited, and mild.

Etiology

Bacteria of the genus *Salmonella* are gram-negative, aerobic, noncapsulated, nonsporulating, generally motile bacilli that are 2 μm to 3 μm × 0.6 μm and grow readily on simple culture mediums. Isolates that fulfill the biochemical prerequisities of the genus fall into three species: *typhi, choleraesuis,* and *enteritidis,* on the bases of distinctive biologic properties.

Serologic classification by means of somatic (O) and flagellar (H) antigens has been carried to maximal refinement with *Salmonella* spp. More than 1400 antigenically distinct serogroups and serotypes have been differentiated. Although names have been assigned, a numerical designation in the form of an antigenic formula would be more appropriate.

The vast majority of *Salmonella* spp. show no particular host preference and multiply in the gastrointestinal tracts of many different animals including humans. However, a few serotypes demonstrate definite adaptation to specific hosts, possibly the best example is *S. typhi,* which is rather strictly adapted to humans, occurring only occasionally as part of the transient microflora of animals. In addition, the serotypes of *S. enteritidis*—called *paratyphi A, paratyphi C,* and *sendai*—show a marked preference for humans. Because *paratyphi B* also produces infection in animals, it appears to be less well adapted to humans than the other serotypes mentioned. Distinct, preference for nonhuman hosts also occurs; for example, *S. enteritidis* serotype *pullorum* is primarily a pathogen of fowl, even though it occasionally causes infections in other animals, including humans.

Although the number of different serologic types is large, just 10 serotypes accounted for about 70% of human salmonellosis in the United States in 1980: *S. enteritidis* serotypes *typhimurium* (including *typhimurium* var. *copenhagen*), *newport, enteritidis, infantis, heidelberg, agona, St. Paul, S. typhi, derby,* and *oranienburg.* Of these, *typhimurium* was by far the most common, accounting for 24% of the isolates. A close correlation exists between the frequency of isolation of specific serotypes from humans and from other animals. In addition, particular serotypes tend to occur in definite regional patterns.

It has been suggested that salmonellas possess an unusual degree of "genetic plasticity" because of the large number of antigenically distinct serotypes, the ease with which mutants can be obtained experimentally, and the demonstration of transferable resistance factors responsible for multiple drug resistance in a relatively large number of strains. Although *Salmonella* spp. exhibit the usual mechanisms for genetic recombination and readily give rise to mutants, there is no sound basis to support the view that they differ significantly in this respect from a number of other microorganisms.

Epidemiology

Humans are infected with salmonellas almost solely by the ingestion of contaminated food or drink. Under quite unusual circumstances, transmission has occurred by direct contact or by inhalation. Although either asymptomatic human carriers or persons with active clinical disease may contaminate food or drink, the greatest single source of salmonellosis in the United States is the vast reservoir of salmonellas in nonhuman animals.

Salmonella spp., other than *S. typhi* and a few other serotypes, occur naturally in many animals, including both homeothermic (fowl—chickens, turkeys, and ducks; mammals—cattle, sheep, swine, horses, dogs, cats, and rodents) and poikilothermic species (reptiles—snakes, lizards, and turtles; insects). One to three percent of all domestic animals are infected with *Salmonella* spp. However, many factors, such as epizootics of infection and crowding of domestic animals, especially before slaughter, favor the spread of infection and account for recovery rates reported to exceed 50% in abattoirs. Overall, domestic fowl, especially chickens (and hen's eggs), turkeys and ducks, constitute the single largest reservoir of infection and the source most often responsible for infection of humans.

The high incidence of infection in domestic animals used as sources of food for humans may be augmented by present methods of processing foods. For example, personnel and tools in a slaughterhouse can contaminate several carcasses after butchering just one infected animal among many in a given slaughter run. As a result, 1% to more than 50% of samples of raw meat purchased in retail markets may be contaminated with salmonellas.

Eggs or egg products are also very common sources of salmonellal infection. The bacilli may be found on the surface of the egg, between the shell and the shell membrane, or in the yolks of eggs from hens with ovarian infection. The incidence of infection may be low, but by pooling large numbers of eggs for freezing or drying, opportunity is provided for the contamination of large quantities of materials. However, with improved technology the rate of contamination has been reduced to around 1 viable bacillus per gram of product.

The probability of infection is decreased, but not eliminated, by cooking meats or eggs from infected animals or meats or eggs contaminated with salmonellas during processing. There are several simple means by which viable salmonellas bypass cooking. Persistence of salmonellas on knives, pans, and tables that have been used in the preparation of the meat before cooking commonly leads to the recontamination of cooked meat. Salmonellas may survive cooking deep inside certain foods, where temperatures may not reach the lethal range, for example, in large turkeys and in soft-cooked eggs.

Foods may also be contaminated by rats, mice, insects, or other vermin harboring *Salmonella* spp. Dried foods, such as egg whites that contain viable salmonellas, may become air-borne and contaminate other food. Dry milk, dry coconut, inactive dry yeast, chocolate bars, and a variety of pharmaceutical products of animal origin have been responsible for salmonellal infections of humans. Pharmaceutical products include carmine dye, pancreatin, pepsin, bile salts, gelatin, vitamins, and extracts of thyroid, adrenal cortex, pancreas, pituitary, liver, and stomach.

In addition to food products, water is occasionally the vehicle responsible for outbreaks of nontyphoidal salmonellal infection. In such instances, water is contaminated by feces or urine from infected human or nonhuman animals.

Household pets may also serve as sources of salmonellal infection. Cases have been traced to contact with infected dogs, cats, turtles, baby chicks, and ducklings.

The numerous by-products of the meat-packing industry, such as fish meal, bone meal, and rendered fat, often contain salmonellas. Because these products are frequently incorporated into foods for domestic animals, they are of particular importance in perpetuating salmonellosis in domestic animals.

Patients convalescing from salmonellal enterocolitis and persons with asymptomatic infections may continue to excrete *Salmonella* spp. for weeks or months, thus serving as sources of infection. The incidence of fecal carriers in the United States has been estimated to be 2 to 50/1000 of the normal population. The carrier rate is higher in food handlers than in other persons, perhaps reflecting more frequent contact with sources of infection. Because *Salmonella* spp. are sometimes present in the upper respiratory tracts of patients with acute salmonellosis, respiratory droplet spread may conceivably be responsible for some instances of salmonellal infection. Pregnant fecal excretors of salmonellae may simultaneously contaminate newborns and delivery rooms. Introduction of infection into the nursery may also result.

During 1980, 33,715 isolations of *Salmonella* spp. from humans were reported to the Salmonella Surveillance Unit of the Centers for Disease Control (CDC), giving a national incidence of 12/100,000 inhabitants. The reported incidence has been relatively constant since 1970. It must be recognized, however, that most cases of salmonellosis go unreported; the incidence of actual infection has been estimated at approximately 2 million cases in the United States per year. The true incidence of salmonellal infections and the opportunity for interstate epidemics of infection have increased during the past 20 years as a result of the increasing frequency of communal meals, the mass production of processed foods, and the increased consumption of poultry products.

Sporadic outbreaks account for approximately 55% of the isolates reported to the Salmonella Surveillence Unit. Family outbreaks account for 20% of the isolates, general outbreaks for 15%, and hospital-associated outbreaks for 10%.

The specific food responsible for infection is rarely identified in investigated sporadic or family outbreaks. This is in contrast to the situation in general outbreaks or epidemics, in which the contaminated food is frequently identified. The foods most commonly verified as responsible for general outbreaks or epidemics of salmonellal infection are poultry and poultry products, including turkeys, chickens, eggs, and egg products.

The incidence of salmonellosis varies with the season. The greatest number of isolates are reported from July through October and the lowest incidence of infection from December through May (Fig. 63–1). Children under 9 years appear to be infected more frequently than older persons.

Pathogenesis and Pathology

Salmonella spp. multiply in the small intestines and colon after ingestion, leading to an inflammation of the lamina propria of the villae. Salmonellas that do not penetrate the epithelial cells and migrate to the lamina propria do not cause disease. The inflammatory response elicited by species other than *S. typhi* and *paratyphi* consists of polymorphonuclear leukocytes, a distinction separating infections limited to the intestine from enteric fevers. In the latter instance, the predominant cells are mononuclear. In both small and large intestines, lymphoid follicles enlarge and may ulcerate; mesenteric nodes are frequently swollen. If the salmonellas are not successfully restrained by mucosal and lymphatic barriers, they will gain access to the bloodstream. The resulting bacteremia may be transient and inconsequential or may lead to metastatic infections giving rise to persistent bacteremia or abscesses.

Modern humans ingest viable salmonellas at relatively frequent intervals. The outcome of this interaction between humans and salmonellas is determined by many factors, including the number of bacilli ingested, their virulence or invasiveness, and the multiple factors that make up normal host resistance. Host factors identified as important include age, the normal flora of the gastrointestinal tract, and the presence of certain noninfectious diseases.

Relatively large numbers of salmonellas must be ingested to produce illness. In volunteers, as many as 100,000 to 1,000,000,000 bacilli have been required to produce disease with certain serotypes. However,

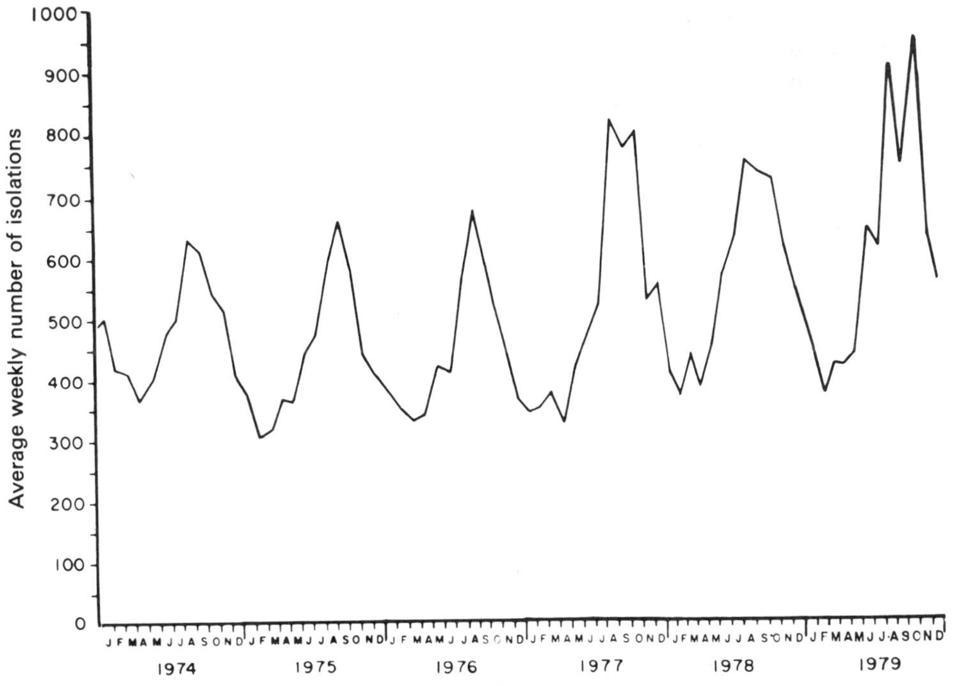

Fig. 63-1. Isolations of *Salmonella* spp. from humans in the United States as reported by the Salmonella Surveillance Unit from 1974–1979. The low point of the seasonal pattern occurs December–May of each year. (Morbid Mortal Suppl. Summary, 1979)

a carrier state can be induced with 10 to 100 times fewer bacteria. In infants and adults with certain underlying diseases, it is probable that a much smaller inoculum produces illness.

Salmonellal serotypes vary markedly in their capacity to cause disease. For example, *S. enteriditis* serotype *anatum* is low in virulence. It usually produces an asymptomatic intestinal infection, occasionally gives rise to manifestations of enterocolitis, and only rarely invades the bloodstream. In contrast, *S. choleraesuis* is highly virulent. It frequently produces bacteremia and the more serious salmonellal syndromes, occasionally causes gastroenteritis, but only rarely gives rise to asymptomatic intestinal infection. *Salmonella enteritidis* serotype *typhimurium* is of intermediate virulence. It sometimes invades the bloodstream, may cause asymptomatic infection, but most often produces colitis. Because it is by far the most frequent isolate, *typhimurium* is the salmonellal serotype most often cultured from nonfecal sources such as blood, urine, or pus. However, if the frequency of isolation of various serotypes from extraintestinal sources is related to the total number of strains isolated, the percentage of nonfecal isolates then becomes relatively greater with *S. enteritidis* types *heidelberg, enteritidis, oranienburg,* and especially with *S. choleraesuis.* About 90% of the isolates of *S. choleraesuis* are from nonfecal sources. Nonfecal isolates are also more frequently recovered in older than in younger persons.

Local factors in the stomach and intestines may be the first line of defense against salmonellosis. Subtotal gastrectomy, gastroenterostomy, and vagotomy predispose humans to salmonellal enterocolitis, perhaps because of reduced bactericidal activity from gastric juice, more rapid passage of salmonellas from the stomach to the site of invasion in the small intestines, or altered intestinal flora. The intestinal flora is an important protective mechanism because the dose of *S. typhi* required to initiate infection by the oral route in humans may be impressively reduced by giving antimicrobics orally before challenge. In other epidemiologic studies, prior antimicrobial therapy has altered the capacity of the human intestinal tract to eradicate salmonellas acquired naturally.

The general depression of resistance to infection seen in hepatic cirrhosis, lupus erythematosus, leukemia, lymphoma, and other neoplastic diseases extends to *Salmonella* spp. because one-third to one-half of patients with salmonellal bacteremia have such diseases. However, the predisposition to salmonellal infection that occurs in acute bartonellosis, the sickle hemoglobinopathies, and malaria is unique because it exceeds general susceptibility to other bacterial genera. The acute hemolytic phase of bartonellosis is complicated by the development of salmonellal bacteremia in as many as 40% of cases. Patients with sickle cell anemia and other sickle hemoglobinopathies are usually susceptible to invasion of the blood by *Salmonella* spp., and there is a strong tendency for localization of infection in bone. In fact, *Salmonella* spp., not staphylococci, account for most cases of osteomyelitis in patients with sickle cell anemia; focalization appears to occur in the areas of ischemia and necrosis of bone so common in sickle cell anemia. Demonstrable defects in the immune system of these patients include defective function of the alternative pathway of complement (associated with deficient opsonizing activity), low levels of the third component of complement (C3), and slightly reduced levels of the fourth component of complement (C4). These abnormalities, plus other defects in the reticuloendothelial system, may result in the strong association of salmonellal infections with sickle cell disease. Other preexisting diseases may provide sites for localization of *Salmonella* spp.: vascular aneurysms, bone compressed by aortic aneurysms, hematomas, areas of infarcation, old suture lines, sites of injection of irritating chemicals, a variety of cysts, and neoplasms located anywhere in the body.

Age is an important determinant in salmonellal infections. In infants between 2 and 4 months of age, the frequency of isolation is greater than 100/100,000 population. With increasing age, this figure decreases to 30/100,000 at 11 months and then to less than 10/100,000 after the age of 5 years, at which frequency it remains in all other age groups.

Among patients in hospitals, salmonellal infections are particularly likely to occur in newborns, in the elderly, and in patients with debilitating diseases that diminish resistance to infection. Various therapeutic measures, special diets, and diagnostic maneuvers may alter susceptibility or enhance the possibility of exposure to salmonellas. Poor sanitation in kitchens and on the wards may be an added factor accounting for the spread of *Salmonella* spp. in certain institutions such as hospitals for mental illness. Salmonellal infection, once established in an institution, may pass from person to person for long periods.

The incidence of salmonellosis in males and females is the same if all age groups are considered together. However, when the occurrence of salmonellal infection is subdivided according to age and sex, there is a significant preponderance of males (5.5:4.5) in patients under the age of 20 years, and a significant preponderance of females (6.0:4.0) in patients over the age of 20 years.

Manifestations

Enterocolitis

Although salmonellal enterocolitis is sometimes referred to as salmonellal food poisoning, it is an infection of the intestinal mucosa, and the ingestion of billions of heat-killed *Salmonella* spp. of the most virulent serotypes will cause no difficulty whatsoever. The typical clinical course of a patient with salmonellal enterocolitis is characterized by fever, abdominal pain, and diarrhea that persists 3 to 5 days. The incubation period is longer than in staphylococcal food poisoning, usually 8 to 24 hours (range, 6–48 hours). Nausea and vomiting are common initial symptoms, but they are rarely as prominent as the colicky abdominal pain and diarrhea that rapidly follow. The abdominal colic and diarrhea are extremely variable in severity. Some patients have a disease that only produces a few loose stools, and others have a fulminating diarrheal disease with the passage of 30 to 40 liquid stools per day. The feces may contain mucus and may be blood-tinged. An initial chill is common during the early phases of illness. The temperature usually ranges from 38°C to 39°C (100.4°F–102.2°F) but may be higher. On physical examination, hyperactive peristalsis and mild to moderate abdominal tenderness are typical. Severe tenderness, even with rebound, occasionally occurs in patients and may lead to confusion with acute appendicitis or acute cholecystitis. Spontaneous subsidence of illness within 5 days is the rule, but in some patients diarrhea and fever continue for as long as 2 weeks.

Several mechanisms may act either alone or in combination to cause diarrhea. A heat-labile enterotoxin, similar to that excreted by enterotoxinogenic *Escherichia coli,* has been isolated from *Salmonella* spp. Direct stimulation of the adenylate cyclase–cyclic AMP system by the toxin would provide the energy needed for secreting chloride ions and inhibiting the absorption of sodium resulting in the outpouring of isotonic liquid. Because the absorptive capacity of the gut cannot keep pace, diarrhea ensues. Prostaglandins capable of activating the adenylate cyclase system may be released from neutrophiles that accumulate in the lamina propria as part of the inflammatory response triggered by the invading salmonellas.

The leukocyte count is usually normal, although some patients may have a moderate leukocytosis. Gram-stained smears of mucoid flecks of diarrheal feces contain polymorphonuclear leukocytes. Early in the course of illness, cultures of the feces always yield *Salmonella* spp. About 59% of patients continue to pass feces positive for salmonellas 2 weeks after the onset of enterocolitis, but only about 10% to 15% remain positive at the end of 4 weeks. During acute enterocolitis, as many as 10^6–10^9 salmonellas may be present per gram of feces. With recovery, the number falls, so that after 3 to 4 weeks, salmonellas frequently cannot be isolated from the feces. A small proportion of patients continue to excrete bacilli after 2 months. Over the ensuing 6 months, cultures usually become negative. Fecal shedding of salmonellas tends to persist longer in infants and young children than in older children and adults. The term "chronic enteric carrier" should be reserved for patients who have persistence of the same species of *Salmonella* in their feces 1 year or more after the original acute enterocolitis has subsided. Chronic enteric carriers of species other than *S. typhi* are exceedingly unusual.

Paratyphoid Fever

Members of the genus *Salmonella* other than *S. typhi* can produce an illness with all the clinical characteristics of typhoid fever—paratyphoid fever. Although any serotype can give rise to paratyphoid fever, the usual causes are *S. enteritidis* serotypes *paratyphi* A and *paratyhpi* B, and *S. choleraesuis.* The clinical features of paratyphoid fever are similar to those of typhoid and are described in Chapter 64, Typhoid Fever. In the individual patient, it is impossible to differentiate typhoid fever from paratyphoid fever on clinical grounds alone. However, when large numbers of patients are compared, it is apparent that the duration of illness is shorter, and the mortality rate is lower in paratyphoid fever than in typhoid fever.

Bacteremia

Nontyphoidal *Salmonella* spp. also occasionally produce a clinical syndrome characterized by prolonged and intermittent fever, chills, anorexia, weight loss, and persistent bacteremia. There are no intestinal complaints, and cultures of feces are frequently negative for *Salmonella* spp. The leukocyte count is normal in most patients.

A prolonged, febrile illness lasting weeks or months and characterized by weight loss, marked anemia, hepatosplenomegaly, and bacteremia with *Salmonella* spp., including *S. typhi,* may complicate hepatosplenic schistosomiasis caused by *Schistosoma mansoni.* Patients with this syndrome have been described in northeastern Brazil and in Egypt.

Localized Infection

Signs of localized infection may appear in any patient with salmonellal bacteremia. Abscesses may form at almost any site; bronchopneumonia, empyema, endocarditis, pericarditis, pyelonephritis, osteomyelitis, or arthritis may develop. There is a striking tendency for *Salmonella* spp. to be localized at sites for preexisting disease. Patients with local infections usually have polymorphonuclear leukocytosis as high as 20,000–30,000/mm^3.

Diagnosis

The definitive diagnosis of salmonellal enterocolitis depends on isolation of the causative microorganism from the feces. Enterocolitis must be differentiated from other causes of acute diarrheal diseases, including staphylococcal food poisoning, shigellosis, campylobacteriosis, infection with enterotoxinogenic *E. coli,* cholera, amebiasis, and enteritis produced by viral agents.

The diagnosis of paratyphoid fever is established by the isolation of *Salmonella* spp. from blood, feces, or other sites. Agglutination tests are occasionally helpful. A fourfold or greater increase in titer of agglutinins against somatic antigens is diagnostic in the absence of a history of recent immunization. The agglutination tests performed in the ordinary clinical laboratory are usually not helpful because only a limited number of antigens are used.

The diagnosis of salmonellal bacteremia or local infection depends on demonstrating the causative microorganism in blood, pus, or other body fluids.

The possibility of an underlying disease should be considered in every patient with a severe salmonellal infection.

Prognosis

The majority of salmonellal infections follow a mild to moderate course without appreciable morbidity or mortality. However, serious illness is common in infants, in the elderly, and in persons with underlying diseases. Dehydration consequent to diarrhea may lead to severe acidosis, electrolyte disturbances, and even death.

The mortality rate from infections caused by *Salmonella* spp. cannot be accurately assessed. The best information has been obtained by studying the case–fatality ratio in outbreaks investigated by the Salmonella Surveillance Unit of the CDC. The mortality rate from 1962 through 1973 was about 0.27% or 65 to 90 per year; deaths occurred primarily in infants, elderly persons, and persons severely ill with other diseases.

Although the information is scanty, it appears that acute, nontyphoidal enterocolitis does not confer immunity. Repeated attacks occur, even with the same serotype.

Therapy

The most important aspects of the management of patients with salmonellal enterocolitis is the prompt correction of dehydration and electrolyte disturbances. Paregoric, diphenoxylate hydrochloride combined with atropine sulfate (Lomotil), codeine, or small doses of morphine may be used sparingly to relieve abdominal cramps and diarrhea. Continuous use of such drugs can lead to prolongation of the disease and fecal carriage of salmonellas. Attention should be focused on supportive and symptomatic therapy, not antimicrobial therapy. Antimicrobial therapy does not exert a beneficial effect on the clinical course of salmonellal enterocolitis. Moreover, the duration of excretion of *Salmonella* spp. in the feces is not shortened; in fact, it may be prolonged by treatment with antimicrobial agents.

Either bacteremia, paratyphoid fever, or serious local infections with systemic manifestations is an indication for treatment with chloramphenicol. After a peroral loading dose of 15 mg–20 mg/kg body wt, treatment should be continued at a dose of 50 mg–60 mg/kg body wt/day, PO, as four equal portions, 6-hourly, for 2 weeks. Defervescence may be slow, requiring 4 to 6 days or longer, in patients with local infections. Surgical drainage of collections of pus is required.

In patients with osteomyelitis or other persistent infections requiring therapy for more than 2 weeks, ampicillin may be used if the infecting strain is susceptible. In addition, ampicillin should always be used in patients with evidence of intravascular infection caused by ampicillin-susceptible *Salmonella* spp. because chloramphenicol may not eradicate bacteria from intravascular sites. Ampicillin should be given by parenteral injection—60 mg–80 mg/kg body wt/day, IM or IV, as four equal portions, 6-hourly. There are many patients in whom neither chloramphenicol nor ampicillin is of value.

Antimicrobial therapy is not indicated in convalescent carriers or in patients with asymptomatic intestinal infection.

The phenomenon of transferable antimicrobial resistance mediated by resistance (R) factors has been described in *Salmonella* spp. isolated throughout the world. The percentage of strains bearing R factors varies remarkably. It is most common with *S. enteritidis* serotype *typhimurium* and least common with *S.*

typhi. Often the resistance acquired involves drugs not useful in the treatment of salmonellal infections. For example, resistance to tetracyclines has increased rapidly during recent years; concomitantly, many strains are also resistant to sulfonamides and streptomycin. Of greater clinical importance is the proportion of strains that are resistant to ampicillin—5% to 20% in most regions of the United States. Resistance to chloramphenicol by this mechanism is unusual and has been of no appreciable clinical significance. The incorporation of antimicrobial agents (*e.g.,* oxytetracycline) into animal feeds may favor the transfer of resistance factors among enteric microorganisms.

Prevention

There is no effective immunization procedure for the prevention of infection by *Salmonella* spp. other than *S. typhi.* Antimicrobial agents are not effective preventives of salmonellosis. In fact, Swedish tourists visiting epidemic areas who took oxyquinolines as a prophylactic measure contracted salmonellosis more often than those who received no antimicrobial therapy (17% versus 28%.)

Because most cases of salmonellosis result from ingestion of contaminated food, the best approach to prevention at present involves the correction of faulty food production and processing methods and the application of better sanitary and hygienic practices. The incidence of salmonellosis in domestic animals used as foods for humans should be reduced. Some European countries have reduced the incidence of infection by heat sterilization of animal feed. Both in industry and in the home, contamination of uncontaminated foods or recontamination after cooking must be prevented. The prolonged incubation of meats at room temperature or in warming ovens should be avoided because this promotes the growth of a few innocuous salmonellas to an infectious inoculum. Food handlers and hospital personnel should observe strict personal hygiene and sanitary practices to minimize person-to-food or person-to-person spread of infection.

Remaining Problems

Control of the reservoir of salmonellosis in domestic animals is the most important step toward control of salmonellosis in humans. This is a difficult problem because *Salmonella* spp. are ubiquitous, and a cycle of salmonellosis is well established in nonhuman animals. Eradication of *Salmonella* spp. from domestic livestock requires the elimination of *Salmonella* spp. from animal foodstuffs.

Other problems of importance include (1) the significance of the genetic variability of *Salmonella* spp., (2) the influence of antimicrobics in animal feeds on the emergence of resistant strains, (3) the lack of effective chemoprophylactic and uniformly effective chemotherapeutic agents, and (4) the lack of an effective vaccine.

Bibliography

Books

CHABBERT YA, BAUDENS JG, BOUANCHAUD DH: Medical aspects of transferable drug resistance. In Wolstenholm EW, O'Connor M (eds): Bacterial Episomes and Plasmids. A Ciba Foundation Symposium. Boston, Little, Brown, & Co, 1969. pp 227–243.

FOSTER EM: An Evaluation of the Salmonella Problem. Washington DC, National Academy of Sciences, Publication 1683, 1969. 207 pp.

Proceedings of the National Conference of Salmonellosis, March 11–13, 1964 Washington DC, Public Health Service Publication 1262, 1965. 217 pp.

Salmonella Surveillance. Annual Summary, 1970. Atlanta, Center for Disease Control, 1971

VAN OYE E (ED): The World Problem of Salmonellosis. The Hague, Dr. W. Junk, 1964. 606 pp.

Journals

ASERKOFF B, BENNETT JV: Effect of therapy in acute salmonellosis on salmonellae in feces. N Engl J Med 281:636–640, 1969

BLACK PH, KUNZ LJ, SWARTZ MN: Salmonellosis: A review of some unusual aspects. N Engl J Med 262:811–817, 864–870, 921–927, 1960

DIXON MS: Effect of antibiotic treatment on duration of excretion of Salmonella typhimurium by children. Br Med J 2:1343–1345, 1965

GILL FA, HOOK EW: Salmonella strains with transferable antimicrobial resistance. JAMA 198:1267–1269, 1966

HOOK EW: Salmonellosis: certain factors influencing the interaction of salmonella and the human host. Bull NY Acad Med 37:499–512, 1961

MENTZING LO, RINGERTZ O: Salmonella infection in tourists. Prophylaxis against salmonellosis. Acta Pathol Microbiol Scand 74:405–413, 1968

SCHROEDER FA, TERRY TM, BENNETT JV: Antibiotic resistance and transfer factor in salmonella, United States, 1967. JAMA 205:903–906, 1968

WAHAB MFA, ROBERTSON RP, RAASCH FO: Paratyphoid A fever. Ann Intern Med 70:913–917, 1969

RICHARD B. HORNICK

64 Typhoid Fever

Typhoid fever is an acute febrile disease caused by *Salmonella typhi* that is unique to humans. It is characterized by fever, headache, apathy, prostration, cough, splenomegaly, rash, and leukopenia. The course of illness is usually severe and prolonged, lasting several weeks if untreated.

Etiology

Salmonella typhi are cytophilic, gram-negative, aerobic, noncapsulated, non-spore-forming, motile bacilli that range in size from 2 μm - 3 μm × 0.6 μm. Glucose is fermented with the production of acid; neither lactose nor sucrose is fermented. Presumptive identification is based on biochemical tests, and definitive identification is established by serologic testing for somatic (O) and flagellar (H) antigens. The subdivision of *S. typhi* into more than 80 definite and stable varieties can be achieved by bacteriophage typing, thus offering epidemiologists a valuable tool for tracing sources of infection.

Epidemiology

The ultimate source of infection with *S. typhi* is a patient with typhoid fever or a carrier of typhoid bacilli. Patients with typhoid fever excrete large numbers of *S. typhi* in feces or urine, and viable bacilli may be present in vomitus, respiratory secretions, and pus. Moreover, chronic enteric carriers, an important source of infection, often excrete 10^6 or more viable bacilli per gram of feces, and urinary carriers void large numbers of bacilli in urine. Typhoid bacilli contaminating the environment can survive for weeks in water, ice, dust, and dried sewage. Food or water contaminated directly or indirectly with human excreta is the usual source of infection. Many epidemics of water-borne typhoid fever have been described in the United States in the past, and they still occur occasionally. Water may be contaminated directly by excreta containing *S. typhi* or by excreta washed down from remote sites or introduced by faulty sanitation or plumbing. Foods for human consumption may be contaminated by excreta from carriers or patients with typhoid, by water containing *S. typhi,* or occasionally by contaminated dust, flies, or other insects. Oysters and other shellfish may be infected in polluted tidal waters and may be responsible for infection of humans. An outbreak was described in 1959 in which water for human consumption was contaminated by droppings from sea gulls that fed on wastes in sewage effluents discharged into the sea. The largest single outbreak of typhoid fever since 1939 occurred in Florida in 1973. Migrant farm workers were exposed to a contaminated water supply, and 222 persons had active disease or evidence of infection. No infections occurred in residents of the area outside the workers' camp.

Typhoid fever is still a disease of major importance in areas of the world that have not attained high standards of sanitation and public health. The progressive decrease in the incidence of typhoid fever, evident since 1900 in the United States, leveled off in the late 1960s; except for the 680 cases in 1973, the incidence has remained constant, varying from 375 to 528 in 1971–1980 (Fig. 64-1).

Typhoid fever now occurs sporadically and in limited outbreaks. About one-half of the cases reported to the CDC are acquired during travel outside the United States. Typhoid fever will continue to occur on a limited scale in the United States because of the existence of a reservoir of chronic carriers, numbering in the thousands, the frequency of typhoid in other areas of the world, and the magnitude of intercontinental travel.

In the United States, there is no difference in the incidence of typhoid fever in males and females. However, the chronic enteric carrier state is much

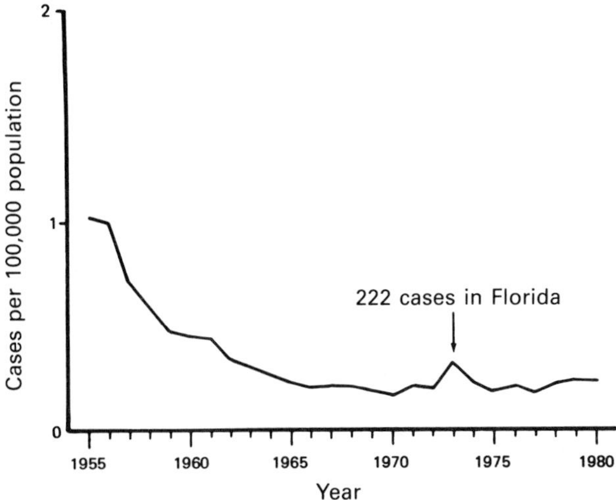

Fig. 64-1. Typhoid fever, reported cases per 100,000 population in the United States by year, 1955–1980. (Morbid Mortal Annual Suppl, Summary, 1980)

more frequent in females than in males, the ratio of reported cases in the United States being 3.65:1. Approximately 85% of the chronic enteric carriers are over 50 years old, whereas approximately 75% of the cases of typhoid fever occur in persons less than 30 years old.

In areas where typhoid fever is common, the incidence of the disease increases during the summer. There is no seasonal variation in the United States.

Pathogenesis and Pathology

The portal of entry of *S. typhi* is almost always the gastrointestinal tract, probably the upper small bowel. The pharynx, once considered a likely site of invasion, has virtually been excluded.

Salmonella typhi, especially in small doses, may be rapidly eliminated from the gastrointestinal tract or may undergo an initial phase of multiplication. Whether or not intraluminal multiplication occurs, typhoid bacilli in the small intestine quickly pass through the intestinal mucosa into the regional lymphatics, where they are phagocytized. Neutrophils are unable to kill ingested typhoid bacilli; the usual burst of oxygen consumption is inhibited. Some bacilli may escape engulfment in the regional nodes, passing to the bloodstream through the lymph and producing an initial, transient bacteremia that is quickly terminated through removal by reticuloendothelial cells in liver, spleen, bone marrow, and lymph nodes. Irrespective of the precise areas of localization, it appears that *S. typhi* rapidly gain access to intracellular sites, in which multiplication proceeds. The incubation period of typhoid fever may correspond to the phase of invasion from the intestines and multiplication within phagocytes; the clinical manifestations of the disease may become evident as bacteria begin to re-enter the blood from intracellular sites. During the phase of sustained bacteremia, infection of the biliary tract occurs regularly and multiplication of typhoid bacilli in bile leads to seeding the intestinal tract with millions of bacilli. Entry of infected bile into the intestine is responsible for the increase in the number of *S. typhi* in the feces during the second and third weeks of the disease. Infection of the gallbladder is usually asymptomatic, although symptoms of cholecystitis occasionally occur.

The proliferation of large mononuclear cells derived from reticuloendothelial tissue is the most prominent feature of the pathology of typhoid fever. Involvement of lymphoid tissue in the intestinal tract, principally Peyer's patches in the terminal ileum, may lead to necrosis and ulceration at these sites. The erosion of blood vessels in the lesions may give rise to intestinal hemorrhage. Although intestinal lesions are usually confined to the mucosa and submucosa, muscular and serosal layers are occasionally penetrated, leading to intestinal perforation. The healing of intestinal lesions does not give rise to appreciable scarring or the formation of strictures.

The liver is enlarged during typhoid fever; there are focal areas of necrosis with cloudy swelling of hepatic cells. The spleen and mesenteric lymph nodes are enlarged, and there is hyperplasia of reticuloendothelial cells. Bronchitis is common and pneumonia is not unusual. The maculopapular skin lesions are infiltrated with mononuclear cells, and there is vascular congestion.

The infectious dose of *S. typhi* for humans is influenced by many factors. Although very little information is available regarding the number of bacilli ingested by patients who develop typhoid under natural circumstances, in volunteers, relatively large numbers of *S. typhi* are required to produce infection. With the extensively studied Quailes strain, the dose producing infection in 50% of volunteers (ID_{50}) was 10^7 viable units given orally; 10^9 viable units caused typhoid in approximately 95% of volunteers, whereas 10^5 viable units produced disease in only 28%. Vi antigen, a surface or shell antigen of some strains of *S. typhi,* apparently interferes with serum bactericidal activity and phagocytosis. It appears to be an important determinant of virulence. Rates of disease in volunteers infected with Vi-positive strains were higher than in those receiving comparable doses of non-Vi strains. Prior administration of streptomycin to volunteers resulted in an increase in susceptibility to infection with *S. typhi;* that is, the normal flora of the intestinal tract may be an important defense against invasion by typhoid bacilli. The applicability of these studies in volunteers to naturally occurring typhoid infection is unknown, but parallels almost certainly exist.

The concept that the endotoxins of *S. typhi* might be important in the pathogenesis of typhoid fever was derived from similarities between the manifestations of typhoid fever and the clinical consequences of injection of bacterial endotoxins in man. Both typhoid fever and endotoxins give rise to chills, fever, headache, myalgias, anorexia, nausea, thrombocytopenia, and leukopenia. Repeated injections of bacterial endotoxins render animals and humans increasingly tolerant to the fever-producing effects of the endotoxins so that even large doses produce no signs or symptoms. Because tolerance to the pyrogenic action of endotoxin was demonstrable in volunteers during the convalescent phase of typhoid, it was thought that biologically active quantities of endotoxin were released during the course of the disease. However, the significance of this observation was placed in doubt when it was subsequently shown that volunteers rendered markedly resistant to endotoxin prior to infection with *S. typhi* developed typhoid fever that was indistinguishable from typhoid fever in nontolerant volunteers. Ultimately, it was shown that tolerance actually persisted during the course of typhoid but that responsiveness to endotoxins seemed to be diminished; that is, the tolerant volunteers reacted to the intravenous injection of endotoxins during the course of typhoid fever but reacted less vigorously than did the nontolerant volunteers with typhoid. As endotoxins cannot be demonstrated in the blood using the limulus gel assay, other mechanisms are implicated in the sustained fever and toxemia of typhoid fever. Perhaps the synthesis and release of endogenous pyrogen from stimulated macrophages and polymorphonuclear neutrophils in local typhoid inflammatory lesions are involved.

In volunteers, vascular hyperreactivity to epinephrine and norepinephrine appears during the febrile phase of typhoid fever and persists into convalescence. Such exaggerated vascular responsiveness is not indicative of endotoxemia but may be related to serotonin released from the diseased bowel.

The studies in volunteers have established conclusively that immunity in typhoid is not related to the presence of antibodies against the common antigens of *S. typhi.* There is no correlation of resistance to natural or experimental infections or the occurrence of relapse with the titer of antibodies to the O, H, or Vi antigens of the typhoid bacilli. Stimulated macrophages seem to be responsible for the resistance in experimental murine typhoid.

Patients with a benign course have stimulated T-lymphocytes, whereas patients with prolonged and severe typhoid disease have suppressor T-lymphocytes.

Manifestations

The incubation period for typhoid fever appears to vary inversely with the size of the inoculum and is usually 8 to 14 days (range, 3–60 days). The clinical manifestations vary markedly from one patient to another. Mild illness may occur and is characterized primarily by fever lasting 1 week or less. Illness may be prolonged if untreated, lasting 8 weeks or more. The duration of illness in a case of average severity is about 4 weeks. In some patients, presumably those ingesting extremely large doses of *S. typhi,* acute gastroenteritis may precede the onset of typhoid fever.

Symptoms

Fever is usually the earliest indication of typhoid disease, rising in a stepwise fashion during the first week. The onset of symptoms is gradual; they include: anorexia, lethargy, malaise, and general aches and pains. Dull, continuous headache is a prominent symptom, and it is frequently confined to the frontal regions. Approximately two-thirds of the patients have a nonproductive cough and symptoms suggesting bronchitis. Approximately 10% of patients have nosebleed. Most patients are aware of vague abdominal pain and discomfort. Constipation is the most common intestinal complaint, although approximately 20% of patients have mild to moderate diarrhea.

During the second week of illness, remission of the fever is less common than in the first week, and the temperature is often sustained around 104°F. The patient is frequently severely ill during this phase of illness; weakness, mental dullness, or even delirium may be prominent. Abdominal discomfort and distention increase, and diarrhea is more common during the second week than during the first. The feces may contain blood.

As the illness extends into the third week, the patient continues to be febrile and becomes increasingly exhausted and weak. If no complications occur, the patient may begin to improve toward the end of the third week. The temperature gradually begins to decline and may reach normal levels by the end of the fourth week.

Signs

During the first week of illness, the only physical signs of disease may be fever and tenderness on palpation of the lower quadrants of the abdomen. Distention is frequently present, and the examiner may experience a sensation of displacing loops of bowel filled with air and fluid on palpation of the abdomen.

During the second or third week of illness, the characteristic physical findings of typhoid fever may develop. The patient appears to be acutely ill. The face is dull and expressionless. In some patients, there is mental confusion. Delirium is relatively common in patients with severe disease. A temperature–pulse disproportion may be evident. Rhonchi and scattered moist rales occur in as many as 50% of patients during this phase of typhoid fever. The abdomen may be quite tender on palpation, and distention may be severe. The incidence of splenomegaly varies, ranging from one-third to three-quarters of the patients. Also during the second and third week of illness, the characteristic rose-colored spots of typhoid fever may appear; they are usually located on the upper abdomen. These are small (2 mm–5 mm) maculopapular lesions that blanch on pressure. The lesions are usually sparse, not exceeding 20 in number. The incidence of rose-colored spots varies markedly from one study to another; some observers rarely see them, whereas others describe them in as many as 80% of patients. Rose spots usually persist 2 to 4 days but may recur in crops.

The signs of illness subside as fever diminishes. Convalescence is slow, and a month or more is often required to regain health.

Laboratory Investigations

During the course of the illness, a normochronic anemia develops that is unrelated to blood loss. However, the anemia may be aggravated by blood loss in the feces. Leukopenia is observed in many cases and is characterized by a relative decrease in the number of polymorphonuclear leukocytes and an absence of eosinophils. The leukopenia is usually moderate, rarely falling below 2500/mm^3. A moderate leukocytosis to 12,000/mm^3 may be observed in some patients. Proteinuria is common during the febrile period of the disease. Melena is common during the third and fourth weeks of illness.

Salmonella typhi can be isolated from the blood in about 90% of patients during the first week of disease and from about 50% of patients at the end of the third week. Positive blood cultures are infrequent after the fourth week. Typhoid bacilli can be cultured from rose spots and may persist in the bone marrow after blood cultures are negative. *Salmonella typhi* can be isolated from feces at any stage of illness, but the greatest incidence of positive results is obtained during the third to fifth weeks, when 85% of patients have positive cultures. Typhoid bacilli can be cultured from urine in about 25% of patients with typhoid fever during the third and fourth weeks of illness. Almost certainly some of the positive urine cultures are related to fecal contamination.

The frequency of positive stool cultures begins to decrease rapidly about 6 weeks after onset of illness. Two or three months after onset, only 5% to 10% of patients continue to excrete bacilli. Additional patients become negative for typhoid bacilli during subsequent months, but 3% continue to excrete *S. typhi* for periods of more than 1 year. Persons with documented excretion of bacilli in feces for 1 or more years are termed chronic enteric carriers. Chronic carriers may continue to excrete bacilli for many years, usually for life, unless efforts are made to terminate the carrier state. The number of typhoid bacilli excreted in the feces of these persons is exceedingly high—always in the range of 10^6 viable units and frequently in the range of 10^9 viable units per gram of feces. Typhoid bacilli enter the feces from the biliary tract. Gallstones are frequently present, or there is nonvisualization of the gallbladder cholecystographically. The chronic enteric carrier state after typhoid fever is more frequently seen in adults than in children, and in women than in men.

An increase in the titer of agglutinins against somatic and flagellar antigens—the Widal reaction—usually occurs in the course of typhoid fever, reaching a peak titer during the third week of the disease. A fourfold or greater increase in titer of O agglutinins, in the absence of typhoid immunization, should be considered highly suggestive of infection; a single high titer is usually not significant in diagnosis. Interpretation of agglutination tests is difficult because of cross-reactions with other enteric bacteria and because agglutinins persist, sometimes in high titer, for many months or years after immunization. Accordingly, in the diagnosis of typhoid, the agglutination reaction is subordinate to direct cultural demonstration of the causative organism.

Diagnosis

Typhoid fever can be confused with a wide variety of infectious diseases characterized by fever. A history of travel in endemic areas or a prolonged febrile illness with or without typical manifestations of typhoid should arouse suspicion. Herpes labialis is rare in typhoid fever, and its presence should lead to the consideration of other diagnoses. The prominence of manifestations of bronchitis may lead to confusion with bacterial, myocoplasmal, or viral pneumonia. Other diagnostic possibilities include systemic infections with other *Salmonella* spp., disseminated tuberculosis, malaria, brucellosis, shigellosis, murine typhus fever, tularemia, Rocky Mountain spotted fever, acute bacterial bronchitis, and Hodgkin's disease.

If typhoid fever is suspected, definitive diagnosis should be sought by attempting to isolate the causative microorganism from the blood, feces, urine, or occasionally the sputum or purulent exudates. A fourfold or greater increase in agglutinin titer, especially against the O antigen, without recent immunization, confirms the diagnosis.

Prognosis

Intestinal Hemorrhage and Perforation

Intestinal hemorrhage may occur during the second or third week of typhoid fever. Severe bleeding occurs in about 2% of patients, although gross blood is present in the feces of 10% to 20% of patients, and a positive test for occult blood is even more common.

Intestinal perforation also occurs during the second or third week of illness. Perforation usually occurs in the lower ileum and develops in about 1% of patients. Intestinal perforation is the most serious of all complications of typhoid fever.

The first sign of hemorrhage or perforation may be a sudden drop in temperature or an increase in pulse rate. Often one or more episodes of bleeding precede a perforation. The perforation is usually associated with acute abdominal pain, tenderness, and rigidity that are most marked in the right lower quadrant of the abdomen. Signs of peritonitis develop rapidly after perforation, and the temperature returns to febrile levels.

Other Complications

Thrombophlebitis, particularly of the femoral vein, occurs in a small proportion of patients. Cerebral thrombosis also develops occasionally. Acute cholecystitis may result in typhoid of the gallbladder. Pneumonia is a well-recognized complication of typhoid fever, occurring in 2% to 3% of patients during the second or third week of illness. Although it is clear that *S. typhi* can produce pneumonia, other bacteria, such as the pneumococcus, may be responsible for the pulmonary complications observed in typhoid fever. *Salmonella typhi* circulating in the blood may localize in any organ and give rise to such local infections as osteomyelitis, meningitis, endocarditis, or abscesses. Encephalopathy, actually a feature of the disease, may be extremely severe in certain patients; it may be associated with deranged mentation persisting 2 to 4 weeks after the other manifestations of typhoid have subsided. Acute circulatory failure, toxic myocarditis, and extreme hyperpyrexia may also complicate the acute phases of typhoid. Alopecia was a well-known sequela of typhoid fever in the preantimicrobic era. The incidence of abortion increases when typhoid fever occurs during pregnancy, especially when it occurs during the first trimester.

Relapse

In 8% to 10% of untreated patients, illness may recur 1 to 2 weeks after defervescence. The signs and symptoms are similar to those observed during the initial illness. Since the introduction of chloramphenicol, the incidence of relapse has increased, ranging from 15% to 20%. The peak incidence of relapse is approximately 2 weeks after the termination of antimicrobic therapy—at a time when the antibody titer is at the highest level. The relapse is usually milder than the initial episode, but it may be quite severe and last for as long as 3 weeks if not interrupted by antimicrobial therapy. Second and even third relapses may occur.

Chronic Carriers

A chronic intestinal carrier state with a site of persistent infection in the gallbladder is observed as a complication of typhoid fever in approximately 3% of cases in the United States and Europe. Chronic urinary carriers are said to be more common than intestinal carriers in areas of the world such as Egypt, where the incidence of infection with *Schistosoma haematobium* is high. Effective treatment of the schistosomiasis results in elimination of chronic urinary carriage of *S. typhi.*

Immunity

Typhoid fever usually confers lifelong immunity, and second attacks, although observed, are rare. Nevertheless, the immunity induced by infection can be overcome by simply increasing the infecting dose of *S. typhi.* Immunity is unrelated to the titer of antibodies against the O, H, or Vi antigens.

Mortality

The fatality rate of typhoid fever before effective antimicrobial therapy varied among socioeconomic groups, averaging about 10%. Death was usually associated with profound toxemia, circulatory failure, intestinal perforation, intestinal hemorrhage, or intercurrent pneumonia. The fatality rate since the introduction of chloramphenicol is 1% to 2% in institutions equipped to provide appropriate supportive care.

Therapy

Chloramphenicol has been employed successfully in the management of typhoid fever since 1948, and it is still the antimicrobial agent of choice. This position of leadership has never been seriously or lastingly challenged by any other antimicrobic. Newer agents are neither more rapid in action nor less toxic.

Strains resistant to chloramphenicol were of no significance despite widespread use in endemic areas until 1972, when a major epidemic of typhoid erupted in Mexico City and the surrounding area. Typhoid bacilli resistant to chloramphenicol appeared and were responsible for the marked increase in the endemic rate of typhoid fever. This strain subsequently has largely disappeared, since as the use of chloramphenicol was curtailed and patients were treated with ampicillin, amoxicillin, or trimethoprim-sulfamethoxazole. Similar chloramphenicol-resistant strains were also isolated from patients in the Middle East and South-east Asian countries. Although a few tourists contracted typhoid caused by these strains, no secondary cases were documented in the United States. The origin of the R factor responsible for chloramphenicol resistance has not been determined.

Comparative trials of chloramphenicol, and ampicillin or amoxicillin, or chloramphenicol, and trimethoprim-sulfamethoxazole demonstrated the slight superiority of chloramphenicol. There was a shorter duration of fever, and there were fewer relapses.

Chloramphenicol is given orally. After a loading dose of 15 mg to 20 mg/kg body wt, treatment is continued at a dosage of 50mg to 60 mg/kg body wt/day, given as four equal portions every 6 hours until the temperature is normal. The dosage is then reduced to 30 mg/kg/day, given as previously, and continued for 2 weeks. The response to treatment is not rapid; fever may persist from 1 to more than 7 days after beginning treatment with chloramphenicol, but is usually normal after 3 to 5 days. Patients generally show some subjective improvement after 1 to 2 days. Hemorrhage and perforation may develop during therapy with chloramphenicol, even in afebrile patients. Response is more prompt when therapy is initiated early in the course of the illness. The response is also more rapid in patients infected with strains of low virulence. Treatment with chloramphenicol does not alter the incidence of the chronic carrier state, but it may result in the suppression of the agglutinin response in patients treated during the early phase of illness. Treatment of a relapse is the same as for the initial episode.

Ampicillin is less effective than chloramphenicol in the treatment of typhoid fever. Fever persists for 6.5 to 8 days in patients treated with ampicillin, but it lasts an average of 5 days in patients given chloramphenicol. Five to ten percent of patients fail to respond during the initial 4 to 5 days of treatment with ampicillin, whereas fewer than 1% of patients have a delayed response to chloramphenicol. Finally, ampicillin offers no advantage over chloramphenicol in reducing the incidence of relapse or of the chronic state. Ampicillin should be given parenterally: 60 mg to 100 mg/kg body wt/day, IM or IV, as four equal portions, 6-hourly.

Amoxicillin is well absorbed from the gastrointestinal tract. A dose of 75 mg to 100 mg/kg body wt/day, given perorally as four equal portions 6-hourly, will be comparable in effectiveness to infected ampicillin. Trimethoprim-sulfamethoxazole has been of therapeutic value, especially in patients infected with chloramphenicol-resistant strains of typhoid bacilli.

Although a number of antimicrobics inhibit *S. typhi* by *in vitro* testing, in patients with typhoid fever, they are either without effect or yield poor results. Antimicrobials in this category include the tetracyclines, cephalosporins, streptomycin, kanamycin, polymyxins, gentamicin, nalidixic acid, sulfonamides, penicillin G in small doses, and furazolidone.

Occasionally a patient with typhoid fever without evidence of suppurative complications shows no evidence of clinical response after 5 to 6 days of antimicrobial therapy. For these patients, and patients with severe toxemia, the use of glucosteroids should be considered. For example, prednisone can be given in a dose of 1 mg/kg body wt during the first day (perorally, four equal portions every 6 hours), 0.6 mg/kg during the second day, and 0.3 mg/kg on the third, final day. In patients treated with glucosteroids, the temperature returns to normal or occasionally decreases to hypothermic levels within hours, and the toxic state rapidly ameliorates. When given in conjunction with antimicrobial therapy, glucosteroids do not seem to increase the risk of complications.

Perforation is usually treated conservatively without surgical intervention. Chloramphenicol should be continued, and additional antimicrobial drugs, for example, gentamicin (5 mg-6 mg/kg body wt/day, as three equal portions every 8 hours by IM or IV injection), should be given.

Patients with typhoid fever are unusually sensitive

to the antipyretic effects of salicylates and may develop profound hypothermia after small doses. Sponge baths with tepid water are effective in lowering temperature and should be used instead of salicylates. Laxatives and enemas should not be used because of the danger of inciting intestinal perforation or hemorrhage.

Cholecystectomy alone results in the cure of the chronic enteric carrier state in about 85% of patients, even in the absence of antimicrobial therapy, although in most series some kind of antimicrobial therapy has been administered at the time of and immediately after cholecystectomy.

Choramphenicol is not effective in the treatment of the chronic carrier state and should not be used for this purpose.

Ampicillin may be of value in certain chronic typhoid carriers. If there is no evidence of gallbladder disease, the prolonged administration of ampicillin is associated with the termination of the carrier state in most patients. Ampicillin should be given in a daily dose of 100 mg/kg body wt/day, PO, as four equal portions every 6 hours, along with probenecid (30 mg/kg body wt/day, PO, as four equal portions 6-hourly for 4 to 6 weeks. Patient compliance is usually poor because of the ampicillin-associated diarrhea and gastrointestinal distress. In patients with evidence of gallbladder disease or gallstones, cholecystectomy is the therapy of choice.

Prevention

Typhoid vaccine is effective in reducing the incidence of disease in properly immunized persons—an effect less evident in adults than children. Although studies in volunteers have documented the protective effect of typhoid immunization, they have also emphasized the relatively minor degree of protection that results from vaccination. Protection is evident only when relatively small numbers of *S. typhi* are used in the challenge; it is easily overcome by increasing the size of the inoculum. There is no correlation between protective effect and titer of agglutinins against O, H, or Vi antigens, or with serum bactericidal activity.

Local discomfort, regional lymphadenopathy, and fever frequently follow the administration of typhoid vaccine. The administration of aspirin (0.3 g every 4 hours) for 1 day beginning with vaccination will eliminate the distress. Alternatively, systemic reactions can be minimized by giving the vaccine intracutaneously in doses of 0.1 ml; the local pain and tenderness may still be severe.

To maintain optimal immunity, it is necessary to repeat immunization with a booster injection of vaccine annually. Typhoid immunization should be given to persons working or traveling in highly endemic areas, laboratory workers exposed to *S. typhi,* and persons residing in areas in which typhoid is prevalent.

Remaining Problems

The control of typhoid fever has a high priority in countries in which there is a high incidence of it. Improving the socioeconomic standards of developing countries is an immediately available method for reducing the incidence of typhoid and many other diseases. Present immunization techniques are not promising as a means of control, and more effective vaccines are needed. Oral vaccines with inactivated or viable bacilli offer some promise.

Other problems include the development of an understanding of immunity in typhoid and the development of effective alternatives to chloramphenicol and ampicillin in therapy.

Bibliography

Book

HUCKSTEP RL: Typhoid Fever and Other Salmonella Infections. London, E & S Livingstone, 1962. 334 pp.

Journals

DINBAR A. ALTMANN G. TULCINSKY DB: The treatment of chronic biliary salmonella carriers. Am J Med 47:236–242, 1969

GARROD LP, JAMES DG, LEWIS AAG: The synergy of trimethoprim and sulfonamides. Postgrad M J (Suppl) 45:1–104, 1969

HORNICK RB, GREISMAN SE, WOODWARD TE, DUPONT HL, DAWKINS AT, SYNDER MJ: Typhoid fever: Pathogenesis and immunologic control. N Engl J Med 283:686–691; 739–746, 1970

KAYE D, MERSELIS JG JR, CONNOLLY CS, HOOK EW: Treatment of chronic enteric carriers of *Salmonella typhosa* with ampicillin. Ann NY Acad Sci 145:429–435, 1967

KAYE D, ROCHA H, EYCHMANS L, PRATA A, HOOK EW: Comparison of parenteral ampicillin and parenteral chloramphenicol in the treatment of typhoid fever. Ann NY Acad Sci 145:423–428, 1967

MERSELIS JG JR, KAYE D. CONNOLLY CS, HOOK EW: Quantative bacteriology of the typhoid carrier state. AM J Trop Med Hyg 13:425–429, 1964

ROBERTSON RP, WAHAB MFA, RAASCH FO: Evaluation of chloramphenicol and ampicillin in salmonella enteric fever. N Engl J Med 278:171–176, 1968

SIMON JH, MILLER RC: Ampicillin in the treatment of chronic typhoid carriers, N Engl J Med 274:808, 1966

WOODWARD TE, SMADEL JE: Management of typhoid fever and its complications. Ann Intern Med 60:144, 1964

CHARLES C. J. CARPENTER

Cholera

65

Cholera is an acute illness caused by an enterotoxin elaborated by *Vibrio cholerae* that have colonized the small bowel. In its most severe form, there is rapid loss of liquid and electrolytes from the gastrointestinal tract, resulting in hypovolemic shock, metabolic acidosis, and, if untreated, death.

Etiology

Vibrio cholerae are short (0.2 μm–0.4 μm by 1.5 μm–4.0 μm), slightly curved, gram-negative rods that are readily seen in gram-stained smears of the watery excreta of patients with cholera. *Vibrio cholerae* grow rapidly on a number of selective mediums, including bile salt agar, glycerine–tellurite–taurocholate agar, and thiosulfate–citrate–bile salt–sucrose (TCBS) agar. Of these, TCBS agar has the advantage of not requiring sterilization before use. On TCBS agar, vibrios can be distinguished from other enteric microorganisms by a distinct, opaque yellow colonial appearance. Distinction between the two major serotypes—Inaba and Ogawa—is made by slide agglutination with type-specific antisera.

Identification of the eltor biotype is important for epidemiologic purposes; it is distinguished from the classic biotype by resistance to polymyxin B, resistance to Mukerjee's choleraphage type IV, and by causing hemolysis of sheep erythrocytes.

Epidemiology

For the past century and a half, cholera has remained endemic in the delta of the Ganges, with annual epidemics in major population centers in West Bengal and Bangladesh. The disease has made periodic incursions into other portions of South and Southeast Asia, and it has given rise to seven major pandemics since 1817. Unlike its predecessors, the seventh and most recent pandemic has made only a modest impact on the Western Hemisphere. Thirteen cases of cholera, all caused by the eltor biotype, were identified in the coastal area of Louisiana in the fall of 1978, and the same *V. cholerae* strain was isolated from shellfish and crabs in several areas of the Louisiana coastal marshes. No further spread of cholera has occurred into North or South America.

Humans are the only documented natural host and victim of *V. cholerae*. Water clearly plays a major role in the transmission of *V. cholerae* in endemic rural areas. During major epidemics, however, the direct contamination of food with infected excreta is also important. Persons with mild or asymptomatic infections (contact carriers) probably play an important role in the dissemination of epidemic disease. The ratio of persons with asymptomatic infection to those with clinical disease varies from 4:1 in certain outbreaks caused by classic *V. cholerae* to more than 20:1 in epidemics caused by the eltor biotype. A prolonged gallbladder carrier state may develop in up to 3% of patients convalescing from cholera caused by the eltor biotype. The gallbladder carrier state is more common in older convalescents, and it has never been observed in the pediatric age group. The role of such convalescent carriers in the transmission of the disease has not yet been clarified. In the endemic areas of Bangladesh and West Bengal, cholera is predominantly a disease of children; attack rates are 10 times greater in the 1 to 5 age group than in those over the age of 14 years. However, when the disease spreads to previously uninvolved areas, the attack rates are initially at least as high in adults as in children.

Pathogenesis and Pathology

All signs, symptoms, and metabolic derangements in cholera result from the rapid loss of liquid from the gut. In the adult with cholera, the feces are nearly isotonic with plasma. As compared with plasma, the concentrations of sodium and chloride are slightly less, bicarbonate is approximately twice as high, and potassium is 3 to 5 times higher. The increased electrolyte secretion is caused, in the absence of morphologic damage to the gut mucosa, by a protein enterotoxin which is elaborated by all pathogenic strains of *V. cholerae.* The enterotoxin has a molecular weight of 84,000 daltons, and consists of a binding (B) moiety and an activating (A) moiety. Five equal subunits of 11,500 daltons each make up the B moiety. On exposure to small bowel epithelial cells, each B subunit rapidly binds to a G_{M1} monosialoganglioside in the gut cell wall (Fig. 65-1). Following binding, the A moiety (composed of two unequal subunits) migrates through the epithelial cell membrane. The A1 subunit (~ 23,000 daltons) contains ADP–ribosyltransferase activity and stimulates, by a catalytic process, the transfer of ADP–ribose from NAD to a GTP–binding protein which regulates adenylate cyclase activity. The ADP ribosylation of the GTP–binding protein inhibits the GTP turnoff reaction and causes a sustained increase in adenylate cyclase activity. The resultant increased intracellular cyclic adenosine 3′, 5′ monophosphate (cyclic AMP) acts at two sites to cause net secretion of isotonic fluid with the small bowel lumen. The increased cyclic AMP inhibits neutral NaCl absorption across the brush border via the cotransport mechanism; it also stimulates active chloride secretion into the gut lumen. Apparently, cyclic AMP exerts a direct chloride secretory action primarily on crypt cells and inhibits neutral sodium chloride absorption primarily in villous cells. The net effect of the increased cyclic AMP is the secretion of isotonic liquid by all segments of the small bowel, at a rate that exceeds the absorptive capacity of the colon. The resultant isotonic, watery feces represents the sum of the secretions of all segments of the small bowel, slightly modified during passage through the colon.

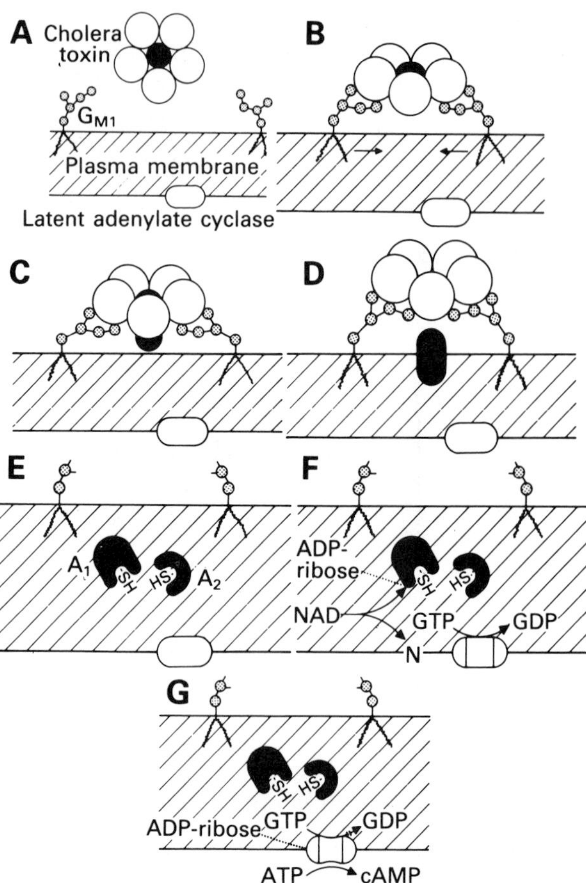

Fig. 65-1. Mechanism of action of cholera enterotoxin. (*A*) Initial situation with enterotoxin free in intestinal lumen. (*B*) Multivalent binding of B subunits of enterotoxin to accessible oligosaccharide chains of G_{M1} monosialoganglioside. (*C*) Conformational change in enterotoxin structure which allows hydrophobic regions in A moiety to interact with mucosal cell membrane. (*D*) Dissociation of enterotoxin components and entry of A moiety into fluid lipid bilayer of membrane. (*E*) Penetration of A moiety into membrane and reduction of disulfide bond to generate active A_1 peptide. (*F*) Cleavage of NAD to nicotinamide (*N*) and ADP-ribose by A_1 peptide. (*G*) Transfer of ADP-ribose to adenylate cyclase complex and its activation by inhibition of GTPase. (Fishman PH: In Field M, Fortran JS, Schultz SG (eds): Secretory Diarrheas. Bethesda, American Physiological Society, 1980)

Manifestations

The clinical onset of cholera is generally that of abrupt, painless, watery diarrhea. In severe cases, several liters of liquid may be lost within a few hours, leading rapidly to profound shock. At varying intervals after the onset of diarrhea, vomiting may ensue. This is characteristically effortless and is not preceded by nausea. In the more severe cases, muscle cramps are almost invariably present and commonly involve the calves.

When first seen by the physician, the patient who is severely ill with cholera is cyanotic and has sunken eyes and cheeks, a scaphoid abdomen, poor skin turgor, and thready or absent peripheral pulses (Fig. 65-2). The voice is high-pitched or inaudible; the vital signs include tachycardia, tachypnea, and low or unobtainable blood pressure. The heart sounds are dis-

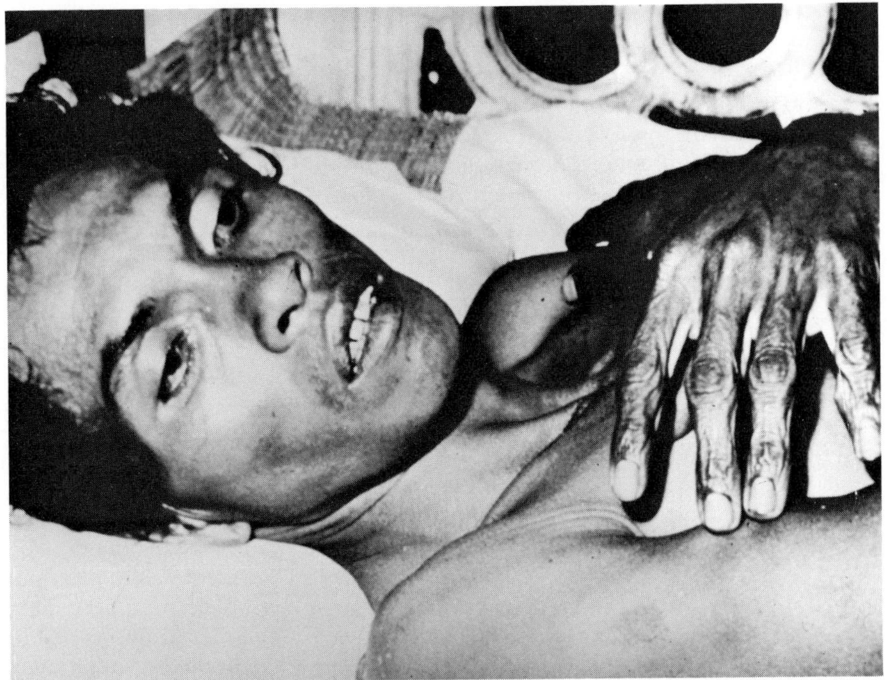

Fig. 65-2. Patient with acute cholera who had a deficit in isotonic fluid of about 10% of his body weight. The "washwoman's hands" are indicative of severe depletion of extracellular fluid. (Gangarosa EJ: Bull NY Acad Med 47:1140–1151, 1971)

tant, often inaudible, and bowel sounds are usually hypoactive. Major alterations in mental status are not common in adults; the patient usually remains well oriented, though apathetic, even in the face of severe hypovolemic shock. As many as 10% of small children may have central nervous system abnormalities that range from stupor to convulsions. In all epidemics, there are large numbers of mild cases in which the loss of liquid from the gut is not severe enough to require hospitalization.

The loss of liquid and electrolytes continues for 1 to 7 days, and subsequent manifestations depend on the adequacy of replacement therapy. With prompt replacement, physiologic recovery is remarkably rapid and uniform despite continuing voluminous diarrhea (Table 65-1). If therapy is inadequate, the mortality rate in hospitalized patients may exceed 50%. The important causes of death are hypovolemic shock, uncompensated metabolic acidosis, and uremia. When renal failure occurs, the characteristic pathologic findings are those of acute tubular necrosis secondary to prolonged hypotension.

Table 65-1. ***Blood Chemical Determinations in 38 Adult Patients With Cholera Before and 4 Hours After Intravenous Fluid Therapy***

	Mean Values ± S.D.	
Blood Chemicals	ON ADMISSION	4 HOURS
Arterial blood pH	7.17 ± 0.6	7.40 ± .05
Plasma bicarbonate (mEq/l)	7 ± 4	20 ± 3
Plasma potassium (mEq/l)	5.6 ± 0.4	3.2 ± 0.3
Total plasma protein (g/dl)	14.2 ± 0.8	7.5 ± 0.6

Diagnosis

In endemic or epidemic areas, the working diagnosis of cholera should be made on the basis of the clinical picture. Liquid and electrolyte replacement therapy should be instituted immediately. Although a cholera-like illness may be caused by microorganisms other than *V. cholerae,* most frequently by enterotoxigenic *Escherichia coli,* the resulting physiologic and metabolic abnormalities are the same, so that identical IV and PO electrolyte therapy should be used in all such cases.

Diagnostic culture techniques are relatively simple. A reliable and practical method consists of direct plating of feces on TCBS agar. Typical opaque yellow colonies appear in 18 hours. Final identification requires agglutination with group- and type-specific antiserums and the demonstration of characteristic biochemical reactions. Rapid tentative diagnosis may be made by the direct observation of the characteristic rapid motility of the comma-shaped bacilli in fresh feces by darkfield microscopy. Group- and type-specific antiserums immobilize homologous strains and clearly distinguish them from other vibrios.

Prognosis

With adequate therapy, the mortality rate approaches zero. Largely because of the mechanical problems inherent in the administration of large amounts of liquid to small children, a mortality rate of 1% to 2% still remains in pediatric patients despite the best current therapy. A single attack of cholera confers only short-lived protection against subsequent infection by *V. cholerae.*

Therapy

Successful therapy demands only prompt replacement of gastrointestinal losses of liquid and electrolytes. A solution for IV infusion which is uniformly effective in adult patients, may be prepared by adding 5 g sodium chloride, 4 g sodium bicarbonate, and 1 g potassium chloride to a liter of sterile distilled water. Alternatively, lactated Ringer's solution can be administered. Either of these isotonic preparations should be given rapidly by IV injection—50 ml to 100 ml per minute—until a strong radial pulse has been restored. Subsequently, the same solution should be infused in quantities equal to gastrointestinal losses, or if these losses cannot be measured accurately, at a rate sufficient to maintain a normal radial pulse volume and normal skin turgor. Overhydration can be avoided by careful observation of the veins in the neck and by ausculation of the lungs. Close observation of the patient is mandatory during the acute phase of the illness. An adult patient can lose as much as 1 liter per hour of isotonic liquid during the first 24 hours of the disease. Inadequate or delayed restoration of electrolyte losses results in a very high incidence of acute renal insufficiency. Serious hypokalemia is rare in the adult, and potassium replacement can usually be carried out by giving PO approximately 15 mEq of potassium chloride for each liter of feces that is produced.

In children, complications are both more frequent and more severe. The most serious include stupor, coma and convulsions (unique to pediatric patients), pulmonary edema, and cardiac arrhythmias that occasionally lead to cardiac arrest. The central nervous system complications may be due to hypoglycemia (observed only in pediatric patients), hypernatremia resulting from the administration of isotonic solutions to the pediatric patient (who, unlike the adult patient, produces feces with a sodium concentration significantly less than that of plasma) or cerebral edema, presumably secondary to rapid shifts during the IV administration of liquids. Pulmonary edema may result if liquid is given intravenously at too rapid a rate, especially in the presence of severe metabolic acidosis. Cardiac arrhythmias may result from potassium depletion in children but occur rarely, if ever, in adults with cholera. Each of these complications can be avoided by the careful IV administration of solutions especially designed to replace the fecal electrolyte losses of children with cholera.

The following solution has been used successfully to correct hypokalemia and hypoglycemia without provoking hypernatremia: sodium 95 mEq/liter, chloride 65 mEq/liter, potassium 15 mEq/liter, bicarbonate 45 mEq/liter, and glucose 20 g/liter. Alternatively, lactated Ringer's solution may be administered, but should be supplemented by the PO administration of water and glucose; one glass (240 ml) of 5% glucose should be given PO, 6-hourly to children who are receiving lactated Ringer's solution by IV injection. Administration of this solution must be carefully monitored, with frequent auscultation of the lungs and inspection of venous filling in the neck in order to avoid overhydration. The outcome in pediatric cholera should be essentially as favorable as that in the adult disease—an overall mortality rate of less than 1%.

When IV liquids are in short supply, PO replacement of water and electrolytes is effective in adults and in children who are alert and able to retain orally administered solutions. Glucose–electrolyte solutions may be given PO in mild cholera throughout the course of illness, and are useful in the more severe cases once the hypovolemic shock has been corrected by initial, rapid IV treatment. Losses from the gut may be replaced by PO administration of an isotonic solution prepared by adding 20 g glucose, 3.5 g sodium chloride, 2.5 g sodium bicarbonate and 1.5 g potassium chloride to a liter of water (see list below). Glucose is an essential component of this solution because the uptake of sodium in the small bowel is enhanced by the presence of intraluminal glucose. If glucose is not available, sucrose (table sugar) may be substituted in a concentration of 40 g per liter; in the small bowel, sucrase splits sucrose into glucose and fructose; that is, half of the sucrose becomes available to facilitate the intestinal sodium absorption. Initially, liquids are given PO in large quantities, for example, 250 ml every 15 minutes in

COMPOSITION OF GLUCOSE-ELECTROLYTE SOLUTION FOR PERORAL THERAPY OF ACUTE DIARRHEAL DISEASES (mEq/LITER)

Sodium	90
Potassium	20
Chloride	80
Bicarbonate	30
Glucose	111

adults, until balance has been restored as gauged by clinical observations. Thereafter, sufficient quantities are administered to balance the output of feces: 1.5 liters of glucose–electrolyte solution should be given PO for each liter of feces. The administration of liquids PO does not decrease the volume of fluid lost through the gut, but provides additional fluids that can be absorbed rapidly enough to counterbalance the enterotoxin-induced secretion of liquid.

Provision of adequate liquid with correction of the attendant biochemical derangements results in rapid recovery in virtually all patients with cholera. However, adjunctive treatment with antimicrobics dramatically reduces the duration and volume of diarrhea and results in the early eradication of vibrios from the feces. Tetracycline in a dose of 30 mg-40 mg/kg body wt/day, PO, as four equal portions, 6-hourly, for 2 days was once uniformly successful. However, in 1979–1980, a number of isolates of *V. cholerae* from patients in Bangladesh and Tanzania exhibited resistance to tetracycline, a phenomenon not yet observed in other areas. Furazolidone and chloramphenicol are also of value, but they are slightly less effective than tetracycline.

Prevention

Immunization using the standard commercial vaccine (containing 10 billion killed vibrios/ml) may provide 60% to 80% protection for 3 to 6 months. Although immunization of experimental animals with toxoid provided highly significant protection, it proved to be no more effective than the standard, whole-cell vaccine in field trials in humans. At present, careful hygiene provides the only sure protection against cholera.

Remaining Problems

Although a uniformly successful replacement regimen has been formulated, the economic, logistic, and educational difficulties in endemic areas are so great that effective therapy is still not available for many patients with cholera. This problem can be bypassed either by developing an immunizing agent that reliably confers long-term immunity on most patients who receive it or by developing an agent that rapidly blocks the action of cholera enterotoxin. On the basis of studies in animals and in volunteers, PO immunization may provide more effective immunity. However, practical means of widespread PO vaccination have not yet been developed, and therefore no field trial of PO immunization has been undertaken. The development of a pharmacologic means of blocking the exotoxin-induced loss of fluid and electrolytes from the gut is under intense study.

Bibliography

Books

BARUA D, BURROWS W: Cholera. Philadelphia, WB Saunders, 1974. 458 pp.

FIELD M, FORDTRAN JS, SCHULTZ SG (EDS): Secretory Diarrheas. Bethesda, American Physiological Society, 1980. 227 pp.

Journals

BLAKE PA, ALLEGRA DT, SNYDER JD, BARRETT TJ, MCFARLAND L, CARRAWAY CT, FEELEY JC, CRAIG JP, LEE JV, PUHR ND, FELDMAN RA: Cholera: A possible endemic focus in the United States. N Engl J Med 302:305–309, 1980

CARPENTER CCJ, MITRA PP, SACK RB: Clinical studies in Asiatic cholera, Parts I–VI. Bull Hopkins Hosp 118:165–245, 1966

GANGAROSA EJ, BEISEL WR, BENYAJATI C, SPRINZ H, PIYARATIN P: The nature of the gastrointestinal lesion in Asiatic cholera and its relation to pathogenesis: A biopsy study. Am J Trop Med Hyg 9:125–135, 1960

GILL M: Mechanism of action of cholera toxin. Adv Cyclic Nucleotide Res 8:85–118, 1977

HIRSCHHORN N, LINDENBAUM J, GREENOUGH WB, ALAM SM: Hypoglycemia in children with acute diarrhea. Lancet 2:128–132, 1966

HOLMGREN L, LONROTH I: Oligomeric structure of cholera toxin. J Gen Microbiol 86:49–65, 1975

MAHALANOBIS D, CHOUDHURI AB, BAGCHI NG, BHATTACHARYA AK, SIMPSON TW: Oral therapy of cholera among Bangladesh refugees. Johns Hopkins Med J 132:197–205, 1973

MOSLEY WH: The role of immunity in cholera. A review of epidemiological and serological studies. Tex Rep Biol Med 27:227–241, 1969

PIERCE NF, KOSTER FT: Priming and suppression of the intestinal immune response to cholera toxin/toxoid by parenteral toxoid in rats. J Immunol 124:307–317, 1980

PIERCE NF. SACK RB, MITRA RC, BANWELL JG, BRIGHAM KL, FEDSON DS, MONDAL A: Replacement of water and electrolyte losses in cholera by an oral glucose–electrolyte solution. Ann Intern Med 70:1173–1181, 1969

WALLACE CK, ANDERSON PN, BROWN TC, KHANRA SR, LEWIS GW, PIERCE NF, SANYAL SN, SEGRE GV, WALDMAN RH: Optimal antibiotic therapy in cholera. Bull WHO 39:239–245, 1968

KERRISON JUNIPER, JR.

66 Amebiasis

Although *amebiasis* actually means infection with amebas, the word is generally construed as infection with *Entamoeba histolytica* because only this species of intestinal ameba causes significant disease. However, *Dientamoeba fragilis* apparently can cause mild intestinal symptoms, and fatal meningoencephalitis may result from nasopharyngeal infection with free-living species of *Acanthamoeba, Hartmannella,* or *Naegleria.*

Etiology

Infection is acquired by ingestion of cysts of *E. histolytica* in contaminated food or water. Excystation occurs in the small intestine, and trophozoites become established in the lumen of the proximal colon in which they often live without causing symptoms. As the contents of the colon solidify and conditions thus become unfavorable, trophozoites develop into cysts which can survive in feces. When diarrhea occurs, trophozoites also may appear in unformed feces. There is no intermediate host.

Entamoeba histolytica must be differentiated from other intestinal amebae, especially *Entamoeba coli* and *Entamoeba hartmanni.* In wet preparations, trophozoites of *E. histolytica* appear as hyaline bodies 12 to 60 μm long; typically they show rapid progressive motility and may contain ingested red blood cells, yeasts, or starch granules. Stained trophozoites have a fine cytoplasm; the nucleus contains a small central karyosome with fine clumps of chromatin evenly distributed on a thin nuclear membrane (Fig. 66–1A). Cysts are 10 μm to 20 μm in size with one to four nuclei; the cytoplasm may contain a large glycogen vacuole and rod-shaped, smooth chromatoidal bodies (Fig. 66–1B).

The trophozoites of *E. coli* are 18 μm to 40 μm in size but do not ingest red blood cells or show rapid motility; the cytoplasm often contains ingested bacteria and other debris. The nuclei of stained trophozoites contain a large eccentric karyosome with coarse chromatin granules irregularly distributed on a thick nuclear membrane. Cysts have 1 to 8 nuclei, and the cytoplasm may contain a large glycogen vacuole and irregular, sticklike chromatoidal bodies.

The morphology of *E. hartmanni* is similar to that of *E. histolytica* but the trophozoites are only 6 μm to 12 μm long, and the cysts are 5 μm to 10 μm in diameter. The trophozoites do not ingest red blood cells, and the cysts do not contain a glycogen vacuole.

Epidemiology

Amebiasis has a worldwide distribution. Infection rates of 50% or more may occur where sanitary conditions are unusually poor, in arctic as well as tropical areas. The infection rate in the United States probably averages 1% to 3% but may be much higher in various institutionalized populations, *e.g.,* mentally defective persons, in whom fecal–oral contamination is common. Common modes of transmission include contaminated fresh vegetables and water. The usual municipal chlorination methods are insufficient to kill amebic cysts in water. Venereal transmission of *E. histolytica* has been reported recently, especially among homosexual men, who may have infection rates as high as 32%.

Pathogenesis and Pathology

Intestinal Disease

In some parts of the world, infections caused by *E. histolytica* are infrequently associated with symptoms; in other areas, especially where sanitation and nutrition are inadequate, amebiasis is a frequent cause of serious disease and even death if untreated.

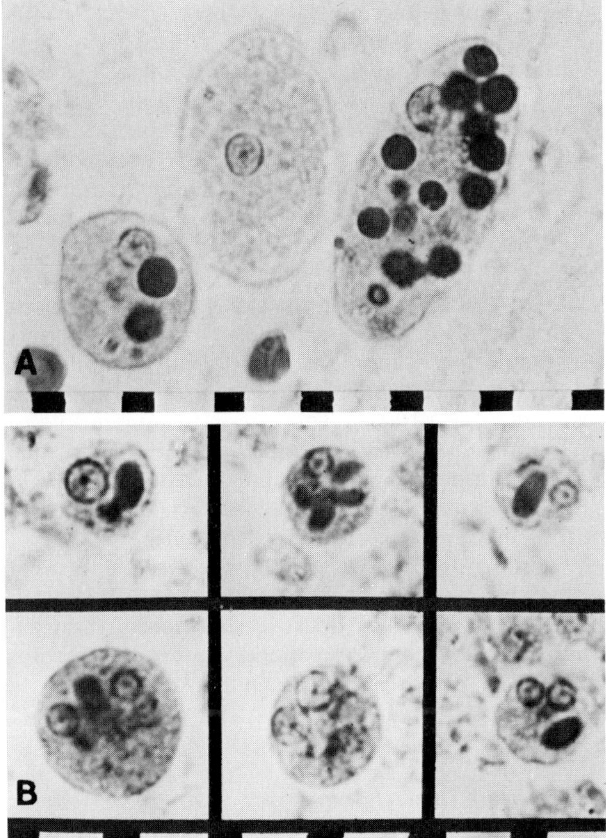

Fig. 66-1. (*A*) Trophozoites of *Entamoeba histolytica.* Note engulfed erythrocytes and characteristic nuclear structure (trichrome stain). Ten-unit micrometer scale shown. (*B*) Cysts of *Entamoeba histolytica* (trichrome stain). Ten-unit micrometer scale shown. (Paulson M (ed): Gastroenterologic Medicine. Philadelphia, Lea & Febiger, 1969)

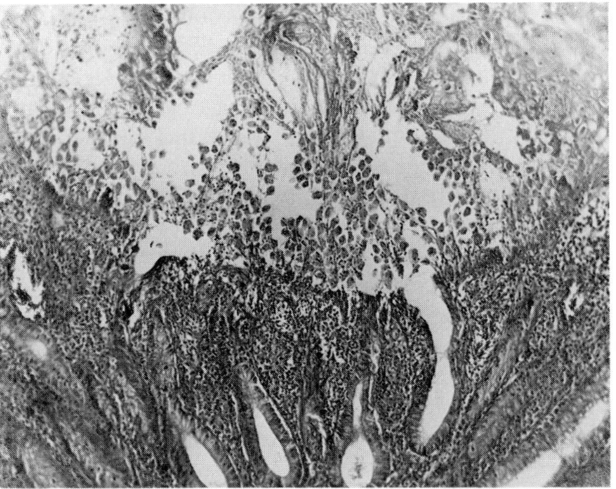

Fig. 66-2. Cross section of biopsy of amebic ulcer in the rectum. Note trophozoites at junction of exudate and viable tissue in base of ulcer. Trophozoites are easily stripped away and lost if exudate is removed from the base of the ulcer. (H&E approximately × 14) (Juniper K Jr, Steele VW, Chester CL: South Med J 51:545–553, 1958)

Because symptoms result from invasion of the colon by trophozoites, the highly variable rate of disease probably reflects the variable pathogenicity of different strains of *E. histolytica* and variable host resistance.

When mucosal resistance becomes lowered, trophozoites can invade colonic epithelium (Fig. 66–2). Ameboid movement and amebic enzymes such as proteases, hyaluronidase, and mucopolysaccharidases, facilitate penetration, either from the surface or within crypts of the mucosa. Microulcers occur in the center of small mucosal nodules caused by tissue reaction to the invading amebae. When cut in cross-section, the flask-shaped area of necrosis typical of these lesions becomes apparent (Fig. 66–3). The invading trophozoites generally do not penetrate muscular layers but spread laterally in the submucosa, undermining the mucosa. Thus, the blood supply to the overlying mucosa is gradually destroyed, resulting in necrosis and sloughing with enlargement of the ulcers to sizes as large as 1 cm–2 cm in diameter.

The invading trophozoites at the periphery of the ulcer induce surprisingly little tissue reaction. There is a narrow border of inflammatory reaction with

Fig. 66-3. Cross section of tiny amebic ulcer in colon at autopsy. Note typical flask shape caused by undermining of mucosa. (H&E approximately × 7)

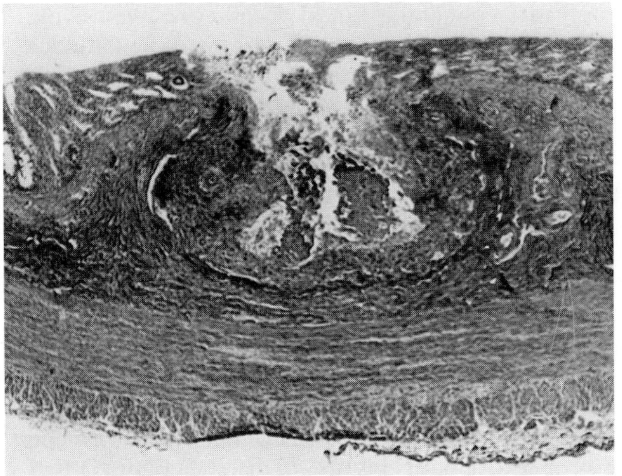

edema and infiltration by plasma cells, eosinophils, and lymphocytes. Neutrophilic polymorphonuclear leukocytes are relatively sparse unless secondary bacterial infection is present. In disease so severe that death results, the amebae may be found in all layers of the colon. Under these conditions neutrophilic infiltration is common and intestinal perforation may occur.

Extraintestinal Disease

The liver is the chief site of extraintestinal amebic disease. Trophozoites gain access to the liver through the portal vein. The frequency of amebic penetration into venules and lymphatics of the colon is unknown, although it is probably common when there is severe amebic ulceration. Also unknown are the factors permitting trophozoites to colonize and initiate necrosis in the liver. Probably few of the amebae that reach the liver survive. Trophozoites induce very little inflammatory response in the liver; so-called amebic hepatitis—attributed to the presence of trophozoites without either necrosis or abscess—is unproven in occurrence and not acceptable as a clinical entity. Only a narrow margin of inflammation is present about an abscess. Solitary abscess is common, but multiple abscesses may occur. Because of the natural channeling of blood within the portal vein (lienal-origin blood goes primarily to the left lobe of the liver; intestinal-origin blood goes primarily to the right lobe), hepatic amebic abscess is commonly located in the right lobe.

Involvement of nonhepatic extraintestinal organs is much less frequent. Trophozoites may disseminate to other organs, especially from a liver abscess, by direct rupture into lung, pleural cavity, or pericardium, or through the bloodstream to lung or brain. Cutaneous lesions may result from direct invasion of macerated epithelium in the perineal area when trophozite-containing liquid feces contaminate the skin, or from subcutaneous invasion from a fistulous tract connecting an abscess or the lumen of the colon to the surface of the body.

Manifestations

Intestinal Disease

Infections caused by *E. histolytica* are often asymptomatic, especially in populations in which nutritional and hygienic conditions are optimum. When present, symptoms result from tissue invasion causing irritation of the colon, leading to diarrhea and associated cramping, and abdominal pain. Symptoms may be mild or severe with episodes of diarrhea lasting 1 to 4 weeks, often recurring several times a year. Periods of diarrhea may alternate with constipation. Less commonly, diarrhea may persist for many weeks. The feces are mushy or watery, foul-smelling, and may contain blood and exudate; defecation occurs 4 to 8 times per day in mild and up to 18 times daily in severe diarrhea. Characteristically, in invasive amebic colitis the feces contain blood-streaked mucus that is shed from the ulcers. Dehydration and electrolyte abnormalities are uncommon because of the small volume of feces. Chronic disease often is associated with weight loss and anemia; less frequently, there is low-grade fever, anorexia, nausea, and vomiting.

Children are more likely to have fever, which often exceeds 38°C (100°F). They are more susceptible to extraintestinal spread of the disease. Infection may occur during the first year of life, but the incidence is highest between 3 and 7 years of age. The mortality rate is higher in children than in adults.

Fulminating amebic colitis with extraintestinal spread has been reported in patients receiving immunosuppressive drugs. Because the mortality rate is high despite antiamebic therapy, amebic infection should be excluded before immunosuppression is undertaken.

Extraintestinal Disease

Liver abscess occurs one-tenth as often as invasive amebic colitis. Only half the patients have a history of diarrhea or a demonstrable intestinal infection with *E. histolytica.* Because the right lobe of the liver is involved in 90% of cases, most patients have pain in the right upper abdomen or right lower chest. The right diaphragm is commonly elevated and moves little if at all (Fig. 66–4). Fever and leukocytosis are present. There may be cough, profuse sweating, anemia, and weight loss. The liver is usually tender and always enlarged, either into the chest or the abdomen. A few patients have only weight loss and a nontender hepatic mass without fever; cancer is often suspected. Jaundice is uncommon but mild when present. Men are afflicted much more often than women. Abscess in the left lobe of the liver produces a tender epigastric mass displacing both stomach and colon. Perforation into the left pleural space, the pericardium, or the peritoneum may complicate a left hepatic abscess.

The lung is the second most common site for extraintestinal amebiasis. The right lower lobe is usually involved by direct extension or rupture of a contiguous liver abscess. Pulmonary infiltration develops, and eventually an abscess may form that may rupture into a bronchus or, less commonly, into the pleural

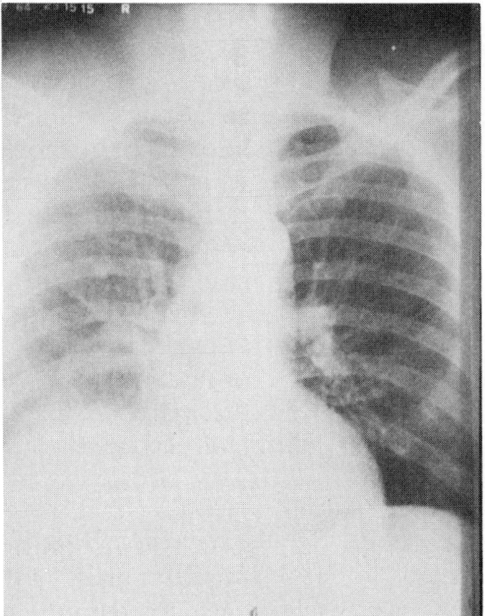
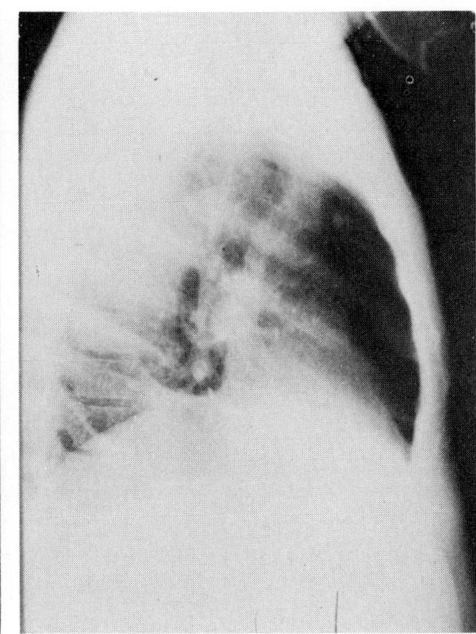

Fig. 66-4. Posterior-anterior and right lateral chest films showing elevation (fixed by fluoroscopy) of the right hemidiaphragm with compression atelectasis of the right lower lobe of the lung resulting from amebic abscess in the right lobe of the liver.

cavity. Chest pain and cough are then aggravated; the purulent sputum may contain trophozoites.

Cutaneous amebiasis constitutes 2% to 3% of invasive amebic disease. In the perineal area, especially perianally, the lesion is well localized and progresses slowly over a period of many months. Lesions are either condylomatous or ulcerative; they are painful and bleed easily. The surface is covered with a grayish yellow exudate, and a serous or semipurulent liquid containing blood and trophozoites exudes from the lesion.

Cutaneous lesions on the thorax or abdomen usually begin by extension from a fistulous tract into the subcutaneous tissues. They are painful and spread rapidly, leaving overhanging edges of necrotic and gangrenous skin. The borders are irregular and elevated, frequently showing a narrow rim of erythema. The base of the ulcer is necrotic (Fig. 66–5). Pus can be expressed from beneath the edges of the ulcer. The mortality is high.

Diagnosis

Intestinal Disease

Amebiasis should always be considered in the differential diagnosis of chronic diarrhea, especially when the feces contains blood-streaked mucus. The diagnosis depends on identification of *E. histolytica* in the feces or in scrapings of rectal ulcers. However, certain substances can render feces unsatisfactory for examination, especially for amebae. Notable in this regard are antidiarrheal preparations containing bismuth or alkaline earths such as kaolin, nonabsorbable antacids, antimicrobics (sulfonamides and antiprotozoal agents), barium sulfate or other heavy metal compounds, oils, and magnesium hydroxide. Substances used for enemas, such as water, soap, irritants, and hypertonic saline solutions, destroy trophozoites and distort cysts. A dependable examination for exclusion of amebiasis cannot be made for a period of 10 to 14 days after the last dose of the interfering substance. This adverse effect also applies to scrapings or biopsies of rectal ulcers. Therefore, it is essential that a careful history of medications be obtained to ascertain the reliability of diagnostic procedures and that these procedures be performed before any interfering substances are given.

Sigmoidoscopy is a valuable diagnostic procedure during an episode of diarrhea. It should be performed without prior preparation of the patient to prevent removal of exudate from ulcers and destruction of trophozoites. Microulcers are difficult to differentiate from prominent mucosal crypts, although each ulcer is often located in the center of a tiny mound of mucosa. Small ulcers may also be very superficial and therefore difficult to detect unless surrounded by a thin rim of mucosal erythema (Fig. 66–6).

Typical well-developed ulcers approach 1 cm to 2 cm in diameter and have rounded or punched-out margins that are elevated from the submucosal inflammatory reaction caused by the advancing trophozoites. The bases of the ulcers are covered by whitish or yellowish exudate (Fig. 66–7). The ulcers may be atypical with irregular margins and bases in 5% to 10% of cases.

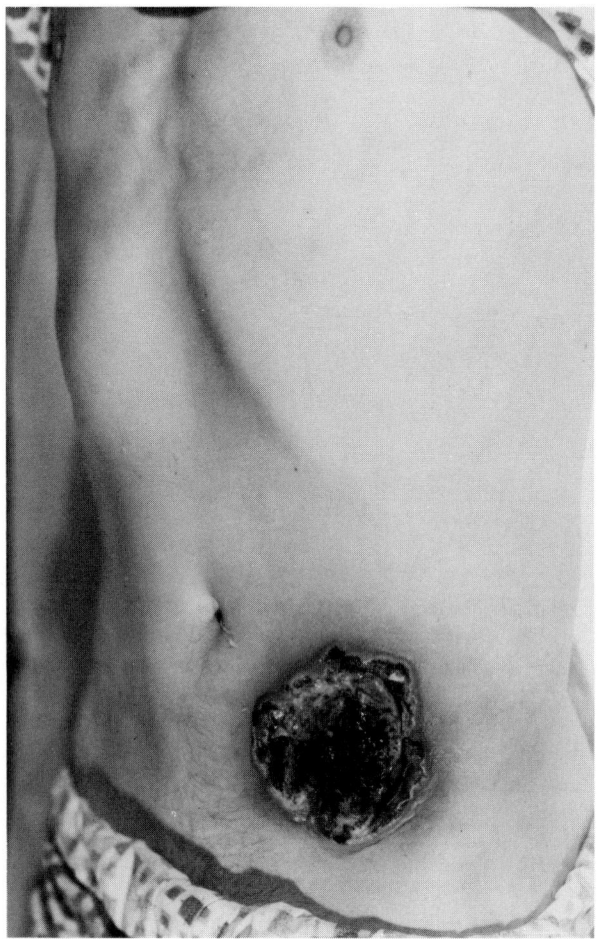

Fig. 66-5. Cutaneous amebic lesion about a colostomy stoma in left lower abdomen. Note necrotic and gangrenous portions of base and elevated irregular margin with surrounding narrow rim of erythema.

A nonspecific diffuse mucosal inflammation commonly occurs in the rectal vault with any type of chronic diarrhea. If such diffuse inflammation is present in amebiasis, there is usually no inflammation in the colon above the rectal vault. However, if diffuse inflammation occurs in the prerectal colon, especially in combination with atypical ulcers, the sigmoidoscopic appearance may be indistinguishable from that of idiopathic ulcerative colitis.

Barium studies of the colon are primarily of value to detect nonamebic causes of diarrhea, such as polyps or cancer, and to identify ameboma. Contrast studies are normal in half the cases of invasive amebic colitis and show distinct ulcerations in only one-fifth of the cases. When ulcers are demonstrated, the roentgenographic changes are not sufficiently characteristic to differentiate amebic from idiopathic ulcerative colitis or other causes of ulceration of the colon.

Various serologic techniques have been successful in detecting antibodies specific for *E. histolytica* when invasive disease is present. However, positive tests can persist for months or even years after cure, and therefore do not necessarily indicate active disease. The tests can be valuable to exclude invasive amebic disease with reasonable reliability in acutely ill patients who have received interfering substances or undergone procedures that compromise diagnosis through examination of the feces. For example, the indirect hemagglutination test will be positive in 94% of patients with invasive amebic colitis.

Extraintestinal Disease

Absolute proof of the diagnosis of amebic abscess of the liver requires demonstration of trophozoites of E. histolytica in the contents of the abscess. In most laboratories, examination of pus is successful in about 50% of cases. Pus must be obtained prior to treatment. Sediment from the last of fractionally collected specimens is most likely to be positive. Also, the yield is increased by adding 10 units of streptodornase to each milliliter of pus, incubating for 30 minutes with shaking, and then examining the centrifuged sediment for trophozoites.

A presumptive diagnosis of amebic abscess can be made if the liquid is an exudate without foul odor and if cultures are negative for bacteria. Amebic abscess

Fig. 66-6. Surface of colon showing early amebic ulcers. Microulcers are located in center of small mounds of mucosa. Larger ulcers are more readily apparent because of narrow rim of erythema about them. (Juniper K Jr. In Paulson M (ed): Gastroenterologic Medicine. Philadelphia, Lea & Febiger, 1969)

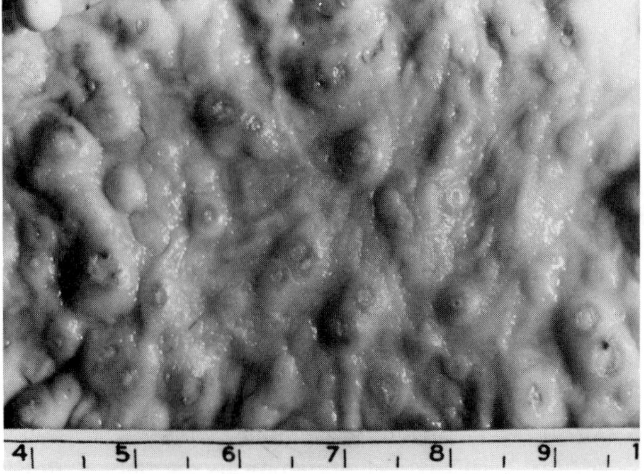

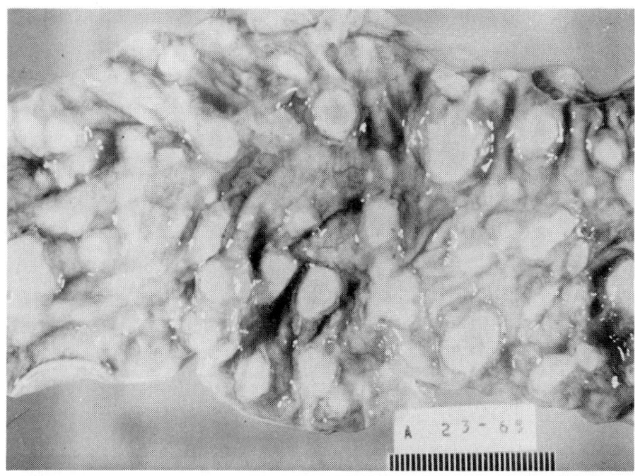

Fig. 66-7. Typical large amebic ulcers with elevated, punched-out margin and white exudate on base. Note normal intervening mucosa.

liquid classically has a brick red or chocolate brown color that results from bleeding into the abscess cavity. However, this color is neither specific nor essential for a presumptive diagnosis, and initial aspiration frequently produces a yellowish or greenish fluid. A presumptive diagnosis of amebic abscess cannot be made when bacteria are present unless trophozoites are also demonstrated.

Roentgenograms of the chest and radioisotope scanning of the liver are of great value in demonstrating hepatomegaly and focal lesions of the liver. Ultrasound examination is useful for differentiating abscesses from cysts and solid tumors. Anemia, leukocytosis, and hypoalbuminemia are present in most cases. Elevation of the serum alkaline phosphatase occurs frequently, whereas the transaminases and bilirubin are usually normal or only mildly elevated. Unfortunately, these laboratory tests are of little help in differentiating amebic and pyogenic abscesses of the liver.

The diagnosis of pulmonary, cutaneous, or other forms of extraintestinal amebiasis requires demonstration of trophozoites in sputum, pleural fluid, exudate, scrapings of skin lesions, or tissue biopsies. Blood-streaked fragments are particularly likely to contain amebae.

Serologic tests are usually positive in extraintestinal amebiasis, for example, in 98% of patients by the indirect hemagglutination test. The titer is generally high, although the magnitude is of no value in differentiating extraintestinal from intestinal disease. Serodiagnosis may be particularly helpful when antiamebic chemotherapy is given prior to examination for amebas. Epidemiologic data and the echinococcal serologic tests are of value in differentiating echinococcal cyst of the liver (Chap. 79, Larval Cestodiasis).

Prognosis

Complications include ameboma, stricture, hemorrhage, intussusception, perforation, and the formation of abscesses. Severe, long-standing amebic colitis uncommonly causes scarring and an irritable colon. Uncomplicated intestinal infections usually respond well to adequate therapy, and the mortality is low. Little protective immunity develops, and reinfection can occur. Recurrent or persistent infection, despite adequate therapy, may result from reinfection, or reflect an incorrect diagnosis. It is possible that rarely a few strains of *E. histolytica* may be resistant to emetine or metronidazole.

The most important complication of liver abscess is extension into adjacent structures, most commonly the right lung. A lung abscess may result and may rupture into a bronchus or the pleural space. A liver abscess may also rupture into peritoneal, pleural, or pericardial cavities. Rupture through the body wall to the surface may give rise to cutaneous amebiasis. The mortality is significant when complications ensue unless early diagnosis leads to early treatment. Brain abscess, a rare complication, usually is fatal.

Therapy

Asymptomatic Intestinal Amebiasis

Opinions vary on the need for treatment of all patients with asymptomatic amebiasis, but most American authorities believe that all such infections in the United States should be treated. Amebic infections are curable except when reinfection is highly likely, and sanitary conditions cannot be controlled. Diiodohydroxyquin or metronidazole are effective in most cases of asymptomatic amebiasis. Metronidazole probably provides a higher cure rate and does not require prolonged administration, but it is more likely than diiodohydroxyquin to cause side effects. Paromomycin and diloxanide are alternative drugs.

Symptomatic Intestinal Amebiasis

Metronidazole is the treatment of choice for symptomatic amebiasis. Tetracycline may be added in critically ill patients when secondary bacterial infection is suspected. Emetine dihydrochloride can be substituted for metronidazole. Emetine dihyrochloride alone will not eradicate intestinal infection, and treatment with metronidazole will eventually be necessary. Metronidazole should be followed by diiodohydroxyquin to cure the few patients who fail with metronidazole alone.

Metronidazole is the drug of choice for ameboma, but emetine dihydrochloride also is effective. The filling defect should disappear within 2 to 4 weeks after treatment is instituted.

Amebic Abscess of Liver

Metronidazole is the drug of choice for the treatment of hepatic amebic abscess because it is less toxic and requires a shorter period of administration than either of the other effective agents, emetine dihydrochloride and chloroquine phosphate. As metronidazole is effective against most anaerobic bacteria, other antibacterial agents are unnecessary unless a specific secondary bacterial infection has been documented. Because treatment with metronidazole has failed in some patients, it may be wise to follow the metronidazole with chloroquine phosphate.

Small abscesses do not require aspiration for treatment, but an initial pretherapy aspiration is advantageous for diagnosis and culture of bacteria. Therapeutic aspiration should be performed if rupture of large abscesses appears to be imminent, or if there is persistent local tenderness or failure of symptoms and signs to remit with drug therapy. As long as 250 ml of liquid is obtained, aspiration of abscesses should be repeated every 3 days. Surgical drainage is necessary only when secondary bacterial infection is present.

Other Forms of Extraintestinal Amebiasis

Pulmonary and cutaneous amebiasis respond to either metronidazole or emetine dihydrochloride. Abscesses may require surgical drainage, but there is no need for resection of lesions. Brain abscesses (1) must be drained surgically, (2) do not respond to emetine dihydrochloride because of poor entry of the drug into the CNS, and (3) should be benefited by use of metronidazole because this drug penetrates the CNS freely.

Use of Drugs

Chloroquine phosphate is not effective for intestinal infections and is used only for the treatment of liver abscesses. The dose of chloroquine base is 15 mg to 17 mg/kg body wt/day, PO, as four equal portions, 6-hourly, for 2 days followed by 7 mg to 8 mg/kg body wt/day, PO, as two equal portions, 12-hourly, for 26 days. Chloroquine is also available for intramuscular use as the hydrochloride salt (same as PO dose in base equivalence). Serious toxic effects may occur with prolonged use but are rare with the above regimen.

Diiodohydroxyquin is effective only against intestinal amebas. It is used primarily to treat asymptomatic infection or to eliminate enteric infection following treatment with metronidazole. The dose is 40 mg/kg body wt/day, PO, as three equal portions, 8-hourly, for 3 weeks.

Diloxanide furoate is an unapproved drug in the United States but it can be obtained from the Parasitic Diseases Division, Centers for Disease Control, Atlanta, Georgia (telephone: 404-329-3311). This drug is not effective in symptomatic amebiasis but is effective in eliminating *E. histolytica* from the intestinal lumen. It can be used in place of diiodohydroxyquin when the latter is contraindicated because of hypersensitivity to iodine, or when halogenated hydroxyquinolines are contraindicated. The dose is 20 mg/kg body wt/day, PO, as three equal portions, 8-hourly, for 10 days. It frequently causes flatulence, and occasionally nausea, vomiting, diarrhea, urticaria, and pruritus.

Emetine dihydrochloride (dehydroemetine dihydrochloride is preferred where available) is effective against trophozoites within tissues but not against intraluminal amebae. It is used for extraintestinal (but nonneural) and severe intestinal disease when metronidazole cannot be given. The dosage of emetine is 1 mg/kg body wt/day (not to exceed 65 mg) by IM or SC injection of two equal portions, 12-hourly, for 10 days; elderly or debilitated patients should receive half as much drug. The dosage of dehydroemetine is 1.5 mg/kg body wt/day (not to exceed 90 mg) by IM or SC injection of two equal portions, 12-hourly for 10 days. The emetine drugs often cause local pain and nausea, and, occasionally, neuromuscular disability. Because of potential adverse cardiovascular effects, patients receiving the emetine drugs should be hospitalized, kept at bed rest and monitored. Electrocardiographic effects such as T-wave changes and prolongation of P-R and Q-T intervals are to be expected. The drugs are excreted slowly, that is, toxic effects can occur several days after the last dose. Despite potential toxicity, few problems arise when the drugs are used correctly.

Metronidazole is given in a dose of 30 mg/kg body wt/day, PO, as three equal portions, 8-hourly, for 10 days for intestinal infections. Lesser doses may be effective for liver abscess, but they do not eliminate intestinal infection and are not recommended. A parenteral form is available for IV injection in the same dose as would be given perorally. The drug is generally well tolerated; headache, anorexia, and nausea are the most common adverse reactions, but occasionally there is vomiting, diarrhea, epigastric distress, and abdominal cramping. Alcohol should be avoided, since it causes flushing, abdominal cramping, nausea, and vomiting. Metronidazole may be teratogenic and should be avoided during pregnancy, especially during the first trimester. Metronidazole is not recommended for children under 4 years of age.

Paromomycin is an aminocyclitol antimicrobic that is sparingly absorbed from the gut. Although it may be effective for invasive intestinal amebiasis, it is generally recommended only for moderately symptomatic or asymptomatic intestinal disease. The dosage is 25 mg to 30 mg/kg body wt /day, PO, as three equal portions, 8-hourly, for 5 to 10 days. Gastrointestinal tract disturbances are common, and it rarely can cause 8th nerve (mainly auditory) or renal damage.

Tetracycline cures about 70% of intestinal amebic infections when given in adequate dosage. It may be used in critically ill patients with intestinal disease in combination with emetine dihydrochloride or metronidazole. Eradication of intestinal infection in adults requires 25 mg to 30 mg/kg body wt/day, PO, as four equal portions, 6-hourly, for 10 days. Newborn infants should receive 10 mg/kg body wt, PO, or 5 mg/kg parenterally daily; older infants and children should be given 20 mg to 40 mg/kg, PO, or 12 mg/kg parenterally/day, as four equal portions, 6-hourly, for 10 days.

Assessment of Therapy

Three fecal specimens should be examined, using both stained film and concentration methods, at intervals of 1, 2, and 3 months after termination of treatment. Ideally, the examination also should be done at 6 months. In areas in which amebiasis is endemic, differentiation of treatment failure from reinfection may be difficult.

Prevention

Control measures, as used for enteric bacterial infections, are effective for amebiasis. Within the hospital, simple precautions to prevent fecal–oral spread are adequate. Use of amebicides by travelers is not recommended.

Remaining Problems

Widespread use of substances that interfere with the detection of amebic infections, such as most antidiarrheal medications and antimicrobics, hampers diagnosis; knowledge of such effects must become commonplace.

Serologic tests have proven useful for exclusion of invasive amebic disease. In the future, fractionation of amebic antigens may enable serologic differentiation between active and cured disease.

The relative importance of strain pathogenicity of *E. histolytica* in causing invasive disease remains to be determined.

Bibliography

Books

JUNIPER K JR: Amebicides. In Miller RR, Greenblatt DJ (eds): Handbook of Drug Therapy. New York, Elsevier, 1979. pp 213–225.

REIMANN HA, JUNIPER K JR: Infectious and Parasitic Diseases of the Intestine; Discussions in Patient Management. New York, Medical Examination Publishing Co, 1977. pp 59–67.

WILMOT AJ: Clinical Amoebiasis. Oxford, Blackwell, 1962. 166 pp.

Journals

BARBOUR GL, JUNIPER K JR: A clinical comparison of amebic and pyogenic abscess of the liver in sixty-six patients. Am J Med 53:323–334, 1972

Drugs for Parasitic Infections. Med Lett 24:5–12, 1982

JUNIPER K JR: Amoebiasis. In Marsden PD (ed): Clinics in Gastroenterology, Intestinal Parasites, vol 7, pp. 3–29, London, WB Saunders, 1978

JUNIPER K JR, WORRELL CL, MINSHEW MC, ROTH LS, CYPERT H, LLOYD RE: Serological diagnosis of amebiasis. Am J Trop Med Hyg 21:157–168, 1972

KEAN BH, WILLIAM DC, LUMINAIS, SK: Epidemic of amoebiasis and giardiasis in a biased population. Br J Vener Dis 55:375–378, 1979

KROGSTAD DJ, SPENCER HC JR, HEALY GR: Current concepts in parasitology, amebiasis. N Engl J Med 298:262–265, 1978

KERRISON JUNIPER, JR.

Nonamebic Protozoal Enteritides 67

Although a number of nonamebic protozoa may inhabit the bowel, only three kinds are pathogens: *Giardia lamblia*, the Coccidia, and *Balantidium coli* can cause gastrointestinal disease. Symptoms should not be ascribed to other protozoa; they are commensals and treatment is not indicated for them.

Giardiasis

Etiology

Giardia lamblia are symmetric flagellates with both trophozoite and cystic stages (Fig. 67-1). The trophozoites are 10 μm to 25 μm in length and are pear-shaped—rounded anteriorly and tapered posteriorly. The ventral side is flattened with a shallow sucking disk on the anterior portion. Trophozoites contain two oval nuclei with central karyosomes, and four pairs of flagella arise from the ventral side. Cysts measure 8μm to 12 μm in length, are oval or ellipsoid, and have 2 to 4 nuclei and four pairs of curved bristle-shaped axonemes containing retracted flagella.

Epidemiology

Humans were thought to be the only hosts for *G. lamblia*. However, beavers and possibly other mammals were recently associated with outbreaks and are consequently implicated as temporary (summer) reservoirs of the organism. Giardiasis occurs worldwide but is more prevalent where sanitary and hygienic conditions are poor. Although the infection is more common in children, a number of outbreaks have occurred in general populations and among tourists traveling both within and outside the United States, usually because of contaminated water supplies. The estimated incidence of giardiasis in the general population in the United States is about 4%, but rates as high as 18% have been reported in special populations such as homosexuals.

Giardiasis is acquired by ingestion of cysts, which rapidly excyst on entering the small bowel. The trophozoites live in the lumen of the duodenum and jejunum, where they can attach to the epithelial surfaces with their sucking disk. Encystation occurs with transit down the colon, and cysts are excreted in formed feces; trophozoites may be found in loose or watery feces when the intestinal transit time is reduced.

Pathogenesis and Pathology

Trophozoites are sometimes found in large numbers in the proximal small intestine, where they can cause mild or moderately severe, patchy villous mucosal abnormalities similar to those of celiac sprue. The trophozoites are capable of superficial invasion of the mucosa, although the frequency and importance of this invasion is uncertain. Symptoms probably result largely from malabsorption.

Manifestations

Light infections with *G. lamblia* often are asymptomatic. Moderate infections can result in chronic recurrent nausea, mild abdominal cramping and distention, flatulence, and mild diarrhea. The feces may contain mucus, but not pus or blood, and number 2 to 10 daily; they may be spruelike and malodorous. Severe infections also may cause vomiting and fever. Chronic symptomatic infection may result in weakness, weight loss, and other manifestations of malabsorption.

Although the trophozoites of *G. lamblia* are occassionally found in bile taken from the gallbadder, the pathologic significance of this finding is uncertain.

Patients with hypogammaglobulinopathies are particularly susceptible to infection with *G. lamblia*, which commonly cause the diarrhea and steatorrhea sometimes seen in these patients. However, the incidence of immunodeficiency is not significantly more common among patients with giardiasis. The inci-

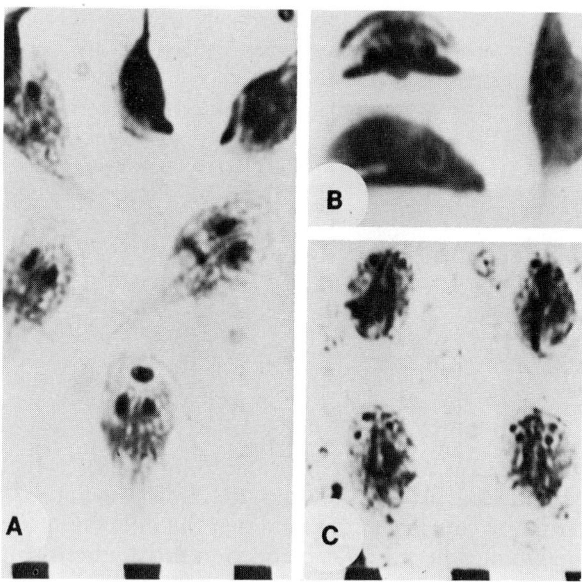

Fig. 67-1. (*A* and *B*) *Giardia lamblia.* Trophozoites in various profiles. (*C*) Cysts. (Trichrome stain, 10-unit micrometer scale shown) (Paulson M (ed): Gastroenterologic Medicine. Philadelphia, Lea & Febiger, 1969)

dence of HLA antigens A1 and B12, and blood group O is higher in patients with giardiasis than in an unselected population.

Diagnosis

Giardiasis should be excluded in all instances of unexplained diarrhea or malabsorption. The diagnosis is made by finding cysts, and occasionally trophozoites, in the feces. However, light infections may be difficult to detect, especially if interfering substances have been given to the patient (Chap. 66, Amebiasis). One-third of infected persons only rarely shed enough organisms for detection by examination of feces; 6 to 12 or more specimens may have to be examined to detect the organism.

Because of the high concentration of trophozoites in the duodenal lumen, examination of duodenal aspirates is the most sensitive diagnostic method. Generally, one aspirate is equal in value to ten fecal specimens, although not every patient with giardiasis may have a positive duodenal aspirate. Mucus adhering to small bowel suction biopsies also can be examined. In wet preparations, trophozoites are usually detected easily because of their rapid motility and large size. Smears of sediment or mucus fixed in Schaudinn's solution and stained with trichrome stain provide the sharpest detail; alternatively, smears may be air dried and prepared for examination with dilute Giemsa's stain.

An immunofluorescent serologic test, using axenically cultured *G. lamblia* for antigen, has shown promise as a diagnostic aid by identifying persons who should have examination of large numbers of fecal specimens and, if necessary, duodenal aspiration. The test has been positive in about 70% of patients with known infections.

Prognosis

Infection with *G. lamblia* does not always result in disease. If disease does occur and goes untreated, there may be episodic waxing and waning of symptoms. Treatment with metronidazole or quinacrine cures about 90% of infections, but sometimes more than one course of therapy is necessary. Apparently protective immunity does not develop, because reinfection occurs.

Therapy

Asymptomatic *G. lamblia* infections should be treated unless sanitary conditions in the area are uncontrollable. The treatment of asymptomatic and symptomatic infections is similar.

Metronidazole is the drug of choice; quinacrine hydrochloride and furazolidone are alternative drugs.

Metronidazole is given in a dose of 10 mg/kg body wt/day, PO as three equal portions, 8-hourly, for 10 days. Adverse effects include nausea, and less frequently, there may be vomiting, diarrhea, epigastric distress, and abdominal cramping. An Antabuse-like effect may result if ethanol is ingested by patients taking metronidazole. Finally, the drug is teratogenic in nonhuman animals and should not be given to pregnant women; it is not recommended for children under 4 years of age.

Quinacrine hydrochloride is effective in a dose of 5 mg/kg body wt/day, PO, as three equal portions, 8-hourly, for 7 days. Untoward effects are mild and include yellow discoloration of the skin and urine, nausea, vomiting, abdominal cramping, diarrhea, and headache. Transient toxic psychosis and exfoliative dermatitis have occasionally been reported. Quinacrine hydrochloride is contraindicated in pregnancy and in patients with a history of psychosis.

Furazolidone is given in a dosage of 5 mg/kg body wt/day, PO, as four equal doses, 6-hourly, for 7 days. The drug occasionally causes nausea, vomiting, headaches, and malaise; it rarely induces an Antabuse-like effect with alcohol, hypotension, urticaria, rash, arthralgia, or blood dyscrasias.

Prevention

In addition to treatment of infected persons, adequate personal and environmental hygiene is fundamental to prevention. Prophylactic medication is not recommended for travelers.

Remaining Problems

Giardiasis is now more widely recognized as an infection of clinical significance than it once was. Because of the high incidence of disease in patients with hypogammaglobulinopathies, immune mechanisms may be more important in preventing or minimizing giardiasis than was previously realized, despite the apparent lack of total protective immunity.

The disease is often difficult to diagnose—microscopic examination of feces is of limited sensitivity. Serologic tests may prove helpful, especially when the disease is symptomatic.

Coccidiosis

Etiology

The Coccidia are sporozoans, two genera of which are known to infect the intestinal tract of humans and cause symptoms: *Isospora* spp. and *Cryptosporidia* spp. Although a number of species of *Isospora* are parasitic in animals, only *I. belli* and *I. hominis* are found in humans. *Isospora* spp. have a life cycle characterized by alternation of generations, one sexual and one asexual. The elliptical oocysts are 20 μm to 33μm in length and are narrowed at one end (Fig. 67-2). The cyst wall is composed of two thin, smooth layers. Unsegmented oocysts contain a clear nucleus within a spherical mass of granules, the sporoblast. The nucleus divides to form two sporoblasts, each developing a cyst wall to become a sporocyst, and finally a spore with a double wall. Further, cell division produces four sporozoites from each spore. The feces usually contain oocysts with an unsegmented sporocyst *(I. belli),* or sporocysts in pairs, or already separated *(I. hominis).*

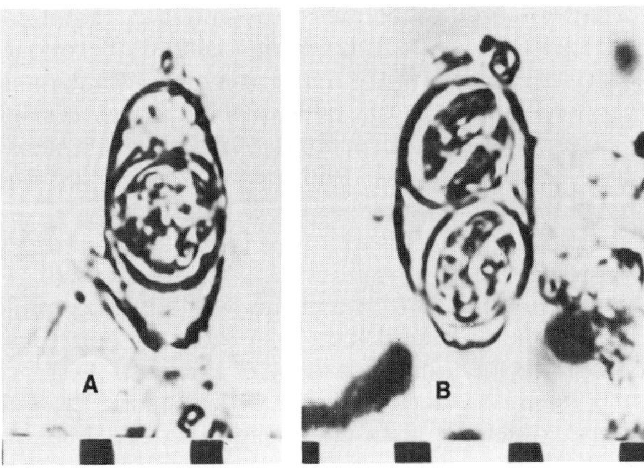

Fig. 67-2. *Isospora belli.* (*A*) Unsegmented sporocyst. (*B*) Segmented sporocyst. (Iron-hematoxylin stain, 10-unit micrometer scale shown) (Paulson M (ed): Gastroenterologic Medicine. Philadelphia, Lea & Febiger, 1969)

The sporozoites enter the epithelial cells where schizogony, the asexual phase, occurs. The dividing schizont releases a number of young merozoites from the host cells. These may then invade other cells and divide asexually, or they may enter the sexual cycle by maturing into a macrogamete (female) or into several microgametes (male). Fertilization produces a zygote that becomes an oocyst after a cyst wall has formed. The oocyst is then shed into the lumen of the gut.

Cryptosporidium spp. differ from *Isospora* spp. because they attach to the microvillar membrane of the intestinal epithelium and do not enter the epithelial cells. *Cryptosporidia* spp. are less commonly found than *Isospora* spp. in nonhuman animals, and only recently have been demonstrated in humans. The tiny 2 μm to 4 μm spherical cells are found attached to the epithelium of the small bowel and rectum. Electron microscopy shows a double host cell membrane surrounding the parasite.

Epidemiology

Coccidiosis is rare in the United States but is more common in the tropics, especially in the Philippines and the southwest Pacific. The infection is acquired by ingestion of ripe oocysts. No reservoir host for the *Isospora* spp. that infect humans is known, although dogs and cats have been suspected. Little is known about the epidemiology of cryptosporidiasis, but infected calves are one source of infection in humans.

Pathogenesis and Pathology

Sporozoites from the oocyst enter the epithelium of the small intestine, in which schizogony occurs. Various developmental forms (schizonts, merozoites, and macro- and microgametes) have been demonstrated in the epithelium of the small bowel (biopsy specimens). The mucosa is patchily involved with lesions of varying severity to give a pattern similar to that of celiac sprue.

Manifestations

Coccidiosis is generally a mild and self-limiting infection. Symptoms appear about 7 days after ingestion of oocysts and last for less than 30 days. However, chronic, symptomatic infections occasionally occur. The onset is usually acute with fever and malaise, followed by diarrhea, abdominal pain, and weight loss. The feces are watery and malodorous, and may contain mucus, but rarely pus or blood. A moderate eosinophilia may occur. On rare occasions, the infection produces an unrelenting, chronic malabsorption.

Diagnosis
The diagnosis of coccidiosis is made by finding oocysts or sporocysts in the feces. Although transparent and easily missed, the cystic forms can be concentrated from specimens of feces. Cystic forms may be absent from feces during the first few days of the diarrhea, and then may be shed for only several days despite continuation of symptoms. Therefore, the diagnosis sometimes is established only by finding various developmental stages of the parasite within the epithelium in biopsies of small bowel. A Colophonium Giemsa stain is helpful for this purpose. Oocysts and sporoblasts also are sometimes found in duodenal aspirates.

Prognosis
Treatment for coccidiosis is not generally required because the infection is usually mild and self-limiting. Documented complications include steatorrhea, hepatic involvement, and, rarely, death.

Therapy
An effective therapy is not known, but one patient with malabsorption improved on combined treatment with pyrimethamine and sulfadiazine.

Prevention
Adequate personal hygiene is essential for prevention of coccidiosis.

Remaining Problems
The true incidence of coccidiosis is probably unknown because of the difficulty of diagnosis. Thus, a specific serologic test would be of clinical and epidemiologic help.

Balantidiasis

Etiology
Balantidium coli, the only ciliate pathogenic for humans has both trophozoite and cystic stages. The trophozoite is oval, 50 μm to 200 μm in length, and is covered with short cilia (Fig. 67-3). One side of the anterior end has a depression ending in a cytostome, and the posterior end has a small opening or cytopyge. The cytoplasm contains many food vacuoles, a large bean-shaped macronucleus and a small, adjacent micronucleus. The round or oval cysts are opaque and 40 μm to 65 μm in diameter. They usually contain colorless, barlike inclusions which disappear on staining.

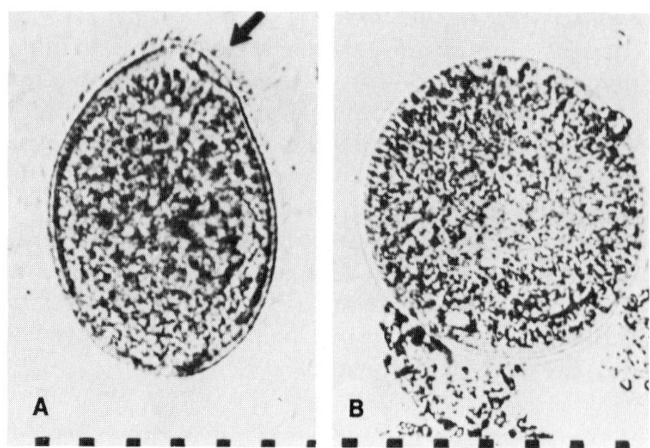

Fig. 67-3. *Balantidium coli.* (*A*) Trophozoite. (*B*) Cyst. (Iron-hematoxylin stain, 10-unit micrometer scale shown) (Paulson M (ed): Gastroenterologic Medicine. Philadelphia, Lea & Febiger, 1969)

Epidemiology
The *B. coli* infection is acquired by ingestion of cysts in contaminated food or water. Hogs, rats, and some primates are common hosts of the parasite, but swine are the typical reservoir for the relatively rare human infections. There is no geographic restriction for *B. coli,* but it is found most frequently in tropical areas.

Pathogenesis and Pathology
Factors that diminish host resistance, such as achlorhydria, are often present in patients who develop balantidiasis. Excystation occurs in the small intestine, and trophozoites become established in the lumen of the colon and terminal ileum, where they may cause ulceration. The rectosigmoid portion of colon is the area most commonly affected, and the pathologic changes are similar to those of amebiasis. Secondary bacterial infection may result in a marked inflammatory reaction. Appendiceal involvement and peritonitis have been described, but extraintestinal lesions do not occur. Cysts are found in formed feces, and trophozoites in watery feces.

Manifestations
Symptomless *B. coli* infections without discernible lesions may occur. Ulcers may develop and cause symptoms identical with those of amebiasis. Diarrhea may be chronic and alternate with constipation. Fulminant dysentery also occurs, especially in delibitated patients. The feces are watery or mushy, have a pigsty odor, and usually contain Charcot–Leyden crystals and mucus, but rarely blood. Endoscopy may show small rectal ulcers or diphtheritic patches 1.5 cm to 3

cm in diameter surrounded by a reddish, swollen mucosa.

Diagnosis
Diagnosis depends on the demonstration of *B. coli* in feces or in scrapings of rectal lesions. Because it is found only sporadically in the feces, repeated examinations may be necessary. The large motile trophozoites are readily detected but may be confused with free-living ciliates that sometimes contaminate feces exposed to air.

Prognosis
Although the infection may be commensal, the mortality in untreated patients, especially debilitated patients, may be appreciable. The infection usually responds to treatment.

Therapy
Symptomless infections may disappear spontaneously. Oxytetracycline, the drug of choice, is given in a dose of 30 mg/kg body wt/day, PO, as four equal portions, 6-hourly, for 10 days. Diiodohydroxyquin also is effective in a dose of 40 mg/kg body wt/day, PO, as three equal portions, 8-hourly, for 3 weeks.

Prevention
Control measures for *B. coli* infections are the same as those applied with any infection spread by the fecal–oral route. Of particular importance is protection against contamination of food and water by porcine feces.

Remaining Problems
The relative infrequency of balantidiasis has hampered its study, and little is known about its immunology.

Bibliography

Book

REIMANN HA, JUNIPER K JR: Infectious and Parasitic Diseases of the Intestine; Discussions in Patient Management. New York, Medical Examination Publishing Co, 1977. pp 67–73.

Journals

Drugs for parasitic infections. Med Lett 24:5–12, 1982 Dec 1979

KEAN BH, WILLIAM DC, LUMINAIS SK: Epidemic of amoebiasis and giardiasis in a biased population. Br J Vener Dis 55:375–378, 1979

NIME FA, BUREK JD, PAGE DL, HOLSCHER MA, YARDLEY JH: Acute enterocolitis in a human being infected with the protozoan cryptosporidium. Gastroenterology 70:592–598, 1978

SMITH JW, WOLFE MS: Giardiasis. Ann Rev Med 31:373–383, 1980

TRIER JS, MOXEY PC, SCHIMMEL EM, ROBLES E: Chronic intestinal coccidiosis in man: intestinal morphology and response to treatment. Gastroenterology 66:923–935, 1975

VISVESARA GS, SMITH PD, HEALY GR, BROWN WR: An immunofluorescent test for detection of anti-Giardia lamblia antibodies. Ann Int Med 93:802–805, 1980

WALZER PD, JUDSON FN, MURPHY KB, HEALY GR, ENGLISH DK, SCHULTZ MG: Balantidiasis outbreak in Truk. Am J Trop Med Hyg 22:33–41, 1973

ALLEN W. MATHIES, JR.

68 Intestinal Nematodiasis

Intestinal nematodes, elongate cylindrical worms, are the most common helminthic parasites of man. The sexes are separate and the female is usually larger. Differential diagnostic characteristics of the seven most common nematodes infecting man are found in Table 68-1. The eggs are shown in Plate 68-1.

Many infections with intestinal nematodes are unapparent, since symptoms are usually associated with large numbers of worms. With occasional exceptions, the worms do not multiply inside the definitive host, and it may be possible to associate finite numbers of worms with clinical syndromes. Knowledge of the life cycle of the nematodes is necessary because avoidance of reinfection is an important adjunct to chemotherapy in the treatment of nematodal infections.

Enterobiasis (Pinworm Infection)

Etiology

Male and female pinworms live in the cecum and ascending large intestine of man. When the female becomes gravid, she migrates the length of the large intestine, exits into the folds of the perianal area (usually at night), and oviposits her burden of approximately 11,000 eggs in this area. The eggs become infectious 4 to 6 hours after deposition. The total life cycle is usually 1 to 2 months. At no time in the normal life cycle does the worm penetrate the intestinal mucosa.

Epidemiology

Enterobius vermicularis is the most cosmopolitan of the nematodes, for it is not restricted in its geographic distribution. Children are more heavily infected than adults, and whites are more frequently infected than blacks. It is estimated that 20% to 30% of all children are infected with pinworms. The infection is acquired primarily by direct hand-to-mouth transmission from the perianal areas. Humans are the only definitive hosts; pets such as dogs and cats do not harbor human pinworms. Indirect transmission, for example, by the ingestion of airborne eggs or retroinfection, occasionally take place. Most eggs are not viable after 2 or 3 days, although under ideal conditions of low humidity and relatively low temperature eggs may remain viable for as long as 1 to 2 months.

Pathogenesis and Pathology

Because the mucosa is not penetrated by *E. vermicularis,* there are no anatomic lesions. In view of the cecal habitat, a possible role in appendicitis has been suggested but remains conjectural. Migration into the vagina occurs but is not associated with lesions. Perianal and perineal excoriations may be inflicted by the patient in response to irritation of these areas from the migration of the female and oviposition.

Manifestations

The major symptom associated with pinworm infection is perianal pruritis. Because the worms migrate at night, sleeplessness is often an associated symptom. In female patients migration of the worm into the genital area may produce vaginitis. Convulsions, enuresis, abdominal pain, behavior disorders, and weight loss have been attributed to pinworm infection, but the relationship is doubtful.

Pinworms are often found in the lumen of the appendix but rarely if ever are they the underlying cause of appendicitis. Occasionally, the pinworm migrates up the female genital tract into the fallopian tubes, where the host attempts to wall off the worm by forming a granuloma. These ectopic foci are rarely associated with symptoms. Eosinophilia is not a com-

Table 68-1. Important Characteristics of Intestinal Nematodes (Roundworms)

Nematode	Adults: Average Size (mm) Male	Adults: Average Size (mm) Female	Adults: Significant Characteristics	Eggs: Embryonal Contents	Eggs: Significant Characteristics
Ascaris lumbricoides	240 × 3	300 × 5	Large, glistening worms; mouth with 3 oval papillate lips; male has curved posterior extremity with 2 spicules; white	Undeveloped embryo (fertile)	Mamillated external coating usually present; bile-stained
				Amorphous, granular (infertile)	Irregular mamillated external coating; bizarre shapes, bile-stained
Enterobius vermicularis	4 × 0.15	10 × 1.4	Male is seldom seen, has coiled posterior extremity; female has anterior cuticular alae, long pointed tail; white	Developed embryo	One side convex, one side flattened; hyaline
Trichuris trichiura	38 × 1.3	42 × 1.7	Narrow whiplike anterior 3/5 of body, more robust posterior 2/5; male has coiled posterior extremity with copulatory spicule; gray white	Undeveloped embryo	Thick shell; translucent polar plugs; bile-stained
Ancylostoma duodenale	10 × 0.45	12 × 0.6	Buccal capsule has 2 ventral pairs of teeth; male has copulatory bursa; female has vulva in anterior half of body; gray white	2–8 cell stage	Thin, transparent shell; hyaline
Necator americanus	7 × 0.3	10 × 0.35	Buccal capsule has 2 semilunar cutting plates; male has copulatory bursa; female has vulva in posterior half of body; gray white	2–8 cell stage	Thin, transparent shell; hyaline
Strongyloides stercoralis	0.7 × 0.04	2.2 × 0.04	Male is seldom seen; filariform parasitic female has single file of eggs in uterus; colorless, transparent	Undeveloped embryo or larva	Thin, transparent shell; hyaline; rarely seen in feces
Capillaria philippinensis	2.7 × 0.025	3.9 × 0.038	Male has long copulatory spicule and very long aspinous sheath; female has vulva immediately behind esophagus, double reflex of oviduct	Undeveloped embryo or larva	Thick shell; translucent flattened polar plugs; shell may be absent

mon manifestation of pinworm infection because the worm does not have a tissue phase.

Diagnosis

There are no physical stigmas of pinworm infection other than the excoriated skin in the perianal area. However, in children the classic symptom of anal pruritis at night is most suggestive. Definitive diagnosis of the infection can be made by observing the female worms migrating at night or by finding the eggs in the perianal area. Because the eggs are deposited outside the intestinal tract, examination of feces is not usually of diagnostic value. The cellulose tape swab technique (Chap. 11, Diagnostic Methods for Protozoa and Helminths) is generally applicable and is most likely to be rewarding if applied before the patient arises in the morning. Approximately 50% of the infections are diagnosed with the first sample; several swabbings may be necessary to establish a diagnosis in all cases.

Prognosis

Reinfection with *E. vermicularis* after apparently successful therapy is common. No protective immunity is engendered by infection.

Treatment

A number of anthelmintics are effective in the treatment of infections caused by *E. vermicularis* (Table 68-2). Mebendazole is the drug of choice because of the absence of side-effects; the dose is 100 mg regardless of the age or weight of the patient.

Much has been made of the need to treat the whole family when pinworm infection is diagnosed in one of the children. This is not necessary with the first symptomatic infection. If the patient is recurrently infected and symptomatic, then therapy for the whole family may be necessary.

Table 68-2. *Anthelmintics for Intestinal Nematodes*

Nematode	Agent	Dosage
Enterobius vermicularis	Piperazine	75 mg/kg body wt/day (not to exceed 3.5 g), perorally as one portion for 7 days
	Pyrvinium pamoate	5 mg/kg body wt (not to exceed 350 mg) perorally as a single dose
	Pyrantel pamoate	11 mg/kg body wt (not to exceed 1 g) perorally as a single dose; repeat after 2 weeks
	Thiabendazole	50 mg/kg body wt/day (not to exceed 3 g) perorally as two equal portions, 12 hourly; repeat after 1 week
	Mebendazole	100 mg perorally as a single dose
Trichuris trichiura	Mebendazole	100 mg perorally every 12 hours for 3 days
Ascaris lumbricoides	Piperazine	75 mg/kg body wt/day (not to exceed 3.5 g) perorally as one portion for 2 days
	Pyrantel pamoate	11 mg/kg body wt (not to exceed 1 g) perorally as a single dose
Necator americanus / *Ancylostoma duodenale*	Mebendazole	100 mg perorally every 12 hours for 3 days
Strongyloides stercoralis	Thiabendazole	50 mg/kg body wt/day (not to exceed 3 g) perorally as two equal portions, 12 hourly, for 2 days
Capillaria philippinensis	Thiabendazole	50 mg/kg body wt/day (not to exceed 3 g) perorally as two equal portions, 12 hourly, for 30 days

Prevention
Improved personal habits and hygiene are the keys to interruption of the anal–oral transfer of eggs.

Trichuriasis (Whipworm Infection)

Etiology
Adult *Trichuris trichiura* live in the cecum and proximal portions of the large intestine. The female lays 3000 to 10,000 eggs per day that are bilestained, barrel-shaped, and plugged at either end (Fig. 68-1). These eggs pass out in the feces and develop in the soil to an infectious stage in 2 to 4 weeks. Upon ingestion, the eggs hatch; the young larvae attach to the mucosa of the small intestine where they undergo several molts. When they become adults, they move downward to the cecum and large intestine where they embed approximately 60% of their length within the mucosa. The adult worms may live for 15 to 20 years.

Epidemiology
The prevalence of whipworm infection is great, particularly in tropical countries. This worm, like many other intestinal nematodes, is spread by the fecal–oral route; it is most common in countries in which sanitation is poor. Factors favoring the development of eggs include heavy rainfall and a warm climate.

Pathogenesis and Pathology
Although the anterior two-thirds of adult *T. trichiura* is embedded in the colonic mucosa, the hemorrhagic lesions that result are considered less important than the mechanical irritation caused by large masses of worms. When infection is heavy, a hemorrhagic colitis may develop and lead to sloughing of the mucosa. Rectal prolapse may occur. Moderate anemia (blood loss, *i.e.,* iron deficiency) may result, but this is less common than mild eosinophilia.

Manifestations
The severity of the symptoms of trichuriasis is directly proportional to the number of worms infecting the patient. Most infections are unapparent. With heavy burdens of worms, patients complain of abdominal pain, localized tenderness, nausea and vomiting, diarrhea, or constipation. In very heavy infections, the characteristic features include microcytic, hypochromic anemia; diarrhea with blood-streaked feces; abdominal pain with tenderness on palpation; weight loss that may lead to cachexia. In very young children, rectal prolapse has occurred.

Diagnosis
Because infection with *T. trichiura* does not evoke a characteristic clinical picture, diagnosis must be based on finding typical eggs in the feces. Peripheral blood eosinophilia is not marked, although a mild eosinophilia in the range 10% to 15% may occur in recently acquired infections.

Prognosis
In light to moderately heavy *T. trichiura* infections, the prognosis is good without specific therapy. In heavy infections (500–4000 worms), severe anemia and abdominal complications can lead to death.

Therapy
Mebendazole given perorally in a dose of 100 mg every 12 hours for 3 days is efficacious in treatment of infections caused by *T. trichiura.* The drug is well tolerated, and the same dose is applicable to all patients, regardless of age or size. In very heavy infections, a second course of therapy may be necessary. Supportive measures, including blood transfusions, may be necessary if the anemia is severe.

Prevention
Treatment of infected persons is part of trichuriasis prevention if it includes an educational program on the proper disposal of feces and improved personal hygiene.

Ascariasis (Roundworm Infection)

Etiology
Ascaris lumbricoides measure 25 cm to 30 cm long and are the largest roundworms found in humans. The adults live in the small intestine, where the female lays approximately 200,000 eggs per day. These eggs are unsegmented when passed in the feces and must reach the soil in order to develop into a stage infective for humans—a process that takes 3 to 4 weeks.

When ingested by humans, the eggs hatch, releasing larvae that penetrate the intestine, entering the venules or lymphatics. The larvae then follow the portal circulation through the liver to the heart and subsequently reach the lungs, where the embryos pass from the circulatory system into the pulmonary alveoli. While in the lungs, the larvae undergo two molts and then migrate up the bronchioles into the larger airways. When they reach the pharynx, they are swallowed and finally pass into the small intestine. It takes about 2 months for maturation from the larval to the adult stage.

Epidemiology

Ascaris lumbricoides is a common parasite of humans both in temperate and tropical regions, wherever sanitation is poor. It is estimated that over 500 million people harbor ascarids. Transmission is by the fecal–oral route, and infection is most prevalent in young children. The eggs are relatively resistant to adverse environmental conditions, although they are susceptible to injury by desiccation.

Pathogenesis and Pathology

The extent of the damage from *A. lumbricoides* is primarily a function of the intensity of the infection. Thus, bleeding is insignificant if only a few larvae penetrate the intestinal wall; subsequently, the pulmonary injury will be correspondingly slight. However, heavy infections may provoke pulmonary inflammation with edema, epithelial desquamation, and focal hemorrhagic pneumonia.

Occasionally, migrating larvae miss the pulmonary tree and are scattered throughout the body by the systemic circulation. The host responds to such errant larvae by forming granulomas.

The adult *A. lumbricoides* usually cause little or no damage to the intestine. However, heavy infections, particularly in children, may lead to volvulus, intussusception, intestinal obstruction, or appendicitis. Extraintestinal incursions are rare, but they may be serious when the biliary tree is invaded (chronic inflammation, fibrosis, obstruction leading to abscess and necrosis), the pancreatic duct is blocked (pancreatitis), or the wall of the intestine is perforated (secondary peritonitis).

Manifestations

Most infections with *A. lumbricoides* go unnoticed by the host until a large worm is passed in the feces. In heavier infections (usually more than 20 worms), both the migrating larvae and the adult worms may cause symptoms. As larvae migrate, patients may complain of itching, wheezing, dyspnea, and angioneurotic edema. Fever and cough, productive of bloody sputum, may occur. A moderate eosinophilia is often present.

The most common complaint of patients with large numbers of adult *A. lumbricoides* is abdominal pain, which may arise from intestinal obstructions (biliary tree, pancreatic ducts). Regurgitation of worms and aspiration may compromise the airway.

Diagnosis

Infection with *A. lumbricoides* cannot be diagnosed by clinical manifestations. Ascarial pneumonia might be suspected in a patient with transient migratory pulmonary infiltrates and eosinophilia. However, a definitive diagnosis is dependent upon identification of the worm or demonstration of characteristic eggs in the feces (Fig. 68-1). During the migratory phase of the infection, eosinophilia may be as prominent as 30% to 40%. Adult worms may also be roentgenographically evident in the intestine as a serendipitous finding during contrast study of the bowel.

Prognosis

In general, infections with *A. lumbricoides* respond promptly to therapy and the prognosis is favorable. In heavy infections, or in those infections in which an ascarid has migrated to an abnormal location, the prognosis may be grave.

Therapy

Piperazine salts or pyrantel pamoate are equally effective drugs against *A. lumbricoides* (Table 68-2). Piperazine paralyzes the worms temporarily through action on the myoneural junction; having no attachment, the worms cannot maintain position in the intestine and are carried out of the body by normal peristalsis. A single dose will cure 80% to 90% of all patients, and two doses (given on 2 consecutive days) increase the cure rate to approximately 95%. Equal cure rates are reported with a single dose of pyrantel pamoate, a drug that is well tolerated and easy to take.

Prevention

Breaking the cycle of fecal–oral transmission is the key to prevention. Although the informational base has long been adequate and available, the socioeconomic barriers to implementation persist.

Hookworm

Etiology

Hookworm infection of humans is caused by either *Ancylostoma duodenale* or *Necator americanus.* Although there are some minor differences in the severity of infection and response to therapy, hookworm infection should be considered a single clinical entity regardless of the specific etiologic agent.

Adult hookworms live in the small intestine. Eggs which are in the 2 to 8 cell stage are passed in the feces (Fig. 68-1). After reaching the soil, the eggs develop to yield larvae within 24 to 48 hours. The rhabdoid larvae (active feeding stage) migrate in the soil and undergo two molts to become filariform larvae that are nonfeeding and infective for man. The filariform larvae penetrate the skin on contact, enter the bloodstream, and are carried to the lungs. In the lungs, the larvae break out of the capillaries into the alveoli and traverse up the tracheobronchial tree; there they are swallowed and subsequently reach the small intestine. After approximately 5 to 6 weeks, the larvae become adults. Most of the worms live for only 1 year, although some live for as long as 5 years. The worms attach to the small intestine by their buccal capsule to obtain blood for nourishment.

Epidemiology

Hookworm infection is found throughout the world but is most common in tropical and subtropical areas. *Ancylostoma duodenale* predominates in the eastern hemisphere, while *N. americanus* is most common in the Western Hemisphere. Environmental features that favor the transmission of hookworms include a sandy soil, moderate moisture (*i.e.,* 30 in of rain per year), and a warm climate. Spread of the infection from man to man is the result of poor sanitation, deposition of feces on the ground, and a population that does not wear shoes regularly. It is estimated that approximately 450 million people in the world are infected with hookworms.

Pathogenesis and Pathology

The piercing of the skin by the filariform larvae may cause a transient rash but does not result in pathology. However, the transpulmonary phase of larval migration often evokes an inflammatory response with pneumonitis, petechial hemorrhages, and epithelial proliferation; it is at this stage of the disease that eosinophilia is most likely to be present and is most intense.

The amount of blood consumed or lost in the gut and the intensity of the enteritis that is provoked are directly proportional to the number of adult worms causing the infection.

Manifestations

The manifestations of hookworm infection are dependent upon the number of worms harbored by the patient and the stage of the disease. Each of the three sequential phases of the infection can produce symptoms. Larval penetration of the skin produces an irritation termed ground itch. The usual form is a localized maculopapular rash, although the site of penetration may become secondarily infected with bacteria and become pustular.

When the larvae break out of the pulmonary capillaries into the alveolar system, hemorrhage and a focal pneumonitis may occur—a process that is less prominent than the similar syndrome caused by *Ascaris lumbricoides.*

In the intestinal phase, a light burden of adult worms can be tolerated by persons taking a diet adequate in iron. Symptoms occur only in those persons who are heavily infected, and the symptoms are primarily the result of the continual loss of blood. Abdominal complaints are not marked although nausea and vomiting, diarrhea, or constipation may occasionally be present. As the blood loss continues and the microcytic hypochromic anemia becomes more severe, the patient may complain of exertional dyspnea, weakness, and dizziness. Secondary cardiomegaly occurs; cardiac failure and anasarca may develop. Infections with *Ancylostoma duodenale* appear to be more severe than those caused by *N. americanus,* corresponding to the relative blood consumption of the two kinds of hookworms (0.2 ml/worm/day and 0.03 ml/worm/day, respectively).

Diagnosis

The clinical picture of a microcytic, hypochromic anemia in a person from a tropical or subtropical area should alert the physician to the possibility of hookworm infection. Eosinophilia may be present at a low level. The specific diagnosis is dependent upon finding the characteristic eggs in the feces. Reliable differentiation of the eggs of *A. duodenale* and *N. americanus* is not generally possible, and it is best to report them simply as hookworm eggs (Fig. 68-1).

Prognosis

Without specific therapy, the outlook for survival for a person with hookworm infection is favorable, although a toll of morbidity is exacted. Despite evidence of an immunologic response, there is no protection against reinfection.

Therapy

In light hookworm infections, treatment with an anthelmintic is usually not necessary, particularly if reinfection is not likely. More important an adequate diet containing sufficient iron prevents the development of severe symptoms. In heavier infections, treatment with mebendazole is suggested (Table 68-2).

Prevention

Wearing shoes will markedly reduce the frequency of occurrence of hookworm infection—particularly if feces are disposed of properly.

Strongyloidiasis

Etiology

The life cycle of *Strongyloides stercoralis* is the most complex of all the intestinal nematodes. Three different life cycles may occur at various times in a single infection. The parasitic female of *S. stercoralis* lives in the small intestine with its anterior end embedded in the intestinal mucosa. Unlike other nematodes, there is no parasitic male and the parasitic female is parthenogenic. The eggs are deposited and hatch within the mucosa, and the rhabdoid larvae pass out in the feces. As in the hookworm life cycle, the rhabdoid larvae develop in the soil into filariform larvae that are infectious. These larvae penetrate the skin of man, reach the bloodstream, and pass to the lungs. There the larvae break out of the capillaries into the alveoli and migrate up the tracheobronchial tree to the pharynx, where they are swallowed.

An alternate life cycle pathway increases the number of infective larvae. Rhabdoid larvae in the soil develop into free-living male and female adults that mate; the eggs they produce hatch into larvae that may become infective for humans.

The third life cycle may take place entirely within the intestinal tract. Rhabdoid larvae molt within the intestinal tract, changing into filariform larvae that are infectious. Humans may be autoinfected with these filariform larvae because they may penetrate the intestinal mucosa or the skin in the perianal areas as they are passed in the feces. Humans are the only definitive host for this infection, and it is difficult to ascertain the life span of the individual parasite because autoinfection may take place. Infections may be perpetuated for 35 to 45 years after the patient leaves an endemic area.

Epidemiology

Strongyloidiasis occurs primarily in tropical areas. Despite the fact that the mode of transmission is essentially the same as with hookworms, the incidence of this infection is much lower.

Pathogenesis and Pathology

There may be a pneumonitis as the larvae pass through the lungs, although it is less severe than that which occurs in hookworm infections. The intestinal lesions from *S. stercoralis,* particularly if aggravated by autoinfection, may rarely lead to necrosis and sloughing of the mucosa. In such severe infections, the gallbladder and liver may also be involved.

Manifestations

As with other infections contracted by penetration of the skin, the presence of a rash characterized by erythematous maculopapular areas with pruritis is an early manifestation of infection with *S. stercoralis.* Pneumonia may occur during the migratory phase. In the intestinal phase, the major manifestation is diarrhea, with frequent passage of watery, bloody feces. If the infection is severe, a malabsorption syndrome may be present, since the patient loses large amounts of fat and protein in the feces. In certain patients, the host–parasite relationship becomes upset, and the parasite undergoes an accelerated autoinfectious cycle. Often, these are patients with malignancies or iatrogenically induced defects of immunocompetence. Bowel lesions resembling ulcerative colitis may develop and lead to systemic manifestations such as toxicity and fever. Fatal, disseminated strongyloidiasis with metastatic lesions has been reported, with and without concurrent bacterial infections.

Diagnosis

The definitive diagnosis of strongyloidiasis depends on finding the rhabdoid larvae in the secretions or excretions of humans. Feces *freshly* passed by an infected patient usually contain active rhabdoid larvae (Fig. 68-1). In older specimens, the presence of larvae does not automatically implicate infection with *S. stercoralis* because any hookworm eggs present in the feces would have had time to hatch, yielding rhabdoid larvae almost identical in appearance. Aspirated duodenal juice should be examined for the presence of larvae in patients suspected of having strongyloidiasis if the examination of feces has been negative. Eosinophilia exceeding 30% is common in infection with *S. stercoralis,* as the worms are in intimate contact with the host's tissues. However, patients with disseminated strongyloidiasis may not be able to respond with a brisk eosinophilia.

Prognosis

Most patients with strongyloidiasis are asymptomatic and the prognosis is good. However, in the heavily infected patient with autoinfection, the debilitation associated with loss of protein makes the prognosis poor. The immunodeficient patient may not be able to confine *S. stercoralis* to the gut.

Therapy

Because of the potential for accelerated autoinfection, every patient with strongyloidiasis should be treated. Thiabendazole should be given for 2 to 3 days (Table 68-2). The drug is quite effective, and the occasional adverse reactions of nausea and vomiting are minimal. Serially examined specimens of feces should be negative for the larvae of *S. stercoralis* if cure has been achieved. Eosinophilia will disappear in 1 to 2 months. In a severely ill patient, supportive measures such as intravenous fluids, blood transfusion, and protein replacement may be necessary. Glucosteroids should be avoided because their use may enhance the ability of the parasite to perpetuate itself by autoinfection, thus favoring dissemination throughout the body.

Prevention

As with hookworms, ensuring that the filariform larvae have no access to the skin depends primarily on proper disposal of feces and wearing shoes.

Capillariasis

Intestinal capillariasis has recently been reported from the Philippines. The infection is characterized by abdominal pain, chronic diarrhea, and a protein-losing enteropathy that may lead to debility and death. *Capillaria philippinensis* are small nematodes that invade the small intestine. The eggs resemble those of *Trichuris trichiura*. However, the life cycle in humans is similar to that of *S. stercoralis*, for eggs hatch within the intestine. Humans are thought to be the only host, acquiring the infection by eating raw fresh water fish. Specific therapy with thiabendazole in high doses for prolonged periods (*e.g.,* 30 days) is reported to be beneficial in this infection; alternatively, mebendazole may be recommended. Supportive measures, such as intravenous feeding and hyperalimentation, are often required for the survival of severely infected patients.

Bibliography

Book

BROWN HW: Basic Clinical Parasitology. New York, Appleton-Century-Crofts, 1975. 355 pp.

Journals

GARCIA FT, SESSIONS JT, STRUM WB, SCHWEISTRIS E, TRIPATHY K, BOLANOS D, LOTERO H, DUQUE E, RAMELLI D, MAYORAL LG: Intestinal function and morphology in strongyloidiasis. Am J Trop Med Hyg 26:859–865, 1977

SCRAGG JN, PROCTOR EḾ: Mebendazole in the treatment of severe symptomatic trichuriasis in children. Am J Trop Med Hyg 26:198–203, 1977

WHALEN GE, STRICKLAND GT, CROSS JH, ROSENBERG RB, GUTMAN RA, WATTEN RH, UYLANGO C, DIZON JJ: Intestinal capillariasis: A new disease in man. Lancet 1:13–16, 1969

ZBIGNIEW S. PAWLOWSKI

69 Intestinal Cestodiases

Several kinds of tapeworms (cestodes) can parasitize the intestines of humans: *Taenia saginata,* the beef tapeworm; *Taenia solium,* the pork tapeworm; *Diphyllobothrium latum,* the fish tapeworm; *Hymenolepis nana,* the dwarf tapeworm; *Hymenolepis diminuta,* the rat tapeworm; and *Dipylidium caninum,* the dog tapeworm (Table 69-1). In addition, some tapeworms of the genera *Bertiella, Inermicapsifer, Mesocestoides,* and *Raillietina* may accidentally infect humans.

Adult tapeworms have a long, flat body consisting of a scolex, a neck, and a strobila—a chain of proglottids. The morphologic similarity of some species, *e.g., T. solium* and *T. saginata,* may create diagnostic problems. The life cycles vary, resulting in different modes of transmission; the sources of infection for humans are either eggs or larvae—the latter from infected beef, pork, fish, or insects. Therefore, the occurrence and prevalence in humans of the various cestodiases vary in different parts of the world, depending on local feeding habits, the level of sanitation, and the intensity of contact with nonhuman animals. Most of the cestodiases of humans are zoonotic infections.

Intestinal cestodiases infrequently provoke serious pathology as a result of ectopic migration of the proglottids *(T. saginata),* secondary cysticercosis *(T. solium),* macrocytic anaemia *(D. latum),* or impairment of intestinal function *(H. nana).* Diagnosis is based on the examination of proglottids or eggs and is not possible in the early stage of infection before the eggs or proglottids are excreted. Treatment of the cestodiases is quite safe. Single-dose therapy is usually effective against most of the tapeworms; only infections caused by *H. nana* require prolonged or repeated treatment.

Taenia saginata taeniasis and *H. nana* hymenolepiasis are the most common cestodiases of humans, but the most serious public health problems are caused by *T. solium* taeniasis and cysticercosis.

Taenia Saginata Taeniasis

Etiology

The adult beef tapeworm is 4 to 10 meters long; the length depends on the number of proglottids (about 2000) and their degree of relaxation. The quadrangular scolex is less than 2 mm in diameter, and has 4 strong hemispherical suckers, which are frequently pigmented. The scolex is usually attached to the mucosa about 50 cm below the duodenal–jejunal flexure. The strobila consists of sexually immature, mature, and gravid proglottids. Gravid proglottids are 22 mm to 30 mm long and 5 mm to 7 mm broad; about 80,000 eggs are enclosed in the uterus which has 18 to 32 lateral extensions on each side. Every day, 6 to 9 gravid proglottids detach singly from the strobila and leave the host, usually passing actively through the anus. Occasionally, a larger piece of the strobila is discharged and the excretion of gravid proglottids is stopped for a time. *Taenia saginata* need 3 to $3\frac{1}{2}$ months to develop a strobila. Infections are usually caused by a single tapeworm, but multiple or mixed (with *T. solium)* infections do occur.

The eggs of *T. saginata* can survive for a few years in the external environment to develop further when ingested by cattle. In this intermediate host, the larva (oncosphere) invades the muscle tissue and within 5 to 6 weeks develops into a bladder larva, the cysticercus. The fully developed cysticercus is an ovoid vesicle (7 mm to 10 mm by 4 mm to 6 mm) filled with an invaginated scolex and liquid; it is a source of infection for man when ingested with raw or semiraw beef.

Epidemiology

Taenia saginata are widespread in most cattle-breeding countries of the world. Taeniasis from *T. saginata* is highly endemic, with a prevalence exceeding 10% of the human population in some regions of Central and East Africa, the Near East, and

Southern USSR. Moderate rates of infection occur in many countries of Europe, Southeast Asia, and South America. In the United States, Canada, and Australia the incidence in man is less than 0.1%. The prevalence of taeniasis in man reflects the extent of the local practice of eating raw beef. The incidence of bovine cysticercosis depends on the proximity of contacts between human carriers and cattle and the degree of contamination of the environment. In highly endemic areas, the incidence of bovine cysticercosis may be as high as 80%; in Europe it is 1% to 5%. In developed countries, the intensity of infection in cattle is usually light; therefore, all infected carcasses cannot be detected by meat inspection. Bovine cysticercosis may occur epizootically in contaminated feed lots.

Pathogenesis and Pathology

Taenia saginata taeniasis more frequently causes changes in motility and secretion of the gastrointestinal tract than local pathologic changes of the intestinal mucosa. Straying *T. saginata* proglottids may sporadically cause appendicitis or cholangitis. Eosinophilia, when it does occur, is usually moderate. The titer of IgE in the serum may be elevated.

Manifestations

Most carriers of *T. saginata* feel some sensation in the perianal area when the proglottids are discharged. Other symptoms differ in individual cases, as they may be of a psychological nature and may appear shortly after the patient becomes aware of being infected with a tapeworm. Vague abdominal pain, nausea, and increase or decrease in appetite and body weight each were recorded in one-third of cases. Abdominal discomfort and a feeling of weakness sometimes occur; allergic reactions and neuroses are rare.

Diagnosis

Tapeworm infection should be considered as a diagnosis in any patient who has eaten raw meat and has vague abdominal symptoms. A history of peranal discharge of proglottids is highly suggestive. The diagnosis of taeniasis is established only by finding *Taenia* eggs in the feces or on an anal swab. Final diagnosis as to species may be difficult and requires parasitologic examination of the scolex or proglottids. The scolex is difficult to find after treatment with niclosamide, paromomycin, or praziquantel, which normally cause disintegration of the proximal part of the strobila. Differentiation between *T. saginata* and *T. solium* is listed in Table 69-1; a proper differentiation between these two is very important for both clinical and epidemiologic reasons.

In the first 3 months of infection, before gravid proglottids are produced and discharged, it is almost impossible to diagnose taeniasis. Serologic tests are of no practical value. A ribbonlike contrast defect in the ileum during roentgenologic examination may be seen in some cases. Searching for proglottids by repeated examinations of fecal material and anal swabs is recommended in patients who have eaten raw beef and have persistent, uncharacteristic abdominal symptoms and signs, and moderate eosinophilia.

Prognosis

Although a large part of the strobila is sometimes discharged, self-cure is exceptional in *T. saginata* taeniasis; *T. saginata* tapeworms may live as long as 40 years.

Therapy

Niclosamide is the drug of choice for the treatment of taeniasis. Adults are given a single dose of 2 g in the morning on an empty stomach, children 2 to 5 years old are given 0.5 g, and older children should receive 1 g of niclosamide. The tablets should be chewed thoroughly. The strobila is usually evacuated within a few hours; if not, a saline purgative is recommended. Treatment is effective in 90% of cases and is safe; side-effects are transient and uncommon (17%). Niclosamide has practically no contraindications, but it is not recommended in the first trimester of pregnancy unless uncontrollable vomiting occurs.

A new schistosomicide, praziquantel, is also highly effective in taeniasis. It is given in a single dose of 5 mg–10 mg/kg of body weight perorally. The side-effects are mostly mild; transient abdominal pain, headache, dizziness, and skin rash are rare. During treatment with praziquantel, as well as with niclosamide,the proximal part of the strobila usually disintegrates and it is difficult to find the scolex. Therefore treatment can be considered successful when no proglottids reappear within 3.5 months after treatment.

Niclosamide and praziquantel have practically replaced the older anthelmintics such as mepacrine, tin compounds, and paromomycin.

Prevention

The best prophylaxis for *T. saginata* is to avoid eating raw or semiraw beef. Prevention at the national level requires proper sewage disposal, better sanitation, and zoohygiene on cattle farms as well as regular inspection of meat with condemnation of heavily infected carcasses and freezing of lightly infected carcasses.

Since humans are the only definitive host of *T. saginata,* early detection and treatment of taeniasis greatly helps to prevent the spread of infection.

Table 69-1. Important Characteristics of Intestinal Cestodes (Tapeworms)

	Adults	
Cestode	AVERAGE SIZE	SIGNIFICANT CHARACTERISTICS
Taenia saginata	4 m–10 m × 12 mm–20 mm	Unarmed scolex has four suckers, about 2000 proglottids; mature proglottids have diffuse testes, discrete bilobed ovary, a vaginal sphincter, irregularly alternate genital pore; gravid proglottid has 18–32 main branches on each side of uterus, contains about 80,000 ova, ivory white
Taenia solium	2 m–4 m × 8 mm–12 mm	Scolex has four suckers and 22–32 hooklets; 800–1000 proglottids have diffuse testes, discrete trilobed ovary, irregularly alternate genital pore; gravid proglottid has 7–12 main branches on each side of uterus, contains up to 50,000 ova, ivory white
Hymenolepis nana	10 mm–40 mm × 0.7 mm	Scolex has four suckers, hooklets, refractile rostellum, up to 200 proglottids; mature proglottid has three round testes, discrete bilobed ovary, unilateral genital pore, and 80–180 ova, ivory white
Diphyllobothrium latum	3 m–5 m × 12 mm	Scolex has two elongate sucking grooves, 3000–4000 proglottids; mature proglottids have ivory white coiled rosettelike uterus, diffuse testes and ovaries, median genital and uterine pores
Hymenolepis diminuta	10 cm–60 cm × 4 mm	Scolex has four suckers, rostellum; 800–1000 proglottid has three round testes, discrete bilobed ovary, unilateral genital pore, ivory white
Dipylidium caninum	10 cm–50 cm × 2.5 mm	Scolex has four suckers, hooklets, refractile rostellum, 60–175 proglottids; mature proglottid has diffuse testes, uterus with nestlike compartments, unilateral genital pore, ivory with red tinge

Table 69-1. (continued)

Eggs	
EMBRYONAL CONTENTS	SIGNIFICANT CHARACTERISTICS
Hexacanth embryo	No operculum, radially striated shell, yellow brown
Hexacanth embryo	Indistinguishable from *T. saginata*
Hexacanth embryo	No operculum, double membrane, four to eight polar filaments, hyaline
Undeveloped embryo	Inconspicuous operculum, small abopercular thickening, light yellow
Hexacanth embryo	No operculum, double membrane, light yellow
Hexacanth embryo	No operculum, packets of 10–25 eggs, brick red

Taenia Solium Taeniasis

Etiology

The adult pork tapeworm, *T. solium,* differs from *T. saginata* in several ways (Table 69-1). It is shorter (average length 2 m–4 m) and has a scolex armed with hooks. The gravid proglottids are smaller, have fewer uterine branches (less than 15 on each side) and fewer eggs (up to 50,000), and are usually expelled passively in groups of 3 to 5 with the feces. *Taenia solium* needs only 2 months to develop a fully grown strobila.

The eggs of *T. solium* are indistinguishable from those of *T. saginata.* They may develop into cysticerci in humans, pigs, monkeys, dogs, and many other domesticated or wild animals. The cysticerci of *T. solium* are larger (up to 20 mm in length) than those of *T. saginata* and are easier to find when meat is inspected. In pigs, cysticerci develop in the muscle tissue; in humans, they show a predilection for the central nervous system, frequently causing cerebral cysticercosis (Chap. 79, Larval Cestodiasis).

Epidemiology

Although *T. solium* may develop in many hosts, the typical cycle is man–pig–man. Taeniasis and cysticercosis caused by *T. solium* occur mostly in rural communities in which pigs feed on human feces and humans eat noninspected, raw, or inadequately cooked pork. The distribution of *T. solium* is limited to certain regions in the world: Central and South America, Central and South Africa, Southeast Asia, and South and East Europe. In highly endemic areas (Mexico, the South African Republic, Zaire, India, Indonesia, and the Republic of Korea), the incidence of cysticercosis in pigs exceeds 1%, and cysticercosis in humans is a serious public health problem. Most of the cases of *T. solium* taeniasis and cysticercosis seen in the United States are imported from other endemic regions.

Pathogenesis and Pathology

The pathology of taeniasis is similar whether it is caused by *T. solium* or *T. saginata* except for the lesions of cysticercosis. About 25% of patients infected with *T. solium* experience autoinvasion—most likely a fecal–oral infection through eggs transmitted on the patient's hands, or possibly intestinal autoinvasion when eggs or proglottids are passed from jejunum to stomach by antiperistalsis.

Manifestations

The manifestations of *T. solium* taeniasis differ from those of *T. saginata* infection in that there is no perianal sensory awareness of the passage of proglottids due to a lack of active movement of proglottids per anus.

Diagnosis

The symptoms of taeniasis are not pathognomonic and the infection may pass unnoticed by the patient unless the discharge of a multiproglottid piece of the strobila is observed. Travel in endemic areas may be an important diagnostic clue in the patient's history. Repeated examinations of the feces may be necessary because the eggs of *T. solium* may remain enclosed in the proglottids and are inconstantly present in the feces. When eggs are present in the feces in the absence of any active discharge of single proglottids, infection with *T. solium* is probable. Species diagnosis is only possible by examination of the scolex or proglottids; neither is easy to find. Accordingly, final diagnosis is often deferred until after treatment when the scolex or strobila become available. Feces that may contain *T. solium* eggs or gravid proglottids are potential sources of cysticercosis and should be handled with maximal care.

Prognosis

Cysticercosis is a serious consequence of undiagnosed or untreated *T. solium* taeniasis; it may be fatal. Self-cure of *T. solium* taeniasis may occur in exceptional cases.

Therapy

Taeniasis caused by *T. solium* should be treated as soon as it is diagnosed or suspected. If species diagnosis was uncertain before treatment, it should be pursued after therapy because knowing the species of the tapeworm is important for prognosis.

A single dose of niclosamide (see *T. saginata)* cures *T. solium* taeniasis even more readily than it cures infection caused by *T. saginata.* Praziquantel is not recommended for *T. solium* taeniasis, since it may cause complications through action of the drug on cysticerci present in the brain or eye. Treatments that may provoke vomiting, for example, mepacrine or saline purgatives, are not recommended in *T. solium* taeniasis. Duodenal intubation must not be done because of the danger of cysticercosis. Successful treatment is confirmed by negative examinations of feces carried out in the second and third months after treatment.

Prevention

The most effective prophylaxis for *T. solium* taeniasis is to avoid eating raw or undercooked pork. The control of *T. solium* taeniasis and cysticercosis is based on education, early detection and treatment of taeniasis in humans, the proper disposal of feces, the practice of sanitation, breeding pigs indoors, inspection of meat and condemnation of infected carcasses, and thorough cooking of all noninspected pork.

Diphyllobothriasis

Etiology

Diphyllobothrium latum, the fish tapeworm, is the longest tapeworm (up to 15 m). As a representative of the order of *Pseudophyllidea,* it differs greatly from the other tapeworms which infect humans. It has an elongated (2 mm–3 mm) scolex with two sucking grooves, and 3000 to 4000 proglottids that are broader than they are long and have a central, rosettelike uterus. Mature proglottids release about one million eggs every day into the intestinal lumen.

The operculated egg embryonates in water and hatches to release a free-swimming larva, a coracidium; the coracidium develops into an elongated larva, a procercoid, in the body cavity of a *Copepoda.* The procercoid develops further into a plerocercoid in the muscle or connective tissue of several species of freshwater fish. The plerocercoid is an invasive stage for humans, for more than 20 species of fish-eating nonhuman animals, and for carnivorous fish (which may serve as transport hosts). The entire cycle outside of humans takes at least 2 months. Eggs are produced 3 to 5 weeks after ingestion of the plerocercoid, and the adult *D. latum* may live up to 30 years.

Epidemiology

Fish tapeworm cestodiasis occurs only in temperate zones of the world around lakes and rivers and in deltas in which suitable *Copepoda* exist. Wild, fish-eating animals are important reservoirs of infection. Whether infection in humans is sporadic or endemic depends on the local habits of eating raw fish. Endemic diphyllobothriasis exists in Finland, Northern U.S.S.R., and Canada; in other parts of the world, infections are sporadic or caused by other species such as *Diphylobothrium pacificum* in Peru. In general, the incidence of diphyllobothriasis in man is declining; however, some new foci of infection continue to appear.

Pathogenesis and Pathology

Diphyllobothriasis provokes little intestinal pathology other than that due to intensive absorption of vitamin B_{12} by the tapeworm. A macrocytic, hyperchromic anemia results in about 2% of cases of diphyllobothriasis. The vitamin B_{12} deficiency is more severe when the tapeworm is located in the proximal part of the jejunum. Lack of vitamin B_{12} in the diet, reduction of the intrinsic factor in the gastric juice, and some genetic factors further enhance the risk of anemia.

Manifestations

Infection with *D. latum* usually causes few abdominal symptoms. There is usually no discharge of proglottids, since they easily disintegrate in the intestine. Occasionally, a large piece of the strobila is evacuated, suggesting a tapeworm infection. In some patients, the symptoms and signs of macrocytic anemia dominate the clinical picture.

Diagnosis

Diphyllobothriasis is easily detected by examination of the feces because eggs of *D. latum* are numerous, relatively large, and discharged constantly. Anemia caused by the infection should be differentiated from other macrocytic anemias; vitamin B_{12} given perorally does not cause haematologic remission in diphyllobothriasis.

Prognosis

Macrocytic anaemia may be a serious complication of diphyllobothriasis, and it cannot be controlled without anthelmintic treatment.

Therapy

Infection caused by *D. latum* responds well to treatment by niclosamide and praziquantel (see *T. saginata* taeniasis). The treatment is deemed successful when fecal examinations are negative for ova 6 to 8 weeks after therapy.

Prevention

Diphyllobothriasis can best be prevented by restricting ingestion of raw, freshwater fish; cooking, frying, hot-smoking, or freezing at home readily kills the plerocercoids. There is no practical way to interfere with the transmission of *D. latum* in nature or with the reservoir of infection in wild animals. However, where diphyllobothriasis in humans is endemic, proper disposal of feces is an important preventive measure.

Hymenolepiasis

Etiology

The dwarf tapeworm, *H. nana* is the smallest cestode that infects humans. It has an armed scolex and a strobila 2 cm–4 cm long, consisting of 200 short proglottids. Localized primarily in the ileum, the adult *H. nana* live for only a few weeks. However, the population is renewed constantly as the life cycle is completed in the intestine. After the eggs leave the disintegrated proglottids in the intestinal lumen, some are evacuated with the feces and are a source of infection for a new host. Other eggs hatch to yield oncospheres which penetrate the intestinal villi and develop into bladder larvae, the cysticercoids. After destroying the villus, the fully developed cysticercoids fall into the intestinal lumen, evaginate, and develop into adult tapeworms. The cycle from egg to egg-producing tapeworm takes 2 to 3 weeks.

Epidemiology

Hymenolepiasis is the most common tapeworm infection in the world; unlike the other cestodiases, *H. nana* parasitizes children more often than adults. The incidence is especially high in warm and arid countries, for example, the Mediterranean region, the near East, the Indian subcontinent, and South America. In some areas, the incidence in children is 5% to 20%. Epidemics may occur in orphanages, institutions for the mentally retarded, and other closed communities where fecal-oral transmission is likely. Humans are occasionally infected by a zoonotic strain *(e.g., H. nana* var. *fraterna)* which is common in rodents and may use fleas and beetles as intermediate hosts.

Pathogenesis and Pathology

The pathologic effect of hymenolepiasis depends upon the number of tapeworms. The population may reach several thousands, but varies periodically and is regulated by many factors, including the immune state of the host and the amount of protein in the diet. The infection usually disappears in adolescence and it is infrequently seen in healthy adults.

Intense infections may cause subacute enteritis from mechanical irritation of the mucosa and damage to the villi. Intestinal absorption may be greatly impaired. It has been suggested that tapeworm metabolites may be neurotoxic.

Manifestations

Light and moderate hymenolepiasis may be asymptomatic. Heavy infections cause nonspecific abdominal symptoms such as anorexia, abdominal cramps, and diarrhea, and usually impair the general health of the infected child. Irritability, dizziness, and even seizures have been observed in some patients but may not be directly related to the infection, since hymenolepiasis is often concomitant with malnutrition and other diseases that impair the immune competence of the host.

Diagnosis

Hymenolepiasis is diagnosed by finding the eggs of *H. nana* in the feces. Flotation techniques are useful, and repeated examination is frequently needed as the egg output may be inconstant.

Prognosis

Hymenolepiasis may be a rather persistent infection with frequent relapses, recrudescences, or reinfections in children. It usually disappears spontaneously in adolescence.

Therapy

Niclosamide and praziquantel are the drugs of choice for hymenolepiasis. Heavy infections need two 5 to 7 day treatments (2 weeks apart) with a full daily dose of 2 g of niclosamide for adults and about 60 mg/kg of body weight for children. The optimal dosage for praziquantel has not been determined, but single doses appear to be effective. Follow-up fecal examinations should be performed every 2 weeks for at least 3 months after treatment. Contemporaneous treatment of all infected family members and inmates of institutions greatly increases the chance of a final cure.

Prevention

As in other fecal–oral infections, personal hygiene and sanitation are the most important preventive measures. Epidemics in institutions may be prevented by examination of all newcomers—inmates and staff—treating all infected persons.

Other Cestodiases

Humans may occasionally be infected with several other cestodes that are natural parasites of nonhuman animals. Most of these cestodiases are benign infections easily cured by a single dose of niclosamide.

Dipylidium caninum, the dog tapeworm, is common in dogs and cats throughout the world. Humans acquire infection by ingesting fleas containing cysticercoids. A few hundreds of cases, mainly in children, have been reported.

Hymenolepis diminuta the rat tapeworm, is common in rodents. Humans acquire infection by ingestion of fleas or beetles containing cysticercoids. Infections are not rare in poor communities plagued by rodents (Iran, Papua, New Guinea).

Several species of *Raillietina,* a cestode infecting rats, have been described in humans in East Asia and South America. *Inermicapsifer madagascariensis* is a tapeworm common in African rodents, which may invade humans in Africa, and is encountered also in Central and South America. *Bertiella studeri* is a tapeworm parasitizing mainly monkeys. Several cases have been reported in humans in Cuba and South America.

Bibliography

Books

VON BONSDORFF B: Diphyllobothriasis in Man. Academic Press, New York, 1977. 189 pp.

PAWLOWSKI Z: Taeniasis and cysticercosis. In Steele JH (ed): Zoonoses, Section C: Parasitic Zoonoses (Handbook Series). Boca Raton, Florida, CRC Press, 1982 (in press)

Journals

GROLL E: Praziquantel for cestode infections in man. Acta Trop 37:293–296, 1980

MOST H, YOELI M, HAMMOND J, SCHEINESSON GP: Yomesan (Niclosamide) therapy of *Hymenolepsis nana* infections. Am J Trop Med Hyg 20:206–208, 1971

PAWLOWSKI Z, SCHULTZ MG: Taeniasis and cysticercosis *(Taenia saginata).* Adv Parasitol 10:269–343, 1972

SCHULTZ MG, HERMOS JA, STEELE JH: Epidemiology of beef tapeworm infection in the United States. Public Health Rep 85:160–176, 1970

Section XII

Infections of the Digestive Glands

Indigenous Microbiota of the Digestive Glands

(None)

WILLIAM S. ROBINSON

Hepatitis A

70

Of the several different viruses that cause acute hepatitis, hepatitis A virus (HAV) is one of the most common. HAV is a small, RNA (picornavirus) that is enteroviruslike in its resistance to acid and in its almost exclusively fecal-oral transmission. The original designation of hepatitis A as infectious hepatitis emphasized the highly communicable nature of HAV and the feature of frequent occurrence in epidemic form. Although molecular and antigenic characteristics of HAV are distinct from those of the other hepatitis viruses, it does not cause acute disease that is clinically distinguishable from that caused by other hepatitis viruses.

Etiology

In 1973, uniformly spherical viruslike particles were first described in the feces of volunteers infected with hepatitis A. Because the particles were precipitated by serum from convalescent but not acutely ill patients, they were thought to be hepatitis A viral antigen (HAAg). Subsequently, similar particles were detected in the feces during natural infections in temporal association with clinical illness. Similar particles have been detected in liver extracts, bile, and serum of HAV-infected marmosets. Their size and appearance in electronmicrographs, and their buoyant density and sedimentation coefficient are similar to those of polioviruses.

The polypeptides of HAAg are similar to those of other picornaviruses with respect to number and size; the RNA is single stranded, measures about the same length as that in other picornaviruses, and contains a polyadenylic acid (poly A) sequence. Since the RNA of HAV has been copied into DNA, incorporated into plasmid vectors, and cloned in bacterial cells, large-scale biosynthesis of HAV antigens may be possible.

The known host range of HAV is restricted to humans, chimpanzees, and several species of South American *Saguinus* marmoset (Tamarin) monkeys. Humans appear to be the only natural hosts. Attempts to infect other nonhuman primates and nonprimates have not been successful. HAV has been propagated in cultures of a variety of human and nonhuman primate cells.

By immunofluorescent staining with anti-HAAg, HAV antigen was found only in the cytoplasm of hepatocytes of infected animals. There was no evidence of synthesis of viral antigens in other tissues, including the bowel mucosa.

The infectivity of HAV for volunteers is destroyed by boiling for 20 minutes, then applying dry heat (160°C) for 60 minutes, but it has survived 60°C for 1 hour. The infectivity of HAV in water is destroyed by chlorination using concentrations that vary with the organic content of the water. HAV is inactivated by ultraviolet irradiation and formalin, but not by ether or acid (pH 3.0 for 3 hours). The virus is also quite stable during storage at 4°C and −20°C.

Epidemiology

HAV is worldwide in distribution, as are some other hepatitis viruses. However, HAV is unlike hepatitis B virus (HBV—Chap. 71, Hepatitis B) in two epidemiologically critical respects: (1) there is no persistent infection with continuous viremia; and (2) HAV is present in the feces of all persons with hepatitis A. The epidemiologic consequences are (1) rare transmission by the parenteral inoculation of blood or blood products, unlike HBV; and (2) ease of fecal-oral spread, often by food or water contaminated with feces. Because there is neither a nonhuman reservoir nor persistent infection in humans, HAV must be maintained by serial transmission from acute cases to susceptibles. In small, isolated populations, HAV disappears after an epidemic that has followed introduction from the outside and reappears years later when HAV is again introduced from outside. Such behavior is similar to that of measles, mumps, rubella, and polio—viruses that do not commonly cause persistent infection in humans and for which no important nonhuman reservoir is known.

The number of cases of viral hepatitis caused by HAV in the United States is not precisely known because viral hepatitis is not a reportable disease, and only a small fraction of cases are actually evaluated by specific HAV serology. However, more than 60,000 cases of acute viral hepatitis are recorded by the Centers for Disease Control (CDC) each year, and approximately 67% are reported to be hepatitis A. The actual number of HAV infections is probably much higher because most primary infections are subclinical and clinically apparent cases are greatly underreported. In the past, the incidence was highest among children and adolescents—both in highly endemic areas and in many epidemics; however, in recent years, the age-specific incidence has clearly changed toward older persons. Males and females appear to be equally susceptible, and the highest seasonal incidence occurs during autumn and winter. Rates of HAV infection are particularly high in populations living under crowded conditions such as schools, military institutions, prisons, and custodial facilities. The secondary attack rate is very high in members (particularly children) of households with an index case.

If the presence of anti-HAAg is taken as evidence of past infection, the highest rates generally occur in developing countries where housing and sanitation are poor. In such regions, antibody appears at very early ages when most infections are subclinical and anicteric. For example, more than 90% of the population of a developing country has antibody by the time they reached adulthood, compared with around 20% in the United States. The incidence of anti-HAAg appears to be independent of sex and race. In developed countries, for example, in the United States, populations of lower socioeconomic status have a higher incidence of anti-HAAg than those of higher socioeconomic status.

Serologic evidence of past infection with both HAV and HBV is relatively low in the United States and Switzerland, whereas in Senegal and Taiwan, the incidence of both is relatively high. In Belgium, Isreal, and Yugoslavia, the rates of infection with HAV are relatively high, whereas the rates of HBV infection are relatively low. Clearly, the factors that determine the rates of infection are not the same for the two viruses.

Most HAV infections appear to be associated with subclinical disease. Of adult populations in the United States, 30% to 50% have serologic evidence of past infection with HAV, but only 3% to 5% of adults can recall an illness suggesting or documented to be hepatitis. Experimental transmission studies have proved that HAV infections may be associated with subclinical and anicteric hepatitis.

From three lines of evidence, it is clear that transmission of HAV usually occurs around the time of onset of symptoms, before the onset of icterus:

1. Cases secondary to contacts in households and institutions, and after ingestion of contaminated water or food, occur approximately one incubation period after the onset of symptoms in the index case.
2. In transmission studies with a limited number of volunteers, infectious HAV was present in the feces 14 to 21 days before to 8 days after the onset of jaundice. No infectious virus was found 28 days or more before, or 19 days or more after, the onset of jaundice. Because the number of subjects in these studies was small, the period of fecal shedding was only approximated. In addition, the quantity of HAV in the feces was not titrated and so the time of maximal risk was not determined.
3. When the time of fecal shedding of HAV was assessed by following HAAg particles by immune electron microscopy or radio-immunoassay, the highest concentrations were found in the late incubation period and at the time of onset of symptoms. In most studies, particles disappeared before the peak of serum transaminase activity or the onset of jaundice, although low levels of particles were sometimes present as late as 10 to 16 days after the onset of icterus.

   Although fecal excretion of HAV may in some patients continue for 1 to 2 weeks after the onset of icterus, transmission is then much less frequent because the titer of infectious virus is lower.

Chronic fecal shedding of HAV is rare if it occurs at all. Disappearance of hepatitis A in small, isolated populations after epidemic infection indicates that shedding ceases or falls to such a low level that transmission is not maintained. Moreover, HAV has never been observed when the feces of experimentally infected humans was assayed for infectious virus or when fecal HAAg was followed during experimental and natural infections.

Fecal shedding of HAV leads to spread of infection by close personal contact and by contamination of water and food. Epidemic and endemic hepatitis A have frequently been associated with ingestion of raw clams contaminated with sewage. Oysters, mussels, and steamed clams are involved less often. Hepatitis A virus transmission by way of milk and other food and drink has been documented, and sometimes a food handler infected with hepatitis A is thought to be the source.

Although small amounts of infectious HAV may at times be present in saliva, respiratory secretions, and urine, there is little evidence that these are important sources of virus for contact transmission.

Some kinds of sexual contact may result in the transmission of HAV. For example, male homosexuals have a markedly increased incidence of anti-HAAg compared with heterosexual controls. The precise mechanism of transmission in these populations is not known.

Transient viremia has been documented repeatedly after HAV infection, but the period of viremia is variable and occurs exclusively during the latter half of the incubation period. Because the incubation period is shorter and there is no persistent infection, the period of viremia in HAV is much shorter than that of HBV. Thus, the percutaneous transfer of blood or blood products is rarely the mode of transmission of HAV, unlike HBV. Sero-epidemiologic evidence supports this view. Children and adult patients who have received several transfusions, as well as staff members of hemodialysis centers have a much higher frequency of anti-HBV than nontransfused controls, but the frequency of anti-HAAg is the same. Studies of posttransfusion hepatitis have failed to reveal cases of hepatitis A by specific serologic testing.

A recent report of six women with serologically documented acute hepatitis A in the second and third trimesters of pregnancy revealed no evidence of transmission of HAV to any of their newborn infants.

Serologically documented cases of hepatitis A following contact with chimpanzees and a few other nonhuman primates have been reported. Animals in captivity that had prior contact with humans have always been involved; that is, the animals were infected by contact with humans rather than with wild nonhuman primates.

Pathogenesis and Pathology

The pathogenesis of the hepatic injury in acute hepatitis A is unclear. It is not known whether HAV is directly cytopathic to infected cells or whether immune injury or some other mechanism is involved. However, in experimental infections in chimpanzees and marmosets, serologic markers of HAV infection can be detected well before the onset of symptoms or evidence of liver disease (Fig. 70-1). The first evidence of viral infection in chimpanzees is the appearance of HAAg detected by immunofluorescent antibody staining in the liver 1 to 2 weeks after infection. At the same time, 27-nm viruslike particles are detectable in vesicles within the cytoplasm of hepatocytes by electron microscopy. HAAg has been observed in the marmoset liver as early as 1 week after infection; within a few days, HAAg can be detected in the feces and the bile by immune electron microscopy and radioimmunoassay. In experimentally infected humans, HAAg may be found in the feces several days before elevation of the SGOT is detectable; usually, the HAAg is maximal at about the time of the first SGOT elevation. In most studies, the fecal HAAg has become undetectable by immunoelectronmicroscopy before the peak SGOT; however, with radioimmunoassay, the antigen has been found up to 16 days after the onset of jaundice in a small fraction of patients. The period when HAAg is detectable in the feces is similar to the period of fecal infectivity. Bile may be the source of fecal HAAg because the antigen has not been detected in bowel mucosa after parenteral or oral infection of chimpanzees, although infection of the bowel mucosa at some time during HAV hepatitis may occur. Antigen has been detected in the blood before the onset of disease, but the time of its appearance and its duration in the blood are not well defined.

HAAg can usually be detected by immunofluorescent antibody in liver longer than by radioimmunoassay in blood or feces. HAAg has been detected in the chimpanzee liver for a period of 4 to 5 weeks, and low levels appear to persist regularly after the SGPT has returned to normal.

The histopathologic changes in acute viral hepatitis include hepatocellular injury, an inflammatory reaction, and hepatocellular regeneration. Focal hepatocellular necrosis may be present and is most common in centrolobular areas; eosinophilic changes in the cytoplasm of hepatocytes (Councilman bodies) and giant multinucleated cells are sometimes present. Fatty infiltration is not observed. The inflammatory response is most intense in the portal areas and consists mainly of mononuclear cells but may include polymorphonuclear neutrophils and eosinophils. Dilated canaliculi and bile plugs are sometimes present.

Histologic lesions may occur in the gastric and small intestinal mucosa, the kidney, and the bone marrow in acute hepatitis. How they may be related to HAV infection is unclear.

Transient arthralgias and occasionally arthritis and

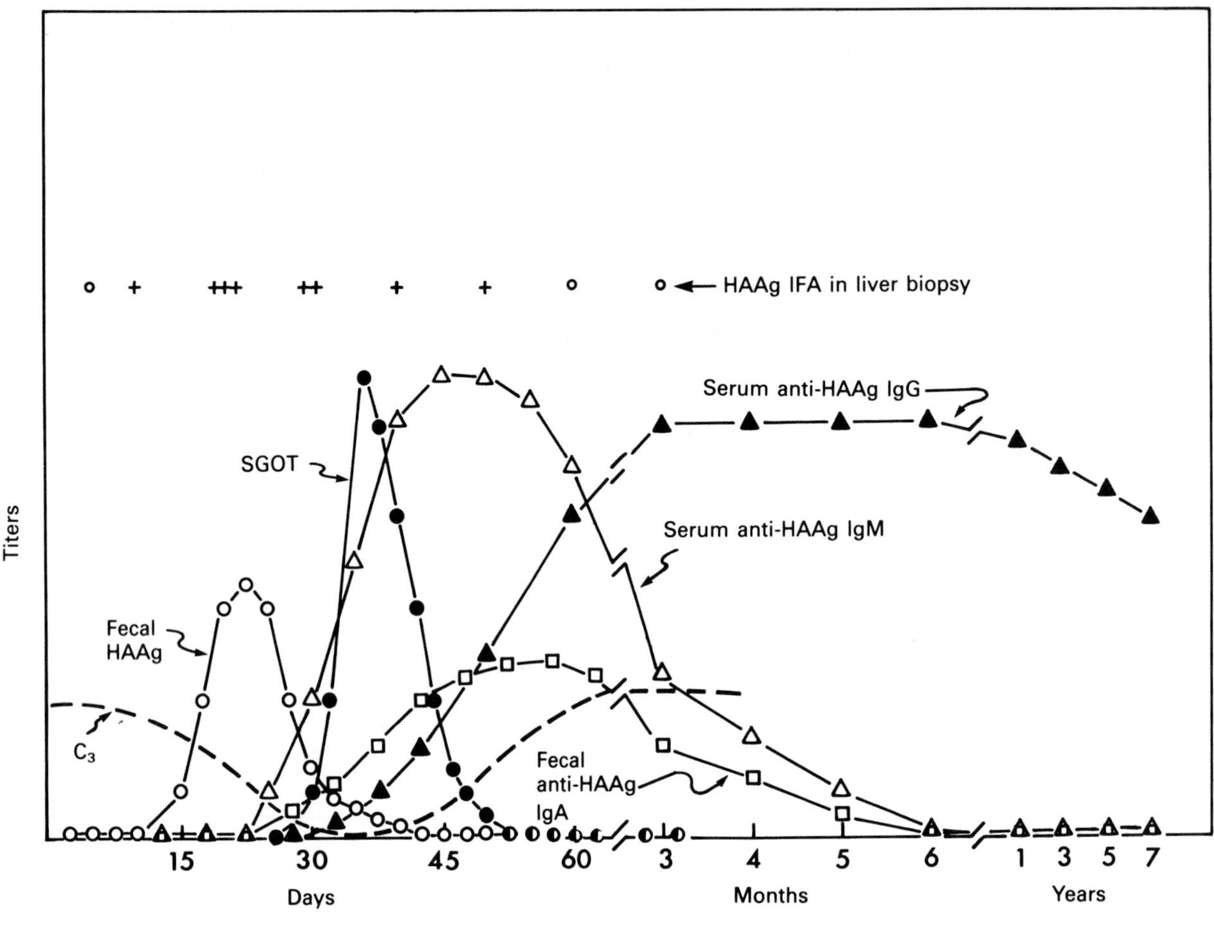

Fig. 70-1. Course of experimental hepatitis A induced in a chimpanzee.

rash occur during the incubation period of hepatitis A, but less frequently than in hepatitis B. The pathogenesis of the joint and skin involvement during HAV infection has not been as extensively studied as in HBV disease. However, HAAg and anti-HAAg may be detected in the same serum, anticomplementary activity occurs during the incubation period, and low C_3 levels are found during an acute hepatitis A illness. These changes are consistent with immune complex formation, but their role in HAV-associated disease has not been proven.

Manifestations

Most primary HAV infections are asymptomatic and are not recognized clinically, although serum transaminase levels are commonly elevated. Of the remainder, many are associated with rather mild, symptomatic but self-limited, icteric or anicteric illness. Acute hepatitis A tends to be milder in children than in adults.

Volunteer studies with infectious hepatitis (most of which was undoubtedly HAV) in the 1940s established an incubation period (the time between exposure and the onset of symptoms) between 14 and 49 days. The incubation period in epidemic hepatitis A (serologically documented) resulting from common-vehicle exposure of humans during brief, defined periods varies from 20 to 45 days with a mean around 28 days. The first symptom is commonly fever (37.5°C–38.5°C); it is followed shortly by malaise, headache, anorexia, nausea, vomiting, and right upper-quadrant pain. In a small fraction of cases, signs of hepatic involvement are preceded by a transient serum sicknesslike illness that may include urticaria and other forms of skin rash, arthralgias, or arthritis, as is more commonly seen in hepatitis B. Elevated serum amino acid transferase activity (*e.g.* SGOT and SGPT) is the most characteristic abnormality of liver function, usually becoming elevated at the time of onset of fever. Hepatomegaly can usually be detected within a few days. If jaundice occurs, it comes on 5 to 10 days after the first elevation of the SGOT following hepatomegaly. The SGOT usually peaks and begins to fall before the onset of jaundice. The maximal values of the SGOT vary from a few hundred to several thousand international units per milliliter, depending on the severity of the disease. The peak concentration of bilirubin in the serum may exceed 20mg/dl. When abnormal, the serum alkaline phosphatase is rarely more than moderately elevated. A relative lymphocytosis with the appearance of atypical lymphocytes is not uncommon. The concentration of the gamma globulins in the serum is commonly elevated and the prothrombin time may be abnormal in severe disease.

During the acute disease, the liver may be moderately enlarged and tender, and there may be scleral and cutaneous icterus. Splenomegaly is detected in 20% of cases, sinus bradycardia may be present in icteric patients, and spider angiomata are observed in some patients.

The average duration of abnormalities in experimentally infected children was 8 days for jaundice and elevated bilirubin, 13 days for hepatomegaly, and 15 days for the elevated SGOT. Hepatitis A is usually more prolonged in adults, and the icteric phase may last for a month or more. In general, the higher the bilirubin, the more prolonged the illness. The SGOT returned to normal within 2 to 3 weeks of the onset of illness in all children in one study, but 20% of college students had elevations of the SGOT for 143 days after exposure, and 50% of Naval recruits had persistent elevations of the SGOT 3.5 weeks after the onset of symptoms, falling to 8% after 14 weeks, with normal values in all patients by 24 weeks. Rarely, HAV infection is associated with hepatic encephalopathy of fulminant hepatitis. Chronic hepatitis has never been shown to follow documented HAV infection. Although acute hepatitis A is generally milder than acute hepatitis B, individual cases cannot be distinguished strictly on the basis of clinical findings.

Anti-HAAg detected by immune adherence hemagglutination rises in titer after acute hepatitis A to a maximum around 10 to 16 weeks after infection (Fig. 70-1). Antibody has been detected earlier in the course of infection by more sensitive tests; anti-HAAg is frequently detected by radioimmunoassay at the time of onset of jaundice or before the peak in SGOT. Most of the anti-HAAg in serum collected during the acute phase (between onset of symptoms and peak of icterus) is IgM, and in convalescent serum it is IgG. Anti-HAAg can be detected for many years after most infections. The presence of serum anti-HAAg indicates immunity and resistance to reinfection. The anti-HAAg IgA present in the feces of patients with acute hepatitis A disappears within a few months. Thus, the intestinal epithelium may be infected by HAV at some time during the course of the acute illness, although no direct evidence has been obtained of HAAg synthesis in the bowel of chimpanzees or marmosets after either parenteral or peroral infection. The possible protective role of such coproantibody is not proven.

Diagnosis

The symptoms, physical findings, and liver function abnormalities that characterize the syndrome of acute viral hepatitis are readily recognized by the clinician. Hepatitis A, however, cannot be distinguished from hepatitis caused by other agents on the basis of these clinical findings.

A specific diagnosis of HAV infection can be made by demonstrating an anti-HAAg response by complement fixation, immune adherence hemagglutination, immune electron microscopy, or radio-immunoassay. The latter two methods are more sensitive than the former two; a highly sensitive and specific radioimmunoassay for total anti-HAAg is commercially available. A fourfold or greater rise in titer between serums collected during the acute illness and 2 or 3 weeks later suggests acute infection (Fig. 70-1). An exception would be a rise due to passive acquisition of anti-HAAg (*e.g.*, by blood transfusion or administration of immune serum globulin). A diagnostic rise in titer is detected in only about half of the cases of acute hepatitis A because many patients already have detectable anti-HAAg by the time the first serum sample can be obtained, and many patients do not provide a convalescent specimen. However, the test is quite useful for identifying persons who are immune (anti-HAAg positive) or susceptible (anti-HAAg negative) to HAV infection.

If the test is refined to detect anti-HAAG IgM, virtually all patients with acute hepatitis A give a positive reaction by the time of onset of jaundice and are negative by 6 months (Fig. 70-1). A sensitive and specific, commercially available radio-immunoassay for anti-HAAg IgM permits accurate diagnosis in 90% to 100% of cases of hepatitis A in clinical settings. Because of its relatively short half-life after HAV infection, anti-HAAg IgM is much less likely to be acquired passively (*e.g.,* by blood transfusion) than is anti-HAAg IgG.

Other diagnostic approaches that are now research procedures include testing fecal specimens for HAAg by immune electron microscopy, enzyme linked immunoassay, or radioimmunoassay. However, fecal HAAg reaches a maximum concentration about the time SGOT first becomes abnormal and is usually undetectable before the peak in SGOT (Fig. 70-1). Thus, examination of feces early in the course of acute, icteric hepatitis A does not ensure finding HAAg particles, and a negative result late in the illness (*e.g.,* after the peak in SGOT) in icteric patients, and at any time after the onset of symptoms in anicteric cases, has little diagnostic significance. In a clinical setting, probably little more than a fourth of the cases of hepatitis A can be identified by examining the feces for HAAg.

Immunofluorescent staining of liver biopsies from HAV-infected chimpanzees revealed HAAg for around 2 weeks after the peak in serum SGPT (Fig. 70-1). Although liver biopsy is not often indicated in acute viral hepatitis, specific diagnosis of HAV hepatitis might be possible in humans much later in the course of the illness than can be accomplished by examination for fecal HAAg.

Because fecal anti-HAAg IgA disappears within a few months after the acute illness (Fig. 70-1), testing the feces for such coproantibodies is currently under evaluation as an aid in diagnosing hepatitis A.

There are many causes of the syndrome of acute hepatitis. In the United States, the list of viruses that must be distinguished from HAV include hepatitis B virus; non-A, non-B hepatitis viruses; Epstein-Barr virus (EBV); and cytomegalovirus. Less often, herpes simplex viruses, herpes zoster virus, measles virus, and coxsackievirus infections may be associated with acute hepatitis, although nonhepatic clinical manifestations frequently permit recognition of infections with these viruses. In other parts of the world, yellow fever, Junin, Machupo, Lassa fever, Rift Valley fever, Marburg, Ebola, and other more exotic viruses may cause the syndrome of acute hepatitis as one feature of more widespread disease. Leptospirosis and malaria occur in the United States and may also be associated with acute hepatitis. When other infectious diseases cannot be distinguished from hepatitis A on clinical grounds, serologic or other testing specific for the infectious agent is required to make a diagnosis. Acute hepatitis caused by hepatotoxic chemicals and drugs such as ethanol, isoniazid, halothane, and benzene must be distinguished from hepatitis A. A history of hepatoxic chemical exposure, assays for toxic chemicals in blood and urine, and liver biopsy may be useful in differentiating chemical hepatitis from hepatitis A.

Prognosis

Most HAV infections are subclinical. Clinically apparent disease is usually mild in children and more severe in adults. Almost all infections are self-limited and resolve. Neither persistent infections nor chronic hepatitis have been demonstrated. Fulminant hepatitis A with high mortality has been documented but is rare and occurs almost exclusively in older age groups. A serum sicknesslike illness sometimes occurs as a prodrome of hepatitis A; it is usually mild and always self-limited.

HAV infections result in immunity and long-standing resistance to reinfection. The presence of anti-HAAg IgG in the serum indicates past infection and immunity, and persists for many years.

Treatment

There is no specific therapy for acute hepatitis A. Relapses and deaths were at one time thought to be increased by severe exercise or even early ambulation. However, controlled studies failed to show deleterious effects from exercise in healthy young adult patients with relatively mild viral hepatitis. In such patients, early ambulation or even light exercise is probably not harmful. For older patients and those with more severe disease, ambulation should be gradual and determined by laboratory surveillance of hepatic function and by the patient's strength and sense of well being. If improvement in the liver disease ceases or appears to be reversed by increasing physical activity, the level of activity should be reduced to determine whether improvement again results. Prolonged bed rest may be deleterious to a patient's overall condition and should be avoided unless required for other medical reasons.

In general, patients with mild viral hepatitis need not be hospitalized. Hospitalization is necessary for those with severe disease and when care at home is inadequate.

No specific diet appears to be beneficial in acute viral hepatitis, with the exception of patients with hepatic failure, for whom restriction of protein and salt may be important. The diet should be determined by the food preferences of the patient so as to maintain the best possible nutritional state. High levels of carbohydrates or protein or other modifications of the diet have no benefit.

The claim that treatment with glucosteroids is beneficial in severe and fulminant acute viral hepatitis was not verified in controlled trials; indeed, the outcome may have been made worse. Likewise, other measures such as exchange transfusion, hemodialysis, and cross-perfusion have not proved to be of value.

Prevention

Prevention of hepatitis A depends upon blocking transmission of virus or making susceptible patients resistant to infection by passive immunization. Successful control must interrupt the spread of HAV from the feces of persons late in the incubation period to susceptibles—most often through household or other close contact, and occasionally through food or water.

The effectiveness of preexposure and postexposure prophylaxis with immune serum globulin (ISG) for modifying or preventing hepatitis A is well established. Moderate doses of ISG reduce the severity of disease without altering the incidence of infection; for example, the frequency of icteric disease is reduced by more than 80% and active immunity appears to follow these mild infections, providing long-term protection. Because higher doses of ISG may prevent both disease and infection, active immunity may not result—an undesirable consequence of high-dose immunoprophylaxis. The administration of ISG in schools and other closed populations will block the spread of HAV both in recipients and nonrecipients of ISG.

IM injection of ISG is safe, and no hepatitis B or other hepatitis is transmitted. Undesirable side-effects include pain and tenderness at the site of injection and the risk of formation of hematomas in patients with bleeding disorders. Severe allergic reactions are rare and occur more frequently after IV than IM administration.

Although all lots of ISG contain clinically useful amounts of anti-HAAg, there are significant differences between the titers of individual lots. With the availability of assays for anti-HAAg, standardization of ISG should be required and the minimum quantity of each preparation necessary for protection against hepatitis A should be designated.

Postexposure immunoprophylaxis with ISG reduces the attack rate of hepatitis A in household contacts by 80% to 90%. Doses of 0.01 to 0.02 ml/kg body wt, IM, appear to offer as much protection as larger doses. The earlier ISG is given after exposure, the more likely it is that protection will result. However, the incubation period of hepatitis A is long, and administration of ISG at any time up to 6 weeks after exposure, if symptoms have not appeared, may provide some protection. However, no benefit results from ISG given after the onset of symptoms.

Household contacts of patients with hepatitis A should be offered postexposure immunoprophylaxis. Although attack rates are highest in children, adults may also develop hepatitis, and ISG should be given to contacts of any age.

ISG is not indicated for school, work, or random contacts of patients with hepatitis A unless there has been direct physical contact with the patient or the patient's secretions. Sharing of toilet facilities is not an indication for ISG. However, in settings in which personal hygiene may be poor, such as in nursery schools or facilities for mentally retarded or psychiatric patients, institution-wide administration of ISG may be indicated when hepatitis A occurs. ISG may also be indicated for common vehicle exposure by way of contaminated food or water, although by the time such single-source outbreaks are recognized, most exposed persons are usually well into the incubation period. Persons known to be anti-HAAg positive are resistant to infection, and they do not need ISG prophylaxis.

Preexposure prophylaxis is most often indicated for susceptible persons living in highly endemic areas of the world. Studies of American missionaries and their dependents have shown annual rates of viral hepatitis of around 0.5% in Japan; 1% to 2% in southern Africa, India, and Southeast Asia; 2% to 3% in Central and South America; and 3% to 8% in North Africa and in the Middle East. Because the high risk may continue for more than 10 years of residence in highly endemic areas, the reduction in the incidence of disease that results from giving ISG, 0.12 ml/kg body wt, IM, every 4 to 6 months, is worthwhile. To avoid needless immunoprophylaxis, testing for anti-HAAg should be carried out before instituting long-term prophylaxis and in persons who developed an intraprophylaxis illness consistent with the viral hepatitis syndrome.

Short-term travelers to highly endemic areas usually have a low risk of developing icteric hepatitis A, and ISG is probably not indicated unless they plan to leave the usual tourist routes.

Other indications for long-term preexposure ISG prophylaxis include persons in institutions such as those for the mentally impaired or in nonhuman primate facilities where a high risk of hepatitis A is shown to continue despite appropriate environmental control measures.

Observing personal hygiene is one of the most important ways to prevent the transmission of HAV. Both patients with hepatitis A and their contacts, including medical personnel, should carry out scrupulous hand-washing after any direct contact with potentially contaminated objects. Although similar measures should be taken by patients and contacts during the late incubation period when patients appear to be most infective, at this stage, infection is not usually recognized.

Strict isolation of patients with hepatitis A in households is usually not necessary because others living in the same household almost always have been fully exposed by the time of onset of symptoms. Personal objects such as eating utensils, toothbrushes, razors, and toys should not be shared; hands should be washed frequently; and objects contacted by patients (particularly objects soiled with feces or blood) should be handled carefully and decontaminated. Patients should not prepare or handle food for others. Thorough washing with soap and hot water is probably sufficient do decontaminate eating utensils, clothes, bedclothes and other household objects that may be contaminated.

Strict isolation of patients with hepatitis A in hospitals is also not necessary, although measures to prevent the spread of virus from feces and blood should be taken until 2 weeks after the onset of jaundice. Objects in direct contact with patients, for example, eating utensils, bed clothes, thermometers, and medical instruments, should be decontaminated before being used for other patients. It is not necessary to confine hepatitis A patients to their rooms or to exclude visitors, although visitors should avoid direct contact with the patient or with contaminated objects.

Patient care personnel should wear gloves while drawing blood and handling feces or objects soiled with excreta. Gowns and masks should be worn during procedures that may involve splashing infected material. Most important is scrupulous hand-washing after direct patient contact or after handling potentially contaminated objects. Blood, feces, and other potentially infected specimens should be labeled infected and handled appropriately.

Patients with hepatitis A whose activities involve direct contact with others (*e.g.,* medical and dental personnel), and food handlers, should cease occupational activities until their illness has completely resolved.

Efforts should be made to reduce the transmission of hepatitis through food by requiring good personal hygiene (*e.g.,* regular hand-washing) on the part of food handlers and minimizing the extent to which food, particularly that to be eaten without further cooking, is handled. ISG should be given to those known to have eaten food that was not cooked after direct handling by an infected person, and to those not yet manifesting symptoms in a food-borne epidemic. Frequently, when food is implicated as a vehicle for HAV, no source of contamination is identified. Contaminated water used to wash uncooked food may be the source. Food should be protected from flies, which may be vectors carrying feces or sewage.

The usual water sanitation standards (Chap. 16, Environmental Factors) provide water free of infectious HAV, but water-borne hepatitis A may result from inadvertant or unrecognized contamination of drinking water with sewage. Correction of the contamination is essential, and ISG should be given to persons exposed but not yet symptomatic.

Material contaminated with HAV can best be disinfected by heat. Boiling for a time as short as 1 minute appears to inactivate HAV in dilute solutions and may suffice to render water free of infectious HAV; more intense heating is required to inactivate HAV in serum or other high-protein or lipid-containing vehicles. The conditions of dry heat, boiling, autoclaving, and chemical disinfection described in Chap. 71, Hepatitis B, are adequate for decontaminating material containing HAV.

Remaining Problems

Sufficient progress has been made in establishing animal models of hepatitis A, propagating the virus in tissue cultures, developing effective diagnostic serology, characterizing the virus, and cloning HAV RNA in bacterial cells to provide a technical basis for development of hepatitis A vaccine. Vaccination of high-risk populations appears to be the best way to push the control of hepatitis A beyond that achieved by public and personal sanitation measures applied in technologically advanced countries such as the United States. Antigenic variation has not been described for HAV, and the development of a HAV vaccine should be feasible, as it was for the similar polio viruses. Control of hepatitis A by application of antiviral chemotherapy appears to be much less likely than development of a vaccine.

Bibliography

Journals

ASHLEY A: Use of gamma globulin for control of infectious hepatitis in an institution for the mentally retarded. N Engl J Med 252:88–91, 1955

BRADLEY DW, MAYNARD JE, HINDMAN SH, HORNBECK CL, FIELDS HA, MCCAUSTLAND KA, COOK EH JR: Serodiagnosis of viral hepatitis A: detection of acute-phase immunoglobulin M anti-hepatitis A virus by radioimmunoassay. J Clin Microbiol 5:521–530, 1977

CHALMERS TC, EKHARDT RD, REYNOLDS WE, CIGARROA JG JR, DEAN N, REIFENSTEIN RW, SMITH CW, DAVIDSON CS: The treatment of acute infectious hepatitis: Controlled studies on the effects of diet, rest and physical reconditioning on the acute course of the disease and on the incidence of relapses and residual abnormalities. J Clin Invest 34: 1163–1235, 1955

CONRAD ME, SCHWARTZ FD, YOUNG AA: Infectious hepatitis: A generalized disease. A study of renal, gastrointestinal and hematologic abnormalities. Am J Med 37:789–801, 1964

DIENSTAG JL, GUST ID, LUCAS CR, WONG DC, PURCELL RH: Mussel-associated viral hepatitis type A: Serological confirmation. Lancet 1:561–564, 1976

DIENSTAG JL, FEINSTONE SM, KAPIKIAN ZG, PURCELL RH: Fecal shedding of hepatitis A antigen. Lancet 1:765–767, 1975

DIENSTAG JL, FEINSTONE SM, PURCELL RH, HOOFNAGLE JH, BARKER LF, LONDON WT, POPPER H, PETERSON JM, KAPIKIAN AZ: Experimental infection of chimpanzees with hepatitis A virus. J Infect Dis 132:532–545, 1975

DIENSTAG JL, SZMUNESS W, STEVENS CE, PURCELL RH: Hepatitis A virus infection: New insights from seroepidemiologic studies. J Infect Dis 137:328–340, 1978

FEINSTONE SM, KAPIKIAN AZ, PURCELL RH: Hepatitis A: Detection by immune electron microscopy of a virus-like antigen associated with acute illness. Science 182:1026–1028, 1973

GILES JP, LIEBHABER H, KRUGMAN S, LATTIMER C: Early viremia and viruria in infectious hepatitis. Virology 24:107–108, 1964

HAVENS WP: Period of infectivity of patients with experimentally induced infectious hepatitis. J Exp Med 83:251–258, 1946

HOLMES AW, WOLFE L, DEINHARDT F, CONRAD ME: Transmission of human hepatitis to marmosets: Further coded studies. J Infect Dis 124:520–521, 1971

KENDRICK MA: Viral hepatitis in American missionaries abroad. J Infect Dis 129:227–229, 1974

KOFF RS, GRADY GF, CHALMERS TC, MOSLEY JW, SWARTZ BL and the Boston Interhospital Liver Group. Viral hepatitis from shellfish. N Engl J Med 276:703–710, 1967

KRUGMAN S, FRIEDMAN MA, LATTIMER C: Viral hepatitis, type A, identification by specific complement fixation and immune adherence tests. N Engl J Med 292:1142–1143, 1975

KRUGMAN S, GILES JP: Viral hepatitis. A new light on an old disease. J Am Med Assoc 212:1019–1029, 1974

KRUGMAN S, GILES JP, HAMMOND J: Hepatitis virus: Effect of heat on the infectivity and antigenicity of MS-1 and MS-2 strains. J Infect Dis 122: 432–436, 1970

KRUGMAN S, WARD R, GILES JP, JACOBS AM: Infectious hepatitis: Studies on the effect of gamma globulin and on the incidence of inapparent infection. JAMA 174:823–830, 1960

KUDZMA DJ, PETERSON EW, KNUDSEN KB: Small intestinal morphology in infectious hepatitis. Arch Intern Med 124:322–325, 1969

MAYNARD JE, BRADLEY DW, GRAVELLE CR, EBERT JW, KRUSHAK DH: Preliminary studies of hepatitis A in chimpanzees. J Infect Dis 131:194–196, 1975

MAYNARD JE, LORENZ D, BRADLEY DW, FEINSTONE FM, KRUSHAK DH, BARKER LF, PURCELL RH: Review of infectivity studies in nonhuman primates with virus-like particles associated with MS1 hepatitis. Am J Med Sci 270:81–85, 1975

MOSLEY JW: The epidemiology of viral hepatitis: An overview. Am J Med Sci 271:253–270, 1975

MOSLEY JW, REDEKER AG, FEINSTONE SM, PURCELL RH: Multiple hepatitis viruses in multiple attacks of acute viral hepatitis. N Engl J Med 296:75–78, 1977

NEFSZGER MD, CHALMERS JC: Treatment of acute infectious hepatitis. Ten year follow-up study of the effects of diet and rest. Am J Med 35:299–305, 1963

PROVOST PJ, WOLANSKI BS, MILLER WJ, ITTENSOLM OL, MCALEER WJ, HILLEMAN MR: Physical, chemical and morphologic dimension of human hepatitis A virus. Proc Soc Exp Biol Med 148:532–539, 1975

RAKELA J, MOSLEY JW, REDEKER AG: The role of hepatitis A virus in fulminant hepatitis. Gastroenterology 69:854, 1975

REPSHER LW, FREEBERN RK: Effect of early and vigorous exercise on recovery from infectious hepatitis. N Engl J Med 281:1393–1396, 1969

SCHULMAN AN, DIENSTAG JL, JACKSON DRE, HOOFNAGLE JH, GERETY RJ, PURCELL RH, BARKER LF: Hepatitis A antigen particles in liver, bile, and stool of chimpanzees. J Infect Dis 134:80–84, 1976

SZMUNESS W, DIENSTAG JL, PURCELL RH, HARLEY EJ, STEVENS CE, WONG DC: Distribution of antibody to hepatitis A antigen in urban adult populations. N Engl J Med 295:755–759, 1976

SZMUNESS W, DIENSTAG JL, PURCELL RH, STEVENS CE, WONG DC, IKRAM H, BAR-SHANY S, BEASLEY RP, DESMYTER J, GAON JA: The prevalence of antibody to hepatitis A antigen in various parts of the world. Am J Epidemiol 106:392–398, 1977

WOODSON RD, CLINTON JJ: Hepatitis prophylaxis abroad: Effectiveness of immune serum globulin in protecting Peace Corps volunteers. JAMA 209:1053–1058, 1969

WILLIAM S. ROBINSON

71 Hepatitis B

Hepatitis B, hepatitis caused by infection with hepatitis B virus (HBV), was also known as serum hepatitis and long-incubation hepatitis—terms that reflected the characteristically high frequency of transmission by percutaneous inoculation with serum, and the continuous viremia. HBV, like hepatitis A virus (HAV, Chap. 70, Hepatitis A), is worldwide in distribution, and is one of the most common causes of acute viral hepatitis in the United States. However, unlike HAV, HBV is a major cause worldwide of chronic hepatitis (which sometimes leads to cirrhosis); hepatocellular carcinoma; and immune-complex diseases such as necrotizing vasculitis (polyarteritis) and glomerulonephritis.

Etiology

HBV and three other very similar viruses, found in woodchucks, ground squirrels, and ducks, form a new virus family called hepadna viruses. The hepadna viruses contain DNA that is partly single stranded and is circular in arrangement, and DNA polymerase. They exhibit a striking tropism for hepatocytes and commonly cause persistent infection with high concentrations of complete and incomplete viral forms present in the blood continuously for many months or years.

The hepatitis B virion is a spherical particle approximately 42 nm in diameter (Figs. 71-1A and 71-2). It has an electron-dense, spherical inner core with a diameter of approximately 27 nm and an outer shell or envelope approximately 14 nm in thickness. The lipid-containing envelope bears the hepatitis B surface antigen (HBsAg) that is contained in a viral genome-specified polypeptide to which virus neutralizing antibody (anti-HBs) is directed.

Detergent treatment of HBV (Figs. 71-1B and 71-2) releases the inner core particles that bear the hepatitis B core antigen (HBcAg) and contain the viral DNA, DNA polymerase, and a protein kinase that phosphorylates the viral genome-specified, major polypeptide of the core.

The third HBV antigen, the hepatitis B e antigen (HBeAg), is soluble and was first detected in serum from patients infected with HBV. Apparently, HBeAg is present in a cryptic form in the core of HBV; not only is it detectable after disruption of core particles by treatment with a detergent, but also the major polypeptide of the core displays serologic identity with HBeAg.

The single-stranded part of the small circular DNA molecules of HBV varies in length from approximately 15% to 60% of the circular portion. Thus, there is a long strand of constant length (3200 nucleotides) and a short strand of 1700 to 2800 nucleotides. The long strand is not actually a closed circle; a nick exists at a unique site to which a protein is covalently attached. By cloning and transformation experiments in *Escherichia coli* and yeasts, the complete nucleotide sequence of the DNA has been determined. Four open-reading frames have been identified in the complete or long DNA strand; that is, HBV may have only four genes.

Little is known of the mechanism of replication of these unique viruses, although the viral DNAs are commonly found to be integrated into the DNA of host cells such as the hepatocytes of infected liver and the malignant cells of hepatocellular carcinomas. The duck hepadna virus DNA has been shown to be synthesized by a reverse transcriptase using a full length RNA intermediate as a template, analogous to the RNA tumor (*i.e.,* retro or oncorna) viruses.

In addition to virions, the serums of patients infected with HBV contains 10^2 to 10^5 times higher concentrations of particles that bear HBsAg. These are small spheres (16 nm–25 nm in diameter) and filaments 22 nm in width and of various lengths (Figs. 71-2 and 71-3). Composed of lipid, protein, and carbohydrate, these particles lack HBcAg, nucleic acid,

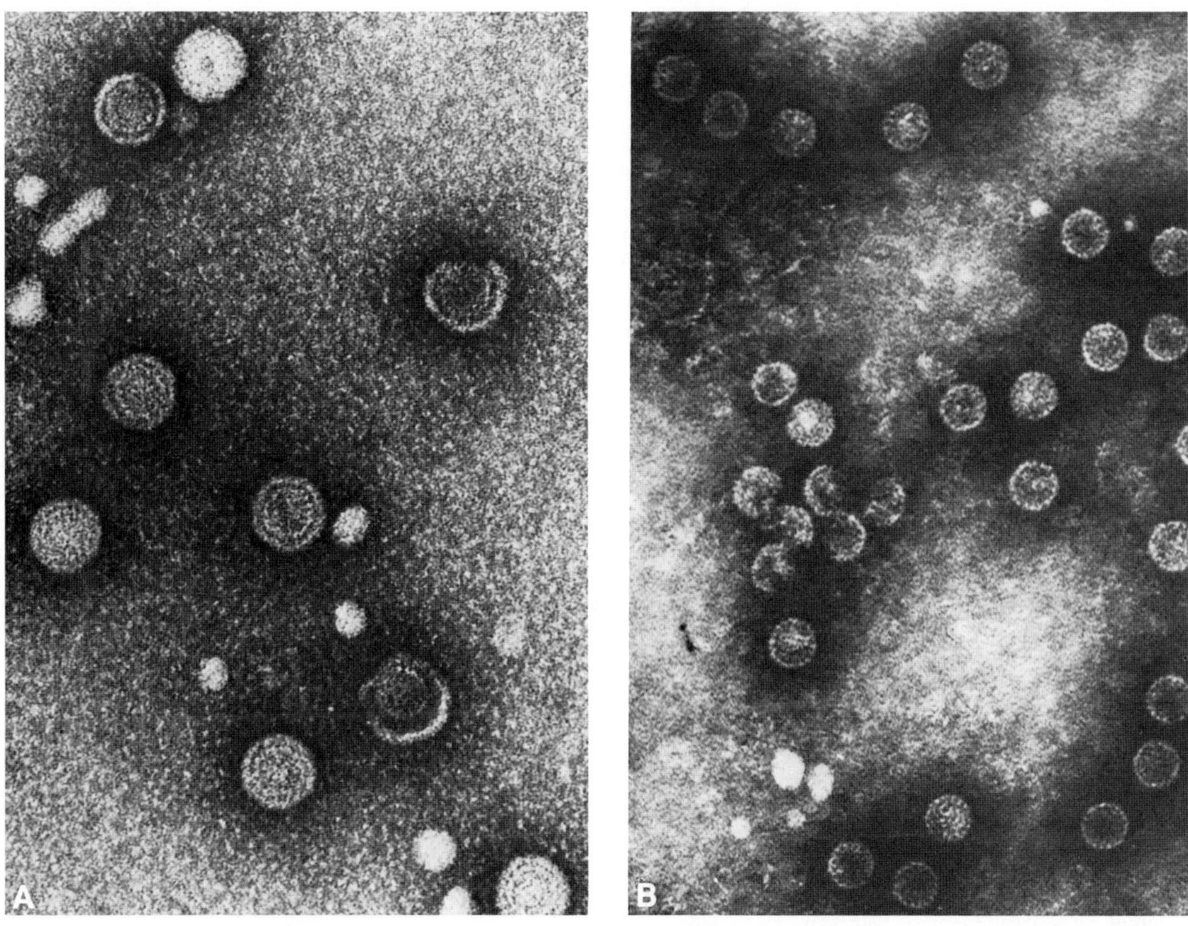

Fig. 71-1. Electron micrographs of (*A*) intact hepatitis B virions (Dane particles) and (*B*) virion cores prepared by detergent treatment of virions. (Original magnification approximately $\times\ 2 \times 10^6$) (Courtesy of June Almeida)

or other components of the core of HBV. Thus, they are incomplete forms of HBV.

Carriers of HBsAg who also carry complete virus may have 10^5 to 10^9 virions/ml serum. There is a rough correspondence between the concentrations of complete virions and infectivity with some serums proving infectious in volunteers at a dilution as high as 10^{-8}. There is a good correlation between the presence of complete virions, HBeAg, and high titers of infectivity in serums.

Using immunofluorescence, a fourth antigen, termed δ-antigen, was found in the nuclei of hepatocytes of some, but not all, specimens obtained by biopsy of carriers of HBsAg. Delta-antigen purified from hepatic tissue is a protein with a molecular weight of approximately 68,000. There may be a higher incidence of δ-antigen in patients with acute and chronic hepatitis than in asymptomatic carriers of HBsAg. Most patients with hepatic δ-antigen have anti-δ antibodies in their serum. The prevalence of anti-δ is high in Italians residing in Italy and elsewhere, in intravenous drug users, and in polytransfused HBsAg carriers. Although δ-antigen has not been found in HBsAg-negative patients, anti-δ was found in low inci-

Fig. 71-2. Schematic representation of the forms of hepatitis B virus in the blood of infected patients.

1. HBsAg (a, d/y, w/r) bearing particles in blood.
2. Virion core with HBoAg on its surface and containing DNA, and DNA polymerase and protein kinase activities.
3. Viral DNA: circular, double-stranded molecule with single-stranded gap up to 50% of circle length. DNA polymerase repairs the single stranded gap making 3200 bp molecule. 5′ end of the long strand has covalently attached protein.
4. HBeAg: Released from virion core by detergent (SDS) treatment and found as soluble antigen in serum.

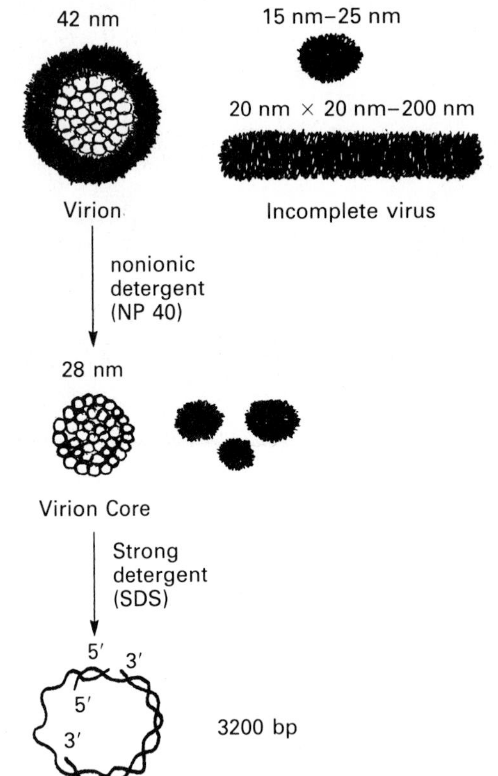

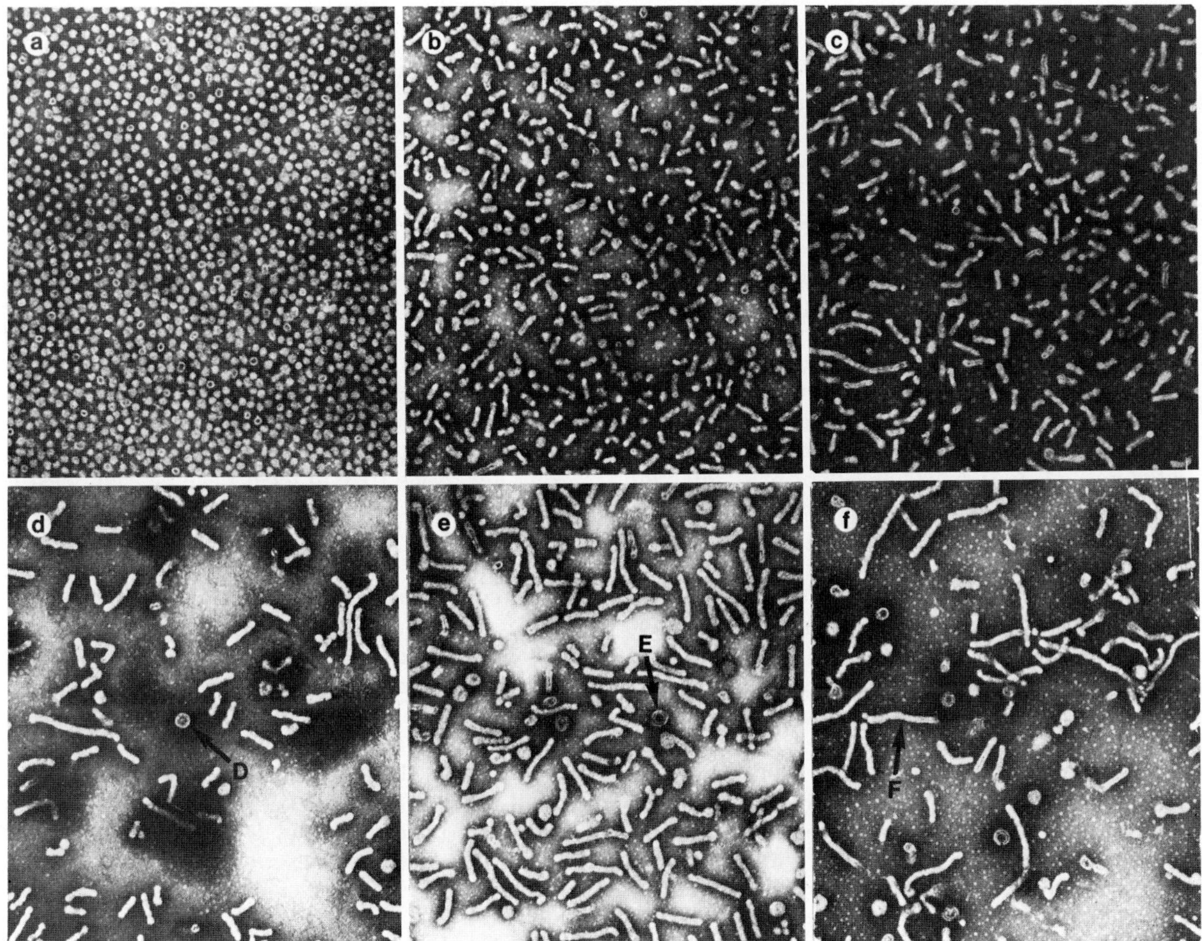

Fig. 71-3. Electron micrographs of the forms of HBsAg in serum after sucrose density gradient sedimentation. (*A*) shows small spherical particles that sediment most slowly; (*F*) shows long filaments (*f*) that sediment most rapidly. (*d*) indicates a complete virion (Dane particle) with an electron dense center; (*e*) is a Dane particle with an empty core. (Original magnification approximately $\times$ 10^5) (Courtesy of John L. Gerin)

dence in polytransfused, HBsAg negative patients, but only those with anti-HBs. The relationship of δ-antigen to HBV and its possible role in disease remain to be determined.

HBV has a narrow host range. In addition to humans, it has been shown to infect only chimpanzees, gibbons, and a few other higher primates. No reproducible infections of tissue culture cells have been reported. The agent retains infectivity for humans for months when stored in serum at 4°C, and for years if frozen at −20°C. Heating to 60°C for 10 hours, or to 98°C for 2 minutes, destroys infectivity for volunteers. Many detergents also appear to inactivate HBV.

Epidemiology

In the United States, most acute hepatitis B occurs in young adults, unlike the younger age distribution of hepatitis A. Also unlike hepatitis A, in which there is no apparent sex difference, more cases of hepatitis B occur in males than females.

The incidence of acute hepatitis B differs in different populations within the United States. At greatest risk are percutaneous drug users; patients receiving blood transfusions and those requiring hemodialysis; laboratory personnel who work with human blood, serum, and blood products; and homosexuals and others with frequent and multiple sexual contacts. Blood donor screening for HBsAg by the most sensitive tests, and a shift away from paid blood donors to use of volunteer donors, greatly reduced, but did not completely eliminate, posttransfusion hepatitis B during the 1970s. The 5% to 10% of cases of posttransfusion hepatitis still caused by HBV occur after transfusion of blood that is negative for HBsAg by the most sensitive tests available.

The incidence of HBV infecton in populations is reflected in the incidence of HBsAg and anti-HBs in the serum. For the most part, the incidence of HBsAg is directly related to the rate of persistent HBV infections (chronic carrier state), and anti-HBs indicates immunity consequent on past infection with HBV.

The rate of carriage of HBsAg in any population is related not only to the incidence of primary infection in that population but also to host and possibly viral factors. That there may be a genetic predisposition to persistent infection has been suggested by family studies in which the chronic carrier state appears to segregate as an autosomal recessive trait; however, there is no association between the chronic carrier state and HLA or blood-group antigens. Persistent infection is probably more common after initial anicteric than icteric acute hepatitis; survivors of fulminant hepatitis B rarely become chronically infected. Anicteric neonatal hepatitis is almost invariably followed by chronic infection. Immunosuppression appears to be associated with milder initial disease and more frequent persistent infection than occurs in immunologically normal persons. Finally, the HBsAg carrier state appears to be more common in patients with certain diseases such as Down's syndrome, lepromatous leprosy, and chronic lymphocytic leukemia than in the general population. The frequency in males is several times higher than in females.

In most areas of the United States, 0.05% to 0.5% of volunteer blood donors have been found to be HBsAg positive, and most of these are HBsAg carriers. The carrier rate in paid donors may be 1% or higher. Among percutaneous drug users, patients in certain hemodialysis centers, and certain homosexual populations, 2% to 5% may be HBsAg positive. The carrier rates in Northern European countries are similar to those in the United States, but they are higher in countries of the Mediterranean littoral such as Greece and North Africa. The highest incidence is in sub-Saharan Africa, parts of Asia, and Oceania, where carrier rates may exceed 10% in some populations. In these populations, there is a very high incidence of primary infection in infancy and childhood, and transmission from carrier mothers to young children is a common route by which HBV is spread. It has been estimated that there are more than 170 million chronic carriers in the world, and most of these are in Asia and Africa.

Although blood and blood products are the best-documented vehicles for transmission of HBV, HBsAg has also been found in other body liquids such as urine, bile, tears, saliva, semen, breast milk, vaginal secretions, cerebrospinal fluid (CSF), and cord blood. The concentrations of antigen in these liquids are always lower than in the serums of infected patients, and sometimes antigen can be demonstrated only after concentration. If infectious virus is also present, its concentration is undoubtedly lower than in serum. Semen and saliva have been documented to contain infectious HBV. Many attempts to demonstrate infectious HBV in feces have proved negative, and there is no evidence of fecal-oral transmission by way of food or water, as is common with HBA.

In the United States, HBV is most often transmitted by percutaneous transfer of, and probably mucous membrane contact with, blood and possibly other body liquids (*e.g.,* saliva), as for example by therapeutic use of blood products or by sharing needles during illicit drug use and by heterosexual and homosexual contacts. In areas of the world where carrier rates are very high, HBV is frequently transmitted from infected mothers to infants at the time of birth or by intimate contact in infancy or early childhood. Crowded or close living conditions, such as occur among family members of the same household and among institutionalized children, appear to favor transmission, although the exact mode of transmission in such circumstances is not known. Transmission is facilitated by the continous presence of high concentrations of infectious virus in blood and the lower concentrations in other body liquids such as saliva and semen during acute and persistent infections.

Transplacental or intrauterine infections are rare if they occur at all, and neonatal infections are the result of transmission at the time of birth, or soon after. In the United States, neonatal transmission occurs more frequently when mothers have acute hepatitis B either in the third trimester or in the first 2 months post-partum than earlier in pregnancy. The risk of transmission of HBV from HBsAg carriers by any route, including neonatal transmission from mothers, is greatly increased if HBeAg or virion DNA polymerase activity is present in the blood.

HBsAg has also been detected in nonhuman sources. Pools of wild mosquitos collected in Africa and the United States contained HBsAg, raising the possibility (not proved) that insects might serve as vectors for HBV. Although HBsAg was found in clams from coastal waters into which untreated sewage drained, outbreaks from such sources were uniformly non–type B hepatitis.

Pathogenesis and Pathology

The histologic features of acute viral hepatitis are described in Chapter 70, Hepatitis A. The changes in acute hepatitis B are very similar, and the severity can vary from mild inflammatory changes in subclinical HBV infections to extensive necrosis in fulminant hepatitis B.

Chronic HBV infection may be associated with a histologically normal liver and normal liver functions. More often, the syndrome of chronic persistent hepatitis occurs; it is not associated with progressive liver disease, although mild abnormalities of histology and liver function are present. Chronic HBV infection may also be associated with chronic active hepatitis (CAH), a chronic inflammatory and fibrosing process in which necrosis may bridge portal triads (bridging necrosis) or involve adjacent lobules, diffusely causing collapse (multilobular necrosis). CAH may not be clinically evident for prolonged periods or may be active with symptoms and progression to cirrhosis.

The pathogenesis of acute and chronic hepatitis B is not certain, but immune injury may play a major role. The specific viral or host antigens that may incite a cytopathic immune response are not known. However, HBsAg may not be implicated because the presence of this antigen in liver and serum does not correlate with active hepatitis, whereas there is a correlation with the presence of HBcAg in liver and HBeAg and virions containing DNA and HBcAg in serum.

Long-standing carriers, mostly those with cirrhosis, develop hepatocellular carcinoma with an incidence that may exceed 300 times that in negative controls. Hepatocellular carcinomas develop in more than two cases per thousand male HBsAg carriers who are 50 years or older in Taiwan and account for more than 40% of all deaths in that age group.

Three extrahepatic manifestations of infection with HBV appear to be related to circulating immune complexes consisting of HBsAg and anti-HBs. 1. A serum sickness–like illness during the incubation period has been associated with HBsAg–antiHBs complexes and diminished complement in synovial fluid from afflicted joints. 2. Polyarteritis nodosa and chronic HBV infection commonly coexist (e.g., among 21 patients with biopsy proven polyarteritis nodosa, 9 were carriers of HBsAg). Moreover, immune complexes and complement were detected in diseased blood vessels by immunofluorescent staining. 3. Membranous glomerulonephritis has been associated with chronic active hepatitis and persistent HBV infection. Nodular deposits of HBsAg, immune globulin, and C_3 were found by immunofluorescent staining in glommeruli and along the subepithelial surface of glomerular basement membranes.

Infantile papular acrodermatitis has been associated with persistent HBV infection in Italy and Japan, and some cases of aplastic anemia occurred during or immediately following acute hepatitis B.

Manifestations

Many primary infections with HBV are subclinical and are detected only by laboratory tests. Of clinically manifest primary infections in adults, most are self-limited and resolve completely within 6 months of onset.

Clinically apparent infections vary in severity from mild to fulminant. The clinical features of acute hepatitis B are similar to those of hepatitis A (Chap. 70, Hepatitis A) except that the incubation period of hepatitis B ranges from 40 to 180 days. Among patients with icteric hepatitis B, as in hepatitis A, 10% to 20% have a serum sickness–like illness with skin rash, urticaria, arthralgias, and (sometimes) arthritis several days to weeks before the onset of clinically apparent liver disease. This syndrome resolves without residual damage after 2 to 7 days.

Following infection with HBV, HBsAg is usually the first viral marker to appear in the blood. When very sensitive methods are used, HBsAg may be detected as early as 1 to 2 weeks and as late as 11 to 12 weeks after infection. Evidence of hepatitis follows the appearance of HBsAg by an average of 4 weeks (usually within 1 to 7 weeks). In self-limited infections (Fig. 71-4), HBsAg remains detectable by complement fixation in the blood for 1 to 6 weeks in most patients, although it may persist for up to 20 weeks. If HBsAg disappears within 7 weeks, symptomatic hepatitis rarely develops. The severity of the hepatitis, as measured by elevation of the bilirubin, correlated roughly with the duration of HBsAg positivity in patients with self-limited, experimental infections. As symptoms and jaundice diminish, the HBsAg titer usually falls and HBsAg becomes undetectable in most symptomatic patients several weeks after resolution of hepatitis. However, in experimental transmission studies,

8% of patients became HBsAg negative even before the onset of symptoms, and 28% were negative by the time symptoms had resolved.

HBeAg is also a regular and early marker of HBV infection, as depicted in Fig. 71-4. Highly sensitive assays have demonstrated that HBeAg is present in all or almost all primary infections, rising and declining in parallel with HBsAg. The titer of HBeAg declines constantly over the first 10 weeks after onset of symptoms. HBeAg usually disappears just before the disappearance of HBsAg in self-limited infections. Patients who remain HBeAg positive for 10 weeks or longer are likely to become persistently infected. In most patients, anti-HBe appears at the time HBeAg becomes undetectable or shortly thereafter. Anti-HBe persists for 1 to 2 years after resolution of infection with HBV.

The third markers in order of appearance are DNA polymerase or DNA-containing virions. These particles can be detected by their DNA polymerase activity or by DNA hybridization. They appear in the blood of most patients soon after the appearance of HBsAg, rise to high concentrations during the late incubation period, and fall with the onset of hepatic disease (Fig. 71-4).

The fourth marker of infection, anti-HBc, appears in most patients before the onset of hepatic injury, some 3 to 5 weeks after the appearance of HBsAg in the blood (Fig. 71-4). Anti-HBc titers usually rise during the period of HBsAg positivity, level off, and eventually fall after HBsAg becomes undetectable. The highest titers of anti-HBc appear in the patients with the longest period of HBsAg positivity. Anti-HBc titers fall threefold to fourfold in the first year follow-

Fig. 71-4. Hepatitis B viral markers in the blood during the course of HBsAg-positive, self-limited HBV infection.

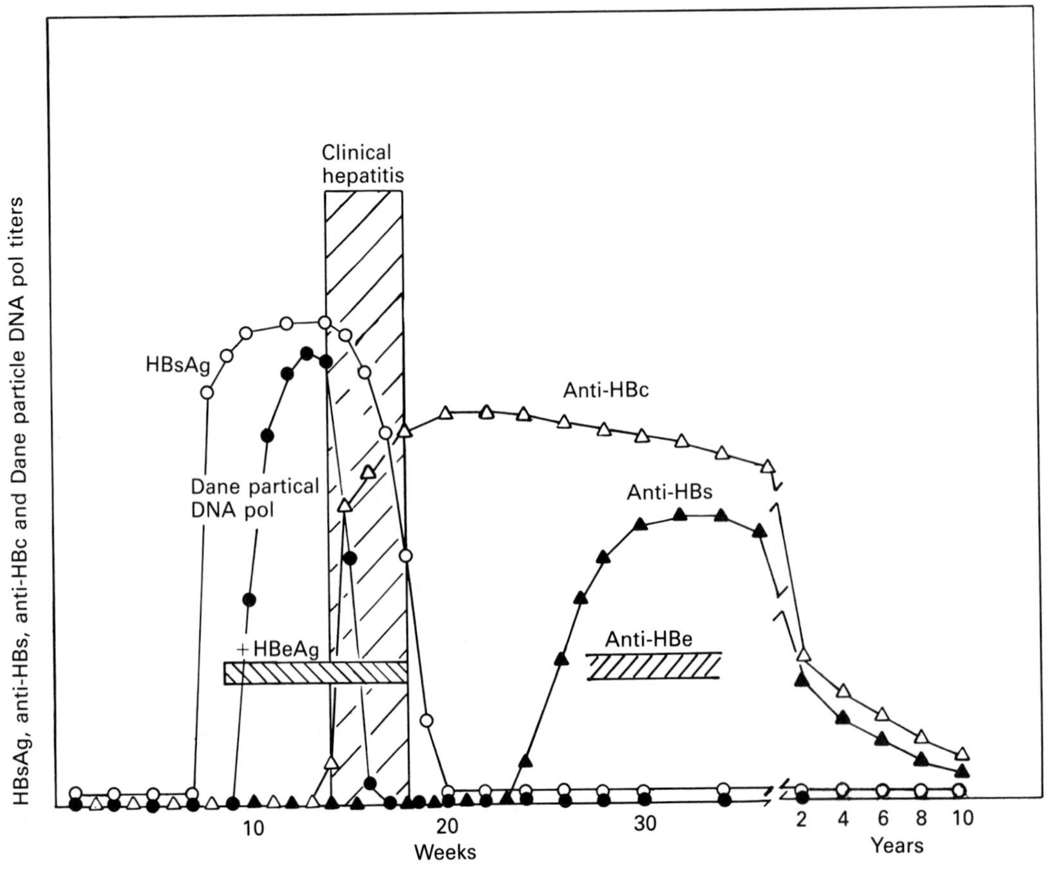

ing acute infection, then decline more slowly, and may still be detected by immunoelectroosmophoresis 5 to 6 years after the acute infection. Although most of the anti-HBc activity is IgG, IgM anti-HBc may be found in almost all patients with acute hepatitis B.

Antibody to HBsAg (anti-HBs) appears during antigenemia before the onset of clinically apparent hepatitis in the 10% to 20% of patients who develop a serum sickness–like prodromal illness in association with immune complex formation. However, HBsAg–anti-HBs complexes have also been detected in patients with acute hepatitis B who do not have an immune complex disease. Generally, anti-HBs can be detected only after HBsAg disappears from the blood, as illustrated in Fig. 71-4. Anti-HBs cannot be detected even by the most sensitive tests in many patients immediately after HBsAg disappears. There is a time interval of up to several months between the disappearance of detectable HBsAg and the appearance of anti-HBs in approximately one-half of patients with self-limited infections. In approximately 10% of patients with transient antigenemia, anti-HBs never appears. In patients with measurable anti-HBs responses, the antibody titer rises slowly during recovery and may still be rising 6 to 12 months after the disappearance of HBsAg. In contrast to the anti-HBc response, the highest titers of anti-HBs appear in the patients with the shortest period of antigenemia. Anti-HBc may persist for years after HBV infection and is associated with protection against reinfection. Self-limited infection in which serum HBsAg is detected transiently, as depicted in Fig. 71-4, is the most common pattern of primary HBV infection, and has been observed in 70% of experimentally infected patients.

The second most common pattern of primary HBV infection is self-limited infection in which HBsAg is never detected in the blood (Fig. 71-5). This pattern is observed in approximately 20% of experimental infections. Anti-HBs usually appears 4 to 12 weeks after exposure to HBV (at about the time HBsAg appears in patients with detectable antigen), and the titer rises rapidly to a high level at which it is sustained. Anti-HBc response is also detectable and includes IgM anti-HBc, but the antibody usually appears only in low titers and may not persist as long as in patients manifesting antigenemia. Infections associated with a primary antibody response without detectable HBsAg in the blood are usually accompanied by asymptomatic disease with only minor elevations in serum transaminase activity. Although the pattern of anti-HBs and anti-HBc response differs in order and relative magnitude, compared with the responses of patients with detectable antigenemia, the fact that both antibodies (including IgM anti-HBc) and liver function abnormalities appear after a period consistent with the incubation period of HBV infection indicates that actual infection with HBV has taken place. DNA polymerase–containing virions and HBeAg have not been studied in such cases.

Patients who remain HBsAg positive for 20 weeks or longer after primary infection are very likely to remain positive for a prolonged period and are designated chronic HBsAg carriers (Fig. 71-6). Such persistent infections follow symptomatic acute hepatitis B in 5% to 10% of adults. A much higher fraction of young infants becomes persistently infected. Virions (Dane particles) can be detected by electron microscopy, and it is possible to demonstrate DNA polymerase activity, HBcAg, or virion DNA in the blood of some persistently infected patients who are positive for HBsAg. By a sensitive assay for virion DNA polymerase, approximately 50% of persistently infected blood donors tested were positive, and 5% to 10% had very high concentrations. All patients with detectable virion DNA polymerase in the blood have HBcAg by immunofluorescence in liver biopsies, and when a highly sensitive assay for virions is used, all patients with HBcAg in liver have been found to have detectable virions in the serum. The duration of the infection and the kind of associated liver disease appear to correlate with the incidence of detectable amounts of virion markers in serum.

Almost all persistently infected patients have high titers of anti-HBc in the blood, as shown in Fig. 71-6. The titers of this antibody are higher during persistent infection than during most self-limited infections or during convalescence. Although most of the anti-HBc is in the IgG fraction, IgM anti-HBc continues to be made and can be detected indefinitely in the serum of most persistently infected patients.

HBeAg can be detected in the serums of almost all patients early in primary infection with HBV, and anti-HBe appears in almost all patients during resolution of the infection. However, in persistent infections, sensitive assays reveal HBeAg in one-fourth to one-half of the patients, and anti-HBe in almost all of the remainder. When less sensitive assays are used, neither marker may be detected in 50% or more of persistently infected patients. There is a very high correlation between the presence in serum of HBeAg and virions detected either by electron microscopy, DNA polymerase activity, or assays for viral DNA.

There is a wide range of HBsAg titers in persistently infected patients, and in general those with the highest titers of infectious virus and detectable virion DNA polymerase activity or HBeAg have the highest HBsAg titers.

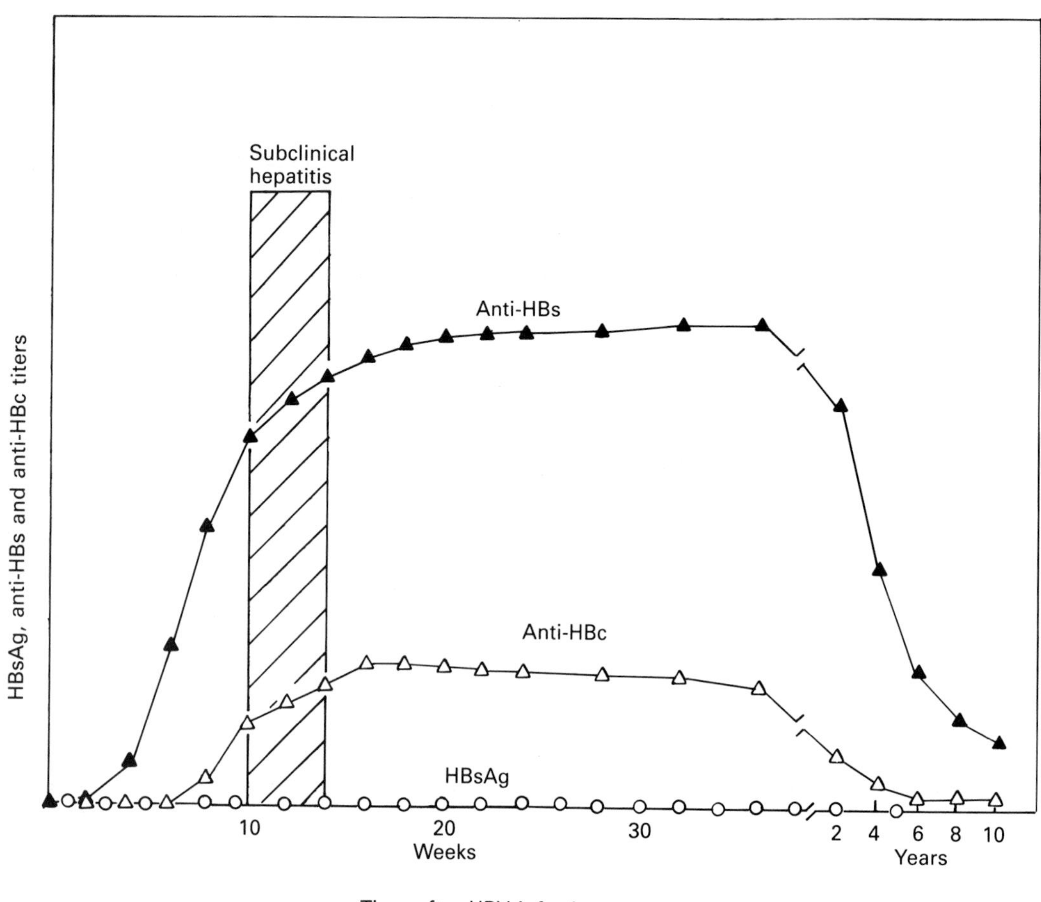

Fig. 71-5. Hepatitis B viral markers in the blood during the course of HBsAg-negative primary HBV infection.

The most sensitive assay for complete virions is undoubtedly infectivity titrations by inoculation into susceptible hosts such as humans or chimpanzees. Although most HBsAg carriers have high titers of infectious HBV in their serum, some carriers appear to have no detectable infectious virus. The highest titers of infectious HBV are found in patients with detectable HBeAg or virion DNA polymerase activity in serum; those without these markers and those with anti-HBe have much lower titers. However, it has been shown that some persistently infected patients who continue to produce HBsAg do not produce detectable amounts of infectious HBV; these are carriers without detectable virion DNA polymerase or HBeAg.

Although immune complexes of HBsAg with anti-HBs are regularly associated with a serum sickness–like prodromal illness, polyarteritis nodosa, and membranous glomerulous nephritis, such complexes are also present in the serums of persistently infected patients with chronic liver disease and in some so-called healthy carriers. That is, anti-HBs is made in many patients in the face of on-going persistent infection and without significant associated disease. Standard assays for anti-HBs rarely detect this antibody in persistently infected subjects because of the great antigen excess in the serum. It is not known whether the anti-HBs response in these patients is diminished in quantity; however, the frequent presence of this antibody, anti-HBc, and anti-HBe during persistent infection with HBV is not consistent with immunologic tolerance to the respective viral antigens as a mechanism for the persistence of the infection.

Very little detailed information is available about

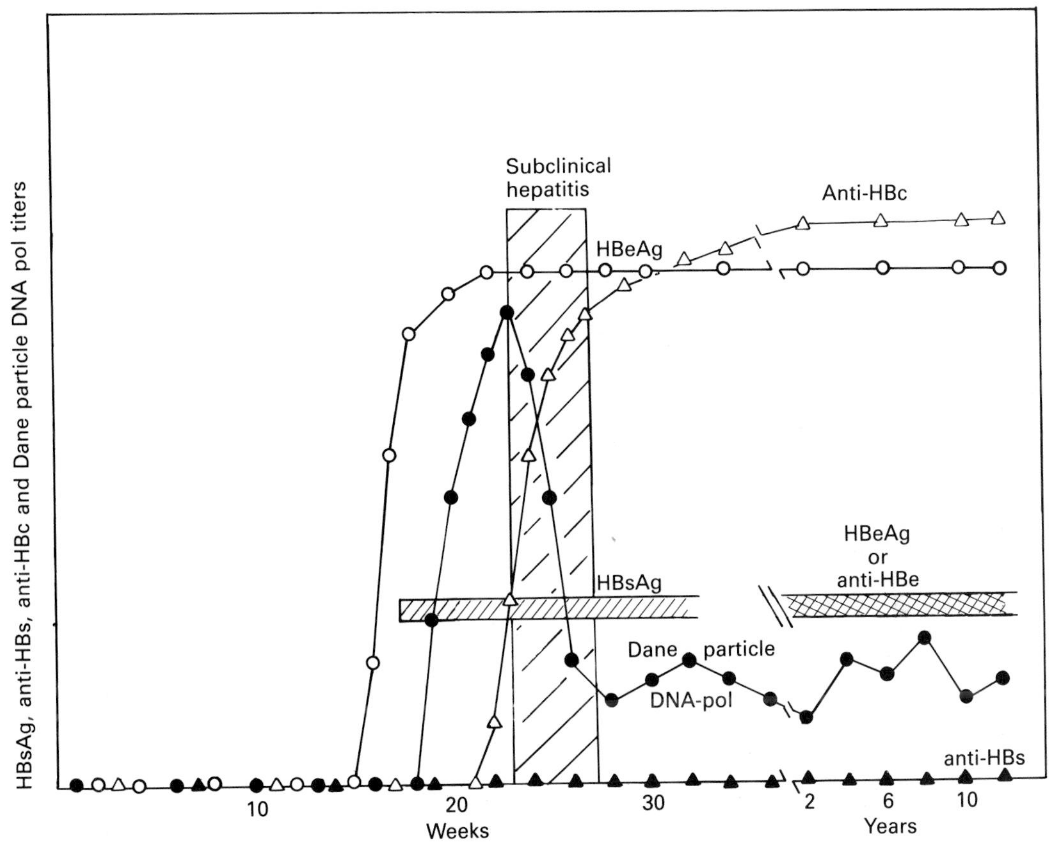

Fig. 71-6. Hepatitis B viral markers in the blood during the course of HBsAg-positive primary HBV infection that becomes persistent.

the long-term natural history of persistent HBV infection in any patient population. Prolonged infection (i.e., for many years) appears to be the rule for chronic carriers. Although titers of HBsAg and virion DNA polymerase are relatively stable over weeks or months, persistent HBV infections tend to regress spontaneously over many months to years with HBsAg titers falling slowly, and virion DNA polymerase and HBeAg titers falling below the level of detection with time. Among persistently infected patients with HBeAg and Dane particles, these markers become undetectable in 10% to 15% per year. Approximately 2% of carriers become HBsAg negative each year.

There is evidence that some patients with persistent infection with HBV do not have detectable HBsAg in their serums. For example, a small fraction of blood donors who are HBsAg negative by the most sensitive tests transmit HBV infection to recipients of their blood. Although some of these donors could be in the incubation period of hepatitis B before the appearance of detectable HBsAg, most probably represent persistently infected patients with concentrations of HBsAg below the level of detection because they have high titers of anti-HBc. Cases of chronic hepatitis without detectable HBsAg have been ascribed to active HBV infection because of persistent high titers of anti-HBc, but proof of active HBV infection is lacking.

Diagnosis

A diagnosis of acute viral hepatitis can usually be made from clinical findings, and a specific viral agent can sometimes be suspected from knowledge of the epidemiologic setting and the incubation period. However, only tests specific for the virus can conclusively establish infection with a virus such as HBV.

Serologic tests for HBsAg, anti-HBs, anti-HBc, HBeAg, and anti-HBe are specific for HBV, diagnostically useful, and commercially available. HBsAg is the most important and commonly used marker for active HBV infection. Presence of HBsAg in serum indicates active HBV infection, except after passive transfer of HBsAg, for example by blood transfusion. HBsAg can be detected in most, although not all, patients with infectious HBV in the blood. Serum or other body liquids containing HBsAg should be considered infective.

If HBsAg is detected in a patient with clinical findings and liver function abnormalities compatible with acute viral hepatitis, the diagnosis is acute hepatitis B, although superimposed acute hepatitis caused by another agent or acute exacerbations of CAH in a patient persistently infected with HBV can give similar findings. Falling titers of HBsAg or rising titers of anti-HBc in such a patient are consistent with acute hepatitis B (see Fig. 71-4). In a few patients with acute hepatitis B, HBsAg can never be detected; in some, HBsAg becomes undetectable before the end of clinical disease; and in a few, it becomes negative even before the onset of disease. In such patients, infection with HBV may be documented only by a rising titer of anti-HBc or the subsequent appearance of anti-HBs.

HBsAg is present without detectable anti-HBc during the first few weeks after infection with HBV and in any infected patient who is unable to make antibody (*e.g.,* in agammaglobulinemia). HBsAg is present with anti-HBc in self-limited infections sometime after the early period (Fig. 71-4) or in persistent infection (Fig. 71-6). Anti-HBc titers are usually higher with persistent infection than during or after self-limited infection.

The presence of anti-HBs and anti-HBc without HBsAg is consistent with past infection with HBV and indicates immunity. In general, the more recent the infection, the higher the antibody titers. The presence of either anti-HBs or anti-HBc alone in low titer is most commonly seen after infection in the distant past in persons who have lost the second antibody. Anti-HBc may be present alone in relatively high titer after the disappearance of HBsAg and before the appearance of anti-HBs (Fig. 71-4), thus indicating a recent infection. Anti-HBc is the only antibody detected after self-limited infection in 10% of patients—persons who never develop detectable anti-HBs.

Infrequently, blood containing high titers of anti-HBc but no detectable HBsAg has been shown to transmit HBV infection to recipients. Low anti-HBs titers frequently occur in patients infected in the distant past and with subsequent loss of anti-HBc. High anti-HBs titers alone may occur after secondary anti-HBs responses after exposure to HBV and HBsAg (*e.g.,* by blood tranfusion or immunization with vaccine) without reinfection (reinfection would result in a rise in both anti-HBc and anti-HBs). Blood containing detectable anti-HBs rarely, if ever, transmits HBV.

Passive transfer of HBsAg, anti-HBs, or anti-HBc can produce any of the patterns described above after transfusion with blood or blood products containing the appropriate serologic activity.

Although analysis of a single blood sample may permit a diagnosis in some cases, more than one sample may be required to document infection with HBV and the stage of infection or convalescence. For example, falling titers of HBsAg in serial specimens is the pattern of resolving acute infection (Fig. 71-4). A fourfold or greater rise in titers of anti-HBc denotes on-going infection (Figs. 71-4, 71-5, and 71-6), whereas a fourfold or greater rise in anti-HBs is consistent with recent infection (Figs. 71-4, 71-5) or a secondary response after exposure to HBsAg without infection (*e.g.,* after receiving HBV vaccine). Persistent infection (*i.e.,* the chronic carrier state) is not established until HBsAg has been shown to be present for at least 6 months.

Complete virion and HBeAg have not been found in serum without detectable HBsAg. High concentrations of HBV-associated DNA polymerase activity or viral DNA, and HBeAg appear regularly in the late incubation period of hepatitis B, and their presence with HBsAg in serums from patients without anti-HBc indicates early infection (Fig. 71-4). The presence of virions and HBeAg during acute or persistent infection identifies patients more likely to transmit HBV to contacts than do infected patients without these markers. The presence of these markers correlates well with transmission of HBV from carriers by way of percutaneous routes, from carrier pregnant women to their newborns, from carriers to sexual contacts, and from medical care personnel, such as dentists, to their patients. Carriers of HBsAg with anti-HBe in their serums appear to transmit infection by these routes much less often. These correlations are not absolute, and blood containing HBsAg and anti-HBe may in some cases contain infectious HBV, although the titer appears to be very much lower than that in blood containing HBeAg. Although these viral markers distinguish infected patients who readily transmit infection from those unlikely to infect others, the correlations are not absolute; the outcome of contacts with infected patients cannot be predicted with certainty. A less clear-cut correlation with HBeAg in persistently infected patients is the presence of chronic hepatitis.

The differential diagnosis of acute hepatitis B is the

same as that of hepatitis A (Chap. 70, Hepatitis A). Chronic persistent hepatitis and CAH may be associated with persistent HBV infection, non-A, or non-B hepatitis agents, or, it may be idiopathic.

Males in Taiwan who are over 40 years of age and are carriers of HBsAg have a very high incidence of hepatocellular carcinomas (HCCs). Testing serum for alphafetoprotein every 6 to 12 months revealed sudden rises to abnormal levels that were regularly associated with HCC as proved by scanning procedures or surgical exploration. Although not proven effective in the United States, such regular screening of long-standing carriers in older age groups, particularly those with cirrhosis, should be considered because the incidence of HBsAg in HCC is much higher among them than among persons without HBsAg. Most HBV infections occur in young adults in the United States and in early childhood in Taiwan; therefore, the highest risk for HCC may be at correspondingly older ages in the United States.

Prognosis

Approximately 200,000 primary infections with HBV occur each year in the United States. About 25% develop acute, icteric disease; of these, 10,000 are hospitalized and 250 die of fulminant hepatitis. Between 6% and 10% become persistently infected (become chronic carries of HBsAg).

The pool of chronic carriers in the United States includes 400,000 to 800,000. Of these, as many as 25% may have chronic active hepatitis, a disease with a prognosis varying from recovery to death—4000 per year may die of cirrhosis, and 800 per year from cancer of the liver. About three-fourths of the chronic carriers of HBsAg have chronic persistent hepatitis, a disease that is not progressive.

Therapy

The treatment of acute hepatitis B is the same as that for other forms of acute viral hepatitis (Chaps. 70, Hepatitis A; 72, Non-A, Non-B Hepatitis). There is no specific therapy for either acute or chronic hepatitis B. Although the progression of chronic active hepatitis in patients without HBV infection may be favorably altered by administration of glucosteroids and azathioprine, patients who are HBsAg positive do not benefit similarly. Indeed, such therapy may be contraindicated because it regularly results in rises in HBsAg, HBeAg, and concentrations of virions in the blood; that is, replication of HBV is promoted.

Patients with persistent HBV infection and chronic hepatitis have been treated with human leukocyte interferon or adenine arabinoside in experimental trials. In a fraction of the patients, some or all viral markers in serum and liver became undetectable, and improvement in liver function and histology occurred. Randomized, blinded, controlled trials are needed.

Prevention

Prevention of hepatitis B requires interruption of the transmission of HBV by environmental barriers, and by rendering susceptible persons resistant to infection by passive or active immunization. Human immune serum globulin with very high titers of anti-HBs (hepatitis B hyperimmune globulin, or HBIG) reduces the incidence of clinical hepatitis B in recently admitted patients and recently hired employees in renal dialysis units; hospital and laboratory personnel accidentally exposed to hepatitis B infections, for example by needle stick; spouses of patients with acute hepatitis B; and newborn infants of HBsAg positive mothers. The principle indication for HBIG is postexposure prophylaxis in the following settings: (1) acute, intense exposure to HBV, as after accidental percutaneous inoculation or mucous membrane exposure to blood or other body liquids, such as saliva, from a HBsAg-positive patient; (2) intimate contact (*e.g.,* cohabitation or sexual contact) with a patient with acute hepatitis B, or one such exposure to a HBsAg carrier, particularly if the carrier is also HBeAg-positive; and (3) newborn infants of mothers with acute hepatitis B in the second or third trimester or the first 2 months postpartum, or HBsAg carrier mothers, particularly if they are also HBeAg positive. The dosage schedule recommended by the United States Public Health Service for children or adults following a single intense exposure such as accidental needle stick or sexual intercourse is 0.05 to 0.07 ml/kg of body wt, IM, as soon as possible within the first 7 days after the exposure, followed by the same dose 1 month later. The most important feature of this schedule is administration of the first dose as soon as possible after exposure because administration of HBIG in the first 48 hours is much more effective than administration 3 to 7 days after exposure. The need for the second dose is not proven.

Because standard immune serum globulin (ISG) contains moderate titers of anti-HBs, it may be as effective as HBIG for some kinds of exposure, and it should be used if HBIG is unavailable. Passive immunoprophylaxis is not indicated for exposed persons known to be positive for HBsAg or anti-HBs.

However, it is probably unwise to delay administration of HBIG or ISG more than a very few hours for testing to determine the immune status of the exposed person. After intimate exposure to a patient with abnormal liver functions who is suspected of having a viral hepatitis, the exposed person should receive ISG as soon as possible after exposure. If subsequent testing indicates that the index case is infected with HBV, HBIG should then be given to the contact if no more than 7 days have passed since the exposure.

Babies born of HBsAg-positive mothers should receive 0.5 ml HBIG within 1 hour of delivery, and the same dose should be repeated at 3 and 6 months postpartum. Lower doses of HBIG, longer time intervals between delivery and the first HBIG dose, and use of standard ISG instead of HBIG provides less protection.

Development of a HBV vaccine enabling active immunoprophylaxis generally makes preexposure passive immunization unnecessary. The currently available HBV vaccine consists of HBsAg particles purified from the plasmas of HBsAg carriers and inactivated with formalin. It has been shown to modify disease and reduce the incidence of HBV infections in sexually active homosexual males. The United States Public Health Service recommends that immunologically normal adults receive 1 ml (20 μg), and children under age 10 years, 0.5 ml (10 μg), repeating the same dose after 1 and 6 months for a total of 3 injections. Anti-HBs responses with this schedule are excellent in well over 90% of patients in all age groups. Although titers fall with time, protective titers persist for at least 2 years. Immunologically impaired persons, such as those undergoing hemodialysis or those with organ transplants, respond less well, and 2 ml (40 μg) of vaccine is recommended.

The vaccine should be offered to persons at high risk of exposure to HBV. This includes some health care workers, particularly those with frequent contact with blood or serum such as laboratory technologists, phlebotomists, hemodialysis and cardiac catheterization staff, dental surgeons, homosexually active males and some males with frequent different sexual contacts, illicit parenteral drug users, hemodialysis patients, regular recipients of certain blood products such as factor VIII or IX, clients and staff of some institutions for the mentally retarded and inmates of some prisons, and household and sexual contacts of carriers. Although in general these groups are at greater risk for HBV infection than others in the population, individual circumstances must be considered in assessing the need for vaccine because all members of all such groups are not at great risk. For example, the risk of HBV infection for particular categories of hospital-based health care workers may be quite different in different hospitals because the incidence of active HBV infection in different patient populations varies widely.

Known side-effects of the vaccine are principally moderate soreness at the site of injection and mild fever in some of the patients. However, the HBV vaccine has been given to only a few thousand patients, and has a unique source and composition. Rare or late adverse effects cannot be ruled out until much larger numbers of patients have been followed for much longer periods.

Although no special ill effects have been associated with vaccination of persons carrying HBsAg or anti-HBs in their serum, vaccination of such persons is of no value. The vaccine is relatively expensive. Yet, assessment of the usefulness of prior serologic screening to avoid vaccinating HBsAg- and anti-HBs-positive persons must take into account not only the actual cost of vaccination, but also the cost of testing and the incidence of HBsAg and anti-HBs in the population. In some circumstances, patients may prefer to bear the cost of serologic testing on the chance that the inconvenience and the (probably small) risk of rare, unknown side-effects of vaccination may be avoided.

Although postexposure vaccination would appear to be logical in some settings, its efficacy in preventing infection or disease resulting from the prior exposure has not been proven. However, vaccination should be considered in conjunction with HBIG for newborns of mothers who are HBsAg carriers or babies who have acute hepatitis B (*i.e.,* HBIG is given at the time of delivery, and vaccination is started at 3 months), sexual or household contacts of carriers or persons with acute hepatitis B, and for health-care workers exposed by needle stick who are at risk of continued reexposure. Immune responses to the vaccine have been shown to be unchanged by concomitant administration of HBIG.

A most important preventive of hepatitis B in the United States has been elimination, in so far as is possible, of donors whose blood contains infectious HBV. Use of volunteers rather than paid donors and testing all donors for HBsAg has reduced hepatitis-B–caused posttransfusion hepatitis to about 5%.

Environmental control measures are important to prevent transmission of HBV from infected persons to their contacts. For example, hospitalized patients who have acute hepatitis B or are chronic carriers of HBsAg (particularly those who are HBeAg positive) should be placed in single rooms, and gloves should be worn by personnel performing venipunctures and carrying out procedures that require intimate contact. Careful hand-washing should follow each contact. Blood, feces, urine, and other body liquids, and any materials that have been wet with such liquids must be properly contained, labeled, handled, and disposed of or decontaminated. Patients need not be confined to their rooms, and precautions to prevent respiratory infection by aerosols are unnecessary. Containment procedures should be followed for at least 3 weeks after the onset of acute hepatitis or until HBsAg is no longer detected in the blood. Isolation of patients confined at home with acute viral hepatitis B is less important because household contacts usually have already been thoroughly exposed during the incubation period.

Under certain circumstances, HBsAg-positive health-care personnel may be the source of HBV infection. Accordingly, all such personnel must take special care to reduce the risk of transmission of HBV to patients, and those that have been implicated in transmission must change their behavior and technique to ensure that further transmission cannot occur—for example, wearing gloves for patient contact. In some cases, authorities have revoked professional licensure to protect the public.

Remaining Problems

Improved testing is required to identify the few HBV-infectious blood donors not detected by currently available methods. Although the recently licensed HBV vaccine represents an important advance in the effort to control HBV, its supply is not unlimited, and the expense is high. Further efforts are needed to solve these problems, for example by developing vaccines through use of prokaryote or yeast cells transformed with recombinant DNA molecules containing viral genes, or by chemical synthesis of HBsAg-reactive polypeptides.

The precise role of HBV in the development of hepatocellular carcinoma must be defined, and methods for early detection of this cancer in carriers of HBsAg must be developed. Methods are needed for terminating persistent HBV infections and suppressing liver disease. This will require a better understanding of the mechanisms that permit persistent infection and the pathogenesis of liver disease, and the development of effective therapy—for example, antiviral chemotherapy or immunotherapy. Finally, in highly endemic areas of the world such as Asia and Africa, effective and economical strategies for interrupting the cycle of mother-to-newborn transmission are badly needed.

Bibliography

Journals

ALMEIDA JD, RUBENSTEIN D, STOTT EJ: New antigen–antibody system in Australia–antigen-positive hepatitis. Lancet 2:1225–1227, 1971

ALTER JH, HOLLAND PV, PURCELL RH: The emerging pattern of posttransfusion hepatitis. Am J Med Sci 270:329–334, 1975

BARKER LF, MAYNARD JE, PURCELL RH, HOOFNAGLE JH, BERQUIST KR, LONDON WT: Viral hepatitis, type B, in experimental animals. Am J Med Sci 270:189–195, 1975

BARKER LF, MURRAY R: Relationship of virus dose to incubation time of clinical hepatitis and time of appearance of hepatitis-associated antigen. Am J Med Sci 263:27–33, 1972

BAYER ME, BLUMBERG BS, WERNER B: Particles associated with Australia antigen in sera of patients with leukemia, Down's syndrome and hepatitis. Nature 218:1057–1059, 1968

BEASLEY RP, LIN CC, WANG KY, HSIEH FJ, HWANG LY, STEVENS CE, SUN TS, SZMUNESS W: Hepatitis B immune globulin (HBIG) efficacy in the interruption of perinatal transmission of hepatitis B virus carrier state: Initial report of a randomized double-blind placebo-controlled trial. Lancet 2:388–393, 1981

BEASLEY RP, LIN CC, HWANG LY, CHIEN CS: Hepatocellular carcinoma and hepatitis B virus: A prospective study of 22,707 men in Taiwan. Lancet 2:1129–1133, 1981

BLUMBERG BS, ALTER JH, VISNICH S: A "new" antigen in leukemia sera. JAMA 191:541–546, 1965

BLUMBERG BS, GERSTLEY BJS, HUNGERFORD DA: A serum antigen (Australia antigen) in Down's syndrome, leukemia and hepatitis. Ann Intern Med 66:924–931, 1967

Immune globulins for protection against viral hepatitis. Morbid Mortal Weekly Rep 30:423–435, 1981

Inactivated hepatitis B virus vaccine. Recommendations of the Immunization Practices Advisory Committee. Ann Intern Med 97:379–383, 1982

DANE DS, CAMERON CH, BRIGGS M: Virus-like particles in serum of patients with Australia-antigen-associated hepatitis. Lancet 1:695–698, 1970

FRANCIS DP, HADLER SC, THOMPSON SE, MAYNARD JE: The prevention of hepatitis B with vaccine: Report of the Centers for Disease Control multicenter efficacy trial among homosexual men. Ann Intern Med 97:362–366, 1982

GOCKE DJ: Extrahepatic manifestations of viral hepatitis. Am J Med Sci 270:49–52, 1975

GOLDFIELD M, BLACK HC, BILL J, SRIHONGSE S, PIZZUTI W: The consequences of administering blood pretested for HBsAg by third generation techniques: A progress report. Am J Med Sci 270:335–342, 1975

GRADY GF, LEE GA: Hepatitis B immune globulin: Prevention of hepatitis from accidental exposure among medical personnel. N Engl J Med 293:1067–1070, 1975

HOOFNAGLE JH, GERETY RJ, BARKER LF: Antibody to hepatitis B core antigen. Am J Med Sci 270:179–187, 1975

KARVOUNTZIS GG, MOSLEY JW, REDEKER AG: Serologic characterization of two episodes of acute viral hepatitis. Am J Med 58:815–822, 1975

KRUGMAN S, GILES GP: Viral hepatitis: New light on an old disease. JAMA 212:1019–1029, 1970

KRUGMAN S, HOOFNAGLE JH, GERETY RJ, KAPLAN PM, GERIN JL: Viral hepatitis, type B: DNA polymerase activity and antibody to hepatitis B core antigen. N Engl J Med 290:1331–1335, 1974

MAZZURE S, BERGERT S, BLUMBERG BS: Geographical distribution of Australia antigen determinants, *d, y* and *w*. Nature 247:38–40, 1974

MCCOLLUM RW: The size of serum hepatitis virus. Proc Soc Exp Biol Med 81:157–163, 1952

MOSLEY JW: Epidemiology of viral hepatitis: An overview. Am J Med Sci 270:253–270, 1975

MOSLEY JW, EDWARD VM, MEIHAUS JE: Subdeterminants *d* and *y* of hepatitis B antigen as epidemiologic markers. Am J Epidemiol 95:529–535, 1972

MULLEY AG, SILVERSTEIN MD, DIENSTAG JL: Indications for use of hepatitis B vaccine, based on cost-effectiveness analysis. N Engl J Med 307:644–652, 1982

SZMUNESS W: Hepatocellular carcinoma and the hepatitis B virus: Evidence for a causal association. Prog Med Virol 24:40–69, 1978

SZMUNESS W, STEVENS CE, ZANG EA, HARLEY EJ, KELLNER A: A controlled clinical trial of the efficacy of the hepatitis B vaccine (Hepatavax B): A final report. Hepatology 1:377–385, 1981

WERNER BG, GRADY GF: Accidental hepatitis-B-surface-antigen-positive inoculations: Use of e antigen to estimate infectivity. Ann Intern Med 97:367–369, 1982

WILLIAM S. ROBINSON

Non-A, Non-B Hepatitis

72

Non-A, non-B (NANB) hepatitis—hepatitis not caused by any known viruses or other identifiable etiologic factors—emerged as an entity in the mid-1970s. By that time, screening blood donors for hepatitis B surface antigen (HBsAg) by sensitive assays, a shift away from paid donors, and greater use of volunteer donors had resulted in a marked reduction in posttransfusion hepatitis B. Still, the overall incidence of posttransfusion hepatitis (PTH) remained high, and it became clear that very few of the cases were associated with infection by any known or serologically identifiable virus. Subsequently, it was shown that many of the cases of hepatitis not related to blood transfusions are also NANB hepatitis.

Etiology

The most important experimental advance in defining the etiology of NANB hepatitis was the transmission of the disease to nonhuman primates. Transmissibility was documented, an animal model became available, and an assay for the causative agent(s) was provided. The disease was transmitted to chimpanzees with plasma from humans with NANB hepatitis and then serially transmitted in chimpanzees using serum or plasma from animals with acute or chronic hepatitis. Subsequently, NANB hepatitis was successfully transmitted to marmosets.

Several lines of evidence make it likely that more than one agent causes NANB hepatitis: (1) at least two episodes of NANB hepatitis have been described in patients with biopsy-proven hepatitis—for example, in patients with hemophilia given multiple doses of Factor VIII; (2) a wider range of incubation periods has been observed for NANB hepatitis than for hepatitis A or B; (3) infectious material from several different patients has consistently produced either nuclear or cytoplasmic untrastructural changes in hepatocytes of experimentally infected chimpanzees; and (4) sequential infections of individual chimpanzees have followed inoculations with specimens from different patients with NANB hepatitis. Although it is probable that there are at least two antigenically different causes of NANB hepatitis, all of the agents in serums from patients with NANB hepatitis are not different, because cross-challenge experiments in chimpanzees have shown cross-protection using serums from patients in different parts of the United States.

Little is known about the physical and chemical properties of the NANB agent(s). However, exposure to formalin inactivated the infectivity of the NANB hepatitis-producing agent in the serum of a patient with chronic NANB hepatitis. This result is interesting because the formalin treatment used in the preparation of vaccine from hepatitis B virus antigen purified from human serums may eliminate the risk of transmission of NANB agents in the vaccine.

Although NANB hepatitis has been transmitted to experimental animals, no virus or other infectious agent has yet been physically identified. Using serums from humans convalescing from NANB hepatitis and from patients who have received several blood transfusions, apparently unique antigen-antibody systems have been detected in patients and chimpanzees with NANB hepatitis. Such results have been difficult to confirm, and none of these tests has successfully identified serums known to contain NANB agents in a panel of serums sent to several laboratories. Immunofluorescent staining of liver tissue with convalescent-phase serums has also been described. The relationship of these antigen–antibody tests to the causes of NANB hepatitis, and their possible diagnostic usefulness, remain to be determined. They may represent autoantigen–antibody or other nonspecific reactions. Also, there may be greater variation in the titer of infectious NANB hepatitis agents in serums than is encountered with hepatitis B.

Viruslike particulate structures have been observed by electron microscopy in the serums and in the livers of humans and chimpanzees with NANB hepatitis. Some were small, cytoplasmic particles resembling picornaviruses, and others (in serum) had the appearance of hepatitis B virions.

Epidemiology

NANB hepatitis is a worldwide problem, having been reported in the United States, Central America, Europe, Australia, India, and Asia. The epidemiologic patterns are protean—sometimes that of classical blood-borne serum hepatitis and sometimes that of infectious hepatitis. Whether these different epidemiologic patterns are manifestations of the same agents or of different agents remains to be seen.

Most studies of posttransfusion hepatitis published since 1975 have shown that only 5% to 10% of patients who develop hepatitis after transfusion with blood that is HBsAg-negative by radioimmunoassay are infected with hepatitis B virus (HBV), less frequently with cytomeglovirus or Epstein-Barr virus, (EBV), and very rarely with hepatitis A virus (HAV). Thus, 90% to 95% of cases of PTH can be designated NANB hepatitis. The source of transfused blood clearly influences the incidence of posttransfusion NANB hepatitis: 6% to 7% of recipients of blood from volunteer donors compared with 17% to 35% of recipients of blood from paid donors. Although these cases meet the exclusion criteria for NANB hepatitis, transmission studies in nonhuman primates were carried out in only a few cases. If infectious NANB hepatitis agents are involved in most or all of these cases, there is a remarkably high incidence of chronic infection in the healthy blood donor population.

NANB hepatitis may occur as sporadic, and occasionally, as epidemic disease. It may be more common in large urban than in rural populations. Although parenteral drug abuse appears to increase the risk of NANB hepatitis, most cases appear to be unrelated to blood transfusion or other forms of parenteral exposure. The criteria for NANB hepatitis are met in about 25% of the cases of sporadic hepatitis seen in some referral hospitals in urban areas, and in small nosocomial epidemics in oncology and plasmaphoresis units. An epidemic of 275 cases of hepatitis in Kashmir, India, resembled HAV hepatitis (apparent fecal–oral transmission—water-borne; characteristic incubation period; lack of progression to chronic hepatitis; and epidemicity with frequent occurrence of secondary cases in households) but met the criteria for NANB hepatitis. Thus, it appears that 25% to 50% of sporadic cases of hepatitis in some settings in the United States and abroad, and some epidemic hepatitis, both in nosocomial and community settings, are caused by NANB agent(s).

Pathogenesis and Pathology

The mechanism of hepatic injury in NANB hepatitis is not known. The spectrum of the acute disease ranges from minimal to fulminant, and the histopathology of NANB hepatitis cannot be distinguished from that of the known viral hepatitides.

Chronic NANB hepatitis does occur and may have the histologic features of chronic persistent or chronic active hepatitis; the latter may lead to cirrhosis. Hepatocellular carcinoma has not been associated with NANB hepatitis.

Manifestations

The incubation period, or time between exposure and onset of symptoms or first detection of abnormal liver function, has been defined in posttransfusion NANB hepatitis. The mean time between transfusion and the first chemical evidence of abnormal liver function (usually elevated concentrations of alanine aminotransferase, or ALT, in the serum) is about 7 to 8 weeks, a period between the incubation periods of hepatitis A and hepatitis B. However, there is great variation, with extremes of 2 to 26 weeks, perhaps reflecting quantitative or qualitative differences in inoculums or other factors.

In a given patient, acute NANB hepatitis is not clinically distinguishable from hepatitis A or hepatitis B. Overall, NANB hepatitis tends to be mild during the acute phase with maximal concentrations of ALT in PTH cases of less than 800 IU/liter in about 33% and 800 to 2000 IU/liter in about 10%; 20% to 30% are icteric. However, NANB hepatitis may be fulminant: (1) of fulminant hepatitis in Los Angeles, nearly as many cases were NANB hepatitis as were caused by HBV; and (2) in Kashmir, India, 12 of 275 cases of epidemic NANB hepatitis were fulminant (6 of 8 cases in pregnant women were fatalities).

NANB hepatitis may be transmitted from pregnant women to their newborn infants. In one study, six of eight neonates of mothers with acute NANB hepatitis in the third trimester of pregnancy developed very mild liver function abnormalities, whereas, in another study, none of three infants whose mothers had NANB hepatitis in the second trimester of pregnancy had any liver function abnormalities.

Diagnosis

Because there is no specific test for NANB hepatitis and there are no pathognomonic clinical features, the clinical diagnosis of the disease is at best tentative. It depends on excluding identifiable hepatitis viruses such as HAV, HBV, EBV, and cytomegalovirus, and other etiologic factors such as hepatotoxic drugs and chemicals. Although inoculation of chimpanzees or marmosets can be used to demonstrate the presence of a transmissible hepatitis agent, such testing is available only in a research setting.

In lieu of a practical, specific test, and because of the urgent need to identify NANB infection in blood donors, several nonspecific tests for chronic hepatitis have been evaluated. It appears that the incidence of NANB PTH is proportional to the concentration of ALT in donor blood. Moreover, an ALT exclusion level for blood donors may be identified that will eliminate 50% or more of NANB PTH without excluding an unacceptable fraction of noninfectious donors. Because the concentration of ALT varies with age, sex, alcohol use, and geographic region, more work is required to define ALT exclusion levels that are cost effective for various donor populations.

Prognosis

Chronic hepatitis is a common sequel of NANB PTH. Abnormalities of liver function may persist for more than 1 year after acute hepatitis in 10% to 60% of patients. The development of chronic hepatitis appears to correlate with the severity of the acute hepatitis. Chronic active hepatitis, documented by biopsy, occurs in 30% to 90% of patients with persistent abnormalities of liver function after PTH NANB hepatitis; cirrhosis develops in some of these patients. Although abnormalities of liver function resolve after 1 to 3 years in a few patients, potentially serious long-term liver disease appears to develop in a significant fraction of patients with NANB PTH. However, the prognosis may be better than that for chronic active hepatitis of other causes, and resolution appears to occur with time in some patients. The relatively common development of chronic active hepatitis after NANB PTH and the relatively high incidence of infectious NANB hepatitis agent(s) in the population suggest that many cases of chronic active hepatitis that are not associated with HBV infection and are now considered idiopathic may in fact be related to infection with NANB hepatitis agent(s).

In addition to the chronic liver disease that commonly develops after acute NANB PTH, transmissibility persists for as long as 6 years in the blood for the few patients studied by inoculation of chimpanzees. The high incidence of NANB PTH is also consistent with frequent persistence of the infectious agents in the blood of apparently healthy donors.

NANB hepatitis not associated with blood transfusion may have a different outcome than that following transfusion; chronic hepatitis has not been observed in NANB disease unassociated with transfusion. Whether the different outcome reflects different infectious agents, differences in doses of infecting virus and severity of initial disease, or other factors remains to be determined.

Therapy

Patients with acute NANB hepatitis should be managed as outlined for acute hepatitis A (Chap. 70) and hepatitis B (Chap. 71). The role of glucosteroid therapy in chronic active hepatitis following NANB hepatitis is not yet known, although as described in Chapter 71, glucosteroids have been shown to affect the course of chronic active hepatitis favorably, particularly in HBsAg-negative cases.

Prevention

Prevention of NANB hepatitis is best approached using general environmental control measures known to be effective for HBV and HAV (Chap. 70, Hepatitis A, and Chap. 71, Hepatitis B).

Use of blood and blood products from volunteer donors rather than commercial donors clearly reduces the incidence of posttransfusion NANB hepatitis, but development of specific serologic tests for blood donor screening is essential to reduce the incidence even further.

Passive immunization with immune serum globulin (ISG) affords some protection against NANB hepatitis following blood transfusion. The greatest effect appears to be a reduction in the incidence of icterus, but prevention of infection and progression to chronic hepatitis may also result. Passive immunization for the prevention of NANB hepatitis transmitted by other routes has not yet been investigated. However, ISG could be administered to persons with puncture wounds, open skin lesions, or mucous membrane exposure to serum or blood of infected patients.

It is arguable whether ISG should be used for prevention of PTH. Although it appears that ISG can provide some protection, the expense and limited supply of this substance would preclude its use in all transfusions. Perhaps the augmented risk of receipt of three or more units of blood justifies passive immunoprophylaxis with ISG.

Remaining Problems

NANB hepatitis is common following blood transfusions and is often encountered as sporadic and epidemic disease. It is emerging as an important factor in chronic liver disease. The most urgent need is for specific diagnostic tests for screening blood donors and for diagnosis in other settings. Further characterizations of the causative agent(s) is necessary to identify antigens and other markers that may be useful in diagnosis, for developing immunoglobulin preparations for passive immunization, and for directing strategies for vaccine development. Because extensive efforts to identify the etiologic agent(s) by standard serologic methods have been unsuccessful, new and innovative approaches are needed.

Bibliography

Book

ALTER HB, PURCELL RH, FEINSTONE SM, TEGITMEIER GE: Non-A, non-B hepatitis: Its relationship to cytomegalovirus, to chronic hepatitis, and to direct and indirect test methods. In Szmuness W, Alter HJ, Maynard JE (eds): Viral Hepatitis: 1981 International Symposium. Philadelphia, Franklin Institute Press, 1982. pp 279–294.

Journals

AACH RD, SZMUNESS W, MOSLEY JW, HOLLINGER FB, KAHN RA, STEVENS CE, EDWARDS VM, MERCH J: Serum alanine aminotransferase of donors in relation to the risk of non-A, non-B hepatitis. N Engl J Med 204:989–994, 1981

ALTER HJ, PURCELL RH, HOLLAND PV, ALLING DW, KOZIOL DE: Donor transaminase and recipient hepatitis: Impact on blood transfusion service. JAMA 246:630–634, 1981

ALTER HJ, PURCELL RH, HOLLAND PV, FEINSTONE SM, MORROW AG, MORITSUGU Y: Clinical and serological analysis of transfusion-associated hepatitis. Lancet 2:838–841, 1975

ALTER HJ, PURCELL RH, HOLLAND PV, POPPER H: Transmissible agent in non-A, non-B hepatitis. Lancet 1:459–463, 1978

BERMAN M, ALTER HJ, ISHAK KG, PURCELL RH, JONES EA: Chronic sequelae of non-A, non-B hepatitis. Ann Intern Med 91:1–6, 1979

DIENSTAG JL, ALAAMA A, MOSLEY JW, REDEKER AG, PURCELL RH: Etiology of sporadic hepatitis B surface antigen negative hepatitis. Ann Intern Med 87:1–6, 1977

DIENSTAG JL, FEINSTONE SM, PURCELL RH, WONG DC, ALTER HJ, HOLLAND PV: Non-A, non-B post-transfusion hepatitis. Lancet 1:560–562, 1977

HOLLINGER RB, GITNICK GL, AACH RD, SZMUNESS W, MOSLEY JW, STEVENS CE, PETERS RL, WEINER JM, WERCH JB, LANDER JJ: Non-A, non-B hepatitis transmission in chimpanzees: Project of the Transfusion-Transmitted Viruses Study Group. Intervirology 10:60–68, 1978

HOLLINGER FB, MOSELY JW, SZMUNESS W, AACH RD, PETERS RL, STEVENS C: Transfusion-transmitted viruses study: Experimental evidence for two non-A, non-B hepatitis agents. J Infect Dis 142:400–407, 1980

HOOFNAGLE JH, GERETY RH, TABOR E, FEINSTONE SM, BARKER LF, PURCELL RH: Transmission of non-A, non-B hepatitis. Ann Intern Med 87:14–20, 1977

KHUROO MS: Study of an epidemic of non-A, non-B hepatitis: Possibility of another human hepatitis virus distinct from post-transfusion non-A, non-B type. Am J Med 68: 818–824, 1980

KNODELL RG,CONRAD ME, GINSBERG AL, BELL CJ, FLAMMERY EP: Efficacy of prophylactic gamma-globulin in preventing non-A, non-B post-transfusion hepatitis. Lancet 1:557–561, 1976

KNODELL R, CONRAD ME, ISHAK KG: Development of chronic liver disease after acute non-A, non-B post-transfusion hepatitis: role of γ-globulin prophylaxis in its prevention. Gastroenterology 72:902–909, 1977

MOSLEY JW, REDEKER AG, FEINSTONE SM, PURCELL RH: Multiple hepatitis viruses in multiple attacks of acute viral hepatitis. N Engl J Med 296:75–78, 1977

PRINCE AM, BROTMAN B, GRADY GF, KUHNS WJ, HAZZI C, LEVINE RW, MILLIAN SJ: Long-incubation post-transfusion hepatitis without serological evidence of exposure to hepatitis B virus. Lancet 2:241–246, 1974

ROBINSON WS: The enigma of non-A non-B hepatitis. J Infect Dis 145:387–395, 1982

TABOR E, APRIL M, SEEFF LB, GERETY RJ: Acquired immunity to human non-A, non-B hepatitis: Cross-challenge of chimpanzees with three infectious human sera. J Infect Dis 140:789–793, 1979

TABOR E, GERETY RJ: Inactivation of an agent of human non-A, non-B hepatitis by formalin. J Infect Dis 142: 767–770, 1980

TABOR E, GERETY RJ, DRUCKER JA, SEEFF LB, HOOFNAGLE JA, JACKSON DR: Transmission of non-A, non-B hepatitis from man to chimpanzee. Lancet 1:463–466, 1978

TONG MJ, THRUSBY M, RAKELA J, MCPEAK C, EDWARDS VM, MOSLEY JW: Studies of the maternal-infant transmission of the viruses which cause acute hepatitis. Gastroenterology 80:999–1004, 1981

VILLAREJOS VM, VISONA KA, EDUARTE CA, PROVOST PJ, HILLEMAN MR: Evidence for viral hepatitis other than type A or type B among persons in Costa Rica. N Engl J Med 283:1350–1352, 1975

YOSHIZAWA H, ITOH Y, IWAKIRI S, KATAJIMA K, TANAKA A, NOJIRI T, MIYAKAWA Y, MAYUMI M: Demonstration of two different types of non-A, non-B hepatitis by reinjection of cross-challenge studies in chimpanzees. Gastroenterology 81:107–113, 1981

THOMAS P. MONATH

73 Yellow Fever

Yellow fever is an acute, mosquito-borne viral infection that occurs in epidemic and endemic form in tropical America and Africa, but not in Asia. In its most severe form, the disease is characterized by fever, jaundice, hemorrhage, and proteinuria. Mild and abortive forms, with or without jaundice, are common. Yellow fever is classified as one of the viral hemorrhagic fevers; however, the severity of the hepatic injury in this disease distinguishes it from other hemorrhagic fevers.

Etiology

Yellow fever virus is the prototype of the flavivirus genus (family Togaviridae). Flaviviruses are small, spherical, enveloped RNA viruses, which share antigenic determinants characteristic of the genus. As a result, the serodiagnosis of yellow fever in endemic zones is often difficult. Strains of yellow fever virus in tropical America and Africa differ in various laboratory markers, but do not clearly differ in the disease they produce in humans. The virus is pathogenic for a variety of cell cultures, infant mice (by intracranial and peripheral inoculation), adult mice inoculated intracranially, and some monkey species (*e.g.,* rhesus, cynomolgus, howler).

Epidemiology

In tropical America, approximately 50 to 300 cases of yellow fever are recognized annually, but the disease is undoubtedly underreported. The virus circulates principally in the Amazon region where it is maintained as an enzootic and epizootic infection of monkeys, which is transmitted by *Haemagogus* spp. mosquitoes. Lethal infections occur in some species of monkeys and deaths herald epizootic spread. If humans come into contact with the jungle transmission cycle and are bitten by *Haemogogus* spp., they may acquire *jungle yellow fever* as an incidental infection. Thus, yellow fever in humans in tropical America is generally a sporadic disease, although small outbreaks (20–50 cases) are not uncommon and dramatic episodes may occur when groups of unvaccinated laborers enter the jungle. Formerly, human–mosquito–human transmission by the peridomestic mosquito, *Aedes aegypti,* was responsible for large epidemics of *urban yellow fever* in the cities and towns of South America, and as late as 1905 in North America (New Orleans). Eradication of *A. aegypti* from urban areas of most South American countries has precluded urban transmission, and the last such outbreak occurred in Trinidad in 1954. However, the recent establishment of *A. aegypti* in areas of Colombia adjacent to the yellow fever enzootic zone and the widespread occurrence of *A. aegypti*-borne dengue in the Caribbean and northern countries of South America, are impressive reminders that yellow fever could again become epidemic in the Western Hemisphere.

Yellow fever is a more important public health problem in Africa. Epidemics of note in the last 25 years include Ethiopia, 1960–1962 (100,000 cases); Senegal, 1965 (2000–20,000 cases); Nigeria–Togo–Ghana–Upper Volta–Mali, 1969–1970 (many thousands of cases); and the Gambia, 1978–1979 (8500 cases). Endemic infection and sporadic disease, as well as unrecognized epidemics, account for much unreported morbidity. The transmission cycles are complex and continue to be the subject of intensive study. In forested areas, enzootic–epizootic circulation of yellow fever virus occurs between monkeys and a variety of *Aedes* spp. Transmission from monkeys to man by wild, tree-hold breeding *Aedes* spp. occurs, but epidemics are sustained by a man–mosquito–man cycle involving wild *Aedes* spp. or domestic *A. aegypti.*

The specific vectors incriminated vary from area to area; important wild species include *A. luteocephalus, africanus,* and *furcifer-taylori* in West Africa, and *A. simpsoni, africanus,* and *vittatus* in East Africa. A major vector of interhuman transmission in West Africa is *A. aegypti,* breeding in water storage jars and other receptacles in and around houses in villages and towns. Transovarial transmission of yellow fever virus has been documented in wild *Aedes* spp. and provides a mechanism for survival of the virus over long dry periods.

Nonimmune persons are equally susceptible, regardless of race, age, or sex. However, the incidence is generally higher in adult males because of greater exposure to mosquitoes during wood cutting or agricultural pursuits. Outbreaks occur during the rainy season or early dry season, that is, times of peak vector populations. The susceptibility of a given population of humans is closely related to the level of immunity to yellow fever (naturally acquired or vaccine-induced) and possibly also influenced by heterologous immunity engendered by closely related, non-yellow fever flaviviruses.

Pathogenesis and Pathology

Early in the infection with yellow fever virus, viral replication, as manifested by cytopathology, is limited to the Kupffer cells. Spread to hepatocytes follows. The resulting injury and death of infected liver cells leads to hepatic failure with the accumulation and appearance in the blood of metabolites normally processed by the liver, and substances normally confined inside hepatocytes.

In all severe cases, some degree of renal failure is present. The pathogenesis is not clear but may be related to primary injury from invasion of kidney cells by yellow fever virus, or renal failure secondary to hepatic failure. The latter mechanism is favored by the finding of a decrease in renal perfusion preceding the development of acute tubular necrosis in monkeys infected experimentally with yellow fever virus.

Circulatory shock, acidosis, and hyperkalemia appear to be late events in fatal yellow fever. Hemorrhage may exacerbate the hypotension. Disseminated intravascular clotting may occur but the significance of this complication remains to be determined.

The histopathologic changes in the liver characteristic of yellow fever include: coagulative necrosis of hepatocytes in the midzone of the liver lobule with sparing of cells bordering on the central vein, eosinophilic degeneration of liver cells (Councilman bodies), intranuclear eosinophilic granular inclusions (Torres bodies), multivacuolar and microvacuolar fatty change, sparing of the reticulin framework, and absence of inflammation. However, this classic array of findings is not always present. The histopathology is frequently atypical or difficult to interpret, especially when death occurs after the 10th day of illness. Other conditions, for example, Lassa, Marburg-Ebola virus infections, and the usual viral hepatitides (see Chaps. 70–72, Hepatitis A; Hepatitis B; Non-A, Non-B Hepatitis) must be differentiated from atypical cases of yellow fever.

Changes in other organs include acute tubular necrosis and fatty vacuolization of the kidneys, depletion and necrosis of the lymphocytic elements in the spleen and lymph nodes, cloudy swelling and degeneration of myocardial fibers, and edema and petechial hemorrhages in the brain.

Manifestations

After an incubation period of 3 to 6 days, clinically evident yellow fever varies from very mild to fatal disease. Mild cases are frequent, occurring in 80% to 90% of those infected. The manifestations include fever, headache, malaise, and lassitude which persist for 2 to 4 days. Since the illness is clinically nonspecific the diagnosis of yellow fever will be suspected only in the setting of an epidemic, and can be confirmed only by laboratory tests.

The classic syndromes of yellow fever occur in 10% to 20% of persons infected. The onset is abrupt, with fever to 40°C (104°F), chills or chilliness, headache, and myalgias. Nausea, vomiting, and minor gingival bleeding or epistsaxis may occur. The patient appears to be in acute distress with flushing of the face and a tongue red at the tip and edges. The pulse is slow in relation to the fever (Faget's sign). This syndrome may last several days and is named the *period of infection* because yellow fever virus is present in the blood. The patient may then have a brief (several hours to 24 hours) *period of remission* of fever and symptoms. This is followed by a *period of intoxication,* during which disease reappears and progresses. Fever increases, with frequent vomiting, epigastric pain, prostration, increasing proteinuria, oliguria, jaundice, and hemorrhage, especially hematemesis. The case–fatality rate in severe cases approaches 50%. Deaths generally occur 7 to 10 days after onset of illness. Hypothermia, hypotension, delirium or stupor, coma, and intractable hiccup are terminal events.

In patients surviving severe yellow fever, convalescence may be prolonged and is associated with aesthenia lasting several weeks. Late deaths, attributed to heart failure or arrhythmias, have been recorded.

Diagnosis

The diagnosis of yellow fever should be considered in nonvaccinated persons with a febrile illness who have a history of travel within endemic areas. Early in the illness, the number of leukocytes and blood platelets is normal or depressed. In severe cases, there is prolongation of the clotting, prothrombin, and partial thromboplastin times. The serum transaminase concentrations are markedly elevated in cases with jaundice, but may or may not be abnormal in mild, anicteric infections. The total and conjugated serum bilirubin concentrations rise simultaneously and may reach 15 mg to 20 mg/dl. The blood glucose may fall preterminally. The urine contains a small amount of protein during the period of infection; the concentration rises abruptly to levels of 3 g to 5 g/1 (occasionally higher) during the period of intoxication. Nonspecific ST-T wave electrocardiographic changes may be present.

Specific diagnosis is achieved by isolating virus from blood taken during the period of infection or by demonstrating a rise in titer of antibody comparing serum obtained as early after the onset as possible with a specimen taken 10 to 14 days later. The hemagglutination-inhibition, indirect fluorescent antibody, complement–fixation, enzyme-linked immunosorbent assay, and neutralization tests are useful. Of these, the neutralization test is the most specific, a matter of some importance as cross-reactions with heterologous flaviviruses may complicate serologic diagnosis. Liver biopsy is not an acceptable means of diagnosis because of the bleeding diathesis. Postmortem examination of the liver may provide a specific diagnosis; tissues other than liver (especially spleen and lymph nodes) should also be subjected to study. Occasionally, the virus may be isolated from the liver.

Other diseases which may be confused with yellow fever include viral hepatitis (Chaps. 70–72, Hepatitis A; Hepatitis B; Non-A, Non-B, hepatitis), falciparum malaria (Chap. 145, Malaria), leptospirosis (Chap. 76, Leptospirosis), typhoid fever (Chap. 64, Typhoid Fever), Rift Valley fever, rickettsial infections (Chap. 96, The Spotted Fevers; Chap. 98, The Typhus Fevers), and surgical and toxic conditions. Argentine and Bolivian hemorrhagic fever (Chap. 90, Epidemic Hemorrhagic Fevers), dengue (Chap. 89, Dengue), Lassa, Marburg, and Ebola virus diseases must also be considered; jaundice is generally not a feature of these infections. Mild yellow fever cannot be distinguished clinically from a large number of febrile diseases.

Prognosis

The case-fatality rate in all patients with clinical illness is probably 2% to 5%; however, in severe cases, it may be as high as 50%. A poor prognosis is augured by the appearance of a period of intoxication, rising proteinuria and bilirubinemia, progressive oliguria, marked prolongation of the prothrombin time, and severe hemorrhage.

Therapy

There is no specific treatment for yellow fever, and the intensive application of nonspecific therapies is largely of unproved value because patients with severe yellow fever are usually cared for in relatively primitive facilities. Yet, it is known that complete hepatic regeneration occurs in patients who survive the acute disease, providing a rationale for vigorous supportive efforts. Thus, nonaspirin analgesics, antiemetics, and water and electrolytes should be administered during the period of infection. During the period of intoxication, intensive care similar to that provided for other forms of acute hepatic and acute renal failure is necessary. Monitoring renal function, for example, by measuring the excreted fraction of sodium (FE_{Na}), and efforts to maintain fluid balance and combat hypotension may be helpful in preventing the progression of uremia. In cases with *documented* disseminated intravascular coagulation, the use of heparin should be considered.

Prevention

The acutely ill patient should be placed under a bed net to prevent contact with mosquito vectors. Care should be taken to prevent accidental infection of others by contaminated needles.

Yellow fever 17D vaccine (a live, attenuated strain of yellow fever virus) is a safe and highly effective means of immunoprophylaxis. Immunity is demonstrable within 10 days after vaccination and provides protection for at least 30 years (probably for a lifetime). The vaccine rarely causes mild systemic reactions. Because the vaccine strain is propagated in chick embryos, it should be used with caution in persons with a history of allergy to hens' eggs. Although no harmful effects on the developing fetus have been documented, the vaccine should not be used during pregnancy unless there is a high risk of natural yellow fever infection. The vaccine now used in the United States contains an avian leukosis viral (ALV) contaminant; a vaccine without ALV is now under investigation.

Prevention of outbreaks mediated by *A. aegypti* depends primarily on elimination of sites suitable for the peridomestic breeding of this mosquito. Infections acquired from wild mosquito vectors can be prevented by vaccinating the human population at risk. If an outbreak does occur, insecticides should be used to kill infected adult female mosquitoes.

Remaining Problems

More information is needed about the ecology of yellow fever to define the factors responsible for the recrudescence of epidemics and the mechanisms that maintain enzootics. The possibility of large *A. aegypti*-borne outbreaks of yellow fever in the Caribbean, southern United States, or even Asia remains a threat.

The pathogenesis and pathophysiology of yellow fever (and other viral hemorrhagic fevers) remain ill-defined. Clarification may lead to improved, specific, and supportive therapies. Presently available intensive care capabilities should be evaluated in experimental yellow fever (preferably in nonhuman primates), and in clinical studies.

Improved methods for rapid and early diagnosis are required. Current vaccine production is inadequate to meet potential pandemic situations of commitments to mass vaccination campaigns in endemic areas, such as West Africa. Modernization of vaccine production by the use of cell cultures for propagation of the 17D virus strain should be investigated as an alternative to the chick embryo.

Bibliography

Journals

BERRY GP, KITCHEN SF: Yellow fever accidently contracted in the laboratory: A study of seven cases. Am J Trop Med Hyg 11:365–434, 1931

CHAMBON L, WONE I, BRÈS P, CORNET M, CIRE LY, MICHEL A, LACAN A, ROBIN Y, HENDERSON BE, WILLIAMS KH, CAMAIN R, LAMBERT D, REY M, DIOPMAR I, OUDART JL, CAUSSE G, BA H, MARTIN M, ARTUS JC: Une epidémie de fièvre jaune au Sénégal en 1965: l'Epidémie humaine. Bull WHO 36:113–150, 1967

DENNIS LH, REISBERG BE, CROSBIE J, CROZIER D, CONRAD ME: The original hemorrhagic fever: Yellow fever. Brit J Haematol 17:455–462, 1969

GERMAIN M, MOUCHET J, CORDELLIER R, CHIPPAUX A, CORNET M, HERVE JP, SUREAU P, FABRE J, ROBIN Y: Epidémiologie de la fièvre jaune en Afrique. Med Mal Infect 2:69–77, 1978

JONES EMM, WILSON DC: Clinical features of yellow fever cases at Vom Christian Hospital during the 1969 epidemic on the Jos Plateau, Nigeria. Bull WHO 46:653–657, 1972

MONATH TP, CRAVEN RB, ADJUKIEWICZ, A, GERMAIN M, FRANCY DB, FERRARA L, SAMBA EM, N'JIE H, CHAM K, FITZGERALD SA, CRIPPEN PH, SIMPSON DIH, BOWEN ETW, FABIYI A, SALAUN J-J: Yellow fever in The Gambia, 1978–1979: Epidemiologic aspects. Am J Trop Med Hyg 29:912–28, 1980

Third Report, World Health Organization Expert Committee on Yellow Fever. WHO Tech Rep Ser No. 479, 1971

TRAPIDO H, GALINDO P: The epidemiology of yellow fever in Middle America. Exper Parasitol 5:285–323, 1956

S. MICHAEL MARCY
SIDNEY KIBRICK

Mumps

74

Mumps is an acute, generalized infectious disease seen primarily in children and young adults. Although painful parotid enlargement is the characteristic clinical feature, mumps encompasses a spectrum ranging from inapparent infection or a mild upper respiratory illness to involvement of multiple organ systems. Meningoencephalitis, epididymoorchitis, and pancreatitis are the most commonly associated manifestations.

Etiology

The mumps virion consists of a tightly coiled, helical, RNA nucleocapsid encased in an envelope composed of protein and lipid. The envelope, derived from altered cell membrane and pinched off during viral release from the cell surface, is roughly spherical and covered with numerous small spikelike projections. Viral particle diameters range from 85 μm to more than 300 μm, with a mean of 140 μm. The internal ribonucleoprotein core represents the soluble (S) complement-fixing antigen, whereas the virus (V) antigen is incorporated into the envelope. Hemagglutinating and hemolytic activity, and receptor-destroying enzyme (neuraminidase), are also structurally associated with the viral envelope.

The virus can be isolated or propagated in cultures of various human and monkey tissues and in embryonated eggs. A member of the family Paramyxoviridae, mumps virus, together with the parainfluenza viruses and Newcastle disease virus, constitute the genus *Paramyxovirus*. These viruses, as well as other Paramyxoviridae (*e.g.,* measles, respiratory syncytial virus) characteristically form multinucleated giant cells (syncytia) in tissue culture.

The infectivity of mumps virus is abolished by exposure to ether, 0.1% formaldehyde solution, β-propiolactone, ultraviolet light, and temperatures of 50°C to 60°C for 20 minutes; however, hemagglutinating activity and CF antigens may persist. Mumps virus is stable at 4°C for several days, at −20°C for weeks and at −70°C for years.

Epidemiology

Laboratory infections can be induced in monkeys, small rodents, and various other animals; however humans are the only known natural hosts. The transmission of mumps occurs through direct contact with infected droplet nuclei, saliva, or contaminated fomites. The virus has been isolated from the saliva of patients from 7 days before, to 9 days after, the onset of salivary gland involvement. The actual period of communicability, however, is probably somewhat shorter. Patients with inapparent infection or with mumps sparing the salivary glands are equally capable of spreading the disease. Transmission through an immune carrier has not been documented.

Mumps is primarily a disease of childhood; almost 95% of cases occur in children under 15 years of age. Cases have been reported in both neonates and the aged; however, placental transfer of passive immunity and the high incidence of childhood infection make mumps exceedingly rare at the extremes of life.

The disease is endemic throughout the year, although most cases occur in the winter and early spring. Periods of greater prevalence, which occur in the general population in cycles of 2 to 4 years, are uncommon in highly immunized populations. Local epidemics usually occur in situations favoring the crowding of susceptible populations, as in institutions, hospitals, boarding schools, and the armed forces. Approximately 80% of adults in an urban–suburban population, with or without a history of clinical mumps, have serologic evidence of immunity to the disease.

Pathogenesis and Pathology

The course of events preceding clinical disease remains unclear. It is believed by some that mumps begins as a direct, ascending infection of the salivary glands, with replication in the glands, followed by a blood-borne dissemination of the virus. However, this theory fails to explain the generalized involvement that may be seen before, or unassociated with, sialitis. Furthermore, experimental studies in humans show that the incubation period following the inoculation of mumps directly into the parotid duct is about one-third as long (5–8 days) as when virus is acquired through the respiratory tract (14–25 days). Therefore, it is likely that replication of the virus in the upper respiratory tract epithelium leads to viremia with dissemination to the salivary glands or other organs. A second viremia from these sites may then further extend the infection to previously uninvolved structures.

Pathologic changes in the salivary glands are nonspecific. Interstitial edema, punctate hemorrhages, and a lymphocytic infiltration with necrosis of acinar cells may be seen in the parenchyma. The ducts are filled with cellular debris and polymorphonuclear leukocytes, with edema and partial destruction of the ductal epithelium. Parenchymal changes similar to those found in the parotids have been described in the pancreas and testes.

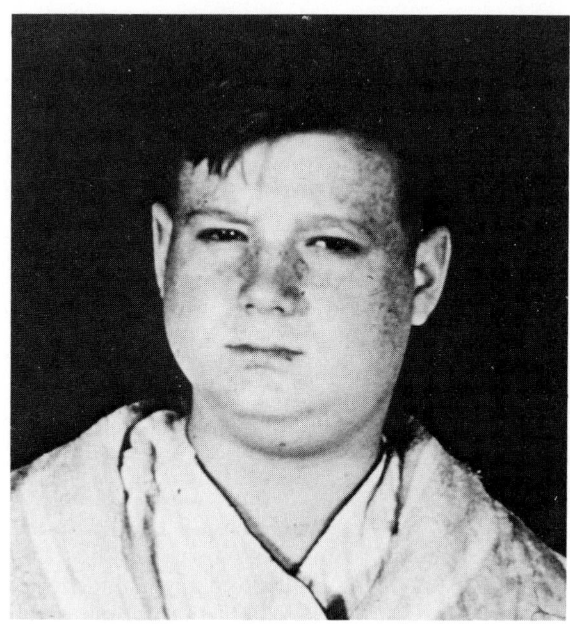

Fig. 74-1. Mumps involving the right parotid and submaxillary glands.

Manifestations

The incubation period of mumps averages 18 days, varying from 14 to 25 days. A prominent feature of infection with mumps virus is the high incidence of clinically unrecognized infections; this varies from 30% to 70% with age. Such infections may cause clinically nondescript, febrile upper respiratory disease, and predominate in infants and preschoolers.

Patients with classic mumps develop enlargement of one or more of the salivary glands (Fig. 74-1). Parotitis is the most common manifestation, but all possible combinations of multiple or single salivary gland involvement have been described. Bilateral parotitis occurs in about 75% of patients, with swelling in one gland usually preceding that of the other side by 1 to 5 days. Isolated submandibular or sublingual gland involvement is quite unusual.

The prodromal symptoms of classic mumps are nonspecific: myalgia, anorexia, malaise, and headache in the presence of a low grade fever. Early parotid involvement becomes apparent within 1 to 2 days in the form of earache and tenderness on palpation over the angle of the jaw. Slight enlargement of the gland is most readily detected as an asymmetry of the profile of the neck when the patient is viewed from behind. As the swelling progresses, the angle between the earlobe and the side of the neck increases, as compared with the unaffected side. When observed from the side, the swelling of the parotid gland covers the angle of the jaw and is bisected by a line through the long axis of the ear. In severe cases it may extend above to the eye, laterally to the mastoid area, and below to the chin and anterior neck. In contrast to cervical adenitis, parotid swelling usually obliterates the angle of the jaw so that it cannot be clearly felt. Palpation of the gland yields a doughy, brawny, nonpitting edematous sensation, which blends into indistinct lateral borders. Direct pressure on involved glands produces either clear mucus or nothing from ducts; purulent material is not seen.

Swelling of the salivary glands generally increases for 1 to 3 days, persists an equal length of time, and then subsides over the next week. Rarely, it may last for 2 weeks or more. As glandular enlargement increases, the orifices of Wharton's or Stensen's ducts often become red and swollen, and pinpoint petechial hemorrhages may be present in and around the openings. Obstruction of these ducts by edema and cellular debris may make chewing or drinking sour liquids extremely painful. The temperature is sometimes normal, but it usually remains around 38°C to 40°C. The fever, pain, and constitutional symptoms usually diminish after swelling has reached its maximum.

The range of manifestations varies widely. In some patients, fever and tenderness to palpation without visible swelling constitute the entire picture; in others glandular involvement may be marked, suggesting the bull-necked appearance described in diphtheria. Presternal or laryngeal edema, probably on the basis of lymphatic obstruction, can occur with severe glandular swelling, especially in cases of bilateral submandibulitis. Sublingual gland involvement may lead to swelling of the tongue and resultant dysphagia.

Although salivary gland infection remains the distinctive clinical feature of mumps, the propensity of the virus to invade glandular and nervous tissue often results in the widespread involvement of seemingly unrelated structures (see list below). Such infections are properly considered manifestations of a general disease rather than complications. *They may occur before, during, after, or without salivary gland involvement.* (Reappearance or persistence of fever after swelling or other signs of the disease have begun to subside may indicate involvement of additional organs.)

SYSTEMIC MANIFESTATIONS OF MUMPS

- Glandular
  - Sialadenitis (70%)
  - Orchitis (20% of postpubertal males)
  - Epididymitis (85% of cases of orchitis)
  - Prostatitis
  - Seminal vesiculitis
  - Oophoritis (5% of postpubertal females)
  - Bartholinitis
  - Pancreatitis (about 5%)
  - Mastitis
  - Dacryoadenitis
  - Thyroiditis
  - Thymus enlargement
- Nervous system
  - Asymptomatic pleocytosis (about 50%)
  - Symptomatic meningitis (about 10%)
  - Encephalomyelitis
  - Postinfectious encephalitis†
  - Myelitis
  - Neuritis of cranial nerves II, III, VI, VII, VIII
  - Polyneuritis (meningoradiculitis)
  - Guillain–Barré syndrome
  - ?Acquired aqueductal stenosis/hydrocephalus
- Other manifestations
  - Upper respiratory illness
  - Labyrinthitis
  - Conjunctivitis/keratitis/iritis
  - Myocarditis/pericarditis (ECG changes in 3% to 15%)†
  - Nephritis†
  - Thrombocytopenic purpura
  - Splenomegaly
  - Arthritis
  - Fetal wastage
  - ?Hepatitis
  - ?Endocardial fibroelastosis (intrauterine mumps?)†
  - ?Exanthem, maculopapular

* Most manifestations may occur before, during, after, or without salivary gland involvement.
† Has been associated with fatalities.

Epididymoorchitis

Approximately 20% of postpubertal males who contract mumps develop an epididymoorchitis. In one-fourth of these males, the orchitis is bilateral. Symptoms begin abruptly, with testicular swelling and tenderness, nausea, vomiting, and a rise in temperature, often accompanied by chills. Rarely, testicular pain is first referred to the right lower quadrant and may mimic appendicitis. The testicle may enlarge to 3 to 4 times its original size before regressing. Pain generally diminishes after 3 to 5 days as the temperature falls, but tenderness and swelling may last for weeks. Epididymitis precedes or accompanies the orchitis in 85% of male patients, but it may also occur without testicular involvement. Approximately 50% of the affected testicles become atrophic to some degree. However, sterility after mumps orchitis is rare.

Some impairment of Leydig-cell function has been described during and after acute orchitis. Nevertheless, no cases of true hypogonadism have been documented. Psychogenic impotence may, however, be associated with testicular atrophy.

Orchitis has been reported in infants as young as 7 months, but must be considered quite rare before adolescence. Follow-up data are too scanty to evaluate the long-term effects of orchitis in prepubertal males.

Meningitis

Mumps is one of the most common causes of aseptic meningitis (Chap. 118, Viral Meningitis). Asymptomatic pleocytosis of the cerebrospinal fluid (CSF) occurs in over half of all cases of mumps, and about 10% of patients have clinical signs or symptoms referable to the central nervous system (CNS). Such clinical manifestations are about 3 times more common in the male.

Symptoms are identical to those seen in other benign viral meningitides: fever, headache, nausea, vomiting, and lethargy predominate. Nuchal rigidity is usually mild to moderate, and Kernig's and Brudzinski's signs are frequently lacking. Fever and symptoms generally subside after 3 to 10 days. Recovery is generally complete.

Encephalitis and Encephalomyelitis

Brain and spinal cord involvement are rare manifestations of mumps, occurring only once in 6000 cases. Encephalitis is seen more frequently in males than in females; the age incidence conforms to that of the uncomplicated disease.

The clinical features suggesting cerebral involvement include convulsions, focal neurologic signs, movement disorders, and profound changes in sensorium. The signs and symptoms of meningitis are usually but not invariably also evident. If myelitis is present, segmental involvement of the spinal cord, primarily in the lower thoracic and lumbar regions, or a paralytic poliomyelitislike syndrome with muscular weakness and loss of tendon reflexes, may be seen. Long-term sequelae after mumps encephalitis are infrequent; however, fatalities have been reported.

On the basis of clinical and pathologic observations, it has been suggested that CNS injury may be caused either by direct viral invasion alone (primary encephalomyelitis) or through an immune response of the host to breakdown products of cells and myelin (postinfectious demyelinating encephalomyelitis).

Pancreatitis

The exact frequency of pancreatitis in mumps is uncertain, but it is probably present in about 5% of patients. A rise in temperature, gastrointestinal complaints, and deep epigastric pain with tenderness on palpation are the most common findings. Complete recovery takes place over 5 to 7 days, but may be delayed for up to 2 weeks in severe cases of necrotizing pancreatitis.

Deafness

Mumps was one of the leading causes of unilateral, neurosensory deafness in childhood. Despite the low incidence of hearing loss (about 1:15,000), many children were afflicted because virtually every child contracted mumps before the vaccine was available. The onset may be sudden or gradual, and it is sometimes preceded by symptoms of acute Ménière's disease. The hearing loss is complete and permanent, but fortunately it is unilateral in 75% of cases. Loss of vestibular reactions may accompany the deafness. Endolymphatic labyrinthitis and acoustic neuritis have been suggested as etiologic factors; however, autopsy data are too limited to enable determination of the exact pathogenesis.

Arthritis

Migratory polyarthritis, monarticular arthritis, or arthralgia occurs at about 2 weeks and chiefly affect the larger joints—most frequently in young adult males. Symptoms persist for periods ranging from several days up to 3 months; however, resolution is spontaneous and complete, and residual joint damage has not been described. Rheumatoid factor (latex fixation) may be transiently elevated.

Myocarditis and Pericarditis

Electrocardiographic changes compatible with myocarditis are seen in 3% to 15% of adults with mumps (Chap. 133, Myocarditis), most commonly resulting in a prolonged atrioventricular (AV) conduction time and, less frequently, these changes are seen with pericarditis (Chap. 132, Pericarditis). Symptomatic involvement is unusual. Complete recovery is the rule, but deaths have been reported.

Oophoritis

Approximately 5% of postpubertal females evidence ovarian involvement. When the right ovary is affected, the symptoms may mimic acute appendicitis. An enlarged, tender ovary may be palpated on pelvic examination. There is no evidence that mumps oophoritis causes impaired fertility.

Nephritis

In one carefully studied series of 20 young adult males with mumps, all had a transient impairment of renal function. The frequency of this manifestation in children is unknown. Severe nephritis leading to death has been reported.

Mumps in Pregnancy

Intrauterine mumps early in pregnancy has been associated with an increased incidence of fetal death and abortion. However, there is no evidence of an increased incidence of congenital malformations as a result of gestational mumps virus infection. A relationship between intrauterine mumps and endocardial fibroelastosis has been postulated but not confirmed.

Clinically apparent mumps infection in neonates is exceedingly rare. However, systemic illness with bilateral pneumonia has been documented in a 7-day-old infant whose mother was febrile with parotitis during delivery.

Other Manifestations

Involvement of various glands, such as the thyroid, lacrimal, and prostate, may be manifested by symptoms associated with swelling at these sites. Thus, prostatitis sufficiently severe to obstruct the urethra has been observed.

Diagnosis

In typical mumps with parotitis, the clinical criteria are generally sufficient for diagnosis, particularly if there is a history of exposure within the preceding 2 to 3 weeks. The peripheral blood leukocytes may be depressed, normal, or elevated in number; lymphocytes usually predominate. Leukemoid reactions have been described. With orchitis, pancreatitis, or aseptic meningitis, the total white cell count may rise to 20,000 or more with a high percentage of polymorphonuclear leukocytes. Slight and transient proteinuria and microscopic hematuria occur when there is an associated nephritis, but urinalyses are otherwise normal.

The CSF in mumps meningitis or encephalitis usually contains fewer than 500 cells per mm^3, with only occasional cell counts exceeding 2000 per mm^3. The cells are almost exclusively mononuclear from the outset; in a small percentage of patients, polymorphonuclear leukocytes may predominate for the first few days. Pleocytosis may continue for several weeks. The CSF concentration of glucose is usually normal, but may occasionally be depressed; the concentration of protein is generally slightly elevated.

In 90% of patients with parotitis, the serum amylase is increased during the period of swelling and for about 10 days thereafter. Prolonged elevations lasting up to 3 weeks may be helpful in establishing a retrospective diagnosis of mumps. Occasionally, this enzyme is also increased in the serums of patients with subclinical parotitis. Because high concentrations of amylase in the serum in mumps generally reflect parotid gland involvement, this test is of no value for diagnosis of pancreatitis; determination of serum lipase or use of pancreatic ultrasonography may be used as alternate indicators. The clinical value of measuring pancreatic versus parotid isoamylases has not yet been determined.

A history, or at least a high index of suspicion, of exposure to mumps is necessary to diagnose any of the general manifestations of mumps without salivary gland involvement. In such instances, virologic or serologic confirmation is necessary.

The diagnosis of mumps can be established by virus isolation using cultures of susceptible tissue such as monkey renal cells. Virus has been isolated from saliva and blood during the acute phase of illness, from urine for 14 days after onset of illness, and from CSF in patients with meningitis for up to 6 days after onset. It has also been recovered from breast milk and infected tissues.

Measurement of complement-fixing antibodies against the S and V antigens is the most useful serologic test. The S antibodies usually rise within the first week of illness, the V antibodies appearing about 1 to 2 weeks later. A presumptive diagnosis of mumps virus infection can therefore be made when elevated S antibodies are found without V antibodies. A fourfold or greater rise in either of these antibodies 2 or 3 weeks later is confirmatory. S antibodies are not measurable after 6 to 12 months, whereas V antibodies persist at low levels for years. Thus, an elevation of V antibodies in the absence of S antibodies suggests previous, but not concurrent, mumps.

The measurement of hemagglutination-inhibition antibodies, although easier to perform, has not proved as reliable as the complement fixation test. Neutralizing antibodies serve as the most reliable index of the immune status of a person; however, their determination is currently impractical as a routine diagnostic procedure. Newer tests, such as enzyme-linked immunosorbent assay (ELISA), radioimmunoassay, and radial hemolysis, may become increasingly useful. These methods are simple and rapid, with a level of accuracy comparable to that of the neutralization test.

The presence of mumps IgM antibodies is indicative of recent infection. These antibodies, which may be detected by the indirect immunofluorescence or by the ELISA technique, generally reach their maximum titers during the first week or two following onset of symptoms. Thereafter, they decline rapidly and are no longer detectable within 6 to 9 months in most patients. Their diagnostic significance, therefore, is analogous to that of the S antibodies demonstrable by complement fixation.

Heterotypic antibody responses frequently occur during infections with parainfluenza and mumps virus, probably on the basis of shared antigenic components in the viral envelopes. Because infection with parainfluenza virus types 1 and 3 may be associated with disease clinically indistinguishable from mumps, serologic data must be carefully evaluated. Ultimately, viral isolation procedures may be necessary for a specific diagnosis.

A mumps skin test antigen using inactivated virus was formerly commercially available for determining immunity to mumps. Because the antigen lacked both sensitivity and specificity, production was stopped.

Rapid diagnosis of paramyxovirus infection has been made through electron-microscopic examination of clinical specimens, including nasopharyngeal secretions and CSF. Immunoflourescent techniques have been used to identify mumps antigen within hours in cells present in the CSF, and within 1 to 2 days in experimentally inoculated cell cultures. These methods are not now generally available.

There are a number of conditions associated with parotid swelling that may closely resemble epidemic parotitis, particularly when acute in onset. Some are characteristically unilateral (*e.g.,* tumors, cysts, obstructive lesions) while others are bilateral (*e.g.,* drug effects and metabolic diseases). Swellings caused by drugs and metabolic abnormalities are generally asymptomatic; infections and obstructive lesions are commonly associated with pain and discomfort. Many of the conditions causing parotid swelling are associated with, or secondary to, an increase or decrease in the rate of salivary secretion. A number of conditions affecting anterior cervical lymph nodes, periauricular skin, or mandibular structures may appear to resemble parotid enlargement on casual observation. A careful physical examination followed by appropriate laboratory studies should serve to differentiate these illnesses from mumps (see list below).

Prognosis

The usual manifestations of mumps are transient, and fatalities are extremely rare (see list on p. 739). After mumps sialitis, healing is complete without residual fibrosis. There is no conclusive evidence to support the suggestion that pancreatic involvement is associated with later development of pancreatic insufficiency or diabetes.

A single attack of mumps generally confers permanent immunity. There have been no virologically and serologically documented second attacks. Inapparent infections, unilateral parotitis, or mumps affecting organs other than the salivary glands, appear to be equally effective in conferring durable immunity. Passive immunity, which may persist 6 to 9 months, is transferred from an immune mother to her infant.

DIFFERENTIAL DIAGNOSIS OF PAROTID SWELLING

- Infections
  - Viral
    - Mumps, parainfluenza types 1 and 3, Coxsackievirus A, echovirus, lymphocytic choriomeningitis, influenza A
  - Bacterial
    - Acute, suppurative parotitis (staphylococcal, anaerobes, occasionally gram-negative enteric bacilli), recurrent parotitis (primarily *Streptococcus viridans*), typical and atypical mycobacterial parotitis
  - Other
    - Trichinosis, actinomycosis, histoplasmosis
- Obstructive
  - Sialolithiasis
  - Papillary trauma (including ill-fitting dentures)
  - Foreign body in Stensen's duct
  - Parotid-masseter hypertrophy-malocclusion syndrome
  - Chronic sialectasis
  - Tumor of duct
- Tumors or cysts
  - Benign and malignant parenchymal tumors
  - Hemangiomas
  - Lymphangiomas
  - Cysts, congenital and acquired
- Drugs—toxic or allergic
  - Iodides ("pyelography mumps")
  - Isoproterenol
  - Phenylbutazone, oxyphenylbutazone
  - alpha-methyl DOPA, Bretylium
  - Bromide, heavy-metal poisoning (lead, mercury)
  - Sulfisoxazole
  - Thiouracil, Thiocyanate
  - Phenothiazines
- Metabolic
  - Malnutrition (protein deficiency?)
  - Rapid refeeding after malnutrition
  - Bulimia
  - Obesity
  - Diabetes mellitus, overt and latent
  - Alcoholism (malnutrition?)
  - Gouty parotitis
  - Uremic parotitis
- Miscellaneous
  - Sarcoidosis (uveoparotid fever)
  - Mikulicz's disease, Sjögren's syndrome, benign lymphoepithelial lesion
  - Waldenström's macroglobulinemia
  - Systemic lupus erythematosus

Fatty atrophy
Menopausal hypertrophy
Excessive starch ingestion
Cystic fibrosis
Fibrous parotitis
Pneumoparotitis (glass blowers, trumpet players)
"Anesthesia" mumps
Conditions resembling parotitis
Intraparotid, anterior cervical, lymphadenitis
Lymphoma
Dental abscess
Severe otitis externa
Caffey's disease (infantile cortical hyperostosis)
Cervicofacial actinomycosis
Masseter hypertrophy (bruxism, excessive gum-chewing)
Branchial cleft cysts
Prominent transverse process of atlas

Therapy

Treatment is symptomatic. Aspirin is useful for the control of fever and pain. The opium alkaloids should be avoided when pancreatitis is suspected because they induce spasm of the sphincter of Oddi. The intravenous administration of fluid and electrolytes may be needed when there has been persistent vomiting. There is no evidence that antimicrobics shorten the course of mumps.

The treatment of severe orchitis with steroids, diethylstilbesterol, or incision of the tunic albuginea has not proven effective in the prevention of testicular atrophy. Cold packs, support of the scrotum with a bridge, and meperidine or morphine may be helpful for relief of pain. Cortisone (75 mg, PO, four times a day for 3–4 days) may also be effective, probably through its antiinflammatory action, but trial of this drug should be limited to patients with severe orchitis.

Prevention

Live attenuated mumps virus vaccine is more than 95% effective in prevention of mumps in susceptible populations. It is available both as a single virus vaccine and in combination with measles and rubella vaccines. Mumps vaccine induces low antibody titers, which provide long-lasting, possibly lifelong protection. The routine immunization of children at about 15 months is recommended. The vaccine should also be given to children approaching puberty, adolescents, and adults, especially those with no history of mumps parotitis. Vaccine should not be given to pregnant women, since the virus has been shown to cross the placenta; however, there are no data to indicate a risk to the fetus. The vaccine virus is not transferred from vaccinees to susceptible contacts.

There is no proven method for protection against orchitis in susceptible adult males who have been exposed to mumps. Hyperimmune mumps immunoglobulin has been used, but it is of questionable value and is not generally available.

It has been suggested that live vaccine be given immediately to susceptible patients who have been exposed to mumps. Because adverse reactions to the vaccine are uncommon, this poses little risk and may be of value in preventing or attenuating the disease. Passive immunoprophylaxis is not ordinarily indicated for children.

Public health authorities generally recommend that patients with active mumps be isolated until parotid swelling or other manifestations have subsided. Because mumps is contagious both during the incubation period and in persons who have subclinical disease, it is highly unlikely that quarantine measures are of any value in preventing dissemination of the disease.

Remaining Problems

It has been suggested that mumps virus may play an etiologic role in congenital or acquired hydrocephalus. Ependymitis, leading to aqueductal stenosis and hydrocephalus, can be induced in suckling hamsters by the intracerebral injection of either wild or attenuated mumps virus. Ependymitis also occurs regularly in mumps meningoencephalitis in humans. In a few patients, mumps infection has been followed after 2 to 27 months by hydrocephalus.

Scattered clinical reports have appeared that purport to link diabetes mellitus with a preceding mumps virus infection, presumably through involvement of the pancreatic islets of Langerhans. Further investigation is necessary to determine whether there is a relationship between mumps and diabetes. The possibility that genetic factors (*e.g.,* specific HLA types) may predispose to such an association should also be examined.

Mumps virus infection in the embryonated hen's egg provides an experimental model for studying the effects of persistent infection with this virus in a fetal host. Chicks hatched from such eggs develop endocardial fibroelastosis at about 1 year. The relevance of this model for infections of the human fetus during pregnancy requires further study.

Bibliography

Books

HOPPS HE, PARKMAN PD: Mumps. In Lennette EH, Schmidt NJ (eds): Diagnostic Procedures for Viral, Rickettsial and Chlamydial Diseases, 5th ed. Washington DC, American Public Health Association, 1979. pp 633–653.

Journals

BEARD CM, BENSON RC JR, KELALIS PP, ELVEBACK LR, KURLAND LT The incidence and outcome of mumps orchitis in Roch ester, Minnesota, 1935–1974. Mayo Clin Proc 52:3–7 1977

Centers for Disease Control: Mumps surveillance, July 1974–December 1976. Issued July 1978. 19 pp.

COONEY MK, FOX JP, HALL CE: The Seattle Virus Watch. VI. Observations of infections with and illness due to parainfluenza, mumps and respiratory syncytial viruses and *Mycoplasma pneumoniae.* Am J Epidem 101:532–551, 1975

LEVITT LP, RICH TA, KINDE SW, LEWIS A, GATES E, BOND I: Central nervous system mumps: A review of 64 cases. Neurology 20:829–834, 1970

Research Unit of the Royal College of Practitioners: Complications of mumps. The incidence and complications of mumps. J R Coll Gen Prac 24:545–551, 552–556, 1974

MEYER MB: An epidemiologic study of mumps: Its spread in schools and families. Am J Hyg 75:259–281, 1962

M. COLIN JORDAN

Cytomegalovirus Infections

75

Cytomegalovirus (CMV) infections are very common throughout the world. Although most are subclinical, disease occasionally results. The most devastating infections occur *in utero* and in the host whose defenses are impaired by underlying disease, immunosuppressive chemotherapy, or both. To a certain extent, the clinical manifestations and outcome depend on the age and health of the host, the route of infection, and whether the infection is acquired exogenously or from activation of virus previously dormant in the host.

In the past two decades, a great deal has been learned about the pathogenesis, epidemiology, and clinical aspects of CMV infection. However, an understanding of basic virus–host interactions at the cellular level has been slow to develop, and information on the social and cultural impact of CMV infection has only begun to accumulate. While experimental work proceeds in an effort to remedy these deficiencies in knowledge, clinicians must deal with the all too frequently tragic outcomes of the viral infection. Thus, preliminary work on vaccines has begun, and means of therapeutic intervention are now under investigation.

Etiology

The cytomegaloviruses are members of the herpes virus group. In addition to CMV in humans, strains have been described and studied as models of infection in the mouse, rat, guinea pig, and monkey. All CMV have a double-stranded DNA genome, an icosahedral capsid containing 162 capsomeres and a lipid-containing envelope. The virions of the CMV of humans have a diameter of 100 nm, and the molecular weight of the genome is 150×10^6 daltons. Replication of the virus *in vitro* occurs almost exclusively in human diploid fibroblast cell cultures, usually derived from fetal lung or tonsil, or from neonatal foreskin. CMV grows slowly *in vitro,* and only small amounts of infectious virus are released into the culture medium. The evolution of cytopathic effects involves cellular swelling and rounding, the appearance of intranuclear and intracytoplasmic inclusions, peripheralization of nuclear chromatin (imparting a characteristic "owl eye" appearance to the cell, Fig. 75-1), and fusion or coalescence of cells. Infectious virus is best preserved at −70°C in the presence of a stabilizer such as sorbitol or dimethyl sulfoxide. Oddly, the virus survives better at 4°C than at −20°C.

In vivo, CMV replication appears to occur predominantly in epithelial cells, although virus inclusions may be found in endothelium or macrophages. As with other herpesviruses, CMV has oncogenic potential at least *in vitro.* The virus stimulates DNA synthesis of human diploid cells in culture, and inactivation of CMV with ultraviolet light can transform hamster-derived fibroblasts into malignant cells.

Epidemiology

Infections with CMV occur commonly throughout the world, and the vast majority are asymptomatic. In general, lower socioeconomic status and crowded living conditions are associated with an increased incidence of infection. The percentage of persons infected as determined by serum antibody surveys also increases with age. Thus, the incidence of infection in adults over 35 years ranges from 38% in Rochester, New York to 99% in Tanzania. Despite the high frequency of infection, however, the means of transmission of most infections has not yet been defined. Presumably, many occur as a result of respiratory spread among asymptomatic persons. Certain groups have a relatively high rate of active CMV infection without symptoms and therefore represent a potentially silent pool of communicability within the population (Table 75-1).

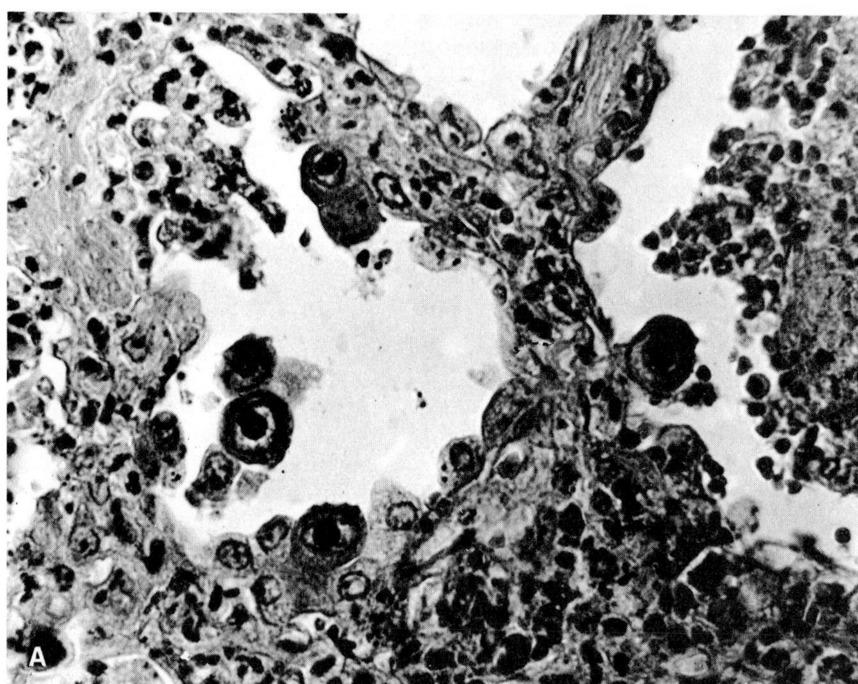

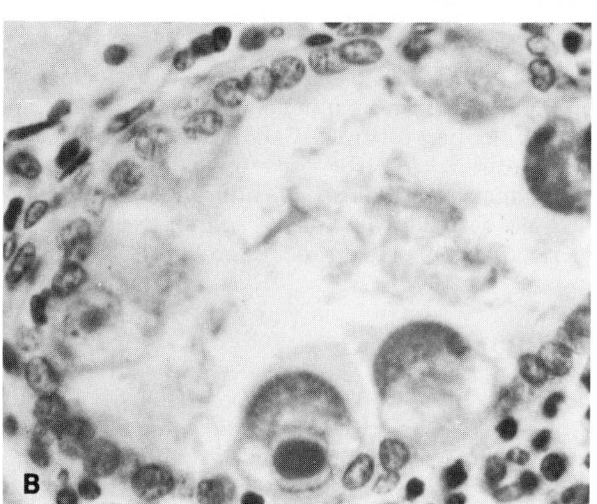

Fig. 75-1. (*A*) Cytomegalovirus inclusion bodies within pulmonary alveolar macrophages from a patient dying after cardiac transplantation (H&E × 500) (Courtesy of Charles Bieber). (*B*) Section from kidney of patient who died with general cytomegalovirus infection. Intranuclear inclusion bodies are present in tubular epithelial cells. (H&E × 800)

Young children in particular, frequently shed infectious virus in the urine or saliva, as do patients convalescing from various clinical syndromes caused by CMV. In the latter instance, the shedding of CMV is often protracted over months or even years, particularly in infants with cytomegalic inclusion disease or adults with CMV mononucleosis. During pregnancy, there is a progressively increasing rate of recovery of CMV from the cervicovaginal secretions of healthy women. Children born of such mothers are often infected during parturition and develop specific anti-CMV antibodies without discernible illness. Occasionally, however, severe interstitial pneumonia develops, presumably due to aspiration of CMV by the infant. Infection of the uterine cervix is rare in the absence of pregnancy except for women examined because of suspected venereal disease. Since CMV may be contained in maternal breast milk, breast feeding may be a means of transmission.

CMV has been recovered from the semen of 6% of

***Table 75-1.** Shedding of Cytomegalovirus From Various Sites*

Patient or Subject	Site	Frequency of Isolation of CMV (%)
Newborn infants	Urine	0.5–3.0
Cytomegalic inclusion disease	Urine	95–100
	Saliva	90–100
Infants < 1 year of age	Urine	3–55
Normal children	Urine	8–28
Young adults	Urine	0
Young women	Urine	0
	Cervix	0
Young women in venereal disease clinic	Cervix	10–15
Men in venereal disease clinic	Semen	3–8
Pregnant women	Urine	1–3
First trimester	Cervix	0
Second trimester	Cervix	5–12
Third trimester	Cervix	12–29
Lactating women	Breast milk	10–27
Patients with CMV mononucleosis	Urine	95–100
	Saliva	70–85
Patients with malignancy, transplants, or immunosuppressive therapy	Urine	20–90

normal young adult males and from several men with CMV mononucleosis; that is, the virus may be sexually transmitted, although the consequences of such infections are not known. Finally, studies of recipients of blood by transfusion disclosed a risk of subclinical CMV infection of 3% to 6% following administration of a single unit of blood; the risk of infection increases in direct proportion to the number of units transfused. Renal allografts may be the source of CMV in transplant recipients given a kidney from a seropositive donor. The incidence of CMV infection is extremely high in recipients of bone marrow transplants, but the source of virus is less clear.

Pathogenesis and Pathology

The pathogenesis of many infections caused by CMV is not yet clearly defined. However, two distinct mechanisms appear to be involved: (1) infection resulting from primary exogenous acquisition of the virus and (2) infection resulting from activation of virus previously latent in the host tissues. Primary infection of the mother (usually asymptomatic) with transplacental passage of virus in the first or second trimester of pregnancy may lead to severe cytomegalic inclusion disease *in utero*. Other manifestations of primary infection include CMV mononucleosis (spontaneous or after blood transfusion), CMV hepatitis in children, Guillain-Barré syndrome, and rare instances of meningoencephalitis.

Consecutive pregnancies that result in infected infants have been described, and may result from reactivation of latent maternal virus in the second pregnancy. The second infected infant appears to be normal at birth.

Severe disseminated disease due to CMV may result from either primary or reactivated CMV infection in the immunocompromised host and in the organ transplant recipient. In general, illness is more likely to be life-threatening when infection develops in the host without previous contact with the virus (*i.e.,* seronegative persons).

The histopathologic lesions of CMV infection consist of enlarged inclusion-bearing cells surrounded by varying degrees of mononuclear cell infiltration, depending on the functional level of the host's immune system (Fig. 75-1*A, B*). Calcification of lesions may occur, especially in the central nervous system of newborn infants. Although any organ may have characteristic lesions, they are especially prominent in the lung, liver, brain, eye, kidneys, and gastrointestinal tract.

The host defense factors that lead to resolution of

the infection are not known. Because virus may continue to be shed in saliva and urine for long periods in spite of high titers of specific serum antibody, it has been assumed that cell-mediated immunity is the most important defense mechanism. However, the issue is far from resolved. Likewise, the site(s) of viral latency has never been demonstrated experimentally in man. Latent CMV has been sought in leukocytes of normal blood donors without success. Similarly, latent virus cannot be demonstrated in renal allograft tissue prior to transplantation into the recipient.

Manifestations

Congenital Infection

Intrauterine infection may result from primary acquisition or reactivation of latent virus in the mother. Of all newborn infants, 1% to 3% have CMV in the urine at birth. Although these infants appear to be normal, the risk of subsequent development of deficiencies in intelligence or sensorineural hearing loss is substantially greater than in matched cohorts. Of infants infected *in utero,* 10% to 15% have classic cytomegalic inclusion disease. Findings include chorioretinitis, microcephaly, intracerebral calcifications, subsequent mental retardation, hepatosplenomegaly, jaundice, and thrombocytopenia with petechiae. Many infants die shortly after birth, while others require institutional care.

Acquired Infections

NEONATES

Infants may become infected with CMV either during delivery by inhalation of cervicovaginal secretions or postpartum from maternal breast milk. These infections are almost always asymptomatic but result in seroconversion and a period of shedding CMV in the urine. Occasionally, interstitial pneumonia results and may be progressive, terminating in death.

CHILDREN

Infection of children with CMV is nearly always asymptomatic. Rarely, liver dysfunction may occur, or progressive hepatomegaly may take place with the development of cirrhosis. Most children simply shed virus in the urine and saliva for several months. Whether CMV causes pharyngitis or other respiratory illnesses has not been clarified.

ADULTS

Infection of adults with CMV is most commonly symptomatic as a mononucleosis syndrome. The disease may be virtually identical with classic heterophil-positive infectious mononucleosis caused by the Epstein–Barr virus (Chap. 137, Infectious Mononucleosis). However, in CMV mononucleosis, the heterophil or mononucleosis slide test is always negative. Sore throat is a common complaint but objective evidence of pharyngitis is often minimal. Pharyngeal exudate is extremely unusual. Fever, marked atypical lymphocytosis, and abnormal liver function tests last for several weeks. Uncommon complications including ascending polyneuritis (Guillain-Barré) syndrome, facial nerve diplegia, granulomatous hepatitis, myopericarditis, thrombocytopenia with hemorrhage, splenic rupture or subcapsular hematoma, interstitial pneumonitis, and hemolytic anemia.

Many laboratory studies often yield positive tests: cold agglutinins, rheumatoid factor, antinuclear antibodies, syphilis serology, Coombs' antibody, and cryoglobulins. As in EBV–mononucleosis, a maculopapular rash frequently follows treatment with ampicillin. Although most patients recover uneventfully, convalescence may be protracted, and symptomatic relapses may occur. An identical illness may appear 3 to 6 weeks after blood transfusion with or without preceding extracorporeal circulation (postperfusion syndrome).

Additional isolated manifestations of infection with CMV may also occur: hepatitis, meningoencephalitis, and possibly pancreatitis.

IMMUNOCOMPROMISED PATIENTS

The immunocompromised patient is at greater risk of infection with CMV acquired either exogenously (blood, granulocyte transfusions, organ transplants, person-to-person) or from activation of latent virus. Treatment with immunosuppressive agents often activates CMV, as indicated by asymptomatic salivary or urinary virus shedding. When disseminated disease develops, involvement of the liver and lung is most likely to be associated with a fatal outcome. Diffuse nodular or interstitial pneumonitis with hypoxemia is usually refractory to therapy and may be complicated by superinfection with *Pneumocystis carinii* (Chap. 45, Pneumocystosis), fungi, or gram-negative bacteria. Febrile episodes in the granulocytopenic patient may be caused by CMV, especially when abnormal liver function tests are noted. In disseminated infection, viremia is usually associated with the polymorphonuclear leukocytes and may precede serious lung or liver involvement. CMV interstitial pneumonia is a major cause of death following otherwise successful bone marrow transplantation.

Diagnosis

Recovery of CMV from tissues or bodily fluids, significant changes in the titer of antibodies in the serum, and characteristic histopathology in tissue obtained by biopsy or at autopsy may be used to aid in diagnosis. Isolation of the virus is best achieved by direct inoculation of fresh specimens into human diploid cell cultures. Urine, saliva, pharyngeal secretions, the buffy coat of blood (leukocytes), cervicovaginal secretions, semen, intraocular fluids, breast milk, and tissue biopsies are appropriate for culture. In patients with suspected CMV interstitial pneumonitis, surgical open lung biopsy may be required for diagnosis. Tissue cultures generally become positive after 5 to 28 days of incubation. Conversion from negative to positive, or a 4- to 8-fold rise in titer of antibodies in the serum is required for serologic diagnosis of active infection. The complement–fixation test is widely available, although other tests may be more sensitive. Infants infected *in utero* give rise to IgM antibodies against CMV which are demonstrable by immunofluorescence using serum from umbilical cord blood.

Prognosis

The outlook in congenital cytomegalic inclusion disease is poor. Death or permanent institutionalization results frequently. In acquired infections, the prognosis depends largely on the integrity of the host's immune system. Previously normal persons usually recover uneventfully. However, the compromised host may succumb from liver involvement, interstitial pneumonitis, or disseminated disease. In general, primary infections in the compromised host are more likely to cause severe disease than are reactivated latent infections.

Therapy

There is currently no specific therapy for CMV infections. Temporary suppression of urinary CMV excretion has been demonstrated during therapy with cytosine arabinoside, adenosine arabinoside, and interferon, but virus reappears when treatment is stopped. In patients receiving immunosuppressive agents, decreased dosage or discontinuation of these drugs may be beneficial by allowing restoration of host defense mechanisms.

Prevention

Passive immunization of patients who receive transplanted organs with anti-CMV globulin prior to immunosuppression is under evaluation in several centers. Studies of the safety and efficacy of live, attenuated CMV vaccine are under investigation in normal subjects and in recipients of transplanted organs. Of major concern is the possible induction of latent CMV infection by the vaccine, or reversion of the vaccine virus to a virulent state. The oncogenic potential of CMV is also of concern. If these problems can be resolved and an effective vaccine developed, women anticipating pregnancy and patients scheduled to receive immunosuppressive therapy or open heart surgery would be among the candidates for vaccination.

Remaining Problems

The pathogenesis of CMV infection, especially congenital infection, needs to be thoroughly investigated. A better understanding of virus–cell interactions and the mechanisms involved in the latent viral state are clearly needed. Efforts to develop and evaluate potentially effective antiviral substances with activity against CMV must continue. Studies of the safety and efficacy of attenuated CMV vaccines and the development of killed or subunit viral vaccines should continue.

Bibliography

Book

GOLD E, NANKERVIS GA: Cytomegalovirus in Viral Infections of Humans: Epidemiology and Control In Evans AS (ed): Viral and Human Epidemiology and Control. Plenum Medical Book Co, 1976. pp 143–161.

Journals

ABDALLAH PS, MARK JBD, MERIGAN TC: Diagnosis of cytomegalovirus pneumonia in compromised hosts. Am J Med 61:326–332, 1976

GLASER JP, FRIEDMAN HM, GUSSMAN RA, STARR SE, BARKER CF, PERLOFF LJ, HUANG ES, PLOTKIN SA: Live cytomegalovirus vaccination of renal transplant candidates: A preliminary trial. Ann Intern Med 91:676–683, 1979

HANSHAW JA: Congenital cytomegalovirus infection: A fifteen year prospective. J Infect Dis 123:555–61, 1971

HO M, SUWANSIRIKUL S, DOWLING JN, YOUNGBLOOD LA, ARMSTRONG JA: The transplanted kidney as a source of cytomegalovirus infection. N Engl J Med 293:1109–1112, 1975

HUANG ES, ALFORD CA, REYNOLDS DW, STAGNO S, PASS RF: Molecular epidemiology of cytomegalovirus infections in women and their infants. N Engl J Med 303:958–962, 1980

JORDAN MC, ROUSSEAU WE, NOBLE GR, STEWART JA, CHIN TDY: Association of cervical cytomegalovirus with venereal disease. N Engl J Med 288:923–924, 1973

JORDAN MC, ROUSSEAU WE, STEWART JA, NOBLE GR, CHIN TDY: Spontaneous cytomegalovirus mononucleosis: Clinical and laboratory evaluation in nine cases. Ann Intern Med 22:624–630, 1973

STAGNO S, REYNOLDS DW, HUANG ES, THAMES SD, SMITH RJ, ALFORD CA, JR: Congenital cytomegalovirus infection in an immune population. N Engl J Med 296:1254–1258, 1977

STAGNO S, REYNOLDS DW, PASS RF, ALFORD CA: Breast feeding and the risk of cytomegalovirus infection. N Engl J Med 302:1073–1076, 1980

WELLER TH: The cytomegalovirus: Ubiquitous agents with protean clinical manifestations. N Engl J Med 285:203–214, 1971

WINSTON DJ, HO WG, HOWELL CL, MILLER JR, MICKEY R, MARTIN WJ, LIN CH, GALE RP: Cytomegalovirus infections associated with leukocyte transfusions. Ann Intern Med 93:671–675, 1980

AARON D. ALEXANDER

Leptospirosis

76

Leptospirosis is an acute septicemic and systemic disease caused by any one of a large number of serologic types (serovars) of *Leptospira interrogans*. The serovars are distributed worldwide in a large variety of wild and domestic animals. Naturally infected animals shed the organisms in their urine. Humans are infected by direct contact with infected urine or by contact with wet soil and waters contaminated with infected urine. The disease in man is characterized in most cases by an abrupt onset, fever, chills, myalgias, severe headache, and conjunctival suffusion; usually, the disease resolves uneventfully in 2 to 3 weeks. Signs of meningitis appear in a large proportion of patients and may dominate the clinical picture. An icteric form of disease with severe kidney and liver dysfunction and hemorrhagic manifestations, the so-called Weil's disease, occurs in a small proportion of cases and may result in death.

Etiology

Leptospires are motile, flexuous, helical bacteria, approximately 0.1 μm in diameter and usually 6 μm to 20 μm long, with characteristic semicircular hooks, usually at both ends but occasionally at one end only (Fig. 76-1). The structure of leptospires as revealed by electron microscopic examination consists of a helicoidal protoplasmic cylinder wound about two flagella that are inserted subterminally at each end with their free ends extending toward the central portion of the cell where they usually do not overlap (Fig. 76-2). The cell wall membrane complex of leptospires is similar to that of gram-negative bacteria. Both flagella and protoplasmic cylinder are enveloped by an outer sheath.

Leptospires appear to be faintly colored in preparations stained by Wright's or Giemsa stains and are not readily observed in gram-stained smears. However, they can be demonstrated by the use of fluorescent antibody or silver deposition techniques. Unstained, leptospires can be seen by darkfield or phase contrast microscopy, but not by bright field. Characteristically, in liquid mediums they move forward and backward as they rotate with their hooked ends spinning in alternate directions along their longitudinal axis. In semisolid mediums, flexuous, boring, and serpentine movements are seen. Leptospires can pass through filters that normally retain bacteria. This attribute, along with the difficulties of detection by microscopy and by the usual culture procedures, has frequently led to the mistaken diagnosis of viral infection for leptospirosis.

Leptospires grow readily in mediums containing serum, for example, 10% rabbit serum, or bovine serum albumin plus long-chain fatty acids, over a pH range of 6.8 to 7.8, and an optimum temperature of 30°C. Growth is usually detected after 6 to 14 days of incubation but may be delayed up to 6 weeks.

Two species of leptospires have been proposed; *Leptospira interrogans,* for the parasitic members, and *Leptospira biflexa,* for the so-called saprophytic leptospires. Strains of *L. biflexa* are omnipresent in fresh waters and occasionally found in salt waters; however, such isolates are not known to be pathogenic for humans or other mammals.

Each species consists of a large variety of serovars. The serovar serves as the basic taxon. Serovars are distinguished on the basis of agglutinogenic properties as disclosed in cross-agglutination and agglutinin-adsorption tests. Serovars within species are otherwise indistinguishable on the basis of morphologic and biochemical characteristics. Approximately 180 different serovars of *L. interrogans* have been identified. The serovars have been assembled into 18 serogroups on the basis of shared major agglutinogens. The serogroup has no taxonomic status but is used as an expedient for selecting antisera or antigens to identify isolates or to test serums for antibodies.

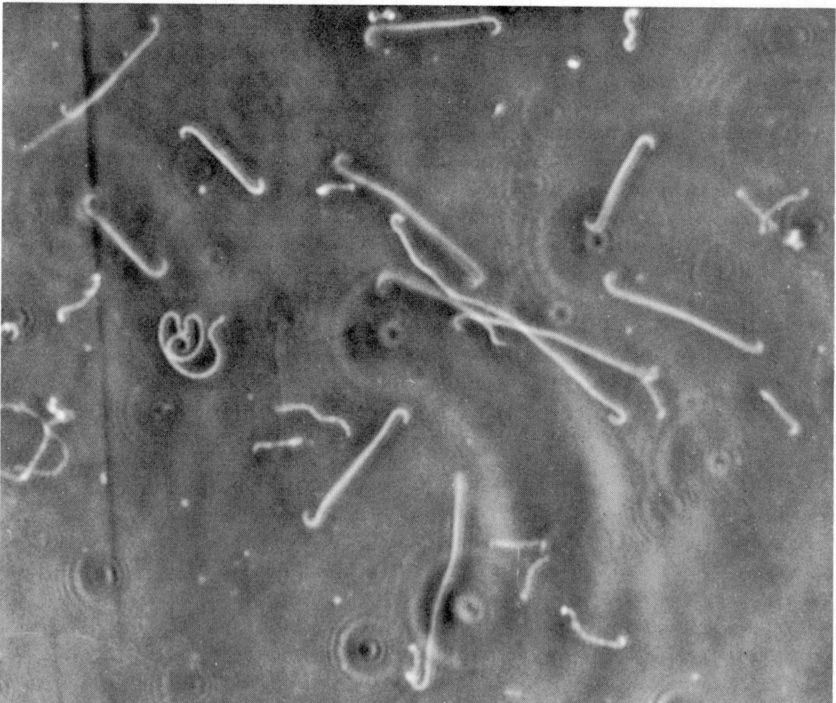

Fig. 76-1. *Leptospira interrogans,* viewed by anoptral phase-contrast microscopy. (Original magnification approximately × 1335)

Epidemiology

Approximately 160 different mammalian species, including domestic animals as well as a large variety of rodents and other mammals, have been found to harbor pathogenic leptospires. The distribution of the various serovars in hosts may vary geographically. The host range of some selected serovars frequently associated with disease in humans in the United States is shown in Table 76-1. Many serovars appear to be preferentially adapted to particular mammalian hosts. Thus, serovar *canicola* is primarily associated with dogs, *icterohaemorrhagiae* with Norway rats, and *pomona* with cattle and swine. The distribution of a particular serovar in a specific host is not exclusive. A specific serovar may be well adapted to more than one host, and conversely a specific animal may be a major maintenance host for two or more serovars. Moreover, various animals may be infected with types primarily adapted to different animal species, and thus may transmit the infection to other mammals, including humans. Infections in natural hosts are usually unapparent but may be morbid. Naturally occurring disease has been observed in dogs, swine, cattle, sheep, and other livestock, and is an important animal health problem in many countries, including the United States.

Leptospires nest in the nephritic tubules of mammalian hosts and are shed with the urine. The duration and amount of shedding vary with the host and the infecting serovar. For example, rodents, such as Norway rats, infected with *icterohaemorrhagiae,* may shed profuse numbers of organisms for the remainder of their natural life. On the other hand, shedding in dogs and domestic animals may be heavy for several months after infection, and then become intermittent for up to 6 months or a year, but rarely longer. Carrier rates in natural hosts may be remarkably high, frequently exceeding 50% in Norway rats and other rodents. Rates of 10% to 50% in other feral mammals and domestic animals have been reported in the United States and many other countries.

Humans acquire leptospires either directly through contact with the urine of animal carriers or by contact with damp soil or natural waters contaminated by animal carriers. Pathogenic leptospires can survive 3 months or longer in neutral, slightly alkaline waters. Organisms enter hosts through abrasions of the skin or through the mucosal surface of the eye, mouth, nasopharynx, or esophagus. Males and females of all ages are equally susceptible.

Infections in humans are accidental and are related to recreational or occupational exposure, or contact with pets or rodents in infested dwellings. Person-

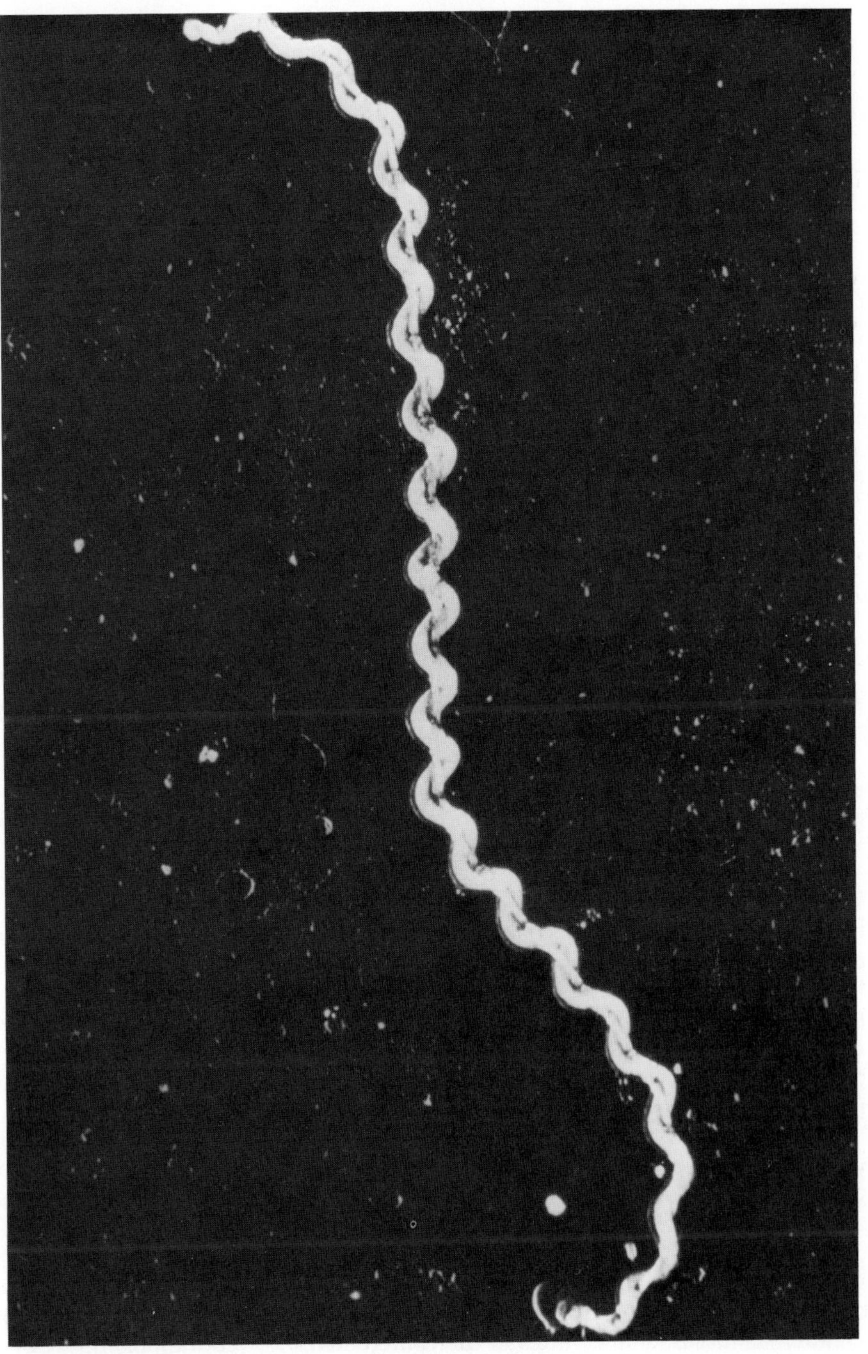

Fig. 76-2. Electron micrograph of leptospire (about × 12,500). (Simpson CF, White RH: J Infect Dis 109:243–250, 1961)

to-person transfer rarely occurs. Sewer workers, fish and poultry processors, butchers, ditch diggers, and others who work or live in rat-infested areas are at risk, as are dairymen, swineherds, abattoir workers, and veterinarians who have contact with livestock. In many countries, sporadic cases or epidemics occur in agricultural workers engaged in raising rice, flax, vegetables, or sugar cane, in rubber plantation workers, and in soldiers exposed to natural waters soiled by carriers. Common source epidemics have occurred

Table 76-1. *Host Range of Leptospiral Serovars Isolated from Humans and Domestic Animals in the United States*

Serovar	Animal Hosts		
	HUMAN	DOMESTIC	WILD
icterohaemorrhagiae	+	Dog, pig, cattle	Rats*, mice, fox, raccoon, muskrat, opossum, skunk, woodchuck, nutria, ape (zoo)
copenhageni	+	Dog	Raccoon, armadillo
canicola	+	Dog*, pig, cattle	Skunk, raccoon
pomona	+	Cattle*, pig*, dog, horse, goat	Skunk, raccoon, fox, opossum, woodchuck, deer, mice, sea lion, armadillo
fort-bragg	+	?	?
grippotyphosa		Cattle, pig	Mole, raccoon, fox, skunk, opossum, muskrat, leopard cat, rabbit, squirrel, bobcat, mice
hardjo	+	Cattle*	
georgia	+		Racoon, opossum, skunk
swarjizak		Cattle	
balcanica		Cattle	

* Known major maintenance host (Leptospiral distribution lists according to host and geographic area. Atlanta, GA, U.S. Dept. of Health, Education and Welfare, Center for Disease Control, 1966 [Supplement 1975])

repeatedly in children and young adults who swam or bathed in ponds or streams located in pastureland. In many Asian, South and Central American countries, sections of Eastern and Southern Europe, Australia, and New Zealand, leptospirosis is an important public health problem. In the United States, leptospirosis is primarily a veterinary medical problem.

The number of cases in humans over the past 20 years rarely exceeded 100 annually, in spite of the great prevalence of carriers in rodents, other wildlife, and domestic animals (Fig. 76-3). The actual number of cases is undoubtedly much higher, but probably still relatively low, reflecting in large measure the high degree of mechanization in agriculture, high sanitary standards, and facilities in the United States.

Pathogenesis and Pathology

There is no inflammatory response at the site of entry of leptospires. During the 10- to 12-day period of incubation, there is spread and multiplication of the organism by means and at sites not yet established. On the basis of findings in experimentally infected animals, leptospires spread from the site of entry through the bloodstream; initial multiplication is believed to occur in the blood and liver. At the time of onset of disease, the organsims are found in the blood and cerebrospinal fluid, and are apparently present in most organs.

The action of a toxin has been postulated in the pathogenesis of leptospirosis because of the marked disparity between the severity of the functional derangement of the kidneys and liver and the histopathology. No toxin(s) has been related to the manifestations of the disease in humans, and it appears that the lesions of leptospirosis result from damage to the endothelial lining of capillaries resulting in increased permeability, hemorrhagic diathesis, and a diminished supply of oxygen to tissues. Although hemorrhagic manifestations occur in nonicteric leptospirosis, they tend to be especially pronounced in icteric disease. The jaundice in severe cases results from dysfunction of liver cells. The histologic changes include dissociation of hepatic cords, variation in the size and the shape of parenchymal cells, increase in

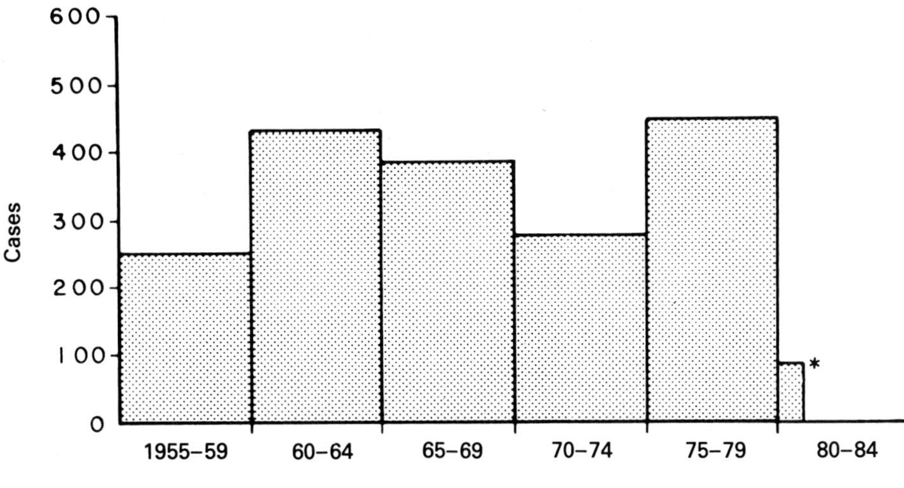

Fig. 76-3. Reported cases of leptospirosis by 5-year periods in the United States, 1955–1980. (Morbid Mortal Week Rep, Annual Summary 1980)

the size and number of Kupffer's cells, proliferation of multinucleated cells, stasis of bile in the canaliculi, and aberration of the mitochondria. Hepatocellular necrosis is sparse. Death from leptospirosis is usually related to renal tubular dysfunction which results from necrosis of tubular epithelial cells. The histopathologic alterations in the kidney and liver are reversible in patients who recover.

The pathogenesis of leptospiral meningitis is undetermined. During the acute phase when leptospires are readily found in cerebrospinal fluid, the signs of meningeal irritation are not present in most cases. Meningeal signs are more likely to be seen after the leptospiremic phase, at which time leptospires are infrequently present in the spinal fluid, and antibodies are detectable in the serum. It has been suggested that leptospiral meningitis is a consequence of an immune complex reaction. The pathologic changes in the meninges are minimal in leptospiral meningitis; similarly, in the cerebrospinal fluid there may be a moderate lymphocytic pleocytosis and an elevated protein, but normal glucose.

Lesions arise in the respiratory tract not from inflammation but as a result of hemorrhagic diathesis, varying from mild bleeding in the mucosa, pleura, and lungs to a hemorrhagic pneumonia. The myalgias and muscle tenderness present in severe cases have been related to transient degenerative changes in striated muscle. Uveitis is a frequent sequel appearing weeks or months after onset and has been associated with the presence of leptospires in the anterior chamber. Generally, leptospires are demonstrable in specimens obtained during the first week of illness. Thereafter, they may be seen only in specimens from the kidney and eye. The persistence of leptospires in brain tissue has also been recognized in naturally infected, feral mammals.

Manifestations

The clinical manifestations of leptospirosis are variable and extend from an asymptomatic infection to a severe icteric hepatorenal disease. The protean manifestations reflect to a certain extent differences in virulence of strains. The severe icteric form, or Weil's disease, has most frequently been caused by strains of a few serovars, for example, *icterohaemorrhagiae.* However, any serovar may provoke the various forms of illness. Severe icteric illness occurs infrequently—probably in fewer than 5% of the cases. Mild, anicteric disease is more characteristic, even in infections caused by the strains with icterogenic tendencies.

The illness appears abruptly after an incubation period of 10 to 12 days (extremes 2–30 days). The signs and symptoms of leptospirosis are nonspecific and include a rising fever, chills, severe headache, myalgia, malaise, and conjunctival suffusion. Leptospiremia usually persists for 6 to 8 days but may continue for more than 10 days. During the leptospiremic period, leptospires may also be found in the spinal fluid. The termination of the leptospiremic period is marked by the appearance of antibodies and, in mild cases, by the abatement of signs and symptoms. During the second, and occasionally the third week following onset, short febrile relapses may occur that are frequently associated with signs of meningeal irritation. In some cases, the meningeal manifestations may be predominant. After the first week of disease, leptospires may be found in the urine; leptospiruria may persist with decreasing intensity, becoming intermittent, for 3 or more months thereafter.

At onset, the fever is usually 39°C to 40°C (102°F–104°F) with extremes of 37.8°C to 41.1°C (100°F–106°F). The duration of fever is usually less than 8 days. The various signs and symptoms in a large series of anicteric and icteric cases is shown in Table 76-2. Frequently associated signs and symptoms include nausea, vomiting, diarrhea or constipation, abdominal pain, muscle tenderness, and retro-orbital pain. Lymphadenopathy, rash, bradycardia, or tachycardia are reported less frequently. The occurrence of pharyngitis, cough, hepatomegaly, oliguria, hemorrhagic pneumonitis, or other hemorrhagic manifestations varies with the severity of disease.

In severe cases, jaundice generally appears in the middle or at the end of the first week, reaching maximum intensity 4 to 5 days later. It is generally accompanied by oliguria or anuria, and hemorrhagic manifestations are common. Central nervous system dysfunction is seen frequently but may be over-

Table 76-2. *Clinical Manifestations of 208 Cases of Leptospirosis in Puerto Rico*

	Percentages		
Symptom or Sign	ANICTERIC (106 CASES)	ITCERIC (102 CASES)	WHOLE GROUP (208 CASES)
Fever	100	99	99
Conjunctival injection	100	98	99
Myalgia	97	97	97
Headache	82	95	91
Chills	84	90	85
Pharyngitis	72	87	79
Nausea	71	81	75
Muscle tenderness	70	79	75
Vomiting	65	75	69
Hepatomegaly	60	80	69
Tachycardia	64	83	64
Jaundice	0	100	49
Burning of eyes	54	38	46
Diarrhea	25	30	27
Oliguria	20	30	25
Cough	15	32	24
Pulmonary findings	11	36	24
Adenopathy	35	12	24
Petechiae and ecchymoses	4	29	16
Hypotension	8	14	11
Stiffness of neck	12	5	9
Hemoptysis	5	14	9
Coma	0	19	9
Conjunctival hemorrhage	2	12	7
Erythema of face	6	9	7
Maculopapular rash	3	10	6
Diastolic hypertension	3	8	5
Bloddy diarrhea	1	6	3
Splenomegaly	2	5	3
Hematemesis	0	6	3
Epistaxis	0	5	2
Herpes labialis	3	2	2

(Diaz–Rivera RS, Hall HE, Ramos–Morales KY et al: Leptospirosis in Puerto Rico. Clinical aspects of human infection. Zoonos Res 2:159–177, 1963)

shadowed by the manifestations of kidney and liver malfunction. Deaths in untreated cases range from 5% to 30% and generally result from renal failure at the end of the second or beginning of the third week of disease.

Diagnosis

The clinical manifestations of leptospirosis are not pathognomonic and have been confused with numerous other diseases. Of over 1000 confirmed cases reported by the Center for Disease Control since 1949, leptospirosis was considered in the initial clinical impression in less than 25% of the cases. The other impressions included a wide variety of diseases such as influenza, viral meningitis, viral hepatitis, gastroenteritis, rickettsial diseases, cholecystitis, and appendicitis.

Leptospirosis should be considered in the differential diagnosis of any febrile illness occurring in a patient with a history of contact with animals, either directly or indirectly through contact with damp soil, waters, work areas, or dwellings contaminated with animal urine. In particular, illnesses characterized by an abrupt onset, chills, rapidly rising fever, myalgia, conjunctival suffusion, marked headache, with nausea and vomiting should suggest leptospirosis. The possibility of a leptospiral etiology in any case of nonbacterial meningitis should be considered, since up to 12% of these patients have leptospirosis.

The clinical laboratory findings in patients with leptospirosis are not remarkable, but may be useful in ruling out specific diseases. Generally, the blood picture may be normal or may range from a mild to a marked neutrophilic leukocytosis, depending on the severity of the disease. Prothrombin, clotting times, and platelet counts are usually normal; erythrocyte sedimentation rates are invariably raised, often markedly. Jaundiced patients may be slightly anemic. Liver function tests in anicteric patients are usually normal. In jaundiced patients, the concentration of the bilirubin in the serum is high, and the SGOT and SGPT values are normal or moderately elevated, in contrast to the findings in viral hepatitis patients. Urinalysis in anicteric patients may be normal but usually discloses proteinuria. When there is jaundice and kidney involvement, the urine contains protein and, depending on the severity, white and red blood cells, granular and hyalin casts, and bile. Azotemia appears when the kidney dysfunction is severe.

Although the clinical laboratory findings may be useful in supporting the clinical impression, the definitive diagnosis of leptospirosis is contingent on the demonstration of *L. interrogans* in tissues or body fluids or by the demonstration of significant titers of antibody in serum.

During the first week of disease, leptospires may be isolated from the blood and cerebrospinal fluid. Culture of leptospires is within the capabilities of an ordinary hospital laboratory. With the use of commercially available mediums, incubation at 30°C, and weekly examination by darkfield microscopy, growth of characteristic leptospires is generally detectable after 5 to 10 days of incubation. After the first week of disease, isolation of leptospires from fresh urine is possible in a large proportion of cases. A midstream sample is collected and diluted 1:10 and 1:100 with medium. Undiluted and diluted samples are cultured. In fatal cases, leptospires may be isolated from triturated kidney, and less frequently, from liver tissue. The use of a minimal inoculum (1–2 drops/5 ml of medium) is recommended for all specimens to rule out growth-inhibitory substances which may be present.

Serologic typing of cultures is available from the Bacteriology Division, Centers for Disease Control, Atlanta, Georgia. Attempts at diagnosis by demonstrating leptospires in tissues and liquids by microscopic examination is not recommended as the sole diagnostic procedure because (1) the concentration of leptospires is small and microscopy will succeed in only a small proportion of cases; and (2) the all too common result is mistaken identification of fibrils or extrusions from cells as spirochetes.

Animal inoculation may be used to isolate leptospires from blood or other materials but offers no advantage over direct culture for recovery of leptospires from aseptically derived specimens. However, if specimens are contaminated, the intraperitoneal inoculation of weanling hamsters and young guinea pigs may be quite useful. Infections range from unapparent to lethal. Heart blood for culture and microscopic examination is obtained whenever signs of disease are present, or at the fourth and sixth days and periodically thereafter to the 20th day after inoculation. Culture of the kidneys of surviving animals provides another opportunity to recover leptospires.

Serologic procedures are used more frequently than isolation to establish a diagnosis either because patients are first seen during a phase of illness when cultural techniques may not succeed or, most likely, because isolation was not attempted. The microscopic agglutination test using live or formalin-treated antigen is the standard procedure. It is highly specific and requires the use of multiple serovars to ensure detection of antibodies which may be provoked by any one of the large number of serovars that may be present. The number of antigens may range from a few to 15 or more, depending on the known occurrence of serovars in specific geographic regions. It is a laborious procedure which is usually restricted to state and federal laboratories. Most hospital laboratories use commercially available macroscopic-agglutination slide tests available as single or pooled antigens.

Agglutinins are detectable by the sixth to tenth day of disease, reaching maximum levels by the third or fourth week. Low antibody titers may be detectable for months or years thereafter. A sensitized erythrocyte lysis test using a "genus-specific" antigen has been used advantageously in areas of multiple-serovar leptospirosis. A modification of this test using fixed, sensitized red blood cells in an agglutination procedure is now in use at the Centers for Disease Control, along with the standard microscopic agglutination test. A genus-specific complement fixation test is used in some European laboratories.

Prognosis

Patients who have anicteric leptospirosis usually recover uneventfully in 2 to 3 weeks, but convalescence may extend for one or more months depending on the severity of the disease. Deaths occur in 5% to 30% of untreated, jaundiced patients, usually of acute renal failure. Today, however, the percentage of deaths can be remarkably decreased by the use of dialysis procedures. Jaundiced patients who survive have an excellent prognosis for complete recovery.

Uveitis syndromes may appear in up to 10% of cases from 2 weeks to 1 year following the onset of disease. The prognosis is generally good; rarely does this condition progress to hypopyon.

Superficially, immunity in leptospirosis is related to the specific agglutinogenic characteristics of serovars. Patients who recover develop long-lasting immunity against the infecting serovar but are susceptible to infection with unrelated serovars.

Therapy

Pathogenic leptospires are susceptible to most of the commonly used antimicrobics except chloramphenicol. Although the various penicillins, cephalosporins, tetracyclines, streptomycin, and macrolide antimicrobics are effective in experimental infections of laboratory animals, the clinical results are contradictory. It is generally believed that antimicrobics are effective if treatment is initiated on the first 2 days of the disease, and possibly on the third and fourth days, but not thereafter. Treatment with penicillin or tetracycline is most frequently recommended, but there is no firm evidence that other drugs are less effective. High doses are used, for example penicillin G (50 mg–70 mg [80,000–110,000 units] /kg body wt/day given IV as six equal portions 6-hourly) or tetracycline (30 mg/kg body weight/day given IV as four equal portions 6-hourly), for 5 to 10 days. Herxheimer-like reactions have been recorded in a few instances in patients treated with penicillin. Supportive treatment is especially important in icteric patients to maintain electrolyte balance and kidney and liver functions. Peritoneal dialysis has been an effective life-saving measure in patients with azotemia.

Prevention

Potential livestock and canine sources of leptospire infection may be reduced by vaccine prophylaxis, although elimination of the urinary carrier stage is not always ensured. Leptospiral vaccines are extensively used in livestock and dogs in the United States. Rodent control in work and living areas is an obvious preventive measure which may be feasible. Control of wildlife reservoirs is usually impractical. The prevalence of leptospires in the general population or even in potentially high risk populations in the United States is low and does not warrant prophylactic measures. In many countries in Europe and Asia in which leptospirosis is highly endemic, vaccine prophylaxis is widely practiced.

Remaining Problems

Current laboratory procedures rarely provide a rapid confirmation during the critically important first stage of leptospirosis when it could best serve the clinician. There is a lack of information on virulence factors and how they relate to pathogenesis and icterogenic tendencies. The relative paucity of histologic changes in organs compared with the profound alteration in functions remains unexplained. There is a critical need for a therapeutic agent that can cure the patient even when given late in the course of disease.

Bibliography

Books

ALEXANDER AD: Leptospira. In Lennette EH, Balows A, Haesler WH Jr, Truant JP (eds): Manual of Clinical Microbiology 3rd ed. Washington, DC, American Society for Microbiology. 1980. pp 376–382.

ALEXANDER AD: Serological diagnosis of leptospirosis. In Rose NR, Friedman H (eds): Manual of Clinical Immunology, 2nd ed. Washington, DC, American Society for Microbiology, 1980. pp 542–546.

ALSTON JM, BROOM JC: Leptospirosis in Man and Animals. London, E & S Livingstone, 1958. 367 pp.

KAUFMAN AF: Epidemiological trends of leptospirosis in the United States, 1965–1974. In Johnson RC(ed): The Biology of Parasitic Spirochetes. New York, Academic Press, 1976. pp 177–189.

Journals

BERMAN SJ, TSAR CC, HOLMES K, FRESH JW, WATTEN RH: Sporadic anicteric leptospirosis in Sout Vietnam: A study in 150 patients. Ann Intern Med 79:167–173, 1973

DIAX-RIVERA RS, HALL HE, RAMOS–MORALES KY, SWISHER JA JR, DEJESUS JA, BENENSON AS: Leptospirosis in Puerto Rico: Clinical aspects of human infection. Zoonos Res 2:159–177, 1963

EDWARDS GA, DOMM BM: Human leptospirosis. Medicine 39:117–156, 1960

FEIGEN RD, ANDERSON DC: Human leptospirosis. CRC Crit Rev Clin Lab Sci 5:413–467, 1975

HEATH CW JR, ALEXANDER AD, GALTON MM: Leptospirosis in the United States: Analysis of 483 cases in man, 1949–1961. N Engl J Med 273:857–864; 915–922, 1965

Leptospiral serotype distribution lists according to host and geographic area. Atlanta, GA, US Dept Health, Education and Welfare, Center for Disease Control, 1966 (Supplement 1975)

MCCRUMB FR JR, STOCKARD JL, ROBINSON CR, TURNER LH, LEVIS DG, MAISEY CW, KELLEHER MF, GLEISER CA, SMADEL JE: Leptospirosis in Malaya. 1: Sporadic cases among military and civilian personnel. Am J Trop Med Hyg 6:238–256, 1957

Morbidity and Mortality Weekly Report. Annual Summary 1980. Center for Disease Control 29:48, 1981

RUTH M. LAWRENCE

77 Pancreatitis and Pancreatic Abscesses

Pancreatitis is an inflammatory condition of the pancreas that may vary from a brief, mild illness characterized by interstitial edema to a fulminant disease associated with widespread hemorrhage and necrosis of the gland.

Etiology

The pancreatic inflammatory process is the result of chemical digestion consequent to the release of enzymes normally contained within the gland. Many inciting factors and associated conditions have been recognized: infectious agents, biliary tract disease, alcoholism, trauma, hyperparathyroidism, and hyperlipidemia. Infectious agents, for example, mumps virus (Chap. 74, Mumps) and Group B coxsackievirus (Chap. 149, Coxsackievirus and Echovirus Infections), cause only a small proportion of all cases of pancreatitis. However, secondary bacterial infection of the diseased gland is not uncommon and can lead to the formation of abscesses.

Between 1935 and 1945 emergency surgical exploration was frequently performed on patients with acute pancreatitis. A variety of aerobic bacteria, including *Streptococcus pyogenes, Staphylococcus aureus, Escherichia coli,* and other enteric bacilli were cultured from the pancreas and surrounding areas of inflammation. These same bacteria were cultured from pancreatic abscesses that were drained surgically during the decade 1963–1973 (Table 77-1). In about half the pancreatic abscesses, more than one kind of bacteria may be cultured. Because adequate techniques for anaerobic culture were either not generally available or not applied, it is likely that anaerobic bacteria were missed both in acute pancreatitis and in pancreatic abscesses. In more recent experience, the preoperative use of antimicrobics effective against anaerobes may account for the paucity of anaerobic bacteria.

Epidemiology

Pancreatitis occurs at any age but is rare during childhood. The sexes are affected equally often, but the underlying or precipitating events vary according to sex. Pancreatitis associated with biliary tract disease is more common in females, whereas association with alcoholism and trauma is more common in males. The true incidence of pancreatitis is difficult to determine. Autopsy series report incidences varying from less than 1% to over 50% because of different pathologic criteria. Of 279 patients who came to autopsy in Philadelphia in 1964, interstitial pancreatitis was present in 15.4%. The process was considered to be acute in less than 3%.

Pathogenesis and Pathology

Autodigestion of the pancreas by activation of precursor proteolytic enzymes contained within the pancreas is believed to be the initial event in pancreatitis. Tissue hypoxia, acidosis, trauma, endotoxins, exotoxins, and other factors convert proenzymes such as trypsinogen and chymotrypsinogen to trypsin and chymotrypsin. These activated enzymes digest cell membranes with subsequent activation of other enzymes (phospholipase, elastase) resulting in extensive tissue damage, interstitial edema, hemorrhage, and necrosis. Histamine and bradykinin are activated and contribute to further vasodilation and edema because of increased vascular permeability. The pancreas becomes swollen and edematous, and usually contains small, yellowish, waxy areas of lipid necrosis. With recurrent attacks of pancreatitis, acinar cells are replaced by collagen, proteinaceous material accumulates in the ducts, and ductal calculi may form.

Pancreatic abscesses result when an area of necrosis becomes infected. The exact route of infection is not known but pancreatic infection may result from

Table 77-1. Bacteriology of 152 Pancreatic Abscesses

Bacteria	Occurrences
Polymicrobial	61
Monomicrobial	67
No growth or unknown	24
Escherichia coli	57
Enterobacter aerogenes	35
Staphylococcus aureus	22
Proteus spp.	22
Enterococcus	12
Pseudomonas aeruginosa	13
Streptococcus spp.	7

hematogenous seeding, from lymphatic spread from the gallbladder or colon, from infected bile, or it may occur transmurally from the adjacent colon. Because of the retroperitoneal location of the pancreas, the infection may involve the lesser omental sac, may spread upward to the subphrenic spaces, pleura, and mediastinum, or may spread downward along the psoas muscles.

Manifestations

Acute pancreatitis is classically manifested by severe epigastric pain that may be referred to the back. The pain may be mild and short-lived, or the attack may be fulminant with severe pain, hypotension, and shock. Frequently, there is a history of recent heavy ingestion of food and alcohol. On physical examination the patient appears anxious and restless. The abdomen is usually tender in the epigastrium with guarding and spasm; bowel sounds may be present or absent depending on the extent of associated ileus. Manifestations of underlying/associated conditions, such as jaundice, xanthomas, or spider angiomas, may be present. The patient's temperature is usually normal early in pancreatitis but rises within the first few days. A leukocytosis (10,000–20,000/mm^3) with increased polymorphonuclear leukocytes is usually present.

Diagnosis

Pancreatitis must be differentiated from a variety of other acute abdominal conditions such as acute cholecystitis, perforated peptic ulcer, and intestinal obstruction. Measurements of the concentration of amylase and lipase in the serum are the most helpful laboratory tests. However, the concentration of amylase in the serum may also be elevated when there is inflammation of the salivary glands and in the presence of other inflammatory intra-abdominal processes. In addition, the serum amylase may fall rapidly despite progressing pancreatitis. Urinary amylase and serum lipase may remain elevated after the serum amylase has returned to normal.

The increased urinary clearance of amylase relative to clearance of creatinine (C_{Am}/C_{Cr}) has been used to separate pancreatitis from other causes of elevated amylase. This ratio, normally less than 4%, is calculated using the formula:

$$\frac{C_{Am}}{C_{Cr}} = \frac{[\text{urine amylase}]}{[\text{serum amylase}]} \times \frac{[\text{serum creatinine}]}{[\text{urine creatinine}]} \times 100$$

The ratio is uniformly elevated in severe pancreatitis but it is still not known whether it is consistently elevated in milder cases of pancreatitis. Isoamylase analysis can be used to differentiate pancreatic from non-pancreatic amylase. The finding of high concentrations of amylase in peritoneal or pleural fluid is helpful in the confirmation of acute pancreatitis.

In severe hemorrhagic pancreatitis, physical signs of the hemorrhage may develop after several days: bluish periumbilical discoloration (Cullen's sign), and blue discoloration in the flanks (Grey Turner's sign). The presence of methemalbuminemia (evidenced by brown discoloration of the serum in severe cases) may help to distinguish hemorrhagic from edematous pancreatitis.

The radiologic signs of acute pancreatitis include widening of the duodenal sweep, edematous thickening of the bowel wall, a single dilated loop of small bowel in the left upper quadrant—the "sentinel loop sign,"—or an abrupt cutoff of colonic gas in the region of the splenic flexure—the "colon cutoff sign." In chronic pancreatitis, radiopaque calcium carbonate calculi may be visible in the region of the gland. A pancreatic abscess should be suspected when a patient with acute pancreatitis has persistent fever and abdominal tenderness or evidences clinical worsening 2 to 3 weeks following initial improvement. Formation of an abscess usually results in spiking fever, leukocytosis, bacteremia, nausea, vomiting, and the presence of a mass or fullness in the region of the pancreas. With the exception of hectic fever and bacteremia, the same features may also accompany formation of a pseudocyst.

By ultrasonic scanning, the normal pancreas is a strong echo-producing organ that is readily distinguishable from nearby loops of bowel. In contrast, the edematous pancreas is nearly devoid of echoes. Pseudocysts are marked by a rounded, echo-free area within the pancreatic region. Because ultrasound examination may not permit differentiation of a

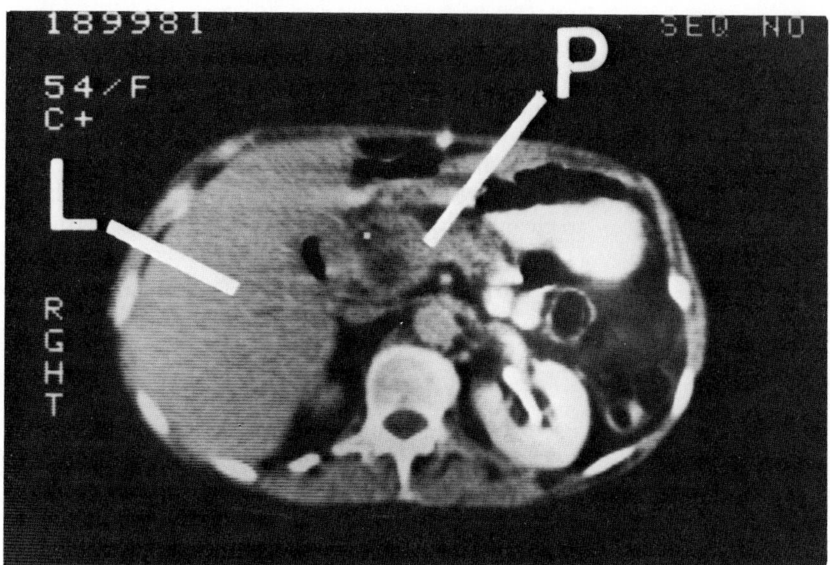

Fig. 77-1. Computed tomographic abdominal scan of a 54-year-old woman. *L* = liver; *P* = pancreas. The head of the pancreas is enlarged and contains multiple, low-density areas which are consistent with either pseudocyst or abscess.

pseudocyst from a pancreatic abscess, percutaneous aspiration of the liquid-filled mass may be required to exclude infection.

With computed tomography (CT), the pancreas can be distinguished from retroperitoneal fat, and lesions within the pancreas may be delineated (Fig. 77-1). The demonstration of gas in the pancreatic parenchyma by CT scan almost always means that infection is present even when an abscess cavity is not defined. By defining the limits of the abscess, CT aids the surgeon in deciding how to achieve drainage.

Prognosis

The mortality of acute pancreatitis varies from 0% to 10% with mild, edematous disease, to 50% to 80% with severe hemorrhagic necrosis. In uncomplicated cases, the edema and inflammation subside over 5 to 7 days. Complications include recurrent bouts of pancreatitis, formation of pseudocysts (collections of uninfected pancreatic liquid within the pancreas), abscesses, and the late complications of chronic pancreatitis, that is, impaired glucose tolerance and malabsorption of dietary fats. About 4% of all patients with acute pancreatitis develop abscesses, and the incidence is highest in those patients with the most severe disease. With surgical drainage, at least two-thirds of patients with abscesses survive. The course may be prolonged and complicated by the need for repeated surgical drainage or by rupture of the abscess into the peritoneal cavity or adjacent structures.

Therapy

Acute pancreatitis is usually treated with analgesics, nasogastric suction, and maintenance of circulating blood volume by intravenous administration of liquids containing crystalloids and colloids. The status of the intravascular volume must be monitored by determination of the hematocrit, urine output, and intravascular pressures by Swan–Ganz catheterization (in severe cases).

In most patients, symptoms resolve rapidly, and gradual increases in the diet over a 5 to 7 day period are tolerated. In mild, alcohol-associated pancreatitis, nasogastric suction does not bring about more rapid recovery and this may not be necessary. When pancreatitis is more severe, decompression of the stomach with a nasogastric tube may provide relief of pain. Of narcotic analgesics, meperidine is preferable for relief of pain because it causes fewer spasms of the sphincter of Oddi than morphine. Antacids may be administered through the nasogastric tube to neutralize gastric acid. Anticholinergic agents are not recommended because their value has not been established and their effects (tachycardia, intestinal ileus) may be confused with the effects of worsening pancreatitis. Histamine antagonists and glucagon have not been of value in acute pancreatitis. Somatostatin remains under clinical investigation but its value has not been established. Aprotinin (Trasylol) is an extract of beef salivary gland that inhibits trypsin and kallikrein *in vitro;* however, its efficacy in the treatment of pancreatitis has not been documented.

The concentrations of glucose and calcium in the

blood should be monitored. If hyperglycemia occurs, it should be treated with insulin; if tetany occurs, it should be treated with intravenous calcium gluconate. In fulminant pancreatitis, removal of extracellular enzymes by peritoneal lavage using a peritoneal dialysis catheter or multiple drains in the pancreatic bed and retroperitoneum may improve survival.

In some patients, surgical exploration may be necessary to exclude other causes of severe abdominal pain and shock.

The dreaded complications of acute pancreatitis are infection, renal failure, and severe pulmonary failure, attributed to the so-called adult respiratory distress syndrome. The pathophysiology remains unclear, but with supportive therapy the hypoxemia can be reversed.

The use of antimicrobics in acute pancreatitis has not been conclusively shown to reduce the incidence of pancreatic abscess or suppuration. Nevertheless, antimicrobics are frequently administered, such as ampicillin 100 mg to 150 mg/kg body wt/day as six equal portions given 4-hourly by IV injection. Although ampicillin is active against some aerobic gram-negative bacilli (*e.g., Escherichia coli*) and enteric streptococci, neither *Staphylococcus aureus* nor many of the nonsporulating anaerobic bacteria are likely to be affected.

Once the diagnosis of pancreatic abscess is established, prompt surgical drainage is required. At surgery, careful search for metastatic abscesses is necessary. Administration of antimicrobics prior to surgery is indicated.

Because polymicrobial infections are so common, two or more drugs are usually given. Gentamicin (or tobramycin or netilmicin), 5 mg to 6 mg/kg/body wt/day as three equal doses injected IV or IM 8-hourly, provides treatment for gram-negative aerobic bacilli and *S. aureus*. Either clindamycin, 20 mg to 40 mg/kg body wt/day as four equal portions injected IV 6-hourly; or chloramphenicol, 30 mg to 70 mg/kg body wt/day as four equal doses injected IV 6-hourly, provides activity against the anaerobic bowel flora and *S. aureus*. Surgical drainage may have to be repeated in about one-third of the patients.

Pancreatic pseudocysts are drained surgically by anastomosis of the cyst wall to the stomach or a loop of small bowel.

Chronic pancreatitis may be extremely difficult to treat because of intractable pain. Low-fat diets and anticholinergic drugs are not always effective. If pancreatic insufficiency with steatorrhea is present, pancreatic extracts (Viokase or Cotazym) 5 to 10 g daily by mouth, or supplements of medium chain triglycerides are useful. Surgery is usually not helpful unless there is a biliary tract lesion or ductal obstruction which can be corrected. Subtotal pancreatectomy may help to relieve pain when the gland is nonfunctional and the patient has intractable pain.

Prevention

Prevention of pancreatitis depends on amelioration of underlying pathology such as cholelithiasis or hyperlipidemia, abstinence from alcohol, and avoidance of trauma. Despite all preventive measures, about 20% of patients have recurrent attacks.

Remaining Problems

The exact sequence of intracellular events that trigger enzyme release and activation remains to be elucidated. The role of bacteria and their toxins has not been defined, nor is it known how either reaches the pancreas.

Bibliography

Journals

ALTEMEIER WA, ALEXANDER JW: Pancreatic abscess. Arch Surg 87:80–98, 1963

CAMER SJ, TAN EGC, WARREN KW, BRAASCH JW: Pancreatic abscess: A critical analysis of 113 cases. Am J Surg 129:426–431, 1975

EVANS FC: Pancreatic abscess. Am J Surg 117:537–540, 1969

FARRINGER JL, ROBBINS LB, PICKENS DR: Abscesses of the pancreas. Surgery 69:964–970, 1966

FREY CF, LINDENAUER SM, MILLER TA: Pancreatic abscess. Surg Gynecol Obstet 149:722–726, 1979

GEOKAS MC, VAN LANCKER JL, KADELL BM, MACHLEDER HI: Acute pancreatitis. Ann Intern Med 76:105–117, 1972

INTERIANO B, STUARD ID, HYDE RW: Acute respiratory distress syndrome in pancreatitis. Ann Intern Med 77:923–926, 1972

ISIKOFF M: Diagnostic imaging of the pancreas. Compr Ther 6:11–17, 1980

KODESCH R, DUPONT HL: Infectious complications of acute pancreatitis. Surg Gynecol Obstet 136:763–768, 1973

LEVITT MD: Clinical use of amylase clearance and isoamylase measurements. Mayo Clin Proc 54:428–431, 1979

REGAN PT: Medical treatment of acute pancreatitis. Mayo Clin Proc 54:432–434, 1979

SMITH FR, BARKEN JS: Complications of pancreatic inflammation. Compr Ther 6:32–36, 1980

WARSHAW AL: Pancreatic abscesses. N Engl J Med 287:1234–1236, 1972

CAROLYN COKER HUNTLEY

78 Visceral Larva Migrans

Visceral larva migrans (VLM) is a syndrome that occurs primarily in young children and is characterized by fever, pulmonary symptoms, hepatomegaly, and marked eosinophilia. It is caused by the migration of larval nematodes of nonhuman animal origin that are unable to complete their life cycles in humans. The classic syndrome, seen in preschool children, is the result of massive infection acquired by eating dirt. Light infections may be asymptomatic and probably occur in all age groups. The diagnosis of VLM is usually made on clinical grounds because the infecting larvae are difficult to demonstrate, even in biopsy material.

Etiology

VLM is most often caused by *Toxocara canis,* the common roundworm of dogs in the United States and the world. Puppies become infected *in utero* and begin to pass ova in the feces by 3 weeks of age. The eggs are 75 μm to 80 μm in diameter, undeveloped, and encased in a finely pitted, light brown shell. Counts of 15,000 ova per gram of feces have been recorded. Ova are passed in large numbers until the pup is 6 months of age, when the adult worms (6 cm–12 cm in length, white to reddish in color) may be passed spontaneously; the animal is less heavily infected thereafter. Humans become infected by the ingestion of ova that have become embryonated after a suitable period of incubation (about 30 days) in the soil.

Other nematodes of nonhuman animal origin occasionally cause the VLM syndrome: *Toxocara cati, Ascaris suum, Toxascaris leonina,* and *Capillaria hepatica. Ascaris suum,* the common roundworm of pigs, is a potential hazard for children exposed to infected swine on farms. The mode of infection of humans is similar to that described for *T. canis. Toxascaris leonina* may be the cause of VLM in northern Canada because it is prevalent in the dog population, whereas *T. canis* is absent. The life cycle of *T. leonina* differs from that of *T. canis,* since prenatal infection does not occur, and there is no migration through the lungs of the dog. Mice may act as transport hosts.

Capillaria hepatica, a common rat liver nematode, requires a second host (usually the cat) before the ova become infective for man. The cat eats the infected rat and passes the noninfective ova in the feces. The ova then become infective for man after embryonation in the soil. Eleven cases of infection in humans with this nematode have been reported. It is not known why infection of man with *C. hepatica* is rare in view of the high frequency of infection in rats.

Continuing reinfection with other worms that are classically parasitic in humans and have a tissue phase may produce similar syndromes. This group of helminths includes *Ascaris lumbricoides, Necator americanus,* and *Strongyloides stercoralis* (Chap. 68, Intestinal Nematodiasis). Tropical eosinophilia due to *Dirofilaria immitis* infection must also be considered in the differential diagnosis.

Epidemiology

Toxocara canis and other nematodes that cause the VLM syndrome occur worldwide in tropical and temperate areas. Soil from public parks commonly contains *T. canis;* for example, 24% of 800 soil samples obtained from public places in Britain were found to contain viable ova of *Toxocara* spp. Because of the ubiquity of the parasite, the true incidence of infection is undoubtedly greater than the number of reported cases indicates, and asymptomatic infections are probably the cause of many cases of unexplained eosinophilia. Boys are infected more often than girls by a ratio of 2:1.

Pathogenesis and Pathology

Following ingestion, the infective ova of *T. canis* hatch in the intestine. The second stage larvae migrate by way of the lymphatics and venules to the portal system and from there are disseminated throughout the body. Because of their small size (0.5 mm long × 0.2 mm in diameter), the second stage larvae of *T. canis* are not trapped in the capillaries of the lungs as are the larger third and fourth stage larvae of *Ascaris lumbricoides* (0.8 mm–1.5 mm long × 0.3 mm–0.5 mm in diameter). Accordingly, in primary infections, larvae of *T. canis* are found in all organs and tissues of the body, including the spinal cord and brain. This pattern is similar to that seen in primary infections in the mouse. In immune animals, larval migration through the liver is delayed, and the majority of the parasites are retained in the liver. In children who have suffered recurrent VLM infections, hepatomegaly is characteristically present.

The tissue reaction to the larvae varies with the site and duration of the infection. Granulomas form about the larvae with lymphocytes and eosinophiles predominating. Larval remnants may be seen within a granuloma or an intact larva may be found some distance away, having escaped from the granuloma. This continuing movement away from the site of tissue reaction explains the difficulty encountered in locating larvae in tissue sections. Very little cellular reaction is engendered in the brain; hemorrhagic tracts mark the path of migration. In the lung, an interstitial pneumonitis with eosinophilia is present in addition to the characteristic granulomas. Larvae do not develop beyond the second stage in man but may live for long periods in the tissues. They have been found to survive in the liver of the rhesus monkey for at least 7 years following infections.

The larvae of *Ascaris suum* migrate to the liver and lung but do not enter the systemic circulation because of their large size. Larvae as large as 4 mm in length have been recovered from sputum, but the worms rarely mature in the gut. Severe pneumonia and asthma may occur, which may lead to cyanosis and respiratory failure if the infecting dose is large.

Capillaria hepatica larvae invade the bowel and migrate to the liver where they mature, mate, and produce large numbers of ova. In fatal cases, the liver is markedly enlarged, and there is an intense inflammatory reaction surrounding the worms and ova. Eosinophils and giant cells are prominent.

Manifestations

Systemic Disease

The most frequently encountered symptoms and signs of VLM are fever, cough, wheezing, rales, and hepatomegaly; a history of pica is common. Less often, there are nausea and vomiting, abdominal pain, weight loss, malnutrition, maculopapular or urticarial skin lesions, splenomegaly, and lymphadenopathy. Muscle pain is an unusual symptom but may be severe. Central nervous system manifestations include ataxia, convulsions, hemiparesis, coma, and in one reported case, Guillain–Barré syndrome. Myocarditis occurs rarely, but may be fatal. Other fatalities have been caused by a bronchiolitislike syndrome and by encephalitis. Viruses may be important in the etiology of central nervous system manifestations associated with VLM.

Biopsy proven cases of VLM may be asymptomatic; the diagnosis may be suspected in such cases after routine blood studies demonstrate eosinophilia. More often, the clinical setting which leads to discovery of the eosinophilia is asthma or a febrile respiratory infection.

A peripheral blood eosinophilia of 30% or greater is an important diagnostic criterion. There is no absolute cutoff point, because the eosinophilia may vary widely from day to day in a given patient. Most patients have a leukocytosis which is sometimes massive (*e.g.*, 100,000/mm^3 or greater), with up to 80% eosinophiles. Iron deficiency anemia is present in at least half the patients.

The immunoglobulins of the blood are increased in concentration, with IgA least changed, IgG and IgM markedly elevated, and IgE showing proportionately the greatest rise. Thus, among 40 patients with VLM (clinical diagnosis supported by demonstration of precipitating antibody to toxocaral or ascarial antigens), the IgE concentrations varied 60 units to 26,400 units/ml with a mean of 2990 units. All but one value was greater than two standard deviations above the normal, age-adjusted mean.

Antibodies to group A and B human red blood cells are often IgG in type, and titers of such antibodies may be extremely high. It has been suggested that *T. canis* infection of pregnant women in tropical countries may contribute to an increased incidence of ABO hemolytic disease of the newborn.

Antihuman gammaglobulin antibodies can be detected by the latex agglutination test in almost half the cases of VLM, while other tests for rheumatoid factors are rarely positive. Antinuclear antibodies have not been found.

Radiographic examination of the chest may disclose no abnormalities, an asthmalike picture, or multiple fluffy infiltrates (Fig. 78-1). Liver function tests may be normal or slightly abnormal.

Ocular Lesions

The ocular lesions of *T. canis* infection rarely occur during the systemic disease syndrome of VLM. In the usual case of ocular toxocariasis, the patient gives either a history compatible with VLM several years previously or no history of VLM at all. The eye lesions are seen in children over 4 years of age and are not associated with abnormalities of immunoglobulins. There are three kinds of lesions: (1) posterior pole granulomas, (2) peripheral choroidal lesions often associated with elevated retinal folds extending to the disk, and (3) diffuse endophthalmitis with retinal detachment.

Diagnosis

VLM should be suspected when hypereosinophilia (greater than 3000 eosinophils/mm^3) is found in a young child who has a dog and eats dirt. If there has been exposure to pigs rather than dogs, VLM caused by *Ascaris suum* should be suspected. The diagnois can be confirmed by finding the larvae of *Toxocara* spp. in the liver. The presence of precipitating antibody to *T. canis* antigens in the patient's serum also confirms the diagnosis; false-positive reactions have not been encountered with this test. Because a high titer of antibody is necessary for a positive reaction, low-grade infections or specimens obtained late in the course of the disease may give negative results. Patients with precipitins to *T. canis* often have precipitins to *A. suum* and to A and B substances of nonhuman animal origin, presumably because of cross-reactivity of the various antigens. Elevated immunoglobulin concentrations and isohemagglutinin titers are suggestive but not diagnostic.

Other tests include bentonite flocculation, hemagglutination, and skin tests. The problem with all these tests is the lack of a specific antigen—all will cross-react with antigens of other helminths and with human A and B blood group substances. The most promising new developments use larval antigens or secretory-excretory antigens from cultures of *T. canis* larvae in various test systems including hemagglutination, fluorescent antibody techniques, enzyme linked immunosorbent assay (ELISA), or radioimmunoassay (RIA). Recently, a macromolecular antigen has been identified in extracts of adult *A. suum* worms, which precipitates the serum from *T. canis*-infected, but not *A. suum*-infected, rabbits and does not cross-react with A or B blood group substances, or Forssman antigen. The preparation of this

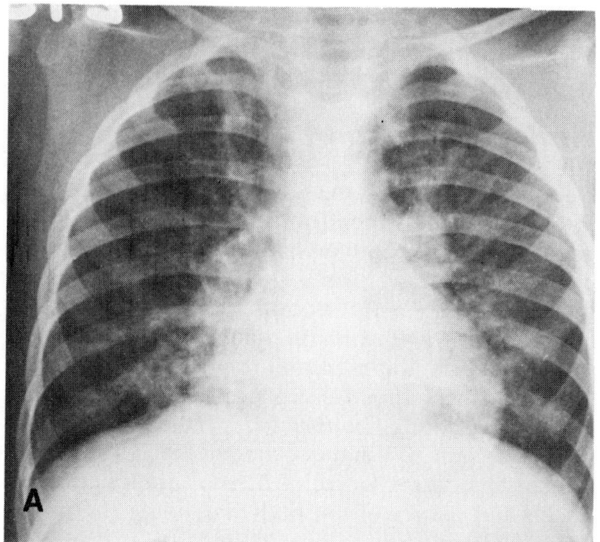

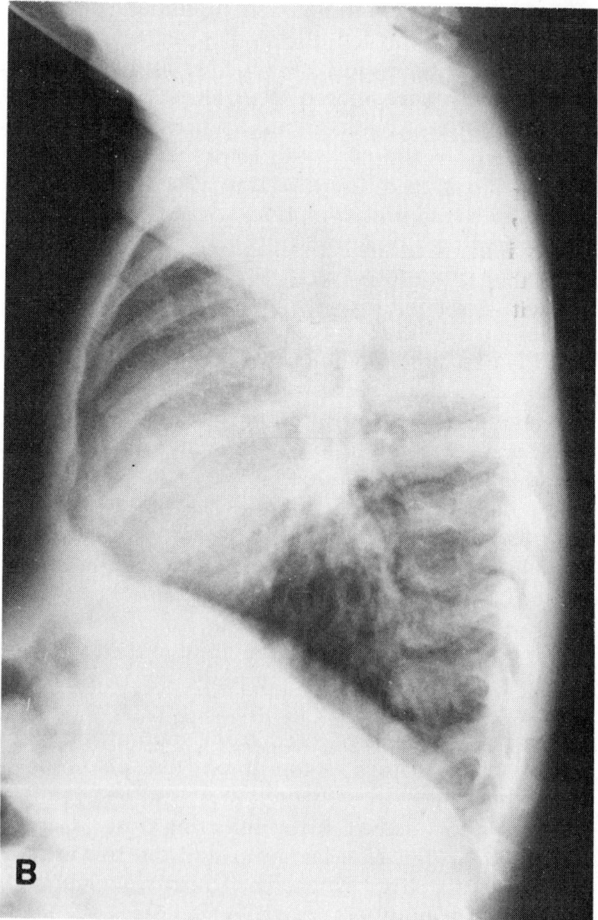

Fig. 78-1. Patient with acute visceral larva migrans. There is hyperaeration and bilateral pulmonary infiltration, primarily involving the lower lobes. (*A*) Posterior–anterior view. (*B*) Left lateral view.

antigen, which apparently is the same as or cross-reacts with an important *T. canis* larval antigen, does not require working with the infective stage of the worm and shows promise for use with ELISA or RIA techniques.

Patients with VLM should always be studied for intestinal helminthic infections because any child with pica may have acquired more than one kind of worm. *Strongyloides stercoralis* larvae, not ova, must be searched for in liquid feces following catharsis using direct, not flotation, techniques. Strongyloidiasis should be suspected in the presence of eosinphilia when gastrointestinal symptoms are marked, in elderly patients, and in patients who have been treated with glucosteroids or immunosuppressive drugs.

Because children with VLM have pica, in addition to eating dirt they may also ingest cigarette butts and many other nonfood materials. Thus, poisoning from hydrocarbon ingestion or lead poisoning may lead to medical consultation, with VLM discovered secondarily.

Eosinophilic leukemia is almost unknown in children. Examination of the bone marrow is usually unnecessary unless thrombocytopenia is present or blasts are found in the peripheral blood. Liver biopsy is not indicated except when immunologic tests for *Toxocara* spp. and ascarids are negative, and hepatomegaly is marked. Liver biopsy should be carried out under these circumstances in order to rule out infection with *Capillaria hepatica*.

Prognosis

The outcome, even in massive VLM infections, is usually good; complete resolution of all symptoms and signs is to be expected. Eye involvement may occur years after the acute illness. The parents should be made aware of the diagnosis so that if eye lesions eventually appear, the ophthalmologist can be informed of the preceding disease.

Very ill patients may die during the acute phase of the disease from pulmonary, myocardial, or CNS involvement. Occasionally, a patient develops chronic liver disease as a consequence of continuing reinfection.

Therapy

There is no convincing evidence that specific drug therapy is of value either in the treatment of acute VLM or in prevention of eye involvement. Studies of experimental infections in mice have shown that diethylcarbamazine (Hetrazan) decreases the number of larvae recoverable from the tissues. Thiabendazole was also tested in mice and failed to kill larvae. If diethylcarbamazine is used, the dosage is, 12 mg/kg body wt/day, PO, as four equal portions, 6-hourly, for 3 weeks. A concomitant infection with *Ascaris lumbricoides* should be treated with piperazine (Chap. 68, Intestinal Nematodiasis) or mebendazole before the use of diethylcarbamazine. (Diethylcarbamazine causes adult ascarids to migrate and possibly cause intestinal obstruction or perforation.) If eye lesions are present, anthelminthics should be given cautiously, if at all, and should be given only in association with glucosteroids. Glucosteriods are helpful in the treatment of endophthalmitis caused by *T. canis*. Patients who are seriously ill with wheezing and respiratory distress should be treated as for asthma with bronchodilators, for example, theophylline ethylenediamine (aminophylline) and glucosteroids. The iron deficiency must be adequately treated, and further pica must be prevented.

Sodium antimonylgluconate has been reported to be an effective treatment for *Capillaria hepatica*.

Prevention

The public health hazard posed by the increasing canine population, most of which is infected during the early months of life, is not appreciated in the United States. Once the soil has become infected, there is no effective method of killing the ova, and it is sometimes necessary for families to move to other locations if pica cannot be prevented. Frequent worming of puppies and proper disposal of canine fecal material are essential to preventing the spread of *T. canis* to humans. As long as puppies are allowed to run free and defecate in areas frequented by children, the incidence and severity of VLM will increase.

Bibliography

Book

LEVINE ND: Nematode Parasites of Domestic Animals and of Man. Minneapolis, Burgess Publishing, 2nd ed, 1980. 477 pp.

Journals

ANDERSON DC, GREENWOOD R, FISHMAN M, KAGAN IG: Acute infantile hemiplegia with cerebrospinal fluid eosinophilic pleocytosis: An unusual case of visceral larva migrans. J Pediatr 86:247–249, 1975

BENCROFT DM: Infection by the dog roundworm *Toxocara canis* and fatal myocarditis. NZ Med J 63:729–732, 1964

COCHRANE JC, SAGORIN L, WILCOCKS MG: Capillaria hepatica infection in man. S Afr Med J 31:751–755, 1957

DAFALLA AA: A study of the effect of diethylcarbamazine and

thiabendazole on experimental *Toxocara canis* infection in mice. Am J Trop Med Hyg 75:158–159, 1972

HUNTLEY CC, COSTAS MC, LYERLY A: Visceral larva migrans syndrome: clinical characteristics and immunologic studies in 51 patients. Pediatrics 36:523–536, 1965

HUNTLEY CC, LYERLY AD, LITTLEJOHN MP, RODRIGUEZ–TRIAS MD, BOWERS GW: ABO hemolytic disease in Puerto Rico and North Carolina. Pediatrics 57:875–883, 1976

MIKHAEL NZ, MONTPETIT VJA, ORIZAGA M, ROWSELL HC, RICHARD MT: *Toxocara canis* infestation with encephalitis. Can J Neurol Sci 1:114–120, 1974

NICHOLS RL: The etiology of visceral larva migrans. II. Comparative larval morphology of *Ascaris lumbricoides,* Necator americanus, *Strongyloides stercoralis* and *Anclystoma* caninum. J Parasitol 42:363–399, 1956

PHILLS JA, HARROLD AJ, WHITEMAN GV, PERELMUTTER L: Pulmonary infiltrates, asthma and eosinophilia due to *Ascaris suum* infestation in man. N Engl J Med 286:965–970, 1972

PIKE EH: Effect of diethylcarbamazine, oxophenarsine hydrochloride and piperazine citrate on *Toxocara canis* larvae in mice. Exp Parasitol 9:223–232, 1960

SILVERMAN NH, KATZ JS, LEVIN SE: Capillaria hepatica infestation in a child. S Afr Med J 47(6):219–221, 1973

SPRENT JFA: Observations on the development of *Toxocara canis.* Parasitology 48:184–209, 1958

WILKINSON CP, WELCH RB: Intraocular Toxocara. Am J Ophthalmol 71:921–930, 1971

PETER M. SCHANTZ

79 Larval Cestodiasis

Most of the larval cestodes that infect humans (Table 79-1) are members of the family Taeniidae (Order: Cyclophyllidea); they have bladderlike larval forms (metacestodes), each with one or more protoscolices. The life cycles of all taeniid cestodes require two hosts; cyclical transmission occurs as a result of the predator-prey relationship existing between hosts. All these infections are zoonoses, and with one exception humans are nonessential (accidental) hosts. For *Taenia solium,* humans are the sole definitive host; however, the role of humans as intermediate hosts to the larval form of this cestode is accidental in the ecologic sense. The metacestode forms of *Echinococcus* spp. characteristically develop numerous protoscolices and are referred to as hydatid cysts or hydatids. Otherwise, *Echinococcus* spp. vary greatly in host specificity, geographic distribution, and the diseases produced.

At least three species of *Echinococcus* infect humans: *E. granulosus, E. multilocularis,* and *E. vogeli;* they cause, respectively, cystic, alveolar, and polycystic forms of hydatid disease. A fourth species, *E. oligarthrus,* occurs in Central and South America, and has not been shown to cause disease in humans.

Humans become infected with taeniid larvae by ingesting the tapeworm eggs passed in the feces of infected, definitive hosts. In the case of sparganosis, the only nontaeniid cestodiasis described in this chapter, humans become infected when they ingest the first or second stage larvae of *Spirometra* spp. in invertebrate or vertebrate intermediate hosts, respectively.

The wide range of pathologic processes and manifestations produced by larval cestodes is mainly related to differences in host-parasite compatibility and localization. Some kinds of larval cestodiasis, such as cystic hydatid disease, and cysticercosis are widespread geographically and are among the major helminthic diseases of humans, whereas others occur only rarely.

Cysticercosis (Taenia solium)

Etiology

Cysticercosis is a disease caused by infection with the metacestode or larval form of *T. solium.* The typical cysticercus is a tiny, ellipsoid bladder with a white translucent membrane that contains a single spherical, invaginated protoscolex bathed in a small amount of clear liquid.

Fully developed cysticerci in the intermuscular tissues or cerebral parenchyma are 1 cm to 2 cm in diameter; when growth is less restricted, for example, in the cerebral ventricles and the subarachnoid space, cysticerci may grow to 3 cm to 6 cm in diameter and sometimes take the form of an acephalic, lobate (racemose) structure with connecting branches.

Epidemiology

The life cycle of *T. solium* involves humans as definitive hosts and swine as natural, intermediate hosts. Humans acquire intestinal taeniasis (see Chap. 69, Intestinal Cestodiasis) by ingesting pork from infected pigs; cysticercosis is contracted by ingesting the eggs of *T. solium* either from the patient's own intestinal infection (autoinfection) or from the feces of other infected persons. Autoinfection is either external—the ingestion of eggs passed in the patient's own feces—or, conceivably, internal—the hatching of eggs transported into the stomach by retroperistalsis of gravid proglottids or loose eggs. It is not known how often internal autoinfection occurs; only about one-third of patients with cysticercosis have a history of taeniasis.

Essential to the propagation of *T. solium* is the practice of eating raw or inadequately cooked pork. The disease is virtually unknown in predominantly Muslim communities in which pork is not eaten. A common characteristic of areas in which *T. solium* is endemic is the practice of allowing pigs to run loose and scavenge. The coprophagic habits of pigs make

Table 79-1. *Larval Cestodes and Some Characteristics of the Infections They Cause in Humans*

Disease	Cestode Agent	Predominant Sites of Localization
Cysticercosis	*Taenia solium*	Muscles, central nervous system, eyes; occasionally other sites
Cystic hydatid	*Echinococcus granulosus*	Liver and lungs; less frequently kidneys, spleen, bones, central nervous system; other sites
Alveolar hydatid	*Echincoccus multilocularis*	Liver; other sites by extension and metastasis
Polycystic hydatid	*Echinococcus vogeli*	Liver and peritoneum
Coenurosis	*Taenia (Multiceps)* spp.	Central nervous system, eyes, subcutaneous tissues
Sparganosis	*Spirometra* spp.	Subcutaneous tissues, eyes

them particularly efficient hosts for this parasite. The highest incidence of cysticercosis is in Mexico, Central and South America (especially Peru, Bolivia, Brazil, Ecuador, Colombia, and Chile), India, and parts of Africa and the Far East. The incidence is lower in eastern European countries, Spain, and Portugal. The infection has all but disappeared from Western Europe and the Soviet Union. In the United States, infections are seen predominantly in Mexicans and Mexican Americans.

Pathogenesis and Pathology

After ingestion, the eggs of *T. solium* hatch in the duodenum. The released embryos (oncospheres) penetrate the intestinal mucosa, gain access to the circulatory system, and distribute to extraenteric sites where they develop as larval cysts. In the pig, the cysticerci of *T. solium* localize most frequently within the lymphatic capillaries of the skeletal muscles and in the brain. In humans, cysticerci also occur most frequently in skeletal muscles, but the manifestations that lead to diagnosis emanate from localization in the central nervous system (CNS). Within the CNS 1 to more than 1000 cysticerci may occur in the meninges, the ventricles, the subarachnoid space, or the brain substance. Less frequently, cysticerci may localize in the eyes, skin, and heart. Unless massive numbers of cysticerci are present, the initial host tissue reaction is minimal. The developing cysticercus affects the surrounding tissues as a slowly growing mass that may cause pressure atropy. Although most live cysts do not engender an inflammatory reaction, an acute response occurs when the cysts die and degenerate—an occurrence that may not take place until several years after the initial infection. The necrotic larvae are partially absorbed, but may become calcified and result in focal scarring.

Manifestations

The manifestations of cysticercosis are determined by the number and location of the cysticerci and by the extent of the inflammatory response of the host. The infection may be asymptomatic, or severe disease may result. Because the manifestations are so variable in kind and severity, the symptoms and signs are rarely diagnostic. The period between initial infection and the onset of symptoms is also variable and may be several months or many years; in a study of 450 cases among British soldiers in India, the average period between arrival in the endemic areas and onset of symptoms was 4.8 years.

Invasion of the CNS by many cysticerci at the time of dissemination may cause seizures in patients who only later develop subcutaneous nodules. In other patients, cerebral cysticercosis may become manifest later in the course of infection in association with the death and destruction of the larvae. Epilepsy is the most common feature and is present in more than 50% of cases. Although strictly focal symptoms may be present, generally there are multiple cysts scattered throughout the brain, and the surgical removal of a single cyst does not usually relieve the focal attacks. In some patients, increasing intracranial pressure may be the earliest sign. Cysticerci in the meninges may cause communicating hydrocephalus, often causing cranial nerve dysfunctions. Cysts within the ventricular system may cause internal hydrocephalus.

Prognosis

Symptomatic cerebral cysticercosis is ultimately fatal in a large proportion of cases. The mortality may be 25% in patients with signs of an intracranial tumor at the outset, and 65% if the initial symptoms were due to internal hydrocephalus. Among patients followed for 30 or more years, 48% improved or became free of symptoms, and 52% remained unchanged or became worse.

Diagnosis

Cysticercosis is relatively difficult to diagnose because the manifestations are nonspecific, and demonstration of the parasite is not usually feasible. Although a history compatible with exposure to the parasite is helpful, the physician might not ask the necessary questions. Roentgenography rarely demonstrates the larval cysts except in advanced cases in which calcification has occurred, whereas contrast studies may reveal avascular masses within the ventricles or brain substance (Fig. 79-1).

The etiology of subcutaneous nodules can often be determined by biopsy. Radiologic demonstration of calcified nodules of characteristic size and shape in the soft tissues also supports the diagnosis.

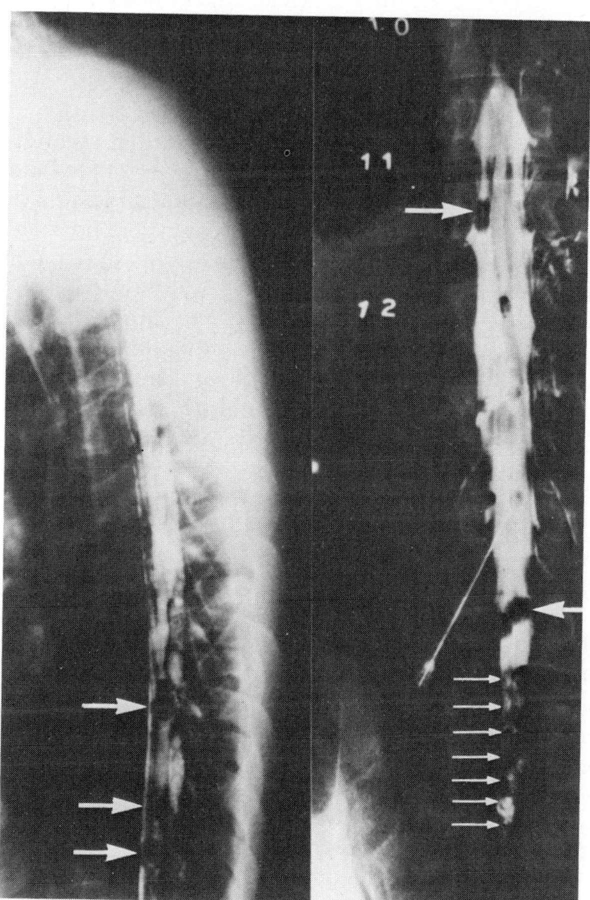

Fig. 79-1. Contrast radiographic examination of the spine of a patient with cysticercosis. Arrows point to filling defects caused by cysticerci. (Carmalt JE, Theis J, Goldstein E: West J Med 123:311–313, 1975)

Computed tomography (CT) scans may reveal the location of cysts, areas of atrophy, and degree of ventricular dilation. Eosinophilia is present only occasionally. The typical findings in the cerebrospinal fluid (CSF) are pleocytosis (with eosinophils), elevated protein, and low glucose. Detection of antibody in the serum supports the diagnosis but is nonspecific, and false negatives are common. Demonstration of antibody in the CSF is more reliable, but the sensitivity of the methods appears to be low.

Therapy

An effective chemotherapy for cysticercosis has not yet been developed. However, praziquantel, an agent shown to be effective in some forms of cysticercosis in nonhuman animals, has been dramatically successful in first trials in humans with cysticercosis. Surgical excision of lesions is curative; however, removal of all the cysticerci is rarely possible and surgery is palliative in most patients. Anticonvulsants are often effective in controlling epileptic episodes, and glucosteroids appear to be useful in the management of symptomatic crises. Persistence in such nonspecific control of symptoms may eventually result in self-cure with minimal residua as larvae die off and are resorbed.

Prevention

Eating only adequately cooked pork helps prevent *T. solium* taeniasis, but does not lessen the possibility of acquiring cysticercosis from carriers of *T. solium* in the endemic areas. The latter requires the assiduous application of hygiene, and particularly, the avoidance of all foods which might be contaminated with human feces.

Control of cysticercosis is always favored by enclosing pigs in pens. However, efficient and carefully regulated meat inspection programs, adequate disposal of infected swine carcasses, and effective health education are also important measures. Mass diagnosis and treatment of tapeworm infections in human populations in the U.S.S.R. was reported to be an effective preventive.

Cystic Hydatid Disease (Echinococcus granulosus)

Etiology

Cystic hydatid disease connotes liquid-filled, spherical, and unilocular cysts which arise in response to

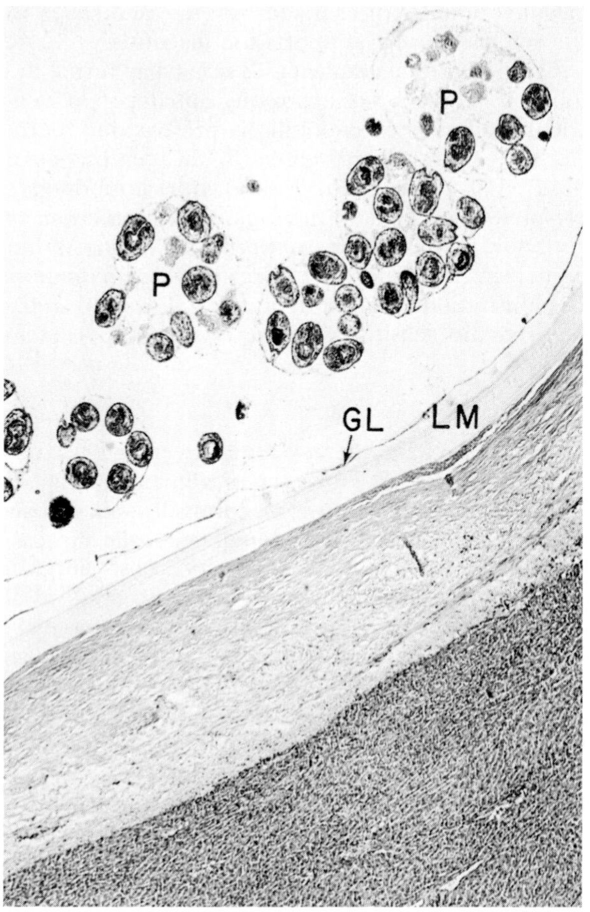

Fig. 79-2. Hydatid cyst of *Echinococcus granulosus* in liver of sheep showing larval protoscoleces (*P*) in brood capsules, germinal layer (*GL*), and laminated membrane (*LM*). (H&E approximately × 350)

infection with larval *Echinococcus granulosus*. Structurally, the cysts consist of an inner germinal layer of cells supported by a characteristic acidophilic-staining, acellular, laminated membrane of variable thickness (Fig. 79-2). Each cyst is surrounded by a host-produced layer of granulomatous adventitial reaction. Small vesicles called "brood capsules" bud internally from the germinal layer and produce multiple protoscolices by asexual division. In humans, the slowly growing hydatid cysts may attain a volume of many liters and contain many thousands of protoscolices.

Epidemiology

The life cycle of *E. granulosus* involves dogs and other canids as definitive hosts, and domestic and wild ungulates as intermediate hosts. At least two geographic strains or races of *E. granulosus* exist with different host ranges. The northern or sylvatic strain is maintained in wolves and wild ungulates (moose and reindeer) in northern Alaska, Canada, Scandinavia and Eurasia. The pastoral strain with greater pathogenicity for humans is maintained in dogs and domestic ungulates throughout the world. Sheep are the most important intermediate hosts, but swine, cattle, goats, horses, and camels are susceptible and assume dominant importance in certain regions.

Certain activities of humans (*e.g.*, the widespread rural practice of feeding dogs with the viscera of home-butchered sheep) facilitate transmission of the pastoral strain and consequently increase the risk that humans will become infected. Dogs infected with tapeworms pass eggs in their feces, and humans become infected through fecal–oral contact, particularly in the course of playful and intimate contact between children and dogs. Cestode eggs adhere to hairs around the infected dog's anus and are also found on the muzzle and paws. Indirect transfer of eggs either through contaminated water and uncooked food or through the intermediary of flies and other arthropods can also result in human infection. Taeniid eggs are extraordinarily resistant to environmental factors and can survive many months under most climatic conditions.

The greatest prevalence of cystic hydatid disease in humans and nonhuman animals is found in countries of the temperate zones including southern South America, the entire Mediterranean littoral, southern and central U.S.S.R., central Asia, Australia, and parts of Africa. In the United States, most infections are seen in immigrants from countries in which hydatid disease is highly endemic, but autochthonous transmission is currently recognized in Alaska, California, Utah, Arizona, and New Mexico.

Pathogenesis and Pathology

Following ingestion, cestode eggs hatch to release embryos in the small intestine. Penetration through the mucosa leads to blood-borne distribution to the liver and other sites in which the development of cysts begins. Most primary infections in humans consist of a single cyst; however, 20% to 40% of patients have multiple cysts or multiple organ involvement. The liver is the most common site of the hydatid cyst of the pastoral strain (more than 65%), followed by the lungs (25%), and the cyst is less frequently seen in the spleen, kidneys, heart, bone, and CNS. However, cysts of the northern sylvatic strain of this cestode localize predominantly in the lungs, and the disease that results is more benign and uncomplicated than that caused by the pastoral strain. The rates of growth of cysts are highly variable and range from 1 cm to 5 cm in diameter per year. The slowly growing hydatid cyst is often well tolerated until it causes dysfunction because of its size. If a cyst ruptures, the sudden release of its contents may precipitate allergic reactions ranging from mild to fatal anaphylaxis. In the lungs, ruptured cyst membranes may be evacuated entirely through the bronchi or retained to serve as a nidus for bacterial infection. Dissemination of protoscolices may result in multiple secondary hydatid disease. Larval growth in bones is atypical; when it occurs, invasion of marrow cavities and spongiosa is common and causes extensive erosion of the bone.

Manifestations

The clinical manifestations of cystic hydatid disease are variable and determined by the site, size, and condition of the cysts. The period between first infection and clinical manifestations is also variable and often prolonged for many years. Most infections are diagnosed in patients between 10 and 50 years old. The signs and symptoms of hepatic hydatid disease may include hepatic enlargement (with or without a palpable mass in the right upper quadrant), right epigastric pain, nausea, and vomiting. Rupture or leakage usually results in acute or intermittent allergic manifestations. Complications that existed at the time of initial presentation in 7% of Australian patients include traumatic or spontaneous rupture, thoracobilia, and biliary fistula. One-fourth of the patients with hepatic cysts also had cysts in the lungs.

Intact hydatid cysts in the lungs may cause no symptoms, but leakage or rupture of the cysts may cause chest pain, coughing, dyspnea, and hemoptysis. Complications which existed in 20% of Australian patients at the time of initial presentation included cyst rupture and secondary bacterial infections. Nearly 40% of patients with pulmonary hydatidiasis have liver involvement as well. The first symptom of cerebral cysts may be elevated intracranial pressure or focal epilepsy. Renal cysts may be manifested by loin pain or hematuria. Cysts in bones are often asymptomatic until pathologic fractures occur.

Diagnosis

The presence of a cystlike mass in a person with a history of exposure to dogs or sheep in areas in which *E. granulosus* is endemic supports the diagnosis of hydatid disease.

Roentgenography permits the detection of hydatid cysts in the lungs; in other sites, calcification is necessary for visualization (Fig. 79-3). Radioisotopic and ultrasonic scanning, computerized axial tomography, and angiography are useful for detecting the avascular cysts in many organs. Closed aspiration of cysts should not be carried out because spillage may cause anaphylaxis or secondary lesions. Protoscolices may sometimes be demonstrated in sputum or bronchial washings; identification of hooklets is facilitated by acid-fast stains. Eosinophilia is present in less than 25% of infected persons.

Serologic tests, including indirect hemagglutination, latex agglutination, and immunoelectrophoresis, are often useful, although some patients with hydatidiasis do not develop a detectable immune response. Hepatic cysts are more likely to elicit an immune response than pulmonary cysts; nearly 50% of patients with intact hyaline cysts of the lungs are

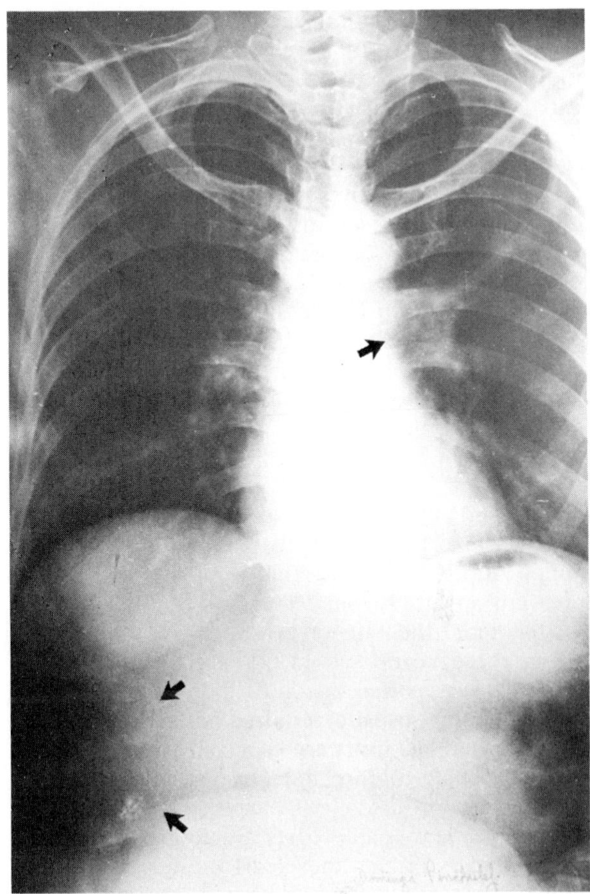

Fig. 79-3. Chest roentgenogram of a woman demonstrating two partially calcified hydatid cysts of the liver and a single cyst of the left lung (*arrows*). (Schantz PM, Williams JF, Posse CR: Am J Trop Med Hyg 22:629–641, 1973)

seronegative. From the fact that fissuring or rupture of cysts is followed by an abrupt rise in titer of antibodies, it appears that the sensitivity of serologic tests is inversely related to the degree of sequestration of hydatid antigens inside cysts, regardless of location. The direct hemagglutination and latex agglutination tests are highly sensitive procedures for the initial screening of serums; specific confirmation of reactivity can be obtained with immunodiffusion tests which detect the *Echinococcus* "arc 5." The sensitivity of skin tests is comparable to that of serologic tests; however, skin tests are less specific.

Cystic hydatid disease must be differentiated from cavitary tuberculosis, mycosis, abscess, and benign or malignant neoplasms.

Prognosis

If diagnosed before rupture, surgical removal of hydatid cysts may be possible with a minimum risk of complications. The case-fatality ratio with surgical intervention varies from 2% to 10%. In one study of 106 patients, the rate of postoperative recurrence within three years was 11%. Extensive secondary hydatid disease often becomes inoperable. Involvement of bones usually requires amputation of the limb. Cysts in the heart are especially dangerous because they may rupture and cause systemic dissemination of the protoscolices, anaphylaxis, and cardiac tamponade. Few viable cysts are found in patients over 60 years of age; therefore, these patients may often be managed without surgery. Nonsurgical treatment is generally adequate for pulmonary infections with the more benign northern sylvatic strain.

Therapy

Surgical removal of the hydatid cyst remains the most effective treatment. The aim of surgery is total removal of the cyst while avoiding the adverse consequences of spillage of cyst contents. Cetrimide (5%), hypertonic saline (20%), and other chemicals are often injected into hydatid cysts at the time of surgical operation to inactivate the protoscolices prior to manipulation of the cyst.

Surgery may not be possible because of the general condition of the patient and the extent or location of the cysts. Under such conditions, treatment with mebendazole may be tried, although the results are unpredictable and adverse reactions have been reported. Pulmonary cysts of *E. granulosus* seem to respond best, hepatic cysts less dramatically, and cysts in other locations, particularly brain, bone, and eye, poorly if at all. For *E. granulosus,* mebendazole 50 mg to 150 mg/kg of body weight/day perorally as a single dose for three months is probably the minimal effective dose; many patients require repeated courses.

Prevention

In endemic areas, preventive measures available include careful personal hygiene, strict dietary regulation of pet dogs to preclude ingestion of sheep offal, and avoidance of dogs that are not so regulated. Prophylactic treatment of pet dogs at intervals might be necessary in some situations. Control measures applicable in communities include limitation of the numbers and movements of dogs, and reductions in the prevalence of *E. granulosus* below levels necessary for continued transmission. In Iceland, New Zealand, Cyprus, and the Australian state of Tasmania, educational, technical, and legislative measures have eliminated or vastly reduced the frequency of infection. However, in less advanced, pastoral societies, a variety of social, economic, and technical factors have prevented the implementation of effective control measures such as health education, regulation of livestock slaughtering in abattoirs and on farms, dog control, and periodic, diagnostic testing of dogs. The absence of effective vaccines and chemotherapy for the larval stages of *E. granulosus* further hinders control efforts.

Alveolar Hydatid Disease (Echinococcus multilocularis)

Etiology

Alveolar hydatid disease results from infection by larval *Echinococcus multilocularis.* In rodents, the natural intermediate hosts, the larval mass proliferates rapidly by exogenous budding of germinative tissue and produces an alveolarlike pattern of microvesicles filled with protoscolices (Fig. 79-4).

Epidemiology

The life cycle of *E. multilocularis* involves foxes and arvicolid rodents, an ecosystem generally separate from humans. However, there is ecologic overlap to humans, since domestic dogs or cats may become infected when they eat infected wild rodents. As a result, exposure of humans to *E. multilocularis* is relatively less common than exposure to *E. granulosus.* Alveolar hydatid disease has been reported in parts of central Europe, throughout much of the U.S.S.R., in the northwestern portion of Canada, and in western Alaska. The incidence appears to be increasing in central North America. Hunters, trappers, and persons who work with fox fur are most fre-

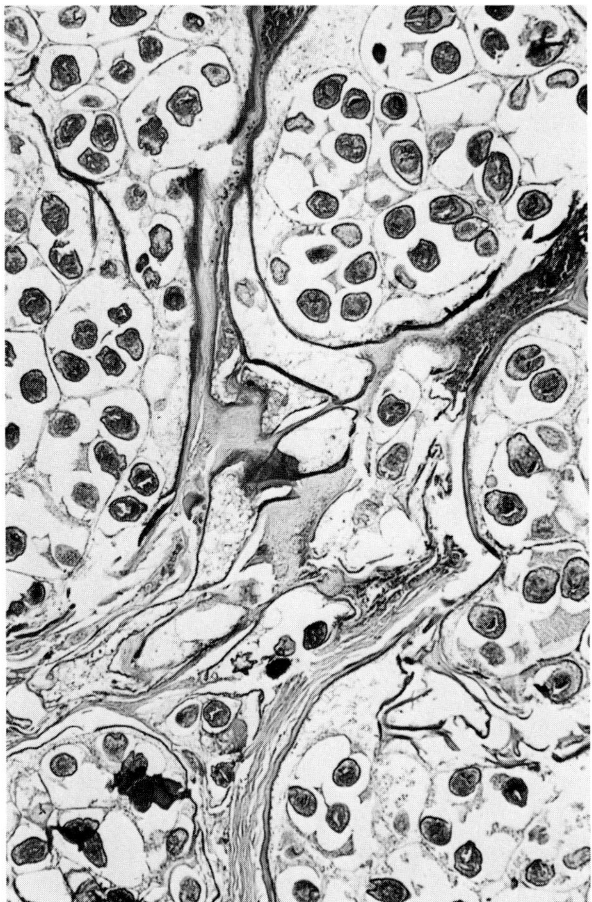

Fig. 79-4. Lesion of larval *Echinococcus multilocularis* in liver of a naturally infected rodent. Note typical alveolarlike microvesicles with protoscolices. (H&E, about × 350)

quently exposed to alveolar hydatid disease. Hyperendemic foci have been described in some Eskimo villages of the North American tundra where local dogs regularly feed on infected commensal rodents.

Pathogenesis and Pathology

The primary localization of the larvae of *E. multilocularis* in humans as well as natural intermediate hosts is the liver. Local extension of the lesion and metastases to the lungs and the brain may follow. The larval mass resembles a malignancy in appearance and behavior, since it proliferates indefinitely by exogenous budding and invades the surrounding tissues. In chronic alveolar hydatid infections, the lesion consists of a central necrotic cavity filled with a white amorphous material and covered with a thin peripheral layer of dense fibrous tissue. The lesion contains focal areas of calcification and is extensively infiltrated by the proliferating vesicles. Protoscolces are rarely observed in infections of humans (Fig. 79-5).

Manifestations

The initial symptoms of alveolar hydatid disease are usually vague. Mild upper quadrant and epigastric pain with hepatomegaly can progress to obstructive jaundice. Occasionally, the initial manifestations are related to metastases to the lungs or brain.

Diagnosis

Alveolar hydatid disease is typically observed in persons of advanced age and closely mimics hepatic carcinoma or cirrhosis. Roentgenography shows hepatomegaly and characteristic scattered areas of radiolucency outlined by calcific rings 2 mm to 4 mm in diameter. Serologic tests are usually positive at high titers; because *Echinococcus* spp. share antigens, serologic tests do not distinguish between cystic and alveolar hydatid disease. Needle biopsy of the liver may confirm the diagnosis if larval elements are demonstrated. Exploratory laparotomy is often carried out for diagnosis and delineation of the extent of the lesion.

Prognosis

With or without treatment, the mortality of alveolar hydatidiasis has been 50% to 75%.

Therapy

In alveolar hydatid disease, the entire larval mass must be resected. This usually requires excision of the entire affected lobe of the liver; when involvement is more extensive, wedge resections of the lesions may be attempted. Because alveolar hydatid disease is often not diagnosed until the disease is well advanced, the lesion is frequently inoperable. Treatment with mebendazole may prolong survival by inhibiting the growth of larval *E. multilocularis;* however, the drug is not larvicidal.

Prevention

Eliminating *E. multilocularis* from its wild animal hosts is not practical. Therefore, contact with dogs and foxes in areas in which the infection is endemic should be avoided. Prevention of infection in the human depends upon education to improve hygiene and sanitation. Patent infections in dogs and cats prone to eat infected rodents can be prevented by monthly treatments with praziquantel.

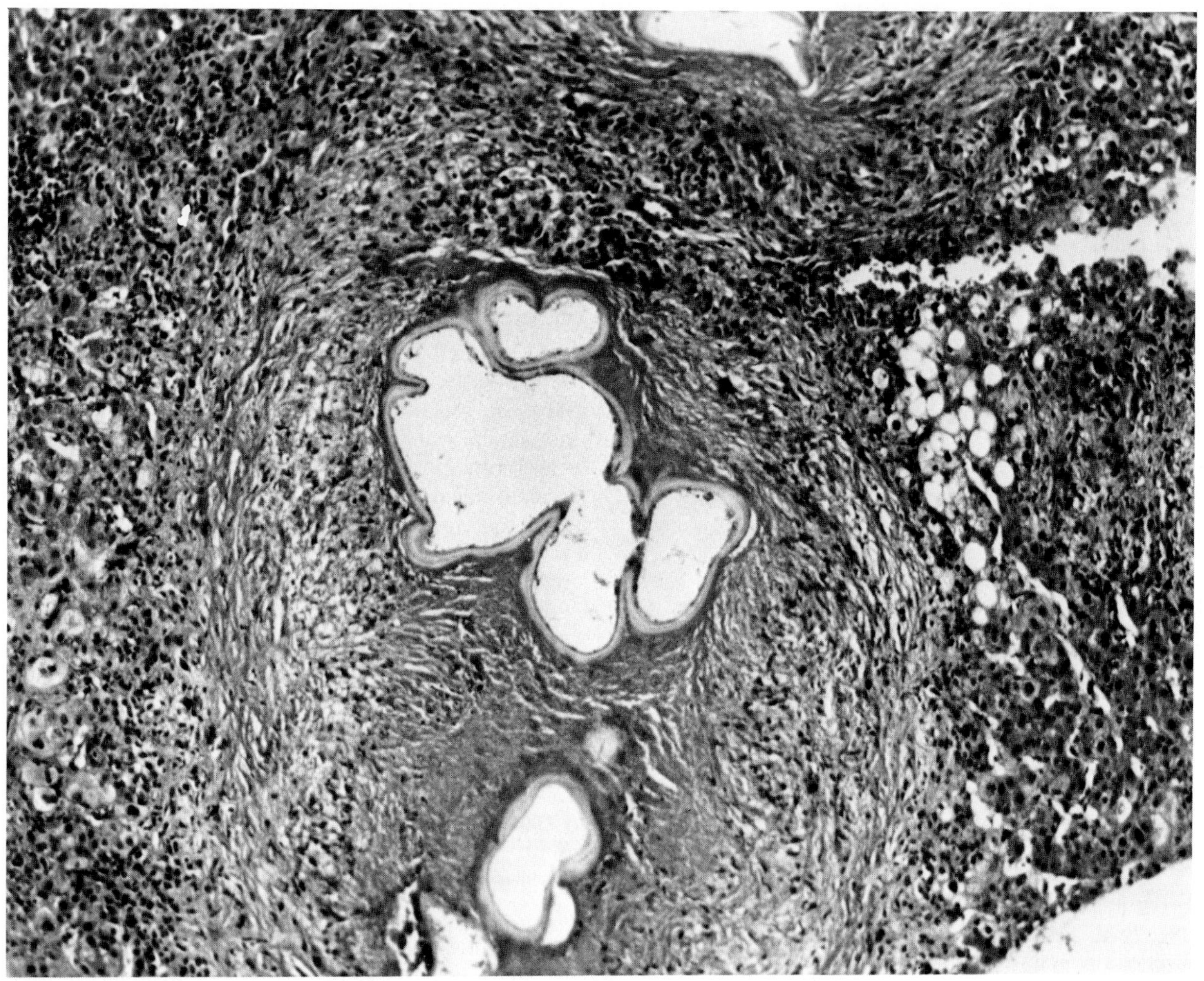

Fig. 79-5. Sterile microvesicles of *Echinococcus multilocularis:* section of a chronic hepatic lesion in a woman. Hematoxylin-eosin stain. (Original magnification approximately × 150)

Polycystic Hydatid Disease (Echinococcus vogeli)

Etiology

A polycystic form of hydatid disease in humans is caused by *Echinococcus vogeli.* The hydatid cyst of *E. vogeli* has a structure similar to that of *E. granulosus.*

Epidemiology

The life cycle of *E. vogeli* involves the bush dog and possibly other wild canids. Domestic dogs are also susceptible. Pacas, agoutis, and spiny rats are the principal intermediate hosts. *Echinococcus vogeli* is indigenous to the humid tropical forests in central and northern South America. Bush dogs are rare and avoid human beings; therefore they play little role in direct exposure to humans. In endemic areas, hunting dogs are often fed the raw viscera of pacas; dogs thus infected may then expose associated humans. Polycystic hydatidiasis has been recognized in humans in Panama, Ecuador, Colombia, and Venezuela.

Pathogenesis and Pathology

Echinococcus vogeli causes a polycystic form of hydatid disease in humans that has characteristics intermediate between cystic and alveolar hydatid disease. The relatively large cysts are filled with fluid and contain brood capsules with numerous protoscolices. The primary localization is the liver, but cysts may spread to contiguous sites. The disease appears to be less vigorously progressive than alveolar hydatid disease.

Diagnosis

Techniques useful for diagnosing cystic or alveolar hydatid disease should also be of value in diagnosing polycystic hydatid disease. Because *E. vogeli* share antigens with the other *Echinococcus* spp., present immunodiagnostic tests do not permit species diagnosis. However, the hydatid cysts of *E. vogeli* differ from the other species in the dimensions of the hooks of the protoscolices.

Therapy

The clinical aspects of polycystic hydatid disease have not been reported in detail. It is probable that the principles of management of cystic and alveolar hydatid disease also apply to polycystic hydatidiasis.

Coenurosis (Taenia [Multiceps] *spp.*)

Etiology

Coenurosis is infection by the larval form of several related *Taenia (Multiceps)* spp. The *coenurus* is a liquid-filled cyst surrounded by a thin, delicate membrane to which are attached invaginated protoscolices arranged in rows or clusters. The coenuroid larvae have distinctly larger protoscolices than those of cysticerci and hydatid cysts. In addition, morphologic differences in the membrane structure of the respective larval forms are usually identifiable.

Epidemiology

The cestodes causing coenurosis have dogs and other canids as definitive hosts; sheep, goats, rabbits, hares, and various rodents are intermediate hosts. Disagreement exists regarding speciation within the genus *Taenia (Multiceps)*. There are several sibling species or geographic strains with different assemblies of intermediate hosts in which the coenuri occur in different parts of the body. Humans become infected by ingesting eggs passed in the feces of infected canids. Of the fewer than 100 reported cases of coenurosis in humans, most occurred in tropical Africa; the coenuri were predominantly subcutaneous. A higher frequency of intracranial localization marked the cases reported from South Africa and other temperate regions.

Manifestations

The manifestations of coenurosis of the brain, eye, or subcutaneous tissues, are similar to those produced by hydatid cysts in the same locations.

Diagnosis

Diagnostic techniques useful for cystic hydatid disease are also useful for coenurosis; etiologic differentiation of the cysts is not usually possible preoperatively.

Prognosis

The prognosis of cerebral coenurosis is similar to cysticercosis and hydatid disease involving the same sites.

Therapy

Coenuri in subcutaneous sites are usually excisable with no sequelae.

Prevention

When coenurosis in humans also occurs in dogs and domestic ungulates, the disease may be controlled by the same measures that are effective against cystic hydatid disease. When coenurosis occurs in wild animal hosts, specific control measures are limited to avoidance of infected carnivores and good hygiene.

Sparganosis (Spirometra *spp.*)

Etiology

Sparganosis is infection by the second stage larvae of cestodes of the genus *Spirometra* (order Pseudophyllidea). The sparganum, or plerocercoid, is a fleshy, motile, elongated (3 cm–50 cm in length) larva, flattened dorsoventrally, with a broad evaginated anterior end that is the future scolex.

Epidemiology

The life cycle of *Spirometra* spp. requires at least three hosts. The definitive hosts of *Spirometra* spp. include a wide variety of wild carnivores. Eggs are eliminated in the feces, and if the feces are dropped into water, the eggs hatch to release free-swimming embryos. After ingestion by the first intermediate host, a copepod, the larvae progress to the sparganum stage only when the infected copepod is ingested by second intermediate hosts—many amphibian, reptilian, avian, and mammalian species. The life cycle is completed when a carnivorous definitive host ingests an infected, second intermediate host. Infection of humans probably occurs most frequently by ingesting infected copepods in unfiltered or untreated water. Ingestion of uncooked tissues of the second intermediate hosts containing spargana may also cause sparganosis, as well as contact with the raw flesh of these animals; the oriental custom of applying the raw flesh of certain amphibians and reptiles to wounds or sores accounts for a relatively high incidence of contact sparganosis in China and southeast Asia. Sparganosis in humans has been reported from throughout the world, but most cases are reported from the Far East. In the United States, most cases are associated with residence in the southeastern states and Puerto Rico.

Pathogenesis and Pathology

The lesion in sparganosis results from invasion of tissues by the motile spargana. The larvae are almost always found in the subcutaneous tissues or those surrounding the eye, where their presence provokes an acute inflammatory response. The usual outcome is death of the larvae followed by absorption or calcification. Occasionally, spargana may invade virtually any tissue including the CNS. Rarely, a proliferative form occurs which is characterized by extensive tissue invasion.

Manifestations

Sparganosis is often manifested as tender or migratory subcutaneous nodules. Painful swelling of the conjunctival, palpebral, periorbital, or retro-orbital tissues is characteristic of ocular sparginosis.

Diagnosis

The diagnosis of sparganosis is based on the clinical manifestations and is usually not confirmed until the sparganum is excised at surgery.

Therapy

During surgical removal of spargana, care must be taken to remove the larvae intact because remnants provoke a painful, inflammatory reaction.

Prevention

Most infections by spargana can be prevented by eschewing untreated or unfiltered water and eating only adequately cooked meat from reptiles or amphibians.

Remaining Problems

Refinement of serologic tests to distinguish reliably between cysticercosis and hydatidiasis, and among the species of *Echinococcus* would enable specific, noninvasive diagnosis.

Currently, surgical removal of the larval cestodes is the only effective therapy. However, by the time cerebral cysticercosis, secondary cystic hydatid disease, and alveolar hydatid disease are recognized, they are often inoperable. The utility of mebendazole and other benzimidazoles in all forms of larval cestodiasis remains to be determined.

Vaccines effective in the prevention of larval cestodiasis in nonhuman animals are very much needed. Drugs practical for the mass treatment of human and canine tapeworm carriers are now available and need to be used more widely in control programs. Other methods of control must also be implemented more widely: good animal husbandry, adequate meat inspection, strict dog control, and proper personal hygiene.

Bibliography

GENERAL

MARCIAL–ROJAS RA (ED): Pathology of Protozoal and Helminthic Diseases with Clinical Correlation. Baltimore, Williams & Wilkins, 1971. 1010 pp.

CYSTICERCOSIS

Book

DIXON HBF, LIPSCOMB FM: Cysticercosis: An analysis and follow-up of 450 cases. Medical Research Council Special Report Series No. 299(London):1–58, 1961

Journals

LAMAS E, ESTEBEZ J, SOTO M, OBRADOR S: Computerized axial tomography for the diagnosis of cerebral cysticercosis. Acta Neurochir 44:192–205, 1978

ROBLES C, CHAVARRIA MC: Presentación de un caso clínico de cisticercosis cerebral tratado médicamente con un nuevo fármaco: praziquantel. Salud Pub Mex 21:603–618, 1980

STEPIEN L: Cerebral cysticercosis in Poland. Clinical symptoms and operative results in 132 cases. J Neurosurg 19:505–513, 1962

HYDATID DISEASE

Book

SCHANTZ PM, KAGAN IG: Echinococcosis (hydatidosis). In Houba V (ed): Immunologic Investigation of Tropical Parasitic Disease. Edinburgh, Churchill Livingston, 1980. pp. 104–129.

Journals

AMIR–JAHED AK, FARDIN R, FARZAD A, BAKSHANDEH K: Clinical echinococcosis. Ann Surg 182:541–546, 1975

D'ALESSANDRO A, RAUSCH RL, CUELLO C, ARISTIZABAL N: *Echinococcus vogeli* in man, with a review of human cases of polycystic hydatid disease in Colombia and neighboring countries. Am J Trop Med Hyg 28:303–317, 1979

GROVE DI, WARREN KS, MAHMOUD AAF: Algorithms in the diagnosis and management of exotic diseases. J Infect Dis 133:354–358, 1976

LITTLE JM: Hydatid disease at Royal Prince Alfred Hospital, 1964 to 1974. Med J Aust 1:903–908, 1976

SCHANTZ PM, VAN DEN BOSSCHE H, ECKERT J: Chemotherapy for larval echinococcosis in animals and humans: Report of a workshop. Z Parasitenkd 67:5–26, 1982

WILSON JF, RAUSCH RL: Alveolar hydatid disease: A review of clinical features of 33 indigenous cases of *Echinococcus multilocularis* infection in Alaskan Eskimos. Am J Trop Med Hyg 29:1,340–1,355, 1980

COENUROSIS

Journal

TEMPLETON AC: Anatomical and geographical location of human coenurus infection. Trop Geogr Med 23:105–108, 1971

SPARGANOSIS

Journal

DALY JJ, BAKER GF, JOHNSON BR: Human sparganosis in Arkansas. J Arkansas Med Soc 71:397–402, 1975

RALPH L. MULLER

80 Liver Fluke Infection

The major liver flukes infecting humans are *Clonorchis sinensis* (clonorchiasis, Chinese liver fluke disease), the closely related *Opisthorchis felineus* and *Opisthorchis viverrini* (opisthorchiasis), and *Fasciola hepatica* (fascioliasis, liver-rot in sheep).

Etiology

The liver flukes that infect humans are flattened, hermaphroditic trematodes, possessing an oral and ventral sucker and living in the bile ducts. *Clonorchis* sp. and *Opisthorchis* spp. are very similar, since they are both elongated and extremely flat, tapering anteriorly and rounded posteriorly. When living they are translucent and pinkish. *Clonorchis* sp. is longer (11 cm–20 cm × 3 cm–4.5 cm) than *Opisthorchis* spp. (7 cm–12 cm × 1.5 cm–3 cm) and has branched rather than lobed posterior testes (adult *O. felineus* and *O. viverrini* cannot be reliably differentiated). *Fasciola* sp. is larger and wider (25 mm × 13 mm) and leaf-shaped; the male and female organs and the gut are all highly branched.

The eggs of the various liver flukes are shown in Plate 68-1, and several characteristics are listed in Table 80-1.

Epidemiology

The life cycles of all liver flukes involve snails as first intermediate hosts, and humans or other mammals as definitive hosts. *Clonorchis* sp. and *Opisthorchis* spp. have fishes as second intermediate hosts, whereas *Fasciola* sp. has a cystic stage on vegetation. The eggs are deposited in the biliary passages of the definitive host and are passed in the feces. On reaching water, the embryonated eggs of *Clonorchis* sp. and *Opisthorchis* spp. are ingested by susceptible aquatic snails (principally *Parafossarulus* sp., or *Bulimus* sp. in northern China), and the miracidia hatch in the snails; on the other hand, the undeveloped eggs of *Fasciola* sp. require about 2 weeks on wet pastures before the miracidia hatch and penetrate the appropriate amphibious snail host (*Lymnaea* sp.). After multiplications within the snail, the emergent cercariae locate the second intermediate host and encyst as metacercariae (*Clonorchis* sp. and *Opisthorchis* spp. in the muscles and subcutaneous tissues of over 80 species of freshwater cyprinoid fishes, *Fasciola* sp. on wet vegetation such as grass and, in human infections, watercress or lettuce).

Following the ingestion of infected, uncooked fish or plants, the metacercariae excyst in the duodenum or jejunum. The immature clonorchid and opisthorchid flukes make their way to the ampulla of Vater and enter the biliary tree. After about a week the young flukes, measuring 1 mm in length, migrate to the distal ducts, and are mature by 4 weeks after infection. The development of fasciolid flukes differ in that the immature worms penetrate the intestinal wall, migrate through the peritoneal cavity, and reach the proximal bile ducts by penetrating the liver capsule and eating their way through the hepatic parenchyma. The flukes mature and lay eggs about 12 weeks after ingestion of the metacercariae.

The life span of the liver flukes is usually around 8 years but may sometimes be as long as 15 to 20 years.

Clonorchiasis is endemic in the Far East, particularly in areas in which commercial fish ponds are fertilized with human feces. It occurs principally in China, Japan, Korea, Taiwan, and Vietnam and is also found in Chinese communities in Hong Kong and Malaysia, with occasionally an imported case in America and Europe. Locally, incidence may be high, 30% in Kwangtung province (China), 47% along Lake Kasumigawa (Japan), 25% in parts of Miao-Li county (Taiwan), 70% around Hanoi (Vietnam), 29% in Yeongsan (Korea), 65% to 80% in Hong Kong

Table 80-1. Important Characteristics of Liver Flukes

	Adults		Eggs	
Fluke	AVERAGE SIZE (mm)	SIGNIFICANT CHARACTERISTICS	EMBRYONAL CONTENTS	SIGNIFICANT CHARACTERISTICS
Fasciola hepatica	25 × 13	Flat, leaflike, conical anterior; scalelike spines; suckers of equal size; brown	Undeveloped ovum	Ovoid, indistinct operculum, uniformly granular contents, yellow brown (140 μm × 80 μm)
Clonorchis sinensis	11–20 × 3–4.5	Flat, elongate, tapering anteriorly; aspinous; ventral smaller than oral; gray (brown when bile-stained).	Differentiated (with miracidium larva)	Distinct operculum, prominent opercular shoulders, abopercular knob, yellow brown (30 μm × 15 μm)
Opisthorchis felineus and *Opisthorchis viverrini*	7–12 × 1.5–3	Flat, elongate, tapering anteriorly; aspinous; ventral sucker smaller than oral; yellow red.	Differentiated (with miracidium larva)	Distinct operculum, prominent opercular shoulders, prominent abopercular knob, (30 μm × 12 μm)

(transmission does not occur in Hong Kong, but the infection is imported in fishes brought in from mainland China). However, the incidence and intensity of infection appear to have fallen in the last few years in China and Japan. Transmission is usually from human to human but fish-eating carnivores can serve as reservoir hosts. In South Fukien province (China), infection is maintained almost entirely by dogs, because the people do not eat raw fish.

Opisthorchis felineus and *O. viverrini* are natural parasites of fish-eating carnivores—the former of cats, dogs, foxes, and pigs, and the latter of the civet and domestic cat and dog. Human infection with *O. felineus* is most common in Russia (Siberia and the Dneiper basin) and eastern Europe; *O. viverrini* occurs in northeastern Thailand (3½ million cases) and Laos.

Fascioliasis is essentially a disease of sheep and cattle. Humans are occasionally infected in sheep- and cattle-raising areas, particularly those with high rainfall. Most cases in humans have been from Central and South America, Cuba, France, Great Britain, and North Africa; epidemics may occur in particularly wet years. The source of fascioliasis is usually infected watercress.

Infections with the cosmopolitan lanceolate liver flukes of sheep (*Dicrocoelium dendriticum* and *Dicrocoelium hospes*) have been reported very rarely in humans, presumably because the infective metacercariae are encysted in ants and not on vegetation. Symptoms are said to resemble hepatitis with flatulence, but most cases have proved to be spurious.

Pathogenesis and Pathology

Clonorchiasis and *opisthorchiasis* are similar in pathology, but the severity varies widely, depending on the intensity of the infection. In the early stages, there is an inflammatory reaction of the bilary epithelium, followed by proliferation of the ducts with increased production of mucus from an increased number of goblet cells. In chronic cases, there is widespread periductal fibrosis which occasionally causes occlusion of the bile ducts; however, there is no periportal fibrosis as is typical of hepatic schistosome infection. A heavily infected liver is readily recognized on gross examination because of the fibrosed, dilated ducts near the surface; if the liver is cut, many shiny, brownish flukes emerge. The hepatic architecture remains normal. Although cirrhosis is present in about 10% of patients with liver fluke infections who come to autopsy, it is probably coincidental or accentuated by an accompanying bacterial infection.

Carcinoma of the intrahepatic bile ducts is related to the presence of clonorchiasis or opisthorchiasis and is particularly prevalent in areas of Thailand in which infections with *O. viverrini* are contracted in childhood. About 1% of all autopsies in a hospital in Bangkok showed the presence of *O. viverrini*, and 44% of these had cholangiocarcinomas.

A recurrent bacterial cholangitis, associated with cholecystitis, is common in Hong Kong. The gallbladder and bile ducts may contain remnants of *Clonorchis* sp. (or sometimes *Ascaris* sp.). A suppurative pancholangitis with hypoglycemic jaundice also occurs, in which the main ducts are obstructed by a mass of dead clonorchid worms.

When there are septic complications with clonorchiasis, eggs may be found in the hepatic parenchyma, but they are not so commonly associated with the formation of pseudotubercles as are the eggs of schistosomes.

Portal hypertension and splenomegaly may occur in heavy infections, and ascites is almost always found in fatal cases, although it is rarely diagnosed during life.

In over one-third of patients with clonorchiasis, flukes are found in the pancreatic ducts. An acute pancreatitis with the formation of a squamous metaplasia is particularly likely to occur in males.

Mature fasciolid flukes may also be associated with adenomatous hyperplasia, and infiltration with plasma cells, lymphocytes, and eosinophils in the periductal tissues; in time, this reaction is replaced by fibrosis causing greatly thickened ducts. Unlike other human liver flukes, the integument of *Fasciola* sp. is covered with spines, and these aid in debridement of the epithelium. As they migrate in the liver parenchyma, the immature fasciolids cause a coagulation necrosis of the hepatic cells with numerous neutrophils, lymphocytes, and eosinophils.

Manifestations

Most *Clonorchis* sp. and *Opisthorchis* spp. infections are light (less than 100 parasites), and over 70% are asymptomatic.

With heavier infections (up to 1000 flukes), there is likely to be abdominal discomfort and diarrhea.

In very heavy infections (the maximum recorded number of *Clonorchis* sp. being 21,000), there is usually intermittent, acute pain in the right upper quadrant, hepatic tenderness and enlargement, edema, anorexia, and loss of weight; that is, the symptoms may stimulate acute hepatitis. Worms may be contracted progressively, with an insidious increase in symptoms over a period; however, it is remarkable how some patients with no symptoms during life have severe liver pathology at autopsy.

Patients with fascioliasis are usually seen by the clinician in the acute phase when young flukes are migrating through the liver tissue. At this time, there is likely to be a sudden onset of high fever, dyspepsia, nausea, and intense, recurrent abdominal pain localized in the right hypochondrium or epigastrium. Diagnosis is difficult because of the absence of eggs. Later, there may be painful hepatomegaly, an obstructive jaundice closely resembling biliary disease, anemia, a neutrophilia, and an eosinophilia of up to 60%.

Occasionally, ectopic fascioliasis occurs in humans with flukes developing in other organs or in the wall of the abdominal cavity.

Diagnosis

Definitive diagnosis of liver fluke infection is based on the identification of eggs in the feces by direct examination or by concentration techniques. Eggs are likely to be numerous in clinically important cases of clonorchiasis or opisthorchiasis. The eggs of *Fasciola* sp. are often scanty or absent (in about 30% of human cases); however, the use of a swallowed, brushed nylon thread in a gelatin capsule, or duodenal aspiration may reveal eggs when fecal examination is negative. Spurious cases with eggs of *Fasciola* sp. in the feces can occur from eating infected sheep livers.

Fever, enlargement of the liver, and a high eosinophilia (40%) are very suggestive of fascioliasis, particularly if accompanied by urticaria in patients with a history of having eaten watercress a few weeks earlier.

The intradermal skin test is usually positive in patients infected with liver flukes, and there is a commercially available skin test kit for fascioliasis (Wellcome Reagents). However, the reaction persists for years in cured infections and there are cross-reactions with *Paragonimus westermani* and *Schistosoma japonicum.* Serologic tests, such as complement fixation, indirect hemagglutination and immunoelectrophoresis, have also been employed with some success.

Prognosis

The prognosis is favorable when infections are light. Heavy infections with *Clonorchis* sp. and *Opisthorchis* spp. have a poor prognosis; however, death is only likely to occur when there is an intercurrent bacterial infection.

Therapy

The treatment of clonorchiasis and opisthorchiasis is often unsatisfactory, particularly in chronic or heavy infections. Hexachloroparaxylol (Hetol), 70 mg/kg body wt/day for 5 days, given perorally as a single dose is effective and still widely used in China and

Russia. However, the drug is no longer commercially available in the West because high doses cause chronic renal disease and blindness in dogs, and anemia in dogs and humans. The risk of treatment would have to be weighed against the fact that infections are usually light. Chloroquine phosphate (250 mg perorally, every 8 hours for 6 weeks) is moderately successful.

Bithionol is the treatment of choice for human fascioliasis. The usual dose is 30 mg to 50 mg/kg body wt/day, perorally, once a day for 10 to 15 days. A single dose of 45 g for an adult (half that for a child) was also successful in one outbreak. Dehydroemetine dihydrochloride (65 mg daily by intramuscular injection for 12 days) is an alternative treatment. Both of these compounds have had only limited success in the treatment of clonorchiasis. Dehydroemetine has been given orally as delayed release tablets (2.5 mg/kg body wt in three doses on alternate days over a 60-day period); in one trial, although there was a reduction in egg count of 47%, little clinical improvement resulted.

In recent clinical trials, praziquantel (25 mg/kg body wt, PO, taken three times in 1 day) was very effective against all liver flukes; it is likely to become the drug of choice for the treatment of liver fluke infections.

Prevention

The obvious method of preventing clonorchiasis and opisthorchiasis is by thorough cooking of fish. However, this requires changes in long-established eating habits. In South Korea, for example, raw fish is eaten traditionally by men at drinking parties to increase thirst.

Fish ponds are commonly fertilized with human feces in many Far East countries. Storage of feces for a few days, or the addition of ammonium sulfate is effective in killing eggs; this simple measure has markedly lowered the incidence in China during the last few years. Industrial pollution of rivers in Japan has served to lower the incidence there.

Fascioliasis can be controlled by preventing people from eating wild watercress and by excluding livestock from the vicinity of cultivated watercress. The growing watercress should be irrigated from spring or well water and not from rivers likely to be contaminated with feces from sheep or cattle.

Remaining Problems

There is still an urgent need for an effective chemotherapeutic agent for clonorchiasis and opisthorchiasis. Research has been hampered by an inability to maintain snail intermediate hosts of *Clonorchis* sp. in the laboratory.

Bibliography

Books

BINFORD CH, CONNOR DH (EDS): Pathology of Tropical and Extraordinary Diseases, Vol II, Section 10, Chaps. 2 and 4. Washington, AFIP, 1976

MARSDEN PD (ED): Clinics in Gastroenterology: Vol 7/1 Intestinal Parasites. Philadelphia, WB Saunders, 1978. 243 pp.

MULLER R: Worms and Disease: A Manual of Medical Helminthology, London, WM Heinemann Medical Books, 1975. 161 pp.

Journals

FLAVELL DJ: Liver fluke as an etiological factor in bile duct carcinoma of man. Trans R Soc Trop Med Hyg 75:814–824, 1981

KHORSAND HO: Obstructive jaundice due to Fasciola hepatica. Bull Soc Pathol Exot Filiales 70:626–628, 1977

KOOMPITOCHANA C, SONAKUL D, CLINDA K, STITNIMANKARM T: Opisthorchiasis: A clinicopathologic study of 154 autopsy cases. Southeast Asian J Trop Med Public Health 9:60–64, 1978

PURTILO DT: Clonorchiasis and hepatic neoplasms. Trop Geogr Med 28:21–27, 1976

THOMAS H. WELLER

81 Schistosomiasis

Schistosomiasis is a disease complex caused by the adult forms of long-lived flukes (trematodes) that belong to the genus *Schistosoma* and reside within the venous plexuses of mammals. The illness may be acute or chronic with slow progression, reflecting the response of the host to the continuing intravascular deposition of eggs and to the continued elaboration of excretions by the worms. Schistosomiasis is usually attributed to three species of schistosomes, subdivided into intestinal (*Schistosoma mansoni* and *Schistosoma japonicum*) or urinary (*Schistosoma haematobium*) types, according to the site preferred by the adult worms. This schema is useful but simplistic. Other species infect man: *Schistosoma mekonqi, Schistosoma intercalatum,* and *Schistosoma matthei.* Moreover, the preferred sites of involvement are relative rather than absolute; for example, eggs of *S. haematobium* are commonly found in the rectal mucosa of an infected person, and in infections with *S. mansoni,* eggs may appear sporadically in the urine.

Etiology

The adult schistosomes are delicate cylindrical worms 1 cm to 2 cm in length that are adapted for existence in venules. They differ from other trematodes in that the sexes are separate; two longitudinal outfoldings of the male form a gynecophoral canal in which the filiform female is clasped *in copula* (Fig. 81-1). Although the species differ morphologically, this fact is not clinically important because a specific diagnosis is derived from the characteristic shape of eggs recovered from the urine, feces, or infected tissues (Plate 68-1).

Epidemiology

Humans are infected with schistosomes through contact with water containing the infective larval stage, the free-swimming cercariae, which penetrate the skin or mucous membranes. The cercariae are 0.4 mm to 0.6 mm long, fork-tailed organisms derived from infected aquatic or amphibious snails. Snails become infected only if eggs of schistosomes passed in the urine or feces of the infected mammalian host reach fresh water and hatch. The minute, free-swimming miracidium thus released lives only a few hours unless it contacts and promptly penetrates a snail suitable as an intermediate host. In this essential intermediate host, the parasite undergoes extensive multiplication within the tissues so that a single infected snail may shed thousands of cercariae into the water over a period of many weeks.

The parasite–snail interaction is highly specific, and only a few species of snail support the cycle. The geographic distribution of schistosomiasis is, therefore, peculiarly focal. For example, appropriate snails are present in Puerto Rico but not in the Virgin Islands or Cuba. They are not present in the United States.

Adult schistosomes are less host-specific. Mammals other than humans can serve to a variable degree as definitive hosts and maintain the infection. *Schistosoma japonicum* is the extreme example; in endemic areas, high rates of this infection may be found in dogs, cats, rats, and cattle, a factor that complicates control of the disease.

The global pattern of schistosomiasis is determined by the distribution of snails appropriate as intermediate hosts, the pattern of discharge into fresh water of egg-containing feces or urine, and the water contact habits of humans. Aptly termed a man-made disease,

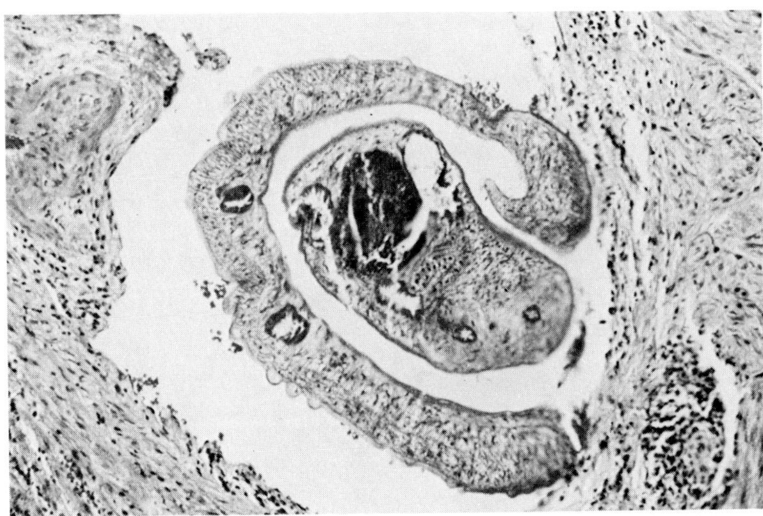

Fig. 81-1. Pair of adult schistosomes in a vein of the cervix; cross section with the female enfolded in the gynecophoral canal of the male. (H&E × 25)

schistosomiasis increases in frequency of occurrence as man-made lakes and irrigation systems are developed in tropical regions.

Manson's schistosomiasis is the only form that occurs in the Western Hemisphere. It is confined to Puerto Rico and some islands in the Lesser Antilles, and to northern South America in Brazil, Surinam, and Venezuela. *Schistosoma mansoni* also occurs across central Africa, in the Nile Valley, Malagasy, and in Yemen. *Schistosoma haematobium* is distributed throughout much of Africa and in some Middle Eastern countries; there is also a focus in India. *Schistosoma japonicum* is highly endemic in parts of the Philippines and is present in Thailand, Laos, Cambodia, and the Celebes. Intensive control activities have virtually eliminated human infections from Japan and have reduced incidence in mainland China.

In endemic areas, more than 90% of adults may be infected. The intensity of infection, that is, the number of worms per person, is of epidemiologic and clinical import. The worm burden can be indirectly estimated in children or in recent infections in adults by counting the eggs passed in the urine or feces. Older children and young adolescents characteristically constitute the age group that excretes the greatest number of eggs in endemic areas.

Pathogenesis and Pathology

Cercarial proteolytic secretions aid rapid penetration of the skin; in the process, the cercariae lose their tails and become schistosomules that measure 0.1 mm to 0.2 mm in length. Some of the larvae are trapped in the skin of previously sensitized persons, inducing a papular pruritic eruption. In the inexperienced host, the majority of the schistosomules move into the lymphatics and venules and migrate through the pulmonary capillary filter. Schistosomules feed on blood and grow rapidly in the intrahepatic portal venous system. Those of *S. mansoni* and *S. japonicum* then migrate into the distal branches of the superior and inferior mesenteric veins around the intestine and rectum, and those of *S. haematobium* migrate through the hemorrhoidal and pudendal veins into the vesical and pelvic plexuses. By this time the worms have mated, and egg laying begins 5 to 12 weeks after cercarial penetration, varying with the species.

The young schistosome rapidly acquires host-derived antigenic materials on its body surface and thus is immunologically camouflaged. Humans do not react to the living worms *per se,* but the secretions and excretions of the worms may engender hypersensitivity and general manifestations of illness.

The most important pathologic consequences of schistosomiasis are egg associated. Because each female worm may lay eggs for years, the disease is slowly progressive. Eggs are deposited in the small venules of the intestine or genitourinary organs; some are trapped locally while others move in the venous stream and lodge at the first sinusoidal or capillary filter, that is , the liver or the lungs. Toxic and antigenic products of a viable miracidium pass through the shell of the egg and cause a minute abscess wherever the egg lodges. An initial acute inflammatory infiltrate with numerous eosinophils is replaced by round cells, giant cells, and epithelioid cells that accumulate around the egg. Fibroblastic activity follows, with the end-result a minute, granu-

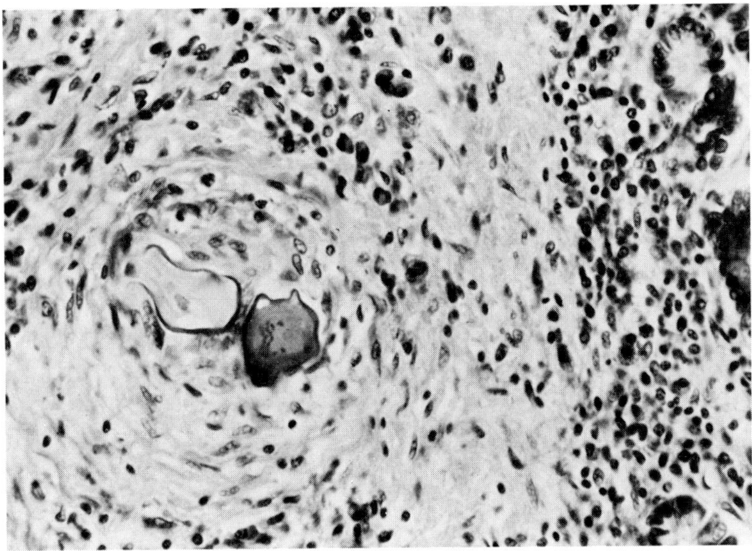

Fig. 81-2. Pseudotubercle reaction around two eggs of *Schistosoma mansoni* lodged in the submucosa of the intestine. (H&E × 65)

lomatous pseudotubercle (Fig. 81-2), the typical defense mechanism of the sensitized host.

In heavy infections, masses of eggs may produce confluent ulcerations: (1) in the intestinal mucosa, resulting in an acute schistosomal dysentery, or (2) in the urinary bladder mucosa, causing an acute hemorrhagic cystitis (Fig. 81-3). Only a small percentage of the eggs which are laid escape in the feces or urine. Those trapped locally induce a fibrotic, irregular thickening of the bowel or bladder wall and formation of abscesses and papillomatous growths (Fig. 81-4). Strictures, adhesions, and fistulas may develop. In infections with *S. haematobium,* calcified eggs may accumulate in the bladder wall, there is functional impairment of the bladder and ureters, and hydronephrosis is common. Additionally, the pelvic genital organs are usually involved. (Fig. 81-5).

Although morbidity is associated with lesions in the intestinal or urinary tract, mortality often reflects circulatory dysfunction resulting from the progressive fibrosis engendered in the liver (Fig. 81-6*A*) or the lungs (Fig. 81-6*B*) in response to trapped, embolic eggs. Hepatomegaly, especially with enlargement of the left lobe, may develop rapidly. In the liver, extensive periportal and perilobular fibrosis occurs; the end-result is the so-called Symmers' pipestem fibrosis—grossly observable white accumulations of fibrotic tissue. An early hyperplasia of splenic reticular tissue is followed by diffuse fibrosis. Portal hypertension may follow, with marked splenomegaly. Collateral vascular pathways become functional, and some eggs are thereby shunted directly to the lungs. In one series of autopsies, one-third of the deaths associated with Manson's schistosomiasis resulted from bleeding from a collateral varix. With *S. haematobium,* the lungs are the primary filter for embolic eggs; pulmonary hypertension with cor pulmonale and right-side failure may be an end-result.

Aberrant migration of worms and deposition of eggs may result in bizarre complications. A flaccid paralysis may follow spinal cord involvement; cerebral egg deposition may lead to epileptiform seizures. Abscesses in the skin may develop following topical egg laying. Indeed, examination of digests of tissues obtained at autopsy reveals that widespread dissemination of eggs throughout the body is common.

Chronic intestinal schistosomiasis may be associated with lesions in the kidney. Glomerulosclerotic changes in infected patients may be the result of deposition of specific schistosomal immune complexes. Antigenic materials elaborated by the worms are demonstrable in the blood and urine of infected persons.

In areas where infections caused by *Salmonella* spp. and *Schistosoma* spp. are both endemic, there may be a synergistic relationship. Patients with urinary schistosomiasis may be urinary carriers of *Salmonella typhi.* Patients with hepatosplenic schistosomiasis may exhibit a chronic salmonellal bacteremia.

Manifestations

Cercarial penetration is often accompanied by a transient, pruritic rash. Subsequently, but prior to egg lay-

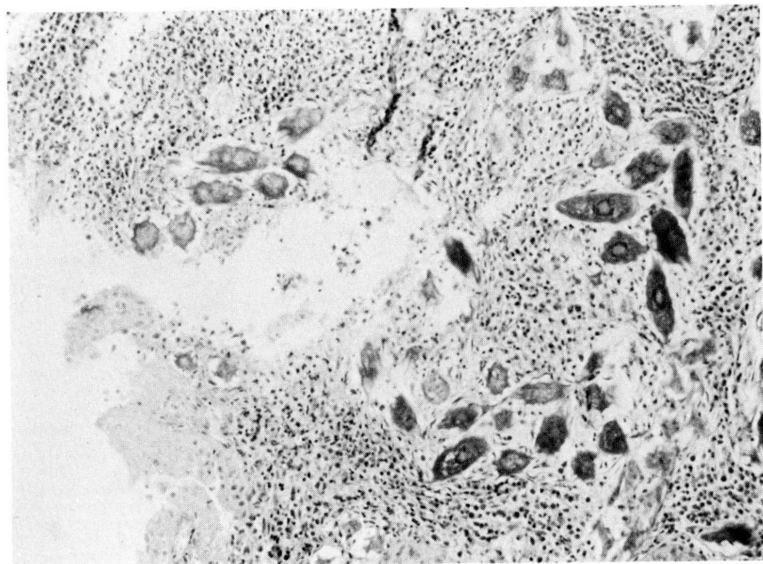

Fig. 81-3. Eggs of *Schistosoma haematobium* escaping into the lumen of the bladder. There is an acute inflammatory reaction with destruction of the epithelium. (H&E × 25)

ing, an acute illness is likely to develop in patients with heavy infections. There may be fever, headache, extreme malaise, cough, abdominal pain, enlargement and tenderness of the liver, and diarrhea; urticaria and eosinophilia (as high as 90%) may also occur.

As the intestinal form of the disease becomes chronic, manifestations vary in severity and may include irregular fever, malaise, weakness, weight loss, abdominal distress, diarrhea, ascites, hepatosplenomegaly, and portal hypertension. Fistulas may develop and papillomatous growths or intestinal strictures may occur. Death is the result of portal or pulmonary hypertension; hematemesis from ruptured esophageal varices, ascites, inanition, and heart failure are also prominent causes of death from schistosomiasis.

In infections with *S. haematobium,* hematuria at the end of micturition, dysuria, and frequency are early symptoms. Ureteral colic often occurs. With the development of fibrosis and of secondary infection, the symptoms of hydronephrosis or pyonephrosis may appear.

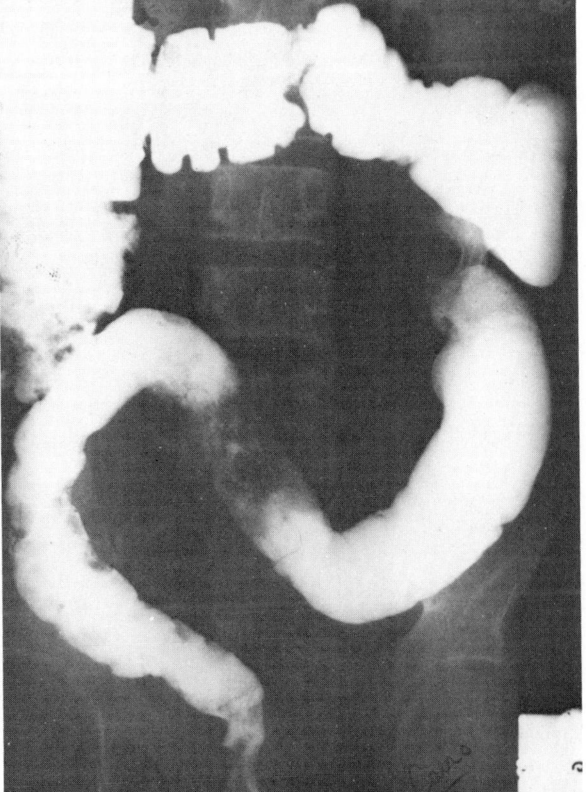

Fig. 81-4. Barium contrast study of the large bowel of a patient with chronic intestinal schistosomiasis. The rectosigmoid colon is narrowed and the thickened wall bears multiple polyps. (Courtesy of Professor PES Palmer, University of California, Davis)

Diagnosis

The patient must have been in a region where schistosomiasis occurs for the diagnosis to be considered. Most infections follow contact with natural or impounded bodies of water in rural areas. However, foci of transmission may occur within tropical cities in

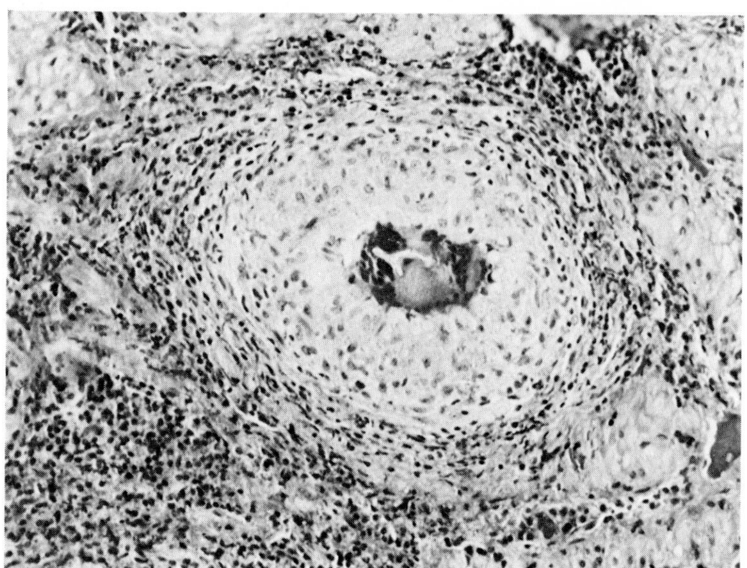

Fig. 81-5. Nodular epithelioid reaction around egg of *Schistosoma haematobium* trapped in the cervix. (H&E × 42)

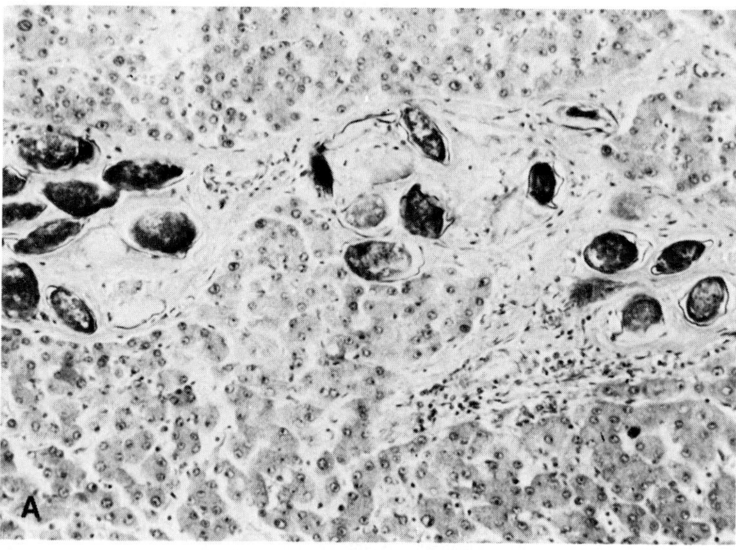

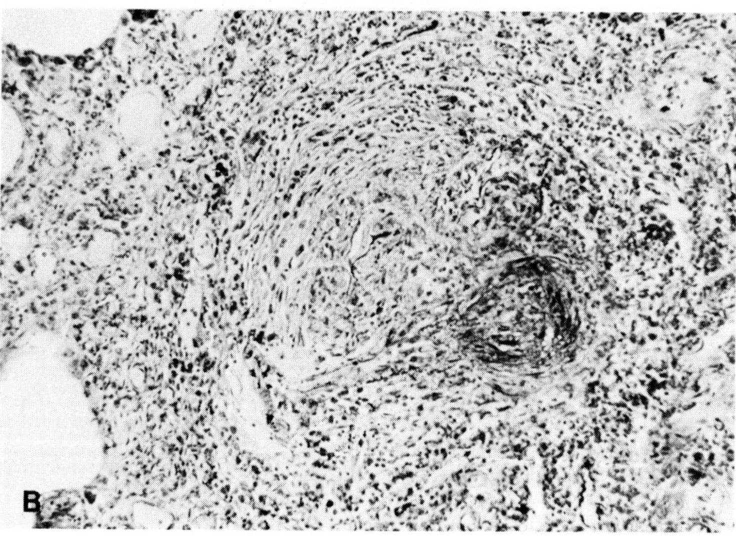

Fig. 81-6. (*A*) Calcified eggs of *Schistoma japonicum* with associated fibrosis of periportal area of liver. (H&E × 33) (*B*) Fibrotic nodule around remnant of an egg of *Schistosoma mansoni* in the lung with an associated occlusive vascular response. (Hematoxylin-Azur II-eosin, × 25)

endemic areas, as in uncontrolled swimming pools, or rarely, even in a motel bathtub.

Schistosomiasis can be diagnosed with certainty only by the microscopic demonstration of the characteristic eggs. Since excretion of eggs may be scanty, it is essential that repetitive examinations be done using appropriate concentration techniques (see Chap. 11, Diagnostic Methods for Protozoa and Helminths). The eggs of *S. mansoni* and *S. japonicum* should be sought by microscopic examination of sediments obtained from feces after processing by a procedure such as the formalin-ether concentration method. The eggs of *S. haematobium* are passed in the urine with a diurnal periodicity; that is, peak excretion occurs between 10 AM and 2 PM. Eggs present in urine collected at this time (or preferably in a 24-hour collection) are concentrated in the apex of a conical container simply by sedimentation. If schistosomiasis is suspected and repeated examinations of feces and urine are negative, then proctoscopy or cystoscopy with biopsy of mucosal lesions is justified; microscopic examination of the fragment after compression will suffice to reveal eggs.

A number of immunologic diagnostic procedures have been introduced; some are available through the Centers for Disease Control. Problems of specificity and sensitivity are such that specific therapy should not be instituted unless the diagnosis can be confirmed by the demonstration of eggs. Because optimal therapy varies with the species of schistosome, a specific diagnosis is essential.

In the initial phase of a severe infection, the high fever, prostration, cough, headache, muscle aches, and abdominal pain may suggest typhoid or other bacteremic states; a developing eosinophilia is then a useful diagnostic clue. With the onset of deposition of eggs by *S. mansoni,* or particularly *S. japonicum,* intestinal involvement may be blatant, with an acute dysentery that requires differentiation from shigellosis, amebiasis, and ulcerative colitis. At the other extreme, if few worms are present, there may be little change in bowel habits. Gross hematuria, with or without symptoms of cystitis, is the characteristic sign of a developing infection with *S. haematobium;* a history of travel in an endemic area and the presence of eosinophilia should lead to a search for eggs.

Prognosis

Specific therapy will terminate or greatly reduce the deposition of eggs and thus halt or reverse an otherwise slowly progressive course of schistosomiasis. The acute, egg-associated inflammatory component of the disease will subside, as evidenced by the disappearance of papillomatous masses in the bladder, the cessation of diarrhea or hematuria, and a reduction of hepatomegaly. However, the fibrotic and stenotic consequences of a long-term infection are irreversible. Therapy will neither restore the functional integrity of the intestinal and urinary tracts nor correct the hepatic periportal fibrosis underlying portal hypertension or the obliterative arteriolitis responsible for cor pulmonale.

Therapy

Treatment of the patient with schistosomiasis involves several considerations. Although no ideal drug is available, any therapy that reduces the burden of worms is of benefit. Schistosomes differ in their response to schistosomicidal drugs; compounds effective for *S. haematobium* may be ineffective for the treatment of *S. japonicum,* the species most refractory to drugs. Further, there are differences in the effectiveness of a particular drug against strains of a single species from different geographic areas.

Schistosomicides exhibit toxicity for the host as well as for the parasite, and the risk of undesirable side-effects may be enhanced by concomitant cardiac, renal, or hepatosplenic disease. Several nonmetallic drugs now in use have been shown to have mutagenic, carcinogenic, or teratogenic activity in microbial and other test systems. Whether these observations justify concern regarding their use in humans is a matter of opinion rather than of fact; yet prudence would proscribe the administration of niridazole, hycanthone, and oxamniquine to the pregnant female. Short-term symptoms, particularly fever, nausea, vertigo, and abdominal pain, may follow use of an effective schistosomicide apparently reflecting the host's response to substances released from degenerating worms.

The patient with active schistosomiasis requires specific therapy. It has been suggested that the asymptomatic patient who apparently harbors few worms (evidenced by low egg counts in the feces or urine) should not be treated because of the potential toxicity of available drugs. This concept is statistically valid. In the individual patient, however, the worm burden cannot be precisely determined, the subsequent evolution of the disease is uncertain, and the possibility that even a single egg-laying female might deposit eggs in a vital area cannot be ignored. Thus, there is justification for treatment of all patients who pass viable eggs.

The treatment of schistosomiasis is in a constructive state of flux. New nonmetallic compounds are replacing the classic antimony-containing drugs. These are less toxic, more effective, and can be given perorally. Certain new drugs that are unavailable commercially may be obtained from the Parasitic Disease Drug Services, Centers for Disease Control (CDC), Atlanta, Georgia 30333 (telephone 404-329-3670). Since the list of available drugs is always changing, consultative advice should be sought. There is a species specificity of the individual drugs.

Metrifonate (obtainable from CDC) is active only against *S. haematobium* and is the drug of choice for the treatment of urinary schistosomiasis. An organophosphorus anticholinesterase compound, it is administered perorally in three doses of 10 mg/kg body wt with 2 weeks intervening between each dose.

Of available compounds, the drug of choice for treatment of Manson's schistosomiasis is oxamniquine (Vansil), a tetrahydroquinolene derivative. Infections with *S. mansoni* acquired in the Western Hemisphere respond well to a single, peroral dose of 15 mg/kg body wt. Oxamniquine has been approved by the Food and Drug Administration for treatment of Manson's schistosomiasis of Western Hemisphere origin and is available in the form of 250-mg capsules from commercial sources. Persons infected with strains of *S. mansoni* acquired in Africa do not respond as well to equivalent doses of oxamniquine; advice should be obtained from the CDC regarding current recommendations on the use of higher doses.

Infections with *S. japonicum* are relatively refractory to therapy. The new drug, praziquantel, a perorally administrable compound which is not related structurally to previously used schistosomicides, appears to be effective. Indeed, praziquantel appears to be effective in the treatment of all three major schistosomal diseases, and is being tested on a global basis under the auspices of the World Health Organization. The Parasitic Disease Services of CDC should be contacted for current recommendations regarding the use of praziquantel for schistosomiasis. Niridazole frequently causes adverse reactions of the central nervous system when it is given to patients with hepatosplenic involvement.

Prevention

Persons planning travel to regions in which schistosomiasis is endemic should be warned of the hazard associated with swimming or wading in fresh water. No chemoprophylaxis is available. In organized societies, effective control can be achieved by prevention of contact by humans with infected water, by collection and treatment of egg-containing excreta, and by control of vector snails through environmental engineering or through the use of molluscicides.

Remaining Problems

Currently, the demonstration of eggs in feces, urine, or tissues is the only method of establishing a specific diagnosis of schistosomiasis. Greater sensitivity and increased ease of diagnosis might be achieved through the preparation of schistosomal antigens that would permit the development of specific serodiagnostic tests. The current search for vaccines to modify or prevent schistosomiasis is likewise being expedited.

Wherever schistosomiasis is endemic, the disease may be controlled by mass chemotherapy, by killing the vector snails, or by providing safe water supplies. Unfortunately, these approaches require economic and scientific resources that most often are not available. Simpler and cheaper methods are needed.

Bibliography

Books

HOFFMAN DB JR, WARREN KS: Schistosomiasis IV. Condensation of the selected literature, 1963–1975. Vols I/II. Washington, Hemisphere, 1978. pp vii and 538.

JORDAN P, WEBBE G: Human Schistosomiasis. Springfield, Ill, Charles C Thomas, 1969. 212 pp.

WARREN KS, HOFFMAN DB JR: Schistosomiasis III. Abstracts of the complete literature, 1963–1974. Vols I/II. Hemisphere Publishing Company (distributed by John Wiley & Sons, New York), 1976. pp vi and 730.

World Health Organization Expert Committee Report. Epidemiology and control of schistosomiasis. Technical Report Series 643. Geneva, WHO, 1980. 63 pp.

Journals

ABRAMOWICZ M (ED): Drugs for parasitic infections. The Medical Letter 24:5–12, 1982

DAVIS A: Clinically available antischistosomal drugs. J Toxicol Environ Health 1:191–201, 1975

DAVIS A, WEGNER DHG: Multicentre trials of praziquantel in human schistosomiasis: Design and techniques. Bull WHO 57:767–771, 1979

WELLER TH: Manson's schistosomiasis: Frontiers in vivo, in vitro, and in the body politic. Am J Trop Med Hyg 25:208–216, 1976

Section XIII

Infections of the Peritoneum

Indigenous Microbiota of the Peritoneum

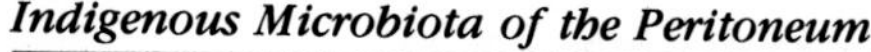

(None)

SYDNEY M. FINEGOLD

Peritonitis

82

Peritonitis is inflammation of the serous lining of the peritoneal cavity. It is a nonspecific response to either microbial agents or chemical irritation.

Etiology

Nonbacterial peritonitis results from introduction into the peritoneal cavity of irritants such as blood, bile, pancreatic juice, gastroduodenal juices, and meconium. Primary or spontaneous bacterial peritonitis is uncommon. It occurs in patients with nephrosis or postnecrotic cirrhosis; in this situation, it is caused by *Streptococcus pneumoniae* or *Streptococcus pyogenes.* More commonly, it is seen in patients with advanced, decompensated cirrhosis with ascites. Pneumococci and group A streptococci may also be involved in such patients, but *Escherichia coli* or other enteric organisms are more common.

Bacterial peritonitis is usually secondary to underlying disease—vascular, obstructive, traumatic, infective, neoplastic, or postoperative. Common predisposing lesions include appendicitis, ruptured peptic ulcer, cholecystitis, diverticulitis, intestinal strangulation, intestinal obstruction, post-operative leakage from the site of an anastomosis, salpingitis, and traumatic injury to abdominal or pelvic viscera. Other causes are mesenteric thrombosis, acute pancreatitis, cancers of the gastrointestinal tract, regional enteritis, rupture of a liver abscess, and parametritis.

The specific microorganisms involved in peritonitis are generally drawn from the flora of the gastrointestinal tract (Table 82-1). Because this flora varies markedly according to the level sampled, the infectious agents involved in peritonitis also vary with site and kind of underlying problem. However, it must be remembered that the enteric flora itself may change with abnormal conditions. For example, bacterial counts are much higher in gastric juice when the pH is above 4.0 and when there is obstruction, impaired motility, or bleeding. The flora of the small intestine is much more profuse and complex in the presence of intestinal obstruction or other processes affecting motility or absorption. Persons receiving antimicrobial agents by injection and by mouth may undergo significant modifications in their enteric flora. Infections related to the female genital tract may involve *Neisseria gonorrhoeae, Streptococcus pyogenes, Escherichia coli,* anaerobic streptococci, and various *Bacteroides* spp. and *Clostridium* spp. Clues to the presence of anaerobes in an infective process have been noted in Chapter 32, Necrotizing Pneumonias and Lung Abscess, along with details characterizing various anaerobic bacteria.

Peritonitis is an excellent example of synergism in infection. It is uncommon to find a single kind of microorganism involved in peritonitis. Characteristically, the more kinds of bacteria that can be isolated from the patient with peritonitis, the more serious the prognosis.

Peritonitis following abdominal surgery often involves *Staphylococcus aureus* and gram-negative bacilli such as *Proteus* spp., *Klebsiella* spp., *Enterobacter* spp., and *Pseudomonas* spp., particularly if the patient has received preoperative bowel preparation and additional antimicrobial agents.

Tuberculosis peritonitis is considered in Chapter 34, Pulmonary Tuberculosis.

Epidemiology

Peritonitis is still a common infection. Although most of the etiologic agents come from the normal and abnormal flora of the gastrointestinal tract, or sometimes from the female genital tract, many infections are caused by microorganisms introduced from outside the body in the course of trauma or surgery. Peritonitis may also follow peritoneal dialysis.

Pathogenesis and Pathology

The healthy peritoneum has a marked ability to resist infection. Two factors are of major importance to the establishment of peritonitis: a continuing source of infection in the peritoneal cavity and foreign material (bile, feces, or necrotic tissue) that protects bacteria from host defense mechanisms. Free hemoglobin facilitates peritonitis in ways not yet explained.

The inflamed peritoneum accumulates plaques of fibrinous material that cause loops of intestine to adhere to one another and to the parietal peritoneum. There is an outpouring of serous fluid containing leukocytes. The greater omentum appears to seek out and adhere to areas of peritonitis. These factors, along with ileus, tend to localize infection to a region of the peritoneal cavity. The ratio of bacteria to available leukocytes is an important factor determining the outcome of peritonitis.

Manifestations

The mode of onset varies according to the precipitating cause. Typical findings are pain, abdominal distention, absence of abdominal respiratory movement, diffuse muscle spasm, tenderness and rebound tenderness, decreased or absent peristalsis, rigidity of the abdominal wall, tenderness on rectal or vaginal examination, and fever. There may also be toxemia and shock.

Pain and muscle spasm may be deceptively absent in the very old or young and in patients with shock. Patients receiving glucosteroids may show none of the typical findings. In such patients, the most important finding is a completely silent abdomen on auscultation. A high index of suspicion is necessary in such patients; the only early manifestation may be an unexplained rise in pulse rate or hypotension. In addition, the signs of peritonitis may be overshadowed

Table 82-1. *Normal Flora of the Human Gastrointestinal Tract*

Site	Mean Count per ml or g of Contents	Flora
Stomach	$<10^3$	Viridans group streptococci; *Lactobacillus* spp. and yeasts
Upper small bowel	$<10^5$	Gram-positive aerobes
Lower small bowel	10^{6-7}	Equal numbers of aerobes (chiefly coliforms) and anaerobes (*Bacteroides* spp. and bifid bacilli, chiefly)
Colon (left)	10^{11-12}	Anaerobes (*Bacteroides fragilis* group*, *Bifidobacterium* spp.*, *Eubacterium* spp.*, *Clostridium* spp., anaerobic cocci*) constitute 99.0%–99.9% of flora. *Escherichia coli,* enterococcal and viridans group streptococci, *Lactobacillus* spp. make up balance of flora

* Predominant microorganisms.

by manifestations of the primary process, for example, trauma to the abdomen. In primary bacterial peritonitis, there is often marked fever and leukocytosis, with typical abdominal findings. However, in patients with an underlying postnecrotic or Laennec's cirrhosis, the disease may be quite insidious.

Diagnosis

The pain of peritonitis must be carefully evaluated. The physician must know the site of origin of the pain, the site of the most intense pain, and the character and radiation of the pain. This information is a great aid in the diagnosis of peritonitis and its underlying causes. It is all-important in differentiating peritonitis from myocardial infarction, tabetic crisis, arachnidism, porphyria, diabetic acidosis, plumbism, pulmonary disease, or renal disease. Fever is quite common in peritonitis; however, when it exceeds 39.4°C (103°F) at the onset of illness, a surgically reparable process is quite unlikely. The blood leukocyte count is usually over 12,000 but counts above 20,000 cells/mm^3 are rare in patients with an acute surgical abdomen. Glycosuria and hyperglycemia may be seen in acute pancreatitis and also in diabetic acidosis, but they are not typical in peritonitis. Hematuria and pyuria usually reflect primary genitourinary tract involvement, but they may reflect no more than adjacent inflammatory disease, such as appendicitis or diverticulitis. Very high concentrations of amylase in the serum are consistent with acute pancreatitis (Chap. 77, Pancreatitis and Pancreatic Abscesses), but lower levels may occur in peritonitis (from virtually any cause), intestinal obstruction, perforated viscus, and uremia, and after the injection of opiates. Films of the abdomen (supine, upright, or left lateral decubitus) may reveal free air in the peritoneal cavity, encapsulated air or gas in an abscess, features of ileus or obstruction, evidence of peritoneal fluid, calcification within the bladder or other organs, and obliteration of the psoas shadow or other peritoneal lines. Examination of the abdomen using ultrasound, computerized tomography, and radiogallium scanning may aid in diagnosis.

Needle aspiration of the peritoneal cavity is often very helpful. The liquid obtained may be turbid, purulent, bloody, or pathognomonic of the digestion of fat—containing free-floating globules of fat. Negative findings are of no diagnostic value. When pus or liquid is encountered, gram-stained smears, and aerobic and anaerobic cultures should be made. Peritoneoscopy or needle biopsy of the peritoneum may occasionally provide useful information.

Prognosis

The mortality rate in diffuse peritonitis declined remarkably with the introduction of antimicrobial chemotherapy. However, the percentage of postoperative residual abscesses is still quite high, and there may still be significant mortality, depending on the underlying cause of the peritonitis. Complications of peritonitis include septic shock, intraabdominal or retroperitoneal abscess, respiratory failure, adhesions, and fistulas.

Therapy

The principles of therapy are (1) to improve vascular perfusion by correcting fluid and electrolyte deficits; (2) to combat the effects of bacteria and their toxic metabolites; (3) to reduce paralytic ileus; (4) to eliminate the primary source of infection by means of excision, closure, or isolation; (5) to aspirate as much of the infected peritoneal exudate as possible and to drain the site of the primary lesion; and (6) to treat local or distant complications as necessary. Conservative treatment is advisable in certain types of peritonitis, appendiceal abscess, and certain cases of perforated peptic ulcer. In most cases of peritonitis, surgical intervention is required for management of an underlying problem and for drainage of purulent collections. Surgery should be performed at the earliest time consistent with adequate preparation of the patient.

Systemic antimicrobial agents should be used before and after surgical therapy. The choice of antimicrobic depends on the microorganisms involved in the peritonitis. Primary bacterial peritonitis involving streptococci is best treated with penicillin G. Postoperative peritonitis should be treated with one of the penicillinase-resistant penicillins or cephalosporins when *S. aureus* is involved, or with gentamicin, tobramycin, or netilmicin (4 mg–6 mg/kg body wt/day, IM or IV, as three equal portions 8-hourly), or amikacin (15 mg/kg body wt/day IV or IM, as three equal portions, 8-hourly), or other agents, depending on the gram-negative bacteria which may be implicated (Chap. 32, Necrotizing Pneumonias and Lung Abscess and 53, Intrarenal and Perinephric Abscess). Cefoxitin (100 mg–150 mg/kg body wt/day, IV, as 6 equal portions, 4-hourly) will often be effective if *Pseudomonas* spp. are absent, and it provides reasonably good coverage for anaerobes as well.

Without previous chemotherapy that may have altered the resident enteric microflora, peritonitis caused by enteric bacteria may be treated with either chloramphenicol (alone or with an aminocyclitol such as gentamicin), or gentamicin plus clindamycin, or metronidazole. Chloramphenicol (succinate derivative) should be injected intravenously in a loading dose of 25 mg/kg body wt and continued at 30 mg–60 mg/kg body wt/day as four equal portions 6-hourly in the adult (exact dose dependent on the severity of the illness). Chloramphenicol is active against *Bacteroides fragilis,* the predominant microorganism in the colon and a major offender in peritonitis, and against all other anaerobic bacteria (Chap. 32, Necrotizing Pneumonias and Lung Abscess). Thus, chloramphenicol is also a potentially useful drug for the management of peritonitis secondary to infection in the female genital tract (Chap. 50, Infections of the Female Genital Tract). Metronidazole may be given IV (30 mg/kg body wt/day as four equal portions, 6-hourly, after a loading dose of 15 mg/kg). Gentamicin and tobramycin (dosage given above) are effective against most gram-negative aerobic and facultative bacteria; clindamycin (25 mg–40 mg/kg body wt/day, IM or IV as four equal portions 6-hourly) is effective against most anaerobes. Amikacin is the aminocyclitol of choice in very ill patients in hospitals in which gram-negative bacilli are frequently resistant to gentamicin. In critically ill patients, penicillin G should be added (150 mg–200 mg [240,000–320,000 units]/kg body wt/day, IV, as six equal portions, 4-hourly) to provide antimicrobial coverage against *Clostridium* spp. and other anaerobes resistant to clindamycin or to metronidazole. Repeated intraperitoneal administration of antimicrobics is neither desirable nor necessary. Peritoneal lavage, with an appropriate antimicrobic in the lavage fluid, has been advocated on a prolonged, intermittent basis in certain patients with diffuse peritonitis in whom it may not otherwise be feasible to effect good drainage. A regimen of this kind should not be used in patients with local peritonitis, because it may actually result in dissemination of the process.

Prevention

Early, appropriate treatment of salpingitis and endometritis lowers the incidence of peritonitis secondary to these conditions. Similarly, definitive surgical therapy of perforated viscera may prevent peritonitis. Postoperative peritonitis is still a very important complication of abdominal surgery. Both the frequency and the severity of peritonitis may be minimized by good surgical technique and careful asepsis. Preoperative bowel preparation with oral neomycin or kanamycin plus tetracycline or erythromycin lowers the incidence of peritonitis or other postoperative infection. Along with appropriate drainage, antimicrobial agents should be given when there has been contamination of the peritoneal cavity with bowel contents. In other situations, such as acute pancreatitis after which there is a 15% incidence of bacterial peritonitis, it is more difficult to judge whether chemoprophylaxis will be helpful; there are no definitive data.

Remaining Problems

Peritonitis is another syndrome in which the prevention of nosocomial infections would be very helpful. Much work has been done in the past on the significance in peritonitis of various bacteria, alone and in combinations. Additional work is necessitated by the availability of new antimicrobial agents and improved techniques in laboratory diagnosis; such studies are in progress.

Bibliography

Books

FINEGOLD SM: Anaerobic Bacteria in Human Disease. New York, Academic Press, 1977. 710 pp.

STEINBERG B: Infections of the Peritoneum. New York, Paul B Hoeber, 1944. 455 pp.

Journals

ALTEMEIER WA: The pathogenicity of the bacteria of appendicitis and peritonitis: An experimental study. Surgery 11:374–384, 1942

CONN HO, FESSEL JM: Spontaneous bacterial peritonitis in cirrhosis: Variations on a theme. Medicine 50:161–197, 1971

PULASKI EJ, NOYES HE, EVANS JR, BRAME RA: The influence of antibiotics on experimental endogenous peritonitis. Surg Gynecol Obstet 99:341–358, 1954

SWENSON RM, LORBER B, MICHAELSON TC, SPAULDING EH: The bacteriology of intra-abdominal infections. Arch Surg 109:398–399, 1974

SYDNEY M. FINEGOLD

Appendicitis and Diverticulitis

83

Appendicitis and diverticulitis connote inflammation, usually acute, involving the vermiform appendix and diverticula of the infragastric enteric tract. The anatomy of the structures involved is different, but as problems of infectious disease, they are reasonably discussed together because they are so alike in pathogenesis and bacterial etiology.

Etiology

Bacterial involvement is a complication of obstruction of the lumen of the appendix and of diverticula. Accordingly, the bacteria that are associated with appendicitis and diverticulitis are those normally present in that portion of the gut with which the afflicted structure(s) communicated. A mixture of microorganisms is the rule, and anaerobic bacteria play a much more important role than is generally appreciated.

Two to seven or more kinds of bacteria are usually present in acute appendicitis. Among the aerobic forms, *Escherichia coli* and *Streptococcus* spp. (enterococcal group and others) are common. Anaerobes are present in large numbers, clearly predominating over aerobes. Of these, the *Bacteroides melaninogenicus–Bacteroides asaccharolyticus,* and *Bacteroides fragilis* groups outnumber the commonly found anaerobic cocci and streptococci. *Clostridium* spp. (including *C. perfringens*) and *Eubacterium* spp. are found in 15% to 25% of cases. Various other anaerobes are found occasionally; details concerning these anaerobes are given in Chap. 32, Necrotizing Pneumonias and Lung Abscess. Rarely, *Streptococcus pneumoniae* and group A *Streptococcus pyogenes* are involved in acute appendicitis following acute respiratory infections.

The bacteria involved in diverticulitis are those normally present at the site of connection of a diverticulum with the gut. The discussion given in Chap. 82, Peritonitis, of the bacterial flora normally present at various levels of the enteric tract is pertinent. The finding of many kinds of bacteria, with predominance of anaerobes, is to be expected because fecal flora is normal in the sigmoid colon, the region most commonly afflicted with diverticula. The bacterial flora of the small intestine is both less profuse and varied, but diverticula occur much less commonly in this part of the gut.

Epidemiology

Acute appendicitis occurs in more than 200,000 persons in the United States each year. There is some evidence that the disease is more common, and perhaps more severe, among those of higher social and economic status. Appendicitis occurs at any age, but most commonly in early life. Between puberty and 25 years of age, males are more commonly affected.

Diverticulosis is uncommon under the age of 40, but it increases in frequency with age so that by the ninth decade, two-thirds of persons are affected. Males and females are affected equally. The longer the patient has had diverticulosis and the older the patient, the more likely diverticulitis becomes. Approximately one-half of patients will have diverticula in the sigmoid area only. Most of the remainder will have them both in the sigmoid and in other areas of the colon. In whites, diverticular disease involves the left colon primarily, whereas in Orientals up to 60% of cases of diverticulitis occur in the right colon. Diverticula of the small bowel are less common and less likely to be involved with diverticulitis. Diverticula of the duodenum are found in approximately 1% and in more distal sections of the small bowel in only 0.1% of all patients studied by upper gastrointestinal contrast radiography.

Pathogenesis and Pathology

Obstruction is the critical event in the pathogenesis of both appendicitis and diverticulitis. With obstruction of the lumen, trapped enteric contents are augmented in volume by secretions. Increased intraluminal pressure develops and is aggravated by peristalsis causing distention, and ultimately, occlusion and thrombosis of capillaries and venules. Infarction, hemorrhage, and pressure necrosis follow; eventually perforation results.

In almost all cases of appendicitis, a fecalith is the cause of obstruction. However, the antecedence of an acute viral infection, notably rubeola, is too common to be merely coincidental.

In diverticulitis, it is possible that the same factors responsible for the development of diverticula also contribute to their distention with fecal material. Diabetes mellitus appears to predispose patients to diverticulitis; however, the same increased intraenteric pressure that forces feces into diverticula causes vascular engorgement, mucosal necrosis, and bacterial penetration. The actual inflammation of diverticulitis results from perforation (usually of a single diverticulum) rather than stagnation.

Inflammation is the characteristic finding on histologic examination. Generally, the response is acute in appendicitis, and often there are edema, hemorrhage, necrosis, thrombosis, and hyperplasia of lymphoid follicles. Granulation tissue and nodular aggregates of lymphoid cells as part of the response in diverticulitis attest to the protracted course so frequent in this disease.

Perforation of an inflamed appendix yields local or general peritonitis. Usually, the process is well-localized, although abscess formation is common. Slow, episodic leakage is typical in diverticular perforation; microabscesses form, and the affected segment of colon becomes thickened and firm.

Manifestations

Abdominal pain, signs of peritoneal irritation, fever, and leukocytosis are the major clinical findings in appendicitis and diverticulitis. There are, however, important differences in the patterns of these manifestations.

Pain is the principal and often the only symptom of uncomplicated appendicitis. The sequence is typical: periumbilical or epigastric reference of pain at onset, followed by a shift to the right lower quadrant after a few hours. Tenderness, muscle spasm, and rebound tenderness do not become prominent until the pain has shifted. Anorexia, nausea, and vomiting occur after the illness has commenced with pain. Atypical clinical presentations occur, particularly in the very young and in the very old. If the appendix is retrocecal, the anterior abdominal reference of symptoms and signs is diminished or absent, although iliopsoas manipulation (hyperextension of the legs, straight leg raising) will elicit signs of inflammation. Pelvic location of the appendix also militates against anterior abdominal manifestations, and findings are generally more impressive on rectal than on abdominal examination. Sudden cessation of pain is often coincident with perforation of the appendix.

The pattern of manifestations is generally less firmly predictable in diverticulitis. The location of the pain depends on the site and extent of the diverticulitis. Increased intraabdominal pressure, as in defecation, aggravates the pain. Spasm of the bowel usually produces constipation, but there may be diarrhea. Nausea and vomiting are not uncommon. Rectal bleeding occurs in one-fourth of patients with sigmoid diverticulitis, and occasionally this is massive. Eventually, it may be possible to feel a tender mass on abdominal examination. Partial obstruction may develop behind the mass.

Diagnosis

The history and physical examination are of paramount importance in diagnosis. In addition, neutrophilic leukocytosis, up to $20{,}000/mm^3$, is typical in appendicitis, although generally less marked in diverticulitis. Urinalysis is helpful because hematuria, pyuria, glycosuria, and bilirubinuria are not typical findings. However, an inflamed appendix or diverticulum juxtaposed to a ureter or the urinary bladder may cause hematuria or pyuria. Although appendicitis itself does not cause characteristic roentgenographic findings, contrast studies may sometimes be helpful; for example, in appendiceal abscess (Fig. 83-1).

Roentgenographic studies are of particular value in diverticulitis. Barium should not be given by mouth because of the danger of obstruction, and barium enemas must be administered with care. Roentgenographic findings diagnostic of diverticulitis include the demonstration of an abscess cavity communicating with the lumen of the colon (Fig. 83-2), and the demonstration of an intramural sinus tract. Other important roentgenographic findings are free air secondary to perforation, evidence of obstruction, and fistulas to adjacent organs. A filling defect of the intestinal lumen produced by an intramural or pericolic

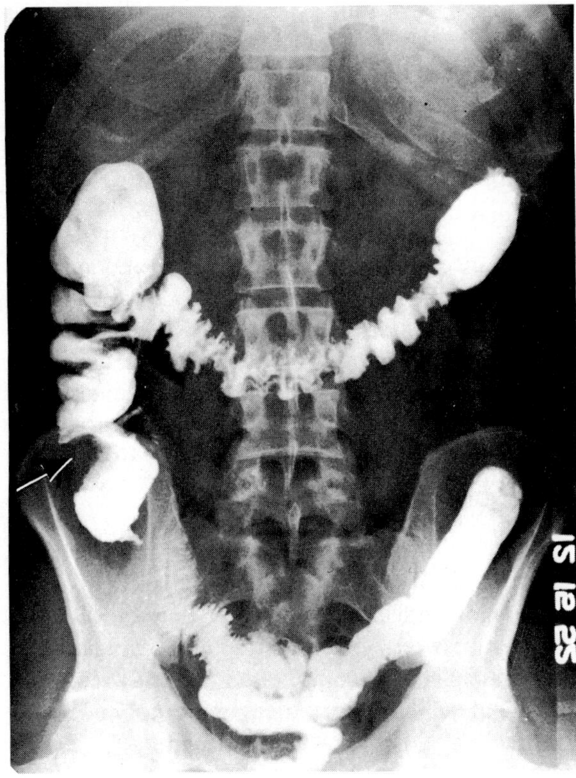

Fig. 83-1. The arrow points to extrinsic compression of the cecum by an appendiceal abscess.

mass strongly suggests acute diverticulitis. Roentgenographic findings of lesser significance include incomplete distention and elongation of a colonic segment, transverse ridging of the colon suggestive of foreshortening of the segment, and persistent colonic narrowing that occasionally relents (suggesting spasm; see Fig. 83-2).

Sigmoidoscopy is very helpful in the diagnosis of diverticulitis, particularly when there is limited mobility of a bowel segment that is normally freely movable, abnormally sharp angulation in the region of the rectosigmoid or higher, narrowing of the lumen of the bowel, sigmoidal sacculation not obliterated by inflation, and an extraluminal mass.

When there is complicating abscess formation, gallium scan, indium-labeled white blood cell scan, computed tomography, and ultrasound examination may be very useful.

Differential diagnosis must include all conditions capable of causing peritonitis, and all medical diseases that simulate acute abdominal inflammation. Of particular importance are gastroenteritis, mesenteric lymphadenitis, mesenteric thrombosis, cholecystitis, incarcerated hernia, infarction of epiploic appendages, regional enteritis, chronic ulcerative colitis, granulomatous diseases of the bowel, perforation of colonic carcinoma, extravasation of urine, cystitis, ruptured ovarian follicle, ovarian tumor, ruptured tubal pregnancy, torsion of an ovarian cyst, acute salpingitis, pelvic inflammatory disease, and endometriosis.

The most difficult problem is that of distinguishing between diverticulitis and carcinoma. The patient's history is often helpful: severe abdominal pain is three times more common in diverticulitis; gross bleeding per rectum is three times more common in carcinoma. Sigmoidoscopy may enable the visualization and biopsy of a carcinoma. The cytologic study of rectal washings for malignant cells should be carried out. Contrast roentgenographic findings that favor the diagnosis of diverticulitis include the involvement of a relatively long segment of bowel with tapered ends above and below the lesion, intact mucosa showing a fringed contour (picket-fence de-

Fig. 83-2. Diverticulitis of the sigmoid colon, with perforation. The large arrow points to barium extravasating through a perforation. The small arrows point to diverticula. Note the spasm of the sigmoid proximal to the point of perforation.

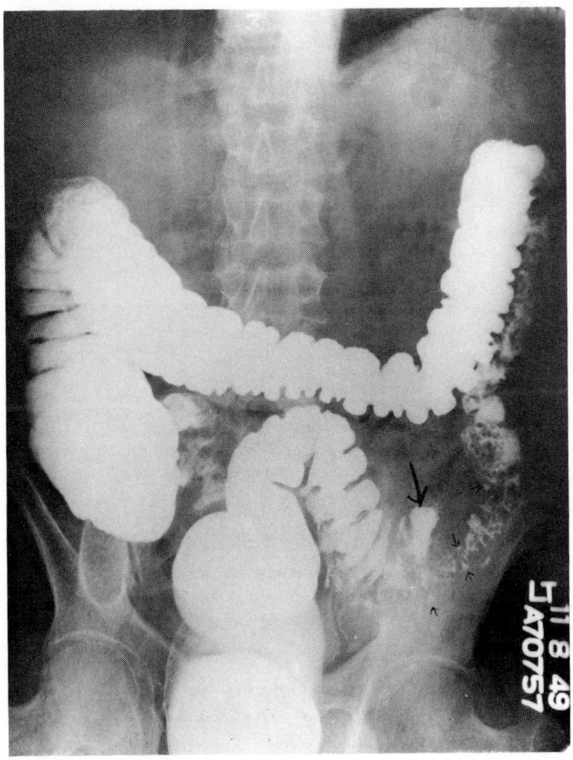

formity), and intestinal spasm. Surgical exploration may be required to make the diagnosis and even at surgery, the gross appearance of diverticulitis and carcinoma can be virtually identical.

Prognosis

Overall, the mortality of acute appendicitis is now less than 1% in the United States; with nonperforated appendices it is less than 0.2%. Rupture, the most common complication, usually leads to periappendiceal abscess, but it occasionally produces general peritonitis, and subsequently, abscesses anywhere in the abdomen. The most serious complication is pylephlebitis, which may cause multiple liver abscesses (see Chap. 84, Pylephlebitis and Liver Abscess). Adhesions may cause difficulties at a later time. Rare complications include gas gangrene, fecal fistulas, acute bowel obstruction, and granulomas.

The mortality rate of diverticulitis is in the range of 2% to 4%. Older patients, particularly those over 70, and diabetic patients have a higher mortality, as do patients requiring emergency operations. Mortality is generally lowest when elective surgery is done in stages. Complications include obstruction, perforation with either abscess formation or peritonitis, hemorrhage, and development of a fistula between the colon and the bladder, the vagina, other viscera, or the abdominal wall. Second or repeated attacks of diverticulitis may occur, even in patients who have had resection of an involved segment of bowel.

Therapy

Early surgery is the treatment of choice in acute appendicitis. Antimicrobial agents have no place in the management of uncomplicated appendicitis and are actually contraindicated because their use may cloud the clinical picture.

If perforation has occurred, delay in primary wound closure after surgery is desirable. In addition to drainage, antimicrobics are useful. The drugs of choice are either chloramphenicol, clindamycin, or metronidazole with gentamicin (see Chap. 82, Peritonitis, for details on the use of these drugs); cefoxitin is also effective. Supportive therapy, such as gastrointestinal intubation and proper management of fluid and electrolyte balance, is important.

Without complications, treatment of diverticulitis is medical. The patient is given nothing by mouth. Morphine should not be given because it may lead to a considerable increase in intraluminal pressure and thus predispose the patient to perforation. Anticholinergic drugs and barbiturates may be helpful. Parenterally administered chloramphenicol, clindamycin, or metronidazole—combined with gentamicin—should be used until the acute febrile attack has subsided. (See Chap. 82, Peritonitis, for details on the use of these drugs). Cefoxitin is also effective. Constipation may be treated by rectal instillations of oil or small enemas. Probably less than 10% of patients who develop diverticulitis require surgery. Indications for elective surgery are recurrent inflammatory episodes, a progressive stenosis of significant degree, a palpable mass with no regression under antimicrobial therapy, refractory dysuria (suggesting the likelihood of colovesical fistula), fistulas of other types, failure to rule out carcinoma, and recurrent significant bleeding. More serious complications, such as obstruction or perforation, require early surgery. In the presence of abscess, peritonitis, or obstruction, primary resection of the diseased colon is not safe. When major complications are not present and it is possible to free up the colon readily so that it may be exteriorized, resection of the diseased tissue may be carried out at the time of the initial surgery. However, rather than attempt primary anastomosis, it is preferable to perform a colostomy and closure or exteriorization of the distal loop. A three-stage operation, involving a colostomy, then resection of the diseased bowel after all inflammation has subsided, and finally reanastomosis of the bowel, may be the preferred procedure in some cases. In the case of acute perforation, drainage may be carried out at the time of the initial colostomy.

Diverticulitis of the cecum often heals spontaneously. If an accurate diagnosis can be made without resort to surgery, conservative treatment is justified.

A low-residue diet is desirable during the acute inflammatory process.

Prevention

Routine appendectomy in the course of other abdominal surgery is a laudable preventive measure if the patient can readily tolerate the extra procedure. Early management of pinworm infestation in children may minimize appendicitis related to this condition.

High-residue diets are now recommended for patients with diverticula to prevent further development of diverticulosis and to minimize the likelihood of diverticulitis. Constipation should be managed without the use of strong laxatives or irritating enemas. Obese patients should reduce to their normal weight.

Remaining Problems

More effective means for diagnosing appendicitis are needed, particularly in patients with an inadequate history.

Information is needed that will enable the prediction of which patients with diverticula will develop diverticulitis. The effect of various medical measures on preventing diverticulitis in patients with diverticulosis is not known with certainty.

Bibliography

Books

BOYCE FF: Acute Appendicitis and its Complications. New York, Oxford University Press, 1949. 487 pp.

LOCALIO SA, STAHL WM: Diverticular Disease of the Alimentary Tract. Part I. The Colon. Part II. The Esophagus, Stomach, Duodenum and Small Intestine. Current Problems in Surgery. Chicago, Year Book Medical Publishers. Part I, Dec 1967, 78 pp; Part II, Jan 1968, 47 pp.

Journals

BRADLEY EL, ISAACS J: Appendiceal abscess revisited. Arch Surg 113:130–132, 1978

LARSON DM, MASTERS SS, SPIRO HM: Medical and surgical therapy in diverticular disease. Gastroenterology 71:734–737, 1976

LEIGH DA, SIMMONS K, NORMAN E: Bacterial flora of the appendix fossa in appendicitis and postoperative wound infection. J Clin Pathol 27:997–1000, 1974

LEWIS FR, HOLCROFT JW, BOEY J, DUNPHY JE: Appendicitis: A critical review of diagnosis and treatment in 1000 cases. Arch Surg 110:677–684, 1975

RODKEY GV, WELCH CE: Colonic diverticular disease with surgical treatment: A study of 338 cases. Surg Clin North Am 54:655–674, 1974

SYDNEY M. FINEGOLD

84 Pylephlebitis and Liver Abscess

Pylephlebitis is acute suppurative thrombosis of one of the tributaries of the portal vein. It is frequently, but not exclusively, the antecedent of pyogenic liver abscess.

Etiology

Bowel flora—anaerobic or microaerophilic streptococci, *Bacteroides* spp. and other anaerobes, *Escherichia coli* and enterococcal group *Streptococcus* spp.—usually predominate in pylephlebitis; *Staphylococcus aureus* may also be found.

Before the availability of antibacterial agents, the microorganisms predominating in pyogenic liver abscess were *E. coli* and *Streptococcus* spp., particularly of the enterococcal and viridans group. In recent years, other aerobic gram-negative bacilli, such as *Klebsiella* spp., *Enterobacter* spp., *Proteus* spp., and *Pseudomonas* spp., have been recovered with increasing frequency. The actual incidence of anaerobic bacteria is not known because in most series adequate anaerobic culture techniques were not used. Anaerobes are important and are clearly involved in at least 50% of cases of pyogenic liver abscess. With proper transport of specimens and suitable anaerobic methodology, anaerobes are the exclusive isolates in two-thirds of the cases yielding anaerobic bacteria. The anaerobes most prevalent in liver abscess are anaerobic and microaerophilic streptococci, *Fusobacterium nucleatum,* and the *Bacteroides fragilis-Bacteroides melaninogenicus-Bacteroides asaccharolyticus* groups. Clues to the presence of anaerobes and the characteristics of various anaerobic bacteria are discussed in Chapter 32, Necrotizing Pneumonias and Lung Abscess.

Epidemiology

Pylephlebitis and liver abscess are uncommon infections. Their incidence varies from 0.05% to 0.5% of all hospital admissions or autopsies. They are seen predominantly in males. There is no apparent racial susceptibility. Multiple abscesses probably outnumber solitary abscesses, and the right lobe is involved much more frequently than the left.

Pathogenesis and Pathology

Pylephlebitis is secondary either to suppurative disease in tissues drained by tributaries of the portal vein or to suppuration in contiguous structures. The most common underlying causes of pylephlebitis are acute appendicitis and biliary tract infections. Other causes include chronic ulcerative colitis, diverticulitis, and carcinoma of the bowel. In pylephlebitis, the portal vein and its intrahepatic radicles show an acute inflammatory reaction and not infrequently contain pus or thrombi. Microscopically, there is round-cell infiltration of the venous wall with leukocytes and cellular debris within the lumen. Adjacent liver cells show varying degrees of inflammation or degeneration.

Most cases of pyogenic liver abscess are secondary to pylephlebitis, and suppurative cholangitis is also common. Embolic abscesses, usually multiple, may originate from foci anywhere in the body by way of the hepatic artery. Direct extension of infection, or extension by way of the lymphatics, may develop from such situations as a perforated gallbladder or duodenal ulcer, pancreatic abscess, perinephric or subdiaphragmatic abscess, or even lung abscess or thoracic empyema. Uncommon causes of liver abscess are retrograde infection through the hepatic vein and infections secondary to penetrating wounds or foreign bodies. In a significant percentage of cases, it is not possible to determine the underlying cause of liver abscess. The pathology of liver abscess is that of any abscess. Adjacent liver cells show varying degrees of inflammation or degeneration.

Manifestations

The manifestations of pylephlebitis include chills, fever, epigastric or right upper-quadrant pain, nausea, vomiting, enlargement and tenderness of the liver, and sometimes splenomegaly. Jaundice is inconstant and usually mild when present. Signs of liver abscess or of acute portal vein thrombosis (abdominal pain, ileus, vomiting, diarrhea; perhaps later, ascites, splenomegaly, and even gastrointestinal infarction) may complicate the picture.

Fever, the most common finding in liver abscess, may be accompanied by chills and sweats. The second most common finding is right upper-quadrant pain. The pain is aching in character, and tends to be localized either over the liver itself or the epigastrium. It may radiate to the right shoulder when it is aggravated by respiration. Percussion of the liver is painful. One may note a local mass beneath the costal margin, or fullness and tenderness of the intercostal spaces. At times there is local, firm edema of the right lateral thoracic wall or the adjacent abdominal wall. Anorexia, nausea, and vomiting are relatively uncommon. The presence of right upper-quadrant pain and tenderness without nausea and vomiting should suggest the possibility of liver abscess. Hepatic enlargement is typically upward and is detected in two-thirds of cases. Weight loss and prostration are common. Abscesses high in the right lobe may involve the diaphragm and pleura, causing cough, splinting of the chest, dyspnea, pleural effusion, and atelectasis. Jaundice is uncommon and probably indicates a poor prognosis. Not uncommonly, the course is more indolent, or an indolent course can be interrupted by acute symptoms.

Diagnosis

Marked leukocytosis (over 20,000/mm^3), with increased numbers of immature neutrophils, is commonly seen in both pylephlebitis and liver abscess. Anemia may develop in long-standing disease. Liver function tests are usually normal, but in liver abscess, the akaline phosphatase level is almost always elevated. Blood cultures are positive in one-third to one-half of the patients. A higher yield would very likely result with adequate anaerobic blood cultures.

Roentgenographic studies are often helpful in diagnosing liver abscess. Elevation, change in contour, and reduced mobility of the diaphragm may be noted. When subphrenic and liver abscesses coexist, there is obliteration of the cardiophrenic angle in the anteroposterior view, and of the anterior costophrenic angle in the lateral view. An isolated subphrenic abscess typically causes obliteration of the costophrenic angle in the anteroposterior view and the posterior costophrenic angle in the lateral view. Abscess of the left lobe of the liver may produce pressure deformities in the barium- or gas-filled stomach, or it may displace the duodenal cap. Pleural effusion or thickening may also be noted, and occasionally a gas-fluid level may be noted within the liver.

Hepatic photoscanning, after the intravenous injection of radioisotope-labeled material, is a most valuable aid in establishing the diagnosis and location of liver abscess (Fig. 84-1). Ultrasonography and computed tomography are also useful. Hepatic arteriography is occasionally useful, as is splenoportography. At times T-tube cholangiography may enable the demonstration of hepatic abscess in patients with ascending cholangitis. Umbilical vein portography may be useful in the diagnosis of liver abscess. Percutaneous aspiration may be undertaken for diagnostic purposes, but preparations must first be made for immediate surgery, if that becomes necessary.

The two conditions that may be most difficult to distinguish from pyogenic liver abscess are amebic liver abscess and subphrenic abscess. Amebic abscess has an insidious onset, the patients are less acutely ill, and there may be a history of previous dysentery; in some patients, the diagnosis may be suggested by finding amebas in the stools or by finding a high titer of antibodies by indirect hemagglutination, latex agglutination, or gel diffusion tests for amebiasis (see Chap. 66, Amebiasis). Subphrenic abscess is discussed in Chap. 85, Subphrenic and Other Intraabdominal Abscesses.

Prognosis

The complications of pylephlebitis include liver abscess, peritonitis, and septicemia. Portal vein thrombosis, occurring either rapidly or slowly, and the development of portal hypertension are rare.

When liver abscess can be diagnosed before the patient becomes gravely ill, the mortality is relatively low. Complications of liver abscess include bacte-

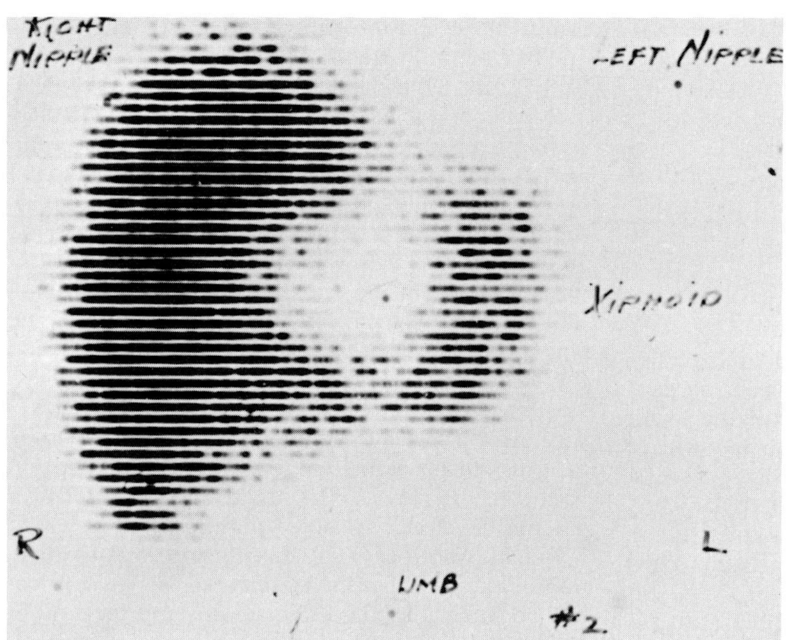

Fig. 84-1. Liver scan showing a large abscess.

remia, empyema, pneumonia, lung abscess, hepatobronchial fistula, rupture into the pericardium, peritonitis, subphrenic abscess, and metastatic abscesses in other organs.

Therapy

Surgical drainage, with or without excision, is usually essential to the elimination of the source for pylephlebitis. In liver abscess, the most important aspect of therapy is surgical drainage.

The transperitoneal approach is now considered best for drainage of liver abscess, since the abdomen may also be explored seeking an antecedent focus of infection that can be treated. If liver abscess is associated with cholangitis, drainage through the extrahepatic bile ducts may be effective. Effective drainage may not be possible when there are multiple abscesses. In this circumstance, the administration of antimicrobics through the umbilical vein has resulted in improvement.

Reports of successful medical therapy by means of antimicrobial agents, with or without percutaneous aspiration drainage of the abscess, are impressive enough to warrant formal evaluation. This approach may be particularly indicated in patients who are poor surgical risks. Ultrasound provides accurate localization for percutaneous needle aspiration and may facilitate the aspiration of multiple abscesses. Ultrasound is also an effective means for monitoring the size of an abscess cavity following drainage.

Of secondary importance to surgery, antimicrobics nonetheless should be given in full dosage, systemically, for an extended period. Clindamycin or metronidazole are active against most anaerobes involved in liver abscess and should be supplemented with an aminocyclitol if Enterobacteriaceae are or may be present. Chloramphenicol is generally effective against all the bacteria encountered in hepatic abscesses; cefoxitin represents another alternative. Tetracycline is less active but may be useful because of the relatively high concentrations that are achieved in hepatic tissue. See Chapters 53, Intrarenal and Perinephric Abscess, and 82, Peritonitis, for details concerning the use of the drugs appropriate for these infections.

Prevention

Appropriate medical and surgical therapy of infections and other conditions that predispose to pylephlebitis and liver abscess will lower the incidence of these conditions.

Remaining Problems

Better techniques are needed for the early diagnosis of pylephlebitis and liver abscess. Umbilical vein administration of antimicrobics should be carefully evaluated because this route of administration appears to be particularly effective.

Bibliography

Journals

MAHER JA, REYNOLDS TB, YELLIN AE: Successful medical treatment of pyogenic liver abscess. Gastroenterology 77:618–622, 1979

OCHSNER A, DEBAKEY M, MURRAY S: Pyogenic abscess of liver: Analysis of 47 cases with review of literature. Am J Surg 40:292–319, 1938

PITT HA, ZUIDEMA GD: Factors influencing mortality in the treatment of pyogenic hepatic abscess. Surg Gynecol Obstet 140:228–234, 1975

RUBIN RH, SWARTZ MN, MALT R: Hepatic abscess: Changes in clinical, bacteriologic and therapeutic aspects. Am J Med 57:601–610, 1974

SABBAJ J, SUTTER VL, FINEGOLD SM: Anaerobic pyogenic liver abscess. Ann Intern Med 77:629–638, 1972

SYDNEY M. FINEGOLD

85 Subphrenic and Other Intraabdominal Abscesses

The chief anatomic sites of intraabdominal abscess are the subphrenic areas (used here to include subhepatic and subdiaphragmatic abscesses), the pelvis, the lumbar gutters, and the intermesenteric folds. Subphrenic abscesses may be divided into three groups—right and left subdiaphragmatic, and subhepatic abscesses. Characteristically, the large spaces above and below the liver become subdivided at about their midpoints by the formation of pyogenic membranes, leading to the designations anterior and posterior.

Subdiaphragmatic abscesses—collections of pus beneath the diaphragm and in direct contact with it—are a special problem. Nationwide, the mortality associated with this disease is close to 50%. Anatomically, there are three subdiaphragmatic areas on each side: the two intraperitoneal areas are anterior and posterior; the one extraperitoneal area lies even further posteriorly. On the right, the extraperitoneal abscesses are in the layer of the crus of the diaphragm and coronary ligament. On the left, they arise above the superior pole of the left kidney.

Etiology

Although the older writings report *Escherichia coli, Staphylococcus aureus,* and various aerobic streptococci as the predominant bacteria of intraabdominal abscesses, in recent years there has been an increase in the number of other aerobic gram-negative bacilli, such as *Klebsiella* spp., *Enterobacter* spp., *Proteus* spp., and *Pseudomonas* spp. However, as anaerobic cultures have been made with increasing frequency, it is now apparent that anaerobic gram-negative bacilli, anaerobic cocci, and clostridia play an important, if not dominant, role in intraabdominal abscesses (Table 85-1). Details concerning classification and identification of anaerobic bacteria are given in Chap. 32, Necrotizing Pneumonias and Lung Abscess.

Epidemiology

Because intraabdominal abscesses are always secondary to infection elsewhere, there is no unique epidemiology. The data concerning antecedent events are most extensive and reliable in regard to subphrenic abscesses. There are three general patterns. The first and most common pattern includes abscesses developing after an intraabdominal operation (Table 85-2). The second group includes abscesses that follow the perforation of a hollow viscus that subsequently seals off and in which the contaminated material is loculated in the subphrenic space, for example, perforated peptic ulcer in 10% of patients and acute appendicitis in about 0.7% of cases. The third category includes abscesses that develop secondary to a remote infection, apparently spreading hematogenously to the subphrenic areas.

Males are much more likely to develop intraabdominal abscesses than females. The highest incidence of subphrenic abscess is in the third to fifth decades of life.

Pathogenesis and Pathology

The underlying lesion in subphrenic abscess is almost always within the abdomen. In recent years, most cases have been related to the stomach and duodenum or the biliary tract, appendicitis being responsible for distinctly fewer cases than previously. A primary source in the lower intestinal tract or the female genitalia is not uncommon. Abdominal surgery or other abdominal trauma is also a relatively common cause of subphrenic abscess. The major route of infection is by direct extension or by way of lymphatic drainage. Because the suprahepatic space is closed and has a negative pressure, enhanced during inspiration, it is much more likely to be infected than the infrahepatic space. Left-sided subphrenic abscess is primarily seen after upper abdominal sur-

Table 85-1. *Bacteriology of 73 Intraabdominal Infections (62 Patients; Chiefly Intraabdominal Abscess or Peritonitis)*

Average number of bacterial isolates per specimen	
Overall average	4.5
Aerobes and facultatives	2.0
Anaerobes	2.5
Range	1–12
General bacteriologic results	
Mixed flora (aerobes and anaerobes)	78%
Aerobic or facultative bacteria only	17%
Anaerobic bacteria only	5%
Anaerobic bacteria recovered	**Number of isolates**
Bacteroides fragilis	57
Other *Bacteroides* spp.	30
Fusobacterium spp.	13
Clostridium perfringens	11
Other *Clostridium* spp.	20
Peptococcus spp.	17
Peptostreptococcus spp.	10
Eubacterium spp.	12
Others	11
Total	181
Aerobic or facultative organisms recovered	**Number of isolates**
Escherichia coli	50
Proteus spp.	18
Klebsiella spp.	18
Pseudomonas spp.	5
Other gram-negative bacilli	9
Group D streptococci	33
Other streptococci	18
Staphylococcus aureus	6
Candida spp.	3
Total	160

Flora DJ, Sutter VL, Finegold SM, at Wadsworth Hospital Center, Veterans Administration, Los Angeles, California, 1973–1975

gery or lesions of the stomach or duodenum.

The most frequent precursors to pelvic abscess are perforated appendix, colonic diverticulitis, and pelvic inflammatory disease. Acute diffuse peritonitis may also localize as a pelvic abscess. Paracolic abscess is more frequent on the right side.

Manifestations

Infection and abscess formation in the abdomen, particularly under the diaphragm, may be an insidious process. The manifestations may be nonexistent, are usually nonspecific, and may be misleading.

Data regarding subdiaphragmatic abscess are presented in Table 85-3. Most patients complain of fever. Although pain may be present, it is referred to the lower chest almost as often as the upper abdomen. Hiccups that may be persistent are notable in some patients.

The findings are commonly those of an intrathoracic rather than an intraabdominal condition. Dyspnea, cough, chest and shoulder pain, and dullness or rales over the lung base may be noted. Tenderness or localized edema, particularly at the costal margin, is common and usually localized directly over the abscess. Pain and tenderness are much less common in subhepatic abscess. Unfortunately, in many patients with subphrenic abscess, the disease is much more insidious. The physician may be faced with a patient who is febrile, losing weight, and just not doing well. This is particularly true when antimicrobial chemoprophylaxis has been attempted. There may be a delay of weeks to more than a year between the time of the inciting event and the overt manifestations of subphrenic abscess. Some patients may have vague pain, general debility, and unexplained fever and anemia; apparently such symptoms can persist for more than 10 years before the diagnosis is finally made.

The symptoms of pelvic abscess are pain, deep tenderness in one or both lower quadrants, fever, urinary frequency, dysuria, and diarrhea with the pas-

Table 85-2. *Surgical Operations Preceding Subdiaphragmatic Abscess*

Surgical Operation	Percentage
Stomach and duodenum	35
Plication of perforated ulcer	20
Gastrotomy	4
Gastric resection (7 with drainage)	68
Vagotomy	4
Duodenal diverticulectomy	4
Biliary tract (all with drainage)	22
Cholecystectomy	46
Cholecystostomy	7
Cholecystectomy with common-duct exploration	33
Common-duct exploration	14
Appendectomy (7 with drainage)	12
Colon	3
Sigmoid resection	3
Small intestine	6
Segmental resection	6
Splenectomy	3
Splenorenal shunt	2
Nephrolithotomy (with drainage)	2
No preceding operation	15

At the New York Hospital–Cornell Medical Center, 1954–1969

Table 85-3. Clinical Manifestations of Subdiaphragmatic Abscess

Clinical manifestations	Percentage
Symptoms	
Chest pain	16
Upper abdominal pain	21
Signs	
Fever	90
Tenderness in upper abdominal quadrant	30
Roentgenographic findings	
Elevated diaphragm	62
Pleural effusion	41
Immobile diaphragm	23
Laboratory data	
Leukocytosis	68
Basis for diagnosis	
Physical examination	26
Roentgenographic findings	65
Unsuccessful (established at autopsy)	9

At New York Hospital–Cornell Medical Center, 1954–1969

sage of mucus in the first stools. Rectal or vaginal examination may reveal tenderness of the pelvic peritoneum and bulging of the anterior rectal wall. Paracolic abscess provokes fever and a tender enlarging mass that may be difficult to palpate. Abscesses forming between or below the folds of the jejunoileal mesentery are typically small, multiple, and difficult to diagnose. There may be fever, malaise, anorexia, vague general pain, or partial obstruction of the small intestine.

Diagnosis

It may be superfluous to point out that consideration of subphrenic or other intraabdominal abscess is the most important step in the differential diagnosis. Unfortunately, it is a diagnosis that is far too often thought of too late.

Most patients exhibit leukocytosis. Roentgenographic examinations are very important in the diagnosis of subphrenic abscess. In suprahepatic abscess, roentgenographic signs are chiefly thoracic. The earliest, most common sign is pleural effusion. Elevation and decreased mobility of the diaphragm are common important signs (Fig. 85-1). Lower-lobe pulmonary infiltrates or atelectasis may be seen. Hoover's sign—unilateral widening of the angle between the chondral arch and the sternum—is another valuable diagnostic clue to subphrenic abscess. Unfortunately, the abnormalities detected in chest films may lead to a mistaken diagnosis of pneumonia, particularly in a postoperative patient. Obliteration of the costophrenic angle in the lateral view has been commented on earlier in Chapter 84, Pylephlebitis and Liver Abscess.

An occasional, very important finding, is the presence of gas bubbles or a gas-fluid level (see Fig. 85-2). An abscess under the left diaphragm may displace the spleen, stomach, colon, or left lobe of the liver, and such displacement may be detected by roentgenographic examination, with or without the use of barium or carbonated drinks. The use of the Trendelenburg position may be very helpful. The fundus of the stomach is normally against the inferior diaphragmatic surface. However, if an abscess is present, the stomach may be displaced. Subdiaphragmatic gas may arise from perforation of a viscus. However, gas may be present under the diaphragm as long as two or three weeks after abdominal surgery. Artificial pneumoperitoneum may be very useful in diagnosing

Fig. 85-1. Subdiaphragmatic abscess on the left in a 9-year-old boy with a ruptured appendix. Note the abdominal distention and elevated diaphragms; the left hemidiaphragm is higher than right.

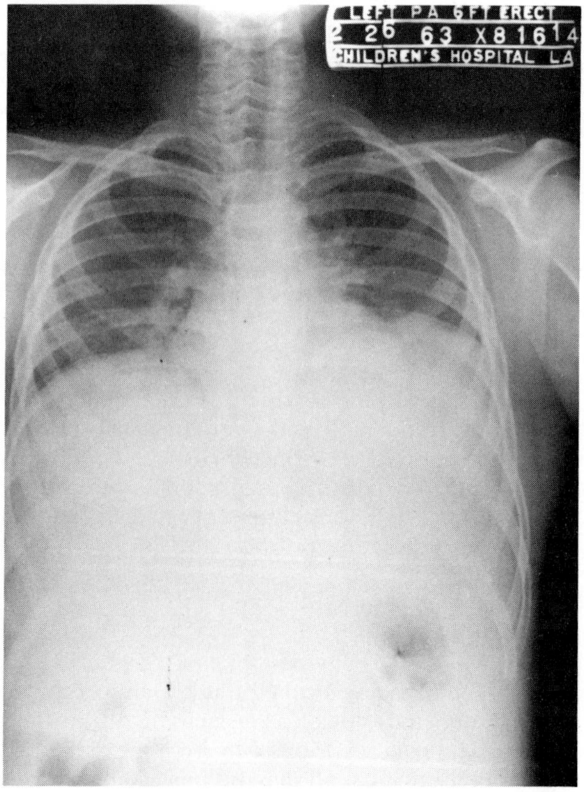

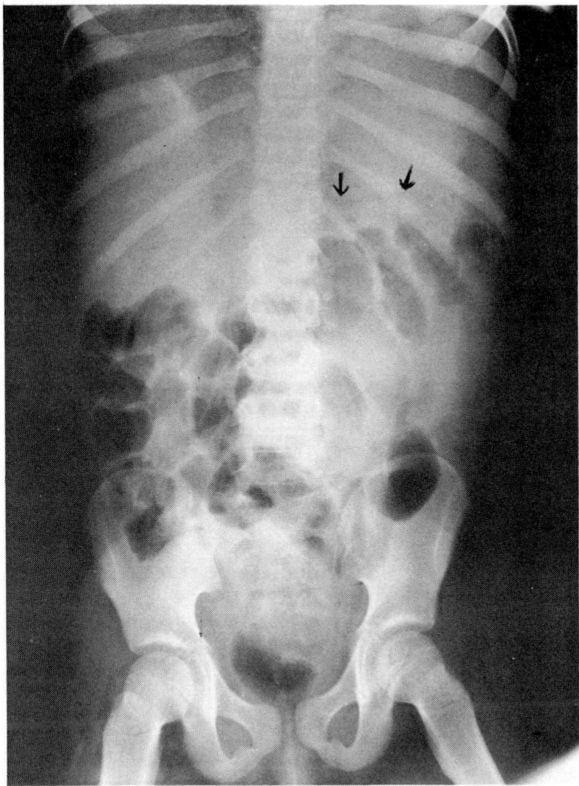

Fig. 85-2. Subdiaphragmatic abscess. Gas in the abscess is noted by arrows.

subphrenic abscess. Other noninvasive techniques which are extremely useful include hepatic photoscanning, combined liver and lung scanning, gallium scanning (Fig. 85-3), ultrasound (Fig. 85-4) computed tomography, and leukocyte labeling with indium-111 oxine. However, in some patients an almost instinctive clinical judgment is ultimately necessary.

Continued fever and leukocytosis after known intraperitoneal suppuration or abdominal surgery must be regarded as a subphrenic or other intraabdominal abscess until proved otherwise.

The differential diagnosis of subphrenic abscess includes pneumonia, pulmonary infarct, atelectasis, other intraabdominal abscess, and lesser sac or retroperitoneal abscess.

Other types of intraabdominal abscess may be more difficult to detect than subphrenic abscess. Again, roentgenographic examination may be helpful. An intraperitoneal abscess may be demonstrable as a space-occupying lesion displacing intestinal loops. An important sign is obliteration of the intermuscular and subperitoneal fat layers of the adjacent abdominal wall. Gas formation in intraperitoneal abscesses may be very difficult to appreciate. However, it may be possible to determine that the gas bubbles are in an area not usually occupied by intestinal loops. At times it is helpful to administer contrast medium by mouth to outline the gastrointestinal tract. In the case of pelvic abscess, the possible presence of a collection of pus may be verified by inserting a long needle through the posterior wall of the vaginal vault or through the anterior wall of the rectum.

Prognosis

The mortality of subphrenic abscess is still about 50%. Patients who are not operated on, elderly patients, and patients with serious underlying diseases have a much higher mortality. The most frequent complications of subphrenic abscess are intrathoracic. Included are serous effusion, empyema, ne-

Fig. 85-3. Ga^{67} scan showing diverticular abscess in left lower quadrant. (Courtesy of Dr. W. Blahd)

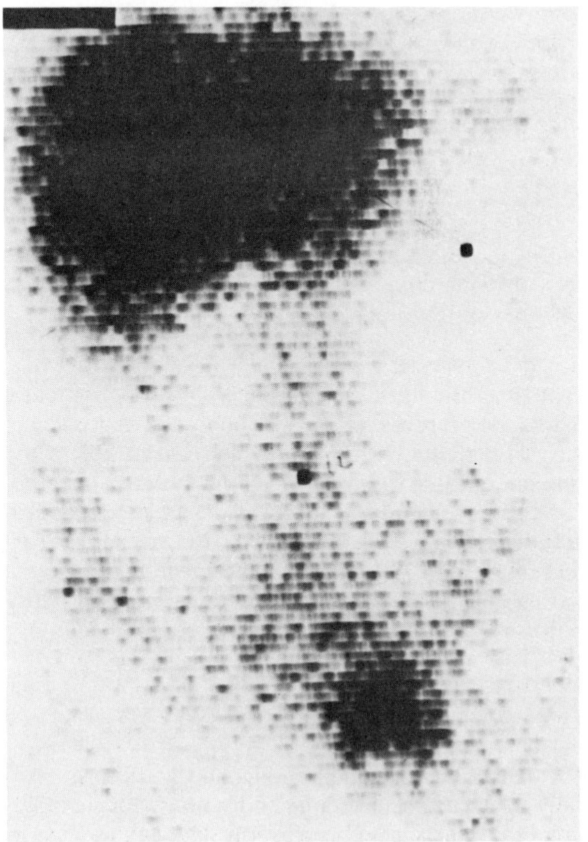

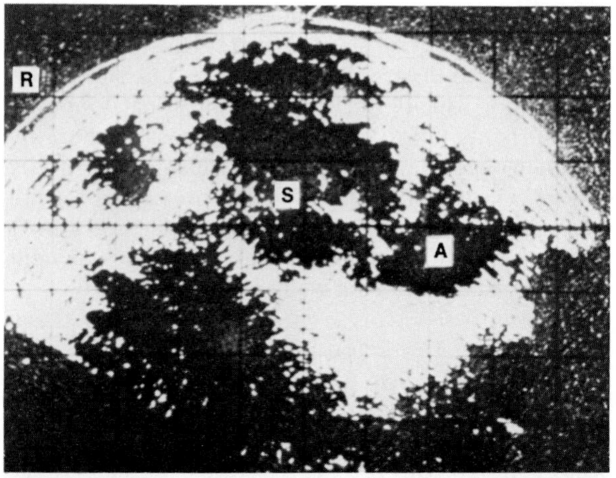

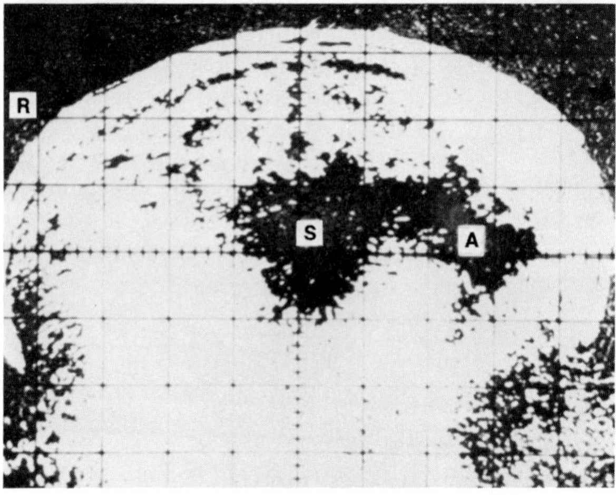

Fig. 85-4. Ultrasonogram, with high and low gain, of abdomen showing psoas abscess. *A* = abscess, *S* = spine, *R* = right. (Courtesy of Drs. M. Winston and W. Blahd)

crotizing pneumonia, bronchial or bronchopleural fistula, pericarditis, mediastinal abscess, and particularly in patients with post-operative strictures of the bile ducts, biliary communications with the intrathoracic cavity. Bronchobiliary fistula is an extremely serious complication because of the necrotizing effect of the bile. Other complications include general peritonitis, perforation into the intestine, and perforation to the outside.

Therapy

The treatment of subdiaphragmatic abscess is basically surgical. The principle of draining a local collection of pus is as valid here as it is with any abscess in any other part of the body. The posterior extraperitoneal approach suffers the disadvantages of delay in drainage due to a two-stage procedure and the risk of not obtaining adequate drainage because of limited exposure. The transperitoneal approach is now used almost exclusively because it enables the complete exploration and drainage of the subdiaphragmatic space while enabling visualization and drainage of the subhepatic space. Many subphrenic abscesses have subhepatic extensions or separate collections of pus. The danger of the transperitoneal approach is that of general peritonitis. The peritoneal cavity must be adequately walled off at the time of drainage to minimize this risk.

The overall mortality of this disease continues to be appalling; it has not improved generally in the past half century. However, recent experience has shown that early surgery significantly reduces the mortality. A reduction from 32 to 14 days in the average elapsed time from the original operation antecedent to infection to the drainage of the complicating abscess reduced the mortality to 18% at the New York Hospital–Cornell Medical Center. It is clear that an aggressive approach is essential to improving the outcome.

Pelvic abscesses are drained by incision through the rectum or vagina. Paracolic abscesses can be drained retroperitoneally through an incision lateral to the abscess. Intermesenteric abscesses are drained by evacuation after gentle separation of the mesenteric folds.

Antimicrobial agents may be of value in the stage of cellulitis, before actual walling off proceeds to abscess formation. Therefore, a patient who may be developing or have an incompletely localized subphrenic abscess or other intraabdominal abscess can be treated with antimicrobial drugs if he is well enough to withstand 3 or 4 more days of illness. However, if a patient is so sick that failure of antimicrobial treatment would be fatal, a trial of antimicrobics is not justified. The judgment that a patient is too sick to have an operation should be deplored as lethal defeatism. A patient can withstand incision and drainage much better than he can tolerate an undrained abscess. Antimicrobial agents are useful adjuncts to surgical management. See Chapter 82, Peritonitis, for details of antimicrobial therapy.

Prevention

Appropriate medical and surgical therapy of predisposing conditions should lower the incidence of intraabdominal abscess. If postoperative drainage is avoided after splenectomy, the incidence of local complications, including abscess, is much lower. Rigid aseptic surgical technique is important in preventing postoperative infection.

Remaining Problems

The major need is for better techniques in the early diagnosis of intraabdominal abscess. Means for preventing nosocomial infections are also needed.

Miscellaneous Intraabdominal Infections

Splenic Abscess

Splenic abscesses are uncommon. They usually arise as a result of hematogenous dissemination of microorganisms. The original focus of infection may be in the skin, respiratory tract, bone, endometrium, endocardium, or other organ. Occassionally there is spread of infection from contiguous organs or direct inoculation related to surgery or trauma. The bacterial etiology is variable and depends on the original lesion. The onset is often sudden, with chills, fever, and left upper-quadrant pain. With involvement of the upper pole, there is commonly left pleuritic pain radiating to the shoulder, elevation of the left diaphragm, and left pleural effusion. Abscess in the lower pole gives rise to signs of peritoneal inflammation. The spleen is frequently palpable and tender, and a friction rub is often audible over it. Roentgenographically, there may be medial compression of the gastric air shadow; displacement of the left colon, stomach, or kidney; extraluminal gas shadows; or associated contiguous infected lesions. Splenic arteriography may show stretching or displacement of intrasplenic vessels. A liver-spleen radioisotope scan may also be positive, as may a gallium-67 or indium-111-labeled white cell scan.

Aerobic and anaerobic blood cultures should always be made. Differential diagnosis includes subphrenic abscess, bland infarct of the spleen, pulmonary infection, and pancreatic pseudocyst. Complications include subdiaphragmatic abscess and diffuse peritonitis. When feasible, splenectomy is carried out; antimicrobial therapy is secondary. An infected splenic infarct is a rare cause of continued bacteremia in bacterial endocarditis, despite appropriate chemotherapy. Splenectomy may be required to achieve a cure.

Phlegmonous Gastritis

Bacterial infection of the stomach is rare. It may arise from hematogenous spread from a distant focus or locally by way of the mucosa. The involvement may be diffuse or local. The typical symptoms are midepigastric pain and vomiting, often of sudden onset. On rare occasions, the vomitus is purulent. The clinical picture is that of an abdominal catastrophe with septicemia. Tenderness is localized to the epigastrium until general peritonitis develops. It has been said that the disappearance of abdominal pain when the patient sits up is specific for the diagnosis of diffuse phlegmonous gastritis. The bacteria involved include streptococci, *S. aureus,* pneumococci, *E. coli* and other gram-negative bacilli, and *Clostridium perfringens.* Mortality is high, but survivals have followed gastrectomy and the administration of antimicrobial agents.

Bibliography

Books

WILSON SE, FINEGOLD SM, WILLIAMS RA: Intra-Abdominal Infection. New York, McGraw–Hill, 1982. 495 pp.

Journals

ALTEMEIER WA, CULBERTSON WR, FULLEN WD, SHOOK CD: Intra-abdominal abscesses. Am J Surg 125:70–79, 1973

CHUN CH, RAFF LJ, CONTRERAS L, VARGHESE R, WATERMAN N, DAFNER R, MELO JC: Splenic abscesses. Medicine 59:50–65, 1980

MAGILLIGAN DJ JR: Suprahepatic abscess. Arch Surg 96:14–19, 1968

OCHSNER A, DEBAKEY M: Subphrenic abscess. Int Abstr Surg 66:426–438, 1938

SCANLON EF: Editorial: The intra-abdominal dead space and abscess formation. Surg Gynecol Obstet 146:789, 1978

WANG SMS, WILSON SE: Subphrenic abscess. The new epidemiology. Arch Surg 112:934–936, 1977

Section XIV

Integumentary Infections

Indigenous Microbiota of the Skin and Its Appendages

Species or Group	General	Feet
Bacteria		
Gram-positive cocci		
Staphylococcus epidermidis	**85–100***	
	2–6/cm^2	
Staphylococcus aureus	**5–24†**	
Anaerobic micrococci	±	
Streptococcus mitis; undifferentiated α and γ streptococci	± to 0	
Streptococcus pyogenes (usually group A unless noted)	**0–4**	
Gram-positive bacilli		
Lactobacillus spp.	**55**	
Aerobic *Corynebacterium* spp.	5/cm^2	
Propionibacterium acnes	**45–100**	
	6/cm^2	
Mycobacterium spp.	+	
Aerobic gram-negative bacilli		
Enterobacteriaceae	±	
Fungi		
Candida albicans	±	±
non-albicans *Candida* spp.	**1–15**	+
Pityrosporon ovale	100‡	
Pityrosporon orbiculare	++	
Dermatophytes		**2–41**
Metazoa		
Demodex folliculorum	+	

± to 0, rare; ±, irregular or uncertain (may be only pathologic); +, common; ++, prominent.

*Boldface values (*e.g.,* **30–60**) = range of incidence in percentage, rounded, in different surveys.

†Associated with nasal carriage.

‡Especially scalp and nasal folds; also other skin areas.

S. MICHAEL MARCY
SIDNEY KIBRICK

Measles

86

Measles is a highly contagious, acute disease characterized by a general maculopapular eruption; it occurs most commonly in children. Characteristically, a prominent prodrome marked by fever, coryza, cough, conjunctivitis, and Koplik's spots (a pathognomonic enanthema) precedes the rash. Complications caused by extensive viral involvement or secondary bacterial invasion are relatively common. Measles remains one of the leading causes of childhood mortality in countries where malnutrition, poor sanitation, and inadequate medical care are prevalent.

Etiology

The disease is the result of infection with the measles virus. The measles virion is a roughly spherical particle, 120 nm to 250 nm in diameter, made up of a coiled helical RNA-nucleocapsid core surrounded by an outer envelope containing lipid, glycoprotein, and other polypeptides. The envelope, which is covered with many short, spikelike projections, appears to be derived from an altered cell membrane that surrounds the nucleocapsid and pinches off as the virus is released from the cell surface (Fig. 86-1). Hemagglutinating, hemolytic, and cell-fusion activities are structurally associated with the envelope; complement-fixing antigens are present in both the envelope and nucleocapsid. There is only one antigenic type. No neuraminidase has been found.

The measles virus is most readily isolated in primary cell cultures of the human or simian kidney, and it can be propagated in a variety of continuous cell lines. The virus has been recovered from the throat, conjunctiva, urine, blood, and other infected tissues. On rare occasions the virus has been isolated from the cerebrospinal fluid (CSF) of patients with measles. A distinctive cytopathogenic effect, characterized by the formation of multinucleated giant cells (syncytia) with eosinophilic intranuclear and cytoplasmic inclusions, is usually produced in tissue culture.

The virus is rapidly inactivated by various agents, including ether, trypsin, formalin, and ultraviolet and visible light. Activity is maintained for several weeks at refrigerator temperature; the half-life at 37°C is about 2 hours. The survival of the measles virus in air is inversely related to the relative humidity (RH): at room temperature and low RH, the virus survives well, but loss of infectivity increases rapidly in the range from 50% to 70% RH. On the basis of common biophysical properties, antigenic components, and histopathologic effects, the measles virus is closely related to the viruses of canine distemper, bovine rinderpest, and *peste des petites ruminants.* These four viruses have been classified in the genus *Morbillivirus* within the family Paramyxoviridae.

Epidemiology

Humans and monkeys are the only natural hosts of measles. The disease is spread to susceptible individuals through direct contact with infected droplets or contaminated fomites. Neither a carrier state nor third-party transmission has been documented. The upper respiratory tract is probably the primary portal of entry, although the conjunctivae may be an important alternate site. Clinical observations indicate that the period of communicability begins during the prodromal phase and continues until 4 to 5 days after onset of the rash. Isolation of virus from the nasopharynx has been achieved from 2 days before to 5 days after appearance of the rash. Viruria may persist a few days longer.

Measles is one of the most contagious of the childhood exanthems. After intimate exposure, the attack rate in susceptible patients is more than 90%. Even brief or casual contact may occasionally be followed by infection.

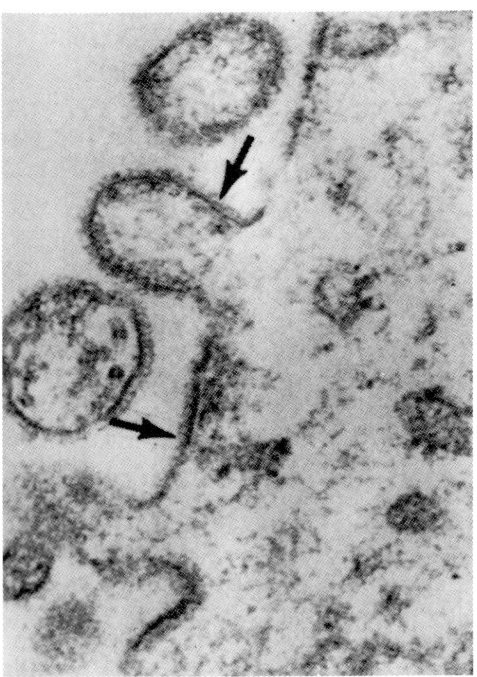

Fig. 86-1. The measles virion is 120 nm–250 nm in diameter. The protein–lipoprotein outer envelope is derived from the host cell (*arrows*). (Nakai M, Imagawa DT: J Virol 3:187–197, 1969)

Measles is worldwide in distribution and has no racial or sex predisposition. It is endemic throughout the year in heavily populated areas, although the peak incidence coincides with the onset of drier weather in the spring. Such seasonal variation probably results from patterns of school attendance among children, but may also indicate the effects of low humidity on the survival of the virus and its communicability. In addition, every 2 to 3 years, when 30% to 40% of children are susceptible, widespread epidemics occur and continue until the pool of susceptible persons has been reduced by about half. In highly immunized populations, this periodicity is lacking. Rather, small outbreaks occur among selected susceptible groups residing within the larger immune population.

The peak age incidence of measles is variable, depending largely on the socioeconomic environment. In areas where populations live under primitive and overcrowded conditions, epidemics occur yearly; most children have acquired measles by the age of 3 years. In rural communities and less crowded urban areas, the average age of attack of 5 to 6 years coincides with the time of increased exposure and crowding as children begin school. With the reduction of natural measles in the general population in the United States, an increasing number of unimmunized or improperly immunized susceptible persons reach adolescence and early adulthood. As a result, more than half of all cases of measles now occur in persons 10 to 19 years of age (Fig. 86-2).

Although measles has been described in neonates born of susceptible mothers, it is rarely seen in infants under 6 months of age because more than 90% of infants acquire maternal antibodies transplacentally.

Pathogenesis and Pathology

Few studies provide direct evidence for the sequence of events after initiation of the infection. However, Fenner's classic observations on ectromelia (mousepox) in the mouse are generally accepted as the model for the pathogenesis of measles and other exanthematous diseases.

By analogy, inoculation of the upper respiratory tract or conjunctival sac with measles is followed by a period of viral replication in the mucosa and in the regional lymph nodes. Shortly thereafter, on the second or third day of illness, a primary viremia disseminates the virus to lymphoid tissues throughout the body, where it multiplies to high titer. A more extensive and prolonged secondary viremia, from the fifth or sixth day onward, is responsible for the widespread, focal infection of the tissues that later show involvement. Multiplication of the virus and inflammation with necrosis progress in involved organs; by the 11th day prodromal symptoms are generally evident. On or about the 14th day, the rash appears. From 24 to 48 hours later, coincident with the appearance of measurable amounts of circulating antibody, viremia ceases and symptoms begin to abate.

During the biphasic viremia, the measles virus seems to be disseminated mainly within leukocytes. Measles has been transmitted to susceptible volunteers through the transfer of washed leukocytes (but not plasma) obtained from patients 6 and 8 days before onset of the rash. Viral multiplication within leukocytes is believed to account for the leukopenia and the increased incidence of chromosomal breaks seen in measles.

The etiology of the rash in measles is not known. However, viral replication in the skin lesions is attested by foci of multinucleated giant cells, characteristic intranuclear inclusion bodies, and the presence of viral antigen demonstrated by immunofluorescent staining. Moreover, the injection of measles hyperimmune serum into the skin prevents the development

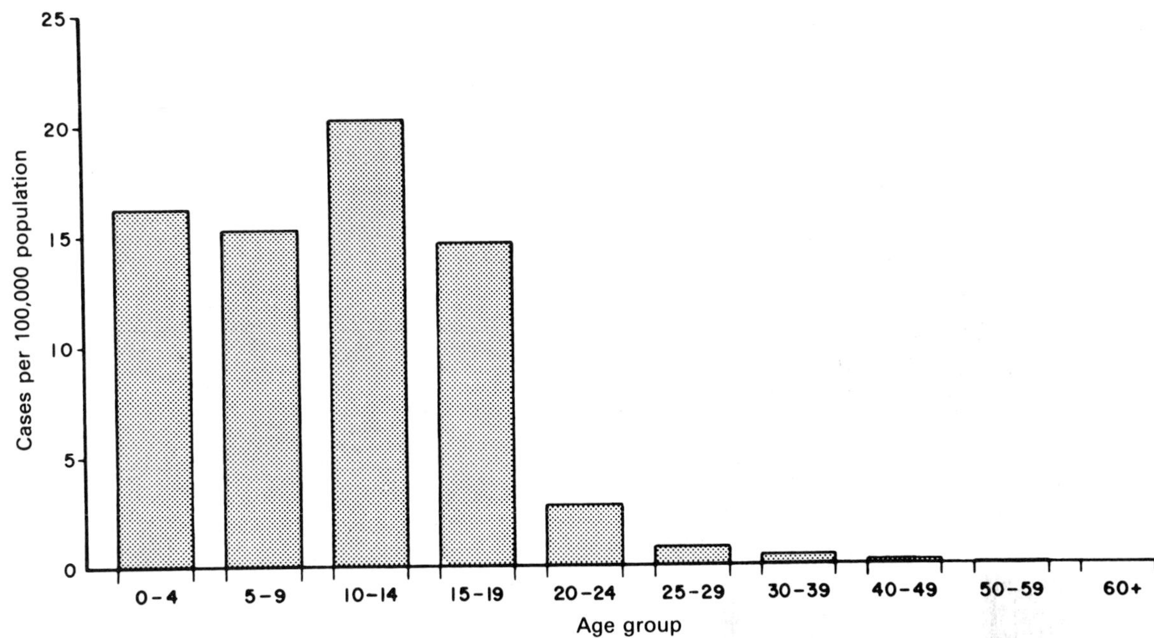

Fig. 86-2. Reported cases of measles by age group in the United States, 1980. (Morbid Mortal Week Rep Suppl, Summary, 1980)

of the rash at the site of injection. The skin lesions may be caused by direct viral damage to the epithelium and vascular endothelium, or they may occur as the result of a general, delayed hypersensitivity response to virus–antibody complexes.

During the prodromal period, hyperplasia of lymphoid tissues is present in various organs, including the lymph nodes, tonsils, adenoids, Peyer's patches, appendix, spleen, and thymus. A more specific finding is the presence of large, multinucleated giant cells (Warthin–Finkeldey cells) that contain as many as 100 nuclei along with cytoplasmic and intranuclear eosinophilic inclusion bodies.

The histologic features of Koplik's spots and skin lesions are similar. Koplik's spots originate in the submucous glands as inflammatory lesions that progress to necrosis and vesiculation. Multinucleated giant cells are prominent. The exanthem begins with hyaline necrosis of epidermal cells followed by endothelial proliferation, exudation of serum, and necrosis of epithelial cells with the formation of minute vesicles that rapidly break down and desquamate. Multinucleated giant cells are also present in these cells. Destructive changes may occur in hair follicles and sebaceous glands.

Multinucleate giant cells are also found in the epithelial lining of the respiratory tract from the nasal to the bronchiolar mucosa (Fig. 86-3). In pneumonitis, there is, in addition, a peribronchial and interstitial mononuclear cell response, with the proliferation of alveolar lining cells and parenchymal giant cells. Identical pathologic changes have been noted in cases of Hecht's giant-cell pneumonia.

When measles causes a postinfectious encephalomyelitis, there are edema, petechial hemorrhages, mononuclear infiltrates, and perivenous demyelination—changes typical of the syndrome, but not characteristic of measles. Direct viral involvement of the central nervous system (CNS) also occurs. Not only are inclusion bodies found in about three-fourths of patients with fatal measles encephalitis, but also measles antigen has been demonstrated in ganglion and glial cells by indirect immunofluorescence. Moreover, infectious virus has been recovered from brain tissue through the use of newer tissue culture techniques.

Mononuclear cells with cytoplasmic inclusions or giant cells have been seen in Bowman's capsule, tubular epithelium, and ureteral and urinary bladder mucosa.

Manifestations

Shortly after infection, at a time corresponding to the primary viremia—during the incubation period but

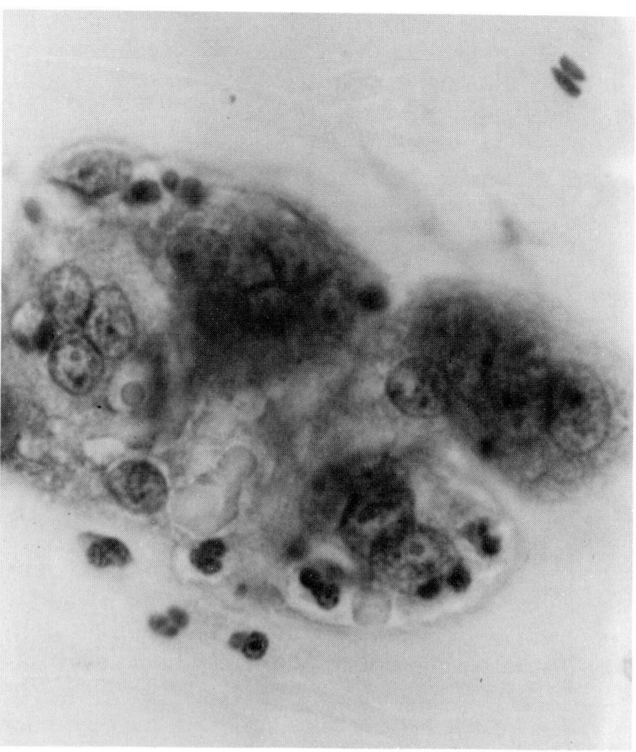

Fig. 86-3. Multinucleated giant cells in the nasal secretions of a patient incubating measles. (Original magnification approximately × 750) (Courtesy of John M Adams, MD)

before the appearance of prodromal symptoms—a mild illness may occur that is accompanied in some instances by a faint rash. Ten to twelve days after infection, the very prominent and characteristic prodromal symptoms appear: coryza; a persistent, barking cough; keratoconjunctivitis, often with photophobia; and fever. General lymphadenopathy and splenomegaly are also frequent at this time. During this period, Koplik's spots, the enanthema of measles, appear on the buccal mucosa. They are generally first seen on the inner lip or opposite the lower molars—in Koplik's words, appearing as "small, irregular spots, of a bright red color. In the center of each spot, there is noted, in strong daylight, a minute bluish white speck." Although few in number and often difficult to find during the early stages of the prodrome, they rapidly spread, involving the entire mucous membrane, resembling at their height small grains of white sand on a red background. These spots are usually gone by the time the skin rash reaches its peak. Similar spots have occasionally been observed on the conjunctivas, and labia, and in the gastrointestinal tract. Although true Koplik's spots are considered absolutely pathognomonic of measles, an enanthema somewhat similar in appearance has been reported in patients with echovirus 9 and coxsackievirus A-16 infections.

The rash of measles appears after a 3- to 5-day prodome (range, 1–8 days), some 14 days (range, 10–19 days) after exposure. It is first evident as faintly pink macules located behind the ears or on the forehead near the hairline. The rash quickly becomes maculopapular and spreads rapidly downward over the face, neck, trunk, and extremities during the next 3 days. As the rash progresses, the areas initially involved develop additional lesions that tend to coalesce, especially on the face. At its height, the eruption has generally deepened to a reddish purple and may be associated with edema of the skin. Thereafter, the fever begins to fall, and systemic manifestations usually diminish over the succeeding several days. The rash fades from above downward, regressing as it evolved. As clearing occurs, the lesions become brown, and a fine, branny desquamation often appears, usually sparing the hands and feet and thus distinguishable from the heavier, flaky desquamation seen in scarlet fever. Although the early rash blanches on pressure, the brown staining that is the residual from capillary hemorrhages does not.

Hemorrhagic measles (black measles) is a severe, often fatal form of measles, characterized by hemorrhages into the skin and extensive bleeding from mucous membranes that may be difficult to control. High fever, pneumonia, and encephalitis are often present. This syndrome does not seem to be caused by a thrombocytopenia; it has been suggested that an unusually severe vasculitis or disseminated intravascular clotting (DIC) may be responsible. Although frequently mentioned in earlier descriptions of the disease, hemorrhagic measles is rarely seen today.

Measles may be prevented or modified after exposure to the disease through passive immunization with pooled, adult gamma globulin. The administration of a modifying dose produces a prolonged incubation period, often 2 to 3 weeks in duration, which is followed by minimal prodromal symptoms of a mild upper respiratory infection. Koplik's spots, when present, are few in number and disappear rapidly. The rash is usually discrete, faint in color, and of brief duration. The complications seen with natural measles are extremely uncommon in the modified disease. A clinical picture similar to the one just described has been seen in infants with partial immunity from passively acquired maternal antibodies.

An atypical form of measles has been described in children who have been exposed to natural measles several months to years after primary immunization with either inactivated or, uncommonly, live measles virus vaccines.

The illness begins with a prodrome of 2 to 3 days, characterized by high fever, headache, myalgia, abdominal pains, and prostration. The exanthem that follows often begins on the wrists and ankles, progressing inward to involve the trunk and extremities, and usually remaining most dense on the feet and legs. It has been described as maculopapular with superimposed petechiae, purpura, urticaria, vesicles, or erythema multiforme. Pruritus, peripheral edema, and marked hyperesthesia have also been associated with the rash. Severe pneumonia, sometimes accompanied by hilar adenopathy and pleural effusion, is a relatively constant feature of this syndrome. Solitary pulmonary nodules 2 cm to 5 cm in diameter may persist in areas of pneumonia for periods up to 30 months and longer. These atypical manifestations are believed to occur as a result of a delayed hypersensitivity response to an antigen common to both the inactivated and live virus. A similar mechanism probably explains the severe local reactions (redness, induration, tenderness, vesicles, fever, adenopathy) that may occur about 5 to 7 days after live vaccine is given to a child who has received killed vaccine in the past.

Measles is a general infection associated with tissue destruction and inflammatory changes that are often intense. The definition of a complication is therefore arbitrary, but it is generally considered to include the manifestations of measles that are due to unusually severe viral involvement, secondary bacterial infection, and possibly, autoimmune reactions. Bacterial superinfection is most often caused by *Streptococcus pyogenes, Streptococcus pneumoniae,* and *Staphylococcus aureus*. In children under 5 years of age, *Hemophilus influenzae* is frequently implicated.

Respiratory Tract

Coryza, tracheobronchitis, and a mild laryngitis (croup) are almost invariably present during the course of natural measles. Roentgenographic evidence of an interstitial, viral pneumonia, and hilar enlargement is present in 20% to 60% of patients. Bronchiolitis is frequently seen in infants. Secondary bacterial pneumonia, the leading cause of death in measles, is probably potentiated by the depressing effects of the viral infection on pulmonary antibacterial activity. The pneumonia is generally associated with increasing respiratory distress, leukocytosis, and a persistence of fever and cough beyond the third day of the rash. When respiratory difficulty is accompanied by progresive hoarseness, inspiratory stridor, retractions, tachycardia, and restlessness, obstructive laryngitis should be suspected. Pneumomediastinum and subcutaneous emphysema have been seen in patients with measles, and the development of unilateral radiolucency of the lung (McLeod's syndrome) is a late complication of measles pneumonitis.

Giant-cell pneumonia (Hecht's pneumonia) is a protracted, fatal, interstitial pneumonitis that may be clinically indistinguishable from uncomplicated measles pneumonia. It is observed most frequently in children with underlying congenital or acquired immunologic disorders, and particularly, those with leukemias or under treatment with immunosuppressive agents. The measles virus persists unduly long in respiratory secretions and tissues—perhaps a reflection of a marked depression in the development of cellular immunity or production of specific measles neutralizing antibodies. The observation that most patients with giant-cell pneumonia fail to develop a rash or other signs and symptoms of measles is consistent with the thought that a defect in the delayed hypersensitivity response may be important in explaining the progressive nature of this form of measles. Recently, parainfluenza 3 virus infection in immunosuppressed patients has been associated with identical clinical and pathologic findings.

Central Nervous System

Acute, symptomatic encephalitis occurs without race, sex, or age preference in 0.1% to 0.2% of patients with measles. The incidence of subclinical involvement of the CNS seems to be far higher because patients with apparently uncomplicated measles have transient electroencephalographic changes (about 50%) and CSF pleocytosis (more than 10 leukocytes/ mm^3) in about 10%.

Symptoms usually begin between the first and seventh days of the rash, although onsets during both the prodrome and the postrash period have been described. The first signs and symptoms are generally drowsiness or irritability, which may progress to coma or convulsions within a few hours. Sudden rises in temperature, meningismus, headache, and vomiting are common additional features. Coma or stupor usually lightens after 1 to 3 days, but may continue for more than a month. The period of recovery that follows is variable in duration, and it is frequently associated with severe behavioral changes. Brief coma or rapid recovery is an excellent prognostic sign. A cerebellar syndrome, myelitis, polyneuropathy, optic neuritis, and retinopathy may accompany cerebral involvement or may rarely appear as isolated phenomena. The cells in the CSF are almost exclusively lymphocytes and usually range from 7 to 250 per mm^3. The protein is normal or increased; the glucose may be normal or slightly increased.

There is great variation in the frequency of death and the incidence of sequelae in measles encephalitis. On the average, death probably occurs in about 5% to 10% of patients, with the highest incidence in children under 4 years of age. Approximately one-half of the patients have a full clinical recovery, although electroencephalographic abnormalities may persist for many weeks or months. The remaining 30% to 35% are left with mild to severe neurologic sequelae. Children under 2 years of age are most commonly affected.

The etiology of acute measles encephalitis is unknown. However, two major hypotheses have been advanced: direct viral invasion and destruction of CNS tissue and an autoimmune reaction against either altered neural tissue or a neural tissue-virus complex. There is evidence to support both explanations, but the definitive answer must await further investigation.

Subacute sclerosing panencephalitis (SSPE; inclusion body encephalitis of Dawson) is a slowly progressing, almost invariably fatal, disease of the CNS of children and young adults. It is characterized by personality changes, mental deterioration, involuntary movements, decorticate rigidity, and death in 6 to 36 months. Several observations support the concept that SSPE is caused by a persistent, temperate measles virus infection of the CNS: (1) SSPE occurs 4 to 17 years after a clinical attack of measles (the age of measles infection in such cases has generally been under 2 years with the mean age of onset of SSPE at about 7 years); (2) there are unusually high levels of measles antibodies in the serums and CSFs of patients with this disorder; and (3) measles virus has been isolated from brain and lymphoid tissue obtained from such patients.

Although patients with SSPE have high titers of humoral antibodies against measles proteins, they do not have antibodies against measles M protein, a component required for assembly of the virus. Thus, SSPE may represent a host cell restriction of measles virus replication in the brain. Because most patients with SSPE had measles at an early age, the host cell restriction may represent a general property of certain types of brain cells at a particular stage of CNS development, with measles infection subsequently manifested by SSPE.

A subacute measles encephalopathy has been described among children with deficient cell-mediated immunity caused by malignancy or chemotherapy. In these patients, neurologic deterioration begins several weeks to months after the measles infection, which is often inapparent. In addition to disturbances of consciousness, intractable seizures, and motor deficits, hypertension and inappropriate antidiuretic hormone secretion have been described as typical clinical features. The CSF is usually normal. Almost all patients die from 2 weeks to 2 months after onset of their symptoms.

A relationship between measles and multiple sclerosis, possibly related to the HLA type of the host, has been postulated.

Otitis Media

Bacterial otitis media occurs in almost 10% of patients with measles, usually children with a history of ear infection. Younger children, who cannot complain of earache, must be closely observed for ear pulling, irritability, aural drainage, and the persistence of fever beyond the third or fourth day of rash. Secondary mastoiditis, although unusual, may follow a delay in therapy or the use of inappropriate antimicrobics for the treatment of otitis media.

Thrombocytopenic Purpura

A transient depression in the platelet count frequently follows vaccination with attenuated live measles virus; however, symptomatic thrombocytopenia is a rare complication of natural measles. The first symptoms are generally sudden epistaxis or purpura appearing 2 to 14 days (mean, 6 days) after onset of rash. Hemorrhage into the mouth, genitourinary tract, gastrointestinal tract, ears, and eyes may follow. Bleeding usually abates after 1 to 2 weeks. However, platelet counts may not return to normal until 2 to 3 weeks later. Fatalities due to CNS hemorrhage have been reported. The thrombocytopenia appears to be secondary to peripheral platelet destruction, possibly caused by antibodies directed against altered platelet antigen or a virus–platelet complex. In contrast, the purpura seen in black measles generally appears somewhat earlier (during the first 3 days of the rash) and is confined to the areas of the skin involved by the rash.

Myocarditis–Pericarditis

Transient electrocardiographic changes have been described during the prodromal and acute phases of measles. The reported incidence of this complication has varied from 0.5% to 33%; conduction defects and arrhythmias constitute the major abnormalities. Clinical cardiac symptoms or fatal myocarditis is exceedingly rare.

Eye

Keratitis (with photophobia) and conjunctivitis are classic features of the prodromal and early eruptive period of measles. After the acute stage of modified or natural measles, slit-lamp examination may reveal signs of a punctate keratoconjunctivitis persisting up to 3 months. More serious complications such as corneal ulceration and pyogenic ocular infection are quite rare.

Gastrointestinal Tract and Liver

General lymphoid hyperplasia affecting the mesenteric lymph nodes may cause nonspecific abdominal pain; symptomatic enteritis or enterocolitis are very uncommon in otherwise healthy children. The incidence of appendicitis is minimally increased, if at all, during measles.

Subclinical hepatitis, associated with transient serum hepatic enzyme elevations, was detected in 14 of 17 young adults with measles.

Tropical Measles

Measles is often a fatal disease among socioeconomically deprived children in tropical countries. An impairment of cell-mediated immunity caused by protein–calorie malnutrition is probably a key factor in many cases. Underlying disease and the high incidence of measles in children under 3 years of age also play a role. Mortality rates of 10% to 15% are common, and the incidence of complications may run as high as 85%. Although viral and secondary bacterial pneumonias are leading causes of death, these children may also be afflicted with enteritis and severe diarrhea persisting for weeks or months. Other complications include ulcerative stomatitis or cancrum oris (noma), severe keratitis, and extensive, protracted desquamation with multiple skin abscesses after the rash. Acute kwashiorkor or marasmus are also common sequelae of this disease.

Measles in Pregnancy

The effects of measles acquired during pregnancy remain a matter of some controversy. In general, epidemiologic evidence implicates maternal measles as a significant cause of fetal death and premature births, but not of congenital malformations. Classic measles has been well documented in newborn infants, the disease having been acquired from a susceptible mother who was exposed to measles shortly before delivery.

Secondary Effects of Measles

An attack of measles is often followed by a transient clinical remission of lipoid nephrosis, infantile eczema, or bronchial asthma. Conversely, measles may be associated with exacerbation of tuberculosis, with serious, even fatal, consequences. The mechanism(s) underlying these effects is not known. The transient depression of cellular (delayed) hypersensitivity, clinically manifested by the loss of tuberculin reactivity for 2 to 6 weeks after the measles infection or live-virus vaccination, may be related to the above phenomena.

Diagnosis

The features of measles are distinctive, and the disease in its characteristic form is usually recognized without difficulty. When modified by maternal antibody (in infants) or by human immune serum globulin, however, the milder disease that results may resemble a wide variety of disorders, including rubella (Chap. 87, Rubella), roseola infantum (Chap. 88, Other Exanthems), enterovirus infection (Chap. 118, Viral Meningitis), toxoplasmosis (Chap. 129, Toxoplasmosis), and drug eruptions. In a severe form with hemorrhagic rash, or when atypical as in previously sensitized children, it may be mistaken for meningococcemia (Chap. 119, Acute Bacterial Meningitis) or Rocky Mountain spotted fever (Chap. 96, Spotted Fevers). Therefore, laboratory tests may occasionally be needed to confirm the diagnosis. Although a lymphocytosis may elevate the total leukocyte count during the incubation period in measles, leukopenia is prominent after onset of the rash.

During the prodromal stage and the first day of the rash, multinucleated giant cells may be demonstrated in stained smears of nasal secretions (Fig. 86-3), sputum, and swabbings from epithelial surfaces such as the pharynx, nasal and buccal cavities, and conjunctivae. Urinary sediments may contain mononuclear cells with cytoplasmic inclusions in addition to the giant cells. The identification of measles virus antigen in these exfoliated cells by direct immunofluorescent methods is an additional rapid and sensitive technique. Immunofluorescent staining of nasopharyngeal cells for measles antigen may be positive from 4 days before, to 10 days after, onset of the rash.

In modified measles or unusual cases in which diagnosis is doubtful, infection can be confirmed by isolation of the virus or by demonstration of a significant (fourfold or greater) rise in measles antibody titer. The measurement of hemagglutination-inhibition (HI) antibodies is most widely used, because it is more rapid and practical than neutralization or complement fixation (CF) techniques. Enzyme-linked immunosorbent assay (ELISA) is promising and may well become the primary method.

Because serum antibody is demonstrable within 1 to 2 days after appearance of the rash, the acute serum specimen must be obtained as early as possible. The convalescent serum should be drawn 2 to 3 weeks later. After infection, neutralizing and HI antibodies persist at measurable levels for prolonged periods, usually for life; CF antibodies, however, may not be detectable after a few years. Although the presence of neutralizing or HI antibodies correlates well with resistance to infection, lack of them does not always indicate susceptibility. Indeed, persons who appear to lack antibodies by the standard tests sometimes show evidence of immunity when enhancing methods are used and display a secondary or recall IgG response to measles virus vaccine.

Prognosis

The prognosis for patients with measles—even for those with complications—is good. Older children fare better than infants. On the average, severe respiratory tract involvement or otitis media occurs in 7% to 10% of cases. Pneumonia or encephalitis are most frequently responsible for the 1 or 2 measles deaths that occur in every 10,000 cases. Although the use of antimicrobial agents has been an important advance in the management of secondary bacterial infections, the decline in measles mortality began long before such agents were introduced; improved social conditions, nutrition, and general health care seemingly are of equal importance. The prognosis in measles is poor for children with leukemia, cystic fibrosis, or deficiencies in cellular immunity. Exacerbations of preexisting tuberculosis may also affect prognosis adversely.

Immunity after measles seems to be solid and lifelong. If second attacks do occur, they are exceedingly rare. No recurrence has been serologically and virologically documented.

Therapy

The treatment of uncomplicated measles is symptomatic. General measures include bed rest, maintenance of fluid intake, and aspirin for fever and headache. Attempts to suppress the cough with cough mixtures containing narcotics or sedatives should be avoided. The use of a vaporizer and an expectorant cough mixture may be of value. A darkened room may provide comfort to the patient with photophobia. Antimicrobic- or steroid-containing ophthalmic ointments are of no value in the treatment of viral keratoconjunctivitis. Obstructive laryngitis may require a tracheostomy. Early tracheostomy performed in the operating room may be life-saving and is safer than an emergency bedside procedure necessitated by undue delay.

The therapy of secondary bacterial complications should be guided by isolation and susceptibility studies. Examination of a Gram-stained smear and culture of sputum or other discharges should be performed before the institution of antimicrobial therapy. For otitis media in children in whom *H. influenzae* is a potential pathogen, amoxicillin should be given. Primary therapy should also include a penicillinase-resistant penicillin or a cephalosporin because complications are frequently caused by *Staphylococcus aureus* (*e.g.,* bacterial pneumonia, skin abscesses, and cancrum oris). Because *Streptococcus pyogenes* and *Streptococcus pneumoniae* are frequently invaders, tetracycline should not be used to initiate the antimicrobial therapy. The prophylactic use of antimicrobics is of no value. Antimicrobial agents do not prevent bacterial complications and may, by selective pressure, increase the risk of severe bacterial superinfections that are difficult to treat.

There is no specific therapy for measles encephalitis; treatment is entirely symptomatic and supportive. The use of glucosteroids or large doses of gamma globulin is of no proven value in the treatment of this complication.

Prevention

Live attenuated measles virus vaccine is currently recommended as one of the routine primary immuni-

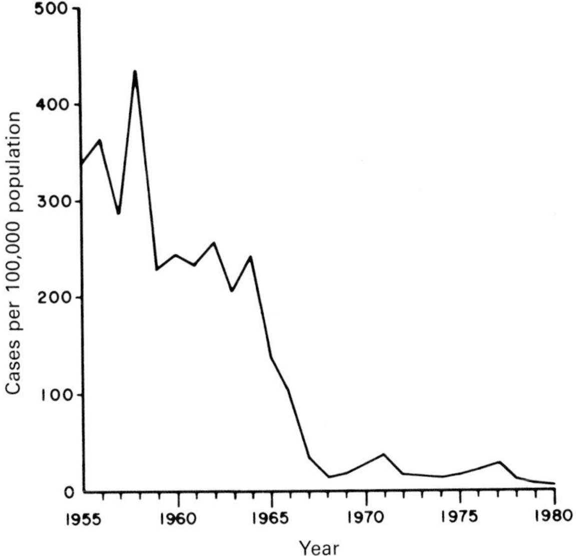

Fig. 86-4. Reported cases of measles in the United States by year, 1955–1980. (Morbid Mortal Week Rep Suppl, Summary, 1980)

zations for all children over 15 months of age. Older children and adults who have not had natural measles or the vaccine should also receive immunization. The attenuated live virus vaccines are highly effective, as shown by the decline in frequency of the disease (Fig. 86-4). Moreover, the vaccines are safe and noncommunicable, and they provoke very few side reactions. Clinical studies and determinations of antibody levels indicate that the protection conferred by a single injection of live vaccine is, in most cases, solid and prolonged. Waning of circulating immunity resulting in typical, modified, or atypical measles after exposure to natural disease, although uncommon, has been described. Transient, reversible electroencephalographic changes may occur after live virus measles immunization, but clinical neurologic complications occur at a rate of only 1 per million immunizations, an incidence far lower than that of the encephalitis associated with natural disease.

Two live attenuated similar measles virus vaccines are available at present. Both were derived from a chick tissue-culture adapted Edmonston B strain of virus by further passage in chick-cell cultures, and are generally referred to as further attenuated measles vaccines (Schwarz and Attenuvax types). With these vaccines, the febrile reactions and rash that were prominent with earlier preparations, have been reduced to 15% or less. Combined, live, bivalent (measles and rubella), and trivalent (measles, mumps and rubella) vaccines are commercially available. Persons receiving a measles vaccine do not transmit live virus to others.

Administration of live measles vaccine is routinely delayed until 15 months of age or later to eliminate possible interfering effects from maternally derived antibody. It has been suggested that the vaccine may be given to younger infants (as early as 6 months) if measles is prevalent or the risk of exposure is high. Because there may be reduced antibody formation following such early immunization, preventive doses of gamma globulin may be more desirable in infants under 12 months of age after known exposure. In such cases, vaccine must be given after 15 months of age to ensure solid, lasting immunity.

Elective use of live vaccine should be delayed for at least 12 weeks after administration of whole blood, plasma, or gamma globulin because the measles antibody content of these preparations may neutralize the vaccine.

Contraindications to live measles virus vaccine include active untreated tuberculosis, pregnancy, leukemia or other general malignancy, diseases and medications that suppress cell-mediated immunity or antibody response, severe febrile illness, and hypersensitivity to neomycin (in the case of Attenuvax). The vaccine appears to contain only minimal amounts of egg albumin and yolk components since egg-sensitive children has been immunized without adverse effect.

Live attenuated measles virus vaccine is usually preventive if given within 3 days of exposure to natural measles. Protection is unreliable when the vaccine is given thereafter.

Immunization with inactivated measles vaccines has been discontinued because they were less effective than live vaccines in preventing natural disease, and required frequent booster injections. All persons previously immunized with an inactivated vaccine should also receive a live vaccine. The hypersensitivity reactions that may follow vaccination or exposure to natural measles in children immunized with killed vaccine have already been discussed (see Manifestations, above).

Pooled adult gamma globulin is effective in preventing or modifying natural measles if given within 6 to 8 days after exposure. During the first 6 days after exposure, measles can be prevented with 0.25 ml/kg. After 6 days and up to 8 days, a dose of 0.25 ml/kg results only in modification. Despite the mild or subclinical nature of modified measles, the development of active immunity comparable to that of natural infection generally follows. The incubation period in such disease is usually prolonged (to 20 days or more), Koplik's spots are generally lacking, and the rash may be sparse and brief. Because patients with modified measles may disseminate virus, persons receiving either a modifying dose of gamma globulin or a supposed preventive dose (when the exact time of exposure is unknown) should be considered a potential risk to susceptible persons for at least 21 days.

With the availability of an effective measles vaccine, there is no indication for inducing modified measles. Exposed, susceptible, normal persons should receive a protective dose of gamma globulin (0.25 ml/kg) as soon as possible after exposure, followed by live vaccine after 12 weeks to induce lasting immunity. Exposed, susceptible, compromised hosts (*i.e.*, patients with leukemia, disseminated malignancy, impaired cell-mediated immunity, or immunosuppression of any cause) should receive 0.5 ml/kg, up to 20 ml to 30 ml of gamma globulin. Live virus vaccine is contraindicated in such patients; indirect protection should be sought through immunizing all measles-susceptible close contacts of this group of patients.

Children should be isolated until 5 days after onset of the rash; however, the widespread dissemination of measles during the prodromal period, before the diagnosis has been established, diminishes the value of isolation and quarantine procedures. The use of gamma globulin for individual, susceptible contacts, combined with mass, live-virus immunization of the childhood population, is far superior in modifying the course of an outbreak of measles.

Remaining Problems

Little is known about the factors that influence the severity and extent of measles in the apparently normal host. The contributions of this disease to subsequent learning and behavioral problems, impaired attention span, and chronic bronchopulmonary disorders have not been clearly defined.

The relative roles of direct viral invasion and delayed hypersensitivity in measles rash and measles encephalitis remain to be determined. The pathogenesis of subacute sclerosing panencephalitis and the possible relationship of measles virus to other disorders (*e.g.*, multiple sclerosis, systemic lupus erythematosus) also require further study.

Additional areas for investigation include the bases for the characteristic progression and distribution of the rash; the mechanism whereby measles temporarily depresses delayed cutaneous hypersensitivity; and the events underlying the remissions that this virus may induce in such disorders as asthma, eczema, and nephrosis. Development of an effective chemotherapeutic agent for use in measles-infected immunosuppressed patients should be pursued.

The persistence of immunity after live attenuated virus vaccination and the role of subclinical reinfections due to wild virus in the maintenance of that immunity require additional study. Development of a vaccine suitable for intranasal administration should be explored. Further development and evaluation of a heat-stable vaccine for use in tropical countries is essential.

Bibliography

Books

GERSHON AA, KRUGMAN S: Measles virus. In Lennette EH, Schmidt NJ (ed): Diagnostic Procedures for: Viral, Rickettsial, and Chlamydial Infections, 5th ed. Washington DC, American Public Health Association, 1979. pp 665–693.

Journals

BREM J: Koplik spots for the record: An illustrated historical note. Clin Pediatr 11:161–163, 1972

BURNET FM: Measles as an index of immunological function. Lancet 2:610–613, 1968

CHRISTENSEN PE, SCHMIDT H, JENSEN O, BANG HO, ANDERSEN V, JORDAL B: An epidemic of measles in southern Greenland, 1951. Acta Med Scand 144:313–322, 430–449, 450–454; 145:126–142, 1953

ENDERS JF: Seminar on the epidemiology and prevention of measles and rubella. Arch Gesamte Virusforsch 16:1–374, 1965

FENNER F: The pathogenesis of the acute exanthems: An interpretation based on experimental investigations with mousepox (infectious ectromelia of mice). Lancet 2:915–920, 1948

FULGINITI VA, ELLER JJ, DOWNIE AW, KEMPE CH: Altered reactivity to measles virus. Atypical measles in children previously immunized with inactivated measles virus vaccine. JAMA 202:1075–1080, 1967

HALL WW, CHOPPIN PW: Measles-virus proteins in the brain tissue of patients with subacute sclerosing panencephalitis: Absence of the M protein. N Engl J Med 304:1152–1155, 1981

KRAUSE PJ, CHERRY JD, DESADA—TOUS J, CHAMPION JG, STRASSBURG M, SULLIVAN C, SPENCER MJ, BRYSON YJ, WELLIVER RC, BOYER KM: Epidemic measles in young adults: Clinical, epidemiologic, and serologic studies. Ann Intern Med 90:873–876, 1979

MORGAN EM, RAPP F: Measles virus and its associated diseases. Bacteriol Rev 41:636–666, 1977

OLDING—STENKVIST E, BJORVATN B: Rapid detection of measles virus in skin rashes by immunofluorescence. J Infect Dis 134:463–469, 1976

S. MICHAEL MARCY
SIDNEY KIBRICK

Rubella

87

Rubella (German measles, 3-day measles) is a moderately contagious disease that begins insidiously and is marked by an acute, exanthematous, maculopapular eruption that lasts 3 days or less. There is usually tender postauricular and suboccipital lymphadenopathy. Although rubella is typically a mild illness in children and young adults, when acquired in early pregnancy it may produce a severe general infection of the fetus, resulting in multiple abnormalities known as the congenital rubella syndrome.

Etiology

Since the initial isolation in tissue culture in 1962, increasing knowledge of the morphologic and biochemical properties of the rubella virus has resulted in frequent reclassification. It is presently classified with certain group A and B arboviruses as a member of the Togavirus family. However, the epidemiologic and clinical features of rubella virus infection are similar to those of the paramyxoviruses. The agent is not antigenically related to any other viruses; only a single serotype is known.

The rubella virion varies in size from 50 nm to 70 nm and consists of a central nucleoid of single stranded RNA surrounded by an envelope that is covered with many short, fine projections (Fig. 87-1). The envelope contains both lipid and protein, and it is derived from altered host-cell membrane that pinches off and surrounds the maturing virus as it buds from the cytoplasmic membrane or into intracytoplasmic vacuoles. A hemagglutinin is associated with rubella virus. Two antigens that evoke complement-fixing antibodies are designated: viral or V antigen, which induces a rapid antibody response, and S antigen, which engenders a response that is both later and lower. Additional components include the precipitinogens *theta* and *iota*. The hemagglutinin, complement-fixing viral antigen, and theta precipitinogen are envelope components; the others are associated with the RNA core.

The rubella virus has been isolated and propagated in several primary tissue cultures and continuous cell lines. In some tissue culture systems, the virus causes a subtle but distinctive cytopathic effect by which its presence can be recognized. In others, it can be detected only by its ability to prevent characteristic cytopathic changes brought about when the tissue culture is superinfected with one of a variety of viruses, the most common of which are echo–11, coxsackie A–9, or sindbis virus. The mechanism of this interference phenomenon is poorly understood, although in some cases it appears to be mediated by interferon.

Viral infectivity is lost on exposure to lipid solvents (ether, chloroform), sodium deoxycholate, or proteolytic enzymes (trypsin). The virus is also inactivated by formalin, β-propiolactone, ultraviolet light, and extremes of pH. Although thermolabile, with a half-life of 1 hour at 37°C, the virus can be stored in protein-containing solutions, for example, 1% gelatin or 0.5% bovine albumin, for 1 or 2 weeks at 4°C and for years at −60°C without significant loss of infectivity. Materials for culture may be stored or transported for several days at 4°C or in wet ice and for longer periods in dry ice (−60°C). Infectivity is quickly lost at freezer temperatures (−10 to −20°C). Amantadine HCl, an antiviral agent that inhibits viral cellular penetration, is effective against rubella virus *in vitro*.

Epidemiology

Humans are the only known natural host of rubella virus. However, experimental infections may be induced in a variety of laboratory animals.

The rubella virus appears to spread through the inhalation of droplet nuclei emanating from the respiratory tract of infected persons. A single, brief exposure to an infected patient is relatively inefficient in

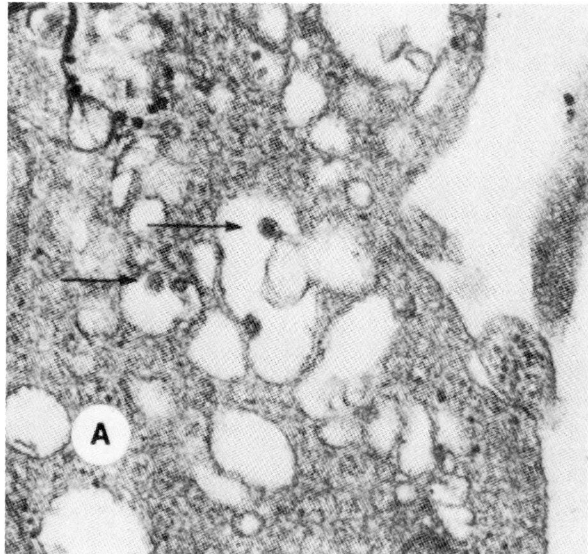

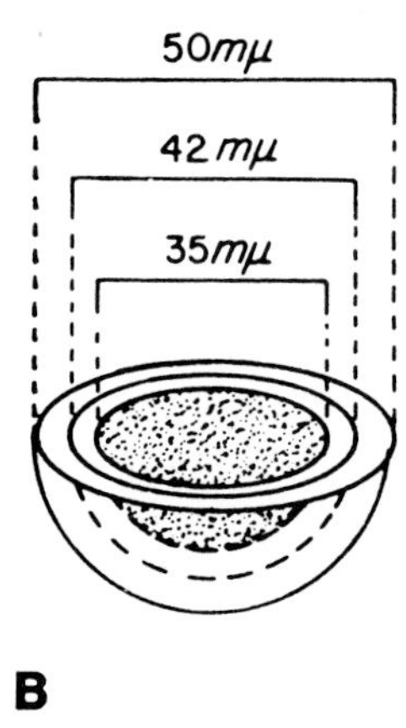

Fig. 87-1. (*A*) Rubella virus particles within cytoplasmic vesicles of infected cells (*arrows*). (B) Diagram of structure of rubella virus particle. (Rawls WE: Int Ophthalmol Clin 12:21–66, 1972; Courtesy of RM McCombs)

transmitting the disease, and in most situations close and prolonged contact seems to be required. The virus has been recovered from nasopharyngeal secretions from 13 days before to more than 21 days after onset of the rash. However, the period of greatest communicability extends from 5 days before to 5 days after the appearance of the rash. Patients with atypical or subclinical infections are equally capable of disseminating the virus.

Although generally considered a childhood disease, rubella is only moderately contagious, and young children often escape the illness. In the United States, where intensive immunization efforts have further reduced the pool of susceptible youngsters, the incidence in adolescents and young adults is now similar to that for young children. Local outbreaks are thus relatively common in colleges, hospitals, and military installations.

Rubella tends to be endemic in most communities throughout the year, although most cases in the Northern Hemisphere occur during the spring. Widespread epidemics have been seen in 6- to 9-year cycles; however, mass immunization programs have reduced or eliminated this characteristic epidemiologic pattern in many countries.

Pathogenesis and Pathology

The incubation period of naturally acquired rubella is about 18 days, with a range of 12 to 23 days. It is believed that initial viral replication occurs in the upper respiratory tract mucosa and in cervical lymph nodes. After multiplication at these sites, the virus is disseminated to other parts of the body through the blood. Viremia can be detected as early as 7 days before the exanthem. During this period or shortly thereafter, enlargement of the lymph nodes commonly appears, perhaps indicating secondary sites of viral replication. Coincident with development of the rash, or within 24 to 48 hours, neutralizing antibodies become detectable and circulating virus disappears from the blood. As in measles, the emergence of rash simultaneously with the initiation of a measurable antibody response has led to the suggestion that the exanthem may represent an inflammatory effect exerted by an antibody–virus complex, rather than direct viral invasion of the vascular endothelium.

The virus has been isolated from affected and unaffected areas of skin biopsied within 24 hours of the appearance of the rash. It has also been recovered from urine during the period of viremia, feces shortly before and after the rash, circulating lymphocytes, uterine cervical secretions, breast milk, and the conjunctivae. More prolonged shedding occurs only from the nasopharynx; usually the virus can be recovered from this site from about 7 days before to 2 weeks after the onset of the rash.

Owing to the generally mild nature of the disease, few histologic studies have been done in postnatal rubella. Nonspecific acute and chronic inflammatory changes have been described in the skin and affected lymph nodes. Acute rubella encephalitis results in nonspecific, perivascular infiltration, edema, and neuronal degeneration of variable severity with a mild meningeal reaction. The demyelination characteristic of measles and varicella encephalitis is not usually seen with rubella, possibly because death prevents evolution of the process.

Manifestations

After the incubation period—1 to 5 days before the rash—a mild prodrome may occur. Often absent in young children, the prodrome is most conspicuous in adolescents and young adults. When it occurs, it is characterized by anorexia, malaise, conjunctivitis, headache, low-grade fever, and minimal respiratory symptoms.

Enlargement and tenderness of the lymph nodes are prominent features of the disease. They usually develop 4 to 10 days before the rash appears, but they may be seen as early as 13 to 18 days before the rash. The postauricular, suboccipital, and posterior cervical lymph nodes are noticeably affected, although mild general lymphadenopathy is frequently also present. Adenopathy is at its height during the rash and generally persists during the following week; on occasion, it may last for months. The tip of the spleen is often palpable, reflecting what is almost certainly general involvement of the lymphoid tissue.

As the rash appears, the prodromal symptoms diminish. The exanthem consists of a discrete, pink, maculopapular eruption that begins on the face, spreads rapidly downward over the trunk and extremities, often within hours, and fades in the same order in which it evolved. By the end of the second day, the face may be clearing and the previously discrete rash on the trunk may be nearly confluent. At this stage, rubella is often confused with scarlet fever, although the exanthem usually remains discrete on the extremities. The rash may persist 4 or 5 days, but it generally disappears by the end of the third day, thus accounting for the name 3-day measles. In severe cases, there may follow a fine, flaky desquamation that spares the hands and feet. A low-grade fever may accompany the rash; rarely, fever may reach 40°C (104°F).

An enanthem (Forchheimer spots) consisting of small, red macules on the soft palate, often precedes or accompanies the rash. These lesions are petechiae induced by a combination of increased capillary fragility and pressure changes due to swallowing. They are in no way pathognomonic and have been described in various other disorders, including scarlet fever, roseola, infectious mononucleosis, and septicemia.

Although prodromal symptoms, lymphadenopathy, and a typical exanthem constitute classic rubella, any one or all of these manifestations may be entirely lacking. The exact frequency of inapparent rubella ranges from 6 in 7 (in military recruits) to 1 in 9 (in random civilian populations). When an exanthem is present, it is almost always accompanied by adenopathy, but it may vary widely in appearance. Thus, proven cases of rubella have been associated with a transient, erythematous flush, and petechial, acneiform, and biphasic exanthems.

Neurologic Manifestations

Symptomatic, acute rubella encephalitis is an infrequent complication, occuring in approximately 1 in 6000 cases. The encephalopathy is more common in children and generally occurs 1 to 7 days after appearance of the rash. As in other viral or toxic encephalitides, the clinical findings are variable and nonspecific, consisting of high fever, convulsions, and alterations in the state of consciousness. An ascending polyneuritis with motor and sensory disturbances including cranial nerve palsies may also occur. In these patients, the cerebrospinal fluid (CSF) may contain up to 300 cells, almost all mononuclear, with normal concentrations of sugar and normal or elevated protein concentrations. Despite a high mortality (20%), careful follow-up studies have shown a low incidence of permanent intellectual or neurologic damage in those who recover. However, EEG abnormalities may persist for months or years. The rubella virus has been visualized by electron microscopy and immunofluorescence in the brain tissues of patients with acute encephalopathy. It has, on a single occasion, been cultured from the CSF.

In contrast to other postviral encephalitides, rubella encephalitis is not associated with demyelination.

Progressive rubella panencephalitis (PRP) is a recently recognized clinical syndrome associated with chronic rubella infection. Six cases have now been reported, but the true incidence is unknown. The disease appears to be primarily associated with congenital rubella and, less commonly, with infection early in life. Initially, the affected children show no evidence of this illness until the second decade of life, when they begin to develop panencephalitis with mental deterioration, seizures, ataxia, nystagmus, and occasionally myoclonus. Serum and spinal fluid antibody titers to rubella are high. Progressive motor and mental deterioration continues over months to years, followed by death. Rubella virus has been recovered in one case by cocultivation of brain tissue. PRP apparently represents a persistence of a suppressed rubella infection from fetal life or the newborn period followed by a subsequent exacerbation with disease.

This syndrome resembles in many respects subacute sclerosing panencephalitis (SSPE), associated with measles virus infection. The mechanisms responsible for PRP remain to be determined.

Arthritis

Involvement of the joints is uncommon in children and adult males, but it occurs in up to 33% of adult women with rubella. The arthritis usually appears with the rash or within 3 days after the eruption, most frequently involving the fingers, wrists, and knees. Symptoms range from a mild, transient arthralgia to overt arthritis, with effusion, redness, and intense pain. Tenosynovitis and parasthesias, most commonly manifest as a carpal tunnel syndrome, often accompany the more severe cases. If several joints are involved in succession, rubella arthritis closely resembles the migratory polyarthritis of acute rheumatic fever. When symptoms persist in the joints initially involved, the condition may be confused with rheumatoid arthritis. Tests for rheumatoid factor may be positive; moreover, the erythrocyte sedimentation rate (ESR) is elevated. However, the synovial fluid contains mononuclear cells; polymorphonuclear cells are almost completely lacking.

Rubella arthritis is self-limited and usually clears without residua within 2 to 30 days, although arthralgia may occasionally persist for several months, and rarely, for years. The virus has been recovered on several occasions from joint effusions.

Hemorrhagic Manifestations

Despite the frequency of transient thrombocytopenia and increased capillary fragility, purpura or hemorrhage is rarely clinically manifest in rubella. When bleeding occurs, it begins abruptly 3 to 4 days after onset of the rash (range, 1–15 days). The skin and mucous membranes are the most common sites of bleeding. Gastrointestinal, renal, subconjunctival, and fatal central nervous system (CNS) hemorrhages have also been described. Thrombocytopenia may persist 6 months, but it usually resolves within 1 to 2 weeks. Because agglutinins for platelets have been demonstrated in the blood of some patients, excessive peripheral destruction of virus–platelet complexes may contribute to thrombocytopenia. In addition, platelet production seems to be decreased, although there are normal or increased numbers of megakaryocytes in the bone marrow.

Other Manifestations

Rubella will inhibit host-cell-mediated immunity for about 4 to 6 weeks. This transient immunosuppression is clinically detectable as a reduction or disappearance of tuberculin skin sensitivity during this period.

Diagnosis

The clinical diagnosis of rubella may be made with assurance only in typical cases occuring during an epidemic. The large number of atypical and subclinical cases of rubella, together with the numerous conditions of an infectious or allergic nature that may be associated with a rubelliform rash make the clinical diagnosis in sporadic cases extremely difficult, if not impossible (Chap. 88, Other Exanthems). Routine laboratory tests are of little value. Leukocyte counts are usually low, but they may be normal. Türk cells, plasma cells (up to 24%), and atypical lymphocytes are frequent, but nondiagnostic, features of the disease.

A specific diagnosis of rubella can be established either by virus isolation in appropriate tissue cultures or by serologic tests. Virus isolation procedures, however, are rarely used for routine diagnosis of this disease because of the lability of the agent. In addition, they are time consuming and technically difficult. Recently, viral antigen has been demonstrated by direct immunofluorescence in cells swabbed from the throats of children with rubella. Further experience may confirm the usefulness of this procedure for rapid diagnosis.

Several methods are currently available for the detection of rubella antibody: hemagglutination inhibition (HI), neutralization, fluorescence (FA), complement fixation (CF); and immunodiffusion testing to detect precipitins to the soluble rubella antigens *theta* and *iota* (structural components of the virion). Of these, the measurement of HI antibodies is most widely used, because it provides a rapid, convenient, and accurate method of demonstrating the immune status of a person or confirming the diagnosis of rubella. HI antibodies are first detectable during the rash, rise rapidly for 1 to 2 weeks, and after 4 to 12 months fall to baseline levels, at which they probably persist for life. Because of the rapid rise in HI antibodies, the titers of serums obtained more than a few days after appearance of the rash may already be near peak values, precluding a diagnostic, fourfold rise in titer in subsequent (convalescent) specimens. If delay in obtaining the initial blood specimen is unavoidable, alternate methods are helpful in establishing the diagnosis.

For serodiagnosis, acute and convalescent serums must be tested at the same time to avoid false differences in titer from variations in technique or sensitivity. Accordingly, serum specimens obtained from pregnant women should be held at least until after delivery to facilitate repeated testing when necessary. A high HI titer in a single, early convalescent serum specimen is not dependable for making a diagnosis of recent rubella infection with this agent. However, a low titer ($\leq$ 1:16) 14 days or more after a suspected infection has some diagnostic value, since it is not generally consistent with a recent infection.

If delay in obtaining the initial blood specimen is unavoidable, alternate methods are helpful in establishing the diagnosis. Because CF antibodies usually appear several days after onset of the rash and do not reach peak levels for 4 to 8 weeks, a short delay does not detract from the diagnostic value of CF testing.

A less useful alternative is based on the fact that the earliest HI antibodies are IgM immunoglobulins. Although it was generally held that these antibodies declined rapidly and became undetectable within 3 to 8 weeks after appearance of the rash, more sensitive techniques have revealed a variable persistence of IgM—usually at very low titer—for 4 to 6 months in some patients. Thus, depending on the method used, finding rubella IgM in the blood may reflect a primary infection within the preceding months rather than weeks. Although the anamnestic or booster response in HI antibodies that sometimes results from heavy exposure of an immune person may give a fourfold or greater rise in titer, the response consists solely of IgG antibodies.

The pattern of neutralizing, FA, and theta responses is similar to that of the HI antibodies, although the titers are 4 to 16 times lower. These antibodies also appear to persist for life. The more slowly rising CF antibodies, however, begin to decrease in titer 8 to 12 months after infection, and they are undetectable in 50% of patients with 10 years. Similarly, *iota* precipitins usually disappear within 1 year. Rubella antibody detected by any of the four methods is a reliable indicator of past infection. Susceptibility to infection is best indicated by the lack of neutralizing or HI antibodies, because the variable persistence of CF antibodies and the weakening of the FA antibody response make interpretation of these tests difficult.

A small percentage of children and adults who are immune to rubella as a result of earlier infection or immunization may have titers too low to be detected by the standard HI tests. Generally, the sera of such persons contain low levels of antibodies that can be demonstrated by neutralization or more sensitive enhanced HI techniques. When challenged with rubella vaccine virus, these persons develop an accelerated rise in IgG antibody titer typical of a booster response rather than of primary infection.

During the past several years, highly sensitive enzyme-linked immunosorbent assay (ELISA), radioimmunoassay, and gel-diffusion methods have been developed for measurement of IgG or IgM rubella antibodies. At present a kit is commercially available for performing at least one of these tests, the ELISA. This assay can also be used to determine or verify immunity in patients who do not have detectable HI antibodies.

Prognosis

The prognosis in postnatal rubella is excellent. Fatalities have been caused either by encephalitis or by thrombocytopenia with cerebral hemorrhage; both of these complications are rare.

A single attack of overt or subclinical rubella generally confers prolonged immunity through induction of nasopharyngeal and serum antibodies. Epidemiologic studies documenting the reinfection of previously immune persons after heavy exposure to rubella have, however, cast some doubt on the lifelong quality of active immunity. In most cases, reinfections are subclinical and, though causing significant increases in antibody titer, are probably not accompanied by a viremia. Such reinfections are believed to be important in maintaining immunity and are most likely to occur in persons with low antibody titers at the time of exposure. Passive immunity lasting 6 to 12 months is transferred from an immune mother to her infant.

Therapy

The treatment of rubella is symptomatic. Aspirin is usually sufficient to relieve the discomfort of lymphadenitis, headache, fever, and arthritis. Severe bleeding associated with thrombocytopenic purpura has been treated with glucosteroids or platelet transfusions; however, no studies are available to substantiate the value of this therapy. Supportive therapy is indicated in rubella encephalopathy. Bacterial complications are rare in rubella. There is no convincing evidence that antimicrobics modify the course of the uncomplicated disease. Although effective *in vitro,* amantadine has not been of therapeutic or prophylactic value in rubella.

Prevention

Several attenuated live rubella virus vaccines have been licensed in the United States since 1969. Recent

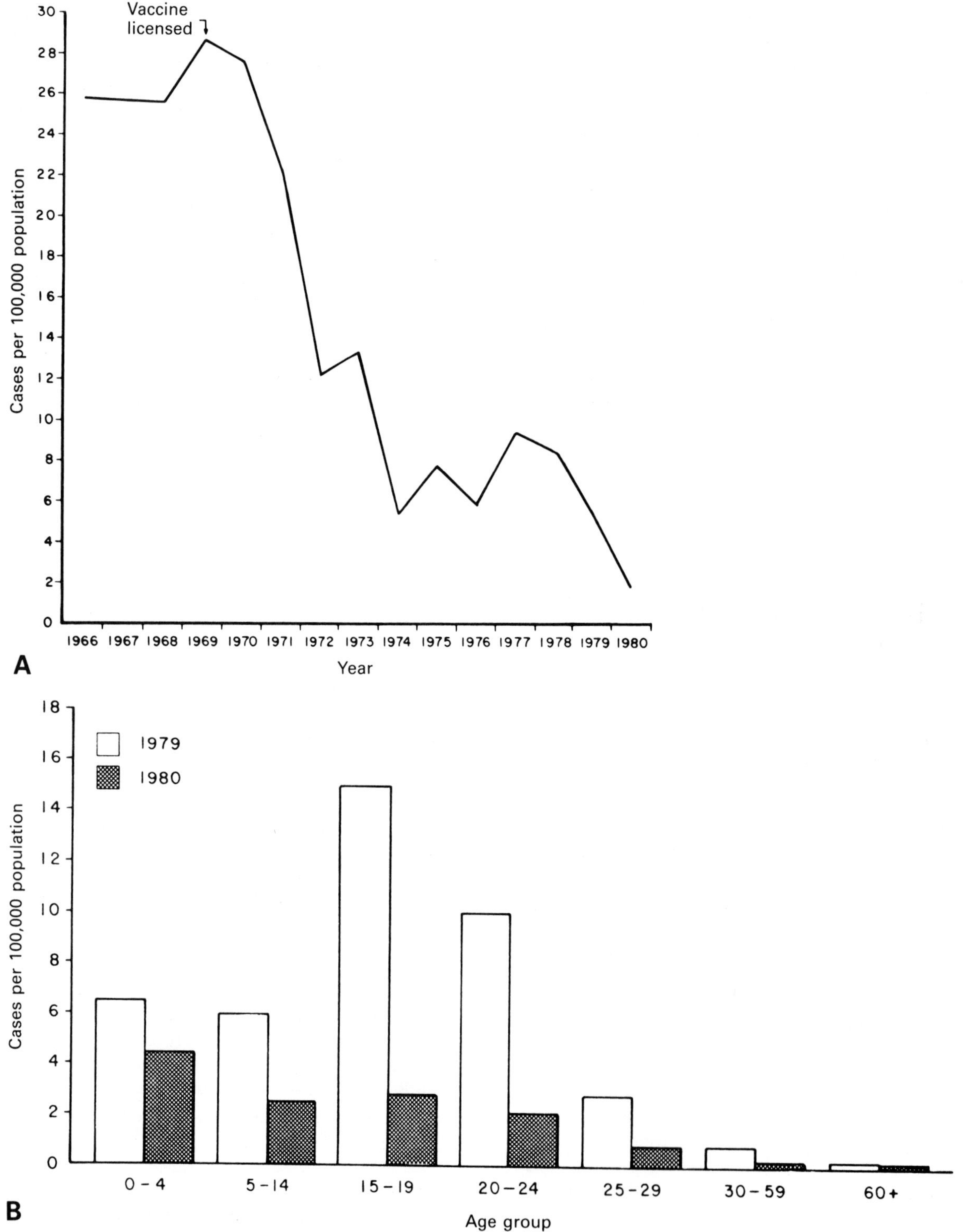

Fig. 87-2. (*A*) Reported cases of rubella in the United States by year, 1966–1980. (Morbid Mortal Week Rep Suppl, Summary, 1980) (*B*) Reported cases of rubella by age group in the United States, comparing 1979 with 1980. (Morbid Mortal Week Rep Suppl, Summary, 1980)

studies have seriously questioned the durability and completeness of circulating and cell-mediated immunity induced by the most widely used of these preparations, the high passage virus 77 (HPV-77) vaccine. Nevertheless, surveillance data seem to indicate that the administration of HPV-77 to a large segment of the childhood population has been associated with a significant reduction in the overall incidence of rubella and a shift in the age-related incidence to the disease (Fig. 87-2). The greatest shift has been the decline in 1980 in the 15- to 19- and 20- to 24-year-old age groups. From 1976 through 1979, more than 70% of the cases were in patients ≥ 15 years old, whereas in 1980, only 47% were in this age group.

Another live attenuated rubella vaccine, RA 27/3, prepared in a human diploid cell line (WI-38), was licensed in 1979 and replaced the HPV-77 strain. It is licensed only for subcutaneous administration and is available as a monovalent vaccine or in combination with measles or mumps vaccines. Following inoculation, it has been shown to (1) induce HI antibodies in over 95% of susceptible subjects, (2) elicit higher antibody titers than previous rubella vaccines, and (3) induce a broader profile of circulating antibodies, simulating natural infection more closely than previous vaccines. Antibody levels have been shown to persist without substantial decline for at least 6 years.

The United States Public Health Service Advisory Committee on Immunization Practices (ACIP) recommends that rubella vaccine be used for the following groups: (1) children between the ages of 12 months and puberty (unless the vaccine also contains measles antigen, in which case it should be delayed up to 15 months to maximize measles seroconversion); (2) adolescent and adult males; and (3) adolescent and adult females who are not pregnant, will not become pregnant within 3 months of vaccination and, when feasible, have been shown to be seronegative.

Studies of women inadvertently immunized with rubella vaccine shortly before or after conception have shown that the vaccine virus can cross the placenta and in some cases, infect the fetus. Although the number of such cases is limited, data on previously and presently available rubella vaccines indicate that the theoretical risk of serious malformations from live rubella vaccine is quite small—0% to 4%. Accordingly the ACIP now believes that rubella vaccination during pregnancy is not a reason for routinely recommending abortion. While the ACIP believes that, "the risk of vaccine-associated malformations is so small as to be negligible," the final decision must rest with each patient and her physician.

RA 27/3 vaccine virus has been recovered from the blood for 3 weeks after vaccination. Small amounts of virus may also be present in the pharynx between the first and third week after immunization. However, the risk of transmission of virus from the pharynx to susceptible contacts appears to be negligible, possibly because of the low titers and the short, irregular persistence of virus.

The incidence of side-effects following rubella vaccination is about 15%. Arthritis and arthralgia, generally beginning 2 to 3 weeks after vaccination and lasting 1 to 7 days, are seen occasionally in adult women and less frequently in children. Additional adverse reactions include signs of rubella such as adenopathy, rash, and fever. As with the disease a transient (4–6 week) suppression of tuberculin skin reactivity generally follows vaccination.

Live rubella vaccine is contraindicated not only during, and in anticipation of, pregnancy, but also in patients with acute febrile illnesses or altered immune states. There is no contraindication to the use of vaccine after exposure to natural rubella, but its value in this circumstance is not known. As with other live-virus vaccines administered parenterally, vaccination should be deferred for at least 3 months following blood or plasma transfusions or administration of immune serum globulin. Postpartum use of anti-Rho(D) immune globulin is not a contraindication to vaccination.

Human immune serum globulin (ISG) has occasionally been employed for the prophylaxis of rubella during the first trimester of pregnancy. Its efficacy in preventing infection, even when given before exposure, has not been clearly established. Administration of human ISG does not interfere with the serologic diagnosis of actual rubella infection. The recommended dose is 20 ml intramuscularly.

The administration of human ISG containing high titers of rubella antibodies and given shortly after exposure may be of some value in preventing fetal infection. Serum antibody titers may rise and persist for several weeks after administration of hyperimmune globulin. Use of either standard ISG or high-titer globulin should be limited to cases in which therapeutic abortion would not be acceptable.

In cases in which virologic or serologic studies confirm the presence of rubella during the first trimester, termination of pregnancy should be considered because of the high risk to the fetus (see Congenital Rubella, below). Rare, isolated cases of rubella reinfection in pregnancy with transmission of the virus to the fetus have been documented.

The prolonged excretion of the virus before clinical illness renders isolation of patients ineffective as a preventive measure. However, during the period of communicability, patients with suspected rubella should avoid contact with women of childbearing age.

Congenital Rubella

In 1941, after an epidemic of rubella in Australia, Gregg noted that children born of mothers who had rubella in the first few months of pregnancy exhibited certain constant features that he believed were related to the maternal infection. These children were small and ill nourished. More than three-fourths of them had congenital cataracts, many with microphthalmia, and over half had evidence of congenital heart disease. Subsequently, he also noted that most of these children seemed retarded in their mental development. Swan, studying a similar group of patients in 1943, confirmed and extended Gregg's original findings. Many children had been of low birth weight and exhibited deaf-mutism, microcephaly, buphthalmos, hypospadias, and clubfoot in a frequency greater than expected. Thereafter, the combination of congenital cataracts, deafness, and heart disease became known as the congenital rubella syndrome.

The extensive epidemic of rubella that took place in 1964–1965 was followed by the birth of affected infants with clinical manifestations not previously associated with the rubella syndrome. An expanded congenital rubella syndrome grew out of this experience. Although some investigators have postulated that the wide spectrum of disease seen in 1964 was due to greater virulence in the infecting strain of rubella virus, there is evidence to indicate that the added features of the expanded syndrome were present but not recognized before 1964.

Epidemiology

Before the 1964 epidemic in the United States, approximately 15% of young women had no detectable rubella antibodies and were susceptible to the disease. Consequently, 4% of pregnancies that occurred in 1964 were complicated by rubella, resulting in 6250 fetal deaths, 5000 therapeutic abortions, 2100 neonatal deaths, and the birth of more than 20,000 children with the congenital rubella syndrome.

The isolation of rubella virus in 1962 made possible prospective epidemiologic studies of the etiology and frequency of the rubella syndrome that were firmly based on viral isolation and serodiagnosis. Although many of the earlier studies had been conducted during epidemics, when a clinical diagnosis of rubella could be established with reasonable certainty, the data were often retrospective and based on questionnaires answered by physicians. Because these reports usually failed to take into account misdiagnosed exanthems, inapparent or atypical maternal rubella, early fetal loss, neonatal deaths, and the manifestations of the rubella syndrome that develop late or remain undetected for many years, it is not surprising that estimates of the risk of acquiring major congenital defects after maternal rubella varied widely, ranging up to 50% in the first month of pregnancy, 30% in the second month, 20% in the third month, and 5% in the fourth month. Although it was generally agreed that the risk of acquiring major abnormalities after the fourth month of gestation was negligible, additional data from the 1964–1965 epidemic resulted in revision of the earlier estimates. Thus, in one prospective study, 90% of surviving infants had some abnormality following maternal rubella during the first 12 weeks of gestation. Nonfatal damage exceeded 50% following rubella in the second trimester and also occurred in the third trimester.

It has also become apparent within the last few years that infants with the congenital rubella syndrome may be contagious for many months after birth. There are many reports of rubella acquired by nursery personnel, physicians, and other contacts of infected infants. Although virus shedding from the nasopharynx may continue for more than 2 years, it is unusual for infants older than 12 to 18 months to disseminate infection.

Pathogenesis

The present concept of the pathogenesis of congenital rubella is shown in Figure 87-3. Maternal viremia leads to placental infection; the virus may then enter the fetal circulation through placental leaks or within emboli of desquamated chorionic tissue. The factors determining whether infection will remain confined to placental tissue or involve the fetus are unknown, although they appear to be related in part to gestational age. Once fetal viremia does occur, the virus is rapidly disseminated and can be isolated from virtually every organ of the fetus. Viral infection may be limited to a relatively small number of cells, however, and it has been estimated that generally no more than 1:1000 to 1:250,000 fetal cells are infected.

Four mechanisms, either singly or in combination, are apparently responsible for the malformations that follow intrauterine infection: (1) persistent infection of fetal tissues, producing mitotic arrest and inhibition of cellular multiplication, which retards the growth of organs so that they contain a subnormal number of morphologically normal cells; (2) vasculopathy of placental and fetal vessels leading to fibromuscular proliferation of the arterial wall and inter-

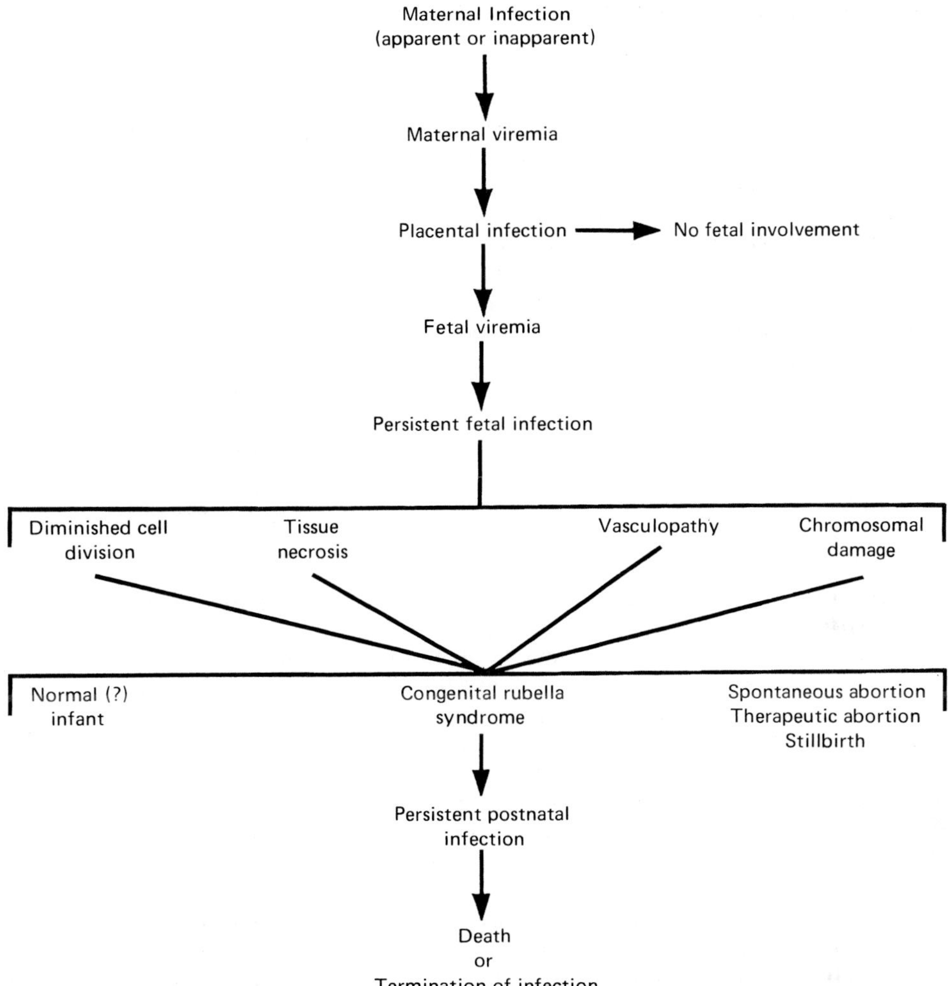

Fig. 87-3. The pathogenesis of congenital rubella.

ference with blood supply of growing tissues; (3) tissue necrosis; and (4) an increased incidence of chromosomal damage.

Persistent cellular infection and the transfer of virus to daughter cells during cell division are believed to be of primary importance in the pathogenesis of the rubella syndrome. Once established, infection is present throughout gestation and after birth. Effects may be expressed in the developing embryo, fetus, or neonate. Serious congenital defects or fetal death may result from direct damage or the retarded growth or primordial cells during periods of rapid differentiation and organogenesis. Whichever mechanism is operative, it is clear that early infection generally produces more widespread involvement than infection acquired later in gestation. However, such a temporal relationship is not invariable. Infected infants with no detectable clinical abnormalities have been born after rubella in the first trimester. Conversely, several instances have been reported in which damage of infants has resulted from maternal rubella acquired as late as the seventh month of pregnancy.

The progression of symptoms and the discovery of previously undetectable abnormalities months to years after birth is consistent with viral persistence well past the intrauterine period. Indeed, the virus can be recovered from the throats of about 85% of infants with congenital rubella in the first month of life, from 60% at 1 to 4 months, 33% at 5 to 8 months, 10% at 9 to 12 months, 3% at 13 to 20 months, and rarely at 30 months. Virus has also been recovered from the urine for up to 30 months, from CSF and middle ear fluid for up to 18 months, from circulating leukocytes for up to 14 months, and from a congenital cataract removed at 3 years of age. Congenital rubella may in some cases be a lifelong infection, for the virus has been isolated from brain tissue and the urine 12 and 29 years, respectively, after acquisition *in utero.* The host factors involved in the establishment and termination of viral persistence are poorly understood. It has been established that the humoral component of immunity is intact. Evidence suggests a defect either in cellular immunity or in interferon response that might be responsible for the prolonged excretion of the virus.

Manifestations

The features of the expanded rubella syndrome are outlined in the list below.

Diagnosis

In view of the high incidence of congenital rubella syndrome associated with maternal infection during the first trimester, the following circumstances should alert the physician to the possibility of this disorder: a history of proven rubella exposure or a rubella-like rash during the first trimester and manifestations consistent with congenital rubella in the infant. Isolation of rubella virus from fluid obtained by amniocentesis should be considered evidence of fetal infection. Because clinical diagnosis is not reliable in nonepidemic situations and because manifestations of congenital rubella may be minimal or lacking at birth, the final confirmation generally depends on viral isolation or serodiagnosis.

In newborns with congenital rubella, the serum usually contains both actively acquired IgM antibodies and passively acquired (maternal) IgG antibodies. The IgM antibodies are short lived and usually disappear during the first year of life. The passively acquired IgG antibodies rarely persist more than 6 months, but they are replaced by IgG antibodies formed by the infant in response to his infection. Accordingly, in the absence of postnatal rubella, the presence of rubella antibodies in infants older than 6 months or the presence of rubella IgM antibodies in early infancy both indicate congenital rubella infection. Because rubella antibodies may not persist in all infants with congenital infection, lack of such antibodies in an older infant does not necessarily rule out this diagnosis.

Congenital rubella may resemble congenital infection caused by cytomegalovirus, toxoplasmosis, herpes simplex virus, coxsackie virus B, or syphilis. However, it should be possible to distinguish rubella by the presence of typical teratologic characteristics (*e.g.,* congenital cataracts or glaucoma, typical congenital cardiac malformations, deafness), viral isolation, or serologic tests.

CLINICAL MANIFESTATONS OF THE EXPANDED RUBELLA SYNDROMES

- General
  - Retardation of intrauterine growth
  - Failure to thrive
- Ocular
  - Retinopathy
  - Nuclear cataracts
  - Microphthalmia
  - Glaucoma
  - Transient corneal cloudiness
  - Iridocyclitis
- Auditory
  - Sensorineural hearing loss
  - Central auditory imperception
  - Otitis media
  - Vestibular dysfunction
- Cardiovascular and Pulmonary
  - Congenital heart disease*
  - Interstitial pneumonitis†
  - Fibromuscular proliferation of arterial intima
    - Stenosis or hypoplasia of pulmonary and systemic arteries
    - Systemic hypertension
  - Myocardial necrosis
- Musculoskeletal
  - Metaphyseal osteoporosis
  - High arched palate
  - Hypoplastic mandible
  - Dental abnormalities
    - Delayed eruption
    - Enamel defects
  - Myositis
  - Minor extremity abnormalities
- Blood and reticuloendothelial system
  - Extramedullary hematopoiesis
    - Hepatosplenomegaly
    - "Blueberry muffin" syndrome
  - Generalized adenopathy†
  - Thrombocytopenic purpura
  - Hemolytic anemia
  - Hypoplastic anemia
  - Thymic hypoplasia
  - Depressed humoral and cellular immunity†
- Central nervous system
  - Meningoencephalitis
  - Psychomotor retardation
  - Spastic quadriparesis

Microcephaly
Chronic progressive panencephalitis (late)
Gastrointestinal
Indirect inguinal hernia
Cholangiolytic hepatitis
Intestinal atresia
Chronic diarrhea†
Giant-cell hepatitis
Interstitial pancreatitis
Skin
Abnormal dermatoglyphics
Chronic rubelliform rash†
Skin dimples
Vasomotor instability
Seborrheic dermatitis
Dyshydrosis
Genitourinary
Cryptorchidism
Anatomic renal abnormalities
Hypospadias
Anatomic vasoepididymal abnormalities
Interstitial nephritis
Metabolic
Early-onset diabetes mellitus
Chronic lymphocytic thyroiditis/hypothyroidism
Growth hormone deficiency

* Patent ductus arteriosus, pulmonary artery or valvular stenosis, and aortic stenosis are most common.

† "Late-onset disease" features often presenting in the 4th to 6th month of life.

Prognosis

The prognosis in congenital rubella is highly variable, depending on the severity of the infection and the structures involved. Prospective studies have shown an overall mortality of 6%; however, thrombocytopenic purpura, congenital heart disease, or encephalitis is often associated with severe general disease and a 20% to 35% mortality in the first year of life. Death may be associated with secondary bacterial sepsis, congestive heart failure (CHF), irreversible CNS damage, or simply failure to thrive. Fatal hemorrhage is quite unusual.

Therapy

At present, there is no specific therapy for this disease. Thrombocytopenic purpura, hemolytic anemia, hyperbilirubinemia, and cardiac failure from congenital heart disease should be treated supportively. Because immediate surgical treatment is indicated for glaucoma, it is important that this condition be distinguished from transient, self-limited corneal cloudiness.

Many older infants with congenital rubella have been labeled mentally retarded when in fact their delayed development was due to defective vision or hearing loss. The use of a hearing aid and enrollment in a program of auditory training should be started promptly after a diagnosis of deafness; no child is too young to participate in such a program. Bilateral cataracts, particularly when associated with hearing loss, should be removed as soon as surgically feasible.

It is imperative that children with either proved or suspected congenital rubella be examined frequently during the first years of life. Glaucoma, ocular lesions, hearing loss, congenital heart disease, hypertension, and orthopedic anomalies may not become clinically detectable for months or years after birth. Hearing loss and psychomotor retardation may be progressive during infancy. As the child grows older, decisions must be made about the repair of surgically correctable defects such as those of congenital heart disease, cryptorchidism, and hypospadias. Proper schooling must be arranged for children with delayed language development or defects in auditory processing. It is essential that both the physician and parents be aware of the dynamic and often subtle nature of the rubella syndrome.

Remaining Problems

The etiology of the rash in rubella and the bases for its characteristic distribution still remain to be determined. It is not yet known whether rubella arthritis represents an immune reaction, invasion of the joint space by virus, or both. The possible role of rubella virus in the pathogenesis of juvenile rheumatoid arthritis remains to be defined. The pathogenesis of both the encephalitis and the thrombocytopenia in rubella is not clear.

The role of antibody and the mechanisms of virus persistence in congenital rubella have not been adequately explained. The mechanism underlying the apparent failure of the virus to cross the placenta late in gestation is still obscure.

The durability of vaccine-induced immunity, the pathogenesis of reinfection, and the incidence of viremia during such reinfection all require further study. The roles of histocompatibility antigens and other genetic factors in determining susceptiblity to rubella and its complications remain to be defined.

An improved technique is needed for the rapid detection of rubella virus or rubella virus antigen in amniotic fluid or desquamated amniotic cells.

Bibliography

Books

HERRMANN KL: Rubella virus. In Lennette EH, Schmidt NL (eds): Diagnostic Procedures for: Viral, Rickettsial, and Chlamydial Infections, 5th ed. Washington DC, American Public Health Association, 1979. pp 725–766.

ALFORD CA JR: Rubella. In Remington JS, Klein JO (eds): Infectious Diseases of the Fetus and Newborn Infant. Philadelphia, WB Saunders, 1976. pp 71–106.

Journals

BORDLEY JE (ed): State of the art report: congenital rubella. Arch Otolaryngol, 98:217–277, 1973

Centers for Disease Control: Recommendation of the Immunization Practices Advisory Committee (ACIP), Rubella Prevention. Morbid Mortal Week Rep 30:37–47, 1981

GREGG NM: Congenital cataract following German measles in the mother. Trans Ophthalmol Soc Aust 3:35–46, 1941

HEGGIE AD: Pathogenesis of the rubella exanthem: Distribution of rubella virus in the skin during rubella with and without rash. J Infect Dis 137:74–77, 1978

HORSTMANN DM: Problems in measles and rubella. Disease-A-Month 24:1–52, 1978

JOHNSON RT: Progressive rubella encephalitis. N Engl J Med 292:1023–1024, 1975

MANN JM, PREBLUD SR, HOFFMAN RE, BRANDING–BENNETT AD, HINMAN AR, HERRMANN KL: Assessing risks of rubella infection during pregnancy: A standardized approach. JAMA 245:1647–1652, 1981

PREBLUD SR, STETLER HC, FRANK JA JR, GREAVES WL, HINMAN AR, HERRMAN KL: Fetal risk associated with rubella vaccine. JAMA 246:1413–1417, 1981

S. MICHAEL MARCY
SIDNEY KIBRICK

88 Other Exanthems

Acute exanthematous diseases may be divided into those characterized by erythematous, maculopapular or punctate lesions, and those in which a vesicular (papulovesicular, vesicopustular) stage predominates. Acute disorders characterized by a vesicular rash are relatively few. They can usually be identified without difficulty by their clinical course, features of the exanthem, histopathology of the lesions (Tzanck smear), or by diagnostic laboratory tests. Those characterized by a generalized vesicular eruption include varicella (Chap. 93, Varicella and Herpes Zoster); the now extinct smallpox (Chap. 92, Smallpox and Other Poxvirus Infections); eczema herpeticum (Chap. 91, Infections Caused by Herpes Simplex Virus); eczema vaccinatum and generalized vaccinia (Chap. 92, Smallpox and Other Poxvirus Infections); hand-foot-and-mouth disease (Chap. 149, Coxsackievirus and Echovirus Infections); and rickettsialpox (Chap. 97, Rickettsialpox). Localized vesicular lesions usually represent manifestations of primary or recurrent herpes simplex (Chap. 91, Infections Caused by Herpes Simplex Virus); herpes zoster (Chap. 93, Varicella and Herpes Zoster); or vaccinial infection (Chap. 92, Smallpox and Other Poxvirus Infections). Other conditions that must be considered include allergic rashes, staphylococcal or streptococcal infection (impetigo—Chap. 100, Staphylococcal Skin Infections; Chap. 101, Streptococcal Skin Infections and Glomerulonephritis); and insect bites (*e.g.,* chiggers—Chap. 115, Trombiculosis).

Clinical differentiation and etiologic identification of the acute maculopapular exanthems are more difficult, since a much wider variety of agents and conditions may produce such eruptions. Often, moreover, the disorders may lack features that are sufficiently characteristic to be helpful in diagnosis. In addition, the frequency with which such rashes occur may vary with the specific agent and with the age of the host. With some agents, the incidence of such exanthems is high; with others, the rash may represent a relatively uncommon portion of a wide spectrum of manifestations.

In the early 1900s an attempt was made to classify these disorders by delineating certain clinical entities from the group on the basis of history, incubation period, prodrome, clinical course, characteristics of the rash, and laboratory findings. On these bases, six specific entities were characterized and numerically designated as first through sixth diseases. In this classification, measles, scarlet fever, rubella, and Dukes' disease became first disease through fourth disease, respectively; erythema infectiosum became fifth disease; and roseola infantum sixth disease. The first three of these exanthems were subsequently defined more clearly after the isolation of their etiologic agents, and the development of specific laboratory tests. Fourth disease (Dukes' disease), a rubellalike illness, has now been discarded from this classification because it is no longer considered a single etiologic entity. The agents responsible for fifth and sixth diseases are still unknown, but the distinctive features of these disorders indicate that they probably are specific entities.

During the past few decades, progress in virologic techniques has made possible a further etiologic classification of these disorders. Numerous, previously unrecognized viruses have been uncovered, primarily by the use of tissue cultures, and it has become evident that some of these newer viruses are responsible for certain acute exanthems that had not been previously characterized.

Two recently recognized acute disorders, staphylococcal toxic shock syndrome and Kawasaki syndrome (mucocutaneous lymph node syndrome), both characterized by rash, are discussed in Chapters 50 and 165, respectively.

In this chapter, roseola infantum (sixth disease) and erythema infectiosum (fifth disease) are described, and the role of certain of the newer viruses as causes of acute disease with rash is considered. A more extensive summary of infectious agents responsible for acute exanthems is found in Table 8-1. Additional data about such disorders may be found in the chapters dealing with the specific agents and their clinical manifestations.

Roseola Infantum

Roseola infantum (exanthema subitum, sixth disease, Zahorsky's disease) is an acute, benign infectious disease of infants and young children. Three to five days of high fever, either sustained or spiking, is followed by a morbilliform rash that appears either as the temperature falls or shortly thereafter.

Etiology

The etiologic agent of this disease has not been identified, but it is most likely a virus. Bacteria-free serum obtained on the third day of fever from an infant with typical roseola induced the disease 9 days after injection into a susceptible infant. In a second study, blood obtained from affected infants on the first day of the rash induced typical roseola in 3 of 14 inoculated subjects aged 2 to 17 months, within 6 to 9 days. However, this agent has not been propagated in the laboratory.

Epidemiology

The mode of transmission and period of communicability are unknown. Cases occur throughout the year, with some increase in autumn and spring. An important distinguishing feature of this disease is its age incidence. Roseola is the most common febrile exanthem seen in infants under 2 years of age. It is very unusual in infants under 6 months, which indicates that maternal antibodies provide passive protection against this disease. Of all cases, 95% occur in children between 6 months and 3 years of age, pointing to an endemic disease of high incidence that engenders lasting immunity. In several small outbreaks, patients with high fever but without rash were observed. Because outbreaks occur infrequently, and presumably susceptible younger siblings of patients rarely acquire the disease, it has been assumed that the infectivity of roseola is less than that of the other common childhood exanthems. However, it is more likely that infectivity is high, and the inapparent cases and cases without rash (especially common among older children and adults) escape detection. About 30% of all children develop the characteristic disease.

Pathogenesis and Pathology

Neither the pathogenesis nor the pathology of roseola is known. Studies on these subjects have been hampered by the benign nature of the disorder and the lack of a specific diagnostic test.

Manifestations

A history of contact exposure is usually lacking in patients with roseola infantum. After an incubation period of 10 to 15 days, there is a sudden onset of fever, ranging from 39°C to 41°C (103°F–106°F). Malaise, mild coryza, and slight reddening of the pharynx and tympanic membrane may be present. Occasionally, some swelling of the eyelids is seen. Typically, the patient is not as severely ill as might be expected from the height of the fever.

The predominant picture is that of a high, generally sustained fever, only transiently responsive to aspirin, and occasionally associated with vomiting, restlessness, and irritability. Less often, the fever is intermittent. In some patients, especially children under 2 years, the sharp temperature rise may be accompanied by convulsions. On the second or third day, the occipital, cervical, and posterior auricular nodes may become palpable; this adenopathy subsides over the following week. After 3 to 5 days of fever, the temperature falls by crisis, sometimes to subnormal levels, and simultaneously the malaise and irritability subside.

The rash appears coincident with or after the defervescence. Resembling rubella in some patients, the rash consists of pale, rose-pink macules or maculopapules that are first evident on the trunk and neck. The exanthem may be limited to this area, or it may be more widely disseminated. However, the face and lower extremities are mostly spared. The rash blanches on pressure, rarely desquamates, and leaves no pigmentation. It may fade in hours or persist for 1 to 2 days. A nonspecific enanthem, consisting of pink specks and representing a lymphoid hyperplasia, may appear in the region of the uvula and soft palate during the first few days of fever, and it persists after onset of the rash.

The complications of roseola are limited to convulsive seizures that occasionally accompany the abrupt rise in temperature and, rarely, encephalopathy. A transient, benign bulging of the fontanel has also been observed. Some cases of encephalopathy may be secondary to anoxia incurred during the course of seizure activity. Neurologic residua such as hemiparesis, cerebral atrophy, and epilepsy have been described but are quite uncommon.

Diagnosis

Roseola must be distinguished from the many other diseases of infancy and early childhood that are characterized by maculopapular eruptions (Chap. 86, Measles; Chap. 87, Rubella; Chap. 149, Coxsackievirus and Echovirus Infections). The diagnosis is based primarily on the sudden onset of high fever and irritability without demonstrable cause; rather mild illness in view of the fever; and the emergence at defervescence of a pink, maculopapular rash on the trunk, spreading to neck, arms, and possibly other sites.

During the preeruptive, febrile period, a tentative diagnosis may be made only after exclusion of other causes of fever.

Prior to eruption of the rash, a marked leukopenia with a relative lymphocytosis develops, persisting until after the appearance of the rash. Uncommonly, a transitory thrombocytopenia manifested clinically by petechiae may occur. Total leukocyte counts may range from 3000 to 5000 cells, with as many as 90% lymphocytes. The cerebrospinal fluid (CSF) remains normal, even in patients with convulsions; however, encephalopathy may occasionally be accompanied by a mononuclear cell pleocytosis.

Prognosis

The prognosis in uncomplicated cases of roseola is excellent. If properly managed, the appearance of general seizures should not alter the outcome.

Therapy

Treatment is symptomatic. Antipyretic therapy may be useful in preventing or minimizing seizure activity and decreasing irritability. Anticonvulsive medication should be used in infants with a history of seizures and as required.

Prevention

The isolation of patients with this disease is not indicated because the agent is apparently widespread, known contact cases are uncommon, and the disease is generally benign.

Erythema Infectiosum

Erythema infectiosum (fifth disease) is an acute benign infectious disease characterized by a specific exanthem that primarily affects children. The rash begins as a marked erythema of the cheeks. This is followed by the appearance of maculopapular lesions on the extremities and trunk. These lesions assume a characteristic reticular pattern as they fade, and they tend to recur with irritation of the skin.

Etiology

The cause of this disease is not known, but it is generally assumed to be a virus.

Epidemiology

Erythema infectiosum is primarily a disease of childhood. Of all patients, 80% are under 15 years in age, and the cases are concentrated in the 2- to 12-year age group. It is mildly contagious, and it is commonly observed in outbreaks that generally coincide with the onset of winter or spring. Spread is believed to occur by droplet infection, and it is greatest among family members, schoolmates, and other close associates. During outbreaks, up to a third of exposed children under 12 years old may develop the typical rash. The duration of infectivity is uncertain. There is no evidence that infection of women during pregnancy is associated with an increase in congenital defects in their offspring.

Pathogenesis and Pathology

The pathogenesis of erythema infectiosum is not known. Because of the benign nature of this disease, study of the morbid anatomy has been limited to biopsies of skin lesions. These show only nonspecific findings, including dermal and epidermal edema, and lymphocytic perivascular cuffing of the smaller vessels.

Manifestations

The incubation period appears to range from 5 to 14 days. A prodrome is frequently lacking, but may consist of 1 to 2 days of low-grade fever and mild malaise. The most striking feature of the disease is the rash. It begins as a markedly erythematous, confluent maculopapular eruption over the cheeks, accompanied by some degree of circumoral pallor. The affected area may have a well-defined border. It is hot but not painful to the touch, and it has a slapped-cheek appearance. In addition, discrete lesions may be present on the forehead and chin and behind the ears. The eruption on the face generally fades within several days.

One to four days after onset of the facial rash, a pink maculopapular eruption that tends to coalesce appears on the extensor surface of the arms and thighs. Over the next few days, the symmetrically distributed rash spreads to the flexor and distal portions of the extremities, to the buttocks, and, to a lesser degree, to the trunk. During this progression, the earlier lesions on the arms and thighs begin to fade in their center, and the faded areas coalesce, giving rise to a characteristic irregular, reticular pattern. The rash is accentuated by exposure to sunlight and may be sharply demarcated where the arms are covered by sleeves. Occasionally, it is associated with a mild pruritus. Several days to weeks (average, 10 days) may be required for the rash to fade completely; generally, it recedes in the order in which it appeared. A characteristic feature of erythema infectiosum is the recurrent and evanescent nature of the rash. After it has faded, it may reappear for varying periods in response to skin irritants such as heat, cold, sunlight, exercise, and excitement.

Erythema infectiosum seems to be innocuous. Transient arthralgia and arthritis of the larger joints of the extremities have occasionally been observed preceding or accompanying the rash, chiefly in adults.

Diagnosis

There are no specific tests for this disease and no significant laboratory findings. Diagnosis is based on the characteristic clinical picture and is supported when outbreaks of such cases occur. During the initial or slapped-cheek phase of the disease, the differential diagnosis may include such conditions as erysipelas, lupus erythematosus, scarlet fever, enteroviral rashes, and drug eruptions. During the disseminated phase, the rash may resemble that of mild measles, scarlet fever, rubella, and a wide variety of other disorders characterized by a maculopapular eruption.

Prognosis

The prognosis is excellent. Rarely, serious complications such as encephalitis, pneumonitis, and hemolytic anemia have been reported, but have not been confirmed.

Therapy

No treatment is indicated.

Prevention

Isolation is not necessary for children with this disease. In the absence of findings other than the characteristic rash, such children need not be excluded from school.

Other Viral Agents

Infection with more than 35 other viruses has been implicated in erythematous, maculopapular, papulovesicular rashes. Because etiologic diagnosis depends primarily on laboratory procedures that are not generally available, illnesses caused by these agents are either undiagnosed or incorrectly attributed to some other cause.

Enteroviruses

Infection with at least 30 coxsackieviruses and echoviruses has been associated with febrile exanthematous disease occurring either alone or in conjunction with aseptic meningitis (Chap. 118, Viral Meningitis and Chap. 149, Coxsackievirus and Echovirus Infections). These enteroviral rashes have most commonly been maculopapular, but erythematous, vesicular, scarlatiniform, petechial, and various mixed eruptions have also been observed. Less commonly, urticarial hemangioma-like lesions with a pale halo, and telangiectasia-like lesions have also been described. In general, enteroviral rashes are variable in extent and distribution, are nonpruritic, do not desquamate, and heal without discoloration. These exanthems are most common in infants and young children. Although adenopathy may be present, it is not generally a prominent feature. Occasionally, the illness is associated with a papular or vesicular enanthem or with small ulcerative or typical herpanginal lesions in the oropharynx. With some of these exanthems, meningeal signs are also prominent. When the infection is associated with a biphasic or triphasic febrile course, the rash may recur with each episode.

Several general patterns of exanthems have been observed with the enteroviruses, in addition to features that may be more specific for certain agents. With some of these viruses, the rash is predominantly maculopapular; has a central distribution (*i.e.,* is most concentrated on the head and trunk); and is associated with fever. This pattern has been noted especially with echovirus 9 and coxsackievirus A9, but has also occurred with other enteroviruses. Thus, in exanthematous diseases caused by echovirus 9, the rash almost always involves the face and chest, but may extend to the extremities, where it tends to be more prominent on the extensor surfaces. On the extremities and trunk it clears rapidly, but on the face, especially the cheeks, forehead, and chin, it often becomes semiconfluent with a violaceous tint and tends to persist (for an average of 5 days). Occasionally, petechiae are present and the rash may resemble that of meningococcemia. In some patients, an enanthem consisting of small yellowish or grayish white lesions may be seen in the oropharynx. A central maculopapular rash with occasional petechiae may occur during infection with coxackievirus A9, B3, and Echovirus 11. By contrast, a peripheral maculopapular rash with petechiae is seen in certain arbovirus and rickettsial infections and also in the atypical measles that sometimes occurs on reinfection with wild virus in previously immunized persons.

Another enteroviral rash is also maculopapular and predominantly central in distribution, but tends to appear as the fever subsides. This is especially characteristic of echovirus 16 disease (Boston exanthem), but is not pathognomonic, since it also occurs in roseola, occasionally in coxsackievirus A4 and B5 infections, and some adenovirus infections.

In certain patients with maculopapular eruptions caused by enteroviruses, some of the lesions may progress to form clear, supeficial vesicles. These subsequently regress without forming pustules or crusting. Infections characterized by such lesions are either primarily central, as is occasionally seen in coxsackievirus A9 infection, or predominantly on the extremities, as is seen in hand-foot-and-mouth disease. This latter syndrome is generally associated with coxsackievirus A16, but may also result from infection with coxsackievirus A10 and A5 and various other enteroviruses. There is an oral vesicular enanthem and a symmetrically distributed maculopapular eruption that usually progresses to vesicles; it affects primarily the hands and feet, but may also involve other parts of the body, namely, the trunk, limbs, face, and, mostly in infants and young children, the buttocks. Lesions on the body may persist as maculopapules.

In temperate zones, enteroviral infections are most prevalent in the summer and fall. Epidemiologic support for a diagnosis of enteroviral exanthematous disease is provided by the occurrence of illness in the season of highest prevalence for these agents, other manifestations of enteroviral infection in close associates of the patient, and documentation of the presence of these viruses in the community.

Adenoviruses

At least 4 of the 33 recognized types of human adenoviruses (Chap. 23, Nonbacterial Pharyngitis), namely types 1, 2, 3, 7, and 7a, have been recovered on one or more occasions from patients (mostly children) with rashes. Cutaneous manifestations have included maculopapular and scarlatiniform eruptions. In several patients, adenovirus infection has been associated with an illness resembling roseola. Erythema multiforme, and in rare instances, a vesicular rash or angiitis with edema and cutaneous necrosis, has also been observed. Generally, but not always, other signs of adenoviral infection have been present, such as conjunctivitis, rhinitis, pharyngotonsillitis, lymphadenopathy, or pneumonia. Rashes have only been encountered in a relatively small proportion of patients during outbreaks of adenovirus disease (2% in one study).

Because of the ubiquity of the adenoviruses, the relationship of these agents to exanthems is still under question. Thus, concomitant adenovirus infections have been found in some infants with roseola and in rubellalike illness, subsequently confirmed as rubella, among military recruits. In addition, adenoviruses have been recovered from patients receiving medications known to produce rashes. On the other hand, the same types of virus (types 1, 2, 3, 7, and 7a) have been recovered by different investigators on several occasions in association with appropriate antibody responses from patients with cutaneous manifestations. Also, adenoviruses may be responsible for some sporadic cases of exanthematous illness that occur in children during the winter.

Reoviruses

A mild to moderate maculopapular rash and in one instance, a vesicular rash, was noted in a small number of children infected with reovirus type 1 or 2. The rash persisted 3 to 9 days and was most prominent on the trunk, neck, and face.

Respiratory Syncytial Virus

Rashes ranging from mild, nonspecific erythemas to heavy maculopapular eruptions have been described in a few infants and young children with respiratory syncytial infection. A mother and her newborn infant displayed a mixed macular and petechial rash. The rashes generally involved trunk, arms, and face and persisted from one to several days.

Cytomegalovirus, Epstein–Barr Virus

Maculopapular, and occasionally papulovesicular, rashes have been inconstant findings (as high as 30% in one report) in acquired cytomegalovirus (CMV) infections (Chap. 75, Cytomegalovirus Infections). These rashes have been observed both in CMV mononucleosis syndrome and in the "postperfusion" syndrome. Infection with Epstein–Barr (EB) virus (Chap. 137, Infectious Mononucleosis), another of the herpesvirus group, may also be accompanied by a maculopapular rash. Such a rash, affecting primarily the trunk and proximal extremities, occurs in about 10% of patients with infectious mononucleosis. Ampicillin or amoxicillin when given to patients with infectious mononucleosis induces or exacerbates a maculopapular eruption. This effect has also been observed frequently in patients with acquired CMV infections. It may not always be possible to differentiate the drug rash from that due to the infection.

Hepatitis A Virus, Hepatitis B Virus

Disease caused by hepatitis B virus (Chap. 71, Hepatitis B) is associated with a transitory, erythematous, maculopapular or urticarial rash in about 10% of cases. Usually it precedes the jaundice. Similar rashes occur even less commonly in hepatitis A disease (Chap. 70, Hepatitis A).

New Acute Syndromes With Rash

Kawasaki Syndrome (Mucocutaneous Lymph Node Syndrome)

An apparently self-limited disease syndrome of infants and young children, Kawasaki syndrome was first described in Japan in 1967. Patients with this disorder have now been recognized in many countries including the United States. In some respects this disease resembles both scarlet fever and the Stevens–Johnson syndrome, but it is sufficiently different that it can be distinguished from these entitites. Although the individual features of Kawasaki syndrome are not diagnostic, taken together they appear to define yet another entity separable from the childhood maculopapular eruptions. A full discussion is given in Chapter 165, Kawasaki Syndrome.

Toxic Shock Syndrome

Toxic shock syndrome (TSS; see also Chap. 50, Infections of the Female Genital Tract) is characterized by a sudden onset with high fever, vomiting, watery diarrhea, and occasionally sore throat, myalgias, headache, and confusion. A nonpurulent conjunctivitis may be present. The disease progresses within 48 hours to hypotension, subcutaneous edema, and in severe cases shock and death. During the acute phase of the illness an erythematous, macular rash appears; this desquamates in 1 to 2 weeks, particularly on the palms and soles.

Laboratory findings may include oliguria; mild pyuria and hematuria; and elevated urea, creatinine, bilirubin and creatine phosphokinase in the blood. Initially, platelet counts are low, and differential blood counts show a marked left shift.

TSS involves, in order of decreasing frequency, gastrointestinal, muscular, mucous membrane, renal, hematologic, hepatic, central nervous system (CNS) and cardiopulmonary systems. Recurrences of this disorder have been noted.

Most cases of this disease have occurred among menstruating women; continuous use of tampons may be an important risk factor. *Staphylococcus aureus* was implicated because it was frequently isolated from the vaginas of patients with TSS. There is evidence that specifically toxinogenic strains of *S. aureus* are involved. The relationship between these organisms and tampons remains to be clarified. TSS has also been reported in men and children who have focal staphylococcal infections, and it appears as a consequence of postoperative staphylococcal sepsis.

Management of patients suspected of having this syndrome includes a pelvic examination with cervical and vaginal cultures and a search for focal staphylococcal infections in nonmenstruating patients. Aggressive fluid replacement therapy and the use of other supportive measures as needed, including ventilatory assistance and vasopressors, is very important. Treatment with β-lactamase-resistant antistaphylococcal antimicrobics should also be initiated. Although the incidence is low, a recurrence rate of up to 30% has been reported, and women who have had TSS should be encouraged to forgo the use of tampons, at least temporarily.

Miscellaneous

Drug rashes may be manifested by a spectrum of eruptions—urticarial, erythematous, maculopapular, vesicular, bullous, petechial, or mixed. Such rashes may at times closely resemble those due to various infectious diseases. In such cases, there is no prodrome or characteristic adenopathy, and a history of drug ingestion or exposure can generally be obtained.

Remaining Problems

The etiologic agents of roseola infantum and erythema infectiosum have not yet been propagated in the laboratory, and there are no specific diagnostic tests for these disorders. As a result, little is known about the epidemiology, pathogenesis, pathology, range of clinical manifestations, and incidence of inapparent infections in these diseases.

It is not known whether the convulsions that sometimes accompany roseola are the result of the fever or an encephalitis induced by the etiologic agent.

Further studies are needed to determine the role of the newer viral agents as causes of acute exanthems; for example, the clinical spectrums induced by these agents, the age groups affected, seasonal prevalence, pathogenesis, and factors predisposing to rash. In many exanthematous diseases, the causes are still obscure. Laboratory studies of acute exanthems might help to uncover new agents and delineate additional characteristic syndromes associated with specific viruses.

The etiology, pathogenesis, and optimal treatment for Kawasaki syndrome are not clear.

The pathogenesis of TSS is not fully understood. If toxinogenic staphylococci are responsible, what is the reservoir, what is the vector, and what is their relationship to tampons? Why is the incidence of this disease so low?

Bibliography

GENERAL

Book

LERNER AM: Exanthems caused by coxsackievirus, echovirus and reovirus infections. In Demis DJ, Dobson RL, McGuire J (eds): Clinical Dermatology, vol 3, Unit 14-19. Harper & Row, 1982. 23 pp.

Journal

WENNER HA: Virus diseases associated with cutaneous eruptions. Prog Med Virol 16:269–336, 1973

ROSEOLA INFANTUM

Journals

BERENBERG W, WRIGHT S, JANEWAY CA: Roseola infantum (exanthem subitum). N Engl J Med 241:253–259, 1949

BURNSTINE RC, PAINE RS: Residual encephalopathy following roseola infantum. Am J Dis Child 98: 144–152, 1959

CLEMENS H: Exanthem subitum (roseola infantum): report of eighty cases. J Pediatr 26:66–77, 1945

ERYTHEMA INFECTIOSUM

Journals

AGER EA, CHIN TDY, POLAND JD: Epidemic erythema infectiosum. N Engl J Med 275:1326–1331, 1966

LAUER BA, MACCORMACK JN, WILFERT C: Erythema infectiosum. An elementary school outbreak. Am J Dis Child 130:252–254, 1976

WADLINGTON WB: Erythema infectiosum. JAMA 192:144–146, 1965

MUCOCUTANEOUS LYMPHNODE SYNDROME

Journals

MELISH ME, HICKS RM, LARSON EJ: Mucocutaneous lymph node syndrome in the United States. Am J Dis Child 130:599–607, 1976

MORENS DM, NAHMIAS AJ: Kawasaki disease: A new pediatric enigma. Hosp Pract 13:109–120, 1978

YANAGIHARA R, TODD JK: Acute febrile mucocutaneous lymph node syndrome. Am J Dis Child 134:603–614, 1980

TOXIC-SHOCK SYNDROME

Journals

CHESNEY PJ, DAVIS JP, PURDY WK, WAND PJ, CHESNEY RW: Clinical manifestations of toxic shock syndrome. JAMA 246:741–748, 1981

GLASGOW LA: Staphylococcal infection in the toxic-shock syndrome. N Engl J Med 303:1473–1475, 1980

SHANDS AN, SCHMID GP, DAN BB, BLUM D, GUIDOTTI RJ, HARGRETT NT, ANDERSON RL, HILL DL, BROOME CV, BAND JD, FRASER DW: Toxic-shock syndrome in menstruating women: Association with tampon use and *Staphylococcus aureus* and clinical features in 52 cases. N Engl J Med 303:1436–1442, 1980

SCOTT B. HALSTEAD

89 Dengue

Dengue fever is a benign, acute febrile syndrome caused by several arthropod-borne viruses; it is generally confined to tropical areas and characterized by biphasic fever, myalgia or arthralgia, exanthem, leukopenia, and lymphadenopathy. The term "dengue" is a Spanish homonym for the African *"ki denga pepo"* introduced into the English literature during an 1827–1828 Caribbean outbreak probably caused by chikungunya virus. Dengue viruses also cause an acute vascular permeability syndrome accompanied by abnormalities of hemostasis (dengue hemorrhagic fever) and, frequently, hypotension (dengue shock syndrome). In the modern era, dengue hemorrhagic fever/dengue shock syndrome (DHF/DSS) has most often involved Asian children. DHF/DSS is thought to have an immunologic basis.

Etiology

Dengue viruses are enveloped RNA viruses classified in the flavivirus group of the family Togaviridae. At least four clearly defined types exist; antigenic and biologic variants of type 3 are found in the American and Asian tropics. Cross comparisons by the plaque reduction neutralization test show the dengue viruses to be an antigenic subgroup within the flaviviruses. All flaviviruses share group antigens best demonstrated by the hemagglutination–inhibition test. Each of the dengue viruses causes closely related clinical illnesses. After a short period of cross-protection, a person is fully susceptible to infection with a different type. This heterotypic infection is accompanied by a secondary type antibody response. Homotypic immunity is lifelong. Nondengue virus causes of the dengue fever syndrome are discussed under Diagnosis.

Epidemiology

Dengue viruses are widely distributed in tropical countries girdling the globe. In 1980, dengue virus was transmitted within the continental United States for the first time in nearly 40 years. This event, plus recent epidemic activity in South China, calls attention to the fact that contemporary demographic and ecologic conditions favor episodic extension of dengue viruses into subtropical areas. Year-round transmission occurs between 25° north and south.

Aedes aegypti, a daytime biting mosquito, is the principal vector in dengue fever. In most tropical areas, *A. aegypti* is highly domesticated, breeding in water stored for drinking or bathing or in any container that collects fresh water. The eggs resist desiccation and hatch following immersion. In some outbreaks, *Aedes albopictus, Aedes polynesiensis,* and *Aedes scutellaris* have been implicated as vectors. Following ingestion of viremic blood, dengue viruses replicate in the gut and eventually infect the salivary glands. This process normally requires 8 to 11 days and constitutes the extrinsic incubation period. *Aedes aegypti* preferentially feeds on human beings. Mosquitoes are infectious for a lifetime. Because female mosquitoes take repeated blood meals, long-lived females have great potency as vectors. Dengue virus may also be transmitted mechanically due to interrupted feeding.

When *A. aegypti* are abundant, the epidemiology of dengue resembles that of respiratory viruses. Transmission is increased in densely populated areas. The virus moves primarily with viremic hosts, because *A. aegypti* has a limited flight range.

The existence of a jungle dengue cycle has been documented in Malaysia, involving canopy-feeding monkeys and *Aedes niveus,* a species which feeds both on monkeys and humans. The full geographic extent of the zoonotic reservoir is unknown. At present, *A. aegypti* and susceptible humans are so numerous that the impact of the jungle cycle is hardly discernible. If urban dengue were eliminated, the jungle reservoir would assume greater importance.

Epidemic DHF/DSS is presently confined to 10 Asian countries (Philippines, Vietnam, Laos, Cambodia, China, Thailand, Burma, Malaysia, Singapore, and Indonesia). Sporadic cases have been reported in Sri Lanka. An isolated outbreak occurred in India. Characteristically, all four types of dengue virus circulate in urban areas of DHF-endemic countries, and there are also dense populations of *A. aegypti.* Sequential infections are common. Clinical and prospective epidemiologic studies have shown that DHF/DSS occurs during second dengue infections in children who are 1 year of age or older and in infants less than 1 year born to dengue-immune mothers. Although third and fourth sequential infections are theoretically possible, age-specific hospitalization data suggest that persons are at risk of DHF/DSS only during their second infection. Repeated attacks of DHF/DSS in the same person have not been reported.

Despite the association in the Asian tropics between DHF/DSS and those with preinfection antibody, no such relationship has been observed in the American tropics. Dengue 3 was established in the Caribbean basin in 1963; after a lapse of six years, dengue 2 became endemic, and since 1977, dengue 1 has been distributed widely. These sequential dengue outbreaks have been associated with only sporadic DHF/DSS cases.

Pathogenesis and Pathology

Although the pathogenesis of human dengue infection is not fully known, observations from experimentally infected rhesus monkeys are instructive. Following intracutaneous inoculation, virus replicates in the skin at the site of inoculation. Viral antigen has been visualized in histiocytes. Within 12 to 24 hours, virus is found in regional lymph nodes where replication is confined to mononuclear cells with abundant cytoplasm. Successively, virus is found in lymph nodes, bone marrow and the spleen, liver, thymus, and Peyer's patches. During this stage, free virus is found in the blood. In humans, viremia, fever, and constitutional symptoms occur simultaneously. At the end of the viremic period, virus-infected monocytes appear in the blood for 1 to 2 days. At about this time, virus is recovered from the skin. Each tissue site that supports viral replication remains infected, producing a cumulative effect resulting in maximal intracellular infection 1 to 2 days after viremia ends. Infected cells are eliminated abruptly by an immunologic mechanism not yet identified. From the data available, the pathogenesis of dengue in humans and monkeys is similar; that is, in primates, virus replicates in cells of mononuclear phagocyte lineage (reticuloendothelial system).

The localization of dengue infection to mononuclear phagocytes is of pathogenetic interest because studies show that flavivirus antisera mediate infection of these cells by dengue viruses. Rhesus monkeys circulating heterotypic dengue antibody acquired actively or passively develop enhanced infections compared with controls when they are inoculated with dengue type 2 virus. A current concept of the pathogenesis of DHF/DSS is that nonneutralizing infection-enhancing heterotypic dengue antibodies amplify infection in mononuclear phagocytes. These cells are known to produce factors that activate the complement and blood-clotting systems and mediate vascular permeability. The hypothesis that the severity of dengue infection is related to the number of infected cells corresponds with the observed clinical continuum between the dengue fever syndrome and DHF/DSS.

On autopsy, the usual observation in DHF/DSS is the absence of sufficiently severe gross or microscopic lesions to explain death. This is consistent with case reports of terminal hyperkalemia. Minimal to moderate hemorrhages are typical in the upper gastrointestinal tract, and petechial hemorrhages are frequently seen in the ventricular septum of the heart, on the pericardium, and on the subserosal surfaces of major viscera. Focal hemorrhages are seen in the lungs, liver, adrenals, and subarachnoid spaces. The liver is usually enlarged, often with fatty changes. Effusions are present in serous cavities in about three-fourths of patients. Retroperitoneal tissues are markedly edematous. Microscopically, there is perivascular edema in soft tissues and widespread diapedesis of red blood cells. Bone marrow megakaryocytes show maturation arrest and increased numbers of them are seen in lung capillaries, renal glomeruli, and liver and spleen sinusoids. In the liver, there is hyperplasia and hyalin necrosis of Kupffer's cells, the appearance in sinusoids of nonnucleated cells with vacuolated acidophilic cytoplasm resembling Councilman bodies, areas of fatty metamorphosis, and focal midzonal necrosis. In thymus, lymph nodes, and spleen, there is marked lymphocytolysis and lymphophagocytosis. Dengue antigen has been demonstrated in Kupffer's cells, and in splenic, thymic, and pulmonary macrophages. Kidney biopsies reveal mild, proliferative glomerulonephritis during convalescence. Presumably this is due to deposition of dengue antigen, antibody and complement.

Denguelike particles have been visualized in glomerular macrophages. Biopsies of skin rash show swelling and minimal necrosis of endothelial cells and subcutaneous deposits of fibrinogen. Dengue antigen is found in extravascular mononuclear cells.

Manifestations

Dengue Fever

Biphasic fever and rash are the most characteristic features of the dengue fever syndrome. Manifestations vary with age and from patient to patient. In infants and young children, the disease may be undifferentiated or characterized by a 1- to 5-day fever, pharyngeal inflammation, rhinitis, and mild cough.

Although a distinctive mean incubation period, duration of illness, and spectrum of clinical findings may characterize infection with each dengue type, this is not fully established. In outbreaks of dengue, a majority of infected adults have most of the findings summarized below.

After an incubation period of 2 to 7 days, there is an abrupt onset of fever that rapidly rises to 39.5°C to 41.4°C (103°F–106°F), usually accompanied by frontal or retro-orbital headache. Occasionally, back pain precedes the fever. A transient, macular, generalized rash that blanches under pressure may be seen during the first 24 to 48 hours of fever. The pulse rate may be slow in proportion to the degree in fever. Myalgia or bone pain occurs soon after onset and increases in severity. During the second to the sixth day of fever, nausea and vomiting are apt to occur, and during this phase generalized lymphadenopathy, cutaneous hyperesthesia, taste aberrations, and pronounced anorexia may develop.

Coincident with, or one or two days after, defervescence, a generalized, morbilliform, maculopapular rash appears, which spares the palms and soles. It disappears in 1 to 5 days. In some cases there is edema of the palms and soles. Desquamation may occur. About the time of appearance of this second rash, the body temperature may become slightly elevated and establish the biphasic temperature curve.

Epistaxis, petechiae, and purpuric lesions, though uncommon, may occur at any stage of the disease. Swallowed blood from epistaxis may be passed by rectum or vomited and may be interpreted as bleeding of gastrointestinal origin. Gastrointestinal bleeding, menorrhagia, and bleeding from other organs have been observed in adults in some outbreaks of dengue fever, apparently without concurrent thrombocytopenia or hypovolemia. Mechanisms of hemostatic abnormalities in these cases are unknown.

Dengue Hemorrhagic Fever/Dengue Shock Syndrome

The incubation period of DHF is unknown, but is presumed to be that of dengue fever. In children, the progression of the illness is characteristic. A relatively mild first phase with abrupt onset of fever, malaise, vomiting, headache, anorexia, and cough is followed after 2 to 5 days by rapid deterioration and physical collapse. The median day of admission to hospital after onset of fever is day 4. In this second phase, the patient usually manifests cold, clammy extremities, warm trunk, flushed face, diaphoresis, restlessness, irritability, and possibly midepigastric pain. Frequently, there are scattered petechiae on the forehead and extremities, spontaneous ecchymoses may appear, and easy bruisability and bleeding at sites of venipuncture are common. The tourniquet test is positive. There may be circumoral and peripheral cyanosis. Respirations are rapid and often labored. The pulse is weak, rapid, and thready, and the heart sounds are faint. The pulse pressure is frequently narrow ($\leq$ 20 mm Hg); the systolic and diastolic pressures may be low or unobtainable. The liver may become palpable 2 to 3 fingerbreadths below the coastal margin and is usually firm and nontender.

Approximately 10% of children manifest ecchymoses or gastrointestinal bleeding. In adults, it appears that the severity of hemorrhagic phenomena is disproportionate to the degree of hypotension. After a 24- or 36-hour period of crisis, convalescence is fairly rapid. The temperature may return to normal before or during the stage of shock.

By definition, a patient with DHF/DSS must exhibit thrombocytopenia (100,000/mm^3 or less) and hemoconcentration (hematocrit $\geq$ 120% of the recovery value). The number and degree of laboratory abnormalities increase with severity of disease. Elevations in transaminases, metabolic acidosis, hypovolemia and hypoproteinemia are common. Roentgenograms of the chest may reveal bronchopneumonia and pleural effusion. Hematologic abnormalities include hypofibrinogenemia, increased fibrin split products, prolonged bleeding and silicone clotting times, moderate prolongation of prothrombin time with deficiencies in factors 5, 7, 9, and 10. Blood levels of Cl_q, C3, C4, C5–9, and C3 proactivator are depressed and C3 catabolic rates are elevated. In children, the degree of complement depletion and level of circulating fibrin split products relate directly to the severity of shock. In adults, disseminated intravascular coagulation may be relatively severe. Hematuria and proteinuria are rarely seen. Acute central nervous system (CNS) findings are of uncertain etiology but may be due to cerebral edema. Occasionally, intracranial bleeding may produce severe and more permanent CNS damage.

Diagnosis

The clinical diagnosis of the dengue fever syndrome derives from a knowledge of the geographic distribution and ecology of viral causes of this syndrome and possible exposure of the patient at an appropriate interval prior to onset of disease.

The differential diagnosis of fever and myalgia includes many viral and bacterial diseases and the early stages of malaria (Chap. 145, Malaria), scrub typhus (Chap. 99, Scrub Typhus), hepatitis (Chaps. 70–72, Hepatitis A; Hepatitis B; Non-A, Non-B Hepatitis) and leptospirosis (Chap. 76, Leptospirosis). Abortive forms of the latter diseases may never evolve beyond a denguelike stage. Three common arbovirus exanthems are denguelike: chikungunya and O'nyong nyong fevers (alphaviruses) and West Nile fever (flavivirus). Three others are denguelike but without rash: Colorado tick fever (Chap. 123, Colorado Tick Fever), sandfly fever, and the mild form of Rift Valley fever. Each of these are acute febrile diseases with an incubation period of a few days. The geographic distribution of these diseases is shown in Table 89-1. Because of the variation in clinical findings and the multiplicity of possible causative agents, the descriptive term denguelike disease should be used until a specific etiologic diagnosis is provided by the laboratory.

In areas endemic for dengue viruses, DHF/DSS should be suspected in persons exhibiting hemoconcentration with thrombocytopenia. Shock, hemorrhagic manifestations including positive tourniquet test, and hepatic enlargement are common accompanying findings. Since many rickettsial diseases, meningococcemia, and other severe illnesses caused by a variety of agents may produce a similar clinical picture, the diagnosis should be made only when epidemiologic or serologic evidence is consistent with a dengue etiology. Hemorrhagic manifestations have been described in other diseases of viral origin (Chap. 90, Epidemic Hemorrhagic Fevers); these include the arenavirus hemorrhagic fevers of Argentina, Bolivia, and West Africa, Ebola and Marburg disease, the tick-borne hemorrhagic fevers of India and the Soviet Union, and hemorrhagic fever with renal syndrome which occurs across northern Eurasia from Scandinavia to Korea.

Etiologic diagnosis can be made by serologic study of properly collected acute and convalescent serum samples or by isolation of the virus. Blood should be obtained during the febrile period, preferably before the fourth day after onset of illness. A second sample should be taken two weeks or more after onset. The acute phase serum or plasma may be frozen, optimally at −65°C or colder, to preserve the specimen for later virus isolation. Serologic diagnosis depends on a fourfold or greater increase in antibody titer by the hemagglutination-inhibition (HI), complement fixation, or neutralization test. It may not be possible to distinguish the infecting virus by serologic methods alone, particularly when there has been prior infection with another member of the dengue subgroup. Sequential infections with dengue and nondengue flavivirus, or *vice versa,* result in the production of type-specific IgM directed to the second infecting virus. At the same time a second antibody is produced, a group-specific IgG. This masks type-specific IgM in whole serum unless special tests are undertaken. Sequential infections with two dengue infections do not produce a type-specific IgM.

Table 89-1. *Denguelike Arbovirus Infections*

Mode of Transmission	Virus and Disease	Virus Group	Geographic Location
With Rash*			
Mosquito-borne	Chikungunya	Alphavirus	Africa, India, Southeast Asia
Mosquito-borne	O'nyong nyong	Alphavirus	East Africa
Mosquito-borne	West Nile fever	Flavivirus	Middle East, Africa, South Asia
Without Rash			
Tick-borne	Colorado tick fever	Orbivirus	Rocky Mountain states to California
Sandfly-borne	Sandfly fever	Bunyavirus	Southern Europe and USSR, Middle East, South Asia
Mosquito-borne	Rift Valley fever	Bunyavirus	Africa

*Sporadic cause of denguelike illness with rash: flaviviruses: Wesselsbron (Africa, SE Asia); Zika (Africa, SE Asia). alphavirus: Sindbis (Africa, Asia). bunyaviruses: Tataguine (Central Africa); Bunyamwera (Africa); Ilesha (Central Africa)

Differentiation of a primary from a secondary type of antibody response may have epidemiologic or pathogenetic significance. With standardized test procedures, a primary response is one in which (1) the HI antibody titer is generally less than 1:20 in a serum obtained on or before the fourth day after onset of illness; or (2) there is antibody present in the acute phase specimen with a fourfold or greater increase in antibody, but the titer in the convalescent serum does not exceed 1:1280. A secondary type of response is one in which (1) HI antibody is detected in a specimen of serum collected before the fifth day after onset, with a fourfold or greater antibody rise; (2) no HI antibody is detected in a serum collected prior to the fifth day after onset, with an antibody rise to a titer of at least 1:2560; or (3) there are high fixed HI antibodies at a titer of 1:1280 or greater in paired sera.

Acute phase serum, mosquito suspensions, or other materials thought to contain dengue virus may be inoculated into suckling mice, several tissue cultures, or mosquitoes (intrathoracic injection) of the *Toxorhynchites* or *Stegomyia* genera. The presence of virus in mosquitoes may be detected by fluorescent antibody, complement-fixation, or inoculation of mosquito suspensions in tissue cultures.

Prognosis

Prolonged asthenia, mental depression, bradycardia, and ventricular extrasystoles are relatively common after dengue virus-caused dengue fever. Chikungunya infections may result in residual polyarthralgia and arthritis. There is evidence that the prognosis in dengue is adversely affected in persons who have experienced prior dengue infection or passively acquired dengue antibody (see Pathogenesis). The relation of other flavivirus infections to DHF/DSS is not known.

Death occurs in 5% to 40% of children with shock. Fatality rates in adults are not known. Survival is directly related to early hospitalization and the intensity of physiologic management. Infrequently there is residual brain damage either from prolonged shock or from intracranial hemorrhage.

Therapy

Dengue Fever

Treatment of patients with dengue fever is supportive. Bed rest is advised during the febrile period. It may be advisable to avoid salicylates because they may cause bleeding or acidosis. Antipyretics or cold sponging should be used to keep the body temperature below 40°C (104°F). Analgesics or mild sedation may be required to control pain. Fluid and electrolyte replacement therapy is required when there are deficits due to sweating, fasting, thirsting, vomiting, or diarrhea.

DHF/DSS

Management of DHF/DSS requires immediate assessment of hemoconcentration and electrolyte imbalance. Close monitoring is essential for at least 48 hours, because shock may occur or recur precipitously. Patients who have labored breathing or are cyanotic should be given oxygen. Rapid intravenous replacement of fluids and electrolytes is frequently sufficient to sustain patients until spontaneous recovery occurs. When elevation of the hematocrit persists after vigorous fluid replacement, plasma or colloid preparations are indicated. Care must be taken to avoid overhydration, which may contribute to cardiac failure. Transfusion of fresh blood may be required, but should not be given during hemoconcentration.

Paraldehyde or chloral hydrate may be required for persons who are markedly agitated. Heparin may be used for those with intractable bleeding, but only if there is objective evidence of disseminated intravascular coagulation. Neither glucosteroids nor the administration of immune serum have any effect on the duration of disease or prognosis.

No vaccines for dengue viruses or other viral causes of denguelike syndromes are commercially available. Control of *A. aegypti* or avoiding mosquito bites are the only available means of protection. Individual measures include destruction of sites suitable for the breeding of *A. aegypti.* Stored water should be protected with a tight-fitting lid or a thin layer of oil to prevent egg laying or hatching. Abate (0, 0′-[thiodi-*p*-phenylene] 0, 0, 0′ 0′-tetramethyl phosphorothioate), available as a 1% sand-granule formulation and effective at a concentration of 1 part per million, may be added safely to drinking water. Ultra-low volume spray equipment mounted on truck or airplane effectively dispenses malathion for rapid intervention by killing adult mosquitoes during an epidemic.

Remaining Problems

Control or eradication of *A. aegypti* on a global scale is a prodigious challenge. Current efforts are centered on the development of a tetravalent dengue vaccine; this may prove to be a difficult and long process. A number of important clinical and epidemiologic research problems remain to be solved: (1) the pathogenesis and pathophysiology of dengue infections in adults which are complicated by severe hemorrhage are not well known and require thorough study; (2) the role that infection-enhancing antibodies play in the pathogenesis of DHF/DSS needs to be evaluated by prospective studies; (3) the mechanisms of vascular permeability and bleeding in DHF/DSS are still unknown, and the contribution of mononuclear phagocytes to the pathogenesis of these phenomena deserves particular attention; and (4) the association of DHF/DSS in persons with preinfection dengue antibody in some but not all dengue endemic areas is a major enigma which can be solved only through comprehensive, comparative epidemiologic studies.

Bibliography

Books

HALSTEAD SB: Immunological Parameters of Togavirus Disease Syndromes. In Schlesinger RW (ed): The Togaviruses. Biology, Structure, Replication. New York, Academic Press. 1980. pp 107–173.

SCHLESINGER RW: Dengue Viruses. Virology Monographs, Vol. 16. New York, Springer–Verlag, 1977. 132 pp.

Journals

BOKISCH VA, TOP RH, RUSSELL PK, DIXON FJ, MULLER-EBERHARD HJ: The potential pathogenic role of complement in dengue hemorrhagic shock syndrome. N Engl J Med 289:996–1000, 1973

EHRENKRANZ NJ, VENTURA AK, CUADRADO RR, POND WL, PORTER JE: Pandemic dengue in Caribbean countries and the southern United States: Past, present and potential problems. N Engl J Med 285:1460–1469, 1971

HALSTEAD SB: Dengue haemorrhagic fever: A public health problem and a field for research. Bull WHO 58:1–21, 1980

HALSTEAD SB: The pathogenesis of dengue: Molecular epidemiology in infectious disease. Am J Epidemiol 114:632–648, 1981

HALSTEAD SB, O'ROURKE EJ: Dengue viruses and mononuclear phagocytes. I. Infection enhancement by non-neutralizing antibody. J Exp Med 146:201–217, 1977

SABIN AB: Research on dengue during World War II. Am J Trop Med Hyg 1:30–50, 1952

KARL M. JOHNSON

90 Epidemic Hemorrhagic Fevers

The term hemorrhagic fever was first used in the 1930s by Soviet and Japanese scientists to describe an acute febrile disease encountered in eastern Siberia and northern Manchuria. This syndrome was subsequently reported from Korea, Bulgaria, Hungary, European Russia, and northern Scandinavia under several labels including epidemic hemorrhagic fever, hemorrhagic fever with renal syndrome and hemorrhagic nephrosonephritis (HNN). Since 1940, nine other nosologic hemorrhagic fevers have been recognized: Omsk hemorrhagic fever (OHF), Kyasanur Forest disease (KFD), Crimean hemorrhagic fever (CrHF), Argentine hemorrhagic fever (AHF), Bolivian hemorrhagic fever (BHF), Lassa fever (LF), dengue hemorrhagic fever (DHF), African hemorrhagic fever (AFHF), and Rift Valley fever (RVF). Omsk hemorrhagic fever occurs in western Siberia, KFD in Mysore State, India, DHF in several large cities in southeast Asia, AFHF in portions of central, eastern, and southern Africa, and RVF in southern and eastern Africa with a major, recent incursion northward into Egypt.

All these diseases are caused by proven or presumptive viruses, and all are loosely united by the fact that hemorrhage is their most conspicuous clinical characteristic. This is not to say that other acute infectious diseases do not produce hemorrhage; for example, severe hemorrhage without jaundice often occurs with yellow fever (Chap. 73, Yellow Fever). Nevertheless, the pattern of acute fever with hemorrhagic diathesis and the general absence of other striking stigmata provide a convenient basis for grouping a variety of diseases into a single broad syndrome, such as pneumonia and nephritis.

Etiology

The etiologic viruses of hemorrhagic fevers are diverse (Table 90-1). Two of the diseases, OHF and KFD, are caused by group B arboviruses, immunologically related to the virus of Russian spring–summer encephalitis (RSSE). All these viruses are members of the so-called tick-borne complex of group B arboviruses. Dengue hemorrhagic fever may be induced by infection with any of at least four distinct dengue viral serotypes, all belonging to the immunologic mosquito-borne complex of group B arboviruses (flaviviruses).

Junin, Machupo, and Lassa viruses are arenaviruses, morphologically indistinguishable from lymphocytic choriomeningitis virus of mice (LCM). The first two are the causative agents of the South American hemorrhagic fevers and are antigenically closely related. Lassa virus shares more antigens with LCM.

Crimean hemorrhagic fever is caused by a tick-borne bunyavirus immunologically indistinguishable from Congo virus, an agent recovered from humans, animals, and ticks in Africa. Rift Valley fever is caused by another bunyavirus thought to be transmitted principally by mosquitoes.

African hemorrhagic fever is caused by two morphologically related agents (Marburg and Ebola), which are structurally reminiscent of rhabdoviruses but which perhaps represent prototypes of a new family of viruses. Hantaan virus, which causes HNN, has not been characterized sufficiently to permit taxonomic classification.

Although the hemorrhagic fever viruses differ somewhat in size, and more so immunologically, and although the properties of many of the agents are incompletely known, two fundamental characteristics appear to be common. (1) All contain essential lipids; that is, they are inactivated by ether and chloroform; and (2) those viruses which have been analyzed possess RNA.

Epidemiology

More is probably known concerning the epidemiology of each of the hemorrhagic fevers than about any other aspect. Certain salient features of the hemor-

Table 90-1. *Etiology of Viral Hemorrhagic Fevers*

Disease	Agent	Classification	Properties
Omsk hemorrhagic fever (OHF)	OHF virus	Tick-borne flavivirus	
Kyasanur forest disease (KFD)	KFD virus	Tick-borne flavivirus	35 nm–50 nm; contains single segment RNA; lipid in envelope
Dengue hemorrhagic fever (DHF)	Dengue virus, types 1–4	Mosquito-borne flavivirus	
Congo-Crimean hemorrhagic fever (CrHF)	Congo-CrHF virus	Bunyavirus, genus nairovirus	85 nm–100 nm; contains three RNA segments; lipid in envelope
Rift Valley fever (RVF)	RVF virus	Bunyavirus, genus phlebovirus	
Argentine hemorrhagic fever (AHF)	Junin virus	Arenavirus	75 nm–250 nm; pleomorphic; contains host cell ribosomes and two RNA segments; lipid in envelope
Bolivian hemorrhagic fever (BHF)	Machupo virus	Arenavirus	
Lassa fever (LF)	Lassa virus	Arenavirus	
African hemorrhagic fever (AFHF)	Marburg virus and Ebola virus	Ungrouped	790 nm–970 nm bacilliform; single RNA segment; lipid in envelope
Hemorrhagic nephrosonephritis (HNN)	Hantaan virus	Ungrouped lipid in envelope	Not yet visualized; lipid in envelope

rhagic fevers are listed in Table 90-2. Although much valuable detail has been sacrificed, this synthesis enables a rapid appreciation of several principal facts.

Hemorrhagic fevers are mainly transmitted from animals to humans. As such, they are strongly focal in occurrence, and their geographic distribution is coincident with that of variously complex biologic systems involving wild animals, domestic animals, and sometimes, arthropods. Not unexpectedly, each disease has a definite seasonal pattern. CrHF, OHF, and KFD are tick-borne; HNN, AHF, BHF, and LF are known or thought to induce chronic infections of wild rodents and are transmitted to man by virus-infected urine or feces; DHF is acquired by mosquito bite.

All but DHF, LF, and, to a much lesser extent, BHF are essentially diseases in which occupational exposure to critical vertebrate or arthropod vectors largely determines attack rates and the age and sex patterns of the disease in humans. In sharp contrast, DHF is urban, is seen almost exclusively in children (no sex difference), and is concentrated in cities in which certain *Aedes* mosquitoes are numerous and infection with more than one type of dengue virus is highly endemic.

Pathogenesis and Pathology

The mechanics by which the viruses of hemorrhagic fevers produce disease are poorly understood. Sophisticated clinical study is often impossible in the rural areas where most cases are seen, and animals resembling humans in response to infection are known only for AHF, BHF, LF, and KFD. With the exceptions of HNN and DHF, however, a general sequence of events may be as follows: The virus enters by blood, lymph vessels, the respiratory, or digestive tracts, and it multiplies in cells of the reticuloendothelial system. In 2 to 14 days, viremia and fever are present, produced either by the virus itself or by a virus-induced host pyrogen. Capillary lesions ensue, leading to the loss of erythrocytes and plasma. The role of coagulation defects and thrombocytes in hemorrhage is uncertain, although mild-to-moderate thrombocytopenia is common. Resolution of the disease is usually by crisis accompanied or followed by the formation of virus-specific antibodies. Pathologic residua of infection are rare. There are few specific changes in autopsied cases. Focal hemorrhages are prominent in the stomach, small intestines, kidneys, lungs, and brain. Characteristically, there is little in-

Table 90-2. *Epidemiologic Characteristics of Viral Hemorrhagic Fevers*

Disease	Recent Annual Incidence	Incubation Period	Seasonal Pattern	Case Pattern	Arthropod Vector	Vertebrate Hosts
Omsk hemorrhagic fever (OHF)	<20 since 1960	3–8 days	Biphasic; (peak, May and August)	Contact with cattle pastures; winter contact with muskrats	Tick *Dermacentor pictus*	Domestic animals (adult ticks); field mouse *Microtus gregalis* (larvae and nymphs)
Kyasanur Forest disease (KFD)	50–400	3–8 days	February–June (peak, April–May)	Contact with forest and cattle	Ticks of genus *Haemaphysalis* (*H. spinigera* most important)	Domestic animals, monkeys, certain birds, and rodents
Dengue hemorrhagic fever (DHF)	5000–>30,000	2–5 days	May–November (peak, June–August)	Urban; nearly all cases in children <14 years	*Aedes aegypti, Aedes albopictus*	Man only known reservoir
Crimean hemorrhagic fever (CrHF)	±1000 since 1953	2–7 days	June–August	Contact with cattle or pastures	Ticks of genus *Hyalomma*	Domestic animals (adult ticks), rooks, crows, hares (larvae and nymphs)
Rift Valley fever (RVF)	500–1,000,000	2–7 days	Late summer, fall	Contact with domestic animals and arthropods	Mosquitos, several genera ? *Culex pipiens* in Egypt	Domestic animals; sheep, cattle, goats, camels
Argentine hemorrhagic fever (AHF)	100–3000	10–14 days	March–July (autumn–winter) (peak, April–May)	Adult males harvesting maize	Probably none	Field mouse, *Calomys laucha laucha;* field mouse, *Calomys musculinus*
Bolivian hemorrhagic fever (BHF)	<20 since 1970	10–14 days	February–September (no marked peak)	Farm work or cattle tending at grassland-forest edge; major house outbreaks	Probably none	Field mouse, *Calomys callosus*
Lassa fever (LF)	500–5000 (estimated)	7–15 days	No marked peak	Rural; no strong association; nosocomial cases occur	None proven	Wild rodent, *Mastomys natalensis*
African hemorrhagic fever (AFHF)	3–300	7–16 days	Not definite	Sporadic, rural with nosocomial secondary cases	Unknown	Unknown
Hemorrhagic nephrosonephritis (HNN)	500–2000	2–4 weeks	May–July and October–November (Asia), September–January (Europe)	Forest contact or hay making (Asia); also autumn house outbreaks (Europe)	Probably none	Field mouse, *Apodemus agrarius;* red vole, *Clethrionomys glariolus*

Table 90-3. *Some Clinical Features of Viral Hemorrhagic Fevers*

Disease	Biphasic Fever	Bradycardia	Hemorrhage	Shock	Neurologic Disturbance	Leukopenia	Hemoconcentration	Proteinuria	Mortality (%)
Omsk hemorrhagic fever (OHF)	+	+	±	±	+	+	±	+	0.5–3
Kyasanur Forest disease (KFD)	+	±	±	±	+	+	±	+	3–10
Dengue hemorrhagic fever (DHF)	–	–	+	{+}	–	–	{+}	–	5–10
Crimean hemorrhagic fever (CrHF)	±	+	{+}	{+}	+	+	+	+	10–50
Rift Valley fever (RVF)	–	±	{+}	{+}	+	{+}	±	+	>50*
Argentine hemorrhagic fever (AHF)	–	+	+	{+}	{+}	+	+	+	5–30
Bolivian hemorrhagic fever (BHF)	–	+	+	{+}	{+}	+	+	+	5–30
Lassa fever (LF)	±	+	+	±	+	+	+	{+}	10–50*
African hemorrhagic fever (AFHF)	–	+	{+}	{+}	–	±	+	{+}	50–90
Hemorrhagic nephrosonephritis (HNN)	–	–	+	{+}	±	–	{+}	{+}	<1–10

+ Common or conspicuous finding; ± not common or not conspicuous finding; – rarely or never reported, { } highly conspicuous in frequency or severity
*Many mild infections seen for each case of HF: mortality for HF cases only

flammatory response. Severe liver damage is a hallmark of AFHF, LF, CrHF, and the hemorrhagic form of RVF, and disseminated intravascular coagulation is highly correlated with death in AFHF.

Careful study of HNN in Korea disclosed a functional capillary lesion in which plasma proteins escape at a much faster rate than erythrocytes. Paradoxically, despite clinical hemorrhage, this leads to a relative hemoconcentration and hypovolemia that are important in the genesis of shock. Patients surviving this phase of HNN frequently experience renal shutdown, a feature peculiar to HNN. At autopsy, kidneys from patients who have died of HNN show extensive medullary congestion and hemorrhage that contrast dramatically with the pale cortex, providing a pathognomonic gross appearance.

The severe form of DHF known as dengue shock syndrome is also unique. The onset is rapid, with fever lasting 2 to 3 days; resolution, by death or recovery, is equally swift. This virus is rarely recovered from the tissues of fatal cases, and isolation of the agent is infrequent from the blood of patients. Most patients in areas of high endemicity for dengue show evidence of a secondary immunologic response with high titers to all dengue viruses and other related group B arboviruses. It has been speculated that DHF is caused by a specific virus(antigen)-antibody reaction requiring a history of one or more previous infections with dengue viruses. Nevertheless, DHF has been documented in several instances in persons undergoing undoubted primary dengue infection.

Manifestations

The outstanding manifestations of viral hemorrhagic fevers are depicted in Table 90-3. Fever is high, unremittent, and sustained for 5 to 8 days in HNN, AHF, and BHF; it is high but shorter in DHF and RVF.

In all the hemorrhagic fevers, patients appear to be toxic and very sick, complaining of severe myalgia. Local abdominal pain has sometimes led to ill-advised laparotomy. Only in CrHF, and less often in HNN, has blood loss *per se* been recognized as directly life-threatening. In addition to melena and hematemesis, bleeding may occur from the nose, uterus, lungs, and gingivae in all syndromes. Petechiae, although sparse, are usually found on the upper chest, shoulders, neck, and palate. Major ecchymotic lesions have been reported in CrHF.

Shock is of minor importance in OHF and KFD. It is, however, a major feature of the eight hemorrhagic fevers with high mortality rates. Typically, 4 to 7 days after the onset of fever, the process begins with a progressive fall in the blood pressure; at this stage, it is reversible. If unrecognized, there is progression to clinical shock, with tachycardia, pallor, and cold, moist skin. This, the condition of true crisis in most hemorrhagic fevers, persists 1 to 2 days, during which time life hangs in the balance.

Encephalitic manifestations are at least as prominent as hemorrhage in OHF and KFD, and a patchy bronchopneumonia is considered part of the primary disease in the former. Neuropathy in AHF, BHF, and LF consists of intention tremor of the tongue and the muscles of the pharynx and larynx. There may be progression to intention tremors of the extremities and general convulsions. In contrast to OHF and KFD, however, the spinal fluid contains neither virus nor cells, and the concentration of protein is normal. Hepatomegaly is conspicuous in DHF.

Distinguishing features of Lassa fever include a stormy, febrile course of 2 to 3 weeks' duration, an exudative pharyngitis, clinical and pathologic evidence of myocarditis and hepatitis, and the frequent occurrence of residual deafness—either unilateral or bilateral.

Diagnosis

In no complex of diseases is an epidemiologic history of greater value. When dealing with a patient who has traveled to any of the known endemic areas, the essential questions relate to the column headings of Table 90-2. Clinically, however, many cases of hemorrhagic fever, particularly those in which hemorrhage is minimal or absent, are difficult to differentiate from such infections as yellow fever (Chap. 73, Yellow Fever), murine typhus (Chap. 98, The Typhus Fevers), Rocky Mountain spotted fever (Chap. 96, The Spotted Fevers), leptospirosis (Chap. 76, Leptospirosis), typhoid fever (Chap. 64, Typhoid Fever), and a variety of arbovirus diseases such as Colorado tick fever (Chap. 123, Colorado Tick Fever), and several encephalitides (Chap. 122, Viral Encephalitides). Because the nonviral infections in this list are specifically treatable, they should be rigorously excluded by appropriate laboratory means in all instances in which the clinicoepidemiologic story is compatible with hemorrhagic fever.

Specific diagnosis can be made in two ways. Blood, throat secretions, urine, spinal fluid, and tissues may yield the causative virus when inoculated into baby mice, baby hamsters, or tissue cultures. Paired acute- and convalescent-phase sera can be tested for virus-specific antibodies using complement fixation, hemagglutination–inhibition, neutralization, or immunofluorescent techniques, depending on the particular virus.

Prognosis

The prognosis varies widely (Table 90-3). Mortality figures are not comparably reliable for all the hemorrhagic fevers. Shock, secondary bacterial infection, and preexistent chronic diseases are the most common autopsy diagnoses. In general, patients surviving the acute manifestations recover completely and seem to be immune thereafter, because antibodies have been demonstrated for several years and *bona fide* second attacks have not been seen.

Therapy

Strict isolation and observance of precautions designed to preclude contact with infectious materials from patients are required for the safe management of patients possibly suffering from CrHF, LF, and AFHF, since these diseases have been repeatedly transmitted as nosocomial infections. Supportive treatment is based on the principles of careful control of fluid and electrolyte balance, the diagnosis and therapy of secondary bacterial infections, and the anticipation of shock (proteinuria, rising hematocrit) with prompt intravenous administration of colloids. Other modalities often employed in the treatment of septic shock caused by bacteria, such as hypertonic saline, selective vasopressors, and high doses of glucosteroids, have not been systematically evaluated in the management of viral hemorrhagic fevers but deserve serious consideration in individual cases. Administration of specific antibodies to Junin virus produces dramatic reduction in mortality of AHF if treatment is begun within 8 days of the onset of disease. Studies in monkeys have demonstrated clearly the value of combined treatment with antibodies and the experimental drug ribavirin in LF; clinical trials of this regimen are in progress.

Prevention

There are as yet no effective vaccines available for any viral hemorrhagic fever. In HNN, LF, AHF, and BHF, simple sanitary standards and specific rodent control measures are adequate where economic and cultural norms permit their maintenance. The prevention of DHF is essentially that long known for the control of yellow fever because the principal mosquito vector is *Aedes aegypti.* Soviet workers have reported success in the control of OHF by using large-scale aerial application of DDT to reduce tick populations. Individual protection is offered by insect repellents used directly on the skin or impregnated into outdoor clothing.

Remaining Problems

There are many problems related to hemorrhagic fevers, and they are of potential value to the understanding of other infectious diseases. For example, what is the pathophysiology of hemorrhage in these diseases? Is disseminated intravascular coagulation a major factor in pathogenesis of many of the epidemic hemorrhagic fevers? What experimental hosts can be found to answer such questions? Is DHF really an antigen-antibody disease? If so, how do these complexes cause bleeding and shock?

How can effective, safe vaccines be made for some of the hemorrhagic fevers? How can present knowledge be better applied to control these diseases by means other than vaccines? What are the minimum practical and safe procedures and facilities required for prevention of nosocomial infection in CrHF, LF, and AFHF?

Bibliography

Books

JOHNSON KM, HALSTEAD SB, COHEN SN: Hemorrhagic fevers of Southeast Asia and South America: A comparative appraisal. In Melnick JL (ed): Progress in Medical Virology, Vol IX. New York, Karger, 1967. pp 105–158.

PATTYN SR (ED): Ebola Virus Hemorrhagic Fever. Amsterdam/New York, Elsevier/North-Holland, 1978. 436 pp.

SMORODINTSEV AA, KAZBINDSEV LI, CHADAKOV VG: Virus Hemorrhagic Fevers. Washington DC, Department of Commerce, Office of Technical Services, 1964. 245 pp.

Journals

CASALS J, HOOGSTRAAL H, JOHNSON KM, SHELOKOV A, WIEBENGA NH, WORK TH: A current appraisal of hemorrhagic fevers in the USSR. Am J Trop Med Hyg 15:751–764, 1966

EARLE DP (ED): Symposium on epidemic hemorrhagic fever. Am J Med 16:619–709, 1954

International Symposium on Arenaviral Infections of Public Health Importance. Bull WHO 52:381–766, 1975

ANDRÉ J. NAHMIAS
DONALD E. CAMPBELL

91 Infections Caused By Herpes Simplex Viruses

The spectrum of disease associated with infections caused by herpes simplex viruses types 1 and 2 (HSV-1 and HSV-2) has widened as a result of the development of laboratory tools for precise diagnosis and expanded clinicopathologic awareness. Descriptions of herpes febrilis were recorded as early as 100 A.D. Herpes genitalis and acute vesicular dermatosis were described in the early 18th century. However, the association of HSV with keratitis, Kaposi's varicelliform eruption, gingivostomatitis, meningoencephalitis, and disseminated disease of the newborn awaited the identification of multinucleated giant cells and intranuclear inclusions in herpetic lesions and the transmissibility of the virus to the rabbit cornea, the chorioallantoic membrane of the chick embryo, and various nonhuman animals (1890–1950).

The pattern continues. With increasing interest in HSV, involvement of the liver, lungs, and dissemination in certain compromised hosts have been documented. Modern laboratory methods, particularly tissue culture, and serologic and molecular techniques, have made feasible investigations of the possible role of HSV in abortions, congenital malformations, allergic reactions, neoplasia, and chronic diseases of the eye and central nervous system.

Etiology

The herpesviruses are double-stranded DNA viruses that are about 180 nm in diameter and have an icosahedral capsid with 162 capsomeres that is surrounded by a lipid-containing envelope. The human herpesviruses include cytomegaloviruses (Chap. 75, Cytomegalovirus Infections), varicella-zoster virus (Chap. 93, Varicella and Herpes Zoster), Epstein–Barr virus (Chap. 137, Infectious Mononucleosis), and HSV-1 and HSV-2.

One or more herpesviruses have been identified from almost every nonhuman animal species examined. So far, only one, *Herpesvirus simiae,* the B virus of macaque monkeys, has been found to cause disease in humans; it is a severe, almost always fatal, encephalitis (Chap. 122, Viral Encephalitides). On the other hand, HSV of human origin has caused fatal infections under natural conditions in gibbons and pet skunks. Under experimental conditions, HSV can produce mild or fatal disease in mice, hamsters, rabbits, guinea pigs, and various nonhuman primates.

It was not until the early 1960s that HSV was found to consist of two antigenic types, HSV-1 and HSV-2, which also differ in their effect on mice, the chorioallantoic membrane of the chick embryo, and various tissue cultures. In addition, differences have been found in the electron microscopic appearance of infected cells, the viral structural and nonstructural proteins, and the DNA of the two types of HSV. Restriction enzyme analyses of the viral DNA enables differentiation of strains within one type. These methods have been exploited to gain knowledge of the clinicoepidemiologic features of infection with the two types.

Epidemiology

Of the several features of infections caused by HSV, those of primary epidemiologic importance are their common prevalence and their tendency to recur. Humans seem to be the definitive reservoir of HSV; no vector has been shown to be involved in transmission. Kissing and sexual relations have been implicated so frequently that herpes has been called the "virus of love." Close body contact, as occurs during wrestling, has been associated with outbreaks of skin herpes (herpes gladiatorum). The higher frequency of HSV antibodies in children of lower socioeconomic groups apparently correlates with close living conditions. There is no evidence of human-to-human transmission by way of inanimate objects such as toilet bowls, even though virus can be recovered from such sites.

Although herpetic infections are most commonly endemic, there have been several reports of outbreaks in families, in institutions for children, and in hospitals. The attack rate in closed populations has varied from 33% to 75%. HSV can be considered a cause of nosocomial infection in view of the many reports of herpetic paronychia occurring in hospital personnel, particularly those attending neurosurgical patients. The virus is acquired in these cases from the infected oral cavities of patients or from contaminated tracheal catheters. Hospital personnel and patients have contracted herpetic infection from other patients, particularly those with eczema herpeticum, and nursery spread has also been documented. The laboratory acquisition of HSV infection has also occurred.

The incubation period of primary HSV infections ranges from 2 to 12 days, with an average of 6 days. It has been difficult to estimate the incubation period of herpetic encephalitis or chorioretinitis, but it has exceeded 12 days on occasion. There may be differences in frequency of herpetic infection according to season. Thus, HSV infections of the skin occur more commonly in the warmer months, whereas HSV infections of the eye and herpes febrilis seem to occur more frequently in the winter months. No seasonal differences have been found with herpetic gingivostomatitis.

Of particular clinical and epidemiologic importance have been the differences in the site of involvement and modes of transmission of HSV-1 and HSV-2. HSV-1 is usually transmitted nonvenereally. Most commonly, in adults and children beyond the newborn age group, it involves nongenital sites, including the mouth, lips, skin above the waist, eyes, and brain. On occasion, as a result of autoinoculation or oral–genital contact, HSV-1 may involve genital sites, although recurrent genital infection is much less common with HSV-1 than with HSV-2.

HSV-2 is most often transmitted venereally in adolescents and adults, causing infection of the genitalia and skin below the waist. HSV-2, and occasionally HSV-1, can also be transmitted from the mother's genitalia to the newborn, in whom any site can be involved (Table 91-1).

In any discussion of the epidemiologic features of HSV infections, serologic responses must be considered because the presence of antibodies to HSV has correlated better with previous subclinical infection than with overt clinical manifestations. Over the past three decades, the generally accepted concept has been that persons who have no detectable antibodies to HSV would develop a primary infection, after which antibodies to the virus would appear in their serum. Despite such circulating antibodies, however, many persons would develop recurrent infections, usually at or close to the site of their initial infection, but sometimes remote from the original site. Many factors are known to trigger recurrences, including physical agents, fever, several infectious diseases, menstruation, and emotional stresses.

Three mechanisms have been postulated to explain the viral aspects of recurrent infections: (1) the oldest concept postulates latent, noninfectious virus remaining in some site, probably the nerves. The isolation of HSV from human sensory and autonomic ganglia lends support to this theory. (2) A second concept envisions a constant, low-grade chronic infection, with the virus persisting in sites such as the lacrimal glands, in a sensitized but still infectious form, that is, virus-coated by antibody but not neutralized by either serum or secretory antibodies. (3) Autoinfection and reinfection, the third concept, explains some, but certainly not all, of the clinical observations in humans. Autoinfection requires transfer of the virus from a manifestly or subclinically infected site to a noninfected site. Reinfection occurs when HSV, either homologous or heterologous, is acquired from an exogenous source.

The persistence of antibodies in the blood at a relatively constant titer has been noted in most recurrent infections. On occasion, however, a rise in antibody titer has been demonstrated in recurrent infections; on the other hand, a fall in antibody titer has also been recorded after a primary infection. Thus, the relatively constant level of antibody observed over long periods is probably maintained by some boosting effect of endogenous or exogenous virus.

Recognition of the two types of HSV renders the terminology of primary and recurrent infection inadequate. For example, what is the appropriate designation for a person who has a recurrent HSV-1 infection, but contracts his first HSV-2 infection? A new terminology and conceptualized scheme of what may occur in persons who lack antibodies to either type of HSV or who already have antibodies to one or both types is given in Table 91-2. Because specific antigens to the two types of HSV are not completely defined, substantiation of the proposed scheme is incomplete. It is based in large part on studies enabling the differentiation of antibodies to one or both types of HSV in the serums of persons with herpetic infections with one or the other type.

When persons with previous HSV-1, HSV-2, or dual antibodies are infected with HSV-2 virus, they are much less severely ill than if they had no antibodies

Table 91-1. *Clinical Spectrum of Infections Caused by Herpes Simplex Viruses 1 and 2 in Newborns and Older Persons and the Type* Isolated From Different Sites and Clinical Conditions*

	Number of Individuals With HSV Type		
	TYPE 1	TYPE 2	TOTAL
Usually Mild to Moderately Severe (persons over 1 month of age)			
Urogenital Infections			
Females (cervix, vulva, vagina, urethra)	36 (7[†])	300 (5[‡])	336
Males (penis, urethra)	7 (1[†])	225 (1[§])	232
Nongenital Infections			
Gingivostomatitis or asymptomatic (mouth)	156	4 (2[‖])	160
Herpes febrilis (lips)	84	0	84
Keratitis or conjunctivitis (cornea and/or conjunctiva)	29	1	30
Dermatitis			
Skin above waist	92 (1[‖])	4	96
Skin below waist	4 (1[†], 1[‖])	85 (6[‖], 1[#])	89
Hands or arms	16 (1[#])	16 (2[#], 2[‖])	32
Latent infections (trigeminal or thoracic ganglia)	21 (1[**])	0	21
(sacral ganglia)	0	5	5
Usually Severe to Fatal (persons over 1 month of age)			
Meningoencephalitis (brain, spinal cord, CSF)	101	2	103
Multiple sclerosis (brain)	0	1	1
Eczema herpeticum (skin, lungs)	12	1	13
Generalized disease (visceral organs)	2	1 (1[††])	3
Newborns—localized or generalized infection (skin, eyes, brain, CSF, visceral organs)	46 (7[‡‡])	92 (25[‡‡])	138
Total	606	737	1343

*Typing is done by microneutralization or direct immunofluorescent tests.
†Simultaneous isolation of similar HSV type from mouth.
‡Simultaneous isolation of HSV-2 from cervix or vulva and HSV-1 from lip or mouth.
§Simultaneous isolation of HSV-2 from penile lesion and HSV-1 from eye.
‖Simultaneous isolation of same HSV type from genitalia.
#Laboratory- or hospital-acquired infection.
**Simultaneous isolation of HSV-2 from sacral ganglia.
††Isolated also from brain.
‡‡Same HSV type isolated from mother's genital tract.

Table 91-2. *Expected Type-Specific Antibody Response in Persons With No Antibodies to Either Type of Herpes Simplex Virus (HSV) or With Prior Antibodies to Type 1, Type 2, or Both Types*

Proposed Classification	**Prior HSV Type Antibodies in Persons**		**Source of Virus**	**Virus Type**	**Antibody Type Response**
	HSV-1	HSV-2			
Primary*					
Initial 1–Ab[†] 0	0	0	Exogenous	1	1
Initial 2–Ab 0	0	0	Exogenous	2	2
Recurrent*					
Recurrent 1–Ab 1	+	0	Exogenous or endogenous	1	1
Initial 2–AB 1	+	0	Exogenous	2	Dual
Recurrent 2–Ab 2	0	+	Exogenous or endogenous	2	2
Initial 1–Ab 2	0	+	Exogenous	1	Dual
Recurrent 1, 2–Ab 1, 2	+	+	Exogenous or endogenous	1	Dual
Recurrent 1, 2–AB 1, 2	+	+	Exogenous or endogenous	2	Dual

*Old classification.
†AB—antibody; "immune" would not be accurate because of the inability of antibodies to convey total immunity.

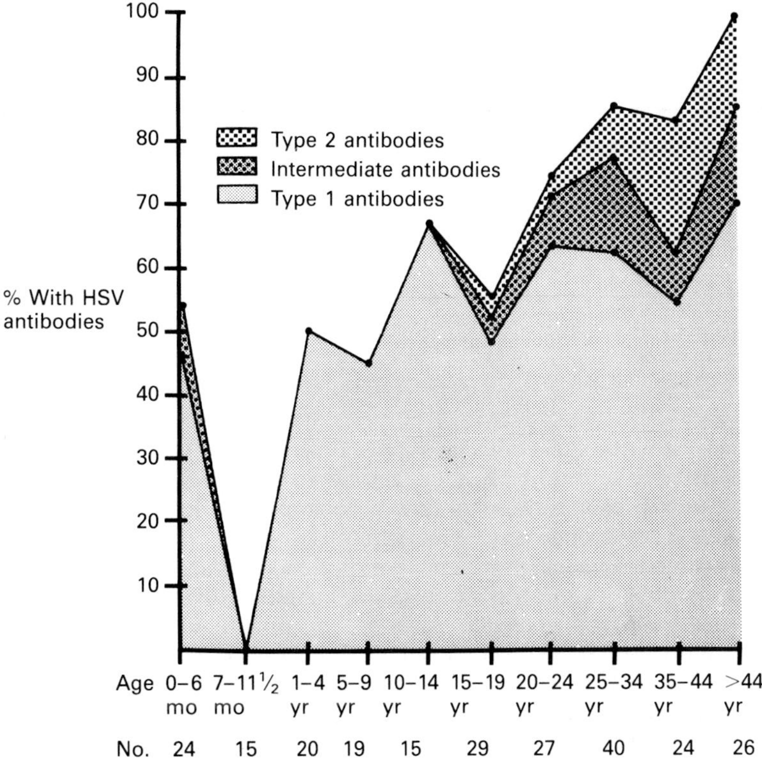

Fig. 91-1. Percent distribution of antibodies to herpes simplex virus type 1, type 2, or intermediate (type 1 and type 2) in 239 persons of varying age groups.

to HSV of either type. However, in certain particularly susceptible hosts (newborns, persons with certain dermatoses or burns, and natively or iatrogenically immunologically defective persons) and in some patients with encephalitis, severe infection can occur despite the presence of circulating (homologous or heterologous) HSV antibodies.

Using neutralization or complement fixation tests, antibodies to HSV have been assayed in various population groups (Fig 91-1). A compilation of several studies enables the following conclusions to be made:

1. Up to about 6 months of age, transplacental antibodies can be detected in the serums of newborns whose mothers had antibodies against HSV.
2. There is a sharp rise in antibodies between 1 and 4 years, primarily in antibodies to HSV-1.
3. From ages 5 through 14 years, there is a slight increase, again mostly in HSV-1 antibodies.
4. After the age of 14 years, there is a more marked rise of antibodies to HSV. This may be explained, in part, by the appearance of HSV-2 antibodies, which gradually increase in frequency until late adulthood.
5. There are striking differences in the overall frequency of adults with antibodies to HSV, depending primarily on socioeconomic status. Only 40% of some population groups, such as medical students and nurses, may show antibodies, whereas 60% to 85% of young adults in lower socioeconomic groups may demonstrate antibodies.

The age distribution of persons with antibodies to HSV appears to correlate to some extent with the site of involvement and the age prevalence of infections caused by HSV. An estimate of the relative frequency of infections caused by HSV according to body site is presented in Table 91-3. Thus, in children 6 months to 4 years of age, the major site of infection is the oral cavity. Gingivostomatitis can be detected clinically in 1% to 15% of children in this age group. In addition, HSV can actually be recovered from the oral cavity in 1% to 20% of subclinical cases. Up to the age of 14 years, other clinically manifest infections are those involving the eye and skin, and much less frequently, the central nervous system and genitalia.

During adolescence, the major new type of herpetic infection is that affecting the genitalia. Genital herpetic infection is primarily a venereal disease (the

Table 91-3. *Incidence of Herpes Simplex Virus Infection According to Age and Site of Involvement*

Clinical Involvement	1–11 Months	1–4 Years	5–14 Years	15–19 Years	20–29 Years	30 Years and Over
Gingivostomatitis	+	++++	++	±	±	±
Labialis	±	±	+	++	+++	++++
Keratitis	±	+	+	++	++	+++
Dermatitis	+	+	+	++	++	++
Genital herpes	±	±	±	+++	+++	++
Encephalitis	+	+	+	+	+	++

*This rough estimate (± very infrequent to ++++ very frequent) is based on several reports. The chart should be read left to right and not up and down because no attempt was made to arrive at the relative proportion of site involvement at any one specific age.

attack rate in sexual contacts is approximately 75%). Accordingly, it is more prevalent among sexually promiscuous persons, those of lower socio-economic groups, adolescents, and young adults.

Older persons are more apt to experience recurrent herpetic infection at various sites, including lips, cornea, skin, and genitalia. Herpetic encephalitis is also more frequently recognized after the age of 30 years. It is of interest that HSV can be recovered from the oral cavity in as much as 5% of asymptomatic adults sampled at random.

One form of disseminated herpetic infection affects primarily grossly malnourished African children, ages 6 months to 4 years, or those with associated infectious processes, such as measles. Another form of severe disease—neonatal herpes—occurs more frequently in infants born to young mothers of lower socioeconomic groups who are primigravidas. Transplacental infection of the fetus has not been demonstrated conclusively in humans.

Pathogenesis and Pathology

In the common focal forms of infection caused by HSV, direct inoculation or local activation at first yields a small patch of erythema that evolves into a thin-walled vesicle filled with clear liquid. Several vesicles may be grouped on an erythematous base to form a plaque. On microscopic examination, the intradermal locus of the vesicle is revealed. Inflammatory cells around the vesicle are associated with edema and congestion. Intranuclear inclusion bodies are present in the epithelial cells, particularly at the margin of the vesicle. The virus is most readily recovered from the vesicle in titers up to 10^7, and is less likely to be demonstrated in crusts after the vesicles have ruptured.

In normal persons, the lesions are limited to the epidermis or superficial mucous membranes, and dissemination of the virus from such focal lesions through the bloodstream has rarely been demonstrated. On the other hand, viremia has been well documented in compromised hosts, including newborns, grossly malnourished children or children with associated infections such as measles, persons with skin disorders, such as atopic eczema or burns, patients receiving treatment with immunosuppressive drugs, and persons with defects in cell-mediated immunity, for example Hodgkin's disease, Wiskott–Aldrich syndrome, and ataxia telangiectasia.

The pathogenesis of the disseminated form of herpetic infection has been well studied in malnourished children. Primary viremia results from spillover of the virus from replication in cells at the portal of entry. Although most susceptible organ sites become infected at this time, histologic evidence of infection is minimal. In the second or progressive stage, the virus disappears from the blood but increases within cells of infected organs, at which time histologic evidence of cell damage can be seen. In the third or florid stage, a secondary viremia occurs as a result of increasing virus production in the organs initially infected, and multiple organ systems are thereby seeded. Histopathologic evidence of cell destruction may be extensive at this stage. In the final stages of regression and recovery, the virus clears from the blood, and diminishing amounts are detectable in involved viscera that are undergoing cellular regeneration. During the course of disseminated disease, the number of organ systems involved and the amount of cellular damage and virus production are quite variable in individual cases, so that the clinical expression of disseminated herpetic infection can be very broad.

The direct spread of HSV to the central nervous system and retina through the peripheral nerves has been demonstrated in experimental animals; however, there is scanty evidence of direct spread in humans. The ineffectiveness of humoral antibodies in the prevention of mild to moderately severe herpetic recurrences, or even severe disease in certain susceptible persons, has remained one of the major enigmas regarding HSV and the other herpesviruses affecting man or animals.

The mechanisms responsible for the activation of herpesvirus, the limiting of virus shedding or the number of lesions, and the determination of the outcome of the primary infection have yet to be understood. Nonspecific mechanisms, such as NK lymphocytes or macrophages, possibly together with interferon, may be particularly important in the control of herpetic infections. When there is a recurrence, there also appears to be an interaction among many immune effector mechanisms that limits spread to other organs. From observations of compromised hosts, immune factors may play a role in the reactivation of virus and in the chronicity or severity of the infection, despite the fact that the diseases of reactivation may not be severe. It is difficult to ascertain which is the important or crucial immune system in host resistance. From preliminary information in nonhuman animals, the effectiveness of mechanisms that control herpesviral infections may be genetically determined.

Manifestations

Mild to Moderate Manifestations

GENITAL HERPES

Genital herpes in women (Chap. 50, Infections of the Female Genital Tract) may involve the vulva, vagina, and cervix (Plate 91-1*E*). As a primary infection with either HSV-1 or HSV-2, the manifestations may include fever, dysuria, leukorrhea, genital soreness, and inguinal adenopathy; there may be extension to the skin of the perineum, buttocks, and thighs. Recurrent disease is particularly frequent with HSV-2. When it involves the cervix, it is usually subclinical and is often undiagnosed.

In males, herpetic vesicles or ulcers are usually noted on the glans penis, prepuce, or shaft of the penis (Plate 91-1*D*) and are less frequently seen on the scrotum and adjacent perineal areas. Primary infections are more commonly associated with tender adenopathy, dysuria, and constitutional signs than recurrent infections. As a result of varied sex practices, genital herpetic infections in males and females can also involve the anus or the mouth. A severe form of herpetic proctitis occurs in male homosexuals and has been associated with Kaposi's sarcoma and pneumocystis pneumonia. The virus may be recovered from the urethra, whether or not symptoms are present. Herpetic urethritis may occur alone or in association with genital lesions. Herpetic cystitis has been reported infrequently. Complications of genital herpes in males and females have included neuralgia, meningitis, and infrequently, ascending myelitis and encephalitis.

The differential diagnosis of genital herpes consists primarily of the venereal diseases: syphilis (Chap. 59, Syphilis), lymphogranuloma venereum (Chap. 54, Lymphogranuloma Venereum), granuloma inguinale (Chap. 58, Granuloma Inguinale), and particularly, chancroid (Chap. 57, Chancroid). Other diseases to be differentiated include herpes zoster (Chap. 93, Varicella and Herpes Zoster), Behçet's syndrome, erythema multiforme, and impetigo (Chap. 100, Staphylococcal Skin Infections).

NONGENITAL HERPES

Oral Manifestations. Like the cervix, the mouth may be involved without any clinical manifestations, although a few lesions may be seen on close, sequential examinations. Gingivostomatitis occurs most commonly in young children (Plate 91-1*A*), but it may also be observed occasionally in older persons. Oral lesions caused by HSV-2 are now more commonly encountered as a result of oral-genital contact. The vesicular and ulcerative lesions may involve both anterior and posterior parts of the mouth, and the tongue. Often inflammation of the gums, cervical adenopathy, and fever are present. Finger-suckers may develop concomitant infections of the fingers (Plate 91-1*A*), and autoinoculation of other sites can occur.

Recurrences of herpetic lesions in the mouth are very infrequent. Painful ulcers that are recurrent are usually aphthous stomatitis. Other lesions of the mouth that might be confused with herpetic stomatitis are Vincent's angina, candidosis (Chap. 39, Candidosis), herpangina or hand-foot-and-mouth syndrome caused by group A coxsackieviruses (Chap. 149, Coxsackievirus and Echovirus Infections), and stomatitis resulting from trauma or associated with drugs or erythema multiforme. If the oral involvement is localized to the pharynx or tonsils, herpetic infections may be misdiagnosed as streptococcal infections (Chap. 24, Streptococcal Diseases), diphtheria (Chap. 25, Diphtheria), or infectious mononucleosis (Chap. 137, Infectious Mononucleosis).

Lips Although occasionally the lips may be the site of a primary infection, by far the most common symptomatic herpetic lip involvement is the recurrent cold sore, or fever blister. Vesicle formation is preceded by 1 to 2 days of hyperesthesia and burning sensations. The lesions last 3 to 10 days, and they may recur either at the identical site or in a neighboring area. The most common sites of affliction are the mucosa of the lower lip and the skin of the upper lip (Plate 91-1*B*), the sites also most commonly associated with cancer of the lip. Almost all strains have been HSV-1.

Eyes. Primary herpetic keratitis may be accompanied by conjunctivitis and tender, enlarged preauricular nodes. Conjunctivitis without keratitis may also be a manifestation of primary infection, and occasionally, recurrent infection. Recurrent keratitis is usually unilateral, but up to 6% of cases may be bilateral. Within a 2-year period, recurrences become manifest in about one-fourth to one-third of patients.

The diagnosis of herpetic keratitis can usually be made with confidence on clinical grounds alone in view of the typical branched, fluorescein-staining, dendritic ulcers (Fig. 162-1*F*) and corneal hypesthesia. Herpetic vesicles on the face, lips, or eyelids occasionally may be detected, and trauma to the cornea, occasionally associated with contact lenses, occurs in 5% to 10% of cases. Stromal corneal involvement has been attributed both to a delayed hypersensitivity mechanism and to inflammation resulting from virus proliferation in the stroma itself. Such diskiform keratitis may progress to interstitial keratitis or to hypopyon keratitis, with or without perforation and associated iridocyclitis. Iridocyclitis may also occur without concomitant corneal disease.

Locally applied glucosteroids may cause deeper ocular involvement. Herpetic bilateral panuveitus, with HSV isolated from the anterior chamber, has been reported in a patient who was not receiving glucosteroids. Chorioretinitis has been described primarily in newborns with HSV-2 infection (Fig. 162-1*H*), raising the question of whether cases of undiagnosed chorioretinitis in older persons may also be caused by infection with HSV-2. Cataracts have also been associated with neonatal herpes.

Skin. HSV can affect the skin of any part of the body, including the face, hands, and feet. In general, viruses isolated from dermal lesions above the waist have been HSV-1, those from herpetic lesions below the waist have been HSV-2, and viruses isolated from the hands or fingers have been either HSV-1 or HSV-2 (Table 91-1). That is, there are many ways in which the finger may become infected, including autoinfection, genital-to-finger contact, or finger-to-mouth contact (*e.g.*, paronychia in hospital personnel).

Primary cutaneous infection may be accompanied by edema of the skin, fever, lymphangitis, and lymphadenopathy. Recurrent infections of the face present an important cosmetic problem, although scarring does not result unless there is secondary infection; however, scarring may occur in newborns infected with HSV. Herpetic skin lesions may be very extensive, and even chronic, in persons with immunologic defects (Plate 91-1*C*) or under treatment with immunosuppressive drugs. Occasionally, trauma to the skin is the obvious way in which a herpetic skin is acquired (*e.g.*, herpes gladiatorum in wrestlers; herpes rugbeiform in rugby players). In some patients, with either nongenital or genital herpetic infections, erythema multiforme has been an occasional complication. This allergic manifestation has been noted in some persons with every recurrence of their herpetic infection, commonly herpes febrilis (Plate 91-1*B*). Such an association may be more common than is appreciated, particularly if the herpetic infection is clinically inapparent.

Cutaneous herpetic infections are most often mistaken for pyoderma, contact dermatitis, or herpes zoster. Particularly difficult to diagnose are the occasional instances of cutaneous HSV infections with a zosteriform distribution.

Severe to Fatal Manifestations

NEWBORNS

The incidence of neonatal herpetic infection has been estimated to range from a minimum of 1 in 30,000 to a maximum of 1 in 2000 deliveries. Manifestations range from subclinical infections to local infections involving the oral cavity, skin, eyes, or central nervous system (CNS) to disseminated infection affecting visceral organs with or without CNS involvement (Plate 91-1*G*). In the past, most cases of neonatal herpetic infection were diagnosed at postmortem examination; now, many who survive neonatal infection are recognized because of improved awareness and diagnostic methods. About half the surviving infants have neurologic or ocular sequelae. With the advent of effective antiherpesviral therapy, it is necessary to diagnose neonatal herpes rapidly.

In only one-half of the reported cases of neonatal herpes could the diagnosis be suspected from vesicles, ulcers, of the skin and mouth, or keratoconjunctivitis. In the remainder, the picture was nonspecific and resembled other perinatal infections, such as cytomegalovirus (Chap. 75, Cytomegalovirus Infections), rubella (Chap. 87, Rubella), and toxoplasmosis (Chap. 129, Toxoplasmosis) (TORCH syndrome), and bacterial meningitis (Chap. 119, Acute Bacterial Meningitis), or septicemia.

Genital herpes in a pregnant woman or her sexual contact(s) should alert the physician to the possible risk of herpetic infection in the newborn. The outcome of pregnancy in women with primary infections may be associated with abortion or prematurity.

IN PATIENTS MORE THAN ONE MONTH OF AGE

Central Nervous System Disease. The encephalitic form of HSV infection is, with rare exceptions, caused by HSV-1 in non-neonatal persons, whereas HSV-2 infection is more often associated with a benign meningitis (that can recur). In the absence of treatment, the fatality rate of HSV encephalitis is about 70%; more than half of the survivors are left with neurologic sequelae. There are several conditions that mimic HSV encephalitis, including treatable fungal (Chaps. 41, Coccidioidomycosis; 120, Cryptococcosis) or tuberculous diseases (Chap. 35, Extrapulmonary Tuberculosis), meningitides, or brain abscesses (Chap. 125, Intracranial Suppuration). Brain biopsy is imperative to avoid missing a treatable disease and to avert needless toxic effects from antiviral drugs. Because HSV involves the temporal lobes primarily, clinical, neuroradiologic, and EEG findings provide the bases for suspecting HSV encephalitis and obtaining a brain biopsy. However, no more than half the biopsies taken from patients suspected of having encephalitis are positive for HSV. Although the coincidence of herpetic skin or mucous membrane lesions with the findings of meningoencephalitis is virtually diagnostic of HSV encephalitis in the newborn, this is not true in older patients. HSV infections may also be manifested by myelitis, radiculitis, and Guillain–Barré syndrome. A possible role of HSV in Bell's palsy, demyelinating disease, and psychiatric disorders merits investigation.

Eczema Herpeticum Kaposi's varicelliform eruption caused by HSV occurs most commonly in persons with atopic eczema or in those with the Wiskott–Aldrich syndrome. It is occasionally found in patients with other skin disorders, such as seborrheic eczema, diaper rash, Darier's disease, and pemphigus. Most often, the disease is a primary infection, but it has also been seen in the recurrent form in either eczematous or intact skin, after the eczema has cleared.

The skin manifestations of eczema herpeticum (Plate 91-1*C*) resemble those of eczema vaccinatum. They are often misdiagnosed as representing either an exacerbation of the underlying skin disorder itself or a bacterial or fungal cutaneous infection. The areas affected in eczema herpeticum are both those with dermatitis and those with apparently normal skin. Initially, vesicles appear that may umbilicate and become pustular, encrusted, confluent, and hemorrhagic. Associated fever and adenopathy are common. The process varies from a transient disease to a fatal disorder (5% to 15% case fatality rate). Fatality may result from disseminated viremia to the brain and visceral organs, or it may be associated with a bacterial or fungal superinfection.

Generalized Disease in Children Only occasionally reported in the United States and Europe, general herpetic infection is not uncommon in Africa. Kwashiorkor or another infection (*e.g.,* measles, pertussis) is the usual setting. Blood-borne viral dissemination results in the involvement of the visceral organs. As in eczema herpeticum, children with this disease commonly die either from their herpetic infection or from a bacterial superinfection.

Recently Recognized Incursions

IMPAIRED IMMUNITY

Certain conditions or drugs that compromise immune competence, particularly cellular immunity, can be associated with increased severity of HSV infections. Either the lesions are more extensive, even disseminated, or they are chronic. The immunosuppressive therapies that are applied in and of themselves may augment the already predisposing effect of organ transplants and such diseases as Hodgkin's disease, other lymphomas, leukemias.

In addition, certain persons with defects of cell-mediated immunity (*e.g.,* immunologic paralysis syndrome) may develop severe forms of herpetic infection.

BURNS

Patients with severe burns may contract disseminated infection with HSV, esophagitis, or a severe form of herpetic pneumonia that is lethal. The frequency of such occurrences remains to be determined.

OTHER

Focal organ involvement with HSV has been implicated on the basis of viral isolations,the demonstration of intranuclear inclusion bodies, or by serologic means in hepatitis, pharyngitis, laryngitis, pneumonitis, arthritis, esophagitis, and gastritis. A causative relationship is becoming better substantiated for these entities.

NEOPLASIA

Various herpesviruses have been associated with the production of tumors in several nonhuman species and in man. Prime suspects in humans are the EB virus in Burkitt's lymphoma and nasopharyngeal carcinoma, and HSV-2 in carcinoma of the cervix.

Diagnosis

Although the appearance of herpetic lesions is often characteristic, even such a presumptive diagnosis is not possible when there is secondary bacterial infection or when certain sites, such as the cervix or CNS, are involved. Microscopic examination of scrapings from skin, mouth, eye, or genital lesions is a readily and rapidly available aid. Microscopy may also help by detection of viral changes in biopsies of the skin, brain, or liver. Fixation of cytologic specimens in 90% ethanol and histologic specimens in Bouin's solution should precede staining and examination for multinucleated giant cells and intranuclear inclusions (Plate 91-1*F* and *H*), which are typical of HSV and of varicella–zoster viruses. Even electron microscopy is not diagnostic, because HSV cannot be distinguished from other herpesviruses on morphologic grounds alone. The direct application of immunofluorescent or enzyme-linked techniques to clinical specimens can aid in diagnosing HSV. However, the sensitivity and specificity of these methods must be monitored carefully.

The isolation of HSV from clinical specimens is most readily accomplished in a variety of tissue cultures. Typical cytopathic changes can be detected in 1 to 4 days. Isolation can also be achieved in embryonated eggs or in mice. The typing of isolates is accomplished by using a variety of serologic techniques, including fluorescent antibody and neutralization tests.

Unless they are epidemiologically related, specific strains may be differentiated within each type by electrophoretic analysis of DNA fragments derived from HSV by various DNA restriction endonucleases. Not only is this method of great epidemiologic value, but also it enables study of the specificity of HSV strains for particular diseases, for example, stromal keratitis.

Monoclonal antibodies appear to have potential for (1) differentiating strains among the two types of HSV according to antigenic differences and (2) preparation of type-specific antigens for detecting particular antibodies in the serums of patients. Currently, identification of virus is of greater clinical use than the measurement of specific immunoglobins. The detection of HSV antibodies in serum or cerebrospinal fluid is neither sufficiently sensitive nor specific for the early diagnosis of HSV encephalitis; brain biopsy is still required for diagnosis.

Prognosis

The outcome of infection with HSV depends on many factors, including the individual characteristics of the patient (age, status of host defenses) and site of infection, and whether the infection is primary or recurrent. Primary infections are usually self-limited and of relatively short duration, but they may occasionally cause local and systemic disease that requires hospitalization (gingivostomatitis, genital herpes). In the normal person, herpetic keratitis and encephalitis are the major threats. Herpetic keratitis may occasionally lead to blindness; herpetic encephalitis may cause death. Indeed, herpetic encephalitis in which coma supervenes may be fatal in 70% of patients, with sequelae the rule in survivors.

In the newborn and in compromised hosts, herpetic infections may sometimes be subclinical or mild. The mortality in newborns is around 50% with devastating sequelae in many survivors. The mortality is also high in disseminated infections in older, compromised hosts. Recurrent herpesvirus infections are debilitating, both emotionally and physically. Ocular involvement is often prolonged. Lesions of the face and genitalia are cosmetically and psychologically distressing. Recurrences every 3 or 4 weeks are tedious, and they may be painful, especially if associated with neuralgias.

Therapy

Iododeoxyuridine, adenine arabinoside (ara-A; vidarabine) and trifluorothymidine are effective in the treatment of most cases of herpetic keratitis without, however, affecting the rate of recurrence. The investigational antiviral drug, acyclovir (ACV), is also clinically effective, and several interferon preparations for ocular herpes are currently being studied.

Systemically administered ara-A reduces the mortality and the morbidity of brain–biopsy proven HSV encephalitis if applied early in the course of the disease; it is also effective in severe forms of neonatal herpes. Because of the potential toxicity of the drug and the importance of diagnosing other treatable conditions that might mimic HSV encephalitis, a brain biopsy is required prior to using ara-A in suspected cases.

Intravenously administered ACV is effective in the prophylaxis of HSV disease in recipients of transplanted organs, and as therapy in the compromised host. ACV is also in comparative trial with ara-A for neonatal herpes. Controlled trials with systemically administered ara-A in immunocompromised patients with HSV infections have also demonstrated the efficacy of this drug.

Systemically administered ACV, as well as the topical form of the drug, is effective in reducing virus shedding, and the duration of some of the clinical manifestations of primary genital herpes. Topically administered ACV decreased virus shedding but had little effect on the clinical manifestations of either recurrent genital herpes or labial herpes. The preventive value of ACV administered during the prodromal phase of recurrent herpes is under evaluation. Other drugs, for example, phosphonoformate and interferon, are also under study.

A variety of other forms of therapy for recurrent herpetic infections have been advocated without documented efficacy. These include ether, photodynamic inactivation, BCG, levamisole, transfer factor, and smallpox (vaccinia virus) inoculation. The latter may be life-threatening in compromised hosts, such as patients with Hodgkin's disease.

Other considerations in the therapy of severe herpetic infections include the restoration of electrolytes and fluid balance. Antibacterial agents may be necessary to combat secondary infections in eczema herpeticum and neonatal herpes.

Prevention

Neonatal herpes might be prevented by cesarean section in women discovered to have genital herpes around the time of delivery. Frequent monitoring by virologic and cytologic methods from 32 weeks of gestation on would assist in detecting asymptomatic cervical infection. The women to be monitored include those with genital herpes before or during pregnancy, those who have had sexual contact with males with penile herpes and those who had herpetic lesions below the waist. Exposed neonates and those with suspected or active herpes, and patients with eczema herpeticum, should be isolated. The topical application of antiviral drugs into the eyes might be preventive in such patients, although such chemoprophylaxis has not been critically evaluated.

Mechanical measures of proved value in other infectious diseases should also be preventive of infections caused by HSV, although there is no proof of their usefulness by controlled studies. Thus, to prevent herpetic paronychia, hospital personnel should wear gloves when using tracheal catheters or carrying out procedures that necessitate putting fingers in a patient's mouth. Persons with active genital herpes should abstain from sexual contact until the lesions are healed. Although not proven, the use of condoms might prevent transmission during asymptomatic periods of shedding of infectious virus from such sites as the cervix or urethra.

Vaccines are under evaluation in experimental animals and humans for the prevention or amelioration of primary or recurrent HSV infections. Because of the potential oncogenicity and latency of herpes simplex viruses, most efforts have been directed at developing vaccines containing immunogenic glycoproteins and lacking viral DNA. Such proteins may be produced by genetic engineering, a methodology that may lead to the construction of viruses lacking the genes associated with potential disease while preserving, if not bolstering, genes coding for immunogenic proteins.

Remaining Problems

Exploration is necessary regarding the possible role of HSV in (1) cervical carcinogenesis and other cancers, (2) fetal wastage and other neonatal disease, (3) neurologic disease—acute and chronic, (4) autoimmune diseases, (5) chronic diseases of the eye and other organs.

Further understanding of latency and immune responses to HSV, as well as genetic aspects of virus and host interactions, is necessary. Basic information is needed to define more specifically the antigens of HSV-1 and HSV-2, both for improved serologic specificity and as possible immunogens.

Continued search should be made to evaluate and develop better preventive measures, and safe, effective, antiherpetic antimicrobal agents. Improved evaluation of presently available systemic drugs is necessary. The comparative aspects of human and nonhuman herpes require more concerted study.

Bibliography

Books

GALASSO GJ, MERIGAN TC, BUCHANAN RA (EDS): Antiviral Agents and Viral Diseases of Man. New York, Raven Press, 1979. 719 pp.

JUEL-JENSEN BE, MACCALLUM FO: Herpes Simplex, Varicella and Zoster: Clinical Manifestations and Treatment. Philadelphia, JB Lippincott, 1972. 194 pp.

JURETIC M: Herpetic Infections of Man. Hanover, New Hampshire, University Press of New England, 1980. 202 pp.

NAHMIAS A: The evolution (evovirology) of herpesvirus. In Kurstak E, Maramorosch (eds): Viruses, Evolution and Cancer. New York, Academic Press, 1974. pp 605–622.

NAHMIAS A, JOSEY W: Epidemiology of herpes simplex viruses 1 and 2. In Evans A (ed): Viral Infections of Humans—Epidemiology and Control, 2nd ed. New York, Plenum Press. (in press)

NAHMIAS AJ, DOWDLE W, SCHINAZI RF (EDS): The Human Herpesviruses: An Interdisciplinary Perspective. New York, Elsevier-North Holland, 1981. 721 pp.

NAHMIAS AJ, VISINTINE AM: Herpes simplex virus infection of the fetus and newborn. In Remington J, Klein JO (eds). Infectious Diseases of the Fetus and Newborn Infant, 2nd ed. Philadelphia, WB Saunders. (in press)

SHORE S, NAHMIAS A: Immunology of herpes simplex viruses. In Nahmias A, O'Reilly R (eds): Immunology of Human Infection. New York, Plenum Press, 1982. pp 21–72.

Journals

BARINGER JR, SWOVELAND P: Recovery of herpes simplex virus from human trigeminal ganglions. N Engl J Med 288:648–650, 1973

BECKER WB, KIPPS A, MCKENZIE D: Disseminated herpes simplex virus infection. Am J Dis Child 115:1–9, 1968

BUCHMAN TG, ROIZMAN B, NAHMIAS AJ: Structure of herpes simplex virus DNA and application to molecular epidemiology. Ann NY Acad Sci 354:279–290, 1980

CRAIG C, NAHMIAS A: Different patterns of neurologic involvement with herpes simplex virus types 1 and 2 from the buffy coat of two adults with meningitis. J Infect Dis 127:365–372, 1973

DODD K, JOHNSTON LM, BUDDINGH GJ: Herpetic stomatitis. J Pediatr 12:95–102, 1938

Herpesvirus and Cervical Cancer (Symposium). Cancer Res 33:1345–1563, 1973

NAHMIAS A, NORRILD B: The oncogenic potential of herpes simplex viruses and their association with cervical neoplasia. In Rapp F (ed): Oncogenic Herpesviruses, Vol 2, pp. 25–46. Boca Raton, Florida, CRC Press, 1980

NAHMIAS A, ROIZMAN B: Infection with herpes simplex viruses 1 and 2. N Engl J Med 289:667, 719, 781, 1973

NAHMIAS AJ, DOWDLE WR: Antigenic and biological differences in Herpesvirus hominis. Prog Med Virol 10:110–159, 1968

OH J (ED): Symposium on herpesvirus infections. Survey Ophthalmol 21:81–216, 1976

SMITH IW, PEUTHETER JF: The incidence of Herpesvirus hominis antibody in the population. J Hyg (Camb) 65:395–448, 1967

STERN H, ELEK SD, MILLAR DM, ANDERSON HF: Herpetic whitlow: A form of cross-infection in hospitals. Lancet 2:871–874, 1959

WHEELER CE, ABELE DC: Eczema herpeticum: Primary and recurrent. Arch Dermatol 93:162–171, 1966

WHITLEY RJ, NAHMIAS AJ, SOONG S–J, GALASSO GG, FLEMING CL, ALFORD CA: Vidarabine therapy of neonatal herpes simplex virus infection. Pediatrics 66:495–501, 1980

WHITLEY RJ, NAHMIAS AJ, VISINTINE AM, FLEMING CL, ALFORD CA: The natural history of herpes simplex virus infection of mother and newborn. Pediatrics 66: 495–501, 1908

J. DONALD MILLAR
JAMES H. NAKANO

Smallpox and Other Pox Virus Infections

92

Smallpox, until recently a terrifying natural infection in man, was the first disease of humans to be eradicated. Vaccinia is an artifically induced infection which prevents smallpox; other pox virus infections are exotic zoonoses. The respective etiologic viruses are physically similar and closely related in antigenic constituency.

Smallpox

Etiology

The smallpox viruses measure 210 nm × 260 nm. Several morphologically indistinguishable strains produce diseases of varying severity and have distinctive temperature-related growth characteristics on the chorioallantoic membrane of the chick embryo. Variola major kills 25% to 50% of humans infected with it. Variola minor, once called alastrim, is lethal in 1% or less of patients. Apparently, there are several intermediate strains that produce illnesses of intermediate severity.

Epidemiology

Natural smallpox occurred only in humans. It was once ubiquitous, and without vaccination it probably would have remained so. Although nonhuman primates may be infected under experimental conditions, they are not natural hosts. Smallpox has exterminated groups of humans not only by lethal infections but also by engendering a self-destructive hysteria. In epidemics in the plains Indians of North America (ca. 1837), entire tribes were destroyed by smallpox itself and by suicides apparently povoked by the utter incomprehensibility of such a catastrophic visitation.

The epidemiologically appropriate use of vaccination with vaccinia virus has, through a global masterwork of international cooperation, eradicated smallpox. The last case of naturally acquired smallpox occurred in Somalia in October 1977; an outbreak of two cases associated with a virologic laboratory occurred in England in 1978. Since that time there has been no smallpox in the world.

The incubation period of natural smallpox was 12 to 14 days (for inoculation smallpox, 7–8 days). Smallpox was spread from person to person, requiring neither vectors nor additional reservoirs. The respiratory tract was the usual portal of entry. Droplets of upper respiratory tract secretions contained virus shed from lesions of the oropharyngeal mucous membrane, and desquamating skin lesions were the source of virus-laden detritus that became airborne. The communicability of smallpox was relatively low in comparison with other viral infections such as measles and chickenpox. Perhaps this related to the rapid settling of the relatively large infective particles.

As a consequence, smallpox, in its latter days, spread in two settings: families and hospitals. In endemic areas, spread occurred chiefly among household members. After World War II, most cases of smallpox in nonendemic areas resulted from hospital transmission to physicians, nurses, orderlies, and other patients. In European outbreaks, spread occurred primarily to persons in intimate contact with patients: nurses and physicians directly involved in patient care; family and friends who kissed or otherwise touched the patients; and those who handled the cadaver when smallpox was lethal. Persons have been infected through airborne transmission of virus over brief distances: from one story of a building to the next in a hospital-associated outbreak in Germany and in the laboratory-associated outbreak in England in 1978.

Patients were not infective before the clinical onset of illness and were generally most infective soon after the appearance of the rash. Infection was followed by recovery or death, the person ceasing to be a source of spread of the disease 3 to 4 weeks after onset. The surviving patient was immune to reinfection virtually for life.

The Global Campaign of Smallpox Eradication

In 1966, the nineteenth World Health Assembly established a 10-year global smallpox eradication program based on favorable epidemiologic features: smallpox spreads only from person to person; the patient is infectious only briefly, and after recovery, is resistant to infection; and vaccination produces long-lasting immunity.

By May 1970, the West and Central African Smallpox Eradication (and Measles Control) Program (extensively supported by the United States) eliminated smallpox from 20 African countries. WHO-sponsored campaigns produced zero incidence of smallpox in Brazil and Zaire in 1971, Indonesia and Afghanistan in 1972, Nepal in 1973, Pakistan in 1974, and India and Bangladesh in 1975.

The last case of naturally acquired smallpox occurred in Merca, Somalia in 1977. A 23-year-old male cook in a hospital in Merca who had been unsuccessfully vaccinated in the past, contracted smallpox when exposed for a few minutes to two patients with smallpox who were being transported to an isolation camp near Merca. The driver of the vehicle stopped, seeking directions to the camp. The cook entered the vehicle and traveled briefly to clarify the directions. In the process, he was infected and developed moderately severe smallpox; the clinical diagnosis was confirmed by the isolation of variola minor. After an uncomplicated course, he recovered and was discharged at the end of November 1977. He remains alive and well in Merca and, as might be expected, has become something of an international celebrity.

The history of the global campaign is a stirring epic of modern public health and enlightened international cooperation. The achievement of eradication required a drastic change from the strategic doctrine of smallpox eradication that existed before 1966. Authorities then believed that the eradication of smallpox would require rapid vaccination of a large majority (probably more than 80%) of the entire populations in all of the smallpox-endemic countries.

An alternative approach was developed by epidemiologists working in West Africa. They suggested that transmission could be interrupted without mass vaccination by prudent exploitation of two epidemiologic aspects of the smallpox, namely: the wide and predictable seasonal variations in incidence; and the focal nature of outbreaks. At the ebb of an annual cycle, smallpox was restricted to a small number of cases in discrete outbreaks in only a few geographic locations. Through aggressive surveillance techniques, such as large scale, house-to-house searches for cases, the whereabouts of the disease was quickly and precisely defined. By concentrating intensive vaccination activities in areas known to be infected, transmission was interrupted even without mass vaccination of populations. This new technique was labeled "epidemiologically directed surveillance and containment" and once forged and tested in West Africa, it became the cornerstone method for eradicating smallpox from the remaining endemic areas of the world.

On May 8, 1980, after a 2-year process of investigation following the last case of smallpox, the 33rd World Health Assembly unanimously accepted the conclusions of the Global Commission for the Certification of Smallpox Eradication that "1. Smallpox eradication has been achieved throughout the world; 2. There is no evidence that smallpox will return as an endemic disease."

Pathogenesis and Pathology

Smallpox virus entered through the upper respiratory tract and spread to regional lymph nodes. Transient viremia followed with dissemination throughout the body. Epithelial cells were particularly vulnerable, although smallpox virus could invade all tissues.

The initial lesion was the *macule,* a focus of edema, congestion, and infiltration with mononuclear and plasma cells, that was most prominent about capillaries and small blood vessels in the papillary bodies. The *papule* represented the evolution of the process, with ballooning degeneration of epithelial cells, that is, an increase in the size of the cells with clearing around the nucleus. Spherical inclusion bodies—the so-called Guarnieri bodies, 1 μm to 4 μm in diameter—appeared in the cytoplasm and juxtanuclear cleared space of degenerating epithelial cells. As interstitital fluid collected and epithelial cells underwent necrosis, the vesicle developed. When viral replication ceased, the vesicle dried and crusted; the lesion healed and scars formed and replaced the destroyed dermal elements. Secondary staphylococcal infection of vesicles was common and probably contributed to the extent of scarring; scars were more likely to persist on the face.

Lesions of the mucous membranes followed the same course as those of the foci of necrosis in other organs. For example, lesions of the testicles and bone marrow also began in the vicinity of the endothelial cells of capillaries and small blood vessels.

The extent of viral replication was a function of several variables, including the immune status and age of the patient, the inoculating dose, and the virulence of the infecting strain of virus. Variola major was much more likely to produce fatal smallpox, whereas variola minor usually caused less severe disease. However, all strains could case both severe and mild disease; that is, clinical differentiation of the infecting strain of virus was impossible.

The very young and the very old were most likely to die of smallpox. The cause of death was not understood; toxicity was generally cited.

Manifestations

In nonvaccinated persons, a distinct, febrile illness occurred that was nonspecific—the prodrome—and lasted 2 to 4 days before eruptive smallpox. About 90% of the patients went on to typical or ordinary smallpox; approximately 10% of cases were either rapidly fatal (fulminant hemorrhagic smallpox) or unusually mild, even free of rash (variola *sine eruptione*).

On clinical bases, five broad groupings could be distinguished: hemorrhagic, flat, ordinary, modified, and variola *sine eruptione*. Hemorrhagic smallpox killed all of its victims and was frequently misdiagnosed as a hemorrhagic blood dyscrasia. The disease began with fever, which persisted throughout the illness. The rash appeared as a dusky erythema of the trunk, leading to scattered petechiae, diffuse purpura, or large ecchymoses of skin and mucous membranes. A vesicular rash did not develop.

Flat smallpox was frequently fatal; the rash failed to mature. Illness began with a fever that could persist after the rash emerged. A dusky erythema appeared on the face, trunk, and arms. Velvety papules developed slowly and sometimes became vesicular after 10 to 12 days. Instead of scabbing, the epidermis peeled away in sheets. Death occurred during the second week.

Ordinary smallpox killed 1% to 50% of patients. The febrile prodrome was of varying severity, but it always occurred. The fever fell before the rash appeared. The lesions, even when sparse, were distributed in a centrifugal pattern; the face, arms, and legs were more heavily involved than the trunk. Appearing as erythematous macules, the lesions became papular and evolved progressively through the vesicular and pustular stages to scabs in about 2 weeks. All lesions were in approximately the same stage of development. The scabs separated, leaving fresh scars that were permanent in half the survivors.

Modified smallpox usually occurred in previously vaccinated persons with residual immunity; it rarely killed. Vaccinomodification altered the rash, but there was little or no change in the prodrome. The rash was sparse, but remained distinctly centrifugal. The characteristics of the lesions were more like those of chickenpox: a shortened period of rash evolution, more superficial placement of lesions, and an increased tendency to cropping. Modified smallpox was particularly significant in the spread of the disease, because the patients remained mobile and could transmit severe smallpox to susceptible contacts. Thus, in an outbreak of smallpox in Stockholm, Sweden in 1963, five of the initial six cases of smallpox involved persons with highly modified disease, retrospectively diagnosed when the epidemic had reached its fifth generation.

Variola *sine eruptione* was smallpox aborted by existing immunity; only the febrile prodrome occurred. Such cases developed only in vaccinated persons who were intensely exposed, for example, while caring for patients with smallpox. In this form, the disease was not contagious.

Diagnosis

Though infrequent, the unusual clinical forms of smallpox posed formidable diagnostic problems, whereas ordinary smallpox consistently yielded to confident clinical diagnosis. Epidemiologists of the Centers for Disease Control based their judgments on four criteria: (1) There was (or was not) a possible exposure to smallpox 2 weeks before onset of illness. (2) There was (or was not) a distinct febrile prodrome. (3) There was (or was not) a visible scar of primary vaccination. (4) The rash did (or did not) conform to smallpox in the distribution, evolution, and characteristics of the individual lesions.

In the posteradication era, any transmission of smallpox must necessarily begin with the escape of smallpox virus from a laboratory. Thus, a person with smallpox must have an appropriate history of exposure to a laboratory containing smallpox virus or must have acquired smallpox from a previously undetected intermediary related directly or indirectly to a laboratory source of smallpox virus. A definable prodromal illness is a highly consistent feature of smallpox. The presence of a vaccination scar (opposed to a history of vaccination) is of distinct diagnostic advantage. From the experience in India, Pakistan, and West Africa, more than 80% of all smallpox cases occurred in persons without primary vaccination scars.

Among conditions confused with smallpox, varicella, and other general herpesvirus infections are by far the most common. Chickenpox and smallpox differ in prodromal illness and in the appearance of the rash itself—distribution, evolution, and characteristics of the individual lesions (stage, border, depth, feel):

1. The prodrome of smallpox is a distinct, febrile illness lasting 2 to 4 days; there is usually no prodrome in chickenpox.
2. The rash of smallpox, even when only a few lesions are present, is centrifugal—more dense on the head, arms, and legs, and less dense on the trunk (Fig. 92-1). In chickenpox, the rash is as dense on the trunk as elsewhere. In both diseases, lesions may occur on the palms, soles, and mucous membranes.
3. The lesions of smallpox appear in a single crop and evolve to scabs and scars. Maturation to the pustular stage requires about a week (Plate 92-1); approximately 2 weeks intervene between onset and scabbing. Chickenpox appears in several crops over 2 to 4 days, with lesions evolving from macule to scabe in 24 to 48 hours. Thus, a second physical examination 6 hours after the first reveals distinct evolution, often with a new crop of lesions (Plate 92-1*C*).
4. The characteristics of the individual lesions are quite helpful: (a) Stage—in smallpox, all lesions are at essentially the same stage of development. In chickenpox, a single area of skin may present lesions in all stages from macule to scab. (b) Shape—the lesions of smallpox are round with smooth borders and display roughly similar configurations. Chickenpox lesions are irregular in shape and size and have crenated borders. (c) Depth—deep lesions, clearly reaching into the dermis, are characteristic of smallpox; the lesions of chickenpox are superficial. (d) Feel—smallpox vesicles feel shotty. Chickenpox vesicles feel soft and collapse easily.

Fig. 92-1. The skin lesions of smallpox characteristically display a centrifugal pattern of distribution. (Courtesy of the World Health Organization)

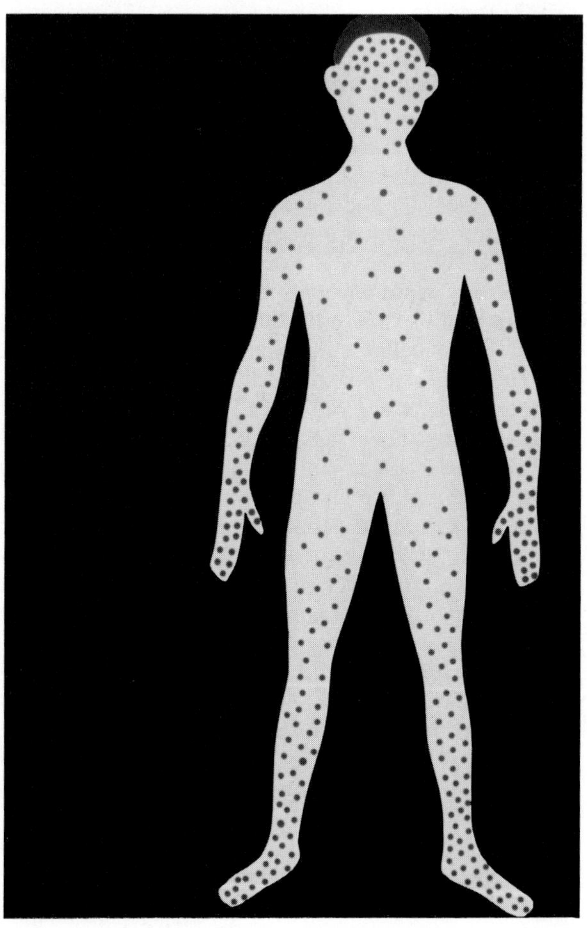

In the laboratory, the classic means for differentiating variola and chickenpox viruses has involved the inoculation of embryonated hens' eggs. Variola, vaccinia, and monkeypox viruses produce pocks on the chorioallantoic membrane 48 to 72 hours after inoculation; varicella virus has no effect. Differentiation can now be accomplished in as little as 1 hour by the examination of material from vesicles, pus, or crusts by electron microscopy. Variola, vaccinia, and monkeypox viruses are not easily distinguished from each other, but they are readily separable on the basis of appearance from herpes and varicella viruses (Fig. 92-2).

If the clinical findings are at all consistent with smallpox, a public health emergency exists, and the local health officer must be informed at once. Other immediate actions include: strict isolation of the patient and identification of his contacts including physicians, nurses, orderlies, and other hospital workers, for vaccination and surveillance.

Prognosis

The prognosis in smallpox depended primarily on the strain of infecting virus, the clinical form of the disease, and the age of the patient. The quality of the medical care made remarkably little difference.

A variety of complications occurred including pneumonitis, corneal destruction, encephalitis, joint effusions, and osteitis. All except pneumonitis were infrequent. Although second attacks of smallpox have been recorded, they were so rare as to be medical curiosities. The immunity following smallpox was, for practical purposes, lifelong.

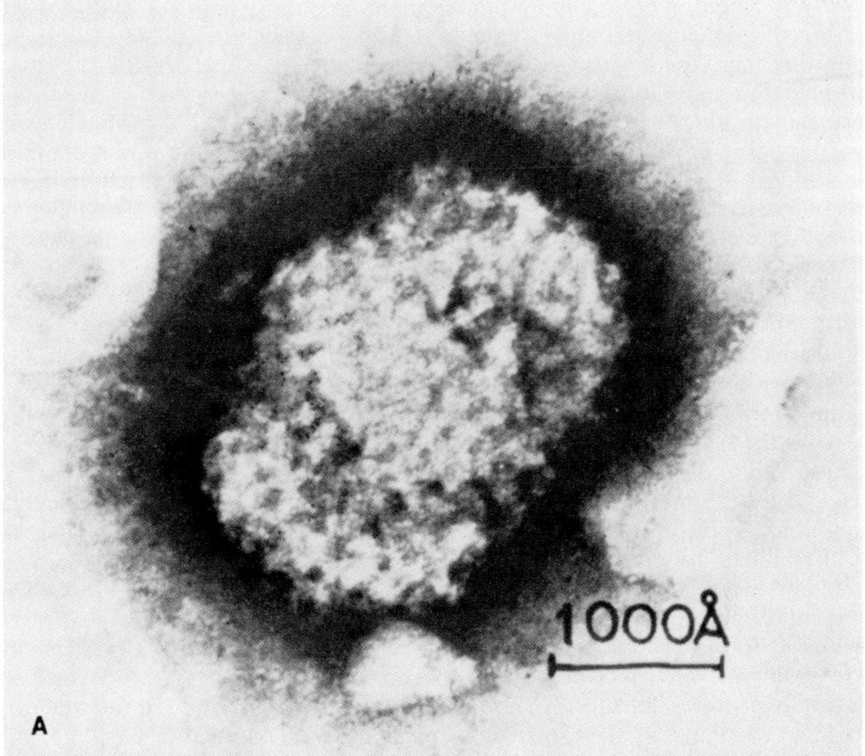

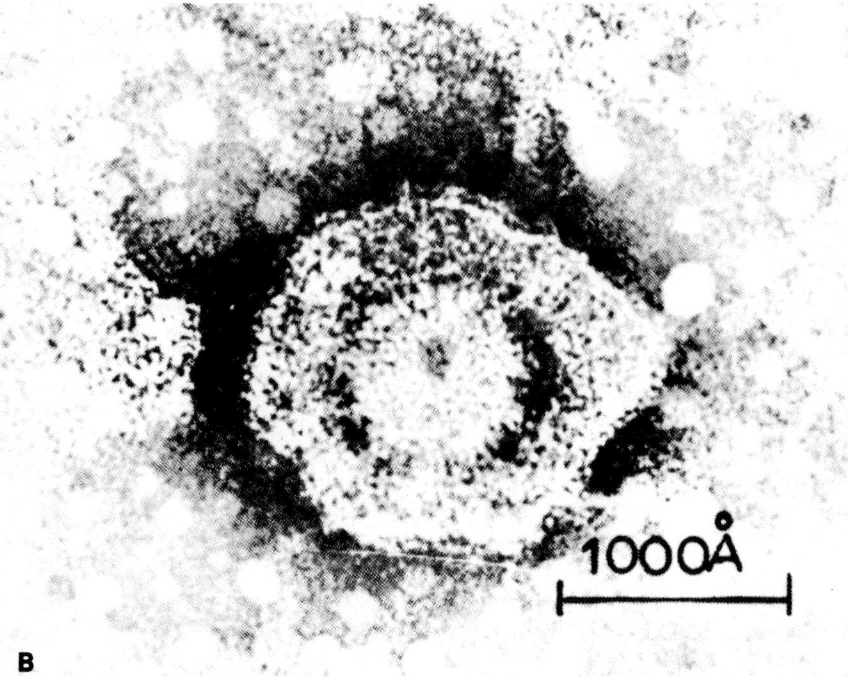

Fig. 92-2. (*A*) Variola virus particles in the crust of a skin lesion. (Original magnification approximately × 40,000) (*B*) Chickenpox virus particles in a smear of vesicular fluid. (Cruickshank JG, Bedson HS, Watson DH: Lancet 1:528, 1966) (Original magnification approximately × 200,000)

Therapy

Although vaccinia immune globulin (VIG) and methisazone (methylisatin-beta-thiosemicarbazone) were shown to be of some prophylactic effect, there was no specific treatment for the patient with smallpox. Support of nutritional and hygienic needs, and treatment of superinfections with antimicrobial agents were all that could be done.

Prevention

Vaccination with vaccinia virus produces immunity to smallpox for a relatively long period. The procedure was introduced by Edward Jenner; on May 14, 1796, in Gloucestershire, England, he inoculated 8-year-old James Phipps with material from a cowpox sore on the hand of Sarah Nelmes, a milkmaid. Vaccination today differs little from Jenner's technique, except in the superiority of the inoculum. Excellent immunity is produced in virtually every person properly vaccinated with a potent vaccine.

Long before Jenner's discovery, prophylaxis was accomplished by dermal inoculation of pus or scab materials from the lesions of smallpox—variolation. The result was far fewer deaths than occurred from naturally acquired smallpox. The practice persisted in modern times among isolated peoples, for religious or magical reasons, as well as for prevention of smallpox. Variolated persons with active lesions were as great a hazard to susceptible persons as patients with naturally acquired smallpox. Intensive investigations by WHO in the certification of smallpox eradication failed to reveal viable virus more than 9 months after the specimen was said to have been originally collected from a patient with smallpox. Hence, the possibility that a smallpox infection might be initiated in the future from some material sequestered by a variolator is extremely remote.

Remaining Problems

The eradication of smallpox has left no unsolved problems which rival those solved in order to eradicate the disease. That smallpox was eliminated before the discovery of a specific therapy, is a pristine example of the transcendent quality of preventive medicine. Thus, remaining problems of smallpox will have relevance only if smallpox virus is somehow reintroduced into human populations.

The WHO has listed the possible sources for such reintroductions as: laboratory stocks of variola virus, the use of variola virus as a biologic weapon in warfare, variola virus in old crusts, and animal reservoirs of variola virus. As a result of the international cooperative efforts of the WHO, the laboratories maintaining stocks of smallpox virus have been reduced to five, of which only one (Centers for Disease Control) is in the Western Hemisphere. Precautions for handling these stocks were prescribed in detail by the WHO with the aim of eliminating any risk of the escape of variola virus. Although treaties barring the use of biologic weapons have been signed by the major powers, the nefarious use of smallpox virus (particularly by terrorists) is conceivable. Since the offending parties would have to breach the security arrangements in one or more of the laboratories in which variola virus is stored, alarm would probably be given. In any case, the relatively slow transmission of smallpox, and its blatant clinical appearance (especially in unimmunized persons) would reveal its presence soon enough to permit restriction of transmission by vaccination to relatively few cases. However, the possibility of the hostile use of smallpox virus emphasizes the need for continued surveillance of febrile illnesses with rash and the prompt investigation of any rumors of smallpox. Also, this possibility, however remote, is one reason for the continued use of smallpox vaccination for active duty military personnel.

Since declaring the world free of smallpox, the WHO has investigated many rumors of smallpox; none has proved to be smallpox and most, as expected, were cases of chickenpox. Because of the limited persistence of viable virus in old crusts, such as those retained by variolators, this is a most unlikely source for reintroduction.

Although nonhuman primate hosts can be infected with smallpox virus, there is no documented instance of smallpox having been transmitted from nonhumans to humans despite intense epidemiologic interest in the possibility for several decades. In recent years, infections of monkeypox in humans have been detected in Africa and thoroughly investigated. The reports of these cases confirm that the existing systems for surveillance of illnesses with skin rashes in countries in which smallpox was previously endemic are effective. The discovery of a variolalike "white pox" virus in tissues from monkeys from Malaysia and Zaire provoked additional questions about the relationships between pox viruses and the potential for their transformation from one species to another. However, the possibility that some other pox virus species might change in variola is so remote that the conceivable risk of reintroducing smallpox in this way must be viewed as only a theoretical construction.

Vaccinia

Infection with vaccinia virus is usually deliberately induced in vaccination to prevent smallpox. Vaccinia virus is not distinguishable from smallpox and other pox viruses by electronmicroscopy. Although vaccinia, variola, monkeypox, and whitepox viruses appear to be closely related to each other, each produces distinctive pocks on the chorioallantoic membrane of the chick embryo.

Vaccinia virus vaccine is prepared by the inoculation of ruminants, usually calves. The pulp that results from confluent dermal lesions is processed to prepare either thermolabile liquid vaccine or thermostable lyophilized vaccine. Minimum potency standards (WHO) specify a titer of 10^8 pock-forming units per milliliter of vaccine. Lyophilized vaccine has virtually replaced lymph vaccine because of its superiority for field use.

Vaccination is performed by various methods. The successful methods include multiple-pressure and multiple-puncture techniques, and intradermal jet injection. The scratch technique, although excellent for primary vaccination, is inferior for revaccination. Rotary lancet vaccination, once used routinely in India and Pakistan, is unacceptable.

In the multiple-pressure technique, 30 strokes are applied through a drop of vaccine with a needle held tangentially to the skin of the lateral aspect of the upper arm. With a special bifurcated needle*, the simpler technique of multiple puncture is carried out with the needle perpendicular to the skin. A bridge between the two forks of the needle prevents deep penetration.

The intradermal jet injection of 0.1 ml diluted vaccine ($10^{6.5}$ plaque-forming units per ml) is rapid and thoroughly reliable, yielding primary take rates consistently in excess of 98%.

Successful primary vaccination by any method produces the typical Jennerian vesicle, which evolves to scabbing in 14 to 21 days (Plate 92-2*A*). Cutaneous responses to successful revaccination include delayed hypersensitivity occurring within 24 to 72 hours (elicited by both impotent and potent vaccines) and induration and vesiculation due to viral multiplication generally evolving 1 to 2 weeks after inoculation (Plate 92-2*B*).

Because there are difficulties in interpreting revaccination responses, the World Health Organization advocates a single examination of the vaccination site 7 days after inoculation. Findings are classified either as a major reaction, indicating viral growth, or an equivocal reaction, which is likely to indicate only hypersensitivity. A major reaction is "one which on examination six to eight days after vaccination presents a vesicular or pustular lesion which may be a scab or ulcer." All other findings are termed equivocal reactions and are presumed to signify failure of revaccination.

Primary vaccination yields protective immunity against smallpox for 3 to 5 years. Protection wanes gradually, with some ameliorating influence on the severity of disease persisting for up to 20 years. For persons who had a distinct risk of exposure, such as travelers to smallpox-infected areas, a successful revaccination every 3 years assured a consistent, high level of protection.

The complications of vaccination, include: postvaccinal encephalitis, eczema vaccinatum, vaccinia necrosum, generalized vaccinia, accidental implantation (especially in the eye), and miscellaneous dermal manifestations. Surveys in the United States indicate one death for each million primary vaccinations. The risks of death among children vaccinated during the first year of life (generally 6 to 12 months of age in the United States) are 4 to 5 per million. Complications after revaccination are dramatically less frequent than those after primary vaccination.

The dermal complications, particularly vaccinia necrosum and eczema vaccinatum, can be successfully treated with vaccinia immune globulin and methisazone. Topical idoxuridine has been useful in treating implantations involving the cornea.

Vaccination poses an increased risk of complications in persons who have (1) eczema or a history of eczema either in the subject or a member of his household, (2) neoplasia involving the hematopoietic–lymphoreticular system, (3) immunologic disorders including therapy with immunosuppressants, (4) pregnancy, and (5) an acute febrile illness. The rigid observance of these contraindications would reduce the complications of vaccination by half.

Because smallpox has been absent from the United States since 1949, the advisability of routine childhood vaccination was increasingly challenged during the 1960s. In 1972, the Public Health Service Advisory Committee on Immunization Practices recommended against the use of smallpox vaccine in routine pediatric immunization schedules. Now that smallpox has been eradicated, vaccination (of civilians) is recommended only for one very small group, laboratory workers directly involved with smallpox or closely related pox viruses.

Although occasionally smallpox vaccination is used as a treatment for recurrent infections with herpes simplex virus, warts, or other skin conditions, there is no documentation of any therapeutic value.

Remaining Problems

Thomas Jefferson in 1806 wrote to Edward Jenner, ". . . future generations will know by history only that the loathsome smallpox has existed." One hun-

*Developed by Wyeth Laboratories, Philadelphia, Pennsylvania.

dred and seventy-five years later, Jefferson's prophecy has come to pass. Over the years vaccinia virus vaccine has proved to be one of the most effective and safest of immunogens. Lyophilization and the development of simple vaccination methods eliminated most of the field problems of vaccination. In the hands of hundreds of thousands of minimally trained vaccinators throughout the world, the vaccine proved adequate for the eradication of smallpox.

In every sense, smallpox vaccine deserves the title "noble" agent. Nonetheless, the vaccine is not perfect and its use entails risks to health. The eradication of smallpox has drastically reduced the need for vaccinia virus vaccination. Though the risks of vaccination are small, only persons with some possibility of exposure to smallpox virus and its close relatives should be subjected to them. Future concerns regarding vaccinia are to assure that the vaccine is used only for this highly selected target group. Stockpiles of vaccine for use in the unlikely event of reintroduction of smallpox in the human population have been arranged by the WHO, the United States, and other national governments.

Monkeypox

In Copenhagen, Denmark, in 1958, an outbreak of an illness with rash occurred among captive cynomolgus monkeys. The causative agent was a new species of poxvirus of the same genus as smallpox and vaccinia. This agent caused other outbreaks in captive Asian monkeys over the subsequent 10 years. In August, 1970, a child in a region in Zaire that had been free of smallpox for over 6 months, developed a smallpoxlike disease; monkeypox virus was isolated from skin lesions of the patient. Since then, this newly detected pox virus has been recovered from 56 persons suffering a smallpoxlike illness. These cases occurred in several West and Central African countries. The symptoms are similar to the intermediate form of smallpox as it occurred in Africa before smallpox eradication. Eight patients died, none of whom had been vaccinated. In four instances, person-to-person transmission occurred among members of the same family with secondary cases developing in about 2 weeks. Transmission beyond the second generation did not occur.

The source of these human infections has been extensively investigated and is, at present, unclear. The populations in which the cases occurred were in frequent contact with monkeys but also with numerous other wild animals. No monkeypox virus has been isolated from wild animals in their natural environment. However, serologic studies of monkeys and rodents in the African areas in which human cases occurred, revealed antibodies to orthopox viruses in a significant proportion of the animals; radioimmunoassay tests confirmed the existence of specific monkeypox antibodies in the monkeys.

Monkeypox is of principle concern because its clinical manifestations are apparently so similar to those of smallpox. The prodrome is a febrile illness of 2 to 4 days' duration, followed by eruption. Lymphadenopathy in the neck and inguinal areas seem to be more prominent than in smallpox. The distribution of the rash, its evolution, and the characteristics of the lesions also resemble smallpox (Plate 92-1*D*). By electron microscopy, the monkeypox virus is morphologically indistinguishable from smallpox and vaccinia. However, it is easily differentiated by the morphology of the pocks it produces on the chorioallantoic membrane of the chick embryo. It can also be differentiated from other viruses by electrophoretic patterns of its solubilized structural protein on polyacrylamide gel, electropherograms of restriction endonuclease, digested DNA fragments, and DNA mappings.

It appears that vaccination can prevent or at least modify monkeypox. Because of the clinical similarity to smallpox, and the fact that the origins of smallpox are unknown, the discovery of monkeypox has heightened interest in the relationships among the pox viruses and the potential for one to transform into another.

Whitepox

Another development on the pox virologic frontier is the discovery of the whitepox or albapox virus, an agent which is remarkably similar to smallpox virus in most of its laboratory characteristics. It was isolated in the Netherlands in 1964 from the kidneys of healthy cynomologous monkeys from Malaysia. Later, the virus was also recovered from the kidneys of four apparently healthy wild animals (one chimpanzee, one sala monkey, and two rodents) in Zaire. These animals were captured in the area in which cases of monkeypox in humans were under intense investigation. During the past 10 years, the surveillance system in Zaire and in the western countries of Africa has been sensitive enough to detect 56 cases of infection in humans caused by monkeypox virus. Yet, in Zaire and elsewhere, there has been no case of smallpoxlike illness in humans that might have arisen by transmission of virus from some wild animals to humans. Whitepox virus has never been recovered from humans and is not known to cause disease in humans.

Cowpox

Cowpox is a pox virus infection of cattle manifested as a vesicular eruption of the udder and teats. The cowpox virus can infect humans; usually it produces lesions on the hands and immunity to smallpox, as Jenner observed in 1796. The virus is antigenically similar to present vaccinia strains; natural cowpox is no longer present in the United States.

Cowpox should not be confused with milker's nodules (pseudocowpox, paravaccinia), a vesicular disease of cattle in the United States. Occasionally, milker's nodules are acquired by persons who milk infected cows. No cross-immunity to vaccinia (or smallpox) is produced. In 1963, a pox virus agent was isolated in bovine cell tissue culture from a 17-year-old male with milker's nodules; the patient had been successfully vaccinated several years previously. The virus is distinctly different from cowpox and vaccinia viruses.

Bibliography

Books

DIXON CW: Smallpox. London, JA Churchill, 1962. 512 pp.

NAKANO JH: Poxviruses. In Lennette EH, Schmidt NJ (eds): Diagnostic Procedures for Viral Rickettsial and Chlamydial Diseases, 5th ed. American Public Health Association, Washington, D.C., 1979. pp 257–308.

RICKETTS TF, BYLES JB: The Diagnosis of Smallpox, London, Cassell, 1908. Vol I (text), 147 pp; Vol II, 121 plates.

Smallpox. In Control of Communicable Diseases in Man. New York, American Public Health Association, 1975. pp 288–297.

World Health Organization. The Global Eradication of Smallpox: Final Report of the Global Commission for the Certification of Smallpox Eradication. Geneva, 1980. 122 pp.

Journals

ARITA I: Virological evidence for the success of the smallpox eradication programme. Nature 279:293–298, 1979

ARITA I, HENDERSON DA: Smallpox and monkeypox in non-human primates. Bull WHO 39:277–283, 1968

ESPOSITO JJ, OBIJESKIE JF, NAKANO JH: The virion and soluble antigen proteins of variola, monkeypox and vaccinia viruses. J Med Virol 1:95–110, 1977

FOEGE WH: Editorial: Should the smallpox virus be allowed to survive? N Engl J Med 300:670–671, 1979

FOEGE WH, MILLAR JD, HENDERSON DA: Smallpox eradication in West and Central Africa. Bull WHO 52:209–222, 1975

FRIEDMAN–KIEN AE, ROWE WP, BANFIELD WG: Milker's nodules: Isolation of a poxvirus from a human case. Science 140:1335–1336, 1963

LANE JM, MILLAR JD: Routine childhood vaccination against smallpox reconsidered. N Engl J Med 281:1220–1224, 1969

NEFF JM, LANE JM, PERT JH, MOORE R, MILLAR JD, HENDERSON DA: Complications of smallpox vaccination. I. National survey in the United States, 1963. N Engl J Med 276: 125–132, 1967

Progress in smallpox eradication. WHO Chron 28(8):359–1363, 1974

RAO AR: Some epidemiological and clinical features of smallpox and its diagnosis. Bull Ind Soc Malaria Other Comm Dis 3:96–112, 1966

SMALLPOX VACCINE: Recommendation of the Immunization Advisory Committee (ACIP). Morb Mort Weekly Report 29:417–420, 1980

S. MICHAEL MARCY
SIDNEY KIBRICK

93 Varicella and Herpes Zoster

Varicella or chickenpox (a name possibly derived from Old English *gican,* "to itch," or from the resemblance of the vesicles of the rash to chick peas [*Cicer arietinum*]) is a highly contagious, acute exanthematous disease that is most common in childhood. It is characterized by successive crops of pruritic lesions that progress rapidly from macules and papules to vesicles, pustules, and crusts. In children, chickenpox is generally a mild disease with few complications. When acquired by adults, however, it is often associated with high fever, severe constitutional symptoms, and pulmonary involvement.

Herpes zoster or shingles (a name derived from Latin *cingulus* "a girdle," to describe the progression of the rash around the body) is caused by the same virus, but it is primarily a disease of adults. It is thought to represent reactivation of a latent varicella infection in a person with waning immunity to this virus.

Etiology

Chickenpox and herpes zoster are both caused by the varicella-zoster (V-Z) virus, a member of the herpesvirus family (Herpesviridae). Other pathogens for humans in this group include herpes simplex viruses (Chap. 91, Infections Caused by Herpes Simplex Virus), the cytomegaloviruses (Chap. 75, Cytomegalovirus Infections), and the Epstein–Barr virus of infectious mononucleosis (Chap. 137, Infectious Mononucleosis). These agents tend to produce a persistent, perhaps lifelong, infection after primary invasion.

The V-Z virion contains double-stranded DNA and is approximately 200 nm in diameter (Fig. 93-1). The DNA core is enclosed in a capsid of icosohedral symmetry that is made up of 162 capsomeres and is contained in a roughly spherical lipoprotein envelope. The envelope contains both virus-specific subunits, particularly glycoproteins, and host cell materials; it is formed by evagination of the inner nuclear membrane, which is altered morphologically and pinched off as it surrounds the nucleocapsids that have been synthesized and assembled in the host cell nucleus. Some particles acquire additional envelope material from the cytoplasm. Both non-virion- and virion-associated complement-fixing (CF) antigens have been demonstrated. Most of the CF activity is non-virion associated. An indirect hemagglutinating antigen is thought to be present in the viral envelope. The V-Z viruses appear to be antigenically homogeneous—there is only one serotype.

None of the common laboratory animals are susceptible to infection with V-Z viruses, with the possible exception of the guinea pig. However, V-Z virus can be isolated and propagated in a variety of primary and cell-line cultures of human or simian origin and in cells from guinea pig embryos. The cytopathic effect in such cultures is characteristically focal, with the formation of large multinucleated giant cells or syncytia containing intranuclear eosinophilic inclusion bodies. Replication proceeds through the direct transfer of viral particles from cell to neighboring cell; infectious virions are not released into the liquid phase of most tissue cultures. Indeed, on electromicroscopic examination, viruses obtained from tissue culture liquid are frequently ragged and misshapen and often have defective cores or membranes.

In contrast, the V-Z viruses obtained from vesicle fluid are intact and infectious. Even though recovery is readily accomplished from vesicles, virus isolation is only occasionally successful from infected tissues and is rare from the blood, nasopharynx, or saliva of patients with chickenpox.

The V-Z virus loses its infectivity rather quickly in the external environment—probably within hours. Infectivity is also abolished by exposure to heat or trypsin. Acycloguanosine, 5-iodo-2-deoxyuridine (IDU), and either cytosine or adenine arabinoside inhibit replication *in vitro*.

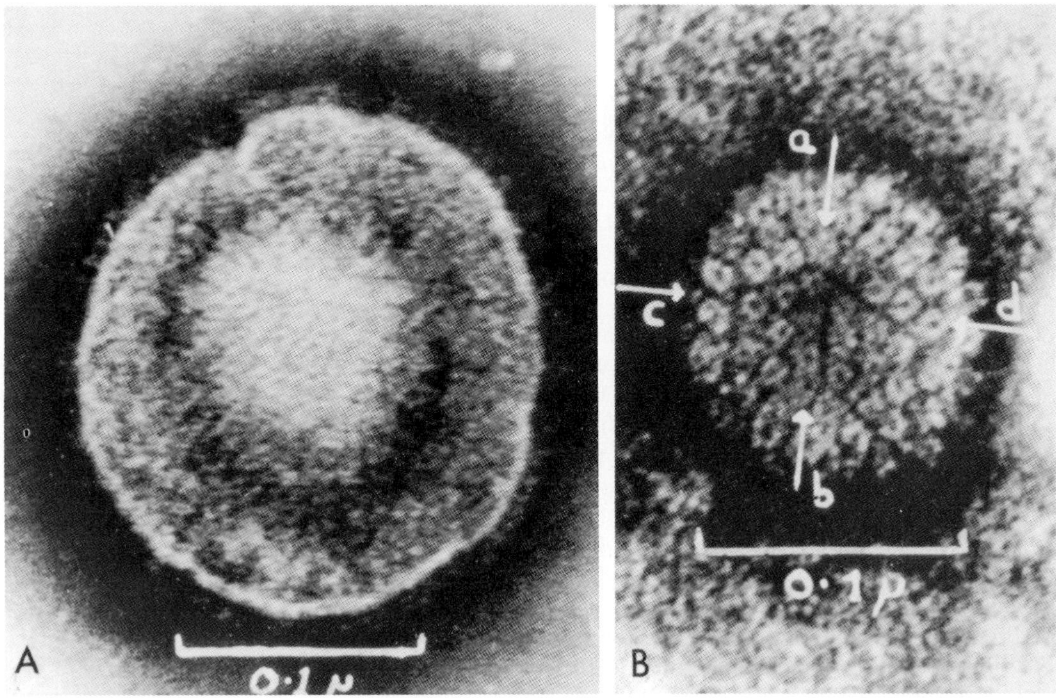

Fig. 93-1. Varicella-zoster virus. (*A*) Intact virus particle. Note surface projections. (*B*) Rupture of the capsule exposes the detailed structure of the capsid. (Original magnification approximately × 200,000) (Almeida JD, Howatson AF, Williams MG: Virology 16:353–355, 1962)

Varicella

Epidemiology

Humans are the only known natural host of chickenpox. Transmission of V-Z virus probably occurs through direct contact, by droplet spread, or within a limited time and distance from an infected person, by indirect spread. Unlike smallpox, crusts do not contain infectious virus.

Despite the apparent lability of the virus, varicella is highly contagious. The virus is transmissible from about 1 day before (rarely, 2–3 days) until 5 days after onset of the exanthem or until all vesicles are dry. Virus has been isolated from vesicles up to 3 days after the appearance of the rash in normal patients; in patients with immunodeficiency disorders such as leukemia or lymphoma, persistence of virus, duration of the eruptive phase, and communicability may all be prolonged.

Chickenpox is primarily a disease of childhood. In temperate zones, the maximum observed incidence is at around 6 years of age and is associated with entering school. Almost 90% of cases occur before the age of 9 years. If spread is limited by the isolation of patients with varicella, as once occurred in certain tropical countries through fear of misdiagnosis of smallpox, the percentage of cases occurring in persons over 20 years of age may be considerably increased. Chickenpox has been reported in neonates and the aged, although the high incidence in childhood makes this disease rare in adults. The placental transfer of passive immunity is usually completely protective, but not always. Varicella has been acquired in the first month of life by infants born to immune mothers.

The disease is endemic throughout the year, although most cases occur in the winter and spring. Epidemics, with a doubling of the attack rate, occur in cycles of 2 to 3 years. Local epidemics are seen mainly in susceptible young children in situations that favor crowding—in institutions, boarding schools, and hospital wards, for example.

Pathogenesis and Pathology

Fenner's classic observations on ectromelia (mousepox) in the mouse (Chap. 86, Measles) are generally accepted by analogy as applicable to the pathogenesis of varicella and many exanthematous diseases. Sufficient data are now available to support this assumption with regard to varicella. Most cases are probably acquired through close contact with infectious lesions or by droplets produced by talking, coughing, sneezing, with the virus entering the respiratory passages or conjunctivae. Occasionally, airborne transmission also occurs. The primary site of replication is uncertain, but it may be the regional lymph nodes and tonsils, or the ductal tissue of the salivary glands. Following 4 to 6 days of replication, a primary viremia ensues, seeding internal organs, including the liver, spleen, respiratory tract, and other organs. Replication at these sites is followed by a secondary, more prolonged viremia, which results in spread of virus to the skin and appearance of the rash at about 14 days after the onset of the infection. The skin lesions appear in crops, consistent with an intermittent viremia and multiple cycles of focal viral replication. One to four days after onset of the rash, coincident with the appearance of measurable amounts of circulating antibody, viremia ceases and symptoms begin to abate. The prolonged and severe eruptions that occur in patients with deficiencies in cellular immunity may testify to the importance of delayed hypersensitivity as a major determinant of resistance to the infection. The concentration of interferon in vesicular fluid is inversely related to the severity of disease. The role of interferon in varicella, however, remains to be determined.

The histopathology of the skin lesions of varicella and herpes zoster is identical, and it is similar to that seen in herpes simplex. The early papular lesions are minute vacuoles surrounded by ballooning degeneration of epithelial cells within the prickle cell (Malpighian) layer of the epidermis. In a few hours, edema fluid accumulates, elevating the stratum corneum to form a clear vesicle, while multinucleated giant cells, containing eosinophilic type A intranuclear inclusions, form among the cells at the edges and base of the lesion (Fig. 93-2). The capillary endothelium and fibroblasts in the corium adjacent to the vesicles may also contain intranuclear inclusions. As the vesicles begin to dry, they become filled with a cloudy, fibrinous fluid containing leukocytes and desquamated epidermal cells; this is followed by crusting along with regeneration of the epithelial cells. Vesicles on mucous membranes develop in a similar manner; however, the roof quickly becomes thickened, edematous, and macerated, and it sloughs to form a shallow ulcer that heals rapidly. Focal lesions may also occur on the serosa of the peritoneal and pleural surfaces and in visceral organs.

In varicella pneumonia, there is a diffuse interstitial and peribronchiolar mononuclear cell response, with scattered areas of focal necrosis, consolidation, and alveolar hemorrhage. Alveoli and bronchioles may be lined or filled with a proteinaceous exudate composed of erythrocytes, fibrin, and inclusion-bearing mononuclear cells. Intranuclear inclusions are also seen within alveolar lining cells, endothelial cells, and fibroblasts, as well as bronchiolar and tracheobronchial epithelium.

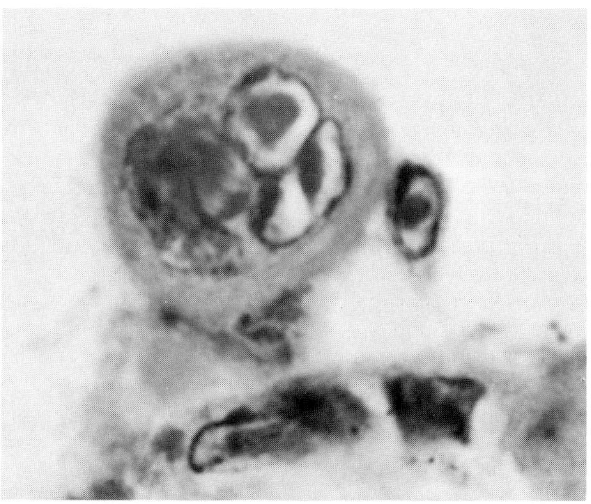

Fig. 93-2. Multinucleated giant cell from base of zoster vesicle. (Original magnification approximately × 1600) (Case Records of the Massachusetts General Hospital. N Engl J Med 294:485–493, 1976)

The pathologic changes of varicella encephalitis are nonspecific, and they are similar to those seen in measles, mumps, and other postinfectious encephalitides—for example, edema, scattered petechial hemorrhage, and perivenous demyelination with round-cell infiltration. Although direct viral invasion of the central nervous system (CNS) is believed to occur, inclusion bodies have been observed in the CNS only once, and V-Z virus has not been isolated from the brain or spinal fluid in varicella encephalitis. In fatal varicella, areas of focal necrosis, with or without characteristic inclusions, have been observed in almost every organ.

Manifestations

Prodromal symptoms are generally lacking in young children; occasionally, slight malaise or low-grade fever is seen. In older children and adults, 1 to 2 days of low-grade fever, myalgia, and mild constitutional symptoms are frequent. A fleeting erythema, occurring just before or coincident with the appearance of the vesicular rash, has been described.

The varicella rash usually appears 14 to 15 days after exposure (range, 10–23 days). Within 12 to 24 hours, individual skin lesions evolve from small red macules to papules, vesicles, then pustules that generally begin to crust.

The vesicles are variable in size and shape. They are filled with straw-colored fluid and are surrounded at the base by an intense red corona of inflammation. They seem to lie on, rather than in, the skin, resembling a small chickpea, or "a dew-drop on a rose petal." As the vesicles dry, septa that have formed within pull down on the roof, producing an umbilicated appearance, and the red areola fades. The crusts that subsequently form may fall off in 1 week, but they often persist 2 to 3 weeks, particularly in lesions that have become secondarily infected. As the crusts separate, they reveal shallow pink depressions that may pass through a stage of depigmentation before disappearing over the ensuing weeks to months. Scar or keloid formation is rare in uncomplicated varicella. Atypical vesicles with relatively thick roofs may occur on the palms, soles, and other exposed areas. Vesicles on the mucous membranes, particularly in the mouth or on the vulva, rapidly become macerated and develop into shallow white ulcers. The exanthem of chickenpox characteristically appears in successive crops for 1 to 6 days. Consequently, lesions in a given area may be seen in all stages of development from macule to crust as the disease progresses (Fig. 92-2*C*). The eruption also tends to have a central concentration, presenting first and in greatest abundance on the trunk, then the neck, face, and proximal extremities. Lesions are sparse on the distal extremities and unusual on the palms or soles. Vesicles often appear early, simultaneously, and in profuse numbers on areas of skin irritation such as diaper rash, sunburn, eczema, and other forms of dermatitis.

There is wide variation in the severity and intensity of the rash. The illness may be limited to several vesicles appearing in a single crop; at the other extreme, thousands of lesions, erupting in five or six crops, may cover the entire body. In general, more vesicles are seen in secondary cases—probably reflecting more intimate and prolonged family contact—and in older persons. There is epidemiologic evidence for the rare occurrence of inapparent infections.

Vesicles on the skin are painless; however, lesions on the tympanum, cornea, or mucosal surfaces may produce great discomfort. Pruritis is extremely common during the first few days of the eruption, probably accounting for the sleeplessness so characteristic of childhood varicella. Nonspecific symptoms, usually more severe in older children and adults, include irritability or listlessness, headache, chilly sensations, anorexia, and myalgia.

Fever normally persists as long as new lesions continue to appear, and it is generally proportional to the severity of the rash. Oral temperatures usually do not exceed 37.8°C to 38.5°C (100°F–101°F). Prolonged fever or a rise in temperature after defervescence is most commonly seen after a secondary bacterial infection or other complications.

Varicella bullosa is a rare, benign manifestation of chickenpox usually limited to children under 2 years of age. Crops of bullae, 2 cm to 7 cm in diameter, develop from single vesicles, leaving denuded areas when the soft, thin-walled, bullae rupture. Healing is rapid and without scarring. Complications are no more frequent than in ordinary varicella. In some cases, the bullous lesions may represent a variant of the staphylococcal scalded skin syndrome, appearing 2 to 5 days after onset of the typical varicella lesions.

PRIMARY VARICELLA PNEUMONIA

Varicella pneumonia is uncommon in normal children. However, 16% to 33% of adults with chickenpox show clinical or roentgenographic evidence of pneumonitis during the course of disease. Symptoms begin 2 days before to 6 days after the onset of the rash, and they vary widely in severity. Approximately one-third of patients have no more than a mild, nonproductive cough. More severe cases begin abruptly with high fevers, often accompanied by chills; inspiratory chest pain, cough, hemoptysis, dyspnea, and cyanosis are common. Auscultation of the chest in such patients usually reveals rales, wheezes, and an increased expiratory phase. Classic signs of consolidation are uncommon.

Recovery is rapid in patients with mild symptoms. Improvement in moderately ill patients is often prolonged over 1 to 2 weeks, although shortness of breath usually diminishes in 2 to 3 days as the rash fades. A few patients show progressive deterioration with increasing tachypnea, dyspnea, cyanosis, and eventual death due to respiratory insufficiency.

Pleural effusions occur in 5% to 10% of cases—presumably as a consequence of focal lesions of the pleura. Additional complications in moderately or severely ill patients include pulmonary edema, subcutaneous emphysema, secondary bacterial infections, and pulmonary abscesses. Persistent pulmonary fibrosis and diffusion abnormalities may occur in adults who have recovered from varicella pneumonia.

Roentgenographic changes are usually far more prominent than either symptoms or physical findings. Subclinical pneumonitis, detectable only roentgenographically, represents the most common form of pulmonary varicella. The typical roentgenogram shows diffuse nodular densities, varying from 2 mm to 20 mm, scattered throughout both lung fields, with a tendency to concentrate at the bases and hilum. Nodules in a given area may disappear on serial examination, whereas others may coalesce to form discrete infiltrates that mimic metastatic carcinoma or areas of consolidation. Roentgenographic changes subside within 5 to 10 days in patients with mild or no symptoms, but the changes may persist 6 to 12 weeks in the more seriously ill, lagging far behind clinical response. Occasionally, small, soft nodules that represent fibrotic scars in areas of focal necrosis persist for months or years. These nodules may gradually calcify after 2 to 5 years, eventually producing a roentgenographic appearance that is indistinguishable from that of healed miliary tuberculosis.

Vesicles on the larynx severe enough to necessitate intubation or cause death have been reported and should be considered in the differential diagnosis of respiratory distress with varicella.

CENTRAL NERVOUS SYSTEM

The incidence of acute, symptomatic involvement of the CNS in chickenpox is unknown. Estimates have varied as widely as 1 in 1000 to 1 in 10,000 cases. Encephalitis is responsible for 90% of the neurologic complications; transverse myelitis, neuritis, and aseptic meningitis compose the remainder. Subclinical involvement of the CNS, as indicated by pleocytosis or transient but significant electroencephalographic changes, occurs in about 10% of patients with varicella.

Varicella encephalitis is twice as common in males as in females. The age distribution of this complication approximates that of varicella in the general population, with a mean age of onset between 5 and 7 years; however, there is epidemiologic evidence that patients 20 years of age and older may be at greatest risk. Symptoms usually begin 3 to 8 days after the appearance of the rash, although preeruptive (up to 2 weeks) and late posteruptive (up to 3 weeks) encephalitis has also been reported.

The clinical manifestations are often similar to those described in other viral encephalitides. However, cerebellar dysfunction is a characteristic feature of varicella encephalitis, occurring in up to 35% of patients with this complication. The onset may be gradual or very sudden. Headache, vomiting, and changes in the sensorium are common early symptoms; fever and signs of meningeal irritation are often lacking. When corticocerebral involvement predominates, convulsions, paralysis, stupor, and sometimes coma may follow the initial nonspecific symptoms. The cerebellar syndrome is usually milder. It is characterized by ataxia, nystagmus, tremors, dizziness, and speech disturbances. A multifocal encephalitis, combining features of both the cerebral and cerebellar forms, may also occur. The period of recovery is variable, generally lasting 1 to 3 weeks.

The cells in the cerebrospinal fluid (CSF) vary in number from normal to fewer than 100 per mm^3 and are almost exclusively mononuclear. The concentration of glucose is normal; the CSF protein is normal or slightly elevated.

The case fatality rate ranges from 5% to 25%. Encephalitis with predominantly cerebellar signs and symptoms is rarely fatal, whereas onset with convulsions or coma is apparently associated with a poor prognosis. Permanent neurologic sequelae, consisting primarily of behavior disorders, mental retardation, and seizures, occur in up to 15% of survivors.

Little is known of the pathogenesis of encephalitis. Both direct viral invasion of the CNS and an allergic response, either to altered CNS tissue or to a virus–CNS tissue complex, may be involved.

ACUTE ENCEPHALOPATHY AND FATTY DEGENERATION OF THE VISCERA (REYE'S SYNDROME).

Reye's syndrome affects primarily children. Of 209 cases reported from December 1980 through October 1981, 35% were 4 years old or younger, 59% were 5 to 14 years old, and 6% were 15 years old or older. The etiology of this disease is unknown, but it seems to be related to an immediately preceding infection by several common viral agents and probably represents a postviral syndrome. Of 203 patients with a known antecedent illness, 60% had an influenzal or other respiratory infection, 30% had varicella, and 10% had diarrheal disease.

Reye's syndrome must be considered in the differential diagnosis of varicella encephalitis or hepatitis. Vomiting, a consistent feature of the disease, begins as the child is recovering from the prodromal illness. This is followed, often rapidly, by signs and symptoms of CNS involvement, usually in the form of altered behavior (lethargy, confusion, irritability, or aggressiveness), as well as spasticity and seizures. Mild to moderate hepatomegaly, elevated serum glutamic-oxaloacetic transaminase (SGOT) and blood ammonia concentrations, and normal or slightly elevated bilirubin concentrations accompany the encephalopathy; jaundice and fever are usually lacking. Hypoglycemia is a frequent finding, and it is likely that early reports of hypoglycemia with chickenpox represent instances of this disorder. The cell count and protein of the CSF are normal. Formerly, 80% of patients died; with earlier recognition of the disease and aggressive supportive treatment, survival rates have improved dramatically, and the mortality rate is now 20% to 30%. Characteristic findings at autopsy include fatty infiltration of the liver, kidneys, and other viscera, and cerebral edema.

In young infants, Reye's syndrome may cause mild vomiting and respiratory disturbances such as hyperventilation or apneic episodes. Seizures are common.

There appears to be a relationship between Reye's syndrome and salicylates, but the nature of this association is not clear. Until more data are available, the Centers for Disease Control have recommended that the use of salicylates be avoided in children with varicella or presumed influenza.

GLOMERULONEPHRITIS

Glomerulonephritis, unassociated with serologic or bacteriologic evidence of a preceding streptococcal infection, has been described as a rare complication of varicella. Proteinuria and microscopic or gross hematuria may appear in a few days before or after onset of the rash. Urinary abnormalities constitute the only evidence of renal damage in most cases. However, progression to azotemia or anuria with edema, hypertension, and death have been reported. Renal tissue obtained by biopsy or at autopsy shows histologic changes similar to those found in poststreptococcal nephritis. Intranuclear inclusions have not been described in renal cells. Hematuria caused by nephritis must be differentiated—by the presence of erythrocyte casts—from bleeding secondary to vesicles in the urinary bladder.

CARDITIS

The frequency of subclinical or mild cardiac involvement in apparently uncomplicated varicella is unknown. Symptomatic myocarditis is a rare manifestation of varicella, although focal inflammatory lesions of the myocardium are a common incidental finding in patients who have died of other complications. Symptoms and electrocardiographic changes, when present, are similar to those described in myocarditis caused by other viral agents. Pericarditis, epicarditis, and endocarditis have also been reported in varicella. Intranuclear inclusion bodies have been described in myocardial muscle cells and cardiac vascular endothelium.

HEMORRHAGIC MANIFESTATIONS

Symptomatic thrombocytopenia, with purpura and bleeding into mucous membranes, is a rare manifestation of varicella. When such bleeding occurs, it usually begins 1 to 2 weeks after onset of the rash, and it may last up to 5 weeks. Peripheral thrombocyte counts often remain depressed for several weeks to months. The etiology of the thrombocytopenia is unclear; however, viral particles were demonstrated within megakaryocytes from a patient with purpura. Thrombocyte production is usually reduced, despite the presence of normal or increased numbers of megakaryocytes in the bone marrow. There may also be increased peripheral destruction of thrombocytes by antibodies directed against altered thrombocytes or a virus–thrombocyte complex.

In addition to thrombocytopenia, a number of ill-defined hemorrhagic syndromes are associated with varicella. A mild, self-limited condition—febrile purpura—usually begins on the first or second day of the eruption, with slight epistaxis, melena, and hemorrhage into vesicles.

In contrast, malignant chickenpox with purpura occurs during the first or second week of the disease, beginning abruptly with high fever, toxicity, and bleeding from the gastrointestinal tract, genitourinary tract, and other mucous membranes. Fatalities are common and result primarily from intractable bleeding, intracranial hemorrhage, or the pneumonia that often accompanies this condition. It is seen most frequently in adults and in children with deficient cellular immunity.

Purpura fulminans is characterized by progressive purpura leading to skin necrosis, and in severe cases to gangrene of an extremity, necessitating amputation. Both purpura fulminans and malignant chickenpox may be forms of disseminated intravascular coagulation with the clinical findings secondary to widespread arterial thrombosis or depression of clotting factors.

VARICELLA IN THE COMPROMISED HOST

Chickenpox is often extremely serious in patients with leukemia, lymphomatosis, or other disorders causing diminished cellular immunity. Fatalities secondary to hemorrhage, pneumonia, disseminated visceral disease, or secondary bacterial infections are common. Unusually severe, prolonged, or hemorrhagic eruptions may also occur. Complications and death in leukemia show a close correlation with hematologic status, occurring most frequently during relapse.

The poor prognosis in these diseases has been attributed to the primary disorders and the associated therapy (steroids, radiation, antimetabolites, alkylating agents) because both suppress host defense mechanisms. Many reports have warned of the seriousness of varicella acquired by patients receiving steroids, and it has been suggested that these drugs exert a direct adverse effect through their lymphocytotoxicity or by the enhancement of viral multiplication and dissemination. Most of these observations, however, have been based on compromised hosts in whom it is not possible to differentiate the effects of the underlying disease, superinfections, or adrenal insufficiency following abrupt withdrawal of exogenous glucosteroids. The extent to which morbidity and mortality can be attributed to glucosteroids is therefore unknown. Until these data become available, patients who are receiving prednisone in a dosage of 2 or more mg/kg body wt/day (or equivalent dosage of another glucosteroid) should be considered to be at increased risk from V-Z virus.

PREPARTUM AND CONGENITAL VARICELLA

Varicella during pregnancy is rare, occurring in only 0.7 pregnancies per 1000. Overall, the incidence of fetal mortality or prematurity is not significantly increased. However, individual cases of prematurity or fetal death, particularly in association with maternal pneumonia and hypoxia, have been described.

Clinical congenital varicella (rash appearing within 10 days after birth) occurs in about 17% of neonates whose mothers acquire varicella 1 to 16 days before delivery. The case fatality rate for neonates with rash developing within the first 5 to 10 days of life is about 14%; deaths have not been reported in neonates whose rash began within the first 4 days of life.

Varicella during the first and early second trimester of gestation may result in a syndrome of congenital malformations, but this is uncommon. At least eight such cases have been described. The major features include low birthweight for gestational age; hypoplasia of a limb; cicatricial scars with a zosteriform distribution (often involving a hypoplastic area); cortical atrophy with seizures or psychomotor retardation; other neurologic deficits; and various ocular lesions, including cataracts and chorioretinitis. Five of these eight infants died. In one additional case, in which the mother had varicella early in the third trimester, the infant had similar dermal lesions on one ankle and a deformity of the affected foot. Infants with no history of varicella but whose mothers had this disease during pregnancy have occasionally developed zoster, indicating that they were infected with V-Z virus *in utero*.

HEPATITIS

Clinical hepatitis has been reported chiefly in immunocompromised patients or in association with varicella pneumonia. Focal hepatic necrosis is present at autopsy of patients with hepatitis and in association with disseminated visceral disease. Clinically apparent hepatitis has occasionally been observed in adults with varicella but it seldom occurs in normal healthy children; however, subclinical hepatic changes are common. Of 39 children with uncomplicated varicella, 49% showed mild elevations of SGOT and 28% showed marked elevations that were occasionally accompanied by vomiting. Other evidence of Reye's syndrome was lacking.

OTHER MANIFESTATIONS

Keratitis and vesicular conjunctivitis are unusual and are generally benign. Individual cases of orchitis, arthritis, and splenic hemorrhage with rupture have also been reported. Tuberculin reactivity may be depressed following varicella (and certain other viral diseases) beginning 2 to 6 weeks after onset of the illness and persisting for up to 2 months. Varicella may also be associated with exacerbations of pulmonary tuberculosis. Biologic false-positive (reaginic) serologic tests for syphilis occur in varicellar infection in 5% of patients.

Diagnosis

Clinical criteria are usually sufficient to establish a diagnosis of chickenpox, particularly when there is a history of exposure within the preceding 2 to 3 weeks. The peripheral leukocyte count is generally normal, although a slight leukocytosis often accompanies varicellar pneumonia. Urinalysis is also normal, except when hematuria and proteinuria occur in association with glomerulonephritis or lesions of the bladder mucosa.

Scrapings from the base of a newly formed vesicle, if stained with the Giemsa or Wright stain (Tzanck smear), will show the multinucleated giant cells characteristic of infection with both V-Z and herpes simplex virus. Fixation with the Bouin, Zenker, or other acid fixative is necessary to demonstrate the intranuclear inclusions within these and other infected cells. Sputum from a patient with varicellar pneumonia may also contain intranuclear inclusions within cells desquamated from the tracheobronchial mucosa. Electromicroscopy has proved useful as a rapid (30 minutes) and reliable diagnostic procedure (Fig. 92-3*B*). By this method, herpesvirus has been identified in lesions from patients with chickenpox, zoster, or herpes simplex infection. Neither electromicroscopy nor the Tzanck smear is capable of distinguishing lesions caused by herpes simplex virus from those caused by V-Z virus.

In addition to isolation of the agent, a number of techniques are available for specific identification of V-Z virus. Viral antigen may be detected through gel-diffusion precipitation studies using the reaction of vesicle fluid, or extracts of vesicle roofs, crusts, or scabs, with human immune zoster serum. Direct fluorescent-antibody staining of cellular material from fresh vesicles has been used in a limited number of cases. Failure of V-Z virus to grow on the rabbit cornea (Paul's test) or on the chorioallantoic membrane of embryonated eggs differentiates it from variola. Failure to infect suckling mice differentiates it from herpes simplex virus.

In atypical or doubtful cases of chickenpox, the demonstration of a significant (fourfold or greater) rise in V-Z antibody titer may be helpful in establishing the diagnosis. Measurement of CF antibodies is most practical and is widely used, although an indirect fluorescent-antibody (FA) technique is also available. Because CF antibodies appear 1 to 4 days after onset of the rash, acute-phase serum specimens should be obtained as early as possible. Convalescent serum should be drawn 2 to 6 weeks later. After primary infection, titers of CF antibodies decline rapidly and may no longer be detectable after 6 to 12 months. The CF test is of little value, therefore, in determining susceptibility of an exposed person to this disease. The use of zoster immune globulin (not pooled human serum immune globulin) may cause a transient rise in antibody that persists for less than 4 to 8 weeks. Neutralizing antibodies persist for life, but their measurement is not generally feasible because of the difficulty of obtaining cell-free infectious virus.

Certain difficulties in interpreting the CF antibody response have been described. Infants with congenital or neonatal varicella may fail to develop detectable amounts of CF antibodies. In addition, significant heterologous increases in CF and FA antibody titers may occur between V-Z virus and herpes simplex virus, probably on the basis of shared minor antigens. Thus, patients with chickenpox or zoster may develop significant increases in CF titers to both V-Z virus and herpes simplex virus; patients with primary herpes simplex may show a rise in CF and FA titers of both herpes simplex and V-Z virus. This heterologous response depends both on age—occurring less frequently in younger age groups—and the presence of preexisting antibodies to the cross-reacting virus. Patients with varicella rarely show heterologous rises in herpes simplex neutralizing antibody titers, a valuable confirmatory test when doubt exists.

Several tests are available for determining susceptibility to varicella. The indirect detection of antibody to membrane antigen by immunofluorescence (FAMA test) is based on the observation that living cells infected with V-Z virus develop a virus-induced membrane antigen; persons whose serum reacts with this membrane antigen are immune to infection with V-Z virus. The enzyme-linked immunosorbent assay (ELISA), immune adherence hemagglutination test, indirect hemagglutination test, and neutralization test have also been used to assess immunity to this virus. An inactivated V-Z skin test antigen has been developed in Japan. A positive response to this antigen also appears to correlate well with immunity.

Smallpox (variola major) is now extinct, but was the most important disease from which varicella, particularly severe varicella, had to be distinguished. Differentiation of chickenpox from variola minor (alastrim) or vaccination-modified forms of variola major (varioloid) may be impossible on clinical grounds alone. These differentiations are thoroughly reviewed in Chapter 92, Smallpox and Other Poxvirus Infections. In conditions other than varicella, zoster, and herpes simplex, the Tzanck smear shows no multinucleated giant cells.

Disseminated herpes simplex (Chap. 91, Infections Caused by Herpes Simplex Virus) generally presents no problem because it is rare in normal persons, occurring most frequently in neonates, the severely malnourished, and persons with immunodeficiency disorders. Moreover, neither the distribution nor the progression of the rash resembles varicella. Also, in eczema vaccination or eczema herpeticum (Kaposi's varicelliform eruption), the lesions in the noneczematous or undamaged areas of skin do not have the characteristic distribution, features, and course of those in varicella. In addition, a history of contact with a vaccinated person or one with recurrent herpes simplex can generally be elicited.

Rickettsialpox (Chap. 97, Rickettsialpox) begins with a primary eschar and prominent prodromal symptoms; the single crop of lesions that follows consists of vesicles that differ from those of varicella in that they are smaller and are located at the very apex of the papule.

The vesicular lesions of the enteroviral exanthems (Chap. 149, Coxsackievirus and Echovirus Infections) are generally smaller than those of varicella, usually fail to crust, occur almost exclusively during the summer months, and may have a characteristic hand, foot, and mouth distribution (*e.g.,* hand-foot-and-mouth disease of coxsackievirus A16, A10, or A5). A pruritic, papulovesicular rash that resembles varicella has been described in Stevens–Johnson syndrome associated with *Mycoplasma pneumoniae,* but this rash evolves far differently from that of varicella. However, mycoplasmal infection should be considered in patients with atypical varicella, especially when there is associated stomatitis, conjunctivitis, or pulmonary symptoms.

The lesions of impetigo (Chap. 100, Staphylococcal Skin Infections and Chap. 101, Streptococcal Skin Infections and Glomerulonephritis) are usually less widely distributed. Moreover, the mucous membranes are spared, the lesions rapidly become pustular, and constitutional symptoms are infrequent. Insect bites may also be very difficult to distinguish from early varicella.

Prognosis

Because varicella is not a nationally reportable disease, the incidence of fatalities is unknown. However, the prognosis for normal children with varicella is excellent. Most deaths occur in adults over 20 years of age and in infants in the first year of life, particularly those with congenital varicella. Adult deaths are generally the consequence of varicellar pneumonia or encephalitis. The prognosis is also extremely guarded for patients with leukemia or lymphoma who contract chickenpox. The risk to patients receiving glucosteroids or other immunosuppressive therapy is assumed to be increased, although specific data are lacking. Exacerbations of preexisting tuberculosis may also affect the prognosis adversely.

Secondary bacterial infection of vesicles with *Staphylococcus aureus* or *Streptococcus pyogenes* is relatively uncommon in normal persons. Although cellulitis, abscesses, or lymphadenitis may occur, the incidence, even before penicillin, was no more than 2% to 3%. Resultant bacteremias with metastatic infections are rare.

A second attack of acquired varicella has never been documented. Recurrences that have been described are probably examples of herpes zoster generalizatus (see Herpes Zoster, below).

Therapy

There is no specific therapy for varicella. Acetaminophen may be useful to control fever, headache, and myalgia. The Centers for Disease Congrol (CDC) have recommended that salicylates not be used pending clarification of a possible etiologic role in Reye's syndrome. Trimming the fingernails and giving daily baths in tepid water with an antibacterial detergent are measures valuable in preventing secondary bacterial infection of lesions. Hot baths potentiate itching and should be avoided. Oral antihistamines are helpful in providing sedation and relief from pruritis. Calamine lotion and cornstarch or baking soda baths may relieve pruritis in mild cases. Local therapy with bacitracin ointment and hot soaks is generally sufficient to control isolated staphylococcal and streptococcal skin infections. In patients with widespread impetigo, bullous varicella associated with bacterial infection, abscesses, or lymphadenitis, systemic therapy with a penicillinase-resistant penicillin should be initiated after appropriate cultures have been obtained.

The treatment of varicella pneumonia is primarily supportive. Bacterial superinfection is most commonly caused by *Streptococcus pneumoniae, Streptococcus pyogenes,* and *Staphylococcus aureus.* However, gram-negative enteric bacteria and fungi may be important in the compromised host; *Hemophilus influenzae* frequently infects children under 5 years of age. Antimicrobial therapy of complicating bacterial infections should therefore be selected on the basis of examination of Gram-stained smears of appropriate specimens and cultures of the sputum and blood. The use of glucosteroids or antimicrobics is of no proven value in altering the course of varicella pneumonia.

The treatment of varicella encephalitis is entirely symptomatic and supportive. Therapeutic measures in Reye's syndrome are aimed at ameliorating the acute hepatic failure and controlling the cerebral edema. The effect of topical IDU, adenine arabinoside (ara A), acyclovir, or trifluorothymidine in the treatment of varicella keratitis has never been adequately evaluated. However, the use of these drugs poses little risk to the patient.

The dosage of glucosteroids should be reduced to physiologic levels (equivalent to 15 mg–20 mg of prednisone/m^2/day, PO) in patients receiving these agents either at the time of exposure to varicella or as soon thereafter as feasible.

Susceptible children with cancer who are exposed to varicella while receiving immunosuppressive drugs should have these medications halted (or at least, the dosage reduced), and they should be given specific hyperimmune globulin. The anticancer therapy may be reinstituted when the varicella has resolved or when it is apparent that the patient has escaped infection.

In a double-blind, collaborative study, ara A was proved to be valuable in the treatment of varicella in patients with lymphoproliferative disorders. The administration of ara A resulted in a decrease in the appearance of new lesions, shortening of the duration of fever, and a lower incidence of pneumonitis; early treatment favored therapeutic success.

Acyclovir is another DNA inhibitor. It is less toxic than is ara A and is highly active against V-Z virus *in vitro*. Clinical trials with acyclovir are underway.

Prevention

An attenuated, live V-Z virus vaccine propagated in tissue culture has been developed and tested in

Japan. It appears to be effective even in compromised hosts. Two preparations derived from this vaccine are under investigation in the United States. Although preliminary results are promising, there has been controversy regarding the long-term consequences and safety of a vaccine prepared with a virus that may establish a latent infection.

Transfer factor has been used successfully to prevent varicella in children with leukemia. Varicella can be attenuated, but not prevented, by giving human immune serum globulin (HISG) to exposed susceptible normal children within 3 days after exposure. Doses ranging to 0.6 ml/kg body wt up to a total volume of 20 ml have generally been used. Prevention is not achieved, however, even by doses as high as 1.25 ml/kg. Such treatment is unnecessary for the exposed normal child, and its value for modification of this disease in high-risk groups is uncertain.

A more potent product is zoster immune globulin (ZIG). Prepared from plasma obtained from patients 7 to 28 days after onset of a zoster rash, it contains high titers of V-Z CF antibodies. When given within 3 days after exposure, ZIG prevents (rather than modifies) varicella in susceptible, normal children. Although it is not as effective in protecting high-risk children, those with underlying conditions that predispose to severe varicella, ZIG has been shown to reduce both the morbidity and mortality of this disease in such patients. Often, however, it is not available.

V-Z immune globulin (VZIG) is as effective as ZIG and is more plentiful because it is prepared from outdated normal blood plasma with high antibody titers for V-Z virus. VZIG should be administered within 96 hours of exposure to newborns and high-risk children. It is distributed by the American Red Cross Blood Services, Northeast Region, through 13 regional blood centers identified in Morbidity and Mortality Weekly Reports 30:15, 1981; requests should be directed to the nearest regional distribution center. Physicians experienced with VZIG are available for consultation at the Immunization Division, CDC.

Guidelines for use of VZIG are given in the list below. In addition to persons meeting the five criteria listed in this table, immunodeficient children and adults with a history of varicella who subsequently receive a bone marrow transplant also qualify for VZIG because they are at unusually high-risk for developing severe and disseminated disease. The dose is based on body weight: the contents of one vial is given for each 10 kg, up to a maximum of five vials.

In view of the limited supply of both ZIG and VZIG and the unpredictability of spread of varicella among hospitalized patients after a case has appeared, it is generally agreed that the index case and as many of the exposed susceptible children as is feasible, should be discharged. If discharge is not medically feasible, known susceptible contacts may be quarantined during the period from 7 to 21 days after exposure. However, high-risk patients who fulfill the criteria for passive immunization should receive ZIG or VZIG. Exposed adults with a negative or uncertain history of varicella hold a low priority, because about 95% are immune. Because tests for determining susceptibility to V-Z virus are now available, patients and hospital employees should be screened and appropriate protective measures initiated. Patients with varicella or herpes zoster should be cared for only by personnel not at risk to prevent spread of V-Z infection.

VZIG has not been shown to be valuable in treatment of (1) established V-Z infection or its sequelae, including progressive varicella and (2) the pregnant woman with V-Z infection to prevent fetal infection, congenital defects, abortion, or miscarriage.

It is generally recommended that children with varicella be isolated until all vesicles are dry. Normally, this takes 5 to 6 days, but it may take longer in patients with altered immune responses. Because varicella is communicable before the appearance of the rash and is preferably acquired during childhood

INDICATIONS AND GUIDELINES FOR THE USE OF VARICELLA–ZOSTER IMMUNE GLOBULIN FOR THE PROPHYLAXIS OF CHICKENPOX (VARICELLA)

- One of the following underlying illnesses or conditions
  - Leukemia or lymphoma
  - Congenital or acquired immunodeficiency
  - Under immunosuppressive treatment
  - Newborn of mother who had onset of chickenpox <5 days before delivery or within 48 hours after delivery
- One of the following types of exposure to chickenpox or zoster patient(s)
  - Household contact
  - Playmate contact (>1 hour play indoors)
  - Hospital contact (in same 2- to 4-bed room or adjacent beds in a large ward)
  - Newborn contact (newborn of mother who had onset of chickenpox <5 days before delivery or within 48 hours after delivery)
- Negative or unknown prior history of chickenpox (see text)
- Age of <15 years, with administration to older patients on an *individual* basis (see text)
- Time elapsed after exposure is such that VZIG can be administered within 96 hours

(Morbid Mortal Week Rep 30:15, 1981)

when it is a mild and uncomplicated disease, isolation from susceptible siblings is generally discouraged as impractical and unnecessary. However, high-risk patients and young infants in whom serious complications may occur should be separated from exposed susceptible persons for the 2 weeks corresponding to the period from day 7 to day 21 after exposure of the susceptible persons.

Herpes Zoster

Herpes zoster (shingles, zona) is an acute infectious disease caused by the V-Z virus and is characterized by the inflammation of dorsal root ganglia, neuralgic pain, and crops of clustered vesicles localized to dermatomes innervated by the affected ganglia. The eruption is usually unilateral and commonly affects a cutaneous area innervated by a single ganglion. The V-Z virus may be recovered from vesicle fluid, CSF, and infected tissues.

Epidemiology

Because herpes zoster results from the reactivation of a latent varicella infection, contact with zoster may produce varicella in susceptible persons. Although zoster has been reported following contact with either varicella or zoster, such cases most likely represent a coincidental reactivation of V-Z virus.

In zoster, transmission of the V-Z virus appears to occur chiefly by direct contact with infected vesicles. It is less readily communicable than varicella, possibly because the lesions usually occur in areas ordinarily covered by clothing and because of the relative infrequency of mucosal lesions. In addition, patients with zoster often have antibodies by the time their rash has developed, and these antibodies may decrease their infectivity by neutralizing virus in the lesions. The varicella attack rate in susceptibles exposed to zoster has been estimated at about 15%.

Although shingles may occur at any age, the maximum observed incidence is between 50 and 80 years of age. Zoster in the infant or child generally results from reactivation of a primary infection with V-Z virus that was acquired either *in utero* or in early infancy and was masked by partial protection due to maternal antibody. Cases diagnosed as neonatal zoster have never been documented by viral isolation, and most cases probably are zosteriform distribution of lesions caused by herpes simplex virus.

Herpes zoster occurs sporadically throughout the year with no seasonal prevalence. It affects both sexes and all races with equal frequency.

Pathogenesis and Pathology

The mechanisms responsible for the appearance of herpes zoster many years after a primary varicella infection are not known. The most widely accepted theory, the Hope–Simpson theory, is derived from epidemiologic and pathologic observations of the natural disease in man.

According to this concept, the V-Z virus enters the cutaneous endings of sensory nerves during the initial varicella infection and migrates centripetally along the nerve fibers to the sensory ganglia, where it is thought to become latent within the neurons. Latency of V-Z virus in sensory ganglia remains to be proved, since the virus has not been detected in ganglia obtained from immune adults with no history of recent zoster. V-Z virus has been isolated, however, from sensory ganglia after acute attacks of zoster. The demonstration that a different herpesvirus, herpes simplex virus, regularly becomes latent in affected sensory ganglia also provides support for this hypothesis. Although the dormant virus retains its potential for full infectivity, reactivation is sporadic and infrequent. The few infectious particles that may escape beyond the limits of the host's neurons are neutralized by circulating antibodies (or perhaps are disposed of by cellular immune responses) before they can replicate to high titers and infect adjacent cells. When host resistance falls below a critical level, the reactivated virus is no longer contained, and it multiplies without hindrance, producing intense inflammation and necrosis of the affected sensory ganglion. This process is usually accompanied by severe neuralgia and is followed by centrifugal passsage of the virus down the sensory nerve into the skin, where it produces the characteristic segmental, vesicular eruption of herpes zoster. Occasionally, spread of the infection to the anterior horn cells and the motor nerve root may cause muscular weakness or paralysis in the corresponding dermatome. Because spontaneous reactivation of the virus is a chance occurrence, simultaneous involvement of more than one ganglion is unusual.

Hematogenous dissemination of the V-Z virus from the affected ganglion stimulates an anamnestic response of host immunologic defense mechanisms that then terminates the infectious process. Should these responses be delayed, however, a general variceliform eruption, occasionally with visceral involvement, may accompany the local eruption (general, or disseminated, zoster)—a phenomenon that may be correlated with delayed interferon production in the skin. In any event, the increase in humoral and cellular immunity that follows an attack of zoster is generally sufficient to restrict multiplication of the reactivated virus. In the normal person, second attacks of shingles are rare.

There is extensive lymphocytic infiltration, focal hemorrhage, and nerve cell destruction in the sensory ganglia involved. After weeks to months, widespread fibrosis follows. The diffuse lymphocytic infiltration, axonal destruction, demyelination, and fibrosis that may occur in peripheral nerves could result either from direct viral invasion, Wallerian degeneration, or both processes. A unilateral, segmental myelitis, resembling anterior poliomyelitis, has also been described. Local leptomeningitis, with a mild cellular infiltrate, often accompanies the ganglionitis. The V-Z virus was demonstrated by immunofluorescence and electron microscopy in the trigeminal nerve and ganglion of a patient with zoster ophthalmicus, and it has been isolated from the spinal cord and dorsal root ganglion tissues of patients with truncal zoster.

The pathologic changes of zoster encephalitis are similar to those seen in varicella. Direct viral invasion of the CNS has been documented by observation of intranuclear inclusions, and electron microscopic demonstration of the virus within oligodendroglia; V-Z virus has been isolated from brain tissue.

The histopathology of the focal lesions of cutaneous and disseminated visceral zoster is identical with that of chickenpox.

Manifestations

In most cases, factors responsible for reactivation of V-Z virus are obscure. A number of conditions have been associated with the appearance of the clinical disease. These include depressed host resistance in Hodgkin's disease, non-Hodgkin's lymphomas, lymphocytic leukemia, or other malignant neoplasia; the use of immunosuppressive agents; irradiation of the spinal column; tumor involvement of the spinal cord, dorsal root ganglion, or vertebral column adjacent to these structures; local trauma; injury or surgical manipulation of the spine; heavy metal (*e.g.,* arsenic, lead) poisoning or therapy. In general, zoster appears within 6 to 12 months after the clinical onset of malignancy or the initiation of irradiation or chemotherapy. Following trauma or spinal surgery, the eruption usually occurs within 3 to 7 days.

The individual cutaneous lesions of zoster, like those of varicella, begin as erythematous maculopapules that evolve over the next 24 to 72 hours to form closely grouped vesicles, pustules, and crusts. In normal persons, new lesions continue to appear in successive crops for 1 to 4 days, occasionally for as long as 7 days. Crusts often persist 2 to 4 weeks and tend to remain in place longer in older patients. The severity and extent of the eruption are variable, ranging from 1 or 2 small vesicles to large, confluent bullae that extend throughout the dermatomal segment. Progress to gangrene is rare. Intense and prolonged eruptions generally occur in older patients.

The typical rash of zoster appears in a unilateral dermatomal distribution corresponding to the area of innervation of the involved sensory nerve. It occurs with greatest frequency in those sensory segments in which the rash of varicella tends to concentrate—that is, thoracic (50%), cervical (15%), facial (15%), and sacral (5%). In most cases, the eruption is strictly unilateral, rarely crossing more than one-half inch over the midline. Generally, a single sensory ganglion is involved, although lesions overlap onto adjacent dermatomes in about 20%. Occasionally, affected dermatomes are widely separated or on opposite sides of the body.

Segmental cutaneous parasthesias or pain of a burning, stabbing, pruritic, or deep aching nature (neuralgia) are characteristic of herpes zoster. Generally, these symptoms accompany the rash, or follow shortly after its onset, but they occasionally precede the eruption by 4 to 5 days. In such patients, prodromal symptoms are easily confused with the pain of angina pectoris, duodenal ulcer, biliary or renal colic, appendicitis, pleurodynia, or early glaucoma. Although the pain of zoster usually remits as the crusts fall off, the disease may produce a prolonged postherpetic neuralgia, particularly in older patients. Typically, children have little local discomfort during or after an attack of zoster.

Regional adenitis with freely movable and nontender lymph nodes is a consistent feature of zoster. Constitutional symptoms such as fever, malaise, headache, or meningismus precede or accompany the rash in about 5% of patients and are seen most frequently in children.

General herpes zoster, often mistakenly reported as "simultaneous zoster and varicella," occurs in approximately 2% to 5% of all patients, most commonly in those with immunologic defects due to underlying malignancy (particularly lymphomas) or the use of immunosuppressive therapy. This complication, which usually begins with the first or second week after onset of the local eruption, may be manifest as a varicelliform eruption of variable intensity, occasionally with widespread visceral involvement and fatal termination. Aggressive immunosuppressive treatment regimens, especially for patients with lymphomas and for organ transplant recipients, are occasionally associated with marked prolongation of zoster with persistence of lesions in the affected dermatome for weeks to months and recurrent cycles of cutaneous dissemination. These manifestations appear to be related to a decrease in the number of T-lymphocytes capable of mounting a cell-mediated immune response.

Rarely, segmental neuralgia of a type associated with zoster may occur without cutaneous vesicles. This entity, referred to as *zoster sine herpete,* has been serologically confirmed in only a single case.

POSTHERPETIC NEURALGIA

Neuralgia persisting after all crusts have fallen off the skin lesions is unusual in patients under 40 years of age, but occurs in approximately 50% of patients older than 60 years. The incidence of this complication does not appear to be influenced by the location of the eruption or the time required for skin lesions to heal, but it may be more common in patients with severe pain during the acute attack. In most cases, it resolves spontaneously within 1 to 3 months, but it may continue for more than 12 months in a small percentage of patients. Prolonged postherpetic neuralgia has been associated with severe depression, narcotic addiction, and even suicide, particularly in the elderly. Although the etiology of the pain is unknown, it is believed to be central, perhaps thalamic, in origin. Avulsion of the affected nerve or infiltration with procaine or ethanol provides no relief from the symptoms.

ZOSTER OPHTHALMICUS

Ocular lesions occur in approximately one-third of patients who have zoster involving the ophthalmic division of the trigeminal nerve. There is a close correlation between the presence of zoster vesicles on the tip of the nose and lesions of the eye, probably as a result of common innervation through the nasociliary branch of the trigeminal nerve.

Although ocular involvement is rare in children and adults under 20 years of age, in older age groups frequency of occurrence is not a function of age. Conjunctivitis is the most common mnifestation, although keratitis and iridocyclitis may also occur. When the keratitis is severe, extensive scarring and significant impairment of vision may follow. Superimposed bacterial infections caused by *Staphylococcus aureus* or *Pseudomonas* spp. may augment tissue destruction unless promptly recognized and treated with appropriate antimicrobial therapy.

A contralateral hemiplegia caused by a segmental granulomatous vasculitis of the CNS is an infrequent complication of zoster ophthalmicus. Usually, it occurs within a few weeks after onset of the rash.

Neuritis of trigeminal sensory fibers may be associated with palsies of the third, fourth, and sixth cranial nerves, leading to partial or complete external ophthalmoplegia, iridoplegia, or ptosis. These symptoms generally follow onset of the eruption by several weeks, but occasionally precede or accompany it. Retrobulbar neuritis, neuroretinitis, glaucoma, and occlusion of the retinal vessels have also been described in association with zoster ophthalmicus.

ZOSTER ENCEPHALOMYELITIS

A lymphocytic pleocytosis, with or without an increase in the concentration of protein in the CSF, occurs in approximately 33% of patients with herpes zoster, most frequently in patients with involvement of the cervical ganglia. Symptoms referrable to meningeal involvement are generally lacking or are limited to slight headache and meningismus. Although CSF changes may persist for several weeks, recovery is generally complete.

The incidence of acute, symptomatic meningoencephalitis in association with zoster is not known, but it appears to be exceedingly low. The age and sex of patients and location of the eruption are comparable to those of zoster in the general population.

The clinical manifestations and CSF findings are similar to those described in varicella encephalitis. Symptoms usually begin 1 to 2 weeks after the appearance of the rash, but they may precede the eruption by several weeks. The mode of onset is generally abrupt and rapid, with signs of meningeal irritation, headache, vomiting, convulsions, or progressive changes in the sensorium. Temperature elevations are variable or lacking. Ataxia and other cerebellar signs frequently dominate the clinical picture. Evidence of a transverse myelitis with spastic weakness or sensory impairment is uncommon.

The incidence of fatalities and neurologic residua is difficult to evaluate because only a few cases have been described, and many of the patients were aged and suffering from serious underlying diseases. Death from meningoencephalitis seems to be uncommon; however, relapsing illness may occur. The etiology of this complication is not completely understood.

MOTOR PARALYSIS

Motor paralysis accompanying herpes zoster is unusual, probably occurring in no more than 1% of patients. The diagnosis must be confirmed by electromyography because pseudoparalysis may result from pain, interruption of the reflex arc as a result of necrosis of the posterior root ganglion, and muscle atrophy secondary to disuse.

The age and sex distributions of motor paralysis in general reflect those of zoster. Paralysis usually occurs within the first 2 weeks after onset of the rash and attains maximal severity within hours or days. It almost always involves muscle groups innervated by nerves arising from the spinal segment corresponding to the rash. Thus, unilateral diaphragmatic paralysis (involvement of the phrenic nerve) may accompany a homolateral cervical eruption.

The paralysis may persist for weeks to months; total or functional recovery occurs in about 75% of patients. The motor paralysis accompanying zoster is often indistinguishable from that caused by intraspinal or paraspinal tumors—neoplasms that may have precipitated the eruption. Accordingly, such tumors must be looked for in all pateints with motor paralysis complicating zoster.

VISCERAL ZOSTER

Extension of viral infection from posterior root ganglia to unmyelinated sympathetic and parasympathetic visceral fibers is probably responsible for the gastrointestinal and genitourinary symptoms and distrubances in visceral function may reflect either irritation (hypertonia, spasm) or destruction (hypotonia, atonia, ileus) of the affected neural tissue. Segmental inflammation of the gastrointestinal tract and unilateral ulcerative lesions of the bladder mucosa have also been described in conjunction with these changes in visceral motility.

Symptoms of irritation, and even effusions, may occur with zoster involving peritoneal, pleural, or synovial surfaces.

HERPES ZOSTER OTICUS (RAMSAY HUNT SYNDROME)

Herpes zoster oticus results from involvement of the facial and auditory nerves (rarely, the ninth and tenth cranial nerves) by V-Z virus. Although originally termed geniculate herpes zoster by Hunt, herpetic inflammation of the geniculate ganglion has never been demonstrated.

The presenting features include either zoster of the external ear or tympanic membrane (herpes auricularis); herpes auricularis with homolateral facial paralysis; or herpes auricularis, facial paralysis, and auditory symptoms.

The facial nerve palsy may result from a viral neuritis, inflammatory edema with compression of the nerve in its bony canal, or a combination of both. Paralysis is usually transient, but it is occasionally permanent. Associated symptoms include loss of taste in the anterior two-thirds of the tongue, disturbances of lacrimation, and a vesicular nasopalatine eruption. Faulty regeneration of facial nerve fibers during recovery may result in profuse tearing during mastication, the crocodile tears syndrome.

Auditory symptoms include mild to severe tinnitus, deafness, vertigo, nausea and vomiting, and nystagmus. Although vestibular symptoms usually disappear, tinnitus and loss of hearing may be prolonged or permanent. Hearing seldom returns to normal if loss during the acute attack was profound.

Diagnosis

The appearance of clustered vesicles in a unilateral segmental distribution, particularly when accompanied by intense neuralgia, is generally sufficient to establish the diagnosis of shingles. Additional information may be obtained, when necessary, using the laboratory methods already described.

A significant (fourfold or greater) anamnestic response in neutralizing, FA, or CF antibody titer usually occurs in patients with zoster, although acute-phase serum samples may contain levels sufficiently high to preclude the demonstration of a further rise in titer. The heterologous antibody responses that take place with V-Z virus and herpes simplex virus have already been outlined. Infants with zoster, like those with varicella, may fail to synthesize detectable amounts of CF antibody to the V-Z virus.

Zosteriform herpes simplex eruptions are frequently impossible to distinguish from herpes zoster by clinical or serologic methods. A history of recurrent appearances of the eruption is common with herpes simplex, but is exceedingly rare in zoster. Isolation of the virus is diagnostic. Vaccinia autoinoculation can be differentiated from zoster by history, lack of neuralgia, a negative Tzanck smear, and isolation of the vaccinia virus. Rarely, localized enteroviral eruptions are mistaken for zoster. When either the course of the illness or the appearance of the skin lesions is atypical, viral cultures should be obtained. The linear dermatoses—lichen striatus, linear psoriasis, lichen nitidus, linear verruca—are generally papular, nonpainful, and nonsegmental. Contact dermatitis does not produce neuralgia or a serologic response to the V-Z virus; the Tzank smear and cultures for V-Z virus are negative. The differential diagnosis of generalized zoster corresponds to that of varicella.

Prognosis

The prognosis for patients with herpes zoster is good. Fatalities are seen most frequently in patients with generalized zoster and are determined primarily by the nature of the underlying disease.

Recurrences of zoster are unusual; of those who develop the disease, 50% do so by the age of 85 years and 1% have two attacks. The interval preceding recurrences is generally 20 to 40 years. Second attacks may be seen with greater frequency in patients with cellular immune deficiencies.

Bacterial infection of ruptured vesicles occasionally occurs and is usually caused by *Staphylococcus aureus* or *Streptococcus pyogenes.* Herpes zoster in pregnancy has not been shown to cause adverse effects in either the mother or the fetus.

Therapy

The neuralgia of herpes zoster can usually be relieved by analgesics such as aspirin or codeine. The prolonged use of narcotics, particularly in patients with postherpetic neuralgia, poses the risk of addiction and should be avoided whenever possible. Treatment with tap-water soaks, calamine, or a similar drying lotion may hasten resolution of the vesicles. A bland ointment may expedite the softening and disappearance of the crusts.

Treatment of postherpetic neuralgia is generally directed at attempts to disrupt the pain cycle for several days by combined use of analgesics, tranquilizers, and soporifics, followed by more limited use of such medications. Tranquilizers are helpful in treating the depression associated with prolonged neuralgia, particularly in elderly patients. In healthy patients over 60 years of age, the early treatment of zoster with large doses of prednisone (*e.g.,* 48 mg/days, PO, as three equal portions for 7 days, then 24 mg/day, PO, as three equal portions for 7 days, and finally 16 mg/day, PO, as two equal portions for 7 days) may decrease the incidence of postherpetic neuralgia without increasing the frequency of complications or of general spread. Not all patients respond. The pain may be relieved by epidural injection of a local anesthetic agent as long as 7 weeks after onset.

The management of persistent, disseminated cutaneous zoster in immunosuppressed hosts consists in reducing the immunosuppression as much as is practical in the hope that lesions will heal. Should this approach fail, a trial of an antiviral agent (*e.g.,* ara A) or interferon should be considered.

The efficacy of glucosteroids in hastening the resolution of facial paralysis in the Ramsay Hunt syndrome has not been established.

Bacterial infection of ruptured vesicles may be treated topically with bacitracin ointment or, if severe, by systemic therapy with appropriate agents. The choice of antimicrobic should be guided by the results of cultures and susceptibility tests.

It is important that ocular infection due to V-Z virus be distinguished from that caused by herpes simplex virus, since the former is treated with glucosteroids to suppress the inflammatory response, whereas glucosteroids are contraindicated in the latter. The treatment of patients with ocular involvement should be directed by an ophthalmologist.

Several antiviral agents are under investigation for the treatment of patients with herpes zoster. Ara A, given parenterally to immunocompromised patients with localized or disseminated zoster, accelerated healing of lesions and expedited clearance of virus from vesicles. In addition, the frequency of cutaneous dissemination was reduced, and the duration of postherpetic neuralgia was decreased. However, no clear effect on mortality or visceral dissemination was observed. Treatment was most effective when started early—within 2 to 3 days of onset. Preliminary studies with acyclovir in such patients have given similar results.

High-dosage interferon treatment has been reported to be effective in limiting cutaneous dissemination and visceral complications in patients with malignancy and early herpes zoster.

Dissemination of herpes zoster lesions has been shown to occur in the presence of high levels of antibody. Administration of V-Z antibody preparations, therefore, would not be expected to affect the course of this disease.

Prevention

Because exposure to zoster occasionally results in varicella, the isolation procedures recommended for varicella are also pertinent to zoster.

Remaining Problems

The form in which V-Z virus persists in the latent state following primary infection is not known. The site of viral persistence also remains to be determined. V-Z virus has been demonstrated in sensory ganglia only during or shortly after the development of zoster. Has it been there in some other form, or has it migrated from some other site?

The mechanism of viral reactivation remains to be determined. What are the respective roles of humoral and cellular immunity in this process? If the mechanism can be determined and inhibitors developed, recurrences might be prevented.

Studies on the pathogenesis of V-Z virus infection are limited by lack of a suitable animal model. How does the virus proceed up the sensory nerve? What is the mechanism of retrograde spread? What organs are affected? What syndromes are produced? How does latency occur? How can it be prevented? These and similar questions could be more easily approached if an animal model were available.

The replicative cycle of V-Z virus is not fully understood. Biochemical studies are hampered by the lack of a tissue culture system that yields high titers of virus for analysis. Such studies might help explain the mechanism whereby V-Z virus in tissue culture is cell associated with only low titers of virus in the extracellular fluid and why virus is easily demonstrable in vesicle fluid but rarely found in the throat.

The relationship between V-Z virus and Reye's syndrome is obscure. The role of aspirin in this disease also remains to be elucidated.

Additional areas for future consideration include further evaluation of the antiviral agents that appear to be effective against V-Z virus, further studies on the use of transfer factor and interferon in V-Z virus infections, and further assessment of the efficacy and safety of the attenuated live V-Z virus vaccines.

Bibliography

Books

EMOND RTD: Color Atlas of Infectious Diseases. Chicago, Year Book Medical Publishers, 1974. pp 136–183.

WELLER TH: Varicella and herpes zoster. In Lenette EH, Schmidt NL (eds): Diagnostic Procedures for Viral, Rickettsial and Chlamydial Infections, 5th ed. Washington DC, American Public Health Association, 1979. pp 375–398.

Journals

DENICOLA LK, HANSHAW JB: Congenital and neonatal varicella. J Pediatr 94:175–176, 1979

EY JL, SMITH SM, FULGINITI VA: Varicella hepatitis without neurologic symptoms or findings. Pediatrics 67:285–287, 1981

GROSE C: Variation on a theme by Fenner: The pathogenesis of chickenpox. Pediatrics 68:735–737, 1981

HOPE–SIMPSON RE: The nature of herpes zoster: A long term study and a new hypothesis. Proc R Soc Med 58:9–20, 1965

National Surveillance for Reye Syndrome, 1981: Update: Reye Syndrome and Salicylate Usage. Morbid Mortal Week Rep 31:53–61, 1982

NIH Conference, Dolin R, Moderator: Herpes zoster–varicella infections in immunosuppressed patients. Ann Intern Med 89:375–388, 1978

PERKINS HM, HANLON PR: Epidural injection of local anes- and steroids for relief of pain secondary to herpes zoster. Arch Surg 113:253–254, 1978

PREBLUD SR: Age-specific risks of varicella complications. Pediatrics 68:14–17, 1981

REULER JB, GIRARD DE, NARDONE DA: The chronic pain syndrome: Misconceptions and management. Ann Intern Med 93:588–596, 1980

BURTON JANIS

94 Molluscum Contagiosum

Molluscum contagiosum is a communicable viral disease of humans that is confined to the skin; it is manifest as umbilicated papules.

Etiology

Molluscum contagiosum virus (MCV) is a DNA virus of the poxvirus group (see Chap. 1, Attributes of Infectious Agents). Brick-shaped and large (300 nm × 230 nm × 100 nm), each virus consists of a dense central core which is dumbbell-shaped in longitudinal section and contains double-stranded DNA with a molecular weight of 160 to 200 daltons × 10^6 daltons. Negative staining of the surface of purified virions reveals a filament 10 nm to 12 nm in diameter that is wound around the central core to give the virus particle the appearance of a ball of yarn (Fig. 94-1). MCV has never been propagated outside the human body. The virus penetrates cells in culture by viropexis, but a full infectious cycle is not initiated.

Epidemiology

Molluscum contagiosum is worldwide in distribution. Data regarding incidence are available from only a few locations, for example, 0.14% to 1.2% in Scotland and 4.5% in Fiji.

Transmission of MCV by direct contact or by fomites is indicated by the occurrence of outbreaks in wrestlers, persons using the same swimming pool, and closely associated persons living under poor hygienic conditions. Intimate direct contact and venereal spread is suggested by a report of lesions on the genitalia, thighs, and pubic area in a group of 55 men who had extramarital coitus within 6 months of the onset of the disease; the consorts of these patients were not examined.

Pathogenesis and Pathology

The basal cell layer of human skin is the site of the earliest or primary interaction of MCV virus and host. Using electron microscopic examination of serial sections of lesions, cores of virions are demonstrable in the perinuclear zone of basal cells, close to the Golgi apparatus. These cores lie within phagocytic vacuoles. Subsequently, a specific and complex set of virus–host cell changes occurs which results in the formation of mature virus in the suprabasal layers. Details of the molecular virology accompanying these morphologic changes are lacking. Intracytoplasmic vacuoles that contain mature virus particles are present in the stratum spinosum—the next external layer. Within the infected cell, the vacuoles are separated by partitioning trabeculae that contain nascent virus. As the cell migrates externally, the virus-filled vacuoles enlarge progressively; the nucleus and the small empty vacuoles within the cytoplasm rim the periphery as they are pushed against the cell membrane. The virus-filled vacuoles are the molluscum bodies, that is, basophilic, Feulgen-positive, intracytoplasmic inclusion bodies as seen with the light microscope. Within the granular cell layer, the molluscum body enlarges further. In the dermis, collections of fibroblasts with bizarre nuclei lie subjacent to epithelial lesions; neither virus nor inflammatory cells are present. The mass of molluscum bodies with their accumulated cellular debris are surrounded by thin shells of fibrous tissues that form firm boundaries that facilitate expressing the core.

The early, close interaction of MCV virus with the basal layers results in the formation of anticellular and virus-specific antibodies. The anticellular antibodies are IgM and appear to be directed against the protein fibrils of MCV; however, they are nonspecific, since they are adsorbed by human myometrium. The virus-specific antibodies are primarily IgG and are present in the molluscum lesions in about 70% of

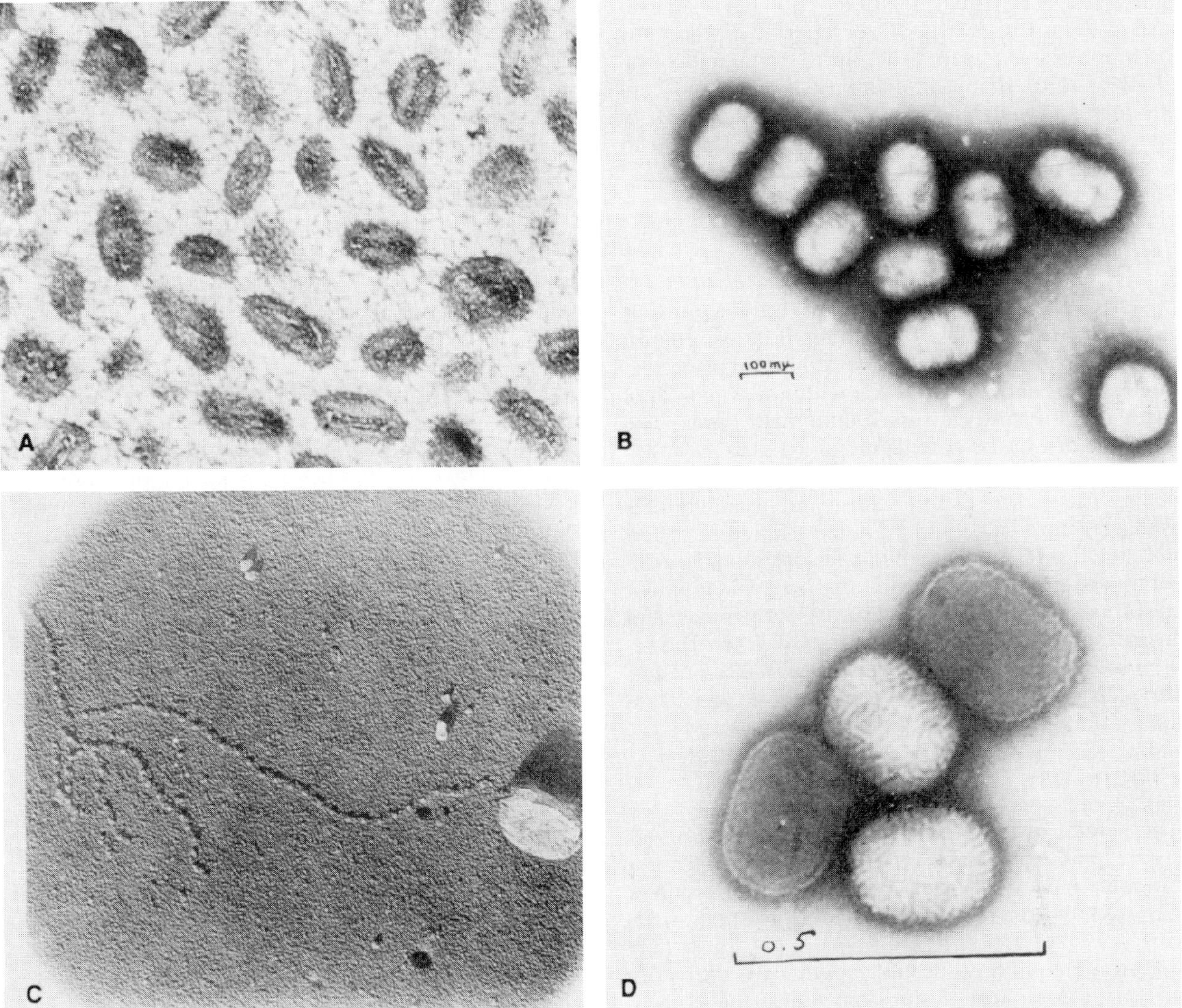

Fig. 94-1. Electron photomicrograph of the molluscum contagiosum virus. (*A*) Mature virus from lesion. (*B*) Viral particles stained with phosphotungstic acid. Note the shape and the ball-of-yarn appearance. (*C*) A shadow cast revealing the beaded appearance of a filamentous structure unwinding from the surface. (*D*) Genitron-treatment with two particles intact and two without external filamentous structures—serrated outer surface. (Courtesy of Charles G. Mendelson, M. D.)

patients. When anticellular antibody is demonstrable, specific antiviral antibody is also detectable. The role played by these humoral antibodies in the pathogenesis and regression of the benign molluscum skin tumors is unknown. Severe MCV infection in a patient with T cell deficiency implicates cell-mediated immunity in the pathogenesis of this condition.

Manifestations

The lesions of molluscum contagiosum are smooth, firm, shiny, flesh-colored to pearly white hemispheric papules with umbilicated centers confined to the skin and mucous membranes. They are found most commonly on the trunk and in the anogenital region, but lesions are also seen on the face, eyelids, scalp, lip, and other mucous membranes. The palms and soles are spared. The incubation period has been estimated to be 1 to 50 days. Over a period of 3 months or more, lesions grow to 1 mm to 5 mm and occasionally up to 10 mm in diameter. Eczema and conjunctivitis may also be present and have been attributed to toxic substances produced by the virus or to a hypersensitivity reaction to the virus.

Diagnosis

When multiple lesions are present, the diagnosis is usually obvious. Single, large atypical lesions are more difficult to identify by inspection and palpation. Such lesions should be nicked with a no. 11 scalpel blade and the core expressed onto a glass slide. The addition of one or two drops of 10% KOH and a coverslip facilitate examination with the light microscope. The presence of the classic molluscum bodies is diagnostic. Small, multiple lesions should be differentiated from flat warts. Solitary lesions should be differentiated from keratoacanthoma, pyogenic granulomas, and basal cell epitheliomas. Syringomas and hydrocystomas should be considered when the lesion is located around the eye; biopsy is often necessary.

Prognosis

The natural history of molluscum contagiosum was studied in Fiji. Although lesions were present from 6 months to 3 years, a given lesion persisted for only 2 months. Natural resolution occurred without scarring.

Chronic conjunctivitis and superficial keratitis occasionally complicate lesions on or near the eyelids. With removal of the molluscum lesions, these associated conditions subsided.

Therapy

Because molluscum contagiosum is a benign disease—the lesions resolve spontaneously without scarring—treatment should be gentle. A small number of lesions can easily be removed by gentle curettage after cyroanesthesia. Larger numbers of lesions have been treated by the application of caustic chemicals such as iodine, podophyllin, trichloroacetic acid, phenol, or cantharidin. These chemicals can cause scarring and should be used cautiously. Two months after therapy, the patient should be examined for new lesions.

Prevention

Good hygienic practice and avoidance of close contact with infected persons probably prevent infection with molluscum contagiosum.

Remaining Problems

A tissue culture system to grow the MCV is sorely needed. Once that has been obtained, more information can be gained about the epidemiology, immunology, and molecular aspects of virus–host cell interactions.

Bibliography

Book

ROOK A, WILKINSON DS, EBLING FJG (EDS): Textbook of Dermatology, vol I, 2nd ed. Oxford, Blackwell Scientific Publications, 1972. pp 586–589.

Journals

HAWLEY TG: The natural history of molluscum contagiosum in Fijian children. J Hyg (Camb) 68:631–632, 1970

LYNCH PJ, MINKIN W: Molluscum contagiosum of the adult: probable venereal transmission. Arch Dermatol 98:141–143, 1968

POSTLETHWAITE R: Molluscum contagiosum. Arch Environ Health 21:432–452, 1970

SHIRODARIA PV, MATTHEWS RS, SAMUEL M: Virus-specific and anticellular antibodies in molluscum contagiosum. Brit J Dermatol 101:133–140, 1979

SUTTON JS, BURNETT JW: Ultrastructural changes in dermal and epidermal cells of skin infected with molluscum contagiosum virus. J Ultrastr Res 26:177–196, 1969

VREESWIJK J, LEENE W, KALSBEEK GL: Early host cell-molluscum contagiosum virus interactions. II. Viral interactions with the basal epidermal cells. J Invest Dermatol 69:249–256, 1977

VREESWIJK J, LEENE W, KALSBEEK GL: Early interactions of the virus molluscum contagiosum with its host cell: Virus induced alterations in the basal and suprabasal layers of the epidermis. J Ultrastr Res 54:37–52, 1976

BURTON JANIS

95

Human Warts

Warts are benign epithelial tumors induced by human papilloma viruses (HPVs).

Etiology

The human papilloma viruses belong to the papova virus group (see Chap. 1, Attributes of Infectious Agents). They are small, icosahedral, DNA viruses similar in morphology, buoyant density, either resistance, and relative thermal stability. They grow slowly in the nucleus of the host cell and produce latent, chronic, and proliferative infections in a variety of hosts. Members of the group include the polyomavirus of mice, the SV-40 virus of monkeys and the Shope papillomavirus of rabbits. The BK virus obtained from the urine of immunosuppressed patients and the JC virus obtained from brains of patients with progressive multifocal leukoencephalopathy are additional human papovaviruses. The viruses of the papova group can be differentiated on the basis of virion size, surface antigen characteristics, and the molecular weight of the DNA. The HPV isolated from human warts is 52 nm to 55 nm in diameter and has icosahedral symmetry with 72 capsomers (Fig. 95-1); the circular double-stranded DNA has a molecular weight of approximately 5×10^6 daltons.

Until recent years, the various morphologic kinds of human warts were thought to be caused by a single virus. On the basis of restriction endonuclease mapping, nucleic acid hybridization, and serology performed with purified virions or purified polypeptide fragments, at least six types of papilloma viruses have been described. The nomenclature of these viruses has been confusing because a name was coined for a virus by the investigator who isolated it without regard to previous isolations. A recent conference resulted in a proposed, standard nomenclature: HPV-1a, HPV-1b, HPV-1c, HPV-2, HPV-3, HPV-4, and HPV-5. The HPV-1 viruses are found in plantar warts, whereas HPV-2 is found predominantly in common skin warts. HPV-3 is found in flat warts and in some patients with epidermodysplasia verruciformis (EV). HPV-4 is found in other patients with EV and is associated with lesions undergoing malignant transformation. It is not clear which type of virus is associated with condyloma acuminata (CA) and laryngeal warts. Condyloma acuminata contain too few virions to be characterized by restriction endonuclease mapping. However, by DNA homology studies it is probable that CA is caused by a distinct type of virus yet to be characterized. Tissue culture growth and characterization of the HPVs has not been reproducible. The use of an epithelioid cell strain (BE cells) and three successive pH stresses appears to be necessary for growth in one tissue culture system.

Epidemiology

Humans worldwide are affected with warts. They are more common in children than in adults. Immunosuppressed patients who have received renal transplants also have a higher incidence of warts. Transmission is probably effected through direct contact, but fomites may also be involved. HPVs infect only humans, and attempts to transmit human warts to other animals have been unsuccessful. Venereal spread is important in the transmission of genital warts.

Pathogenesis and Pathology

Facts about the pathogenesis of human warts are scant. Although incubation periods of 1 to 20 months were reported from human transmission experiments, the location of the virus during this time and the events responsible for the formation of warts are unknown. In a tissue culture system using NHP cells,

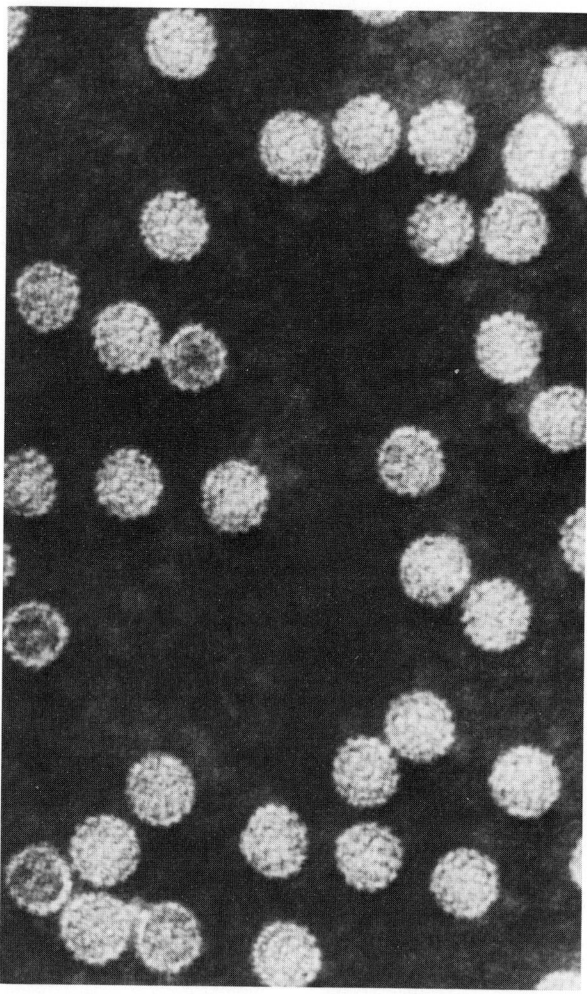

Fig. 95-1. Human papillomavirus isolated from human warts. Cesium chloride banding, negatively stained with phosphotungstic acid. (Original magnification × 170,000)

the gene sequences of HPVs were detected in normal-appearing cells 11 months after infection. Although the gene sequences of HPVs have not been reported in the normal-appearing basal cells of warts, such an occurrence could cause a latent, persistent infection that might precede the formation of warts.

The presence of an immune response against the HPVs depends on the length of time that the person has had warts. Both humoral and cellular immune responses are more evident in patients with regressing warts or with a history of warts than in patients with recently overt warts. Investigators have speculated that the locations of the HPVs in the outer layer of the epidermis keeps the virus sequestered from the immune system. A cell-mediated immune response has been postulated and corroborated histologically as being the first regression event. As a result, virus reacts with antibody-forming cells; virus-specific IgM and IgG subsequently appear.

The histopathologic features of hematoxylin- and eosin-stained warts include hyperkeratosis, parakeratosis, papillomatosis, acanthosis, and elongated rete ridges. Large, vacuolated cells located in the stratum spinosum and granular layer are a characteristic feature, but they may be absent from older warts. Two types of intranuclear inclusions are seen: an eosinophilic inclusion representing degenerated keratin; and a basophilic, Feulgen-positive inclusion representing viral nucleoprotein. Electron microscopic and fluorescent antibody studies corroborate the virus-containing nature of these basophilic inclusions.

Genital warts are less cornified and contain far fewer virus particles than the usual papilloma of human skin.

Manifestations

The appearance of human warts varies with their location on the body: (1) verrucae vulgaris, or common warts—usually 1 mm to 5 mm in diameter, raised from the skin, with a rough, keratotic surface; (2) verrucae plana, or flat, plane, or juvenile warts—smooth-surfaced, smaller, and more numerous than common warts, often involving the face, forehead, and knees or shins; (3) filiform warts—horny excrescences on the face, especially around the eyelids and nares; (4) verruca plantaris—localized on the weight-bearing regions, for example, the heels and soles, where they frequently cause large, painful, mosaiclike plaques; (5) condyloma acuminata or genital warts—large, soft, fleshy excrescences that occur around the vulva, anus, labia, vagina, glans penis, urethral orifices, and perineum; and (6) laryngeal warts—usually multiple occurring in children and young adults.

Diagnosis

The different clinical forms of warts are usually easy to identify by their gross appearance. Serologic diagnosis is strictly a research procedure. If there is doubt regarding a lesion, it should be excised and examined histologically or by electron microscopy. Conditions that mimic warts vary with the kind of wart and its location: granuloma annulare and seborrheic keratosis may be confused with verrucae vulgaris; seborrheic keratosis and cutaneous horn may simulate filiform warts; the micronodular forms of lichen planus or lichen nitidus or molluscum contagiosum (see Chap 94, Molluscum Contagiosum) might be mistaken for flat warts; EV may be mistaken for multiple flat warts; corns may look very much like plantar warts; and syphilitic condyloma or condyloma lata (see Chap. 59, Syphilis) should be differentiated from condyloma acuminata.

Prognosis

Although warts may persist for many years, two-thirds of untreated warts resolve within 2 years. The presence of warts is not harmful unless pain or discomfort results, as with plantar warts, subungual and periungual warts, or genital warts. Malignant transformation occurs in three settings: (1) very rarely in CA, (2) in patients with EV who have HPV-4, and (3) rarely in elderly patients with solitary laryngeal papillomas.

Therapy

The therapy of warts has run the gamut from hypnosuggestion to destructive treatment, immunotherapy, and chemotherapy. Because most warts resolve spontaneously within 2 years, therapy should be offered only to patients with warts that inflict pain or discomfort. The major therapies are destructive: excision, cryotherapy, electrocautery, curettage, and the application of chemicals such as trichloroacetic acid or podophyllin. New insight into the nature of the immune response in wart regression has resulted in the publication of numerous reports about the efficacy of immune modulating agents and autogenous vaccines in treating warts.

Prevention

The diagnosis of wart virus infection is an indication for examination of the other members of the family. Until more is known about the epidemiology, rules of prevention cannot be formulated.

Remaining Problems

The progress made in the last 5 years in understanding the biology of HPVs has opened new areas for investigation. Remaining problems involve further elucidation of the molecular virology and replicative cycle of the HPVs and the events in the virus–keratinocyte interaction that result in the formation and resolution of clinical warts. Studies should be instigated and interpreted in the light of what is known of the oncogenic potential of other papovaviruses. In addition, more information is needed about the immunologic and epidemiologic aspects of HPV infections. Also, a reliable *in vitro* system is needed for cultivation of HPVs.

Bibliography

Journals

ADLER A, SAFAI B: Immunity in wart resolution. J Am Acad Dermatol 1:305–309, 1979

BRIGGAMAN RA, WHEELER CE, JR: Immunology of human warts. J Am Acad Dermatol 1:297–304, 1979

EISINGER M, KUCAROVA O, SARKAR NH, GOOD RA: Propagation of human wart virus in tissue culture. Nature 256:432–434, 1975

GISSMANN L, PFISTER H, ZUR HAUSEN H: Human papilloma viruses (HPV): Characterization of four differet isolates. Virology 76:569–580, 1977

GOLD S: The enigma of viral warts. Practitioner 211:583–592, 1973

JABLONSKA S, ORTH G, JARZABEK–CHORZELSKA M, RZESA G, OBALEK S, GLINSKI W, FAVRE M, CROISSANT O: Epidermodysplasia verruciformis versus disseminated verrucae planae: Is epidermodysplasia verruciformis a generalized infection with wart virus? J Invest Dermatol 72:114–119, 1979

LANCASTER WD, MEENKE W: Persistence of viral DNA in human cell cultures infected with human papilloma virus. Nature 256:434–436, 1975

MELNICK JL: Papova virus group. Science 135:1128–1130, 1962

ORTH A, FAVRE M, JABLONSKA S, BRYLAK K, CROISSANT O: Viral sequences related to human skin papilloma virus in genital warts. Nature 275:334–336, 1978

ORTH G, JABLONSKA S, BREITBURD F, FAVRE M, CROISSANT O: The human papillomaviruses. Bull Cancer 65:151–164, 1978

PASS F: Progress toward a new wart biology. J Invest Dermatol 72:109, 1979

ROWSON KEK, MAKY BWJ: Human papova (wart) virus. Bacteriol Rev 31:110–131, 1967

Workshop on Papilloma Viruses and Cancer. Cancer Res 39:545–546, 1979

CHARLES L. WISSEMAN, JR.

96 Spotted Fevers

The spotted fevers (tick-typhus fevers) are acute, self-limited infectious diseases caused by rickettsias transmitted to humans by the bite of infected ticks. Rocky Mountain spotted fever (RMSF), caused by *Rickettsia rickettsii,* is the most severe disease of this group and is confined to the Western hemisphere. The other diseases of this group also have distinct geographical distributions (Table 96-1). However, as tests with greater specificity have been applied, it has become clear that the ticks of the major land masses harbor a variety of rickettsias of the spotted fever group, which vary from avirulent to highly virulent for humans. All of the spotted fever rickettsias exist in enzootic cycles involving ticks and vertebrate hosts (mammals). The human is an accidental, dead-end host.

Rocky Mountain Spotted Fever

Etiology

Rickettsia rickettsii, the cause of Rocky Mountain spotted fever, shares many properties with other members of the genus *Rickettsia* (Chap. 98, Typhus Fevers). Members of this species are slightly larger than *R. prowazekii,* stain with the Gimenez stain, have an outer envelop that resembles that of gram-negative bacteria ultrastructurally, and are obligate intracellular parasites that grow free in the cytoplasm of host cells. In common with the other spotted fever rickettsias, *R. rickettsii* may enter and grow within the nucleus of host cells and may exit from host cells without destroying them, producing *in vitro* an infection that spreads rapidly throughout the culture. All members of the spotted fever group possess cross-reacting, major antigenic components, and *R. rickettsii* shares at least one antigenic determinant with the typhus group (Chap. 98, Typhus Fevers).

Epidemiology

Rocky Mountain spotted fever is widely distributed throughout the temperate and tropical zones of the western hemisphere. First recognized in the western United States, it has been reported from most of the contiguous states of the United States, as well as from Mexico, Central America (Panama, Costa Rica), and South America. During the past decade, the number of cases per year has increased in the United States for unknown reasons (Fig. 96-1). Although a record total of 1163 cases was reported in 1980, the incidence of 0.52 per 100,000 has not changed since 1977. RMSF is now reported most often from the southern Atlantic states (709 cases, 61%) with North Carolina reporting more cases (321 cases, 28%) than any other state in 1980. The highest incidence is in the 5- to 9-year-old age group. Overall, the mortality rate is 5% to 10%; however, both morbidity and mortality increase with age. Most cases occur in the spring and early summer, the seasons of maximum tick activity, but cases occur in all months of the year in the southern states.

RMSF exists in nature in an enzootic cycle involving ticks and a variety of mammals. In the United States, the most important vectors of *R. rickettsii* for humans are *Dermacentor andersoni* (the wood tick of the West), *Dermacentor variabilis* (the dog tick of the East), and *Amblyomma americanum* (the Lone Star tick of the South).

Dermacentor spp. are three-host ticks: The larvae feed on small rodents (*e.g.,* deer mice), the nymphs feed on larger rodents (*e.g.,* rabbits, hares), and the adults feed on medium to large nonrodent mammals (deer, dogs). All stages are capable of transmitting *R. rickettsii.* Because the ticks transmit the rickettsias transovarially, they not only serve as vectors but also are the major reservoirs; mammalians serve primarily as amplifying hosts.

Table 96-1. *Summary of Certain Important Epidemiologic and Clinical Characteristics of Rickettsial Diseases*

Disease	**Epidemiologic features**			**Usual Incubation Period in Days (Range)**	**Rash**		
	GEOGRAPHIC OCCURRENCE	USUAL MODE OF TRANSMISSION TO MAN	RESERVOIR		ESCHAR	DISTRIBUTION	TYPE
Spotted fever group							
Rocky Mountain spotted fever	Western hemisphere	Tick bite	Ticks Rodents	3–4 (2–12)	None	Extremities to trunk; palms and soles	Macular, maculopapular, petechial
Tick typhus	Mediterranean littoral, Africa, Asia	Tick bite	Ticks Rodents	12 (7–18)	Frequent	Trunk, extremities, face, palms, soles	Macular, maculopapular, petechial
Rickettsialpox	USA, Russia, Korea	House mouse mite bite	Mites Mice	12 (9–24)	Usually present	Trunk, face, extremities	Papular, vesicular
Typhus group							
Primary louse-borne typhus	Worldwide	Infected louse feces rubbed into broken skin or as aerosol to mucous membranes	Man	12 (8–15)	None	Trunk to extremities	Macular, maculopapular
Brill–Zinsser disease	Worldwide	Recrudescence months or years after primary attack of louse-borne typhus	—	—	None	Trunk to extremities	Macular, maculopapular
Murine typhus	Scattered pockets worldwide	Infected flea feces rubbed into broken skin or as aerosols to mucous membranes	Rodents	12 (6–14)	None	Trunk to extremities	Macular, maculopapular
Scurb typhus	Japan, SE Asia, W and SW Pacific	Mite bite	Mites Rodents	11 (6–11)	Frequent	Trunk to extremities	Macular, maculopapular, evanescent
Q Fever	Worldwide	Inhalation of dried dusts from environment of infected animals	Ticks Mammals	14 (9–20)	None	None	None

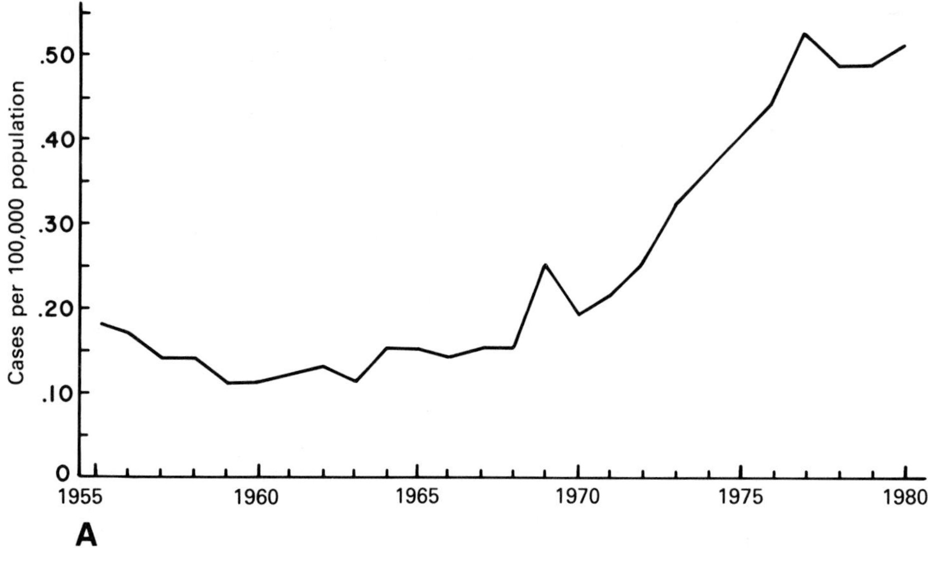

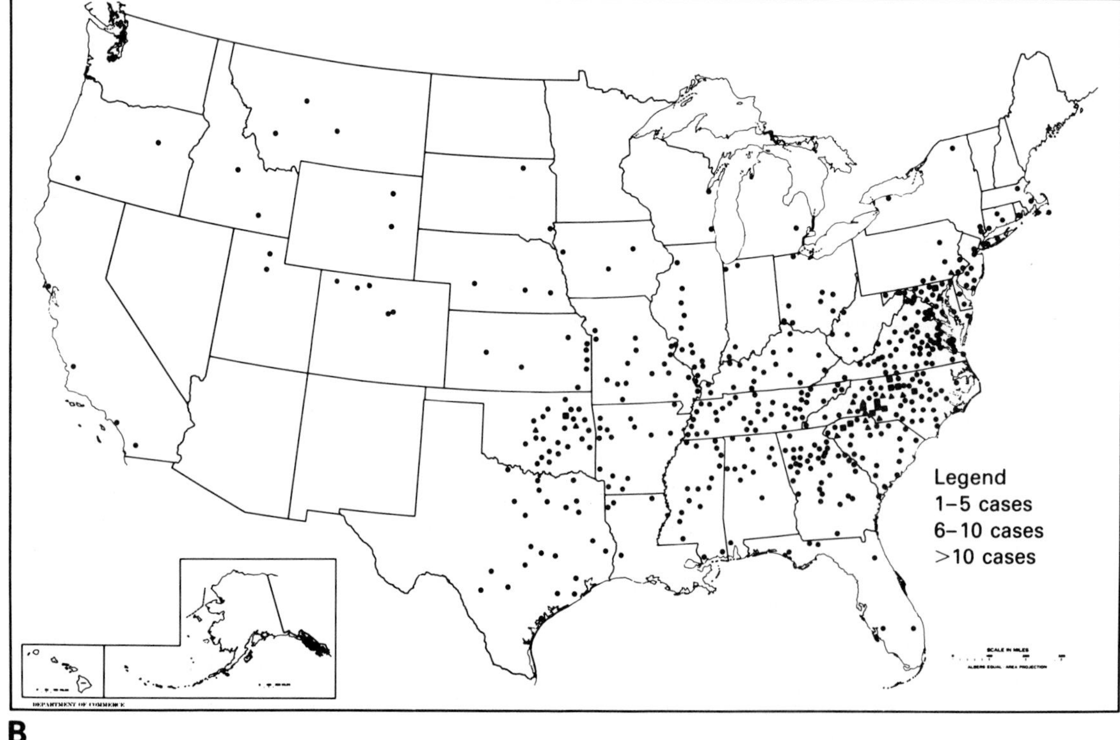

Fig. 96-1. (*A*) Cases of Rocky Mountain spotted fever reported in the United States, 1955–1980. (Morbid Mortal Week Rep, Suppl Summary, 1980) (*B*) Cases of Rocky Mountain spotted fever reported by county in the United States, 1980. (Morbid Mortal Week Rep, Suppl Summary, 1980)

Because *R. rickettsii* is transmitted to humans by the bite of infected ticks, humans must enter into the habitats of ticks to become infected. Thus, RMSF is primarily a disease of rural and suburban areas, the latter extending into previously wooded and agricultural areas, and is associated with those who engage in certain activities, both recreational and occupational (*e.g.,* ranchers, farmers, rangers, telephone and electrical lineworkers, road workers). A history of potential exposure is extremely important in alerting the physician to suspect RMSF early in the undifferentiated, acute febrile stage when the administration of appropriate, specific antimicrobial therapy will reduce mortality virtually to zero.

Pathology and Pathogenesis

RMSF is a vasculitis that afflicts small blood vessels, causing focal lesions that may be widespread and very severe. Both endothelial and smooth muscle cells are invaded; there is marked cell damage and destruction, permitting leakage of plasma as well as red cells. The extravascular fluid volume is increased, as may be reflected by clinically apparent edema. Fibrin-platelet thrombi, containing varying numbers of leukocytes, develop at sites of endothelial damage, often occluding the lumen of the blood vessel. A perivascular cellular infiltrate develops that contains some polymorphonuclear leukocytes (early) but consists largely of mononuclear cells (monocyte-macrophage series, lymphocytes, plasma cells). In rapidly fatal cases, the characteristic perivascular cellular infiltrate may be lacking. The vascular lesions occur in virtually all organs, including the brain, where vascular occlusion may also produce microinfarcts.

Manifestations

The usual incubation period is 5 to 7 days (variation, 2–12 days); severe disease tends to be associated with a shorter incubation period. If present, prodromes consist of anorexia, irritability, malaise, feverishness, and chilly sensations. The disease may be so mild that the patient remains ambulatory, or it may be so severe that the patient dies 3 to 6 days after onset. Typically, the onset of disease is fairly sudden, with the development of severe headache, chills, fever, prostration, nausea and occasionally vomiting, myalgia (especially of the back and the legs), abdominal pain, conjunctival injection, and photophobia. The temperature attains 39°C to 40°C (102°F–104°F) in the first 2 days, is unremittant for about 2 weeks, and falls by lysis over 3 to 4 days.

Although a prodromal rash may be present at the onset, the characteristic rash (Fig. 96-2) appears after 2 to 6 days—at first on the wrists and ankles, then extending over the limbs and body (including palms, soles, face, and mucous membranes of the oropharynx). The lesions soon darken, become fixed, and develop a papular component. They may become petechial or hemorrhagic. The rash begins to recede with defervescence and disappears slowly.

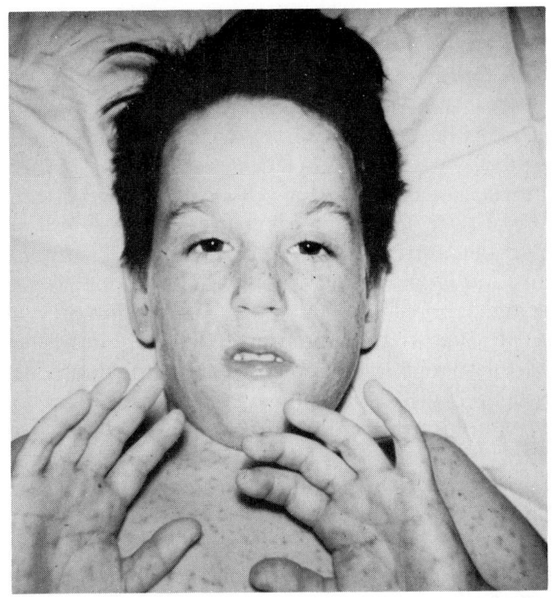

Fig. 96-2. Typical Rocky Mountain spotted fever rash occurring on face and palms. (Hazard GW, Ganz RN, Nevin RW, Nauss AH, Curtis E, Bell WJ, Murray ES: N Engl J Med 280:57–62, 1969)

When the vascular lesions are widespread, the manifestations of RMSF involve several organ systems to varying degrees, with a strong cardiovascular component. Early in the disease, the pulse is full, regular, and elevated in proportion to the fever; later, it becomes more rapid and feeble. The electrocardiogram may show minor S-T deflections and prolonged P-R intervals. Hypotension of some degree is common and shock may occur. The skin may become necrotic over bony prominences and pressure points. Gangrene of the fingers, toes, ears, or genitalia may develop. There may be bleeding from the nose, gastrointestinal tract, or kidneys. Edema may become apparent.

The manifestations of central nervous system (CNS) involvement may include restlessness, insomnia, delirium, stupor, and in severe cases coma. Transient deafness is common; cranial nerves serving other senses are involved with variable frequency. Tremors, athetoid movements, convulsions, and muscular rigidity may occur. Electroencephalographic changes may persist for months. Sequelae may include behavioral disturbances and learning disabilities.

Thrombocytopenia is common. Other disturbances of the clotting mechanism may occur, and occasionally the syndrome of disseminated intravascular coagulation (DIC) appears (Chap. 7, Manifestations of Infectious Diseases). Serum enzyme and isoenzyme determinations frequently reveal evidence of damage to liver, skeletal muscle, myocardium, and lung. Indeed, interstitial pneumonitis with varying degrees of pulmonary dysfunction is common. Proteinuria is common. Oliguria, anuria, and azotemia occur in severe cases and probably reflect the degree of hypotension rather than primary kidney pathology. Severe hypotension, tachycardia, respiratory distress and a falling temperature are grave prognostic signs. Convalescence may take weeks to months.

Diagnosis

The clinical diagnosis of RMSF is essential on two counts: (1) laboratory tests diagnostic of RMSF are not positive at the onset of disease and (2) a favorable outcome depends on early initiation of specific therapy. Because RMSF is at first an acute, undifferentiated, febrile disease with no pathognomonic signs, all circumstantial evidence must be heeded: the finding of an attached tick; a history of a tick-bite or handling ticks from dogs; exposure to endemic (recreational, occupational) areas is also quite important information, since many patients give no history of finding or seeing ticks; a normal to low blood leukocyte count with or without a depressed platelet count; severe headache and myalgia. As the disease progresses, typical manifestations appear: rash, sustained high fever, intractable headache, change in mental status, low blood pressure. However, measles, meningococcemia, and rash-producing enteroviral infections must be considered even in endemic areas.

In many patients, a specific diagnosis can be made quickly by demonstration of *R. rickettsii* using specific fluorescent antibody and frozen sections of a punch biopsy of the rash, even if the patient has already received tetracycline or chloramphenicol for 24 to 48 hours. It may become possible to detect rickettsial antigen in urine by sensitive tests, such as the enzyme-linked immunosorbent antibody (ELISA) test (Chap. 14, Immunologic Diagnosis).

The antibody response is relatively slow in RMSF and may be further delayed (as long as 4–6 weeks after onset) by early chemotherapy. Hence, serologic tests for antibody are used to confirm the diagnosis, but are not useful in making a specific diagnosis at the critical time when decisions about chemotherapy must be made. Indeed, antibodies may never be detectable in rapidly fatal cases, and the histopathology may not be diagnostic. The most useful specific serologic test is the indirect fluorescent antibody test; it is available through local health departments, the Centers for Disease Control, and the World Health Organization Rickettsial Reference Laboratories. The complement fixation (CF) and microagglutination tests may also be used. Nonspecific but still useful because of general availability is the Weil–Felix test using Proteus OX-2 and OX-19 antigens (Table 98-1).

On the basis of serologic evidence, some of the RMSF-like disease encountered in the region of Fort Bragg, North Carolina, was caused by *Rickettsia canada,* tick-borne rickettsias that cross-react with the typhus group rickettsias. Similarly, and RMSF-like disease reported in California may be caused by new rickettsias of the spotted fever group. It is unknown how many, if any, of the growing number of spotted fever group rickettsias isolated from ticks in the United States and other parts of the world actually cause disease in humans. The occurrence of sporadic, flying-squirrel-associated infections with *R. prowazekii* in the eastern United States reinforces the need to submit to an appropriate reference laboratory blood drawn as early as possible in the disease for isolation of the many rickettsial agents suspected or recently recognized as causes for disease in humans.

Prognosis

Early, prompt administration of specific antirickettsial antimicrobics is the single most important factor in reducing morbidity and mortality. If treated early and appropriately, RMSF responds surprisingly rapidly and presents no special problems. Delay in instituting specific therapy is associated with increased risk of serious pathophysiologic changes that are difficult to manage, prolonged convalescence, various complications, and death.

Although RMSF varies from mild to fulminant, increasing age is the one known determinant of the severity of the disease. On epidemiologic bases, strains of *R. rickettsii* were once thought to vary in virulence, a suggestion that has not been confirmed.

Therapy

Unlike the other rickettsioses, within a few days (as early as 2–3 days in fulminant cases) after the onset of RMSF, pathophysiologic changes may occur that do not respond to antirickettsial therapy, are difficult to correct medically, and may lead rapidly to death. *Delay in administering appropriate, specific antirickettsial therapy is the single most important factor making for a continuing fatality rate of 5% to*

10% in RMSF. A suspected case of RMSF must be considered a medical emergency. Only the tetracyclines and chloramphenicol are effective. Erythromycin is unreliable. The penicillins, cephalosporins, aminocyclitols, sulfonamides, and trimethoprim-sulfamethoxazole are ineffective. If it is reasonable to suspect that a patient is suffering from RMSF, it is reasonable to initiate specific therapy as soon as specimens have been taken for the laboratory diagnosis of other possible causes of the illness.

Tetracycline in a dose of 25 to 50 mg/kg body wt/day, PO, as four equal portions, 6-hourly, is adequate; if parenteral treatment is necessary, 25 to 30 mg/kg body wt/day, IV, as four equal portions, 6-hourly, is sufficient. Doxycycline is also effective, in a dose of 100 mg every 12 hours, either PO or IV.

Chloramphenicol is equally effective: 50 to 75 mg/kg body wt/day, PO, as four equal portions, 6-hourly, for adults and children (no more than 25 mg/kg body wt/day for premature or neonatal infants) or as the succinate derivative, 50 to 60 mg/kg body wt/day, IV, as four equal portions, 6-hourly for adults and children (no more than 25 mg/kg body wt/day for premature or neonatal infants).

Neither the tetracyclines nor chloramphenicol are rickettsiacidal; they do not eradicate the organism from the body. Cure depends on inhibiting the further growth of the rickettsias until an adequate immune response develops. Hence, the duration of antimicrobial therapy depends somewhat on the length of the period from onset of disease to commencement of therapy. The antimicrobial therapy should be continued for at least 6 days and until the patient has been afebrile for at least 48 hours. Patients who relapse should be treated again using the same regimen applied initially.

If there are no complications and treatment was begun early in the course of the disease, patients with RMSF usually become afebrile within 48 to 72 hours and require little special care. However, the seriously ill patient whose disease has progressed for several days often requires multifaceted, individualized, and intensive care. For example, the parenteral administration of fluids must be slow so as not to tax the potentially labile cardiovascular system; the quantities and electrolyte content must take into account the presence of oliguria or anuria and the fact that excesses may contribute to general and pulmonary edema. Albumin may be used to combat hypoproteinemia and packed red cells to correct anemia. Management of peripheral vascular collapse is empirical and generally unsatisfactory: (1) oxygen; (2) judicious use of salt-poor, concentrated albumin as a plasma expander and to reduce edema; (3) vasopressor drugs; and (4) glucosteroids (*e.g.,* dexamethasone). Pulmonary edema and congestive heart failure have been treated with digitalis. Treatment of DIC has been generally unsatisfactory; the use of heparin is controversial.

In seriously ill patients, nursing care is essential. Stuporous or comatose patients should be turned frequently to avoid pressure necroses and hypostatic pneumonia. Proper oral hygiene may reduce the risk of suppurative parotitis.

Prevention

There is no vaccine for immunoprophylaxis against RMSF. The vaccines once used did prolong the incubation period and modify the disease, but were unreliable as preventives.

Avoidance of ticks and tick bites is preventive, that is, tick-infested areas should not be entered. If such areas must be gone into, protective clothing impregnated with tick repellents may be effective but may not be tolerable in a hot climate. Frequent inspection of the body for ticks is important, since ticks usually crawl about for some time prior to attaching and can be removed easily before they attach. Persons living in tick-infested rural or suburban areas should routinely inspect themselves and their children at evening bath time—a very practical and effective measure. Ticks that are attached should be removed promptly because the transmission of rickettsias is inefficient during the first few hours of attachment. Although many methods for removal of attached ticks have been proposed, the most reliable is gentle steady traction with forceps (to prevent contamination of the hands with rickettsias), taking care that the mouth parts of the tick are removed in the process of detachment.

Dogs readily become infested with ticks and may bring them into the house or yard. The use of repellent-impregnated collars may reduce the number of ticks on dogs. Attached ticks may also be removed periodically with the aid of forceps.

The management of an afebrile person from whom a tick has been removed warrants special comment. Although the actual risk varies from place to place, the possibility is remote that a particular tick taken from a person is infected with *R. rickettsii* and has actually transmitted the organism. Chemoprophylaxis is unwarranted. Infection may not have occurred; if it has, the administration of a rickettsiastatic antimicrobic during the incubation period would only delay the onset of disease, not prevent it. Instead, a report of malaise, fever, or other indication of illness during the 2 to 3 weeks following removal of the tick should be evaluated by the physician prior to giving early chemotherapy.

Tick Typhus Fevers

In addition to RMSF, three other tick-borne rickettsioses of the spotted fever group have been recognized on clinical, epidemiologic and geographic grounds: (1) Siberian tick typhus (North Asian tick-borne rickettsiosis) caused by *Rickettsia sibirica;* (2) Queensland tick typhus caused by *Rickettsia australis;* and (3) tick-borne rickettsioses, putatively caused by *Rickettsia conorii,* and given numerous local names, which are widely distributed in the Mediterranean, Black and Caspian Sea littorals (fievre boutonneuse, Marseilles fever), continental Africa (Kenya tick typhus, South African tick typhus), and Southern Asia (Indian tick typhus). Though similar in many respects to RMSF, these diseases are milder, are rarely fatal, and characteristically exhibit an eschar at the site of the infecting tick bite that is associated with regional lymphadenopathy. All respond readily to treatment with a tetracycline or chloramphenicol.

The present classification and etiology of the tick-typhus fevers is probably simplistic; discriminating studies by modern methods may reveal multiple agents for the tick-typhus spotted fevers. For example, South African investigators have long claimed that the agent of South African tick bite fever differs from classical *R. conorii.* Also, new spotted fever group rickettsias, tentatively named *R. israelii,* have been reported to be associated with disease more severe than that usually ascribed to *R. conorii* in parts of Israel. In ticks in Pakistan, *R. sibirica* have been found along with *R. conorii* and several new spotted fever group rickettsias. Tick-borne spotted fever group rickettsioses have been reported in humans in southeast Asia, but the agent(s) have not been identified.

Bibliography

Books

BURGDORFER W, ANACKER RL (eds): Rickettsiae and Rickettsial Diseases. Academic Press, New York, 1981. 650 pp.

Center for Disease Control: Rickettsial Disease Surveillance Report No. 1, 1975–1978. September 1979. 15 pp.

KAPLOWITZ LG, FISCHER JJ, SPARLING PF: Rocky Mountain spotted fever: A clinical dilemma. In Remington JS, Swartz MN (eds): Clinical Current Topics in Infectious Diseases. New York, McGraw–Hill, 1981. pp 89–108.

ZDRODOVSKII PF, GOLINEVICH HM: The Rickettsial Diseases. New York, Pergamon Press, 1960. 629 pp.

Journals

HATTWICK MAW, O'BRIEN FJ, HANSON, B: Rocky Mountain spotted fever: Epidemiology of an increasing problem. Ann Intern Med 84:732–736, 1976

PHILIP RN, CASPER EA, MACCORMACK JN, SEXTON DJ, THOMAS LA, ANACKER RL, BURGDORFER W, STEWART V: A comparison of serological methods for diagnosis of Rocky Mountain spotted fever. Am J Epidemiol 105:56–67, 1977

WALKER DH, CAIN BG, OLMSTEAD PM: Laboratory diagnosis of Rocky Mountain spotted fever by immunofluorescent demonstration of *Rickettsia rickettsii* in cutaneous lesions. Am J Clin Pathol 69:619–623, 1978

WOODWARD TE, PEDERSEN CE, OSTER CN, BOGLEY LR, ROMBERGER J, SNYDER MJ: Prompt confirmation of Rocky Mountain spotted fever: Identification of rickettsiae in skin tissues. J Infect Dis 134:297–301, 1976

PAUL D. HOEPRICH

Rickettsialpox

97

First described in 1946, rickettsialpox is a benign disease that is caused by *Rickettsia akari* and transmitted to man by the mouse mite, *Allodermanyssus sanguineus.* Additional features include an eschar at the site of inoculation, a vesiculopapular rash, leukopenia, and the lack of Weil–Felix agglutinins.

Etiology

Rickettsia akari are typical members of the spotted fever group of rickettsias, as confirmed by cross-reactions with other rickettsias of the group in serologic (soluble antigen) and protection tests.

The rickettsias isolated in 1949 in the southern Ukraine and designated *Dermacentroxenus murinus* by Soviet authors, are identical with *R. akari.* Although the vector and the disease are also identical and consistent with the findings in the United States, the rat has been implicated as the major rodent host in the Ukraine.

As with other rickettsias, *R. akari* are quite susceptible to chloramphenicol and the tetracyclines.

Epidemiology

The mouse mite is the arthropod host. Because *R. akari* does not cause disease in mites and is passed transovarially, *A. sanguineus* is a reservoir, even as the house mouse, *Mus musculus,* is the definitive, preferred host of *A. sanguineus.* In addition, the mite is the vector of rickettsialpox. After taking a blood meal, the mite drops off its host, ordinarily remaining in or near nesting areas; it does not seek a new provider until it is again hungry, a period that may be as long as 24 hours. Humans are involved only if available to infected mites that have come on hard times. That is, rickettsialpox is virtually limited in occurrence to urban settings when the depletion of murine hosts (reduced food supplies, disease, poisoning, trapping) forces mites infected with *R. akari* to feed on humans. Persons of any age and either sex may be infected.

The range of *A. sanguineus* in the United States is known to extend from the Atlantic Coast at least as far west as Utah; however, it is probably present wherever there are mice. Infections have been reported in greatest numbers from New York City; cases have also been reported from Boston, and as far west as Salt Lake City. Curiously, there has been a dearth of reports of rickettsialpox in the United States since the 1950s. In part, this may be related to improved rodent control. However, it is possible that the replacement of *A. sanguineus* by the tropical rat mite *(Ornithonyssus bacoti)* as the dominant ectoparasite of house mice in New York City may also be important, because *O. bacoti* is not an efficient vector of *R. akari.*

In addition to the Russian experience, disease clinically consistent with rickettsialpox has been described in Africa. Moreover, isolation of *R. akari* has been reported from a wild Korean field mouse, and the Korean vole. Thus, the arthropod–rodent cycle of parasitism may be maintained independent of human-associated rodents.

Pathogenesis and Pathology

The inoculation of humans with *R. akari* occurs through the oral secretions of the mite that are injected as a blood meal is obtained. The reaction is most intense at the site of the bite—the primary lesion. In this respect, the disease resembles scrub typhus. Regional lymphadenopathy may occur. This, and isolation of *R. akari* from vesiculopapular lesions (secondary lesions), attests to lymphohematogenous spread from the primary lesion.

Because the disease is benign, there are no

reports of postmortem examination. However, in biopsy specimens of the eschar of inoculation, inflammation is intense in the deeper layers of the dermis, where there is actual necrosis. Thrombosis and necrosis of capillaries, intercellular edema, and infiltration with mononuclear cells are the principal features. The vesiculopapular lesions display much the same histopathologic features, but the reaction is less intense and more superficial. Rickettsias are not usually seen in either primary or secondary lesions.

Manifestations

Because the bite of *A. sanguineus* is not usually noted by the patient, the lapse of time from inoculation to the appearance of the primary lesion of rickettsialpox is not known with certainity, but it appears to be 1 to 2 weeks. The primary lesion may not be noticed by the patient, although it is detected on physical examination in 95% of patients. Virtually any area of the body may be involved. Beginning as a firm, reddened papule, the primary lesion soon enlarges to 1 cm to 1.5 cm in diameter, and it is surrounded by erythema as central vesiculation occurs about 2 days after onset. When it dries, it forms a brownish crust, followed by evolution to a blackened eschar that sloughs in about 3 weeks and leaves a scar. Although the primary lesion is asymptomatic, regional nodes are usually enlarged and may be tender.

Four to seven days after the primary lesion has appeared, there is an abrupt onset of illness with chills (2 or 3 times a day), fever (remittent, to 40°C–104°F), sweats, headache, backache, and malaise. Without specific therapy, symptoms may persist 7 to 10 days.

Accompanying the onset of illness, or 1 to 2 days later, discrete maculopapular lesions appear that are smaller than the primary lesion. There is quick progression to central vesiculation. The vesicles are small, and they appear to be embedded in the papule. The rash may involve any part of the body, but is rarely present on the palms, soles, or oropharyngeal mucous membranes. Over the course of a week, the vesicles dry, the lesions scab, and the scabs fall off, leaving a brownish discoloration. Scarring does not result. Hepatosplenomegaly does not occur, and there is neither clinical nor roentgenographic evidence of cardiopulmonary involvement.

Leukopenia is usual, without distortion of the differential count. Serum agglutinins do not appear, either for bacterial pathogens or for the strains of *Proteus* spp. used in the Weil–Felix reaction.

Diagnosis

The clinical manifestations and course of illness of rickettsialpox may suggest the correct diagnosis. However, confirmation is usually achieved through the demonstration of a rise in titer of specific complement-fixing antibodies in the weeks after the illness. Serums obtained during the acute illness are nonreactive, whereas titers of 1:16 or more are found 4 to 6 weeks after the onset of illness.

Isolation of *R. akari* has been accomplished by the inoculation of mice, guinea pigs, and embryonated hens' eggs. The clot from blood drawn during the acute, febrile illness and the liquid aspirated from vesicles may yield the parasite.

Chickenpox (Chap. 93, Varicella and Herpes Zoster) is the usual misdiagnosis, although chickenpox is usually a disease of children, whereas rickettsialpox occurs more often in adults. Also, the skin lesions differ. There is no primary eschar in chickenpox. Moreover, the entire papule, down to the base, is committed to the vesicle in chickenpox. Fever does not ordinarily precede the rash of chickenpox, and it usually continues as long as new lesions form.

Patients with smallpox (Chap. 92, Smallpox and Other Poxvirus Infections) are much more seriously ill than those with rickettsialpox. Again, there is no primary eschar. The lesions are distinct and characteristically pustulate.

Although fever and a general vesicular skin rash may occur with cytomegalovirus (Chap. 75, Cytomegalovirus Infections), coxsackievirus and echovirus (Chap. 149, Coxsackievirus and Echovirus Infections) infections, the epidemiologic features and manifestations readily permit distinction from rickettsialpox.

Nearly all other rickettsioses (Chap. 96, 98, and 99, Spotted Fevers; Typhus Fevers; Scrub Typhus) are more severe than rickettsialpox. None yields vesicular lesions. However, the rashes of both scrub typhus and boutonneuse fever are heralded by a primary lesion that progresses to an eschar identical with that of rickettsialpox. The geographic distribution of these diseases is unique. Moreover, serologic distinction is readily made.

Prognosis

Rickettsialpox is benign, subsiding within 10 days without antimicrobial therapy. Defervescence and the termination of symptoms follow within 12 to 24 hours after the institution of appropriate chemotherapy.

Therapy

The tetracyclines are the agents of choice for treatment of patients with rickettsialpox. Tetracycline (15 mg/kg body wt/day, PO, as four equal portions, 6-hourly, for 1 week) is uniformly effective. Chloramphenicol should be equally effective.

Prevention

The ultimate preventive of rickettsialpox is the elimination of rodent infestation of human habitations.

Bibliography

Journals

BARKER LP: Rickettsialpox: Clinical and laboratory study of twelve hospitalized cases. JAMA 141:1119–1123, 1949

GREENBERG M: Rickettsialpox in New York City. Am J Med 4:866–874, 1947

LACKMAN DB: A review of information on rickettsialpox in the United States. Clin Pediatr 2:296–301, 1963

ROUCHE B: Reporter at large: Alerting of Pomerantz. The New Yorker 23:28–37, 1947

WONG B, SINGER C, ARMSTRONG D, MILLIAN SJ: Rickettsialpox. Case report and epidemiologic review. JAMA 242:1998–1999, 1979

ZDRODOVSKIJ PF: Les rickettsioses en URSS. Bull WHO 31:33–43, 1964

CHARLES L. WISSEMAN, JR.

98 Typhus Fevers

Of the three typhus fevers, primary louse-borne typhus and Brill–Zinsser disease are caused by *Rickettsia prowazekii,* whereas murine flea-borne typhus is caused by *Rickettsia typhi* (formerly *Rickettsia mooseri*). Clinically and pathologically these three diseases are very similar, but each displays unique epidemiologic features.

Primary Louse-Borne Typhus

Primary louse-borne typhus is an acute infectious disease usually transmitted to humans by the body louse (*Pediculus humanus humanus*—Chap. 114, Pediculosis). The disease is known also as epidemic typhus, typhus exanthematicus, tabardillo, fleckfieber, and classic typhus.

Etiology

Rickettsia prowazekii consists of obligate intracellular parasites that grow in the cytoplasm of the host cell and reproduce by binary fission. The optimum temperature for growth is 35°C. They are typical gram-negative bacilli in ultrastructure, possess a slime layer, display endotoxic actions, and conduct a complex array of independent metabolic activities. The DNA genome (about 10^9 daltons) hybridizes to about 70% with that of *R. typhi,* with which it shares some serologically cross-reacting polysaccharide and polypeptide antigens. Although the live organisms can penetrate nucleated host cells, they may cause lysis from without. Also, they are capable of hemolyzing the erythrocytes of several mammals and causing a toxic death in mice that is associated with increased vascular permeability.

Although the morphology of *R. prowasekii* is protean, coccobacillary forms predominate, varying in length from about 0.3 μm to 0.8 μm, with a diameter of 0.3 μm. The typical forms are diplobacilli that have slightly pointed ends with a transparent band between the paired bacilli. The rickettsias stain red by the Gimenez method (Chap. 9, Microscopic Examinations). Although *R. prowazekii* is easily killed by common antiseptics and dies in a few hours at room temperature, viability is retained for several days in blood at 5°C, and for many years by quick-freezing and storing at or below −70°C.

Epidemiology

Louse-borne typhus is perhaps best known in temperate zones for devastating epidemics recurrent over centuries in association with war and famine. In the present century, epidemics have resulted in more than 30 million cases in eastern Europe between 1918 and 1922, and several million cases during World War II in eastern Europe (among Yugoslav partisan forces), North Africa, and Central Asia.

Currently, typhus is endemic in the mountains of Central and South America, parts of Africa, South Asia (Afghanistan, Himalaya Mountains) and probably northern China. Influenced by a complex variety of factors, louse-borne typhus in endemic zones may occur as inapparent infections, sporadic cases, sharp village outbreaks, and even large epidemics.

The occurrence of typhus in a population and the epidemiologic pattern of the disease depend on (1) the presence of lice and conditions conducive to infestation (*e.g.,* prolonged wearing of the same clothing because of war, natural disaster, depressed socioeconomic conditions, climate, cultural factors); (2) the ways in which people exchange lice (crowded conditions, prisons, markets, festivals); (3) the availability of *R. prowazekii* (introduced, endogenous recrudescent); and (4) the immunity of the population (an attack of typhus usually confers solid and long-lasting, but nonsterile immunity). Because typhus is transmitted from person to person only by human body lice, a deloused and bathed person cannot transmit typhus. However, when conditions favor the occurrence of typhus, humans serve as both (1) amplifying hosts during acute disease and (2) the major interepidemic reservoir—through persisting, latent infections after convalescence. Indeed, until recently, humans were thought to be the only reservoir. However, the discovery of a natural enzootic cycle of rickettsias indistinguishable from *R. prowazekii* in flying squirrels in the eastern United States has introduced a new dimension to the epidemiology of typhus. There is need to explore this possible reservoir, since sporadic cases of apparently typical typhus have occurred in persons living in close association with flying squirrels.

Human body lice acquire *R. prowazekii* by feeding on the blood of a person with primary or recrudescent typhus (Brill–Zinsser disease) during the acute febrile (rickettsemic) period. In lice, *R. prowazekii* proliferate in the cells of the midgut, and after 5 to 10 days rickettsias appear in the feces. Lice do not inject rickettsias as they bite; however, they defecate as they feed, and infected feces are rubbed into bite wounds during scratching. Dried feces may become airborne and infect through the conjuctivae or the respiratory tract. Lice usually die of the infection, and there is no transovarial transmission. Because lice prefer a temperature of 29°C to 30°C, after feeding they retreat to the clothing where they breed. They leave both the febrile patient and the cooling corpse. Lice move readily from person to person.

Pathogenesis and Pathology

Rickettsia prowazekii multiplies preferentially in the endothelial cells of small blood vessels, leaving the smooth muscle layers intact. Foci of vasculitis result and are found in all organs but are most numerous in the skin, subcutaneous tissues, and central nervous system (CNS). Several days after the appearance of the skin rash, the lesions consist of damaged or swollen endothelial cells, fibrin–platelet–leukocyte thrombi that partially or completely occlude the lumina of vessels, and a perivascular infiltrate of mononuclear cells (primarily monocyte–macrophage cells, a few lymphocytes, and some plasma cells). Diffuse mononuclear cell infiltrates may be present in the myocardium and lungs.

Manifestations

Typhus may begin with vague symptoms such as evening malaise and fatigue, and go on to clinically inapparent infection, mild illness, or rapidly fatal disease. However, classical typhus is marked by a fairly abrupt onset of fever, headache, and malaise; there is increasing prostration as the fever mounts rapidly and is sustained at 39°C to 41°C (102°F–106°F). The conjunctivae become injected. Headache becomes severe, constant, and intractable; pain and tenderness of the back and legs may be severe.

Violent delirium is frequent, especially at night. Tinnitus with or without progression to deafness is frequent. Dysphagia, dysphonia, and slurring of the speech may occur. Changes in mental status are common, as the name typhus (from the Greek *typhos,* "smoky or hazy") implies. Typically, the patient lies motionless, staring without expression at the ceiling, responding only to strong verbal or painful stimuli. Severely ill patients may become stuporous or fall into coma, have general seizures, become incontinent, or develop a plastic kind of rigidity.

A rash develops about 5 to 7 days after onset; it appears first on the trunk (often most easily seen in the axillary folds), and then it spreads to the extremities. Initially, it is macular and blanches on pressure; it then develops a papular component and may become fixed, petechial, or ecchymotic.

At onset, the pulse may be slow relative to the fever, but it increases as the disease progresses (to 120–140 beats per minute) and may become weak and irregular. The systolic blood pressure frequently falls to 80 to 90 mm Hg; episodes of severe hypotension may occur. As patients approach an uncomplicated death, they develop cold extremities, a weak rapid pulse, and severe hypotension; since there is no evidence of cardiac failure and since peripheral vascular lesions are widespread, it is thought that death is due to peripheral vascular collapse. Gangrene of the extremities may develop, as may hemiplegia consistent with a major vascular occlusion. Pressure necroses are common.

Defervescence is by lysis over a period of several days. Depending upon the severity of the disease, the resolution of abnormalities may be rapid or prolonged, but ultimately it is usually remarkably complete.

In marked contrast to Rocky Mountain spotted fever, adequate, specific antirickettsial chemotherapy and appropriate supportive measures may halt the disease process at almost any stage, often even in patients who would have been classed as moribund.

Diagnosis

An acute, undifferentiated, febrile disease at onset, typhus is difficult to diagnose on clinical grounds alone. Even as it evolves into a more typical form it may be confused with typhoid fever, measles, meningococcemia, malaria, and relapsing fever.

Routine clinical laboratory data are not of great diagnostic value. The leukocyte count may be normal or low at the onset and then rise to normal, or become moderately elevated, as the disease progresses. A normochromic anemia may develop and then resolve in convalescence. The serum albumin may be depressed, whereas globulin levels may increase. Liver function abnormalities, such as increased transaminase levels, frequently appear early in the disease, but jaundice is rare. Oliguria and azotemia are common and are especially prominent in severely hypotensive patients. Minor changes in the electrocardiogram are common.

Rickettsias have been identified in stained sections of biopsies of skin lesions and, as with Rocky Mountain spotted fever, examination of biopsy specimens presumably could be made more sensitive and specific by staining with specific fluorescent antibody. However, the diagnosis is usually made by serologic tests. Antibodies tend to appear around the end of the first week of disease. Despite its nonspecificity, the Weil–Felix test, an agglutination test depending on polysaccharide antigens common to certain strains of *Proteus* and certain rickettsias, retains popularity because of its ready availability (Table 98-1). The Weil–Felix test has been adapted for bedside use as a rapid slide agglutination test.

A variety of serologic tests employing rickettsial antigens exists, although rickettsial antigens are not commercially available. Consequently, these tests are usually performed by local or state health departments, by the Centers for Disease Control (on reference of specimens by the local health department), or by the World Health Organization Reference Laboratories. The most useful antigen-based test is the indirect fluorescent antibody test. It is sensitive for both IgG and IgM antibodies, enabling differentiation of recent from past infections, and primary typhus from recrudescent typhus (Brill–Zinsser disease). It can be modified to be species specific so that murine and epidemic typhus are distinguished. The more cumbersome complement fixation (CF) test, the standard of the past, is still useful and provides for the detection of both group antibodies and specific antibodies. The rickettsial microagglutination test requires larger quantities of antigen and does not reliably differentiate between murine and louse-borne typhus in humans, but can be carried out in the field with minimal equipment.

The isolation of *R. prowazekii* from blood or tissues may be accomplished in guinea pigs or directly in cell cultures. It is not a routinely available procedure because it is too hazardous for inexperienced personnel.

Because typhus fever often occurs in areas where other serious infectious diseases are common, the physician must remain alert to other possibilities. For example, typhoid fever may be confused with typhus—today as it was in the past; of the drugs now available for the treatment of typhoid fever, only chloramphenicol is also effective against rickettsial infections. In malarious regions, patients with typhus may also have malaria. Cerebral malaria (Chap. 145, Malaria) is a medical emergency, and it may mimic the coma of severe typhus. Thus, in such regions, blood smears from all patients suspected of having typhus should be examined for *Plasmodium* spp.

Table 98-1. *Complement Fixation and Weil–Felix Reactions in Rickettsioses*

		Rickettsial Complement Fixation (CF)			**Weil–Felix (WF) Agglutination**		
		GROUP ANTIGEN TYPE			*PROTEUS* STRAIN		
Group	**Disease**	TYPHUS	RMSF	Q FEVER	OX19	OX2	OXK
I	Primary louse-borne typhus	+++*	±	0	+++	+	0
	Brill–Zinsser disease	+++	±	0	0 or +++	0	0
	Murine typhus	+++	±	0	+++	+	0
II	RMSF	±	+++	0	+++†	+++†	0
	Tick typhus	±	+++	0	+++†	+++†	0
	Rickettsialpox	±	+++	0	0	0	0
III	Scrub typhus	0	0	0	0	0	+++
IV	Q fever	0	0	+++	0	0	0

*+++ = Strong reactions in CF, 1:40 to 1:1280; strong reactions in WF, 1:160 or greater. + = OX2 reactions relatively weaker than OX19. 0 = Negative at 1:5 dilution in CF; negative at 1:40 dilution in WF. ± = Cross reactions between the typhus and RMSF groups occur frequently.

†In RMSF or tick typhus, agglutinins to either OX19, or OX2, or both can be present in either high or low titer.

Prognosis

The prognosis of untreated typhus is closely related to age. The disease tends to be less severe and more often atypical in children under 10 years, whereas the mortality may exceed 50% in patients over 60 years. Specific antirickettsial chemotherapy in patients without other serious complicating disease reduces the mortality almost to zero and even in late, almost moribund patients is dramatically effective. Abortion is uncommon in pregnant women who receive specific treatment promptly.

The rapid response to specific chemotherapy has largely eliminated the secondary bacterial infections (*e.g.,* parotitis, otitis media, hypostatic pneumonia) formerly seen in untreated patients. Occasionally, gangrene of the extremities, hemiplegia and thrombophlebitis occurs in a patient who appears to be responding to antimicrobial therapy; tinnitus and deafness may progress before resolving. Otherwise, recovery is usually remarkable and without residua.

Immunity after infection is extraordinarily solid and longlasting in most cases, despite its nonsterile nature. However, a small, unquantitated fraction of persons convalescent from primary louse-borne typhus develop recrudescent disease (see Brill–Zinsser Disease, below) months to many years later. Predisposing factors are unknown.

Therapy

The prompt administration of specific antirickettsial chemotherapy (*i.e.,* one of the tetracyclines or chloramphenicol) is the single most important therapeutic measure. A single peroral dose of 100 mg of doxycycline hyclate cures most adults, and 50 mg cures most children under the age of about 10 years, even if given very early in the disease. When oral administration is not possible, the same dose injected IV is suitable. The patient usually becomes afebrile 48 to 72 hours (average, about 60 hours) after treatment, even if the therapy was initiated in the second week of the disease. If a definite response is not evident within 48 hours, a vigorous search for some other cause for the illness is necessary.

Tetracycline and chloramphenicol are equally effective, but daily treatment must be continued until the patient has been afebrile for 2 to 3 days, or longer if the treatment was started very early in the disease. Details of dosage and route of administration are described in Chapter 96, Spotted Fevers, under Rocky Mountain Spotted Fever.

The available antirickettsial drugs are primarily rickettsiastatic, and cure depends upon an adequate immune response. Premature cessation of antirickettsial chemotherapy may be followed by a relapse. If necessary, relapses may be retreated with the same drug, since naturally occurring resistance has not been recognized, though it has been produced in the laboratory.

Practical concentrations of the β-lactam and aminocyclitol antimicrobics are ineffective. Similarly, sulfonamides and trimethoprim-sulfamethoxazole are ineffective.

The rapid response to specific chemotherapy has markedly simplified the management of typhus patients. Delirium is still common, and delirious patients must be protected from self-injury. However, problems of hydration and nutrition, decubitus ulcers, and secondary bacterial infections are minimal, though gangrene may occur in the defervescing patient. Heart failure, secondary bacterial infections, and gangrene are treated in conventional ways.

Prevention

Delousing and louse control are highly effective for interrupting the transmission of typhus and are measures essential to control of acute outbreaks or epidemics of typhus. Delousing is most readily accomplished by the application of insecticide dusts to the clothing of the louse-infected population, but older methods, such as heat, may be useful under some circumstances. Ten percent DDT dust is especially effective because it kills lice rapidly and persists long enough to kill larval lice as they hatch. Unfortunately, resistance to DDT is widespread, as is resistance to lindane (1% gamma HCH). Malathion (1% dust) and 2% temephos (Abate) are effective in most areas, and the carbamate insecticides are held in reserve. Susceptibility tests with WHO kits should be performed to ensure that the lice are susceptible to the insecticides intended for use in any given situation. Long-term control of lice in populations whose living conditions predispose to endemic louse infestation is difficult. Insecticides do not substitute for improvement in the standard of living, level of hygiene, and health education.

Active immunization is an effective preventive and control measure. However, the killed typhus vaccine of yolk sac origin that partially protects against disease and significantly reduces both severity and mortality, is no longer commercially available. The attenuated E strain of *R. prowazekii,* when used as a living vaccine, induces adequate protection, but may cause some reactions; it is not generally available, and its use is restricted. New vaccines are under development.

Although chemoprophylaxis is possible in special groups under close professional supervision, persons who may have been exposed to typhus but who are not ill should not be given doxycycline in a misguided attempt at prevention.

Brill–Zinsser Disease

Brill–Zinsser disease is a recrudescence of louse-borne typhus months to years after the primary attack. Factors that predispose to recrudescence of infection by the persisting *R. prowazekii* are unknown. The disease is milder, briefer, and associated with a lesser mortality than primary typhus. The rash may be fleeting or lacking altogether. Rickettsemia does occur; however, it is less intense than in primary infection, though it may be sufficient to infect body lice. The Weil–Felix reaction is often negative. However, specific rickettsial serologic tests (*e.g.,* the indirect immunofluorescence test) show a secondary type of dominantly IgG early antibody response, which differentiates it from primary typhus. The treatment is the same as for primary louse-borne typhus. No preventive measures are known.

Murine Typhus

Murine typhus is also called flea-borne typhus, urban or shop typhus and endemic typhus. Endemic typhus is inappropriate because louse-borne typhus can also be endemic. Before murine typhus and recrudescent louse-borne typhus were recognized and differentiated, both diseases were often called Brill's disease. Murine typhus is a zoonosis involving rats and their ectoparasites and is sporadically transmitted to humans by the rat flea, *Xenopsylla cheopis.* It is widely distributed in temperate and tropical regions of the world.

Etiology

The etiologic agent, *Rickettsia typhi,* is similar to *R. prowazekii* in morphology, staining properties, and metabolic activities, but differs in growth pattern in cell culture, and in host range. The two organisms also possess some common polysaccharide and polypeptide antigenic determinants.

Epidemiology

The basic enzootic cycle of *R. typhi* appears to involve rodents of the genus *Rattus* and their ectoparasites, namely, fleas—notably *X. cheopis,* lice, and perhaps certain mites. In some areas, other rodents, including mice and shrews, and occasionally other small mammals may also participate in the enzootic cycle. During acute infection, the rat shows no signs of illness, but has rickettsemia, which leads to infection of the rat's ectoparasites. The oriental rat flea, *X. cheopis,* has received the greatest attention, but it is likely that other fleas and rat lice are also involved in the intramurid enzootic cycle. The rickettsiae multiply in the cells of the flea's midgut and are excreted in the feces for the life of the flea. There is no transovarial transmission. Although *X. cheopis* feeds preferentially on rats, it does bite man. When feeding, an infected flea deposits a droplet of rickettsia-containing feces, which may contaminate the bite wound or a scratch, or may be transferred to the conjunctiva or respiratory tract. Man is a dead-end host and does not participate in the perpetuation of *R. typhi.*

The enzootic cycle appears to be confined to buildings, such as houses, shops, warehouses, graneries, or supply dumps, and humans usually contract the disease in such sites. Thus, murine typhus may be occupational. About 70 to 80 cases are diagnosed each year in the United States (Fig. 98-1); in 1980, 61 cases (75% of those reported) were in Texas.

Foci of murine typhus are distributed more widely than is commonly recognized, since they occur throughout tropical and temperate zones of the world. Murine typhus fever in humans is probably a grossly underestimated component of the acute fevers of the world. For example, in regions where diagnosis is largely a clinical exercise and the treatment of typhoid fever is routine chloramphenicol, specific laboratory diagnostic procedures have identified many cases of previously unrecognized murine typhus.

Pathogenesis and Pathology

Because of the low mortality, few postmortem studies have been performed on humans who died of murine typhus. The lesions observed in experimentally infected animals are similar to those produced by *R. prowazekii,* and hence, it has been assumed that the pathogenesis and pathology of the infection in humans are generally similar to, but perhaps milder than, louse-borne typhus.

Manifestations

The clinical features of murine typhus are similar to those of primary louse-borne typhus, but on the average are relatively milder. The headache, myalgias, and severe malaise are similar. Usually, the rash is not as prominent and the mortality rate is lower (<5% in untreated cases). Although truly mild cases do occur and fewer untreated patients die, murine typhus is "mild" only relative to the more severe louse-borne typhus fever. Untreated, it can be a serious, debilitat-

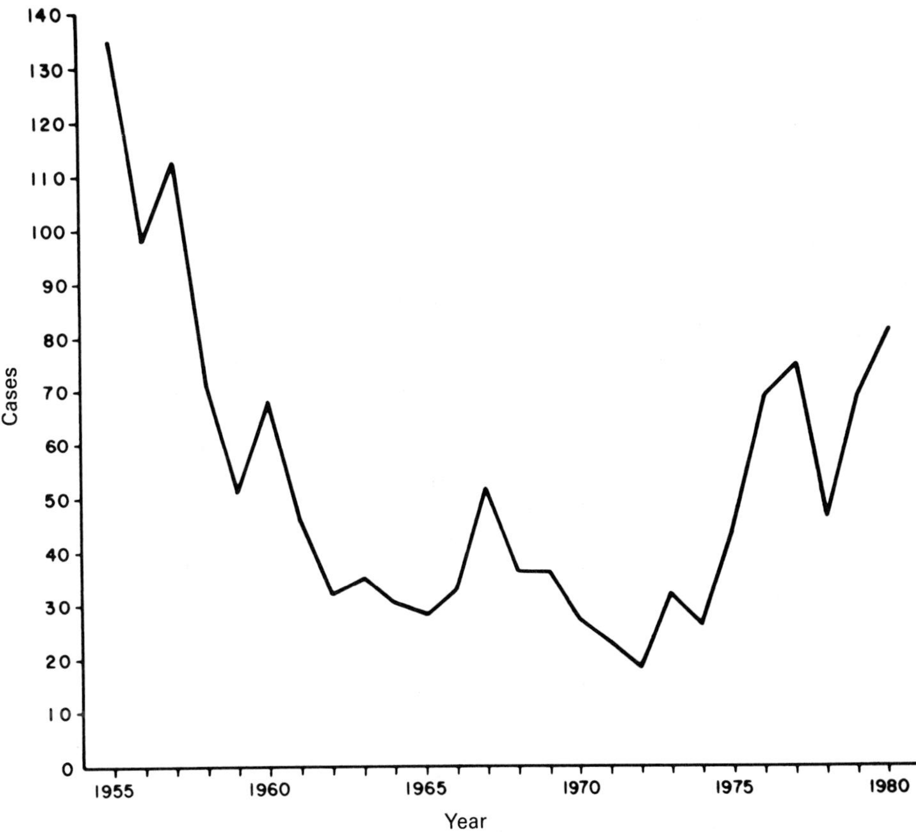

Fig. 98-1. Reported cases of murine (flea-borne) typhus in the United States by year, 1955–1980. (Morbid Mortal Week Rep, Suppl Ann Summary, 1980)

ing disease, requiring 2 to 3 months to regain strength and lost body tissue. Gangrene does not occur.

Diagnosis

Because murine typhus occurs sporadically and has no clearcut, distinguishing clinical features, tests are necessary for the identification of cases. Thus, the simple introduction of specific laboratory diagnostic methods may reveal murine typhus previously unrecognized among the patients in a fever ward. Or, the substitution of ampicillin, amoxicillin, or trimethoprim-sulfamethoxazole for chloramphenicol in the treatment of clinically diagnosed enteric fevers may, by failure of clinical response, identify patients subsequently proved to have murine typhus on further investigation.

Prognosis

The prognosis of untreated murine typhus is good. The mortality is low, and after convalescence (which may be lengthy), the residua are insignificant. With prompt, adequate, specific antirickettsial chemotherapy, the mortality is reduced almost to zero, and convalescence is accelerated remarkably.

Therapy

Murine typhus responds regularly to treatment with the tetracyclines or chloramphenicol given as described for louse-borne typhus. Limited experience suggests that murine typhus is not readily cured by a single dose of doxycycline. Doxycycline is highly effective if administered as 100 to 200 mg per day according to the same schedule used for tetracycline and chloramphenicol in the treatment of louse-borne typhus and Rocky Mountain spotted fever.

Prevention

A vaccine is not available. Prevention and control of murine typhus rely on rodent and flea control. Dusting rat runs and burrows with an appropriate insecticide as determined on the basis of the insecticide resistance patterns of fleas in a given locality (insecticide resistance among fleas is a growing problem) sharply reduces the transmission of murine typhus. The control of rodents must be preceded or accompanied by flea control. If rodenticides are used for rodent control, insecticides can be placed at the entrances to the poison bait tubes.

Bibliography

Books

HORSFALL FL, TAMM I (eds): Viral and Rickettsial Infections of Man, 4th ed. Philadelphia, JB Lippincott, 1965. pp 1059–1094.

WISSEMAN CL JR: Concepts of louse-borne typhus control in developing countries: The use of the living attenuated E strain typhus in epidemic and endemic situations. In Kohn A, Klingberg MA (eds): Immunity in Viral and Rickettsial Diseases. New York, Plenum, 1972. pp 97–130.

WOLBACH SB, TODD JL, PALFREY FW: The Etiology and Pathology of Typhus. Cambridge, Harvard University Press, 1922. 222 pp.

ZDODOWSKII PF, GOLINEVICH HM: The Rickettsial Diseases. New York, Pergamon Press, 1960. 629 pp.

ZINSSER H: Rats, Lice and History. Boston, Little, Brown & Co, 1935. 301 pp.

Journals

BREZINA R, MURRAY ES, TARIZZO ML, BOGEL K: Rickettsiae and rickettsial diseases. Bull WHO 49:433–442, 1973

MURRAY ES, BAHR G, SHWARTZMAN G, MANDELBAUM RA, ROSENTHAL N, DOANE JC, WEISS LB, DOHEN S, SNYDER JC: Brill's disease. I. Clinical and laboratory diagnosis. JAMA 142:1059–1066, 1955

MURRAY ES, O'CONNOR JM, GAON JA: Differentiation of 19S and 7S complement fixing antibodies in primary versus recrudescent typhus by either enthanethiol or heat. Proc Soc Exp Biol Med 119:291–297, 1965

ORMSBEE RA, PEACOCK M, PHILIP R, CASPER E, PLORDE J, GABRE–KIDAN T, WRIGHT L: Serologic diagnosis of epidemic typhus fever. Am J Epidemiol 105:261–271, 1977

Pan American Health Organization: Proceedings of the International Symposium on the Control of Lice and Louse-Borne Diseases, No. 263. Washington DC, Scientific Publication, 1972

NEWHOUSE VF, SHEPARD CC, REDUC MD, TZIANABOS T, MCDADE JE: A comparison of the complement fixation, indirect fluorescent antibody, and microagglutination tests for the serological diagnosis of rickettsial diseases. Am J Trop Med Med Hyg 28:387–395, 1979

SMADEL JE: Status of the rickettsioses in the United States. Ann Intern Med 51:421, 1959

TRAUB R, WISSEMAN CL JR, FARHANG–AZAD A: The ecology of murine typhus: A critical review. Trop Dis Bull 75:237–315, 1978

CHARLES L. WISSEMAN, JR.

Scrub Typhus

99

Scrub typhus is an acute, typhuslike infectious disease that is endemic in rural Asia and is transmitted to humans by the bite of larval mites (chiggers) of the genus *Leptotrombidium.*

Etiology

The etiologic agent is *Rickettsia tsutsugamushi*—small pleomorphic, often bipolar-staining bacilli that grow free in the cytoplasm of host cells. They differ from the rickettsias of the typhus and spotted fever groups in the ultrastructure of outer envelopes, lack of dependence on CO_2 in the atmosphere of infected cell cultures, and some tinctorial properties (accommodated by a modification of the Gimenez staining method—Chap. 9, Microscopic Examinations). Multiple serotypes exist that display only limited cross-immunity. Thus, scrub typhus may be contracted more than once as a result of infection with different serotypes. Strains may vary widely in virulence for mice.

Epidemiology

Scrub typhus is widely distributed in eastern and southern Asia and the islands of the western Pacific—from as far north as Hokkaido in Japan and the Primorye region of Asian Soviet Russia, as far south as the northern tip of Australia, and as far west as Pakistan and Tadzhikistan. It is a zoonosis; humans are nonessential, dead-end hosts who accidentally intrude into the enzootic cycle when they are bitten by infected, larval trombiculid mites (chiggers). Four elements are constant features of endemic foci: (1) wild rats, especially of the subgenus *Rattus;* (2) chiggers of the *Leptotrombidium deliense* group; (3) transitional vegetation (cleared forest areas, fringe vegetation, abandoned agricultural areas); and (4) *R. tsutsugamushi.* Suitable habitats are distributed from tropical to temperate zones and encompass disturbed rain forests, semideserts, alpine meadows, and seashores. The larval stage of the mite (chigger) is the vector because this is the only stage during which the chigger feeds on rodents and humans. Because *R. tsutsugamushi* is transmitted transovarially with high efficiency, the mite serves also as the main reservoir. In temperate zones, the chiggers are usually active at some time during the warm months, although *L. scutellare*-transmitted winter scrub typhus occurs in certain Japanese islands. In tropical and subtropical regions, the disease may be more prevalent at one time of the year than another because of rainfall, flooding, and other factors.

Best known from outbreaks in groups of nonimmune humans entering endemic areas (soldiers, roadbuilders, agricultural developers), scrub typhus is now recognized as a major cause of disease in human populations indigenous to endemic areas. The latter illnesses may be atypical (no eschar; no *Proteus* OX-K agglutinins), possibly as a result of prior infections with different serotypes.

Pathogenesis and Pathology

During the incubation period (usually 9–12 days, with extremes of 6–18 days), *R. tsutsugamushi* multiply primarily at the site of inoculation into the skin. A focal lesion results, which may go on to necrosis, yielding the characteristic black, crusted eschar (2 mm–10 mm in diameter). Although regional lymphadenopathy also develops during the incubation period, *R. tsutsugamushi* are seldom restrained; instead, they disseminate widely to form focal lesions of the small blood vessels similar to those described for typhus (Chap. 98, Typhus Fevers). Compared with louse-borne typhus and Rocky Mountain spotted fever, vascular thrombosis is less frequent in scrub typhus, but general lymphadenopathy (cervical, axillary, inguinal) is more prominent.

Blood leukocyte patterns, reversal of the serum albumin–globulin ratio, occasional clotting distrubances, and elevation of serum transaminases are much as described for typhus (Chap. 98, Typhus Fevers). Proteinuria is common; oliguria, isosthenuria, and azotemia may occur.

Manifestations

An eschar develops in about 70% of patients with full-blown untreated primary scrub typhus and in a substantially lower proportion in second infections. Prodromes of headache, malaise, and anorexia may occur. The onset of disease is usually acute, with a progressive rise in fever to about 39.5°C to 40.5°C (103°F–105°F) accompanied by severe headache, ocular pain, conjunctival injection, anorexia, nonproductive cough, increasing malaise, prostration, and apathy. The fever is unremittant. Toward the end of the first week of illness, a macular to maculopapular rash appears first on the trunk and then on the extremities. Signs of multiple, complex organ involvements appear. Apathy gives way to delirium and restlessness, stupor, and weakness and, and in severe cases, to coma, convulsions, and tremors. Varying degrees of deafness and papilledema are common. Signs of diffuse and focal myocarditis may appear, but classical congestive failure is rare. Peripheral circulatory failure may appear in varying degrees: increasing pulse rate; falling blood pressure (commonly below 100 mm Hg systolic); rapid, shallow respiration; cyanosis; sweating; and cold, clammy skin. Gangrene is rare, but edema may be overt in some cases. Oliguria or anuria may occur in some patients. Spontaneous diuresis is fairly common late in the febrile phase or in early convalescence. Defervescence occurs by lysis after about 10 to 14 days (up to 21 days or more in very severe cases). Convalescence is prolonged. Most of the abnormalities are reversible, though deafness, personality changes, and cardiovascular instability may persist for weeks to months. Long-term (10 years or more) follow-up has failed to reveal any significant residua. Specific chemotherapy promptly halts the progress of the disease.

Mild or atypical cases of scrub typhus may be common in some areas.

Diagnosis

A typhuslike illness in a person from an area that is endemic for scrub typhus should alert the physician to the possibility of the disease. Finding an eschar, with or without associated regional lymphadenopathy, is especially helpful, although both may sometimes occur in tick typhus. Mild or atypical cases must be associated with a high index of suspicion to merit the support of serodiagnostic laboratory procedures. Other diseases, such as typhoid fever and murine or tick typhus, may be especially confusing. Malaria may be present concurrently.

Although *R. tsutsugamuschi* can be isolated readily from the blood by mouse inoculation, the most frequently used and the most practical laboratory diagnostic methods are serologic. The Weil–Felix test with *Proteus* OX-K antigen (Table 98-1) is commonly employed because of general availability; however, it is not positive in many cases of scrub typhus, and may be positive in other infections, such as relapsing fever and leptospirosis. At the present time, the indirect fluorescent antibody test using multiple serotypes of *R. tsutsugamushi* is the most reliable method.

Prognosis

Untreated, the mortality of scrub typhus varies from zero to more than 30%. If promptly applied, specific antimicrobial therapy reduces mortality virtually to zero.

Therapy

Scrub typhus responds rapidly to treatment with the tetracyclines or chloramphenicol given as described for typhus (Chap. 98, Typhus Fevers). A single dose of 200 mg of doxycycline hyclate has been reported to be curative.

Prevention

A scrub typhus vaccine is not available. Chemoprophylaxis with carefully spaced doses of chloramphenicol or doxycycline is feasible and may be appropriate under special conditions. However, prevention of scrub typhus relies heavily on personal protection against chiggers by wearing repellant-treated clothing (dimethyl or dibutyl phthalate or benzyl benzoate) and applying repellents (*e.g.,* diethyltoluamide) to the exposed skin. Chigger populations in and around campsites or in other limited areas may be reduced by (1) treating the area intensively with appropriate acaricides; (2) destroying the vegetation (bulldozing, burning, herbicides); and (3) reducing the rodent population by poison bait campaigns. Decisions on the use of these measures must be tempered by appropriate and relevant environmental, medical, and ecologic considerations.

Bibliography

Book

HORSFALL FL, TAMM I (eds): Viral and Rickettsial Infections of Man, 4th ed. Philadelphia, JB Lippincott, 1965. pp 1130–1143.

Journals

BOZEMAN FM, ELISBERG BL: Serological diagnosis of scrub typhus by indirect immunofluorescence. Proc Soc Exp Biol Med 112:568–573, 1963

BROWN GW, ROBINSON DM, HUXSOLL DL: Scrub typhus: A common cause of illness in indigenous populations. Trans R Soc Trop Med Hyg 70:444, 1976

BROWN GW, SAUNDERS JP, SINGH S, HUXSOLL DL, and SHIRAI A: Single dose doxycycline therapy for scrub typhus. Trans Royal Soc Trop Med Hyg 72:412–416, 1978

DELLER JJ JR, RUSSEL PK: An analysis of fevers of unknown origin in American soldiers in Vietnam. Ann Intern Med 66:1129, 1967

LEY HL JR, DIERCKS FH, PATERSON PY, SMADEL JE, WISSEMAN CL JR, and TRAUB R: Immunization against scrub typhus. IV. Living Karp vaccine and chemoprophylaxis in volunteers. Am J Hyg 56:303–312, 1952

OLSON JG, BOURGEOIS AL, FANG RCY, COOLBAUGH JC, DENNIS DT: Prevention of scrub typhus: Prophylactic administration of doxycycline in a randomized double blind trial. Am J Trop Med Hyg 29:989–997, 1980

SHEEHY TW, HAZLETT D, TURK RE: Scrub typhus: A comparison of chloramphenicol and tetracycline in its treatment. Arch Intern Med 132:77–80, 1973

TRAUB R, WISSEMAN CL JR: Ecology of chigger-borne rickettsiosis (scrub typhus). J Med Entomol 11:237–303, 1974

L. JOSEPH WHEAT
ARTHUR WHITE

100 Staphylococcal Skin Infections

Furunculosis, carbuncles, and pyoderma are the major skin infections associated with *Staphylococcus aureus.* Staphylococcal skin infections frequently complicate trauma or surgical incisions of the skin.

Etiology

Staphylococci are gram-positive, aerobic (facultatively anaerobic), nonmotile bacteria that are approximately 0.8 μm in diameter and tend to grow in clusters (Fig. 100-1). Most of the staphylococci isolated from skin infections are *S. aureus;* that is, they produce coagulase and usually elaborate a golden pigment and a number of exotoxins including α-hemolysin. Also, the nuclease of *S. aureus* is singular in its resistance to heat—hence the designation of thermonuclease. Only rarely do *Staphylococcus epidermidis,* the coagulase-negative (generally nonpigmented, nonhemolytic) staphylococci, cause skin infections, although *S. epidermidis* do occasionally cause infective endocarditis (Chap. 134, Infective Endocarditis).

The cell walls of coagulase-positive staphylococci contain protein antigen A and teichoic acid antigens differentiating them from the coagulase-negative staphylococci and *Micrococcus* spp. The teichoic acids of coagulase-positive staphylococci are acetylglucosaminyl ribitol teichoic acids, which may cross-react serologically with antigens of other bacteria, including acetyglucosamine antigenic determinants in the mucopeptides of many other bacteria, surface antigens of *Streptococcus* bovis, ribitol of type b Haemophilus influenzae, and antigens present in extracts of diphtheroids. These cross-reactions are infrequently encountered when serums from infected patients are used.

The cell walls of *S. aureus* also contain peptidoglycan, a mucopeptide material much like that found in cell walls of other bacteria. However, in contrast to the mucopeptides of other bacteria, the mucopeptides of *S. aureus* contain pentaglycine bridges binding the tetrapeptide chains. Pentaglycine is efficiently hydrolyzed by the enzyme lysostaphin; thus, the susceptibility of *S. aureus* to lysis by lysostaphin is a unique property.

Perhaps the most subtle characteristics of staphylococal cell walls are the fine structures that are the receptors specific for particular viruses parasitic on *S. aureus,* the staphylococcal bacteriophages (Fig. 100-2). These cell wall receptors are genetically stable characteristics which vary sufficiently from strain to strain to enable differentiation of most isolates of *S. aureus* according to patterns of susceptibility/resistance to lysis by a series of 22 specific bacteriophages (Chap. 13, Bacteriophage Typing).

The cell wall substances of *S. aureus* are antigenic in man, and most adults have detectable humoral antibodies. Moreover, reactions of delayed hypersensitivity may be evoked with one or more of these antigens.

Epidemiology

Coagulase-positive staphylococci are normal components of the microbiota resident in the lower colon and can be found in the anterior nares of virtually all children and about 50% of adults. The frequency of isolation from the skin is a function of skin conditions, the site of sampling, and the density of colonization in the rectum and nose.

The nasal reservoir appears to be the major source for dissemination of *S. aureus* and infection. However, in some persons the perineum is the major reservoir for multiplication and dissemination onto the skin and into the air. Selective treatment of the anterior nares with topically applied antimicrobial agents not only temporarily depresses the proliferation of nasal staphylococci, but also markedly reduces the frequency with which *S. aureus* can be isolated from

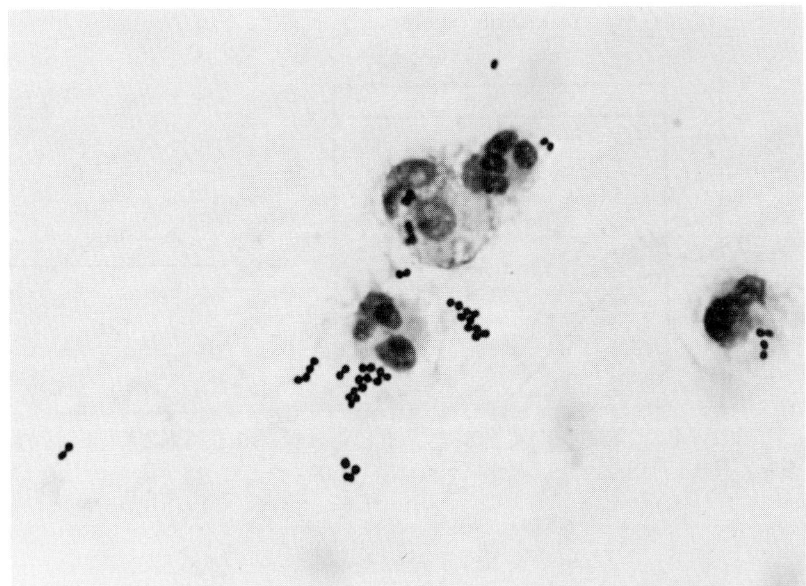

Fig. 100-1. *Staphylococcus aureus,* both intracellular and extracellular, with numerous white cells in an exudate. (Gram's stain, original magnification approximately × 650)

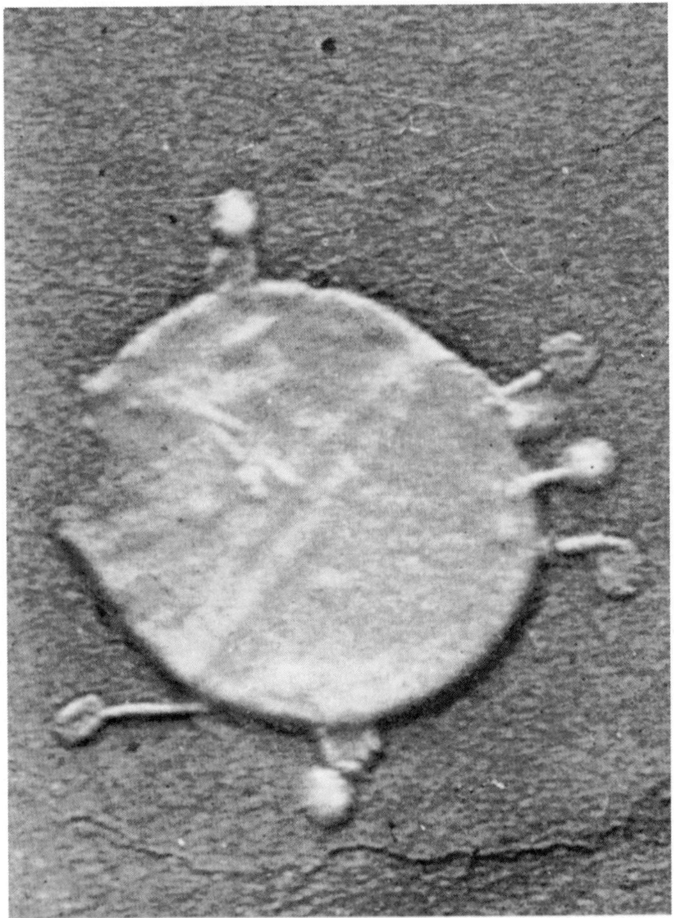

Fig. 100-2. Bacteriophages attach to specific strains of *Staphylococcus aureus* using genetically stable cell receptors. (Original magnification approximately × 65,000) (Hotchin JE, Dawson IM, Elford WJ: Brit J Exp Path 33:177–182, 1952)

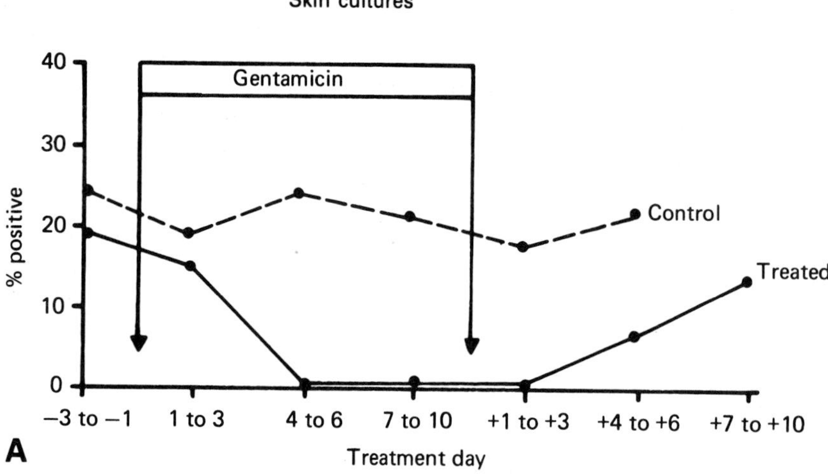

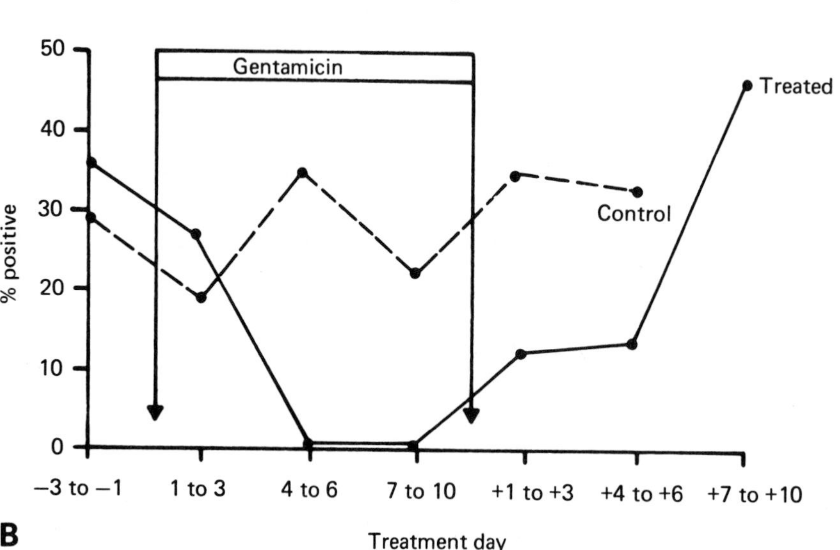

Fig. 100-3. Suppression of skin and aerial staphylococci in nasal carriers by selective treatment of the nose with topical gentamicin. (*A*) Skin cultures. (*B*) Air samples. (White AC: Am J Med Sci 248:52, 1964)

the skin and the air around the treated carriers (Fig. 100-3).

In hospital environments, most of the staphylococci isolated from patients who have received antimicrobics are resistant to penicillin G, the tetracyclines, and erythromycin. If a patient enters the hospital carrying drug-susceptible staphylococci and is treated with antimicrobial agents, the susceptible staphylococci in the nose are rapidly suppressed and are usually replaced with drug-resistant *S. aureus.* Thus, the total carrier rate in hospitalized patients is not lowered but may be increased, and the carried strains will have changed from drug-susceptible to drug-resistant. These changes are a replacement phenomenon. The staphylococci which are acquired differ both in bacteriophage type and in susceptibility to antimicrobial agents. In patients and in hosptial personnel who do not receive antimicrobics, the replacement or acquisition of drug-resistant staphylococci from the hospital environment is a much slower process.

The actual number of coagulase-positive staphylococci that can be isolated from carriers varies from only a few to more than 10^7 per swab. Quite reasonably, carriers of large numbers of *S. aureus,* either in the anterior nares or in the perineal area, are more efficient disseminators onto the skin and into the air than are carriers of just a few *S. aureus.* Patients with staphylococcal furunculosis or with postoperative staphylococcal wound infections usually carry large numbers of *S. aureus.*

Staphylococci are rapidly disseminated from the skin into the air around persons who are heavily colonized. After burns, exfoliative dermatitis, surgery, minor cuts, or scratches, the skin may become infected with *S. aureus* originally derived from the nose. In healthy skin, the intradermal injection of more than 10^6 staphylococci is required to initiate a pus-producing lesion. When foreign material is present (*e.g.,* a suture), an inoculum of only a few hundred staphylococci produces a clinical infection. There does not appear to be a measurable variation in virulence among strains of *S. aureus* from lesions and from carriers of various phage types, and of differing susceptibility to antimicrobics.

Pathogenesis and Pathology

Most adults are continuously exposed to staphylococci, but overt infection is infrequent. Approximately 5% of the population has one symptomatic staphylococcal infection per year, but these infections are usually minor. Because the minimal infecting dose is quite large, there must be a considerable degree of resistance to infectious diseases caused by *S. aureus* in humans. Observations of persons with a variety of abnormalities in host defense mechanisms have helped to explain some of the factors responsible for this resistance.

Selected defects in white cells are associated with an increased frequency of staphylococcal infections, including staphylococcal skin abscesses. In chronic granulomatous disease, the white cells phagocytize but do not kill catalase-positive organisms, including *S. aureus,* because of defects in myeloperoxidase and superoxide production by the white cells. An uncommon but similar syndrome occurs in children with eczema associated with high levels of IgE specific for staphylococci or candidas. In these patients, there is inhibition of chemotaxis of white cells by these organisms, and there is a high frequency of staphylococcal skin disease.

In patients with congenital or acquired hypogammaglobulinemia, there is a markedly increased frequency of clinically significant infections caused by a variety of gram-positive bacteria, including staphylococci. Correction of the deficit by injection of human gammaglobulin largely corrects the increased susceptibility to clinical infection.

Testing *in vitro* indicates that maximal destruction of staphylococci requires both opsonins (IgG) to promote phagocytosis and granulocytes to destroy the phagocytized staphylococci. Antibodies against a portion of the mucopeptide appear to be important opsonins. Most adults also have antibodies specific for α-hemolysin, β-toxins, teichoic acids, and other antigens of *S. aureus,* but no protective roles for these antibodies have been demonstrated.

Patients with diabetes mellitus are particularly prone to recurrent episodes of furunculosis. The high osmolarity associated with hyperglycemia appears to prevent effective granulocyte function. Also, abnormally high concentrations of ketone bodies inhibit the intraleukocytic killing of engulfed *S. aureus.*

Manifestations

The clinical manifestations of infections of the skin caused by *S. aureus* may vary from a small pimple, in which coagulase-positive staphylococci are present, to a very large furuncle or carbuncle with rapid destruction of skin and extension of infection into the subcutaneous tissues. If noninfectious skin diseases, such as exfoliative dermatitis or burns, are complicated by infection with *S. aureus,* there will be exudation of pus and occasionally bacteremia.

Bullous impetigo is characterized by superficial blebs of skin that may cover large areas. This kind of impetigo is almost exclusively caused by staphylococci, usually phage type 71.

Impetigo may appear as small macules that rapidly develop into vesicles, become pustular, and then encrust. Impetigo may be due to either streptococci or staphylococci, and the two kinds of cocci may be cocontributors. With streptococcal impetigo, regional adenitis and cellulitis are prominent signs.

Unusual manifestations of staphylococcal skin disease include the scalded skin syndrome or toxic epidermal necrolysis in which often unapparent staphylococcal infections are associated with elaboration of exfoliative toxin whic causes cleavage high in the dermis. The syndrome usually occurs in children under the age of two, but occasionally has been reported in adults.

A toxic shock syndrome has been associated with infection or colonization by certain exotoxin-producing staphylococci. Although the syndrome occurs in children and adults with staphylococcal skin disease, osteomyelitis, and postoperative wound infections, it has attained prominence as an affliction of menstruating women who use vaginal tampons. Accordingly, the syndrome is discussed in Chapter 50, Infections of the Female Genital Tract.

Diagnosis

Furunculosis is almost exclusively a staphylococcal disease. Occasionally, lesions of sporotrichosis (Chap. 108, Sporotrichosis), swimming pool granuloma (Chap. 36, Nontuberculous Mycobacterioses), or skin infiltration with neoplastic cells may mimic furunculosis. These can be differentiated by failure to demonstrate staphylococci on culture or Gram stain, by culturing *Sporothrix* spp. or *Mycobacterium marinum,* or by demonstrating leukemic or other neoplastic cells on biopsy.

Pyodermas following cuts or scratches are usually caused by staphylococci or by group A *Streptococcus pyogenes* (Chap. 101, Streptococcal Skin Infections and Glomerulonephritis). Rapid development of cellulitis and lymphangitis is more typical of streptococcal involvement.

Other kinds of bacteria, particularly obligate anaerobes, may play a more important role in chronic skin ulcers, decubiti, or soft-tissue abscesses around the neck or perineal area. With adequate Gram stains, and aerobic and anaerobic cultures, these infections can be differentiated from lesions caused by staphylococci.

High levels of antibodies against staphylococcal teichoic acids can be demonstrated by use of either simple agar gel diffusion or counterimmunoelectrophoresis. These methods are more rapid than cultures and can be applied in patients from whom isolation of staphylococci may be difficult because of relative inaccessibility of the lesions or treatment with antimicrobics. Examples include deep-seated abscesses, bacteremias, osteomyelitis, meningitis, and especially infective endocarditis.

In addition to allowing the diagnosis of staphylococcal infections earlier than cultures and in patients in whom cultures might be negative because of previous therapy, teichoic acid antibodies are also useful in differentiating bacteremia which results in endocarditis or metastatic infections from transient staphylococcal bacteremia without metastatic disease. Ninety percent of patients with staphylococcal bacteremia who develop endocarditis or other metastatic disease have elevated concentrations of teichoic acid antibodies. Patients with staphylococcal bacteremia without dissemination rarely develop elevated concentrations of teichoic acid antibodies.

Prognosis

Most small furuncles recede without specific therapy. However, lesions that contain large quantities of pus often require surgical drainage for prompt healing. A small number of patients without discernible, predisposing, noninfectious diseases tend to have repeated episodes of furunculosis over a period of years.

Pyodermas of various types, particularly abscesses around scratches or cuts, may require no therapy beyond drainage. More extensive infections, particularly those associated with burns or exfoliative dermatitis, have an ominous prognosis when accompanied by bacteremia. Staphylococcal bacteremias from these sources, as from other sources, have mortality rates of 30% to 40%.

Therapy

Large collections of pus in the skin are abscesses; surgical drainage is required for optimal therapeutic response. However, it is clear that the addition of systemic antimicrobial therapy increases the rate of healing of large pyodermas and furuncles.

Specific treatment for staphylococcal diseases is complicated by the marked propensity of these bacteria to become resistant to an antimicrobial agent within a relatively short time after the agent is introduced into general clinical use; such resistance is not related to coagulase activity. Thus, after the introduction of penicillin G, strains of *S. aureus* were isolated that were resistant through elaboration of a β-lactamase (penicillinase) that inactivates penicillin G. In patients infected with such penicillinase-producing staphylococci, therapy with penicillin G was ineffective. Shortly after the tetracyclines and erythromycin were introduced, only a small proportion of staphylococcal isolates were resistant to these antimicrobics. Yet about a decade later, almost all staphylococci isolated from hospitalized patients were resistant to penicillin G, the tetracyclines, and erythromycin.

Many of the semisynthetic penicillins and related compounds were developed because they are relatively nonsusceptible to the action of staphylococcal β-lactamase. The first of these, methicillin, was soon followed by other semisynthetic, penicillinase-resistant penicillins, including oxacillin, nafcillin, cloxacillin, and dicloxacillin. The cephalosporin antimicrobics, including cephalothin, cephalexin, and cefazolin are also resistant to staphylococcal β-lactamase.

Staphylococcus aureus resistant to all of the penicillins and the cephalosporins has been isolated from patients throughout the world. Frequently termed "methicillin"-resistant, such staphylococci are usually susceptible only to vancomycin, clindamycin, fusidic acid, gentamicin (and other newer aminocyclitols), rifampin, and cycloserine. In the late

1960s, more than 20% of patient isolates from some hospitals in Europe were methicillin-resistant strains, a situation which has spontaneously improved. Relatively few infections were caused methicillin-resistant staphylococci in the United States; however, there were epidemics in burn units in which 80% of the staphylococcal infections were caused by methicillin-resistant staphylococci.

Some strains of *S. aureus* are inhibited but not killed by concentrations of β-lactam antimicrobics that are usually bactericidal for other strains of staphylococci. These tolerant strains appear to lack an autolytic enzyme. The concentrations of penicillins or cephalosporins that are required to kill tolerant staphylococci are at least 16-fold higher than the concentrations required to inhibit growth. In patients with endocarditis caused by tolerant organisms, there is a decreased rate of cure with nafcillin, and cephalosporins. In patients with serious staphylococcal infections caused by tolerant staphylococci, the addition of gentamicin, rifampin, or vancomycin has resulted in high titers of bactericidal activity in the serum and in clinical response in patients. It is not known whether patients with localized skin infections caused by tolerant staphylococci also respond less favorably.

There is marked variability in the susceptibility of staphylococci to the available, commonly used antimicrobial agents. Thus, in all serious infections, the responsible staphylococci must be isolated and tested for susceptibility to antimicrobics.

In the treatment of infections caused by staphylococci that do not produce β-lactamase, the most effective and least expensive antimicrobial is penicillin G. Therefore, infections caused by staphylococci susceptible to penicillin G should not be treated with either semisynthetic penicillins or cephalosporins. However, in seriously ill patients with signs and symptoms of bacteremia, penicillinase-producing staphylococci are isolated so frequently that the initial therapy must include a penicillinase-resistant penicillin, or a cephalosporin in patients who are allergic to the penicillins. The bases for preferring nafcillin (150 mg–200 mg/kg body wt/day, as six equal portions IV every 4 hours) or cefazolin (75 mg–100 mg/kg body wt/day, as four equal portions IV every 6 hours) are presented in Chapter 18 (Antimicrobics and Anthelmintics for Systemic Therapy. If the causative *S. aureus* is found to be penicillinase-negative, penicillin G should be substituted in a dose of 150 mg to 200 mg (240,000–320,000 units)/kg body wt/day, IV, as six equal portions, 4-hourly.

In patients with impetigo or with a few small furuncles, peroral treatment with either penicillin V (15 mg–20 mg/kg body wt/day, as four equal portions, 6-hourly), or erythromycin (same dosage) has been successful when the infecting bacteria are susceptible to these drugs. With penicillinase-producing staphylococci, a semi-synthetic, penicillinase-resistant penicillin that is reliably absorbed (*e.g.,* cloxacillin or dicloxacillin) should be given in a dose of 20 mg to 30 mg/kg body wt/day, PO, as four equal portions, 6-hourly. Cephalexin or cephradine are orally administrable alternatives (same dose as for cloxacillin) for use in patients who are allergic to the penicillins.

Prevention

Various methods have been applied to preventing staphylococcal infections. These include control of the nasal reservoir, replacement of virulent staphylococci in the nose with a strain presumed to be less virulent, vaccination to increase antibody responses, control of hypersensitivity by vaccines, and introduction of physical or chemical barriers between the reservoir and the susceptible host.

No measures yet devised have been completely successful in suppressing nasal carriage of staphylococci. Thus, the logical step of eliminating the reservoir is not feasible with *S. aureus.* However, suppression of the nasal reservoir has been achieved by the topical application of antimicrobial agents in patients with frequent and recurring furunculosis. Ointments containing neomycin or bacitracin have been successful in the past, but many staphylococci in hospitals are resistant to neomycin. In the hospital environment, gentamicin ointment is the preferred agent. Few strains of *S. aureus* are resistant to gentamicin, and tri-daily application to the anterior nares markedly reduces both the frequency of isolation and the numbers of staphylococci that can be cultured from the nose, skin, and the immediate vicinity of carriers. Treatment must be continued for at least 3 months, because recurrences of both nasal staphylococci and furunculosis are very common after shorter courses. Recently, rifampin has been reported to be effective in eradicating staphylococci from 80% of nasal carriers. However, 20% of the subjects acquired a staphylococci of a different phage type within 12 weeks after therapy was discontinued.

Another approach has been to replace the *S. aureus* originally carried in the anterior nose with a presumably less virulent strain—reacquisition of the original infecting strain is prevented through bacterial interference. In newborns who have not yet been colonized with bacteria, the 502 A strain of *S. aureus* can be directly implanted in the nose and umbilicus. In this manner, epidemics of staphylococcal disease in newborn nurseries have been controlled. In older patients with staphylococci already present in the nose, the original resident strain must be eradicated by the topical application of gentamicin and the oral administration of cloxacillin or dicloxacillin (60 mg–70 mg/kg body wt/day, as four equal portions, 6-hourly, for 10 days) before the 502 A strain can be implanted. This procedure appears to have been successful in families with recurrent staphylococcal infections. However, 502 A has caused severe disseminated disease. Moreover, the 502 A strain is eliminated rapidly if other antimicrobics are given.

Although immunization with staphylococcal antigens appears to be reasonable, it has not been successful in the prevention of staphylococcal infections, possibly because of inadequate knowledge of which antigen or antigens are important in inducing a protective immune response or in promoting phagocytosis. Similarly, although hypersensitivity to whole staphylococci increases the susceptibility of experimental animals to staphylococcal skin lesions, the antigen(s) important to this phenomenon are not known. The use of vaccines made from the patient's own infecting staphylococci is also of unproved value. There are no data from controlled studies clearly demonstrating increased phagocytosis, decreased hypersensitivity, or reduction in the frequency of furuncles following the use of autologous vaccines.

The prevention of staphylococcal infections in hospitals requires the removal of personnel with lesions from contact with susceptible patients. A number of staphylococcal epidemics have occurred in surgical units or newborn nurseries in which the single source of infecting staphylococci was surgeon or a nurse with an open, draining, staphylococcal skin lesion.

Newborn infants differ from older children and adults in that they rapidly acquire staphylococci in the nose and umbilicus, even though they are not receiving antimicrobial agents. In the hospital, endemic strains of staphylococci are often transmitted from infant to infant by the hands of personnel.

Remaining Problems

Several important aspects of staphylococcal diseases are poorly understood. About one-third of all adults are long-term nasal carriers of coagulase-positive staphylococci, whereas the remaining two-thirds of adults are carriers for only brief periods or are not carriers at all. A better understanding of other differences between these two groups should lead to a reduction in the number of those who carry staphylococci and, therefore, the incidence of staphylococcal disease.

Although most adults have considerable resistance to staphylococcal infections, no significant differences in immunity have been demonstrated between those who do not acquire staphylococcal infections and those who have multiple furuncles. Only a very small proportion of patients with recurrent furunculosis have diabetes mellitus, grossly abnormal immunoglobulins, or leukocyte abnormalities. The remaining patients do not have abnormalities that can be readily identified as defects in host defenses. A clearer understanding of the specific antigen(s) responsible for the production of opsonins and the antigen(s) involved in delayed hypersensitivity should enable a more logical approach to the specific immunity important in preventing staphylococcal disease.

Some patients with severe staphylococcal infections have circulating antigens detectable by enzyme-linked immunosorbent assays or radioimmunoassays. The great sensitivity inherent in these methods may allow earlier, specific diagnosis of staphylococcal disease.

Bibliography

Books

BAYER AS, GUZE LB: Staphylococcus aureus Bacteremic Syndromes: Diagnostic Therapeutic update. Disease-a-Month. Chicago, Year Book Medical Publishers, 1979. 42 pp.

ELEK SD: *Staphylococcus pyogenes* and Its Relation to Disease. London, E & S Livingstone, 1959. 767 pp.

Journals

CROSS AS, STEIGBIGEL RT: Infective endocarditis and access site infections in patients on hemodialysis. Medicine 5:453–466, 1976

DAVIS JP, CHESNEY PJ, WAND PJ, LAVENTURE M: Toxic-shock syndrome. N Engl J Med 303:1429–1442, 1980

DOBKIN JF, MILLER MH, STEIGBIGEL NH: Septicemia in patients on chronic hemodialysis. Ann Intern Med 88:28–33, 1978

IANNINI PB, CROSSLEY K: Therapy of *Staphylococcus aureus* bacteremia associated with a removable focus of infection. Ann Intern Med 85:558–560, 1976

KLIMEK JJ, MARSIK FJ, BARTLETT RC, WEIB B, SHEA P, QUINTILIANI R: Clinical, epidemiologic and bacteriologic observations of an outbreak of methicillin-resistant *Staphylococcus aureus* at a large community hospital. Am J Med 61:340–349, 1976

MUSHER DM, MCKENZIE SO: Infections due to *Staphylococcus aureus.* Medicine 56:383–409, 1977

NOLAN CM, BEATTY HN: *Staphylococcus aureus* bacteremia-current clinical patterns. Am J Med 60:495–500, 1976

RAJASHEKARAIAH KR, RICE T, RAO VS, MARSH D, RAMAKRISHNA B, KALLICK CA: Clinical significance of tolerant strains of *Staphylococcus aureus* in patients with endocarditis. Ann Int Med 93:796–801, 1980

SABATH LD, LAVERDIERE M, WHEELER N, BLAZEVIC D, WILKINSON BJ: A new type of penicillin resistance in *Staphylococcus aureus.* Lancet 1:443–447, 1977

TUAZON CU, SHEAGREN JN, CHOA MS, MARCUS D, CURTIN JA: *Staphylococcus aureus* bacteremia-relationship between formation of antibodies to teichoic acid and development of metastiatic abscesses. J Infect Dis 137:57–62, 1978

WALDVOGEL FA, MEDOFF G, SWARTZ N: Osteomyelitis: Review of clinical features, therapeutic considerations and unusual aspects. N Engl J Med 282:198–206, 1970

WATANAKUNAKORN D, BAIRD IM: *Staphylococcus aureus* bacteremia and endocarditis associated with a removable infected intravenous device. Am J Med 63:253–256, 1977

WHEAT LJ, KOHLER RB, WHITE A: Solid-phase radioimmunoassay for immunoglobulin G *Staphylococcus aureus* antibody in serious staphylococcal infection. Ann Intern Med 89:467–472, 1978

WHEAT LJ, KOHLER RB, WHITE AL, WHITE A: Effect of rifampin on nasal carriers of coagulase-positive staphylococci. J Infect Dis 143:177, 1981

HUGH C. DILLON, JR.

101 Streptococcal Skin Infections and Glomerulonephritis

Streptococcus pyogenes of Lancefield's group A are associated with distinct forms of skin and soft-tissue infection including pyoderma, suppurative infection of burns and wounds, cellulitis, and the now rare erysipelas. Pyoderma, which includes impetigo and secondarily infected dermatoses, is particularly common. Cellulitis may accompany any of the forms of skin infection but also occurs in the absence of an obvious cutaneous portal of entry.

In early studies, it was noted that streptococcal infections of either the skin and soft tissues or the respiratory tract may be antecedent to acute glomerulonephritis (AGN) but not rheumatic fever. In contrast, streptococcal pharyngitis, with or without scarlet fever, might be followed by either glomerulonephritis or rheumatic fever. This intriguing difference in the locus of the antecedent streptococcal infection has remained of epidemiologic and perhaps pathogenetic significance. Pyoderma is a common form of streptococcal infection preceding nephritis found in certain parts of the United States and in other parts of the world, for example, Trinidad.

Etiology

Streptococcal skin infections are almost always caused by group A *S. pyogenes,* with only occasional isolations from pyodermas of groups B, C, and G. All further references to streptococci in this chapter can be taken to mean group A beta-hemolytic streptococci unless a specific group is designated. The characteristics of *S. pyogenes* are described in Chapter 24, Streptococcal Diseases.

More than 70 types of streptococci have been differentiated on the basis of the specific M antigen found in the coccal cell wall. However, certain limitations compromise the value of the M typing as an epidemiologic tool. M antisera are difficult to prepare and maintain for a number of types, including many associated with pyoderma. This may reflect quantitative variation in the production of M antigen, differences in immunogenicity among strains, instability of M-precipitin antibody, or combinations of these factors. Among given collections of strains from either skin or throat infections, 50% or more may be M non-typable.

T antigens, also found in the coccal cell wall, permit classification by agglutination reactions of over 90% of strains whether or not M antigen is detectable. However, T antigens are less specific than M antigens; multiple agglutination reactions resulting in T patterns are common, especially among pyoderma strains. Commonly, T antigens or patterns are shared by members of several different M serotypes. In a few cases, the same M antigen may be found in strains of different T patterns. M and T typing systems are complementary, and a fair degree of correspondence between M and T antigens makes preliminary typing with T antisera useful in selecting antisera for M typing. Several of the more common M and T antigen relationships are summarized in Table 101-1. There is a considerable dichotomy between M types that commonly cause pharyngitis and those usually responsible for pyoderma.

Staphylococcus aureus often colonize in skin lesions of streptococcal origin. Because lesions that yield both kinds of bacteria do not otherwise differ from those yielding group A *S. pyogenes* alone, the staphylococci are of doubtful significance. Bullous impetigo lesions, as commonly caused by *Staphylococcus aureus* of phage type 71, are seldom superinfected by group A streptococci. Certain of the bullous impetigo staphylococci produce a bacteriocin inhibitory for streptococci. However, primary staphylococcal pyoderma, followed by mixed infections resulting in typical streptococcal lesions, are occasionally seen. In burns (Chap. 157, Infections Following Burns) and in wound suppuration (Chap. 158, Infections Following Surgical Operations), *S. aureus*

Table 101-1. Relationships of Streptococcal M and T Antigens

T Antigen or Pattern	Corresponding M Serotypes and Predominant Site of Infection	
	SKIN	THROAT
1	68*	1, 3
2		2
3, 13, B3264†	33, 39, 41, 43, 52, 53, 56	1, 3, 13, 67,* 69,* 71*
4	60, 63*	4, 24, 26, 29, 46, 48
6		6
8, 25, Imp. 19†	2, 55, 57, 58, 65*	8, 25
11, 11/12	59, 61	11
12	66*	12, 22, 62
14, 49	49	14, 51
15, 17, 19, 23, 47	54	15, 17, 19, 23, 30, 47
T-28 (± others)		70*

*Denotes provisional number; epidemiologic information is incomplete on most types above 65; over 70 M types have been identified.
†3, 13, B3264, and 8, 25, Imp. 19 were T agglutination patterns originally associated with impetigo streptococci.

and *S. pyogenes* should both be regarded as pathogens when they are found together because bacteremia may result from either.

Epidemiology

The epidemiologic features of streptococcal pyoderma and pharyngitis are contrasted in Table 101-2. In general, the epidemiology of AGN parallels the epidemiology of the antecedent infection.

In Figure 101-1, the seasonal distribution of endemic and epidemic AGN following streptococcal pyoderma is depicted. Clearly, hot and humid climatic conditions favor the occurrence of pyoderma and AGN.

The mode of transmission of streptococcal pyoderma is not completely understood, but direct contact with infected material is important. Multiple cases of impetigo frequently occur in siblings within a short span. When caused by nephritogenic streptococci, multiple cases of nephritis may also occur within the family.

Humans are the most important reservoir for streptococci that cause pyoderma. Evidence of respiratory infection is normally lacking, and the numbers of streptococci recovered from the nose and throat are usually small. However, wound or soft-tissue infections and impetiginous lesions about the nose and mouth may complicate streptococcal respiratory infection.

In Trinidad, it was found that flies (*Hippelates* spp.) carried viable streptococci for prolonged periods after feeding on infected lesions. Such flies could possibly transfer an infective dose of streptococci to the skin of uninfected persons.

There is a strong association between mosquito bites and subsequent streptococcal impetigo. Direct evidence that mosquitoes either transmit or transfer infective doses of streptococci to the skin of susceptible patients is lacking. However, minor trauma and itching associated with mosquito bites is of considerable importance in predisposition to or perpetuation of infected lesions.

A limited number of serotypes are associated with AGN, regardless of the site of the antecedent infection. Referred to collectively as nephritogenic streptococci, the strains of known importance are related to the usual site of infection in Table 101-3.

The dichotomy in serotypes responsible for pyoderma and pharyngitis (Table 101-1) also holds true in strains with nephritogenic potential.

Type 49, the original Red Lake strain, is of worldwide importance in causing nephritis after pyoderma. This type has been repeatedly associated with epidemic nephritis in widely separated areas and may occasionally cause nephritis after infection of the throat; moreover, it appears to be more likely to cause pharyngitis than other common pyoderma–nephritis strains. Additional pyoderma–nephritis strains of primary importance include M types 2, 55, 57, and 60. Type 55 has been a major epidemic strain in Trinidad, where it was first identified. The type 2 pyoderma–nephritis strains share in common with types 55 and 57 the T pattern 8/25/Imp.19. Recently, M 2, T 2 streptococci have caused nephritis after pharyngitis. The difference in T antigen that relates to site of infection is an interesting but unexplained characteristic of the nephritogenic type 2 streptococci. Type 60 is widespread in distribution, causing nephritis in the United States, Trinidad, and Israel. As type 49, type 60 has also been associated with nephritis following either pyoderma or pharyngitis. The M 12 streptococcus is a common, widely distributed serotype that causes pharyngitis. Major epidemics of AGN following respiratory infection have most often been associated with type M 12 and less frequently with type 1 (Table 101-3). Relatively few reports of nephritis following type 12 infection have been described in recent years, although type 12 remains a common pharyngeal strain. Neither type 12 nor the other nephritogenic M serotypes appear to be uniformly capable of inducing nephritis. The role of specific M antigen or related properties in causing nephritis are as yet unexplained.

Table 101-2. *Comparison of Epidemiology of Streptococcal Pyoderma and Pharyngitis*

Feature	Site of Infection	
	PYODERMA	PHARYNGITIS
Age	Common in infants and young children	Common during early school years
Sex	Similar distribution	Similar distribution
Race	Probably similar (see text)	Similar distribution
Climate*	Warm, humid, tropical	Temperate, cool
Geography	Appears related to climate	Related to climate
Seasonal incidence	Summer–Fall	Winter–Spring
Predisposing illness	Minor trauma, insect bites, poor hygiene	Preceding illness uncommon
Family spread	Common	Common
Mode of transmission	Direct contact with infected material; insects may be mechanical vectors	Direct spread by respiratory droplets
Streptococcal serotypes	Certain types common in pyoderma (see Table 101-1)	Certain types common in pharyngitis (see Table 101-1)
Average latent period, infection to AGN	21 days	10 days

*According to recent epidemiologic data, streptococcal pharyngitis is common in many warm or tropical climates.

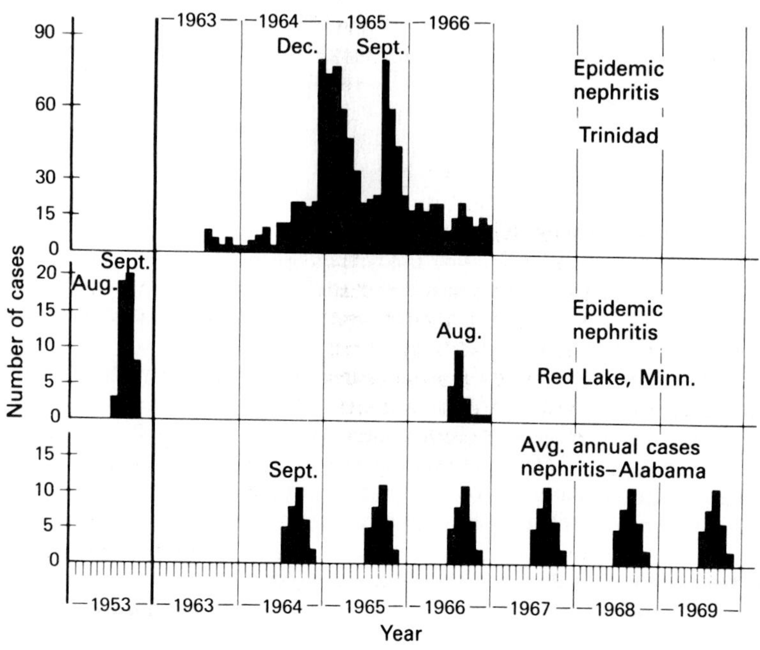

Fig. 101-1. Seasonal distribution of acute glomerulonephritis following pyoderma observed in three widely separated areas. The cases reported in Alabama were averaged for peak months, 1964–1969. Two epidemics separated by 13 years, both caused by type 49 streptococci, occurred at Red Lake, Minnesota. The seasonal incidence of cases in Alabama and Minnesota followed a similar pattern; during the summer in both areas the weather is hot and humid, and mosquitoes abound. In contrast, epidemic nephritis in tropical Trinidad during the years 1964–1966 followed an irregular pattern, with major peaks in September and December. Different serotypes were encountered during epidemic peaks.

Table 101-3. Nephritogenic Serotypes of Recognized Importance

T and M Antigens		Usual Site of Antecedent Infection	
T	M	SKIN	THROAT
1	1		+
2	2		+
4	4		+
4	60	+	+
6	6		+
12	12		+
14, 49	49	+	+
8, 25, Imp. 19	2, 55, 57	+	

Pathogenesis and Pathology

Pyoderma strains of *S. pyogenes* can colonize or survive on normal skin surfaces for extended periods. Epidermal carriage or acquisition appears to be the initial event predisposing to the development of impetigo in most patients. Following acquisition on the normal skin, minor trauma seems to be a prerequisite for initiating infection. Pyoderma strains of *S. pyogenes* produce the gamut of extracellular substances considered in relation to virulence and infectivity in Chapter 24, Streptococcal Diseases. Hyaluronidase and DNase B are uniformly produced, the latter provoking marked antibody responses. The elaboration of large quantities of cell wall membrane lipid is also characteristic and may favor survival in skin lesions.

Strains that commonly cause impetigo have also been incriminated in erysipelas and wound infections. Inflammation and suppuration are more acute in wound infections than in superficial pyoderma. Host factors may account in part for apparent differences in the virulence of streptococci causing these more severe forms of infection.

The initial lesion of streptococcal impetigo is a small pustule in the superficial epidermis; capillary dilation and infiltration with leukocytes occur in the upper cutis. Older lesions are frankly purulent, and ecthyma is characterized by an ulcer crater with thickened margins. Lymphatic channels and regional lymph nodes are involved; lymphangitis is more common in cellulitis and deeper wound infections. Bacteremia may result from pyoderma, but it is more likely in erysipelas or deeper, suppurative infection.

It is generally accepted that the most likely pathogenetic mechanisms involved in poststreptococcal nephritis resemble those demonstrated in experimental immune complex disease, serum sickness nephritis, and the nephritis of lupus erythematosus. Nephritis resembling that in humans was produced by serial infection of rabbits with nephritogenic streptococci. Immunopathologic studies in man have revealed glomerular deposition of IgG, complement, fibrin, and occasionally in early, acute lesions, products and components of streptococcal cells. A decrease in complement occurs prior to or in the absence of hematuria in patients infected with nephritogenic streptococci, including persons who go on to develop clinical nephritis. A hyperimmune response to streptococcal antigens has also been demonstrated in patients with pyoderma-nephritis.

Properdin may also be involved as an activator of complement in the abscence of either antibody or antigen–antibody complexes. Not only is the concentration in the serum decreased, but also properdin is deposited in the glomeruli of patients with poststreptococcal nephritis. Thus, definitive proof of a particular, precise mechanism for nephritis is still lacking and perhaps more than one mechanism may be responsible for the development of this disease. Light and electron microscopic studies have defined the pathologic picture of poststreptococcal nephritis. The humps and lumps seen by the latter technique presumably represent deposition of immune products and fibrin. Differences in the pathology and natural history of poststreptococccal nephritis in children and adults have been described and progressive changes are more often observed in the adult. Nephritis after pyoderma is infrequent in adults.

The continued search for "nephritic factors" has led to recent reports of an extracellular protein thought to be unique to nephritogenic streptococci, as well as a different antigen called endostreptosin; neither of these observations has yet been confirmed.

Manifestations

The typical crusted and pustular lesions of impetigo are illustrated in Figure 52-4G. Systemic manifestations are minimal or absent. The lesions begin as pustules with little erythema. They rapidly progress and are subsequently covered with thickened, yellow crusts with thin pus beneath. Such lesions commonly occur over exposed areas, especially on the extremities. Itching is frequent. Satellite impetigo lesions may develop along scratch lines. Urticaria or erythema multiforme occasionally develops. Scarlet fever may accompany streptococcal pyoderma or wound infection (surgical scarlet fever). Transient lymphadenitis occurs, and significant regional lymphadenopathy is characteristic of streptococcal impetigo.

Secondary infection of dermatoses, such as eczema and seborrheic dermatitis, results in the development of confluent, purulent, crusted lesions with concomitant lymphatic involvement.

Redness, heat, edema, and streaking lymphangitis are hallmarks of the more acute, toxic forms of streptococcal skin and wound infections. Chills and fever commonly accompany such illnesses. Erysipelas is characterized by acute toxicity; the typical lesion is a raised, demarcated, bright red area of dermal and subcutaneous inflammation, which advances as the disease progresses. Erysipelas has been observed to follow chickenpox.

Diagnosis

The etiologic diagnosis of streptococcal pyoderma is confirmed by the isolation of *S. pyogenes* in cultures of material from typical lesions. Underlying skin diseases that predispose to streptococcal pyoderma, such as tinea capitis and eczema, may become more apparent as secondary streptococcal infection is treated and improved. Embolic pustular lesions are occasionally seen in seriously ill patients with septicemias caused, for example, by *Pseudomonas aeruginosa* and *S. aureus.* The underlying diseases, the typical clinical manifestations of general sepsis, smears, and cultures from the lesions, usually enable the separation of such patients from those with streptococcal pyoderma.

Serologic Responses to Dermal Streptococcal Infections

The immune response to streptococcal skin infection differs in several respects from that observed following pharyngitis. The relative behavior of several antibody tests is shown in Table 101-4. Anti-DNase B is especially useful in studies of streptococcal skin infections because the titers are more often elevated and the magnitude of the response is much greater than that seen with antistreptolysin O (ASO). The antihyaluronidase response is also superior to the ASO in pyoderma and nephritis; less is known of this response in pharyngitis–nephritis. In contrast, anti-NADase, although useful as an indicator of postpharyngitis nephritis, is of limited value in pyoderma; presumably, strains that commonly cause pyoderma and nephritis produce little, if any, NADase.

The feeble or erratic ASO response in pyoderma and pyoderma–nephritis is best explained by inhibition of the streptolysin O antigen by lipids in the skin. The marked differences in the various antibody responses (to extracellular antigens) that relate to the site of infection are of primary consideration in the selection of appropriate serologic tests. Generally, higher antibody titers occur in nephritis than occur in uncomplicated infections, as demonstrated in particular with anti-DNase B responses in pyoderma–nephritis. Data are limited on the type-specific immune response in patients with skin infection, including those with AGN, but antibody responses to either M type 2 or M type 49 were infrequently demonstrated in a study of nephritic patients.

Acute Glomerulonephritis

The major clinical and laboratory manifestations of acute poststreptococcal glomerulonephritis are listed in Table 101-5. Acute nephritis encompasses a broad clinical spectrum, ranging from minimal disease to death. Acute nephritis with normal urinary findings has been documented by biopsy. The finding of a low C3 level not only confirms the clinical diagnosis of acute glomerulonephritis, but also is of value in the detection of subclinical or asymptomatic cases of nephritis. The typical self-limited course of poststreptococcal nephritis, with the return of urine abnormalities—proteinuria, hematuria, and cylindruruia (Fig. 52-4*D, F*)—and complement to normal within days to weeks after onset of the disease, distinguishes AGN from other nephritides. The triad of

Table 101-4. *Relative Value of Streptococcal Antibody Tests in Acute Glomerulonephritis in Relation to Antecedent Site of Infection*

	Average Frequency % Elevated Titers			
Site of Infection	ASO*	ANTI-DNASE B†	ANTI-HYALURONIDASE	ANTI-NADASE‡
Pharyngitis–AGN	80–85	80		>80
Pyoderma–AGN	50	90	>80	<25

*Antistreptolysin O.

†Antideoxyribonuclease B.

‡Anti-nicotinamide-adenine-dinucleotidase (formerly anti-DPNase).

Table 101-5. *Clinical and Laboratory Manifestations of Poststreptococcal Acute Glomerulonephritis*

Clinical Features	Laboratory Findings
Abrupt onset	Hematuria, cylindruria
Headache, malaise	Proteinuria
Edema, oliguria, dark urine	Azotemia
	Low complement (acute)
Hypertension, congestive failure, encephalopathy	Elevated streptococcal antibody titer
Diuresis, weight loss, clinical recovery	Positive streptococcal culture

documented streptococcal infection, self-limited illness, and transient low complement is diagnostic of acute poststreptococcal nephritis.

Prognosis

Streptococcal pyoderma tends to be a benign, indolent disease. In untreated cases, old lesions may persist for weeks or even months while new lesions develop. In patients with predisposing conditions, recurrent pyoderma is common. Suppurative complications occasionally occur—purulent lymphadenitis, soft-tissue infection, and cellulitis. Cellulitis may be painfully disabling, and hospitalization is often required. The possibility of bacteremia in these forms of infection is real; prompt and vigorous therapy is indicated.

On the basis of limited data, it appears that type-specific (anti-M) antibody develops less often in patients with pyoderma than in patients with untreated pharyngitis. Furthermore, the development of anti-M antibody may vary considerably in relation to the specific M type. Certain pyodermal M types appear to be relatively poor antigens, as evidenced by difficulty in preparing and maintaining suitable M antisera. The role of type-specific immunity (specific serum opsonin), in preventing skin infections has not yet been clearly delineated. Cellular immunity and secretory antibody fractions have not been determined.

In epidemic nephritis in children and military recruits, the prognosis for complete recovery exceeds 95%. In older adults, the prognosis is worse; in general, the more severe the illness, the less likely complete healing becomes. Failure of the glomerular changes to regress and the continued development of abnormalities in glomerular basement membranes are characteristic of cases that show progression. The mechanisms of production of more severe nephritis in adults remain unexplained. True recurrences of acute glomerulonephritis are infrequent in either age group, probably because of the limited number of streptococcal serotypes capable of provoking this reaction.

Therapy

Streptococcal skin and soft-tissue infections are best treated by the systemic administration of antimicrobial agents. Deeper infections and those with cellulitis require more vigorous initial treatment than do uncomplicated pyodermas. Topical antimicrobics, such as bactracin, are recommended only for patients with small numbers of lesions or as supplemental therapy for residual unhealed lesions after systemic antimicrobic therapy. The antimicrobics and regimens given in Chapter 24 are generally suitable. However, if large numbers of penicillinase-producing staphylococci are present in lesions with streptococci, healing may be retarded despite peroral administration of penicillin. Erythromycin has proven to be quite effective for streptococcal and mixed streptococcal-staphylococcal forms of pyoderma. Seven days of treatment is usually adequate to ensure clearing of the lesions, but for extensive infections, 10 days of therapy is recommended.

Prevention

Hygienic skin care minimizes the likelihood of streptococcal skin infections. Once skin infection is present, however, improved skin hygiene alone is insufficient to eradicate the infection. The reduction of minor skin trauma through the control of biting insects appears to be important to the prevention of impetigo. Because pyoderma is especially common in patients at lower socioeconomic levels, improvement in living conditions, health care, and possibly nutrition should reduce the incidence of streptococcal skin infection.

Prompt treatment of streptococcal infections has not always resulted in the prevention of acute nephritis, unlike the excellent results obtained in the prevention of acute rheumatic fever. The shorter latent period of nephritis (average, 10 days) following respiratory infection probably accounts for this discrepancy. Although the latent period of nephritis following skin infection may be twice that of respiratory nephritis, there is usually a corresponding delay in seeking medical attention that negates this potential advantage.

Therapy with penicillin is effective in aborting streptococcal epidemics of either the skin or the respiratory tract. Stopping or limiting the spread of nephritogenic strains of streptococci is an important preventive measure. In selected situations, such as families in which an index case of nephritis occurs, chemoprophylaxis in contacts may prevent additional cases of nephritis. For contacts who are not yet infected, penicillin V by mouth (25 mg/kg body wt/day, as four equal portions, every 6 hours for 2–3 days) taken during the time the index case is simultaneously treated usually prevents streptococcal infection.

Chemoprophylaxis is not the optimal means for preventing poststreptococcal glomerulonephritis; yet, proven streptococcal vaccines do not exist. Too little is known about the role of type-specific antibody in the prevention of streptococcal skin infections to indicate that vaccines would be effective, if they become available. Recurrences of poststreptococcal nephritis are rare. Continuous chemoprophylaxis for patients who have had glomerulonephritis is unnecessary.

Bibliography

Books

AHMED U, TRESER G, JACKSON JJ, CARLO DG, LANGE K: The relation of a recently identified streptococcal antigen (endostreptosin) to renal diseases. In Parker MT (ed): Pathogenic Streptococci. Surrey, England, Reedbooks, 1979. pp 137–139.

DILLON HC, DERRICK CW: Type specific antibody response after pyoderma and acute glomerulonephritis: types 2 and 49. In Parker MT (ed): Pathogenic Streptococci. Surrey, England, Reedbooks, 1979. pp 92–93.

DILLON HC, MADDOX S, WARE JC: Pathogenesis and prevention of streptococcal impetigo. In Nelson JD, Grassi C (eds): Current Chemotherapy and Infectious Disease, Vol II. Washington, DC, American Society of Microbiology, 1980. pp 1190–1192.

DILLON HC: Streptococcal infections of the skin and their complications: impetigo and nephritis. In Wannamaker LW, Matsen J (eds): Streptococci and Streptococcal Diseases. New York, Academic Press, 1972. pp 572–586.

MICHAEL F, HOYER R, WESTBURG NG, FISH AJ: Experimental models for the pathogenesis of acute poststreptococcal glomerulonephritis. In Wannamaker LW, Matsen J (eds): Streptococci and Streptococcal Disease. New York, Academic Press, 1972. pp 481–500.

POON-KING T, POTTER EV, ACHONG J, SVARTMAN M, BURT EG, BRAY JP, SHARRETT AR, ORTIZ JS, FINKLEA JF, EARLE DP: The epidemiology of acute poststreptococcal nephritis in South Trinidad. In Haverkorn MJ (ed): Streptococcal Disease and the Community. Amsterdam Excerpta Medica. 1974. pp 292–300.

VILLARREAL H JR, VAN DE RIJN I, FISCHETTI VA, MAHABIR RN, ZABRISKIE JG: An extracellular protein unique to nephritogenic streptococci. In Parker MT (ed): Pathogenic Streptococci. Surrey, England, Reedbooks, 1979. pp 135–137.

WANNAMAKER LW: Epidemiology of acute glomerulonephritis. In Metcoff J (ed): Acute Glomerulonephritis; 17th Annual Symposium on the Kidney. Boston, Little, Brown, 1967. pp 39–67.

WIDDOWSON JP, MAXTED WR, NORLEY CM, PINNEY AM: Type-specific and M-associated antibody response to different serotypes of Group A streptococci. In Haverkorn MJ (ed): Streptococcal Disease and the Community. Amsterdam, Excerpta Medica, 1974. pp 116–125.

Journals

DERRICK W, DILLON HC: Impetigo contagiosa. Am Fam Physician 4:75–81, 1971

DERRICK CW, REEVES MS, DILLON HC: Complement in overt and asymptomatic nephritis after skin infection. J Clin Invest 49:1178–1187, 1970

DILLON HC JR: Post-streptococcal glomerulonephritis following pyoderma. Rev Infect Dis 1:935–943, 1979

DILLON HC JR: Topical and systemic therapy for pyodermas. Internat J Dermatol 19:443–451, 1980

DILLON HC: Impetigo contagiosa: suppurative and non-suppurative complications. Am J Dis Child 115:530–541, 1968

DILLON HC, DERRICK CW, DILLON MS: M-antigens common to pyoderma and nephritis. J Infect Dis 130:257–267, 1974

DILLON HC, REEVES MSA: Streptococcal immune response in nephritis after skin infection. Am J Med 56:333–346, 1974

FERRIERI P, DAJANI AS, WANNAMAKER LW, CHAPMAN SS: Natural history of impetigo. I. Site sequence of acquisition and familiar patterns of spread of cutaneous streptococci. J Clin Invest 51:2851–2861, 1972

FISH AJ, HERDMAN RC, MICHAEL AF, PICKERING RJ, GOOD RA: Epidemic acute nephritis associated with type 49 streptococcal pyoderma. II Correlative study of light, immunofluorescent and electron microscopic findings. Am J Med 48:28–39, 1970

KAPLAN EL, BASCOM FA, CHAPMAN SS, WANNAMAKER LW: Epidemic acute glomerulonephritis associated with type 49 streptococcal pyoderma. I. Clinical and laboratory findings. Am J Med 48:9–27, 1970

KAPLAN EL, WANNAMAKER LW: Streptolysin O: Suppression of its antigenicity by lipids extracted from skin. Pro Soc Exp Biol Med 146:205–208, 1974

PARKER MT: Streptococcal skin infection and acute glomerulonephritis. Br J Dermatol (Suppl) 81:37–45, 1969

POTTER EV, SIEGEL AC, SIMON NM, MCANINCH J, EARLE DP, POON–KING T, MOHAMMED I, ABIDH S: Streptococcal infections in South Trinidad. J Pediatr 72:871–884, 1968

RAMMELKAMP CH JR, WEAVER RS: Acute glomerulonephritis: The significance of the variations in the incidence of the disease. J Clin Invest 32:345–358, 1953

WANNAMAKER LW: Differences between streptococcal infection of the throat and of the skin. N Engl J Med 282:23–31, 78–85, 1970

W. CHRISTOPHER DUNCAN

Erythrasma and Trichomycosis Axillaris

102

Erythrasma and trichomycosis axillaris are both caused by bacteria of the genus *Corynebacterium*. Both diseases are, in addition, rather benign and often chronic. Yet, there are differences, particularly in epidemiology and pathogenesis.

Erythrasma

Erythrasma is usually a mild, chronic, localized superficial infection of the body folds and clefts characterized by well-defined areas of dry and scaly or finely wrinkled skin. At times, the involved area may be inflamed, and weeping can ensue—a development more common in occlusive, intertriginous areas.

Etiology

Erythrasma is caused by infection with *Corynebacterium minutissimum*. Potassium hydroxide preparations may enable the visualization of the bacilli in scales; however, stained preparations (Gram, Giemsa) examined with the oil immersion lens are preferable. *Corynebacterium minutissimum* are nonmotile, gram-positive rods (1.5 μm–2 μm in length) and filaments; granules are frequently visible in the cytoplasm. The isolation and identification of *C. minutissimum* are not performed routinely in most laboratories. When grown in tissue culture medium 199 containing 20% fetal bovine serum and gelled with agar, small colonies of *C. minutissimum* can be obtained within 12 to 24 hours. These colonies and the surrounding medium fluoresce coral red when examined in ultraviolet (Wood's) light.

Epidemiology

All age groups may be affected, but erythrasma is much more common in adults than in children. The overall incidence has declined significantly during the past decade. This is in all probability a result of the widespread use of antibacterial bar soaps that are effective in treatment of the clinical disease.

A generalized form of the disease is more common in tropical and subtropical areas than it is in temperate or arctic regions. A variety of erythrasma that affects the trunk and the genitocrural folds extensively is particularly common in middle-aged black women. The disease as it affects the toe clefts is common, with a reported incidence of 14% to 84%. In many cases, there is an associated tinea pedis. *Corynebacterium minutissimum* is widespread among nonhuman animals, and it is commonly found on both normal and abnormal human skin.

Pathogenesis and Pathology

The infection begins as a proliferation of *C. minutissimum* on the surface of the skin. Invasion of the upper third of the stratum corneum follows; there the bacteria are found both extracellularly and intracellularly in the keratinized cells. A mild round-cell response is sometimes present in the subjacent dermis.

Manifestations

The groins, pubis, axillae, intergluteal folds, and inframammary and periumbilical areas are commonly affected in erythrasma (Fig. 102-1). Patches of involvement are irregular in shape, dry and scaly, and initially pink, although they later become brown. New lesions are smooth, but older patches tend to show fine epidermal wrinkling (Fig. 102-2). Scaling, if not obvious, can be demonstrated by scratching the surface. Although most lesions are asymptomatic, there may be a mild irritation in the groins, where scratching may lead to thickening and lichenification. The hair in the affected area is normal. In the two lateral toe clefts, scaling, fissuring, and a slight maceration are the most common findings. However, erythrasma of the toe webs is often symptom-free, and of little importance to the patient. Extensive ery-

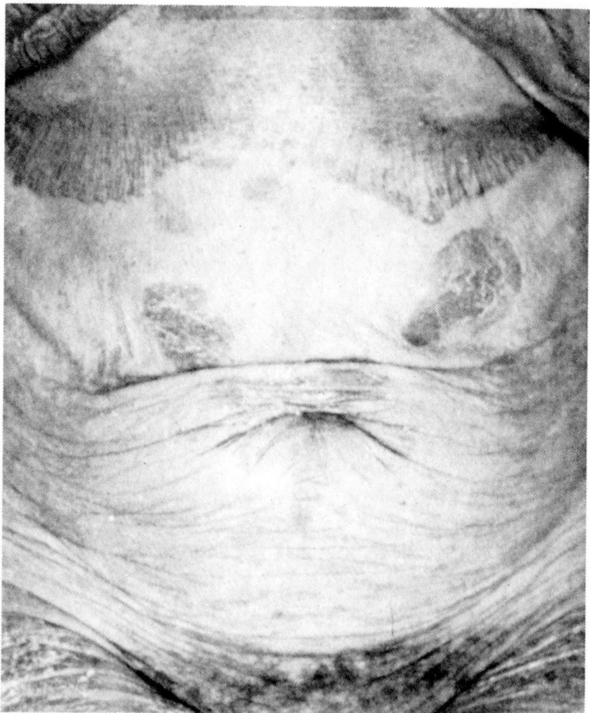

Fig. 102-1. Extensive erythrasma with inframammary and genitocrural involvement in a diabetic.

Fig. 102-2. Erythrasma. Sharply demarcated patch with scaling and fine wrinkling.

thrasma, however, may be important as a sign of diabetes mellitus; concomitance with diabetes has been reported as high as 47%. It may be the presenting manifestation of adult-onset diabetes of and is in this way similar to candidosis.

Diagnosis

Diagnosis of erythrasma is based on finding scaly patches in intertriginous areas. Examination using a Wood's light, preparation of gram-stained smears, and cultures of scrapings enable confirmation of the diagnosis. Wood's light is of inestimable diagnostic value because the lesions of erythrasma glow with a coral red fluorescence that is probably due to a porphyrin.

Tinea versicolor may be confused with erythrasma, but it does not localize in the body folds. On the thighs, groins, and pubic area, tinea cruris and candidosis may be simulated. However, in erythrasma there is relatively little inflammation, no vesiculation or satellite lesions and no active border. It is exceedingly difficult to differentiate erythrasma of the toe clefts from mild tinea pedis, but the presence of coral red fluorescence under Wood's light is diagnostic. Because many patients have both tinea pedis and erythrasma or tinea cruris and erythrasma, mycologic examination of scales is still important.

Prognosis

Without treatment, erythrasma tends to persist indefinitely.

Therapy

In mild to moderately severe cases of erythrasma, one of the antibacterial bar soaps should be tried initially. If the infection does not respond to a regimen of bidaily washing, systemic erythromycin, in a dose of 15 mg/kg body wt/day as four equal portions, given perorally once every 6 hours, should be used for 5 days. In widespread disease or in patients who are very uncomfortable, both therapeutic approaches should be insitituted simultaneously. Diabetics with extensive erythrasma may require treatment with erythromycin for 2 to 3 weeks.

Prevention

There is no known specific preventive measure for erythrasma. An ancillary benefit of maintaining control of diabetes mellitus and good hygienic practice seems to be the decreased likelihood of developing erythrasma.

Trichomycosis Axillaris

Trichomycosis axillaris is a superificial bacterial infection of axillary, and occasionally, pubic hair, or both that results in the formation of adherent yellow, red, or black nodules or cylindric sheaths on the hair shaft.

Etiology

The term trichomycosis is inappropriate because the causative agent is not a fungus, as was once believed. Bacteria are recognized as the etiologic agent. However, the designation *Corynebacterium tenuis* is probably not tenable because at least three species of *Cornyebacterium,* judged by colonial morphology, can penetrate the cuticle of hair during growth.

Gram stains of infected hairs reveal dense masses of gram-positive material that appear to be homogeneous. After soaking overnight in water, the masses become gelatinous, and staining effectively demonstrates gram-positive, pleomorphic filaments and rods in the meshwork of frayed hair cuticle. Culture on blood agar results in a reversion of the filaments of some species to the characteristic short, gram-positive rods typical of diphtheroids.

Epidemiology

Trichomycosis axillaris occurs in both temperate and tropical climates, and it is not limited by race or sex. The incidence of trichomycosis, as that of erythrasma, has declined since the antibacerial bar soaps have come into common usage.

Corynebacterium tenuis is frequently found as part of the resident bacterial flora in the axilla without evidence of clinical disease.

Pathogenesis and Pathology

Growth of *C. tenuis* in naturally infected hairs is limited to the cuticle of the hair. There is invasion of the soft keratin of the cuticle, but not the hard keratin of the hair cortex. Reproduction *in vitro* of typical bacterial nodules on hairs has been accomplished by incubating normal sterile hair with pure cultures of *C. tenuis* in broth.

Manifestations

Trichomycosis axillaris is usually asymptomatic, and the patient is often totally unaware of it. However, complaints of colored hair, stained clothes, offensive odor, or colored sweat may be voiced.

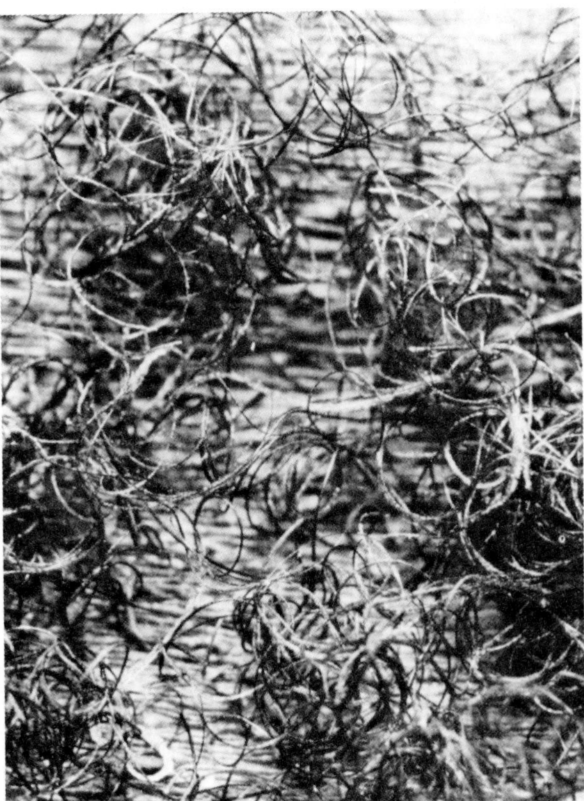

Fig. 102-3. Trichomycosis axillaris.

Diagnosis

Yellow, red, or black concretions that are hard or soft, nodular or diffuse, are present on the hair shaft (Fig. 102-3). The skin is unaffected. The axillary sweat may be yellow, red, or black, according to the color of the concretions. Yellow is most common; black is rare. Clothing may take up the stain. Persons with trichomycosis have a characteristic (and virtually diagnostic) axillary odor.

In differential diagnosis, pediculosis pubis, which may affect axillary as well as pubic hair, and piedra should be considered. Differentiation is accomplished by the microscopic examination of involved hairs.

Therapy

The regular use of one of the antibacterial bar soaps or liquid skin cleansers usually clears the infection in 1 to 2 weeks. Erythromycin or clindamycin, applied topically, are effective. Shaving the affected hair is rarely necessary.

Bibliography

ERYTHRASMA

Journals

BURNS RE, GREER JE, MIKHAIL G, LIVINGOOD CS: The significance of coral red fluorescence of the skin. Arch Dermatol 96:436–440, 1967

DODGE BG, KNOWLES WR, MCBRIDE ME, DUNCAN WC, KNOX JM: Treatment of erythrasma with an antibacterial soap. Arch Dermatol 97:548–552, 1968

MONTES LF, DOBSON H, DODGE BG, KNOWLES WR: Erythrasma and diabetes mellitus. Arch Dermatol 99:674–680, 1969

SARKANY I, TAPLIN D, BLANK H: The etiology and treatment of erythrasma. J Invest Dermatol 37:282–290, 1961

TRICHOMYCOSIS AXILLARIS

Journals

CRISSEY T, REBELL GC, LASKOS JJ: Studies on the causative organism of trichomycosis axillaris. J Invest Dermatol 19:187–197, 1952

FREEMAN RG, MCBRIDE ME, DUNCAN WC, WAND C: Pathogenesis of trichomycosis axillaris. South Med J 62:78–80, 1969

MCBRIDE ME, FREEMAN RG, KNOX JM: The bacteriology of trichomycosis axillaris. Br J Dermatol 80:509–513, 1968

PAUL D. HOEPRICH

Erysipeloid

103

Erysipeloid, an uncommon, acute but slowly evolving, self-limited infection of the skin, is the most common clinical incursion of *Erysipelothrix rhusiopathiae* in humans. Endocarditis (Chap. 134, Infective Endocarditis) and arthritis (Chap. 151, Septic Arthritis) are additional, rare forms of disease.

Many nonhuman animal species may be infected, including both vertebrates (mammals, birds, fish) and invertebrates (shellfish, insects). Diseases caused by *E. rhusiopathiae* in pigs (swine erysipelas [diamond back], acute septicemia, polyarthritis, endocarditis) are of great economic importance, since they may cause death or lead to condemnation of carcasses.

Etiology

The genus *Erysipelothrix* contains but one species: *rhusiopathiae*—once known as *insidiosa.* They are gram-positive, nonmotile, noncapsulated, nonsporulating bacilli (0.5 μm–2.5 μm long × 0.2 μm–0.4 μm in diameter), which are aerobic but flourish with reduced O_2 and increased CO_2 tensions. On initial isolation, they form tiny (1.0 mm–1.5 mm in diameter), smooth, transparent colonies which display a bluish iridescence. On subculture, they tend to form rough colonies made up of long filaments (4 μm–15 μm), chains, or masses of pleomorphic bacilli that may become gram-negative and develop granules as the culture ages.

In 1884, Rosenbach, in culturing *E. rhusiopathiae* from a skin lesion of a patient not only achieved the first isolation from a human but also named the disease erysipeloid and proved that *E. rhusiopathiae* was the etiologic agent by self-inoculation. Loeffler had previously documented the relationship of *E. rhusiopathiae* to swine erysipelas in 1886 and Koch had cultured *Erysipelothrix* from mice 6 years earlier.

Erysipelothrix spp. grow on the usual, nonselective culture mediums. Although they are nonhemolytic, they may produce a greening reaction on blood (horse, sheep) agar. They display no singular biochemical or metabolic properties, but are quite distinct from *Listeria monocytogenes.*

Differentiation of *E. rhusiopathiae* from *L. monocytogenes* (Chap. 51, Listeriosis) and *Corynebacterium* spp. (Chap. 25, Diphtheria) is accomplished by proving lack of motility, lack of catalase, failure of hemolysis, inability to hydrolyze esculin, and relative inability to reduce triphenyltetrazolium chloride. In addition, the intraperitoneal inoculation of mice leads to a general infection with septicemia, severe conjunctivitis, and death in 3 to 5 days. On the other hand, the conjunctival inoculation of *Erysipelothrix* spp. in the rabbit, hamster, or guinea pig does not lead to a progressive ocular infection. Serologic differentiation is also possible but is a research or reference laboratory procedure. There is no host specificity among the several serotypes.

Capable of a nonparasitic existence, erysipelothrix tolerate 0.2% phenol, 0.5% potassium tellurite, and the food preservation maneuvers of salting, pickling, and smoking. These bacteria are highly susceptible to penicillin G (minimal inhibitory and lethal concentrations of about 0.0025 μg/ml and 0.025 μg/ml, respectively), erythromycin, the tetracyclines, and chloramphenicol, but they are resistant to the sulfonamides and polymyxins.

Epidemiology

Widespread in nature, *Erysipelothrix* sp. may be primarily saprophytic. Infection in humans is virtually restricted to persons who handle dead animal matter in their work, either edible (meat, poultry, fish, shellfish) or nonedible (bones, shells). Erysipeloid occurs most often in the summer and early fall, also the seasonal peak of swine erysipelas. Curiously, however, pig handlers do not commonly develop erysipelas. Men are afflicted more often than women. There are no vectors, and the infection is not contagious.

Pathogenesis and Pathology

The traumatic inoculation of *E. rhusiopathiae* is prerequisite to the development of erysipeloid; that is, the skin of the fingers and hands is most often involved. Failure of localization to the skin is unusual, but bacteremia has apparently followed the ingestion of undercooked pork from pigs infected with *E. rhusiopathiae.* If bacteremia occurs, infection of normal or previously damaged heart valves or of joints may result.

The histopathology of erysipeloid is that of intense inflammation in the dermis. The bacilli are extracellular, and are located deep in the corium where they are scattered about the capillaries.

Manifestations

Two to seven days after injury—the site of inoculation may already have healed—the lesion of erysipeloid becomes evident as an area of purplish red, nonvesiculated inflammation that is sharply defined by an irregular, raised border. Particularly with lesions of the fingers, the swelling may be sufficient to limit the movement of nearby joints. The lesions itch and burn, but usually there is no lymphangitis or lymphadenitis, nor are there symptoms or signs of systemic illness. As the initial, oldest part of the lesion heals, a slow (1 cm/day), centrifugal spread may occur. Although the fingers and hands (distal to the wrists) are usually involved, the terminal phalanges typically are spared.

The manifestations of infective endocarditis and septic arthritis caused by *E. rhusiopathiae* are in no way unique. If erysipeloid was the source, the skin has usually healed completely by the time endocarditis becomes manifest; that is, etiologic diagnosis depends on isolation of *E. rhusiopathiae* from the blood.

Diagnosis

The clinical appearance of erysipeloid is unique; once seen, the disease will always be recognized when encountered again. Microbiologic diagnosis is most often successful when a full-thickness biopsy of skin taken from the advancing edge of a lesion is cultured in glucose-containing broth. The aspiration of sterile, bacteriostat-free 0.9% sodium chloride solution after injection into the periphery of an advancing lesion less often produces an inoculum from which *Erysipelothrix* sp. are recovered. Abrasion of a florid lesion followed by culture of the exudate may be productive of etiologic diagnosis.

Erysipelas typically afflicts the face and scalp with bright red, hot, tender lesions of acute inflammation that spread relatively rapidly. Regional lymphadenopathy is common, and systemic illness is evident. Other dermatoses, such as eczema and the erythemas are not migratory, and they are not typically localized to the hands and fingers.

Prognosis

Erysipeloid is usually self-limited, subsiding spontaneously in about 3 weeks. However, relapses may occur. Lasting protective immunity apparently does not occur after recovery from erysipeloid, although specific agglutinins may appear during convalescence.

Therapy

Penicillin is the agent of choice for treatment of patients with erysipeloid. One injection of 600,000 units of benzathine penicillin into each buttock (adults) generally brings about cure. In persons hypersensitive to penicillins, erythromycin (15 mg/kg body wt/day, PO, as four equal portions, 6-hourly, for 5–7 days) is satisfactory.

The treatment of endocarditis and arthritis depends on the use of penicillin (Chaps. 134 and 151, Infective Endocarditis and Septic Arthritis).

Prevention

There are no known preventive measures for erysipeloid that are applicable in humans. Vaccines and antiserums have been used with variable success as preventives of swine erysipelas.

Bibliography

Journals

GRIECO MH, SHELDON C: *Erysipelothrix rhusiopathiae.* Ann NY Acad Sci 174:523–532, 1970

NELSON E: Five hundred cases of erysipeloid. Rocky Mt Med J 52:40–42, 1955

STUART MR, PEASE PE: A numerical study on the relationships of Listeria and Erysipelothrix. J Gen Microbiol 73:551–565, 1972

PHILIP S. BRACHMAN

Anthrax

104

Anthrax, a zoonotic disease, occurs in three forms in humans: cutaneous, accounting for 95% of cases seen in the United States; inhalation, accounting for 5%; and gastrointestinal, which has never been reported in the United States. The breakdown of cases throughout the world is probably similar; the few gastrointestinal cases reported have occurred in Asia and Africa. Meningitis and septicemia may be complications of any form.

Etiology

Bacillus anthracis are gram-positive, nonmotile, capsulated bacilli (1–1.3 μm × 3–10 μm) that produce central or paracentral oval spores which do not cause significant swelling of the rods. In smears from growth on ordinary artificial mediums, the bacilli lie in long, parallel chains. In clinical specimens, they occur singly or in short chains containing two or three square-ended or slightly rounded bacilli that are encapsulated. A specific fluorescent antibody conjugate stains the bacteria brilliantly.

The spores are formed under aerobic conditions, and they are relatively resistant to destruction by disinfectants and heat. They reportedly persist for years in the soil and in some animal products.

On ordinary culture mediums such as nutrient agar, after 18 hours at 37°C, colonies are round, approximately 5 mm in diameter, gray to white, and slightly rough-textured, and have a ground glass appearance. Comma-shaped outgrowths may project from the edge of the colony (medusa head or comet tail). Additionally, on 5% sheep blood agar, colonies are nonhemolytic.

Bacillus anthracis colonies are tenacious; if an inoculating needle is drawn through a colony, the disturbed part of the colony stands up like beaten egg whites. Capsule production may be helpful to presumptive identification in laboratories that do not have special reagents: cultures are grown under increased carbon dioxide concentration on bicarbonate-containing mediums: smooth, mucoid colonies result with *B. anthracis.* Three exotoxins are elaborated by vegetative *B. anthracis.*

Lysis of isolates by a specific anthrax gamma bacteriophage may be used to identify *B. anthracis* tentatively. Laboratory mice and guinea pigs die 2 to 5 days after inoculation with an agar-grown suspension or washed broth culture of *B. anthracis.*

Epidemiology

The average number of cases of anthrax reported annually in the United States has declined from 127 (1916–1925) to 2.5 (1970–1980) (Fig. 104-1). Of the 231 cases reported between 1955 and 1980, 20 were fatal. The worldwide annual number of cases in humans has been estimated to be approximately 2000, although the actual number could be ten times higher.

Anthrax is classified as industrial, agricultural, or laboratory-acquired. Industrial cases, which account for 80% of cases in the United States, result from contact with such animal products as goat hair, wool, hides, skins, and bones originating principally in Asia, the Middle East, and Africa. Agricultural cases result from contact with diseased animals, primarily cattle, swine, and horses, and occasionally from the inadvertent self-inoculation of veterinary anthrax vaccine. The sources of infection of 231 cases of human anthrax reported from 1955 through 1980 are shown in Table 104-1.

Within involved industries, persons who work in the early processing stages, where contamination is heaviest, are more frequently infected. The inhalation of *B. anthracis* occurs when aerosols are created during the processing of infected materials. Cutaneous infections have resulted from contact with contami-

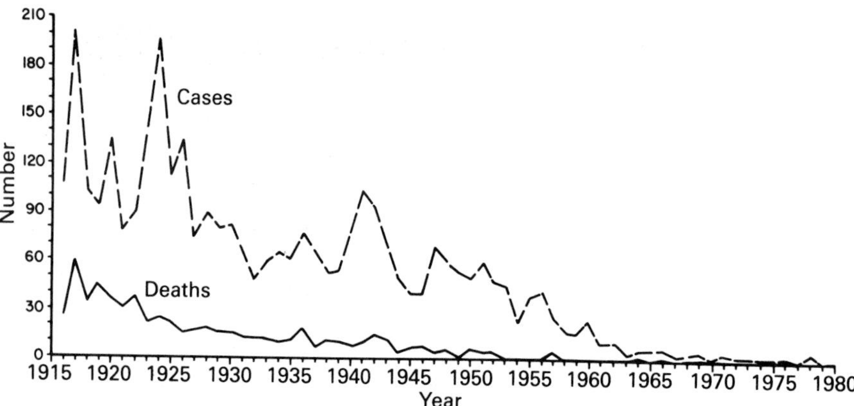

Fig. 104-1. Anthrax in humans (all forms) in the United States, 1916–1980.

Table 104-1. *Source of Infection in 231 Cases of Anthrax in Humans in the United States, 1955–1980*

Industrial		**Agricultural**	
Goat hair	112	Animal	40
Wool	34	Vaccine (veterinary)	2
Goat skin	16	Unknown	8
Meat	3		
Bone	4		
Unknown	12		
Total	181		50

nated finished products, such as flight helmets, wool coats, shaving brushes, and yarn. Some cases have resulted from contact with work clothes contaminated, when a member of the household worked in a high-risk area. There have been no reports of human-to-human transmission.

Pathogenesis and Pathology

Cutaneous anthrax follows the deposition of *B. anthracis* spores under the epidermis, where they germinate, multiply, and produce toxin. Local lesions are evidence of the ability of the body's defenses to confine the infection. The black eschar associated with cutaneous anthrax results from the action of the toxin on tissues causing necrosis; healing requires the developemnt of scar tissue. The bacilli or the toxin may be distributed locally, as a consequence of regional lymphangitis or lymphadenopathy, or systemically through the blood and lymph, to cause bacteremia and systemic manifestations.

Inhalation anthrax results from the alveolar deposition of air-borne particles contaminated with *B. anthracis* spores. After phagocytosis, the spores are carried to the regional lymph nodes before germination takes place. With replication, there is toxin production. Septicemia, general toxemia, and death may result. The severe illness is primarily caused by general intoxication; however, the necrotic, hemorrhagic, edematous mediastinal nodes that result from the local action of the toxin may actually compress the respiratory passages. Direct toxic depression of the respiratory centers of the central nervous system may also be a factor. Primary pneumonia is not typical of inhalation anthrax, although secondary pneumonia may occasionally result after extension from the mediastinal process. The immediate cause of death in the typical case may be respiratory failure secondary to pulmonary capillary thrombosis. Perhaps this is the result of a direct toxic effect on capillary endothelium, as has been demonstrated on electron microscopy of lung tissue in experimental anthrax in rats and monkeys.

Gastrointestinal anthrax results when spores (or possibly, vegetative cells are ingested, pass through the intestinal mucosa, germinate, multiply, and produce toxin in the submucosal tissue. As in cutaneous anthrax, the toxin causes a necrotic, ulcerative lesion—most frequently in the terminal ileum or cecum—that may lead to hemorrhage. Extension to regional lymph nodes may occur.

Manifestations

Cutaneous Anthrax

After an incubation period of 1 to 7 days (usually 2–5 days), a small papule develops; the papule progresses to a vesicle over the next few days. The initial lesion may consist of a small ring of vesicles that coalesce to form a single large vesicle. Erythema and nonpitting

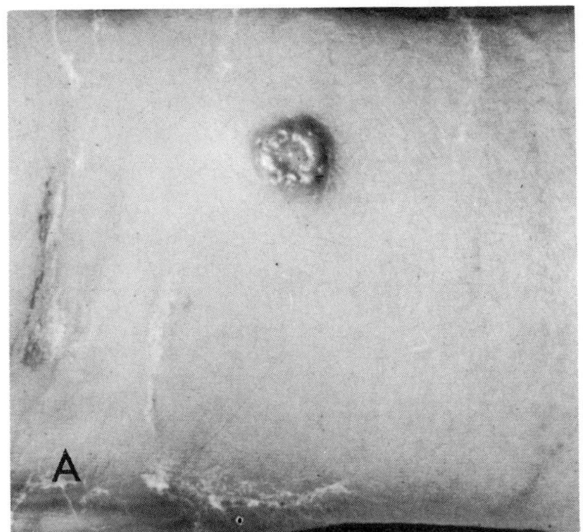

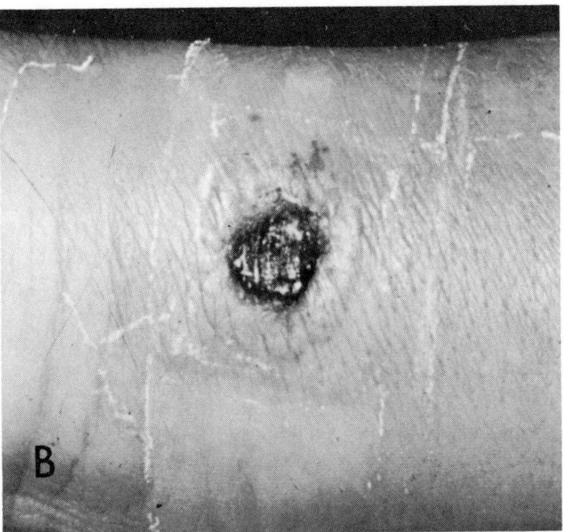

Fig. 104-2. Evolution of cutaneous anthrax in a 38-year-old goat hair carder. The lesion (left volar wrist) began as a pruritic papule from which a hair was extracted. Both penicillin and tetracycline were given; evolution of the lesion was unaffected and recovery was uneventful. (*A*) Fourth day. A central depressed area is ringed by vesicles and surrounded by nonpitting edema. (*B*) Fourteenth day. The firm, depressed, black central eschar is demarcated by dried vesicular tissue.

edema may surround the vesicle. The initial symptom is usually pruritus without pain. In a few days, the clear vesicular fluid becomes dark, typically blue-black. When ruptured, the vesicular tissue reveals a sharp-walled depressed ulcer crater with a black eschar developing in the center (Fig. 104-2A).

There may be mild systemic symptoms, a degree or two of fever, malaise, and occasionally, regional lymphangitis and lymphadenopathy. Further progression to general toxemia and septicemia is rare.

The typical eschar, when fully developed 7 to 10 days after onset, is round and 1 cm to 3 cm in diameter (Fig. 104-2B). With no secondary infection, the edges begin to separate from the crater. Eventually the eschar loosens and falls off. Healing continues by granulation, resulting in scar tissue.

Lesions occur primarily on exposed parts of the body, such as the face, neck, and arms (Fig. 104-3). Rarely, multiple, simultaneously evolving cutaneous lesions have been reported. These probably are the result of simultaneous multiple inoculations.

Lesions in the perioribital area are frequently associated with extensive edema that may involve the entire face, extend down to the neck and upper chest, and impinge on the trachea. Similarly, lesions of the neck and upper chest may also give rise to extensive edema of the surrounding tissues.

Fig. 104-3. Sites of cutaneous lesions of industrial and agricultural anthrax in 220 infections in humans in the United States, 1955–1980.

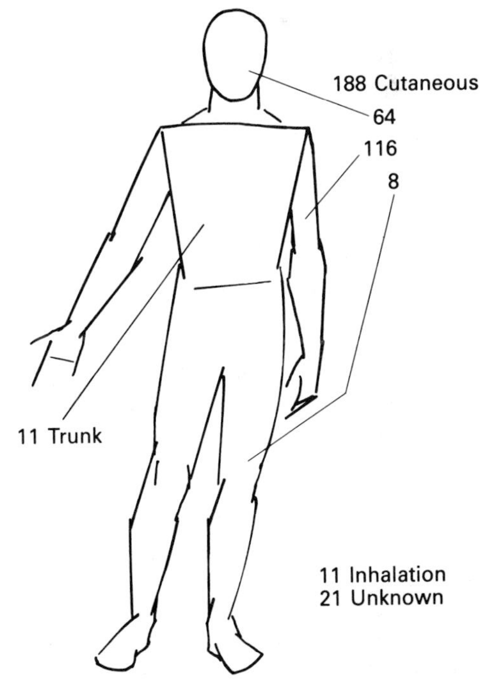

Malignant edema is the term used to describe cutaneous anthrax associated with significant local reactions such as multiple bullae, extensive edema, induration, and with systemic illness resulting from general toxemia.

Inhalation Anthrax

Inhalation anthrax has a biphasic clinical pattern; the initial stage begins after an incubation period of 1 to 5 days as a nonspecific illness, with malaise, fatigue, myalgia, mild fever, nonproductive cough, and infrequently, a sensation of precordial oppression. Rhonchi may be heard. The illness is frequently diagnosed as a respiratory infection. Within 2 to 4 days, symptoms may improve, but soon the second stage is heralded by the sudden development of severe respiratory distress, with dyspnea, cyanosis, stridor, and profuse diaphoresis. Subcutaneous edema of the chest and neck may develop. The pulse, respiratory rate, and temperature are elevated. There are moist, crepitant rales and possibly signs of a pleural effusion. Roentgenographic examination may disclose widening of the mediastinum. The leukocyte count may be moderately elevated. Death usually follows within 24 hours after onset of the acute phase; it is sometimes preceded by shock. Meningitis may be a complication.

Gastrointestinal Anthrax

Symptoms of gastrointestinal anthrax develop 2 to 5 days after the ingestion of contaminated meat; they consist of nausea, vomiting, anorexia, and fever. Progression of the disease is evidenced by abdominal pain, hematemesis, and in some cases, bloody diarrhea. The clinical course is similar to that seen in an acute surgical condition of the abdomen.The leukocyte count may be moderately elevated, with abnormal numbers of immature forms. The disease may progress to generalized toxemia, shock, cyanosis, and death.

Ingestion of contaminated meat has also caused a clinical picture characterized by fever, anorexia, and cervical lymphadenopathy or submandibular edema. Also, primary anthrax of the pharynx has been described and may possibly arise from ingestion of contaminated meat.

Meningeal Anthrax

Anthrax meningitis may complicate cutaneous, inhalation, or gastrointestinal anthrax, although it occurs in less than 5% of patients. In one report of 70 cases of anthrax meningitis, the primary focus of infection was the skin in 53% of cases, the lungs in 23%, and the intestine in 9%; no primary focus was identified in 12% of these cases. The onset of meningeal symptoms was noted simultaneously with the occurrence of the primary lesion or within several days. The symptoms are those of hemorrhagic meningitis; death occurs in 1 to 6 days. Meningeal encephalomyelitis and cortical hemorrhages have also been reported.

Diagnosis

Cutaneous anthrax should be considered whenever a painless, pruritic papule on an exposed part of the body progresses through a vesicular stage to become a black, depressed eschar, regardless of antimicrobial therapy. The recovery of *B. anthracis* from vesicular fluid or exudate from the ulcer confirms the diagnosis. Staphylococcal skin lesions, (Chap. 100, Staphylococcal Skin Infections), tularemia, (Chap. 139, Tularemia), plague (Chap. 140, Plague),milker's nodules (Chap. 92, Smallpox and Other Poxvirus Infections), and contagious pustular dermatitis (ecthyma contagiosum or orf) must be considered. The source of the anthrax bacilli should be identified if at all possible.

Most likely, it is a history of exposure to an aerosol containing *B. anthracis* that leads to the consideration of inhalation anthrax in the prodromal phase of mild illness. Identification of the microorganism in pleural fluid and evidence of mediastinal widening may aid in diagnosis. Anthrax in this early stage must be differentiated from such mild respiratory infections as influenza and bronchitis. The succeeding acute stage, which usually lasts 24 hours or less, resembles any disease in which shock and acute respiratory distress are seen.

Gastrointestinal anthrax is not clinically unique. A history of gastrointestinal symptoms following ingestion of inadequately cooked meat that may have been contaminated should alert the clinician.

A fourfold rise in titer (indirect hemagglutination) in paired serum specimens confirms the diagnosis of anthrax. In anthrax meningitis, *B. anthracis* has always been recovered from the cerebral spinal fluid.

Prognosis

Untreated *cutaneous anthrax* results in death in 10% to 20% of cases; with effective antimicrobial therapy, fewer than 1% of patients will die. Regardless of the kind or intensity of systemic antimicrobial therapy, cutaneous lesions progress through the classic changes. Adequate antimicrobial therapy, however, reduces local reactions, such as edema and erythema. A scar in proportion to the size of the cutaneous lesion remains.

Protective immunity appears to result, although there are reports of patients who have had two cutaneous infection, years apart. In none of these patients was there laboratory confirmation of both infections.

Inhalation anthrax is virtually always fatal, even with antibacterial therapy. *Gastrointestinal anthrax* is associated with a 25% to 50% fatality. The case–fatality ratio in cases of anthrax meningitis is also high, although nonfatal cases are occasionally reported.

Antibodies in serums from industrial workers and immunized persons have been detected with agar gel diffusion, complement fixation, and hemagglutination techniques. Because antibody increases have been found in employees of goat hair mills who have no history of anthrax, subclinical infections must occur. Persisting titers in immunized workers have been demonstrated.

Therapy

Cultures must be taken within 24 hours of starting treatment for anthrax because specific therapy may inhibit the recovery of *B. anthracis*. The drug of choice in cutaneous anthrax is penicillin. In mild disease, peroral treatment with potassium penicillin V is suitable (30 mg/kg body wt as four equal portions, given every 6 hours for 5–7 days). With extensive lesions or in systemic illness, intramuscular procaine penicillin (20 mg–25 mg [34,000–42,500 units]/kg body wt/day as two equal portions should be given every 12 hours for 5–7 days). Many other agents are also effective, including tetracycline (15 mg/kg body wt/day as four equal portions, given perorally every 6 hours for 5–7 days).

Excision of cutaneous lesions is not recommended because it may lead to an intensification of the symptoms and possibly to the spread of infection. The local application of ointments containing antimicrobics has no effect. The cutaneous lesions should be kept clean and covered; soiled dressings should be bagged (polyethylene) until incinerated. If hospitalized, the patient should be handled with secretion precautions. Glucosteroids (systemically) are said to reduce significantly the morbidity and mortality of severe cutaneous anthrax (malignant edema).

The therapy of inhalation anthrax is based on empirical knowledge and extrapolation from animal experiments. Massive doses of penicillin G by intravenous infection (50 mg[80,000 units]/kg body wt as a loading dose given in the first hour; with a maintenance dosage of 200 mg[320,000 units]/kg body wt/day) should be used. Streptomycin (7 mg–15 mg/kg body wt as a loading dose and 15 mg–30 mg/kg body wt/day as the maintenance dose, given intravenously to assure proper blood levels) may also be used. Specific antitoxin may be of value; however, there is no domestic source of this material at the present time. Supportive therapy should be given, for example, volume expanders and vasopressor agents to combat hypotension and oxygen for respiratory distress. With encroaching cervical edema, tracheal intubation should be carried out. If hospitalized, the patient should be placed in strict isolation.

In addition to fluid replacement and other supportive therapy, patients with gastrointestinal anthrax should be given penicillin by intravenous injection according to the regimen described for treating inhalation anthrax. Tetracycline has been reported to be effective in treating some cases; the recommended dosage is 1 g intravenously every 24 hours.

With anthrax meningitis, the regimen described for treating inhalation anthrax should be used in addition to supportive therapy.

Prevention

Individual awareness of the danger of potentially contaminated materials is the key to prevention of anthrax. Control programs should include (1) the education of employees in involved industries; (2) the effective and regular cleaning of equipment and work areas; (3) the decontamination of potentiallly contaminated raw materials, if possible and practical; and (4) adequate provision for hand washing, showering and storing clothing. Adequate health facilities should be available so that a physician or nurse can examine employees and immediately obtain cultures if lesions or illness consistent with anthrax is detected. Cuts and abrasions should be kept clean and covered. A cell-free anthrax vaccine suitable for use in humans is available, and it should be given to employees in high-risk industries. Unimmunized visitors should not be allowed in contaminated areas. Workers in dusty contaminated areas should be given respirators and urged to use them, but ways must be found to control the production of contaminated aerosols. All confirmed and highly probable cases of anthrax must be reported to local public health authorities.

Persons exposed to *B. anthracis* should be placed under surveillance for 7 days, the maximum expected incubation period of anthrax. Prophylactic antimicrobics are not indicated unless there is a history of ingestion of contaminated meat, or injection with virulent bacilli through the skin. In the former case, penicillin V, as recommended for cutaneous infections, should be given for 7 days; in the latter situation, intramuscular penicillin, as recommended for extensive cutaneous lesions, should be given for 7 days. In both situations, the patient should be placed under surveillance for 10 days.

Agricultural anthrax can be controlled by good animal husbandry, including vaccination in endemic areas and the proper disposal of carcasses. Contaminated feeds or fertilizers must not be used. The diagnosis should be confirmed in all animals suspected of having died of anthrax.

Bibliography

Books

BRACHMAN PS: Anthrax. In Evans AS, Feldman H (eds): Bacterial Infections of Humans: Epidemiology and Control. (In press)

BRACHMAN PA, FEELEY JC: Bacillus anthracis. In Blair JE, Lennette EH, Truant JP (eds): Manual of Clinical Microbiology. Bethesda, American Society for Microbiology, 1970. pp 106–111.

Journals

ALBRINK WS, BROOKS SM, BIRON RE, KOPEL M: Human inhalation anthrax: A report of three fatal cases. Am J Pathol 36:457–471, 1960

AMIDI S, DUTZ W, KOHOUT E, RONAGHY HA: Anthrax in Iran. Z Troppenmed Parasitol 24:250–255, 1973

BRACHMAN PS: Inhalation Anthrax. Ann NY Acad Sci 353:83–93, 1980

BRACHMAN PS, FEKETY FR: Industrial anthrax. Ann NY Acad Sci 70:574–584, 1958

BRACHMAN PS, GOLD H, PLOTKIN SA, FEKETY FR, WERRIN M, INGRAM NR: Field evaluation of a human anthrax vaccine. Am J Public Health 52:632–645, 1962

BRACHMAN PS, PLOTKIN SA, BUMFORD FH, ATCHISON MM: An epidemic of inhalation anthrax: The first in the Twentieth Century. II. Epidemiology. Am J Hyg 72:6–23, 1960

DUTZ W, KOHOUT E: Anthrax. Pathol Annu 6:209–248, 1971

GLASSMAN HN: World incidence of anthrax in man. Public Health 73:22–24, 1958

HAIGHT TH: Anthrax meningitis: Review of literature and report of two cases with autopsies. Am J Med Sci 224:57–69, 1952

LINCOLN RE, KLEIN F, WALKER JS, HAINES BW, JONES WI, MAHLANDT BG, FRIEDMAN RH: Successful treatment of rhesus monkeys for septicemic anthrax. Antimicrob Agents Chemother 4:759–763, 1964, 1965

NORMAN PS, RAY JG JR, BRACHMAN PS, PLOTKIN SA, PAGANO JS: Serologic testing for anthrax antibodies in workers in a goat hair processing mill. Am J Hyg 72:32–37, 1960

PLOTKIN SA, BRACHMAN PS, UTELL M, BUMFORD FH, ATCHISON MM: An epidemic of inhalation anthrax: The first in the Twentieth Century. Am J Med 29:992–1001, 1960

LOUIS LEVY

105

Leprosy

Leprosy is a disease that results from infection with *Mycobacterium leprae* in a small proportion of humans exposed and presumed to be infected with this microorganism. The disease is chronic, ordinarily progresses if untreated, and exhibits a broad spectrum of manifestations, ranging from the limited process in patients with a brisk response (tuberculoid leprosy) to the disseminated disease characteristic of patients with a minimal response (lepromatous leprosy). Although *M. leprae* has heretofore been considered pathogenic only for humans, a similar process associated with an organism that cannot be distinguished from *M. leprae* has recently been encountered among armadillos captured in Louisiana and contiguous portions of Mississippi and Texas.

Etiology

Mycobacterium leprae, the etiologic agent of leprosy, is an acid-fast bacillus (AFB). After fixation and staining by carefully standardized techniques, viable *M. leprae* stain both brightly and uniformly. Dead bacilli stain irregularly and usually predominate in material obtained from lesions, thus accounting for the frequent characterization of the organism as pleomorphic. In common with other mycobacteria, *M. leprae* fluoresce after treatment with phenolauramine O. Treatment with periodic acid caused the organism to stain more intensely with carbol fuchsin, whereas extraction with pyridine brings about loss of acid-fastness; both properties are probably characteristic of dead *M. leprae.* Leprosy bacilli have not been cultivated in cell-free mediums and have not been grown consistently in cell cultures. However, *M. leprae* appear to incorporate ^{3}H-thymidine and ^{3}H-dihydroxyphenylalanine when exposed to these substances in cultures of human peripheral blood monocytes or in short-term, cell-free cultures.

The optimal temperature for multiplication of *M. leprae* is lower than 37°C. This is consistent with the predilection of lesions to form on the cooler parts of the body, and with the results of experimental infection of rodents, for example, limited multiplication in the hind footpad of immunologically competent mice. Following the inoculation of 5000 organisms and a lag phase of indeterminate duration, *M. leprae* multiply to a maximum of 1 to 2 million bacilli in the course of 4 to 6 months, with a doubling time during logarithmic growth of 11 to 13 days (Fig. 105-1). Thereafter, the number of organisms changes very little, while the viable organisms are killed as the mouse mounts an effective cell-mediated immune response. Gross lesions of the infected footpad are never seen. The ability of immunosuppressed rodents (adult-thymectomized, lethally irradiated, and bone-marrow-reconstituted mice; neonatally thymectomized rats; congenitally athymic "nude" mice and rats) to limit multiplication of *M. leprae* is greatly impaired, and gross lesions occur regularly in experimentally infected nude mice. Experimental leprosy of the armadillo is now well established and has provided the immense numbers of organisms required for biochemical and immunologic studies and for the development of a vaccine.

Epidemiology

Although *M. leprae* was the first bacterial pathogen of humans to be recognized, progress in understanding the epidemiology of leprosy has been obstructed by the inability to cultivate the organism *in vitro* and by the tenacious doctrine that leprosy is feebly contagious and transmitted by prolonged, direct skin-to-skin contact. Patients with multibacillary (*i.e.,* lepromatous and near-lepromatous) leprosy are the most important sources of infection. The existence of healthy carriers has been claimed, but no evidence of their infectiousness has been produced. No non-

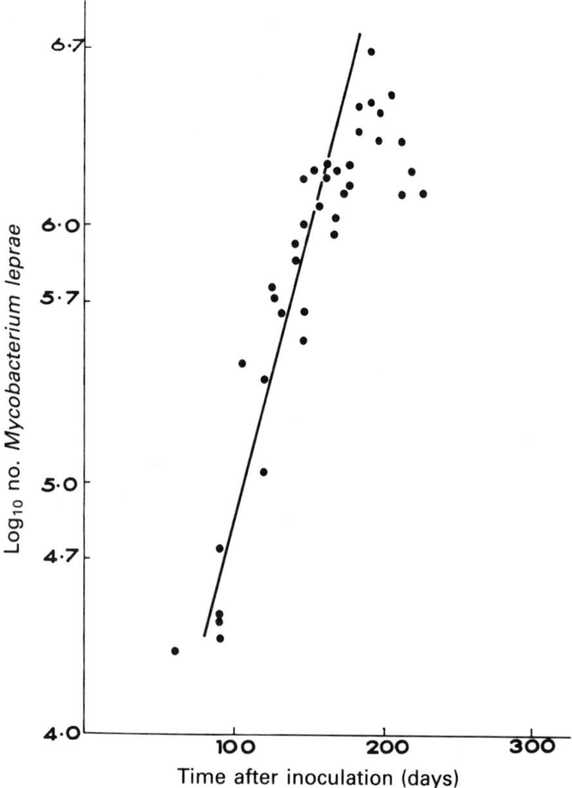

Fig. 105-1. Multiplication of *Mycobacterium leprae* in the mouse foot pad as a function of time after inoculation. Each point represents the harvest of *M. leprae* from a pool of four foot pads. The solid line, the straight line that best fits the experimental data and represents the phase of logarithmic multiplication, has a slope equivalent to a doubling time of 13 days.

human reservoir of infection is known; although *M. leprae* infection of feral armadillos has been demonstrated, no association between contact with armadillos and human leprosy has been shown.

According to World Health Association estimates, there are in the world more than 10 million patients with leprosy. The majority of these patients reside in Southeast Asia, India, sub-Saharan Africa, and Latin America (Fig. 105-2).

Untreated patients with lepromatous leprosy may have extensive involvement of the nasal mucous membranes with consequent shedding of large numbers of viable *M. leprae* in the sputum and in nasal secretions. Moreover, survival of leprosy bacilli outside the body for hours, if not days, has been demonstrated. In fact, there appears to be a close analogy between leprosy and tuberculosis in terms of both the numbers of organisms broadcast into the environment and the attack rates among household contacts. Thus, *M. leprae* is probably transmitted by the respiratory route.

The possibility of an arthropod vector has been suggested by the recovery of viable *M. leprae* from laboratory-reared mosquitos and bedbugs permitted to feed on untreated patients with lepromatous leprosy, but infection of humans by the bite of these arthropods has not been demonstrated.

Finally, there exist a few recorded cases of transmission by injection, that is, by presumably contaminated tattoo needles.

The inability to cultivate *M. leprae* has delayed the preparation of pure antigens, thus delaying the development of methods to detect subclinical leprosy and making it difficult to define a contact. Nevertheless, it appears that of those persons infected with *M. leprae,* relatively few develop disease.

The factors that determine who will exhibit clinical leprosy are not known. However, intercurrent viral infections may increase susceptibility to *M. leprae;* thus, an epidemic of leprosy occurred on the Pacific island of Nauru shortly after the conclusion of World War I, following pandemic influenza in which 30% of the islanders died. Currently, there is also considerable interest in the possibility that susceptibility to leprosy may be HLA-linked.

Pathogenesis and Pathology

Both histopathologically and clinically, the manifestations of leprosy appear to vary continuously from the tuberculoid to the lepromatous end (pole) of the spectrum (Table 105-1). Tests of delayed type hypersensitivity (DTH) and cell-mediated immunity *in vitro* demonstrate a continuous decrease of reactivity from the tuberculoid toward the lepromatous pole of the spectrum. Patients with lepromatous and near-lepromatous leprosy regularly exhibit deficient DTH reactions to the antigens of *M. leprae,* whereas their reactions to other thymus-dependent antigens may or may not be deficient. During prolonged treatment, reactivity to antigens other than those of *M. leprae* is often recovered, whereas reactivity to the antigens of *M. leprae* is not. On the other hand, the concentrations of antibodies, both specific and nonspecific, increase toward the lepromatous pole, and in general humoral immunity appears to be uncompromised.

There is little evidence that the macrophages of patients with lepromatous leprosy are intrinsically defective. The numbers of T cells reactive to *M. leprae* in the blood are profoundly suppressed in lepromatous leprosy through mechanisms that remain ob-

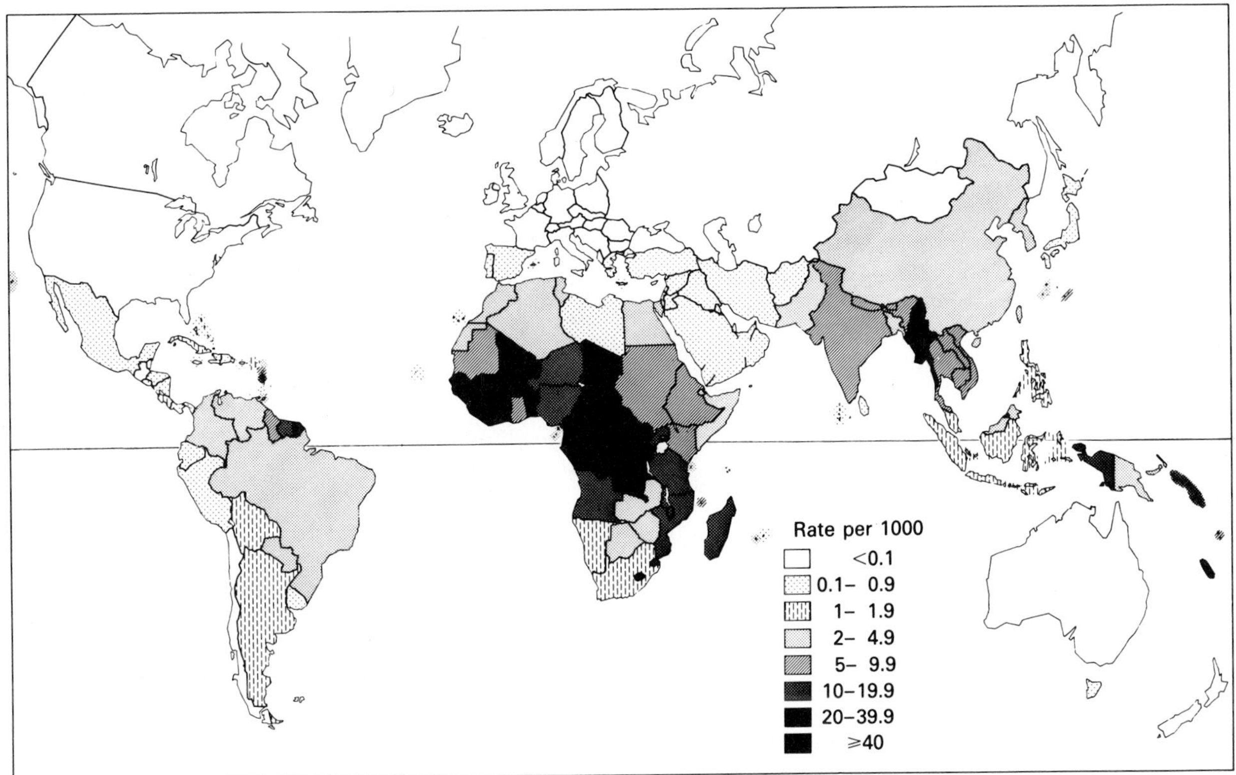

Fig. 105-2. Distribution of leprosy in the world (rate of estimated cases). (After Bechelli LM, Martinez Dominguez: Bull WHO 34:811, 1966)

Table 105-1. Histopathologic Features of Leprosy According to the Ridley-Jopling Classification

	Class*					
Feature	TT	BT	BB	BL	LLs	LLp
Epithelioid Cells	++	++	++	±	0	0
Nonvacuolated giant cells	0−++	±	0	0	0	0
Histiocytes or foamy macrophages	0	0	0	++	++	++
Small vesicles	0	0	0	0−++	0−++	0−++
Vacuolated giant cells	0	0	0	0	0−++	±
Giant vacuoles	0	0	0	0	0−+	0−++
Lymphocytes	+−++	0−++	±	+−++	±	±
Dermal nerve (maximal diameter in μm)	1000	400	250	200	200	80
Onion-skin perineurium	0	±	±	0−++	0−++	0
Clear subepidermal zone	±	0−++	++	++	++	++
Erosion of epidermis	0−++	±	0	0	0	0
Acid-fast bacilli in granuloma†	0−1	0−2	3−4	4−5	5−6	5−6

*TT = polar tuberculoid; BT = borderline tuberculoid; BB = borderline; BL = borderline lepromatous; LLs = subpolar lepromatous; LLp = polar lepromatous.

†Bacteriologic Index, Ridley DS: In Cochrane RG, Davey TF (eds): Leprosy in Theory and Practice. Baltimore, Williams & Wilkins, 1964. pp 620–622.

(After Ridley DS: Bull WHO 51:451–465, 1974)

scure; either they are not produced or they are selectively retained in lymphoid tissues. Moreover, circulating suppressor cells—both macrophages and T cells—have been recognized in patients with lepromatous and borderline leprosy.

Additional aspects of the pathogenesis of leprosy include the possibility of genetic factors in the host, environmental factors favoring transmission, the relatively low temperature optimal for the growth of *M. leprae,* and the unique predilection for localization of *M. leprae* in peripheral nerves. Totally unexplained are the long incubation period and the varied distribution of patients in the clinical spectrum of leprosy. Among Americans exposed to leprosy during military service in endemic areas, the average interval between overseas service and clinical onset varied from 2 to 5 years for tuberculoid and 9 to 12 years for lepromatous leprosy. The proportion of patients with the lepromatous form of the disease has been found to range from 3 per 100 in Nigeria to 10 times that ratio in the Philippines.

The earliest lesions—those of indeterminate leprosy—are characterized by lymphocytic and histiocytic infiltrations around skin appendages, dermal nerves, and blood vessels; proliferation of Schwann cells; and the presence of AFB in dermal nerves, erector pili muscles, or the subepidermal zone. With the passage of time, the indeterminate lesions regress spontaneously, remain unchanges, or evolve into lesions typical of the tuberculoid, borderline, or lepromatous forms of the disease. The salient histopathologic features of the major forms of leprosy are summarized in Table 105-1. The number of *M. leprae* present in the patient varies across the spectrum—sparse in tuberculoid and innumerable in lepromatous leprosy. In the latter form, continuous bacteremia has been demonstrated with as many as 10^4 bacilli per ml peripheral venous blood. Leprosy bacilli may be found in every organ, including the dental pulp, but excluding the central nervous system.

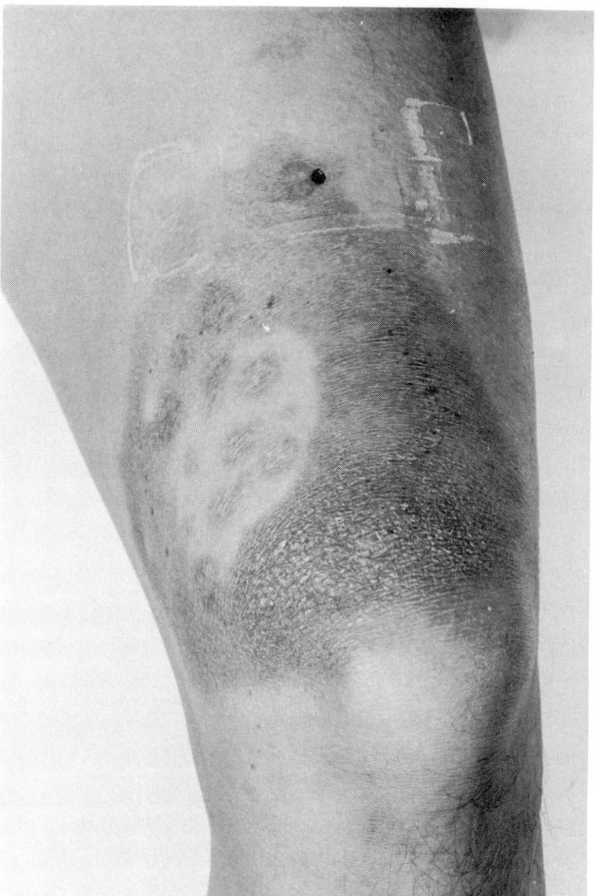

Fig. 105-3. Tuberculoid leprosy. This sharply marginated erythematous lesion surrounds a slightly eccentric area of central clearing. Within the clear zone are scars from moxibustion (a traditional Asian folk remedy). The punch biopsy scar at the top of the lesion indicates the proper site (just within the advancing margin) for obtaining biopsies of suspected tuberculoid lesions.

Manifestations

Indeterminate Leprosy

The earliest clinical manifestation of leprosy is one or more ill-defined, hypopigmented macules that are characteristically hypesthetic. Although these lesions may be recognized readily in areas in which leprosy is endemic, the disease may not be suspected in a nonendemic area, unless the physician is alerted by a history of contact. The histopathologic features of such macules are not diagnostic, unless involvement of dermal nerves or the presence of AFB (typically only a few) can be demonstrated.

Tuberculoid Leprosy

The sparse lesions of polar tuberculoid leprosy are macular or raised and usually display loss of pigmentation, sweating, and tactile sensation. A dermal nerve may be palpable near the lesion, and characteristically there is tender induration of a major peripheral nerve serving the area of the lesion. A typical lesion is shown in Figure 105-3. The lesions of borderline tuberculoid leprosy resemble those of the polar tuberculoid form, but are usually multiple and smaller. Enlarged cutaneous sensory nerves are less commonly found, but enlargement of major peripheral nerves is common.

Borderline (Dimorphous) Leprosy

The lesions of borderline leprosy differ from those of tuberculoid disease in that they are more numerous, symmetrically distributed, and erythematous or hypopigmented. The characteristic borderline lesion is circular, with a raised, fairly well-defined erythematous margin and an atrophic, hypesthetic center. Enlargement of peripheral nerve trunks may be widespread.

Lepromatous Leprosy

The skin lesions of lepromatous leprosy are numerous and symmetric, consisting of small hypopigmented macules or erythematous papules. Nodules develop later in the course of the disease, and even later, the skin becomes diffusely infiltrated and thickened. Characteristic late lesions include enlarged, sometimes pendulous, ear lobes; thinned eyebrows, eyelashes, facial and body hair; and destruction of the nasal cartilages with obstruction of the nasal passages and typical deformity of the nose (Fig. 105-4). Nerve damage is diffuse and symmetric, and involves dermal nerves and nerve endings more than major nerve trunks. The features typical of advanced lepromatous leprosy are summarized in Table 105-2.

Fig. 105-4. Lepromatous leprosy. Diffuse bacillary infiltration of the skin has coarsened this patient's features. Loss of eyebrows and massive enlargement of the ears are especially apparent.

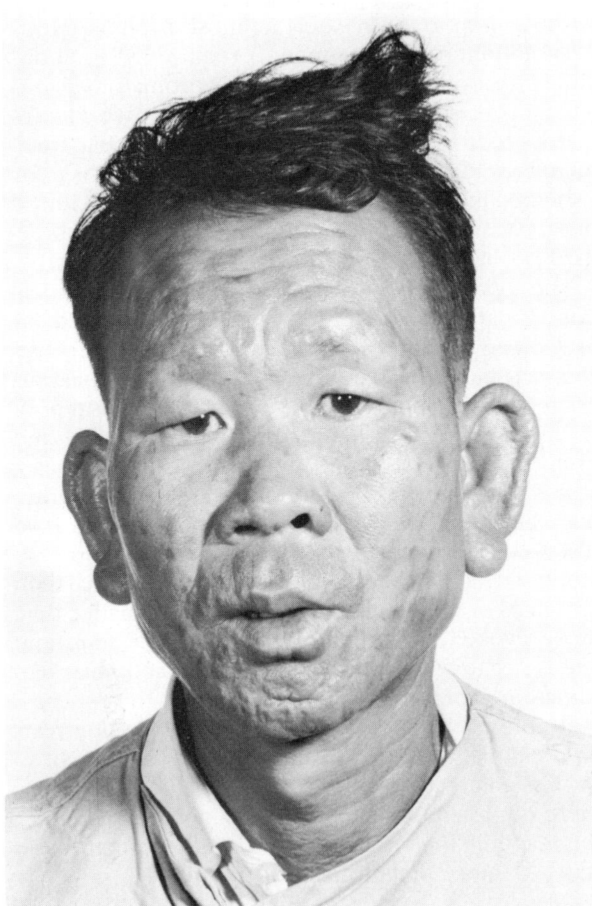

Reactions

The course of leprosy may be punctuated from time to time by reactions—bouts of relatively acute inflammation in lesions that are not associated wth secondary infection or trauma.

BORDERLINE (REVERSAL) REACTIONS

Borderline reactions are characterized by intracutaneous hyperemia, edema, and infiltration occurring in old or new lesions; they are sometimes accompanied by severe neuritis. These reactions typically occur during treatment in patients with forms of leprosy that are neither polar tuberculoid nor lepromatous. They are also termed reversal reactions, reflecting association with some recovery of cell-mediated immune responses, that is, a shift from a position nearer the lepromatous pole to one nearer the tuberculoid pole.

ERYTHEMA NODOSUM LEPROSUM

Erythema nodosum leprosum (ENL) occurs only in patients with multibacillary leprosy, especially early in the course of effective antimicrobial treatment, and appears to be a consequence of killing *M. leprae.* The name derives from the commonest manifestations, namely, painful, erythematous, subcutaneous nodules. The appearance of the nodules is frequently associated with fever, and sometimes with neuritis, orchitis, iridocyclitis, arthritis, lymphadenopathy, or proteinuria. The histopathology is very similar to that of an Arthus reaction. Deposits of immunoglobins and complement have been described, and circulating immune complexes have been found in a large proportion of patients with ENL. Patients with recurrent ENL appear to be particularly prone to develop glomerulonephritis and secondary amyloidosis.

Peripheral Nerves

Damage to peripheral nerves that leads to loss of sensation, deformity, and mutilation is characteristic of leprosy. The patterns of damage vary across the

Table 105-2. *Clinical Features of Advanced Lepromatous Leprosy*

Site	Symptoms
Skin	Symmetrically distributed macules, papules, plaques, and nodules (lepromas); loss of eyebrows (especially outer third) and eyelashes; rarely, loss of scalp hair; leonine facies (accentuation of features by infiltration and nodules); thickened pendulous ears; spider telangiectases; edema of extremities (invasion of lymphatics)
Eyes	Conjunctival and episcleral nodules; beading of corneal nerves; superficial punctate keratitis, interstitial keratitis with pannus formation; chronic plastic iridocyclitis
Upper respiratory mucous membranes	Nasal stuffiness, coryza, epistaxis (infiltration of mucous membrane); ulcers of uvula and tonsils, loss of teeth (oropharyngeal infiltration); septal perforation, nasal collapse (destruction of cartilaginous septum), hoarseness, stridor, asphyxia (laryngeal infiltration)
Other organs/systems	Hepatomegaly, splenomegaly, lymphadenopathy, testicular invasion and destruction, gynecomastia, cystic bone changes in the distal phalanges, and skeletal muscle invasion. Kidneys are spared in the absence of immune complex nephritis or amyloidosis.
Serum	Hypergammaglobulinemia (polyclonal), elevated immunoglobulins (especially IgG), biologic false-positive serologic tests for syphilis, antithyroglobulin antibody, rheumatoid factor, positive LE cell preparations, cryoglobulinemia.

spectrum of leprosy. Toward the tuberculoid pole, the process is usually asymmetrically distributed in superficial portions of one or more major nerves (Table 105-3). Toward the lepromatous pole, the process is usually more diffuse and symmetric, involving smaller ramifications of sensory nerves and the sensory endings themselves.

Diagnosis

The diagnosis of leprosy rests on the demonstration of *M. leprae* in association with characteristic histopathologic changes; it is established by histopathologic examination of tissue obtained by biopsy of a lesion. The biopsy specimen should include all of the layers of the skin. If properly prepared sections are stained with a carefully standardized, room temperature, acid-fast stain, AFB will be found. The number of bacilli may be very small in polar tuberculoid and indeterminate forms of the disease, requiring intensive search of many sections. Observing histopathology that is in any way suggestive of leprosy should lead to the preparation of sections stained for AFB. The diagnosis of leprosy should never be excluded *a priori* because of the absence of a history of contact.

Prognosis

Indeterminate leprosy probably heals spontaneously without important residua in most patients. However, antimicrobial treatment is required to limit disability in both tuberculoid and lepromatous forms and to reverse infectiousness in patients with lepromatous leprosy. Because effective antimicrobial treatment is available, reversal of communicability is to be expected in virtually all patients, and arrest of clinical progression is possible in the majority of patients regardless of the form of leprosy.

The lepromin skin test is useful for the classification of patients in the spectrum of leprosy and for prognosis; *it is not a diagnostic test.* Because lepromin is an autoclaved homogenate of lepromatous tissue that is standardized according to its content of *M. leprae,* it contains antigens from *M. leprae* and from the host–histocompatibility antigens. The reaction is usually read after 3 or 4 weeks; a papule larger than 3 mm in diameter is considered to be a positive reaction. Most normal adults react to lepromin. Moreover, a "lepromin" prepared from normal skin provokes reactions that are similar but smaller than those evoked by standard lepromin. The lepromin test is negative with near-lepromatous and polar lepromatous leprosy, and positive toward the tuberculoid pole of the spectrum. Its prognostic value rests on the belief that indeterminate leprosy is thought to be less likely to evolve to lepromatous leprosy if there is a reaction to lepromin. Generally, the larger the reaction, the closer the patient is to a tuberculoid state—a more benign form of the disease.

Table 105-3. *Sites of Peripheral Nerve Enlargement and Damage in Leprosy in Approximate Descending Order of Frequency**

Nerve	Site of Enlargement	Major Sequelae
Ulnar	Elbow and several inches above	Clawing of 4th and 5th fingers, wasting of intrinsic hand musculature
Posterior tibial	Between medial malleolus and heel	Clawing of toes, plantar anesthesia
Superficial peroneal	Winding around neck of fibula	Foot drop
Greater auricular	Crossing sternocleidomastoid muscle in neck	Cosmetic importance only
Median	Antecubital fossa or just proximal to carpal tunnel in wrist	Thenar wasting, loss of apposibility of thumb, palmar anesthesia
Radial	Winding around radius at wrist	Wrist drop (unusual)
Facial	Crossing zygoma or near stylomastoid foramen	Relatively selective damage to temporal and zygomatic branches, resulting in inability to close the eye (lagophthalmos)
Trigeminal	Emerging from respective foramina	Anesthesia of face, cornea, and conjunctiva
Supraorbital	Above the eyes	Cosmetic importance only

*Early manifestations of leprosy may include local paresthesias or dysesthesias. Anesthesia to heat and cold are lost before other modalities. Late sequelae of nerve damage include vasomotor and trophic changes, infection and ulceration of anesthetic parts, pyogenic osteomyelitis, muscle wasting, and resorption of soft tissue and bone.

Therapy

Antimicrobial Therapy

Specific antimicrobial therapy for leprosy was introduced in 1941 when glucosulfone (Promin) was first given at the U.S. Public Health Service Hospital in Carville, Louisiana. Subsequently, the modern therapy of leprosy evolved through three well-defined phases.

The first phase lasted two decades and was devoted to measuring the efficacy of treatment with dapsone (4,4′-diaminodiphenylsulfone, DDS) and related drugs, the sulfones. Response was assessed in lepromatous leprosy by registering the clinical status and the number of AFB in scrapings of lesions. Because these were indirect measures of effectiveness, the early clinical trials required the observation of large numbers of patients for long periods.

The second phase (1960–1975) was occupied largely by evaluation of the antileprosy activity of a number of drugs administered individually, using the technique of cultivation of *M. leprae* in the footpads of normal mice. This method permitted at least qualitative assessment of a drug during a few months of clinical trial. The efficacy of several drugs, including dapsone, clofazimine, diacetyldapsone, ethionamide, and prothionamide was demonstrated. However, the footpads of normal mice are a relatively insensitive culture medium. For example, before treatment, a patient with lepromatous leprosy might well carry 10^{11} *M. leprae* of which 10^{10} were viable by morphologic criteria; after 3 months of treatment with dapsone, there would be a loss of infectivity for normal mice, although more than 10^7 (but $<10^8$) viable *M. leprae* could still be present in the patient (Table 105-4). By using immunosuppressed mice, the threshold for detecting viable *M. leprae* is reduced to about 1 in 10^5 organisms; as a result, the persistence of viable, fully drug-susceptible *M. leprae* was demonstrated in the tissues of patients after treatment with dapsone for 10 years, diacetyldapsone for 4 or 5 years, rifampin for 2 years, and dapsone plus rifampin for 6 months.

In addition, relapse of lepromatous leprosy associated with the emergence of dapsone-resistant strains of *M. leprae* was observed, and the development of lepromatous leprosy in patients originally infected with dapsone-resistant *M. leprae* was documented. Also, relapses with rifampin-resistant strains were reported. Thus, it has become clear that monotherapy of multibacillary leprosy with dapsone, or with any other single drug, is not adequate. On the other hand, it appears sufficient to treat patients with paucibacillary leprosy with dapsone monotherapy for two years beyond the time of apparent clinical resolution of lesions; however, there may be combined drug regimens that permit considerable shortening of the duration of therapy.

The third, current phase of antimicrobial therapy is aimed at the development of practical, combined-

Table 105-4. *Course of Events in a Typical Patient With Lepromatous Leprosy Who Responded to Treatment With Dapsone*

	Findings			Interpretation	
Period of Treatment (Months)	BI*	MI† (%)	MOUSE INOCULATION	TOTAL *MICOBACTERIUM LEPRAE*	VIABLE *MICOBACTERIUM LEPRAE*
0	4+	10	positive	10^{11}	10^{10}
1	4+	1	positive	10^{11}	10^{9}
2	4+	<1	positive	10^{11}	10^{8}
3	4+	<1	negative	10^{11}	$<10^{8}$
12	3+	<1	negative	10^{10}	$<10^{7}$
24	2+	<1	negative	10^{9}	$<10^{6}$

*Bacteriologic index
†Morphologic index—% brightly and solidly stained

drug regimens of finite duration that prevent relapse of multibacillary leprosy with either drug-resistant *M. leprae* during therapy, or with drug-susceptible or drug-resistant organisms after cessation of therapy. This evolution in therapy is essential to the control of leprosy in leprosy-endemic regions, a goal is based logically on suppression of the infectiousness of source (multibacillary) cases. Perhaps the most interesting regimen, one that can be almost fully supervised, is dapsone, self-administered in an oral dose of 100 mg daily, plus diacetyldapsone, 225 mg administered intramuscularly every 2 months, plus rifampin, 600 mg orally on each of 2 consecutive days per month (at least the first dose to be administered under supervision), plus clofazimine, also administered orally in a dose of 600 mg on each of 2 consecutive days monthly (at least the first dose supervised). This regimen includes three bactericidal drugs and appears to be both safe and reasonably cheap; it should be effective and should prevent relapse with drug-resistant bacilli.

This same regimen should also be useful for the treatment of patients with multibacillary leprosy in nonendemic regions. However, clofazimine may be less well accepted in the nonendemic situation because of the pigmentation that accompanies its use. Because the toxic potential of ethionamide (or its equivalent, prothionamide) might be more readily managed, either ethionamide or prothionamide, administered orally in a daily dosage of 500 mg, could be substituted for clofazimine.

A similar, two-drug regimen (two-drug, because diacetyldapsone slowly releases dapsone) has also been recommended: rifampin, 600 mg, and dapsone, 100 mg each administered by mouth, daily, for an initial 1- or 2-week period, accompanied by an initial intramuscular injection of 225 mg of diacetyldapsone; this is followed by rifampin, 600 mg perorally and diacetyldapsone, 225 mg intramuscularly, each administered once monthly under supervision, together with self-administered oral dapsone in a 100 mg daily dose.

Management of Reactions

Severe borderline (reversal) reactions require aggressive treatment with glucosteroids to minimize important and permanent nerve damage. Less severe borderline reactions are best treated symptomatically.

ENL responds dramatically to the administration of thalidomide in an oral dose of 100 mg to 400 mg daily, and is held in abeyance by maintenance therapy with 50 mg to 100 mg/day. The mechanism of this action of thalidomide has not been elucidated. In fertile female patients, two alternatives exist: (1) clofazimine, 100 mg–300 mg/day, and (2) glucosteroids, such as, prednisone, 15 mg–25 mg/day. Mild ENL may be treated symptomatically using either trivalent antimonials (traditional, but of doubtful value) or antimalarials (apparently not of value).

Prevention

Leprosy is best prevented by blocking transmission of *M. leprae* in the community. In a very few leprosy control programs, the incidence and prevalence of leprosy appear to have been reduced with long-term application of dapsone monotherapy of source cases coupled with aggressive case-finding; however, the overall picture is one of failure. The failures appear to occur because patients do not take their medication regularly. Dapsone monotherapy is not curative, and maintenance of suppression by lifelong treatment is an impossible burden.

Leprosy may also be prevented by prophylactic antimicrobial therapy. Logically, only the subclinically infected should be treated; however, they cannot yet be identified. Community-wide prophylactic treatment is preventive of leprosy as was shown by administering diacetyldapsone (225 mg intramuscularly every 11 weeks) to all members of the community for 3 years.

Isolation of patients presumed to be infectious appears to be illogical as a preventive measure. Most contacts have probably already been infected by the time the patient comes to diagnosis and treatment. Also, effective chemotherapy promptly renders the patient noninfectious.

There is no vaccine for the prevention of leprosy.

Remaining Problems

Efforts to develop a vaccine from heat-killed *M. leprae* harvested from experimentally infected armadillos offer great promise.

Work is also going forward on the development of means to detect subclinical infections with *M. leprae*. Preparation of an antigen specific for *M. leprae* is key to candidate procedures: two serologic methods, and one lymphocyte transformation method.

The cultivation of *M. leprae in vitro* still appears to be an elusive goal.

Bibliography

Books

COCHRANE RG, DAVEY TF (EDS): Leprosy in Theory and Practice, 2nd ed. Baltimore, Williams & Wilkins, 1964. 659 pp.

GODAL T, LEVY L: *Mycobacterium leprae*. In Kubica GP, Wayne LG (eds): Mycobacteria: A Source Book. New York, Marcel Dekker. (in press)

TURK JL, WATERS MFR: Leprosy. In Samter M (ed): Immunological Diseases, 3rd ed. Boston, Little, Brown, 1978. pp 627–638.

WORLD HEALTH ORGANIZATION: Fifth report of the Expert Committee on Leprosy. WHO Tech Rep Series 607, 1977. 48 pp.

Journals

COMMITTEE ON EXPERIMENTAL CHEMOTHERAPY: Experimental chemotherapy in leprosy. Bull WHO 53:425–433, 1976

ELLARD GA: Combined treatment for lepromatous leprosy. Lepr Rev 51:199–205, 1980

GODAL T: Immunological aspects of leprosy-present status. Prog Allergy 25:211–242, 1978

REES RJW: Enhanced susceptibility of thymectomized and irradiated mice to infection with *Mycobacterium leprae*. Nature (London) 211:657–658, 1966

RUSSEL DA, WORTH RM, JANO B, FASAL P, SHEPARD CC: Acedapsone in the prevention of leprosy: Field trial in three high prevalence villages in Micronesia. Am J Trop Med Hyg 28:559–563, 1979

SHEPARD CC: The experimental disease that follows the injection of human leprosy bacilli into foot-pads of mice. J Exp Med 112:445–454, 1960

SHEPARD CC, MCRAE DH: A method for counting acid-fast bacteria. Int J Lepr 36:224–227, 1968

D. JOSEPH DEMIS
PAUL D. HOEPRICH

106 *Nonsyphilitic Treponematoses*

Yaws, pinta, and bejel are known as the nonsyphilitic treponematoses. They are discussed in this chapter, whereas the fourth treponemal disease of humans, syphilis, is the subject of Chapter 59. All four are communicable diseases for which humans are at once reservoirs, vectors, and hosts. They are caused by treponemes that cannot be distinguished morphologically or immunologically, and it has been suggested there is but one species pathogenic for humans, namely *Treponema pallidum.* According to this view, environmental factors such as geographic isolation and prevalent temperature and humidity are the basic determinants of the geographic regionalism and the clinical features that differentiate the treponematoses of humans.

However, the nonsyphilitic treponematoses are (1) nonvenereal; (2) usually transmitted before puberty; (3) seen primarily in subtropical or tropical areas, afflicting primitive, isolated, and economically underdeveloped peoples (Fig. 106-1); (4) rare causes of disease involving internal organs; (5) generally nonfatal, but debilitating, often causing social ostracism; and (6) rapidly diminishing in incidence under the impact of penicillin and soap. These epidemiologic and pathologic differences can be accommodated by naming variants: *T. pallidum* var. *pallidum* (the cause of syphilis and bejel), *T. pallidum* var. *pertenue* (the cause of yaws), and *T. pallidum* var. *carateum* (the cause of pinta).

Yaws

Yaws (also known as frambesia, pian, buba, and bouba) is an ancient disease thought to have arisen in the Afro-Asian land mass in approximately 10,000 B.C., presumably as a mutant of pinta. The disease apparently was carried to the Caribbean and the Americas by African slaves in the 16th century, and in this hemisphere it has remained largely restricted to populations of African heritage.

Etiology

The causal organism, *T. pallidum* var. *pertenue,* is 8 µm to 16 µm long × 0.2 µm wide and has some 8 to 16 regular spirals. Only a handful of experts can differentiate this microorganism from the nonpathogenic treponemes, particularly those found in the mouth (*e.g., T. microdentium*). In tissue preparations; they are best seen with silver staining, but identification can be made with relative certainty only by an expert.

Treponema pallidum var. *pertenue* has not been cultivated in nonliving mediums. However, it readily infects laboratory animals, including monkeys, rabbits, and hamsters, and it causes subclinical infections in others, including rats, mice, and guinea pigs. The replication time is apparently 30 to 33 hours.

Survival of *T. pallidum* var. *pertenue* outside the body is quite brief, although virulence is retained for years when stored at −70°C. Susceptibility to penicillin G, erythromycin, and other antimicrobics is marked.

Epidemiology

Yaws is a disease of rural populations. Formerly, in many tropical countries, incidence of active disease of more than 10% was not uncommon in certain populations, and positive serologic tests for syphilis resulting from yaws were found in more than 80% of the adult population. In general, for every patient with active yaws there were 2 to 5 infected persons in the latent stage with no visible lesions. In children and young adolescents with yaws, many with latent infection relapse to produce infectious lesions.

From 1900 to 1925, yaws was most prevalent in Africa, although recession had already begun elsewhere. Improvements in the standard of living greatly reduced the transmission and prevalence of early yaws and the prevalence and destructiveness of the late lesions. Thus, recession of the disease had begun in many countries before mass treatment with penicillin. As with other drugs in other infectious dis-

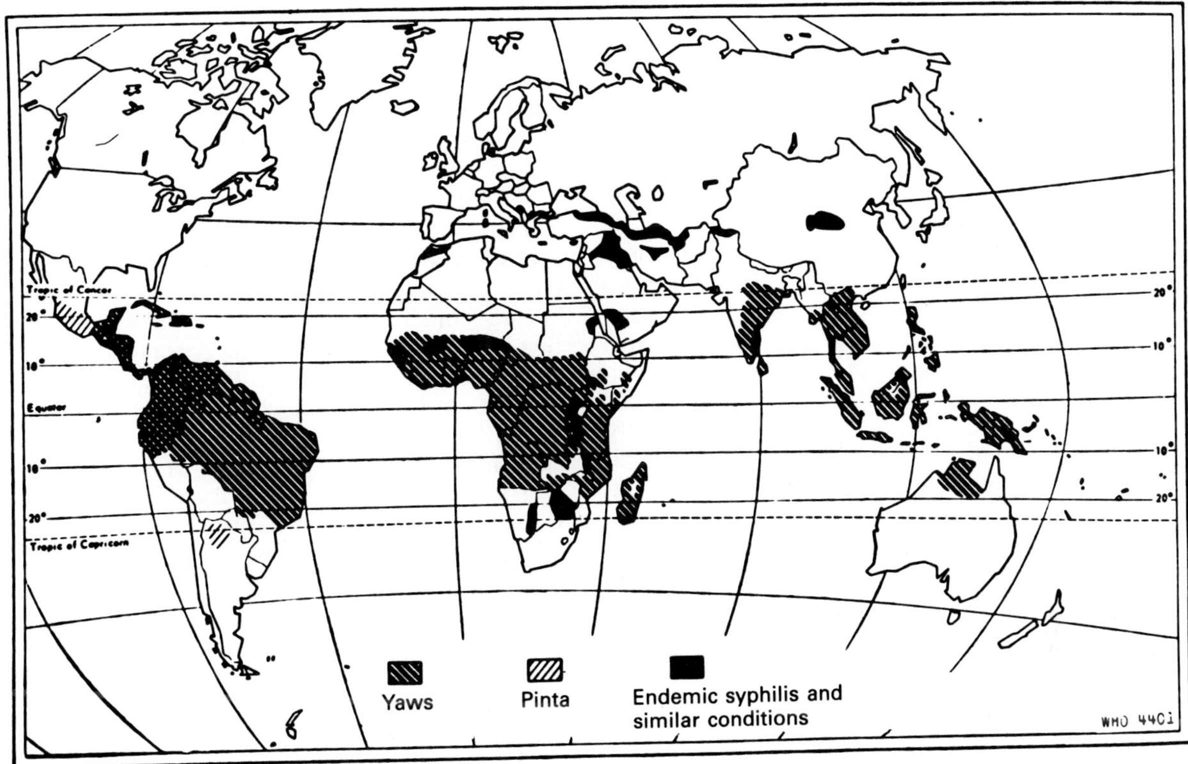

Fig. 106-1. Distribution of the nonsyphilitic (nonvenereal) treponematoses. (Guthe T: Acta Derm-Venereol 49:343–368, 1969)

eases (*e.g.,* antituberculosis drugs), penicillin greatly hastened an already apparent trend.

Beginning in the early 1950's, a number of mass treatment and eradication campaigns were carried out. Before these campaigns, infectious yaws in children and destructive lesions in adults were common in areas where careful surveys subsequently failed to reveal any active lesions. Unfortunately, there was a resurgence of yaws and bejel in West Africa in the 1970s; the application of penicillin by mobile teams in the early 1980s appeared to interrupt the increasing prevalence.

In South America, yaws has a curious distribution. In addition to being limited to the tropical countries, it is found almost exclusively on the coasts because of its limitation to persons of African ancestry. In India, its limited distribution can be attributed to certain previously isolated aboriginal tribes.

Yaws affects both sexes equally. Rural populations of warm, humid districts of developing countries are attacked. It is widely agreed that yaws is not transmitted by sexual contact, nor do cases of congenital yaws occur, presumably because infection occurs so long before sexual maturity that during pregnancy the patient is no longer infectious. There is little reason to suspect that contact with inanimate objects plays a role in the transmission of the disease, and there is no convincing evidence of nonhuman vectors or reservoirs.

The infection is usually contracted beginning at the age of 2 or 3 years, and by age 15 most of the population of endemic areas has been infected. Susceptible children are presumed to be infected by contact with children from other households rather than their own siblings, because their older siblings have latent, noninfectious lesions.

Pathogenesis and Pathology

Most early lesions of yaws occur on the exposed areas and are particularly prevalent below the knee. Trauma may be important if it causes a break in the skin. Presumably, treponemes are then introduced by direct contact because the early lesions usually teem with treponemes. Soon after infection, *T. pallidum* var. *pertenue* enters the bloodstream and is distributed to all tissues.

The pathology of yaws has not been adequately documented. However, it is apparent that the early skin lesions show epithelial hyperplasia with edema of the upper corium and a nonspecific exudation of inflammatory cells. Many treponemes are present in the epidermis and upper corium. There is little destruction, and these lesions usually heal with minimal scarring. The skin lesions of late yaws contain few treponemes. They bear a close similarity to the lesions of venereal syphilis, and histologic differentiation is usually not possible. Vascular changes, particularly the endarteritis that often characterizes venereal syphilis, is minimal or lacking in late yaws; otherwise, differentiating features are minimal. The bone lesions of late yaws include hypertrophic periostitis, gummatous periostitis, osteitis, and osteomyelitis with nodular or even general involvement of the bones of the limbs, hands, feet, and occasionally, calvarium. Destructive ulceration of the nose and mouth (gangosa or rhinopharyngitis mutilans) occurs in all populations in which yaws is highly endemic, and it may result in extensive destruction of the nose and palate. Amazingly prominent juxta articular nodules, which in reality are fibrous nodes, may occur over bony prominences. Enlargement of the prepatellar bursa and ganglion of the tendon sheath may also occur.

Manifestations

Yaws appears to attack only skin and bones.

EARLY STAGE

The early stage of yaws extends 4 to 5 years after infection, and it is characterized by multiple, nondestructive lesions. Initial lesions, as they occur in about 80% of patients, are large papillomas of the exposed skin (Fig. 106-2). They are especially likely to occur on the leg below the knee or on the foot. The lesion is elevated and somewhat warty across the surface, generally measures 2 cm to 5 cm in diameter, and usually heals spontaneously after several months, generally with depigmentation but only mild scarring. Such a lesion may be thought of as analogous to the chancre of venereal syphilis.

Some weeks or months after the appearance of the initial lesion, a general eruption is usually noted (Fig. 106-3). The primary lesion may or may not have healed. These secondary lesions generally are widely dispersed small papules, usually associated with extensive lymphadenopathy and occasionally with some malaise. Most of the papules disappear spontaneously; others develop into papillomas that are usually described as characteristic of yaws. There may be only a few large papillomas or there may be hundreds, each measuring up to 1 cm in diameter. These papillomatous lesions are circular, with a raised, granular surface. They are reddish yellow and frequently exude a clear yellowish serum. In time, a black scab tends to form, and after a few months, the general eruption heals with little or no scarring. Many patients complain of bone pain at this time. Pain is usually most prominent in the long bones, especially of the lower extremities, and it may be associated with roentgenographic evidence of periostitis.

Without treatment, several relapses of the early lesions may occur. In general, with each relapse there are fewer lesions, but there is a tendency for the palms and soles to be involved eventually.

Early bone lesions are frequent and include periostitis, osteitis, and osteomyelitis, particularly involving the shafts of the long bones. These are usually painful but not destructive; on healing there is little bony alteration. Polydactylitis (Fig. 106-4) is a frequent and often characteristic finding, as is bilateral swelling of the frontal processes of the maxilla (goundou). Goundou has at times been observed in as many as 15% of African patients, but it has almost never been seen on other continents.

LATE STAGE

After an asymptomatic period of 3 or more years, the late stage of yaws is usually heralded by papillomatous lesions on the hands and feet (Fig. 106-5). The late lesions are characteristically destructive and solitary, and they are most frequently observed in older adolescents and adults. They have occasionally been reported in children as young as 10 years. Without therapy, they may disappear and reappear, but at longer intervals than those between appearances of the early lesions.

Plantar and palmar hyperkeratoses, often with painful fissures (crab yaws), are the most common late lesions and are the last to occur (Fig. 106-6). The cutaneous papillomas tend to break down, yielding either small and superficial or deep extensive ulcers. Subcutaneous nodules also tend to ulcerate. Healing leads to depigmentation. Scarring is almost invariable, and it may lead to contractures that limit motion.

The late bone lesions include gummatous periostitis, hypertrophic periostitis, osteitis, and osteomyelitis. These are often associated with nodular or general involvement of the bones and the limbs, hands, and skull. The lesions are usually single and often ulcerate through the skin. On healing, a bony thickening that is prominent both clinically and roentgenographically usually results. Late bone lesions of yaws have been reported in some 10% of patients. Despite the extreme destruction often associated with these lesions, spontaneous fractures are not frequent. Impressive destructive ulceration of the nose and palate (gangosa) may occur (Fig. 106-7).

Fig. 106-2. Early lesions of yaws.

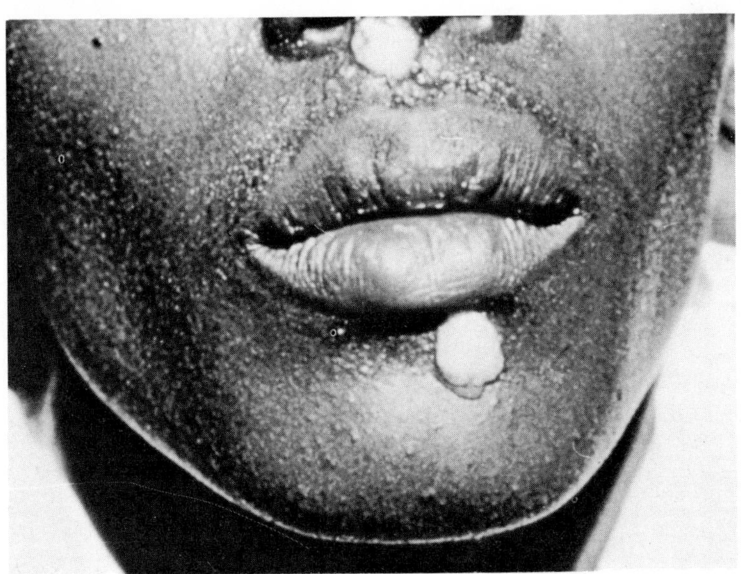

Fig. 106-3. General eruption of early yaws.

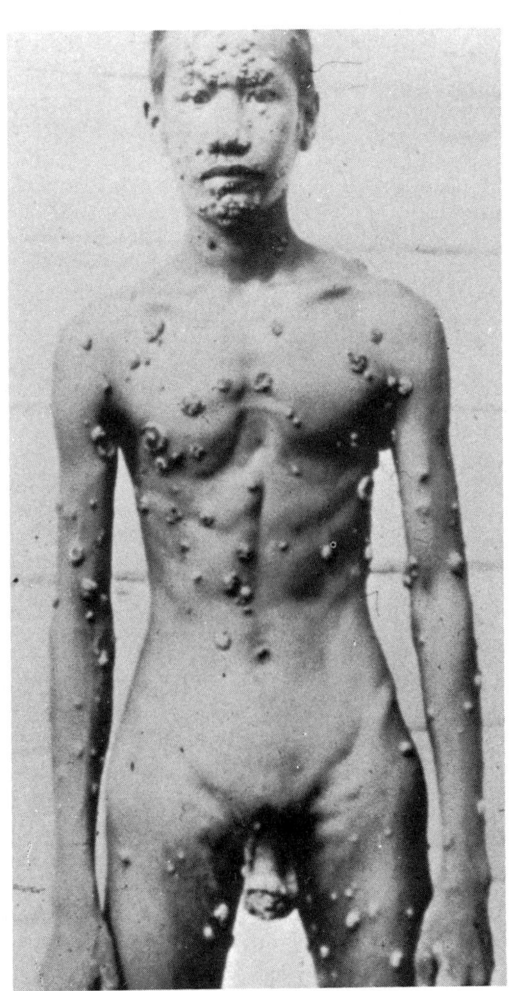

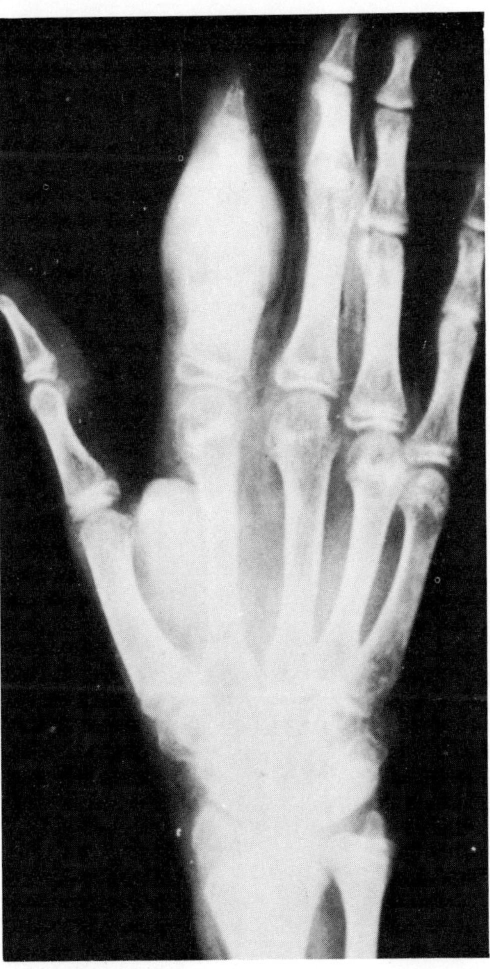

Fig. 106-4. Roentgenographic appearance of polydactylitis of early yaws.

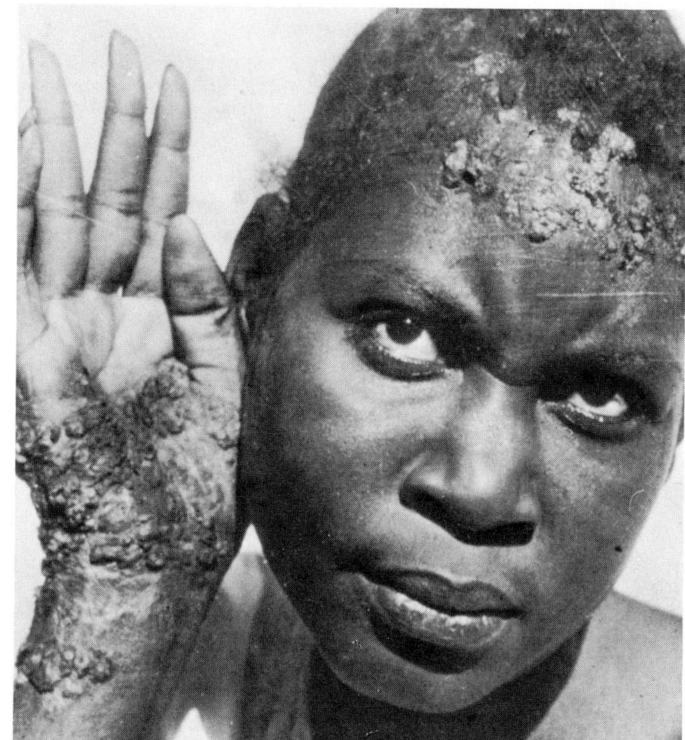

Fig. 106-5. Papillomatous lesions of late yaws.

Fig. 106-6. Plantar hyperkeratosis with fissuring—early crab yaws, the most common late lesion of yaws.

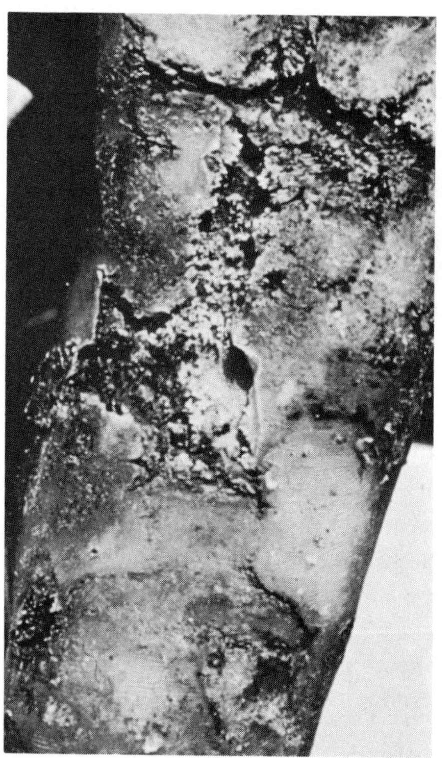

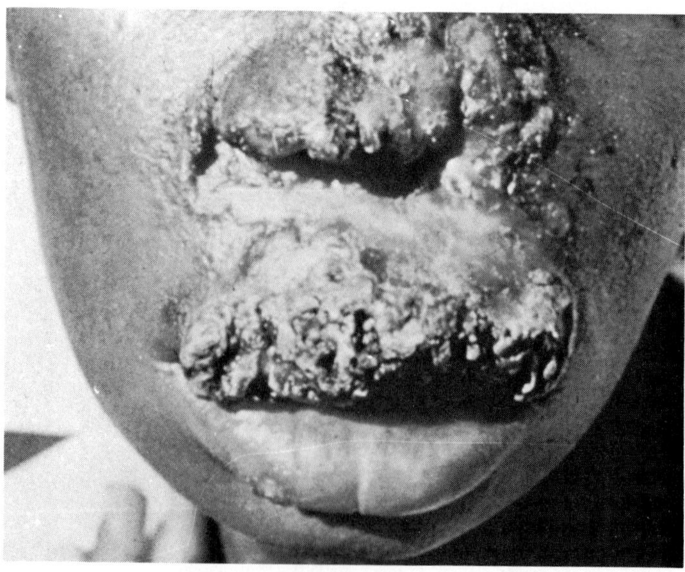

Fig. 106-7. Destructive ulcerations of the nose and face in late yaws—early gangosa.

Diagnosis

Only in endemic areas are clinicians likely to be alert to the possibility of yaws. In nonendemic areas—most of the world—yaws may go undiagnosed for a long time. Such was the case in London in the early 1960s, when there was an influx of immigrants from endemic areas.

The appearance of the early lesions and the darkfield microscopic demonstration of treponemes in the exudate establish the diagnosis. A strong note of caution must be sounded: few microscopists now have sufficient training and experience to be expert in identifying treponemes in darkfield preparations. Several of the recent "epidemics" of venereal and endemic syphilis and of yaws have resulted from the misinterpretation of darkfield preparations by incompetent microscopists. Moreover, the late lesions of yaws are usually darkfield-negative. Serologic tests for syphilis become reactive within a few weeks of infection with yaws. These tests are clearly not diagnostic of yaws. The final distinction between venereal syphilis and yaws rests primarily on the clinical history, epidemiologic findings, and other nonlaboratory criteria.

Biologic false-positive tests for syphilis, when found on routine serologic tests performed in areas endemic for yaws, may be confusing because a number of tropical diseases may activate the VDRL, particularly in children. The simplified FTA-ABS test is of practical differentiating value.

Prognosis

Yaws may undergo spontaneous clinical and serologic cure at any stage of the disease. However, cures without specific therapy seem to be much less frequent than in syphilis. Most cases progress from early to late lesions, and many patients develop debilitating, if not crippling, sequelae. Periarticular ulcers may produce contractures. Contractures of the hands may accompany palmar hyperkeratoses. Gangosa may be hideously disfiguring. Occasionally, discharging sinuses may follow secondary bacterial infection leading to osteomyelitis.

As is true of venereal syphilis, infection with yaws apparently protects the patient from reinfection manifesting an earlier stage. Yaws provides strong protection, if not total immunity, from venereal syphilis. There are few areas in the world in which yaws has existed in close juxtaposition with either pinta or bejel, and the question of cross-immunity remains indeterminate.

Therapy

Penicillin G is the treatment of choice. As in all treponematoses, there has never been a clinical or laboratory demonstration of resistance of *T. pallidum* var. *pertenue* to penicillin. It is exquisitely susceptible to penicillin G, and a single injection of 600,000 units of procaine penicillin in aluminum monosterate (PAM) 2% is probably adequate to cure the disease. The current recommendation of the World Health Organization (WHO) is 1.2 million units for adults and 600,000 units for patients under 15 years of age. In general, half these doses are administered to patients with latent infections.

The response to these small doses of PAM is excellent and sometimes virtually unbelievable. Early lesions become noninfectious within a few days and are healed within 1 to 2 weeks. Subsequent relapses are few and are sometimes thought to represent reinfection. In many of the mass treatment campaigns, one injection of PAM was given and 1 year later approximately 10% of the population received a second injection because of some evidence of active lesions. Subsequent follow-up 1 year later revealed less than 2% of the original group with any evidence of yaws.

Seropositive patients, when treated in the early stages, frequently become seronegative. However, patients with late yaws often remain seropositive for a long period, if not for life. The use of larger doses of penicillin given over a longer period seems to increase the number of cases that become seronegative.

Prevention

The incidence of yaws has been decreasing since the 1920s, primarily because of better standards of living. Simply introducing the use of soap and water into a primitive society has regularly been followed by a diminution in the number of cases of yaws. Mass treatment with penicillin has in 2 or 3 years reduced the number of cases to an extent that previously required 20 or more years to achieve. Yaws has in fact become so uncommon that mass treatment teams, after the first or second resurvey, generally carry out mass measures against other communicable diseases.

Remaining Problems

The factors responsible for the transmission of yaws have never been clearly defined, and it now seems likely that the true mechanisms will never be discovered.

Pinta

Pinta (also known as mal del pinto and carate) existed in tropical South and Central America before the Spanish conquest. A factual description of the disease was provided by Cortez in a letter to King Charles V of Spain. Unfortunately for the Indians, the Spaniards regarded this disease as a variant of leprosy, and those afflicted were shot on sight. Thus, the disease was carried by affected tribes into the remote portions of the jungle in an effort to avoid contact with the Spaniards. Although the disease is neither fatal nor crippling, it is severely disfiguring, and affected persons have been ostracized by outsiders and other members of their tribes. The achromic, characteristic late lesions are often described as "dead white," and although the lesions are not associated with scarring, patients are usually unable to adjust to anything but a primitive rural life.

Etiology

Pinta is caused by *T. pallidum* var. *carateum,* (microorganisms morphologically and immunologically identical with the other variants of *T. pallidum.* Shortly after infection, the VDRL becomes positive, and soon thereafter the treponemal serologic tests are also reactive.

The fragility of the treponeme outside the body of the host and its susceptibility to antimicrobial agents are the same as those of the other varieties of *T. pallidum.*

Epidemiology

Pinta is limited to tropical Central and South America. The disease tends to be endemic in certain river basins, and in particular, the upper reaches of the Amazon and the Balsas River in Mexico. In the early 1960s, it was estimated that some 500,000 cases existed in Latin America. That number is certainly vastly diminished now, and persons with active infections are becoming quite rare.

The disease is found almost exclusively in remote, primitive, rural areas, generally in close-knit Indian communities, where inhabitants live in close proximity to one another. Blacks living under similar conditions in or near these communities may also be involved, but fewer cases usually occur in whites. In all probability, the disease has never existed in the United States.

Pinta has been found at elevations as high as 7300 feet in Colombia, although most cases occur at lower elevations in the river valleys. It is curious that pinta is not endemic to coastal areas of South America (areas in which yaws has been endemic).

The populations in which pinta occurs have a characteristic lack of interest in bathing and virtually all aspects of personal hygiene; invariably, they exhibit numerous insect bites, many with accompanying excoriations. Males and females are almost equally affected, and all races seem susceptible, although South American Indians and blacks are most commonly affected. In most surveys, 40% to 60% of patients were under 16. The percentage of children with pinta in a population is often thought to be a good index of the communicability of the disease within the group. Pinta is not transmitted congenitally.

Pinta was first transmitted experimentally by the Cuban physicians Latapi and Leon y Blanco in 1939. They described the stages of the disease after inoculation of material obtained from an early lesion of pinta into normal volunteers. Transmission appears to require a break in the skin, and most authorities believe that transmission occurs as a result of intimate contact with infected persons.

The possible direct role of biting insects in the transmission of the disease has often been postulated, although never proved. There are many graphic accounts describing the frequency of insect bites in patients with pinta. For example, clouds of blackflies (*Simuliidae*) have been observed to follow groups of Mosetene Indians in Bolivia; by direct count, there were well over 1000 bites on the four extremities. Despite these observations, the evidence is compelling that household contact between persons with large areas of excoriated skin favors personal contact as the primary method of transmission. In this connection, there is an interesting traditional account of a tribal ritual among the Puru-puru Indians of the Amazon basin, among whom affected adults and noninfected youths are alternately whipped in order to transmit the disease among tribal members.

Pathogenesis and Pathology

The pathologic changes of pinta are restricted to the skin. *Treponema pallidum* var. *carateum* is present in the epidermis and upper corium in early lesions. Later, they are found in small numbers only in the epidermis and occasionally in the pilosebaceous follicles.

Pigmentary changes, although the most prominent feature of late lesions, are minimal in early lesions. Early lesions are characterized by relatively nonspecific changes, including moderate acanthosis, slight spongiosis, and a mild inflammatory infiltrate in the upper corium. As opposed to venereal syphilis, the blood vessels do not show proliferation or obliteration. Older lesions may show hyperkeratosis, some parakeratosis, and varying degrees of pigment deposition in the basal cell layer. in the late achromic lesion, the pigment has disappeared. Electron-microscopic study reveals a lack of basal epidermal melanocytes, topographic substitution of basal melanocytes by

Langerhans' cells with hyperplasia of Langerhans' cells in the malpighian layer, and melanin granules within the lysosomes of the Langerhans' cells.

The pathophysiologic mechanism by which treponemes produce changes so prominent in the pigment layer is unknown. Although other treponemal diseases may lead to hyperpigmentation, this change can be extraordinarily striking in pinta, producing a so-called blue man in the early (usually secondary) stages of the disease, only to be followed by the complete obliteration of pigment from the skin in the late stages.

Manifestations

Pinta is traditionally described as an evolution of lesions that are sometimes categorized as primary, secondary, and tertiary, but these lesions can better be thought of as early and late lesions. The stages are not well delineated, particularly the early stages. Any of these stages may not appear, or any or all may be present simultaneously.

EARLY STAGES

The primary lesions appear from 3 days to 2 months after inoculation, beginning as small, erythematous papules that are slightly scaly and indurated. In 1 to 3 months, these papules increase in size, gradually enlarging to 1 cm to 3 cm in diameter, often coalescing with surrounding, developing satellite papules. As the lesions progress, they may form scaly or even psoriasiform plaques that can ultimately achieve a size of up to 10 cm. These primary lesions may disappear after a few months or may persist for several years. In infants, they are most commonly observed in areas of continual contact with their mothers; the sites most often involved are thus the gluteal regions, posterior thighs, and trunk. In older children, primary lesions are usually found on the extremities, especially the wrists, forearms, dorsa of the feet, and ankles. In adolescents and adults, primary lesions have been described in almost all other body areas except the genitalia. After healing, the initial lesion may leave residual depigmentation, or, more commonly, there is no striking pigment alteration.

The secondary lesions are associated with dissemination, and frequently it is impossible to determine which lesions are primary and which developed later. The disseminated lesions, often called secondaries or pintids, can affect almost any area of the skin (Fig. 106-8). They tend to occur on uncovered surfaces, particularly areas exposed to the sun, and thus they are more frequently observed on the arms, legs, face, and neck. With further development of the secondary stage, more lesions appear in these areas, although

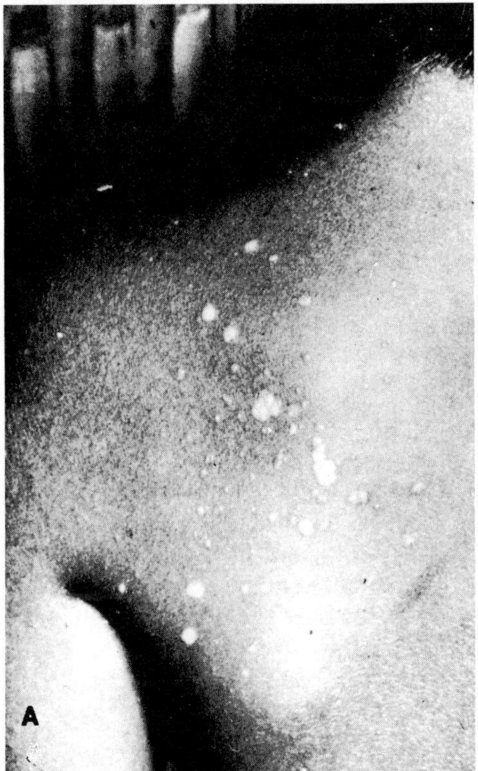

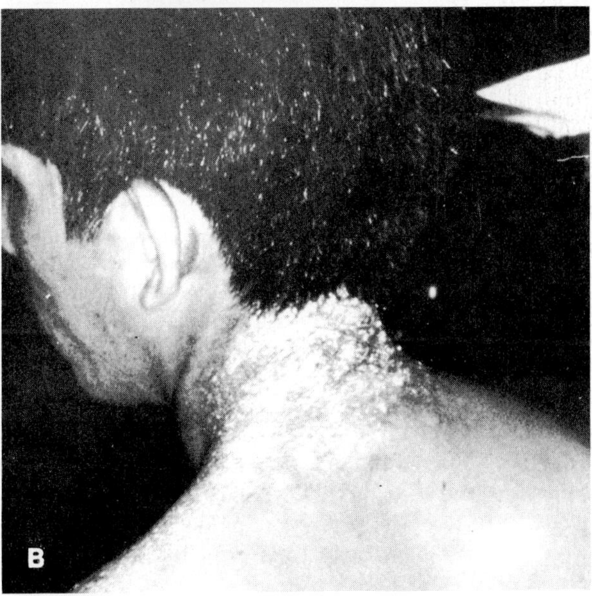

Fig. 106-8. (*A*) Secondary pintids on the shoulder of a young girl. (*B*) Secondary pintids on the neck of a boy.

eventually much of the body may be covered. The individual pintids usually are small, scaly papules that gradually enlarge and may even coalesce.

A very curious aspect of the early lesions, and particularly of the secondary lesions, is the variety of colors that may occur. The earlier lesions tend to be red to violaceous; later lesions, particularly those on the face and neck, may be slate blue, gray, or black. Extensive, dark blue lesions of the face and neck, although now rare, can be most striking; no other clinical entity exactly mimics this curious blue color. Lesions of the legs tend to be yellow brown or dark brown.

LATE STAGE

The tertiary stage is heralded by the development of depigmented areas that usually appear first over body prominences. Particularly characteristic is the depigmentation of the inner aspects of the wrists, elbows, and ankles (Fig. 106-9), although depigmentation may follow earlier lesions at any site. Lesions exhibiting a loss of color usually appear several years after the initial lesions. However, they may begin to develop as early as 3 months after the onset of pinta, or they may not be noted until some 10 years after the appearance of the pintids. Initially, these achromic areas are interspersed with earlier and often recurrent dyschromic lesions, so that patients frequently appear mottled, having light spots and dark spots often in close proximity.

A hyperkeratosis that differs from the lesions of yaws often develops on the palms and soles of Cubans with pinta. Fungi have not been isolated from such lesions.

Early and late latent stages of pinta have been shown to occur. Thus, the observations of a relapsing course in untreated patients are entirely reasonable.

Diagnosis

The diagnosis of pinta depends primarily on clinical suspicion; a positive darkfield examination for treponemes is supportive as long as it is kept in mind that *T. pallidum* var. *carateum* cannot be differentiated morphologically from *T. pallidum* var. *pallidum*. Seroconversion is very slow compared with syphilis or yaws and may not occur for as long as 4 months after the appearance of the primary lesion of pinta. However, the tests usually remain positive for life and frequently do not become negative after adequate therapy, though the titer may decline very slowly.

Prognosis

Untreated pinta produces dyschromic changes of the skin. Ultimately, most patients who receive no treatment develop prominent white areas of the skin that

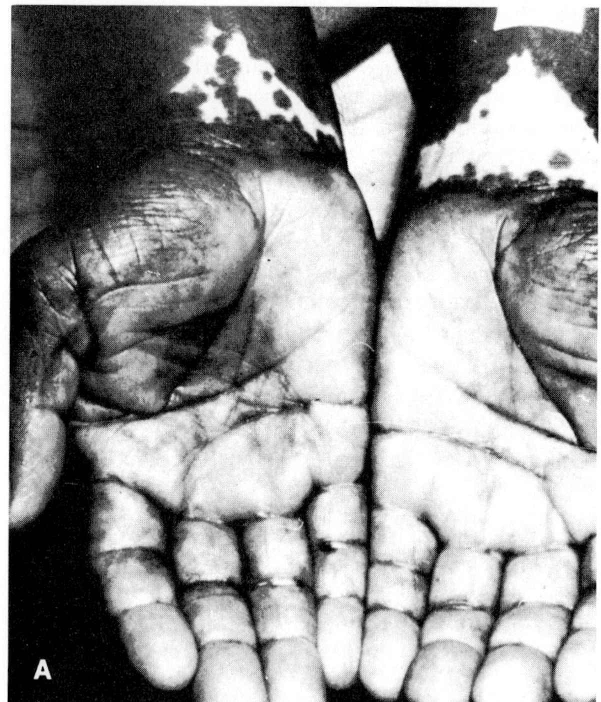

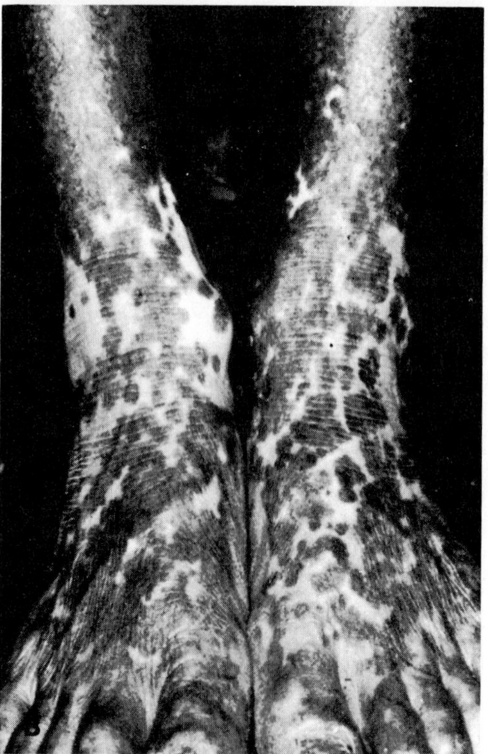

Fig. 106-9. (*A*) The depigmentation of skin on the wrists in late pinta. Note the characteristic triangular pattern. (*B*) Mottled hypopigmentation of skin on the ankles in late pinta.

may vary in size from small triangles (characteristically, 2 cm–5 cm on a side) of the inner wrists to extensive depigmented areas. Without treatment, relapses are common, and a latent stage may occur.

Although patients with untreated pinta seem to be immune to reinfection, it is not known whether immunity is perpetuated after adequate treatment. Pinta provides no protection against yaws or veneral syphilis.

The major complication of pinta is social. Victims of this disease are often ostracized by members of their own group, and they are not accepted by other (usually urban) societies. As a consequence, rehabilitation after appropriate treatment has been largely ineffective.

Therapy

Penicillin G is the treatment of choice. The recommended adult dose is 1.2 million units of a long-acting penicillin (*e.g.*, benzathine penicillin G). Children should receive 300,000 to 600,000 units. Small children may be treated with repeated doses of intramuscular procaine penicillin rather than be subjected to the intramuscular injection of benzathine penicillin.

The tetracyclines and chloramphenicol are effective in the treatment of pinta. The dosage schedules recommended for venereal syphilis are appropriate (Chap. 59, Syphilis). In most patients, both clinical and serologic responses to treatment are notably slow. Lesions treated before the skin color begins to fade often heal without residual hypopigmentation; hypopigmented lesions usually leave a residual lightened area. The treatment of patients with achromic areas of long duration usually fails to produce any evidence of repigmentation on long-term follow-up.

Prevention

Pinta was also disappearing before the advent of antimicrobial therapy, though penicillin has accelerated the process. Possibly, the simple addition of bathing with soap and water in endemic communities would ultimately have eliminated pinta.

Remaining Problems

Pinta may well be the archtypal disease from which all of the treponematoses of humans arose. The clinical and laboratory studies that may support this hypothesis should be carried out before pinta disappears.

Bejel (Endemic Syphilis)

Bejel is a nonvenereal treponematosis commonly acquired in childhood. It has no relationship to human sexual activity.

The origin of bejel is uncertain. There seems to be little doubt that numerous endemic foci have existed in Africa since antiquity. Epidemics of what seems to have been this disease occurred during the fifteenth century, apparently when conditions were favorable for extravenereal transmission of the infection in childhood. Thus, sibbens of seventeenth century Scotland and radesyge of the eighteenth century in Norway are generally accepted to be descriptions of endemic, nonvenereal syphilis. Presently endemic in several eastern Mediterranean countries, bejel is also called endemic syphilis of the Bedouins.

Etiology

The etiologic agent of bejel is morphologically indistinguishable from the microorganisms found in the other treponematoses of humans, and it is considered to be *T. pallidum* var. *pallidum* (sometimes designated *T. pallidum* II). The lesions induced in experimental animals by injecting strains from bejel are said to be intermediate in severity between those resulting from strains of venereal origin (which are more severe) and from yaws (which are less severe). All of the serologic tests for syphilis become positive in bejel.

Epidemiology

Bejel once seemed to be disappearing more rapidly than any other treponemal disease. Endemic active foci once existed in several areas of Africa (*e.g.*, Bechuanaland, Sudan, southern Zimbabwe, and Equatorial Africa). Although no active cases were found in South Africa in 1970, large numbers of cases were reported in several countries of West Africa in the late 1970s. Formerly endemic areas of Bosnia–Herzegovina, Yugoslavia were free of disease when surveyed in 1970. Small foci were known in the Middle East, although in 1964 no active cases were found in Saudi Arabia, eastern Iran, and western Afghanistan. Areas of Southeast Asia, the Western Pacific, and Australia are also said to contain endemic foci.

Bejel occurs predominantly in children, usually before puberty. Both sexes are equally affected. Up to 25% of the infections occur before age 6, and some 50% to 60% occur before age 16 in areas with active foci. Bejel is found exclusively among rural populations with low standards of personal hygiene.

Unlike yaws, bejel apparently spreads within the household so that simultaneous infections of several members of the family may produce lesions that are virtually identical in appearance. Common drinking vessels, which pass treponemes from mouth to mouth, may be most important as the mode of transmission.

Mass treatment campaigns with penicillin G have

been successful in eliminating new infections in children. Similar success has followed a general improvement in the standard of living—as with yaws and pinta.

Pathogenesis and Pathology

The pathologic and histologic changes of bejel are virtually identical to those of venereal syphilis.

Manifestations

Primary lesions in bejel have only rarely been encountered in the field in the past, and they are now almost never seen. Most primary lesions have been observed in children, and the lesions seem to result from contact with the mouth. A primary lesion has occasionally been reported on the nipple of a previously uninfected mother as a result of nursing an infected infant.

In most cases, the primary lesion is lacking or goes unobserved, presumably because of the small inoculum of treponemes. A large inoculum may result in a chancre that is very similar to the chancre of venereal syphilis. However, most authorities think that repeated transfer of small numbers of treponemes is the rule of bejel, resulting in no clinically apparent primary lesion.

The lesions most commonly observed occur during the secondary stage. These consist primarily of mucous patches on the lips, tongue, palate, and larynx. Angular stomatitis is not uncommon, and condylomas of the anogenital area are commonly seen in children.

The late manifestations of bejel are qualitatively very similar to those of venereal syphilis, although the severe late sequelae are rare. Gummas may affect the skin, and the nasopharyngeal area is most commonly involved. Ulceration, with tissue destruction and marked disfigurement, particularly of the nose, may be produced. Cutaneous gummas often extend laterally, with marked ulceration.

Involvement of the bones is relatively common. Osteitis with gumma formation and periostitis are the lesions most frequently observed. The tibia is most commonly affected. The joints are often involved with bilateral synovitis, especially the knee joints.

Late gummatous lesions may develop in childhood, sometimes even before puberty. Cardiovascular and neural late lesions are very rare, but they are accepted as a part of bejel. Neurosyphilis from bejel, when it occurs, is usually relatively mild.

If it ever occurred, congenital bejel was quite rare, and now it is apparently nonexistent. Its rarity is explained, as in the case of yaws, by the early age at which bejel is usually contracted. By the time a woman becomes pregnant, the active infection is over, even without therapy.

Diagnosis

The diagnosis of bejel is difficult under the best of circumstances. Because transmission is nonvenereal, an understanding of the mores of the afflicted societal unit is important to diagnosis. It is probably fair to say that the diagnosis cannot be made with certainty outside of an endemic setting. In an endemic setting, a patient with lesions clinically consistent with bejel who has a positive darkfield examination and positive serologic tests for syphilis may well have the disease. The final diagnosis remains presumptive until cases are found among children and young adolescents. High titers of the various serologic tests for syphilis are frequent in children with overt bejel and in latency because the disease is apt to be contracted early in life.

Prognosis

The prognosis of any patient with untreated bejel is uncertain. Although cardiovascular and neural late sequelae may develop, these are generally quite mild. The most common late sequelae are gummatous lesions of skin and bones, and these may be disfiguring and disabling. Active infection seems to provide essentially complete immunity to reinfection and to yaws; data are lacking for pinta.

Therapy

Penicillin G is the treatment of choice and is usually administered as benzathine penicillin given in a single dose of 1.2 million units. No laboratory or clinical evidence of resistance to penicillin has been reported. In mass treatment campaigns administered by WHO, this dose has led to the eradication of bejel in many countries.

Prevention

Endemic syphilis is easily prevented by improving the general level of personal hygiene and the standard of living. Mass treatment programs have been extremely successful in eradicating the disease. However, there are no data that enable any conclusions to be made about the long-term efficacy of mass treatment programs when practiced without attempting to raise the standard of living. To date, however, resurveys have failed to demonstrate the recurrence of bejel in areas where treatment has been carried out.

Remaining Problems

As with the other treponematoses, bejel should be eradicated from the world by the application of available technology.

Bibliography

GENERAL

Book

WHO Scientific group: Treponematosis Research. Geneva, World Health Organization, 1970. 91 pp.

Journals

GJESTLAND T: The Oslo study of untreated syphilis. Acta Dermatovener 35(Suppl 34):1–368, 1955

GUTHE T: Treponematoses as a world problem. Br J Vener Dis 36:67–77, 1960

HACKETT CJ: On the origin of the human treponematoses. Bull WHO 29:7–41, 1963

HACKETT CJ: Treponematosis and antrhopology. Ann Intern Med 58:1037–1048, 1963

HARDY PH: Death knell for the *Treponema pallidum* immobilization test. Sex Transm Dis 7:145–148, 1980

HOLLANDER DH: Treponematosis from pinta to venereal syphilis revisited: Hypothesis for temperature determination of disease patterns. Sex Transm Dis 8:34–37, 1981

HUDSON EH: Treponematosis and anthropology. Ann Intern Med 58:1037–1048, 1963

TURNER TB, HOLLANDER DH: Biology of the treponematoses. WHO Monogr Ser 35:1–310, 1957

YAWS

Books

HACKETT CJ: Yaws. In Demis DJ, Dobson RC, McGuire J (eds): Clinical Dermatology, Vol 3, Unit 16-23. New York, Harper & Row, 1980. 19 pp.

Journals

FURTADO T: Some problems of late yaws. Int J Dermatol 12:123–130, 1973

GUTHE T: Clinical, serological and epidemiological features of frambesia (yaws) and its control in rural communities. Acta Derm-Venereol 49:343–368, 1969

HACKETT CJ: An international nomenclature of yaws lesions. WHO Monogr Ser 35:1–310, 1957

PINTA

Books

EDMUNDSON WF: Pinta. In Demis DJ, Dobson RC, McGuire J (eds): Clinical Dermatology, Vol 3, Unit 16-24. New York, Harper & Row, 1980. 12 pp.

Journals

EDMUNDSON WF, DENNIS DJ, BEJARINO G: A clinicoserologic study of pinta in the Alto Beni region, Bolivia. Dermatol Int 6:64–76, 1967

HASSELMANN CM: Studien über die Histopathologie von Pinta, Frambosie and Syphilis. Arch Klin Exp Derm 201:1–8, 1955

LATAPI F, LEON Y BLANCO F: Las lesiones de principio del mal del pinto. Med Rev Mex 20:315–358, 1940

RODRIGUEZ HA, ALBORES–SAAVEDRA J, LOZANO MM: Langerhans' cells in late pinta. Arch Pathol 91:302–306, 1971

BEJEL

Books

GRIN EI: Endemic syphilis (bejel). In Demis DJ, Dobson RC, McGuire J (eds): Clinical Dermatology, Vol. 3, Unit 16-25. New York, Harper & Row, 1980. 7 pp.

Journals

GRIN EI: Endemic treponematoses in the Sudan. Bull WHO 24:229–238, 1961

GRIN EI, GUTHE T: Evaluation of a previous mass campaign against endemic syphilis in Bosnia and Herzegovina. Br J Vener Dis 49:1–19, 1973

MCFADZEAN JA, MCCOURT JF, WILKINSON AE: Treponematoses in Gambia, West Africa. Trans R Soc Trop Med Hyg 51: 169–181, 1956

World Health Organization: Endemic treponematoses. Wkly Epidem Rec 56:241–244, 1981

HENRY E. JONES

107 Superficial Fungus Infections of the Skin

Of the fungi capable of causing diesase in man, more than half are termed dermatophytes because the infect only the skin and its appendages. The essentially extracorporal existence of these parasites in the keratinized and cornified layer of the skin, hair, and nails belies the fact that they can cause severe and disabling disease that may be difficult to prevent and treat. The superficial infections that they cause are known as dermatophytosis.

In addition, two fungi not included among the dermatophytes often cause superficial skin infections. One is *Pityrosporum orbiculare* (formerly called *Malassezia furfur*), which always remains exquisitely superficial; the other, *Candida albicans,* is capable of causing much deeper infections that may progress to fatality (see Chap. 39, Candidosis).

Etiology

Mycology is the oldest of the microbiologic sciences. In 1841, Gruby proved that a fungus could cause a disease in humans (favus) by culturing it from lesions and reproducing the infection by reinoculation with the resulting material.Thus he anticipated by some 40 years what later became known as Koch's postulates.

During the next century a multitude of fungal isolates were reported as different pathogenic species. The list soon became too complex for the classification to be clinically useful. Although the taxonomic advances provided by the description of the perfect state of many of the dermatophytes has removed them from the Fungi Imperfecti and placed classification on a much firmer basis, the same complexity exists today. As a result, the clinical–anatomic syndromes themselves became and remain the basis for classification. Thus, infection by any member of the genera, *Epidermophyton, Microsporum,* and *Trichophyton* is called dermatophytosis or tinea; to tinea, an adjective is added to designate the anatomic area involved, for example, tinea pedis. The fundamental differences among the various clinical–anatomic syndromes are more appropriately attributed to the characteristics of the skin involved than to differences in the various etiologic agents.

The clinical forms of disease that may be caused by the two nondermatophytic fungi that cause superficial infections of the skin are not always distinguishable clinically. They may produce lesions that resemble dermatophytosis. Pityriasis versicolor is probably caused by *Pityrosporum orbiculare,* and was called tinea versicolor until recently. The several kinds of superficial infection caused by *Candida* spp. are referred to as candidosis.

The microorganisms that cause dermatophytosis, pityriasis versicolor, and candidosis are easily distinguished microbiologically (Table 107-1).

Dermatophytes

There are approximately 30 species of dermatophytes, all of which grow in lesions as hyphae that are 2 μm to 3 μm in diameter (Fig. 107-1*A*). In cultures, all grow in a similar, nondistinctive filamentous form that may or may not produce distinctive, identifiable vegetative or spore structures. Precise identification requires considerable expert knowledge. The assignment of genera and species is made on the basis of color, morphology of the hyphae, macroconidia, microconidia, and chlamydospores. However, final identification may rest on growth characteristics observed in special mediums.

Fortunately for the clinician, most infections are caused by 11 species, and in the United States, a mere 7 species cause more that 95% of all dermatophytosis. The clinical-anatomic syndromes and the characteristics of these 7 dermatophytes are compared in Table 107-2. A presumptive speciation of these few pathogens can be made with knowledge of the source of the culture, the nature of the lesion, the

Table 107-1. *Major Categories of Superficial Fungal Infection and Various Etiologic Agents*

Type of Infection	Synonyms	Causative Organism	Microscopic Appearance in Smears From Lesions	Growth on Sabouraud's Dextrose Agar
Dermatophytosis	Tinea capitis, ringworm	*Trichophyton, Microsporum, Epidermophyton* spp.	All have branched, septate hyphae	2–3 weeks as filamentous molds*
Candidosis	Candidiasis	*Candida* spp.	Branched septate hyphae ± budding yeast forms	1–3 days as moist yeasts†
Pityriasis versicolor	Tinea versicolor	*Pityrosporum orbiculare* ?	Short, curved hyphae plus clumps of spores	No growth‡

*Slow growth producing white to tan thallus, often with colored obverse.
†Differentiation of *Candida albicans* from other species requires further tests.
‡Growth occurs when lipid (*e.g.,* olive oil) is added to agar.

Table 107-2. *Common Dermatophytes, Their Microbial Characteristics, and the Clinical–Anatomic Syndromes They Produce*

Genus and Species	Primary Source in Nature	Frequency of Isolation	Characteristic Morphology on Sabouraud's Dextrose Agar		Common Clinical–Anatomic Syndromes				
			COLONY	MICROSCOPIC	CAPITIS	CORPORIS	CRURIS	PEDIS	UNGUIUM
Trichophyton rubrum	Humans	Very, very common	White cotton; red reverse	Sparse	—	+	+	+	+
Trichophyton mentagrophytes	Humans, animals	Moderate	White cotton, or cream to tan powder	Microaleuriospores	Ectothrix	+	+	+	+
Epidermophyton floccosum	Humans	Moderate	Fuzzy; tan, yellow, green	Fanlike macroaleuriospores	—	+	+	+	+
Trichophyton tonsurans	Humans	Moderate	Flat, powdery, or suedelike; yellow	Sparse	Endothrix	+	—	—	—
Microsporum canis	Dogs, cats	Moderate	Woolly, yellow white	Typical macroaleuriospore	Ectothrix*	+	—	—	—
Microsporum audouinii	Humans	Low	White, tan, silky to furry	Sparse	Ectothrix*	+	—	—	—
Trichophyton verrucosum	Cattle, other nonhuman animals	Low	Folded, heaped; gray white	Branched, antlerlike hyphae	Ectothrix	+	—	—	—

*Involved hair fluoresces a brilliant green.

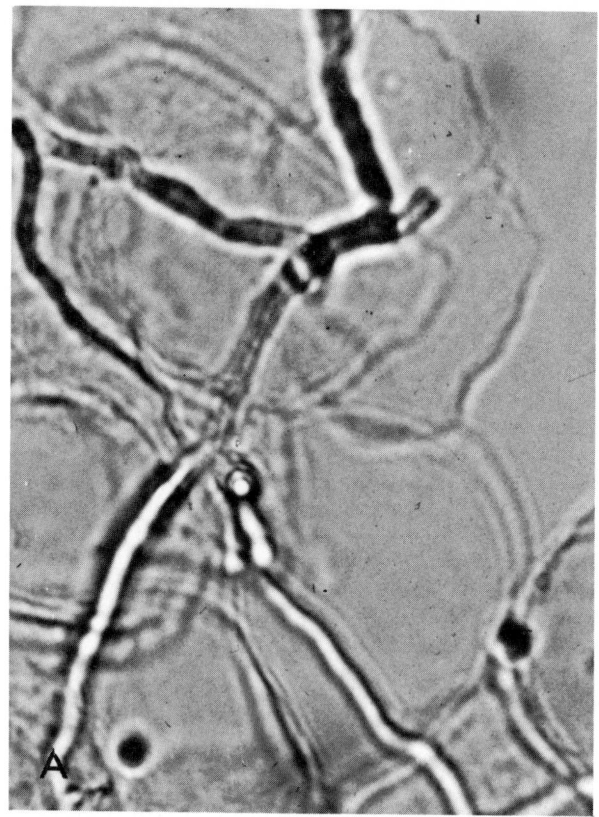

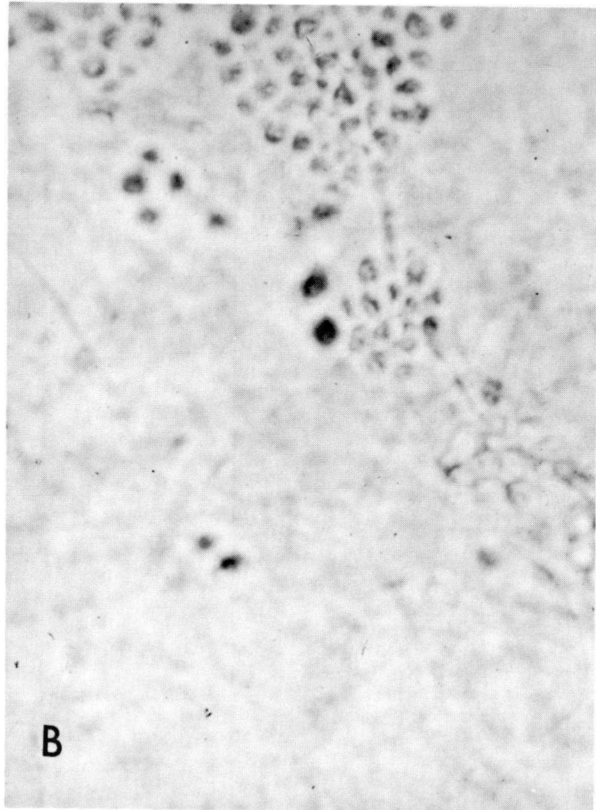

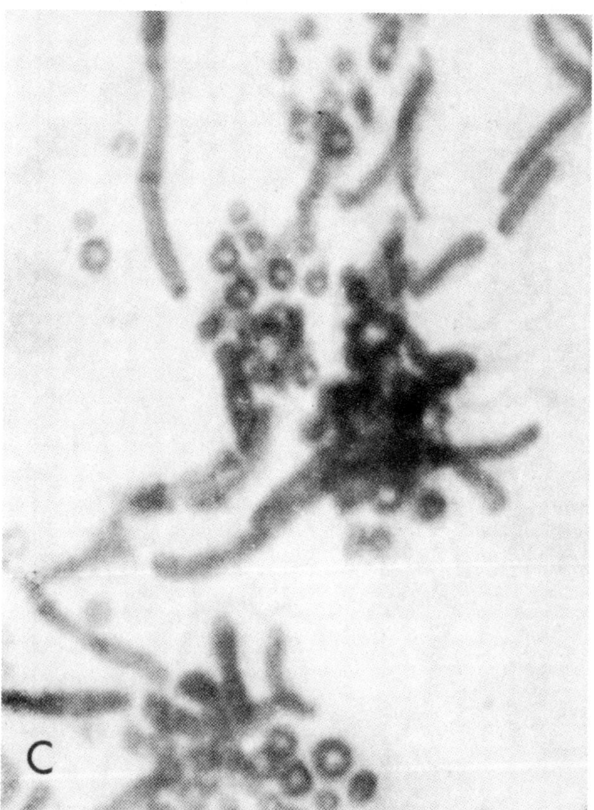

Fig. 107-1. Skin scrapings from patients with superficial fungus infections. (*A*) Dermatophytosis—note the septate hyphae. (*B*) Pityriasis versicolor—typical clusters of spores and short, thick hyphae. (*C*) Candidal infection—both the hyphal and budding yeast forms of this dimorphic fungus are present. (Courtesy of J Walter Wilson, MD) (KOH preparations, original magnification about × 1500)

gross and microscopic appearance of the organism on Sabouraud's agar, and, in the case of scalp infections, the presence or lack of fluorescence with 360 nm of ultraviolet light.

For example, cultures obtained from the groin or feet usually yield one of three species, each of which has a characteristic colonial morphology and color. *Epidermophyton floccosum* is yellowish green when viewed from the culture surface and brown when viewed from the reverse through the agar. Colonies of *Trichophton mentagrophytes* are white and cottony, although sometimes they are powdery, and appear brown when viewed through the agar. *Trichophyton rubrum* is also white and cottony, but examination of the culture through the agar reveals a characteristic red to purplish wine color.

Many of the less common dermatophytes may be identified similarly, especially with the aid of microscopic examination. Precise identification may require subculture on special mediums, plus consultation with an expert. Exact identification of the dermatophyte species is of little direct clinical significance because all species respond to the same therapies. However, speciation should be carried out when there is an epidemic, when the diagnosis of dermatophytosis is questionable, when therapy fails, or when there is an investigation. In this regard, the perfect states of several species of the genera *Trichophyton* and *Microsporum* have been identified. Knowledge of the ascigerous genera and species of the dermatophytes has proven valuable, and already the use of mating pairs is helpful in defining the perfect state and species of isolates that are difficult to identify.

Nondermatophytes

PITYRIASIS VERSICOLOR

In pityriasis versicolor (formerly called tinea versicolor), the direct microscopic examination of scales of skin treated with potassium hydroxide (KOH) reveals the hyphal form of *Pityrosporum orbiculare* (formerly called *Malassezia furfur*; see Figure 107-1*B*). The characteristic picture of short, curved 5 μm in diameter hyphae having round ends, admixed with clumps of spherical, budding, thick-walled blastospores, approximately 3μm to 8 μm in diameter, is specific. This pattern establishes the diagnosis. Culture is not necessary for clinical purposes.

CANDIDOSIS

Cutaneous candidosis is usually caused by *Candida albicans.* The mycelial, and occasionally the yeast, form of this dimorphic fungus may be seen in skin or mucosal lesions. Typically, the mycelial form dominates in lesions although the yeast form is present. The yeast phases of *Candida* spp. are frequently normal inhibitants on moist mucous membranes and intertriginous skin. Therefore, recovery of *Candida* spp. in cultures from lesions in such areas does not document an etiologic role. However, the demonstration of the mycelial form in a lesion greatly heightens the probability of etiologic significance.

Smears from lesions contain septate hyphae that may bear clumps of 2 μm to 4 μm in diameter blastospores or small (2 μm–4 μm), ovoid, thin-walled budding cells (Fig. 107-1*C*). Growth of candida at 37°C on Sabouraud's agar is rapid (1–3 days), yielding round, opaque, moderately large, creamy colonies that give off a yeasty odor.

Testing for the formation of germ tubes and chlamydoconidia is usually sufficient (see Chap. 39, Candidosis) to differentiate *C. albicans* from other species of *Candida.*

Epidemiology

Fungi that cause superficial infections are worldwide in distribution. Certain species of *Candida* and some dermatophytes afflict not only humans but also domestic and wild animals. Recently, the National Health Survey provided data attesting to the incidence of cutaneous fungal infections; approximately 9% of a population of 227 million (roughly 20 million Americans), may be infected. Thus, fungal infections are the most prevalent kind of cutaneous infection.

Dermatophytes

The incidence of cutaneous fungal infection in the general population is unknown, since only a few special population groups, such as soldiers in the United States Army, have been studied. In these studies, the incidence was very high. It can probably be assumed that there is a high incidence in the general population, because dermatophytosis is the most prevalent cutaneous infection.

Of patients who have significant skin pathology caused by fungi, 85% have some form of dermatophytosis. The most common clinical-anatomic syndromes are tinea pedis (45%), tinea cruris (25%), and tinea unguium (10%). All other clinical-anatomic syndromes together account for the remaining 5%.

The incidence of dermatophytosis is not equal in all age groups or in both sexes. In fact, there are interesting differences in the incidence of certain clinical–anatomic infection syndromes that have a complex relationship to both age and sex (Fig. 107-2*A* and *B*).

All forms of dermatophytosis have a very low incidence during the first decade of life. This is also true of tinea capitis, yet most of the cases of this disease occur before puberty, and boys and girls are equally affected. After puberty, the incidence of all forms of dermatophytosis except tinea capitis increase dramatically. Tinea pedis and tinea cruris are the most common, and all forms of dermatophytosis are much more prevalent in the male. In later life, the incidence of tinea unguium in women increases to approximately half of that found in men.

The source of cutaneous fungal infection may be other humans (anthropophilic fungi), infected nonhuman animals (zoophilic fungi), or even the soil (geophilic fungi, Table 107-2). Zoophilic fungi have traditionally been thought always to produce highly inflammatory infections, whereas anthropophilic fungi have been thought incapable of producing inflammatory infections. This axiom must now be reconsidered because it has been demonstrated that

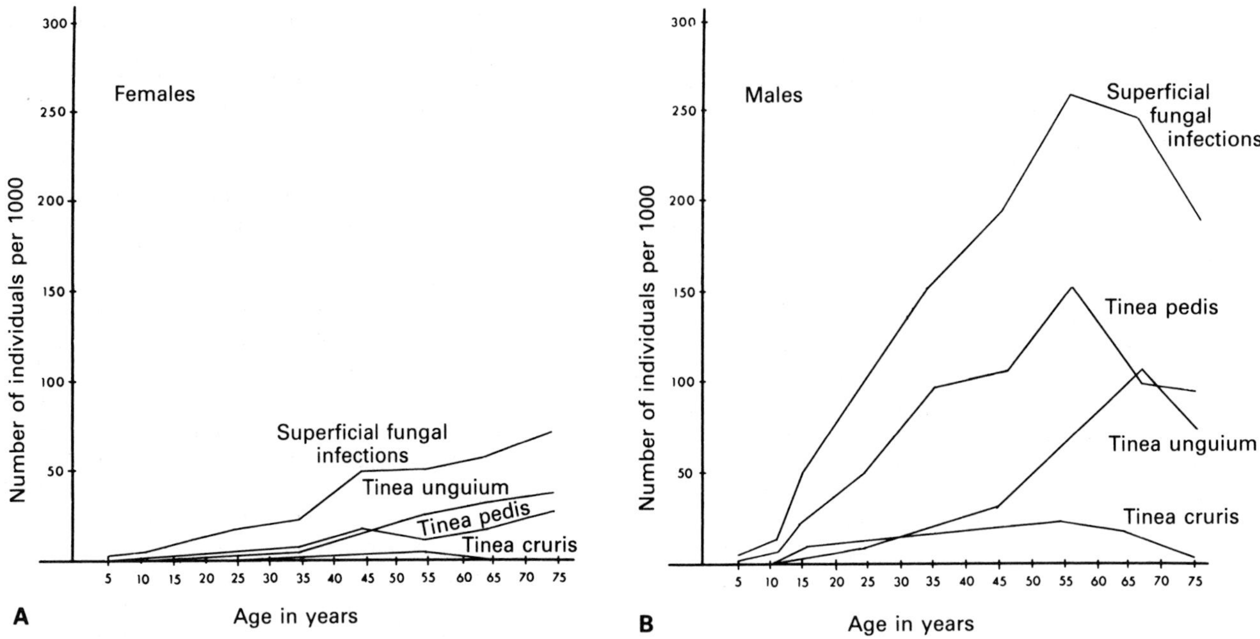

Fig. 107-2. Prevalence of cutaneous fungal infection among residents of the United States 1–74 years of age.

the immune response of the host to dermatophyte group antigen (trichophytin) is the major factor that determines the degree of inflammation in infected skin.

Social, occupational, and environmental factors also appear to affect the incidence of infection as well as the clinical manifestations thereof. For example, inner city ghetto children experience much more tinea capitis than their affluent suburban counterparts. Most ringworm due to *Trichophyton verrucosum* occurs in farmers on exposed body surfaces, such as arms and legs. The role of environment in dermatophytosis has never been clearer than in the tropical monsoon climate of Southeast Asia in which a very high incidence of inflammatory dermatophytosis has been documented in European and American soldiers.

The various clinical–anatomic syndromes caused by dermatophytes account for approximately 5% to 7% of the dermatology patients seen in large clinics throughout the world. As in prevalence and incidence studies, tinea pedis is also the most common form of infection seen by physicians. The proportional rates for the other clinical–anatomic syndromes are in decreasing order of frequency: tinea cruris, tinea unguium, tinea corporis, tinea manuum, and tinea capitis. In the past 20 years, tinea capitis has been controlled to the point at which it is now the least common of the various clinical–anatomic syndromes.

Some dermatophytic infections are acute and self-limited, while others are chronic and last a lifetime. More than 90% of all males will have experienced at least one infection by middle life, whereas far fewer adult women will have had a dermatophytic infection. Approximately 15% of the adult male population will have a chronic, stabilized form of tinea pedis. The fact that the spouses of patients with chronic stabilized infections become infected less frequently than genetically related offspring implies that genetic or hormonal factors are more important than the presence of the etiologic agent.

Nondermatophytes

PITYRIASIS VERSICOLOR

Apparently unique to man, pityriasis versicolor is most commonly observed in the tropics. The putative etiologic agent, *Pityrosporum orbiculare,* is harbored by many people and may cause disease in susceptible persons under the appropriate environmental conditions.

CANDIDOSIS

Candida albicans are part of the resident microbiota of the oral cavity, pharynx, large intestine, vagina, and anogenital skin.

Pathogenesis and Pathology

It is remarkable that fungi that invade only the dead, cornified layers of the skin, hair, and nails can produce such protean manifestations and cause so much morbidity. Most of the resulting pathology is caused by the host's reaction to the infecting fungus. The fungus alone has only a minimal capacity to damage skin directly.

Dermatophytes

The fundamental pathogenic mechanisms of dermatophytosis involve two distinct phases: (1) colonization and (2) host–parasite interaction (Fig. 107-3).

An experimental infection of the skin of a human can be initiated with an inoculum of only one spore. However, the quantity and form of the fungus required to initiate a natural infection is not known. In any event, when the requisite microenvironment and inoculum are present on the surface of the skin, invasion begins. Dermatophytes grow in typical filamentous form within the stratum corneum. The downward extension of these hyphae is apparently restricted because certain micronutrients, principally iron, are not available below the stratum corneum. The iron present in the living cell layers of the epidermis and dermis in which the dermatophytes fail to penetrate is firmly bound to transferrin. The presence of unsaturated transferrin in living tissues assures that the quantity of unbound or available iron is considerably below the minimum requirement of dermatophytes.

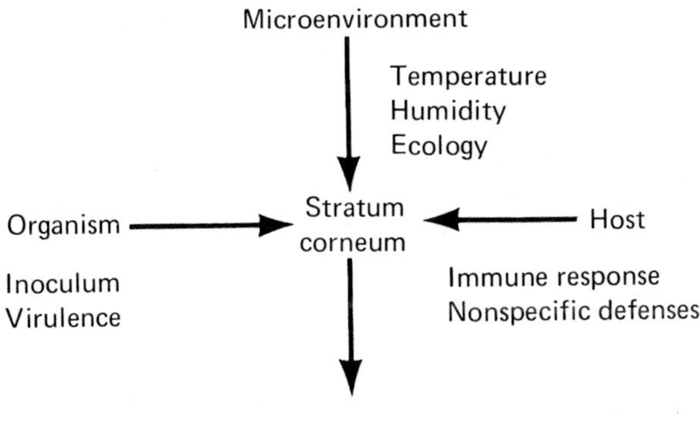

Fig. 107-3. The two phases in pathogenesis of dermatophytosis. I. Colonization—invasion is limited to dead stratum corneum and therefore produces no clinical symptoms or signs. II. Host–parasite interactions—a symptomatic period accompanied by inflammation and skin damage, (*i.e.,* a ringworm is produced by the host's reaction to the fungal organism).

Lateral expansion of the microcolony within the stratum corneum continues for approximately 10 to 35 days, during which time the infected skin appears to be either normal or only very slightly inflamed. That is, dermatophytes do not produce diffusible irritants or toxins that directly damage the skin. After 2 to 3 weeks, the advancing border of the infection may become inflamed (ringworm lesions).

During the colonization phase, the host begins to respond immunologically by undergoing sensitization to soluble fungal antigens (trichophytin). The first detectable immune response in experimental dermatophytosis is cell-mediated immunity (CMI), which is characterized in colonized skin as an intense inflammatory process and demonstrated at the site of a trichophytin skin test by a delayed or tuberculin-type reaction. The genesis and expression of CMI to dermatophytic antigen in an experimental infection occurs between the 10th and 35th days and heralds the beginning of the second distinct period in pathogenesis, the host–parasite interaction phase.

During the host–parasite interaction phase, CMI produces most of the pathology as an acute inflammatory type of dermatophytosis. The immune inflammation that results extends in a spectrum from erythema and edema of the dermis and epidermis (spongiosis) to the formulation of vesicles and pustules). Epidermal integrity is breached; oozing and weeping of tissue fluid occur. Invasion of hair follicles results in inflamed nodules, deep seated pustules, and abscesses.

Cell-mediated immune damage to the skin is not entirely without benefit to the host. The inflammatory damage to the epidermis may internalize what began as an essentially extracorporal fungal colony. The parasitized stratum corneum is now exposed to the internal host defense mechanisms (Fig. 107-4). Several of the host defense mechanisms that are critical for resistance to other microbial pathogens do not appear to be important either in limiting the invasion of dermatophytes or in eradicating them. There is no evidence that either antibody or lymphocytes (*e.g.,* lymphokine) can directly retard fungal growth. Phagocytes surely cannot dissect out and engulf the long fungal filaments that arborize through the compact stratum corneum.

It seems plausible, however, that unsaturated transferrin could diffuse into the stratum corneum and bind iron, rendering this essential micronutrient unavailable for fungal utilization. In any event, the net effect of damage to the skin from CMI is that lateral spread of the colony is abruptly halted, and within 1

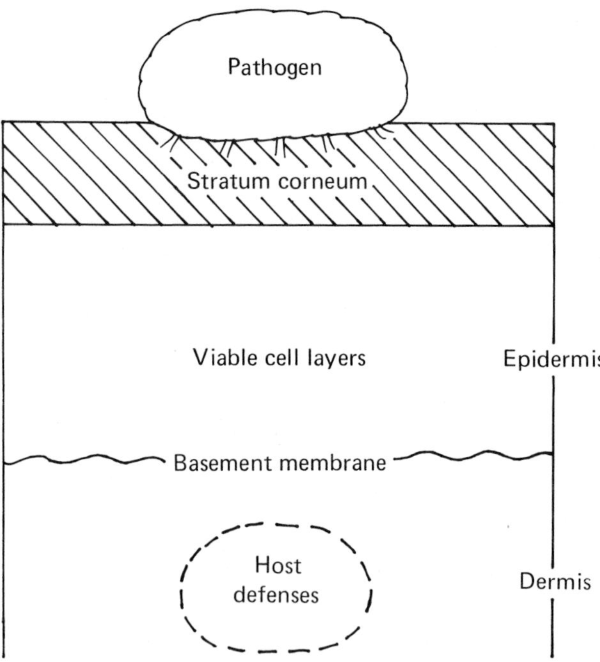

Fig. 107-4. During colonization of the dead, cornified epidermis, fungi are not exposed to the host defense mechanisms that patrol the internal milieu of the body. When the integrity of the epidermal structures that form the skin barrier are damaged by immune inflammation (CMI), the fungal colony is directly exposed to certain host defense mechanisms.

to 2 weeks the pathogen can no longer be recovered from the lesion. The outward growth of the epidermis, which may be accelerated by the inflammation, probably aids in elimination of the infection.

If CMI to dermatophyte antigen does not develop or is suppressed by immune regulation or modulation, the skin will not become sufficiently inflamed to reject the infection. In patients who cannot express CMI to dermatophytic antigens, the chronically infected skin is only minimally inflamed. The result of minimally inflamed, chronic infection is dryness, erythema, scaling, pruritus, fissures, and cracks.

Thus, there are two basic types of dermatophytic infection (Table 107-3). The acute or inflammatory type of infection is associated with CMI to the fungus and generally heals spontaneously or responds nicely to treatment. The chronic or noninflammatory type of infection is associated with a failure to express CMI to the fungus at the site of infection and relapses or responds poorly to treatment.

Several conditions predispose to dermatophytosis. Recurrent colonization is favored by moisture, as provided by the high humidity of the tropics or in certain anatomic sites (intertriginous areas). It is also favored when the skin is frequently bombarded by a heavy fungal inoculum. Any condition that impairs the expression of CMI in the skin, such as congenital immunodeficiency disorders, atopy, reticular malignancy, antimetabolic or glucosteroid therapy (even topical), will lead to chronic infection once colonization has occurred.

Nondermatophytes

In all probability, colonization and host–parasite interaction also play a role in the other two superficial fungal infections. They are not distinct, however, for reasons peculiar to each infection.

PITYRIASIS VERSICOLOR

Almost nothing is known about the pathogenesis of the superficial fungal infection pityriasis versicolor. Susceptibility to infection appears to be influenced by the environment and varies not only according to the individual but also according to the anatomic site.

Observation of the density and topographic distribution of *P. orbiculare* in the skin reveals that spores are abundant in and near the pilosebaceous follicles, whereas hyphae dominate in the interfollicular stratum corneum. When cultured, no microorganism grows on simple agar, but if the agar is fortified with lipid, yeast phase *P. orbiculare* are frequently recovered, whereas hyphal growth is uncommon. There

Table 107-3. *Comparison of Fundamental Types of Dermatophyte Infection*

	Types of Infection	
Parameters	ACUTE	CHRONIC
Inflammation	4+	1+
Depth of invasion	Stratum corneum	Stratum corneum
Symptoms	Vesiculation, oozing tenderness	Pruritus, fissures, scaling
Area of infection	Localized	Extensive
Microscopic examination	+ → ±	4+
Culture	+ → ±	+
Clinical course	Short	Chronic
Response to therapy	Excellent	Poor
Immune response	CMI	None or IgE ± CMI

appear to be qualititative/quantitative requirements for lipid that are important in pathogenesis.

In pityriasis versicolor, colonization is poorly understood, and even less is known of the host–parasite interaction. Inflammation never progresses to the vesicular or pustular stage; if immunologic reactivity exists, it is low grade.

The pathogenesis of the clinical lesions is obscure. Inflammation, manifested as mild erythema and scaling, is the most common finding. Pigmentary changes may be dramatic. Some unidentified substance produced by the organism may affect melanogenesis, causing either hypo- or hyperpigmentation. The accumulation of organismal bulk and debris in follicules can produce small keratotic papules.

Endogenous and exogenous glucosteroids, as well as the application of certain natural lipids to the skin, predispose to tinea versicolor.

CANDIDOSIS

The pathogenesis of candidal cutaneous lesions, unlike dermatophytosis, cannot be clearly divided into a colonization and a host–parasite interaction phase. Colonization occurs rapidly. Previously uninfected neonatal mice develop lesions within hours after inoculation of *C. albicans* onto their skin. This alone indicates that immune reactivity does not produce the lesions because there was insufficient time to permit sensitization. The lesions are apparently produced by host–parasite interactions that involve complement fixation but do not require specific antibody or T cells.

In neonatal mouse skin, the hyphal tips penetrate the depths of the stratum corneum, if not the living cell layers. Apparently, within the viable epidermis, hyphal penetration causes alternative pathway fixation of complement (zymosan effect) that results in chemotaxis of polymorphonuclear leukocytes. This mechanism nicely explains the formation of pustules, so characteristic of certain types of candidosis.

The role of cellular immunity, the mononuclear phagocyte, antibody,and transferrin in the pathogenesis of the clinical lesions and host resistance to *Candida* spp. remains to be clarified. The elegant neonatal mouse studies have not been extended to humans. Deficiencies of CMI are common in patients with chronic mucocutaneous candidosis; that is, this host defense mechanism may be of some value in limiting candidal invasion. CMI defenses may be important for intracellular killing of the fungi.

Certain conditions predispose to candidosis, Obesity, wetness, maceration, antibacterial therapy, and cellular immune deficiency are examples.

Manifestations

Dermatophytes

Clinical manifestations of dermatophytosis may be classified according to the anatomic site infected, the source of the pathogen, for example, zoophilic, or the specific immune status of the host (Table 107-3). The intensity of the host CMI response to soluble dermatophyte antigen determines the intensity of inflammation in infected skin, and in large part determines the outcome of the host–parasite struggle.

TINEA PEDIS

The feet are infected with dermatophytes more frequently than any other anatomic area. Infection occurs on the skin of the interdigital web space and on the plantar skin. Dermatophyte infection of the web spaces must be differentiated from the more common athlete's foot syndrome, which consists of intertrigo and mixed infection by several kinds of bacteria. Minimal dermatophytosis of the third and fourth interdigital web space is common, transient but frequently recurrent, and often of the acutely inflammatory. Trichophyton rubrum, T. mentagrophytes, or *E. floccosum* are usually isolated from web space infections.

Dermatophytosis of plantar skin may be either acute and inflammatory or chronic and noninflammatory. The acute type is characterized by focal involvement with inflammatory vesicles and even bullae. Noninflammatory dermatophytosis of the plantar skin is characterized by contiguous involvement in a so-called sandal distribution. The majority of chronically infected patients will have this type of infection. It is an extremely chronic, minimally to moderately inflammatory, hyperkeratotic, scaly process. This kind of infection is extremely difficult to eradicate, probably because of the deficiency of dermatophyte-specific CMI. *Trichophyton rubrum* is usually isolated; however, *T. mentagrophytes* or *E. floccosum* may be recovered in some patients.

TINEA CRURIS

Infection of the groin is also very common. Tinea cruris is often asymmetric with a raised vesicular, actively progressing border that extends beyond the edges of the area of skin-to-skin contact. The skin of the thigh is almost always involved, yet the adjacent scrotal skin remains free of dermatophyte infection. This is in contrast to candidal infection of the same region in which the scrotal skin is not spared. *Trichophyton rubrum* and *E. floccosum* are most frequently isolated from crural dermatophytosis.

TINEA UNGUIUM

Tinea of the nails (onychomycosis) sometimes occurs alone, but there is often involvement of the skin adjacent to the nails. The tip of the nail is affected first. The process, as caused by dermatophytes, slowly moves proximally, causing loss of luster, discoloration, and an accumulaiton between the nail and its bed of dry detritus that resembles sawdust. *Trichophyton rubrum* is commonly isolated.

TINEA CORPORIS

Clinically, each spot begins as an invisible colony that spreads peripherally to form a disk, then a ring of visible inflammation with a healing center—hence, the name ringworm. The involved skin is scaly, erythematous, often vesicular, and even pustular. Itching is usually bothersome. In some patients, invasion of follicles leads to formation of papules, pustules, and abscesses (Majocchi type infection) that may be persistent.

TINEA MANUUM

Isolated infection of the palmar skin is uncommon unless the feet are also infected. When this occurs, the infection is almost always the chronic noninflammatory type. Often, both feet and only one hand are infected in a stabilized state that may persist for decades without the other hand becoming colonized. Obviously, local conditions and not the immunologic state are responsible for the enigma of this two-foot, one-hand syndrome.

TINEA CAPITIS

At present, tinea capitis is one of the least common types of dermatophytosis. Fungal infections of the scalp occur in several different clinical types, each of which is usually, though not invariably, caused by its own species (or group of species) of dermatophyte (Table 107-1).

The noninflammatory, childhood type of tinea capitis is now usually caused by *Trichophyton tonsurans.* A few years ago, *Microsporum auduinii* accounted for more than 90% of all scalp infections, but it is now only rarely isolated from tinea capitis. The inflammatory type of tinea capitis is caused most often by *Microsporum canis.* The clinical picture is similar to that of the noninflammatory, childhood form except that inflammation is found in every conceivable degree from mild reactions to the formation of extensive, subcutaneous abscesses called kerions.

DERMATOPHYTIDS

The concept of dermatophytids is well established in dermatology. Ids are sterile, allergic manifestations of dermatophytosis that occur at sites remote to the focus of infection. They can be predicted and related in a given patient to the type of specific immune response that is present (*i.e.,* CMI or IgE-mediated). Ids can be reproduced experimentally with sterile dermatophyte antigen.

Nondermatophytes

PITYRIASIS VERSICOLOR

Little anatomic change in the skin results from infection with *P. orbiculare,* although erythema is occasionally evident. Pruritus or burning are the only manifestations, aside from the pigmentary disturbance. An unsightly mottled appearance of the skin is the usual reason for seeking medical aid. The round or oval scaling patches are prominent because they differ in color from the surrounding skin. The patches vary in size from a few millimeters to several centimeters and may be either hypopigmented or hyperpigmented. Sometimes both shades coexist in the same patient. Common locations are the upper portion of the trunk; the arms, shoulders, and lower face and neck. However, bizarre patterns may be present in uncommon locations.

CANDIDOSIS

The most common cutaneous manifestation of candidosis is transient intertriginous infection that is clinically similar to intertrigo. Moisture, maceration, and other complex ecologic effects of occlusion that occur where two skin surfaces are held in contact, for example, the gluteal cleft, are the setting for infection. Pustules are characteristic features of this form of candidosis. Drying of the involved area may be enough to clear such transient or incidental infections.

Mucosal infection and paronychia, two other incidental forms of candidosis are also quite common. Infants, patients receiving antimicrobics, and the aged often develop thrush—oropharyngeal mucosal candidosis that commonly involves the tongue and buccal mucosa. In older persons, there is frequently involvement at the angles of the mouth (perlèche). Vaginitis, the other common form of mucosal candidosis, is a common complication of antimicrobic therapy. There is often local spread with the development of intertriginous infection. Paronychia is often seen in persons who must frequently wet their fingers. Often onycholysis also involves the same nail.

Chronic mucocutaneous candidosis (CMC) is not incidental or transient in nature but occurs in persons with defects in their immunologic defenses (principally CMI). The clinical pathology is severe, and without therapy the disease remains stabilized for years. Involvement occurs in the same areas that are prone to develop incidental candidosis. In addition, the glabrous skin may be involved in this granulomatous process. In many patients, the lesions are hyperkeratotic and verrucous. The vocal cords and esophagus are commonly involved. Scarring of the oral cavity and esophagus is common.

Diagnosis

Clinical diagnosis of superficial fungal infections hinges, as in all dermatologic diagnosis, on observation of the morphology of individual lesions and delineation of the anatomic distribution of the infection. Many, but not all, superficial fungal infections can be recognized by an experienced dermatologist on clinical grounds alone. Several skin conditions can closely resemble mycotic infection. Secondary syphilis (Chap. 59, Syphilis), pityriasis rosea, psoriasis, nummular eczema, lichen planus, alopecia areata, trichotillomania, dyshidrosis, and contact dermatitis are the most commonly encountered, confusing disorders.

Differentiation of superficial fungal infections from these nonfungal dermatoses is made easy by demonstration or culture of the mycotic agent. The microscopic examination of potassium hydroxide(KOH)-treated skin scales from a lesion usually resolves the differential diagnosis. The dermatophytes, and *P. orbiculare* can be distinguished with this technique (Fig. 107-1*A, B, C* and Table 107-1). Candidas may grow in tissues as hyphae that are devoid of spores and indistinguishable from dermatophytic hyphae. Definite distinction between candidas and dermatophytes using only the KOH smear is impossible; culture may be necessary to distinguish the candidas from the dermatophytes. Speciation of *Candida* and the dermatophytes is more difficult (see Etiology).

Prognosis

Superficial fungua infections may cause considerable morbidity, but they have little potential for mortality. The infections do, however, disfigure, cause discomfort, and cause considerable medical costs. The septic form of candidosis is a threat to life. Some of the dermatophytes have been reported to be rare causes of death.

Noninflammatory dermatophyte infection (Table 107-3) and chronic mucocutaneous candidosis (CMC), regardless of the anatomic sites infected, have no tendency to heal spontaneously. Even with the appropriate antifungal therapy, the prognosis is guarded because the underlying immune defect that predisposes to infection persists and will, if not corrected, foster reinfection or relapse.

Therapy

Once the nonfungal dermatoses have been eliminated from the differential diagnosis and the mycotic etiology of the lesion is satisfactorily established, appropriate therapy can be instituted. A few general rules of cutaneous therapy must be observed. The state of the infected skin must be considered. For example, an acutely inflamed denuded area or infection near the eye, genitalia, or anal area cannot be treated with strong or irritating topical medications. Secondary pyogenic infection must be controlled. Inflammatory infections on dependent portions of the body (*e.g.,* lower legs and feet) must be elevated to promote healing.

Dermatophytosis

Essential to the treatment of a dermatophytosis is recognition of the clinical–anatomic syndrome afflicting the patient, and recognition of the natural course of that particular form of disease. The concepts portrayed in Figure 107-3 must also be considered. Acute, highly inflamed infections have a tendency to heal spontaneously. Minimally inflamed infections tend to be chronic and require more aggressive therapy. Thus, if spontaneous healing can be predicted and especially if evidence of healing is already evident, then potentially irritating, expensive topical or oral medications can be avoided.

If specific antifungal therapy is deemed necessary, it is important to select the best antifungal agent, a formulation appropriate to the clinical-anatomic syndrome to be treated, and a method of application that will achieve the desired therapeutic effect. There are numerous topical antifungal agents and formulations, some available over the counter and others requiring a prescription. Whitfield's ointment, one of the original topical antifungal preparations, has survived the test of time to become a standard against which other topical antifungal agents are compared. Although tolnaftate is quite potent by assays *in virto,* it has not proven to be highly effective in treating infected patients. Haloprogin appears to be as effective as tolnaftate and has the added advantage of being active against *C. albicans.*

In recent years, miconazole and clotrimazole have both been found to be more effective topical agents for treating dermatophytosis. In addition, each is active against *C. albicans* and *P. orbiculare,* which makes these two imidazoles the most versatile of the topical antifungal agents. They are available in several formulations for use in different anatomic areas. Minimally inflamed, extensive dermatophytic infections of the feet, glabrous skin, or scalp are best treated by topical application of either clotrimazole or miconazole. When these infections are extremely hyperkeratotic, keratolytics or debriding agents such as vitamin A acid, urea, or salicylic acid may be helpful if used judiciously in conjunction with topical imidazole. If the topical treatment fails, then systemic therapy, such as peroral griseofulvin, should be added to the therapeutic regimen.

Extensive infection, failure to respond to topical therapy, or adverse effects from the application of a topical formulation warrants systemic therapy. Also, systemic therapy, with or without topical treatment, may be justified in certain acute, inflammatory infections, especially those accompanied by an id eruption. The inflammatory kerion of tinea capitis is an example. When the kerion is accompanied by a dermatophytid eruption, systemic peroral antifungal therapy is indicated. In addition, such patients may benefit from a short course of glucosteroids for symptomatic control of the generalized allergic dermatitis.

Griseofulvin, the first orally effective antifungal antimicrobic, was introduced in 1958. It was found to be of great value in treating tinea capitis, especially in epidemics among children. Initially, the dosage of griseofulvin was 1000 mg/day for an adult. Subsequently, griseofulvin became available in a microsize particle form and more recently, in an ultramicrosize form that facilitates absorption. Consequently, it has been possible to reduce the daily dosage for an adult to approximately 250 mg of the ultramicrosize form of griseofulvin. For patients whose infections do not respond, the dosage may be increased to 1000 mg (or more) per day, provided there are no adverse reactions.

However, there are clinical failures even when aggressive treatment with griseofulvin is supplemented with topical therapy in the clinical–anatomic syndromes of erythrodermic, hyperkeratotic, moccasin tinea pedis; the dry, scaling type of tinea capitis; extensive tinea corporis; tinea manuum; and tinea unguium—especially when the toenails are affected. These infections are all minimally inflamed, usually quite extensive, and characterized by a chronic or relapsing course. With better understanding of the immunology of dermatophytosis, it has become clear that these patients have defective host resistance. In addition, failures to respond to treatment with griseofulvin appear to correlate with relative resistance according to testing *in vitro.* However, absolute resistance may occur since some isolates grow in 18 mg/ml of griseofulvin, the upper limit of solubility in aqueous culture mediums. The molecular basis of the resistance of dermatophytes to griseofulvin is unknown, but it may involve demethylation of the drug.

Griseofulvin is delivered into the keratinized and cornified layers of the skin, hair, and nails by two separate routes: (1) from the blood to the tissues that generate keratinizing tissues and (2) from eccrine sweat (*i.e.,* stratum corneum wherever there are eccrine sweat glands). In instances of relative griseofulvin resistance, the delivery of griseofulvin into the stratum corneum may be aided by augmenting sweating and promoting evaporation by exposure to warm, dry air. This process enhances the concentration of griseofulvin in the stratum corneum and may, in some instances of relative resistance, contribute to therapeutic success. Considering that griseofulvin is delivered to the stratum corneum by means of eccrine sweat, it is an enigma why the drug is not equally efficacious when applied topically.

The results of clinical trials with ketoconazole have created considerable interest in this agent. Ketoconazole is an imidazole derivative that differs from predecessor drugs such as clotrimazole and miconazole in being soluble in water, and absorbed from the gastrointestinal tract. After peroral administration, the concentrations of ketoconazole in the blood exceed the minimal inhibitory concentration for many of the pathogenic fungi. Apparently, there is no induction of degradative microsomal enzymes in the liver, as occurred with clotrimazole.

Ketoconazole is effective in all the superficial fungal infections and is promising in many systemic, deep fungal infections. For dermatophytosis, the most compelling evidence of efficacy is the demonstration of microbial and clinical clearing of extensive cutaneous infections that had been present for decades despite aggressive treatment with griseofulvin and topical agents. Even in the difficult problem of tinea unguium, a dermatophytosis in which topical preparations are ineffective, ketoconazole appears to be at least as effective as griseofulvin. Ketoconazole, given in a dose of 200 mg to 400 mg/day for periods as long as 2 years, appears to be well tolerated. In view of the broad spectrum, peroral administration, and efficacy, ketoconazole holds promise for the treatment of dermatophytic, and possibly other, mycoses. Ketoconazole-associated hepatotoxicity has been observed in approximately 30 patients (1 in 5,000–10,000 treated patients). Apparently, the hepatotoxicity is idiosyncratic and is reversible if early changes in hepatic enzymes are heeded by stopping treatment.

Nondermatophyte Infections

PITYRIASIS VERSICOLOR

Although not difficult to treat, infections caused by *P. orbiculare* are frequently recurrent, particularly in the susceptible person who resides in a warm, moist climate. A host of topical agents can be used. Selenium sulfide has produced good results; however, it may cause irritation of the skin in the body folds and should be avoided in those areas. One or two overnight applications to the affected area per week for 4 weeks produces clearing. Several weeks or months may be required for the pigmentation to return to normal. Infections that do not respond to selenium sulfide may be treated with miconazole nitrate or clotrimazole; however, the cost of therapy is greater and recurrences are frequent. Ketoconazole appears to be effective in the treatment of pityriasis versicolor but its role, if any, has not been delineated.

CANDIDOSIS

Incidental candidal infections usually respond to general supportive measures (especially drying of the area) and specific topical therapy. Nystatin has been the drug of choice, although amphotericin B has also been used topically with equally good results. Recently, miconazole cream has won wide acclaim in treating candidal vaginitis. Topically applied clotrimazole has also been reported to be effective in candidal infections.

The therapeutic problem presented by chronic mucocutaneous candidosis is complex and difficult. Systemic antifungal therapy is essential, but unless immunocompetence is restored recurrences are common. Furthermore, parenteral therapy with amphotericin B is plagued by problems of serious toxicity that may necessitate the termination of treatment (see Chap. 39, Candidosis). The administration of transfer factor is experimental, not readily available, and of unproved efficacy. Trials using miconazole by intravenous injection appear to be promising from the point of view of efficacy, but this drug also has several side-effects. Ketoconazole appears to offer distinct advantages over IV administration of miconazole or amphotericin B as the antifungal of choice in the treatment of chronic mucocutaneous candidosis. Ketoconazole also appears to be effective in candidal vaginitis and other forms of candidal infection.

Prevention

Because superficial fungal infections are located on the body surface, there are no barriers preventing the access of pathogens to the stratum corneum. Given the pathogen and the appropriate microenvironment, colonization will occur. This can only be prevented if an inhibitory concentration of an appropriate antifungal is present over the entire surface of the body. That is, prevention does not appear to be feasible.

Remaining Problems

The host resistance mechanisms operative in defense of the skin against *Candida* spp., *P. orbiculare,* and the dermatophytes must be better understood. Some of these mechanisms are nonspecific and others are immunologically specific. Investigations with the dermatophytes and dermatophytosis in humans indicate that acquire immunity of the cell-mediated type is critical to intact skin defense. It may be of value to mobilize cell-mediated defenses by means of an immunization program, to prevent or ameliorate dermatophytosis.

Bibliography

Books

HILDICK–SMITH G, BLANK H: Fungus Diseases and their Treatment. Boston, Little, Brown, 1964. 494 pp.

JOHNSON M–LT: Skin Conditions and Related Need for Medical Care Among Persons 1–74 Years. U. S. Dept. HEW, Series 11, #212, DHEW Pub. # (PHS) 79-1660, November, 1978. 72 pp.

JUNGERMAN PF, SCHWARTZMAN RM: Veterinary Medical Mycology. Philadelphia, Lea & Febiger, 1972. 200 pp.

RIPPON JW: Medical Mycology: The Pathogenic Fungi and the Pathogenic Actinomycetes. Philadelphia, WB Saunders, 1974. 587 pp.

WILSON JW, PLUNKETT OA: The Fungus Diseases of Man. Berkeley, University of California, 1965. 428 pp.

Journals

AJELLO L: Natural history of the dermatophytes and related fungi. Mycopathol Mycol Appl 53:93–110, 1974

ARTIS WM, JONES HE: The effect of human lymphokine on the growth of *Trichophyton mentagrophytes.* J Invest Dermatol 74:131–134, 1980

ARTIS WM, ODLE B, JONES HE: Griseofulvin-resistant dermatophytosis correlates with *in vitro* resistance. Arch Dermatol 117:16–19, 1981

FAERGEMANN J: Experimental tinea versicolor in rabbits and humans with *Pityrisporon orbiculare.* J Invest Dermatol 72:326–329, June, 1979

GRAPPEL SF, BISHOP CT, BLACK F: Immunology of dermatophytes and dermatophytosis. Bacteriol Rev 38:222–250, 1974

GRAYBILL JR, HERNDON JH, JR, KNIKER WT, LEVINE HB: Ketoconazole treatment of chronic mucocutaneous candidiasis. Arch Dermatol 116(10):1137–1142, 1980

GREEN F, III, BALISH EE: *Trichophyton mentagrophytes* dermatophytosis in germfree guinea pigs. J Invest Dermatol 75:475–480, 1980

HAY RJ: Failure of treatment in chronic dermatophyte infections. Postgrad Med J 55:608–610, 1979

JONES HE: The atopic-chronic-dermatophytosis syndrome. Acta Dermatol 92:81–85, 1980

JONES HE, REINHARDT JH, RINALDI MG: Acquired immunity to dermatophytes. Arch Dermatol 109:840–848, 1974

JONES HE, REINHARDT JH, RINALDI MG: Immunologic susceptibility to chronic dermatophytosis. Arch Dermatol 110: 213–220, 1974

JONES HE, REINHARDT JH, RINALDI MG: Model dermatophytosis in naturally infected subjects. Arch Dermatol 110:369–374, 1974

JONES HE, SIMPSON JG, ARTIS WM: Ketoconazole (R41400): An effective oral agent against cutaneous mycotic infections. Arch Dermatol 117:129–134, 1981

KING RD, KHAN HA, FOYE JC, GREENBERG JH, JONES HE: Transferrin, iron and dermatophytes. I. Serum dermatophyte inhibitory component definitely identified as unsaturated transferrin. J Lab Clin Med 86:204–212, 1975

LEPPER AWD: Immunologic aspects of dermatomycoses in animals and man. Rev Med Vet Mycol 6:435–446, 1969

RASMUSSEN JE, AHMED AR: Trichophytin reactions in children with tinea capitis. Arch Dermatol 114:371–372, 1978

RAY TL, WUEPPER KD: Recent advances in cutaneous candidiasis. Int J Dermatol 17:683–690, 1978

RESTREPO A, STEVENS DA, UTZ JP, ET AL: Progress report on ketoconazole. Rev Infect Dis 2(4):519–699, 1980

ROBERTS SOB: Pityriasis versicolor: A clinical and mycological investigation. Br J Dermatol 81:315–326, 1969

SHAH VP, EPSTEIN WL, RIEGELMAN S: Role of sweat in accumulation of orally administered griseofulvin in skin. J Clin Invest 53:1673–1678, 1974

ZAIAS N: Onychomycosis. Arch Dermatol 105:263–274, 1972

JOHN P. UTZ

Sporotrichosis

108

Sporotrichosis is a systemic infectious disease caused by the fungus *Sporothrix (Sporotrichum) schenckii.* Generally, acquisition by accidental implantation of the fungus into the skin results in a chronic, benign, cutaneous-lymphatic disease. In some patients, more widespread diseases, such as infectious polyarthritis or pneumonia, occur with out the distinctive skin lesions.

Etiology

Sporothrix schenckii is a fungus that exists in two forms. In tissues it is either a round (8 μm in diameter), or a cigar-shaped (2 × 8 μm) yeast. On appropriate culture mediums (*e.g.,* Sabouraud's glucose agar) at 30°C, it forms a mold (mycelium) with a mixture of vivid colors from white to yellow to black. Microscopically, the mold is composed of septate filaments (hyphae) that measure approximately 2 μm in diameter. Slender conidiophores branch off hyphae at right angles to bear multiple oval conidia that are 2 μm to 4 μm × 2 μm to 6 μm (Fig. 108-1).

Sporothrix schenckii are not known to elaborate toxins, enzymes, or chemicals that produce disease. However, after intraperitoneal injection into the male mouse, orchitis develops within 10 days. Isolates that grow at 37°C are associated with more progressive disease in humans and disseminate more frequently in experimental infections in mice.

Epidemiology

Sporotrichosis is worldwide in distribution. There was an historic outbreak, to the extent of almost 3000 cases, in the gold mines of Witwatersrand, South Africa in the 1940s. France has been labeled "a land of endemic sporotrichosis," and in Mexico sporotrichosis is the most common systemic or subcutaneous mycosis. In Louisiana, according to delayed cutaneous hypersensitivity testing, the frequency of positive reactions was far greater in nursery workers with more than 10 years' experience (58%) than in prison inmates and hospital patients (11%).

Sporothrix schenckii grows best at a temperature of 26°C to 27°C and at a relative humidity of 92% to 100%. Hence, it is not surprising that the fungus is readily isolated from soil, decaying vegetation, gardening supplies such as sphagnum moss, and the timbers in mines. The mode of entry is almost always by accidental implantation into the skin by a thorn from a barberry or rose bush, or by a vocational or avocational injury. In some instances, infection has occurred through the respiratory tract.

Because infections caused by *S. schenckii* are not encountered in patients who have had renal transplants or in patients with leukemias or other malignant neoplasms, it is not recognized as an opportunistic microorganism. Patients with compromised defense mechanisms are in no way immune to sporotrichosis; rather, they have a minimal risk of accidental inoculation with *S. schenckii.*

Pathogenesis and Pathology

Cutaneous inoculation of *S. schenckii* can occur in minor or unrecognized injuries. Sometime later, a small ulcer or subcutaneous nodule appears, usually with erythema and fluctuance. Secondary nodules develop to mark the course of lymphatic spread.

The response of the body to *S. schenckii* is both suppurative and granulomatous. Microabscesses, surrounded by lymphocytes and plasma cells are present. In nearby areas, there are also nodular lesions consisting of central necrotic tissue with a few neutrophils, eosinophils, and monocytes. Surrounding the necrotic area are epithelioid cells and occasional Langhans' giant cells. Peripheral fibrosis, increased

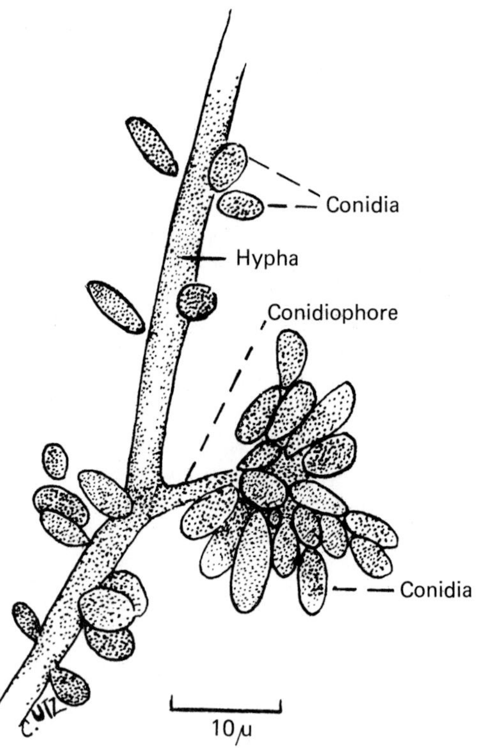

Fig. 108-1. Vegetative form of *Sporothrix schenckii.*

vascularization, lymphocytes, and plasma cells complete the picture.

The asteroid body, also seen in coccidioidomycosis and aspergillosis, is a striking histologic feature of sporotrichosis. The lesion is about 10 μm in diameter and is characterized by amorphous eosinophilic material radiating from a central fungal cell; it is attributed by some workers to an antigen–antibody reaction.

Manifestations

Although interrelationships are not clarified, it is possible to discern three rather distinct forms of sporotrichosis.

Cutaneous-Lymphatic Form

Characteristically, the lesions of sporotrichosis occur on the upper extremity, usually beginning on the hand or finger (Fig. 108-2). Neither drainage, local therapy, nor systemic antibacterial treatment has any remarkable effect on the initial lesion. As multiple subcutaneous nodules appear along the course of the draining lymphatics, they may become discolored and drain spontaneously. Occasionally, cordlike lesions can be palpated between these nodules (Fig. 108-3). Quite in contrast with the bacterial pyogenic lymphangitides, cutaneous-lymphatic sporotrichosis causes little pain, disability, or systemic manifestations of illness. Indeed, most patients continue their usual activities.

Pulmonary Form

Of about 40 patients reported to have pulmonary sporotrichosis, only a few have had other foci of disease. In all but two, cough and sputum production have been the most prominent symptoms; fever or other evidence of sepsis has been absent. The range of pulmonary lesions includes cavities, hilar adenopathy, pleural effusion, nodules, fibrosis, and even a fungus ball. Tuberculosis or sarcoidosis were underlying diseases in many patients. Also, some patients were greenhouse laborers, gardeners, or vegetable produce workers.

Fig. 108-2. The cutaneous-lymphatic form of sporotrichosis with indurated, reddened, crusted, draining lesions (primary on finger, secondary on dorsum of the hand).

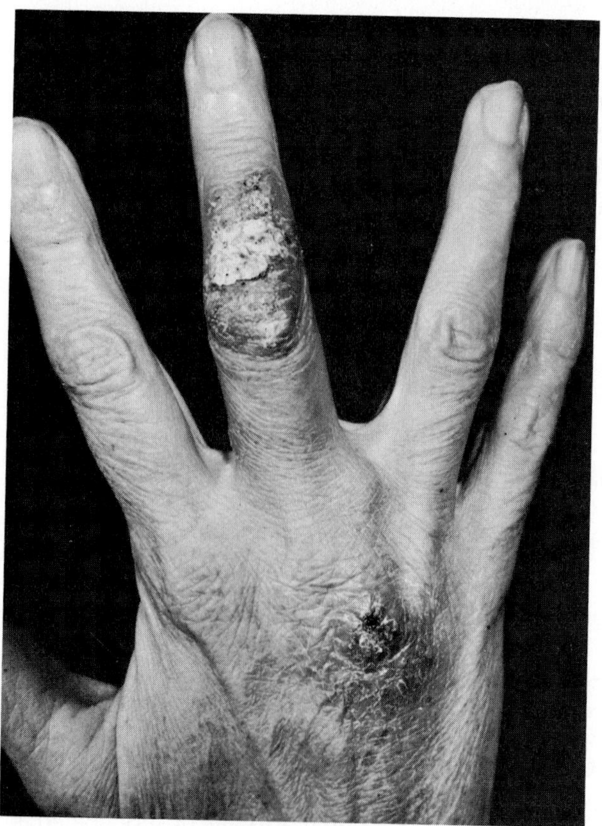

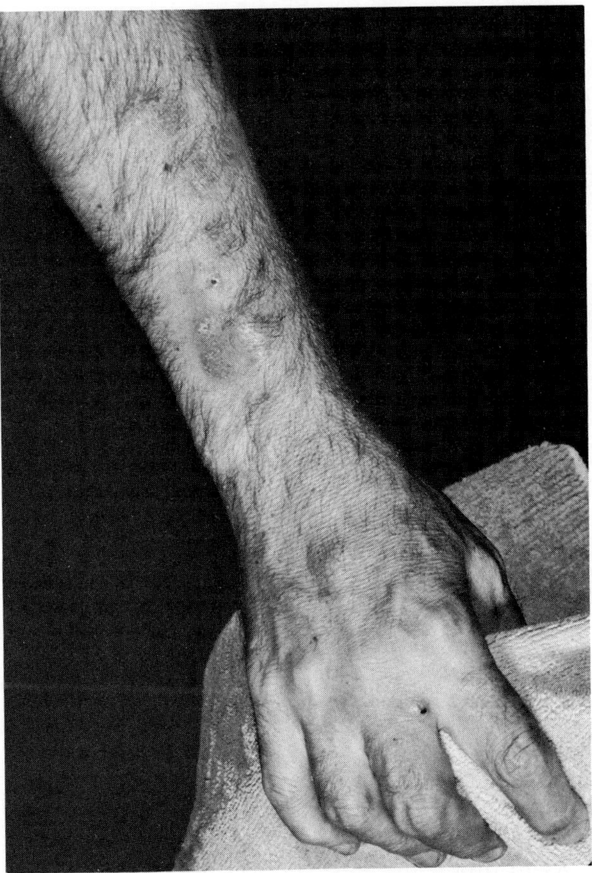

Fig. 108-3. Cutaneous-lymphatic form of sporotrichosis with multiple lymphatic lesions. Involvement of the web of the second and third fingers, the dorsum of the hand, and the forearm was secondary to a primary cutaneous lesion (not visible) on the ventral surface over the middle phalanx of the third finger.

Disseminated Form

In one study of 30 patients with sporotrichosis, there were multifocal lesions consistent with hematogenous dissemination. The disease may have spread from the skin in most of these patients, and in one instance, from the lung. However, in at least six patients, the mode of entry of the fungus was not clear. Eighty percent had synovial or bony lesions.

The onset of disease is usually insidious; in most patients, anorexia and weight loss are evidence of a chronic illness. Signs of acute sepsis—fever, shaking chills, night sweats, and delirium—are characteristically lacking. Similarly, leukocytosis is either absent or only mild. Bone (in descending order of frequency of involvement: metacarpal, phalangeal, and tibial), periosteum, and synovium were involved in approximately 80% of patients with dissemination (Fig. 108-4). Involvement of the eye may mimic ocular zygomycosis.

Diagnosis

All forms of sporotrichosis are unequivocally diagnosed by the isolation and identification in culture of the causative fungus, *S. schenckii.* Although frequently present in the environment, the fungus is virtually never a commensal of man. The presence of *S. schenckii* in the sputum, pus, or drainage from bony lesions is evidence of a causative relationship. On rare occasions, the fungus has been isolated from the blood, bone marrow, and cerebrospinal fluid.

Histopathologic diagnosis is difficult in sporotrichosis, unlike other systemic fungus disease. Only occasionally are the characteristic oval to cigar-shaped, yeast-phase cells of *S. schenckii* found in human tissues by using the Gridley stain (see Chap. 9, Microscopic Examinations). Although the asteroid body is highly indicative, many sections may have to be cut and studied before even one can be found.

Immunologic methods, for example, the application of delayed cutaneous hypersensitivity, and serologic tests, are at present purely research tools.

The classic form of cutaneous-lymphatic sporotrichosis can virtually always be diagnosed at sight. Nevertheless, it is surprising how long patients may be followed by a physician before a specimen is obtained and cultured for fungi. If multiple cutaneous blastomycotic lesions occur in proper alignment, the disease might be misdiagnosed until the fungus is cultured. The photochromogenic *Mycobacterium marinum* (see Chap. 36, Nontuberculous Mycobacterioses) may spread from a cutaneous site of inoculation, for example, a finger, through the lymphatics to give a clinical picture that is identical with that of cutaneous-lymphatic sporotrichosis. Only rarely do bacterial diseases (*e.g.,* tularemia and staphylococcal lymphangitis) run so prolonged a course.

Virtually all patients with pulmonary sporotrichosis are suspected of having tuberculosis. Sarcoidosis and other fungal infections also mimic the pulmonary form of sporotrichosis.

Disseminated sporotrichosis resembles tuberculosis, osteomyelitis, and neoplasia.

Prognosis

Death from sporotrichosis is uncommon. The course of all forms of the disease is so slow that diagnosis and

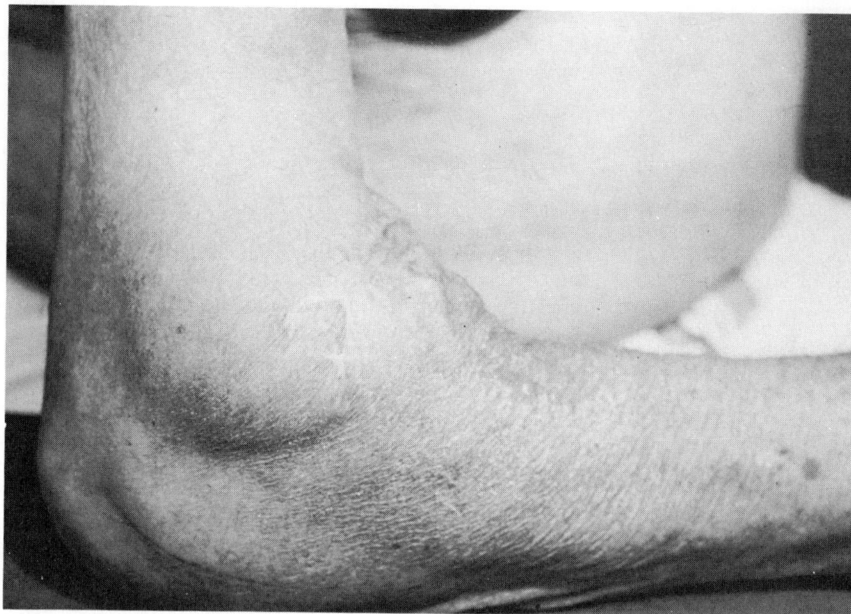

Fig. 108-4. The disseminated form of sporotrichosis with cystic multiloculated lesions of the lateral and antecubital space, contiguous to the synovium of the elbow. A similar lesion was present in the knee.

therapy are virtually always possible. The manifestations of sporotrichosis are usually striking and cause the patient to seek medical attention. Although it is clear that in some patients the disease has worsened or spread, there has been no consistent pattern of progression from one form to another. Relatively little is known about the immune status of patients. However, cutaneous-lymphatic disease almost never relapses, whereas new lesions may appear after otherwise successful therapy in disseminated disease.

Therapy

The cutaneous-lymphatic form of sporotrichosis virtually always responds to potassium iodide therapy; pulmonary and disseminated diseases are only occasionally benefited. A saturated solution (1 g/ml) of potassium iodide is given in a dosage of 9 g to 12 g/day (3 g–4 g every 8 hours). Treatment should be continued for 1 month after the disappearance of cutaneous lesions or after the stabilization of pulmonary or disseminated lesions. Adverse effects of iodine therapy include nausea, vomiting, parotid swelling, acneiform rash, coryza, sneezing, swelling of the eyelids, and occasionally, depression. Most of these side-effects can be controlled by stopping the drug for a few days and reinstituting therapy at a slightly reduced dosage.

When iodide therapy fails, amphotericin B is recommended. Details regarding the use of amphotericin B are given in Chapter 39, Candidosis. Total doses of 1.5 g to 2.5 g have been employed. There is no reported experience with the low daily dose, 10-week regimen. The aromatic diamidines (*e.g.,* hydroxystilbamidine isethionate) are not recommended. It is possible that ketoconazole will be of value.

As in other mycoses, surgical drainage of osteomyelitic and synovial lesions is occasionally of crucial therapeutic importance. In patients with cavitary pulmonary lesions, surgical resection has been curative.

Prevention

Little work has been done on the preparation of vaccines in sporotrichosis. No work has been done on the control of the fungus in the environment.

Remaining Problems

In endemic areas, such as South Africa, France, and Mexico, the possible role of humidity and temperature remains to be investigated. The relationship of disseminated disease to inhalation of the fungus is not known.

In sporotrichosis, as in other fungal diseases, the striking association with sarcoidosis is a mystifying and unexplained phenomenon.

Sporothrix schenckii can grow in a 10% solution

of potassium iodide; why and how is potassium iodide therapeutically useful?

The selective involvement of bones and joints in disseminated sporotrichosis in man and in experimental infections in the mouse deserves further investigation. After immunization with a formalin-killed suspension of *S. schenckii,* mice resist subsequent challenge. Work with vaccines should continue.

Bibliography

Books

MARIAT F: The epidemiology of sporotrichosis. In Wolstenholme GEW, Porter R (eds): Systemic Mycoses. London, J & A Churchill, 1968. pp 144–159.

Journals

CROUT JE, BREWER NS, TOMPKINS RB: Sporotrichosis arthritis. Clinical features in seven patients. Ann Intern Med 86:294–297, 1977

KWON–CHUNG KJ: Comparison of isolates of *Sporothrix schenckii* obtained from fixed cutaneous lesions with isolates from other types of lesions. J Infect Dis 139:424–431, 1979

LURIE HI, STILL WGS: The "capsule" of *Sporotrichum schenckii* and the evolution of the asteroid body. Sabouraudia 7:64–70, 1969

MOHR JA, GRIFFITHS W, LONG H: Pulmonary sporotrichosis in Oklahoma and susceptibilities *in vitro.* Am Rev Resp Dis 119:961–964, 1979

WILSON DE, MANN GG, BENNETT GE, UTZ JP: Clinical features of extracutaneous sporotrichosis. Medicine 46:265–279, 1967

ROBERTO G. BARUZZI
LUIZ F. MARCOPITO

109 Jorge Lobo's Disease

Jorge's Lobo's disease (lobomycosis, Lobo's mycosis, keloidal blastomycosis), is a fungal disease of the New World. It is characterized by polymorphic cutaneous lesions without involvement of the mucosa or internal organs. It is a chronic disease with a slow evolution of fresh lesions.

Etiology

In 1931, the Brazilian physician, Jorge Lobo, examined a patient from the Amazon Basin who had nodular, confluent skin lesions over the lumbosacral region. On histologic examination of the lesions, a new fungus pathogenic for humans was detected which was named *Paracoccidioides loboi* on the basis of morphologic similarity to the etiologic agent of paracoccidioidomycosis (*Paracocidioides brasiliensis,* Chapter 42, Paracoccidioidomycosis). The name *Loboa loboi* was also proposed, and firm classification and definite nomenclature await cultivation and characterization of the fungus.

In the tissues, *P. loboi* are readily visible as round, birefringent, double-walled microorganisms measuring 5 μm to 12 μm in diameter. They are frequently disposed in small chains and are also present in much greater numbers than the fungi of paracoccidioidomycosis. Initially, it appeared that only humans were susceptible to natural infection with *P. loboi;* however, the fungus was found in lesions on the back and tail of a dolphin caught off the East Coast of Florida. The infection was successfully transmitted from dolphins to irradiated mice. Of experimental animals, the armadillo *(Euphractus sexcintus)* appears to be the most sensitive to infection by inoculation.

In the absence of specific antigen(s) for *P. loboi,* other fungal antigens, as obtained from *P. brasiliensis, Histoplasma capsulatum,* and *Blastomyces dermatitidis,* were used for serologic testing; the results were not of value. Skin tests with histoplasmin, sporotrichin, and leishmanin have not elicited significant differences in reactivity between cases and controls.

There appear to be no marked deficiencies in the cellular immune responses of the few patients studied to date. In addition to normal delayed skin test hypersensitivity with a variety of antigens, lymphocyte transformation in the presence of phytohemagglutinin is normal.

Epidemiology

Jorge Lobo's disease has been observed in whites, blacks, and American Indians. It is more common in males than in females. Persons working out doors in close contact with dense vegetation in areas of high temperature and humidity run a higher risk of contracting the disease, for example, farmers, rubber tappers, and prospectors.

Prior to 1981, a total of 213 cases of Jorge Lobo's disease were recorded. The geographic distribution was Brazil, 139; Surinam, 30; Venezuela, 13; French Guiana, 12; Colombia, 8; Panama, 5; Costa Rica, 4; Mexico, 1; and Peru, 1.

All the Brazilian cases were reported from the Amazon Region. A notably high incidence was observed among the Caiabi, a tribe of about 400 Indians living in Central Brazil, among whom 53 cases were reported from 1957 to 1981. It appears that Lobo's mycosis has been present among the Caiabi for a long time, because older Indians refer to the presence of the disease among their forefathers. Also, in 1915, an expedition crossing the former territory of the tribe noted and described skin lesions in many Indians which were probably Jorge Lobo's disease.

Apparently, human-to-human transmission of *P. loboi* does not occur, since no case has been documented in immediate family members. In spite of the high incidence in Caiabi Indians, there have been no cases of Jorge Lobo's disease in neighboring tribes.

Pathogenesis and Pathology

From observation of accidental and experimental inoculations in humans, the skin appears to be the portal of entry for the fungus. Some patients recall an initial skin insult (*e.g.,* an insect bite or trauma), but in view of the frequency of such injuries in the forest this is difficult to evaluate. However, the importance of local trauma favoring the entry of *P. loboi* gains credence from the observation that non-Indians who often carry burdens on their shoulders frequently have lobomycosis of the external ear, whereas Indians who carry nothing on their shoulders rarely have disease of the external ear.

The incubation period of lobomycosis appears to be long, perhaps 1 to 2 years, as is suggested by accidental and experimental inoculations in humans.

The immune response of the host to *P. loboi* appears to be variable, for patients may have disseminated skin lesions or only a small localized lesion. Dissemination may take place through the blood or by autoinoculation. Infection with *P. loboi* does not appear to alter the immune response to other agents.

Manifestations

The lesions of lobomycosis are virtually restricted to the skin; that is, infection of regional lymph nodes is

Fig. 109-1. Isolated lesion of Jorge Lobo's disease in two women from the Caiabi tribe (Central Brazil).

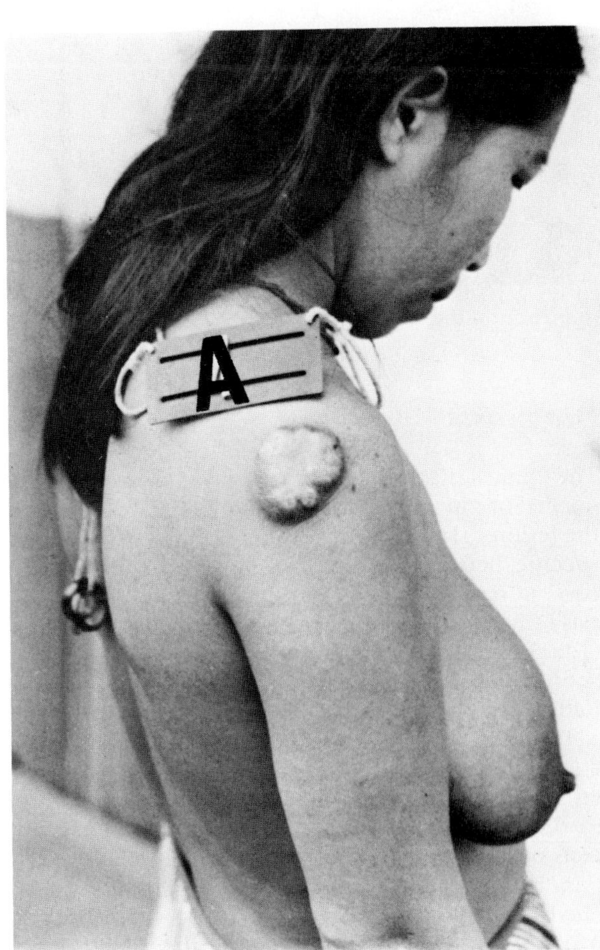

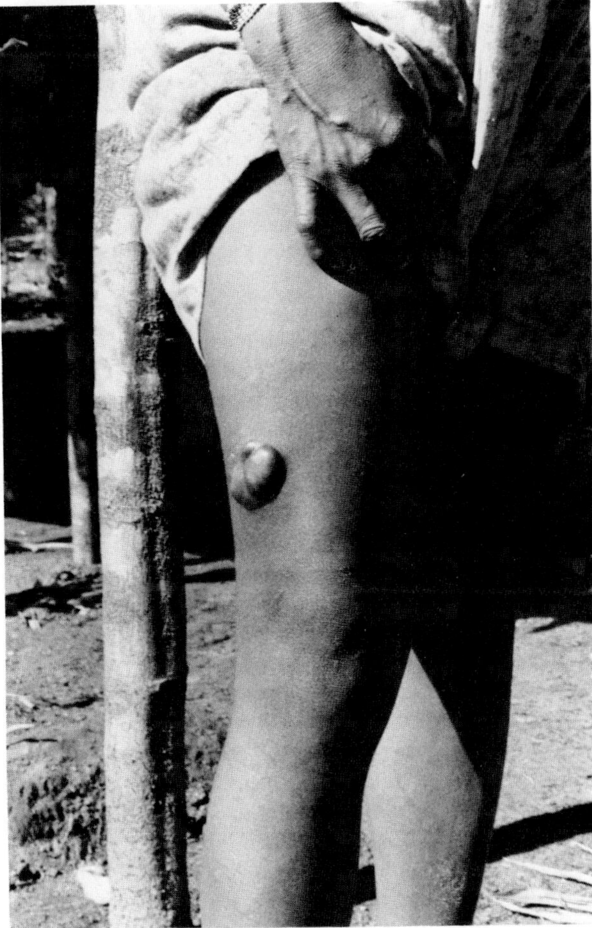

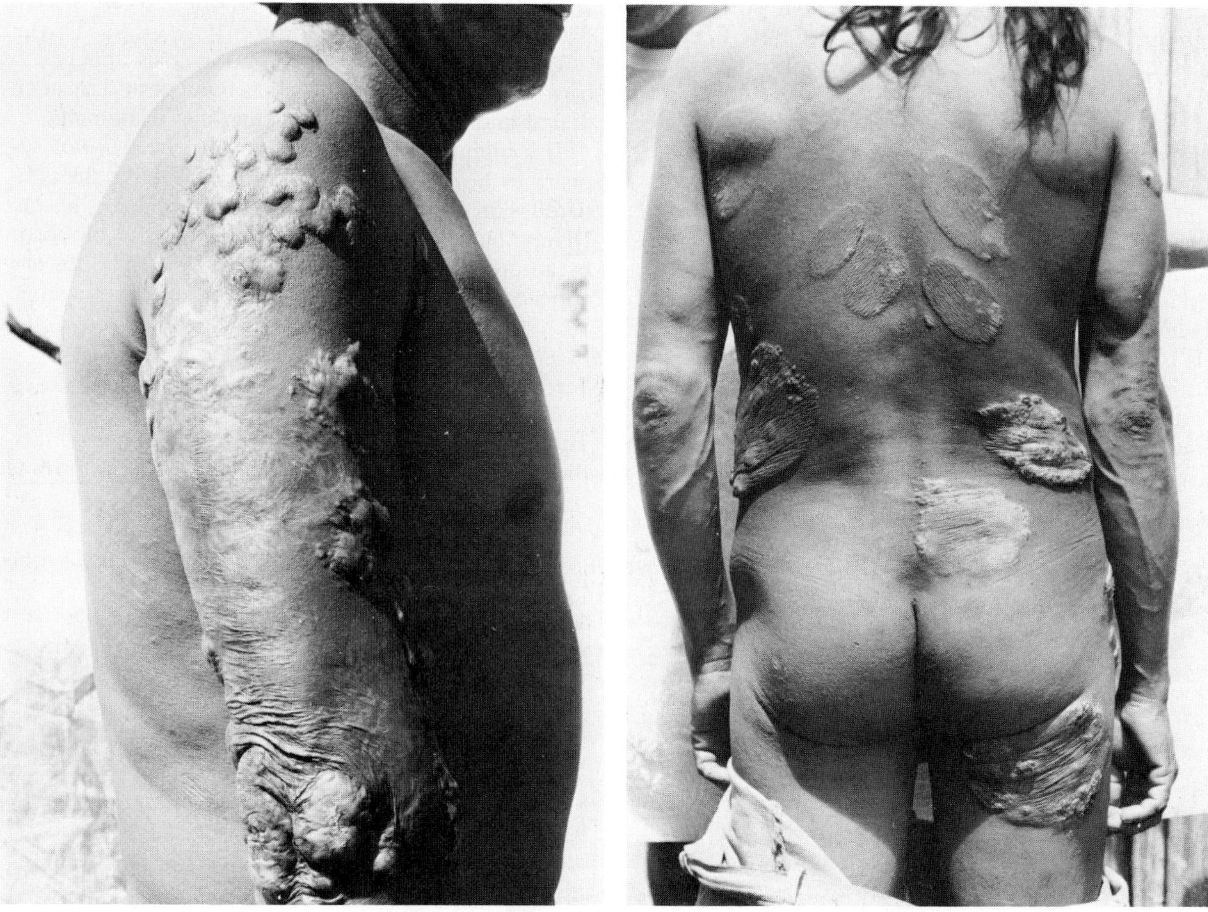

Fig. 109-2. Disseminated lesions of Jorge Lobo's disease in two men from the Caiabi tribe (Central Brazil).

extremely rare. Over many months a single lesion may spread locally to produce satellite lesions.

The lesions are polymorphic, and several different forms may be present at the same time in the same patient. The most common lesions are macules, papules, infiltrated plaques and hard, fibrotic nodules that resemble keloids. Fibrosis does not indicate healing, and in very fibrotic lesions the fungus is easily demonstrated. Rarer forms include gummatous, verrucous, and ulcerative skin lesions. With time, ulceration becomes increasingly common.

Various classifications of the skin lesions of lobomycosis have been proposed. Most useful is a simple, practical distinction between isolated lesions that may be removed surgically and disseminated disease (Figs. 109–1, 109–2).

The major complaints of lobomycosis are pain and itching referred to the lesions. The disease seems to be less severe in women.

Diagnosis

The clinical diagnosis of Jorge Lobo's disease is based on the origin of the patient and the appearance of the lesions. However, the lesions themselves are nonspecific, because they may resemble tuberculoid leprosy (Chap. 105, Leprosy), cutaneous leishmaniasis (Chap. 147, Leishmaniasis), chromblastomycosis (Chap. 110, Chromoblastomycosis), fibrosarcoma, sporotrichosis (Chap. 108, Sporotrichosis), or keloids.

The infection is localized deep in the dermis and the diagnosis is confirmed by skin biopsy which reveals a lesion rich in fungi. These fungi may be free in the tissues or enclosed in multinucleated giant cells or macrophages (Fig. 109-3). Often, the epithelium is intact although the dermal papillae are shortened. Polarized light, PAS, and Grocott's stain enhance definition of the parasite but the fungi can be

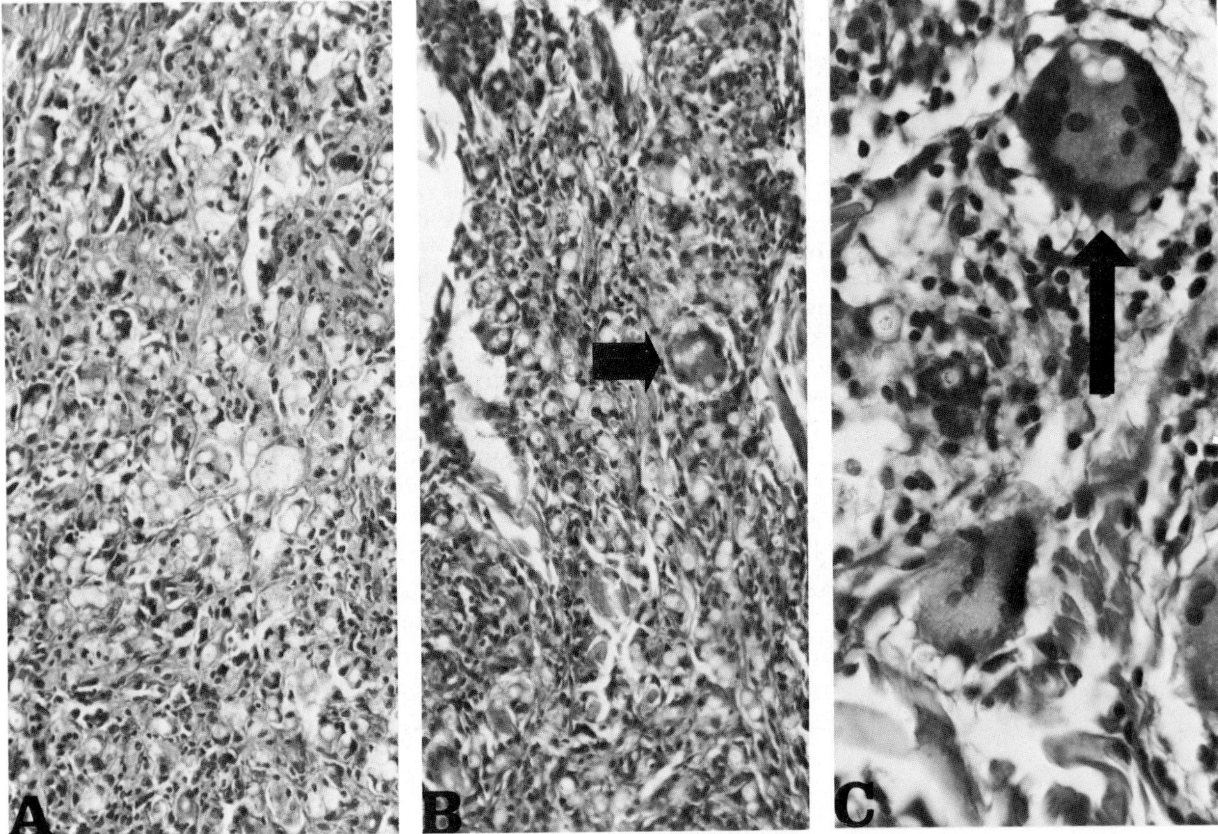

Fig. 109-3. Photomicrographs of a skin lesion in Jorge Lobo's disease). (*A*) Parasites are seen as round, light bodies distributed through the field. (Original magnification approximately × 120) (*B*) Giant multinucleated cell (*arrow*) with enclosed parasites. (Original magnification approximately × 240) (*C*) Fungi inside giant cell (*arrow*) showing birefringent wall (H&E, original magnification approximately × 800) (Courtesy of Dr. N. Michalany)

seen easily in routine hematoxylin–eosin stained sections. Material from lesions may also be examined fresh after suspension in saline, or in gram-stained smears. No immunologic diagnostic tests are sufficiently reliable for routine use.

Prognosis

Patients should be told that lobomycosis has a long course and is not dangerous. Persistent activity of the disease has been documented for 20 to 30 years, and spontaneous cure does not occur. This emphasizes the value of surgical removal of restricted lesions as therapeutic and prophylactic measures. The disease is not communicable.

Therapy

Excision of early lesions offers the best hope of cure. Removal with a margin of normal tissue, minimizes recurrence in the scar that may occur months afterward. Local excision does not preclude the possibility of the development of a lesion at a distant site.

In extensive disease, various drugs have been tried but none has proved satisfactory, including the sulfonamides and amphotericin B. A few patients were said to have improved after clofazimine therapy. Recently, ketoconazole has been tried but with results very inferior to those obtained in paracoccidioidomycosis. In extensive forms, secondary infections of ulcerated lesions may be improved by treatment with long-acting sulfonamides.

Prevention

So little is known of the reservoir of the fungus and the mode of transmission that no firm recommendations can be made for prevention of Lobo's mycosis.

Remaining Problems

Propagation of the etiologic agent in cultures is essential to the characterization of *P. loboi.* Also, the development of methods for serodiagnosis would be greatly aided by success in culture of the fungus.

There is need for an inexpensive, orally administrable, safe and effective antimicrobic for the treatment of lobomycosis.

Bibliography

Book

LACAZ C DA S: Micologia Médica: fungos, actinomicetos e algas de interesse médico, 6th ed. São Paulo, Sarvier, 1977. 569 pp.

Journals

BARUZZI RG, LACAZ C DA S, SOUZA FAA DE: História natural da doenca de Jorge Lobo: Ocorrência entre os índios Caiabi (Brasil Central). Rev Inst Med Trop São Paulo 21:302–338, 1979

BARUZZI RG, MARCOPITO LF, MICHALANY NS, LIVIANU J, PINTO NRS: Early diagnosis and prompt treatment by surgery in Jorge Lobo's disease (keloidal blastomycosis). Mycopathologia 74:51–54, 1981

CALDWELL DK, CALDWELL MC, WOODARD JC, AJELLO L, KAPLAN W, MCCLURE HM: Lobomycosis as a disease of the atlantic bottle nosed dolphin (*Tursiops truncatus,* Montagu 1821). Am J Trop Med Hyg 24:105–114, 1975

DIAS LB, SAMPAIO MM, SILVA D: Jorge Lobo's disease: Observation on its epidemiology and some unusual morphological forms of the fungus. Rev Inst Med Trop São Paulo 12:8–15, 1970

FONSECA OJ DE M, LACAZ C DA S: Estudo de culturas isoladas de blastomicose queloidiforme (Doença de Jorge Lobo): Denominação de seu agente etiológico. Rev Inst Med Trop São Paulo 13:225–251, 1971

JARAMILLO D, CORTES A, RESTREPO A, BUILES M, ROBLEDO M: Lobomycosis: Report of the eight Colombian case and review of the literature. J Cutan Path 3–4:180–189, 1976

SAMPAIO MM, DIAS LB: The Armadillo *"Euphractus sexcintus"* as a suitable animal for experimental studies of Jorge Lobo's disease. Rev Inst Med Trop São Paulo 19:215–220, 1977

WIERSEMA JP, NIEMEL PL: Lobo's disease in Surinam patients. Trop Geogr Med 17:89–91, 1965

PEDRO LAVALLE
MARGARITA SILVA–HUTNER

Chromoblastomycosis

110

Chromoblastomycosis is a localized, chronic, granulomatous fungal infection of the skin. Typically, one of the lower extremities is involved, but in some patients, the upper extremities, the trunk, or the head are also afflicted. The disease is characterized clinically by nodules and, especially, by verrucous or vegetating lesions.

The term chromoblastomycosis is misleading. The prefix *chromo-* might be taken to mean that the lesions have a special color; they do not, although the fungal cells in the tissues are dark brown. The *-blasto-* portion of the word is erroneous as the etiologic fungi do not form blastoconidia (buds) in the tissues but multiply by a splitting process. Nevertheless, chromoblastomycosis has become firmly established as the name of a distinct disease entity.

Etiology

Five species of fungi are accepted as causes of chromoblastomycosis, and a sixth may or may not prove to be causative. Their current nomenclature, taxonomic status, and some of their synonyms are listed in Table 110-1. All are dematiaceous (dark-colored) Hyphomycetes (filamentous fungi lacking a known or verifiable, consistent, method of sexual reproduction). None has been shown to have a yeast form (they are not "black yeasts"); their unicellular, parasitic form in infected tissues consists of spherical sclerotic bodies that are 5 μm to 15 μm in diameter, thick walled, and copper colored. These parasitic cells reproduce by internal septation to form small multicellular clusters resembling mulberries (muriform cells) or *Fumago* (fumagoid cells).

Perhaps the only monomorphic species that causes chromoblastomycosis, *Phialophora verrucosa* produces masses of conidia arising semiendogenously through an ostiole (opening) surrounded by a collarette at the constricted tip of an ampulliform (or vial-shaped) conidiogenous cell (a phialide, hence the name *Phialophora*). In *P. verrucosa,* the collarette (2 μm–3 μm × 2 μm–3 μm) is conspicuous and V-shaped (Fig. 110-1*A*).

Cladosporium carrionii are characterized by production of branching chains of ellipsoid blastoconidia borne acropetally (terminally) and aerially on erect conidiogenous cells, the chains attaining a length of 12 to 15 blastoconidia (Fig. 110-1*B*). However, some isolates display a *Phialophora* sporulation, particularly on certain mediums.

Fonsecaea pedrosoi has been the subject of considerable controversy because of polymorphism and variation in methods of conidiation according to environmental conditions. This genus/species is best characterized by complex conidiophores exhibiting successive layers of sympoduloconidia (Fig. 110-1*C*). In addition, blastogenic conidia may be produced in branching chains such as those of *Cladosporium* and phialoconidia on phialides resembling those of *P. verrucosa.*

Fonsecaea compacta also produces successive series of conidia in sympodial conidiogenous cells and continues to fit well into *Fonsecaea.* It differs from *F. pedrosoi* in having subglobose conidia attached to its neighbors in the series by a broad septum resulting in a more compact head (Fig. 110-1*D*).

Rhinocladiella (*Acrotheca*) *aquaspersa* was originally placed in *Acrotheca* because of the presence of long, unbranched conidial apparatuses that produce conidia sympodially, as do *Rhinocladiella* spp. In addition, clusters of conidia are also produced terminally on phialides without collarettes (Fig. 110-1*E*). This species is unquestioned as an agent of chromoblastomycosis.

The status of several isolates originally assigned to *Wangiella dermatitidis* is currently under scrutiny to determine if the group is homogeneous and whether or not any of the isolates have caused chromoblastomycosis. They have been isolated from subcutaneous (Fig. 110-1*F*), pulmonary, and cerebral phaeohyphomycoses.

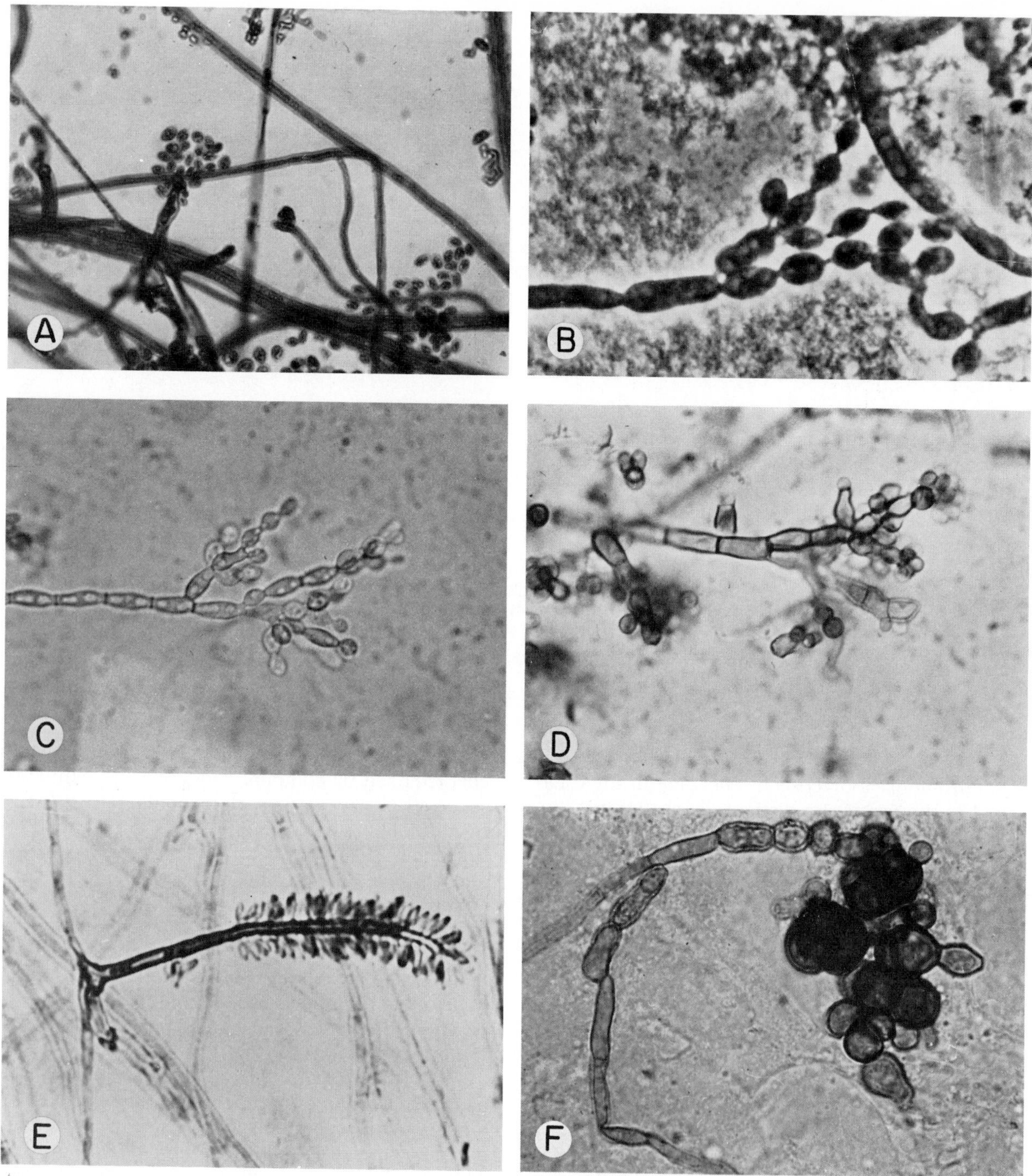

Fig. 110-1. Microscopic appearance of fungi that cause chromoblastomycosis. (*A*) *Phialophora verrucosa,* wet mount. (Original magnification approximately × 48) (*B*) *Cladosporium carrionii.* (Original magnification approximately × 100) (*C*) *Fonseca pedrosoi.* (Original magnification approximately × 45) (*D*) *Fonseca compacta.* (Original magnification approximately × 45) (*E*) *Rhinocladiella aquaspersa.* (Original magnification approximately × 45) (*F*) Fumagoid cells and filaments in skin scrapings (probably *Wangiella dermatitidis;* KOH preparation) (Panels *B* and *E* were kindly supplied by Professor Dante Borelli, Universidad Central de Venezuela; panel E is reproduced with permission from Borelli D: *Acrotheca aquaspersa* n. sp. agente de cromomicosis. Acta Cientifica Venezolena 23:196, 1972).

Table 110-1. *Current Taxonomy and Nomenclature of the Fungi That Cause Chromoblastomycosis*

Genus and Species	Distinctive Conidial Form (Anamorph)	Supplementary Anamorphs
Phialophora verrucosa	*Phialophora*	None (monomorphic genus)
Cladosporium carrionii	*Cladosporium*	*Phialphora* (50% of isolates)*
Fonsecaea pedrosoi	*Fonsecaea*† (series of sympodial conidiogenous cells bearing one-celled holoblastic conidia on denticles	*Cladosporium: Phialophora*
Fonsecaea compacta	Modified *Fonsecaea*†	*Cladosporium*-like *Phialophora*
Rhinocladiella aquaspersa	*Rhinocladiella*‡	Spore clusters borne on phialids without collarettes (hence not *Phialophora*)
Wangiella dermatitidis	Polymorphic species	The ability of this species (or species complex) to cause chromoblastomycosis, phaeohyphomycosis, or both, is currently under investigation.

*Personal communication from Honbo S, Padhye A, Ajello L.
†See text.
‡Schell WA, McGinnis MR, Borelli D: *Rhinocladiella aquaspersa*, a new combination for *Acrotheca aquaspersa*. Mycotaxon. (In press) 1982

Epidemiology

Chromoblastomycosis has been reported from all of the land masses of the world save Antarctica (see list on p. 995). It is more common in warm, humid climates than in cooler climates, 80% of the cases occurring in tropical or subtropical regions and only 20% in temperate regions. For example, in Mexico, chromoblastomycosis is reported almost exclusively from the warm, humid Gulf and Pacific coasts rather than the cooler, drier interior regions.

Chromoblastomycosis is a disease of adults, usually beginning between the ages of 20 and 50 years (with extremes of 3 to 76 years). Over half the cases (56%–96%) occur in males, a predominance attributed to their greater contact with soil containing the fungus; however, even in countries where women labor in the fields equally with men, the disease remains more common in men. It has been suggested that sex hormones may play a role in susceptibility to chromoblastomycosis (and other fungal infections).

The fungi that cause chromoblastomycosis are normally saprobes associated with plant materials—for example, *C. carrionii* is isolated from wooden fence posts, *F. pedrosoi* from decaying palm wood, and *P. verrucosa* from wood pulp. No endogenous reservoir has been demonstrated, and chromoblastomycosis is not communicable.

Pathogenesis and Pathology

Although subclinical pulmonary infection could theoretically lead to the cutaneous lesions characteristic of chromoblastomycosis, the portal of entry is usually a puncture from a thorn or splinter. The fungi inoculated into the skin may produce disease if they survive and proliferate despite the cellular and tissue reaction of the host. A slow evolution takes place with the development of a nodule and satellite lesions by way of the superficial lymphatics or by autoinoculation through scratching.

The histopathologic findings in chromoblastomycosis (Fig. 110-2) are those of nonspecific, extremely polymorphic, infectious granulomas; the only pathognomonic finding is the presence of the fungi. Epidermal changes include intensive hyperkeratosis, irregular acanthosis with pseudoepitheliomatous hyperplasia, and, at times, the formation of microabscesses. The conspicuous changes are mainly in the upper dermis and consist of hyperplasia of the papillary corium, infiltration with leukocytes that is usually intense and may take the form of microabscesses, and follicles or nodules composed of irregularly distributed epithelioid cells bordered by inflammatory cells—mostly lymphocytes and plasma cells. Giant cells, both Langhans' and foreign body, are usually seen in the center of nodules, whereas the changes of chronic fibrosis are found in the stroma between the follicles. The parasitic fumagoid cells may be found in the centers of microabscesses or even within giant cells in the nodules.

Manifestations

Chromoblastomycosis is first manifest as a nodule that gradually forms at the site of inoculation about

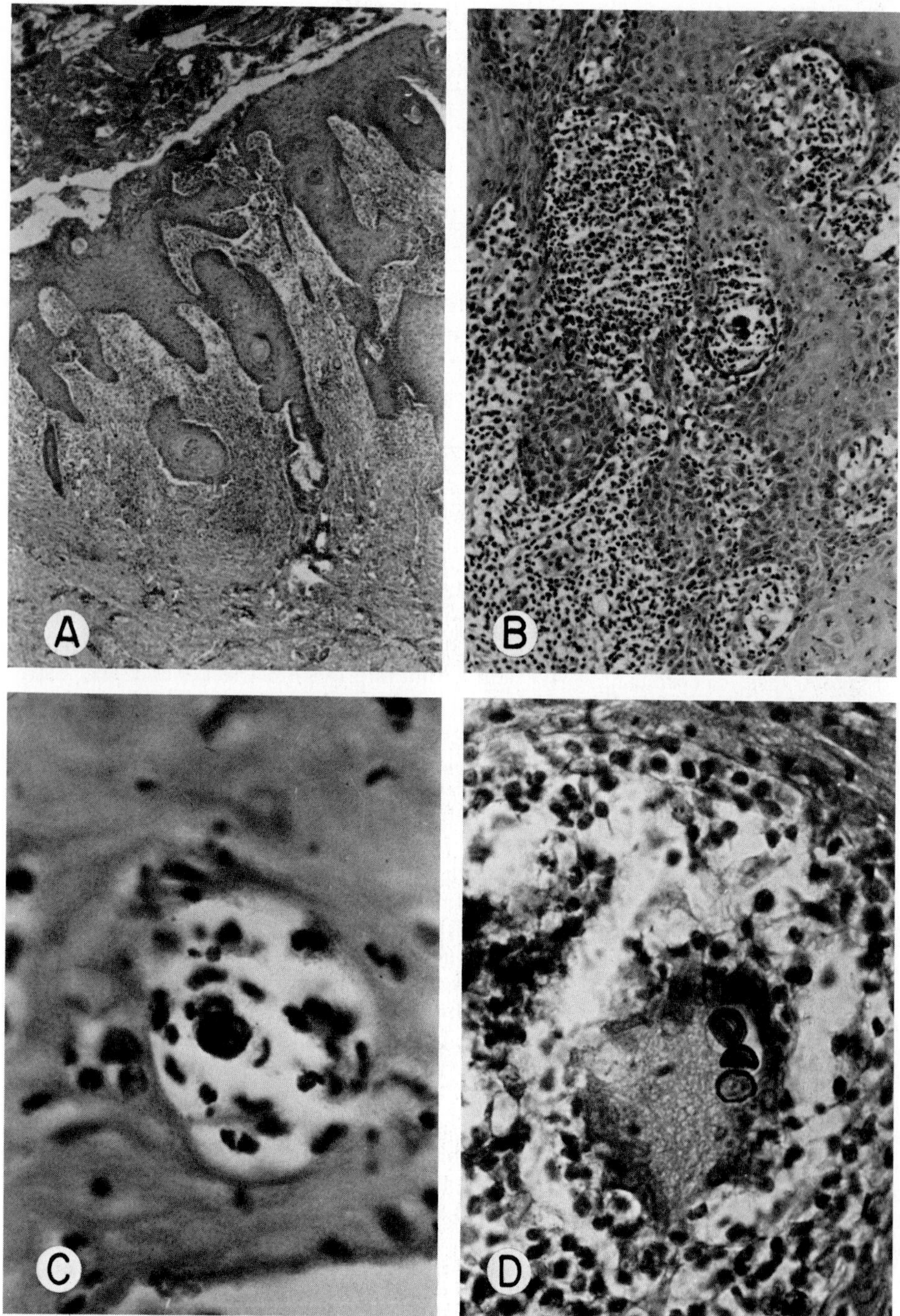

Fig. 110-2. Histopathologic findings in chromoblastomycosis. (*A*) Panoramic view with pseudoepitheliomatous hyperplasia and granulomatous infiltrate (tuberculoid granulomas with giant cells) in the dermis (H & E, approximately × 4) (*B*) Microabscess in a papilla with a group of fumagoid polymorphonuclear, and epitheloid cells (H & E, approximately × 10) (*C*) High-power view of the microabscess in *B,* containing a group of fumagoid cells (H & E, approximately × 100) (*D*) Typical fumagoid cells within a giant cell (H & E approximately × 100)

Fig. 110-3. Typical appearance of chromoblastomycosis. (*A*) Extensive lesions of the lower limb. (*B*) Cauliflowerlike lesions and edema of foot and leg. (*C*) Extensive ulceration in a case of 16 years' duration. (*D*) Crusty and oozing lesions due to secondary bacterial infection. (*E*) Deformity of the hand caused by the fibrotic process of cicatrization. (*F*) Typical elephantiasis in a case of long duration.

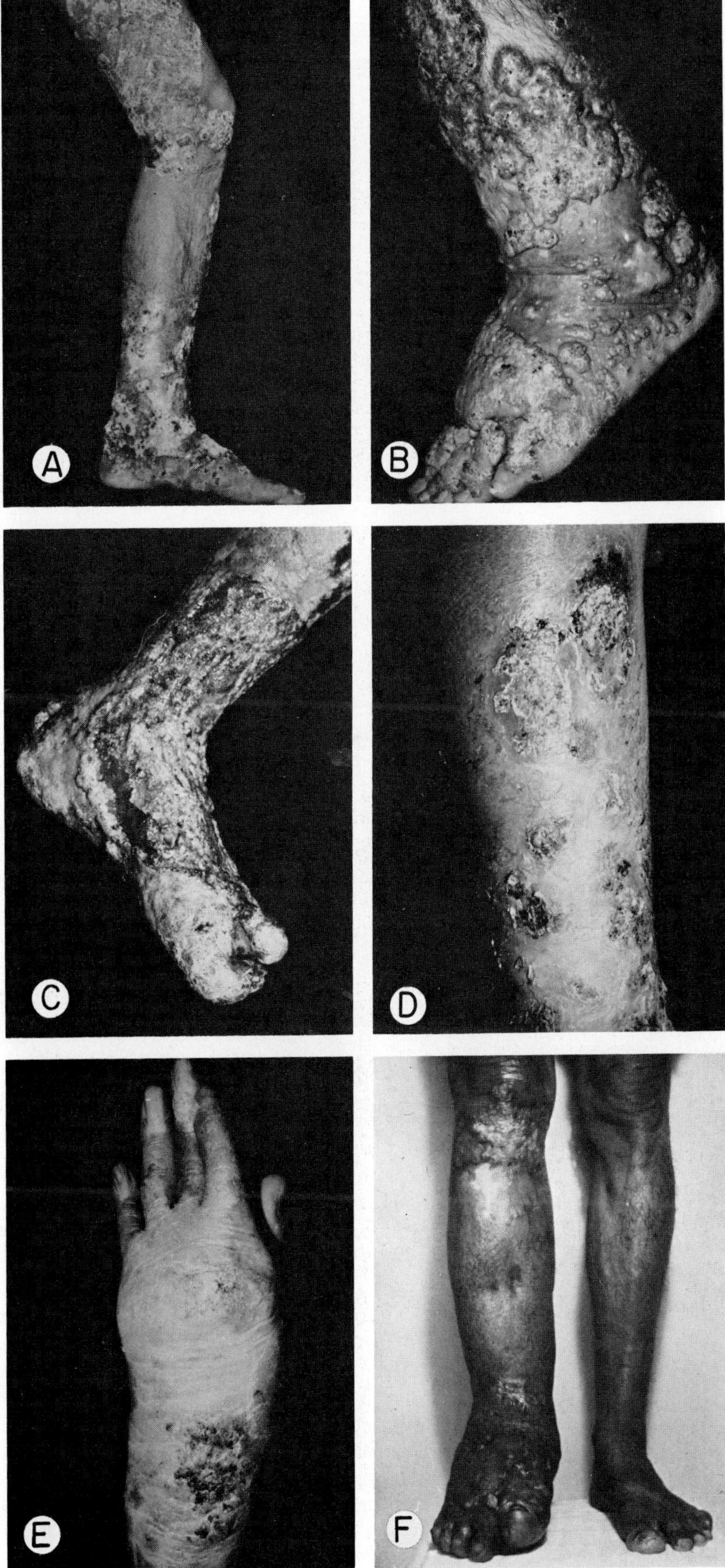

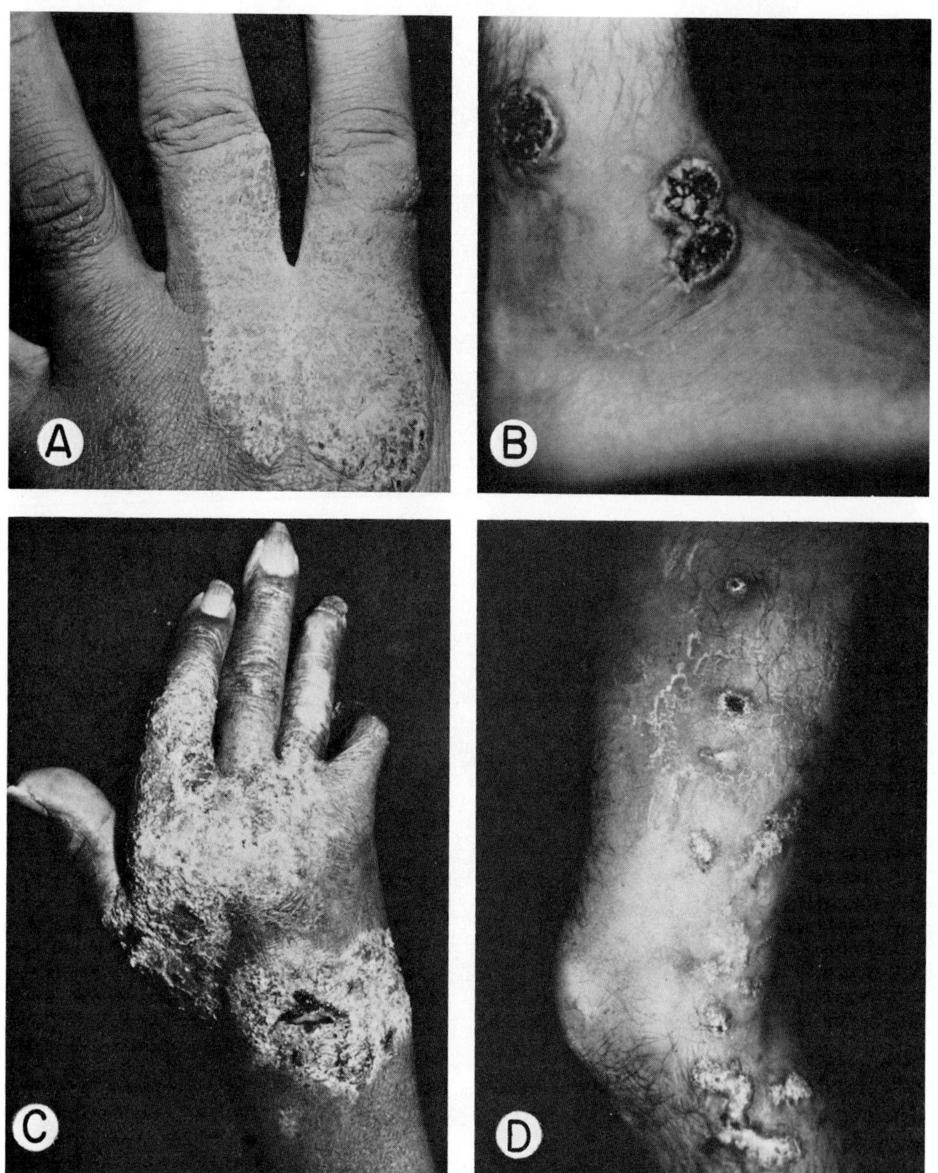

Fig. 110-4. Uncommon forms of chromoblastomycosis. (*A*) Verrucous plaque lesions of hand. (*B*) Very early "syphiloid" lesions of ankle. (*C*) Lesions of the hand with involvement of the fourth finger and its nail. (*D*) 'Sporotrichoid" distribution of lesions on lower extremity.

40 days after introduction of the fungus. The areas first involved are those exposed to trauma—in descending order of frequency, feet (dorsum, instep, heel); legs (ankle, knee); arms (hand, wrist, elbow); thighs; buttocks; face; ears; shoulder–trunk; and perineum. As the nodule grows, it becomes papillomatous and transforms into a vegetating or verrucous lesion. If new, satellite lesions appear, they undergo the same slow transformation into verrucous lesions. The lesions may be classified as either plaque or nodular (see list on p. 995). Although both kinds of lesions may be present, in advanced disease the lesions of the upper extremity, trunk, face, and upper leg are almost exclusively in the plaque form, whereas on the foot and ankle the lesions are nodular.

Plaque lesions arise from the coalescence of verru-

REPORTED GEOGRAPHIC OCCURRENCE OF CHROMOBLASTOMYCOSIS

South America	Argentina, Brazil,* Chile, Columbia, Ecuador,* French Guiana,* Paraguay, Peru, Uruguay, Venezuela*
Central America	Costa Rica,* Cuba,* Dominican Republic,* El Salvador, Guatemala, Honduras, Jamaica,* Panama,* Puerto Rico*
North America	Canada, Mexico,* United States
Africa	Algeria, Cameroon, Canary Islands, Equatorial Africa (various countries), Madagascar, Mozambique, Reunion, South Africa, Zaire, Zimbabwe
Europe	Czechoslovakia, Finland,* Hungary, Soviet Union
Asia	Burma, Ceylon,* China, India, Indonesia, Japan
Oceania	Australia,* New Zealand

*Countries with highest incidence.

CLINICAL CLASSIFICATION OF CHROMOBLASTOMYCOSIS

Plaque form—smooth or verrucous (may be either localized or disseminated)
- *Tuberculoid*—verrucous appearance with central scarring
- *Syphiloid*—serpiginous border, extensive healing
- *Psoriasiform*—slightly infiltrated, scaly
- *Mycetomatoid*—heavily infiltrated with fistuloud prominences

Nodular or pseudotumor form (may be either localized or disseminated)
- *Sarcoidlike*—wine-red, isolated nodules

(After Bopp C: Cromoblastomicose. Doctoral Thesis, Universidad do Rio Grande do Sul, Porto Alegre, Brasil, 1969. pp 101–258.)

cous lesions and consist of flat areas 3 cm to 10 cm in diameter that are raised 1 mm to 5 mm above the surrounding normal skin (Figs. 110-3*A* and 110-4*A*). The surface of a plaque may be verrucous with firmly adherent crusts and scales; pressure, or lifting crusts, may result in exudation of small amounts of pus or caseous or bloody material. Some plaques are uniformly infiltrated, dry, and scaly—that is, psoriasiform. Others are marked by a central, smooth, rose-colored, or achromic scar with prominent borders (the tendency to heal by fibrosis is reflected in the central scarring); these lesions are called tuberculoid, or syphiloid (Fig. 110-4*B*) if the borders are serpigenous. Plaques may remain localized or extend directly to involve contiguous skin. After 6 to 20 or more years, the region of involvement may extend from the foot to the buttock in the lower extremity (Fig. 110-3*A*) and from the hand to the shoulder in the upper extremity.

The nodular or pseudotumor form of chromoblastomycosis consists of lesions that do not coalesce but grow separately as rounded elevations with either a vegetative/verrucous surface (cauliflower-like—Fig. 110-3*B*), or a smooth, hard surface (keloidlike). These lesions also tend to heal after several years and may produce extensive fibrotic scars.

Secondary bacterial infections frequently complicate chromoblastomycosis, especially the nodular form. The lesions ulcerate and ooze abundant quantities of malodorous pus, though they are partially covered with serosanguineous crusts (Fig. 110-3*C* and *D*). Erysipelas is common and contributes to lichenification. As fibrosis advances, two complications are common: (1) impairment of the flow of lymph, resulting in elephantiasis (Fig. 110-3*F*), or the mossy foot syndrome, and (2) contractures of tendons with deformities of the extremities, resulting in limited and difficult movement (Figs. 110-3*E* and 110-4*C*). Lymphangitic spread (Fig. 110-4*D*), and dissemination through the blood is rare in chromoblastomycosis. However, involvement of the brain, but not the thoracolumbar viscera, has been reported.

Diagnosis

The clinical diagnosis of chromoblastomycosis is readily made when verrucous lesions have been present for many years on the lower limbs (Fig. 110-3*A*). Also helpful is rural origin of the patient from an endemic region and a history of trauma. However, demonstration of the causative fungi in tissue sections is essential to diagnosis because other dermatoses may cause a similar clinical picture. Thus, leishmaniasis (Mexico; Central and South America) may cause nodular lesions but involves the mucous membranes, unlike chromoblastomycosis. Verrucous tuberculosis (Mexico, United States); the fixed form of sporotrichosis (Mexico, Central America; Dominican Republic); blastomycosis (United States); and paracoccidioidomycosis (South America) may also mimic chromoblastomycosis. Elephantiasic chromoblastomycosis may be confused with filariasis, leprosy, and recurrent pyogenic lymphangitis, cutaneous tuberculosis, or sporotrichosis. Mycetomatoid chromoblastomycosis must be distinguished from true mycetoma. Plaque forms with serpiginous borders and ulcerated nodes resemble late syphilis, other forms of vegetating pyodermatitis, bromide and iodide hypersensitivity, and rarely, neoplasms.

Laboratory diagnosis depends on demonstration of the parasitic form of the fungus in the lesions by direct microscopic examination of either KOH preparations (Chap. 9, Microscopic Examinations) of crusts or pus, or stained (hematoxylin and eosin—Fig. 110-2) histologic sections. Biopsy specimens should include healthy skin as well as the lesion; staining with hematoxylin and eosin provides contrast and specificity because of the natural brown pigment of the fumagoid cells (both periodic acid–Schiff and Gomori silver methenamine stains decolorize the fungi.

Specimens for primary culture should be planted at multiple spots on the surface of plates or tubes of Sabouraud glucose agar containing gentamicin or chloramphenicol and cycloheximide, and incubated at 30°C. Slide subcultures must be prepared for laboratory identification of genus and species. Because the fungi that cause chromoblastomycosis exist in nature, isolation from specimens must be complemented by demonstration of sclerotid bodies in the same specimens.

Prognosis

Chromoblastomycosis is rarely fatal and generally does not produce systemic disease. Usually benign, it may become morbid if lymphangitis and elephantiasis set in, or if lesions extend and incapacitate a limb. Surgical excision may eradicate early stages of the disease but no known form of therapy completely eradicates the fungus in advanced stages. Widespread hematogenous dissemination has been reported in patients with impaired immunity. Although both humoral and cell-mediated immunologic responses have been demonstrated in patients with chromoblastomycosis, the protective value of such immunity is not known.

Therapy

Many forms of treatment have appeared to be clinically effective in clearing the lesions of chromoblastomycosis. However, the disease recurs either because the fungus is not completely eradicated or because the patient is reinfected from the environment. Thus, the initial enthusiasm for many therapies is dissipated when the same patients are examined five or more years later. Actual cures have resulted only in patients treated in the very early stages of the disease, or, in more advanced cases, by amputation. To date, there is no specific, effective therapy for chromoblastomycosis.

Local

Surgical removal followed by skin grafting is the best treatment for early, localized forms of the disease. Amputation of an extremity may be necessary in very extensive disease with secondary infection, elephantiasis, or ulcerations complicated with squamous cell carcinoma; the regional lymph nodes must also be excised if there is any evidence that they are involved. Intralesional injections of amphotericin B may be effective but are painful and are not suitable for widespread disease.

Electrocoagulation, dessication, iontophoresis, irradiation, and topical heat have been applied with testimonial assertion of good effect.

Systemic

Many drugs have been given in systemic treatment of chromoblastomycosis, but very few merit retention. For example, systemic administration of amphotericin B by IV injection (Chap. 39, Candidosis) gives striking results. However, almost all patients relapse within 2 to 4 months after treatment, and amphotericin B is now used only in combination with other drugs.

Calciferol (600,000 units, PO, once a week for 4–6 months, then once every 2 weeks for 6 more months) is well tolerated and is inexpensive. In Mexico, about half of the patients treated with calciferol are cured.

The administration of thiabendazole (25 mg/kg body wt/day, PO, as a single dose, for 6 weeks to 22 months) results in clinical cure in 40%, improvement in 50%, and no detectable change in 10% of the patients. The major adverse effects are nausea and headache that respond to treatment with antihistamines and analgesics.

Flucytosine (100 mg/kg body wt/day, PO, as 4 equal portions, 6-hourly, for 2–3 months) brings about dramatic improvement. Unfortunately, resistance develops that is clinically apparent and documented by susceptibility testing *in vitro.* Treatment using flucytosine in combination with either amphotericin B or thiabendazole appears to be clinically effective and may prevent the development of resistance.

Ketoconazole (400 mg/day, PO, as a single dose, for a period yet to be determined) is under trial in the treatment of chromoblastomycosis; remission is induced in about 55% of patients. However, ketoconazole is a fungistatic agent that may have to be given in large doses for long periods to avoid relapse—posing the problems of toxicity and cost.

Prevention

No practical measures are known for preventing chromoblastomycosis. Close follow-up of persons who have sustained puncture or abrasive wounds with materials likely to be contaminated with fungi should prevent chronic, disfiguring, or disabling disease if surgical excision is carried out as soon as a lesion is proved chromoblastomycotic.

Remaining Problems

Delivery of immediate medical attention and subsequent follow-up to persons with puncture wounds in rural areas is a pressing social and public health problem. Persons working in the wood pulp industry or those working in gardens in urban areas may fare better if physicians are informed about the pathogenesis and treatment of this disease.

Improved capability in laboratory diagnosis of the fungi that cause chromoblastomycosis is needed.

Bibliography

Books

AL—DOORY Y: Chromomycosis. Foreword by Arturo L. Carrión. Missoula, Mont., Mountain Press, 1972. 203 pp.

BORELLI D: Causal Agents of Chromoblastomycosis. In Proceedings of the Fifth International Conference on Mycoses. Washington, DC, Pan American Health Organization, Scientific Publication No. 396, 1980. pp 334–338.

CARRIÓN AL: Chromoblastomycosis. In Seligson D, Von Graevenitz A (eds), CRC Handbook Series in Clinical Microbiology, Section E, Clinical Microbiology II. Cleveland, Ohio, CRC Press, 1977. pp 3–11.

CARRIÓN AL, SILVA—HUTNER M: Chromoblastomycosis. In Demis DJ, Dobson RL, McGuire J (eds): Clinical Dermatology. Philadelphia, Harper & Row, 1982. Vol. 3, unit 17–23, pp 1–15.

EMMONS CW, BINFORD CH, UTZ JP, KWON—CHUNG KJ: Medical Mycology, 3rd ed. Philadelphia, Lea & Febiger, 1977. pp 386–405.

LAVALLE P: Chromomykose. In Jadassohn (ed): Handbuch der Haut und Geschlechskrankheiten, IV/4. Berlin, Springer-Verlag, 1963. pp 367–435.

LAVALLE P: Chromoblastomycosis in Mexico. Proceedings of the Fifth International Conference on Mycoses. Washington, DC, Pan American Health Organization Scientific Publication No. 396, 1980. pp 235–247.

MCGINNIS MR, SCHELL WA: The genus *Fonsecaea* and its relationship to the genera *Cladosporium, Phialophora, Ramichloridium,* and *Rhinocladiella.* In Proceedings of the Fifth International Conference on Mycoses. Washington, DC, Pan American Health Organization, Scientific Publication No. 396, 1980. pp 215–234.

SILVA—HUTNER M, CARRIÓN AL: Differential characteristics of the fungal agents chromoblastomycosis. Washington, DC, Pan American Health Organization, Scientific Publication No. 304, 1975. pp 118–125.

Journals

SCHELL WA, MCGINNIS MR, BORELLI D: *Rhinocladiella aquaspersa,* a new combination for *Acrotheca aquaspersa.* Mycotaxon. (In press) 1982

CAROLYN COKER HUNTLEY

111 Cutaneous Larva Migrans

Cutaneous larva migrans is an intensely pruritic, migratory skin eruption caused by the percutaneous invasion and subsequent migration of nematode larvae.

Etiology

Often referred to as creeping eruption, the disease is caused by the third stage or infectious larval form of hookworm species that produce intestinal infections in dogs and cats. *Ancylostoma braziliense* is the most important pathogen, although *Ancylostoma caninum* has been implicated in some cases. The human-associated hookworms (*Necator americanus* and *Ancylostoma duodenale,* Chap. 68, Intestinal Nematodiasis) may produce a similar rash, commonly called ground itch, which is of shorter duration than the infections caused by the hookworms of nonhuman origin. Intestinal infections with *Strongyloides stercoralis* (Chap. 68, Intestinal Nematodiasis) may be associated with a perianal larva migrans syndrome called larva currens because of the rapidity of larval migration. This disease is an autoinfection caused by penetration of the perianal skin by infectious larvae as they are passed in the feces.

Epidemiology

Cutaneous larva migrans occurs primarily in the southeastern United States. The parasite thrives in shaded areas where the soil is sandy and moist, and where the climate is warm. The largest number of cases is reported from Florida and Georgia, followed by Alabama, South Carolina, and North Carolina, but the disease is found in all of the southern states from Texas to Virginia. It is an occupational disease of plumbers, pipefitters, and anyone who must work under buildings and in crawlways—situations making for direct contact between skin and soil. Beaches, parks, and sandboxes are also likely locations for acquiring the infection.

Infected dogs and cats deposit fecal material containing *A. braziliense* ova in the soil. IF the temperature, consistency, and moisture content of the soil is optimal, the eggs hatch. The larvae then progress and molt, developing into the infectious third stage larval form within 3 to 4 days.

Pathogenesis and Pathology

The *A. braziliense* larvae penetrate the skin of the human host with the aid of collagenaselike enzymes. They then migrate within and beneath the epidermis, since they are generally unable to penetrate the dermis. Although they may move 1 to 2 cm per day, their path is erratic, seldom winding more than a few centimeters from the point of penetration. The larvae ordinarily remain in the skin; however, cases of pulmonary infiltrates with eosinophilia have been documented. In one patient, *A. braziliense* larvae were repeatedly demonstrated in the sputum. The symptoms and pathologic changes may in large part be the result of the development of hypersensitivity to the worms.

Manifestations

The sites most commonly involved are the hands and feet, buttocks, and genital areas. The appearance of the cutaneous larva migrans lesions is usually diagnostic (Fig. 111-1). Serpiginous tracts with advancing margins are associated with an inflammatory reaction that varies, depending on the degree of hypersensitivity of the host. Papules, which are the sites of resting larvae, may be present. Itching is intense, and scratching may lead to eczematization or secondary infection.

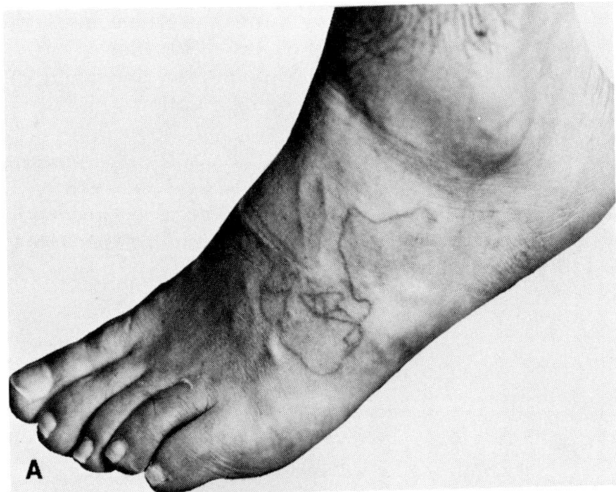

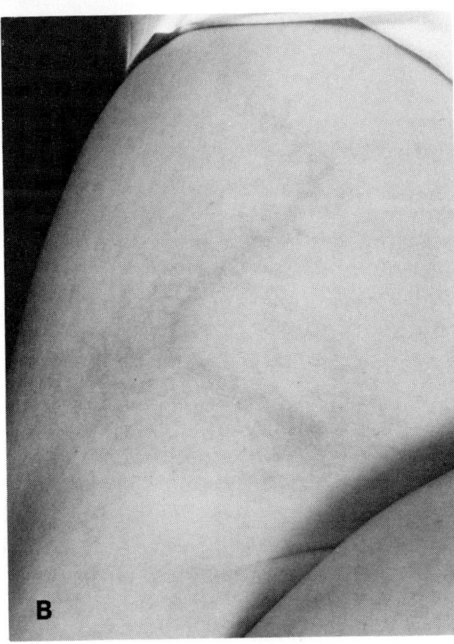

Fig. 111-1. (*A*) The sharply demarcated serpiginous tracts on the foot are typical of infection caused by *Ancylostoma braziliense*. (Morehead RP: Human Pathology. New York, McGraw–Hill, 1965) (*B*) A large urticarial wheel surrounds the larval tract—cutaneous larva migrans of the external aspect of the upper arm.

Diagnosis

The diagnosis of cutaneous larva migrans is usually made by the clinical appearance of the lesions. Motile larvae are located in front of the advancing edge of the burrow, so a biopsy from this area may demonstrate the culprit.

Prognosis

Infections are self-limited but may persist as long as a year, with periods of quiescence alternating with migration, if untreated. Despite the development of apparent hypersensitivity, there is no evidence of protective immunity.

Therapy

Local treatment of patients with cutaneous larva migrans should be directed toward clearing secondary infection, controlling inflammation and itching, and eliminating the parasite. Nonspecific treatment should include aluminum acetate soaks if oozing and crusting are prominent. A 1:20 solution of aluminum acetate can conveniently be made by dissolving one Domeboro tablet (Dome Laboratories) in a pint of water. A 1:40 solution is more practical for soaking large areas. Topical anesthetic remedies such as lidocaine-containing ointments may be desirable if itching is intense; systemic antimicrobics may be indicated for bacterial infection.

Specific treatment involves killing the larvae. In mild infections ethyl chloride spray directed to the advancing edge of the burrow and beyond may be curative. It is necessary to freeze the top layers of the epidermis so that a blister will form and the larvae will be shed with the desquamating skin. Mild infections may respond to thiabendazole suspension rubbed into the lesion four times daily for 10 days. If the lesion is widespread or if larva currens is being treated, thiabendazole by mouth is the treatment of choice. The dose is 50 mg/kg body wt/day, PO, as two equal portions, 12 hourly, for 2 days with a maximum daily dose of 3 g. If necessary, the treatment may be repeated in a few days, or local treatment may be combined with systemic treatment. Adverse reactions to thiabendazole include nausea and vomiting, drowsiness, and rarely, hematuria.

Prevention

Placing plastic sheets over potentially contaminated soil before workers go under buildings or into crawlways will prevent infection. Children's sandboxes should be covered at night to prevent access by stray animals. Better animal control and periodic deworming of all dogs and cats would bring about a sharp decline in the incidence of cutaneous larva migrans.

Bibliography

Books

LEVINE ND (ED): Nematode Parasites of Domestic Animals and of Man, 2nd ed, Minneapolis, Burgess Publishing, 1980. 477 pp.

SHIRKEY HC (ED): Pediatric Therapy, 6th ed, St. Louis, CV Mosby, 1980. 1321 pp.

Journals

BEAVER PC: Parasitological reviews: Larva migrans. Exp Parasitol 5:587–621, 1956

FULLER CE: A common source outbreak of cutaneous larva migrans. Public Health Rep 81:186–190, 1966

MUHLEISEN JP: Demonstration of pulmonary migration of the causative organism of creeping eruption. Ann Intern Med 38:595–600, 1953

STONE OJ, NEWELL GB, MULLINS JF: Cutaneous strongyloidiasis: Larva currens. Arch Dermatol 106:734–736, 1972

WRIGHT DO, GOLD EM: Löffler's syndrome associated with creeping eruption (cutaneous helminthiasis). JAMA 128:1082–1083, 1945

PHILIP D. MARSDEN

Cutaneous Filariasis

112

Two agents of cutaneous filariasis are true filariae: *Onchocerca volvulus* and *Loa loa*. The third, *Dracunculus medinensis*, is a threadlike, tissue nematode, but it differs in being larviparous through a unique, self-destructive delivery. Some of the characteristics of cutaneous filariasis are given in Table 112-1.

Onchocerciasis (River Blindness)

Onchocerciasis, cutaneous filariasis caused by *O. volvulus*, is characterized clinically by skin irritation, corneal opacities, and skin nodules.

Etiology

The threadlike adult worms lie tangled together in fibrous nodules in the subcutaneous tissues or fascial planes. Microfilariae produced by the females become widely distributed in the surrounding skin. Female blackflies (buffalo gnats), species of the genus *Simulium*, ingest these larvae while taking a blood meal. After 1 week of development in the fly, the larvae are infective to humans and are deposited when the fly next bites. In humans, the larvae take more than one year to mature, mate, and produce microfilariae. Adult worms live 7 to 15 years.

Epidemiology

Onchocerciasis is found in humans on the west coast of Africa from Sierra Leone to the Congo and in the east from Sudan to Malawi. It also occurs in Guatemala, Mexico, eastern Venezuela, northern Brazil, and Surinam. Larvae and pupae of *Simulium* spp. are usually found in rapidly running, highly oxygenated water. The patient should be asked if he has been fishing or living near such water. The adult flies are but 3 mm long. They bite low on the legs in Africa and usually around the head in Central America, perhaps accounting for the high incidence of nodules on the heads of people in the latter locality. In East Africa, *Simulium neavei* larvae and pupae evaded detection for many years, but were eventually found on the shells of fresh-water crabs.

Pathogenesis and Pathology

An initial inflammatory reaction around the adult worm is followed by a foreign body granulomatous reaction and the formation of a fibrous capsule (Fig. 112-1). The nodules are literally the graveyards of the adult worms because the worms eventually die and degenerate, sometimes causing abscesses to form. The microfilariae in the surrounding subcutaneous tissues promote a low-grade inflammatory reaction with lymphocytes, plasma cells, and eosinophils. Thickening of the epidermis and dermis due to fibrosis eventually occurs and is accompanied by the destruction of elastic fibers and sometimes a reduction in pigmentation.

Microfilariae that migrate into the tissues of the eye produce important inflammatory lesions that may result in blindness. Punctate keratitis is associated with death of a microfilara in the cornea; if multiplied sufficiently, permanent corneal scarring and opacification may result. A low-grade iritis and iridocyclitis result in pupillary distortion and even occlusion. Choroidoretinitis also occurs.

Manifestations

Any patient who has a persistent, itching skin rash or visual disturbances and has been in one of the areas endemic for *O. volvulus* may have onchocerciasis. More rarely, the complaint is deep-seated muscular pain or subcutaneous nodules. The early skin lesions generally take the form of an erythematous, macular, pruritic rash, with altered pigmentation as the first objective change. In heavy infections, definite thickening with formation of papules (intraepithelial granulomas containing one or more microfilariae) may occur—craw-craw or crocodile skin. Lichenification,

Table 112-1. Some Characteristics of Cutaneous Filariids

	Onchocerca volvulus **Onchocerciasis**	***Loa loa*** **Loiasis**	***Dracunculus medinensis*** **Dracunculiasis**
Vector	*Simulium* spp.	*Chrysops* spp.	*Cyclops* spp.
Location in tissues of humans			
Larvae	Skin and subcutaneous tissues	Blood during day	Intestinal visceral connective tissue
Adults	Nodules in skin, subcutaneous tissue, and fascial planes	Subcutaneous tissues and fascial planes	Subcutaneous tissues, joints and joint cavities
Major manifestation	Rash, thickening, hyperkeratosis of skin; corneal opacities; nodules	Calabar swelling	Ulcer with worm protruding–site of emergence of adult worm
Laboratory diagnosis	Motile microfilariae from skin shavings	Sheathed microfilariae with nuclei to tip of tail, in blood during day	Not needed
Treatment available	Diethylcarbamaizne, suramin, nodulectomy	Diethylcarbamazine (curative)	Gentle traction, niridazole, thiabendazole

drying, scaling, and uneven pigmentation—with persistent itching—has been called "lizard skin" (Fig. 112-2). Rarely, late complications include depigmentation and pendulous bags of skin in the groins containing sclerosed lymph nodes.

Nodules vary greatly in size, from 1 cm–8 cm in diameter. They are frequently detected over bony prominences such as the greater trochanter, along the iliac crest, the olecranons, ribs, and occiput (Fig. 112-2). Often the adults are located deep in the fascial planes and no nodules are palpable. The small, milky dots of punctate keratitis lie near the limbus and become visible when a strong pencil of light is directed obliquely across the cornea. Signs of iritis may be present. Microfilariae may be visible in the aqueous humor by slit-lamp examination. Funduscopic examination may reveal the much rarer posterior segment lesions.

Diagnosis

To demonstrate microfilariae, thin sections of the superficial skin are removed with a razor blade without drawing blood (see Chap. 11, Diagnostic Methods for Protozoa and Helminths). It is important to avoid contamination with blood in case there is a coexistent microfilaremia. After mounting the skin sections in saline solution, they are teased apart and examined. Many motile microfilariae 0.2 mm to 0.3 mm in length emerge from these snips within 1 hour after they have been made. If there is a definite site of skin irritation, shavings should be taken from this area. In lightly infected patients, multiple shaving may be necessary to detect the microfilariae. Quite often, however, microfilariae are not found.

An eosinophilia is present, and the filarial complement fixation test may be positive. A test dose of 50 mg diethylcarbamazine (Mazzotti's test) usually provokes an exacerbation of the itching rash.

Scabies (see Chap. 116, Scabies) and superficial mycoses (see Chap. 109, Superficial Fungus Infections of the Skin) are the most common irritant skin rashes of the tropics; they must be differentiated from onchocerciasis. Streptocerciasis, infection with the rare, closely related filariid *Dipetalonema streptocerca,* causes a similar irritating but otherwise inconsequential skin rash. The dipetalonemal microfilariae are recognizable because of a characteristic crook in the tail.

Prognosis

Although onchocerciasis is not a mortal disease, the recurrent, irritant rash can be most distressing. Severe ocular lesions may cause total blindness—thus the name, the blinding filariid.

Therapy

Wherever practical, all nodules should be excised; this simple measure reduces the load of adult worms.

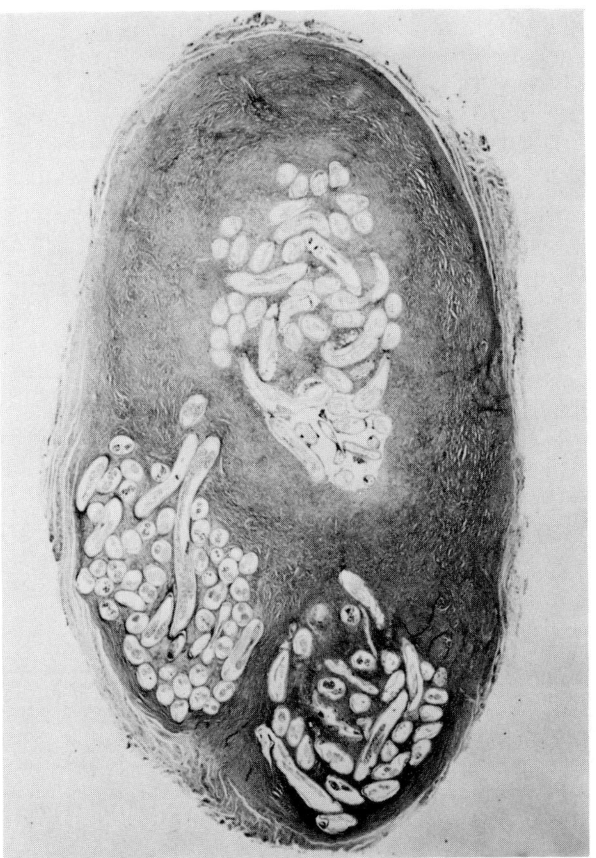

Fig. 112-1. Onchocercal nodule with several coiled adult *Onchocerca volvulus* encased within hyalinized scar tissue. (Morvar stain, original magnification approximately × 8) (Courtesy of Daniel H Conner, MD, Armed Forces Institute of Pathology. AFIP 69-3639)

Fig. 112-2. Scaling, thickened skin with altered pigmentation—"lizard skin." Note onchocercal nodules. (Courtesy of Daniel H Connor, MD, Armed Forces Institute of Pathology. AFIP 69-9769)

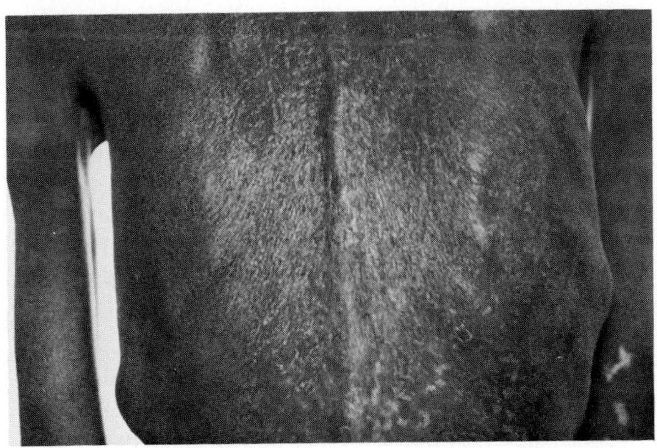

Suramin is effective in killing adult worms. The side-effects and method of administration of this drug are given in Chapter 130, African Trypanosomiasis. A suitable course for onchocerciasis consists of six weekly intraveous injections of 17 mg/kg body wt as one dose. The drug is potentially nephrotoxic; if proteinuria exceeds 30 mg/100 ml, treatment should be stopped.

Diethylcarbamazine (Hetrazin, Banocide) is effective in killing microfilariae but not adult worms. In sensitized persons, death of microfilariae provokes intense skin irritation, cutaneous edema, fever, headache, and malaise. Acute inflammation of the eye may endanger sight. Because these reactions are dose-related, it is usual to start therapy with 0.5 mg/kg body wt by mouth, building up to 6 mg/kg body wt/day (three equal portions, one given every 8 hours) in the course of 3 to 4 days. Treatment is continued at this level for 3 to 4 weeks. Ocular inflammation can be controlled with cortisone acetate 1% eye drops. The systemic manifestations of hypersensitivity often respond to antihistamines, although severe reactions warrant the use of a glucosteroid.

Prevention

Black fly larvae and pupae are very sensitive to small concentrations of DDT in river water (less than one part per million); this has been the most effective form of control of the insect vector. Personal prophylaxis is possible to a limited extent by avoiding the places where biting *Simulium* spp. are numerous.

Loaiasis

Infection with *L. loa* is characterized by transient, inflamed, edematous swellings of the skin. Appearing mainly on the limbs, these Calabar swellings are thought to be the migration sites of adult worms in the subcutaneous tissue. A worm occasionally crosses the eye.

Etiology

The male adult worm is 30 mm long; the female, 70 mm. They live for many years after gaining access to the body through the proboscis of biting flies (deerflies of the genus *Chrysops*). The adult worms seem to be in a state of continuous migration in the subcutaneous tissues of the body. It is not clearly understood how the sexes locate each other, but they meet and mate. The female produces microfilariae that appear in the blood during the day (diurnal periodicity), when they are infectious to the insect vector.

Epidemiology

Humans are the only reservoir host for *L. loa,* with the possible exception of monkeys. Human loiasis is restricted largely to the west coast of Africa, where it occurs from Sierra Leone to the Cameroons, extending into the heart of Africa in the region of the Congo basin.

Pathogenesis and Pathology

The Calabar swellings may result from hypersensitivity to the adult worm or to materials elaborated by it.

Manifestations

The major clinical manifestations of loiasis are repeated occurrences of hot, erythematous swellings (5 cm–10 cm or more in length) in the skin, called Calabar swellings after the endemic area of the Calabar River in southeast Nigeria. Afflicting the upper limbs particularly, they are pruritic and subside in a few days. Similar swellings occur around the eye when the adult worm crosses the eye beneath the conjunctiva. The patient notices the worm in his line of vision ("like a submarine, Doctor"), and it is worth inquiring for such a history. Roentgenography of patients in endemic areas often reveals calcified, dead worms lying between the metacarpals (Fig. 112-3). Rarely, neurologic symptoms may be associated with the infection if the Calabar swelling involves a peripheral nerve. Also, the parasite has been found in the cerebrospinal fluid in patients with meningoencephalitis.

Diagnosis

The initial diagnosis is usually based on a history of Calabar swellings in a patient who comes from an endemic area. Examination of blood taken during the day reveals sheathed microfilariae with a characteristic distribution of caudal nuclei. In early loiasis, microfilariae may not be detected in the blood even by concentration techniques. Eosinophilia as high as 50% to 70% is encountered at this stage. A positive filarial complement fixation test is usually obtained. Occasionally, the adult worm can be extracted as it crosses the eye. It is possible that another filarial nematode, *Dipetalonema perstans* (transmitted by biting midges, *Culicoides* spp.), may also cause Calabar swellings.

Prognosis

Ordinarily, loiasis is of little serious consequence. Symptoms are of most concern to the patient when the eye is involved or, rarely, when a peripheral nerve or the central nervous system is involved. These disturbances are transient.

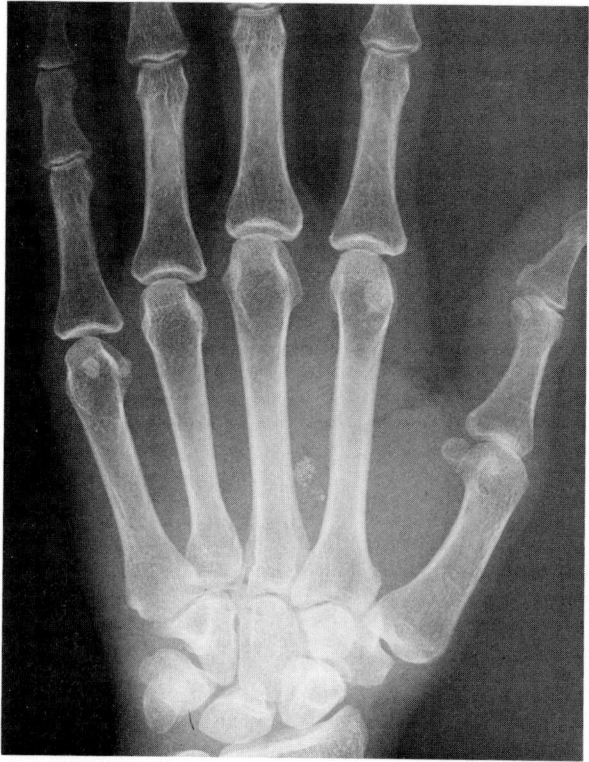

Fig. 112-3. Calcified adult *Loa loa.* (Courtesy of Stanley Bohrer, MD, Professor of Radiology, University of Ibadan)

Therapy

Diethylcarbamazine kills both adults and microfilariae. One course of 12 mg/kg body wt/day, PO, as three equal portions, 8-hourly, for 14 days, is all that is necessary. Adverse reactions are rare.

Dracunculiasis (Guinea Worm Infection)

Infection with the guinea worm (*Dracunculus medinensis*) usually becomes evident as an ulceration of the skin at the site where the adult female worm emerges.

Etiology

Water fleas (*Cyclops* spp.) are infected when they ingest larvae discharged into fresh water from an infected human or other mammal. After development in the hemocoeles of water fleas, the larvae become infective for a final mammalian host. Humans are infected by ingesting infected water fleas while swallowing water from shallow wells or ponds. As the fleas are digested, the infective larvae are freed, penetrate the intestinal walls, and mature in the loose connective tissue. The male is small and dies soon after copulation. The fertilized female requires a year for maturation, developing a thin (2 mm in diameter), meter-long body filled with millions of active, first-stage larvae. When ready to discharge the larvae, she comes to the surface of the skin, possibly selecting regions that are likely to be immersed in cold water. If the protruding worm is wet with cold water, the anterior end ruptures, releasing the tightly coiled first-stage larvae that are infective for *Cyclops* spp.

Epidemiology

Humans are probably the major final host of *D. medinensis,* although natural infection apparently occurs in dogs, wolves, foxes, cats, minks, raccoons, monkeys, baboons, hares, cattle, and leopards. Infection in humans is widespread in the tropics, occurring in local distributions in West Africa, the Nile valley, the Middle East, India and Pakistan, the Caribbean Islands, and Guyana.

Pathogenesis and Pathology

As the adult female *D. medinensis* worm approaches the skin surface, a blister is produced in reaction to a toxic substance secreted from the anterior end of the worm. The blister breaks down to form an ulcer a few centimeters across, and the anterior end of the worm intrudes into this ulcer preparatory to discharging the microfilariae (Fig. 112-4). Secondary infection of the ulcer with resultant cellulitis is common. Eosinophils are prominent in the cellular infiltrate in tissues, and eosinophilia is often found in the peripheral blood.

Manifestations

General allergic symptoms may occur before the blister forms or when surgical removal of the worm is attempted. Multiple infections are common. The lesion is usually on the lower leg, but it may occur on the genitalia, buttocks, or upper limbs. In water carriers, lesions have been observed on the back; that is, the worm appears to be positively hydrotropic.

Rarely, the adult worm involves serous cavities, the extradural space, or joints. Guinea worm arthritis seems to be due to the presence of the adult worm or larvae in the joint.

Diagnosis

The diagnosis of dracunculiasis usually depends on observing the female worm protruding from an ulcer in the skin. A microscopic diagnosis can be made by finding embryos in the exudate from the guinea worm ulcer after exposing it to a few drops of water.

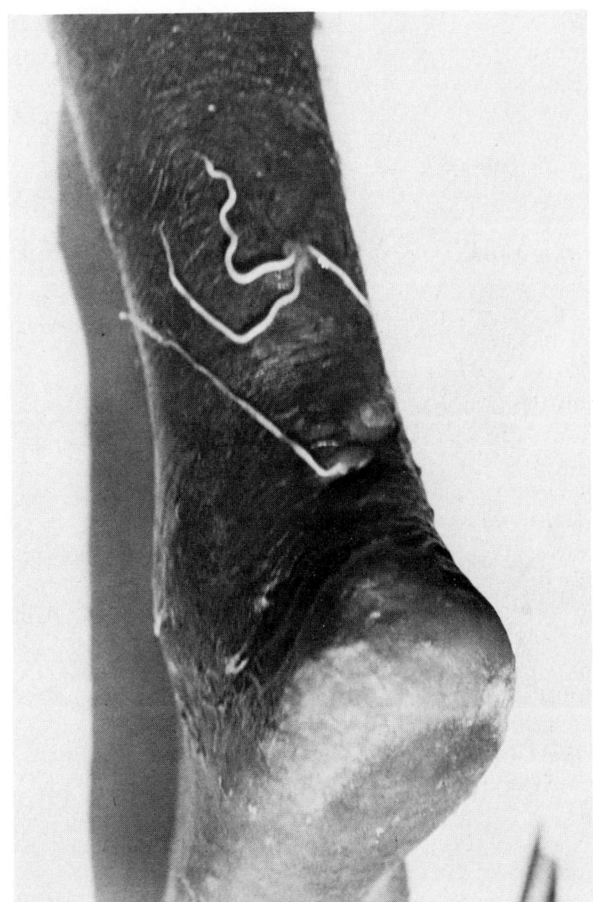

Fig. 112-4. Adult female *Dracunculus medinensis* extruding from ulcers on leg. (Courtesy of Philip ES Palmer, FRCP (Ed), FRCR, Professor of Radiology, University of California, Davis)

Prognosis

The mature female may never reach the surface of the body but may be absorbed or may calcify in the tissues. The roentgenographic appearance is pathognomonic because the worm is so large (Fig. 112-5). If a gravid worm dies *in situ* or is broken during extraction, cellulitis and secondary infection often occur. These may give rise to septicemia and contractures. Also, *Clostridium tetani* may contaminate the wound, and tetanus may result.

Therapy

Gradually winding the guinea worm out of the ulcer by turning it on a stick a few centimeters a day is still common practice. Surgical extraction is also practiced. Recently, niridazole (Ambilhar) has been reported to be lethal to the adult worm. After a course

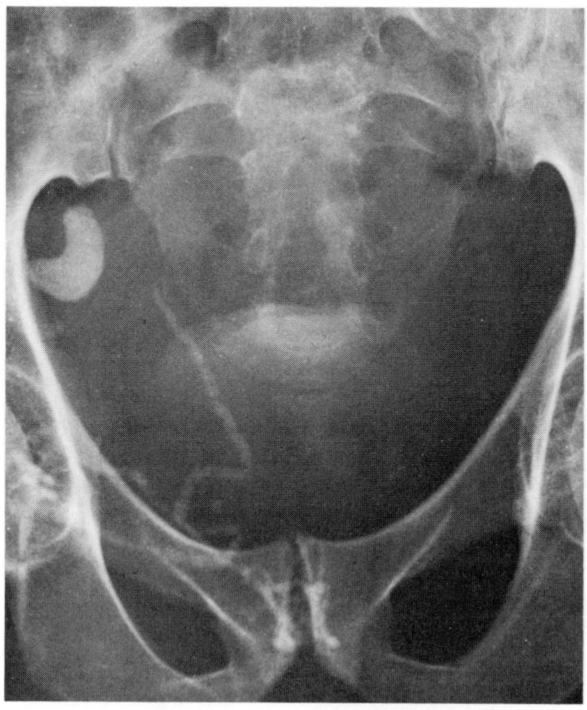

Fig. 112-5. Calcified, adult female *Dracunculus medinensis* lying in the pelvis. (Courtesy of Stanley Bohrer, MD, Professor of Radiology, University of Ibadan)

of 25 mg/kg body wt/day PO for 7 days, the worm can be withdrawn readily. Thiabendazole has also been shown to be effective.

Prevention

Prevention of dracunculiasis involves constructing water sources that cannot be contaminated by humans or other mammals and killing cyclops by chlorination or boiling potable water.

Bibliography

ONCHOCERCIASIS

Books

BUCK AA (ED): Onchocerciasis. Symptomatology, Pathology, Diagnosis. Geneva, World Health Organization, 1974. pp 1–80.

NELSON GS: Onchocerciasis. In Dawes B (ed): Advances in Parasitology. New York, Academic Press, 1970. pp 174–224.

Journals

DUKE BOL: Onchocerciasis. Br Med J 4:301–307, 1968

Expert committee on onchocerciasis. WHO Tech Rep Ser 335:1–92, 1966

LOAIASIS

Book

WOODRUFF AW: Loaiasis. In Fairley NH, Woodruff AW, Walter JH (eds): Recent Advances in Tropical Medicine, London, JA Churchill, 1961. pp 178–194.

DRACONTIASIS

Book

MULLER R: Dracunculus and dracunculiasis. In Dawes B (ed): Advances in Parasitology. Vol IX, New York, Academic Press, 1971. pp 73–151.

Journals

ODUNTAM SO, LUCAS AO, GILLES HM: Treatment of dracontiasis with niridazole. Lancet 2:73–75, 1967

REDDY CRRM, SIVARAMAPPA M: Guinea worm arthritis of the knee joint. Br Med J 1:155–156, 1968

ROGER W. WILLIAMS

Cutaneous Myiasis

113

Cutaneous myiasis is an infestation by the larvae of flies—maggots. Existing wounds and ulcers may be secondarily involved through the deposition of eggs or larvae (traumatic myiasis). With some species, the larvae can penetrate apparently normal skin (furuncular myiasis).

Etiology

The typical maggot is a segmented, cylindrical, legless organism, usually with a tapered, anterior head end with mouth hooks, and a broader, truncate posterior end with spiracles (breathing pores), which may be mistaken for eyes by the untutored (Fig. 113-1).

Epidemiology

Wherever man and flies coexist, there is myiasis. Warm temperatures and humid climates favor the breeding and mobility of flies—hence, the occurrence of myiasis. Socioeconomic deprivation is not necessarily a factor setting the stage for this disease, but nevertheless it often is. Elderly diabetics, living along, are prone to traumatic myiasis. During the summer months, the umbilicus of newborn infants may become infested while they are still in the hospital.

The more commonly involved genera in traumatic myiasis are the larvae of blowflies, the metallic blue, green, copper, and black flies of the family Calliphoridae, and the larvae of the black and gray, often checkered, flies of the family Sarcophagidae. Occasionally larvae of the house fly, *Musca domestica,* and the stable fly, *Stomoxys calcitrans,* may be involved. Wounds with a pH of from 6.9 to 7.3 are most attractive to adult blowflies. Wounds that produce a watery discharge are exceedingly attractive to gravid blowflies.

Some of the genera that cause furuncular myiasis are *Dermatobia* from South and Central America and Mexico, *Wohlfahrtia* and *Cuterebra* of the United States and Canada, and *Cordylobia* of Africa. As a result of rapid air travel, patients infested with the exotic larvae are also seen in the United States. A few larvae, such as *Hypoderma* of cattle, infrequently infect humans and migrate under the skin.

Pathogenesis and Pathology

Just as some flies are attracted by dead and decaying animal and vegetable matter, others are attracted by exudate, pus, and necrotic material in wounds and ulcers (Figs. 113-2 and 113-3). Depending on the kind of fly, either eggs or larvae that have hatched inside the adult female are deposited in wounds or body openings.

If the larvae confine their activities to diseased tissue and act as scavengers, they may be beneficial. However, when maggots burrow below superficial necrotic tissues, destructive pathology may be so extensive that amputations may be required. Indeed, fatalities may result when larvae that produce traumatic myiasis find their way from the nasal passages into the brain or lungs. Serious disease may arise from aural and ocular myiasis, as well as from involvement of the anal region and the lower intestinal tract, and the vagina and the lower urinary tract.

Furuncles form when larvae either penetrate the unbroken skin or enter through minute perforations and hair follicles. Each furuncle has an external opening that allows the larva within to breathe. Usually furuncle-producing larvae do not cause death, but *Dermatobia* spp. have been found in the brains of infants at necropsy.

The inflammatory response to furuncular myiasis consists of hyperemia and slight edema. There is infiltration with neutrophilic and eosinophilic granulo-

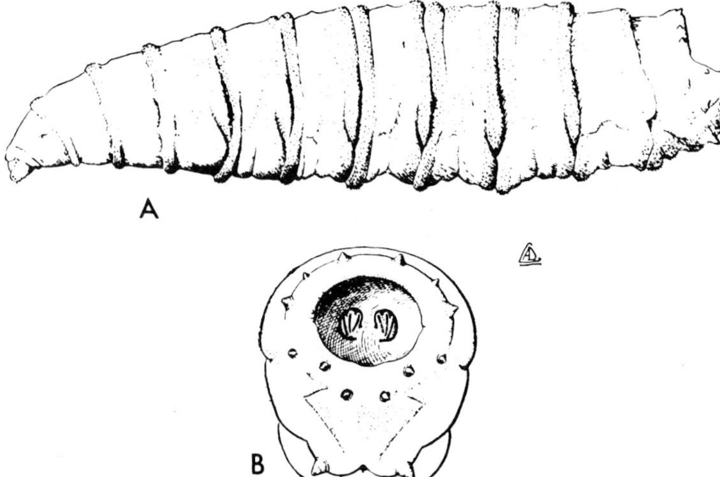

Fig. 113-1. Mature *Sarcophaga* larva. (*A*) Lateral aspect. (*B*) Posterior aspect of last abdominal segment, showing spiracles. (James MT: USDA Miscellaneous Publication No. 631, 1947)

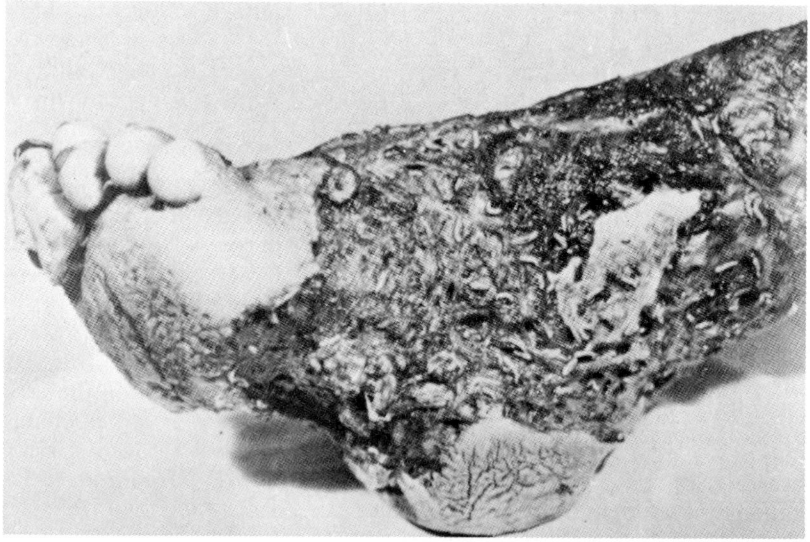

Fig. 113-2. Cutaneous myiasis of the foot and leg. (Kerdel–Vesges F: In Andrews GC, Domonkos AN: Diseases of the Skin, 6th ed. Philadelphia, WB Saunders, 1971)

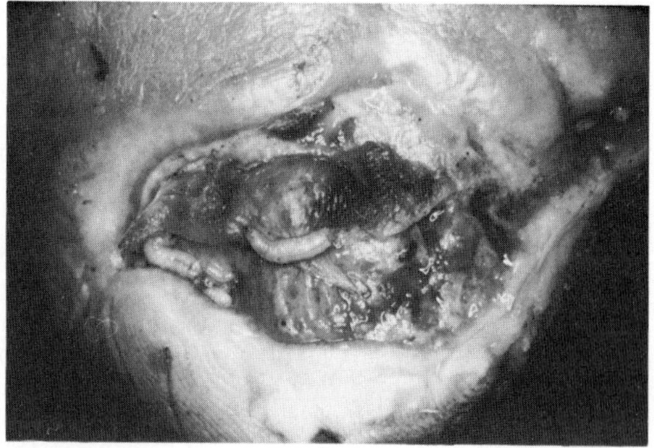

Fig. 113-3. Myiasis in a diabetic following amputation of toes. (Courtesy of the United States Public Health Service).

cytes and plasma cells. There may be small foci of necrosis in the dermis, and edema, even vesiculation, may be evident in the epidermis. Occasionally, cross sections of excised masses show a dense fibrous capsule surrounded by granulation tissue and chronic inflammatory cells—primarily plasma cells, lymphocytes, and eosinophils.

Manifestations

As scavengers, maggots do not cause disease. When living tissues are attacked, disease results. The seriousness of an infestation depends on the species of fly involved, the number of maggots present, the depth and extent of damage, and the area affected. The furuncular form of myiasis is usually painful and may become secondarily infected.

Diagnosis

The diagnosis of myiasis is evident on inspection of the afflicted areas.

Therapy

Prompt removal of the maggots causing traumatic myiasis is imperative. Chloroform (5%–10%) in a light vegetable oil applied either by douching for 30 minutes or by saturated dressings is helpful in stimulating the outward migration of maggots from areas where they cannot be reached easily. Infestations of the nose, sinuses, ears, and other areas may require surgery.

Large maggots may be removed from furuncles with forceps. Small maggots and those with recurved spines (*Dermatobia*) may work their way backward through the opening of the furuncle if petrolatum, grease, or paraffin is applied to this opening and placed into contact with the larval spiracles, thus cutting off the air supply. As they back out, they may be grasped and removed.

Prevention

The use of screening to protect against all types of flies is important. The proper treatment and covering of open wounds and the frequent changing of dressings aid in preventing traumatic myiasis. The destruction of animal carcasses, modern sanitary practices, and, secondarily, the use of insecticides will reduce the number of myiasis-producing flies.

Bibliography

Book

JAMES MT: The Flies That Cause Myiasis in Man. Washington, U. S. Department of Agriculture, Miscellaneous Publication No. 631, 1947. 175 pp.

Journals

HOREN WP, GREGORY GA, KARLSBERG RC: Furuncular dermal myiasis from *Dermatobia hominis.* JAMA 195:787–788, 1966

IANNINI PB, BRANDT D, LAFORCE FM: Furuncular myiasis. JAMA 233:1375–1376, 1975

RICE PL, GLEASON N: Two cases of myiasis in the United States by the African Tumbu Fly, *Cordylobia anthropophaga* (Diptera, Calliphoridae). Am J Trop Med Hyg 21:62–65, 1972

ROGER W. WILLIAMS

114 Pediculosis

Pediculosis is a skin infestation caused by blood-sucking lice.

Etiology

Three varieties of lice attack humans: *Pediculus humanis* var. *capitis* (head louse), *P. humanis* var. *corporis* (body louse), and *Phthirus pubis* (pubic or crab louse) (Fig. 114-1). These dorsoventrally compressed, wingless, oval, grayish insects measure 1 mm to 4 mm in length and become reddish when engorged with blood. The thoracic segments are fused and the one-segmented tarsi are fitted with a single prominent claw for clinging to hairs. Although the head and body louse are sometimes regarded as distinct species, it is preferable to view them as two varieties or subspecies of *P. humanis* because they can be induced to change from one to the other in the course of a few generations in the laboratory. However, only the body louse is the vector of infectious disease, such as epidemic typhus and trench fever (Chap. 98, The Typhus Fevers), and louse-borne relapsing fever (Chap. 143, Relapsing Fever).

Epidemiology

Both the head louse and the crab louse attach their shiny, operculate eggs (nits) to hairs. The head louse usually attaches to head hairs, although it has been found on other hairy parts; the crab louse usually attaches to pubic and perianal hairs, although it sometimes is associated with the hairs of the head, eyebrows, eyelashes, axillae, breast, and beard. The body louse, more often associated with aged people and those living under congested conditions, lays most of its eggs in the seams of clothing. A single female of the head or body louse may have about 2000 descendants during her 30-day life.

Contact with infested clothing and bedding is probably the most common method of acquiring lice. However, lice are very active and crawl on walls of rooms and vehicles of public transportation. They migrate from a person with a fever and can survive 10 days without a blood meal. Head lice are readily spread from head to head when there is close contact, by means of hats and scarfs hung close together in schools and public places, and through the fitting of headgear in millinery stores and haberdasheries. Hair from persons infested with lice is often shed and may be the vehicle for the transmission of lice.

Crab lice can survive only for about 2 days off humans. Spread occurs during coitus, through bedding, by use of common or stacked bath towels, undergarments and gym suits, and from toilet seats.

Pathogenesis and Pathology

Adult and nymphal lice are hematophagous. As they feed, saliva is introduced into the site of puncture, causing an erythematous papule within hours. The papules itch, and as a consequence of scratching, secondary bacterial infection may occur.

On microscopic examination, edema, infiltration with lymphocytes, and the extravasation of erythrocytes are found. A residual pigmentation of the skin from bleeding and scratching is characteristic of lesions from long-continued infestations, particularly with crab lice.

Manifestations

Head lice may be seen, but frequently only the nits are visible, most commonly on hair above the ears or on the occiput an inch or so from the scalp. Intense pruritus of the scalp is common, and affected hairs may become lusterless and dry. Because of scratch-

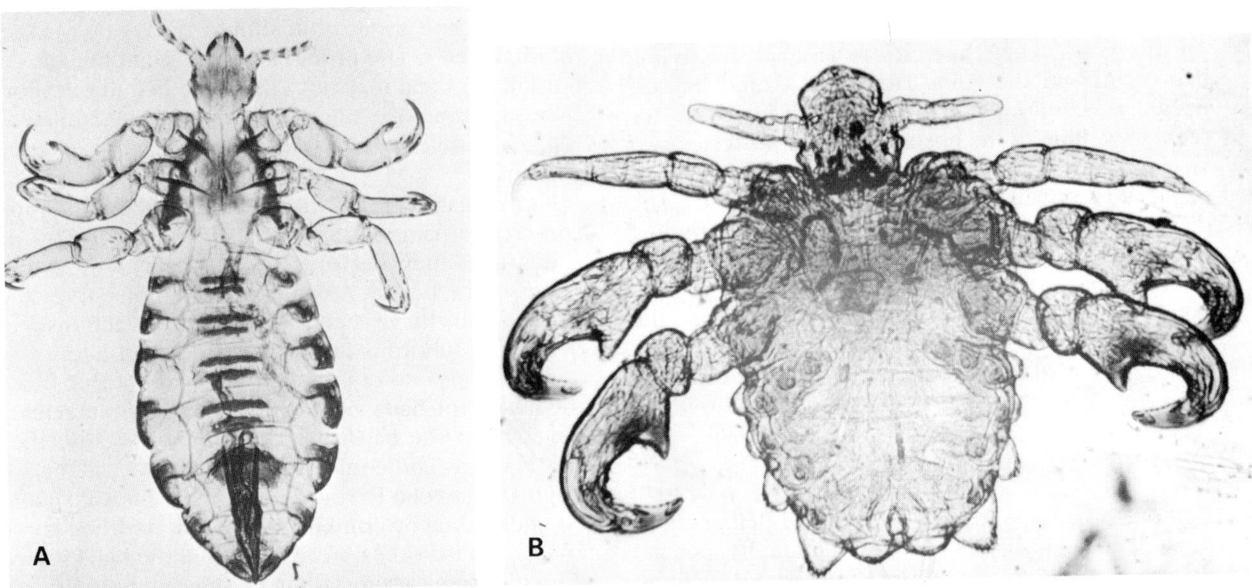

Fig. 114-1. (*A*) Adult male head louse. (Original magnification approximately × 17) (*B*) Adult crab louse. (Original magnification approximately × 20)

ing, secondary complications with impetigo and furunculosis are common and may cause the cervical lymph nodes to enlarge. Pustular eczema may occur (Fig. 114-2). In extremely severe infestations, a condition known as plica polonica may develop; in this condition, the hair may become matted with exudate from pustules, nits, and parasites, forming a fetid carapace in which fungi may proliferate and beneath which many lice may be found. Temporary alopecia may occur (Fig. 114-2).

Body lice live chiefly in the seams of clothing, particularly where there is close contact between garment and wearer, in such places as the waistline, axillae, and shoulders. The bites cause general pruritus, erythematous macules, urticarial wheals, and excoriated papules. A pigmented thickening of the skin with parallel linear scratch marks from continued rubbing and scratching is often observed. Secondary furuculosis is common. In heavy infestations, a tired feeling in the calves of the legs and along the shin bones and the soles of the feet may be so intense that normal sleep is prevented. An irritable and pessimistic state of mind develops.

Symptoms caused by crab lice range from slight discomfort to intolerable pubic itching that may lead to secondary infections from scratching. Pale, bluish gray maculae mark the sites of the bites.

Fig. 114-2. Pustular eczema and temporary alopecia caused by head lice. (McCarthy L: Diagnosis and Treatment of Diseases of the Hair. St. Louis, CV Mosby, 1940)

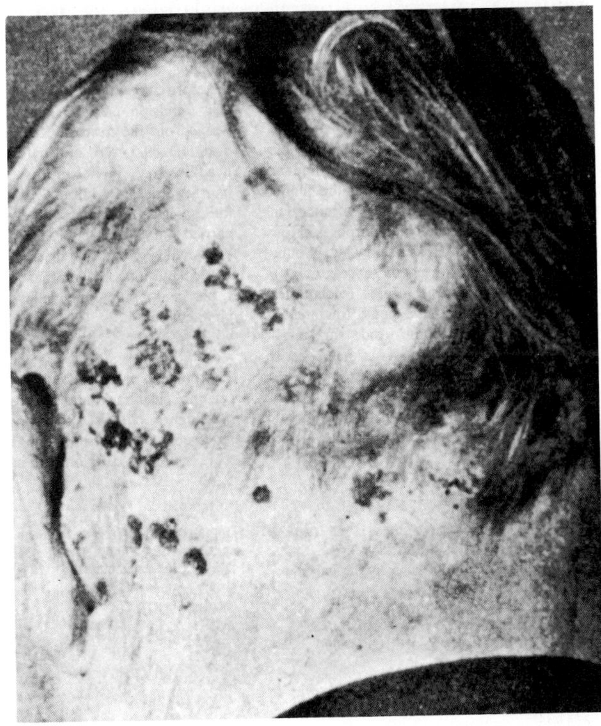

Diagnosis

The diagnosis of head and crab lice is made by finding lice or nits on the hairs. Head lice should be suspected in children with impetigo, furunculosis, or tender swelling of the postauricular or posterior cervical lymph nodes. Lice and eggs are absent in pityriasis sicca or pustular eczema from other causes. The diagnosis of body lice can be confirmed by finding the lice and nits in the seams of clothing, particularly underclothing. Erythematous macules that are accompanied by hyperpigmentation occur on the shoulders and around the axillary region and waist. The center of the back is usually free of eruptions.

Prognosis

Without broad application of chemical delousing to the individual, his family, and his community, persistence of infestation and reinfestation are virtually inevitable.

Therapy

In some countries outside the United States, body lice have shown resistance to DDT, lindane, and malathion. In other areas, including the United States, the use of DDT is being curtailed, though not as yet for medicinal purposes. However, malathion, as a 1% powder, and Abate (a preparation containing 2% temephos, an organophosphorus insecticide) are effective against all stages of the body louse in the United States and in most areas of the world. Because of their ovicidal action, a single treatment is adequate when applied to the inside surface of clothing, particularly the undergarments, with special attention to seams and folds. Dichlorvos plastic strips (No-Pest Strips) are recommended for fumigating clothes in plastic bags.

Head and crab lice infestations are efficiently treated with modern, chemical insecticides. Shearing long-haired persons is not necessary except in the most extreme infestations. In the United States, NBIN emulsion (Topicide) and lindane (Kwell) shampoos, lotions, and creams are available, as well as nonprescription preparations (A-200 Pyrinate, Cuprex, Bornate). Because NBIN emulsion may not kill all the 8- and 9-day-old eggs even after a 10-minute exposure, a second application should always be made 3 to 4 days later. The products that contain lindane do not kill eggs and may not kill all the lice in the short exposure time of a single application. Unfortunately, repeated use may give rise to a dermatitis in some persons.

Not available in the United States, malathion lotion and cream shampoos are extensively used in Europe and Africa; they kill the eggs as well as the other stages of the lice. In African children, poisonings and even deaths have been attributed to the use of organophosphorous insecticides for head lice.

Insecticides do not dissolve the cement that binds the nits to the hairs, both dead and empty nits remain attached to the hairs after treatment. Because they are unsightly and confusing to those who cannot distinguish between live and dead nits, removal should be undertaken by combing with a fine-toothed comb (teeth less than 0.3 mm apart) while the head is covered by a rich creamy lather; rinsing and repetition of the process a number of times is necessary.

Lice and nits on eyelashes are best treated with ophthalmic ointment containing 0.25% physostigmine.

Prevention

The prevention of pediculosis consists largely of personal cleanliness and the frequent washing and pressing of clothes. No amount of cleanliness, however, can prevent a temporary infestation if there is close association with infested persons.

Bibliography

Books

Proceedings of the International Symposium on the Control of Lice and Louse-borne Diseases. Washington, DC. Pan American Health Organization Scientific Publication No. 263, 1973. 311 pp.

Journals

ACKERMAN A: Crabs: the resurgence of *Phthirus pubis.* N Engl J Med 278:950–951, 1968

COATES KG: Control of head louse infestation in schoolchildren. Community Med 126:148–149, 1971

KEH B: Answers to some questions frequently asked about pediculosis. Calif Vector Views 26:51–62, 1979

ROGER W. WILLIAMS

Trombiculosis

115

Trombiculosis (chigger infestation) is an infestation with larval mites of the family Trombiculidae, creatures that can cause more torment for their size than most other living things.

Etiology

Often orange red in color, these mites are arachnids that are 0.15 mm to 0.25 mm in size and up to 0.60 mm when engorged. They possess three pairs of hairy legs. Their oral secretions cause intense pruritus, provoking severe scratching that often results in secondary infections.

Epidemiology

About 20 species of chigger mites cause a dermatitis in humans or are vectors of infectious agents (*e.g.*, scrub typhus, see Chap. 99, Scrub Typhus). Among the former are the chiggers or red bugs of the New World, the harvest mite of Europe, and the scrub-itch mites of the Orient and Australia. *Trombicula (Eutrombicula) alfreddugèsi* is the most widespread trombiculid mite attacking humans in the Western Hemisphere in a range that extends from Canada to South America and the West Indies. This distribution overlaps two other species that attack humans in the southeastern states. The season of activity in the United States varies from July and August in Minnesota and Massachusetts to around the year in southern Florida. Chigger mites are most abundant in second-growth, cutover areas, around wild berry bushes, bush thickets, meadow and low marshy land, transition areas between forest, and grassland. In addition, they have been found in city lots, parks, lawns, and in the rough or golf courses, where they attach to feed on any passing reptile, amphibian, bird, or mammal.

Attachment is favored in body areas in which clothing prevents the free movement of mites, such as ankles, inguinal area, waistline, axillae, and beneath garters or suspenders.

Pathogenesis

The chigger does not burrow but merely pierces the epidermis as deeply as possible, frequently at a hair follicle or sweat gland. Its oral secretions liquefy epidermal cells which, with tissue debris and fluid, are aspirated for nourishment. Only incidentally and rarely is blood ingested. A "stylostome" lined with cornified epithelium is formed by powerful glandular secretions that cause the dermal reactions and characteristic pruritic manifestations (Fig. 115-1). The inner layer of cells of the stylostome become necrotic and appear to be digested. There is a noticeable round-cell infiltration within this tubelike structure, and there is evidence that such cells are sucked into the tube from the surrounding dermis and subcutis, digested extraorally, and then ingested by the chigger. Two to four hours after invasion, a slight tingling may be noted. The larva may be seen as a barely visible red speck centered in an anemic 2-mm to 3-mm macule. During the next 10 to 16 hours the macule increases in size and becomes slightly raised. By 20 to 30 hours, the central area becomes hyperemic, usually taking the shape of a low, spherical, or parabolic papule, or sometimes a markedly acuminate, conical papule. At this stage, the itching has reached its full intensity. As a result of increased serous exudation, the lesion becomes larger and a vesicle usually forms near the apex, eccentric to the central axis of the papule (Fig. 115-2). The hyperemic area becomes hemorrhagic, and involution sets in and wanes over several weeks. Occasionally, the papule may give rise to a nodule that may persist for months, and a hemorrhagic stain that may persist for years.

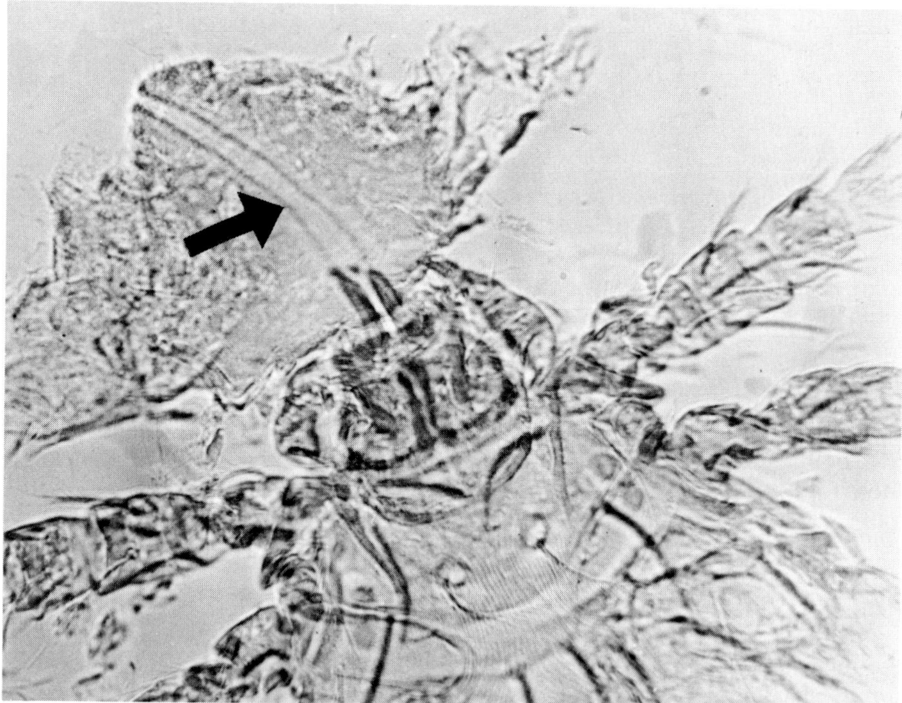

Fig. 115-1. An attached chigger showing "stylostome" formation (*arrow*). Original magnification approximately × 440 (Courtesy of CB Philip)

Fig. 115-2. An eccentric vesicle on a papule, characteristic of chigger bites. (Courtesy of GW Wharton)

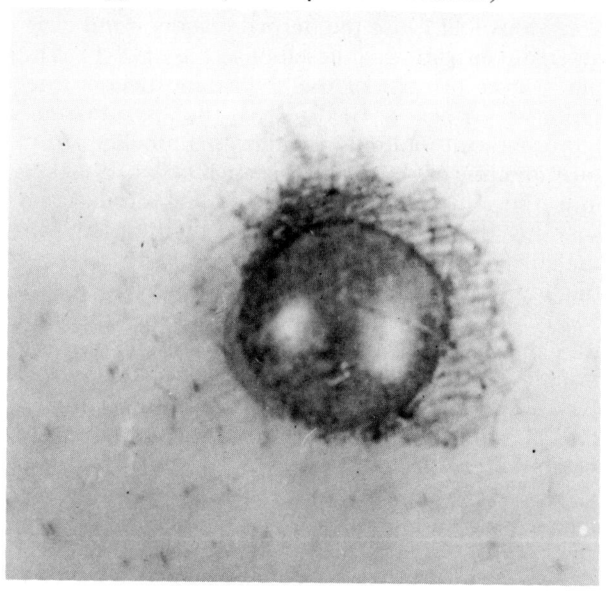

Diagnosis

If examined early, the mite larvae may be found attached near the center of the lesions. The bites of many insects often resemble the early stages of chigger bites, but they are frequently less numerous and are more commonly located on exposed parts of the body. They are usually perceived immediately and are seldom hemorrhagic. Dermatitis caused by schistosomal cercariae may present a picture of pruritic papules that become pustules, a condition unusual with chigger bites. The nettling of certain plants, though rarely found in the same locaton on the body as chigger bites, may produce vesicles that are always centrally located on papules. Infestations of other mites are not typically confined to body areas in which the clothing fits snugly—grocer's itch from handling figs, dates, and prunes; copra mites; and grain itch mites produce pruritic, papulovesicular, urticarial, or vesicopustular eruptions on the hands, face, arms, chest, and back.

Prognosis

If not scratched out or destroyed, chiggers may remain attached for 3 to 5 days. Even if destroyed, the salivary secretions continue to act on the epidermal cells, and the irritation continues. In infants and elderly persons with numerous lesions, there may be systemic reaction with fever, headache, and at times, proteinuria. Pruritus often interferes with sleep. Secondary infections derived from scratching are frequent. An acquired immunity may develop in some persons after repeated exposure.

Therapy

Because pruritus is the first indication of infestation, first measures are aimed at securing relief. The following mixture is helpful as a palliative treatment when applied to each bite with cotton: benzocaine, 5%; methyl salicylate, 2%; salicylic acid, 0.5%; ethyl alcohol, 73%; and water, 19.5%. Repeated application may be necessary. Fingernail polish (nonallergenic) applied to the bites is said to be helpful. Secondarily infected lesions may be treated with antimicrobic (bacitracin–neomycinpolymyxin B) lotions or ointments, or 30% ammoniated mercury ointment.

Prevention

Bathing and a change of clothes within 2 hours of exposure to chiggers considerably decrease the infestation. Almost complete freedom from chiggers may be obtained by treating the clothing with one of the following: dimethyl phthalate, dibutyl phthalate, benzyl benzoate, *N,N*-diethyl-*m*-toluamide (DEET or Off), and *N,N*-diisopropyl-*p*-toluamide. These repellent materials can be applied as a half-inch barrier around the tops of socks, waist, and neck; and by rubbing 4 to 5 ounces or spraying 1 to 2 ounces over the clothing. M-1960, an emulsifiable concentrate—containing by weight 30% benzyl benzoate (protects against mites), 30% *N*-butyl acetanilide (protects against ticks), 30% 2-butyl-2-ethyl-1, 3-propandiol (protects against mosquitoes), and 10% Tween 80 (the emulsifier)—is effective even after several washings if applied to clothing as directed. It should be noted that some synthetic fabrics may be harmed by the repellents. However, powdered sulfur applied in to the areas where clothing fits tightly, is also very effective.

Area control may be carried out by spray or dust treatment with dioxathion, malathion, propoxur, or diazinon used in accordance with the labeled directions. Careful attention should be given to avoiding application to ponds, streams, and other water courses and their adjacent margins.

Dimethoate (0.2%) in rodent baits is an effective systemic acaricide when used for 3 months or longer. It would be useful in reducing chigger populations in parks, permanent campsites, and construction sites in areas in which chiggers are active throughout the year.

Remaining Problems

The development of an effective treatment for the intense itching and discomfort produced by chigger bites is badly needed.

Bibliography

Journals

GOUCK HG: Protection from ticks, fleas, chiggers and leeches. Arch Dermatol 93:112–113, 1966

WILLIAMS RW: A contribution to our knowledge of the bionomics of the common North American chigger, *Eutrombicula alfreddugesi* (Oudemans) with a description of a rapid collecting method. Am J Trop Med Hyg 26:243–250, 1946

ROGER W. WILLIAMS

116 Scabies

Scabies is an infectious disease of the skin produced by the mite *Sarcoptes scabiei,* which burrows in the stratum corneum, depositing eggs in tunnels and causing a characteristic, pruritic skin eruption through sensitization. Various biologic strains are found in a wide variety of domestic and wild animals in which they cause mange.

Etiology

The adult female *S. scabiei* is 300 μm to 400 μm in length and has four pairs of short legs—the posterior pairs terminating in long bristles (Fig. 116-1; Fig. 9-1*A, B*). The male is somewhat over half the size of the female and has a long bristle extending from only the third pair of legs.

Epidemiology

Scabies is characteristically an infestation of closely associated persons, such as in a hospital or business establishment; it can spread rapidly. Person-to-person transmission of mites may also take place at night during the course of prolonged skin-to-skin contact. Transmission through bedding and clothing may occur. The main infective stage is thought to be the newly fertilized female.

In adult males with scabies, about 65% had mites burrowing between the fingers and on the wrists, forming clinically characteristic macroscopic lesions (Fig. 116-2). Other areas of the body were less frequently infested. The distribution of parasites in females and children has not been as thoroughly studied. During the first year of life, infection occurs anywhere on the body, although the soles of the feet, palms, head, and neck seem to be more the commonly infested areas. Not until about the fifth year are most lesions found on the hands and wrists. Children are prone to bulbous lesions, causing this infestation to be mistaken for pemphigus or bulbous pemphigold.

Pathogenesis and Pathology

A vesicle or pustule may be present at the point of entry into the skin. As the gravid female burrows in the skin, she produces a slightly elevated, tortuous tunnel, measuring a few millimeters, in which she has deposited eggs and pellets of feces (scyballa). The larvae that hatch out in 3 to 4 days leave the burrows and appear on the skin surface. They find food and shelter by temporarily entering hair follicles, where both larvae and nymphs may be found. The adult stage is reached in 4 to 6 days. After mating in a burrow, the females generally emerge and wander on the surface until they find a site suitable for burrowing into the cuticle of the skin to repeat the cycle. Initial infections may reach population peaks of 50 to 500 adult mites over a period of 2 to 4 months, during which time sensitization begins. Infiltration with lymphocytes and eosinophils occurs around the tunnels. Eosinophilia may vary from 5% to 15%. There may be an association between epidemic scabies and acute glomerulonephritis.

Occasionally, reddish brown nodules may persist following cure of scabies, particularly in children. Although the nodules may resemble a malignant lymphoid neoplasm, they are composed of lymphocytes and histocytes deep in the corium.

Norwegian scabies, or crusted scabies, ocurs most frequently in persons with poor hygiene or whose appreciation of, or reaction to, itching is impaired, for example, through mental illness, or other concerns or illnesses that override sensations of itching. Where immunosuppressants are being given there is evidence that freshly acquired scabies does not produce hypersensitivity or itching and the mites multiply

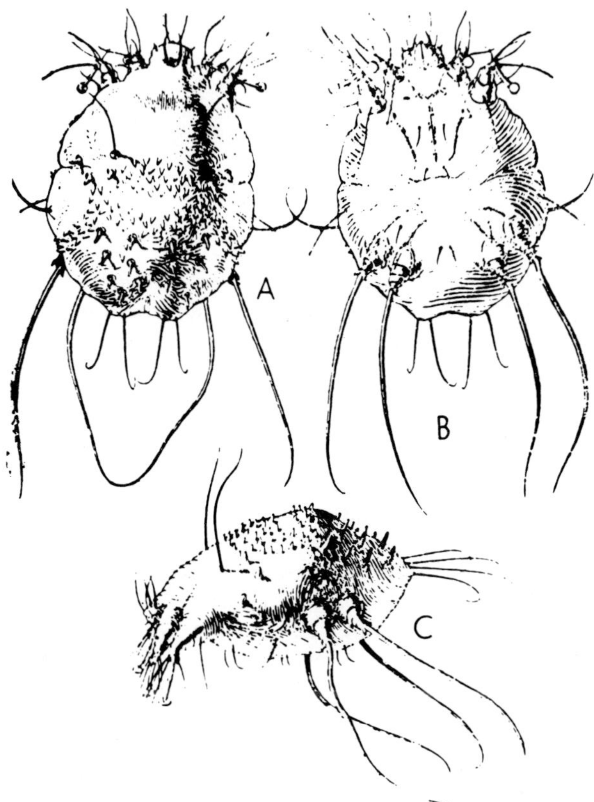

Fig. 116-1. Female *Sarcoptes scabiei.* (*A*) Dorsal aspect. (*B*) Ventral aspect. (*C*) Lateral aspect. (Mellanby K: Scabies. London, Oxford University Press, 1943)

uninterrupted in a favorable environment resulting in a severe condition of crusted scabies. Distinct burrows are not formed, although the same *S. scabiei* is involved. There is extensive ulceration and crusting of the skin to form hyperkeratotic plaques which may occur on any part of the body, including the face, scalp, and subungual areas. As many as 10,000 parasites per mm^2 may be sequestered under such crusts. Crusted scabies frequently serves as a source for other cases of classic scabies.

Manifestations

It is only when hypersensitivity has developed, 1 or more months after infection has occurred, that symptoms of scabies appear. An itching, irritating, erythematous, papular eruption appears that bears no relation to the number of mites or their location (Fig. 116-3). The patient must scratch continually. Excoriations result, and secondary infections in the form of pustules and impetigo may develop, masking the scabies.

Initially, the eruption occurs most commonly in the axillary region, around the waist, on the inner thighs, and on the backs of the arms and legs. It may spread from these areas to more or less cover the whole body. In reinfections, the number of adult female mites is usually less than six, although the typical irritating allergic rash is present.

Mange, scabies in nonhuman animals, is caused by species distinct from those that prefer to parasitize humans. However, mange-causing species, most frequently the canine form, may cause symptoms in humans. For example, persons who work with or handle dogs or who allow them to sit in their laps for long periods, frequently develop papulovesicular, erythematous, itchy, eruptions, usually without burrows, on the arms or around the waist. In these cases, it is very difficult to find mites; they apparently do not multiply in human skin. The infestation is self-limiting, rarely lasting longer than 3 weeks. Treatment for scabies eradicates the eruption and shortens the period of symptoms.

Fig. 116-2. Burrows of scabies mites between fingers. (Andrews GC, Domonkos AN: Diseases of the Skin, 6th ed. Philadelphia. WB Saunders, 1971)

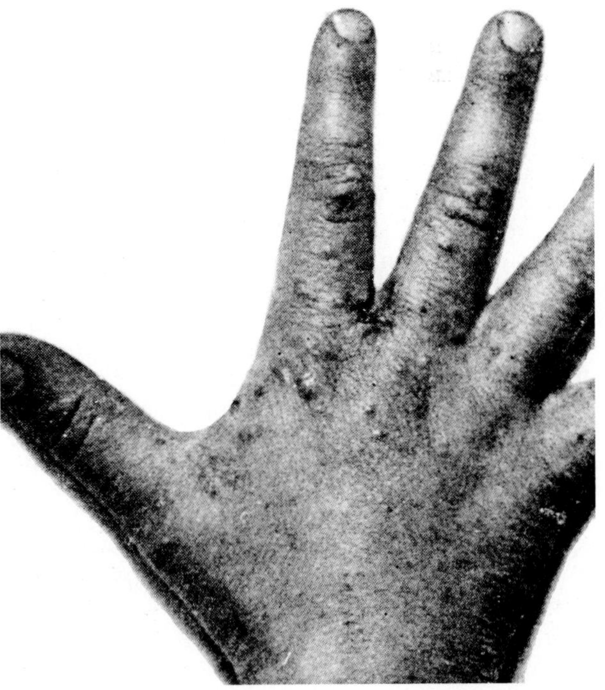

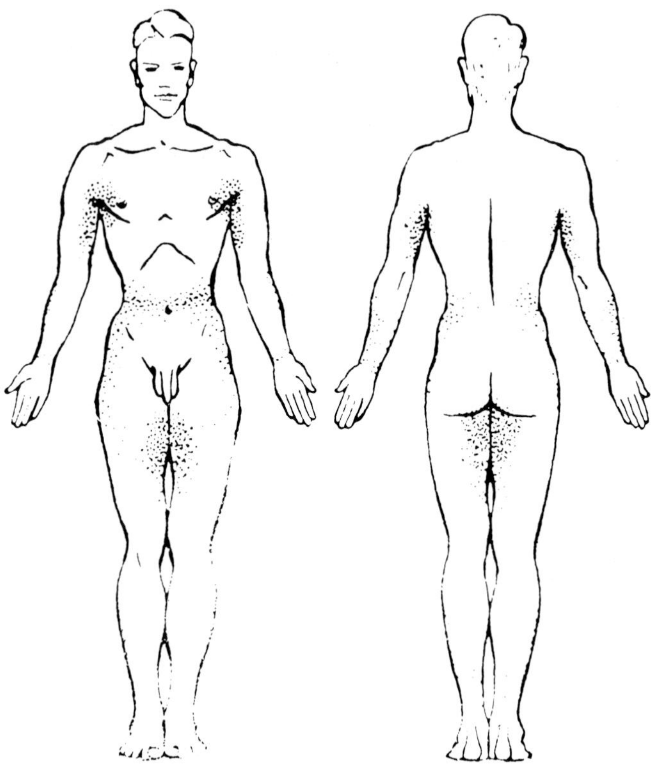

Fig. 116-3. Locations of the typical scabies rash. The rash does not correspond with the sites of election of the mites. (Mellanby K: Scabies. London, Oxford University Press, 1943)

Diagnosis

Because some cases of scabies may not present a typical appearance, positive diagnosis is made by finding the mites, eggs, scyballa, or portions thereof. The secret of finding the *Sarcoptes* sp. is to know where and what to look for, and not to search blindly over the body surface. With a watchmaker's lens, an inhabited burrow may be found between the fingers or around the wrists. The mite will be visible at its anterior end as a whitish oval body with dark pigmentation at the front. The parasite may be extracted on a needle point, placed on a slide, coverslipped, and observed with about 40× magnification. Some prefer to scrape the area of the vesicle and burrow with a sterile, sharp scalpel upon which a drop of sterile mineral oil has been placed. The material is placed on a slide, coverslipped and examined for eggs, mites, or scyballa. The use of mineral oil is superior to using KOH to dissolve tissue cells since the mites tend to float out alive, the difference in refraction is greater, and it does not dissolve the typical fecal compactions.

Prognosis

Left untreated, particularly in the crusted form, scabies may persist for decades. With proper treatment, a given infestation can be eliminated. Reinfection, however, is quite possible.

Therapy

Good medical practice calls for the examination and treatment of all family members and others in close contact with the scabies patient. The classic remedy, a sulfur ointment, is 97% to 100% effective. In some persons, a sulfur dermatitis may develop. After the patient has had a bath, 3 oz of 3% to 10% sulfur (depending on age and condition of the skin) in lanolin or vanishing cream is applied over the entire body. Two or more applications are suggested either on succeeding days or within a period of a week. Self-treatment is possible, but there may be failure of compliance because of the malodor.

Emulsions containing 20% to 25% benzyl benzoate are nearly completely effective. Antimicrobics (bacitracin-neomycin-polymyxin B) can be added to the emulsion to combat secondary bacterial invaders. After the patient has had a bath, the emulsion is applied with a 2-inch wide paint brush, from the neck downward, covering the entire body. At least 24 hours should elapse before bathing. A second treatment is usually given the next day or within a week to allow for inefficiency or other possible sources of failure. The crusted lesions of Norwegian scabies should be removed with sulfur and salicylic acid cream before the application of benzyl benzoate.

Lindane, 1% in vanishing cream (Kwell ointment), applied at the rate of 30 g to 50 g or sprayed on the skin in a 1% emulsion, is very effective against all types of scabies.

Three to five daily applications of crotamiton (Eurax) cream or lotion is effective. The cream is particularly useful for infants under 2 years of age because it possesses both antipruritic and antibacterial properties. This is important because children are very susceptible to superficial bacterial infections of the skin as a result of scratching.

Tetraethylthiuram monosulfide (Tetmosol) has been used with good results, particularly in young children who may not tolerate benzyl benzoate well. Three or more treatments, 24 hours apart, are recommended. Tetmosol has also been incorporated in bath soap to be used as a treatment and prophylaxis.

All the preceding remedies are effective, and some practitioners feel that the technique of application is more important than the specific acaricide.

Prevention

Prevention of scabies depends on the avoidance of prolonged skin-to-skin contact with infected persons and the avoidance of infected bed linen and towels.

Bibliography

Book

MELANBY K: Scabies, 2nd ed. London, Oxford University Press, 1972. 81 pp.

Journals

MULLER G, JACOBS PH, MOORE NE: Scraping for human scabies: A better method for positive preparations. Arch Dermatol 107:70, 1973

PATERSON WD, ALLEN BR, BEVERIDGE GW: Norwegian scabies during immunosuppressive therapy. Br Med J 4:211–212, 1973

SYARTMAN M, POTTER EV, FINKLEA JF, POON–KING T, EARLE DP: Epidemic scabies and acute glomerulonephritis in Trinidad. Lancet 1:249–251, 1972

ROGER W. WILLIAMS

117 Necrotic Arachnidism

Less than 1% of the more than 100,000 species of spiders in the world are capable of inflicting poisonous bites to humans. The relatively few that are potentially hazardous include about 70 species of the genus *Loxosceles,* found in Africa, Europe, and the New World. Bites by either sex are toxic, and some may cause severe cutaneous necrosis.

Etiology

Among important New World species are *L. laetae, L. arisonica, L. devia, L. reclusa, L. refescens,* and *L. unicolor;* all are found in the United States. All are about half an inch long and possess six eyes in a semicircle. The first four species have a characteristic violin-shaped marking on the carapace (Fig. 117-1). The venom of *Loxosceles* contains levarterenol, hemolysins (sphingomyelinase D), and a spreading factor that act with other agents as powerful neurotoxins, hemotoxins, and cytotoxins.

Epidemiology

The bite of *L. laetae* from South America is the most severe. This species has gained entrance into the United States on a number of occasions and has been found in rather large numbers in several communities in Los Angeles County, California. In the United States, *L. reclusa,* the brown recluse or fiddler spider, is the most common agent of necrotic arachnidism. It is found from central Illinois to the Gulf coast and from Oklahoma and Kansas to Georgia. It has also been reported from Ohio, New Jersey, and Wyoming. These spiders can survive northern winters only indoors. *Loxosceles unicolor* is probably the most common species in California, Arizona, Utah, and Nevada while *L. arizonica* is found largely in Arizona, New Mexico, and Texas, and has been reported from California. *Loxosceles devia* is most common in the southern half of Texas, while *L. rufescens* has been reported from Texas, Louisiana, and Georgia. The bites of these species are thought not to be as serious as that of *L. reclusa.* These spiders are shy, sedentary, and most active at night. They spin a large, irregular web, with thick, sticky threads in some dark location in which they usually remain. They are found in barns, chicken coops, garages, storage sheds, and human dwellings where they may be under furniture, in crevices in floors and walls, in closets, bureau drawers, under picture frames, and in clothing hanging on the wall. They bite only when molested.

Pathogenesis and Pathology

The action of the venom of *Loxosceles* spp. may be only local, or both local and systemic. Locally, the venom may cause necrosis by forming hemostatic plugs—microthrombic aggregates of leukocytes and platelets—in venules and arterioles, or a mild cutaneous reaction without necrosis. Eosinophils make up the primary cellular infiltrate following envenomation.

Manifestations

Discomfort referred to the site of the bite may occur immediately after envenomation. The local lesion frequently appears white with an erythematous halo. Blisters may appear, accompanied by severe pain and pronounced edema. The subsequent course of the lesion can be predicted according to its size at 12 hours after the bite: if ≤ 4 cm across (not including ecchymoses around the lesion), local manifestations without necrosis or systemic disease are typical; if $>$ 4 cm, local necrosis and systemic manifestations are the rule. As the lesion evolves, the skin turns purple, then black as gangrene develops (Fig. 117-2*A*). In

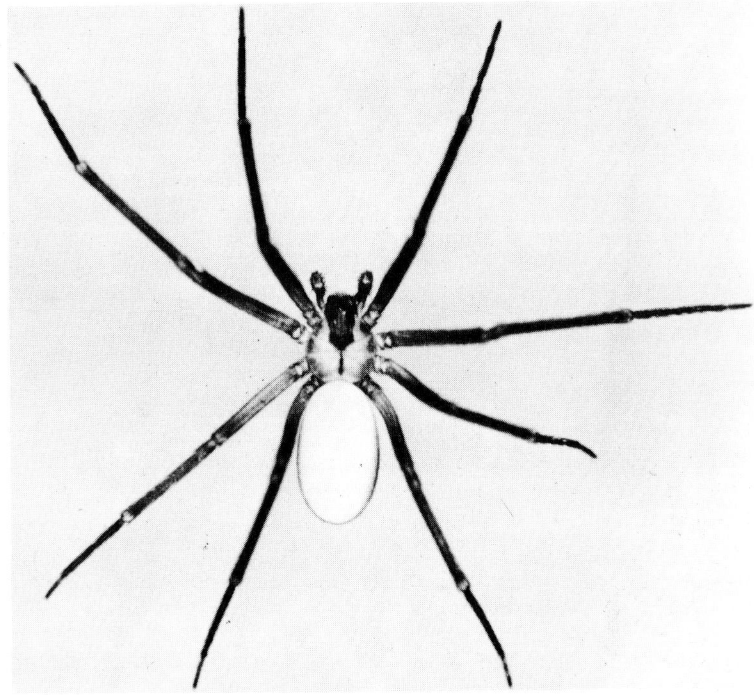

Fig. 117-1. *Loxosceles reclusa.* Note the violin-shaped marking on the cephalothorax. (Courtesy of PN Morgan)

about 2 weeks, the eschar sloughs away leaving an ugly, depressed ulcer (Fig. 117-2*B*) that gradually fills with scar tissue (Fig. 117-2*C*).

Systemic manifestations may include chills, fever, malaise, weakness, nausea, vomiting, joint pains, and at times, a general pruritic, morbilliform, and petechial eruption. There may be marked biochemical alterations with acute thrombocytopenia, leukocytosis, hemolytic anemia, hemoglobinemia, hemoglobinuria, hematuria, proteinuria, and bilirubinemia. Confusion, disorientation, coma, shock, and death may ensue.

Diagnosis

Early diagnosis of necrotic arachnidism is desirable. To this end a passive hemagglutination-inhibition test has been developed. It is based on the ability of venom to inhibit the antiserum-induced agglutination of venom-sensitized human group O erythrocytes.

Therapy

An antivenin to *L. laetae* has been developed in South America, but it is not generally available elsewhere. In the United States, a supply is kept in the collection of antivenins of the Los Angeles County–University of Southern California Medical School. Early surgical excision of the involved tissue, within 4 to 6 hours, appears to some to be the most practical treatment. Local injections of glucosteroids into the site of the bite are of unproved value; they may be contraindicated because they could result in liberation of the toxin into the bloodvascular system. The systemic administration of a glucosteroid as soon as possible after a bite may be the treatment of choice; if delayed 48 hours or more, steroids are unlikely to have any effect on restricting the spread of the toxins. Benefits have not been uniformly recorded.

A regimen recommended for the treatment of the adult begins with the intramuscular injection of 80 mg methylprednisolone acetate immediately after diagnosis. The same dose is repreated every other day for two to three doses. According to the response, the dose is gradually reduced to 40 mg, 20 mg, and then 10 mg every other day to complete an 8- to 10-day course of therapy. Heparin may benefit severe coagulation disorders. Antihistamines and antimicrobics may also be given in severe reactions complicated by secondary infection. Fibrinolysin and deoxyribonuclease (combine, bovine) has produced rapid healing in some cases.

The acute systemic reaction, especially in children,

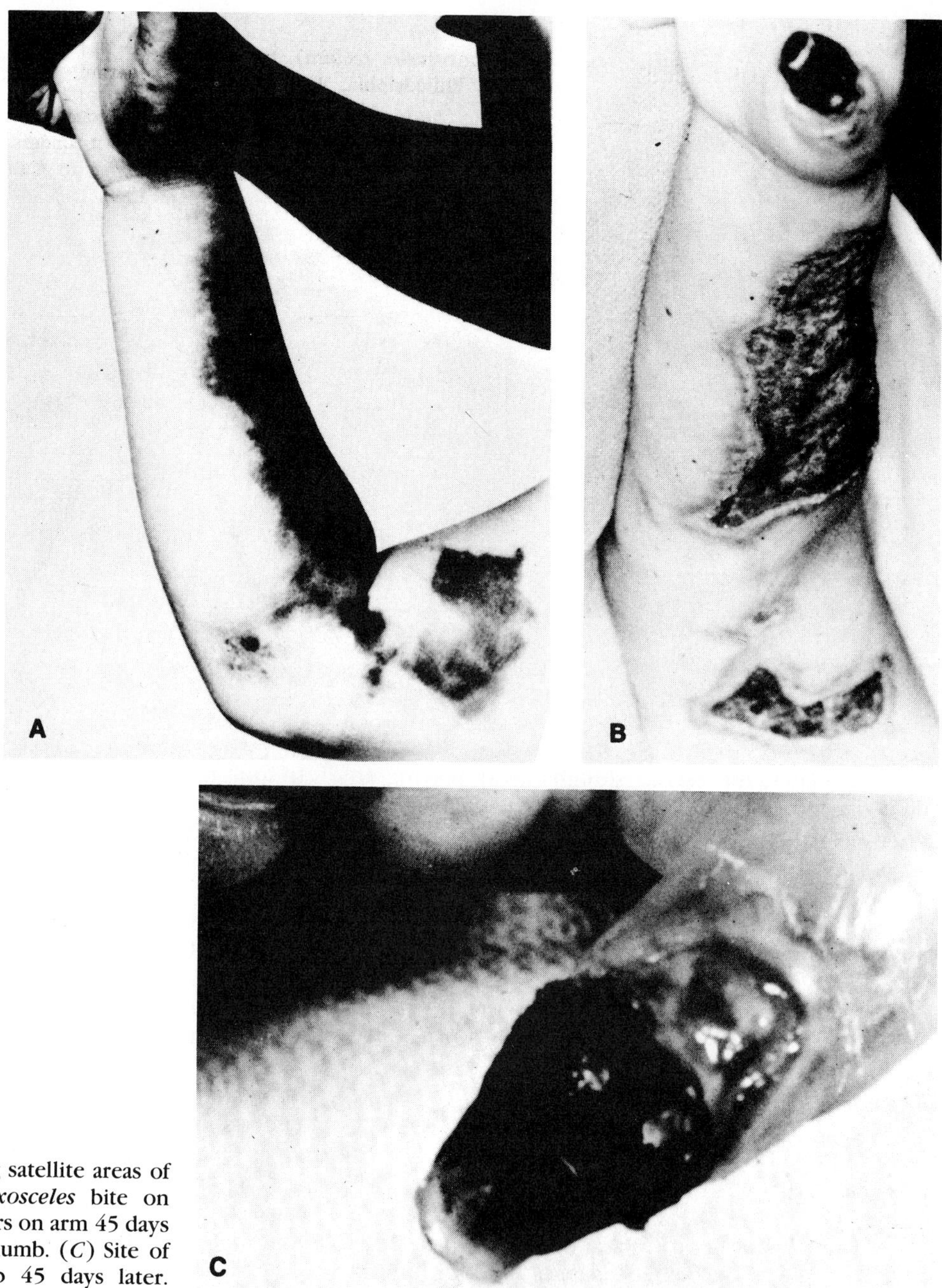

Fig. 117-2. (*A*) Spreading satellite areas of necrosis 5 days after *Loxosceles* bite on thumb. (*B*) Depressed ulcers on arm 45 days after *Loxosceles* bite on thumb. (*C*) Site of *Loxosceles* bite on thumb 45 days later. (Courtesy of B Cosman)

requires hospitalization. A glucosteroid (*e.g.,* 80 mg methylprednisolone sodium succinate, or an equivalent amount of another steroid) should be given by intravenous injection to initiate therapy. For continuation of steroid treatment, intramuscular injections can be given, as stated previously. If hemolysis and thrombocytopenia are severe, fresh, whole blood transfusion may be necessary. When tissue necrosis is extensive and renal failure coexists, peritoneal dialysis or hemodialysis may be necessary to control hyperkalemia. Skin grafting is required to repair the effects of local necrosis. Recovery from the bite is said to give a solid immunity.

Prevention

Lindane, malathion, dichlorvos (DDVP), and paradichlorobenzene are recommended for the control of the spider, but good housekeeping is the essential control technique indoors. Airtight boxes or bags containing plastic strips impregnated with paradichlorobenzene or DDVP should be used for storing clothes and bedding. If not so stored, these articles should be shaken out and aired before use. Unnecessary articles in basements and attics should be discarded. All storage areas, dead space behind mirrors, pictures, behind and under furniture, particularly beds, should be cleaned periodically with a vacuum cleaner.

Remaining Problems

Too often the spider responsible for a necrotic bite is never seen. When one is caught, identification requires a very skilled taxonomist. Quite possibly, the common assumption that the combination of six eyes and a "fiddle" marking on the carapace corresponds to *L. reclusa* is in error, and in reality it is another species. Little is known about the toxic reactions caused by the non-*reclusa* species, but it is thought that the effects are not as severe as those caused by *L. reclusa.* Further studies on the toxicity of the bites of various species should be conducted as well as studies with male spiders to ascertain whether their bites are as toxic as those of females. Such studies might throw light upon what appears to be nonuniformity of toxicity from *L. reclusa.* The distribution of *Loxosceles* spp. in the United States is not well defined and it would be helpful if the distribution was accurately known. Improvement in therapy is needed.

Bibliography

Books

ASEL ND: Spider bites (Loxosceles reclusa). In Conn HF (ed): Current Therapy. Philadelphia, WB Saunders, 1970. p 805.

SCHMAUS JW: Bites of spiders and other arthropods. In Conn HF (ed): Current Therapy. Philadelphia, WB Saunders, 1970. pp 803–804.

Journals

ANDERSON PC: Brown spider bites: An update. J Kentucky Med Assoc 76:172–173, 1978

BERGER RS: The unremarkable brown reculse spider bite. JAMA 225:1109–1111, 1973

FINK JH, CAMPBELL BJ, BARRETT TJ: Serodiagnostic tests for *Loxosceles reclusa* bites. Clin Toxicol 7:375–382, 1974

FOIL LD, NORMENT BR: Review article: Envenomation by *Loxosceles reclusa.* J Med Entomol 16:18–25, 1979

MADRIGAL GC, ERCOLANI RL, WERYL JE: Toxicity from a bite of the brown spider (*Loxosceles reculusa*). Clin Pediatr 11:641–644, 1972

RUSSELL FE, WALDRON WG, MADON MG: Bites by the brown spiders *Loxosceles unicolor* and *Loxosceles arizonica* in California and Arizona. Toxicon 7:109–117, 1969

WALDRON WG, MADON MAB, SUDDARTH T: Observations on the occurrence and ecology of *Loxosceles laeta* (Araneae Scytodidae) in Los Angeles County, California. Calif Vector Views 22:29–36, 1975

Section XV

Infections of the Leptomeninges

Indigenous Microbiota of the Leptomeninges

(None)

HERBERT A. WENNER

Viral Meningitis

118

Viral meningitis is characterized by fever, headache, vomiting, hyperesthesia, myalgia, and stiffness of the neck. It is a common syndrome caused by diverse infectious agents. Some degree of involvement of neural tissue is common, although it is generally unapparent clinically.

Etiology

The viruses most constantly associated with the viral meningitis syndrome are the mumps virus (Chap. 74, Mumps), enteroviruses (Chap. 121, Poliomyelitis and Chap. 149, Coxsackievirus and Echovirus Infections), and arboviruses (Chap. 122, Viral Encephalitides). Others may be encountered periodically: herpes simplex virus (Chap. 91, Infections Caused by Herpes Simplex Viruses and Chap. 122, Viral Encephalitides), lymphocytic choriomeningitis viruses, and encephalomyocarditis viruses (Table 118-1).

Louping ill, pseudolymphocytic meningitis, and hepatitis viruses (Chap. 70–72 Hepatitis A; Hepatitis B; Non-A, Non-B Hepatitis) may cause viral meningitis. Adenoviruses (mainly types 1, 2, 5, 6, and 7—see Chap. 23, Nonbacterial pharyngitis) and one of the rhinoviruses (Chap. 21, The Common Cold) may also be associated with the syndrome; however, their position among the viruses responsible for meningitis has yet to be fully defined. With some 30% to 40% of meningitides presumed to be of viral origin, etiologic diagnosis has not been readily accomplished despite the application of modern techniques.

Epidemiology

Enteroviruses, the mumps virus, and herpesvirus type 1 are transmitted from person to person either by fecal-oral, oral-oral, or respiratory routes. Enteroviruses, the mumps virus, and arboviruses periodically cause epidemics that may sometimes be clinically inapparent; for example, echovirus 7. During interepidemic periods, reservoirs of virus persist, either through the recruitment of susceptible persons or within extrahuman hosts (*e.g.,* arboviruses). Herpesvirus is ubiquitous among humans, recruiting susceptible infants and children without notable periodicity.

The epidemiologies of the mumps virus, arboviruses, and herpesviruses (venereal transmission) are discussed in Chapters 74, Mumps; 122, Viral Encephalitides; and 91, Infections Caused by Herpes Simplex Virus, respectively.

Enteroviruses

Humans are the only known natural hosts of the polioviruses, coxsackieviruses, and echoviruses. Direct, person-to-person spread occurs by the transfer of infected respiratory secretions or feces. These viruses are occasionally disseminated by flies, cockroaches, and possibly other vectors with access to human excrement.

Enteroviruses are seen worldwide. In temperate climates, the incidence of infection from one or more serotypes rises sharply during the summer—the seasonal pattern observed in reported cases of aseptic meninigitis (Fig. 118-1). In tropical climates, infection rates have prevailing endemicity rather than epidemicity. Age-specific attack rates emphasize the risk of youth. The attack rates in children often exceed those in infants, but not invariably. During some outbreaks, for example, echovirus type 11 rates for infants exceed those of young children. Attack rates in young adults may rank with those of children. When introduced into a family or nursery unit, these viruses disperse rapidly to susceptible persons in residence (Table 118-2). Coxsackieviruses and echoviruses have been known to spread widely and quite silently within a community. Because of the many

Table 118-1. *Some Properties of Viruses Often Associated With Meningitis*

Virus		Properties						Types of infections					
		ANTIGENIC		PHYSICAL		TRANSMISSION							
		GROUPS	TYPES	SIZE (nm)	NUCLEIC ACID	PERSON-TO-PERSON	VECTOR*	SILENT†	SYSTEMIC	MENINGITIC	ENCEPHALITIC	MYELITIC	MEM‡
	Polio		3	~25	RNA‖	+	0	+	+	+	0	+	0
Enteroviruses§	Coxsackie	A,B	29	~28	RNA	+	0	+	+	+	+	+	+
	Echo		32	17–28	RNA	+	0	+	+	+	?#	+	?
Mumps			1	85–300	RNA	+	0	+	+	+	+	±	±
Arboviruses		A,B,C	Many	25–50	RNA**	0	+	+	+	+	+	+	+
Herpes simplex virus			⩾2	180	DNA#	+	0	+	+	+	+	±	±
Lymphocytic choriomeningitis			1	40–60	RNA	+	+	?	+	+	±	+	?
Encephalomyocarditis			?	27–28	RNA	?	+	+	+	+	?	?	?

*Arthropod vectors predominantly.

†No specific illness may be recognized.

‡Meningoencephalomyelitis.

§Overlapping characteristics of enteroviruses have made it very difficult to subgroup some serotypes as either polio-, coxsackie-, or echoviruses. In 1970, a numbering system was proposed whereby new members are enumerated beginning with type 68. At least four new serotypes (68, 69, 70, and 71) have been identified.

Entries in the table provide a score of 64 rather than 67. Coxsackievirus A23 and echovirus 9 are identical; echovirus types 10 and 18 have been reclassified as reovirus type 1 and rhinovirus type 1.

‖Ribonucleic acid core.

#Data not clearly interpretable, or as yet unavailable

**Deoxyribonucleic acid core

distinct serotypes, solid immunity is rare in a given population.

The incubation period of enteroviruses varies widely. Estimates for poliomyelitis range 3 to 35 days; for coxsackieviruses type A9, 2 to 12 days; for types A21 and B5, 3 to 5 days; and for most echoviruses, 3 to 8 days. Enteroviruses are readily found in feces and oropharyngeal secretions. Excepting the polioviruses, many have been recovered from cerebrospinal fluid (CSF). During the early stages of illness, enteroviruses may be found in the blood of infected persons.

Table 118-2. *Age-Specific Rates of Recovering Echovirus 6 in Index Patients and Family Associates*

Age (years)	Index cases		Family associates	
	NUMBER EXAMINED	% POSITIVE	NUMBER EXAMINED	% POSITIVE
0–4	16	44	21	52
5–9	53	68	17	41
10–14	29	66	11	9
15–19	12	67	4	0
20 and over	17	47	57	17
All ages	127	61	110	26

*After Winkelstein: Am J Public Health 47:741–749, 1957

Lymphocytic Choriomeningitis (LCM) Virus

The LCM virus was isolated in 1934 from a monkey that had been inoculated with central nervous system (CNS) tissues obtained at necropsy of a patient who was thought to have died of St. Louis encephalitis. A year later, LCM virus was recovered from the CSF of two patients with viral meningitis. Subsequently, the mouse was identified as the definitive host of the LCM virus, both in breeding colonies and in wild populations. The virus is worldwide in distribution.

Mice may shed the LCM virus in nasal secretions, feces, urine, and semen. Viremia is a feature of the murine disease. Guinea pigs, hamsters, dogs, and monkeys may acquire infection. Lice and ticks may harbor the virus.

In humans, the frequency of infection is greatest among young adults, with highest incidence in the winter and spring. The incubation period ranges from 6 to 13 days. The disease has a wide spectrum of clinical expression, one of which is meningitis. In several studies, LCM accounted for approximately 8% of viral infections of the CNS. Outbreaks of LCM have been reported in families with new pet hamsters and among persons exposed to infected hamsters in animal care units.

Encephalomyocarditis Viruses

The several kinds of EMC viruses are alike in pathogenicity and also frequently exhibit antigenic kinship. The MM strain was recovered from hamsters inoculated with CNS tissue from a man who died of an illness resembling poliomyelitis. An EMC virus was isolated from a chimpanzee with myocarditis. The Mengo encephalomyelitis virus was recovered from a paralyzed rhesus monkey. EMC viruses may be recovered from rodents (particularly rats) and occasionally from sick swine, calves, and horses.

EMC viruses have been isolated from feces, throat washings, CSF, and the blood of infected persons. Viremia has been detected as early as the first day of illness, before the onset of meningitis. The frequency of detection of antibodies in human serums varies 5%

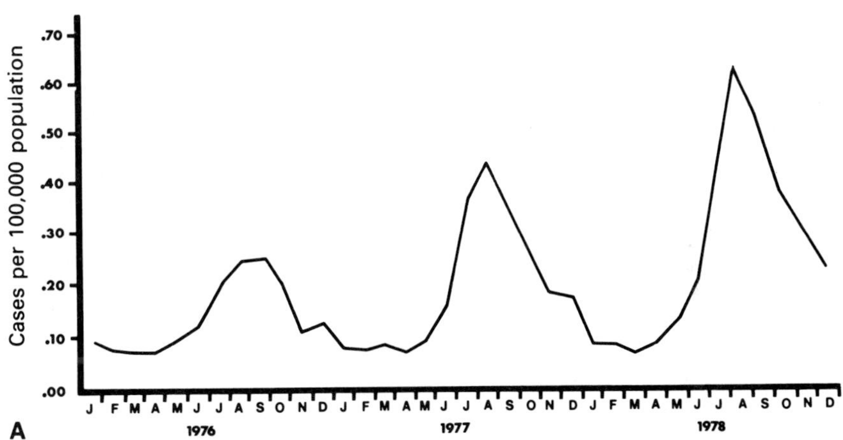

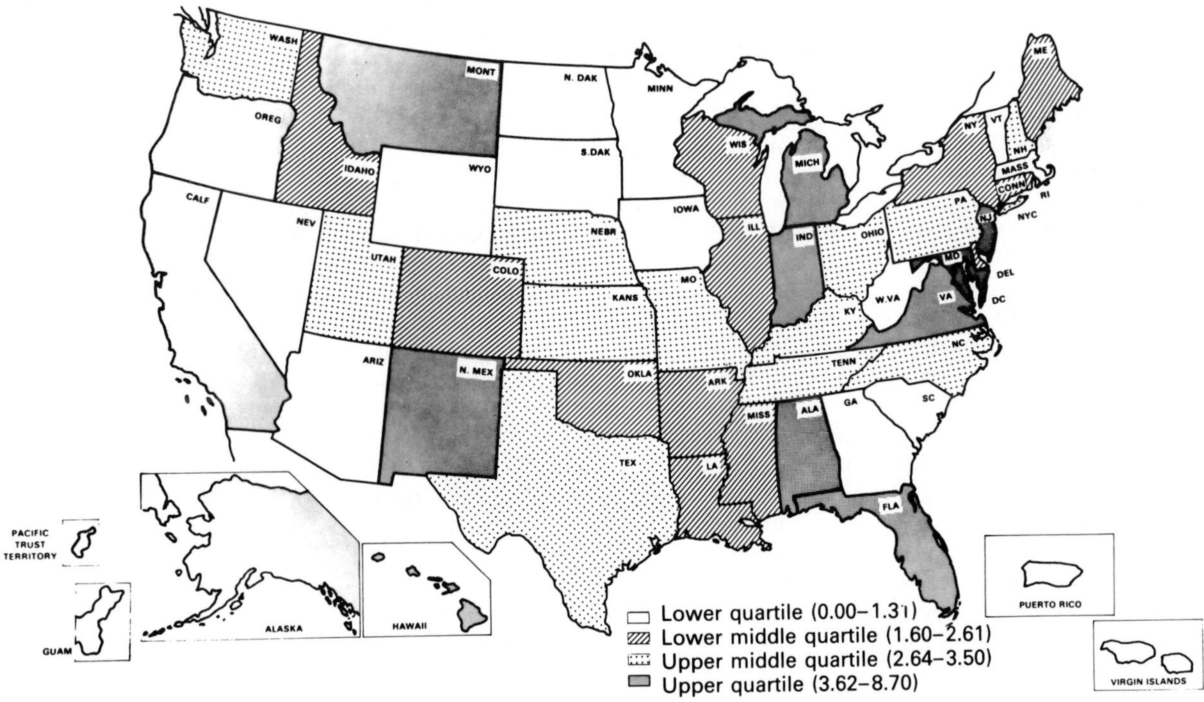

Fig. 118-1. Reported case rates for aseptic meningitis in the United States (*A*) Rates by month, 1976–1978. (*B*) Rates per 100,000 population by state, in 1978. Center for Disease Control, Atlanta, Georgia: Reported morbidity and mortality in the United States, 1978. Morbid Mortal Week Rep 27 (Suppl) 1979. Public Health Service, U.S. Department of Health, Education and Welfare.

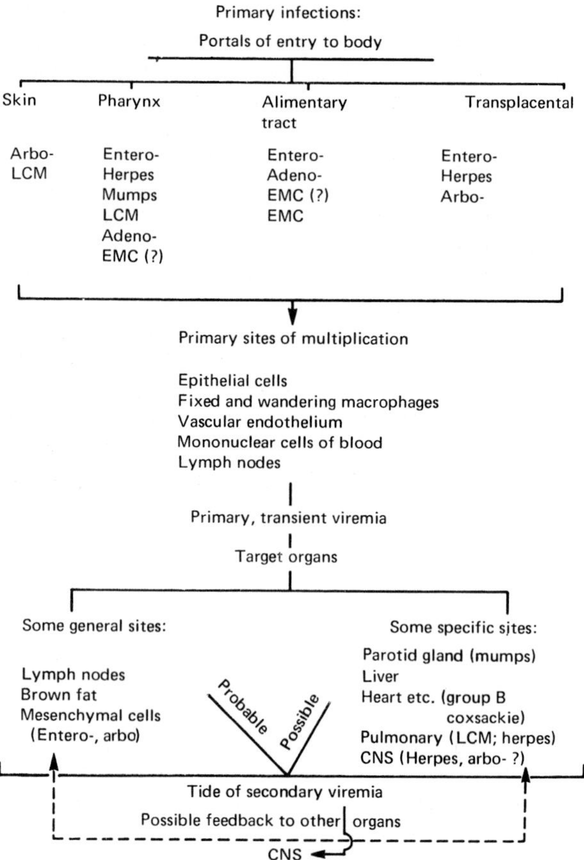

Fig. 118-2. Potential pathogenesis of viral meningitis. Viral agents that cause meningitis typically replicate in areas near the portal of entry before causing a primary viremia during which other organs are seeded. The meninges become infected during a secondary viremia that originates in the secondary organ sites of multiplication. Viruses such as herpes simplex virus type 1 may reach the central nervous system by neuronal pathways.

to 20%. Of serums from persons with poliomyelitislike diseases, 20% to 30% neutralize EMC viruses. Antibodies to EMC viruses are detectable in 13% to 87% of rodent populations.

Infections in humans range from mild, febrile illnesses, so-called 3-day fever, to severe encephalomyelitis. Myocarditis is not a recognized feature in man. A laboratory infection with Mengo virus has resulted in meningitis after an incubation period of 5 to 8 days. The mode of infection with EMC viruses is unknown in humans. Although the presence of virus in pharyngeal washings and in feces is consistent with person-to-person transmission, epidemiologic characteristics are in keeping with other means of transmission. EMC viruses have been recovered from the ectoparasites of rodents and from mosquitoes.

Pathogenesis and Pathology

The sequence of events in humans from the time of virus implantation to the onset of CNS disease is known only in part. A pathogenetic scheme is presented in Figure 118-2. Viral replication probably occurs in sites regional to the portals of entry before the primary viremia that is an early feature of infection. Target organs outside the CNS are infected as a consequence of this primary viremia. Further replication results in continued or secondary viremia in which there is the passage of the virus from the blood to the CNS, where it penetrates susceptible cells and once again multiplies.

Penetration of either the blood–CSF or the blood–brain barrier may be accomplished by means of virus-laden phagocytes migrating through blood vessels of the meninges or brain, or by passage of virus particles through the choroid plexus or other areas of preferential permeability (*e.g.,* the area postrema). Once within the CSF, movement of the virus across meningeal and ependymal cells might occur from the infection of these cells or by diffusion across them. Cells with membranes that are capable of absorbing virus and that permit viral penetrance must also contain a milieu suitable for uncoating viral nucleic acid prior to the replication of fully infectious viral particles. The manifestations of viral meningitis that ensue, with or without clinical encephalomyelitis, depend on the number and kinds of cells involved. At this point in the course of the infection, the viremia usually terminates, coincident with the appearance of circulating interferon and specific humoral antibody.

This hypothesis leaves many questions unanswered. Actually, the principal sites of primary virus multiplication in humans are not known with certainty. Even less is known of the cells intermediary to an upsurge of viremia and the further dissemination of the virus to target organs. Nevertheless, there is a growing appreciation that all of these viruses have extraneural sites of growth before involvement of the CNS.

Autopsy reports of patients with uncomplicated viral meningitis are very few. In fatal cases, an encephalomyelitis has usually intervened. Involvement of the motor neurons of the brain stem and spinal cord is characteristic of enteroviral infections (polioviruses; coxsackieviruses, types A7 and B5; and some echoviruses, types 2, 4, and 11). Group B coxsackieviruses may involve both white and gray matters of the CNS. In infants, the disease tends to involve the brain stem, especially the inferior olivary nuclei.

There is no real characteristic pattern or unique feature to the changes wrought by the arboviruses (see Chap. 122, Viral Encephalitides). Actual necrosis of CNS tissue is prominent in eastern equine, Japanese B, and Far Eastern tick-borne encephalitis. The involvement of the leptomeninges consists of infiltration with small lymphocytes and mesothelial cells; leukocytes are found in perivascular sheaths.

Meningoencephalitis caused by herpes simplex virus may cause a profound hemorrhagic necrosis. Often there is a great destruction of temporal, occipital, and parietal cortical tissues. Laminae of the cortex are occupied or replaced by mononuclear cells. Inflammatory infiltrates and neuronophagic nodules are present in the midbrain, pons, and medulla. The spinal cord is usually spared. Acidophilic intranuclear inclusions in neurons and astrocytes provide evidence of the nature of the infection.

The pathologic features of mumps meningoencephalitis consist of a leptomeningitis similar, but usually less intense, than that engendered by arboviruses. Blood vessels in the white matter of the brain, midbrain, pons, medulla, and cord may be sparsely infiltrated with mononuclear cells. Demyelination may also occur in these same areas.

There are no valid studies of the pathology of LCM virus infection in humans because is has never been proved that LCM virus causes fatal infections. In animals, the choroid plexus is densely infiltrated by mononuclear cells, the meninges are involved to a lesser extent, and the brain substance is relatively uninvolved. Interstitial bronchopneumonia is a common feature of infection.

Fatal infections of humans with EMC viruses have not been documented.

Manifestations

The signs and symptoms of viral meningitis are variable. Typically, the onset of illness is sudden, with intense frontal or retroorbital headache that is particularly pronounced in adults. The fever is generally undulating and seldom rises above 40°C (104°F).

Occasionally, with echovirus 9 or LCM, it may be diphasic or triphasic. At the onset of fever, or shortly thereafter, malaise, drowsiness, sore throat, myalgia, nausea, and vomiting may intervene. Less often, there are also photophobia, tinnitus, vertigo, chest and abdominal pain, and paresthesias. Nuchal rigidity develops, and there is almost always stiffness of the back and pain on flexion. The Kernig and Brudzinski signs may or may not be elicitable. Both the duration and the intensity of these manifestations are inversely related to age.

The leukocyte count in the peripheral blood is generally within normal limits, although it may fluctuate widely during arbovirus infections. A leukopenia may accompany mumps. Anemia is not a notable feature of viral meningitis. The peripheral blood count is usually not helpful in diagnosis.

The CSF is usually transparent but may be slightly turbid; that is, there are usually fewer than 500 leukocytes per mm^3. The early predominance of neutrophils gives way to that of mononuclear cells, usually within 48 hours. There are exceptions, in the leukocytosis persists for longer intervals. The total leukocyte count diminishes gradually, reaching 0 to 15 per mm^3 10 to 14 days after onset of the illness. As the cellular response diminishes, the CSF protein concentration rises from normal to as much as 120 mg/dl. Except for depression in mumps, LCM, and systemic lupus erythematosus, the CSF glucose is normal in concentration (compared with the glucose concentration in simultaneously obtained blood).

Diagnosis

The exact cause of the viral meningitis syndrome in a given patient cannot be determined on clinical grounds alone. However, in some patients, clinical findings not referable to the CNS are of value (*e.g.,* parotitis). Also, the kind of agent involved may sometimes be inferred from epidemiologic associations; for example, epidemic occurrence during the warm months is consistent with enterovirus or arbovirus infection.

The onset and early course of the viral meningitis syndrome may be simulated by other diseases, for example, the onset of meningitis caused by nonviral infectious agents of moderate virulence such as *Haemophilus influenzae* (Chap. 119, Bacterial Meningitis), *Brucella* spp. (Chap. 138, Brucellosis), *Listeria monocytogenes* (Chap. 51, Listeriosis), *Leptospira* spp. (Chap. 76, Leptospirosis), *Mycobacterium tuberculosis* (Chap. 34, Pulmonary Tuberculosis), and *Mycoplasma pneumoniae* (Chap. 30, Nonbacterial Pneumonias). The early course of viral meningitis is also simulated by bacterial meningitides that were inadequately treated. A mononuclear cell pleocytosis in the CSF, generally with an increase in the concentration of protein, may occur in syphilis (Chap. 59, Syphilis), lymphogranuloma venereum (Chap. 54, Lymphogranuloma Venereum), typhus (Chap. 98, Typhus Fevers), *Mycoplasma pneumoniae* infection (Chap. 30, Nonbacterial Pneumonias), and protozoal meningitides. It may also occur after the intrathecal administration of antimicrobial, antimitotic, alkylating, or other agents. Meningeal involvement with or without encephalitis may occur in leukemias, Hodgkin's disease, metastatic carcinomatosis, benign infectious lymphocytosis, cat-scratch fever (Chap. 166, Cat-Scratch Fever), pemphigus, benign myalgic encephalomyelitis (epidemic neuromyasthenia; Chap. 170, Epidemic neuromyasthenia) and plumbism.

In about 3% of patients with infectious mononucleosis, the findings of viral meningitis are prominent, and there is a mononuclear pleocytosis in the CSF. Usually, other features are also present, including exudative pharyngitis, lymphadenopathy, hepatosplenomegaly, and exanthema. Development of heterophil and Epstein–Barr virus antibodies support the diagnosis (Chap. 137, Infectious Mononucleosis).

Postinfectious encephalopathies, caused by varicella–zoster, vaccinia, rubeola, and rubella viruses, seldom cause meningitis, but they take the form of acute, disseminated encephalomyelitis (respectively, Chaps. 93, 92, 86, and 87). In Behçet's syndrome, meningeal signs are associated with recurrent oral and genital ulcerations, and relapsing ocular lesions, including uveitis, iridocyclitis, and retinal hemorrhages.

Bacterial and viral infections of the CNS may develop concurrently in the same person. Such episodes have been reported for *H. influenzae* (type b), echovirus 9, enteroviruses, and arboviruses.

An exact etiologic diagnosis requires the aid of the laboratory. Both virus isolation techniques and serologic methods must be used. With adequate, properly collected specimens, an etiologic diagnosis can be made in about two-thirds of patients with clinically manifest viral meningitis.

Viral Isolation

Many viruses commonly associated with viral meningitis can be recovered from the CSF (Table 118-3). Herpes simplex virus type 2 may be cultured when meningitis develops in young adults. The exceptions relate largely to the arboviruses. The earlier in the course of the meningitis that collection is made, the more probable successful virus isolation becomes. Viruses should also be sought in the feces (enterovi-

Table 118-3. *Synopsis of Laboratory Aids in Diagnosis of Viral Meningitides*[*]

	Kinds of virus						
Category	ENTEROVIRUS	MUMPS	ARBOVIRUS	HERPESVIRUS	LCM	EMC	ADENOVIRUS
Samples yielding virus							
Feces	+	−	Rarely	+	#[†]	+	+
Pharynx	+	+	#	+	#	+	+
Blood	(+)[‡]	(+)	(+)	±	+	+	Selected serotypes
CSF	(+)	(+)	Rarely	(+)	+	+	±
Vesicle fluid	+	−	−	+	−	−	−
Urine	(+)	+	#	?	(+)	#	+
Tissures, CNS, etc.	+	#	+	+	+	+	#
Means of recovery							
Mice							
Infant	+[§]	+	+	+	+	+	0
Young adult 1	−	±	+	+	+	+	0
Embryonated eggs	−	+	+	+	+	+	0
Tissue cultures	+	+	+	+	+	+	+
Antibody development							
Complement fixation	+[‖]	+	+[‖]	+[‖]	+	+	+[‖]
Hemagglutination inhibition	Selected serotypes	+	+	+[**]	#	+	+
Neutralization	+	+	+	+	+	+	+

[*] Other techniques for isolating viruses, chiefly using rodents, are not listed. Also, newer serologic techniques, such as immunoprecipitin labeling of infected cells with fluorescein-conjugated antibody, and immunoenzymatic methods are not listed.

[†] Little or no critical data for interpretations.

[‡] Virus isolation may be difficult because of timing in pathogenesis or other factors.

[§] Principally group A coxsackieviruses; many strains propagate poorly, if at all in cell cultures

[‖] Group cross reactions sometimes occur.

[**] Using sensitized erythrocytes.

ruses, herpesvirus), urine (mumps), saliva (herpesvirus, mumps), and throat washings (enteroviruses, LCM, herpesvirus). Because viremia occurs before the onset of meningitis, isolation from the blood need not be attempted.

The search for viruses is most rewarding when clinicians and virologists work as a team. Proper specimens are as important as the choice of methods of virus and antibody detection. The time required for virus identification is a handicap. Speedier methods include visualization of viruses by electron microscopy (particularly in feces) and of virus-infected cells in the CSF with fluorescent-labeled antibody, or immunoenzymatic (*e.g.,* ELISA, see Chap. 14, Immunologic Diagnosis) methods. The latter techniques are generally available only in research laboratories.

Antibody Response

Three major test systems are used to measure antibody response: complement fixation (CF), hemagglutination–inhibition (HI), and serum neutralization (SN). The CF and HI tests are applicable in mumps, herpesvirus, and some enterovirus serotypes. Other methods such as the ELISA system may be used also.

Because infection (primary target) often precedes the onset of CNS disease (secondary target), antibodies may already have developed to maximum titers in the first serum sample obtained, when meningitis has become overt. As a rule, CF and HI antibodies appear during the first week of disease, rise to maximal levels during the ensuing several weeks, and usually disappear within months. Occasionally, they persist for years, for example, CF *versus* herpes simplex or echovirus 16, and HI *versus* eastern equine encephalomyelitis virus. SN antibodies often appear later than either CF or HI antibodies, but they endure and may be detectable many years after meningitis.

Both HI and CF antibodies develop during the first week of infection from mumps virus. CF antibodies reactive with soluble (S) antigen have been detected by the second day of disease, whereas antibodies against the viral (V) antigen usually develop 7 to 14 days after onset of the infection. Anti-V antibodies persist for months, whereas anti-S antibodies decline and disappear in weeks. In regions of high endemicity for group B arboviruses, a serologic diagnosis may be difficult because of overlapping responses evoked by heterologous members of the group. Such blanket responses are unusual in residents of the continental United States. However, repatriation after residence in foreign endemic areas may obfuscate serodiagnosis.

Prognosis

Classically, recovery from viral meningitis begins after a few days of illness, and with few exceptions, it is complete within days or weeks. Yet, viremia must have occurred before meningitis, and it is not surprising that other organs and systems are sometimes involved. Among infants, some enteroviruses cause disseminated visceral disease with fatal outcome. Persistent enterovirus infections of the CNS, sometimes fatal, occur in agammaglobulinemic persons.

Orchitis may be encountered during mumps, enterovirus, and herpesvirus infection. Pancreatitis, pleurodynia, grippelike syndromes, and various types of exanthemas may intervene during infection from enteroviruses, mumps virus, and LCM virus. Infants and children with enteroviral meningitis may have transitory weakness of skeletal muscles (*e.g.,* the truncal musculature).

Nerve deafness, most often unilateral, is not an uncommon event during mumps.

Therapy

Patients with viral meningitis usually require only bedrest, analgesic drugs, and the repletion and conservation of fluids and electrolytes. Infants and children often appear fully recovered within a few days. Because muscular impairment may follow infections caused by enteroviruses, the physician is obligated to implement programs of graded activity and follow-up examinations for residual weakness.

Specific antiviral drugs are not available for treating the viral infections which cause meningitis. The thymidine analogues and adenosine arabinoside used in treating CNS infections caused by herpesviruses are discussed in Chapter 91, Infections Caused by Herpes Simplex Viruses. Their value in treating meningitis uncomplicated by encephalitis is doubtful. The use of interferon or interferon inducers is of dubious value also, for meningitis is normally a late expression of a systemic viral infection.

Prevention

Unlike the vaccine for poliomyelitis, no means are now available to control echoviruses and coxsackieviruses. The diversity of serotypes precludes the early development of vaccines. Practical public health measures that might afford control (isolation and quarantine) are unlikely to affect channels of virus dispersion because these viruses are truly ubiquitous. Breaking the epidemiologic chain of transmission by sanitary control (*e.g.,* treatment of sewage) is unlikely to alter the disease incidence because a family, or other grouping, apparently is exposed as a unit. Nevertheless, educational efforts directed at upgrading personal hygiene and sanitary practices in hospitals and public gathering places should be continued.

Mumps meningoencephalitis has declined in frequency following widespread immunization with live attenuated mumps virus. The control of mice or other animal carriers and the maintenance of high standards of sanitation may help to secure abatement of infection from LCM and EMC viruses.

Remaining Problems

The clinical characteristics commonly shared among different viruses associated with viral meningitis challenge clinical acumen. Epidemiologic factors may sometimes help, but in general these factors fail to break the chain of transmission, although risks of disease have been significantly reduced for several viruses, for example, mumps and polioviruses. The search for antiviral compounds effective in modulating viral biosynthesis continues; however, the effective use of such compounds, when available, requires the development of techniques for rapid identification to enable proper usage.

Bibliography

Book

FOX JP, HALL CE: Viruses in families. In Infections with Echoviruses and Coxsackieviruses. Littleton, MA, PSG Publishing Company, 1980. 441 pp.

Journals

ALBRECHT P: Pathogenesis of neurotropic arbovirus infections. Curr Top Microbiol Immunol 43:44–91, 1968

BIGGAR RJ, WOODALL JP, WALTER PD, HAUGHIE GE: Lymphocytic choriomeningitis outbreak associated with pet hamsters. JAMA 232:494–500, 1975

FARMER TW, JANEWAY CA: Infection with the virus of lymphocytic choriomeningitis. Medicine 21:1–63, 1942

GAJDUSEK DC: Review article: Encephalomyocarditis virus infection in childhood. Pediatrics 16:902–906, 1955

GEAR JHS, MEASROCH V: Coxsackievirus infections of the newborn. Prog Med Virol 15:42–62, 1973

JOHNSON RT, MIMS CA: Pathogenesis of viral infection of the nervous system. N Engl J Med 278:23–30, 84–91, 1968

KRAUS HG, DIETZMAN D, RAY CG: Fatal infections with echovirus types 6 and 11 in early infancy. Am J Dis Child 126:842–846, 1973

MEYER HM, JOHNSON RT, CRAWFORD IP, DASCOMB HE, ROGERS NG: Central nervous system syndromes of "viral" etiology. Am J Med 29:334–347, 1960

OLSON LC, BUESCHER EL, ARTENSTEIN MS, PARKMAN PD: Herpesvirus infection of the human central nervous system. N Engl J Med 277:1271–1277, 1967

WEIBEL RE, BUYNAK EB, WHITMAN JE, LEAGUS MD, STOKES J JR, HILLEMAN MR: Jeryl Lynn strain live mumps vaccine, durable immunity for three years following vaccination. JAMA 207:1667–1670, 1969

WENNER HA, BEHBEHANI AM: The ECHO viruses. Monogr Virol 1:1–72, 1968

WILFERT CM: Mumps meningoencephalitis with low cerebrospinal fluid glucose, prolonged pleocytosis and elevation of proteins. N Engl J Med 280:855–858, 1969

WILFERT CM, BUCKLEY, HG, MOHANAKUMAN T, GRIFFITH JF, KATZ SL, WHISNANT JK, EGGLESTON PA, MOORE M, TREADWELL E, OXMAN MN, ROSEN FS: Persistent and fatal central-nervous-system ECHO virus infection in patients with agammaglobulinemia. N Engl J Med 296:1485–1489, 1977

YOLKEN RH: Enzyme-linked immunosorbent assay (ELISA): A practical tool for rapid diagnosis of viruses and other infectious agents. Yale J Bio Med 53:85–92, 1980

GARY D. OVERTURF
PAUL D. HOEPRICH

Bacterial Meningitis

119

Bacterial meningitis is inflammatory disease of the central nervous system caused by the growth of bacteria in and adjacent to the leptomeninges; there is always some degree of concomitant encephalitis. The infecting bacteria usually reach the leptomeninges by the bloodstream. Occasionally, however, infection extends to the meninges directly from other intracranial foci or it results from traumatic inoculation of extradural bacteria.

Spread throughout the subarachnoid space, involving the leptomeninges, brain, and spinal cord, may be exceedingly rapid in acute bacterial meningitis. Rarely, death may ensue after a clinical course measured in hours. However, there is usually time to apply antimicrobial therapy, and cure is possible if treatment is instituted early in the course of the disease.

Chronic bacterial meningitis is exemplified by tuberculous meningitis (Chap. 35, Extrapulmonary Tuberculosis). It is also mimicked by the fungal meningitides (Chap. 41, Coccidioidomycosis; Chap. 120, Cryptococcosis), and chronic meningitis caused by leptospires (Chap. 76, Leptospirosis), viruses, (Chap. 118, Viral Meningitis), and protozoa (Chap. 66, Amebiasis; Chap. 129, Toxoplasmosis; Chap. 130, African Trypanosomiasis). Nontuberculous, chronic bacterial meningitis is quite unusual, but may occur with *Listeria monocytogenes* (Chap. 51, Listeriosis) and *Nocardia asteroides* (Chap. 37, Nocardiosis).

Etiology

The cause of acute bacterial meningitis varies with the age group considered and the clinical setting under which the infection occurs. Although many kinds of bacteria have been reported to cause meningitis, *Neisseria meningitidis, Haemophilus influenzae, Streptococcus pneumoniae,* and *Escherichia coli* cause most of the cases (Table 119-1). The characteristics of *H. influenzae, S. pneumoniae,* and *E. coli* are reviewed in Chapters 26, (Epiglottitis, Laryngitis, and Laryngotracheobronchitis), 31, (Bacterial Pneumonias), and 48, (Urethritis and Cystitis), respectively.

Meningococci are gram-negative, nonmotile, nonsporulating cocci that are spherical or oval, and 0.6 μm to 0.8 μm in diameter. Most strains are capsulated. In smears prepared either from clinical specimens or from cultures, meningococci are commonly arranged in pairs. The adjacent sides of such diplococci appear to be flattened, giving a biscuit or bean shape, which is also characteristic of *Neisseria gonorrhoeae* (Chap. 56, Gonococcal Infections). In smears of exudates, diploid meningococci are frequently found within phagocytes.

The smooth, glistening, amorphous colonies are grayish and translucent at outgrowth. After 48 to 72 hours of incubation, many strains elaborate a yellowish pigment. Weak hemolysis is evident with most strains after 2 to 4 days of incubation. Meningococci are oxidase-positive, as are other species of *Neisseria, Pseudomonas* spp., certain of the Enterobacteriaceae and diptheroids, and some yeasts. Autolytic enzymes are activated in cultures only 24 hours old.

Meningococci are aerobic. However, they grow best in the presence of 5% to 10% CO_2 in a humid atmosphere at 37°C and a pH of 7.4 to 7.6. Glucose and maltose are fermented, and acid is produced (no gas). The nutritional requirements of meningococci have not been completely defined, and the use of complex culture mediums (Thayer–Martin VCN, chocolate, blood, Mueller–Hinton agars) is advisable for isolation. Many of the additives used in culture mediums (starch, charcoal, hemoglobin powder, blood) act as adsorbents of substances inimical to the growth of meningococci, for example, unsaturated fatty acids contributed by almost any botanical product, including agar.

Serogroups of *N. meningitidis*—designated A, B, C, D, X, Y, and Z—are differentiated on the basis of

Table 119-1. *Correlation of Cause of Acute Bacterial Meningitis With Age Group and Direct Inoculation**

	Premature and Neonatal (%)	2–60 Months (%)	5–40 Years (%)	>40 Years (%)	Extension from Intracranial Focus‡ (%)	Skull Fractures† (%)	Penetrating Injuries Shunts† (%)	Post Neurosurgical
Neisseria meningitidis	—	~20 (~5)	~40 (~5)	~10 (~25)	—	—	—	—
Haemophilus influenzae	~5 (~50)	~60 (~5)	~5 (~0)	~2 (~0)	~25 (~5)	~10 (~5)	—	—
Escherichia coli	~40 (~40)	—	—	~10 (~50)	occasional	occasional	~5 (~60)	~20 (~50)
Other Enterobacteriaceae	~20 (~60)	—	—					~30 (~50)
Streptococcus pneumoniae	~5 (~50)	~15 (~10)	~30 (~30)	~50 (~45)	~40 (~15)	~80 (~10)		
Staphylococcus spp.	~2 (~60)	—	~10 (~50)	~13 (~40)	~10 (~25)	occasional	~80 (~25)	~45 (~25)
Streptococcus spp.‡	~25 (~40)	~2 (~25)	~5 (~40)	~5 (~45)	occasional	occasional	~5	—
Others (including *Listeria monocytogenes*)	~3 (~40)	~3 (~2)	~10 (~15)	~10 (~50)	~20 (~15)	~5 (~25)	~10 (~25)	~5 (~50)

*The approximate fatality rate with presently available treatment in parentheses.
†Antimicrobial therapy mitigates the immediate threat of acute bacterial meningitis, but appropriate surgical procedures (drainage of abscesses, excision of infected bone, repair of defects in the leptomeninges, removal of foreign bodies) are, in most cases, essential to cure.
‡Includes group B *Streptococcus* spp.

specific, acidic polysaccharides, for example, the group C polysaccharide is polymerized η-acetyl neuraminic acid. The polysaccharides are clearly capsular with groups A and C, as they are with the much less common groups X, Y, and Z. Although groups B and D are usually not capsulated by microscopic examination, group-specific reactants have been isolated from liquid cultures. Purified group A and group C capsular polysaccharides are immunogenic and nontoxic in laboratory animals and in humans. Injection of dead or lysed *N. meningitidis* results in an endotoxinlike effect.

Multiple physical (drying, moist heat to 55°C, ultraviolet light) and chemical agents (1% phenol, 0.1% $HgCL_2$) are rapidly lethal to meningococci. Although a variety of antibacterial agents are active against *N. meningitidis,* a significant clinical problem appeared in the mid-1960s with the ascendancy of sulfonamide-resistant strains of serogroup B, then C, and most recently A, as causes of disease in humans.

Epidemiology

The leptomeninges are usually infected by bloodborne bacteria; that is, the epidemiology of acute bacterial meningitis is primarily the epidemiology of bacteremia. There are peculiarities, however. For example, *Staphylococcus aureus* and various of the Enterobacteriaceae are the most common causes of bacteremias in man, but they are not the most common causes of meningitis. Moreover, the clinical entity of meningococcemia does not invariably give rise to meningococcal meningitis.

The bacteria that commonly cause acute meningitis are generally acquired from other persons, or they are drawn from the microbiota resident on or in the afflicted person. Accordingly, acute bacterial meningitis is worldwide and is seen wherever humans dwell. Males are affected approximately twice as often as females.

The Enterobacteriaceae, group B *Streptococcus* spp. and *S. aureus* exemplify normal bacterial flora that may cause meningitis, particularly in premature and neonatal infants. Direct transfer to the infant from the mother, hospital personnel, or the hospital environment appears to be implicated in the spread.

Upper respiratory tract carriage of *Streptococcus pyogenes* and *S. pneumoniae* is quite common, particularly in the colder seasons of the year, *H. influenzae* and *N. meningitidis* are frequently part of the microflora of the upper respiratory tract. The latter three kinds of bacteria are obligate parasites of humans that have neither nonhuman hosts, reservoirs, nor vectors. Spread is from person to person by way of air-borne droplets.

Neonatal Meningitis

The incidence of neonatal meningitis is 40 to 50/100,000 live births, with about two-thirds of the cases occurring in hospitals. Factors that facilitate the development of meningitis are: (1) maternal—traumatic delivery, prolonged labor, prolonged rupture of the membranes, perinatal infections, antimicrobial therapy that selects for resistant bacteria; (2) fetal—prematurity, low birth weight (<2500 g), general sepsis (bacteremia is present when meningitis is diagnosed in one-third to one-half of infants), lack of immunologic experience or competence; (3) environmental—contaminated equipment (humidification, respiratory assistance personnel who are carriers; and (4) virulence factors that invest microorganisms with a special ability to invade the neonate; for example, 84% of the *E. coli* isolated from neonates with meningitis possess the Kl capsular polysaccharide that is immunochemically identical with meningococcal group B polysaccharide, and enhances lethality for mice 60 to 100 times.

The etiology of meningitis in neonates has changed substantially over the past several years. From 1932 to 1960, gram-negative pathogens predominated, with *E. coli* accounting for the majority of the isolates. At present, approximately 75% of cases of meningitis that occur during the first 14 days of life are caused by gram-negative bacteria. In contrast, about 66% of the cases in infants beyond 14 days are caused by gram-positive bacteria. Overall, the Enterobacteriaceae cause 60% of meningitis cases and *E. coli* alone are isolated in about 40% of patients. Group B streptococci are second, accounting for 20% to 45% of the cases. Many cases of group B streptococcal infections occur during the postpartum weeks after discharge from the hospital; these cases represent spread from sites of colonization such as the gut, the throat, and the umbilical cord, which were established in the hospital.

Haemophilus influenzae **Meningitis**

About 60% to 75% of the postneonatal bacterial meningitis in children is caused by *H. influenzae* type b. The incidence is maximal at 6 to 8 months of age, and declines slowly after 12 months so that haemophilan meningitis is seen about as frequently as meningococcal and pneumococcal meningitis in 2-year-old children. There is a temporal relationship of the onset of vulnerability to disease with the waning of maternally acquired humoral antibody that is bactericidal for *H. influenzae.* Pharyngeal carriage of type b *H. influenzae* is highest in children under 5 years of age. Outbreaks of disease caused by *H. influenzae,* including meningitis, have been recognized in families and day-care centers. Virulent *H. influenzae* may be carried in nearly 65% of family members of patients, and may persist for as long as 3 months. The risk of secondary cases of severe haemophilan infections among household contacts is 0.5% in children under 6 years of age, and 0.6% in children under 12 months. The period of risk extends for several months following the occurrence of disease caused by *H. influenzae.* Characterization of the surface membrane proteins of *H. influenzae* has enabled subgroup categorization; apparently, relatively few serotypes are involved in epidemic situations.

Over the past several years, there has been an unexplained increase in disease (including meningitis) caused by *H. influenzae* type b in the United States. The overall incidence of bacterial meningitis in the United States is 3 in 100,000, with an estimated annual 29,000 cases. The cumulative probability of meningitis caused by *H. influenzae* during the first 5 years of life is 180.2 in 100,000, or 0.18%. The incidence is higher among children from socioeconomically deprived areas.

Meningococcal meningitis

As with all infections caused by *N. meningitidis,* meningococcal meningitis occurs sporadically and in epidemics, with highest incidence during the late winter and early spring (Fig. 119-1). At present, meningococcal meningitis appears to be declining in the United States and in the United Kingdom, whereas there has been an increase in Finland and in Brazil. Most epidemics of meningococcal meningitis are caused by group A strains, but small outbreaks have occurred with both group B and group C strains. Sporadic cases caused by group B, group C, and group Y strains are the rule, with groups B and C alternating in predominance. Whenever group A strains become prevalent, the incidence of meningitis increases markedly.

Meningococcal meningitis has long been associated with military camps and barracks. Recruits apparently suffer a far higher incidence of clinical disease than do experienced military personnel. Overcrowding and fatigue are thought to be the major determinants related to the onset of disease in these situations.

Although the meningococcal carrier rate ranges from 2% to 38%, depending on the population studied, the relationship between meningitis and carriage is still poorly defined. It has been suggested that carriers, not patients, are the foci for the spread of men-

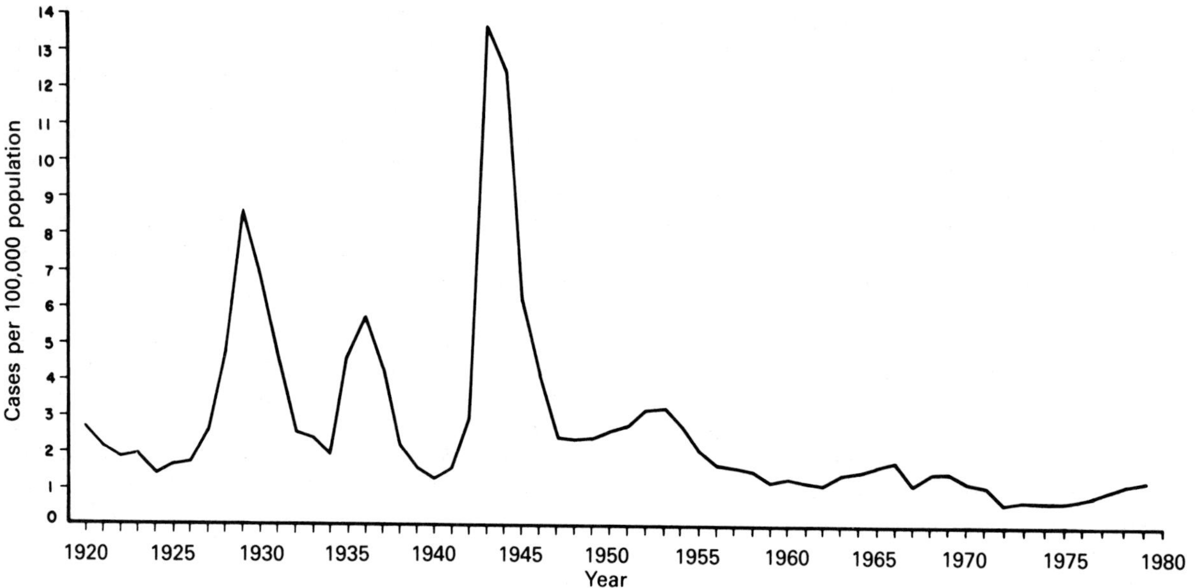

Fig. 119-1. Annual meningococcal attack rate in the United States, 1920–1979. (Morbid Mortal Week Rep Suppl Summary, 1979)

ingococcal meningitis, because epidemics are likely to occur when the carrier rate exceeds 20%. However, carriers of meningococci are usually over 21 years of age, but the attack rates of disease are highest in children: with group B, children ≤ 5 years old; with group C, children 4 to 14 years old.

Clearly, meningococcal disease does arise from association with patients, for the attack rate in household contacts is 4–10.4/1000, or about 500–800 times that of the general population. Since cases rarely occur among school or job contacts, chemoprophylaxis is needed only for intimate contacts of patients.

In this regard, the phenomenon of emergence of sulfonamide-resistant strains as cause for disease is of extreme importance. Resistance was documented in the laboratory with strains of serogroups B and C in the 1940s. However, it was not until 1962 that group B, sulfonamide-resistant *N. meningitidis* were encountered as the cause of epidemic meningitis (San Diego and Fort Ord, California). By 1968, sulfonamide-resistant group C (United States) and group A (Greece, Africa) meningococci were documented as causes of sporadic and epidemic meningitis. The current epidemic strains (group A) in Brazil and Finland are also resistant to sulfonamides. At present in the United States, about 25% of clinical isolates of *N. meningitidis* are resistant to sulfonamides, and rifampin is the chemoprophylactic agent of choice.

Pathogenesis and Pathology

Blood-borne Infection

Meningitis of hematogenous origin is essentially a metastatic infection. The factors that result in meningeal localization of blood-borne bacteria are not known in each case. The typical antecedent infections are lobar pneumonia, otitis media, and endocarditis with *S. pneumoniae;* otitis media and respiratory tract infections with *H. influenzae;* furunculosis, osteomyelitis, and postoperative wound infections with *S. aureus;* and bronchial pneumonia and severe pharyngitis with *Streptococcus pyogenes.* It is in meningococcal meningitis that the antecedent, initial localization is most often covert. Classically, there is an asymptomatic or mildly symptomatic nasopharyngeal carrier state, or a mild rhinopharyngitis.

Blood-borne bacteria appear to settle along the walls of the venous sinuses and other regions of slow blood flow in the low pressure vascular system. Subsequently, bacteria may penetrate the dura and enter the subarachnoid space from which they are cleared through the arachnoid villi. If clearance is deficient, an inoculum capable of producing disease may attain. Bacterial clearance may be aided by macrophages present in the arachnoid. Furthermore, the central nervous system (CNS) appears to have some ability to clear minimal inocula of bacteria; otherwise, bacteremia would commonly lead to meningitis, and experimental meningitis should regularly follow the induction of bacteremia in animals.

The extent of morbid changes in the CNS is determined primarily by the duration of the meningitis before death. Inflammation of the meninges leads to increased vascular permeability and failure of the so-called barriers that ordinarily exclude blood-borne substances from the CNS and the cerebrospinal fluid (CSF). The rise in CSF protein that occurs in meningitis results in part from increased entry of plasma proteins and in part from destruction of CNS tissue. As the infection continues, an exudate consisting of bacteria, leukocytes, and proteinaceous material forms in the subarachnoid space—most prominently around the base of the brain in haemophilan meningitis, over the cerebral convexities in pneumococcal meningitis, and diffusely in meninogococcal meningitis. As the exudate fills the subarachnoid space, it may seriously impede the flow of the CSF, and the drainage channels of the arachnoid villi may become blocked with protein and necrotic material. The resultant disruption of the normal flow of the CSF and the cerebral edema that inevitably accompanies meningitis combine to cause increased intracranial pressure. In some patients, the rise in pressure may be severe enough to cause herniation and death. Vigorous inflammation in the CNS may also have late ill effects if reestablishment of the drainage system by reabsorption of the inflammatory debris is delayed or incomplete.

When the course of meningitis has been fulminant, there may be only slight flattening of the gyri and polymorphonuclear leukocytosis in sections of the meninges and brain. If, as is usual, 6 to 10 days elapse before death, the leptomeninges are congested and acute vasculitis with fibrin deposition involves the smaller vessels. Although the exudate may not involve the brain directly, the changes in vascular flow and the increased intracranial pressure produce diffuse injury to the brain. Ventriculitis is commonly present in neonatal meningitis. Also, in experimental meningitis induced in nonhuman primates with *H. influenzae,* ventriculitis was common.

When meningococcemia is associated with fulminant disease (sudden onset of fever, malaise, abdominal pain, with pupura, cyanosis, hypotension, and death within 6–24 hours), both clinical and pathologic evidences of meningitis may be minimal or absent. The classic finding at necropsy is extensive hemorrhage into both adrenal glands—the anatomic component of the Waterhouse–Friderichsen syndrome. However, an identical clinicpathologic picture can be evoked in patients infected with *S. pneumoniae, S. pyogenes, Staphylococcus* spp., *H. influenzae, Pseudomonas aeruginosa,* and several of the Enterobacteriaceae; septicemic adrenal hemorrhage is, therefore, a preferable designation. Despite the striking pathology of the adrenal glands, the occurrence of the syndrome as a consequence of infection with gram-positive cocci casts doubt on endotoxin shock as the mechanism. It has been suggested that disseminated intravascular coagulation is the common pathogenetic mechanism, a possibility yet unproved but consistent with the observed histopathology.

Widespread vasculitis involving the arterioles and capillaries is actually the major lesion in patients with septicemic adrenal hemmorhage. Vasculitis afflicts the heart, causing diffusely distributed foci of myocarditis and focal involvement of the conduction system. An explanation of the hypotension and vascular collapse is thereby provided that is preferable to the postulated, but unproven, acute adrenal insufficiency—the cortisol concentration in the plasma is usually above normal. Acute vasculitis leads to plugging of the vessels with fibrin, resulting in focal myocardial necrosis with associated hemorrhage and neutrophilic infiltration. Such lesions are present in more than three-fourths of patients who die of meningococcal infections. Pulmonary edema and congestion consequent to acute myocarditis are present in 78% of the fatal cases, and 30% of these have pleural effusions.

Purpura is also a consequence of acute vasculitis, with meningococci in endothelial cells, necrosis of vessel walls, and fibrin-plugged arterioles and capillaries. The mucous membranes of the oral cavity, the conjunctival and serosal surfaces, and occasionally, the glomeruli and adrenal glands, may be similarly afflicted. Hemorrhage and necrosis of the adrenal glands were found in 48% of 200 fatal meningococcal infections. The lesions occur much more frequently with group C than with group B or group A *N. meningitidis.*

Ordinarily, the bacteria involved are *S. pneumoniae* and *H. influenzae;* rarely, *S. aureus,* anaerobes, and *S. pyogenes* may also be implicated. Paracranial osteomyelitis may be part of the pathogenesis either by direct extension or by causing septic thrombophlebitis of the great dural veins. In addition, septic thrombophlebitis secondary to infections of the face, nose, and pharnyx may lead to meningitis—usually with *S. aureus*—although staphylococcemia rarely leads to meningitis.

Trauma

Injuries that breach the bony and membranous coverings of the CNS provide avenues of ingress for the resident microbiota. In simple fractures, the opening through the bone is not in and of itself sufficient to lead to meningitis. Exudate that clots, thereby plugging cracks, also provides an excellent culture medium for the ingrowth of bacteria, causing meningitis. *Streptococcus pneumoniae* is by far the most common bacterium, followed by *H. influenzae, S. aureus,* and *S. pyogenes.*

Missile-inflicted injury to the CNS also leads to acute bacterial meningitis. The outgrowth of bacteria implanted during a penetrating injury is favored by foreign bodies, fragments of bone, clots, and devitalized tissue. *Staphylococcus aureus* is commonly involved. Iatrogenic meningitis, resulting from inadequately sterilized instruments, contaminated solutions, or faulty technique, is frequently caused by *P. aeruginosa.*

Neurosurgery

The insertion of shunting devices into the CNS is followed in 25% to 30% of children by infections caused by *Staphylococcus epidermidis* (50%), *S. aureus* (25%), or other bacteria (enterococci, *S. pyogenes,* meningococci, pneumococci, *Haemophilus* spp., *Bacillus subtilis,* and diphtheroids). If these infections occur within 2 months of surgery, it is thought that the infecting bacteria were introduced during the operative period. Later infections are assumed to be hematogenous in origin.

Infections following other neurosurgical procedures are caused by *S. aureus* or Enterobacteriaceae–*E. coli* and *Klebsiella* spp. in 75% of the patients. Multiple neurosurgical procedures in the presence of extraneural infections are associated with an increased frequency of meningitis.

Enteric Meningitis

Overall, gram-negative enteric bacilli cause 4% to 5% of bacterial meningitis. Of this percentage, 60% are related to neurosurgery, 30% occur in newborns, and 10% to 12% develop in patients with miscellaneous underlying diseases such as diabetes mellitus, urinary tract infections, and systemic diseases with bacteremia. *Pseudomonas aeruginosa* may cause meningitis in patients with malignancies.

Manifestations

The manifestations of acute bacterial meningitis are largely independent of the cause. They result first from infection, and second from increased intracranial pressure. Chills, fever, malaise, and headache are the usual manifestations of infection; headache, vomiting, and rarely, papilledema, may result from increased pressure. Signs of meningeal inflammation are also present. The onset may be abrupt or insidious.

The infant with meningitis rarely displays signs of meningeal irritation. Irritability and refusal to take food are typical; vomiting occurs early in the disease and repeated emesis may lead to dehydration. Fullness of the fontanel is a variable sign, but when present reliably predicts increased intracranial pressure. Fever is typically absent in children under 2 months of age. Hypothermia is more common in neonates. As the disease progresses, apneic episodes, seizures, disturbances in motor tone, and coma may develop.

In older children and adults, specific symptoms and signs are usually present in bacterial meningitis, with fever and altered mental status the most consistent findings. Fever is present in more than 80% of patients and may attain 40°C to 41°C (104°F–106°F). Headache is an early, prominent complaint and is usually very severe, bursting in character, unremitting, and diffuse or localized, often radiating down the neck into the back. Many patients have antecedent disease of the respiratory tract, sinus, ear, or pharynx. Nausea, vomiting and photophobia are also common symptoms that may reflect increased intracranial pressure or cerebellar inflammation.

A wide variety of neurologic signs may be present with bacterial meningitis; approximately one-third of the patients have convulsions or coma when first seen by a physician. Localizing neurologic signs are usually manifestations of cerebritis, but may be caused by a focal process such as vascular thrombosis, infarction, abscess, subdural effusion, or empyema. Signs of meningeal irritation are common: (1) cervical rigidity—passive anteflexion of the head meets with resistance and causes pain (Brudzinski's sign); (2) thoracolumbar rigidity—in its extreme form, there is fixed hyperextension; (3) hamstring spasm—passive extension of the knees with the hips flexed meets with resistance and causes pain referred to the hamstring muscles and the lower back (Kernig's sign); and (4) exaggerated reflexes—symmetric, exquisitely sensitive, deep tendon reflexes. Opisthotonos is hyperextension of the spine so rigidly held that the patient can be pulled up from supine to sitting by his head alone with articulation restricted to the hips; this is the extreme manifestation of meningeal irritation. In order to maintain a sitting posture, the patient throws his arms out and back to form a tripod.

The mental state of the patient varies according to the stage and progress of the disease, and the age of the patient. Delirium is common in the early stages, but may be followed by drowsiness, then stupor, and eventually, coma. Photophobia and a general hyperesthesia to all forms of stimuli are present. Venous congestion of the ocular fundi is common. Papilledema is uncommon at initial examination; indeed, if it is found when the patient is first seen, brain abscess or other intracranial disease must be suspected. The pupils may be unequal and react sluggishly; they may even become dilated and fixed as the disease progresses. Squint and diplopia with ptosis are common. Any of the ocular muscles may be paralyzed—most frequently, one or both external recti. Swallowing may be difficult due to cranial nerve involvement. Although muscular power in the limbs is usually well preserved, slight incoordination and tremor are common, and muscular hypotonia occurs quite regularly. Meningitis may be localized for a time to one hemisphere or the other, cause jacksonian convulsions, hemiparesis, or even hemianopia.

In old or very debilitated patients, meningitis may be insidious in onset. The earliest manifestations often are alterations in mental status that may range from confusion or lethargy to stupor. Signs of meningeal irritation are also quite variable and are frequently confused by the concomitant presence of cervical osteoarthritis. Frequently, there is an associated infection, especially in the lungs or the urinary tract. These patients are often thought to have a cerebrovascular accident, an organic brain syndrome, or coma of unknown etiology. Early meningitis may also be misdiagnosed as a trivial illness with fever, headache, and minimal stiffness of the neck ascribed to myalgia. If there is a history, supported by physical or other findings, consistent with otitis media, mastoiditis, sinusitis, or cavernous sinus thrombosis, secondary meningitis must be suspected. Similarly, patients with pneumonia, osteomyelitis, bacteremia from any cause, or head trauma with or without rhinorrhea or otorrhea, must be carefully studied for evidence of meningitis.

Petechiae, or purpuric or hemorrhagic manifestations, occur from the first to the third day of illness in 30% to 60% of patients with meningococcal disease, with or without meningitis. There is no characteristic distribution of the rash, but hemorrhagic and petechial manifestations may be more prominent in areas of the skin subjected to pressure such as the axillary folds, the belt line, or the back. At least five different lesions have been described in meningococcal infections: (1) a fleeting maculopapular rash occurring during the early hours of the disease, (2) discrete, pleomorphic, raised, petechial lesions ranging from 1 mm–5 mm in diameter, (3) hemorrhagic, purpuric lesions with a geographic border, (4) hemorrhagic lesions evolving into bullae, and (5) lesions of erythema nodesum occurring on the anterior surfaces of the lower extremities. Meningococci can be demonstrated by smear and culture of scrapings in 30% to 50% of early lesions. Hemorrhagic and petechial lesions may be present in the mucous and synovial membranes. Involvement of the synovium occurs in less than 5% of patients with meningococcal disease, appearing typically after the fourth or fifth day of disease, well after the illness has been controlled.

Diagnosis

Examination of the CSF is the key to the definitive diagnosis of acute bacterial meningitis. The CSF should be examined in every patient in whom the clinical findings are consistent with even the possibility of meningitis, however minimal the manifestations. This approach is essential because (1) untreated bacterial meningitis is a lethal infection that may devolve with catastrophic speed; (2) bacterial meningitis treated early with appropriate antibacterial agents is curable, and (3) the selection of appropriate antimicrobics often requires etiologic diagnosis and may depend on susceptibility testing *in vitro*.

The necessity for planning before lumbar puncture is carried out cannot be overemphasized. The diagnostic value of prompt, appropriate examination of the CSF is maximal only if the physician has clearly in mind what tests are necessary.

A portion of the specimen of CSF must be cultured, and blood must also be obtained for culture, prior to the administration of any antimicrobics. Unfortunately, treatment that is not curative has been given before appropriate efforts at etiologic diagnosis were carried out in as many as 50% of patients who eventually were proved to have bacterial meningitis. Such prior therapy is inimical to diagnosis by reducing the yield of cultures of the CSF if the antimicrobic used penetrates efficiently into the CSF through the inflamed meninges and is highly active against pneumococci and meningococci, for example, penicillin G. Drugs that penetrate poorly, such as erythromycin, cause little difficulty. Success in the isolation of *H. influenzae* is usually unaffected by prior therapy. Neither smear diagnosis nor the concentrations of protein, glucose, or lactic acid are likely to be affected by prior therapy, since the dynamics of change of these indices of meningitis extend over several days.

In acute bacterial meningitis, the CSF is usually turbid, containing more than 1000 leukocytes per mm^3, the majority of which are polymorphonuclear

Table 119-2. Characteristic Changes of the Protein, Leukocytes, and Glucose in the Cerebrospinal Fluid (CSF)

CSF Protein (Normal, <50 mg/dl)	**Leukocytes (Normal, 0–5 mononuclear/ml)**	**CSF GLUCOSE (Normal, >50% serum glucose)**
INCREASED (55 MG to 1000 MG/DL)	POLYMORPHONUCLEAR LEUKOCYTE PREDOMINANCE	NORMAL
Any meningitis Viral encephalitis Syphilis Degenerative disease Neoplasia (primary, metastatic) Abscess (intracerebral, osteomyelitis) Hemorrhage, subdural hematoma Polyneuropathies (diphtheria) Myxedema, diabetes mellitus Hyperparathyroidism	Acute bacterial meningitis Subdural empyema Ruptured brain abscess Early viral meningitis (mumps, enteroviruses) Chemical meningitis (hemorrhage, spinal anesthesia)	Viral meningitis Encephalitis Metabolic encephalopathy Toxic encephalopathy
MARKED INCREASE (>1000 MG/DL)	MONONUCLEAR LEUKOCYTE PREDOMINANCE	MARKED INCREASE
Some fungal, tuberculous meningitides Spinal–subarachnoid block Guillain—Barré syndrome	Late viral meningitis Tuberculous meningitis Cryptococcal and other fungal meningitides Meningeal carcinomatosis Osteomyelitis (parameningeal) Syphilis (other spirochetes) Sarcoid Systemic lupus erythematosus Viral encephalitis	Hyperglycemic coma
INCREASED GAMMA GLOBULINS	INDETERMINATE LEUKOCYTIC PREDOMINANCE	20 MG TO 50 MG/DL
Subacute sclerosing panencephalitis Multiple sclerosis Tuberculosis Tabes dorsalis Multiple myeloma	Brain abscess Epidural abscess Septic emboli Coccidioidal meningitis	Early tuberculous or fungal Bacterial (early) Meningeal carcinomatosis Severe hemorrhage Systemic hypoglycemia
		<20 MG/DL
		Late tuberculous or fungal Bacterial (advanced) Ruptured abscess Diabetic ketoacidosis Cysticercosis Reyes syndrome

leukocytes (Table 119-2). In fulminant meningitis, the CSF may contain few leukocytes but many bacteria. In other specimens, there may be many leukocytes and very few bacteria. However, bacteria are readily found by microscopic examination of a gram-stained smear of the sediment collected by centrifugation of the CSF in about 75% of patients. Characteristically, the concentration of glucose in the CSF is less than 50% of the concentration in concomitantly collected serum; also, the concentration of protein is usually greater than 100 mg/dl. These indices are distinctly less reliable than microscopic examination of the gram-stained smear and culture of the sediment obtained by centrifuging the CSF. Thus, at first examination of the CSF in patients proved to have bacterial meningitis, about 20% had more than 60 mg of glucose/dl and 40% had less than 1000 leukocytes per mm^3. Moreover, the CSF from patients with viral meningitis (Chap. 118, Viral Meningitis) may, at initial examination, have more than 1000 leukocytes per mm^3 with more than 75% neutrophiles; a second specimen obtained 8 to 24 hours later will disclose a significant drop in the proportion of neutrophiles in 85% of such patients.

An exact etiologic diagnosis can sometimes be made quite promptly by demonstrating capsular swelling (quellung) on exposure of bacteria concentrated by centrifuging CSF to specific antiserums. This technique is useful with *H. influenzae, N. meningitidis* (groups A and C), and *S. pneumoniae.* Diagnostic serums of high antibody titer are necessary, and controls must be set up to enable proper interpretation.

The capsular polysaccharides of *H. influenzae, N. meningitidis,* and *S. pneumoniae* can be detected by counterimmunoelectrophoresis (CIE; Chap. 14, Immunologic Diagnosis). However, only 60% to 90% of culturally proved cases of bacterial meningitis yield positive results; CIE is best with haemophilan and poorest with pneumococcal infections. Latex particle agglutination appears to be more sensitive than CIE—detection of 0.5 ng *versus* 1.0 ng of capsular polysaccharide per ml, respectively. Since latex particle agglutination can be carried out at the bedside, it may prove to be useful in the early diagnosis of severe infections caused by *H. influenzae* and meningococci.

Many nonspecific tests for differentiating bacterial from nonbacterial meningitis have been advocated. These include assays for endotoxin and the measurement of lactic acid dehydrogenase, glutamic acid-oxaloacetic transaminase, isocitric dehydrogenase, amylase, and volatile acids in the CSF. Of these, perhaps the most valuable is detection of lactic acid; concentrations equal to or greater than 35 mg/dl are indicative of bacterial meningitis.

Brain abscess juxtaposed to the meninges may evoke changes in the CSF that are virtually identical with those of acute bacterial meningitis, with the exception of smears and cultures without bacteria. Early in the course of acute viral meningoencephalomyelitis, there is polymorphonuclear leukocyte response; however, the glucose is usually normal and there are no bacteria by smear or culture.

A traumatic lumbar puncture is characterized by clearing of bleeding after initial entry into the subarachnoid space, clotting only in the first specimens with the most blood, and the absence of xanthochromia in the supernatant liquid after centrifugation. Early in the course of subarachnoid hemorrhage, there may be a predominance of neutrophiles as in bacterial meningitis, and depression of the concentration of glucose as low as 20 mg/dl.

Tuberculous, fungal, leptospiral, and protozoal meningitides are generally insidious in onset. Brudzinski's and Kernig's signs are usually absent, and there may be only slight stiffness of the neck. The cellular response is usually less intense than in bacterial meningitides, and the cells are predominantly mononuclear. In tuberculous meningitis, depression of the chloride concentration (the plasma chloride must be determined simultaneously) is particularly valuable because the glucose may be nearly normal. Xanthochromia of the CSF is relatively common in leptospiral meningitis, and conjunctivitis is frequently present.

Meningismus—meningeal irritation that is clinically evident but not associated with the CSF abnormalities beyond a slightly elevated protein—is typically found in patients who have one of the acute, specific, febrile illnesses of childhood. Other acute infections may also cause meningismus: influenza, pneumonias (upper lobar and central), typhoid fever, and acute rheumatic fever, acute pharyngeal abscess, disease of the cervical spine, the mastoids, and cerebral vessels.

Prognosis

Untreated acute bacterial meningitis is fatal in 70% to 100% of patients. With appropriate antibacterial therapy, the case fatality rate has been greatly reduced (Table 119-1), with death occurring principally in the very young, the very old, or those with potentially lethal underlying diseases. These are the very patients in whom the manifestations of meningitis may be obscure, thus delaying antibacterial therapy. These are also the very patients in whom meningitis is likely to be caused by bacteria that are resistant to many antimicrobics.

Cerebral abscess may complicate acute bacterial meningitis caused by *S. aureus* and enteric bacteria, particularly when the meningitis follows traumatic inoculation or direct extension. Surgical treatment should be delayed until the meningitis is under control and the abscess has localized.

Subdural effusions may form in 6% to 50% of pediatric patients and are especially likely to complicate meningitis caused by *H. influenzae* and occasionally by *S. pneumoniae.* The manifestations include recurrent fever following initial defervescence, convulsions, persistence of signs of meningeal irritation, increased tension of the fontanel, and other signs of increased pressure such as vomiting or focal neurologic signs. The diagnosis requires (1) daily transillumination and neurologic examination, (2) daily measurement of the fronto-occipital circumference, and (3) computed tomographic (CT) scanning to evaluate abnormalities of (1) or (2). Initial subdural paracentesis is necessary to exclude empyema; repeated paracenteses may be considered for relief of specific symptoms or alleviation of large midline shifts. Surgical procedures are rarely required.

Other abnormalities are frequently observed in CT scans of children with bacterial meningitis: cerebral swelling, 9%; ischemic infarcts, 19%; ependymitis, 14%; enhancing basal meninges, 5%; focal spinal cord necrosis, 9%; and ventricular widening, 67%.

Various forms of hydrocephalus may develop months to years after recovery from acute bacterial meningitis. Although the incidence is quite low, the premature–neonatal age group is most often afflicted. Most commonly, an adhesive arachnoiditis, probably consequent to the organization of exudate, involves the basilar cisterns of the brain, occluding the foramina of Luschka and Magendie to cause an internal hydrocephalus. Corrective neurosurgery is frequently necessary.

Other late complications include the persistence of ocular nerve palsies, blindness, and deafness. These are quite uncommon.

Fully 50% of neonates recovering from bacterial meningitis may exhibit either motor or intellectual impairment. These defects may be very minor and may be overlooked at the time of discharge from the hospital. For this reason, it is important to determine the neurologic status of children at regular intervals for at least 1 to 2 years after the acute disease so that proper rehabilitative measures can be planned. The importance of counseling and early attention to defects cannot be overstressed.

Therapy

Supportive Care

When death occurs during the first 24 to 48 hours of bacterial meningitis, it is usually caused by difficulties in care other than the specific treatment of the infectious process. As a result, antimicrobial therapy has had minimal impact on early death. A combination of fever, dehydration secondary to vomiting and decreased fluid intake, with or without shock, may predispose patients, especially young children, to seizures. Respiratory arrest or airway obstruction may follow. If significant CNS or myocardial hypoxia occurs, fatal cardiac arrhythmias or brainstem damage may result. Beyond the correction of fluid and electrolyte deficits and the provision for adequate oxygenation, cardiovascular function must be carefully and continually evaluated. In addition to pulse and arterial blood pressure, the central venous pressure should be monitored by means of an indwelling central venous catheter. The use of a cardiac-active glycoside (*e.g.,* digoxin) may be necessary, and dopamine may be required if shock is refractory to the administration of fluids.

Acute cerebral edema may be life-threatening in bacterial meningitis. Three mechanisms are contributory: (1) vasogenic edema—increased permeability of the capillaries of the brain, (2) cytotoxic edema—cellular swelling with concomitant reduction of the space available for the brain and extracellular fluid, and (3) interstitial edema—an increase in the water and sodium content of the periventricular white matter as occurs in obstructive hydrocephalus. Several treatments have been advocated to control acute cerebral edema: (1) osmotic agents, such as mannitol (1 dose of 0.5 g–2.0 g/kg body wt, IV, over 30 min), appear to exert temporary benefit; the blood pH and electrolytes must be monitored carefully, and there is danger of a rebound increase in intracranial pressure after the hypertonic agent has been excreted. (2) glucosteroids are neither advantageous nor detriental in patients under 16 years of age; however, their use may be associated with a significantly increased risk of death in older patients, particularly in pneumococcal meningitis. (3) controlled ventilation following elective tracheal intubation with maintenance of the pCO_2 at 25 to 30 torr may reduce markedly increased intracranial pressure; and (4) other modalities such as hypothermia and cefazolamide have not been used in patients with bacterial meningitis. Continuous monitoring with an intraventricular catheter or subarachnoid bolt have not been evaluated prospectively in bacterial meningitis.

The treatment for disseminated intravascular clotting (DIC) is at best empiric, and often unsuccessful (Chap. 7, Manifestations of Infectious Diseases). The primary therapy is that directed at curing the meningitis. Treatment with heparin has been advocated but either has had no effect or has caused worsening of the disease. Vigorous treatment of the shock of DIC with adequate fluids or pressor agents appears to enhance survival.

Inappropriate secretion of antidiuretic hormone is an invariable consequence of CNS infections. Fluids should be restricted to about 60% of normal maintenance requirements for the first 48 to 72 hours of therapy. However, if hypotension caused by septic shock or dehydrating hypovolemia is present initially, fluid replacement is mandatory.

Seizures occur in about 30% of children and 10% of adults with bacterial meningitis. Initial management should include the use of diazepam or phenobarbital, and should be followed by maintenance therapy with phenobarbital or dilantin. If seizures are confined or controlled by 72 hours, there is usually no liability for seizures as a long-term sequela; that is, long-term maintenance anticonvulsant therapy is not required. Repeated, prolonged, complicated seizures, and those persisting after the third or fourth day of treatment, are usually predictive of seizures as persistent sequelae of meningitis; chronic suppressive therapy may be required.

Antibacterial Therapy

The initial selection of antibacterial therapy should always be made before the results of cultures are available. If bacteria are found on examination of smears prepared from the CSF, the information used should be used along with knowledge of the patient's age and other data from the history and physical examination. In Table 119-3, regimens of initial antibacterial therapy are recommended for use in the absence of etiologic diagnosis. When etiologic diagnosis has been accomplished, after susceptibility studies have been completed (if indicated), and if the patient's course warrants change, the regimens set out in Table 119-4 should be adopted.

Some aspects of antimicrobial chemotherapy merit further comment. Intravenous injection is recommended for all agents throughout the course of therapy. It is essential to deliver antibacterial agents promptly and reliably; hypotension and coma compromise absorption from the gut or intramuscular depots. Because most antimicrobics enter the CSF and CNS inefficiently (exceptions include sulfonamides, chloramphenicol, cycloserine, isonicotinic acid hydrazide, ethambutol, rifampin, flucytosine, fosfomycin, trimethoprim, and metronidazole), a high gradient from blood to CSF is critical to adequate treatment; that is, intravenous injection of large doses is necessary. The facilitating effect of meningeal inflammation on the entry of antimicrobics decreases if treatment is effective; accordingly, maintenance of a high gradient remains essential as treatment is continued. Moreover, intravenous injection is the humane mode of therapy; the patient who recovers after treatment by repeated intramuscular injections is a mass of misery from chemical myositis. A proved exception to the foregoing is PO administration of chloramphenicol to complete a 10 to 14 day course of treatment after an initial period of IV administration; serum and CSF concentrations are equivalent following IV and PO administration.

Loading doses are recommended. When the decision is made to treat, gradients in concentration favoring passage of antimicrobics from blood into the CSF and CNS should be established quickly.

Alternative agents are listed—in most instances, for use in patients with documented hypersensitivity to the penicillins. The original cephalosporins were not acceptable substitutes since they entered the CNS/CSF poorly or were too toxic for high dose administration. Of the newer cephalosporins, moxalactam according to preliminary reports, has been curative of meningitis caused by gram-negative enteric bacteria.

Staphylococcus aureus should always be presumed to be β-lactamase producers, that is, resistant to penicillins G, V, ampicillin, amoxicillin, carbenicillin, ticarcillin, and the acylureidopenicillins. Although *S. aureus* resistant to the β-lactamase-resistant penicillins and the cephalosporins are not a major problem in the United States, meningitis caused by such staphylococci requires alternative antimicrobics. Vancomycin does not attain high concentrations in the CSF; however, it is bactericidal at low concentrations and it may be injected intrathecally (5 mg every 12–24 hours in the adult). Gentamicin, tobramycin, metilmicin, or amikacin by intrathecal injection, or systemic rifampin may be given to augment the activity of the vancomycin.

Some strains of *S. epidermis* are resistant to many antimicrobics including the penicillins and the cephalosporins. Susceptibility testing is essential for selecting agents for treatment.

Of *H. influenzae* isolated from patients with meningitis in the United States and several other countries, 10% to 30% are resistant to the penicillins and some of the cephalosporins. Therefore, treatment is begun with both ampicillin and chloramphenicol in children more than 4 to 8 weeks of age or in any adult thought to be infected with *H. influenzae*

Table 119-3. *Antimicrobial Therapy of Presumed Bacterial Meningitis Prior to Etiologic Diagnosis*

Clinical feature	Antimicrobic		
	OF CHOICE	ALTERNATE	COMMENT
Premature and neonatal infants	Ampicillin: Loading—50 mg/kg body wt, IV, in first 30 min of therapy (→0.13 mEq Na^+/kg body wt). Maintenance—200–400 mg/kg body wt/day, IV (→0.42–0.93 mEq Na^+/kg body wt) and Gentamicin or tobramycin: Loading—1.7 mg/kg body wt. Maintenance—2.5 mg/kg body wt; every 12 hours in infants less than 1 wk, every 8 hours in older infants	Chloramphenicol (succinate derivative): Loading—25 mg/kg body wt/IV, in first hour of therapy. Maintenance—25 mg–50 mg/kg body wt/day, IV Amikacin: Loading—25 mg/kg body wt, IV, in first hour Maintenance—7.5 mg/kg body wt/day, IV, every 12 hours	In premature infants and neonates under 1 week, the dose of chloramphenicol should not exceed 25 mg/kg/day. Chloramphenicol is not bactericidal for many pathogens; response to therapy must be monitored carefully. Simultaneous mixed meningitis caused by two or more distinct kinds of bacteria is most common in this age group (5%–15% of cases). Foci of infection outside the leptomeninges must be sought, *e.g.,* paranasal sinuses, mastoids, middle ear. Moxalactam, and other newer cephalosporins may be alternatives; dosage not yet evaluated; it will probably be 150 mg–200 mg/kg body wt/day. Treatment should be continued for 14 days or until afebrile for 7 days.
2–60 Months	Ampicillin: Loading—50 mg/kg body wt, IV, in first 30 min of therapy (→0.13 mEq Na^+/kg body wt). Maintenance—300 mg–400 mg/kg body wt/day, IV (→0.42–0.93 mEq Na^+/kg body wt)	* Chloramphenicol (succinate derivative): Loading—25 mg/kg body wt, IV, in first 30 min of therapy. Maintenance—100 mg/kg body wt/day, IV	Moxalactam and other newer cephalosporins may be alternatives; dosage probably ~200 mg/kg body wt/day. Treatment should be continued for 14 days or until afebrile for 7 days.
5–40 Years	Penicillin G: Loading—50 mg (~80,000 units) kg body wt, IV, in first 30 min of therapy (→0.13 mEq K^+/kg body wt). Maintenance—150 mg (~240,000 units) kg body wt/day, IV (→0.4 mEq K^+/kg body wt)	* Chloramphenicol (succinate derivative): Loading—25 mg/kg body wt/day, IV, in first hour. Maintenance—60 mg–75 mg/kg body wt/day, IV	Foci of infection outside the leptomeninges must be sought, *e.g.,* paranasal sinuses, mastoids, middle ear. Treatment should be continued for 14 days, or until afebrile for 7 days.
>40 Years	Penicillin G: Loading—50 mg (~80,000 units)/kg body wt, IV, in first 30 min of therapy (→0.13 mEq K^+/kg body wt). Maintenance—150 mg (~240,000 units)/kg body wt/day, IV (→0.4 mEq K^+/kg body wt)	* Chloramphenicol (succinate derivative): Loading—25 mg/kg body wt, IV, in first 30 min. of therapy. Maintenance—60 mg–75mg/kg body wt/day, IV	Foci of infection outside the leptomeninges must be sought, *e.g.,* paranasal sinuses, mastoids, middle ear. Moxalactam and other newer cephalosporins may be alternatives; dosage probably ~200 mg/kg body wt/day. Treatment should be continued for 14 days, or until afebrile for 7 days.

Extension from intracranial focus	Penicillin G: Loading—50 mg (~80,000 units)/kg body wt, IV, in first 30 min of therapy (→0.13 mEq K^+/kg body wt). Maintenance—150 mg (~240,000 units)/kg body wt/day, IV (→0.4 mEq K^+/kg body wt)	*Chloramphenicol (succinate derivative): Loading—25 mg/kg body wt, IV, in first hour. Maintenance—75 mg–100mg/kg body wt/day, IV (not to exceed 4.0 g/day)	Treatment should be continued during and for at least one week after neurosurgery.
Skull fractures	Penicillin G: Loading—50 mg (~80,000 units)/kg body wt, IV, in first 30 min of therapy (→0.13 mEq K^+/kg body wt). Maintenance—150 mg (~240,000 units)/kg body wt/day, IV (→0.4 mEq K^+/kg body wt)	*Chloramphenicol (succinate derivative): Loading—25 mg/kg body wt/day, IV, in first hour. Maintenance—60 mg–75mg/kg body wt/day, IV	Neurosurgical repair of the defect in the leptomeninges is usually necessary to prevent relapse.
Penetrating injuries, shunting prostheses, endocarditis, leukemias, lymphomas	Nafcillin: Loading—50 mg/kg body wt, IV, in first 30 min of therapy (→0.11 mEq Na^+/kg body wt). Maintenance—200 mg/kg body wt/day, IV (→0.45 mEq Na^+/kg body wt)	Chloramphenicol (succinate derivative): Loading—25mg/kg body wt, IV, in first hour. Maintenance—60 mg–75mg/kg body wt/day, IV or Vancomycin: Loading—20 mg/kg body wt, IV, first hour (not to exceed 1.0 g total). Maintenance—20 mg–40 mg/kg body wt/day, IV (not to exceed 2.0 g/day)	Although antimicrobics will abate the meningitis, removal of the foreign body, if present, is essential to cure. With *S. epidermis,* susceptibility testing *in vitro* is particularly important because other agents may be necessary.

*Chloramphenicol may be given to patients allergic to the penicillins, although moxalactam or cefotaxime may prove to be preferable.

Table 119-4. *Antimicrobial Therapy for Bacterial Meningitis of Known Etiology*

Bacterial etiology	Antimicrobic		
	OF CHOICE	ALTERNATE	COMMENT
Neisseria meningitidis; Streptococcus pneumoniae; Streptococcus pyogenes, groups A, B, C, G	Penicillin G: Loading—50 mg (~80,000 units)/kg body wt, IV, in first hour (→0.13 mEq K^+/kg body wt). Maintenance—150 mg (~240,000 units)/kg body wt/day, IV (→0.4 mEq K^+/kg body wt)	Chloramphenicol (succinate derivative). Loading—25 mg/kg body wt, in first hour. Maintenance—25 mg–100 mg/kg body wt/day, IV	Particularly with *S. pneumoniae,* foci of infection outside the leptomeninges must be sought, *e.g.,* paranasal sinuses, middle ear, mastoids, lungs, heart valves. For group B streptococci, use penicillin G, 400 mg/kg/day with gentamicin, tobramycin, or netilmicin: 2.5 mg/kg body wt, every 12 hours (infants < 1 wk), every 8 hours (infants > 1 wk). Treatment should be continued for at least 1 week after defervescence (3 wk in neonates and prematures).
Haemophilus influenzae	Ampicillin: Loading—50 mg/kg body wt, IV, in first hour (→0.13 mEq Na^+/kg body wt). Maintenance—300 mg/kg body wt/day, IV (→0.76 mEq Na^+/kg body wt)	Chloramphenicol (succinate derivative). Loading—25 mg/kg body wt, in first hour. Maintenance—25 mg–100 mg/kg body wt/day, IV	Use ampicillin + chloramphenicol at the outset, deleting one drug according to β-lactamase capability of isolate. Foci of infection adjacent to the leptomeninges must be sought, *e.g.,* the middle ear. In prematures and neonates under 1 week, the dose of chloramphenicol should not exceed 25 mg/kg/day.
Staphylococcus aureus	Nafcillin: Loading—50 mg/kg body wt, IV, in first hour (→0.11 mEq Na^+/kg body wt). Maintenance—200 mg/kg body wt/day, IV (→0.45 mEq Na^+/kg body wt)	Vancomycin: Loading—20 mg/kg body wt, IV, in first hour (not to exceed 1.0 g total). Maintenance: 20 mg–40 mg/kg body wt/day, IV (not to exceed 20 g/day).	Initial therapy must always be predicated on the possibility that β-lactamase-producing *S. aureus* is the cause of meningitis. If *in vitro* tests indicate susceptibility to penicillin G, change to regimen for this drug as given above. With strains resistant to β-lactamase-resistant drugs, vancomycin may be necessary. Foci from which *S. aureus* metastasized to the CNS must be identified and drained surgically or excised.

Escherichia coli or other enteric gram-negative bacteria	Ampicillin: Loading—50 mg/kg wt, IV, in first hour (→0.13 mEq Na^+/kg body wt). Maintenance—400 mg/kg body wt/day, IV (→0.93 mEq Na^+/kg body wt); perhaps with gentamicin, tobramycin, or netilmicin. Loading—1.7 mg/kg body wt, IV, in first hour. Maintenance—5 mg—6 mg/kg body wt/day, IV. As aminocyclitols enter the CSF poorly, lumbar intrathecal or intraventricular injection of preservative-free preparations (5 mg/12 hours each dose in 3 ml–5 ml 0.9% NaCl solution) may be necessary.	An acylureidopenicillin: Loading—100 mg/kg body wt, IV, in first hour (→0.14 mEq Na^+/kg body wt). Maintenance—300 mg/kg body wt/day, IV (→0.42 mEq Na^+/kg body wt). Moxalactam or other newer cephalosporins may be the best alternatives in a dose of 200 mg/kg body wt/day, IV (→0.76 mEq Na+/kg body wt).	Ampicillin is usually less active than the acylureidopenicillins; use either one if the MLC is <5 μg/ml. Resistant isolates are sometimes susceptible to chloramphenicol, and usually to gentamicin, tobramycin, netilmycin, moxalactam, and other newer cephalosporins. As chloramphenicol is frequently ineffective and the aminocyclitols enter CSF poorly, moxalactam or cefotaxime (200 mg/kg body wt/day, IV) may be preferable.
Pseudomonas aeruginosa	Gentamicin, tobramycin, or netilmicin. Loading—1.7 mg/kg body wt, IV, in first hour. Maintenance—5 mg–6 mg/kg body wt/day, IV, plus lumbar intrathecal or intraventricular (preservative-free preparation): 5 mg every 12 hours, each dose in 3 ml–5 ml 0.9% NaCl. Carbenicillin: Loading—100 mg/kg body wt, IV, in first hour (→0.47 mEq Na^+/kg body wt). Maintenance—300 mg–500 mg/kg body wt/day, IV (→1.41–2.35 mEq Na^+/kg body wt)	Amikacin: Loading—25 mg/kg body wt, IV, in fist hour. Maintenance—50 mg/kg body wt/day, IV or Polymyxin B: Loading—1.0 mg/ kg body wt, IV, in first hour. Maintenance—2.5 mg/kg body wt/ day, IV. Intrathecal: 0.03 mg/kg body wt/day, each dose dissolved in 3 ml–5 ml 0.9% NaCl. Intracisternal injection is preferable to injection into the lumbar subarachnoid space.	*P. aeruginosa* strains natively and independently resistant to gentamicin, tobramycin, netilmicin, amikacin, and acylureidopenicillins do exist. However, the combination of an aminocyclitol plus acylureidopenicillins is synergistic against about two-thirds of the clinical isolates. If resistance to this combination is demonstrated by *in vitro* testing, polymyxin B should be substituted. Even in meningitis, the aminocyclitols and polymyxin B enter the CSF poorly, and intrathecal injection of a preservative-free preparation is necessary.

*Intravenous injection is necessary in these seriously ill patients.

(gram's stain, quellung reaction, CIE, or latex particle agglutination). The regimen is changed when microbiologic data become available from laboratory studies. Alternatively, all children under 5 years of age are given chloramphenicol alone because it is also effective for most strains of pneumococci and meningococci. Isolates of *H. influenzae* should be tested routinely for β-lactamase activity, since this is the mechanism for resistance. Unlike *H. influenzae*, clinical isolates of pneumococci are rarely resistant to penicillin G, and there are no reports of the isolation of resistant meningococci from patients with meningitis. Resistance in pneumococci (MIC $\geq$ 1 μg penicillin/ml) is not mediated by β-lactamases; vancomycin is probably the alternative of choice.

Therapy in the neonate with bacterial meningitis is usually initiated with penicillin G, ampicillin, or, occasionally, carbenicillin, combined with either gentamicin, tobramycin, metilmicin, or amikacin. Unfortunately, the infecting bacteria are frequently resistant to ampicillin alone, and the aminocyclitols enter the CSF erratically and poorly after either IM or IV injection. This deficit is not compensated by intrathecal injection, since translumbar therapy does not reduce the duration of positive CSF cultures, and intraventricular treatment may augment morbidity and mortality. Of the newer cephalosporins, moxalactam administered intravenously attains concentrations in the CSF that are lethal to most enteric gram-negative bacilli, and has been curative of meningitis in preliminary experience. Because chloramphenicol is not often or consistently bactericidal, it should not be employed routinely without laboratory confirmation of lethal capability.

Group B streptococci have remained susceptible to inhibition by penicillin G, but it is clear that many stains are tolerant to the penicillins. Since killing is facilitated by the addition of an aminocyclitol, gentamicin, tobramycin, or metilmicin, should be given with a high dose of penicillin until the isolate has been examined in the laboratory.

The rationale for combination therapy (e.g., penicillin G plus tobramycin) in the treatment of infections, including meningitis, caused by *Listeria monocytogenes* is discussed in Chapter 51, Listeriosis.

In most patients, treatment with antimicrobial agents can be discontinued about 1 week after defervescence; the average period of therapy is 10 to 14 days. Additional criteria for terminating therapy, such as requiring fewer than 50 leukocytes per mm^3 in the CSF, a CSF/blood glucose ratio of 0.5, and a reduction of the protein to $<$ 100 mg/dl in the CSF, are not necessary. Lumbar punctures should be performed after 24 to 36 hours of treatment and near the end of therapy to assess the patient's progress. In the case of infections complicated by the placement of foreign bodies, antimicrobic therapy should be extended for at least 2 weeks after cultures of the CSF have become negative.

Other underlying diseases are indications for prolonged antibacterial therapy: endocarditis, leukemia, and lymphoma. If surgery is needed (drainage of abscesses, excision of infected bone or other lesions, repair of defects in the leptomeninges, removal of foreign bodies), antibacterial agents should be continued into the postoperative period.

Prevention

Vaccines

With the ascendancy of sulfonamide-resistant meningococci as a cause of meningitis, attention was directed once again to the active immunoprophylaxis of infection with *N. meningitidis*. Modern methods of purification resulted in the preparation of group A and group C capsular polysaccharides that are immunogenic in man without provoking adverse reactions. Thus far, however, group B has remained a difficult problem. Apparently, meningococci of group B are either not capsulated or sparsely capsulated, or they bind the capsule quite tightly to the cell wall. The preparation of an immunogenic polysaccharide specific for group B has not yet been accomplished. Groups X, Y, and Z apparently are capsulated, and it may be possible to prepare specific polysaccharides that are immunogenic.

The rationale, composition, and use of multitypic pneumococcal capsular polysaccharide vaccine is described in Chapter 31, Bacterial Pneumonias. Although it is not known whether the vaccine provides protection against meningitis, it should do so by reducing the frequency and severity of pneumococcal pneumonia, thus decreasing the incidence of pneumococcal bacteremia.

Much more important in terms of meningitis in the United States is the prevention of infection with *H. influenzae*. Capsulated type b strains cause virtually all the clinically significant infections, and they are responsible for over half the cases of postneonatal pediatric bacterial meningitis. Thus far, efforts at the development of a vaccine effective in young children have not been successful. There is basis for hope, however, because humoral immunity is present in most persons by the age of 5 years.

Antimicrobics

The value of chemoprophylaxis in preventing meningococcal disease has been proved only in the special

Table 119-5. *Regimens for Chemoprophylaxis on Exposure to* Neisseria Meningitidis *or* Haemophilus Influenzae *Type b.*

Indication	Age	Antibiotic Regimen
Meningococcal disease		
Household contacts	3–12 months	Rifampin*, 5 mg/kg body wt, PO, every we hours for 4 doses
	Children	Rifampin*, 10 mg/kg body wt, PO, every 12 hours for 4 doses
	Adults	Rifampin*, 600 mg, PO, every 12 hours for 4 doses
Close contacts†	Adults	Procaine penicillin G, 600,000 units, IM, every 8 hours for 6 doses; followed by penicillin V, 500 mg, PO, every 8 hours for 8 days
Haemophilan disease		
Household or day-care center contacts	Children less than 6 years of age	Rifampin, 20 mg/kg body wt/day, PO, for 4 days

*Alternate regimen for rifampin-allergic patients: minocycline 1.0 mg/kg body wt, PO, every 12 hours for 5 days or sulfadiazine (for proven susceptible strains) 1.0 g every 12 hours for 4 doses for adults or 500 mg every 12 hours for 4 doses for children.

†Close contacts include only those persons known to have suffered mucosal splash by infected secretions or oral-to-oral contact.

setting of military groups. There is no proof of comparable value in the civilian setting, for example, a decrease in secondary cases among household contacts.

Sulfonamide chemoprophylaxis of meningococcal infections depends on the susceptibility of *N. meningitidis* to $\leq$ 1.0 µg/ml. Because the currently predominant strains are resistant to the sulfonamides, a number of antimicrobics have been evaluated. Of these, rifampin and minocycline have proved to be effective if given for 5 days (Table 119-5). Frequent symptoms of dizziness, nausea, and vomiting associated with minocycline have limited its use in the United States.

Although there is a significant risk of secondary cases of haemophilian disease among young household contacts, it is not clear whether chemoprophylaxis can eliminate the carrier state and thereby interrupt transmission of infection to susceptible hosts. Among children in day-care centers with disease caused by type b *H. influenzae,* the carrier rate is 32% to 56% compared with $<$ 1% in centers without disease. In preliminary studies, rifampin in a dose of 20 mg/kg body wt/day, PO, for 5 days, eradicated *H. influenzae* from more than 85% of carriers. Although rifampin has been recommended for use in group outbreaks, it is not certain that it will be successful in preventing secondary cases, and it has not been evaluated in household outbreaks.

Group B streptococci can be isolated from 65% to 70% of neonates born to women colonized with group B streptococci. Genital/anal colonization rates of mothers coming to term vary from 4% to 40% with a modal incidence of about 23%. Despite the high colonization rates, the attack rate for early onset infection in colonized neonates is about 1% to 2%. In view of the marked disparity between rates of colonization and disease, treating the colonized mother to prevent disease in her infant is not appropriate. It may be that the administration of a single dose of 50,000 units of aqueous penicillin 10 minutes after birth will reduce the frequency of group B streptococcal infections in neonates. Because this has not been proved, the routine administration of penicillin to newborns is not recommended.

Remaining Problems

Further work on preventive measures, specifically the development of a generally applicable vaccine for type b *H. influenzae,* is urgent.

The interrelationships, if any, of acute vasculitis, intravascular coagulation, hypersensitivity, endotoxin, and septicemic adrenal hemorrhage need to be clarified.

The remarkably high mortality of pneumococcal meningitis remains a challenge.

New antimicorbics therapeutically effective against meningococci should be developed. With the appearance of β-lactamase-producing *H. influenzae* in 1974 and gonococci in 1976, the possibility of a similar change in meningococci should be anticipated.

The pathogenesis and management of acutely increased intracranial pressure and cerebral edema in bacterial meningitis are incompletely understood.

Bibliography

Journals

ADAMS RD, KUBICK CS, BONNER FJ: Clinical and pathological aspects of influenzal meningitis. Arch Pediatr 65:354–376, 408–441, 1948

BENSON P, NYHEN WL, SHINIZU H: The prognosis of subdural effusions complicating pyogenic meningitis. J Pediatr 57:670–683, 1980

CHERUBIN CE, MARR JS, SIERRA MF, BECKER S: Listeria and gram-negative bacillary meningitis in New York City, 1972–1979. Am J Med 71:199–209, 1981

DALTON HP, ALLISON MJ: Modification of laboratory results by partial treatment of bacterial meningitis. Am J Clin Pathol 49:410–413, 1968

DODGE PR, SWARTZ MN: Bacterial meningitis-A review of selected aspects. II. Special neurologic problems, postmeningitic complications and clinicopathologic correlations. N Engl J Med 272:954–960, 1003–1010, 1965

FEIGIN RD, DODGE PR: Bacterial meningitis: Newer concepts of pathology and neurologic sequelae. Pediatr Clin North Am 23:541–556, 1976

GEISLER PJ, NELSON KE, LEVIN S, REDDI KT, MOSES VK: Community-acquired purulent meningitis: A review of 1,316 cases during the antibiotic era. 1954–1976. Rev Infect Dis 2:725–745, 1980

HARBIN L, HODGES GR: Corticosteroids as adjunctive therapy for acute bacterial meningitis. South Med J 72:977–981, 1979

HODGES GR, PERKINS RL: Hospital-associated bacterial meningitis. Am J Med Sci 271:335–341, 1976

KAPLAN SL, FEIGIN RD: Rapid identification of the invading microorganism. Pediatr Clin North Am 27:783–803, 1980

LANDESMAN SH, CORRADO ML, SHAH PM, ARMENGAUD M, BARZA M, CHERUBIN CC: Past and current roles for cephalosporin antibiotics in treatment of meningitis: Emphasis on use in gram-negative meningitis. Am J Med 71:693–703, 1981

MCCRACKEN GH, MIZE SG: A controlled study of intrathecal antibiotic therapy in gram-negative enteric meningitis of infancy. J Pediatr 89:66–72, 1976

MCCRACKEN GH, MIZE SG, THRELKELD N: Intraventricular gentamicin therapy in gram-negative bacillary meningitis of infancy. Lancet 1:787–793 April 12, 1980

MCGEHEE WG, RAPAPORT SI, HJORT PF: Intravascular coagulation in fulminant meningococcemia. Ann Intern Med 67:250–260, 1967

Meningococcal Disease Surveillance Group: Analysis of endemic meningococcal disease by serogroup and evaluation of chemoprophylaxis. J Infect Dis 134:201–204, 1976

OLSON DA, HOEPRICH PD, NOLAN SM, GOLDSTEIN E: Successful treatment of gram-negative bacillary meningitis with moxalactam. Ann Intern Med 95:302–305, 1981

SELL SHW, MERRILL RE, DAYNE EO, ZIMSKY EP JR: Long-term sequelae of Hemophilus influenzae meningitis. Pediatrics 49:206–211, 1972

Series of papers regarding infections of infants with Group B Streptococcus spp.: J Pediatr 89:183–204, 1976

SCHOEBAUM SC, GARDNER P, SHILLITO J: Infections of cerebrospinal fluid shunts: Epidemiology, clinical manifestations and therapy. J Infect Dis 132:543–552, 1975

SWARTZ MN, DODGE PR: Bacterial meningitis-A review of selected aspects. I. General clinical features, special problems and unusual meningeal reactions mimicking bacterial meningitis. N Engl J Med 272:725–731, 779–787, 842–848, 898–902, 1965

UNDERMAN AE, OVERTURF GD, LEEDOM JM: Bacterial meningitis: 1978. Disease-a-Month. Vol 24, February 1978, 63 pp.

PAUL D. HOEPRICH

Cryptococcosis

120

Cryptococcosis refers to infection of humans and other mammalians with *Cryptococcus* species. There are at least seven species in the genus *Cryptococcus,* but disease is virtually always caused by *C. neoformans* (yeastlike, anamorphic [asexual, imperfect], haploid fungi; of which *Filobasidiella neoformans* is the basidiomycetous, teleomorphic [sexual, perfect], diploid form); the rare forms of cryptococcal disease caused by either *albidus* or *laurentii* are not specifically discussed in this chapter. Apparently *Cryptococcus* spp. are saprobes, and mammalians are nonessential, dead-end hosts. Moreover, cryptococcosis is not contagious. The development of disease in humans may signal an aberration in host defenses. Central nervous system (CNS) involvement is the classic form of cryptococcal disease and is the localization most likely to cause death.

Etiology

Cryptococcus spp., as seen by microscopic examination of clinical specimens and as isolated in the clinical laboratory, are yeastlike, globous fungi (3.5 μm–7.0 μm × 3.7 μm–8.0 μm) that reproduce by forming 1 to 2 blastoconidia (buds) that are typically connected to the parent cell by a narrow pore (Fig. 120-1). However, they are not true yeasts but are related to the rust and smut fungal pathogens of higher plants, a kinship discovered through the observation of sexual reproduction by conjugation and formation of basidiospores—the teleomorph of the fungus.

Encapsulation of *C. neoformans* varies in extent with the strain and the milieu of growth. It is minimal, if evident, when they are saprobic, minimal to large in various laboratory culture mediums, and invariably evident when they are parasitic in tissues (Fig. 120-1).

Because capability for capsulation appears to be the prime determinant of virulence, experimental infection of mice is useful in the laboratory diagnosis of *C. neoformans.* Two mice are inoculated by intracerebral injection of a cryptococcal isolate. Whether swelling of the head is apparent or not, one mouse is sacrificed for examination 1 week after injection; the second is sacrificed 2 to 3 weeks later if examination of the first was inconclusive. Smears of brain tissues are stained with lactophenol cotton blue or nigrosin (Chap. 9, Microscopic Examinations); the finding of encapsulated budding yeast forms (Fig. 120-1*B* is diagnostic of *C. neoformans,* because the other species of *Cryptococcus* are not pathogenic for mice.

Colonial morphology varies according to capsulation: the white to tan colonies are mucoid and glistening if composed of encapsulated cryptococci, dry and dull if made up of noncapsulated forms. Although cryptococci grow on corn meal agar, pseudohyphae are rarely formed.

Sugars are not fermented, but carbon is assimilated from glucose, galactose, sucrose, maltose, inositol, dulcitol, and inulin, but not from lactose. Some dicarboxylic acids are utilized by serotypes B and C, but not by serotypes A and D (Table 120-1). Nitrogen is not obtained from nitrates, but is assimilated from several amino acids and from urea and creatinine. *Cryptococcus neoformans* are urease positive and possess phenol oxidases. These latter enzymes oxidize certain phenols, yielding melanin or polymers of melaninlike pigments. Thus, a culture medium containing inositol (a source of carbon), urea (a source of nitrogen), caffeic acid and ferric citrate (formation of pigment), and gentamicin (suppression of bacteria) favors both the selective growth and the detection of *Cryptococcus* spp. in contaminated specimens.

The capsules are polysaccharides—polymers of xylose, mannose, and glucuronic acid, which are free of nitrogen and sulfur. They are antigenic, and four serotypes (A–D) are recognized that do not differ appre-

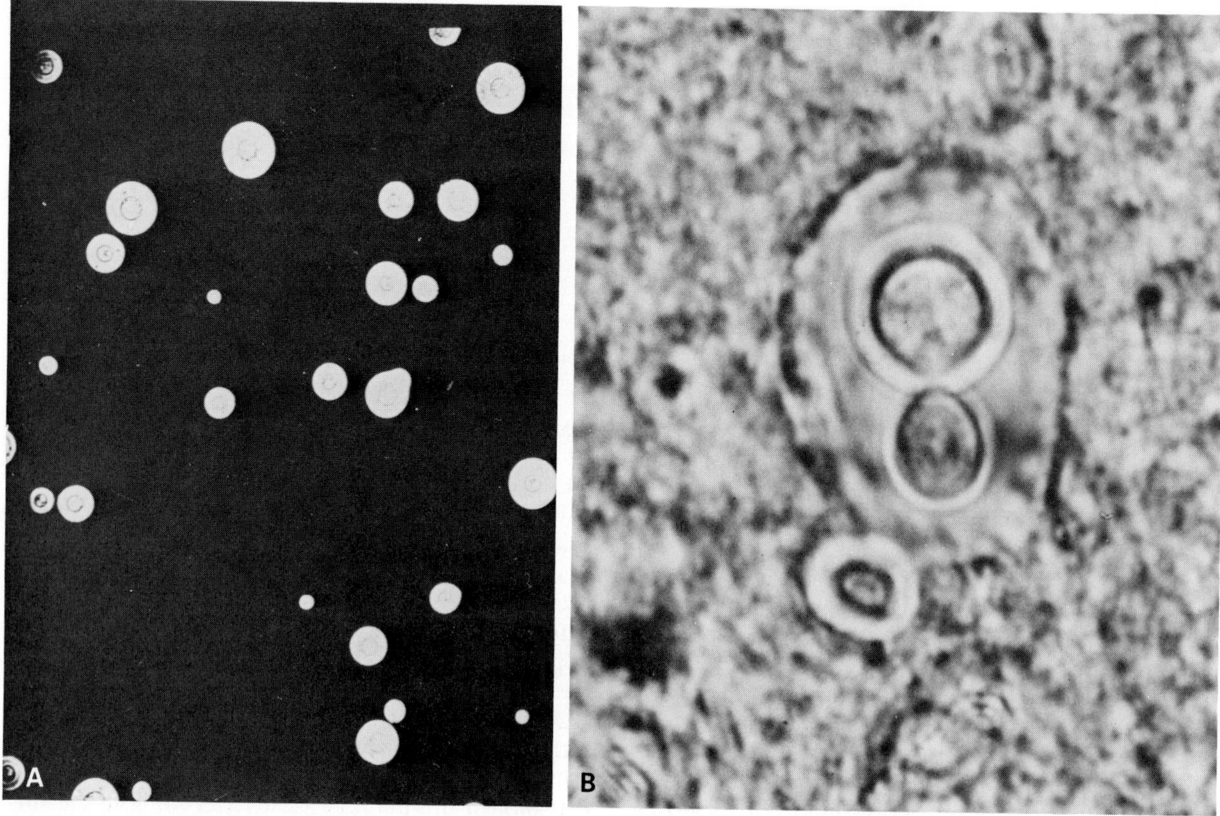

Fig. 120-1. *Cryptococcus neoformans.* (*A*) India ink preparation of sediment from cerebrospinal fluid of a patient with cryptococcal meningoencephalitis. Note the thin pore connecting daughter to parent cell in the right lower field. (Original magnification approximately × 500) (*B*) Crush preparation of brain of a mouse inoculated by intracerebral injection 5 days earlier. (Lactophenol cotton blue, original magnification approximately × 1000)

ciably in virulence, but do correlate with other properties that enable presumptive separation of types A and D from types B and C (Table 120-1). Indeed, a glycine(sole carbon source)-cycloheximide or canavanine (serogroups B and C are relatively resistant) culture medium appears to be useful for this purpose. Moreover, in humans, disease caused by types B and C may be less amenable to conventional therapy than that caused by types A and D.

Special stains are necessary to enable recognition of *C. neoformans* in fixed tissues (Chap. 9, Microscopic Examinations). Mayer's mucicarmine stain is particularly helpful, since the capsules are colored a deep rose red, and neither *Blastomyces dermatididis* nor *Histoplasma capsulatum* takes up this stain. The Masson–Fontana stain is virtually specific through reaction with melaninlike compounds to reveal dark brown–black cryptococci against a pink background. The periodic acid–Schiff (PAS) and methanamine silver stains are less specific. Cryptococci often appear to be haloed in tissue sections; the capsule shrinks as an artifact of fixation.

Epidemiology

Although serologic typing is not routinely carried out, it appears that type A is global in distribution, and it is the most common serotype in the United States and elsewhere. Types B and C are generally uncommon as causes of cryptococcosis but are frequently isolated in southern California and have been isolated from patients in southeastern Oklahoma. Cryptococcosis caused by type D is not common in the United States, but is frequently the cause of cryptococcosis in Europe.

The association of types A and D *C. neoformans* with avian feces is worldwide and has received the

Table 120-1. *Some Characteristics of* Cryptococcus neoformans.*

	Serotypes A and D	Serotypes B and C
Distribution	A—global D—uncommon in the United States, common in Europe	Both rare, except in southern California and southeastern Oklahoma
Reservoir	Bird feces, especially pigeon	Unknown
Dicarboxylic acids	Not assimilated	*l*-malic, fumaric, and succinic utilized
Relative resistance to		
cycloheximide	Susceptible	Resistant
canavanine	Susceptible	Resistant

*Although *C. neoformans* constitutes a valid species, the relationship between serotypes and properties has led to the proposal to designate varieties: *C. neoformans* var. *neoformans* (serotypes A and D); *C. neoformans* var. *gattii* (serotypes B and C).

most careful study and the greatest notoriety with regard to pigeon droppings (although *C. neoformans* is also known to be present in feces from other avians: parakeets, budgerigars, canaries). The cryptococci may be isolated from the contents of the gut of the pigeon and from freshly passed feces, though the pigeon is not apparently ill. In the feces, replication occurs to densities as great as 5×10^7 per g; the cryptococci remain viable for as long as 2 years (drying and exposure to sunlight are inimical). Because they are the predominant fungus in pigeon feces (a few *Geotrichum* spp., *Candida* spp., and *Rhodotorula* spp. may also be present), it has been suggested that the high concentrations of creatinine favor cryptococcal outgrowth. However, pigeon feces are an alkaline, hyperosmolar environment rich in many nitrogen-containing compounds in addition to creatinine. In the laboratory, creatinine is neither markedly nor uniformly stimulatory to growth, although it is utilized more rapidly by types B, C, and D than by type A. Possibly, few other microorganisms find pigeon feces as hospitable, and *C. neoformans* of serotypes A and D may be unable to compete as successfully in other environments (*e.g., C. neoformans* disappears when pigeon feces are mixed with soil, although a stable soil-dwelling status has been described). It appears that *C. neoformans* in pigeon feces occupies an ecologic niche, just as *H. capsulatum* does in starling feces; the niche of serotypes B and C cryptococci has yet to be discovered.

Infections of human and nonhuman mammalians are thought to occur primarily through the inhalation of particles containing live *C. neoformans;* that is, the vector appears to be air currents. There is no proof of this reasonable construction, and even circumstantial evidence is lacking: there is no clustering of cases: a history of known exposure to pigeon feces is rarely obtained; typically, there is no history of a respiratory affliction (with or without pulmonary abnormalities in chest films). The fungus is not an airborne contaminant in clinical laboratories. Although *C. neoformans* has not been recovered from the feces of normal humans, it is found, though rarely, in the interdigital spaces. There is no evidence that human-to-human, or nonhuman animal-to-human transmission of cryptococci occurs.

The frequency of occurrence of cryptococcosis is not known. Rough estimates place meningitis at 200 to 300 cases per year in the United States; about 15,000 cases of subclinical pulmonary cryptococcosis per year are thought to occur in New York City alone. Save infrequency before puberty, there is no relation to age (although most patients are 30–60 years old) or to occupation; whites appear to be infected more often than blacks. Cryptococcosis occurs more often in males than in females (by a ratio of 3:1). Persons with noninfectious diseases that in some way compromise host defenses are predisposed to cryptococcosis. Thus, patients who have malignant neoplasms (particularly of the lymphoreticular system); collagen–vascular diseases (particularly disseminated lupus erythematosus); sarcoidosis; and diabetes mellitus (perhaps also chronic alcoholics and pregnant women)—whether they are under treatment with glucosteroids or not—are at increased risk of developing cryptococcosis. However, a majority of patients with cryptococcosis have no detectable underlying disease.

Pathogenesis and Pathology

When aerosols containing cryptococci are inhaled, it is assumed that the infected particles are engulfed by pulmonary alveolar macrophages. In normal persons, the cryptococci either fail to survive intracellularly or are quickly contained so that either no disease or mild, subclinical illness occurs. Proliferation leading to disease is favored by infection with a capsulated strain, an infecting dose so large that normal cellular defenses are overwhelmed, and the presence of an underlying disease that has crippled host defenses. Spread to extrapulmonary organs may result, with the CNS a preferred target. The course tends to be chronic, particularly in otherwise normal patients, but it may be acute in compromised patients.

The growing cryptococci do not elaborate toxins or engender hypersensitivity. They appear to cause disease by compression of surrounding structures as an infected focus enlarges. Because the lungs are readily compressible, pulmonary infection with *Cryptococcus* spp. is not often clinically manifest, even when lesions are radiographically evident.

Early pulmonary lesions are gelatinous, mucinous nodules composed of encapsulated, budding cryptococci. There is little inflammatory response—a few macrophages, lymphocytes, plasma cells, and occasional giant cells.

If lesions persist, they may become firm and rubbery, resembling granulomas. On histologic examination, cryptococci are less abundant in such lesions and are primarily intracellular. The cellular response is little changed in kind, but may be increased. Some fibroblasts are present, but there is no fibrous encapsulation of lesions. Only rarely does caseation, cavitation, or calcification occur.

If the cryptococci are not successfully restrained in the pulmonary parenchyma, they will pass to the hilar nodes. Again, there is minimal response—typically, there is no hilar node enlargement in the presence of roentgenographically demonstrable parenchymal disease. If cryptococci become blood-borne, they may lodge in any organ or tissue where they may give rise to lesions, which may evolve after the fashion of the predecessor pulmonary lesions.

Central Nervous System

CNS involvement is at once the most commonly diagnosed and the most often lethal form of extrapulmonary cryptococcosis. There is no satisfactory explanation for the apparent predilection of *Cryptococcus* spp. for the CNS. In about half of the patients with CNS cryptococcosis, there is a detectable impairment of host defense mechanisms.

Deep, space-occupying lesions are most likely to form in the grey matter around the ventricles and aqueduct and in the basal ganglia, cerebral white matter, and cerebellar dentate nucleus. Presumably, infection of the meninges leads to seeding of the cerebrospinal fluid (CSF) and spread throughout the subarachnoid space. A greyish, mucinous exudate accumulates most often at the base of the brain and over the cerebellum; leptomeningitis is most pronounced in the same areas, and the adjacent convolutions may be flattened. In most patients, there are lesions both in the brain and the meninges—meningoencephalitis.

Integumentary

If *C. neoformans* lodges in the skin or mucous membranes, it may survive, grow, and accrete to form nodules. Necrosis of the overlying epithelium may lead to ulceration. There is little inflammatory response.

Skeletal

Destruction of bone results as clusters of fungi enlarge. There is not reactive osteogenesis.

Manifestations

The course of cryptococcosis is typically indolent and protracted with symptoms waxing and waning for weeks or months before the diagnosis is made. The patient may feel unwell, lose some weight, and have no other symptoms. There may be no fever, or low-grade fever no higher than 39°C (102°F). In previously normal persons, a subclinical, mild course is usual; the severity of the disease is probably more a function of the infecting dose than the intrinsic virulence of the *C. neoformans.* In the compromised host, the course may be either acute or chronic, and spread to the CNS and other organs is said to occur in at least half such patients.

Pulmonary

Although pulmonary cryptococcosis is probably the most common form of the disease, it is diagnosed less often than meningoencephalitis because it is usually transient and not severe. If there is cough, the production of sputum is minimal (hemoptysis is rare). Mild pleuritic pain may occur; intrapleural effusion is rare.

CENTRAL NERVOUS SYSTEM

The manifestations of cryptococcosis of the brain or spinal cord are those of a slowly growing, space-occupying lesion; about one-fourth of patients are subjected to a neurosurgical procedure before the diagnosis is known.

Cryptococcal meningitis is archetypal of chronic meningitis, for it is insidious in onset and slowly progressive. Although 10% to 15% of patients have no symptoms referable to the CNS, most patients have a mingling of the manifestations of encephalitis and meningitis. Headache is the most common feature, occurring in more than 75% of patients; initially episodic, it becomes more frequent and more severe as the disease progresses and may be frontal, temporal, or retroorbital in distribution. In more than 50% of patients, the gamut of mental aberrations (from simple irritability to psychosis and lethargy to coma); motor abnormalities (from altered reflexes to paralyses), cranial nerve dysfunctions (aphasia, visual disturbances, hearing loss); cerebellar signs; and evidences of increased intracranial pressure are found. Fever is present in at least one-third of patients. Meningismus is not prominent, but is detectable in about half of the patients.

Integumentary

Although integumentary lesions are also secondary to blood-borne dissemination of *Cryptococcus* spp., they may be the first evidence of cryptococcosis. Because they are not painful and cause neither lymphangitis nor lymphadenitis, they are often ignored by the patient. The skin is involved in 10% to 15% of patients. Lesions occur most often on the face and scalp as erythematous papules, acneiform pustules, or abscesses that sometimes break down to form ulcers (not indurated, but often with thickened, slightly undermined edges). Mucosal lesions are detected in fewer than 5% of patients as nodules or ulcers.

Skeletal

In 5% to 10% of patients, discrete, slowly destructive osseous lesions occur, favoring prominences of long bones, cranial bones, and vertebrae. Joints are only rarely involved.

Other

Quite uncommonly, cryptococcosis is manifested as prostatitis, orchitis, endocarditis, pericarditis, nephritis (abscess), and hepatitis. The adrenals, spleen, and lymph nodes are spared.

Diagnosis

Because the manifestations of cryptococcosis are nonspecific, the diagnosis is often backed into after neoplastic diseases, tuberculosis, and other fungal infections have been excluded. Recognition of a state of vulnerability because of an underlying, noninfectious disease and diligent inquiry about possible exposure to avian (particularly pigeon) feces may be rewarding.

Routine laboratory studies of blood and urine are characteristically normal. Even in extensive infections, the blood leukocyte count, hematocrit, and sedimentation rate remain normal.

The isolation of *C. neoformans* from clinical specimens remains the single best diagnostic tool. Whenever possible, specimens should be concentrated by centrifugation (CSF, urine). Culture mediums must not contain cycloheximide (Actidione), because this antimicrobic is inhibitory to many strains of cryptococci. With contaminated specimens (expectorated sputum, sinus drainage, urine), it is important to inoculate a selective culture medium. Aerobic incubation at 37°C should be continued for 4 to 6 weeks before cultures are discarded as negative. Communication between clinicians and laboratory personnel is essential to optimal culture. The major identifying criteria include demonstration of assimilation of inositol, urease and phenol oxidase activities, lack of pseudomycelia when grown on corn meal agar, growth at 37°C, and pathogenicity for mice.

The most useful serodiagnostic modality seeks to identify cryptococcal antigens rather than antibodies, because the host is often not immunocompetent. Moreover, an antibody response may be masked if antibodies react with antigen as quickly as they are formed. Of presently available tests, latex agglutination (latex particles coated with anticapsular polysaccharide antibody) is the most valuable. Antigen can be detected and titrated by serial dilution using CSF, serum, and urine.

Pulmonary

Cultures of expectorated sputum, bronchial washings, or transtracheal aspirates may sometimes yield *Cryptococcus* spp. In all patients seriously suspected of having, or proven to have, pulmonary cryptococcosis, the CSF, bone marrow, urine, and expressed prostatic secretions should also be cultured for cryptococci.

Roentgenographic findings are variable, but multiple centers of relatively dense infiltration (2 cm–7 cm in diameter) in the lower lobes are most common. Diffuse infiltration, peribronchial infiltrates, and even miliary lesions sometimes occur. Hilar adenopathy is uncommon. Coin lesions, cavitation, pulmonary collapse, pulmonary effusions, fibrosis, and calcification are rare. Thin-walled cavities, held to be classic for fungal pneumonias, do not occur in pulmonary cryptococcosis.

A major diagnostic problem is separation of malignancy, either primary or metastatic to the lung, from pulmonary cryptococcosis. Examination of tissue obtained by open pulmonary biopsy is most likely to be definitive; a portion of such a specimen must be cultured. Expectorated sputum from patients with pulmonary malignancies or nonmalignant but chronic pulmonary diseases (including tuberculosis) may yield *Cryptococcus* spp. when there is no clinical evidence of cryptococcosis. If such isolates are capsulated, or encapsulate after intracerebral inoculation in mice, it should not be assumed that they simply betoken endobronchial colonization. Rather, cultures should be obtained from the common sites of extrapulmonary cryptococcosis, and cryptococcal antigen should be sought in the CSF, serum, and urine.

Central Nervous System

In about 90% of patients with symptomatic cryptococcal meningoencephalitis, the CSF is under increased pressure, the protein is elevated in concentration, and there are 40 to 400 leukocytes per mm^3 (mononuclear cells predominate). The concentration of glucose in the CSF is decreased (*i.e.,* less than 45% of the simultaneously obtained blood sugar) in at least half of the patients. However, the CSF may be entirely normal (except for the growth of *C. neoformans* in cultures) in patients with asymptomatic CNS cryptococcosis, a localization that is discovered when the CSF is examined as a routine measure in patients who have cryptococcosis of other organs.

Cryptococcus spp. are found by microscopic examination of India ink or nigrosin preparations of the CSF in at least 50% of patients with CNS cryptococcosis. The sensitivity of this simple test is increased by centrifuging at least 5 ml of CSF before mixing a drop of the sediment on a microscope slide with an equal volume of nigrosin reagent, which is preferable to India ink (see Chap. 9, Microscopic Examinations). After a coverslip has been set in place, newsprint should barely be visible through the preparation. Although the typical cryptococci are easy to identify (Fig. 120-1*A*), artifacts such as other microorganisms, agglutinated carbon particles, and leukocytes or tumor cells (which are less troublesome with nigrosin reagent) may be confused with cryptococci. Confirmation by culture is obligatory.

Arteriography and pneumoencephalography may demonstrate symmetric dilation of the cerebral ventricles. However, computed tomography (CT) is a superior method of study. Not only is it very helpful in evaluating ventricular dilation, but also it may allow detection of focal, intracerebral collections of cryptococci often missed by electroencephalography or radioisotope brain scanning. The injection of radioisotopic material into the lumbar CSF may show impaired transit of the isotope over the cerebral convexities, with or without retrograde filling and stasis within the lateral cerebral ventricles—so-called low-pressure hydrocephalus.

Success in isolation of *C. neoformans* is favored by (1) culturing the sediment from 5 ml to 10 ml of CSF collected on 3 to 5 different occasions and (2) culturing sediment from CSF collected from the cisternal subarachnoid space, rather than either the lumbar space or the cerebral ventricles. Urine and sputum (as well as bone marrow and expressed prostatic secretions) should also be cultured from patients without evident abnormalities of the urinary or respiratory tracts. Blood cultures are positive for *Cryptococcus* spp. only in the most extensively infected patients.

About 90% of patients with cryptococcal meningoencephalitis have antigen detectable in their serum or CSF. The titer reflects the severity of the infection. Although confirmation by culture is desirable, there are circumstances in which therapy should be undertaken without the isolation of *C. neoformans,* for example, an antigen titer (latex agglutination) in the CSF ≥ 1:8 in a vulnerable patient in whom there is lack of support for other diagnostic possibilities.

The several serologic tests for anticryptococcal antibody are less valuable than tests for cryptococcal antigen. Not only are there false-positive reactions, but also many patients (roughly half—those with predisposing, defense-crippling, underlying, noninfectious diseases) are unable to mount a detectable humoral antibody response because of inadequate production or reaction with antigen. There is no skin test of proved usefulness.

The several causes for nonbacterial meningoencephalitis must be considered in patients who may have CNS cryptococcosis. Epidemiologic and clinical considerations are helpful, but the results of cultures and serologic tests are more likely to be definitive. CNS malignancies may be difficult to differentiate, and craniotomy may be necessary—for example, a patient with headache, papilledema, abnormal CSF, and no localizing signs by neurologic examination. Uncommonly, either a brain tumor or intracerebral cyptococcosis gives rise to such a picture, but only the latter process is associated with cryptococcal antigen in the CSF and serum.

Integumentary

Because the clinical manifestations of cryptococcosis of the skin and mucous membranes are not unique, biopsy should be undertaken whenever the nature of skin lesions is in doubt. Histologic diagnosis should be confirmed by isolation of *Cryptococcus* spp. from cultures of a portion of the specimen.

Skeletal

As seen in roentgenographic examination, the lesions of osseous cryptococcosis are round and lytic, and they are not associated with marginal sclerosis. Because such a picture could result from other causes (tuberculosis, certain neoplasms), biopsy with culture and assay of serum for cryptococcal antigen should be carried out.

Prognosis

Pulmonary cryptococcosis usually heals slowly without antifungal therapy, leaving a residual fibrosis in some patients.

Extrapulmonary cryptococcosis is typically chronic with alternation of remissions and exacerbations for periods as long as 16 to 20 years. Integumentary lesions may resolve spontaneously.

Although long-term survival (≥ 3 years) has been documented in several patients with CNS cryptococcosis who did not receive antifungal antimicrobics, the untreated disease is almost always lethal within 3 years of diagnosis (80%–90% within 1 year, 70% within 3 months). Death may result from brain-stem compression from cerebral edema, with or without hydrocephalus. Coma, or the complications of coma, may be lethal. Sequelae include optic atrophy, deafness, ataxia, obstructive (low-pressure) hydrocephalus, chronic brain syndrome, and personality changes. Irritability, nervousness, and lethargy may persist for years.

Although relapse is common in cryptococcosis with or without antifungal therapy, there is no proof of exogenous reinfection. Yet, it is not possible to assert that there is protective immunity in survivors.

Therapy

Amphotericin B given by intravenous injection as described in Chapter 39, Candidosis, is the treatment of choice. *Cryptococcus* spp. are quite susceptible (Table 120-2), and native resistance to amphotericin B apparently does not occur among clinical isolates of *C. neoformans.* Total doses of 30 to 45 mg/kg body wt (2 g–3 g) are usual, but in some patients, as when relapse requires retreatment, larger doses have been given in an effort to control the disease.

Pulmonary cryptococcosis need not be treated in immunocompetent patients if (1) there are no extrapulmonary lesions; (2) cultures of the CSF, bone marrow, urine, and expressed prostatic secretions are negative; (3) cryptococcal antigen cannot be detected in the CSF, and the titer in the serum is lacking or low, or stable or falling; and (4) the pulmonary lesion(s) are small, few, regressing, or stable. Observation every 2 to 3 months for at least 1 year is acceptable management of these patients.

Treatment is necessary in immunocompetent patients with pulmonary cryptococcosis complicated by extrapulmonary lesions. Immunosuppressed patients with pulmonary cryptococcosis should be treated even if no extrapulmonary lesions are found.

CNS cryptococcosis requires treatment with amphotericin B injected IV as described in Chapter 30, Candidosis, to a total dose of 30 to 45 mg/kg body wt (2 g–3 g). The presence of intracerebral mass lesions is not a clear-cut indication for an alternative therapy. Although a favorable response is obtained in about 75% of patients, cure may be claimed in about 60%. Moreover, a significant toll in morbidity is exacted by this therapy, both temporarily and permanently—most often as irreversible nephropathy. Failures of response and relapses are not unexpected in view of the virtually complete exclusion of amphotericin B from the CSF after IV injection. Accordingly, amphotericin B has been injected directly into the subarachnoid space, with or without concurrent IV administration; the value of such topical therapy in cryptococcal meningoencephalitis is not proved. Intrathecal injection of amphotericin B is generally reserved for patients whose meningoencephalitis remains active despite the IV administration of

Table 120-2. *Peak Concentrations in the Serum of Humans, and Geometric Mean Minimal Inhibitory Concentrations (MICs) for* Cryptococcus *spp. of Four Systemically Administrable Antifungal Antimicrobics**

Antimicrobic	Geometric Mean MICs (μg/ml)	Peak Concentrations in Serum (μg/ml @ minutes after dose)
Amphotericin B	0.9	2.5 @ 5
Flucytosine	111†	100 @ 60–90
Miconazole	0.4	5.5 @ 5
Ketoconazole	0.5	3.5 @ 120

*See also Chap. 18, Antimicrobics and Anthelmintics for Systemic Therapy.

†Since some strains are natively highly resistant, the geometric mean MIC is quite high; susceptible strains are inhibited by ≤ 25μg/ml.

amphotericin B and for patients with severely reduced renal function. In experienced hands, intracisternal injection appears to be the route of choice, for the drug is delivered directly to the site of most intense meningitis; however, loss of hearing and arachnoiditis may develop. Intraventricular injection by means of a subcutaneous reservoir-catheter offers ease of injection but carries a definite morbidity during insertion and use: the catheter connecting the reservoir to the ventricle may be malpositioned, or it may become clogged, or infected—usually with *Staphylococcus epidermidis,* but even with the causative *Cryptococcus* spp. The morbidity associated with lumbar intrathecal injection is probably even higher, but use of a hyperbaric vehicle for the amphotericin B (*e.g.,* 10% glucose solution) with Trendelenberg's positioning may (1) minimize exposure of the lumbar CNS to high concentrations of amphotericin B and thus minimize arachnoiditis; (2) lower the concentration of the drug leaking extradurally and so diminish radiculitis. Regardless of route, the dose of amphotericin B is increased slowly from 0.05 mg per injection to a maintenance dose of 0.5 mg on a biweekly schedule (Chap. 41, Coccidioidomycosis).

Because of the several shortcomings of amphotericin B and the advent of other antifungal antimicrobics, alternative therapies have been explored. Flucytosine (5-fluorocytosine) is an orally administrable antimicrobic that readily penetrates into all body water, including that of the CNS and CSF. The majority of pretreatment isolates are susceptible to $\leq$ 25 μg/ml by testing *in vitro,* but native resistance does occur (Table 120-2). The response of cryptococcal meningitis to flucytosine used by itself is essentially the same as that of amphotericin B alone, namely, about two-thirds of patients are cured, albeit without permanent damage from the drug. At least three factors contribute to failures: (1) inadequate dosage—both in terms of daily dose and duration of treatment—particularly as was done in early trials of the drug; (2) failure of recognition of native resistance prior to commencing therapy (testing the susceptibility of isolates *in vitro* before treatment is essential); and (3) the development of resistance during therapy. A proper regimen will yield peak concentrations (1 hour after a peroral dose) of 80 to 100 μg/ml of serum. If renal function is normal, 200 mg/kg body wt/day, as four equal portions, 6-hourly, is usually adequate; if there is renal failure, the dose should be decreased in direct proportion to the diminution of the creatinine clearance (confirmation of the dose by measurement of the concentration in the serum is desirable). Treatment should be continued for 6 to 12 months. Occasionally, profound leukopenia or thrombocytopenia have been attributed to flucytosine, usually in patients simultaneously treated with antineoplastic agents, irradiation, and other antimicrobics including amphotericin B, or in patients with renal dysfunction. Hepatotoxic reactions (primarily increases in the transaminases in the serum) have been less frequent and have resolved completely on withdrawal of the drug.

Combined therapy for 6 weeks, consisting of amophotericin B (0.3 mg/kg body wt/day, IV) and flucytosine (150 mg/kg body wt/day, perorally as four equal portions, 6 hourly), was suggested in the hope that the combination would act additively or synergistically, and might shorten the duration of treatment. The low dose of amphotericin B should be less toxic than conventional doses, but by itself it would be ineffective—that is, it would exert virtually no antifungal activity in the CSF or the CNS. In contrast, the dose of flucytosine recommended for combined therapy has, by itself, cured patients of cryptococcal meningitis. Combination therapy, as described above, appears to be at least as successful as single-agent therapy. Because this success is highly dependent on the action of the flucytosine component of the combination, failures will occur in patients infected with strains of *C. neoformans* that are relatively resistant. Moreover, it is possible that the amphotericin B component of the combination augments the concentration of flucytosine in the body by impairing renal excretory capacity. The relatively high frequency of occurrence of adverse reactions attributable to 5-fluorouracil (arising from oxidative deamination of 5-fluorocytosine by intestinal bacteria) supports this construction.

Two imidazole derivatives that have antifungal activity have been considered for the treatment of cryptococcal meningoencephalitis:

1. Miconazole is a fungistatic, water-insoluble imidazole derivative that is inhibitory *in vitro* to *Cryptococcus* spp. at concentrations well below those attainable in the serum of patients by IV injection of an aqueous suspension of the drug. Although miconazole is neither nephrotoxic nor dependent on the kidneys for excretion, it is eliminated by hepatic catabolism and penetrates into the CSF scarcely at all. Adverse reactions include pruritus, skin rash, nausea, vomiting, anemia, thrombocythemia, hyponatremia, and hyperlipidemia. It is difficult to discern a place for miconazole in the treatment of cryptococcosis.
2. Ketoconazole, a relatively water-soluble imidazole derivative, is sufficiently well absorbed from

the gut to permit peroral therapy. It is also fungistatic, again at concentrations much lower than those attained in the serum of patients under treatment. Nonnephrotoxic, ketoconazole is also eliminated by hepatic catabolism. Concentrations in the CSF are 15% to 20% of contemporaneous specimens of serum. Adverse reactions include nausea, vomiting, skin rash, gynecomastia, and hepatitis. Experience is too limited to permit assessment of the usefulness of ketoconazole in the treatment of cryptococcosis; however, the lack of fungicidal capability may prove to be a serious limitation.

Whatever regimen of antifungal drug therapy is used, surveillance is an essential part of treatment. While antimicrobics are given, the CSF should be examined at least weekly by culture, microscopy (nigrosin and cell count with differential), and determination of the concentrations of glucose and protein. Cultures should become sterile promptly although forms consistent in appearance with *Cryptococcus* spp. may still be observed in India ink preparations. Diminution in the number of leukocytes, fall in the concentration of protein, and rise in the concentration of glucose are usual changes with successful therapy. More meaningful is a fall in the CSF (and serum) antigen—the titers should decrease at least two twofold dilutions during therapy. As changes in titer do not occur rapidly, assays need not be performed more often than every 3 to 4 weeks. With successful therapy, the CSF will become entirely normal within 3 months of termination of treatment. Surveillance by examination of the patient and the CSF at 2 to 3-month intervals is necessary for at least 1 year following therapy.

Prevention

Possibly, recognition of the urban pigeon as a hazard to public health would be preventive.

Remaining Problems

The use of selective culture mediums and routine speciation with serotyping of clinical isolates of *C. neoformans* should aid in elucidating the epidemiology of cryptococcosis.

Refinement of diagnostic capabilities is needed. Exploitation of rapid methods such as counter immunoelectrophoresis and application of gas—liquid chromatography are but two examples.

There is need for a fungicidal antimicrobic that enters the CNS/CSF freely after oral administration.

Bibliography

Books

FETTER BF, KLINTWORTH GK, HENDRY WS: Mycoses of the Central Nervous System. Baltimore, Williams & Wilkins, 1967. 214 pp.

MCGINNIS MR: Laboratory Handbook of Medical Mycology. New York, Academic Press, 1980. 661 pp.

RIPPON JW (ED.): Cryptococcosis and other yeast infections. In Medical Mycology. The Pathogenic Fungi and The Pathogenic Actinomycetes. Philadelphia, WB Saunders, 1974. pp 205–223.

Journals

BENNETT JE, DISMUKES WE, DUMA RJ, MEDOFF G, SANDE MA, GALLIS H, LEONARD J, FIELDS BT, BRADSHAW M, HAYWOOD H, MCGEE ZA, CATE TR, COBBS CJ, WARNER JF, ALLING DW: A comparison of amphotericin B alone and combined with flucytosine in the treatment of cryptococcal meningitis. N Engl J Med 301:126–131, 1979

BENNETT JE, KWON—CHUNG KF, HOWARD DH: Epidemiologic differences among serotypes of *Cryptococcus neoformans.* Am J Epidem 105:582–586, 1977

BUTLER WT, ALLING DW, SPICKARD A, UTZ JP: Diagnostic and prognostic value of clinical and laboratory findings in cryptococcal meningitis. N Engl J Med 270:59–67, 1964

CAMPBELL CC: (Philosophical) review of air currents as a continuing vector. Ann NY Acad Sci 353:123–139, 1980

CAMPBELL GD, CURRIER RD, BUSEY JF: Survival in untreated cryptococcal meningitis. Neurology 31:1154–1157, 1981

FUJITA NK, REYNARD M, SPAICO FL, GUZE LB, EDWARDS JE JR: Cryptococcal intracerebral mass lesions. Ann Intern Med 94:382–388, 1981

HEALY ME, DILLAVOU CL, TAYLOR GE: Diagnostic medium containing inositol, urea, and caffeic acid for selective growth of *Cryptococcus neoformans.* J Clin Microbiol 6:387–391, 1977

HORN JR, GIUSTI DL: The pharmacokinetics of flucytosine in cryptococcal meningitis. Drug Intelligence Clin Pharm 9:180–188, 1975

KWON—CHUNG KJ, BENNETT JE, THEODORE TS: *Cryptococcus bacillisporus* sp. nov.: Serotype B-C of *Cryptococcus neoformans.* Int J System Bacteriol 28: 616–620, 1978

KWON—CHUNG KJ: A new genus, Filobasidiella, the perfect state of Cryptococcus neoformans. Mycologia 67:1197–1200, 1975

UTZ JP, GARRIGUES IL, SANDE MA, WARNER JF, MANDELL GL, MCGEHEE RF, DUMA RJ, SHADOMY S: Therapy of cryptococcosis with a combination of flucytosine and amphotericin B. J. Infect Dis 132:368–373, 1975

YOSHIKAWA TT, FUJITA N, GRINNELL V, EDWARDS JE JR, FELDMAN RA: Management of central nervous system cryptococcosis: Teaching Conference, Harbor–UCLA Medical Center, Torrance, and VA Wadsworth Medical Center, Los Angeles (Specialty Conference). West J Med 132:123–133, 1980

Section XVI

Infections Involving Neural Tissue

Indigenous Microbiota of the Nervous System

(None)

VINCENT A. FULGINITI

121

Poliomyelitis

Infection by one of the polioviruses may result in asymptomatic infection, a mild febrile illness, aseptic meningitis without paralysis, or paralytic disease involving various levels of the central nervous system. In the United States and other countries that have used active immunization, natural poliomyelitis has been reduced to negligible occurrences. Natural infection has been supplanted by very rare paralytic disease occurring typically in recipients or contacts of recipients of live, attenuated poliovirus vaccine.

Etiology

The three serologically distinct groups of polioviruses have characteristics in common that place them into the Picornaviridae family (Chap. 1, Attributes of Infectious Agents). They are small (28 nm in diameter), ether-insensitive, RNA-containing viruses. The RNA is single-stranded. The viruses have cubic symmetry with a nonenveloped capsid composed of repeating protein subunits.

In nature, polioviruses are restricted to humans. Certain simian species can be infected in the laboratory. The viruses have been adapted *in vitro* to a variety of cell culture systems. They replicate in the cell cytoplasm following specific receptor-linked attachment and penetration. Human cell receptors appear to be genetically determined and the genes are located on chromosome 19.

The three serotypes of polioviruses are labeled types 1, 2, and 3. The complement-fixing antigen of each type is cross-reactive, whereas the type-specific antigens determine the specificity of precipitating and neutralizing antibody. Repeated exposures probably lead to heterotypic responses of low level, but primary contact evokes type-specific antibodies.

Two type-specific antigens have been isolated: the N (native) antigens and the H (heated) antigens. Native antigens represent whole, intact virions containing RNA. H antigen is derived from RNA-empty capsids. H antigen evokes primary antibody responses in the human followed by an N antigen response; anti-H antibody declines rapidly and the ultimate antibody response is purely anti-N.

Several markers have been used to differentiate wild (natural) poliovirus types from attenuated (vaccine) types. Tests to detect markers are difficult to perform and interpret and may result in indeterminate status for any given isolate. On the other hand, some isolates can be identified as vaccinelike and others as wildlike.

Epidemiology

Polioviruses occurred worldwide in ubiquitous fashion prior to the introduction of vaccines. In countries that have used either killed or live vaccine in widescale and consistent fashion, the circulation of wild polioviruses has diminished or disappeared; concomitantly, paralytic poliomyelitis has become a rare disease. In contrast, where poliovaccines have been little used or sporadically administered, wild polioviruses and clinical poliomyelitis still occur.

Most poliovirus infections are transmitted from human to human by direct or indirect fecal-oral spread. In tropical countries, the disease occurs throughout the year; in temperate zones, it appears most frequently in the summer and fall. Sources of infection other than human excreta and secretions are uncertain. Certain species of flies may be virus-positive in heavily infected areas, and sewage and water supplies have yielded polioviruses in the same regions.

Poor personal hygiene, inadequate disposal of human fecal wastes, poor sewage management, and opportunities for cross-contamination of water supplies and food are reflected in wide dissemination of wild virus and maintenance of poliomyelitis in the

Table 121-1. *Paralytic Poliomyelitis in the United States, 1969–1979*

Description	Reported Cases and % of Total		
Vaccine-associated*	74 (40%)		
Recipients of live, attentuated vaccine perorally (OPV)		43	
Contacts of vaccinees		31	
Household contacts			25
Nonhousehold contacts			6
Epidemic cases (1970, 1972, 1979)	43 (23%)		
Other (sporadic, imported, unknown)	70 (37%)		
Total	187 (100%)		

* Over the decade 1969–1979, the proportion of cases reported annually as vaccine associated varied from 21% to 80%. (Center for Disease Control: Annual Summary, 1979. Reported Morbidity and Mortality in the United States, USDHHS,PHS 28:64–65, 1980)

population. In such settings, infection occurs very early in life, and most clinical disease is observed in infants. Adults in these regions have usually become immune by late childhood as a result of asymptomatic or nonparalytic infections; hence, paralysis is rare in this age group. If sanitation is improved, fewer persons are infected early in life, and the age incidence of disease shifts toward late childhood and ultimately toward adult life. Thus, in areas free or relatively free of poliovirus, paralysis may occur at any age.

In areas of high endemicity, paralytic disease was believed to be associated with such procedures as tonsillectomy (bulbar poliomyelitis) and injections (poliomyelitis in the injected limb).

Vaccine-associated paralytic poliomyelitis is a rare occurrence in well-immunized populations (Table 121-1 and Figure 121-1). Paralysis is more frequent (though very rare) in immunodeficient infants and children and in nonimmunized, nonimmune adults who are household contacts of immunized infants and are residents in a community in which oral poliovaccine is employed. Even more rarely, recipients of attenuated poliovirus vaccine who are otherwise normal may develop paralysis. For reasons that are unclear, it appears that adults older than 18 years may be more susceptible to vaccine virus-associated paralytic poliomyelitis than younger persons. Wild poliovirus disease is exceedingly uncommon in immunized populations; when it occurs, it tends to affect (1) immigrants incubating the disease, (2) nonimmunized groups within the larger population (*e.g.,* certain religious sects that refuse immunization), and (3) sporadic, local, endemic foci following introduction of a case.

Studies in various populations prior to the availability of poliomyelitis immunization procedures yielded estimates of the occurrence of paralysis of 1 in 60 to 1 in 1000 infected persons. In the United States, the overall incidence of paralytic disease among those infected was probably 0.1% or less. Clinically apparent but nonparalytic illness occurred in approximately 5% of all infections. The remainder, more than 90% of all infections, were asymptomatic or unapparent.

The incubation period of poliovirus from contact to initial clinical symptoms is difficult to determine

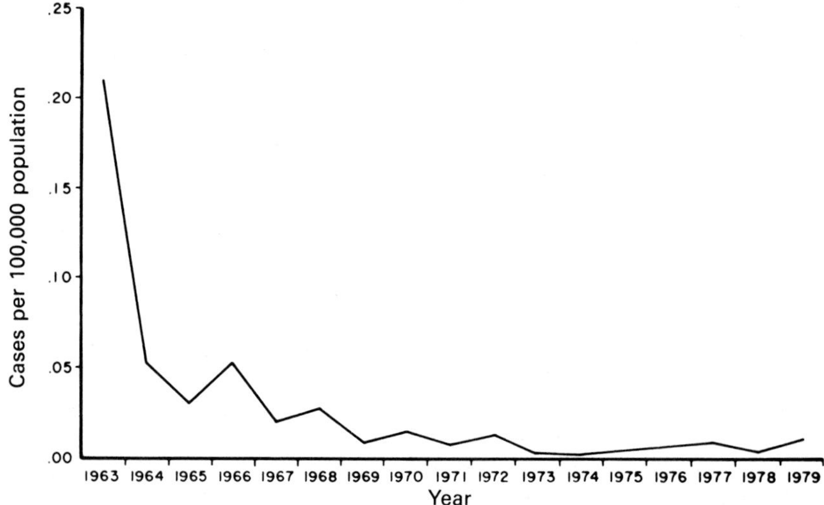

Fig. 121-1. Case rates of paralytic poliomyelitis reported in the United States 1963–1979. (Morbid Mortal United States, September, 1980)

but is usually considered to be 8 to 12 days. A range of 5 to 35 days has been reported, but determination of this interval is complicated by multiple exposures in an area of high endemicity. Paralysis appears later, usually 3 to 8 days after initial symptoms. Poliovirus has been isolated from the feces 2 or more weeks prior to paralysis and several weeks after the onset of symptoms.

Pathogenesis and Pathology

Polioviruses infect cells by adsorbing on to specific, genetically determined receptors. The virus penetrates the cell and then is uncoated and releases RNA, which stimulates the production of viral components in the host cell. These components coalesce to form mature virus particles which are released into the environment by disruption of the cell.

In the contact host, polioviruses gain entry through the respiratory and gastrointestinal tracts. The primary site of replication may be in respiratory mucosa of the upper airway or in the intestine, or both. Regional lymph nodes are infected and a primary viremia results after 2 to 3 days. The virus seeds multiple sites including the reticuloendothelial system, the brown fat deposits, and the central nervous system. Access to the central nervous system is probably through the bloodstream rather than along peripheral nerves, as was once believed. With the first appearance of noncentral nervous system symptoms, a secondary viremia probably occurs as a result of enormous replication in the reticuloendothelial system.

The exact mechanism of entry into the central nervous system is not known. However, once entry is gained, the virus may traverse neural pathways, and multiple sites within the central nervous system are often affected. However, the effect on motor and vegetative neurons is most striking and correlates with the clinical manifestations of infection.

A mixed inflammatory lesion (polymorphonuclear leukocytes and lymphocytes) is located perineuronally and associated with extensive neuronal destruction. Petechial hemorrhages and considerable inflammatory edema also occur in areas of poliovirus infection.

The distribution of the neuronal infection in paralytic disease is strikingly consistent. The gray matter of the spinal cord (anterior horn) and motor areas of the hindbrain (pons and medulla) are involved in an irregular, patchy fashion. Despite this localization and its correlation with clinical findings, involvement of the midbrain, cerebellum, and portions of the cerebral cortex and dorsal root ganglia may also be evident, with permanent damage to some neurons and recovery in others.

Apart from the histopathology of the central nervous system, inflammatory changes occur generally in the reticuloendothelial system. Inflammatory edema and sparse lymphocytic infiltration are prominently associated with hyperplastic lymphocytic follicles.

The pathology of vaccine-associated poliomyelitis mimics that of the natural disease.

Manifestations

Approximately 10% of persons infected with polioviruses develop clinical manifestations that form a spectrum of illnesses. In approximately 5% of patients, a nonspecific influenzalike syndrome occurs 1 to 2 weeks after infection; this is termed *abortive poliomyelitis*. Fever, malaise, anorexia, and headache are prominent features. The patient may complain of a sore throat and abdominal or muscular pain. Vomiting occurs irregularly. The illness is short-lived, (up to 2–3 days), and the physical examination may be normal or may reveal nonspecific pharyngitis, abdominal or muscular tenderness and weakness. Recovery is complete and no neurologic signs or sequelae are present.

In about 1% of all infected patients, the signs of abortive poliomyelitis are present but nuchal stiffness or rigidity is also detected. There is a moderate pleocytosis, usually with predominance of mononuclear cells, and normal concentrations of glucose and protein in the cerebrospinal fluid (CSF). This syndrome is termed *nonparalytic poliomyelitis* and is indistinguishable from *nonbacterial meningitis*, which may be caused by other viruses and by some nonviral agents.

Paralytic poliomyelitis affects fewer than 1 per 1000 of those infected with polioviruses. There are three clinically recognizable syndromes which represent a continuum of infection differentiated only by the portions of the central nervous system most severely affected. These are (1) spinal paralytic poliomyelitis, (2) bulbar poliomyelitis, and (3) polioencephalitis.

Spinal paralytic poliomyelitis may occur as the second phase of a biphasic illness, the first phase of which corresponds to abortive poliomyelitis as described above. The patient then appears to recover and feels better for 2 to 5 days following which severe headache and fever occur with exacerbation of the previous systemic symptoms. Severe muscle pain is noted and sensory and motor phenomena may be observed (paresthesias, hyperesthesias, fasciculations, and spasms). Single muscles, groups of muscles or multiple muscles may be involved in any pattern. Within 1 to 2 days, either flaccid paralysis or paresis occurs in an asymmetric pattern. Examination at this point may reveal nuchal stiffness or rigidity, muscle tenderness, initially hyperactive deep tendon reflexes (for a short period) followed by absent or diminished reflexes, and paresis or flaccid paralysis. Sensation is intact. Sensory disturbances, if present, should suggest a disease other than poliomyelitis.

The paralytic phase of poliomyelitis is extremely variable from patient to patient; some patients progress during observation from paresis to paralysis whereas others recover, quickly or slowly. The extent of paresis or paralysis is directly related to the extent of neuronal involvement; hence, in almost all patients the muscles to be affected are obvious during this phase. That is, the extent of involvement is usually obvious within 1 to 2 days, and only rarely does progression occur beyond this interval. Paralysis of the lower limbs may be accompanied by bowel and bladder dysfunctions ranging from transient incontinence to paralysis with obstipation and urinary retention.

The onset and course of paralysis are variable and age-related. Infants and young children most frequently manifest the biphasic course with prominent prodromal symptoms. Older persons may have a single phase in which prodromal symptoms and paralysis occur in a continuous fashion. Rarely, patients may present initially with paralysis. The degree and duration of muscle pain are also variable. Some patients have none; others complain for days or weeks. Spasm and increased muscle tone with a transient increase in deep tendon reflexes occur in some patients whereas in others flaccid paralysis and decreased reflexes are initially apparent. Weakness may precede paralysis for a few hours or days or paralysis may occur abruptly. Once the temperature returns to normal, no further paralytic manifestations are noted in most patients.

Paralysis is classically asymmetric. Involvement of one leg is most common, followed by involvement of one arm. The proximal areas of the extremities tend to be involved to a greater extent than the distal areas.

Little recovery from paralysis is noted in the first days or weeks but it is usually evident within 6 months if it is to occur. The return of strength and reflexes is slow and may continue as long as 18 months after the acute disease.

Lack of improvement from paralysis within the first several weeks or months after onset is usually evidence of permanent paralysis. Atrophy of the limb, failure of growth, and deformity are common and are especially evident in the growing child. Respiratory paralysis may occur in the spinal form of the disease, but is more common with bulbar involvement. Lesions in the high cervical and thoracic cord may lead to intercostal or diaphragmatic paralysis, with increased dependence on accessory muscles of respiration. Respirations become shallow, the voice may be dysphonic, and effective coughing is lost. Respiratory paralysis is a relatively late manifestation and may be incomplete; recovery is also variable in extent.

Bulbar poliomyelitis may occur as a clinical entity without apparent involvement of the spinal cord. Yet, the infection is a continuum, and designation of the disease as bulbar implies only dominance of the clinical manifestations by dysfunctions of the cranial nerves and medullary centers. Difficulty with swallowing and phonation, facial paralysis, diplopia and ocular paralysis, laryngeal paralysis with stridor, weakness of the respiratory muscles, and vasomotor instability may occur singly or in various combinations. Uncommonly, bulbar disease may culminate an ascending paralysis (Landry type) in which there is progression cephalad from initial involvement of the lower extremities.

Hypertension is common in bulbar involvement and may persist for a week or more or may be transient. Occasionally, hypertension is followed by hypotension and shock and is associated with irregular or failed respiratory effort, delirium, or coma. This kind of bulbar disease may be rapidly fatal.

The course of bulbar disease is variable; some patients die as a result of extensive, severe involvement of the various centers in the medulla, others recover partially but require ongoing respiratory support, and others recover completely. Cranial nerve involvement is seldom permanent. Atrophy of muscles may be evident, patients immobilized for long periods may develop pneumonia, and renal stones may form as a result of hypercalcemia and hypercalciuria secondary to bone resorption.

Polioencephalitis is a rare form of the disease in which higher centers of the brain are severely involved. Seizures, coma, and spastic paralysis with increased reflexes may be observed. The manifestations are common to encephalitis of any cause (Ch. 122, Viral Encephalitides) and can only be attributed to polioviruses by specific viral diagnosis.

Diagnosis

Abortive poliomyelitis cannot be differentiated from many other viral illnesses unless poliovirus happens to be isolated from the patient.

Paralytic disease may be suspected as being poliomyelitis on clinical grounds—a possibility that is enhanced by finding changes in the CSF that are classic for any nonbacterial meningitis or encephalitis. Pleocytosis is usually present, that is, fewer than 500 cells per cubic millimiter. If the spinal fluid is examined early in the disease, polymorphonuclear leukocytes may predominate or equal the numbers of mononuclear cells. Ultimately, lymphocytes are the predominant cell form. Protein and glucose concentrations are also usually normal during the acute phases of illness. However, 1 to 2 weeks after the onset of paralysis, mononuclear cells predominate and the protein concentration becomes elevated. In polioencephalitis, the CSF may remain normal or show minor changes.

The electroencephalogram and other tests of neurologic function give nonspecific results and are not useful in the diagnosis of poliomyelitis.

Specific diagnosis of poliomyelitis is accomplished by the isolation of poliovirus from throat swabs, rectal swabs, or specimens of feces. The CSF should also be submitted for culture of virus, although the recovery of poliovirus is uncommon from this source. Neutralizing antibody in the serum should be measured against the patient's isolate using specimens obtained during the acute phase of illness and 1 to 3 weeks later; a fourfold or greater increase in antibody titer is diagnostic. All viral isolates should be submitted to a reference laboratory (such as the Centers for Disease Control in the United States) for identification and characterization, especially if there is a question of vaccine association. Viral recovery should be attempted at any point within a month after the onset of paralysis. Ideally, specimens should be obtained as soon as the diagnosis is entertained, since polioviruses may be isolated from 80% to 90% of acutely ill patients, whereas less than 20% may yield the virus within 3 to 4 weeks after onset of paralysis.

Isolation of poliovirus alone is not sufficient to establish the diagnosis of poliomyelitis, especially in areas in which the oral vaccine is in constant use. Poliovirus may be excreted as a result of prior immunization or contact with an immunized person, these isolates may have no association with the neurologic disease observed in the patient. Serologic confirmation of poliovirus infection should be attempted in all persons from whom polioviruses are isolated. In recipients of vaccine, both isolation of the virus and 4-fold or greater rises in antibody are typical. Therefore, great care must be exercised in attributing a noncompatible clinical disease to poliomyelitis even when isolation of virus and serologic response have been found.

In lethal infections, specimens of central nervous system tissue should be obtained from areas that correlate with the clinical manifestations. Both attempted viral isolation and histopathology should be carried out on such specimens. If death ensued during acute illness, specimens of reticuloendothelial tissues should also be cultured for viruses. In addition, specimens should be taken for viral isolation from the respiratory tract and from the contents of the intestinal tract.

Prognosis

The ultimate outcome in unapparent, abortive, and aseptic meningitis syndromes is uniformly favorable. Death in aseptic meningitis is exceedingly rare, and long-term sequelae have not been recognized.

The outcome in paralytic disease is determined primarily by the degree and severity of central nervous system involvement. The mortality in severe bulbar poliomyelitis may be as high as 60%, with death following an acute fulminant course within days after the onset of paralysis. Less severe bulbar involvement and most forms of spinal paralytic poliomyelitis may lead to death in 5% to 20% of patients, generally from causes other than the poliovirus infection.

In part, the prognosis depends on clinical complications secondary to the neurologic involvement. For example, severe pulmonary or cardiac disabilities may occur secondary to medullary involvement and may lead to respiratory or cardiovascular death.

In addition, certain risk factors appear to enhance morbidity and mortality of poliomyelitis. In general, male children are more likely to become paralyzed, whereas female adults more often suffer paralysis. The age incidence is dependent on the immune status of the population. In the United States, severe disease in infants is now uncommon, whereas in nonimmunized populations, infantile disease is common and often severe and lethal. In vaccine-associated paralytic disease acquired by contact with vaccines in the United States during the past decade, more adults have been affected than children.

It has been estimated that immunodeficient persons run a risk of developing vaccine-associated paralytic disease which is approximately 10,000 times that of the normal population. A similar risk is probably encountered in the natural disease, although this is difficult to sort out from epidemiologic studies conducted during a time when many of the immunodeficiencies were unknown or undiagnosed. Specific B cell and T cell deficiencies, and combinations thereof, have been implicated. Not only is the risk of disease increased, but also the illness is of longer duration, more often beset by complications, and more frequently fatal. As many as 40% of immunodeficient children with paralytic poliomyelitis die of the disease or disease-related complications.

Pregnancy is associated with both an increased risk of paralytic disease and a slightly increased risk of mortality. Tonsillectomy and injections (subcutaneous, intramuscular) may enhance the risk of acquisition of bulbar or localized disease, respectively.

Other factors cited as increasing the risk of paralytic disease include the status of activity during the early phase of the illness (increased physical activity, exercise, and fatigue), a familial tendency to develop paralysis, and poverty and malnutrition.

Finally, the type, and even the strain, of poliovirus is important. It has been clearly demonstrated that type 1 poliovirus has the greatest propensity for natural poliomyelitis, and type 3 for vaccine-associated disease. Wild strains vary in their capacity to induce neurologic disease in experimental animals, a fact that may in part account for the variation in the severity of epidemics in different parts of the world and in a given area at different times.

The most intriguing aspect of prognosis is the concept that susceptibility to infection is determined by the nature of cell surface receptors that are genetically prescribed. Human chromosome 19 contains a gene that determines the presence of such receptors. More recently, several histocompatibility types (HLA 3 and HLA 7) have been found to be associated with an increased risk of paralysis. It is conceivable that paralytic disease is largely determined by host susceptibility rather than by the neurovirulence of the poliovirus.

Therapy

There is no antiviral therapy effective against polioviruses. Successful management of patients with poliomyelitis includes intensive care during the acute disease and extensive rehabilitation afterward. Hospitalization and bedrest are mandatory for acute paralytic disease because physical activity may exacerbate paralysis. The severe muscle pain of the acute paralytic disease may be mitigated by analgesics which do not suppress respiratory effort, and physical measures such as a stiff mattress, elevation of bed clothes from tender muscles, and hot, wet packs.

Acute intensive care measures to support respiratory and cardiovascular functions are critical in bulbar and bulbospinal poliomyelitis. Life-saving initially, these efforts may ultimately prevent excessive pulmonary morbidity. Expert nursing care is critical to avoid strangulation, and aspiration of secretions.

Rehabilitative efforts should be planned as soon as the extent of paralysis is recognized and muscle spasm has decreased sufficiently to permit passive manipulation.

Prevention

Prior to the development of specific poliomyelitis immunoprophylaxis, prevention consisted largely of hygienic measures and sanitary practices. The initial development of human immune globulin was stimulated by the possibility of passive immunization against poliomyelitis as well as other diseases. The clear demonstration that administration of human immune globulin would in fact prevent poliomyelitis was eclipsed by the widespread application of active immunization using either killed or attenuated live virus vaccines.

Beginning in 1955 and extending through the early 1960s, massive use of formalin inactivated poliovirus vaccine (IPV) resulted in a marked diminution in the occurrence of natural poliomyelitis in many areas of the world. For example, in the United States in 1952, more than 21,000 cases of paralytic poliomyelitis were reported nationally. By 1962, only 691 cases were recorded (Fig. 121-2). Similar striking de-

Fig. 121-2. Decline in case rates of paralytic poliomyelitis reported in the United States during the period 1951–1963. The times of introduction of poliovirus vaccines are indicated by the arrows. (Morbid Mortal United States, September, 1980)

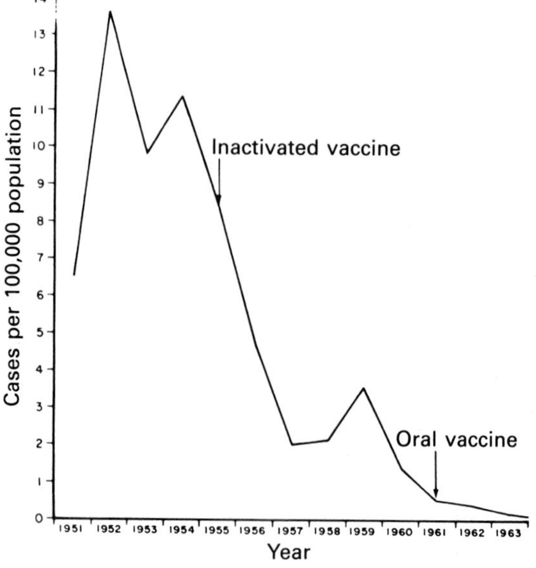

creases were observed in Canada, Sweden, Finland and many other parts of the world.

Inactivated poliovirus vaccine of the kind employed prior to 1970 had several intrinsic disadvantages. The immunogenicity of the vaccine was so low that multiple initial doses and periodic booster doses, presumably throughout life, were required. To some extent, incorporation of IPV into the standard infant diphtheria, tetanus, and pertussis vaccine (DPT) provided a means for the routine initial immunization of the vast majority of the infants in technically advanced societies. However, the requirement for the injection of multiple doses inhibited universal immunization in the United States. In contrast, in Finland more than 95% of the population received and has continued to receive IPV with continuous reduction and eventually, elimination of paralytic disease.

However, IPV is not effective in containing epidemics. Since IPV does not evoke secretory IgA antibody in the respiratory or gastrointestinal tracts, wild or live vaccine virus may replicate in and be transmitted by persons fully immunized with IPV. Theoretically, wild virus could be sustained in an IPV-immunized population, a possibility not substantiated by the Finnish experience.

Further reduction in the incidence of paralytic poliomyelitis accompanied the widespread introduction and use of the perorally administered, live attentuated virus vaccine (OPV) in the United States in the 1960s. By 1972, only 22 cases of paralytic disease were reported (Fig. 121-2). From approximately 1965 onward, IPV became unavailable and only OPV was used in the United States; during the last several years, fewer than 10 cases of paralytic poliomyelitis have occurred annually. Most of these cases were vaccine-associated, and the question whether IPV should again be the primary vaccine was raised.

Although it is apparent that OPV reduced the incidence of poliomyelitis even beyond that associated with the use of IPV, it is possible that the application of IPV for the entire period since it was introduced in the 1960s would have brought about a similar reduction. It is also possible that IPV would not have been as widely employed in the United States as it was in the Scandinavian countries, and as a result a significant portion of the population would remain unimmunized. For these reasons and because of the other disadvantages of IPV, the major advisory bodies in the United States recommended the retention of OPV as the primary vaccine to be used in the routine immunoprophylaxis of poliomyelitis. In 1977, the Institute of Medicine convened a special committee to consider the issue; again, the retention of OPV as the major immunizing biological was recommended; however, areas in which IPV might be used were pointed out, and another review was suggested for 1982 or at a time when 95% of the population was immunized—whichever comes first.

Legal issues have developed as a result of liability suits, completed or in process, directed against manufacturers of OPV, public health agencies, recommending bodies, and individual physicians and health care personnel. The range of issues varies from inadequate discussion of the potential harmful effects of OPV to the intrinsic risk of paralysis associated with OPV. At the present time, these issues have not been resolved, and modifications in recommendations will probably occur as functions of time and experience.

OPV is the preferred immunization for routine immunoprophylaxis against poliomyelitis in infants and children. Ordinarily, it is administered in two or three doses in infancy (2, 4, and 6 months of age) with subsequent doses at 18 months of age and just prior to entry into school. Two doses at 2 and 4 months are preferred by most physicians in the United States. However, in areas of the country in which poliomyelitis is still imported from neighboring countries, for example, the Southwest, a third dose at 6 months can and should be administered in order to convert some of those who were nonreactors to the first two doses against all 3 types of poliovirus. It should be understood that a single feeding of OPV may immunize a recipient against all 3 types of poliovirus. However, for the population as a whole, optimal rates of immunization (more than 95% for each of the 3 types) only occurs after 3 feedings. The reasons for failure are not always clear but include the presence of other enteroviruses in the intestine that inhibit the replication of polioviruses, variable infectivity among the three types, and regurgitation of the dose. In the tropics, a much lower rate of immunization is observed, possibly because of a higher incidence of nonpolio enteroviruses and factors related to malnutrition.

Persons not immunized in infancy who are under 18 years of age may be given two doses of OPV separated by 1 to 2 months and a third dose one year later.

Nonimmunized persons over the age of 18 should not be given OPV electively. If exposure is likely and time permits, IPV should be used as two to three doses separated by one month, with a booster dose one year later. If exposure is imminent, OPV may be offered after adequate explanation of the risks and benefits of vaccine *versus* exposure to natural disease.

All persons or guardians of infants who are to receive OPV or IPV should take part in a discussion concerning the risks and benefits of both the disease and the specific vaccine. After a patient or guardian has a full understanding of the risks and benefits, the appropriate vaccine should be offered, and given with the patient's consent. A special subcommittee of the Institute of Medicine suggested that it is appropriate to give IPV to a person who has been informed of the risks and benefits involved and requests IPV. When a clinician encounters parents and other adults in close household contact with an infant about to be immunized, he may do one of two things. He may choose to ignore the immune status of these adults and administer OPV. This is the common practice in the United States at the present time. Alternatively, the physician may choose to immunize adults who are susceptible and who will be contacts. Two doses of IPV are injected one month apart in the adults prior to giving the infant OPV; at the same time the adult receives a third monthly dose of IPV when the infant receives OPV. The purpose of this procedure is to avoid exposure of any nonimmunized adult contacts in the child's immediate environment to live vaccine virus excreted by the infant. It is recognized that intestinal passage of oral attenuated polioviruses can result in some reversion toward neurovirulence, particularly for type 3. This phenomenon is believed to account, at least in part, for the cases that occur among contacts of infant vaccinees—usually adults.

Oral poliovaccine is not contraindicated in pregnancy but should not be given electively to pregnant women. There is no known association of receipt of OPV and congenital anomalies or disturbances in pregnancy. Thus, if a pregnant, susceptible female is about to be exposed, as might occur with travel and residence in an area of high endemicity, OPV may be administered if time does not permit the administration of IPV.

Immunodeficient persons and contacts of immunodeficient persons should not be immunized with OPV. For these persons, it may be wise to administer IPV to both the immunodeficient person and his or her contacts, despite the fact that the immunologic response in the immunodeficient person may be suboptimal. On the other hand, if a person does not have complete absence of B cell function, neutralizing antibody may develop in response to IPV.

Laboratory workers who handle polioviruses should be adequately immunized. Those over 18 years of age should receive IPV electively. Alternatively, they may be offered OPV after full discussion of its benefits and risks.

OPV can be administered simultaneously with a variety of other vaccines. The most commonly employed combination is to administer DPT by injection and OPV orally in the young infant at the prescribed times. OPV has also been combined with measles vaccine administration and more recently has been administered orally at the same time that MMR (measles, mumps, rubella) virus combinations are administered subcutaneously. At the present time it is uncertain whether OPV, DPT, and MMR should be administered simultaneously. A limited number of children have received all nine antigens without adverse effect and with adequate immunologic response to each. In populations in which medical contact is limited or compliance is diminished, it may be desirable to use this combination.

Remaining Problems

The major problems confronting health care practitioners are (1) maximum use of poliovirus vaccines to eradicate naturally occurring paralytic disease and the wild virus from the world, (2) resolution of the risk benefit ratio for OPV *versus* IPV and selection of the appropriate vaccine and regimen to be employed in immunization, and (3) further development of OPV to the point of reduced capacity to reversion to neurovirulence with maintenance of immunogenicity.

Universal immunization against poliomyelitis is more difficult to achieve than it was against smallpox. Polioviruses are ubiquitous in certain populations and under certain socioeconomic conditions, and it is difficult to reach entire populations in some parts the world. Local strife, revolution, and other social upheavals inhibit the application of adequate immunization to all persons. In the United States, marked success at increasing the level of poliovirus immunization has been achieved with school immunization laws that require proof of poliovirus immunization prior to entry into school or as a condition for continuation in school. This has resulted in more than 90% of persons reporting adequate poliovirus immunization in the school age population. However, those who have not yet entered school still represent an inadequately immunized population. In young infants and children, large percentages of certain subpopulations in the United States fail to receive regular medical care, including poliovirus and other immunizations.

Current IPV products are stated to be more potent than those used in the 50s and 60s. As a result, it has been argued that fewer doses are necessary and booster doses may be unnecessary. Furthermore, experience with vaccines of this type in Europe suggests that disease can be eradicated provided a sufficiently large proportion of the population is immunized. If these contentions are proved, it may be possible to eliminate OPV entirely. However, based on prior experience with IPV, there is basis for skepticism.

Basic investigation with polioviruses is at a standstill because the current OPV strains are thought to represent a satisfactory balance between efficacy in eradicating poliomyelitis and the occurrence of adverse consequences. It is conceivable that vaccines might be developed from strains that have very little or no potential for neurovirulence or reversion that still retain immunogenicity. Laboratory investigation of genetic susceptibility will continue, and someday we may be able to identify those persons who are at greater risk of paralysis either from natural disease or oral poliovaccine.

Bibliography

Books

American Academy of Pediatrics: Report of the Committee on Infectious Diseases (Redbook), 19th ed. Evanston, IL, AAP, 1982. pp 207–211.

PAUL JR: A History of Poliomyelitis, New Haven, CT, Yale University Press, 1971. 486 pp.

Journals

AULD PAM, KEVY SV, ELEY RC: Poliomyelitis in children: Experience with 956 cases in the 1955 Massachusetts epidemic. N Engl J Med 263:1093–1100, 1960

Center for Disease Control: Poliomyelitis prevention: Recommendation of the Public Health Service Advisory Committee on Immunization Practices. Morbid Mortal Rep 28:510–520, 1979

DAWSON KE, LABOCCETTA AC, TORNAY AS, SILVERSTEIN A: Acute poliomyelitis. J Pediatr 40:71–84, 1952

FAGREUS A, BOTTIGER M: Polio vaccination in Sweden. Rev Infect Dis 2:274–276, 1980

FOX TP: Eradication of poliomyelitis in the United States: A commentary on the Salk reviews. Rev Infect Dis 2:277–281, 1980

FULGINITI VA: Problems of poliovirus immunization. Hosp Pract 8:61–67, 1980

LUCCHESI PF: Poliomyelitis: a study of 410 patients at the Philadelphia Hospital for Contagious Diseases. Am J Med Sci 4:515–523, 1934

MELNICK JL: Advantages and disadvantages of killed and live poliomyelitis vaccines. Bull WHO 56:21–38, 1978

MILLER DA, MILLER OJ, DEV VG, HASHMI S, TANTRAVAHL R, MEDRANO L, GREEN H: Human chromosome 19 carries a poliovirus receptor gene. Cell 1:167–170, 1974

NATHANSON N, MARTIN JR: The epidemiology of poliomyelitis. Am J Epidemiol 110:672–692, 1979

NIGHTINGALE EO: Recommendations for a national policy on poliomyelitis vaccination. N Engl J Med 297:249–253, 1977

SABIN AB: Poliomyelitis vaccination: Evaluation and direction in continuing application. Am J Clin Pathol 70:136–140, 1978

SALK D: Eradication of poliomyelitis in the United States. I. Live virus vaccine-associated and wild poliovirus disease. II. Experience with killed poliovirus vaccine. III. Poliovaccines practical considerations. Rev Infect Dis 2:228–242; 243–257; 258–273, 1980

SALK JE, BENNETT BL, LEWIS LJ, WARD EN, YOUNGNER JS: Studies in human subjects on active immunization against poliomyelitis. I. A preliminary report of experiments in progress. JAMA 151:1081–1098, 1953

SCHONBERGER LB, MCGOVIAN JE, GREGG MB: Vaccine-associated poliomyelitis in the United States, 1961–1972. Am J Epidemiol 104:202–211, 1976

RALPH L. DOHERTY

122 Viral Encephalitides

Encephalitis caused by mosquito-borne viruses occurs in epidemics in rural areas of many parts of the world. The causative agents are members of a large group of arboviruses (*arthropod-borne* viruses), some of which are closely related. Distinct arboviruses are specific to certain geographic areas, for example, St. Louis encephalitis in the United States, Japanese B encephalitis in eastern Asia, and Murray Valley encephalitis in Australia. Some of the same viruses are also the causes of endemic encephalitis in several tropical areas (*e.g.,* St. Louis encephalitis in Central America), and other mosquito-borne arboviruses cause sporadic encephalitis in the tropics (*e.g.,* Ilhéus virus in Trinidad). Arboviruses transmitted by ticks cause encephalitis in focal areas in Europe, Asia, and North America.

Arbovirus encephalitides are uncommon in urban communities, with the notable exception of some epidemics of St. Louis encephalitis in the United States. Some urban encephalitides are caused by enteroviruses (see Chap. 121, Poliomyelitis, and Chap. 149, Coxsackievirus and Echovirus Infections), mumps virus (see Chap. 74, Mumps), adenoviruses (see Chap. 30, Nonbacterial Pneumonias), and herpesvirus (see Chap. 91, Infections Caused by Herpes Simplex Viruses), or they are demyelinating diseases following measles (see Chap. 86, Measles), varicella (see Chap. 93, Varicella and Herpes Zoster), rubella (see Chap. 87, Rubella), mumps (see Chap. 74, Mumps), or vaccination (see Chap. 92, Smallpox and Other Poxvirus Infections). Etiologic diagnosis is not accomplished in many cases.

In addition, slow virus infections of the central nervous system (CNS), that is, viral infections of the CNS that have an incubation period of years, have been recognized in humans. Four such infections appear to be established: (1) subacute sclerosing panencephalitis, caused by measles virus (see Chap. 86, Measles), (2) progressive multifocal leukoencephalopathy, a demyelinating disease with progressive neurologic abnormalities which occurs in elderly patients with lymphomas, other chronic diseases, or in association with immunosuppressive therapy, and with viruses of the papovavirus group, (3) Jakob–Creutzfeldt disease (a presenile dementia), and (4) kuru, an affliction of primitive Fore tribesmen of the New Guinea highlands. The last two infections will be discussed in this chapter.

Although in this chapter, consideration is restricted to the arbovirus, herpesvirus, and slow virus encephalitides, some perspective of the frequency of encephalitis associated with various agents, identified and not identified in reported cases in the United States, can be gained from Figure 122-1.

Etiology

More than 350 viruses of at least 46 antigenic groups are included as arboviruses on the basis of their ability to multiply in both vertebrates and arthropods. The arboviruses presently recognized as causes of encephalitis represent several distinct taxonomic entities, the togaviruses (including alphaviruses, formerly group A arboviruses, and flaviviruses, formerly group B arboviruses), and the bunya viruses (including the California group and other groups of arboviruses) (Table 122-1). These viruses all contain RNA, all have a lipoprotein envelope, and thus all are sensitive to such lipid solvents as ether and sodium deoxycholate.

The diameters of the flaviviruses are about 50 nm, the alphaviruses about 70 nm, and the bunyaviruses about 90 nm. By electron microscopy, the togaviruses mature in association with cytoplasmic membranes; there is an electron dense core, and some evidence of cubical capsid symmetry with spikes on the envelope. The bunyaviruses have segmented genomes and helically symmetric nucleocapsids. Gel electrophoresis has shown that alphaviruses, flaviviruses, and bunyaviruses each contain three major virion proteins.

Togaviruses and bunyaviruses multiply to high titers in the brains of infant mice, but various cell cultures (especially Vero cells from the African green monkey, BHK21 cells from the hamster, and PS cells from the pig) and embryonated eggs are also much used as susceptible hosts. Mosquitoes of several species (*e.g., Toxorhynchites* spp.) have been found to be highly susceptible hosts for isolation of several arboviruses and will undoubtedly find application with viruses causing encephalitis. Hemagglutinin for goose and other erythrocytes can be obtained for the viruses associated with encephalitis, most often by the extraction of infected mouse brain with acetone in the presence of sucrose. Three serologic tests—hemagglutination inhibition, complement fixation, and neutralization—are commonly used; they give results that vary among virus groups with regard to specificity and duration of antibody response. The neutralization test is generally viewed as being most useful for surveys of antibody to a specific virus; the complement fixation test is best for the serologic diagnosis of disease. Other serologic techniques (*e.g.,* immunofluorescence and enzyme-linked immunosorbent assay or ELISA) are also available.

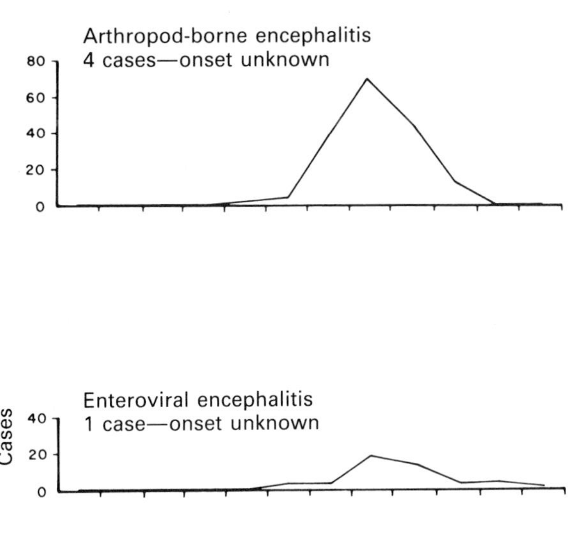

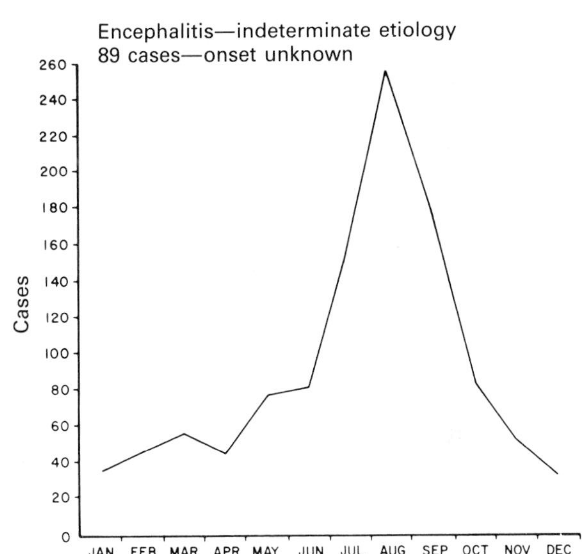

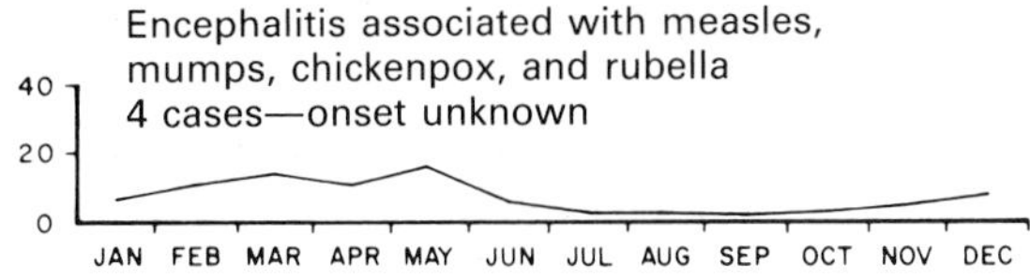

Fig. 122-1. Number of cases of encephalitis reported in the United States in 1979 by month. (Morbid Mortal Week Ann Suppl, 1980)

Table 122-1. Major Epidemic Arbovirus Encephalitides

Disease	Causative Virus	Geographic Distribution	Arthropod Vectors	Vertebrate Hosts (Indicator Hosts)*
Eastern equine encephalitis	Alphavirus	Eastern USA, Central America and Caribbean Islands, Brazil, Guyana, Argentina	*Culiseta melanura, Aedes sollicitans, Aedes vexans, Culex nigripalpus, Culex teniopus*	Birds (horses)
Western equine encephalitis	Alphavirus	USA, Canada, Central America, Guyana, Brazil, Argentina	*Culex tarsalis, Culex quinquefasciatus, Culiseta melanura*	Birds, small mammals, snakes (horses)
Venezuelan equine encephalitis	Alphavirus	Northern South America, Central America, Florida, Texas	*Psorophora confinnis, Aedes sollicitans,* and various other *Aedes* and *Culex* mosquitoes	Horses, other equines, rodents of genera *sigmodon, Peromyscus, heteromys, Zygodontomys,* and *Oryzomys*
St. Louis encephalitis	Flavivirus	Western, central, and southern USA, Canada, Central America and Caribbean Islands, Colombia, Brazil, Argentina	*Culex tarsalis, Culex pipiens* complex, *Culex nigripalpus*	Birds
Japanese B encephalitis	Flavivirus	Siberia, Korea, Japan, China, Taiwan, Philippines, Burma, Vietnam, Laos, Cambodia, Malaysia, Singapore, Thailand, India, Sri Lanka, Indonesia	*Culex tritaeniorhynchus, Culex gelidus, Culex vishnui* complex	Birds, pigs (horses)
Murray Valley encephalitis	Flavivirus	Australia, New Guinea	*Culex annulirostris*	Birds
Sao Paulo encephalitis	Flavivirus (Rocio)	Brazil	Unknown	Birds
Tick-borne encephaliti-des:				
Far-Eastern and Central European forms	Flavivirus	USSR, eastern Europe	*Ixodes persulcatus, Ixodes ricinus*	Small mammals, domestic mammals, especially goats
Louping ill	Flavivirus	Great Britain	*Ixodes ricinus*	Small mammals, sheep, grouse
Negishi	Flavivirus	Japan	Unknown	Unknown
Powassan	Flavivirus	Canada, northern USA	*Ixodes marxi, Ixodes cookei*	Small mammals, especially groundhogs
California encephalitis	Bunyavirus USA, Canada		Various *Aedes* and *Culex* mosquitoes	Small mammals, including *Lepus, Citellus, Peromyscus*

*Indicator hosts are not considered important in virus survival.

The herpesviruses (see Chap. 91) are DNA viruses. Enveloped in lipoproteins and therefore sensitive to lipid solvents, they consist of an icosahedral capsid approximately 110 nm in diameter, made up of 162 capsomeres.

Herpes simplex virus, the agent of herpes febrilis and of herpes encephalitis, has double-stranded DNA with a total molecular weight of 96×10^6 daltons. It has a wide host range, with the embryonated egg, various cell cultures (especially primary rabbit kidney and human amnion), and the infant mouse most often used for propagation. Herpes simplex virus does not agglutinate erythrocytes, but complement fixation and neutralization tests are available for antibody detection. Two distinct types have been demonstrated that are distinguishable antigenically and by a characteristic cytopathic pattern in cell culture. Most strains from herpes meningoencephalitis are type 1, but strains of type 2 (usually from genital herpes) may be isolated from herpes infections of the newborn. *Herpesvirus simiae* (B virus) is a simian counterpart to herpes simplex and can cause encephalomyelitis in man. Although the two viruses are antigenically related, immunity to herpes simplex gives little protection against B virus.

The causative agents of kuru and Jakob–Creutzfeldt disease have been transmitted to primates of several species. They have not been characterized, but are believed to resemble the agent of scrapie, a subacute encephalitis of sheep. The apparent small size of the scrapie agent (measured by resistance to radiation) and its resistance to heat suggest an entity distinct from any known virus, hence the suggested designation, proion (see Chap. 1, Attributes of Infectious Agents.)

Epidemiology

The arbovirus encephalitides are zoonoses, with the virus surviving in infection cycles involving biting arthropods and various vertebrates, especially birds and rodents. Infection of the arthropod vector is a biologic process with multiplication in the gut, dissemination in the hemolymph, and ultimately, at the end of the extrinsic incubation period, infection of the salivary glands coinciding with the ability to transmit the virus. Humans are infected when they come in contact with the zoonotic cycles, and they can be viewed as incidental terminal hosts playing no part in the natural history of the viruses (although humans act as important vertebrate hosts for other arbovirus infections, notably dengue and urban yellow fever; see Chap. 73, Yellow Fever, and Chap. 89, Dengue). As a consequence, multiple household infections are unusual, and secondary cases within affected households do not occur. Most infections of humans are subclinical, and immunity develops without disease.

The proportion of infections manifested as disease in humans can sometimes be determined by antibody surveys after an epidemic, with results varying according to the virus and from epidemic to epidemic: in eastern equine encephalitis in infants, 1 in 10; in Murray Valley encephalitis, 1 in 1000. The extent and distribution of disease in place and in time depend on the various parameters of zoonotic cycles. Notable are the density of the arthropod vector and its biting behavior, the size of the vertebrate reservior, and the closeness of its association with humans. For example, temperate zone epidemics of arbovirus encephalitis occur in summer, when arthropod populations are high, and they may be associated with particular climatic conditions such as heavy rain and flooding. Eastern equine encephalitis in the United States must be limited by the disinclination of the major vector in nature, *Culiseta melanura,* to bite humans. Tick-borne encephalitis in Europe and Asia is an occupational hazard of forest workers who enter areas that are foci of virus-infected ticks.

In the tropics, and in summer epidemics in the Temperate Zone, survival of the virus may be adequately explained by chains of transmission from viremic vertebrate to arthropod to susceptible vertebrate. However, in areas in which winter interrupts the breeding of arthropods, survival of the virus through the winter is more diffcult to explain.

Several hypotheses have been advanced to explain virus maintenance over adverse periods, for example, survival of infected vectors, transovarian transmission of virus in the vector, latent infection of vertebrate hosts, and annual reintroduction of virus by hosts (especially birds) or vectors. Evidence exists for several of these mechanisms. For example, transovarian transmission has been demonstrated for tick-borne encephalitis viruses in Eurasian ticks and for California group viruses in *Aedes* mosquitoes in North America. Western equine encephalitis virus has been shown to survive over winter in hibernating snakes in an experimental system. Western equine encephalitis virus has also been recovered from organs of birds up to 234 days after infection, although such chronically infected birds have not been shown to be able to infect mosquitoes. Even so, the relative importance of these mechanisms of virus survival over adverse seasons remains uncertain.

Transmission to humans by means other than arthropod bites is possible, but is relatively unimportant. Examples of nonarthropod transmission include the ingestion of infected goat's milk with tick-borne encephalitis viruses, person-to-person contact with Venezuelan equine encephalitis, and inhalation of a number of viruses in laboratory infections.

Epidemiologic details of the arbovirus encephalitides are summarized in Table 122-1. The individual diseases may be described briefly.

Eastern Equine Encephalitis

First recognized in 1933, eastern equine encephalitis has caused epidemics in the eastern United States from New Hampshire to Texas (*e.g.,* Massachusetts in 1938, 1956, and 1973, New Jersey in 1959, and Louisiana in 1947), in the Dominican Republic in 1948 and 1978, and in Jamaica in 1962. In the United States, the virus survives in rural cycles involving birds and *Culiseta melanura,* with infection of humans and horses possibly occasionally due to that mosquito, but more commonly due to other mosquitoes, probably including *Aedes sollicitans* and *Aedes vexans. Culex taeniopus* and *Culex nigripalpus* may be important vectors in the Caribbean area. The virus has been isolated from several areas in Central and South America; strains from those areas are antigenically distinguishable from North American strains; that is, reintroduction from the tropics is therefore an unlikely explanation of survival over the winter in the northeastern United States.

Western Equine Encephalitis

Western equine encephalitis was first recognized in 1930. Epidemics occurred in the north central United States and adjoining areas of Canada in 1941. Cases have since been diagnosed over all of the United States west of the Mississippi River and in adjoining provinces of Canada. The infection is endemic in the Central Valley of California.

Summer epidemic cycles involve birds and *Culex tarsalis,* with horses and man acting as indicator hosts. It seems likely that other mosquitoes, especially *Culex quinquefasciatus,* may be important in Texas and *C. melanura* in rural cycles in the eastern United States. Various mechanisms of survival over the winter have been suggested, as previously discussed. The virus has been isolated in Guyana, Brazil, and Argentina. The disease has been diagnosed in humans in Brazil; according to antibody surveys, the infection is common in humans in both Brazil and Argentina.

Venezuelan Equine Encephalitis

First recognized in horses in 1938, Venezuelan equine encephalitis occurs in northern South America and in Central America. The causative virus has been isolated in Florida, and in Texas where 110 laboratory-confirmed cases occurred in the summer of 1971. Both endemic and epidemic infection occurs in Venezuela. Although there were over 30,000 cases in an epidemic in 1962–1964, only a minority developed encephalitis. Epidemic (IA, IB, and IC) and nonepidemic (ID, IE, II, III, IV) strains can be distinguished antigenically. Nonepidemic strains appear to survive in cycles involving rodents and several species of mosquitoes. Epidemics depend on horses and other equines as hosts and a wide range of mosquitoes, especially *Psorophora confinnis* and *A. sollicitans,* as vectors.

St. Louis Encephalitis

Although epidemic St. Louis encephalitis may have occurred in 1932 in Illinois, it was first definitely recognized in 1933 in St. Louis, Missouri. The virus is endemic in the Central Valley of California, where 235 cases were recorded in the period 1945–1953. Cases have occurred in west central and southern United States, Canada, Panama, and Trinidad. Virus isolation from humans or from mosquitoes has confirmed that the virus is active in Central and South America. Important epidemics have occurred in urban communities (*e.g.,* Florida in 1962 and Houston in 1964). Widespread outbreaks in the United States and Canada in 1975 involved 2131 cases confirmed by laboratory studies, including the largest urban epidemic described, with over 700 confirmed or suspected cases in the Chicago metropolitan area.

Transmission involves birds and *C. tarsalis* (in the western United States), *C. nigripalpus* (in Florida), or the *C. pipiens* complex elsewhere in the United States.

Japanese B Encephalitis

Although Japanese B encephalitis occurs from Siberia to India, it has been most thoroughly studied in Japan. It was in Japan that the disease was recognized as a clinical entity in 1871, and the virus was isolated in 1934. Annual epidemics in Japan have involved as many as 8000 cases with particularly large epidemics in 1924, 1935, and 1948.

Epidemic occurrence has been recorded in Korea, Taiwan, Thailand, and Bengal, with more sporadic occurrence elsewhere in eastern Asia.

The major cycle of virus passage involves birds (especially herons and egrets in Japan) and culicine mosquitoes (*C. tritaeniorhynchus* over much of the area, *C. gelidus* in Malaysia and Singapore, and the *C.*

vishnui complex in India). In addition, pigs are raised in large numbers in several areas where they may act as an important amplifying host.

Murray Valley Encephalitis

Formerly known as Australian X disease, Murray Valley encephalitis has occurred as epidemics in 1917, 1918, 1922, 1925, 1951, 1956, 1971, and 1974. The case fatality among the 320 cases that were described exceeded 50%, but fell to 20% in the most recent epidemic. Most cases occurred in the Murray–Darling basin in southeast Australia, but no evidence has been found of virus persistence in that area. The virus has been isolated from *Culex annulirostris,* the suspected vector, during the 1974 epidemic in southern Australia, and on several occasions from 1960–1975 in northern Australia; it has also been isolated from humans and mosquitoes in New Guinea. It seems likely that the virus survives in bird–mosquito cycles in northern Australia and New Guinea and is reintroduced into southern Australia, perhaps by way of the migration of birds.

São Paulo Encephalitis

An epidemic of encephalitis in São Paulo State, Brazil, in 1975–1976 was found to be caused by a previously undescribed flavivirus (Rocio Virus). The virus was isolated from humans, birds, and sentinel mice, but the vector and natural history are not yet known.

California Encephalitis

The prototype strain of California encephalitis group was isolated in 1943, and several cases of mild meningoencephalitis were diagnosed by serologic testing in 1943–1945. No further cases were diagnosed until 1960, when an additional member of the group, the La Crosse virus, was isolated from the brain of a patient who died of the disease in Wisconsin. Since then, the California encephalitis group of viruses has been found to be an important cause of meningoencephalitis that is usually mild. Five hundred and four cases of encephalitis in the United States were shown to be caused by California group viruses in 1963–1971. More recently cases have been diagnosed in Quebec Province, Canada. It seems likely that the virus survives in cycles involving small mammals of the genera *Lepus* (rabbits, hares), *Citellus* (squirrels), and *Peromyscus* (field mice), and several species of mosquitoes including *C. tarsalis, Aedes melanimon, A. atlanticus, A. infirmatus,* and *A. taeniorhynchus.* Overwinter survival can occur in the eggs of *Aedes* spp.

Tick-Borne Encephalitis

Encephalitis syndromes first recognized in Siberia in 1934 were shown to be caused by a tick-borne virus in 1937. Closely related viruses and syndromes were later found in European Russia and in other countries of eastern Europe. Louping ill, first recognized in sheep in Scotland in 1929, should also be considered in this group.

Cases of tick-borne encephalitis occur when humans contact or disturb endemic cycles of infection that normally involve small mammals (moles, shrews, field mice) and ixodid ticks (usually *Ixodes ricinus* or *Ixodes persulcatus*). Although there is transovarian passage of the virus in ticks, this is a relatively inefficient means for survival of the virus. Goats and sheep may also be infected and develop disease, with transmission to humans through contact with infected carcasses (as in louping ill). The virus is shed in goat's milk, and an epidemic of 600 cases in Czechosolvakia is believed to have been milk-borne.

Other members of the tick-borne encephalitis group include the Negishi virus, known only from two cases in Japan in 1948; and the Powassan virus, isolated from the brain of a patient with a fatal case in Canada in 1958 and since shown to survive in cycles involving small mammals, especially the groundhog (*Marmota*), and ixodid ticks, especially *I. marxi* and *I. cookei.*

Herpesvirus Encephalitis

The epidemiology of herpesvirus infection is described in Chapter 91, Infections Caused by Herpes Simplex Viruses. Person-to-person spread occurs by direct or indirect contact. Exposure is common in childhood and may result in subclinical infection but often evokes a gingivostomatitis. Almost all adults have antiherpes antibody; yet, many have recurrent herpetic lesions, especially around the mouth. Herpetic infection of the central nervous system can occur as a primary infection. However, some adult patients with herpes encephalitis have had febrile herpes; central nervous system involvement in these cases may represent recrudescent infection.

Herpesvirus simiae appears to spread and survive similarly in monkeys, and epidemics have been described in captive groups. Humans are infected most commonly by a bite, but cases have also been ascribed to the inhalation of monkey saliva and to contact with infected monkey cell cultures.

Kuru

The age and sex distribution of kuru, and its decline in recent years after ritual cannibalism was curtailed in the Fore area of New Guinea, led to the currently accepted hypothesis that the agent was transmitted by ingestion of, or contact with, undercooked human brain. No cases have occurred outside the Fore linguistic area. In contrast, the similar Jakob–Creutzfeldt disease occurs (rarely) throughout the world. The manner in which Jakob–Creutzfeldt disease spreads is unknown; however, the possibility of direct transmission is supported by the occurrence of the disease in families, and in neurosurgeons, neurosurgical patients, and recipients of corneal grafts.

Pathogenesis and Pathology

In experimental infections with arboviruses, an initial viremia is followed by localization in the central nervous system—a sequence that is believed to occur in humans. In fatal cases, there is little histopathologic change outside the nervous system, possibly excepting renal involvement in St. Louis encephalitis. On gross examination, there are varying degrees of meningitis, cerebral edema, congestion, and hemorrhage in the brain. Microscopic examination confirms a leptomeningitis with round-cell infiltration, small hemorrhages with perivascular cuffing, and nodules of leukocytes or microglial cells. Neuronal damage is seen as chromatolysis and neuronophagia. Areas of necrosis may be extensive, especially in eastern equine encephalitis, Japanese B encephalitis, and the Far Eastern form of tick-borne encephalitis. In patients who survive the initial illness, there are varying degrees of repair, which may include calcification. The pattern of distribution of lesions in the brain is rarely sufficiently specific to enable the identification of the infecting virus. However, the lesions in eastern equine encephalitis are concentrated in the cortex, in western equine encephalitis in the basal nuclei, and in St. Louis encephalitis in substantia nigra, thalamus, pons, cerebellum, cortex, bulb, and anterior horn cells. European forms of tick-borne encephalitis, including louping ill, commonly show a polioencephalomyelitis, with extensive involvement of the anterior horn cells mimicking poliomyelitis pathologically (and clinically).

Herpesvirus encephalitis in infants may be part of a general infection that produces focal necrotic lesions with typical intranuclear inclusions in many organs. In the adult and in some children, lesions are confined to the brain. Necrotic foci may be macroscopically evident as softenings. Inclusion bodies are readily found in the margins of areas of necrosis; focal perivascular infiltration and neuronal damage are evident. The temporal cortex and pons are commonly involved, but the lesions may be widespread.

In kuru and Jakob–Creutzfeldt disease, there is a progressive vacuolation in the dendritic and axonal process of the neurons, and to a lesser extent, in the astrocytes and oligodendrocytes. Extensive astroglial hypertrophy and proliferation occur, and a spongiform change, or status spongiosus, of gray matter is observed.

Manifestations

Infection with arboviruses is usually subclinical. Clinically evident infection varies in severity from a mild, aseptic meningitis to a rapidly fatal, necrotizing encephalitis. Typically, arbovirus encephalitides begin with the acute onset of fever, headache, and vomiting, progress to signs of meningeal involvement (stiff neck and back), and go on to show evidence of neuronal damage (drowsiness, coma, paralysis, convulsions, ataxia, organic psychoses).

The age distribution of disease varies with the causative virus, relating also to its endemicity in the area. Thus, before 1952 western equine encephalitis was most common in children in the Central Valley of California where the virus is endemic and subclinical infection of humans is common. On the other hand, recent epidemics of St. Louis encephalitis have occurred in areas with little previous exposure to this virus (*e.g.,* Houston, Texas). The age distribution of disease has been characteristic of the virus, with the highest attack rates occurring in the older age groups.

Cerebrospinal fluid (CSF) pleocytosis is typical, with up to 1000 leukocytes/mm^3. Mononuclear cells usually predominate, although early in fulminant encephalitis, polymorphonuclear leukocytes predominate. Glucose and chloride concentrations in the CSF are normal, and the protein is increased. The peripheral blood commonly shows a moderate polymorphonuclear leukocytosis.

Individual arbovirus encephalitides have some characteristic clinical features, although, as with histopathology, it is rarely possible to make a specific diagnosis on clinical evidence alone. Eastern equine encephalitis has the highest case fatality rate of the four arbovirus diseases encountered in the United States. Although benign infections without central nervous system involvement are caused by the eastern equine encephalitis virus, with overt encephalitis the mortality approaches 80%. In contrast, case fatality rates of 5% to 15% have been reported in western equine encephalitis and 2% to 20% in St. Louis encephalitis. Most cases of California virus encephalitis take the course of a benign, aseptic meningitis.

Venezuelan equine encephalitis causes fever lasting 1 to 4 days. Actual encephalitis is rare, and the fatality rate in the large epidemic in Venezuela in 1962–1964 was 0.6%.

The tick-borne encephalitides of Europe and Asia are commonly seen as poliomyelitislike syndromes, with flaccid paralysis and aseptic meningitis. Biphasic meningoencephalitis—characterized by an initial febrile illness, an asymptomatic period of several days, and a second meningitic illness that may progress to serious brain involvement—is seen frequently in the Central European form of the disease.

Herpes simplex virus infection of the central nervous system is frequently lethal, although the clinical presentation may vary from an aseptic meningitis to an acute encephalitis. Beyond clinical features common to other encephalitides, there frequently is intrusion of focal signs (disturbance of smell or taste, local electroencephalographic abnormalities) and increased cerebrospinal fluid pressure. Herpesvirus has also been described as the cause of a relapsing disease with progressive neurologic deterioration.

Infection with *H. simiae* may take the form of an acute encephalitis, or more frequently, a progressive myelitis. The outcome is virtually always death.

Kuru is characterized by a progressive ataxia with tremors exaggerated by emotion or muscular exertion, dysarthria, emotionalism, and deterioration to death within 6 to 9 months, rarely longer. Jakob–Creutzfeldt disease is a presenile dementia with involuntary movements and often ataxia.

Diagnosis

During epidemics, viral encephalitis is readily diagnosed on clinical grounds. However, sporadic cases are often difficult to distinguish from other febrile illnesses (*e.g.,* a child with gastroenteritis, dehydration, and convulsions) or from intoxications. Other infectious processes that must be considered include meningitis and meningoencephalitis caused by enteroviruses, mumps, *Leptospira* spp., *Naegleria* spp., bacteria, fungi, and the postinfectious encephalitides that follow measles, varicella, rubella, or vaccination.

The specific laboratory tests available give only a retrospective diagnosis in most cases. The serologic tests depend on the occurrence of a rise in antibody titer. However, the early detection of specific IgM antibody may assist early diagnosis.

Arboviruses can be isolated by inoculation of infant mice; recovery of the virus is most likely to be successful from specimens of brain tissue; it is rarely accomplished from blood or cerebrospinal fluid.

Herpesvirus can be isolated by the inoculation of brain or vesicle fluid into eggs, infant mice, or cell cultures. Encephalitis caused by recrudescence of latent herpesvirus may provoke rising titers of complement-fixing antibody. Recent attempts to treat herpesvirus encephalitis by chemotherapy accent the need for rapid diagnosis. The demonstration of inclusion bodies by immunofluorescence, and the isolation of the virus have been described from brain taken by needle biopsy after localization of the affected areas by electroencephalography.

Diagnosis of kuru and Jakob–Creutzfeldt disease depends on clinical features and histopathology.

Prognosis

Secondary bacterial infections of the respiratory and urinary tracts are major complications of acute encephalitis. They vary in severity directly with the severity of the encephalitis and generally decline in importance as the acute illness passes.

With recovery from acute viral encephalitis, evidence of neuronal injury and death becomes apparent as residual neurologic defects, impairment of intelligence, and psychiatric disturbances. The severity of these sequelae apparently varies according to the causative virus. Thus, after western equine encephalitis, sequelae are uncommon in adults, but frequent in children; recurring convulsions with motor or behavioral changes afflict more than half the children infected before they are 1 month old. With eastern equine encephalitis, most adults over the age of 40 who survive, do so unscathed; children under 5 years in age have crippling sequelae consisting of mental retardation, convulsions, and paralysis. Permanent sequelae after St. Louis encephalitis are uncommon.

Sequelae are reported in only 3% to 10% of cases of Japanese B encephalitis in Japan. Yet, 25% to 30% of young adult males of the armed forces of the United States in World War II had sequelae (including neuroses) 6 months after infection. In addition, 10 of 25 cases of Japanese B encephalitis on Guam, seen in 1948, had neurologic or intellect defects 10 years later.

Observers of the 1951 epidemic of Murray Valley encephalitis noted some instances of incomplete recovery.

Several syndromes of chronic central nervous system disease have been described following tick-borne encephalitis; it has been suggested that they may indicate continuing infection.

Therapy

There is no specific treatment for the arbovirus encephalitides. Accordingly, supportive care is of paramount importance, requiring devoted attention to the airway, bladder function, fluid and electrolyte balance, nutrition, prevention of bed sores, secondary pulmonary infection, and hyperpyrexia. Various chemotherapeutic agents (*e.g.,* 5-iodo-2-deoxyuridine, cytosine arabinoside, adenine arabinoside) have been given systemically to patients with herpesvirus encephalitis; the results with the latter agent are encouraging.

Prevention

Killed virus vaccines have been produced experimentally for several arboviruses. There has been wide use of only one such vaccine, a Japanese B virus preparation made from formalinized mouse brain; users of this vaccine in Japan claim it gives a high degree of protection. Limited use (*e.g.,* in exposed laboratory workers) has been made of Venezuelan equine encephalitis and tick-borne encephalitis virus vaccines. Passive immunization of laboratory workers exposed to a known virus in a laboratory accident has been accomplished with immune (human) serum or gamma globulin.

Control of the mosquito vector has been used with apparent good effect on several recent epidemics. Aerial spraying of insecticides to kill adult mosquitoes, if combined with measures to suppress the breeding of mosquitoes, is more likely to be effective in the urban–suburban breeding areas of the *C. pipiens* complex (*e.g.,* in the southern United States) than in rural habitats of *C. tarsalis, C. tritaeniorhynchus,* or *C. annulirostris*. However, reduction in the population of *C. tarsalis* has been achieved in some areas of California. Tick eradication, most often using DDT, has been found effective in the foci of tick-borne encephalitis in the U.S.S.R. Control of essential vertebrate hosts, for example, the small mammals important to the survival of tick-borne encephalitis viruses, is presently only a theoretic possibility. The immunization of nonhuman amplifying hosts has been used (*e.g.,* of horses against Venezuelan equine encephalitis in the United States) or suggested (*e.g.,* of pigs against Japanese B encephalitis in Japan).

Infection of humans with *H. simiae* can be prevented through care in the handling of monkeys and their tissues. Suitable codes of practice are given in the references.

Remaining Problems

The arbovirus encephalitides present a number of problems in the further study of (1) epidemiology—especially to complete our understanding of the natural cycles of infection, including virus survival between epizootics; (2) therapy—to find effective antiviral agents; and (3) prevention—to develop efficient vaccines and to devise effective and acceptable means for control of the vectors and nonhuman hosts.

Herpesvirus encephalitis also requires further study to make available rapid diagnostic methods and to develop effective chemotherapy. There is also need for more intensive investigation of the large number of patients diagnosed as having encephalitis in metropolitan areas in whom no etiologic diagnosis is presently established.

Our understanding of the agents of kuru and Jakob–Creutzfeldt disease, and of the mechanisms by which they produce disease, is still fragmentary.

Bibliography

Books

HORSFALL FL, TAMM I (eds): Viral and Rickettsial Infections of Man, 4th ed. Philadelphia, JB Lippincott, 1965. Chaps. 25–28, 41.

RHODES AJ, VAN ROOYEN CE (eds): Textbook of Virology, 5th ed. Baltimore, Williams & Wilkins, 1968. Chaps. 2/3, 3/10, and 3/11, and Section b.

SULKIN SE, PIKE RM: In LENNETTE EH, SCHMIDT NJ (eds): Diagnostic Procedures for Viral and Rickettsial Infections, 4th ed. New York, American Public Health Association, 1969. Chap. 2.

Journals

Arboviruses and human disease. Geneva, WHO Technical Series No. 369, 1967

CREECH WB: St. Louis encephalitis in the United States, 1975. J Infect Dis 135:1014–1016, 1977

HAYES CG, WALLIS RC: Ecology of western equine encephalomyelitis in the eastern United States. Adv Virus Res 21:37–83, 1977

MILLER JD, ROSS C: Encephalitis. Lancet 1:1121–1126, 1968

MONATH TP: Arthropod-borne encephalitides in the Americas. Bull WHO 57:513–533, 1979

POWELL KE, KAPPUS KD: Epidemiology of St. Louis encephalitis and other acute encephalitides. Adv Neurol 19:197–213, 1978

REEVES WC: Overwintering of arboviruses. Prog Med Virol 17:193–220, 1974

SMITH CEG: Arbovirus vaccines. Br Med Bull 25:142–147, 1969

SUDIA WD, NEWHOUSE VF: Epidemic Venezuelan equine encephalitis in North America: a summary of virus-vector-host relationships. Am J Epidemiol 101:1–13, 1975

ZIGAS V, GADJUSEK DC: Kuru: clinical study of a new syndrome resembling paralysis agitans in natives of the eastern highlands of Australia and New Guinea. Med J Aust 2:745–754, 1957

ALAN G. BARBOUR
SPOTSWOOD L. SPRUANCE

Colorado Tick Fever

123

Colorado tick fever (CTF) is a viral disease that is transmitted by ticks and occurs in the Rocky Mountain area and Pacific slope of the United States and Canada. There is a characteristic clinical course consisting of the biphasic appearance of fever, headache, and myalgias.

Etiology

Physicians in the newly settled Rocky Mountain region of the United States noticed a mild, tick-borne disease that was distinct from Rocky Mountain spotted fever. Subsequently, Florio was successful in transmitting the disease to volunteers and to hamsters by the injection of serum from patients. The agent was able to pass through filters that retained bacteria, and the causative organism was subsequently shown to be a double-stranded RNA virus. CTF virus is presently classified in the genus *Orbivirus* of the family Reoviridae. Isolates of CTF virus from humans have been of one major serotype. The virus is relatively stable at room temperature and is capable of infecting many types of mammalian cells in tissue culture.

Epidemiology

CTF occurs almost exclusively in the area of distribution of the wood tick *Dermacentor andersoni* (Fig. 123-1) and is acquired from the bite of virus-infected ticks. The virus has been recovered from other ticks in the Rocky Mountain and Pacific Slope areas, but *D. andersoni* is the only tick known to transmit the disease to man. Infection of persons who are transient in endemic areas may lead to the appearance of the disease outside of Western North America.

Dermacentor andersoni, a hard-body tick, is especially abundant in areas where small mammals share habitats with wild and domestic large mammals. Female ticks lay their eggs under dead vegetation. Larvae emerge and feed during the summer on small mammals, particularly rodents, rabbits, and hares. The larvae develop into nymphs and hibernate. In the spring, the nymphs feed on small mammals, fall off and molt into adults. The newly emerged adults take a blood meal and may mate, but more commonly hide under debris near the surface of the soil for a second winter. They then come out of hibernation when the snow melts and climb to the tips of low vegetation (Fig. 123-2), where they have the opportunity to transfer to animals brushing past. Adult ticks usually feed on wild and domestic large mammals or, accidentally, on humans. Female ticks attach and feed for 6 to 13 days, drop off to lay eggs, and die. The male may feed for only a few hours before seeking an attached female. CTF virus is acquired by the larvae and nymphs from feeding on small mammals that are viremic. The virus survives the winter in hibernating nymphs (or adults). The nymphs transmit the infection to other small mammals in the spring, thereby perpetuating a reservoir of the virus.

Although most patients with CTF report possible exposure to ticks while working, hiking, or camping, only one-half are aware of a tick bite or attachment. Males between the ages of 20 and 39 years contract CTF more often than other subgroups of the population, probably reflecting more frequent exposure to ticks. Thus, as many as 15% of forest rangers in endemic areas may possess neutralizing antibody against the virus.

The peak incidence of CTF in humans is in April and May at low altitudes, and in June and July at higher elevations—periods when adult *D. andersoni* are most active. The rare exceptions to this seasonality bespeak nontick transmission as in accidental inoculation of laboratory workers or the transfusion of blood-containing the virus.

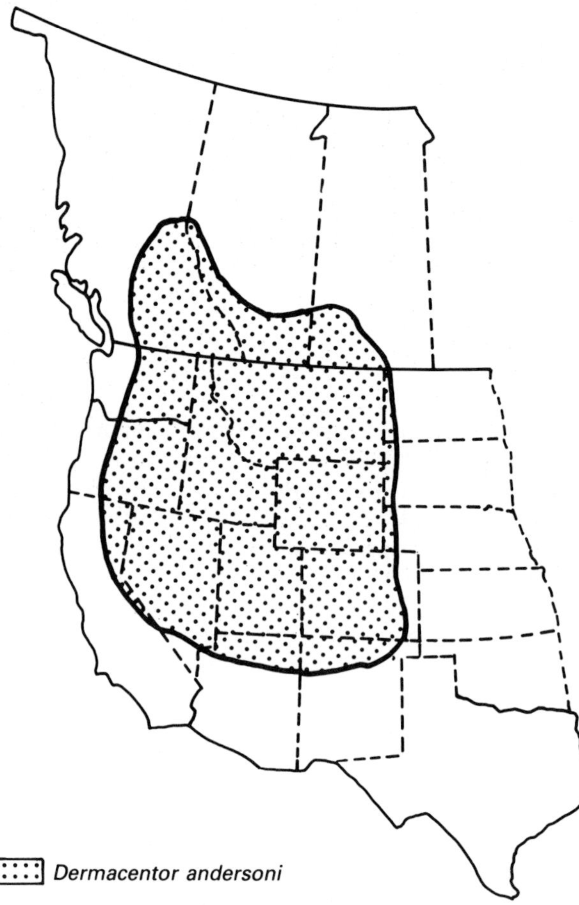

Fig. 123-1. Distribution of *Dermacentor andersoni* in the Western United States and Canada. (After Eklund CM, Kohls GM, Brennan JM: Distribution of Colorado Tick Fever and virus-carrying ticks. JAMA 157:335–337, 1955)

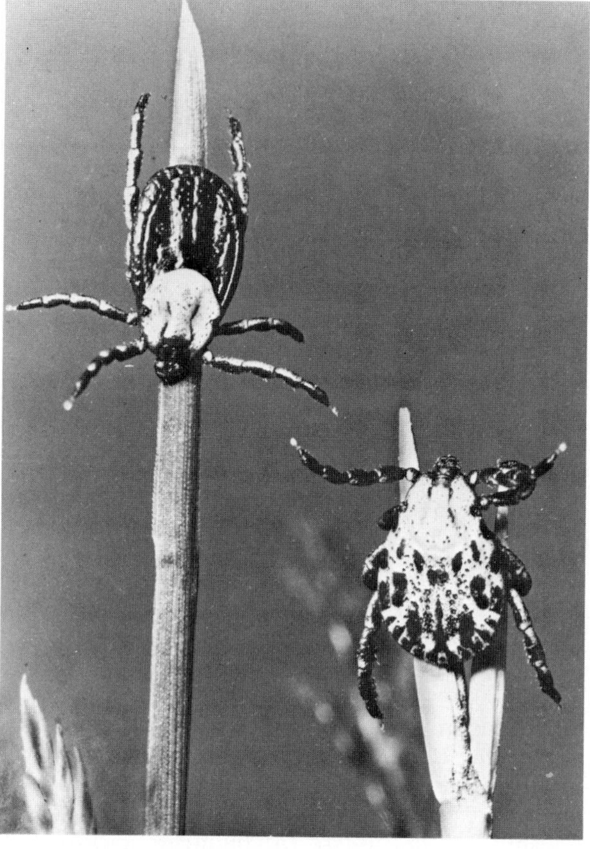

Fig. 123-2. An adult female (left) and male (right) *andersoni* are shown on vegetation. The ticks are waiting to transfer to a mammalian host. (Photograph courtesy of the Rocky Mountain Laboratories, NIAID, NIH, Hamilton, Montana)

Pathogenesis and Pathology

Viremia is almost always found in patients with CTF and in animals experimentally infected with the virus. CTF virus can be recovered from the plasma during the first week of illness and from the blood clot for up to 120 days after onset of the disease. The virus persists inside red cells long after all signs and symptoms have abated, and the duration of viremia corresponds with the normal life span of circulating erythrocytes (Figs. 123-3 and 123-4). The mature erythrocyte lacks functional ribosomes essential to virus replication, and entry of virus into mature erythrocytes has not been demonstrated. It is likely, then, that infection of red cells begins in hematopoietic cells, a hypothesis that is supported by the demonstration of virions and virus replication within erythrocyte precursors in the bone marrow.

Leukopenia is a characteristic finding during the course of CTF. The white cell count typically reaches its nadir during the second febrile episode, and may continue to be depressed for up to 7 days after clinical recovery (Fig. 123-4). Although both polymorphonuclear leukocytes and lymphocytes are decreased in absolute numbers, the percentage of polymorphonuclear cells may increase along with an increase in the proportion of immature neutrophils in the peripheral blood. Bone marrow examinations have revealed a maturation arrest in the neutrophil series.

In the rare hemorrhagic form of the disease, thrombocytopenia and disseminated intravascular coagula-

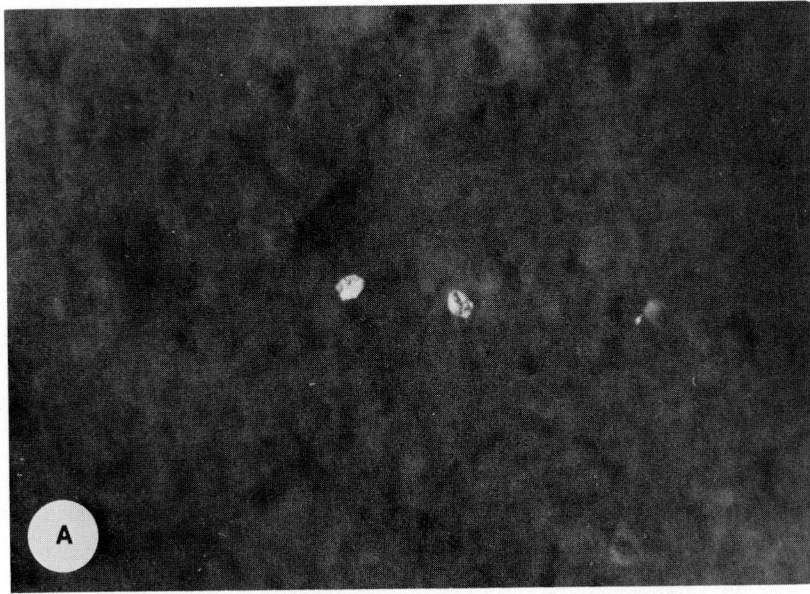

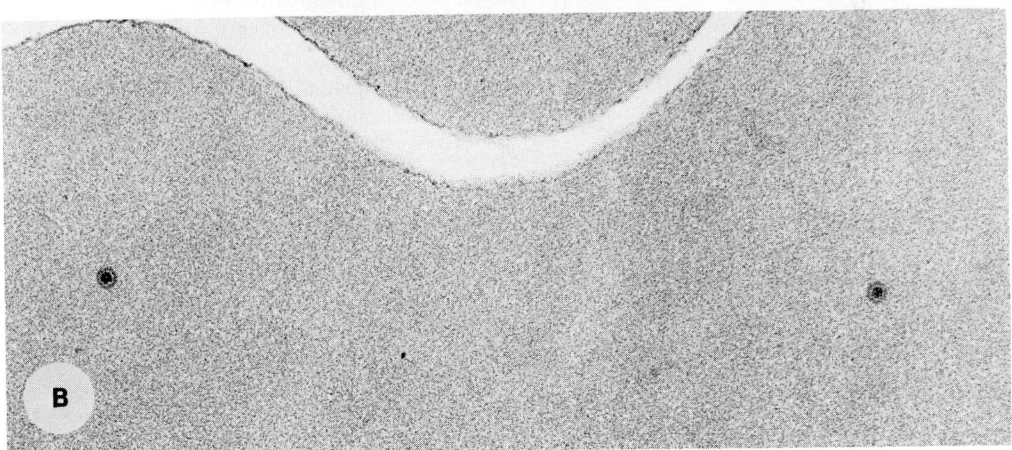

Fig. 123-3. Location of CTF virus in human erythrocytes. *A.* Immunofluorescence of erythrocytes from a patient with CTF. *B.* CTF inside erythrocyte. (original magnification × 50,000) (Emmons RW, Oshiro LS, Johnson HN, Lennette EH: Intraerythrocytic location of Colorado tick fever virus. J Gen Virol 17:185–195, 1972)

tion (DIC) were shown to occur, and there was endothelial swelling with focal necrosis of capillaries in a fatal case.

The rare occurrence of encephalitis and meningitis in CTF probably results from viral invasion of the brain and meninges. The virus was recovered from the cerebrospinal fluid of one patient with encephalitis as well as from that of experimentally infected subjects who had no neurologic symptoms. Intracytoplasmic inclusion bodies were seen in neurons and Purkinje cells of the midbrain in one fatal case of encephalitis.

Manifestations

The incubation period is usually 3 to 5 days, occasionally as long as 14 days. The onset is sudden. Symptoms are commonly maximal within a few hours. Patients often report chilliness, but true rigors do not occur. The usual symptoms are fever, headache, and myalgias, notably of the back and legs. The muscle pains can be severe. Retroorbital pain and pain on ocular movement are commonly reported. Diarrhea is infrequent, but approximately 20% of patients have abdominal pain or vomiting.

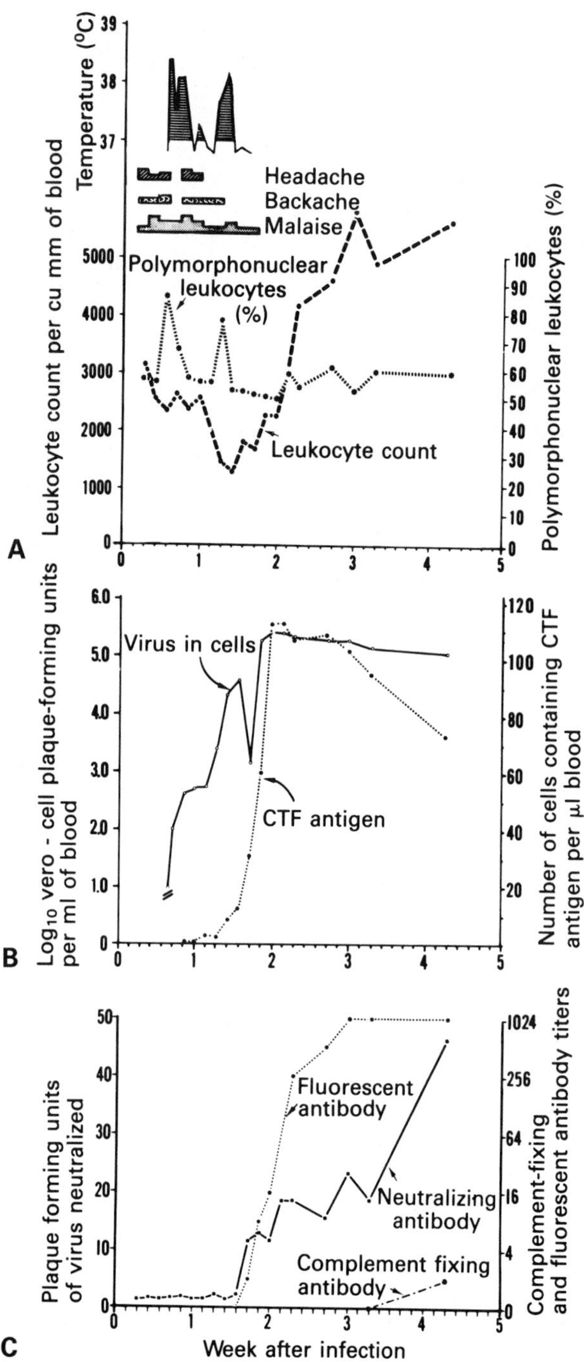

Fig. 123-4. Time course of a laboratory-acquired case of CTF. *A* Oral temperature, clinical manifestations, total leukocyte count, and percent polymorphonuclear leukocytes in the blood. *B* CTF virus in the peripheral blood by virus culture and CTF antigen on red cells by fluorescent antibody staining. *C* Fluorescent antibody, neutralizing antibody, and complement-fixing antibody to CTF virus. (Courtesy of Dr. R. N. Philip, Rocky Mountain Laboratories, NIAID, NIH, Hamilton, Montana)

Most patients experience a characteristic biphasic or "saddle back" fever in which a 2 to 3 day febrile period is followed by a 1 to 2 day remission. This is followed in turn by another 2 to 3 day febrile period (Fig. 123-4). The remaining patients have either a single febrile episode or, less frequently, three bouts of fever.

Physical findings are usually few. A mild, transient rash may be seen in approximately 10% of patients. The rash may be petechial, macular, or maculopapular in character. Flushed facies, conjunctival injection, pharyngeal erythema, tachycardia, and a palpable spleen are other signs that may be observed. An imbedded tick should be sought by examination of the entire body, including the scalp.

Complications of CTF are rare and are usually limited to children. Meningitis, encephalitis, meningoencephalitis, and a hemorrhagic state resembling the hemorrhagic syndrome of dengue have occurred (see Chap. 90, Dengue). The coincidence of rash and central nervous system (CNS) involvement may make distinction from Rocky Mountain spotted fever difficult (see Chap. 96, Spotted Fevers). In adults, pericarditis and myocarditis have occurred in association with CTF. Other unusual complications have been epididymo-orchitis, arthritis, pleuritis, chorioretinitis, and pneumonitis.

Diagnosis

Fever, myalgias, and leukopenia occurring in late spring or summer and associated with recent exposure to ticks in the mountains of the Western United States or Canada should suggest CTF. A biphasic clinical course is a highly specific feature, although biphasic fever also occurs with dengue. Dengue can usually be excluded on epidemiologic grounds; however, the recent migration of dengue to northern Mexico heralds the possibility for confusion between these two diseases. Influenza is also characterized by fever and myalgias, but usually occurs in the fall or winter and in associated with symptoms of respiratory tract involvement (see Chap. 28, Influenza).

In the Western United States, confusion between CTF and Rocky Mountain spotted fever was once common. Rocky Mountain spotted fever can usually be distinguished from CTF by the progressive rash that appears 2 to 6 days after onset, a tendency to leukocytosis, and a more severe course. Although *Rickettsia rickettsii,* the agent of Rocky Mountain spotted fever, may still be recovered from *D. andersoni,* this disease is less frequently reported in the Western United States. Simultaneous infections with both Rocky Mountain spotted fever and CTF have occurred, and ticks that carry both CTF virus and *R. Rickettsii* have been found.

Relapsing fever, a disease caused by spirochetes of the genus *Borrelia* and transmitted by soft-body ticks, also occurs in the endemic areas of CTF (see Chap. 143, Relapsing Fever). In this disease, the leukocyte count is commonly normal and the spirochete can often be seen in smears of peripheral blood.

Tularemia may rarely be tick-borne in the Rocky Mountain area (see Chap. 139, Tularemia). Regional lymphadenopathy and ulceration at the site of the tick bite are typical. The agglutination test for tularemia is reactive after 10 to 14 days.

The leukopenia accompanying CTF may be striking enough to provoke concern about hematopoietic diseases. Leukocyte counts of 1,000 to 3,000 per cubic mm are observed. The lowest values occur during the second febrile period; at the outset, the leukocyte count may be normal. "Toxic" neutrophils and atypical lymphocytes may also be found, and mild to moderate thrombocytopenia is often seen.

The diagnosis of CTF can be confirmed by isolation of virus from blood, identification of the agent in erythrocytes by fluorescent antibody staining, or serology (Fig. 123-4). The titer of virus may be higher in the plasma than in the cellular fraction of the blood during the first few days of illness—until neutralizing antibody appears in the serum. For these reasons, whole blood should be examined during the first 3 days after onset, the blood clot on days 4 to 10 of illness, and a washed blood clot thereafter. The virus is stable, and specimens can be sent by mail. The direct fluorescent antibody examination of a blood clot is positive in virtually all cases from 5 days to about 2 months after onset. False-negative tests may occur during the first few days of the disease. For virus isolation, red cells are homogenized and injected into suckling mice. After 3 to 4 days, the heart blood of the mouse is examined by fluorescent antibody staining. A fourfold rise in neutralizing antibodies, complement-fixing antibodies, or antibodies in the indirect immunofluorescence assay is also diagnostic. However, these tests are rarely needed when the suckling mouse and direct fluorescent antibody tests are available. Diagnostic tests for CTF are available at most state health department laboratories in the endemic area.

Prognosis

Only one death from CTF has been reported. Many patients, especially those over 30 years of age, complain of malaise and weakness during a prolonged convalescence. There is no apparent association between the duration of viremia and the length of convalescence. Although there is one documented case of reinfection, immunity generally appears to be lifelong.

The CTF virus crosses the placenta and is teratogenic in laboratory animals. In six women who had CTF while pregnant, the outcome was as follows: four normal babies, one spontaneous abortion, and one infant with multiple congenital abnormalities.

Therapy

Because there is not specific therapy, the treatment is symptomatic. Analgesic and antipyretic drugs are usually adequate for control of headache and myalgias. In a patient with petechiae or other evidence of a hemorrhagic syndrome, salicylates should not be used. When a pateient appears to be seriously ill and there is a history of exposure to ticks, the possibility of other treatable tick-borne diseases such as Rocky Mountain spotted fever, relapsing fever, and tularemia may warrant administration of a tetracycline until the diagnosis becomes certain.

Prevention

Avoidance of tick bites is the cornerstone of prevention. Persons going into an area likely to have ticks should wear clothing that fits tightly at wrists, ankles, and the waist. The application of repellants to the clothing and the skin is helpful (see Chap. 115, Trombiculosis). Because ticks seldom attach during the first few hours of contact, inspection of the clothing, hair, and skin twice daily is usually sufficient.

Attached ticks should be removed. Lighted cigarettes or open flames should not be applied because of the danger of inflicting burns. A 10-minute application of alcohol, nail polish remover, ether, acetone, or benzene to a tick using a saturated pledget of cloth will aid in detachment. Gentle, straight traction backwards should then be applied with the fingers or with forceps. Care should be taken not to crush the tick because this might contaminate the wound with potentially infectious liquid. The tip of a needle may be inserted under the imbedded head of the tick before applying traction. If these maneuvers fail, or if mouth parts are left in the skin, the hypostome-bearing skin should be excised.

An experimental vaccine prepared from inactivated virus was successful in producing high titers of neutralizing antibody in volunteers. Possible use of a vaccine would appear to be justifiable only for laboratory personnel working with the virus and outdoor workers in highly endemic areas.

The patient with CTF does not pose a risk of contagion and need not be isolated. However, the patient's blood should be considered potentially hazardous and should not be used for transfusion for at least 6 months after the illness.

Remaining Problems

The mechanism of the leukopenia seen in CTF remains to be determined. Infection of precursor cells in the bone marrow or suppression of such cells by high concentrations of interferon has been suggested.

Another unresolved question is the prognosis for the fetus when a woman has CTF during the early stages of pregnancy. Further information on the outcomes of such pregnancies will permit more adequate counseling of patients.

Our understanding of CTF would be much enhanced if we learned those features of the host–parasite relationship that result in the biphasic clinical course of the illness.

Bibliography

Books

EMMONS RW: Colorado tick fever. In Beran G (ed): CRC Handbook of Zoonoses, Section B, Viral Zoonoses, Vol. I. Cleveland, CRC Press, 1979. pp 113–124.

PHILIP RN, CASPER EA, CORY J, WHITLOCK J: The potential for transmission of arboviruses by blood transfusion with particular reference to Colorado tick fever. In GREENWALT TJ, JAMIESON GA (eds): Transmissible Diseases and Blood Transfusion. New York, Grune & Stratton, 1975. pp 175–195.

Journals

EKLUND CM, KOHLS GM, BRENNAN JM: Distribution of Colorado tick fever and virus-carrying ticks. JAMA 157:335–337, 1955

EMMONS RW, DONDERO VS, DEVLIN V, LENNETTE EH: Serologic diagnosis of Colorado tick fever: A comparison of complement-fixation, immunofluorescence, and plaque-reduction methods. Am J Trop Med Hyg 18:796–802, 1969

EMMONS RW, LENNETTE EH: Immunofluorescent staining in the laboratory diagnosis of Colorado tick fever. J Lab Clin Med 68:923–929, 1966

FLORIO L, STEWARD MO, MUGRAGE ER: The experimental transmission of Colorado tick fever. J Exp Med 80:165–187, 1944

GOODPASTURE HC, POLAND JD, FRANCY DB, BOWEN GS, HORN KA: Colorado tick fever: Clinical, epidemiologic, and laboratory aspects of 228 cases in Colorado in 1973–1974. Ann Intern Med 88:303–310, 1978

HARRIS RE, MORAHAN P, COLEMAN P: Teratogenic effects of Colorado tick fever virus in mice. J Infect Dis 131:397–402, 1975

OSHIRO LS, DONDERO DV, EMMONS RW, LENNETTE EH: The development of Colorado tick fever virus within cells of the haemopoietic system. J Gen Virol 39:73–79, 1978

SPRUANCE SL, BAILEY A: Colorado tick fever: A review of 115 laboratory confirmed cases. Arch Int Med 131:288–293, 1973

THOMAS LA, PHILIP RN, PATZER E, CASPER E: Long duration of neutralizing-antibody response after immunization of man with a formalinized Colorado tick fever vaccine. Am J Trop Med Hyg 16:60–62, 1967

GEORGE L. HUMPHREY
DENNY G. CONSTANTINE

Rabies

124

Rabies is primarily a viral infection of nonhuman carnivores. Transmission to man is rare and is usually effected through a bite. Clinical evidence of involvement of the central nervous system (CNS) appears after an extremely variable period of incubation. A deep-seated fear of rabies is typical despite the actual rarity of the infection in humans—reflecting knowledge of the near certainty of death once disease is overt.

Etiology

On the bases of morphology, host range, tissue tropism, and susceptibility to chemical reagents, the rabies virus is classified with the rhabdoviruses. In infected tissues, the virions are nonpleomorphic, bullet-shaped particles about 75 nm in diameter × 180 nm in length. At the center of each there is a helical ribonucleo-protein capsid 50 nm in diameter, which contains a single strand of RNA. A dense, lipoprotein-containing membrane surrounds the virion; accordingly, lipid solvents inactivate the virus. The membrane is covered by surface projections, 6 nm to 8 nm long, each with a knoblike structure at the distal end; an indentation at the flat end of the particle is free of surface projections. These morphologic features are shown in Fig. 124-1.

Sunlight, ultraviolet irradiation, air, heat, bichloride of mercury, formalin, and strong acids and bases are all destructive to the rabies virus. The virus is resistant to putrefaction in infected brain tissue; it is also resistant to phenol and bacteriostatic concentrations of thimerosal. Glycerol preserves the infectivity of infected tissues. Accordingly, specimens (brain or other tissues) for laboratory examination may be shipped by mail when placed in a 50% neutral glycerol-saline solution.

Rabies virus has been propagated in a wide variety of cell culture systems and in embryonated chicken and duck eggs. Viruses propagated in cell cultures and eggs are widely used in the production of rabies vaccines for animals and man. Mammals are susceptible to rabies, but the degree of susceptibility varies widely.

Immunization against rabies produces neutralizing, hemagglutination-inhibiting, complement-fixing, and lytic antibodies. Neutralizing antibodies are stimulated by the glycoprotein antigens in the virion envelope, and are of primary importance in evaluating the immune state.

Epidemiology

Rabies occurs worldwide in wildlife, causing widespread, migrating, cyclic epidemics alternating with periods of endemicity. The urban occurrence of rabies in dogs is an aberrant, man-made cycle resulting from development of the urban complex and domestication of the dog as an urban companion. No true reservoir host of rabies (as a latent, silent, nonfatal infection) has been found in nature. However, on the basis of epidemiologic and ecologic reasoning, members of the Mustelidae (weasel–skunk) and Viverridae (civet–ferret) families seem to be the most likely sources of rabies virus, initiating the migrating epidemics of rabies observed in wildlife periodically. In Australia, New Zealand, the islands of the South Pacific, and Hawaii, where mammals of these two families were not part of the natural fauna, there was no rabies.

Although rabies occurs naturally in wildlife, dogs continue to be the principal vector of rabies in Africa, Latin America, Asia, Greece, Spain, and Yugoslavia. Wild animals are presently the main vectors of rabies in other countries in Europe, Canada, and the United States. Foxes are primarily involved in Europe, skunks and foxes in Canada and the United States, and the mongoose in Grenada and Puerto Rico. Rabies in

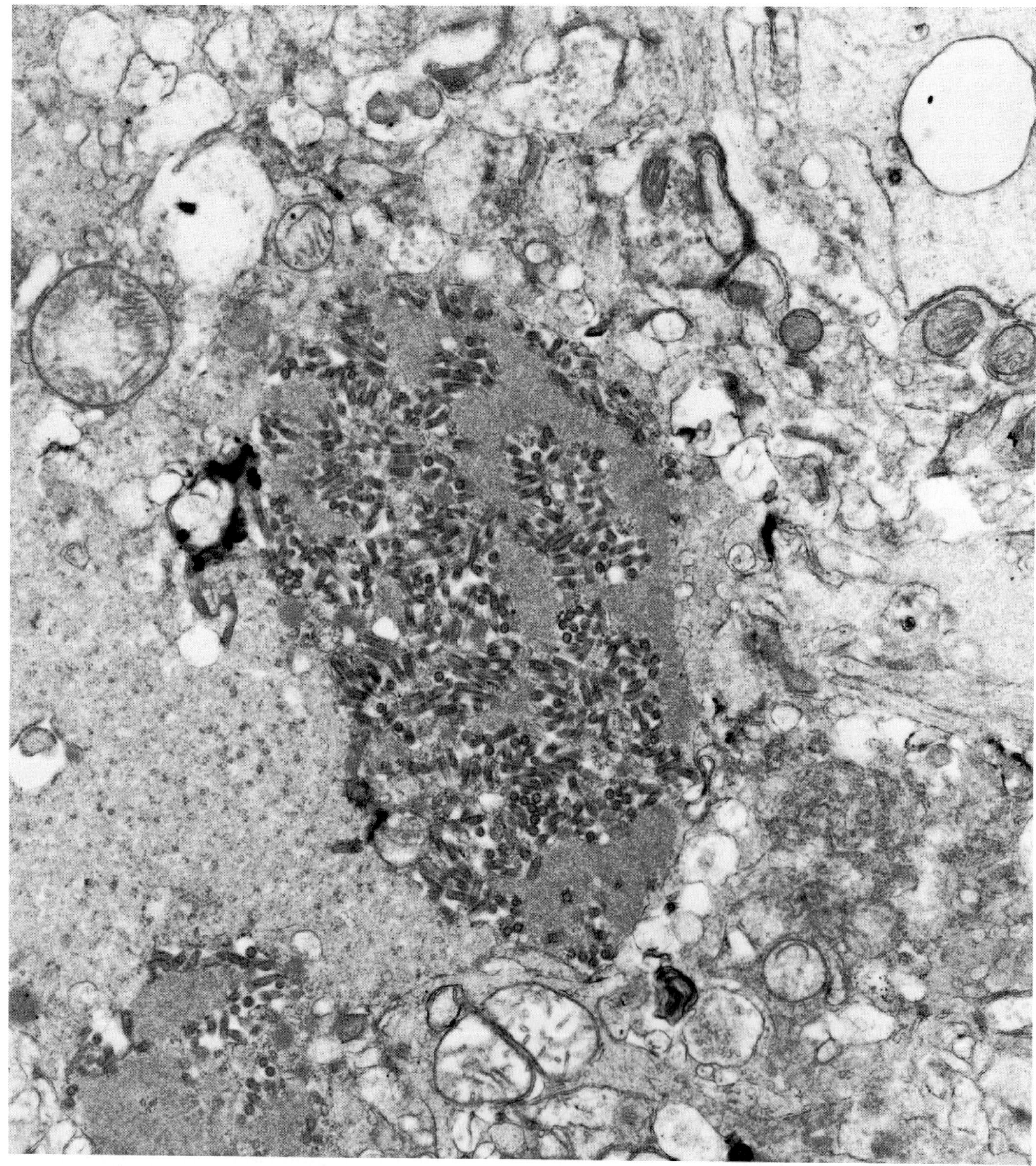

Fig. 124-1. Electron micrograph of rabies virus in mouse brain. (Original magnification approximately × 30,480) (Courtesy of CS Callaway)

Table 124-1. *Breakdown of the 5,150 Cases of Rabies Reported to the Centers for Disease Control in the United States in 1979**

Animal	Number	Percentage
Man	5	0.1
Dogs	196	3.8
Cats	156	3.0
Livestock	284	5.5
Skunks	3031	58.9
Foxes	145	2.8
Bats	756	14.7
Raccoons	543	10.5
Other wild species	34	0.7

*of the reported cases, 4509 (87.5%) occurred in wildlife.

vampire bats results in heavy losses of livestock from Mexico to Argentina. Occasionally, rabies in humans results from exposure to vampire bats. Jackals are the chief vectors of rabies in India and Israel, and wolves in Iran.

In the United States during 1979, 4504 (87.6%) of the 5145 cases of nonhuman animal rabies were reported in wildlife (Table 124-1). The occurrence of rabies in livestock and in dogs—the usual vector for humans in the United States—generally parallels the disease in wildlife (Fig. 124-2A).

Since rabies was first recognized in insectivorous bats in Florida in 1953, it has been identified in 30 of the 39 species of free-living and colonial bats native to the United States. Only Alaska and Hawaii of the 50

Fig. 124-2. (*A*) Reported cases of rabies in wild and domestic animals by year in the United States 1953–1979. (Morbid Mortal Week Rep Suppl, Summary, 1979) (*B*) Reported cases of rabies in humans by year in the United States, 1951–1979. (Morbid Mortal Week Rep Suppl, Summary, 1979)

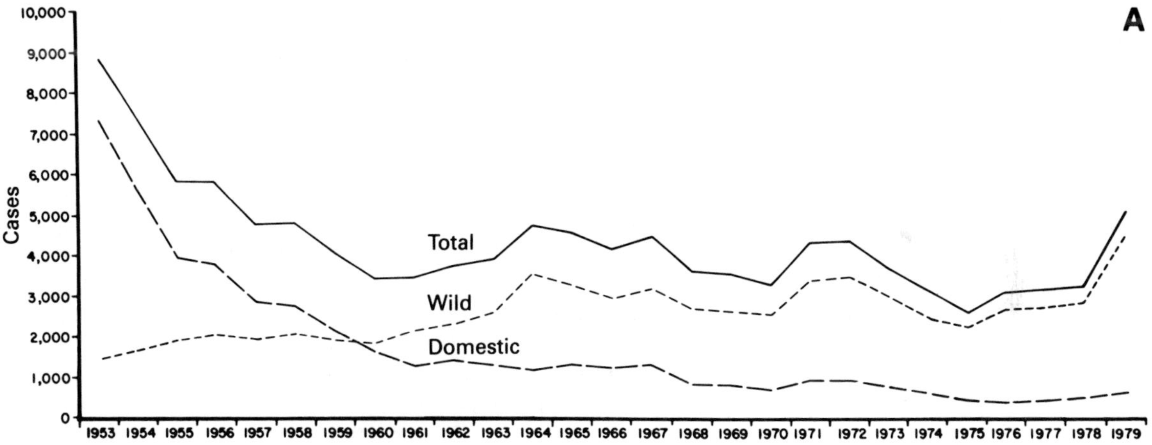

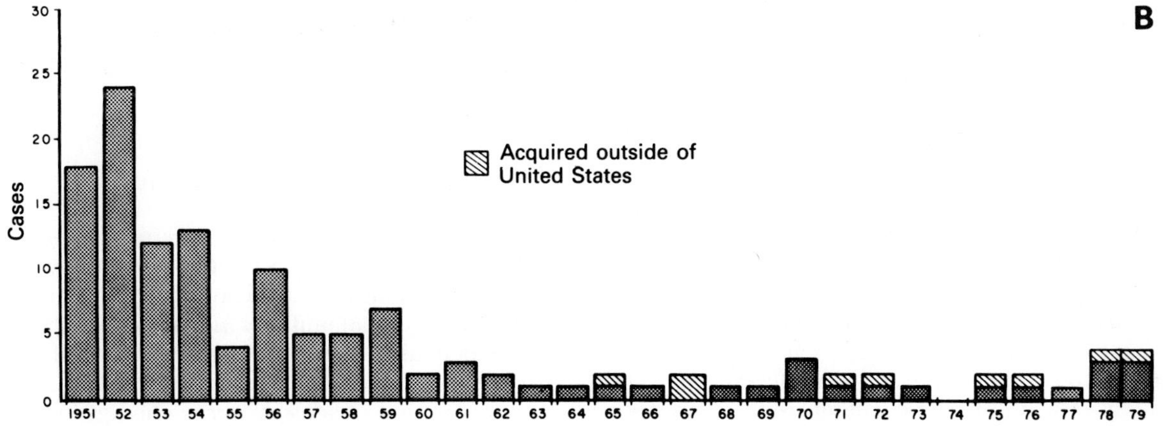

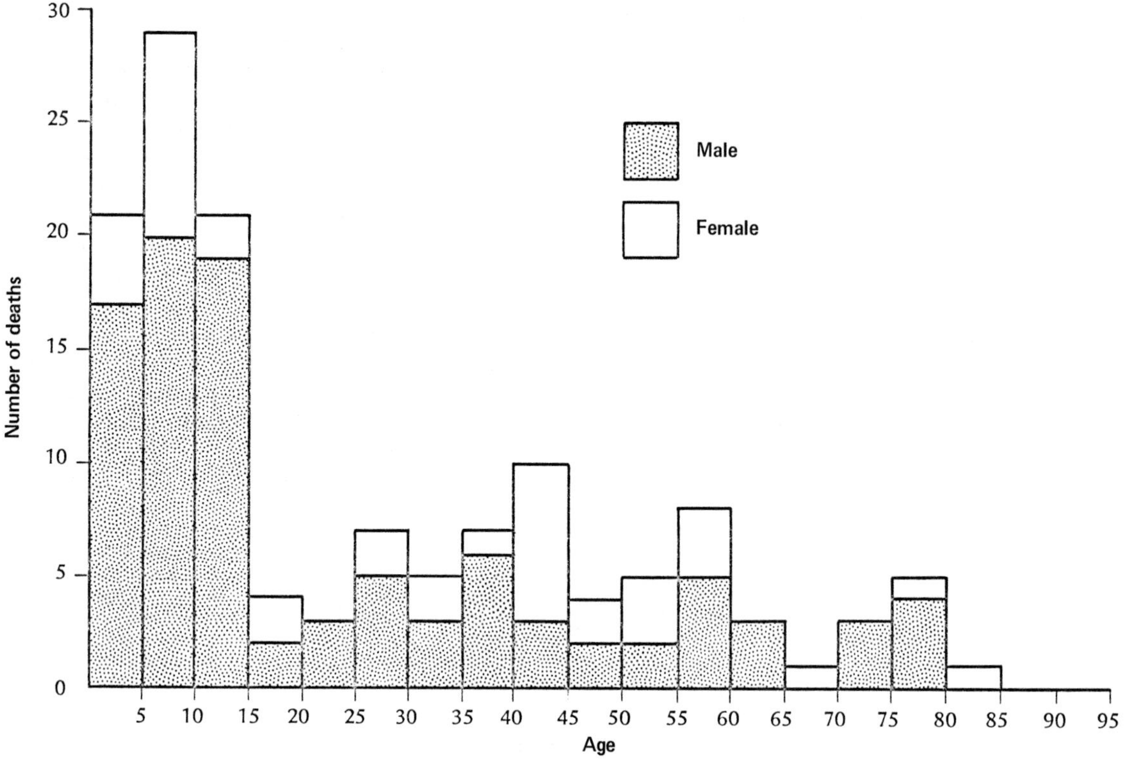

Fig. 124-3. Deaths from rabies in the United States 1950–1973, according to age and sex. (Courtesy of WG Winkler)

states have not reported rabies in bats. A relatively high proportion of the cases reported in bats have been found in the Pacific Coast states; 1653 cases were reported in bats in California between 1954 and 1979.

There is no evidence that insectivorous bats have been involved in the transmission of rabies to terrestrial nonhuman mammals. However, humans have been infected when bitten by rabid bats.

Two persons who entered Frio Cave, Texas, which harbored millions of *Tadarida b. mexicana* bats, subsequently died of rabies, although no bites where sustained. Rabies was known to be present in these bats; infection apparently occurred through the respiratory tract. Subsequently, when rabies developed in coyotes and foxes held in Frio Cave for 24 to 30 days in bat-proof, insect proof cages, air-borne transmission was proved. The rabies virus has also been isolated from the air of Frio Cave by using a mechanical air sampler.

There is a marked variation in the efficiency of mammals as vectors of rabies, perhaps as a function of efficiency of viral replication in salivary glands. Definitely of highest risk of infectivity in the United States are the bites of the skunk, fox, bobcat, bat, badger, and coyote. Intermediate risk is associated with bites inflicted by the dog, raccoon, and cat. Lowest risk, seldom, if ever, requiring antirabies prophylaxis, attends bites from gophers, various squirrels, wild rats and mice, pet rats and mice, guinea pigs, moles, and chinchillas.

In the past two decades, fewer than five cases of rabies per year have been reported in humans in the United States (Fig. 124-2B). Males are infected more often than females with persons under 15 years more often involved than older persons (Fig. 124-3).

Pathogenesis and Pathology

The rabies virus is usually transmitted to humans by a bite that implants saliva containing an infective dose of virus in muscle and near nerve tissue. It appears that the virus can multiply in muscle tissue at the site of inoculation. The virus travels along the nerves from the point of inoculation to the CNS. The dense concentration of sensory nerve endings in the head, face, neck, and fingers accounts for the higher fatality rate observed when these areas are exposed. Similarly, the more extensive or severe the bite wounds, the higher the mortality, because more nerve tissue is exposed to an infective dose of rabies virus. The deposition of saliva on intact skin or on scabbed-over cuts or scratches at least 24 hours old does not require antirabies treatment. The rabies virus, however, is apparently capable of infecting through mucous membranes; such exposure should be handled in the same manner as exposures by bites.

Rabies virus inoculated intramuscularly in animals rapidly falls off in titer but can persist for 24 hours at the site of inoculation and in some instances up to 96 hours. After either intramuscular or intracerebral injection of rabies virus in animals, a period occurs during which the virus cannot be detected. However, the virus will be detected subsequently in the portion of the CNS into which it was injected. After entering the CNS, the virus replicates in the neurons of gray matter before traveling centrifugally along nerves from the CNS to invade a variety of organs and tissues.

Baby mice dying of experimental rabies pass the disease on to the mother if she eats them. The role of ingestion in the transmission of rabies in nature, however, is not known.

The transplacental transmission of rabies did not occur in a pregnant woman with rabies, nor has it been observed in pregnant bats dying of rabies. The young of all species, however, are extremely susceptible to rabies, and it is not uncommon for a rabid female dog or skunk to infect her entire litter before dying of the disease. The route of transmission is not precisely known, but transmucosal infection could occur as the infected mother licks her offspring. The possibility of transmission from an infected mother to her nursing young through lactating mammary glands has not been excluded.

There are marked differences between species in susceptibility to rabies. Also, the susceptibility of a given host has been observed to vary with the origin of virus used in the experimental studies; for example, foxes are apparently more susceptible to strains of virus derived from foxes than are skunks.

Environmental studies in bats show that a lowering of temperature extends the incubation period. Temperature may thus play a role in the pathogenesis of rabies in bats, because their body temperature at rest approximates that of the environment, reducing metabolism and slowing the development of rabies infection.

Adrenocorticotrophic hormone, stress due to crowding, and probably stress from intercurrent infection are capable of activating latent or incubating rabies virus to produce clinical disease.

The rabies virus has been isolated from a variety of organs of naturally infected animals. The virus replicates in the salivary glands to attain titers that often exceed those found in the brain. Rabies virus has been isolated from the kidneys, lactating mammary glands, lungs, pancreas, lacrimal glands, salivary glands, adrenals, brown fat, nasal mucosa, and muscle tissue in naturally infected animals. However, rabies virus has not been isolated from any of these sites in the absence of the virus in the CNS.

Animals dying of natural rabies, or so-called street rabies virus infection, commonly exhibit characteristic intracytoplasmic inclusion bodies in the neurons of the brain; these are called Negri bodies. The presence of Negri bodies has been regarded as pathognomonic of rabies infection, but lack of them does not exclude the infection. The development of Negri bodies relates directly to the host species, the viral strain, and the duration of the clinical illness and probably depends on the establishment of numerous and extensive foci of virus synthesis. The Negri bodies are probably composed of matrices of both viral components and entrapped cellular organelles.

In humans who have died from rabies, Negri bodies are prominent in ganglion cells, particularly in the hippocampus and cerebellum. Other changes also present in the CNS include edema, hemorrhage, congestion, and perivascular cuffing in all parts, but most severe in the pons and medulla. In the cranial, spinal, and sympathetic ganglia, there are actual foci of necrosis with neuronophagia and infiltration with lymphocytes. The severity of the histopathologic changes in the spinal cord often corresponds to the site of the bite; for example, the lumbar cord is extensively affected when the bite is on the foot. Gross changes are inconspicuous.

Fixed rabies virus, that is, virus that has been serially passed intracerebrally in laboratory animals (usually the rabbit), exhibits a loss of infectivity on peripheral inoculation, a greatly shortened incubation period on intracerebral injection, loss of ability to produce Negri bodies, increased virus titer in the brain, and a loss of ability to invade the salivary glands. Strains of virus originating from wildlife differ in their capacity to produce Negri bodies. Other characteristics exhibited by some wildlife strains are extended incubation periods in inoculated mice, the production of a low titer of virus in brain tissue, a pathogenicity for infant mice nearly as great by intraperitoneal or intramuscular inoculation as by intracerebral injection, and the invasion and multiplication of the virus in salivary glands, lungs, kidneys, pancreas, and muscle tissue. Some strains may produce spastic paralysis in adult mice on intracerebral injection with a high rate of recovery.

Manifestations

The clinical phases of rabies are generally the same in all species including humans: prodromal, excitation (or furious in dogs), and paralytic (or dumb in dogs). In humans, until advance to the paralytic phase, mental faculties are, unfortunately, well preserved. The incubation period in humans is usually 1 to 3 months, but is extremely variable, ranging from 10 to 300 days.

Prodromal Phase

The onset of clinical rabies in humans includes 2 to 4 days of prodromal manifestations, most of which are nonspecific. A degree or two of fever, malaise, headache, anorexia, nausea, and sore throat are common. There may also be increasing nervousness, anxiety, irritability, depression and melancholia, with or without a sense of impending death. Hyperesthesia, an increased sensitivity to bright light and loud noise, excessive salivation, lacrimation, and perspiration have been noted. The general muscle tone may be increased, and facial expression can be overactive. Dilated pupils, an increased pulse rate, and shallow respirations are seen. However, by far the most significant symptoms are abnormal sensations referred to the site of inoculation; noted by 80% of patients, these include pain (local or radiating), burning, a sensation of cold, pruritus, and tingling.

Excitation Phase

The excitation phase begins gradually and may persist until death. It may be punctuated at any time by depression and paralysis. There usually are increasing anxiety, apprehension, and a sense of impending doom. Although the tone of the somatic musculature is increased, there may be weakness of the muscle groups around the location of the bite. Cranial nerve malfunctions result in ocular palsies with strabismus and incoordination of the extraocular muscles; dilation or constriction of the pupils that may be asymmetric and associated with hippus, nystagmus, or diplopia; lack of corneal reflexes; weakness of the facial muscles; and hoarseness. There may be tachycardia or bradycardia, cyclic respiration, urinary retention, and constipation.

Hydrophobia, the classic diagnostic manifestation of rabies, is an affliction of the excitatory phase of the disease. When the patient attempts to swallow liquids, forceful, painful expulsion occurs as a consequence of spasmodic contraction of the muscles of swallowing and respiration. Once experienced, the sight, sound, or smell of liquids may provoke the syndrome. The ensuing choking may cause severe apnea and cyanosis. Death frequently occurs during the course of such a convulsive attack. Hydrophobia is observed only in humans. Paralysis of muscles of swallowing occurs commonly in animals, but the hydrophobic contractions observed in humans are lacking. Dehydration is a common consequence.

Paralytic Phase

Hydrophobia, if present, disappears and swallowing becomes possible, although difficult, as the paralytic phase of rabies sets in. A progressive, general, flaccid paralysis develops—rarely in the pattern of Landry's ascending paralysis. Apathy shades into stupor, progressing to coma. There is urinary incontinence. Peripheral vascular collapse ensues and death follows.

Diagnosis

Where there is a history of bite by a known rabid animal and the bitten person shows typical symptoms, the clinical diagnosis of rabies is usually evident. In many instances, a history of exposure is lacking, and the diagnosis of rabies may be missed unless revealed by postmortem laboratory tests.

Clinical laboratory findings are of no value in the diagnosis. There may be a leukocytosis and slight proteinuria, but the cerebrospinal fluid is normal.

Other conditions possibly confused with rabies are poliomyelitis, other viral encephalitides, and paralysis resulting from rabies vaccine containing nerve tissue. After a clear-cut exposure to rabies, the bitten person may develop rabiesphobia or hysteria, and may simulate convulsive seizures.

A definitive diagnosis of rabies in animals and in humans depends on laboratory procedures. Virus isolation should be attempted during the clinical course of the disease from saliva or throat swab specimens, spinal fluid, urine, and conjunctival and nasal secretions. In one instance, rabies was confirmed by a fluorescent rabies antibody (FRA) test of brain tissue obtained by craniotomy before death (San Diego County, California, 1969). Rabies virus could not, however, be recovered after death, 133 days after the onset of illness.

Possible postmortem sources of virus include brain, spinal cord, submaxillary salivary glands, lacrimal glands, muscle tissue, lung, kidney, pancreas, and adrenal glands. All specimens secured during life, and postmortem tissues, should be frozen as soon as possible to ensure suitable preservation for the subsequent inoculation of mice. For FRA testing or mouse inoculation, brain tissue should be immersed in 50% neutral glycerol-saline solution or frozen. For preparation of paraffin sections, the brain tissue should be fixed in Zenker's fluid containing 5% glacial acetic acid.

Brain tissue for examination for Negri bodies is best kept refrigerated but not frozen. If delay in examination or if shipping is necessary, brain tissue for Negri body examination can be placed in 50% neutral glycerol-saline solution. Paraffin sections can also be stained for Negri bodies, but cannot be used for the FRA test. Formalin-fixed brain sections may be rendered suitable for staining by the FRA technique by carefully controlled trypsin digestion.

The FRA test is the most sensitive and accurate means of examining for rabies that is available. In an experienced laboratory, it is rapid (overnight in the California Department of Health Services and in a few hours when urgently needed), and the reliability (99.95%) is such that a negative report weighs heavily in the decision not to treat a bitten person.

Fecal specimens should be obtained for isolation of enteroviruses. Also, acute and convalescent sera should be collected for serologic studies.

Prognosis

Clinical rabies is usually considered to be invariably fatal, because rabies virus has never been isolated from a patient with manifest rabies who subsequently recovered. It is important, in the rare human cases that occur, to obtain adequate specimens early in the illness for animal inoculation and for serologic tests so that apparent recovery from rabies can be verified. Thus, for the first time in 1971, virus was isolated from a throat swab, saliva, an eye swab, urine sediment, and cerebrospinal fluid obtained from a 6-year-old boy in California prior to death.

Antemortem diagnosis has been accomplished in some advanced cases in humans by FRA demonstration of viral antigen in the neural structures of facial or posterior nuchal skin and corneal cells collected by pressing a slide against the cornea. These techniques have resulted in some false-positive readings.

An occasional experimental animal inoculated intramuscularly with rabies virus shows clinical symptoms of rabies and then recovers. There have been no isolations of the rabies virus from the saliva of such animals. However, saliva would not be examined until recovery or clinical improvement was evident, by which time the salivary glands and brain would be expected to be negative. Thus, attempts at isolation of the virus have not been carried out on specimens from nonhuman animals and humans that show symptoms and subsequently recover. However, cerebrospinal fluid rabies antibody titers have been used to diagnose the infection in recovered humans and nonhuman animals.

Therapy

There is no specific therapy for overt rabies. The only means proven useful are preventive and must be initiated as quickly as possible after exposure.

The patient with clinical rabies should be made as comfortable as possible. Barbiturates, phenothiazines, and paraldehyde are used symptomatically. Morphine is contraindicated; small doses may actually increase excitement. Intensive care with particular attention to continuous pulmonary and cardiac monitoring from the outset of clinical illness may be lifesaving in view of recent reports of the extended survival in three laboratory-confirmed cases of clinical rabies (64 days in Kansas, 1968; 133 days in San Diego, 1969; 28 days in Oakland, 1971); the recovery of probable cases (Lima, Ohio, 1970; Argentina, 1973; and New York, 1977).

With the complete recovery of a human with rabies in 1970 and survival with severe sequellae in 1973 and 1977, it is clear that aggressive intensive care should begin early in the disease and be maintained. Prevention of complications such as hypoxia, hypotension, and superinfection is most important.

Prevention

Management of persons potentially exposed to rabies requires the least possible delay in deciding whether to treat, because the longer treatment is postponed, the less likely it is to be effective. Always, the risk of infection must be balanced against the risk of prophylactic treatment. Treatment consists of local measures applied to wounds, the administration of immune globulin, and the inoculation of rabies vaccine. The following recommendations are drawn largely from the 1980 rabies prevention report of the Immunization Practices Advisory Committee (ACIP), United States Department of Health and Human Services, modified according to subsequent recommendations of the ACIP and information from the Centers for Disease Control. References to the duck embryo vaccine (DEV) were deleted because it is no longer available. Also deleted were recommendations for routine serologic testing of persons who received human diploid cell rabies vaccine (HDCV) preexposure or postexposure prophylaxis because of the efficacy of the vaccine (*e.g.*, 510 persons who had preexposure, and 1299 of 1300 persons who had postexposure prophylaxis developed protective levels of antibody). The ACIP also discouraged routine serologic testing after booster doses of HDCV for persons given the recommended primary HDCV vaccination of those shown to have had an adequate antibody response to primary vaccination with other rabies vaccines. Serologic testing was recommended for persons whose immune response might be diminished by drug therapy or other causes. Finally, an unlicensed but ACIP-recommended method of HDCV administration by intradermal inoculation was included under preexposure immunization.

Globulins

Rabies immune globulin (RIG), human, is gamma globulin concentrated from the plasma of hyperimmune human donors. Each milliliter contains 150 IU of neutralizing antibody. It is supplied in 2-ml (300-IU) and 10-ml (1500-IU) vials for pediatric and adult use, respectively.

Antirabies serum (ARS), equine, is refined, concentrated serum from hyperimmune horses. Each 5-ml vial contains 1000 IU. Both products are effective, but RIG is the product of choice, because is rarely causes adverse reactions, whereas over 40% of adults given ARS develop serum sickness.

Rabies Vaccine

Human diploid cell rabies vaccine (HDCV) is supplied as 1-ml, single-dose vials of lyophilized vaccine with accompanying diluent. It is prepared from fixed rabies virus grown on WI-38 cells and inactivated by tri-n-butyl phosphate, or on MRC-5 cells and inactivated with β-propiolactone.

The Decision to Treat

Each possible exposure to rabies should be evaluated individually by the physician, who should consult local or state public health officials if questions arise about the need for rabies prophylaxis. Several factors should be considered before specific antirabies prophylaxis is initiated in the United States (Table 124-*2A*).

Wild carnivorous mammals (especially skunks, foxes, coyotes, raccoons, and bobcats) and bats are the most commonly infected animals and have caused most of the cases of rabies in humans in the United States since 1960. Postexposure prophylaxis should be initiated upon bite or nonbite exposures to one of these animals, and the treatment should be discontinued if the animal is tested and proves to be negative for rabies infection. The need for postexposure prophylaxis following exposures to dogs or cats varies from region to region according to the likelihood that these species are infected. Rodents and rabbits are rarely infected with rabies, they have never caused human rabies in the United States, and their bites almost never call for specific antirabies treatment.

The circumstances of a biting incident are important. An unprovoked attack is more likely than a provoked attack to indicate that the animal is infected with rabies virus. Bites experienced when feeding or handling an apparently healthy animal are usually considered provoked.

Exposures are categorized as either bite or nonbite. The former is any penetration of skin by teeth. Nonbite exposures are scratches, abrasions, open wounds, or mucous membranes contaminated with saliva or other potentially infectious matter such as brain tissue from an infected animal, or inhalation of aerosolized virus. Airborne infection of two persons (probable) and of sentinel animals (proved) occurred only in the presence of millions of bats in densely populated caves. Two laboratory workers were infected by rabies aerosols that leaked from faulty, aerosol-creating laboratory apparatus.

Management of biting animals is critical and differs according to species and circumstances (Table 124-*2A*). The local health department should be notified. Healthy dogs or cats should be confined and observed for 10 days, and at the first sign of illness the health department should be notified and the animal evaluated by a veterinarian. At the development of rabieslike signs, the animal should be killed and its head shipped under refrigeration for rabies testing in a laboratory designated by the local or state health department. Stray or unwanted dogs or cats should be killed and tested without delay. Similarly, wild animals should be killed and tested at once, because the signs of rabies cannot be reliably interpreted in these species. If the brain is negative for rabies by the FRA test, one can assume that the saliva did not contain rabies virus, and the bitten person need not be treated.

Postexposure Prophylaxis

Postexposure antirabies treatment includes (1) local treatment of wounds; (2) globulin—preferably RIG—administered only once at the beginning of therapy; and (3) vaccine (Table 124-2*B*). However,

Table 124-2A. Rabies Postexposure Prophylaxis Guide[*]

	Animal	Condition of Animal at Time of Attack	Treatment of Exposed Person[†]
Domestic	Dog and cat	Healthy and available for 10 days of observation	None, unless animal develops rabies[‡]
		Rabid or suspected rabid	RIG[§] and HDCV[″]
		Unknown (escaped)	Consult public health officials. If treatment is indicated, give RIG[§] and HDCV[″]
Wild	Skunk, bat, fox, coyote, raccoon, bobcat, and other carnivores	Regard as rabid unless proven negative by laboratory tests[#]	RIG[§] and HDCV[″]
Other	Livestock, rodents, and lagomorphs (rabbits and hares)	Consider individually. Local and state public health officials should be consulted on questions about the need for rabies prophylaxis. Bites of squirrels, hamsters, guinea pigs, gerbils, chipmunks, rats, mice, other rodents, rabbits, and hares almost never call for antirabies prophylaxis.	

[*] These recommendations are only a guide. In applying them, take into account the animal species involved, the circumstances of the bite or other exposure, the vaccination status of the animal, and presence of rabies in the region. Local or state public health officials should be consulted if questions arise about the need for rabies prophylaxis.

[†] All bites and wounds should be immediately and thoroughly cleansed with soap and water. If antirabies treatment is indicated, both rabies immune globulin (RIG) and human diploid cell rabies vaccine (HDCV) should be given as soon as possible, regardless of the interval from exposure.

[‡] During the usual holding period of 10 days, begin treatment with RIG and HDCV at first sign of rabies in a dog or cat that has bitten someone. The symptomatic animal should be killed immediately and tested.

[§] If RIG is not available, use antirabies serum, (ARS) equine. Do not use more than the recommended dosage.

[″] Local reactions to vaccines are common and do not contraindicate continuing treatment. Discontinue vaccine if fluorescent-antibody (FA) tests of the animal are negative.

[#] The animal should be killed and tested as soon as possible. Holding for observation is not recommended.

(After Morbid Mortal Week Rep, June 30, 1980)

persons previously given HDCV or with an adequate antibody titer from previous immunization with a different rabies vaccine should not receive globulin.

LOCAL TREATMENT OF WOUNDS

As soon as possible after exposure, bite wounds or scratches should be thoroughly washed with soap and water, swabbed, and copiously flushed. This is probably the most effective measure for preventing rabies. Deep wounds should be flushed by injection with a 20% green soap solution using a blunted needle attached to a large syringe. Also, repeated, vigorous swabbing to the depths of the wound should be carried out using cotton-tipped applicators soaked in the wash fluid. Immune globulin should be infiltrated into the tissues under the wound, supplementing IM administration. Tetanus prophylaxis and measures to control bacterial infection should be given as indicated. The immediate suturing of bite wounds is not recommended.

Table 124-2B. Rabies Immunization Regimens

Pre-Exposure Pre-exposure rabies prophylaxis for persons with special risks of exposure to rabies, such as animal-care and control personnel and selected laboratory workers, consists of immunization with human diploid cell rabies vaccine (HDCV), according to the following schedule.

Rabies Vaccine	No. of 1-ml Doses	Route of Administration	Intervals Between Doses
HDCV	3	Intramuscular	1 week between 1st and 2nd; 2–3 weeks between 2nd and 3rd*

Postexposure Postexposure rabies prophylaxis for persons exposed to rabies consists of the immediate, thorough cleansing of all wounds with soap and water, administration of rabies immune globulin (RIG) or, if RIG is not available, antirabies serum (ARS), equine, and the initiation of HDCV, according to the following schedule.†

Rabies Vaccine	No. of 1-ml Doses	Route of Administration	Intervals Between Doses
HDCV	5‡	Intramuscular	Doses to be given on days 0, 3, 7, 14, and 28*

*Serum for rabies antibody testing should be collected 2–3 weeks after the last dose from persons whose immune responses may be diminished by drug therapy or for other reasons. If the titer is inadequate (<1:16 by the rapid fluorescent-focus inhibition test at CDC), give an additional booster dose and collect serum for testing 2–3 weeks later. If no antibody response is evident, consult the state health department or CDC.

†The postexposure regimen is greatly modified for someone who has previously received recommended preexposure or postexposure regimens of HDCV or with previously demonstrated rabies antibody from any rabies vaccine.

‡The World Health Organization recommends a 6th dose 90 days after the 1st dose.

(After Morbid Mortal Week Rep, June 30, 1980)

GLOBULIN

One dose of RIG (or ARS if RIG is unavailable) is given at the start of antirabies immunization to provide antibodies until the patient produces his own in response to vaccine (which should occur by the eighth day of treatment). Therefore, if RIG inadvertently was not given when vaccination was started, it can be given up to the eighth day after the first dose of vaccine, but not later. The dose of RIG is 20 IU/kg of body weight; when ARS must be used, the dose is 40 IU/kg. Ideally, up to half the dose of globulin is infiltrated in the tissues around the wound, and the remainder is given intramuscularly. No more than the recommended dose should be given, because the immunoglobulin may partially suppress production of antibody.

VACCINE

HDCV should be given in conjunction with globulin, preferably RIG. The Centers for Disease Control (CDC) found that one dose of RIG and five doses of HDCV produced excellent antibody response, and none of 77 persons bitten by infected animals and so treated developed rabies. The World Health Organization (WHO) performed a similar successful study wherein six instead of five doses of HDCV were used. The CDC recommends that five 1-ml doses be given intramuscularly. The first dose should be given as soon as possible after exposure; an additional dose should be given on each of days 3, 7, 14, and 28 after the first dose (WHO recommends a sixth dose 90 days after the first). For persons with diminished immune competence, the titer of rabies antibody in the serum should be measured on day 28 to determine if treatment was effective or if additional vaccine is needed. At least 2 ml of serum (recovered promptly after 5 ml of blood has clotted) should be delivered (refrigerated or frozen) to the laboratory for testing, as can be arranged by the state health department. An antibody titer ≥ 1:16 by the rapid fluorescent-focus inhibition (RFFI) test is an adequate response to vaccination according to the CDC.

Pre-Exposure Immunization

Frequently undertaken by persons in high-risk groups (certain laboratory workers, veterinarians, animal handlers, mammalogists, and persons entering countries where rabies is a constant threat), pre-exposure immunization guards against inapparent infection and anticipated delay in starting immunization, eliminates the need for immunoglobulin following exposure, and decreases the number of doses of vaccine needed.

HDCV is given intramuscularly as three 1-ml injections, on days 0, 7, and 21 or 28. For persons with diminished immune competence, blood should be tested for antibody 2 to 3 weeks after the last injection; HDCV has consistently produced antibody. However, if the antibody response is inadequate, a booster dose should be given, and blood should be collected for antibody testing 2 to 3 weeks later.

Persons with continuing risk of exposure should receive a 1-ml booster dose of vaccine every 2 years. Persons who work with live rabies virus in research laboratories or vaccine production facilities and are at risk of high-dose, inapparent exposure should receive a booster dose every 6 months or be tested for rabies antibody and vaccinated when their antibody titer falls below 1:16 as measured by the RFFI test.

The ACIP has recommended an as yet unlicensed alternate method of preexposure immunization: three 0.1-ml inoculations of HDCV are given intradermally in the lateral aspect of the upper arm over the deltoid on days 0, 7, and 21 or 28; booster doses may be required, as described for IM administration of the vaccine. Licensure awaits appropriate packaging and labeling changes by the manufacturer.

Following exposure to rabies, a person properly vaccinated with HDCV or with previously demonstrated rabies antibody following vaccination with a different rabies vaccine should receive two doses of HDCV (one at once and one 3 days later); immunoglobulin should not be given. A person who has been vaccinated previously with a vaccine other than HDCV but whose immune status has never been determined should be considered fully susceptible and should receive complete postexposure antirabies treatment, including immunoglobulin. However, if antibody can be demonstrated in serum taken before immunization, treatment can be discontinued after two doses of HDCV. Blood may be taken for serum antibody testing 2 to 3 weeks after the last dose.

Accidental Inoculation With Modified Live Rabies Virus (MLV) Vaccines

Insufficient data exist to assess the risk of needle stick or spray exposure of persons to any of the MLV vaccines. Consequently, persons who frequently administer these products should receive and maintain pre-exposure immunization. There have been no reported human cases from exposure to any of the two attenuated strains of rabies virus used in animal rabies vaccines in the United States (high egg passage Flury strain and Street Alabama Dufferin strain; however, an unknown proportion of exposed persons had prior immunization or postexposure treatment. Because these vaccines have been in use more than 10 years without associated cases in humans, the CDC does not recommend treatment following exposure to them. However, both strains may have produced rabies in domestic carnivores, and rabies has resulted in humans from accidental exposure to aerosols of laboratory-altered SAD as well as to the challenge virus standard (CVS) strain.

Adverse Reactions

Reports issued by the CDC on rabies prophylaxis in the United States indicate that adverse reactions to HDCV are markedly fewer and generally less serious than those associated with earlier vaccines. Local reactions (*e.g.,* pain, erythema, and swelling or itching at the injection sites) were reported in about 25% of recipients, mild systemic reactions (*e.g.,* headache, nausea, abdominal pain, muscle aches, and dizziness) were reported in about 20%, and systemic allergic reactions (from hives to anaphylactic shock) in about 0.16%. No neuroparalytic reactions were attributed to HDCV. A single, nonfatal case of Guillain–Barré syndrome was temporarely associated with the use of HDCV in Europe, but a cause–effect relationship was not established. Other inactivated rabies vaccines are used in many developing countries. Inactivated nerve tissue vaccine reportedly causes neuroparalytic reactions in 1 in every 2000 recipients; the rate for inactivated suckling rodent brain vaccine is about 1 in 8000.

RIG administration may be followed by local pain and low-grade fever. Adverse reactions (angioneurotic edema, nephrotic syndrome and anaphylaxis) have rarely been associated with the use of immune serum globulin, but a causal relationship is unclear; it is possible that similar reactions may rarely be seen with the use of RIG. ARS should be used only when RIG cannot be obtained. ARS causes serum sickness in about 40% of adults and fewer children; because it may produce anaphylactic reactions, the patient should be tested for sensitivity to equine serum.

Management of Adverse Reactions

Local or mild systemic adverse reactions are insufficient cause to interrupt or discontinue rabies prophylaxis and are usually controlled with anti-inflammatory and antipyretic drugs (*e.g.,* aspirin). Antihistamines may be given when a person with a history of hypersensitivity must be given rabies vaccines Anaphylactic reactions may be counteracted with epinephrine.

Because anaphylactic reactions rarely develop during the administration of HDCV (or neuroparalytic reactions during the use of other rabies vaccines available outside the United States), the physician must weigh the risk of developing rabies against the risk of discontinuing treatment. If glucosteroids are used to treat neuroparalytic reactions, the development of active immunity to rabies may be inhibited: it is important to test the patient's serum for rabies antibodies. Serious adverse reactions should be reported to the state health department.

Pregnancy is not thought to be a contraindication to postexposure prophylaxis as fetal abnormalities have not been associated with rabies vaccination.

Remaining Problems

There is need for investigation of ingestion as a means of transmitting rabies infection and the possible role ingestion may play in nature.

Knowledge of the pathophysiologic changes in affected nerve tissue during the passage of rabies virus from the site of exposure to the CNS is lacking. A more complete understanding of what is involved may enable the blocking of virus travel from the site of exposure to the CNS. The prolonged incubation periods sometimes observed in rabies remain a biologic mystery, and raise major questions about latency and the rabies virus–host cell relationship. The mechanism of stress in converting latency to overt disease is unknown.

Research should continue on interferon, which is produced in response to some live and some inactivated rabies vaccines. Exogenous or synthetic interferon, given at the time of exposure, is protective in animals, and interferon inducers with vaccine may be more protective than vaccine alone.

There is a need for quantification of evidence that distinct rabies virus strains exist in nature almost exclusively within particular host species. A monoclonal antibody technique, recently applied in rabies strain differentiation studies, should supplement earlier methods of strain characterization. As a result, sources of infection might be disclosed, revealing epidemiologic patterns and links that should be broken to effect maximal control.

Bibliography

Books

BAER GM (ED): The Natural History of Rabies, Vol. I and II. New York, Academic Press, 1975. 454 pp and 387 pp respectively.

CONSTANTINE DG: Rabies Transmission by Air in Bat Caves. U. S. Public Health Service Publ 1617. Washington D. C., U. S. Government Printing Office, 1967. 51 pp.

CONSTANTINE DG: Bats in relation to the health, welfare, and economy of man. In Wimsatt WA (ed): Biology of Bats. Vol. II. New York, Academic Press, 1970. pp 319–449.

International Association of Biological Standardization (eds): Joint HWO/IABS Symposium on the Standardization of Rabies Vaccines for Human Use Produced in Tissue Culture (Rabies III). Develop Biol Standard Vol. 40. BASEL, S KARGER, 1978. 292 pp.

JOHNSON HN: Rabies virus. In HORSFALL FL, TAMM I (eds): Viral and Rickettsial Infections of Man, 4th ed. Philadelphia, JB Lippincott, 1965. pp 814–840.

JOHNSON HN: Rabies virus. In LENNETTE EH, SCHMIDT NJ (eds): Diagnostic Procedures for Viral and Rickettsial Infections, 5th ed. New York, American Public Health Association, 1979. pp 843–877.

NAGANO Y, DAVENPORT FM (eds): Rabies. Tokyo, University of Toyko Press, 1971. 406 pp.

Expert Committee on Rabies, Sixth Report. WHO Technical Report Series No. 523. Geneva, World Health Organization, 1973. 55 pp.

Journals

BHATT DR, HATTWICK MAW, GERDSEN R, EMMONS RW, JOHNSON HN: Human rabies: Diagnosis, complications, and management. Am J Dis Child 127: 862–869, 1974

HUMPHREY GL: Rabies: Suggested indications for treatment of exposed persons. Calif Med 107: 363–377, 1967

MURPHY FA, BAUER SP, HARRISON AK, WINN WC: Comparative pathogenesis of rabies and rabies-like viruses: Viral infection and transit from inoculation site to the central nervous system. Lab Invest 28: 361–376, 1973

MURPHY FA, HARRISON AK, WINN WC, BAUER SP: Comparative pathogenesis of rabies and rabies-like viruses: Infection of the central nervous system and centrifugal spread of virus to peripheral tissues. Lab Invest 29:1–16, 1973

Public Health Service Advisory Committee on Immunization Practices: Rabies prevention. Morbid Mortal Week Rep 29 (23):265–280, June 13, 1980

Public Health Service Advisory Committee on Immunization Practices: Supplementary statement on rabies vaccine and serologic testing. Morbid Mortal Week Rep 30:535–536, 1981

Public Health Service Advisory Committee on Immunization Practices: Supplementary statement on pre-exposure rabies prophylaxis by the intradermal route. Morbid Mortal Week Rep 31:279–280, 285, 1982

MAURY E. MULLIGAN
SYDNEY M. FINEGOLD

Intracranial Suppuration

125

Localized suppurative infection within the cranium may occur as brain abscess (within the brain parenchyma itself), subdural abscess or empyema (in the subdural space between the dura mater and the arachnoid), or epidural or extradural abscess (in the potential space between the dura and the overlying skull). Brain abscess is the most common, but subdural empyema carries the greatest threat to life.

Brain Abscess

Etiology

The etiologic agents of intracranial suppuration vary primarily with the site and kind of antecedent infection, and to a lesser extent, with predisposing factors. The common isolates are anaerobic bacteria (including anaerobic cocci, *Bacteroides* spp., *Fusobacterium* spp., *Actinomyces* spp., and less often *Clostridium* spp.) and aerobic gram-positive cocci (*Staphylococcus aureus, Streptococcus pneumoniae, Streptococcus pyogenes,* and viridans group *Streptococcus* spp.). Fastidious bacteria such as *Actinobacillus actinomycetemcomitans* and *Haemophilus aphrophilus* may also be found. Two or more microorganisms are detected in approximately 30% of positive cultures.

Brain abscesses that arise as a direct extension of infection from the middle ear, mastoids, sinuses, or oropharynx frequently yield anaerobes, although aerobes, such as the various streptococci, *S. aureus, Haemophilus influenzae,* and occasionally Enterobacteriaceae (*e.g., Proteus* spp.), may be encountered. In the compromised host, however, unusual pathogens must be considered. For example, in rhinocerebral zygomycosis (see Chap. 128, Zygomycoses) direct extension of fungal infection of the nasopharynx may lead to intracranial abscess.

Brain abscesses following hematogenous spread from a preceding lung abscess or other pleuropulmonary infection are commonly caused by anaerobic pathogens. *Nocardia* spp., *Aspergillus* spp., and the Zygomycetes may also be found in this setting, especially in the compromised host.

Staphylococcus aureus may cause brain abscess in association with endocarditis, and is the most likely pathogen in brain abscess that follows accidental or surgical trauma to the head. In patients with congenital heart disease, brain abscesses are most often caused by aerobic and anaerobic cocci. Additional, uncommon causes of brain abscess include various Enterobacteriaceae such as *Klebsiella* spp. and *Enterobacter* spp., and *Pseudomonas* spp., which may originate from primary genitourinary or intraabdominal infections; *Haemophilus* spp., *Neisseria meningitidis,* and *Listeria monocytogenes,* which are usually associated with meningitis; *Mycobacterium* spp.; various fungi such as *Candida* spp. and *Phialophora* spp.; and protozoa, including *Entamoeba histolytica.*

Epidemiology

The introduction and widespread application of antibacterial agents have not changed the incidence of brain abscess. Brain abscesses continue to occur most commonly in the first four decades of life, but there are peaks in the 0- to 20-year and 50- to 70-year age groups; there is an unexplained higher incidence in males than in females.

Many of the bacteria involved, particularly the anaerobes, are drawn from the normal flora of the body. Other infectious agents, such as *S. aureus* and some of the gram-negative aerobic bacilli, may be nosocomial in origin.

Pathogenesis and Pathology

Except for the few cases that follow penetrating injuries to the head or intracranial operations, brain abscesses are always secondary to a focus of infection elsewhere in the body. Spread by direct extension or by retrograde procession along veins, usually with septic thrombophlebitis and venous infarction, occurs with infections of the middle ear, mastoid, and paranasal sinuses. Chronic otitis media and mastoiditis are the most common sources, usually leading to a single abscess most often in the temporal lobe, less frequently in the cerebellum, and occasionally in another intracranial site. Frontal and sphenoidal sinusitis may be antecedents of brain abscesses involving the frontal and temporal lobes, respectively.

Brain abscesses are frequently metastatic from distant sites of infection. With the exception of abscesses secondary to congenital heart disease, metastatic brain abscesses tend to be multiple, in contrast to otogenic and rhinogenic abscesses. Metastatic abscesses are most likely to occur at the junction of the gray and white matter.

The most important sources for metastasis are lung abscess, pneumonia, empyema, and bronchiectasis. Abscesses secondary to pleuropulmonary disease are often multiple, affecting the frontal, parietal, and occipital lobes with equal frequency, but only rarely involving the temporal lobes or the cerebellum. Intracranial abscess is also associated with congenital cardiac defects and other conditions in which a right-to-left shunt causes a short-circuiting of the pulmonary circulation. Brain abscess rarely complicates the course of endocarditis. Other sources of metastatic abscess include septic abortion, septicemia after dental extraction, infections of the face or scalp, tonsillitis, and soft-tissue infections.

The early reaction to bacterial invasion of the brain consists of cerebritis with local inflammation; in septic thrombosis of blood vessels, necrosis intervenes. Within a few weeks or months, there is encapsulation of the pus and liquefied brain. The capsule consists of fibroblasts and granulation tissue, and increases in thickness with time. The leptomeninges adjacent to the abscess are infiltrated with neutrophils, lymphocytes, and plasma cells.

Manifestations

The clinical picture of brain abscess is dominated by the manifestations of a space-occupying lesion. The course is often indolent but may be fulminant. Although patients with brain abscess often have a modest fever, many are afebrile, particularly with chronic, well-encapsulated abscesses. Severe headache is the most common and earliest symptom; it may be present for days to weeks in spite of symptomatic therapy and may be severe enough to be distinct from the headache of an underlying sinusitis or otitis. Other symptoms, in decreasing order of frequency, are altered mental status (drowsiness, irritability, confusion, and stupor); nausea and vomiting; general or focal seizures; and focal motor, sensory, or speech disorders. Physical examination may reveal only lethargy and low-grade fever. Localizing neurologic signs reflecting the location of the abscess tend to occur relatively late in the course of the illness unless the lesion is strategically located. Papilledema and nuchal rigidity are less commonly present. In short, the manifestations of brain abscess are often nonspecific, consisting of headache, lethargy, and low-grade fever and associated perhaps with nausea and vomiting or a focal neurologic deficit.

Clinical features that may occur with brain abscess but are much more frequent with subdural empyema are nuchal rigidity, seizures, and focal neurologic signs. Subdural empyema is a neurosurgical emergency and must be considered in any patient with manifestations of intracranial infection (see below).

Diagnosis

The history and physical examination are invaluable in obtaining evidence of a predisposing condition (such as underlying disease of the ear, sinus, lung, or heart). In contrast, routine laboratory tests are rarely helpful. Polymorphonuclear leukocytosis is usual but nonspecific.

Once the possibility of intracranial infection is considered, decision must be made as to the need for immediate lumbar puncture. Lumbar puncture should be considered urgently if purulent meningitis is suspected, but the procedure is contraindicated if intracranial abscess is present because it may precipitate herniation of the brain. Thus, in the patient with papilledema, seizures, or focal neurologic signs, noninvasive procedures (computed tomography or radionuclide brain scan) are mandatory as emergency procedures to search for a mass lesion. Although papilledema is infrequent in meningitis, it is a relatively late sign of intracranial abscess; thus, the presence of papilledema is a contraindication to a lumbar puncture, but the lack of it is much less helpful. Focal neurologic findings are more common in intracranial abscess, but cranial nerve deficits are not rare in meningitis.

The cerebrospinal fluid (CSF) of patients with intracranial suppuration without meningitis may be entirely normal, but (more commonly) abnormalities are detected that are not diagnostic. Usually, the pressure is moderately increased. The leukocyte count is almost always elevated (25–300 cells) with variable numbers of neutrophils and mononuclear cells, although, rarely, in case of deep metastatic brain abscesses, the spinal fluid does not show pleocytosis. The concentration of protein is usually elevated, but the concentration of glucose is normal. Although

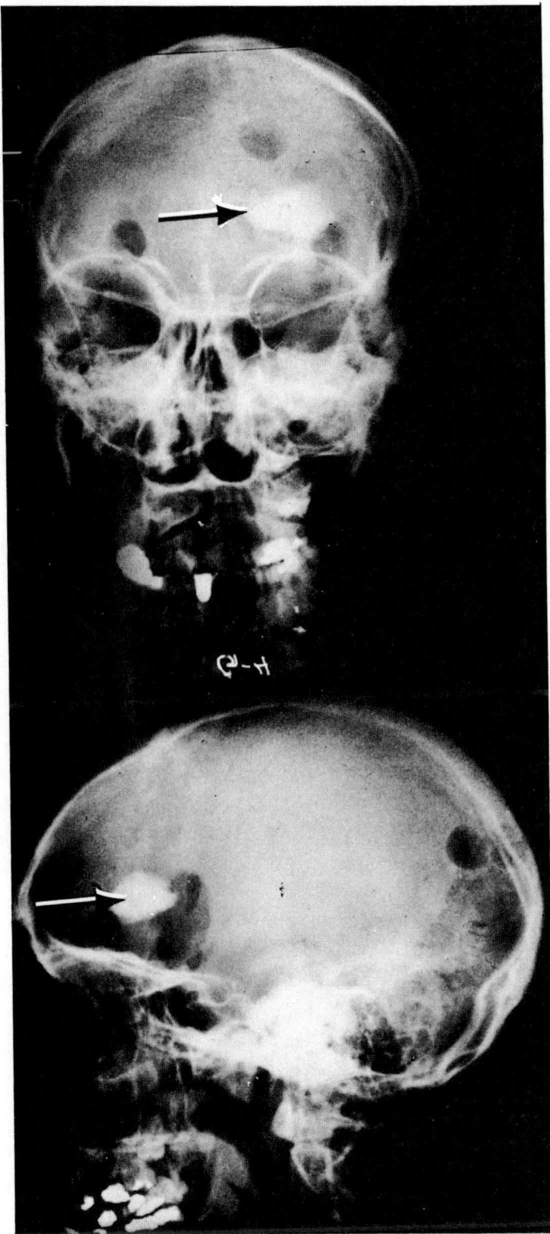

Fig. 125-1. Anteroposterior and lateral views of skull. In this study, the cavity of the brain abscess is outlined with thorotrast.

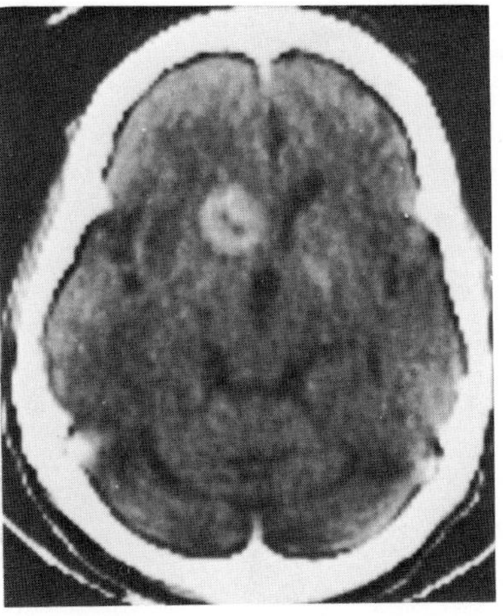

Fig. 125-2. Computed tomography of intracerebral abscess. Computed tomographic scan of the brain after injection of contrast material demonstrates a mass in the right frontal lobe that has obliterated the anterior portion of the frontal horn. A thick rim of contrast enhancement surrounds the mass. (Courtesy of Judith G. Rose, M.D.)

gram's stains and cultures are rarely positive unless the abscess has ruptured into the subarachnoid space or ventricles, the CSF (if obtained) must be cultured for anaerobic and aerobic bacteria, fungi, and acid-fast bacilli. Direct smears and cultures of material from likely portals of entry and sources of metastasis should be made; blood cultures should be obtained.

Useful diagnostic procedures include skull films, computed tomography (CT), radionuclide brain imaging, electroencephalography, and angiography. Air-contrast studies and ventriculography are rarely needed.

Plain skull radiographs, with the addition of special views of the mastoids and sinuses (Fig. 125-1), frequently provide useful information. These films may demonstrate shifting of the normally calcified intracranial structures, evidence of increased intracranial pressure, erosion of bone as a result of osteomyelitis, or inflammation of sinuses or mastoids. Rarely, gas within an abscess cavity is identified.

CT, performed before and after injection of contrast material, is the diagnostic procedure of choice because it permits assessments of the specific intracranial location of an abscess, the presence of multiple foci, the degree of mass effect, and possible extension of the process into a ventricle. On CT (without contrast), an intracranial abscess commonly appears as a focal area of low absorption accompanied by a faint dense ring with a surrounding lucent zone. With the IV administration of contrast material, enhancement of the dense ring occurs, casting in relief the surrounding edema as a region of lower density outside the area of enhancement. The ring represents the capsule of the abscess (Fig. 125-2). The administration of glucosteroids may reduce the degree of enhancement. Other intracranial pathology may yield a similar appearance on CT: primary and metastatic

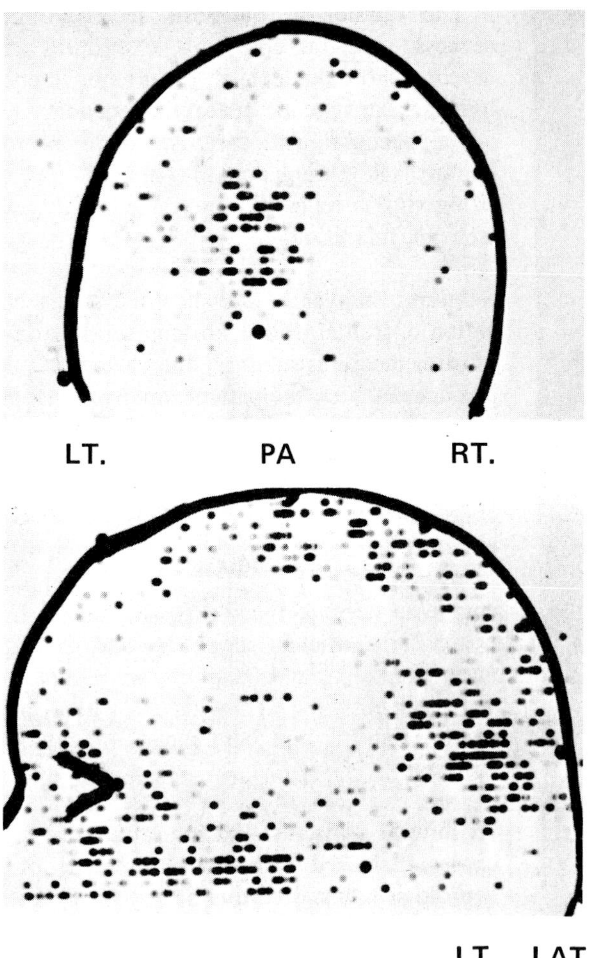

Fig. 125-3. Brain scan showing an occipital lobe abscess.

brain tumors, granulomas, infarction, and certain postoperative conditions. The findings must therefore be considered with the clinical picture if a correct diagnosis is to be obtained.

Radionuclide brain imaging is indicated in specific circumstances (Fig. 125-3). If CT is not available or if the patient has a history of allergy to iodine, radionuclide imaging may be useful. In addition, because the early stages of cerebritis (prior to the formation of the capsule) may be demonstrated by this technique, some authorities advocate the addition of radionuclide brain imaging if CT does not disclose a lesion.

Electroencephalography is not needed in most cases. The usual finding is a focus of high-voltage slow activity that often lateralizes an abscess correctly, but is only about 50% accurate in localization. The electroencephalogram (EEG) is usually not helpful in the diagnosis of multiple brain abscesses. Angiography is generally less informative than CT and thus is usually unnecessary unless clinical information, combined with findings on CT and radionuclide scanning, does not provide a diagnosis. Air studies and ventriculography are much more hazardous procedures that are rarely, if ever, indicated.

The differential diagnosis of brain abscess includes subdural abscess or empyema, epidural abscess, cerebral thrombophlebitis, focal embolic encephalomalacia or mycotic aneurysm secondary to infective endocarditis, acute necrotizing hemorrhagic encephalopathy, primary or metastatic brain tumor, necrotizing viral encephalitis, and occasionally, massive ischemic infarction. In addition, purulent meningitis must be considered, although the clinical picture is usually sufficiently distinctive.

Prognosis

In patients treated with surgery and antimicrobial therapy, the mortality has been approximately 20%, but when cases diagnosed only at autopsy are considered, the overall mortality has been as high as 50%. However, in recent years, mortality as low as 5% to 10% has been reported—an improvement attributed to the ease and accuracy of CT as a method of diagnosing and following brain abscesses. Other factors that make for a better prognosis are early diagnosis, single abscess, younger age, relatively indolent course, lack of severe underlying disease, and lack of serious neurologic deterioration (such as coma) prior to diagnosis.

The major complication of brain abscess is rupture into a cerebral ventricle or into the subarachnoid space. Sequelae include neurologic deficits, most commonly focal seizures.

Therapy

In the stage of acute suppurative encephalitis or cerebritis prior to the formation of an abscess, prolonged, intensive antimicrobial therapy may be curative without surgical intervention. In addition, certain carefully selected patients with fully formed abscesses for whom the risk of surgery is prohibitive may be best treated with antimicrobial therapy alone. Close observation of such patients is obligatory using serial imaging procedures with monitoring for signs of a decreasing level of consciousness and developing focal neurologic deficits.

In most patients, once the abscess has become localized, surgical drainage is necessary. Although some abscesses may be cured by repeated aspiration and intensive antimicrobial therapy, it is generally agreed that excision is preferable. Whenever possible, excision should be carried out immediately after the initial aspiration at the time of exploration. If the abscess is deep, poorly encapsulated, or located in a strategic motor or speech area, repeated aspiration is usually preferable to excision. Abscess cavities require many weeks to close because the brain is relatively rigid and relatively avascular (abscesses often originate at the junction of the white and gray matter, a poorly vascularized area; increased intracerebral pressure may further compromise blood flow).

The regimens of antimicrobial therapy are generally those used to treat meningitis (Chap. 119, Bacterial Meningitis). Treatment must be started early, involve high doses, and be maintained for prolonged periods. The choice of antimicrobics depends on the infecting microorganism(s). The doses must be adjusted for renal (and, in some cases, hepatic) dysfunction. Penicillin G, 200 mg to 300 mg (320,000–480,000 units)/kg body wt/day (injected IV as six equal portions, 4-hourly) is appropriate. With the exception of *Bacteroides fragilis* and a few strains of other gram-negative anaerobic bacilli, most anaerobes would be susceptible. Penicillin G is, of course, active against meningococci, group A *S. pyogenes*, viridans group streptococci, and many strains of *Haemophilus* spp. The succinate derivative of chloramphenicol may also be used initially in a dose of 50 to 60 mg/kg body wt/day (injected intravenously as four equal portions, 6-hourly) in adults and older children. Chloramphenicol is active against essentially all anaerobes, meningococci, *Haemophilus* spp., many of the aerobic gram-negative bacilli, virtually all the aerobic streptococci, and some strains of staphylococci.

Metronidazole is another agent that has excellent effectiveness against virtually all strict anaerobes and readily achieves therapeutic concentrations in the central nervous system. In view of these features and its consistently excellent bactericidal activity, metronidazole is a drug of choice for anaerobic brain abscesses (except for those involving *Actinomyces* spp. and *Arachnia* spp., which are often resistant). Metronidazole should not be used as a single agent if pathogens other than anaerobic bacteria are suspected. The combination of penicillin and metronidazole should be ideal therapy for the majority of brain abscesses.

An antistaphylococcal antimicrobic should be included in the initial therapy for brain abscess following accidental or surgical trauma to the head, or if staphylococcal bacteremia may have preceded the abscess. A penicillinase-resistant penicillin (*e.g.*, nafcillin) is needed in a dose of 200 to 250 mg/kg body wt/day injected intravenously as six equal portions, 4-hourly. In the patient with serious allergy to the penicillins, vancomycin, 25 to 30 mg/kg body wt/day injected intravenously as three or two equal portions, 8- or 12-hourly, may be substituted, or given in combination with rifampin (15–30 mg/kg body wt/day, given perorally as four equal portions, 6-hourly).

Antimicrobics such as gentamicin, tobramycin, netilmicin, and amikacin, although very active against many of the aerobic gram-negative bacilli, are often not effective, even when used in maximum dosage, because of poor penetration into the central nervous system. The acylureidopenicillins, moxalactam, and perhaps other newer β-lactams may be useful in this situation.

The older cephalosporins and clindamycin should not be used in the treatment of infections of the nervous system. Drugs useful for the treatment of infections caused by mycobacteria, fungi, and protozoa are discussed in other chapters.

Antimicrobial therapy should be continued for at least 6 to 8 weeks, with serial CT or radionuclide imaging as an aid to monitor healing.

Anticoagulation is contraindicated in the presence of brain abscess because of the danger of intracranial hemorrhage. Measures to decrease intracranial pressure may be necessary.

Prevention

Early, intensive, appropriate treatment of extracranial sepsis, which might lead to brain abscess, should be preventive. Careful aseptic technique in patients undergoing craniotomy should reduce the number of postoperative infections.

Remaining Problems

With the diagnostic tools, surgical expertise, and antimicrobial agents presently available, intracranial abscess is potentially curable. Earlier consideration of the diagnosis is the one factor that would probably help to decrease further the morbidity and mortality.

Subdural Empyema and Epidural Abscess

Subdural empyema and epidural abscess within the cranium usually result from direct extension of contiguous infection. The predominant etiologic agents include aerobic gram-positive cocci (including streptococci and *S. aureus*), anaerobic bacteria, and a variety of gram-negative organisms (including *Haemophilus* spp. and the Enterobacteriaceae). Uncommon pathogens may be present, especially in the compromised host.

Subdural empyema develops when infection extends to the space between the dura and arachnoid by way of small veins traversing this space, by extension of contiguous infection such as osteomyelitis of the skull that also involves the potential space between bone and dura, following trauma to the head, or when a subdural hematoma becomes infected. In children, subdural empyema is most often a complication of meningitis. Once the subdural compartment has been breached, the infection may spread but still behaves as a confined, expanding mass lesion. The location depends upon the location of the underlying infection, which is most often a frontal sinusitis. An inflammatory exudate within the subdural space is often associated with focal osteomyelitis and epidural abscess, sometimes with septic thrombophlebitis, and occasionally with extension to the subarachnoid space, leading to purulent meningitis.

Intracranial epidural abscess, unlike spinal epidural abscess, is almost always associated with overlying focal osteomyelitis developing as a result of sinusitis, mastoiditis, or craniotomy. Extension to the subdural space is a common, serious occurrence.

The clinical manifestations of subdural empyema may be indistinguishable from those of brain abscess, but it is important to recognize this potentially life-threatening emergency that can progress rapidly to transtentorial or tonsillar herniation. Fever, headache, altered mental status, and vomiting are features common to both brain abscess and subdural empyema. High fever, signs of meningeal irritation, seizures, and focal neurologic signs are appreciably more frequent with subdural empyema. Papilledema is present in less than half the patients, probably because of the rapid progression of the disease. In infants, the size of the head may increase and there may be bulging of the fontanelles. In any patient with very rapid evolution of signs and symptoms of central nervous system infection, suddural empyema should be considered.

In contrast, the initial symptoms of intracranial epidural abscess may merge with those of a preceding sinusitis or otitis. Initial local pain and fever which do not resolve may be followed by generalized headache, alteration of mental status, focal neurologic signs, and seizures with signs of increased intracranial pressure a late development. Early recognition is important to prevent the development of subdural empyema.

In the presence of subdural empyema, lumbar puncture is even more dangerous than in brain abscess. Skull films often demonstrate sinusitis or otitis and may show a shift of the pineal body. CT is the best diagnostic procedure and may be supplemented by angiography in some patients. Surgical drainage must be performed as an emergency procedure to relieve pressure in subdural empyema and, in the case of epidural abscess, to prevent progression to subdural empyema. Measures to decrease intracranial pressure are often needed. For the adult, the initial antimicrobial therapy should be effective against anaerobes, streptococci, and *S. aureusi;* that is, at least chloramphenicol and a penicillinase-resistant penicillin should be included. Vancomycin may be substituted for the latter if there is allergy to the penicillins. Additional drugs may be indicated in certain clinical settings, especially if the bacteriology of the primary infection is known. (*e.g.,* in a patient with sinusitis or endocarditis) In children, initial antimicrobial therapy should be the regimen that is appropriate for the bacterial meningitides of the child's age group.

In subdural empyema, the prognosis is good if appropriate treatment is instituted early, but the overall mortality is 25% to 45%, and permanent neurologic deficits are not uncommon.

Bibliography

Journals

BELLER AJ, SAHAR A, PRAISS I: Brain abscess: Review of 89 cases over a period of 30 years. J Neurol Neurosurg Psychiat 36:757–768, 1973

BREWER NS, MACCARTY CS, WELLMAN WE: Brain abscess: A review of recent experience. Ann Intern Med 82:571–576, 1975

DANZIGER A, PRICE H, SCHECHTER MM: An analysis of 113 intracranial infections. Neuroradiology 19:31–34, 1980

HANDEL SF, KLEIN WC, KIM YWK: Intracranial epidural abscess. Radiology 111:117–120, 1974

HEINEMAN HS, BRAUDE AI: Anaerobic infection of the brain. Observations on eighteen consecutive cases of brain abscess. Am J Med 35:682–697, 1963

KAUFMAN DM, MILLER MH, STEIGBIGEL NH: Subdural empyema: Analysis of 17 recent cases and review of the literature. Medicine 54:485–498, 1975

ROSENBLUM ML, HOFF, JT, NORMAN D, EDWARDS MS, BERG BO: Nonoperative treatment of brain abscesses in selected high-risk patients. J Neurosurg 52:217–225, 1980

ROSENBLUM ML, HOFF JT, NORMAN D, WEINSTEIN PR, PITTS L: Decreased mortality from brain abscesses since advent of computerized tomography. J Neurosurg 49:658–668, 1978

VAN ALPHEN HAM, DREISSEN JJR: Brain abscess and subdural empyema. Factors influencing mortality and results of various surgical techniques. J Neurol Neurosurg Psychiat 39:481–490, 1976

WHELAN MA, HILAL SK: Computed tomography as a guide in the diagnosis and follow-up of brain abscesses. Radiology 135N 3:663–671, 1980

JEFFREY D. BAND
JOHN V. BENNETT

Tetanus

126

Tetanus is an intoxication manifested primarily by neuromuscular dysfunction. It is caused by tetanal toxin (tetanospasmin), an extraordinarily potent exotoxin elaborated by *Clostridium tetani.* The disease can be prevented by immunization with tetanal toxoid.

Etiology

Proliferating cells of *C. tenani* produce tetanal toxin, a water-soluble, diffusible protein with a molecular weight of about 67,000. It has been estimated that as little as 130 μg of purified tetanospasmin may be lethal for humans.

Clostridium tetani are obligate anaerobes. They are bacillary (0.5μm × 2–5 μm), gram-positive, motile, and noncapsulated, and form terminal spores that resemble drumsticks. The spores are survival structures that are relatively resistant to drying and disinfectants. Autoclaving is lethal; boiling is not. Ethylene oxide is sporicidal (see Chap. 17, Sterilization, Disinfection, and Sanitization.)

Spores of *C. tetani* are ubiquitous. They have been cultured from soil, house and operating theater dust, fresh and salt water, and gun wads. Vegetative *C. tetani* are present in the feces of animals and the intestinal contents of about 25% of humans.

Epidemiology

Although tetanus occurs worldwide, the disease is most frequently encountered in developing countries. In these nations, neonatal tetanus (tetanus occurring in the first 28 days of life) may account for up to 10% of neonatal deaths. Historically, the disease has often been recognized as a complication of septic abortions and war injuries.

In the United States, both the incidence (Fig. 126-1) and mortality of tetanus have dropped approximately tenfold over the last 25 years. The case–fatality ratio has decreased in recent years and is currently 35% to 40%. About 60% of all cases occur from April through September. Attack rates are highest in the southern states: on a national basis, the incidence is 0.04 cases per 100,000 per year. Incidence (Fig. 126-2) and mortality rates are substantially higher for neonates and persons over 50 years of age than for other age groups. The median age of non-neonatal patients in the United States is 64 years. According to recent trends, females are about as likley to be affected as males. There is no difference in susceptibility, but males may run a greater risk of exposure. The fivefold lesser frequency of tetanus in whites is most likely attributable to lower immunization levels in nonwhites.

Wounds are the usual portal of entry of *C. tetani* (Table 126-1). About two-thirds of all injuries leading to tetanus occur in the home, and about 20% take place on farms and in gardens. Nearly 10% of the cases reported in 1979 occurred in elderly persons with advanced peripheral vascular disease complicated by decubiti, ulcers, or gangrene.

Six cases of neonatal tetanus were reported in the United States in 1979. The incidence of neonatal tetanus in the 5-year interval of 1975–1979 was about one case per million live births; in nonwhites, it was 20 per million live births. Males and females are affected with equal frequency, and there is no seasonal variation in the distribution of cases. The typical neonate with tetanus is born outside the hospital to an unimmunized mother and is delivered by a midwife who has used unsterile technique in managing the umbilical cord—the portal of entry.

Pathogenesis and Pathology

Spores of *C. tetani* that gain entry to tissues at the time of injury cannot germinate and elaborate tetano-

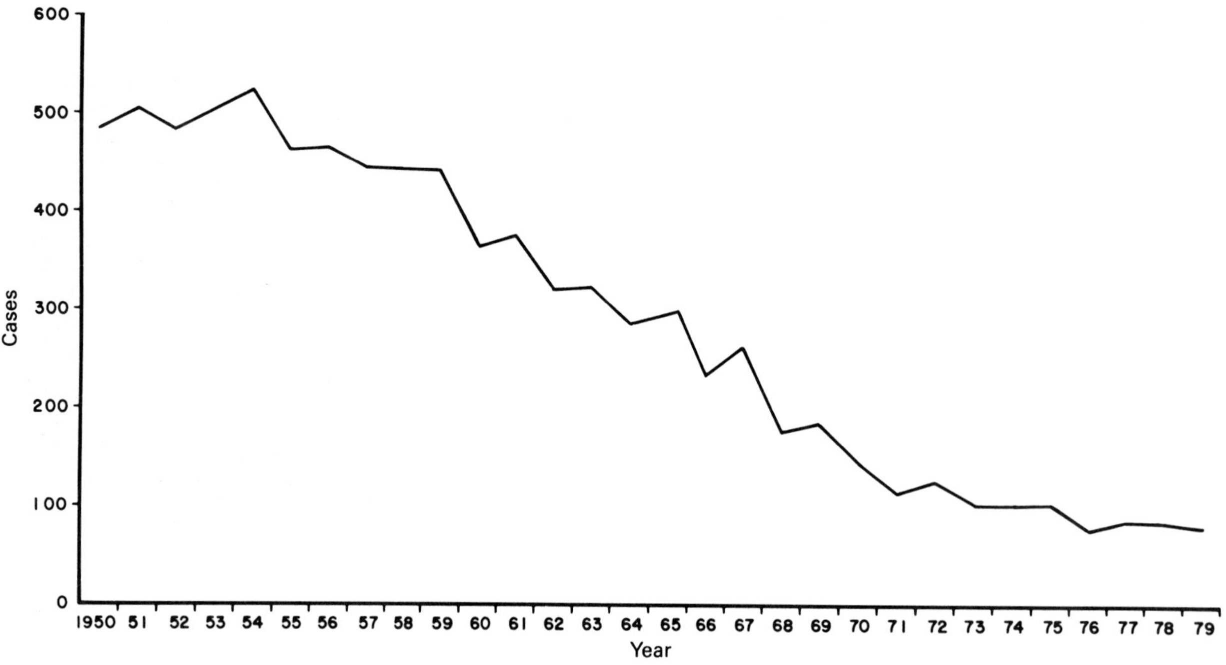

Fig. 126-1. Reported cases of tetanus in the United States, 1950–1979. (Morbid Mortal Week Rep Suppl, Summary, 1979)

Fig. 126-2. Reported cases of tetanus in the United States in 1979 by age groups. (Morbid Mortal Week Rep Suppl, Summary, 1979)

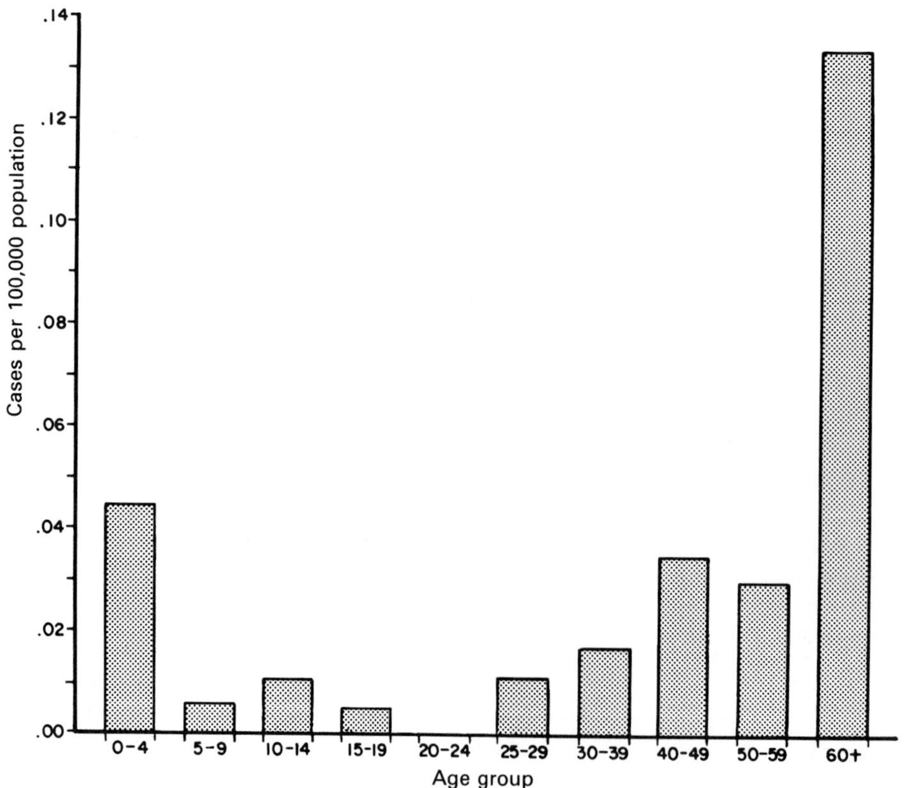

Table 126-1. *Portals of Entry of* Clostridium Tetani *in Patients With Clinical Tetanus in the United States.*

Portal	Frequency (%)
Wounds	
Punctures	27
Lacerations	24
Abrasions	17
Crush	3
Obstetrical & surgical	2
Injections	2
Ulcers (varicose, decubitus)	8
Other wounds	3
None found	5

spasmin unless oxygen is depleted. Such focal anaerobic conditions are most likely to occur in wounds with tissue necrosis, foreign bodies, or infecting aerobic microorganisms. Spores may persist in normal tissues for several months or years, only to germinate at a later time when another injury provides anaerobic conditions. Infections with *C. tetani* remain localized and inconspicuous, with minimal local reaction unless complicated by the presence of other infecting microorganisms. Suppuration and gangrene are not caused by *C. tetani.*

Tetanospasmin is elaborated by proliferating cells of *C. tetani.* Two routes have been suggested for the spread of toxin from the infected site to the central nervous system (CNS): (1) adsorption at myoneural junctions followed by migration through perineural tissue spaces of nerve trunks to the CNS: and (2) passage from tissue spaces to lymphatics, to blood, to the CNS. Despite controversy and debate regarding these modes of spread, it seems likely that both mechanisms are important.

Regardless of the route of ingress, tetanal toxin becomes bound to gangliosides within the CNS. The molecular details of the interaction are not known, but the physiologic action of tetanospasmin is clearly similar to that of strychnine. Both substances suppress inhibitory influences on the motor neurons and interneurons without directly enhancing synaptic excitatory action. Additional actions of tetanospasmin are evident in the neurocirculatory, neuroendocrine, and vegetative nervous systems. It has also been postulated that the toxin directly affects electrolyte flux in the sarcotubular system of muscles and synaptic transmission at myoneural junctions.

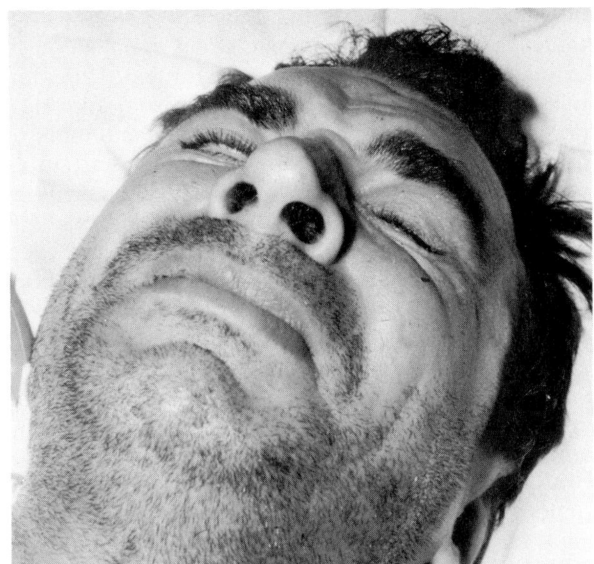

Fig. 126-3. Risus sardonicus. (Courtesy of E Erikson, Karolinska Sjukhuset, Stockholm)

Manifestations

The incubation period of tetanus extends from less than 48 hours to more than 3 weeks. A wound may or may not be present when manifestations of infection first appear. Early symptoms and signs often consist of irritability, restlessness, headache, and low-grade fever. Patients remain alert.

Two basic forms of tetanus may be distinguished: local and general. Local tetanus consists of spasm and increased muscle tone confined to muscles near a wound; there are no systemic signs. General tetanus is far more frequent. Almost all neonatal tetanus is the general form. The first sign is difficulty in sucking, beginning 3 to 10 days after birth and progressing to total inability to suck.

The most characteristic complaint of adult patients with general tetanus is lockjaw or trismus, the inability to open the mouth because of spasm of the masseter muscles. Spasm of the facial muscles leads to a grotesque, grinning expression termed *risus sardonicus* (Fig. 126-3). Spasms of the somatic musculature in general tetanus may be widespread, resulting in opisthotonos and boardlike rigidity of the abdomen. Acute, paroxysmal, incoordinate, widespread spasms of the muscles are characteristic of moderate and severe tetanus. Such tonic convulsions occur intermittently, irregularly, and unpredictably, persisting for a few seconds to several minutes. Initially mild and separated by periods of relaxation, paroxysms tend to become painful, severe, and exhausting as they continue. Paroxysmal spasms may occur spontaneously or may be precipitated by a variety of external stimuli, such as drafts of cold air, the noise from shutting a door, turning on the lights in the room, attempts to move or turn the patient, and the patient's attempts to drink. Paroxysms may also be precipitated by internal triggers, such as a distended bowel or bladder, or mucous plugs in the bronchi. Cyanosis and even sudden death from respiratory arrest may result from these spasms. The work associated with the spasms of tetanus is, at least in part, responsible for a hypermetabolic state, and hyperhidrosis is common.

Three gradations of severity, based on symptoms and signs, are indicators of the appropriate therapy and the prognosis of general tetanus.

Mild cases have an incubation period of 10 days or longer, and slow development of symptoms and signs for 4 to 7 days. Initially, there is local rigidity of the muscles near the wound, which progresses to a general rigidity. Stiffness of the neck and jaws develops insidiously and results in mild trismus. True dysphagia and paroxysmal spasms are not present. Once fully developed, these signs tend to plateau for about a week. Gradual and complete recovery occurs during the next 2 to 4 weeks.

Moderately severe cases have incubation periods of less than 10 days, and symptoms and signs develop in 3 to 6 days. Severe trismus, dysphagia due to pharyngeal muscular spasm, and general muscle rigidity are present. At first, paroxysmal spasms are mild and short, but they progress slowly for several days, becoming frequent, painful, and violent. They are not associated with dyspnea or cyanosis.

Severe cases have incubation periods of less than 7 days; serious illness evolves rapidly in 3 days or less. Muscular hypertonicity is so pronounced, general, and severe that interference with breathing, opisthotonus, and boardlike abdominal rigidity are evident. The paroxysmal spasms are frequent, violent, prolonged, and asphyxial. Patients surviving longer than 1 week experience a gradual reduction in the intensity and frequency of the spasms. A reduction in the general rigidity and a decrease in residual stiffness occur later. Complete recovery takes place in 2 to 6 weeks. In severe cases, autonomic dysfunction is evidenced by sudden changes in heart rate, blood pressure, and central venous pressure that occur either spontaneously or in response to extrinsic stimuli.

Diagnosis

The diagnosis of tetanus is made on the basis of clinical manifestations. The typical, fully developed case is easily recognized. Such patients commonly give no clear history of previous tetanal toxoid immunizations, and the vast majority have evidence of a wound that has occurred within the previous 2 weeks. In addition to trismus, a physical examination may reveal marked hypertonicity of muscles, hyperactive deep tendon reflexes, clear mentation, low-grade fever, and lack of sensory involvement. Local or general paroxysmal spasms may be observed.

Laboratory studies show a moderate leukocytosis. The cerebrospinal fluid is normal in patients with tetanus, but the pressure may be elevated by muscle contractions. Neither electroencephalography (normal) nor electromyography is helpful in the diagnosis. Only about one-third of all wound cultures are positive for *C. tetani* in patients who have clinical evidence of the disease. It must be remembered that the isolation of *C tetani* from contaminated wounds does not mean that the patient has, or will contract, tetanus. The frequency of isolation of *C. tetani* from wounds of patients with clinical tetanus might be improved by heating one set of specimens to 80°C for 15 minutes to destroy the vegetative forms of nonsporulating competing microorganisms before culture mediums are inoculated.

One must be cautious in diagnosing tetanus in persons with reliable histories of having received two or more injections of tetanal toxoid in the past. Serum specimens should be obtained for assaying antitoxin by hemagglutination and, preferably, mouse-neutralizing tests. The presence of 0.01 IU of antitoxin per ml of serum is generally considered protective.

The most common local condition that results in stiffness of the jaw is alveolar abscess. A careful history and physical examination, in conjunction with roentgenographic studies, should enable differentiation. Purulent meningitis can be excluded by an examination of the cerebrospinal fluid (see Chap. 119, Acute Bacterial Meningitis). Encephalitis is occasionally associated with trismus and muscle spasms; however, the sensorium of patients with this disorder is clouded (see Chap. 122, Viral Encephalitides). The muscular spasms of rabies occur early in the course of the disease, and they involve the muscles of respiration and deglutition. Trismus is not present, and the spinal fluid may be pleocytotic. The history of an animal bite is not diagnostic of rabies, for tetanus also occurs after bites. The incubation period of rabies is much longer than that of tetanus (see Chap. 124, Rabies). Abdominal rigidity in tetanus may suggest an acute intraabdominal process requiring surgery. Although physical examination should reveal early trismus and rigidity of the neck, tetanus occasionally results from obstructions and perforations of the intestinal tract. Hysterical conversion reactions and phenothiazine reactions also need to be considered. The former are most likely to occur in nurses or paramedical personnel who have tended a patient with tetanus. In such persons, signs may disappear in response to suggestion, and positive evidence of an underlying hysterical personality may be uncovered. Phenothiazine reactions can cause trismus, but the associated tremors, athetoid movements, and torticollis should alert one to this possibility. Strychnine poisoning may closely mimic tetanus. However, in strychnine poisoning, the possibility of homicide or suicide may be evident from the history, trismus tends to appear late, and symptoms and signs develop much more rapidly than in tetanus. In children less than 2 years of age, tetany must be considered. However, the typical posturing of the hands and feet, the lack of trismus, and a low serum calcium enable this entity to be differentiated from tetanus.

Prognosis

The quality of the supportive care determines the prognosis. This is attested by the contrast between the overall case–fatality rate of 40%, with rates as low as 10% in centers where tetanus is frequent. The prognosis is best for the 10 to 19-year age group and worst for neonates and persons over 50 years. Incubation periods of 10 days or longer are associated with a significantly better prognosis in persons less than 50 years of age. Paroxysmal spasms, whether present on admission or later, are associated with a substantially greater mortality. In general, the more rapid the evolution of symptoms and signs, the worse the prognosis. High fever or a rising temperature is an ominous sign.

Death in tetanus is mainly due to asphyxiation during a muscular spasm or a complicating infection such as bacterial pneumonia or bacteremia. Other complications include atalectasis (inspissated secretions and exudates); aspiration pneumonia; pulmonary emboli; acute gastric ulcers; fecal impaction; urinary retention and catheter-related urinary infections; decubiti; serum sickness; and anaphylaxis from the administration of heterologous antiserum. The intensity of paroxysmal spasms is sometimes sufficient to result in the spontaneous rupture of muscles and intramuscular hematomas. Compression fractures or the subluxation of vertebrae may occur, usually affecting thoracic vertebrae. Persons surviving to the convalescent phase recover completely.

Second attacks of tetanus have occured months or years after recovery from tetanus in persons who were not given tetanal toxoid after the first attack. Apparently, an amount of tetanospasmin sufficient to cause clinical tetanus may not be immunogenic; alternatively, therapeutic doses of exogenous antitoxin may interfere with the immune response to the toxin.

Therapy

The three objectives of therapy are (1) to provide supportive care until the tetanospasmin that is fixed to nervous tissue has been metabolized, (2) to neutralize circulating toxin, and (3) to remove the source of tetanospasmin. The best results follow aggressive and intensive therapy applied to all but mild cases. This is a matter of critical importance because patients who survive the acute phase of the disease recover completely.

Supportive Care

Total, continuous, and expert medical and nursing care is essential, with special attention to the respiratory tract. Transfer of the patient to centers where such care is possible should be carried out under the supervision of competent personnel after therapy with muscle relaxants has been instituted. A respirator, oxygen, and suction and tracheotomy equipment must be at hand for immediate use.

The patient should be weighed daily; the intake and output of fluids and vital signs should be measured frequently. The patient should be turned frequently to avoid bedsores and pulmonary stasis. Extrinsic stimuli that might trigger paroxysmal spasms can be minimized by a quiet, darkened room and infrequent examinations. An intravenous (IV) portal must be maintained. A decrease in drug intake is often required in addicts, and the use of methadone is frequently necessary. Electrolyte and blood gas studies are essential to guide therapy. Tap water enemas and digital evacuation of fecal impactions are frequently necessary. Retention of urine is common. Because an indwelling catheter may act as a visceral trigger, intermittent catherization is preferable in some patients.

Mild cases can usually be managed with supportive care and a combination of muscle relaxants and sedatives.

Moderate and severe cases require more intensive supportive care. Tracheostomy should be carried out before it becomes an emergency procedure, and total paralysis with curarelike compounds should be induced if facilities and personnel are adequate to provide total continuous respiratory care. Such therapy generally must be continued for at least 1 week; some patients may require total maintenance for 3 weeks. Because neither tenanus nor curare affects mentation, sedatives must be given. Concomitant anticoagulant therapy may prevent thromboembolism.

Muscle relaxants should be given to all patients with tetanus, whether mild, moderate, or severe. Agents such as meprobamate and diazepam are exceptionally safe over a wide range of doses, and they are free of significant side-effects (*e.g.,* respiratory depression). Both drugs are also tranquilizers and sedatives at doses smaller than those necessary to abolish muscle rigidity and spasm. The latter effect is not necessary when a curarelike agent is given at the same time. Optimal doses of either meprobamate or diazepam must be determined empirically for each patient and adjusted to accommodate the clinical course of the patient. Two to six weks of IV, intramuscular (IM), or oral therapy may be needed.

Adults may receive 400 mg of meprobamate intramuscularly every 2 to 4 hours. Children 2 to 5 years of age can be given 100 to 200 mg every 3 to 4 hours; infants may receive 50 to 100 mg per dose. Trismus, abdominal rigidity, and opisthotonos diminish or disappear within 10 minutes after dosage. During convalescence, oral doses of 400 to 800 mg meprobamate every 4 hours are usually sufficient initially and may be reduced as the patients improves.

Diazepam is a suitable alternative to meprobamate. In mild cases in adults, peroral doses of 10 mg may be repeated as needed. In moderate and severe cases, diazepam is best given by continuous IV drip in a dose of approximately 120 mg per day using 5% glucose solution for injection containing 120 mg per liter. The drug may also be administered through a nasogastric or gastrostomy tube.

The effect of both meprobamate and diazepam can be prolonged by the judicious addition of phenobarbital in doses too small to depress respiration. In adults, such a dose would be 1 mg per kg of body weight every 4 to 6 hours by IM injection, not to exceed 500 mg total per day. Other seadtives (*e.g.,* paraldehyde) have been advocated.

Maintenance of adequate nutrition by parenteral hyperalimentation may be necessary.

Physical therapy should be instituted early in the convalescent phase of the disease. If curare or a similar drug is used in the treatment, passive movements of the patient's arms and legs should begin during therapy. However, any patient who has had long-continued severe spasms should have spinal roentgenography before being allowed out of bed.

Neutralization of Toxin

One of the first therapeutic manuevers should be the administration of tetanal immune globulin (TIG) of human origin in a total dose of 500 to 3,000 units. If the higher dose is used, it should be injected IM as three equal portions into three sites. Currently available TIG should not be given IV because severe hypotension may result. Unlike tetanal antitoxin of nonhuman origin, neither allergy, anaphylaxis, nor other adverse reactions attend the IM use of TIG. Moreover, TIG produces higher, more persistent titers of antitoxin than heterologous antitoxin. Protective levels are attained rapidly, reach a maximum 48 to 72 hours after administration, and decline slowly with a half-life of about 25 days, that is, repeated doses are not necessary. TIG neutralizes uncombined tetanal toxin in body liquids, but it does not penetrate the blood–brain barrier, and it has no effect on toxin already fixed to nervous tissue.

Active immunization should be started at the same time. Intramuscularly injected toxoid does not interfere with the efficacy of TIG, and TIG does not nullify the immunogenicity of the toxoid.

Eradication of the Infected Site

Thorough débridement of wounds should be undertaken after antitoxin has been given. All devitalized tisue must be excised, all foreign bodies removed, and the wound left open. The wound should be irrigated three times a day with undiluted 3% hydrogen peroxide after the operative procedure.

Antimicrobial agents are of doubtful value in the therapy of tetanus. Any situation in the body that is suitable for the growth of *C. tetani* must be devoid of an adequate blood supply—that is, antimicrobics penetrate poorly into sites of tetanal toxin production. Nevertheless, antimicrobics are generally given. *Clostridium tetani,* like all species of *Clostridium,* are susceptible to penicillin G. Large doses should be given in an effort to favor the diffusion of penicillin into devitalized areas—for example, 200 to 400 mg (319,000–638,000 units) per kg of body weight per day by IV infusion for at least 10 days, if the patient is allergic to penicillin, cefazolin (half the dose of penicillin G) or tetracycline can be substituted (15–20 mg/kg body wt/day, given perorally as four equal portions, one every 6 hours). With mixed infections, identification and susceptibility testing is the best guide to the selection of additional antimicrobial agents.

Prevention

All breaks of the skin surface are potential portals of entry for *C. tetani.* However, the term *tetanusprone* should be reserved for compound fractures, gunshot wounds, burns, crush injuries, wounds with retained foreign bodies, deep puncture wounds, wounds contaminated with soil or feces, wounds untended for

Table 126-2. Guide to Tetanus Prophylaxis in Wound Management

History Tetanus Immunization (Doses)	Clean, Minor Wounds		All Other Wounds	
	Td	TIG	Td	TIG
Uncertain	Yes	No	Yes	Yes
0–1	Yes	No	Yes	Yes
2	Yes	No	Yes	No*
3 or more	No†	No	No‡	No

*Unless wound more than 24 hours old.
†Unless more than 10 years since last dose.
‡Unless more than 5 years since last dose.

more than 24 hours, wounds infected with other microorganisms, wounds with devitalized or avascular tissue, and abortions induced with unsterile equipment. Immediate, thorough surgical treatment of wounds is imperative; this is the single most important maneuver in tetanus prophylaxis.

The prophylactic administration of a single 250-unit dose of TIG should be reserved for patients with major, contaminated wounds (Table 126-2) and either no previous immunization, only one dose of tetanal toxoid, or unreliable histories of immunization. The same dose of TIG is also appropriate with wounds more than 24 hours old in patients who have received only two or fewer doses of tetanal toxoid. TIG does not guarantee protection; nearly 5% of cases seen in the United States occur in persons given TIG at the time of injury.

Previously unimmunized persons with wounds who merit TIG prophylaxis should at the same time be given alum-absorbed toxoid injected IM in a different site. A second dose of tetanal toxoid should be given approximately 1 month after the first dose. Despite slight interference in the development of immunity when toxoid and antitoxin are given simultaneously, active protective levels will usually be reached 8 to 10 days after the second dose of toxoid.

All persons with wounds who are not fully immunized but who have received one or two doses of tetanal toxoid in the past should be given a dose of toxoid immediately, and arrangements should then be made for additional doses suficient to achieve and maintain full immunization. An anamnestic antibody response occurs in such persons, even though the last dose may have been given in the distant past. TIG is not needed in the management of these patients if the wound is clean and minor, and receives adequate surgical care.

Tetanus virtually never occurs in fully immunized persons; the failure rate is less than 4 per 100 million. Protective levels of antitoxin will be present if the most recent dose of toxoid was given within 10 years of injury. However, if the wound is in the tetanus-prone category and several years have elapsed since toxoid was last given, a booster dose of toxoid should be injected. Prophylactic TIG is not indicated for fully immunized patients with wounds.

Neonatal tetanus can be prevented entirely by providing at least two doses of tetanal toxoid to pregnant women, training midwives in aseptic technique, and administering TIG to infants born under unsterile conditions to unimmunized mothers.

Routine immunization of all infants should begin at 1 to 3 months of age, using combined immunogens for tetanus, diphtheria, and pertussis (DPT). Three doses of DPT should be given at 4 to 6 week intervals, with booster doses 1 and 4 years later. Immunity to tetanus can be maintained by one dose of toxoid given every 10 years thereafter. For the routine immunization of adults, two doses of alum-precipitated diphtherial-tetanal toxoid given IM 1 month apart should be followed by a booster dose after 1 year and one dose every 10 years thereafter. The immunologic response seems to be superior when the toxoid is given IM. Alum-absorbed tetanal toxoid is superior to liquid toxoid.

Tetanal toxoid is an exceptionally safe and effective immunizing agent. Reactions to toxoid are uncommon, and they are most freqeuntly seen in those who have received too many doses in the past. Local reactions consisting of edema, erytherma, pain, and fever start a few hours after the injection and resemble an Arthus phenomenon. Although such reactions may occur in as many as 30% of persons who have received toxoid previously, the discomfort is trivial for the most part. Incapacitation for a day or so is probably no more frequent than 0.3%.

Delayed hypersensitivity to tetanal toxoid has been observed 6 to 7 days after administration, with pain, discomfort, and local irritation at the injection site. This hypersensitivity resembles a reaction to tuberculin, and it is totally different from the immediate urticarial reaction. Neither sluffing of tissue nor death has been reported from the administration of tetanal toxoid.

Whether susceptibility is universal among persons who have not been inoculated with toxoid is not entirely certain. The questiona rises because protective levels of antitoxin have been found in some persons with no history of ever having received toxoid. Although direct clinical proof of such naturally acquired immunity will probably never be obtained, it is a matter of interest. A means for natural immunization was suggested by the development of protective levels of antitoxin in guinea pigs after repeated ingestion of tetanal spores, presumably because sublethal doses of tetanospasmin were released in the gastrointestinal tract. If repeated ingestion of spores is also capable of inducing immunity in humans, it is most likely to occur in underdeveloped countries where tetanal spores may be more prevalent in man, animals, and the environment. Whether or not naturally acquired immunity truly occurs in humans, the only certain way to assure protection against tetanus is by administration of tetanal toxoid.

Remaining Problems

The continuing high mortality from tetanus, even in special treatment centers, lends emphasis to the need for further work on the therapy of this disease. The intrathecal administration of tetanal antitoxin was abandoned several years ago because of associated severe reactions. Neonates have been treated intrathecally with equine antitoxin that has been dialyzed to remove the formalin preservative; although experience is limited, such therapy has not been associated with sequelae and has been strikingly effective. Further controlled studies along these lines with a suitable preparation of TIG are clearly indicated.

The rapid access of large quantities of TIG to unbound toxin seems to be desirable in the management of tetanus. Because the available form of TIG cannot be given IV, a preparation suitable for IV use should be developed.

It has been demonstrated that humans can tolerate immense doses of tetanal toxoid. Although toxoid does not have the same affinity as toxin for the gangliosides in the CNS it might be possible to saturate binding sites and competitively displace fixed toxin by massive doses of tetanal toxoid given early in the disease. Such therapy in experimental animals has enabled the animals to withstand several lethal doses of tetanospasmin before antibody formation.

Bibliography

Books

Proceedings of the II International Conference on Tetanus, Bern, Switzerland, July 15–19, 1966. Bern & Stuttgart, Hans Huber, 1967. 577 pp.

Proceedings of the III International Conference on Tetanus, Sao Paulo, Brazil. August 17–22, 1970. Washington DC, Pan American Health Organization, Scientific Publication No. 253, 1972. 138 pp.

Proceedings of the IV International Conference on Tetanus. Dakar, Senegal, April 6–12, 1975. Foundation Merieux, Lyon, France, 1975. 973 pp.

Journals

BLAKE, PA, FELDMAN RA, BUCHANAN TM, BROOKS GF, BENNETT JV: Serologic therapy of tetanus in the United States, 1965–1971. JAMA 235:42–44, 1976

BROOKS VB, CURTIS DR, ECCLES JC: Mode of action of tetanus toxin. Nature 175:120–121, 1955

FRASER DW: Preventing tetanus in patients with wounds. Ann Intern Med 84:95–97, 1976

LAFORCE FM, YOUNG LS, BENNETT JV: Tetanus in the United States: Epidemiologic and clinical features. N Engl J Med 280:569–574, 1969

PERLSTEIN MA, STEIN MD, ELAM H: Routine treatment of tetanus. JAMA 173:1536–1541, 1960

Public Health Service Advisory Committee on Immunization Practices: Diphtheria and tetanus toxoids and pertussis vaccine. Morbid Mortal Weekly Rep 26:401–402, 407, 444, 1977

RUBBO SD: A re-evaluation of tetanus prophylaxis in civilian practice. Med J Aust 2:105–113, 1965

J. GLENN MORRIS, JR.
CHARLES L. HATHEWAY

Botulism

127

Botulism is a neuroparalytic syndrome resulting from the action of heat-labile toxin produced by *Clostridium botulinum.* Three forms are currently recognized: (1) food-borne botulism, acquired by eating food containing toxin; (2) wound botulism, caused by infection of a wound with *C. botulinum* with production of toxin *in vivo;* and (3) infant botulism, resulting from colonization of the infant gastrointestinal tract by *C. botulinum* with production of toxin *in vivo.*

Etiology

Clostridium botulinum are anaerobic, gram-positive bacilli that produce heat-resistant spores. There are seven recognized types of *C. botulinum* (types A–G) based on antigenic differences in the toxins produced; these differences are readily demonstrated by neutralization with type-specific antitoxins. Although designated a single species, *C. botulinum* is really a collection of four different groups of clostridia that have in common the ability to produce neurotoxins with the same unique affinity and mode of action regardless of immunotype. The key characteristics for the four groups are shown in Table 127-1. Toxins of types B and F are produced by bacilli of both groups I and II. Botulism in humans is caused almost exclusively by group I and II strains; types C and D botulism occur in animals and birds, whereas illness caused by type G has not been documented in any species.

Widely distributed in the environment, *C. botulinum* may be isolated from soils and marine sediments, the surfaces of vegetables and fruits, and fish and other seafoods. Although the toxins are readily inactivated by heat, the spores produced by *C. botulinum* are resistant and can survive ordinary cooking temperatures. They do not germinate and grow unless certain requirements are met: anaerobic conditions (restricted oxygen and sufficiently low Eh); adequate nutrients; low acidity (pH >4.6); sufficient availability of water (low solute concentrations; Aw >0.85); suitable temperature (may be as low as 4°C for some group II strains); and lack of inhibiting substances.

Botulinal toxins were previously believed to be exotoxins, elaborated by cells as they grow and divide; it now appears that the toxins are cytoplasmic proteins that are released as cells lyse. The toxic moiety has a molecular weight that varies from 135,000 to 170,000 (depending on the type of toxin), and consists of a large (MW $\sim$ 100,000) and a small (MW $\sim$ 50,000) peptide joined together by a single disulfide bond. The toxins are synthesized as prototoxins or slightly active progenitor molecules that appear to be single peptide chains with an intrachain disulfide linkage. Activation results when a proteolytic enzyme cleaves a peptide bond in the chain between the cysteine residues that comprise the disulfide bridge yielding the two-peptide structure. Endogenous enzymes carry out the activation of toxins in the proteolytic strains, but the action of an exogenous enzyme such as trypsin is necessary to activate fully the toxins of nonproteolytic strains.

Botulinal neurotoxins are the most poisonous substances known. For a mouse, a lethal intraperitoneal dose (i.p. LD_{50}) of chromatographically purified type A toxin is about 10 picograms (10×10^{-12} g), which represents only a few million molecules; for mice and other experimental animals, the lethal oral dose may be from 100 to 10,000 times the lethal intraperitoneal dose. The dose of botulinal toxins lethal for a human after ingestion has been estimated to range from less than 100,000 to 500,000 mouse i.p. LD_{50}, with 7,000 mouse i.p. LD_{50} probably sufficient to cause disease in humans. Botulinal toxins are antigenic, and neutralizing antibodies (antitoxin) are readily formed after exposure to properly inactivated toxins (toxoid). However, in limited studies in natu-

Table 127-1. *Differential Characteristics of Four Groups of* Clostridium botulinum.

Group	Toxin Types	Fermentation of GLUCOSE	Fermentation of MANNOSE	Milk Digestion	Lipase	Trimethoprim Resistance	Volatile Metabolic acids*
I	A, B, F	+	−	+	+	+	A, IB, B, IV
II	B, E, F	+	+	−	+	−	A, B
III	C, D	+	−	−	+	+	A, P, B
IV	G	−	−	+	−	+	A, IB, B, IV

*A = acetic; IB = isobutyric; B = butyric; P = propionic; IV = isovaleric

rally occurring outbreaks of botulism, antibodies have not been demonstrated in the serums of patients who have recovered. That is, no immune response takes place at the level of exposure to toxins encountered in the illness; it may be said that the immunogenic dose is greater than the lethal dose.

Food-borne Botulism

Epidemiology

Outbreaks of food-borne botulism have been reported from all parts of the world. In the United States, between 1950 and 1979, 324 outbreaks (involving 763 persons) were reported to the Centers for Disease Control (Fig. 127-1). Of food-borne outbreaks in the United States in which the type of toxin was determined 58% were type A, 25% were type B, and 17% were type E; there was 1 type F outbreak. In accordance with the observed distribution of botulinal spores in the environment, 87% of outbreaks occurring west of the Mississippi were caused by *C. botulinum* type A, whereas 65% of outbreaks occurring east of the Mississippi were caused by type B; type E outbreaks have usually been associated with fish or seafood and in the United States have been reported primarily from Alaska. Although food-borne botulism is traditionally associated with multiperson outbreaks, 52% of the outbreaks in the United States since 1950 (and 71% of outbreaks since 1975) have involved only one person.

The name *botulism* is derived from the Latin *botulus* (sausage); early outbreaks were often associated with sausage or other preserved meats. In the United States since 1950, home-canned or home-processed foods have been implicated in approximately 90% of outbreaks; home-canned green beans or peppers were the foods most commonly involved, accounting for 10% and 9%, respectively, of outbreaks of known etiology. The diagnosis of botulism should not be excluded, however, just because a patient has not eaten home-canned products: in 1978, 34 persons contracted the disease after eating bean or potato salad at a private club in New Mexico, and 8 became ill after eating potato salad prepared in a restaurant in Colorado.

Pathogenesis and Pathology

Preformed botulinal toxin ingested in food is absorbed primarily from the small intestine, and is distributed generally by way of the lymphatic and circulatory systems. The toxin acts on the peripheral nervous system where it inhibits the release of acetylcholine at cholinergic synapses, probably by impairing Ca^{++}-induced exocytosis. Blockage of neuromuscular transmission involves several steps: there is an initial, rapid-binding step in which toxin attaches to the external surface of the nerve membrane; this is followed by translocation of the toxin molecule (or some portion of it) through the membrane; finally, there is a slow paralytic step that may be at least partially dependent on temperature and neuronal activity. The entire process is essentially irreversible, although during the initial binding step the toxin remains partially susceptible to inactivation by antitoxin. The central nervous system is believed to be unaffected by the toxin. Death results from respiratory paralysis; gross and histologic changes on postmortem examination are inconsistent and nondiagnostic.

Manifestations

Symptoms and signs of the disease may begin as soon as 6 hours or as late as 8 days after ingestion of contaminated food; the usual interval is 12 to 72 hours. Generally, persons with an early onset of clinical illness (within 24 hours) are most severely affected.

The illness is characterized by symmetrical impairment of cranial nerves, followed in a descending pattern by weakness or paralysis of muscles of the extremities and trunk. Common presenting complaints include dysphagia, blurred vision, dysarthria, dry mouth, and fatigue (Table 127-2); in more severe cases, there may be complaints of dyspnea. Paresthesias have been reported in up to 14% of cases. Often nausea and vomiting, and sometimes diarrhea, pre-

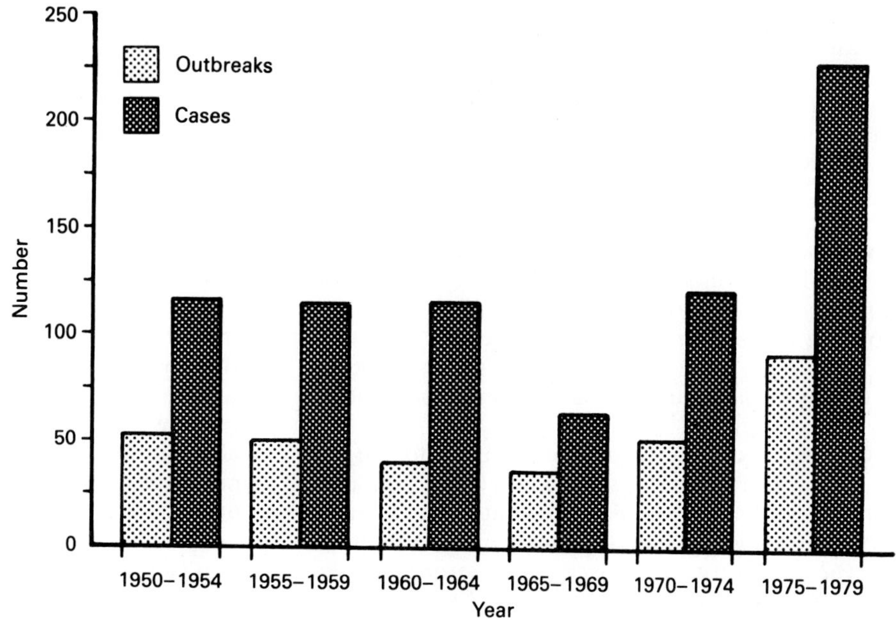

Fig. 127-1. Number of outbreaks and cases of food-borne botulism reported to the Centers for Disease Control from the United States, 1950–1979.

cede or accompany neurologic manifestations; constipation may occur after neurologic signs appear.

On physical examination, ophthalmoplegia and ptosis of the eyelids are usually prominent, along with a decreased gag reflex and facial weakness. Frequently, upper- or lower-extremity weakness is demonstrable; however, respiratory insufficiency may occur before weakness of the arms or legs. Characteristically, patients with botulism are afebrile and have no sensory deficits. The mental status is usually normal, although there may be lethargy. Fixed or dilated pupils are seen in fewer than half of the cases and are significantly more common in type B than in type A botulism. Deep tendon reflexes are normal in most cases but may be hypoactive or lacking. Nystagmus and ataxia have been reported in 22% and 17% of the cases, respectively.

Electromyographic abnormalities are frequently present, although a normal electromyogram (EMG) does not rule out botulism. Characteristic EMG findings include diminution of the amplitude of muscle action potentials after a single supramaximal nerve stimulus and facilitation of the action potential when paired stimuli are delivered at an interval of 2.5 msec or repetitive stimuli are applied at rates of 20 to 50 per second (also seen with the Eaton–Lambert syndrome). Nerve conduction studies are usually normal. The blood cell counts, urinalyses, serum electrolytes, cerebrospinal fluid, and blood enzymes are normal unless there are complications.

Table 127-2. *Frequency of Symptoms in Food-Borne Botulism (From a Review of 55 Cases of Food-Borne Botulism in the United States, Reported to the Centers for Disease Control, 1973–74)*

Symptoms	% of Cases
Dysphagia	96
Dry mouth	93
Diplopia	91
Dysarthria	84
Fatigue	77
Upper extremity weakness	73
Constipation	73
Lower extremity weakness	69
Dyspnea	60
Vomiting	59
Dizziness	51
Diarrhea	19
Paresthesias	14

Hughes JM, Blumenthal JR, Merson MH, Lombard GL, Dowell VR, Gangarosa EJ: Clinical features of Types A and B foodborne botulism. Ann Intern Med 95:442–445, 1981

Diagnosis

The diagnosis of botulism is confirmed by demonstrating botulinal toxin in the patient's serum or feces, culturing *C. botulinum* from feces, or identifying toxin in incriminated food. Botulinal toxin is identified using mouse toxin-neutralization tests, which may require 24 to 96 hours to complete; because of this delay and the need to institute therapy rapidly in suspected cases, the initial diagnosis must generally be based on clinical and electromyographic findings. Laboratory testing requires 10 ml to 15 ml of serum and 25 g to 50 g of feces; after notifying the laboratory, these specimens, as well as a specimen of the implicated food, should be sent to the nearest laboratory capable of testing for botulinal toxin and isolating *C. botulinum.* Such services are available through many state health department laboratories, as well as from the botulism laboratory at the Centers for Disease Control in Atlanta, Georgia.

Diseases most often confused with botulism include the Guillain-Barré syndrome (GBS), myasthenia gravis, cerebrovascular accidents (CVAs), and food poisoning and other types of acute gastroenteritis. The GBS is usually an ascending motor paralysis, although in occasional cases signs may be confined to cranial nerves (Miller Fisher variant); a history of an antecedent viral illness, the presence of paresthesias or other sensory abnormalities, or an elevated spinal fluid protein helps to distinguish this disease. Myasthenia gravis can usually be differentiated by the accentuation of muscular fatigability during exercise and the positive response to edrophonium (although positive responses to edrophonium have been reported in cases of botulism). CVAs generally cause localizing signs. The lack of cranial nerve involvement is usually sufficient to distinguish food poisoning and other forms of acute gastroenteritis from botulism.

Chemical food poisonings sometimes cause neurologic manifestations, but their incubation periods are short—usually within 1 hour and often within minutes of consumption of contaminated food. Carbon monoxide poisoning, an illness frequently mistaken for botulism because it may affect more than one person concurrently, does not affect the cranial nerves. Paralytic shellfish poisoning, ciguatera, and other types of fish and shellfish poisonings are also rapid in onset and have characteristic patterns of paresthesias. The lack of fever in botulism helps to exclude infectious diseases, including poliomyelitis, meningitis, and encephalitis. Certain antimicrobics (*e.g.,* the aminocyclitols, the polymyxins, bacitracin, and combinations of these agents) may rarely induce symmetric, flaccid paralysis, as has been described at surgical laparotomy after intraperitoneal application of these antimicrobics. Idiosyncratic reactions to phenothiazine drugs have been confused with botulism.

Prognosis

The case–fatality rate for botulism between 1975 and 1979 was less than 10%, compared with a rate of approximately 70% between 1910 and 1919 (Fig. 127-2). The improvement can be attributed primarily to advances in general medical care, including the widespread availability of long-term, mechanical ventilatory support. Deaths now occur either because the diagnosis is not considered (and consequently the patient is not properly monitored) or because of problems encountered in providing respiratory care over an extended period.

The severity of illness in a given outbreak is generally related to the quantity of contaminated food eaten; however, persons have died after tasting only a small quantity of food containing botulinal toxin. The duration of illness is related to its severity. For patients requiring mechanical ventilation, the average duration of respiratory support is approximately 1 month (although cases requiring up to 7 months of mechanical ventilatory support have been reported). Recovery is usually complete.

Therapy

Asymptomatic persons who have eaten food that possibly contains botulinal toxin (*i.e.,* food eaten from a swollen can without prior cooking, improperly preserved home-canned foods) should be observed carefully for the development of neurologic signs and symptoms; unless there is a high degree of suspicion that botulism is involved, such observation can frequently be done at home. Induction of vomiting and administration of a cathartic is usually advisable. Since very few patients of this category actually turn out to have botulism, additional treatment, including therapy with antitoxin, is generally not recommended.

Patients with signs and symptoms compatible with botulism, or patients who are known to have eaten food shown by laboratory testing to contain botulinal toxin, should be admitted to an intensive care unit to permit monitoring of respiratory and cardiac function. Airway patency should be guaranteed by insertion of an endotracheal tube or tracheostomy before bulbar or respiratory impairment becomes severe. Induction of vomiting or gastric lavage is recommended if exposure has occurred within several hours. Unless there is paralytic ileus, purgation is advisable, even after several days, to facilitate possible elimination of unabsorbed toxin from the gastrointestinal tract; alternatively, high enemas may be used.

Trivalent (ABE), equine-origin botulinal antitoxin is available on a 24-hour basis from the Centers for Disease Control, Atlanta, Georgia (telephone 404-

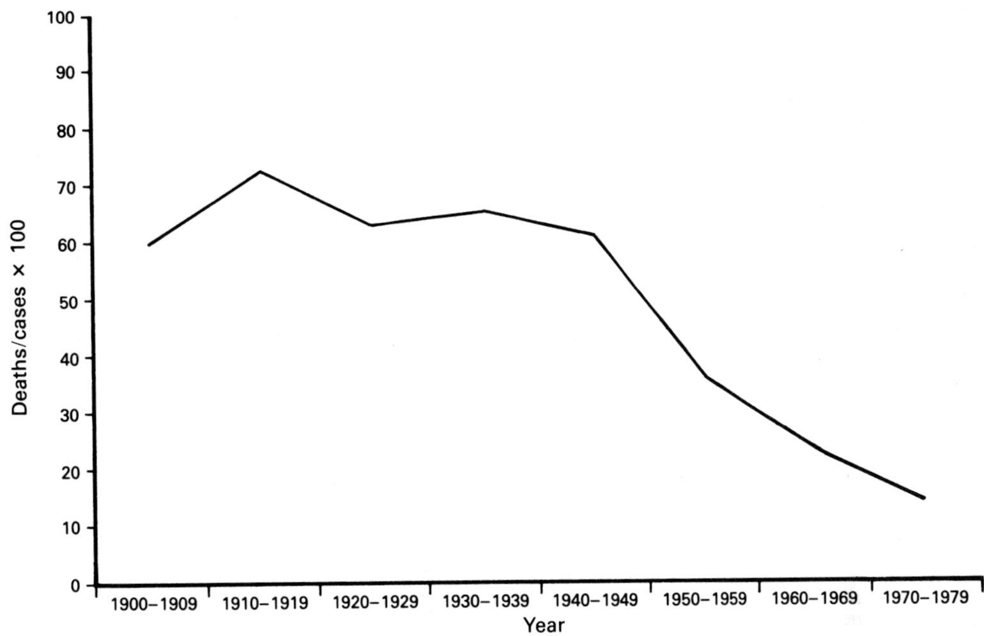

Fig. 127-2. Case–fatality ratio of botulism by ten-year intervals, 1900–1979.

329-3756 days; 404-329-3644 nights and weekends) and from some state health departments. Although data on efficacy in humans are limited, antitoxin is clearly efficacious in nonhuman animals; however, efficacy is directly related to how early in the course of the disease the antitoxin is administered. The decision to use antitoxin should be made quickly, but also with care; because botulinal antitoxin is of equine origin, there is a high risk of adverse reactions associated with its use: anaphylaxis in approximately 2% of cases, and serum sickness in 4% of cases. Instructions for skin testing or conjunctival testing of the antiare included in the package insert.

Guanidine hydrochloride has been given to a number of patients with botulism based on its theoretical benefit in increasing release of acetylcholine from nerve terminals after arrival of the action potential. Response to the drug has varied and its efficacy is equivocal; in a recent controlled study involving patients with type A botulism, treatment with guanidine did not enhance recovery. Other drugs, including 4-aminopyridine, have been used occasionally, but should be regarded strictly as investigational agents.

Prevention

Food-borne botulism is best prevented by stressing careful adherence to proper home-canning techniques, including the importance of using appropriate containers, and adhering strictly to time and temperature guidelines for processing as specified in the recipe being followed. In addition, any home-canned food should be brought to a full boil (not just rewarmed) before it is eaten. Current quality control measures in the food processing industry have minimized the risk of botulism associated with commercially canned products; however, any rusty or swollen can should be discarded, without tasting of the contents.

When botulism is suspected, local, state, and federal authorities should be notified promptly so that an investigation may be conducted. This will permit identification of other persons who may have been exposed to the contaminated food and who may still be asymptomatic, as well as identification of food still in distribution. Such notification is required by law in many states.

Remaining Problems

Outbreaks of botulism continue to occur in which extensive investigation fails to implicate a specific food as the cause of the disease. It is possible that pathophysiologic mechanisms other than ingestion of preformed toxin (such as production of toxin *in vivo* as in infant botulism) may be involved in these cases. Since 1978, such cases have been recorded by the Centers for Disease Control as cases of "undetermined classification," rather than as food-borne cases, in order to determine whether the two groups differ epidemiologically. These cases raise a number of questions about our basic understanding of the pathophysiology of botulism, and should receive increased attention during the next few years.

The problems posed by the high reaction rate to equine botulinal antitoxin have prompted efforts to develop antitoxin of human origin, and it is possible that within the next decade such material will be available. In addition, further work is necessary with drugs (such as the aminopyridines) which may counteract the effect of botulinal toxin.

Wound Botulism

Epidemiology

Between 1942, when the syndrome was first recognized, and the end of 1979, 21 cases of wound botulism were reported in the United States. The median age of the patients was 19 years (range 6–44 years); 81% were male. The wounds were usually deep and contained avascular areas; nine patients had compound fractures, and four had extensive crush injuries of the hand. The median incubation period was 7 days (range 4–21 days).

Manifestations

The clinical manifestations of wound botulism are similar to those of food-borne botulism. However, fever may be present, whereas acute gastrointestinal symptoms are lacking.

Diagnosis

Wound botulism should be considered in any patient with a wound who has the characteristic clinical features of botulism. Laboratory confirmation of the diagnosis requires the isolation of *C. botulinum* from an infected wound or the detection of botulinal toxin in the patient's serum. Tetanus, rabies, and myonecrosis should be included in the differential diagnosis.

Prognosis

Among the 21 cases of wound botulism reported in the United States, 4 deaths occurred, with the last fatal case occurring in 1971. As with food-borne botulism, the prognosis is good if adequate respiratory support is available for the patient; of the three cases reported in 1979, all required respiratory support for 1 to 2 months.

Therapy

Thorough debridement, drainage, and irrigation of the wound are essential to treatment, and should be carried out after botulinal antitoxin has been administered. Antimicrobial agents are generally recommended, with penicillin the drug of choice (Table 127-3). However, most of the patients with wound botulism were under treatment with antimicrobics (including penicillin in some cases) at the time they developed signs and symptoms of botulism. That is, antimicrobics may not penetrate into areas of wounds that are sufficiently avascular to provide conditions suitable for the growth of *C. botulinum.*

Infant Botulism

Epidemiology

Infant botulism was first recognized as a distinct clinical entity in 1976; cases have been identified retro-

Table 127-3. *Minimal Inhibitory Concentrations (μg/ml) of Several Antimicrobics for 174 Strains of* Clostridium botulinum *at the 50%, 90%, and 100% levels*

	Type A			Type B		
Antimicrobic	50	90	100	50	90	100
Penicillin	≤.5	≤.5	4	≤.5	±.5	2
Cephalothin	≤.5	1	32	≤.5	1	32
Chloramphenicol	2–4	4	8	2	4	16
Clindamycin	≤.5	≤.5	16	1–2	4	16
Gentamicin	128	>128	>128	128	>128	<128

*Numbers tested: *C. botulinum* type A—109 strains; *C. botulinum* type B—65 strains.

Swenson JM, Thornsberry C, McCroskey LM, Hatheway CL, Dowell VR: Susceptibility of *Clostridium botulinum* to 13 antimicrobials. Antimicrob Agents Chemother 18:13–19, 1980

spectively, however, and it is likely that the disease has been present for many years. Cases have been reported from the United States, Canada, Great Britain, Australia, and Czechoslovakia. In the United States, 120 cases were reported to the Centers for Disease Control between 1976 and 1979 (Fig. 127-3). Of these cases, 65 (54%) involved *C. botulinum* type A and 54 (45%) involved *C. botulinum* type B; 1 case was caused by *C. botulinum* type F. As with food-borne botulism, the geographic distribution of cases by toxin type correlates roughly with the distribution of botulinal spores in the environment, with 66% of cases occurring west of the Mississippi caused by *C. botulinum* type A and 88% of cases occurring east of the Mississippi caused by type B. Cases occur most commonly in the second month of life (Fig. 127-4); 97.5% of cases were in infants 6 months of age or younger. Infant botulism has been reported most frequently from California (58 of 120 cases), although the case rate per 100,000 live births is highest in Utah (10.3 cases/100,000 live births, 1976–1979) (Fig. 127-5). The number of cases appears to be somewhat greater in the fall, with 62% of cases having occurred in the last 6 months of the year.

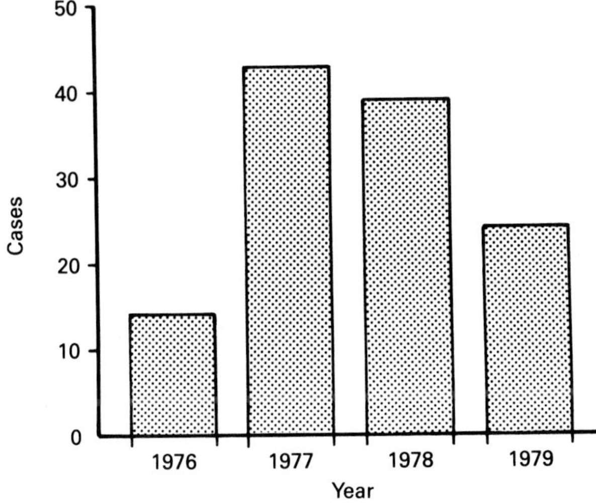

Fig. 127-3. Number of cases of infant botulism reported to the Centers for Disease Control from the United States, 1976–1979.

Pathogenesis

Infant botulism results from colonization of the infant's intestinal tract by *C. botulinum* (in quantitative studies, as many as 10^8 *C. botulinum* per g of feces have been identified in specimens obtained from affected infants), followed by production of toxin *in vivo* and absorption. The actual physiological mechanisms that permit colonization and absorption to occur in the infant gut are still poorly understood. Excretion of *C. botulinum* has been shown to occur for as long as 4 months after discharge of infants from hospital; toxin has been detected in the feces for over 3 months after discharge from hospital.

Animal models of the disease exist. An intestinal

Fig. 127-4. Age distribution of infant botulism cases reported to the Centers for Disease Control from the United States, 1976–1979.

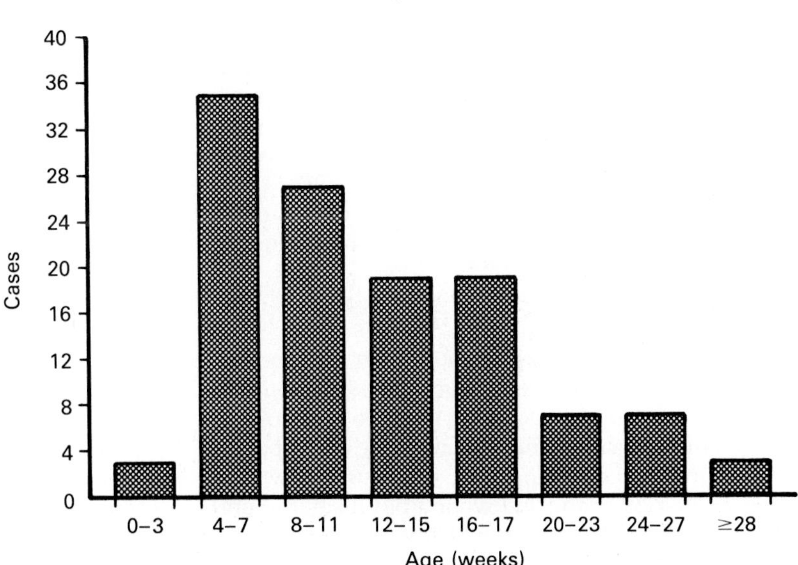

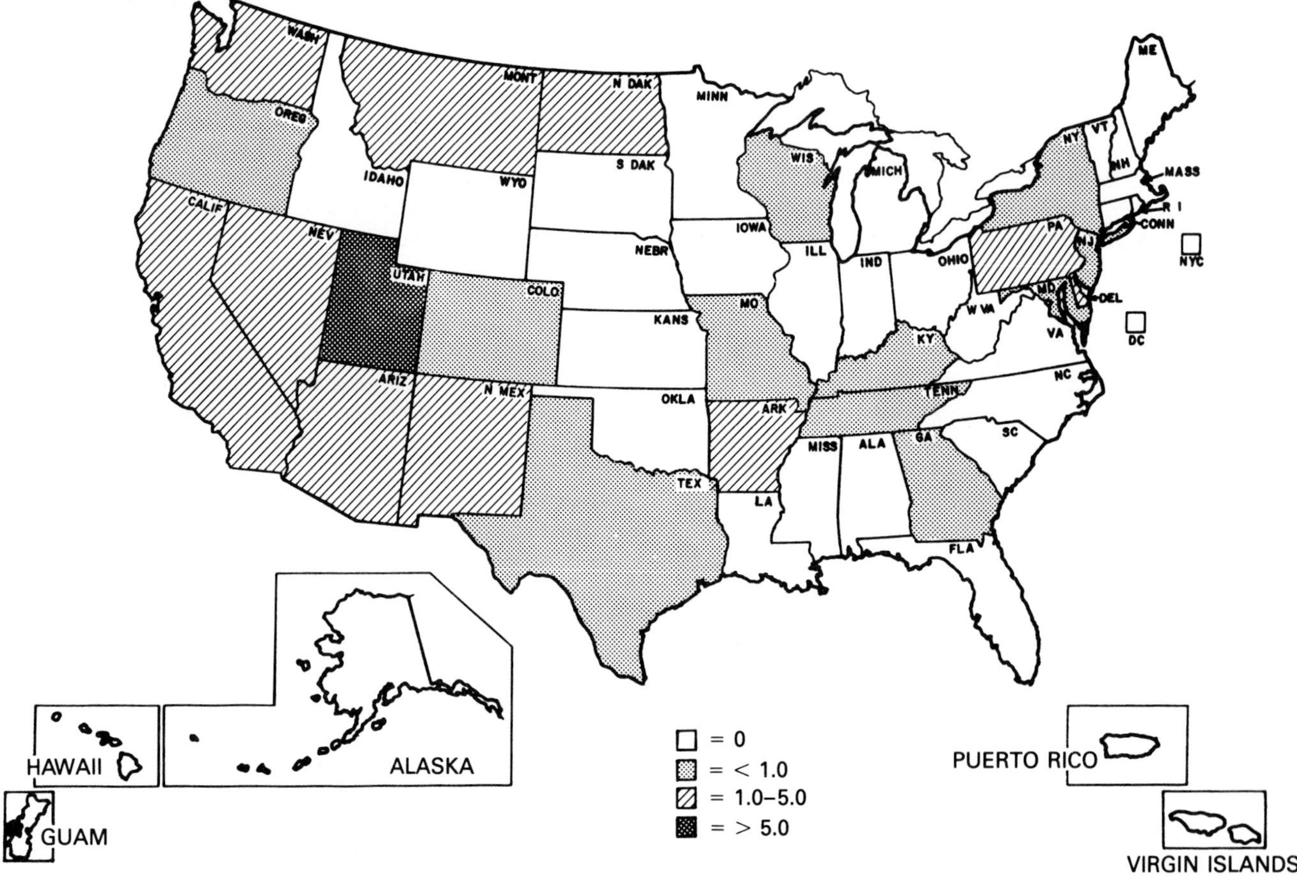

Fig. 127-5. Number of cases of infant botulism reported to the Centers for Disease Control per 100,000 live births in the United States, 1976–1979.

infection with *C. botulinum* can be produced by endogastric administration of spores of *C. botulinum* to conventionally-reared mice 7 to 13 days old, but not in younger or older mice. Although toxin was produced in such mice, absorption was insufficient to cause disease. In colts, the syndrome known as the shaker foal is thought to be analogous to infant botulism; the clinical syndrome is compatible with botulism, and *C. botulinum* has been cultured from the feces of affected animals.

Manifestations

Constipation (defined as 3 or more days without defecation) is usually the first sign of illness, although it is frequently disregarded by parents. Neurologic signs may begin simultaneously with the constipation or may not become apparent until several weeks later. As in food-borne and wound botulism, the cranial nerves are usually the first involved; a progressive, symmetrical, descending paralysis follows. In infants, the characteristic signs of ptosis, ophthalmoplegia, and flaccidity of the facial muscles may be overlooked; the babies are often brought for medical attention only after they exhibit an inability to suck or are irritable and lethargic.

A spectrum of clinical illness is associated with infant botulism, ranging from mild, virtually asymptomatic cases to severe cases in which there is respiratory paralysis necessitating mechanical ventilatory support. Infant botulism may be responsible for up to 5% of cases of sudden infant death syndrome (SIDS). Theoretically in such cases, flaccidity of the tongue and pharyngeal muscles could impede air flow, and cause hypoxia; alternatively, rapid absorption of botulinal toxin could cause respiratory paralysis before the usual clinical syndrome is recognized.

Electromyographic changes have also been described in association with infant botulism: diminution of muscle action potentials after a single supramaximal nerve stimulus; facilitation of the action potential with rapid repetitive stimulation; and the presence of brief, small, amplitude-abundant motor unit potentials (BSAPs). Other laboratory studies are normal unless there are complications.

Diagnosis

The diagnosis of infant botulism is established by demonstrating botulinal toxin in, or by culturing *C. botulinum* from, the infant's feces. Between 1976 and 1979, botulinal toxin was identified in the serum in only one case using the mouse toxin neutralization test.

Included in the differential diagnosis of infant botulism are sepsis (including meningitis and pneumonia), GBS, congenital myasthenia gravis, intoxications (including those caused by organic phosphates and heavy metals), Werdnig–Hoffman disease, and various types of electrolyte imbalances or metabolic encephalopathies. Fever and leukocytosis may help to differentiate sepsis. Meningitis is evidenced by pleocytosis in the spinal fluid. In GBS, the concentration of protein in the cerebrospinal fluid is frequently increased. Myasthenia gravis may respond to edrophonium. Intoxications and metabolic encephalopathies can usually be identified by appropriate blood tests.

Prognosis

The prognosis in hospitalized infants with botulism is excellent; only 3 deaths have been reported in 120 cases. Recovery is complete. However, the hospital course may be as long as 1 to 2 months.

Therapy

Meticulous supportive care, including mechanical respiratory assistance when necessary, is the mainstay of treatment. Antitoxin is not routinely used because of the generally good prognosis and of the risks of using equine antitoxin. There are theoretical considerations both for and against using antimicrobics active against *C. botulinum* in infant botulism. Penicillin has been used in some patients but has not been shown to affect the course of the disease. It has been suggested that aminocyclitols (which are not active against *C. botulinum*) may exacerbate the illness by potentiating the neuromuscular blockade, or by favoring the outgrowth of *C. botulinum* by suppressing enteric competitors.

Prevention

At this time, there is no method for preventing infant botulism. Botulinal spores are ubiquitous and are almost certainly consumed by most infants without apparent adverse effects. One food that has been implicated as a possible high-risk source of botulinal spores is honey; approximately one-third of the infants with botulism were fed honey prior to onset of illness; in a matched, case-control study in California, consumption of honey was shown to be associated with the development of botulism. Concomitant laboratory studies revealed *C. botulinum* spores in approximately 10% of the specimens of honey tested. Consequently, honey is not recommended as a food for infants under the age of 1 year.

Remaining Problems

Much remains to be learned about the epidemiology and physiology of infant botulism. The incidence and distribution of the disease are incompletely known, and undoubtedly a number of unrecognized cases occur. While it appears clear that infant botulism is caused by production of toxin *in vivo,* it is not clear why some infants develop illness and others do not. Much work needs to be done on the pathogenesis of the disease and the possible association of SIDS with infant botulism.

Bibliography

GENERAL

Books

Center for Disease Control: Botulism in the United States, 1899–1977: Handbook for epidemiologists, clinicians, and laboratory workers. May 1979. 41 pp.

SMITH LD: Botulism: The organism, its toxins, the disease. Springfield, IL, Charles C Thomas, 1977. 236 pp.

Journals

BLACK RE, GUNN RA: Hypersensitivity reactions associated with botulinal antitoxin. Am J Med 69:567–570, 1980

DOWELL VR, MCCROSKEY LM, HATHEWAY CL, LOMBARD GL, HUGHES JM, MERSON MH: Coproexamination for botulinal toxin. JAMA 238:1829–1832, 1977

MORRIS JG, HATHEWAY CL: Botulism in the United States: 1979. J Infect Dis 142:302–305, 1980

SUGIYAMA H: *Clostridium botulinum* neurotoxin. Microbiological Rev 44:419–448, 1980

SWENSON JM, THORNSBERRY C, MCCROSKEY LM, HATHEWAY CL, DOWELL VR: Susceptibility of *Clostridium botulinum* to 13 antimicrobials. Antimicrob Agents Chemother 18:13–19, 1980

FOOD-BORNE

Journals

CHERINGTON M: Botulism: Ten-year experience. Arch Neurol 33:432–437, 1974

DOLMAN CE, IIDA H: Type E botulism: Its epidemiology, prevention, and special treatment. Can J Public Health 54:293–308, 1963

HUGHES JM, BLUMENTHAL JR, MERSON MH, LOMBARD GL, DOWELL VR, GANGAROSA EJ: Clinical features of types A and B foodborne botulism. Ann Intern Med 95:442–445, 1981

WOUND

Journal

MERSON MH, DOWELL VR: Epidemiologic, clinical and laboratory aspects of wound botulism. New Engl J Med 289:1005–1010, 1973

INFANT

Journals

ARNON SS: Infant botulism. Ann Rev Med 31:541–560, 1980

ARNON SS, MIDURA TF, DAMUS K, THOMPSON B, WOOD RM, CHIN J: Honey and other environmental risk factors for infant botulism. J Pediatr 94:331–336, 1979

FELDMAN RA (ed): A seminar on infant botulism. Rev Infec Dis 1:611–700, 1979

JOHNSON RO, CLAY SA, ARNON SS: Diagnosis and management of infant botulism. Am J Dis Child 133:586–593, 1979

L'HOMMEDIEU C, STOUGH R, BROWN L, KETTRICK R, POLIN R: Potentiation of neuromuscular weakness in infant botulism by aminoglycosides. J Pediatr 95:1065–1070, 1979

JOHN E. EDWARDS, JR.

Zygomycosis

128

Fungi of the class Zygomycetes are characterized by the production of zygospores. The class is subdivided into three orders: Mucorales, Entomophthorales, and Zoopagales. Only the orders Mucorales and Entomophthorales contain fungi pathogenic for humans. The subdivision of the orders Mucorales and Entomophthorales into families is shown in Table 128-1, and the pathogenic species are listed within these families. The term zygomycosis refers to infection caused by any of the fungi of the class Zygomycetes.

Etiology

Of the Zygomycetes, the family Mucoraceae is the most important because it contains the genera *Rhizopus, Absidia,* and *Mucor* which cause the classical syndrome of rhinocerebral zygomycosis (formerly mucormycosis) and most of the additional, recently recognized forms of zygomycotic infection. It has become apparent that the Zygomycetes are important causes of diseases in immunocompromised patients (especially those with hematopoietic lymphoreticular malignanceis) as well as in patients with acidosis (especially diabetic ketoacidosis). The fungi of the order Entomophthorales (genera *Basidiobolus* and *Entomophthora*) are mainly found in tropical areas and infect previously healthy persons forming chronic, indolent, subcutaneous masses. In contrast to the family Mucoraceae, dissemination of the Entomophthoraceae is unusual. Within the family Mucoraceae, speciation is based on the morphology of the asexual reproductive structures called sporangiophores. Figure 128-1 diagramatically illustrates the structures that distinguish the pathogenic genera *Rhizopus, Absidia,* and *Mucor,* and Table 128-2 summarizes the morphologic features of these three genera.

The characteristic broad (6 μm–50 μm in diameter), nonseptate, thick-walled hyphae that branch nearly at right angles (Fig. 128-2) can be seen on microscopic examination of clinical specimens; yeastlike forms are virtually unseen in material from patients. Either unstained, alkali-cleared preparations, or stained sections are suitable for examination (see Chap. 9, Microscopic Examinations). The Zygomycetes grow in most routine laboratory culture media. However, cyclohexamide as used in some media to inhibit nonpathogenic fungi may also inhibit the Zygomycetes. When zygomycosis is suspected, a medium without antimicrobics should also be used (*e.g.,* Sabouraud's dextrose agar).

Epidemiology

The fungi of the class Zygomycetes are ubiquitous and are found most frequently on decaying organic material. They grow rapidly, are resistant to temperature changes, and produce numerous spores that disperse easily into the air. Occasionally, they have been isolated from normal persons with no evidence of infection. Zygomycetes of the order Entomophthorales (genera *Basidiobolus* and *Entomophthora*) are found in tropical and subtropical regions; they are thought to infect otherwise healthy persons through insect bites and minor puncture wounds.

Pathogenesis and Pathology

With rare exceptions, the Zygomycetes that gain access to humans are contained by phagocytosis. When infection ensues, the organism is found virtually exclusively as hyphae—possibly because host defenses readily dispose of yeastlike cells, whereas hyphae may survive. Hyphal growth is favored by a pH of 7.4 and by cyclic 3′, 5′- adenosine monophosphate, hexose, oxygen, and possibly a morphogenic hormone.

When host defenses were examined in rabbits

*Table 128-1. Pathogenic Members of the Class Zygomycetes**

Order Mucorales†		
Family	**Species‡**	**Synonyms**
Mucoraceae	*Rhizopus oryzae*	*Rhizopus arrhizus*
	Rhizopus rhizopodiformis	*Rhizopus cohnii, Rhizopus equinus*
	Rhizopus microsporus	
	Absidia corymbifera	*Absidia ramosa*
	Mucor circinelloides	
	Mucor pusillus	*Rhizomucor pusillus*
	Mucor miehei	*Rhizomucor miehei*
Mortierellaceae	*Mortierella wolfii*	
Cunninghamellaceae	*Cunninghamella elegans*	
	Cunninghamella bertholletiae	
Saksenaeaceae	*Saksenaea vasiformis*	
Syncephalastraceae	*Syncephalastrum* spp.	

Order Entomophthorales	
Family	**Species**
Entomophthoraceae	*Entomophthora coronata*
	Basidiobolus haptosporus

*Howard DH: Classification of the Mucorales, pp 93–94. In Lehrer RI (moderator): Mucormycosis. Ann Intern Med 93:93–108, 1980

†Several other members of the order are capable of growth at 37°C and thus represent potential pathogens of warm-blooded animals. A few examples include *Rhizopus oligosporus, Rhizopus homothallicus, Absidia hyalospora, Mucor rouxii,* and *Syncephalastrum racemosum.* (Scholer HJ, Muller E, Schipper MAA: The Mucorales. In Howard DH (ed): The Fungi Pathogenic to Humans and Animals: Biology, Pathogenicity and Detection. New York, Marcel Dekker, (In press)

‡Other species reported as pathogens were misidentifications or have been reduced to synonomy.

Table 128-2. Morphologic Features That Distinguish Potentially Pathogenic Genera in the Family Mucoraceae

	Morphologic Feature		
Genus	RHIZOIDS	APOPHYSES	COLUMELLAE
Mucor	None	Rare	Shape not distinctive
Absidia	Not directly beneath sporangiophore	Definite	Pear-shaped
Rhizopus	Directly beneath sporangiophore	Present	Ovoid

Howard DH: Classification of the Mucorales, pp 93–94. In Lehrer RI (moderator): Mucormycosis. Ann Intern Med 93:93–108, 1980

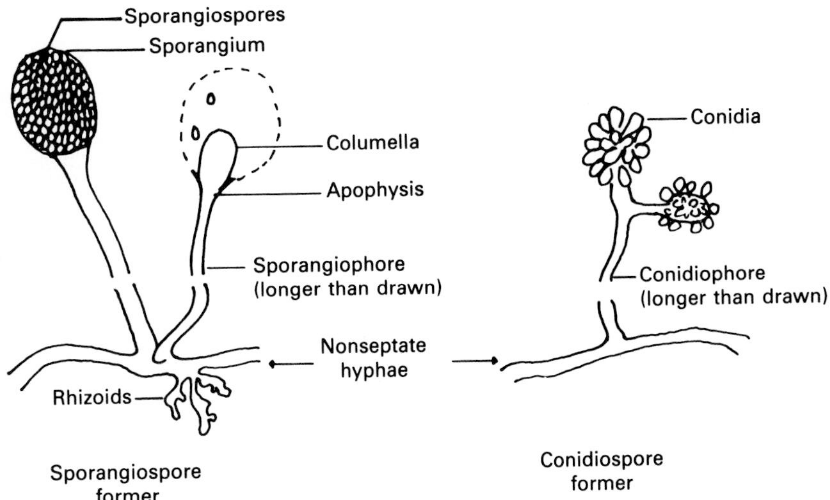

Fig. 128-1. Diagrammatic representation of morphologic features used to distinguish between pathogenic Mucorales. Some authorities do not recognize conidia among the Zygomycetes but consider the spores so labeled above as a sporangium with a single sporangiospore. The only family that displays conidia is Cunninghamellaceae; the others all produce sporangiospores within sporangia. (Howard DH: Classification of the Mucorales. In Lehrer RI: moderator: Mucormycosis, pp. 93–99. Ann Int Med 93:93-108)

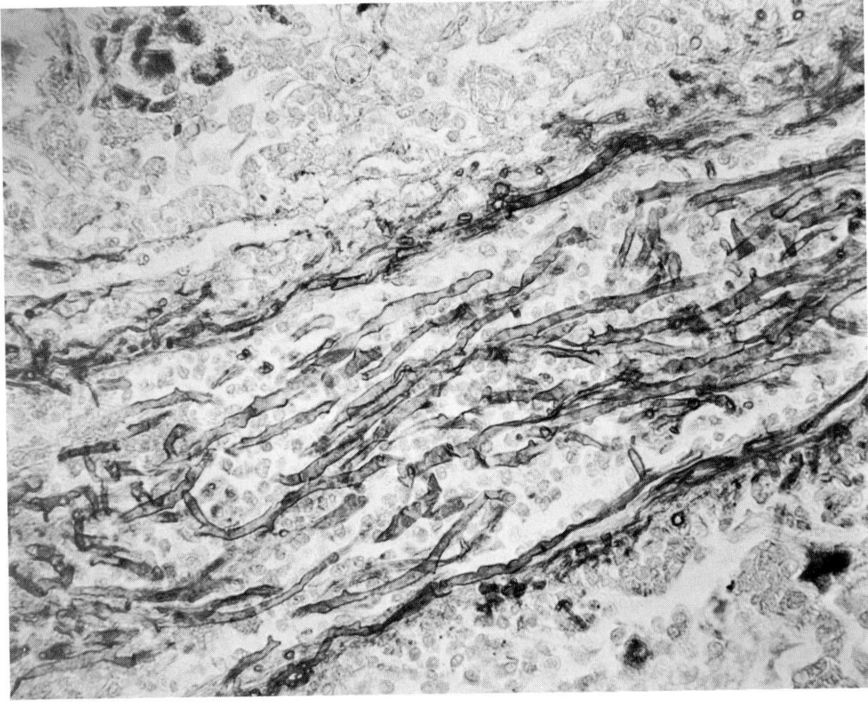

Fig. 128-2. Proliferation of large (8–15 μm) nonseptate hyphae within a pulmonary vein. The patient died of myelogenous leukemia. (H&E, × 300) (Courtesy of C Bieber)

using inocula of conidia of *Rhizopus arrhizus,* it was found that the neutrophil is capable of damaging hyphae. Ketoacidotic rabbits were much more susceptible to invasion than were rabbits that were hyperglycemic but not acidotic. The major difference between ketoacidotic rabbits and controls was the attenuation of the intense neutrophil response. Diminished chemotaxis is said to accompany diabetic ketoacidosis in humans.

Humoral factors may inhibit the growth of *R. arrhizus.* For example, heat-stable, dialyzable factors in normal serum inhibit the growth of spores, whereas the serum of a patient with diabetic ketoacidosis enhances growth.

Control of germination *of Rhizopus* spp. *in vivo* appears to be important in host defense, although the precise mechanisms for control are not known.

The pathologic hallmark of zygomycosis is the direct invasion of vascular channels by hyphal elements (Fig. 128-2). Thrombosis and hemorrhagic infarction of tissues results, and in turn, provokes an intense polymorphonuclear inflammatory cell response. This pathogenetic sequence is unique among fungi (except for *Aspergillus* spp.; see Chap. 44, Aspergillosis). It accounts for the acute and fulminant clinical picture that results from infection with the Mucoraceae and contrasts sharply with the chronic disease processes associated with the Entomophthoraceae and most other systemic mycoses. Common sites of initial invasion are the paranasal sinuses, lungs, and gastrointestinal tract.

Infections caused by the family Entomophthoraceae are marked by an eosinophilic, granulomatous tissue reaction in which hyphae are not abundant and vascular invasion is exceedingly rare. Amorphous periodic acid-Schiff-positive granular debris composed of collagen fragments and degenerating cellular organelles (the Splendore–Hoeppli phenomenon) surrounds the few hyphae. The finding is pathognomonic of subcutaneous zygomycosis and is never seen in invasive zygomycosis.

Manifestations

The clinical manifestations of zygomycosis may be categorized as rhinocerebral, pulmonary, widely disseminated, gastrointestinal, cutaneous, and miscellaneous. Rhinocerebral (particularly in patients with diabetic ketoacidosis) and pulmonary (most often in patients with leukemia or lymphoma) are the most common forms.

Zygomycotic infections are frequently manifested by two clinical characteristics: (1) infarction secondary to direct invasion of vessel walls; and (2) production of black, necrotic material in exudates.

Rhinocerebral

While the majority of patients with rhinocerebral zygomycosis have diabetes mellitus (particularly complicated by acidosis), some patients have had leukemia as an underlying disease. However, most of the patients with leukemia have also had diabetes or have been treated with glucosteroids. The infection usually begins in the nasal sinuses, spreads to the paranasal sinuses, and may extend through the ethmoid sinus into the retroorbital region. Further extension through the apex of the orbit into the brain is the most serious complication. In some immunocompromised patients the infection begins on the palate and extends upward into the nasal sinuses (Fig. 128-3). Early identification of an indolent lesion on the palate, particularly in immunocompromised patients, may enable prevention of extension into the sinuses. Rhinocerebral zygomycosis may be either indolent and slowly progressive or may advance rapidly and result in death within a few days after onset.

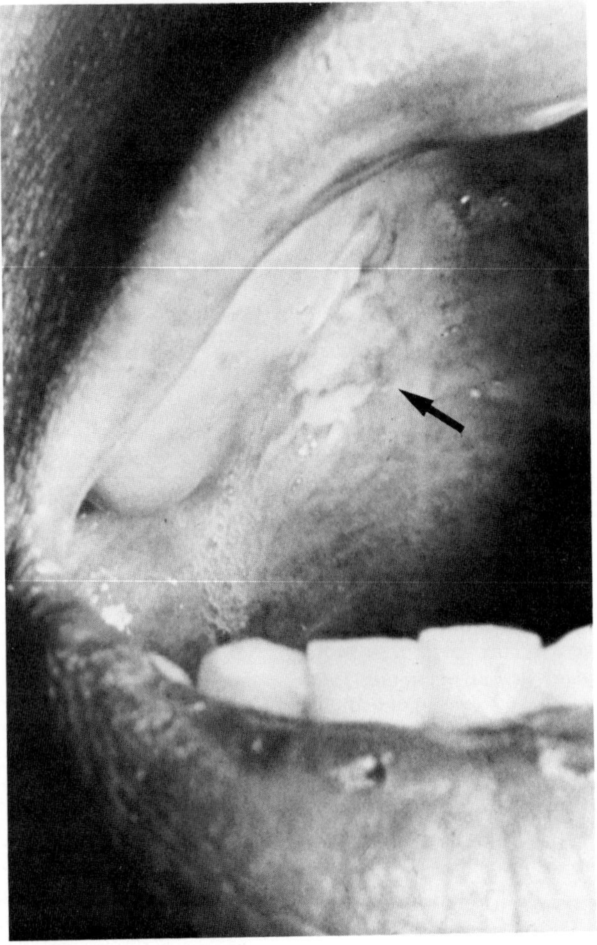

Fig. 128-3. Zygomycotic lesion on the palate of an immunocompromised patient. (New H: Opportunistic Infections. Famous Teachings in Modern Medicine. New York, Medcom, 1973)

The most common initial signs and symptoms of rhinocerebral zygomycosis include lethargy, headache, loss of vision, impaired ocular movement, proptosis, and periorbital cellulitis. Because of the tendency of the fungus to invade the walls of blood vessels, both cavernous sinus thrombosis and internal carotid artery thrombosis are frequent complications. Extension into the globe may occur. Radiographic manifestations are nonspecific: nodular thickening of the mucosa of the sinuses, clouding of the sinuses without air-liquid levels, and spotty destruction of bone in the walls of sinuses. Unusual complications of rhinocerebral zygomycosis include myocardial infarction (occlusion of coronary arteries by fungi), septic abortion, acute subdural hematoma, and thrombosis of the jugular vein.

Because the early manifestations of rhinocerebral zygomycosis are nonspecific, this diagnosis should be considered in patients with diabetic ketoacidosis and obtundation that does not resolve with amelioration of the acidosis and electrolyte abnormalities. Such patients should be evaluated carefully for intracerebral zygomycosis. Unfortunately, the cerebrospinal fluid (CSF) may be entirely normal, or may have a modest leukocytic pleocytosis (approximately 50% polymorphonuclear), with some erythrocytes. Hypoglycorrhachia is uncommon. Computed tomographic examination (CT scan) of the head may be of value.

Pulmonary

Although pulmonary zygomycosis is seen in patients with diabetes mellitus, renal failure (with immunosuppresive therapy), or burns and in normal persons, the most common setting is leukemia, lymphoma, or severe neutropenia. Vascular thrombosis with pulmonary infarction is common. Particularly in immunocompromised patients, a primary bacterial infection may be complicated by Zygomycetes as a superinfection. The pulmonary radiographic findings include patchy, bronchopneumonic infiltrates, consolidation, cavitation, and pleural effusion. Fungus balls may develop in some cavitary lesions. Complications include fatal pulmonary hemorrhage, perforation of the bronchus, broncho-pleural and broncho-cutaneous fistulae, pulmonary infarctions, and granulomatous mediastinitis.

Disseminated

By far the most common setting for widespread disseminated zygomycosis is immunoincompetence, particularly as associated with leukemia and lymphoma. Invasion of the walls of blood vessels producing infarctions in various organs is characteristic. The lungs are involved most commonly; other organs include the spleen, kidney, heart, duodenum, liver, pancreas, stomach, omentum, and brain. Renal vein thrombosis and hepatic artery thrombosis (yielding a clinical picture resembling that of hepatitis) are unusual consequences of dissemination.

Gastrointestinal

Gastrointestinal zygomycosis is exceptionally rare without underlying disease of the gut. Associated abnormalities include gastric ulcers, amebic colitis, salmonellal intestinal infection, pellagra, kwashiorkor, nasogastric suction, and the administration of multiple antimicrobics. In order of decreasing frequency, the regions of involvement are the stomach, the large bowel, and the ileum (dissemination may occur from a gastrointestinal site). Gastrointestinal zygomycosis is not frequent in immunocompromised patients. Complications include obstruction, perforation, and secondary peritonitis.

Cutaneous

Cutaneous zygomycosis may take the form of primary skin involvement, burn-wound zygomycotic gangrene, nodular lesions of hematogenous seeding, and cutaneous lesions associated with use of Elastoplast (Beiersders Inc., Norwalk, Connecticut). In addition, there may be infection along the tract of a renal biopsy, cutaneous infection at the site of intraocular glycosteroid injection, infection along needle tracts into mammary-gland polyethylene implants, and cutaneous lesions resembling ecthyma gangrenosum in a severely immunocompromised patient. The appearance of these cutaneous lesions is nonspecific. Widespread dissemination may originate in a cutaneous site. Black material in the pus and invasion of vessels with infarction may be helpful clues.

Two forms of cutaneous zygomycosis of tropical and subtropical regions are distinct from disease caused by organisms of the order Mucorales. These are infections caused by *Entomophthora coronata* and *Basidiobolus haptosporus* of the order Entomophthorales. Rhinoentomophthoromycosis is caused by *E. coronata* and is characterized by swelling of the nasal mucosa. If the submucosa becomes involved, obstruction of the nasal sinuses may result and lead to formation of a gradually expanding intranasal mass. This intranasal zygomycosis is less fulminant than the rhinocerebral form of zygomycosis caused by the fungi of the order Mucorales; it is associated with an eosinophilic sheath around the hyphae, and it is not associated with vascular invasion. Additionally, the organism does not stain well with either the periodic acid Schiff stain or with methenamine silver. The infection responds to potassium iodide and may regress spontaneously.

Children are most commonly infected with *B. haptosporus.* The process begins as a subcutaneous nodule that gradually expands into a firm and indurated mass involving virtually the entire extremity. Extension onto the trunk may also occur. The histopathology is similar to that elicited by *E. coronata* with respect to the accompanying eosinophilic sheath and poor staining. The treatment is iodides or amphotericin B.

Miscellaneous

Zygomycotic endocarditis has occurred both *de novo* and associated with cardiac surgery. As with other fungal endocarditides, the vegetations are large. Zygomycotic infection has occurred in venous grafts. Hematogenous osteomyelitis has been reported. One patient has been described with a large renal cyst caused by Zygomycetes. Zygomycotic ear infections have also been described.

Diagnosis

The diagnosis of zygomycosis depends upon demonstrating tissue invasion by fungi which have the morphology of the zygomycetes. Unfortunately, in many instances, biopsy of a visceral organ is required. Simply culturing a zygomycete is not enough to establish a diagnosis because these fungi are ubiquitous, may colonize in normal persons, and may be laboratory contaminants. There is no reliable serological test, and skin tests are not helpful.

Virtually all clinical manifestations of zygomycosis are nonspecific. Tumor, pyogenic, retroorbital or intraorbital infection, neurologic disease, Graves' ophthalmopathy, and infection by other fungi should all be considered in the differential diagnosis of rhinocerebral zygomycosis. With intracerebral infection, examination of the CSF is generally not helpful.

The pulmonary findings of zygomycosis are often consistent with a bronchopneumonia caused by bacteria, or infection by other fungi (particularly *Aspergillus* spp.). Fungus balls may form in a variety of pulmonary fungal infections.

The diagnosis of disseminated zygomycosis is difficult because the patients are usually severely ill from multiple diseases, frequently have drug toxicities, and virtually always have negative blood cultures. If there is evidence of infarction in multiple organs, this diagnosis should be considered. However, aspergillal infection may be associated with an identical clinical picture. When disseminated zygomycosis is suspected, a careful search should be made for a hematogenous cutaneous lesion that on biopsy might lead to the diagnosis.

The signs and symptoms of gastrointestinal zygomycosis are nonspecific. Frequently, the diagnosis is made through endoscopic visualization and biopsy of a suspected area. The signs and symptoms of endocarditis caused by zygomycetes are also nonspecific. However, large vegetations may occur, and evidence of arterial emboli may be present.

Whenever zygomycosis is suspected, the clinical laboratory should be alerted because of the possible inhibition of growth of the zygomycetes by media containing cycloheximide. The routine cultures of sputum, feces, urine, cerebrospinal fluid and swabs of infected areas are frequently negative.

Prognosis

The overwhelming majority of zygomycotic infections are fatal despite the use of amphotericin B. The usual delay in diagnosis may be responsible in part for failure of cure with amphotericin B. It is not possible to determine the fatality rate for disseminated disease because only a few patients have been diagnosed prior to death. Immunity to the infection does not develop during the course of primary infection.

Therapy

Successful treatment of zygomycosis depends upon appropriate use of antifungal medication, surgical excision, and control of underlying, predisposing factors. The importance of combined medical and surgical therapy cannot be overemphasized. Of all the fungal diseases, zygomycosis most urgently requires adequate surgical management.

Amphotericin B remains the antifungal agent of choice for zygomycosis. Newer antifungal agents, particularly 5-fluorocytosine, clotrimazole, and miconazole have had inconsistent *in vitro* and *in vivo* effects on the zygomycetes and should not be used alone. While synergy with amphotericin B has been claimed for 5-fluorocytosine, rifampin, the tetracyclines, and other antimicrobics against other fungi, there is no evidence of such an effect with the zygomycetes.

Susceptibility testing for fungi is not a standardized procedure. Results have varied widely with *Rhizopus* spp., for example, inhibition of growth by concentrations of amphotericin B from 0.1 to 5,000 μg/ml. Hence, it is not surprising that success in therapy appears to be neither related nor correlated with susceptibility *in vitro*. Despite the problems with susceptibility testing *in vitro*, amphotericin B remains agent of choice; susceptibility studies as generally reported are of limited value in predicting the utility of therapy with this agent.

Because zygomycosis may be a rapidly lethal infection, amphotericin B should be given so that therapeutic levels are reached as soon as possible. See Chapter 39, Candidosis, for detailed regimens for the use of amphotericin B. The duration of treatment and the total amount of amphotericin B needed for cure are not known; each patient requires evaluation on an individual basis. In most patients with serious zygomycotic infections, a total dose of 30 mg/kg body wt (about 2.0 g) has been given.

While surgical excision alone has been curative in some patients, early and thorough surgical removal of infected tissue while the patient is receiving amphotericin B is the treatment of choice. The amphotericin B is adjuvant; it is given to aid the host in overcoming fungi that escape from the focus of infection by way of the blood and lymph at the time of surgery and to attack fungi that were not removed by the surgical operation. Examples of extensive surgical procedures include excision of sinuses, drainage of abscesses, enucleations, paletectomies, lobectomies for pulmonary zygomycosis, amputations of burned extremities infected with zygomycetes, craniotomies, gastrectomies, nephrectomies, curettage of bones, and replacement of valves. If the zygomycosis recurs or progresses, additional surgery may be necessary.

In addition to amphotericin B and surgery, other therapeutic considerations deserve comment. In the case of diabetic ketoacidosis, correction of the acidosis is of primary importance in the management of the zygomycotic infection. Although there is no definitive, substantiating evidence, as great a reduction of immunosuppressive therapy as is possible should facilitate the management of the infection.

Other therapeutic approaches that have been used include desensitization with autologous vaccines and anticoagulation (no longer used). Hyperbaric oxygen and granulocyte transfusions have also been used, but their efficacy has not been proved.

Prevention

Minimizing factors predisposing to zygomycosis is frequently difficult because the predisposing factors are usually necessary therapeutic modalities (such as cytotoxins for leukemias). Selective and appropriate use of immunosuppressive agents and the proper control of diabetes mellitus are important for preventing zygomycosis. Because the spores of the zygomycetes are spread about in the air, consideration should be given to a filtered ventilation system in hospitals where patients predisposed to both zygomycosis and aspergillosis are present in large numbers (*e.g.,* cancer treatment centers). The use of occlusive dressings, for example Elastoplast bandages, should be avoided.

Remaining Problems

The pathogenesis of infection caused by the Zygomycetes is only partially understood. It is necessary to define the precise role of the individual components of the immune system in order to delineate further, and then obviate, predisposing factors.

Means to earlier diagnosis are badly needed; detection of antigens or other components or metabolites that are specific for the Zygomycetes may be most appropriate.

There is a great need for development of compounds more active against the Zygomycetes and less toxic than amphotericin B.

Bibliography

Books

RIPPON JW: Entomophthoromycosis. In Rippon JW (ed): Medical Mycology, the Pathogenic Fungi, and the Pathogenic Actinomycetes. Philadelphia, WB Saunders, 1974. pp 268–274.

HASSELTINE CW, ELLIS JJ: Mucorales. In Ainsworth GC, Sparrow FK, Sussman AS (eds): The Fungi: An Advanced Treatise, Vol. IVB. A Taxonomic Review with Keys: Basidiomycetes and Lower Fungi. New York, Academic Press, 1973. pp 187–217.

BENJAMIN RK: Zygomycetes and their Spores. In Kendrick B (ed): The Whole Fungus: The Sexual–Asexual Synthesis, Vol. 2. Proceedings of the Second International Mycological Conference held at the Environmental Science Center of the University of Calgary, Kananaskis, Alberta, Canada. Ottawa, National Museums of Canada 1979. pp 573–621.

KONEMAN EW, ROBERTS GD, WRIGHT SE: Practical Laboratory Mycology, 2nd ed. Baltimore, The Williams & Wilkins Co., 1978. 41–102.

Journals

ADER P: Mucormycosis and entomophthoromycosis: A bibliography. Mycopathologia 68:67–99, 1979

AGGER WA, MAKI DG: Mucormycosis: A complication of critical care. Arch Intern Med 138:925–927, 1978

BARTRUM RJ JR, WATNICK M, HERMAN PG: Roentgenographic findings in pulmonary mucormycosis. Am J Roentgenol Radium Ther Nucl Med 117:810–815, 1973

DIAMOND RD, KRZESICKI R, EPSTEIN B, JAO W: Damage to hyphal forms of fungi by human leukocytes *in vitro:* A possible host defense mechanism in aspergillosis and mucormycosis. Am J Pathol 91:313–328, 1978

ECHOLS RM, SELINGER DS, HALLOWELL C, GOODWIN JS, DUNCAN MH and CUSHING AH: Rhizopus osteomyelitis: A case report and review. Am J Med 66:141–145, 1979

EISENBERG L, WOOD T, BOLES R: Mucormycosis. Laryngoscope 87:347–356, 1977

GARTENBERG G, BOTTONE EJ, KEUSCH GT, WEITZMAN I: Hospital-acquired mucormycosis (Rhizopus rhizopodiformis) of skin and subcutaneous tissue: Epidemiology, mycology and treatment. N Engl J Med 229:1115–1118, 1978

LEHRER RI, HOWARD DH, SYPHERD PS, EDWARDS JE JR, SEGAL GP, WINSTON DJ: Mucormycosis. Ann Intern Med 93:93–108, 1980

MEDOFF G, KOBAYASHI GS: Pulmonary mucormycosis. N Engl J Med 286:86–87, 1972

MEYER RD, ARMSTRONG D: Mucormycosis: changing status. CRC Crit Rev Clin Lab Sci 4:421–451, 1973

MEYER RD, KAPLAN MH, ONG M, ARMSTRONG D: Cutaneous lesions in disseminated mucormycosis. JAMA 225:737–738, 1973

MEYER RD, ROSEN P, ARMSTRONG D: Phycomycosis complicating leukemia and lymphoma. Ann Intern Med 77:871–879, 1972

MEYERS BR, WORMSER G, HIRSCHMAN SZ, BLITZER A: Rhinocerebral mucormycosis: Premortem diagnosis and therapy. Arch Intern Med 139:557–560, 1979

SCHULMAN A, BORNMAN P, KAPLAN C, MORTON P, ROSE A: Gastrointestinal mucormycosis. Gastrointest Radiol 4:385–388, 1979

SHELDON DL, JOHNSON WC: Cutaneous mucormycosis: Two documented cases of suspected nosocomial cause. JAMA 241:1032–1034, 1979

STRAATSMA BR, ZIMMERMAN LE, GASS JDM: Phycomycosis: A clinicopathologic study of fifty-one cases. Lab Invest 11:963–985, 1962

BENJAMIN J. LUFT
JACK S. REMINGTON

Toxoplasmosis

129

Infection of humans with *Toxoplasma gondii* is one of the most common host–parasite interactions the world over. In both congenital and acquired forms, the infection may be subclinical or may produce a variety of clinical manifestations. *Chronic infection* refers to persistence of the cyst form of the protozoan in the tissues without provoking clinical manifestations. *Chronic toxoplasmosis* refers to active infection that causes persistent or recrudescent clinical manifestations.

Etiology

Toxoplasma gondii is an obligate intracellular protozoan—considered to be coccidian because of an enteroepithelial cycle—and is presently classified among the Sporozoa in the suborder Eimerina. Three forms exist in nature: tachyzoites (trophozoites), tissue cysts, and oocysts (Fig. 129-1).

Tachyzoites

Crescent to oval in shape (approximately 3 μm × 7 μm), tachyzoites stain well with either Wright or Giemsa stain (Fig. 129-1*A*). This form is seen in the acute stage of infection and invades all mammalian cells except nonnucleated erythrocytes. Multiplication is by endodyogeny (*i.e.,* two daughter cells are formed within each parent). Division continues until the host cell lyses or a tissue cyst forms. Desiccation, freezing and thawing, and digestive juices are lethal to tachyzoites. They may be propagated in the laboratory in the peritoneum of mice, in tissue cultures, or in eggs. Tachyzoites are used in the Sabin–Feldman dye test, the Fulton agglutination test, and the fluorescent antibody test; antigens derived from tachyzoites are used in the complement fixation (CF) test, the hemagglutination test, and the enzyme-linked immunosorbent essay (ELISA).

Tissue Cysts

Varying in size from 10 μm to 100 μm and containing as many as 3000 organisms, tissue cysts are formed within host cells and stand out when the periodic acid–Schiff stain is applied (Fig. 129-1*B*). This form is associated with the chronic (latent) phase of infection and with transmission. However, in the experimental animal, cysts have been noted to be present as early as 7 days after the inception of the acute infection. They are associated with transmission because they may be present in tissues ingested by carnivores, including humans. Disruption of the cyst wall by peptic or tryptic digestion liberates viable *T. gondii,* which survives several hours of exposure to these digestive enzymes and thus is capable of invading the host through the digestive tract. Freezing and thawing, heating to 60°C, or desiccation destroys tissue cysts. The cyst may also be the source of recrudescent infection in the immunocompromised host and in older children and adults who develop chorioretinitis. Cysts exist in virtually every organ, although the brain and the skeletal and heart muscles are the most common sites.

Oocysts

Ovoid in shape and 10 μm to 12 μm in diameter, oocysts (Fig. 129-1*C*) have been found only in members of the cat family (Fig. 129-2). After ingestion of either tissue cysts or oocysts, *T. gondii* is released and invades the epithelial cells of the feline small intestine. An enteroepithelial asexual cycle (schizogony) is followed by a sexual cycle (gametogony), resulting in the development of the noninfectious, unsporulated oocyst. Depending on the form of the organism that infects the cat, oocysts are excreted 3 to 24 days after the initial infection. Millions of oocysts are excreted in the feces of the cat each day for approximately 2 to 3 weeks. Sporogony occurs outside the body, requires 2 to 21 days (depending on the ambient temperature), and results in an infec-

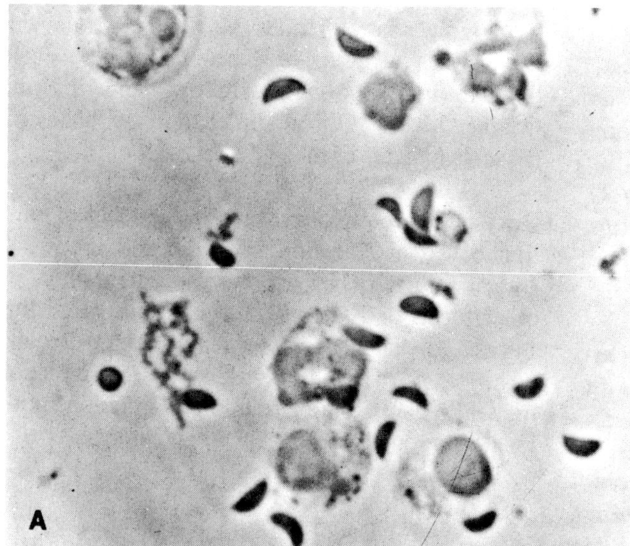

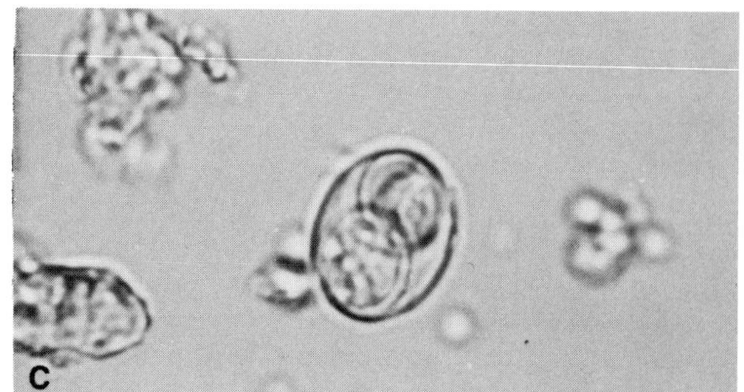

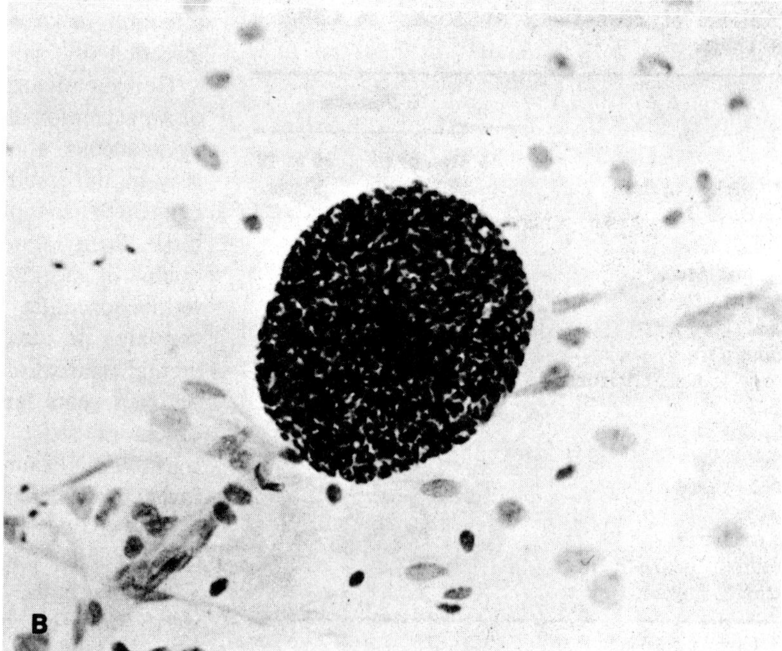

Fig. 129-1. Forms of *Toxoplasma gondii.* (*A*) The tachyzoite (proliferative) form from mouse peritoneal fluid. (Giemsa stain, original magnification approximately × 1000). (*B*) The tissue cyst form in the brain. (Periodic acid–Schiff stain, original magnification × 1000). (*C*) The oocyst form. (Original magnification approximately × 1000).

tive oocyst. Because ingestion of oocysts can lead to infection, it is probable that they play a major role in the transmission of toxoplasmosis. The importance of fecal–oral transmission is also favored by the fact that oocysts are the most tolerant form of *T. gondii* to extrahost environments; under favorable conditions (*e.g.,* warm, moist soil), they may remain infectious for several months to more than 1 year). However, exposure to boiling water or dry heat (over 66°C) renders oocysts noninfectious.

Epidemiology

Toxoplasma gondii are ubiquitous in nature and infect herbivorous, omnivorous, and carnivorous animals, including all orders of mammals, some birds, and probably some reptiles. Members of the family Felidae, including both domestic and feral cats, appear to be the definitive hosts in the life cycle (Fig. 129-2). No other animal has been found to shed oocysts. Coprophagous invertebrates, such as cock-

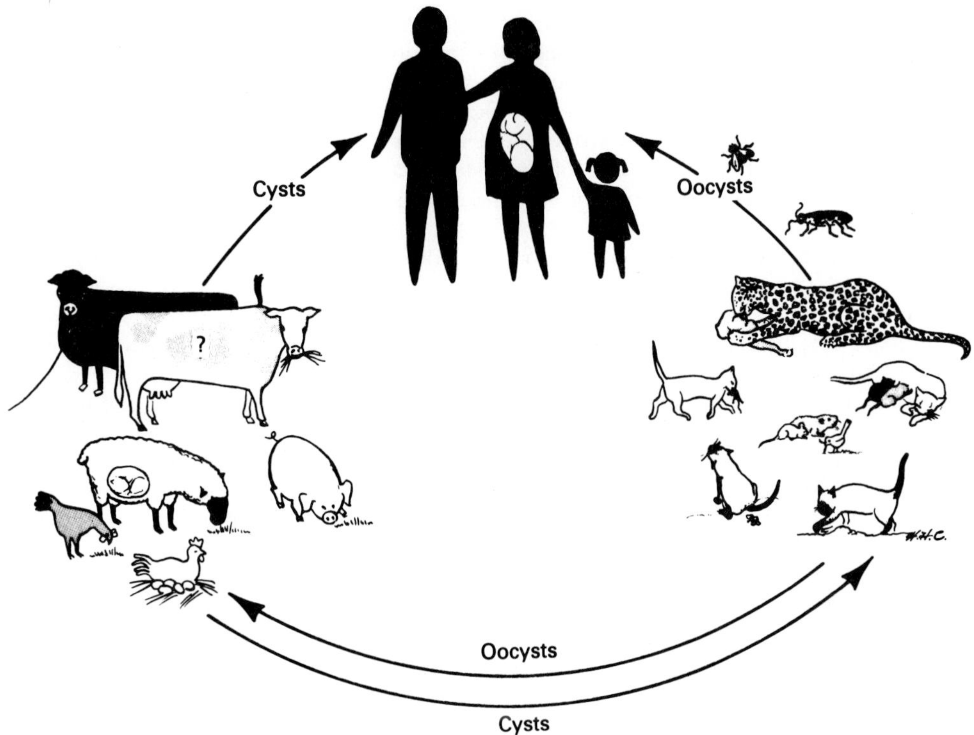

Fig. 129-2. The life cycle of *Toxoplasma gondii.* The cat appears to be the definitive host. (Swartzberg JE, Remington JS: Am J Dis Child 129:777–779, 1975).

roaches and filth flies, may serve as transport hosts for the oocyst form. The life cycle in nature also includes intermediate hosts such as small mammals, especially rodents, and birds, which may become infected either by congenital transmission, carnivorism, ingestion of oocysts, or ingestion of transport hosts. Though it is possible that the life cycle of *T. gondii* can be perpetuated without cats (*i.e.,* through congenital transmission and carnivorism), it appears that the presence of felids is of primary importance in the transmission of toxoplasmas in nature in most areas of the world.

In man, there is an increasing prevalence of positive serologic reactions with increasing age; there is no significant difference between sexes. Geographic variations exist. Prevalence rates for a number of locations are listed in Table 129-1. According to epidemiologic surveys, there is generally less infection in humans in cold regions, in hot and arid areas, and at high elevations. Thus, low rates of toxoplasmosis prevail in Iceland, northern Sweden, and Arizona, whereas rates are high in Tahiti, Trinidad, and other tropical islands or coastal areas. Exceptions do exist. For example, Eskimos, once thought to be free of toxoplasmosis, have been found to have prevalence rates of 13% to 46%, and some isolated tropical communities have little or no toxoplasmosis. Interestingly, these latter communities do not have known exposure to domestic or feral cats. However, there are also infected populations without known exposure to cats. The variation from area to area cannot as yet be explained.

Table 129-1. *Prevalence of Toxoplasma Antibodies* in Children and Adults*

	% Positive	
Origin of Sera	6–120 MONTHS	30–40 YEARS
Portland, Oregon	7	26
St. Louis, Missouri	6	33
New Orleans, Louisiana	21	42
Pittsburgh, Pennsylvania	8	45
Southern California	10	27
Arizona (Navajo Indians)	0	5
Tahiti	45	77
Trinidad	29	45
El Salvador	40	93
Paris, France	33	87
Austria	7	62
Tokyo, Japan	0	13
Helsinki, Finland	6	27
Sheffield, England	2	2

*Dye test titer ≥ 1:16.

The two major routes of transmission of *T. gondii* in man are oral and congenital. Meat used for human consumption may contain tissue cysts (*e.g.,* 10% of mutton, 25% of pork, and 10% of beef samples), thus serving as a source of infection when eaten raw or undercooked. Whether ingestion of oocysts is a major means of transmission of *T. gondii* to man is not yet clear, but this appears to be likely. Thus, laboratory personnel working with oocysts have become infected, and coprophagous insects apparently can contaminate human food with oocysts. However, epidemiologic studies attempting to correlate prevalence of toxoplasmosis with exposure to cats (and thus, presumably, to oocysts) have yielded conflicting results.

There is no evidence of direct human-to-human transmission other than from mother to fetus. Women who acquire the acute infection during pregnancy expose their fetuses to the risk of infection with *T. gondii;* overall, transplacental transmission occurs in about 33% of acute infections. Infection of the fetus may be manifest as a stillbirth, spontaneous abortion, or birth of a symptomatic or an asymptomatic infant. The incidence of fetal infection and the severity of the infection are related to the trimester in which maternal infection occurred. During the first trimester, transplacental infection occurs in approximately 17% of infants, but the disease tends to be severe. During the third trimester, transplacental infection occurs in approximately 65% of infants but the disease tends to be asymptomatic during the neonatal period. It is believed that fetuses are at risk of infection only when the mother has acquired the infection during that particular gestation. Evidence that chronic infection with *T. gondii* in the pregnant woman may lead to congenital infection in her full-term infant has been reported but has not been substantiated. If such transmission does occur, it must be rare. However, *T. gondii* has been recovered from abortuses of women with chronic infection. The importance of chronic infection as a cause of spontaneous abortion has not been fully evaluated.

Infection with *T. gondii* may be acquired through blood or leukocyte transfusion as a result of persistent parasitemia in a normal asymptomatic donor. Transmission may also occur in laboratory workers by accidental self-inoculation of tachyzoites. Infection has also been transmitted by the transplantation of organs.

Pathogenesis and Pathology

Humans are most commonly infected after ingesting raw or undercooked meat contaminated with cysts. Digestive enzymes disrupt the cyst wall, thereby liberating organisms that invade the intestinal wall and spread through both the vascular and lymphatic systems. Because the tachyzoite is capable of infecting all cells except nonnucleated red blood cells, cysts may be found in every organ and tissue.

After multiplication at the site of entry, *T. gondii* disseminates through the blood and may invade all organs and tissues. Proliferation of the tachyzoites usually results in the death of the invaded cells producing foci of necrosis surrounded by an intense cellular reaction. The outcome of the acute process depends primarily on the immune response of the host. Both humoral and cell-mediated immunity are important; however, cell-mediated immunity is of particular consequence. If the host is immunodeficient, the acute infection may persist to cause potentially lethal local or diffuse lesions such as acute, necrotizing encephalitis, pneumonitis, or myocarditis.

With the development of an appropriate immune response, the tachyzoites disappear from the tissues, and the formation of tissue cysts takes place. The tissue cyst form of *T. gondii* (1) is characteristic of chronic or latent toxoplasmosis; (2) provokes little or no inflammatory response; (3) may be domonstrable in histologic sections as early as the eighth day of infection; and (4) persists in a viable, latent state for the life of the host. The brain, skeletal muscles, and cardiac muscle are the most common sites, but tissue cysts may be found in every organ. Some tachyzoites may remain viable inside immune monocytes and macrophages—perhaps the source of the recurrent parasitemias that sometimes occur in asymptomatic patients with chronic infection.

The histopathologic changes in toxoplasmic lymphadenitis are frequently distinctive. Typically, a reactive follicular hyperplasia with irregular clusters of epitheloid histiocytes encroaching upon and blurring the margins of the germinal centers is associated with focal distention of sinuses with monocytoid cells. Giant cells are not present, and only on rare occasions can *T. gondii* be demonstrated.

In the central nervous system (CNS) there may be an acute focal or diffuse meningoencephalitis with cellular necrosis, microglial nodules, and perivascular mononuclear inflammation associated with both intracellular and extracellular tachyzoites. Occasionally, there is thrombosis of blood vessels causing large areas of coagulation necrosis that may mimic mass lesions. Cysts may be present during the acute infection or be indicative of more chronic infection. Periaqueductal and periventricular necrosis, a feature unique to severe, congenital toxoplasmosis, may lead to obstruction of the aqueduct of Sylvius or the foramen of Magendie and foramina of Luschka, resulting in internal hydrocephalus. The areas of necrosis may undergo calcification.

Infection of the eye results in an acute retinochoroiditis that begins in the retina with severe inflammation and necrosis and is accompanied by exudation into the vitreous. The cellular infiltrate consists of mononuclear phagocytes, lymphocytes, and plasma cells. Granulomatous inflammation of the choroid is secondary to the necrotizing retinitis. Single or multiple foci occur with a distinct predilection for involvement of the macular/perimacular area. Both tachyzoites and tissue cysts may be found in the retinal lesions. Rupture of tissue cysts is presumed to cause acute lesions as a result of the release of protozoa and the intense inflammation generated by the immune response. The course is one of episodic flares of retinochoroiditis. There is no systemic reaction, but each episode is accompanied by destruction of irreplaceable retinal elements. Glaucoma, iridocyclitis, and cataracts may develop as a result of the retinochoroiditis.

Interstitial pneumonitis may occur in congenitally infected infants, in immunocompromised hosts, and rarely in normal adults. Histopathologic examination reveals thickened and edematous alveolar septae which are infiltrated (along with peribronchial areas) with mononuclear cells, occasional plasma cells, and rare eosinophils. Vasculitic changes may occur in which the walls of small blood vessels are infiltrated with lymphocytes and mononuclear cells, and organisms may be seen in the endothelial cells. Necrosis within granulomatous foci is a prominent feature in some patients with disseminated toxoplasmosis and malignancy. Toxoplasmic pneumonitis may also occur concurrently with other opportunistic infections. In many cases, there is some degree of bronchopneumonia, often caused by superinfection.

Myocarditis may be manifest in congenitally infected infants, in immunocompromised patients, and rarely in seemingly normal patients with severe acute toxoplasmosis. Cysts and tachyzoites are found within muscle fibers. Foci of inflammatory cells are associated with hyaline necrosis and fragmentation of myocardial cells. Hemorrhagic pericarditis has been reported in some patients. The kidney may be involved with necrosis of both glomeruli and tubules. Glomerulonephritis has been reported as a result of infection with deposits of antigen–antibody complexes. Benign monoclonal gammopathy may occur in infants with congenital toxoplasmosis.

Evidence of infection has been reported in all organ systems and tissues. Pathologic changes may consist of foci of necrosis and organisms, organisms without associated inflammation, and cysts with or without associated inflammation. Skeletal muscle may be prominently involved with focal or diffuse areas of myositis and necrosis, or muscle fibers may be parasitized without histopathologic changes. There is a propensity toward involvement of the pancreas in the immunocompromised patient.

Manifestations

Toxoplasmosis is conveniently considered to be divided into three categories in immunologically normal patients: congenital, acquired, or ocular (either congenital or acquired), and as it occurs in immunodeficient hosts (either acquired toxoplasmosis or reactivation of latent infection). Both congenital and acquired infections are usually asymptomatic. Clinically apparent infection, either in children or adults, may result from a newly contracted infection or from reactivation of a latent infection originally either congenital or acquired. Diagnosis cannot be established in any form of the infection by clinical means alone, because the signs and symptoms of toxoplasmosis may mimic those of a variety of other diseases.

Congenital Toxoplasmosis

Clinical manifestations of acute infection with *T. gondii* occur in 10% to 20% of women during pregnancy. However, the fetus is at risk whether the infection in the mother is symptomatic or asymptomatic. Infants with clinically apparent disease at birth may have any combination of the following: hydrocephalus, microcephalus, cerebral calcification, seizure disorders, psychomotor retardation, microophthalmia, strabismus, cataracts, glaucoma, retinochoroiditis, optic atrophy, deafness, lymphadenopathy, pneumonitis, myocarditis, hepatosplenomegaly, fever, hypothermia, vomiting, diarrhea, jaundice, and rash. At birth, 8% of newborns with congenital toxoplasmosis will have severe impairment of the CNS or eyes; 75% will be asymptomatic. The incidence of untoward sequelae in the asymptomatic population has been studied prospectively and has been found to be over 85%. Prominent later manifestations include sensorineural hearing loss, retinochoroiditis, hydrocephalus, seizures, blindness, delayed psychomotor development, and mental retardation. Laboratory test abnormalities associated with congenital toxoplasmosis include anemia, thrombocytopenia, eosinophilia, monocytosis, and abnormal cerebrospinal fluid (CSF) with xanthochromia, mononuclear pleocytosis, and high protein.

Acquired Toxoplasmosis

The spectrum of acquired toxoplasmosis ranges from subclinical lymphadenopathy to fatal, acute, fulminating disease. Asymptomatic lymphadenopathy is the most common manifestation. The nodes are usually discrete and vary in tenderness and firmness; however, they do not suppurate. The lymphadenopathy may be localized or generalized and involve any group of nodes, although the cervical nodes are the ones most commonly enlarged. The mesenteric or retroperitoneal nodes may be involved and associated with abdominal pain and fever. The lymphadenopathic form of the disease is usually self-limited, but lymphadenopathy has been documented to recur for months. Asymptomatic lymphadenopathy has been mistaken for lymphoma. Lymphadenopathy may be accompanied by fever, malaise, myalgias, sore throat, headache, maculopapular rash, hepatosplenomegaly, and atypical lymphocytosis; infectious mononucleosis (Chap. 137, Infectious Mononucleosis) or cytomegalovirus infection (see Chap. 75, Cytomegalovirus Infections) is frequently mimicked. Rarely, a severe illness occurs with the predominating signs and symptoms referable to the organ system involved: myocarditis, pericarditis, hepatitis, polymyositis, pneumonitis, or encephalitis. Retinochoroiditis rarely occurs in acquired toxoplasmosis.

Ocular Toxoplasmosis

Toxoplasmosis is said to account for about 35% of all retinochoroiditis. The characteristic lesion in both congenital and acquired toxoplasmosis is a focal necrotizing retinitis. Less commonly, a panuveitis and papillitis with optic atrophy may occur. Isolated anterior uveitis due to toxoplasmosis has never been proven. The vast majority of cases of ocular toxoplasmosis are congenital in origin; thus, episodes of toxoplasmic retinochoroiditis in adolescents and young adults usually represent reactivation of latent congenital infection. Retinochoroiditis has been estimated to occur in approximately 1% of patients with acute acquired infection.

Active retinochoroiditis may cause blurred vision, scotomas, pain, photophobia, and epiphora; impairment or loss of central vision occurs when the macula is involved. Careful ophthalmologic examination is essential in the newborn suspected of having infection with *T. gondii* because symptoms may be difficult to elucidate and involvement of the eye may be the only clinical sign of infection. Signs of systemic infection in adults and children with ocular involvement are uncommon. As inflammation subsides, vision improves, frequently without complete recovery of acuity. By ophthalmoscopic examination, the acute lesions appear as yellowish-white, cottonlike patches that have elevated, indistinct margins surrounded by a zone of hyperemia. The inflammatory exudate in the vitreous may obscure the fundus. Older lesions are atrophic, whitish-gray plaques with distinct borders and black spots of choroidal pigment. The lesions may be single or, more commonly multiple and are usually located near the posterior pole of the retina, although they may be peripheral. Lesions of varying age may be seen, indicating episodic flares of activity. Multiple recurrences may result in glaucoma.

Acute Toxoplasmosis in the Immunodeficient Host

Although immunodeficient hosts are more susceptible to serious disease when they become infected with *T. gondii,* it is likely that clinically apparent toxoplasmosis in these patients is most often a consequence of reactivation of latent infection. The manifestations of toxoplasmosis in the immunodeficient host are not unique and may mimic those seen with other opportunistic pathogens. Signs and symptoms may include any or all of those noted in immunocompetent hosts with acquired toxoplasmosis. However, because necrotizing encephalitis, myocarditis, or pneumonitis are the most frequent findings seen at autopsy, the most common clinical manifestations reflect involvement of these organ systems. In more than 50% of these cases, there are signs and symptoms referable to the CNS, including disturbances of consciousness, motor impairment, seizures, headache, and focal neurologic deficits. The findings generally reflect an encephalitis, a meningoencephalitis, or a mass lesion. There is usually a mononuclear pleocytosis, a mild elevation of protein, and a normal glucose in the CSF. Radionuclide and computed tomographic (CT) scans may reveal a lesion with the characteristics of a brain abscess. The electroencephalogram may have diffuse or focal slowing depending on whether there is a diffuse encephalitis or a mass lesion. Biopsy of the brain or aspiration of material from an intracerebral abscess may reveal free tachyzoites. Immunocompromised patients with particular susceptibility to severe toxoplasmic infection include those receiving chemotherapy for lymphoproliferative (especially Hodgkin's disease) and hematologic malignancies, and those receiving immunosuppressive therapy to prevent rejection of a transplanted organ.

Diagnosis

The diagnosis of toxoplasmosis may be established by: (1) isolation of *T. gondii;* (2) demonstration of the protozoa in tissue sections, smears, or body fluids; (3) characteristic histopathology in lymph nodes; and (4) serologic methods.

Isolation Procedures

Body fluids; the buffy coat from centrifuged, heparinized blood; and tissue specimens should be inoculated intraperitoneally into mice or tissue cultures. Body fluids should be processed and inoculated immediately; tissues and blood may be stored at 4°C overnight if necessary. Specimens must not be frozen or placed in formalin, since such treatment kills the parasite. The peritoneal fluid of the mouse should be examined for the presence of tachyzoites 6 to 10 days after inoculation. Mice surviving for 6 weeks should be tested for antibody to *T. gondii* in their serums. If antibody is present, the mouse brain should be examined for cysts in order to make a definitive diagnosis.

Isolation of *T. gondii* from body fluids reflects the acute stage of infection, as does isolation from the blood in most patients. However, recurrent parasitemia has been described rarely in asymptomatic persons with latent infection and more commonly in patients with chronic myelogenous leukemia. Isolation from tissues (*e.g.,* skeletal muscle, lung, brain, eye) obtained by biopsy or at autopsy may reflect only the presence of tissue cysts and thus is not proof of acute infection.

Histologic Diagnosis

Demonstration of tachyzoites in tissue sections or smears (*e.g.,* brain biopsy, bone marrow aspirate) or body fluids (*e.g.,* CSF, amniotic fluid) establishes the diagnosis of acute toxoplasmosis. Unfortunately, it is difficult to visualize the tachyzoite form when stained by ordinary methods. Direct or indirect fluorescent antibody methods and peroxidase:antiperoxidase methods have been used successfully in identifying the antigen or organisms in histologic tissue sections. Demonstration of the tissue cyst establishes the diagnosis of toxoplasmic infection, but does not differentiate between acute or chronic infection. In characteristic cases, histologic criteria alone are probably sufficient to establish the diagnosis of toxoplasmic lymphadenitis. The presence of cysts in the newborn infant establishes the diagnosis of congenital infection.

Serologic Tests

Of the many serologic tests described for the diagnosis of toxoplasmosis, the Sabin–Feldman dye test (DT), the indirect fluorescent antibody (IFA) test, and the indirect hemagglutination (IHA) test are most often employed. The DT is sensitive and specific with no known cross-reactions in humans.

The IFA test is the most widely available procedure and appears to measure the same antibodies as the DT; the titers in both tests tend to be parallel. The antibodies detected by the DT and IFA tests usually appear within 1 to 2 weeks after acute infection, reach high titers (≥1:1000) in 6 to 8 weeks, and then gradually decline over months to years; low titers (1:4–1:64) commonly persist for life. The level of the antibody titer cannot be correlated with the severity of the illness.

The IHA test measures different antibodies than the DT and IFA tests. The IHA test often becomes positive somewhat later and may persist for years. It should not be employed for the diagnosis of congenital toxoplasmosis or for the acute acquired disease in adults, since it has been negative in proven cases. Because of this problem and the wide variations in titers between laboratories, the IHA test cannot supplant the DT or IFA test.

The complement fixation test and the precipitin test have proven value in certain situations, but are performed mainly in research laboratories and are not standardized for general use. The CF antibodies appear several weeks later than the DT antibodies and may persist for years. Thus, a positive CF test titer does not mean the infection is acute and a negative CF test titer does not exclude toxoplasmosis. A significant rise in the CF or IHA test (*i.e.,* two serial dilutions performed in parallel on serums obtained several weeks apart) may establish a diagnosis of recent infection even after the DT has peaked. The direct agglutination (AG) test has been used extensively in France. As a result of modifications in the preparation of the antigen and in the processing of the serums, the AG test is accurate and sensitive and has great potential for use as a screening test.

The IgM-fluorescent antibody (IgM-IFA) test is based on the earlier appearance (as soon as 5 days after infection) and disappearance of IgM antibodies as contrasted with IgG antibodies (the main antibodies measured by the DT and IFA test). The presence of IgM antibodies in the neonate represents synthesis *in utero* by the infected fetus because IgM does not pass the placental barrier, as does IgG. In some immunodeficient patients with acute toxoplasmosis, some patients with isolated active ocular toxoplasmosis, and some infants with congenital toxoplasmosis, IgM antibodies against *T. gondii* may not be demonstrable. The presence of antinuclear antibodies may cause false-positive results in both the IFA and IgM-IFA tests, as can rheumatoid factor in the IgM-IFA test. Rheumatoid factor may be present in the newborn. This is thought to be due to an IgM antibody response to passively transferred maternal antibody. The IgM-IFA test is further limited by the significant rate of negative results in patients with acute acquired toxoplasmosis and in approximately 75% of infants with congenital infection. In adults, this has been shown to be due to the presence of blocking IgG antibodies to *T. gondii* that directly interfere with the IgM-IFA test. A double-sandwich ELISA for IgM—the IgM-ELISA test—circumvents this problem. It is more sensitive and accurate for the diagnosis of both congenital infections (approximately 75% of infected newborns are positive) and acute acquired infections (approximately 97% are positive). The IgM-ELISA is not limited by false-positive results in serums containing rheumatoid factor or antinuclear antibody.

Guidelines for the interpretation of serologic tests are given in Table 129-2. The presence of a positive titer (except for the rare false-positive results noted above) in any of the serologic tests establishes the diagnosis of toxoplasmic infection. A negative DT or IFA test, performed on undiluted serum, virtually excludes the diagnosis of toxoplasmosis unless a prozone is present. To diagnose acute toxoplasmosis by serology, it is necessary to demonstrate a rising titer in serial specimens (either seroconversion from negative to a positive titer or shift from a low to a high titer). Although suggestive of acute infection, a single high titer in either the DT, IFA, IHA, or CF test is not diagnostic. The most useful test for the diagnosis of acute toxoplasmosis is the IgM-ELISA. Based on data from a number of laboratories, the following guidelines appear to be valid: (1) a DT or IFA test titer of ≥ 1:1000 in the presence of a positive IgM-IFA (≥ 1:64) or a positive titer in the double-sandwich ELISA test result and a characteristic clinical syndrome are compatible with a diagnosis of acute toxoplasmosis and (2) a high DT or IFA test titer (1:1000–1:16000) with a high IgM-IFA or IgM-ELISA test titer is probably diagnostic of recent acute infection with or without symptoms. Although in most cases IgM antibodies rise rapidly and thereafter fall to low titers or disappear within a few weeks or months, in some patients they remain positive at low titers for as long as several years. For practical purposes, in immunologically normal patients with positive titers in the DT or IFA test, lack of IgM antibodies excludes the diagnosis of acute infection. The DT or IFA test usually reaches maximum levels (≥ 1:1000) by 6 to 8 weeks after acquisition of infection. Therefore, if the DT or IFA test titer is stable at ≥ 1:1000, the infection was acquired at least 4 weeks earlier and probably more than 8 weeks before the initial serum was obtained. Serologic testing may also be performed on body fluids such as the CSF or aqueous humor. A very high titer in either, compared to the serum titer, reflects local antibody production signifying acute CNS or ocular infection. The following formula is useful in assessing the significance of local antibody production:

$$C = \frac{\text{antibody titer in body fluid}}{\text{antibody titer in serum}} \times \frac{\text{concentration of } \gamma\text{-globulin in serum}}{\text{concentration of } \gamma\text{-globulin in body fluid}}$$

If the concentration coefficient (C) is ≥ 8, it indicates local antibody production. This assessment is not usually useful if the serum DT titer is ≥ 1:1000.

In order to diagnose toxoplasmic infection in the pregnant patient, women who intend to become pregnant should be screened serologically for previous toxoplasmic infection. If a woman is seronegative, she should be followed for possible seroconversion during pregnancy. Guidelines for the interpretation of maternal antibody titers in mothers who have just delivered a child suspected of having congenital toxoplasmic infection are provided in Table 129-3.

The diagnosis of acute toxoplasmosis in the neonate is based on finding either persistent or rising titers in the DT or IFA test or a positive IgM-IFA or IgM-ELISA test (at any titer) without a placental leak or rheumatoid factor if the IgM-IFA test is used. If a placental leak of maternal blood has occurred, the IgM-IFA or IgM-ELISA test titer in the neonate will drop significantly within a week, because the half-life of IgM is approximately 3 to 5 days. Depending on the original titer, passively transferred maternal IgG antibodies may require 6 to 12 months to disappear from the infant's serum. Synthesis of toxoplasmic antibody in the infected infant is usually demonstrable by the third or fourth month, but may be delayed to the sixth to ninth month in the treated infant.

The diagnosis of ocular toxoplasmosis in older children and adults is difficult because the titer of antibody in the serum does not necessarily correlate with the activity of the infection. Indeed, low serologic test titers are usual in patients with active toxoplasmic retinochoroiditis. Toxoplasmic retinochoroiditis is probably excluded if serologic tests are negative when performed on undiluted serum. If the retinal lesion is characteristic and the serologic test is positive, the diagnosis of toxoplasmosis can be made with a high degree of confidence. If the retinal lesion is atypical and the serologic test is positive, the diag-

Table 129-2. *Guidelines* for Interpretation of Commonly Employed Serologic Tests for Diagnosis of Toxoplasmosis*

Test (Abbreviation)	**Positive Titer**	**Peak Titer in Acute Infection**	**Titer in Chronic (Latent) Infection**	**Duration of Elevation of Titer**	**Special Considerations**
Sabin–Feldman dye test (DT)	1:4 undiluted†	≥1:1000	1:4 to 1:2000	Years	(1) There are no known cross-reactions or false-positives in humans. (2) The World Health Organization has recommended titers be expressed in IU/ml.
Conventional indirect fluorescent antibody (IFA) test	1:10‡	≥1:1000	1:8 to 1:2000	Years	(1) The World Health Organization has recommended titers be expressed in IU/ml. (2) Antibody measured is the same as that measured in the dye test. (3) Antinuclear antibodies may cause false-positive results.
Indirect fluorescent antibody test for IgM Toxoplasma antibodies (IgM-IFA)	1:2 infants‡ 1:10 adults‡	≥1:80	Negative to 1:20	Weeks to months; occasionally years	(1) Either antinuclear antibodies or rheumatoid factor (IgM) may cause false-positive results. (2) Rheumatoid factor may be absorbed from serum with heat-aggregated IgG. (3) High-titer IgG antibodies may cause false-negative results.
IgM-enzyme linked immunosorbent assay (IgM-ELISA)§	≥2	6 to 10	Negative	Months and occasionally years	(1) Avoids false-negative results due to IgG antibody to *Toxoplasma gondii.*§ (2) Avoids false-positive reactions due to antinuclear antibodies and rheumatoid factor.
Indirect hemagglutination (IHA) test	1:16‡	≥1:1000	1:16 to 1:256	Years	(1) Not useful for diagnosis of congenital toxoplasmosis. (2) Antibodies by IHA test rise later than antibodies measured by dye test and IFA test. This test may be especially useful when a rising IHA test titer can be demonstrated.
Complement fixation (CF) test	1:4‡	Varies among laboratories	Negative to 1:8	Years	(1) Antigen preparations used for this test have not been standardized. (2) See (2) under IHA test.

*These guidelines are useful in the interpretation of test results, but exceptions may occur.
†In some cases of eye disease, the dye test may be positive only in undiluted serum.
‡These values are representative, but normal values for each laboratory may differ significantly.
§As described by Naot and Remington (1980, 1981). The frequency of false-positive results in the conventional IgM-ELISA precludes its use.

Table 129-3. ***Guidelines for Interpretation of Antibody Test Titers in Mothers Who Have Just Delivered a Child Suspected of Having Congenital Toxoplasmic Infection***

Congenital Infection in Child	Serologic Test Results in Mother	
	DYE TEST*	IgM-FLUORESCENT ANTIBODY TEST OR IgM-ELISA
Most often present	300 to 3000 IU/ml (1:1200–1:12,000)	Positive
Often present	1000 to 3000 IU/ml (1:4000–1:12,000)†	Negative
Seldom present	300 to 1000 IU/ml (1:1200–1:4000)†	Negative
Possible‡	<300 IU/ml	Positive
Excluded	<300 IU/ml	Negative

(After Remington JS, Desmonts G: Toxoplasmosis. In Remington JS, Klein JO (eds): Infectious Diseases of the Fetus and Newborn Infant, 2nd ed, Philadelphia, WB Saunders, 1983)

*Figures in parenthesis represent approximate titers expressed as reciprocal of serum dilution that correspond to the titers expressed in international units.

†There is no information about interpretation of high dye test titers in a mother just delivered of a child suspected of having congenital toxoplasmosis in regions where a significant number of infected mothers have high dye test titers (*e.g.,* Central America).

‡Usually present if maternal dye test is rising after delivery; usually lacking if maternal dye test is not rising.

nosis of toxoplasmosis is only presumptive because the high prevalance of antibodies in the population precludes the assumption of a causal relationship.

Infection of the immunocompromised host with *T. gondii* may be difficult to diagnose. The antibody response may be atypical in view of the compromised state. Clinical suspicion of toxoplasmosis along with use of newer serologic methods (*e.g.,* assay for antigenemia, IgM-ELISA) may allow for an earlier diagnosis. The ELISA for toxoplasmic antigen may be particularly useful in this regard for identification of antigen in the CSF and amniotic fluid of newborns and in the serum of acutely infected adults. The assay was found to detect antigen in 65% of 23 serums from patients with the lymphadenopathic form of toxoplasmosis.

A toxoplasmin skin test that elicits delayed hypersensitivity has been useful in epidemiologic surveys. Because it usually becomes positive months after infection, it is of no value in diagnosing acute infection with *T. gondii.* Lymphocyte transformation to toxoplasmic antigen has been found to be a specific indicator of previous infection in adults; in these cases, however, lymphocyte transformation may not be observed for as long as 3 to 7 months after the onset of clinical infection. Lymphocyte transformation has been found to be a highly sensitive (85%) and specific (100%) test for the diagnosis of congenital toxoplasmic infection.

Congenital toxoplasmosis must be differentiated from erythroblastosis with hydrops fetalis and from congenital infection with rubella virus (Chap. 87, Rubella), herpesvirus (Chap. 91, Infections Caused by Herpes Simplex Viruses), cytomegalovirus (Chap. 75, Cytomegalovirus Infections), *Treponema pallidum* (Chap. 59, Syphilis), and other causes of encephalopathies in the newborn. A markedly elevated CSF protein is a hallmark of both subclinical and overt congenital toxoplasmosis. The differential diagnosis of toxoplasmic lymphadenitis includes lymphoma; infectious mononucleosis (Chap. 137, Infectious Mononucleosis); cytomegalovirus "mononucleosis" (Chap. 75, Cytomegalovirus Infections); cat-scratch disease (Chap. 166, Cat-Scratch Fever); sarcoidosis (Chap. 168, Sarcoidosis); tuberculosis (Chap. 34, Pulmonary Tuberculosis); tularemia (Chap. 139, Tularemia); metastatic carcinoma; and leukemia. A major diagnostic confusion occurs with Hodgkin's disease and other lymphomas. Toxoplasmic lymphadenitis may simulate infectious mononucleosis with atypical lymphocytosis and splenomegaly, but the heterophil test is negative. Acute acquired toxoplasmosis associated with multiple organ involvement may mimic other causes of pneumonitis, hepatitis, myocarditis, or polymyositis. Toxoplasmic retinochoroiditis may resemble the posterior uveitis of tuberculosis, syphilis, or leprosy (Chap. 105, Leprosy). Acute infection of the CNS by *T. gondii* must be differentiated from meningoencephalitis caused by other infectious agents, cerebral hemorrhage, multifocal leukoencephalopathy, and tumor. In immunodeficient patients, CSF mononuclear pleocytosis and high protein concentration without bacteria or fungi warrants consideration of toxoplasmosis.

Prognosis

The outcome of toxoplasmosis is related to the virulence of the infecting strain of *T. gondii* and the immunologic capacity of the infected person, rather than to a postulated tissue tropism peculiar to a certain strain. Nevertheless, the extent and severity of involvement of the vital organs governs the mortality of clinical toxoplasmosis.

Serious sequelae are a threat to all congenitally infected infants. When clinical signs of infection are present at birth, mental retardation, epilepsy, spasticity, and palsies may occur in 80% and severely impaired vision in 50% of infants. Hydrocephalus or microcephalus occurs in about 5% of infants with manifestations of toxoplasmosis involving the CNS. Toxoplasmosis that is subclinical at birth will result in delayed yet serious overt manifestations of the disease months to years later in a significant number of infants (Congenital Toxoplasmosis, above). Women who deliver an infant with congenital toxoplasmosis can be assured that they will not transmit *T. gondii* to the fetus in subsequent pregnancies.

In adults, multiple organ involvement is extremely serious, especially in immunodeficient patients; data are inadequate for calculation of mortality. The lymphadenopathic form of acquired toxoplasmosis is usually self-limited and rarely requires specific therapy. However, lymphadenopathy may persist, or fluctuate in severity, with or without constitutional symptoms for months. True reinfections as a cause of clinical illness have not been recognized. Ocular toxoplasmosis is characterized by frequent relapses.

Therapy

The tissue cyst form of *T. gondii* in the brain is resistant to presently available antimicrobics. Pyrimethamine (Daraprim), a diaminopyrimidine, and sulfonamides are both active against the tachyzoite and are synergistic when used in combination, producing a sequential blockade at different points in the synthesis of nucleic acids (Chap. 18, Antimicrobics and Anthelmintics for Systemic Therapy). Pyrimethamine is lipid soluble, readily absorbed from the gastrointestinal tract, and apparently capable of free entry into all cells and body compartments. Concentrations in the CSF have been found to be 10% to 25% of simultaneous plasma concentrations. Controlled clinical trials of treating toxoplasmosis in humans with this combination are lacking; nevertheless, clinical experience confirms their efficacy. Trimethoprim, also a diaminopyrimidine, is ineffective in treating toxoplasmosis in experimental animals. Sulfamethoxazole, the sulfonamide that is used in combination with trimethoprim, is active in animal models and probably accounts for the activity of the combination. That is, trimethoprim alone or in combination with a sulfonamide has no apparent place in the treatment of toxoplasmosis. Sulfadiazine, sulfapyrazine, sulfamethazine, and sulfamerazine have been found to be equally effective, whereas other sulfonamides have been found to be less effective. Both pyrimethamine and the sulfapyrimidines are used in treatment when indicated, except during the first trimester of pregnancy.

A loading dose of 100 mg to 200 mg pyrimethamine (given orally, as two equal portions) is recommended for the first day of treatment in adults. The maintenance dosage for all ages is 1 mg/kg body wt/day, PO, as a single dose, with a maximum of 25 mg/day. In young children, twice the daily dose (2 mg/kg body wt) should be given as a loading dose for the first 2 to 3 days of treatment. Administration at 3- to 4-day intervals has been suggested in neonates and infants in view of the half-life of 4 to 5 days. Pyrimethamine is available only in tablet form. Because pyrimethamine is a folic acid antagonist, it produces a dose-related, reversible, and usually gradual depression of the bone marrow. Thrombocytopenia is the most serious consequence; leukopenia and anemia also occur. All patients treated with pyrimethamine should have platelet and peripheral blood cell counts twice a week. Folinic acid (calcium leucovorin) may be given either intramuscularly or orally in dosages of 2 to 10 mg/day to prevent suppression of the bone marrow by pyrimethamine. Folinic acid therapy, 6 to 10 mg/day, is mandatory when the platelet count is less than 100,000/mm^3. Bakers' yeast (3–4 cakes a day) is of additional value in preventing toxicity due to pyrimethamine. Unlike folic acid, neither folinic acid nor Bakers' yeast inhibits the action of pyrimethamine on *T. gondii,* although it reduces the toxicity of the drug to humans.

Sulfadiazine or a trisulfapyrimidine mixture (*e.g.,* equal parts of sulfadiazine, sulfamerazine, and sulfamethazine) are the most active sulfonamides against *T. gondii* and should be given in conjunction with pyrimethamine. Other sulfonamides, including sulfisoxazole (Gantrisin), are less active and *should not be used.* The usual dosage of sulfadiazine or trisulfapyrimidines in adults is 75 to 100 mg/kg body wt/day, PO, as four equal portions, 6-hourly after a loading dose of 50 to 75 mg/kg body wt/day, PO, as four equal portions. The dosage in infants is 100 to 150 mg/kg body wt/day, PO, as four equal portions 6-hourly, after a loading dose of 75 to 100 mg/kg body wt. Appropriate dosage of sulfonamides yields concentrations of 10 and 15 mg/dl in the blood predose and 1 hour postdose, respectively. The potential toxicity of sulfonamides (*e.g.,* crystaluria, hematuria, rash) is well known (Chap. 18, Antimicrobics and Anthelmintics for Systemic Therapy).

The optimum duration of combined chemotherapy has not been determined. Evaluation of treatment is difficult because of the extremely variable course and severity of toxoplasmosis. Acute acquired toxoplasmosis should be treated only if the infection is severe or if the patient is immunodeficient. Immunodeficient patients may require therapy for at least 4 to 6 weeks, perhaps for 6 to 12 months, after resolution of all clinical manifestations of active infection. Infections acquired in laboratory accidents or through transfusions may be more virulent than naturally acquired infections and probably should be treated.

Pyrimethamine plus a sulfonamide, or spiramycin (a macrolide antibiotic available in Western Europe, Mexico, and Canada but not in the United States), appear to decrease the incidence of congenital toxoplasmic infection when administered to women who acquire the infection during pregnancy. Pyrimethamine is teratogenic and should not be used until after the first trimester. At present, there is no optimal medical therapy available in the United States for treating women with acute toxoplasmosis who are in their first trimester of pregnancy. However, sulfadiazine or trisulfapyrimidines should be used during the first trimester, since sulfonamides alone are effective in acute toxoplasmosis in animal models. If spiramycin can be obtained, pregnant women acutely infected in the first trimester may be treated until term with 50 to 100 mg/kg body wt/day, PO, as two equal portions, 12-hourly, for 3-week-long courses alternating with 2-week drug-free intervals.

After the first trimester, women with acute toxoplasmosis should be treated with sulfonamides plus pyrimethamine. In one study, application of the combination for 2 weeks, followed by one or two courses of sulfonamide alone or in combination with pyrimethamine (3 to 4 weeks without drugs intervening between courses of antimicrobics), resulted in a decrease in transplacental infection from 17% to 5%.

Although the risk of transmission of the infection to the fetus is low in the first trimester, the probability of severe damage from infection early in fetal life is so high that therapeutic abortion should be considered. There is no proof that pregnant women with a history of habitual abortion who are seropositive for toxoplasmosis will benefit from treatment. Clinically abnormal or normal infants with congenital toxoplasmosis should be treated in an effort to prevent further tissue destruction (see list below).

Because hypersensitivity may play a significant role in the pathogenesis of ocular toxoplasmosis, glucosteroids are often added to the therapeutic regimen. There is no doubt of the rapid good effect and short-term value of glucosteroids, and they are generally given when vision-threatening lesions of retinochoroiditis involve the macula, maculopapillary bundle, or optic nerve. Small peripheral lesions usually subside spontaneously, leaving scars that generally

GUIDELINES FOR THERAPY OF CONGENITAL TOXOPLASMOSIS

- Drugs
  - Pyrimethamine + sulfadiazine or trisulfapyrimidines—21-day course
    - Pyrimethamine—1 mg/kg body wt, PO, every two to three or even four days (the half-life of pyrimethamine is 4–5 days)
    - Sulfadiazine or trisulfapyrimidines—50–100 mg/kg body wt/day, PO, as two equal portions, 12-hourly
    - Spiramycin[†]—50–100 mg/kg body wt/day, PO, as two equal portions, 12-hourly
  - Glucosteroids (prednisone or methylprednisolone)—1–2 mg/kg body wt/day, PO, as two equal portions, 12-hourly. Continue until the inflammatory process (*e.g.,* high CSF protein, retinochoroiditis) has subsided; the dose is then decreased progressively to nil.
  - Folinic acid—5 mg, PO, twice weekly during pyrimethamine treatment
- Indications
  - Overt congenital toxoplasmosis—Pyrimethamine + sulfadiazine or trisulfapyrimidines + folinic acid—21 days. During the first year of life, the child is given 3 to 4 courses of pyrimethamine + sulfadiazine or trisulfapyrimidines, separated by 30 to 45 days. No treatment is usually given after 12 months of age.
  - Overt congenital toxoplasmosis with evidence of inflammatory process (chorioretinitis, high CSF protein content, generalized infection, jaundice)—as for overt congenital toxoplasmosis + glucosteroid treatment
  - Subclinical congenital toxoplasmosis—As for overt congenital toxoplasmosis
  - Healthy newborn in whom serologic testing has not provided definitive results but whose mother acquired infection during pregnancy—one course of pyrimethamine + trisulfapyrimidines for 21 days, then wait for laboratory evidence for diagnosis.

(Courtesy of Dr. Jacques Couvreur, Laboratoire de Serologie Neonatale et de Recherche sur la Toxoplasmose, Institut de Puericulture, Paris; after Remington JS, Desmonts G: Toxoplasmosis. In Remington JS, Klein JO (eds): Infectious Diseases of the Fetus and Newborn Infant. Philadelphia, WB Saunders, 1983)

* If spiramycin is not available, use pyrimethamine–sulfonamide for the total period of therapy.

do not cause significant loss of vision; such lesions may be followed without specific therapy.

Although therapy may be effective against *T. gondii* and induce a beneficial response clinically, it may not eradicate the infection.

Prevention

The prevention of congenital and acquired toxoplasmosis requires further knowledge of the epidemiology of *T. gondii.* Adequate cooking of meat at temperature in excess of 60°C (which destroys the tissue cyst form of the parasite) is recommended. Freezing meat to −20°C for 24 hours or more will kill the cyst form, but many freezers in the United States will not reach this temperature. To minimize the chance of becoming infected by handling raw meat, the hands should be thoroughly washed following contact with meat; touching the mucous membranes of the mouth and eyes with the hand while handling meat should be avoided. Fruits and vegetables may have oocysts on their surfaces and should be washed before ingestion. Cleanliness and the avoidance of areas contaminated with cat feces may prove to be important preventive measures. Specifically, pregnant women should avoid contact with cat feces.

It is conceivable that transmission of *T. gondii* by transfusion of leukocyte-rich blood products may occur with sufficient frequency to warrant rejection of antibody-positive persons as leukocyte donors for immunosuppressed recipients. Indeed, it may be advisable to exclude persons who are (or were, in the case of cadavers) seropositive for toxoplasmosis as donors of organs for transplantation to seronegative recipients.

Remaining Problems

Because maternal immunity appears to prevent congenital transmission of *T. gondii,* the development of a vaccine for use in nonimmune women of childbearing age should be explored. Vaccines that prevent oocyst development in household cats could prove to be of value in interrupting the life cycle of *T. gondii.* Specific antimicrobial agents are needed that are nontoxic, nonteratogenic, and effective against both the tachyzoite and tissue cyst forms of *T. gondii.*

Bibliography

Books

FRENKEL JK: Toxoplasmosis: Parasite life cycle, pathology, and immunology. In Hammond DM, Long PL (eds): The Coccidia: Eimeria, Isospora, Toxoplasma, and Related Genera. Baltimore, University Park Press, 1973. pp 344–410.

REMINGTON JS, DESMONTS G: Toxoplasmosis. In Remington JS, Klein JO (eds): Infectious Diseases of the Fetus and Newborn Infant, 2nd ed. Philadelphia, WB Saunders, 1983. pp 191–332.

Journals

CAREY RM, KIMBALL AC, ARMSTRONG D, LIEBERMAN PH: Toxoplasmosis. Clinical experiences in a cancer hospital. Am J Med 54:30–38, 1973

DESMONTS G, COUVREUR J: Congenital toxoplasmosis: A prospective study of 378 pregnancies. N Engl J Med 290:1110–1116, 1974

FELDMAN HA: Toxoplasmosis. N Engl J Med 279:1370–1375, 1431–1437, 1968

NAOT Y, DESMONTS G, REMINGTON JS: IgM enzyme-linked immunosorbent assay test for the diagnosis of congenital toxoplasma infection. J Pediatr 98:32–36, 1981

NAOT Y, REMINGTON JS: An enzyme-linked immunosorbent assay for detection of IgM antibodies to *Toxoplasma gondii:* Use for diagnosis of acute acquired toxoplasmosis. J Infect Dis 142:757–766, 1980

RUSKIN J, REMINGTON JS: Toxoplasmosis in the compromised host. Ann Intern Med 84:193–199, 1976

Symposium on toxoplasmosis. Bull NY Acad Med 50:197–240, 1974

WELCH PC, MASUR H, JONES TC, REMINGTON JS: Serologic diagnosis of acute lymphadenopathic toxoplasmosis. J Infect Dis 142:256–264, 1980

WILSON CB, REMINGTON JS: What can be done to prevent congenital toxoplasmosis? Am J Obstet Gynecol 138:357–363, 1980

WILSON CB, REMINGTON JS, STAGNO S, REYNOLDS DW: Development of adverse sequelae in children born with subclinical congenital Toxoplasma infection. Pediatrics 66:767–774, 1980

PHILIP D. MARSDEN

130 African Trypanosomiasis

Trypanosoma gambiense and *Trypanosoma rhodesiense* are morphologically identical causes of African trypanosomiasis in humans. At first, they may cause a mild systemic illness, later becoming apparent as a meningoencephalitis that is usually fatal without treatment.

Etiology

Trypomastigotes (trypanosomes) are motile hemoflagellates. A single flagellum originates in a kinetoplast situated posterior to the nucleus. As it passes anteriorly in contiguity with the body of the parasite, the flagellum delimits a protoplasmic excrescence called the undulating membrane. As it projects beyond the body of the parasite, the activity of the flagellum pulls the trypomastigote along.

In the peripheral blood of mammals, trypomastigotes vary greatly in size (10 μm–20 μm × 3 μm–5 μm) and in shape (both broad and slender forms are present—Fig. 130-1). The broad forms have a better developed mitochondrial structure and a more complete form of carbohydrate metabolism. They are thought to be the only forms infectious to the tsetse fly.

Reproduction in the vertebrate host involves longitudinal binary fission. In the fly, a cycle of development occurs that requires approximately 21 days from the time infected blood is ingested until metacyclic forms (infective for mammals) are present in the saliva. The intratsetse cycle is not completed in more than 90% of flies that ingest trypomastigotes. The flies successfully parasitized do not seem to be affected.

Epidemiology

Trypanosoma gambiense and *T. rhodesiense* are morphologically identical with *Trypanosoma brucei,* a protozoan noninfectious to humans but capable of causing disease in cattle and game animals. All three species probably evolved from a common ancestor, and conversion from one to the other remains a possibility. All three are transmitted by tsetse flies (Fig. 130-2), which are *Glossina* spp.

There are some 20 species of *Glossina,* all restricted to Africa. About twice the size of an ordinary housefly, tsetse flies have a forward projecting, biting proboscis. Both sexes feed on mammalian blood, are aggressive, and inflict painful bites. They are viviparous and lay mature larvae that pupate in sandy soil or under the bark of trees. It is not possible, therefore, to destroy eggs and larvae as a means of control. Transovarial transmission of *Trypanosoma* spp. does not occur.

Many of the points used to differentiate *T. gambiense* and *rhodesiense* are epidemiologic (Table 130-1). Overlap of the distribution of the two species occurs in some areas (*e.g.,* Uganda). A few flies around a water hole in a dry season may infect many people visiting the site. Infections caused by *T. rhodesiense* are more rapidly progressive than those caused by *T. gambiense,* possibly as a consequence of nonhuman mammalian passage in bushbucks, pigs, and cattle.

Pathogenesis and Pathology

The initial invasion of trypomastigotes at the site of inoculation is accompanied by infiltration with inflammatory cells, particularly lymphocytes, and interstitial edema. Lymphocytic and histiocytic proliferation occur in the lymph nodes and spleen. Later, fibrosis occurs. Leukocytes contain erythrocytes, fragmented cell debris, and trypomastigotes. The liver shows fatty degeneration, hyperplasia of the Kupffer cells with erythrophagocytosis, and lymphocytic infiltration of the portal tracts.

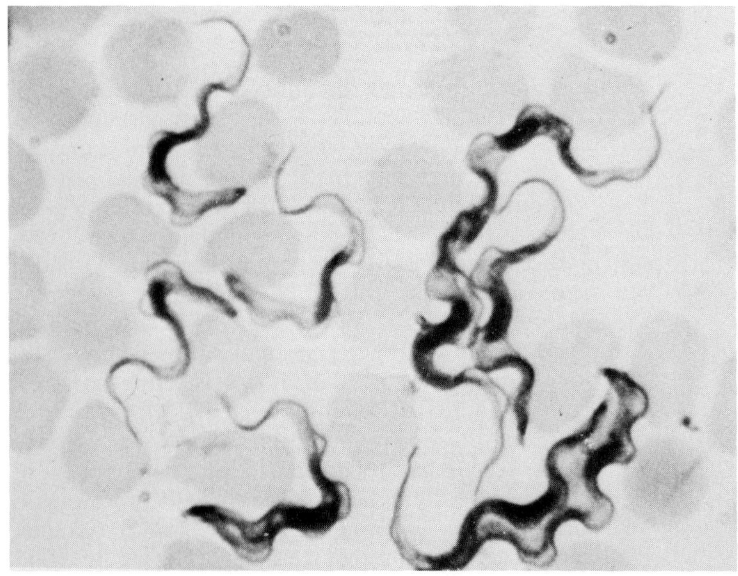

Fig. 130-1. Trypomastigotes (trypanosomes) in peripheral blood. (Giemsa, × 1500) (Courtesy of the Wellcome Museum of Medical Science, London)

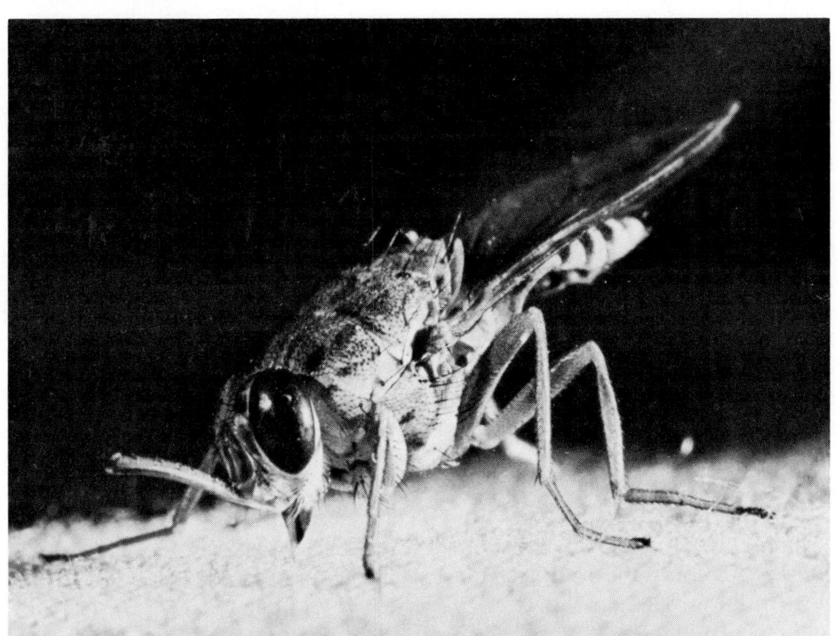

Fig. 130-2. A tsetse fly in the act of biting. (about × 15) (Courtesy of the Wellcome Museum of Medical Science, London)

Table 130-1. ***Differences Between*** Trypanosoma gambiense ***and*** Trypanosoma rhodesiense

	T. gambiense	***T. rhodesiense***
Vector species of *Glossina*	*palpalis* group	*morsitans* group
Distribution	West and Central Africa	East Africa
Animal reservoirs	Rare	Common (bushbuck, pig)
Location	Riverine and around water holes	Savannah and recently cleared bush
Development in laboratory rodents	Poor	Good

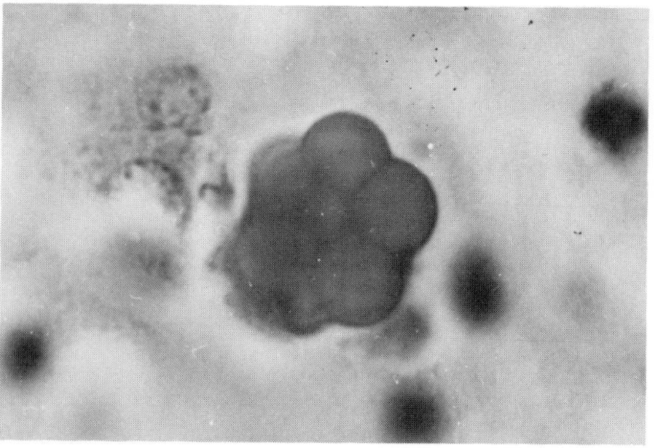

Fig. 130-3. Morular cell of Mott in the brain. (H&E × 2000) (Courtesy of Wellcome Museum of Medical Science, London)

In other viscera, a common lesion is endarteritis of the small vessels. Perivascular cuffing with plasma cells and lymphocytes results. This perivascular cuffing is common in the brain, where it is associated with neurological proliferation. Both become more severe the longer the duration of the illness. A distinctive cell—the morular cell of Mott—is seen in the inflammatory infiltrate. It is a modified plasma cell (9 μm–12 μm in diameter) distorted with a large, eosinophilic inclusion (Fig. 130-3). Demyelination has been observed in the brain and peripheral nerves. Degeneration of nerve cells occurs secondary to destruction of nerve fibers. Ocular nerve involvement with papilledema may lead to subsequent optic atrophy. Iridocyclitis may occur. Edema, hemorrhages, and granulomatous lesions occur in the brain. Thrombosis, as a result of endarteritis, is a major cause of cerebral degeneration.

The heart may be affected, with small pericardial effusions associated with intracardiac hemorrhages, edema, loss of striation of muscle fibers, and mononuclear infiltrates. When *T. rhodesiense* is the infecting agent, cerebral infiltrates are less florid, effusions into serous cavities are more common, and cardiac involvement may be severe. A patchy glomerulonephritis has also been noted.

Manifestations

Patients often remember being bitten by tsetse flies. A dusky red, indurated nodule (the trypanosomal chancre) with an area of edema may appear 1 to 2 weeks after the bite. Serous exudate from this lesion may contain trypomastigotes. The phase of local multiplication is succeeded by a phase of bloodstream dissemination and reticuloendothelial activation. This so-called second stage occurs within a few weeks of inoculation of *T. rhodesiense,* but it may be delayed for months with *T. gambiense*.

Intermittent fever, headaches, and transient edematous swellings may be initial complaints. A circinate, erythematous rash (readily seen in whites), fades within a week. The enlarged lymph nodes are spongy, discrete, and sometimes tender; as fibrosis sets in, they become firm. Lymphoadenopathy in the posterior triangle of the neck is known as Winterbottom's sign. A soft hepatosplenomegaly may occur at this stage, and there may be mild jaundice. Although the leukocytes are usually normal in total numbers, there is a relative lymphocytosis. A mild normocytic normochromic anemia is associated with reduced marrow activity. There is a fall in plasma albumin and a rise in serum globulins (IgG, IgA, IgM). IgM, in particular, is markedly increased and remains elevated throughout the course of the infection.

East African trypanosomiasis (*T. rhodesiense*) may progress to central nervous system (CNS) involvement in a few months, whereas the West African disease (*T. gambiense*) may take years. Persistent headache, inability to concentrate, and a feeling of oppression are early signs. As cerebral damage progresses, apathy and somnolence appear. The speech is slow and mumbling, the gait shuffling, and there are fine tremors of the tongue and limbs. Finally, a phase of continuous sleep blends into true coma. Death is often brought on by malnutrition or intercurrent infection. Localizing signs of disease of the CNS, in the form of cranial nerve palsies and long-tract signs, are uncommon. Peripheral neuritis may occur. The cerebrospinal fluid (CSF) is under increased pressure, up to 2000 mononuclear cells per cubic mm are present, and morular cells may be noted. The higher the concentration of protein in the cerebrospinal fluid, the worse the prognosis.

Diagnosis

Because the clinical picture is not specific, the demonstration of trypomastigotes is important (see Chap. 11, Diagnostic Methods for Protozoa and Helminths). Trypomastigotes are seen more readily in the peripheral blood in *T. rhodesiense* infections because of dense parasitemia. Lymph node puncture is particularly helpful in *T. gambiense* infections; liquid aspirated from a node is placed on a glass slide, stained, and examined for trypomastigotes. The inoculation of blood into rats and mice is frequently positive in *T. rhodesiense* infections. The CSF should be centrifuged and the sediment examined for trypomastigotes; they may be difficult to find. Blood culture is possible, but it is more difficult than with *Trypanosoma cruzi* and is not practical as a field procedure.

Serologic tests have recently been reevaluated. A complement fixation test and indirect fluorescent antibody test are available. The fluorescent antibody test is usually positive on the CSF of affected patients. Of the immunoglobulins, IgM is particularly high in concentration in serum and CSF (up to 15 times normal), a finding of diagnostic value.

The early phase of the disease may resemble syphilis, tuberculosis, Hodgkin's disease, and infectious mononucleosis. Heterophil antibodies are sometimes present early in African trypanosomiasis. Late-stage African trypanosomiasis must be distinguished from CNS syphilis and, particularly, other causes of meningitis with a mononuclear cell response. False-positive reaginic tests for syphilis may occur. As a general rule, African sleeping sickness must be considered in any patient coming from equatorial Africa who has a markedly changed personality or other cerebral symptoms. Tourists on game safari may be at special risk in a tsetse fly area.

Prognosis

The prognosis is good if the CSF is normal at the beginning of treatment. A high CSF protein is a poor prognostic sign—for example, when the concentration exceeds 40 mg per 100 ml, some patients fail to respond even to treatment with Mel B.

Trypomastigotes may develop resistance to almost every known drug, both in the laboratory and in clinical practice. Humans possess some natural resistance, particularly to small inocula of *T. gambiense*. Acquired immunity also occurs, and the periodic disappearance of trypomastigotes from the blood is the result of destruction by trypanolysins. However, no real protection results because immunity is highly type-specific, and the trypomastigotes readily change in antigenic structure.

Therapy

Before CNS involvement has occurred, suramin (Antrypol, germanin, Bayer 205), a complex, nonmetal containing, organic compound, is effective against both *T. gambiense* and *T. rhodesiense* infections. One gram of the drug is dissolved in 10 ml sterile water for each intravenous (IV) injection. A test dose of 0.2 g should be injected intravenously on the first day; if no untoward effect occurs, 0.8 g is given on the next day. The therapeutic dose for adults (17 mg/kg body wt IV, every fourth day) is continued to a total dose of 10 g. Side-effects include papular eruptions, photophobia, peripheral neuritis, and agranulocytosis. More serious are signs of kidney damage with protein, erythrocytes, and casts in the urine. The drug is contraindicated in renal disease, and the urine should be tested for protein before each injection.

Pentamidine isethionate is an alternative drug for the treatment of early African trypanosomiasis, but it is less active against *T. rhodesiense* than suramin. The dose is 4 mg per kg body weight given every other day by intramuscular (IM) injection for a total of 10 injections. Neither suramin nor pentamidine attains effectively antitrypanosomal concentrations in the CSF.

When the CNS is involved, melarsoprol (Mel B, Arsobal) is the drug of choice. It is trivalent arsenic, in the form of melarsen oxide, combined with dimercaprol (BAL, to ameliorate toxicity), dissolved in propylene glycol in a concentration of 3.6 g per 100 ml. The total dose is 20 mg per kg of body weight, injected IV as three incremental courses consisting of three daily doses; the courses are separated by rest periods of 7 days. One day's dose must not exceed 180 mg. Thus, a 60-kg patient would receive a total dose of 1,260 mg (35 ml): first course—90 mg (2.5 ml), 90 mg (2.5 ml), and 108 mg (3 ml); second course—108 mg (3 ml), 144 mg (4 ml), and 180 mg (5 ml); third course—180 mg (5 ml), 180 mg (5 ml), and 180 mg (5 ml). The adverse reactions are those associated with heavy-metal intoxication: exofoliative dermatitis, toxic hepatitis, nephritis, agranulocytosis, and most serious of all, arsenical encephalopathy. A direct toxic effect, arsenical encephalopathy is quite different from the reactive encephalopathy that occurs early in treatment, apparently as a result of the massive death of trypomastigotes in the brain. For debilitated patients, smaller doses of melarsoprol may be necessary. Tryparsamide, a pentavalent arsenical used for many years, has been superseded by melarsoprol. Melarsonyl potassium (Mel W) is water soluble and is suitable for IM injection, but it does not seem to be as effective as melarsoprol.

Nitrofurazone (25 mg/kg body wt/day as three equal portions, given perorally, once every 8 hours for 10 days) has some therapeutic effect and has been used in drug-resistant cases in combination with melarsoprol. Peripheral neuritis is a serious toxic effect, and hemolytic anemia occurs in the presence of glucose-6-phosphate dehydrogenase deficiency.

When using these toxic drugs, the importance of adequate nutrition and the concomitant treatment of intercurrent infections must be kept in mind. In the

United States, both suramin and melarsoprol are available by special arrangement with the Centers for Disease Control, Atlanta, Georgia.

In *T. gambiense* infections, the CSF must be examined every 6 months for 2 years to detect failures of therapy. Infections caused by *T. rhodesiense* usually relapse within months if cure is not achieved.

Prevention

Medical surveillance with mobile teams diagnosing and treating infected patients will reduce the incidence in endemic areas, but permanent control requires that the cycle of human–fly contact be broken. Such measures as the selective clearing of vegetation to destroy tsetse habitats, the restriction of population movement through transmission areas, and in the case of *Glossina morsitans,* selective game destruction have met with some success. DDT and dieldrin are insecticides effective against the tsetse fly, and both are sufficiently persistent to cover the 8-week phase of pupal maturation. The difficulties lie in spraying thoroughly enough to make sure the tsetse comes into contact with the insecticides, and in the cost.

Both suramin and pentamidine have a prophylactic effect in humans by virtue of their slow excretion. Pentamidine isethionate prevents clinical illness in an adult for 6 months after a single IM dose of 4 mg per kg body wt, but it may merely mask infection with *T. rhodesiense.* Accordingly, chemoprophylaxis should be given only to persons exposed to a high risk of infection for a short period.

Bibliography

Books

MULLIGAN HW, POTTS WH (eds): The African Trypanosomiases. London, George Allen & Unwin, 1970. 950 pp.

World Health Organization: African trypanosomiasis. WHO Tech Rep Series No. 434, 1969. 79 pp.

Journals

APTED FC: Sleeping sickness in Tanganyika, Past, present and future. Trans R Soc Trop Med Hyg 56:15–29, 1962

DUGGAN AJ, HUTCHINSON MP: Sleeping sickness in Europeans: A review of 109 cases. J Trop Med Hyg 69:124–131, 1966

LUMSDEN WHR: Trends in research on the immunology of trypanosomiasis. Bull WHO 37:167–175, 1967

ROBERTSON DHH: Chemotherapy of African trypanosomiasis. Practitioner 188:80–83, 1962

World Health Organization: Trypanosomiasis. Bull WHO 28:537–836, 1963

ROGER W. WILLIAMS

Tick Paralysis

131

Tick paralysis is usually manifest as an ascending flaccid paralysis that occurs in humans and other mammals when toxin-secreting ixodid (hard) ticks remain attached for several days. Removal of the tick or ticks results in a cure.

Etiology

Adult ticks are typical eight-legged, saclike arachnids measuring about 2 mm to 6 mm in length in the unengorged state. The female increases in size many times as she engorges and eggs develop (Fig. 131-1).

On a worldwide basis, 10 genera and 43 species of ticks are known to be toxinogenic. The chief offenders in North America are *Dermacentor andersoni* in the West and *Dermacentor variabilis* in the East. In Australia, the toxic fraction was found in an extract of ground *Ixodes holocyclus* that could be used to immunize dogs. The resultant antiserum protected mice against a fatal dose of the toxic fraction.

Epidemiology

Only certain individual female ticks (rarely males, because they do not remain attached as long) and not every tick of a given species seem to be capable of causing the syndrome. The site of attachment is unimportant. Less than 500 cases in man have been reported in the United States and Canada. The fatality rate varies from 3% in the East to 12% in the West. Although the disease occurs in adults, it is more common in children, particularly in the 2- to 5-year age group.

Pathogenesis and Pathology

It was formerly thought that the toxin(s) from all ticks impaired muscle-stretch reflexes and prevented the liberation of acetylcholine at the neuromuscular junction, thus causing a conduction block in the somatic motor fibers. Apparently, this is true of the paralysis caused by *I. holocyclus;* the amplitudes of nerve compound action potential do not change and the muscle response and endplate potential show temperature-dependent differences and an increased concentration of $MgCl_2$. However, the toxins of other ticks produce a motor polyneuropathy with strong functional impairment, particularly of the rapidly conducting motor fibers. There is pharmacologic evidence that the site of neuromuscular blockade is presynaptic and electrodiagnostic evidence of involvement of peripheral nerves rather than neuromuscular blockade.

At postmortem examination, there are no significant pathologic changes.

Manifestations

Irritability and mild diarrhea may occur early in the illness, followed by areflexia and ataxia resulting in poor control of the legs, staggering, and falling. Sensory changes are usually lacking, but there may be hyperesthesia and paresthesia in the affected extremities. Flaccid paralysis soon develops and ascends in 1 or more days to involve the trunk, arms, neck, tongue, and pharynx. There is little or no stiffness of the neck or back. With the appearance of bulbar involvement, the voice becomes thick and nasal, and the patient is unable to swallow and chokes on pharyngeal secretions. Nystagmus and strabismus are sometimes noted. In infants, terminal convulsions may occur. Respiration becomes abdominal, shallow, rapid, and finally irregular. Restlessness gives way to stupor, and death results from paralysis of the respiratory muscles or from respiratory obstruction due to aspirated material. Severe myocarditis has been reported and may also be a cause of death. The temper-

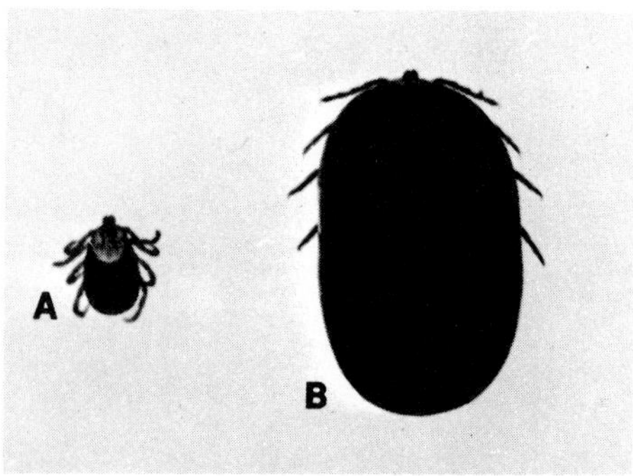

Fig. 131-1. *A* Unengorged female *Dermacentor andersoni* (magnification × 2). *B* Engorged female *Dermacentor andersoni* (magnification × 2).

ature rarely exceeds 100°F unless there is secondary infection. The leukocyte count is usually normal. The spinal fluid is almost always normal. The erythrocyte count, hemoglobin, and urine show no changes. The only abnormality in biochemical tests thus far reported has been a 10-day elevation of plasma creatine phosphokinase, present during and after the paralytic stage.

In France, paralysis does not set in until 2 to 8 weeks after the tick has dropped off. Facial paralysis is frequent and the central nervous system (CNS) may become involved. In Africa, cases fall into two groups: generalized progressive muscular weakness and regional paralysis at the site of tick attachment—the latter frequently caused by male ticks.

Diagnosis

Poliomyelitis (see Chap. 121), polyneuritis, myelitis, infectious neuronitis, syringomyelia, spinal cord tumor, botulism (see Chap. 127), and Guillian–Barré syndrome should be considered in the differential diagnosis. Such diagnoses can be dismissed when a tick is found and prompt recovery follows its removal. *Failure to search through the hair at the base of the skull might result in an unnecessary death.*

Prognosis

Recovery is complete in 1 to 5 days if the tick or ticks are removed before the appearance of bulbar signs. To avoid leaving the mouthparts of the tick at the site of attachment, a cloth soaked in ether, acetone, or benzene should be wrapped around the tick. The tick will loosen in about 10 minutes.

Alternatively, piercing the tick with a hot needle or touching with a lighted cigarette may cause release. Gentle, straight traction on the tick is more effective than a twisting motion. If these maneuvers fail, the skin should be excised, using the cutting edge of a No. 18 needle or a small scalpel. The mouthparts with its hypostome must be removed to ensure freedom from secondary infection.

Therapy

If the patient cannot swallow and is choking on secretions, the foot of the bed should be elevated and the head turned to the side to promote drainage. The pharynx should be aspirated frequently. Nothing should be given by mouth until the patient is able to swallow normally. Parenteral fluids should be given. Sedatives and narcotics should be avoided. Penicillin, given parenterally, may be useful if aspiration pneumonia occurs. Oxygen may be necessary. When the diaphragm and intercostal muscles are paralyzed, a respirator may be life-saving. If no respirator is available, other methods of artificial respiration should be tried. Patients with puddling of pharyngeal secretions should not be placed in a respirator unless they are actually unable to breathe because there is considerable danger of aspiration into the tracheobronchial tree. An apparently moribund patient may show striking improvement in respiration within a few hours after removal of the tick.

Prevention

Dogs and other household pets should be manually "deticked" or treated with a systemic insecticide. Children who play in grassy or partially wooded areas should be examined twice a day for ticks and repellents applied to the skin or clothing (*N, N*-diethyl-*M*-toluamide [Off], dimethylcarbamate, dimethylphthalate, benzyl benzoate). In summer, the hair should be kept short and washed frequently.

Remaining Problems

There is great confusion about the site of action of the toxin(s). The nature of the toxin(s) remains to be determined. Periodically work is published on these subjects, but the results seem to lead to greater mysteries rather than to clarification.

Bibliography

Journals

ABBOTT KH: Tick paralysis: A review. I. Proc Mayo Clin 18:39–45, 1943

ABBOTT KH: Tick paralysis: A review. II. Proc Mayo Clin 18:59–64, 1943

CHERINGTON M, SNYDER RD: Tick paralysis: Neurophysiological studies. N Engl J Med 278:95–97, 1968

GOTHE R, KUNZE K, HOOGSTRALL H: Review article: The mechanisms of pathogenicity in the tick paralyses. J Med Entomol 16:357–369, 1979

HILLER GC, PATERSON DC: Tick paralysis: A case report with emphasis on neurological toxicity. Am J Dis Child 124:915–917, 1972

KAIRE GH: Isolations of tick paralysis toxin from *Ixodes holocylus.* Toxicon 4:91–97, 1966

MCLENNAR H, OIKAWA I: Changes in function of the neuromuscular junction occurring in tick paralysis (caused by *Dermacentor andersoni* Stiles). Can J Physiol Pharmacol 50:53–58, 1972

MURNAGHAM MG: Site and mechanism of tick paralysis. Science 131:418–419, 1960

Section | *XVII*

Cardiovascular Infections

Indigenous Microbiota of the Cardiovascular System

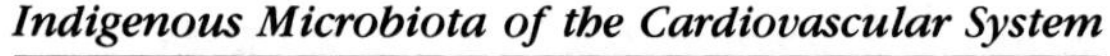

(None)

CHARLES B. SMITH

Pericarditis

132

Pericarditis—inflammation of the pericardium—may be caused by virtually every kind of infectious agent and by a wide variety of noninfectious processes, including neoplastic diseases. *Acute serofibrinous pericarditis* is the commonest form and is associated with enteroviral infections, myocardial infarction, or systemic inflammatory diseases such as rheumatoid arthritis; the course is usually benign. *Acute purulent pericarditis* is usually bacterial in origin and is often rapidly fatal owing to cardiac tamponade. *Chronic granulomatous* or *fibrosing pericarditis* is typically caused by tuberculous or fungal infection and may lead to circulatory failure from constrictive pericarditis.

Etiology

Virtually any infectious agent that reaches the myocardium or pericardium is capable of causing pericarditis (see list below). Enteroviruses are the most common infectious causes of *acute serofibrinous pericarditis.* Substantial evidence for the role of coxsackie and echo viruses in pericarditis includes isolation of the organism from diseased myocardial and pericardial tissues. Many other viruses have been associated with pericarditis by isolating the virus from noncardiac sites or by serologic methods. By these less definitive criteria, common viral pathogens such as influenza viruses, hepatitis viruses, childhood exanthem myxoviruses, and members of the herpes group of viruses have been associated with pericarditis. It is important to remember that occasional cases of acute serofibrinous pericarditis may be caused by potentially treatable infectious agents such as *Mycoplasma pneumoniae, Chlamydia psittaci* and *Coxiella burnetii.* There is a large number of noninfectious causes of pericarditis (see list below).

INFECTIOUS CAUSES OF PERICARDITIS

- Viruses
  - Coxsackievirus
  - Echovirus
  - Influenza virus types A and B
  - Adenovirus
  - Vaccinia virus
  - Hepatitis viruses types A and B
  - Colorado tick fever virus
  - Mumps virus
  - Rubeola virus
  - Rubella virus
  - Cytomegalovirus
  - Varicella-zoster virus
  - Epstein–Barr virus
  - Lymphocytic choriomeningitis virus
- Bacteria
  - *Staphylococcus aureus*
  - *Streptococcus pneumoniae*
  - *Streptococcus pyogenes* and other streptococcus species
  - *Haemophilus influenzae*
  - *Neisseria gonorrhoeae* and *meningitidis*
  - *Salmonella* spp.
  - Enteric gram-negative bacilli
  - Anaerobic gram-negative bacilli and cocci
  - *Actinomyces* and *Nocardia* spp.
  - *Mycobacterium tuberculosis*
  - Nontuberculous *Mycobacterium* spp.
- Fungi
  - *Histoplasma capsulatum*
  - *Coccidioides immitis*
  - *Cryptococcus* spp.
  - *Blastomyces dermatitidis*
  - *Candida* spp.
  - *Aspergillus* spp.

Mycoplasmas
- *Mycoplasma pneumoniae*

Chlamydia
- *Chlamydia psittaci*

Rickettsias
- *Rickettsia rickettsii*
- *Coxiella burnetii*

Protozoa
- *Toxoplasma gondii*
- *Entamoeba histolytica*

Helminths
- *Trichinella spiralis*
- Filaria
- *Echinococcus granulosus*

Acute purulent pericarditis is most often caused by common bacterial pathogens such as staphylococci, pneumococci, streptococci, *Hemophilus influenzae* and meningococci (Table 132-1). Less commonly, gram-negative bacilli such as *Escherichia coli, Klebsiella* spp., *Salmonella* spp., and several kinds of anaerobic bacteria may be etiologic agents. Occasionally, fungi such as *Candida* spp. and *Aspergillus* spp. may cause acute purulent pericarditis. Amebic pericarditis may present initially as an apparently benign serous pericarditis, but if left untreated, it usually progresses to acute purulence with death from tamponade.

Chronic pericarditis is classically caused by *Mycobacterium tuberculosis* or by fungi such as *Coccidioides immitis* or *Histoplasma capsulatum.* The clinicopathologic picture of fibrous–constrictive pericarditis may also result from such noninfectious causes as nonsurgical trauma, cardiotomy, neoplasm, and autoimmune diseases (see list entitled Noninfectious Causes of Pericarditis, above).

NONINFECTIOUS CAUSES OF PERICARDITIS

- Injury
  - Myocardial infarction
  - Trauma (penetrating or nonpenetrating)
    - Postinjury, postpericardiotomy, Dressler's syndrome
    - Irradiation
  - Connective tissue diseases
    - Rheumatic fever
    - Systemic lupus erythematosus
    - Periarteritis nodosa
    - Scleroderma
    - Dermatomyositis
    - Giant cell aortitis
  - Metabolic
    - Uremia
    - Chronic dialysis
    - Myxedema
  - Allergy or Hypersensitivity
    - Serum sickness
    - Giant urticaria
    - Pulmonary infiltrate with eosinophilia syndrome
    - Drugs—procainamide, hydralazine
  - Neoplasm
    - Primary—mesothelioma
    - Metastatic—lung, breast, lymphoma, leukemia
  - Other
    - Chronic anemia
    - Sarcoidosis
    - Atrial septal defect
    - Familial Mediterranean fever
    - Aneurysm
    - Chyle
    - Cholesterol
    - Pancreatitis

Table 132-1. *Causes of Acute Purulent Pericarditis*

	U.S. Adults Post-1960 (%)	U.S. Children Post-1950 (%)	Nigerian Children Post-1967* (%)
Staphylococci	15–30	44	31 tuberculosis
Pneumococci	8–25	6	31
Streptococci	4–13	1	8
Hemophilus influenzae	2–5	22	0
Enteric gram-negative bacilli	5–30	8	27
Meningococci	3–9	9	0
Anaerobes	3–11	1	0
Fungi (acute)	5–20	0	0

*Includes all infectious pericarditis patients.

Epidemiology

Pericarditis is generally an unusual complication of common infectious diseases, and the occurrence of pericarditis reflects the epidemiologic characteristics of the primary infections. For example, enteroviral acute serofibrinous pericarditis occurs most commonly in the late summer and early fall in the United States. Although surveillance for pericarditis has been mostly retrospective, it appears that enteroviral infections are important causes of acute pericarditis in all age groups and in all areas of the world. Acute purulent pericarditis in children in the United States is usually caused by staphylococci or *H. influenzae,* whereas in developing and tropical countries, such as Nigeria, staphylococci *E. coli* or *Salmonella* spp. are the common causes (Table 132-1).

Tuberculosis is no longer the leading cause of nonviral pericarditis in adults in developed countries, but it continues to be a common problem in developing countries. In the United States, an increasing frequency of enteric gram-negative bacilli and fungi such as *Candida* spp. and *Aspergillus* spp. as causes of acute purulent pericarditis reflects an increasing number of patients who are immunosuppressed, have an underlying noninfectious pericarditis such as uremic pericarditis, or who have experienced recent thoracic or heart surgery.

Pathogenesis and Pathology

Microorganisms reach the pericardium by the blood, lymph, direct extension from pulmonary or myocardial foci of infection, or direct inoculation during surgery, other invasive procedures, or penetrating trauma. Viral infections are usually blood-borne and often infect the myocardium as well as the pericardium (see Chap. 133, Myocarditis). Pneumococci or other primary pulmonary pathogens usually infect the pericardium by extension from an adjacent pneumonitis; the common causes of bacteremias—staphylococci, meningococci and *H. influenzae*—are more likely to reach the pericardium through the bloodstream. A pre-existing, noninfectious pericarditis, as is seen with uremia or following cardiac surgery, may increase susceptibility to hematogenous bacterial pericarditis. The endocardium or myocardium may serve as the initial source of bacteria; for example, pericarditis is present in about one-half of the 20% to 30% of patients who have myocardial abscesses complicating staphylococcal endocarditis. Amebic pericarditis may develop as a result of direct extension from amebic liver or subdiaphragmatic abscesses. Echinococcal pericarditis occurs by extension from myocardial echinococcal cysts.

The intensity of the pericardial inflammatory reaction reflects the pathogenicity of the etiologic agent. Viral infections typically produce a relatively mild inflammatory reaction that is associated with focal damage to the adjacent myocardium. The response varies from a small amount of serous fluid with mononuclear cells and fibrinogen to a large, neutrophil-rich, bloody effusion. The tissue damage in viral perimyocarditis is the result of direct cellular damage by the infecting virus. Virus-infected cells may also be destroyed by sensitized T-lymphocytes reacting with viral antigens on the cell surface or by antibody dependent, cell-mediated cytotoxicity. The development of pericarditis following acute viral or mycoplasmal illnesses is consistent with a postinflammatory, autoimmune response provoked by persisting viral or host antigens—a construction used to justify treating viral pericarditis with glucosteroids. Clinical and therapeutic studies in humans have not been adequate either to support or to refute this hypothesis.

Mild fibrosis and occasional adhesions between visceral and parietal pericardial surfaces may mark the healing of viral pericarditis. However, such a fibrotic reaction rarely gives rise to a constrictive pericarditis.

Acute, purulent, bacterial pericarditis as caused by *Staphylococcus aureus* is typically a rapidly progressive disease. The mortality exceeds 50% and is related to general sepsis, myocardial damage and rapidly progressive cardiac tamponade. In patients who survive, healing is associated with extensive fibrosis that may progress to a chronic, constrictive pericarditis requiring pericardiectomy.

Pericardial involvement has been detected at necropsy in approximately 5% of patients with fatal pulmonary tuberculosis. Pericardial inoculation may occur through the blood in primary tuberculosis or subsequently through the lymph from adjacent pulmonary or mediastinal nodes. The early granulomatous stages of tuberculous pericarditis are associated with large pericardial effusions ($\geqslant$300 ml) that are typically serosanguinous and contain monuclear cells. If the effusion accumulates rapidly, acute or subacute cardiac tamponade may result, leading to circulatory failure. As the disease evolves, the inflammatory process becomes chronic; fusion of the parietal and visceral pericardium may result, yielding constrictive pericarditis and circulatory failure.

In cardiac tamponade, pericardial pressure is increased and equilibrates with diastolic ventricular filling pressures, reducing effective ventricular filling pressure and ventricular stroke volume. As an increase in the heart rate fails to compensate, cardiac output falls. Thus, the clinical manifestations of tamponade are associated with low cardiac output, and increased atrial and venous pressures consequent to the increased compensatory end-diastolic ventricular filling pressure.

The hemodynamic lesion in constrictive pericarditis is also due to restriction of ventricular filling and stroke volume. However, unlike the situation in cardiac tamponade, in constrictive pericarditis early diastolic ventricular filling pressures are normal, and it is only in the late phases of ventricular filling that diastolic relaxation and expansion of the ventricle is inhibited by the constricting pericardium. At this point, the diastolic filling pressure rapidly increases to equal that of the atria (Fig. 132-1). As with cardiac tamponade, the systemic venous pressure rises in constrictive pericarditis and leads to prominent physical signs. In constrictive pericarditis the restriction on right ventricular filling equals that on the left ventricle; as a result, pulmonary venous pressure does not increase and there are no signs and symptoms of pulmonary congestion.

Manifestations

Symptoms

Chest pain in acute pericarditis is typically rapid in onset, persists for several hours to days, and is worse during inspiration and recumbency but improves with leaning forward. The pain in usually precordial and may be sharp, dull, constricting, or crushing, making clinical differentiation from myocardial infarction difficult. Radiation of pain to the left trapezius ridge is particularly characteristic of pericarditis. Other symptoms of acute viral pericarditis include fever and malaise. Often there is a history that suggests a preceding acute respiratory or gastrointestinal viral illness.

In acute bacterial pericarditis, fever and chills are prominent and stem from the severe underlying infection; dyspnea, agitation, orthopnea and cough arise from early development of cardiac tamponade. Chest pain is not a prominent symptom in nearly 67% of patients—too often leading to a delay in considering the diagnosis of pericarditis.

Tuberculous pericarditis is not usually an acute process. Hence, the symptoms relate to the tuberculosis (fever, night sweats, weight loss, fatigue) and progressive circulatory failure (slowly progressive dyspnea, ascites, edema).

Signs

GENERAL

Often, clues to the diagnosis of infectious pericarditis are nonspecific and relate to disturbances of cardiac function. The patient with acute pericarditis and impending cardiac tamponade may have the sudden onset of cool extremities, a weak, rapid pulse, falling blood pressure, pulsus paradoxus, a quiet precor-

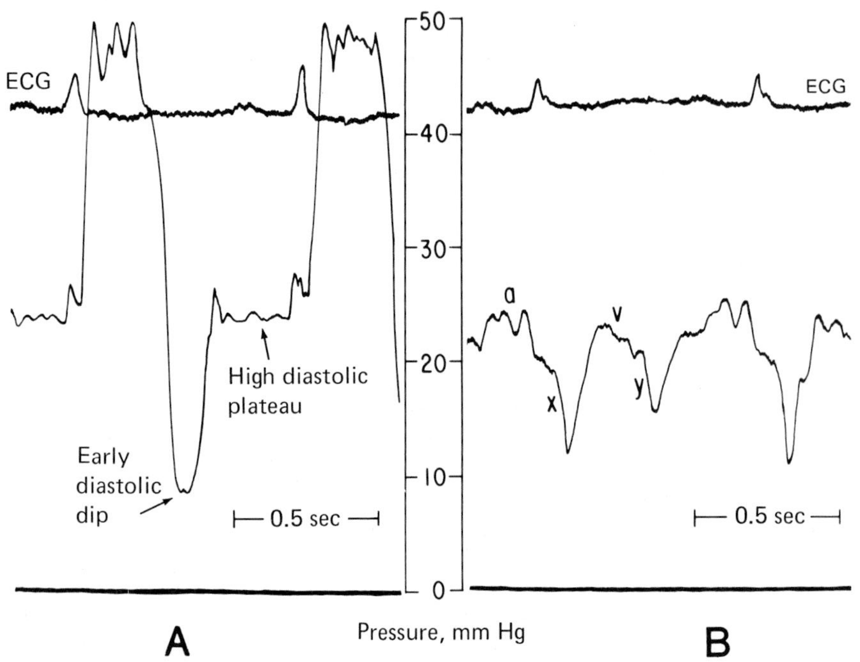

Fig. 132-1. Characteristic pressure tracings in constrictive pericarditis caused by tuberculosis. (*A*) Right ventricular tracing—normal early diastolic filling pressure with abnormally rapid rise in mid to late diastolic filling pressure as the constrictive pericarditis limits ventricular expansion. (*B*) Right atrial tracing—an elevated pressure with prominent *x* descent corresponding with rapid atrial filling during ventricular systole and a rapid *y* descent corresponding with early diastolic filling.

dium with distant heart sounds, and prominent evidence of systemic venous hypertension. These signs in a patient with bacterial endocarditis or bacterial sepsis should lead to serious consideration of acute purulent pericarditis, even when a pericardial friction rub is not present.

The findings in patients with tuberculous chronic constrictive pericarditis may be particularly misleading. Chronic systemic venous hypertension may present with prominent signs of hepatic failure including jaundice and ascites, or in rare cases, with proteinuria and edema suggesting the nephrotic syndrome. Systemic venous hypertension, as evidenced by distended neck veins and signs of poor cardiac output, without an enlarged heart and pulmonary congestion, should immediately suggest constrictive pericarditis.

PERICARDIAL FRICTION RUB

A pericardial friction rub is one of the most helpful signs in making a diagnosis of pericarditis. It is found in most patients with acute viral pericarditis; however, it is lacking in more than 50% of patients with acute purulent pericarditis and in most patients with constrictive pericarditis. Pericardial rubs are usually best heard at the left sternal border, and they may be accentuated when the patient is leaning forward or on hands and knees. The classical pericardial rub is close to the ear, and its quality is scratching and sandpaperlike or resembles the crunch of footsteps on cold snow. Other rubs may be muffled or distant, and their intermittancy may lead to controversy among examiners. The pericardial friction rub usually has three components; less often a biphasic or a single systolic component is heard. The friction rub may become more prominent with either inspiration or expiration, and an associated pleural friction rub may complicate the auscultation. Although pericardial rubs often diminish with the appearance of effusions, this is not always the case, and some patients with large effusions may also have pericardial rubs.

OTHER ABNORMAL HEART SOUNDS

In the presence of pericarditis, the normal heart sounds may be muffled by the effusion, fibrosis, or myocardial failure. Systolic clicks associated with pericardial disease occur in mid to late systole. A loud, abnormal, early diastolic (0.10 to 0.15 sec after the second sound) pericardial knock may be heard in patients with constrictive pericarditis.

PERICARDIAL EFFUSION

When pericardial effusion develops rapidly, relatively small amounts of fluid (200 ml–300 ml) that do not lead to detectable increases in the cardiac silhouette are capable of causing cardiac tamponade. The prominent findings in this situation are elevated venous pressure, decreased systemic pressure, and decreased cardiac output. When pericardial fluid develops gradually, large volumes may be well tolerated hemodynamically. In this situation clinical clues to the presence of fluid include decreased or muffled heart sounds and an area of cardiac dullness that extends beyond the point of maximal impulse. Occasionally bronchial breathing and an area of dullness to percussion may be heard at the tip of the left scapula (Ewart's sign), indicating compression of the lung from a large pericardial effusion.

PULSUS PARADOXUS

The systolic blood pressure normally falls 8 to 10 mm Hg during inspiration because of increased systolic afterload and increased venous return to the right ventricle causing decreased left ventricular filling. With pericarditis and tamponade and with constrictive pericarditis there is increased venous pressure, which accentuates the effect of inspiration on right ventricular filling. Moreover, the increased pericardial pressure causes intrusion on the left ventricular space by displacement of the intraventricular septum consequent on enlargement of the right ventricular chamber. The net effect is a fall in systolic blood pressure of greater than 10 mm Hg on inspiration in most patients with pericarditis and tamponade, and in approximately 30% of patients with constrictive pericarditis (pulsus paradoxus). Other conditions that can also produce pulsus paradoxus include respiratory obstruction, asthma, emphysema, and restrictive cardiomyopathies.

The cervical venous pressure may increase paradoxically with inspiration (Kussmaul's sign) in pericarditis. This finding is not specific for pericarditis and can be found with obstruction of the vena cava, and congestive heart failure from other causes.

Diagnosis

In acute pericarditis, the electrocardiogram (ECG) usually reflects diffuse subepicardial inflammation and injury. The S-T segment vector parallels the QRS vector and S-T elevations are seen in leads I and II and the precordial leads V_3 to V_6. Reciprocal S-T segment depression occurs in leads aVR and V_1. Subepicardial atrial injury may also be manifested by P-R segment depressions in leads II, aVF, and V_4 to V_6. During the resolving phase of pericarditis the S-T changes return to normal, and T waves in leads that showed S-T changes may become flattened or inverted. These changes may persist in patients with chronic pericarditis. Irritation of the atria during acute pericarditis is associated with an increased incidence of atrial arrhythmias including atrial fibrillation. Decreased voltage may be noted in the presence of effusions, and electrical alternans may occur with pericarditis.

Documenting the presence of pericardial effusions in patients with pericarditis is necessary to provide material to aid in etiologic diagnosis. Monitoring the size of the effusion should permit pericardiocentesis before florid signs of tamponade develop. The chest roentgenogram is usually normal in patients with acute pericarditis and may remain normal in patients who develop pericardial tamponade rapidly. The cardiac silhouette is increased with effusions larger than 300 ml. An increasing cardiac silhouette with clear lung fields in a patient with peripheral venous congestion is highly suggestive of tamponade.

Currently, the echocardiogram is the most accurate noninvasive method for detecting and monitoring pericardial effusions. As little as 50 ml of effusion may be detected by observing a sonolucent space between the posterior left ventricular epicardial and the pericardial echoes. As pericardial fluid increases to greater than 300 ml, a similar sonolucent space may be seen anteriorly in the recumbent patient. False-negative studies are unusual; false-positive studies may occur in the presence of a large epicardial fat pad and in patients with left pleural effusions or pulmonary masses. The risk involved in pericardiocentesis may be reduced when passage of the needle is guided by an echocardiographic monitor.

The two-dimensional echocardiogram may also be helpful in the diagnosis of cardiac tamponade and constrictive pericarditis. A marked inspiratory increase in right ventricular volume and a reciprocal decrease in left ventricular volume may be seen in some patients with tamponade. Loculated pericardial effusions, adhesive pericardial bands, and thickened pericardium detected by this technique have led to an increased awareness of the subacute effusive–constrictive form of pericardial disease. Abnormalities of ventricular wall motion detected by echocardiography may also suggest constrictive pericarditis.

The most important decision facing the clinician caring for patients with pericarditis is when to obtain pericardial fluid or biopsy the pericardium to make a definitive etiologic diagnosis. If the manifestations and course of the pericarditis are totally consistent with a viral pericarditis, or if there is an underlying myocardial infarction, rheumatic fever, or uremia, it is reasonable to temporize and observe. On the other hand, the slightest suggestion that the pericarditis is atypical should lead to more aggressive diagnostic tests. When the setting is classic for acute bacterial pericarditis (*i.e.,* patients with bacteremia or bacterial pneumonia who have high fever, leukocytosis, rapidly progressing illness and general toxicity), there should be no delay in obtaining pericardial fluid.

More confusing are patients who have noninfectious diseases that may cause pericarditis who are also at increased risk of developing bacterial pericarditis. Hemodialysis or peritoneal dialysis may be the site for bacterial invasion leading to bacterial pericarditis complicating uremic pericarditis. Glucosteroid therapy may coincide with reactivation of tuberculosis or histoplasmosis, which may be mistaken for lupus pericarditis. Transient benign pericarditis commonly follows pericardiotomy and cardiac surgery. Occasionally, however, the pericardium is the first site of a postoperative infection, and the usual fulminant clinical picture may be masked by administration of antimicrobics. In these situations, pericardial fluid obtained by needle aspiration should be examined by Gram stains and acid-fast stains, and cultured for aerobic, anaerobic, and acid-fast bacteria. If bacteria are not seen on the Gram stain, fungal and viral cultures should also be done. Pericardial tissue obtained by open surgical biopsy is more likely to yield a diagnosis of either tuberculosis, histoplasmosis, or coccidioidomycosis than is examination of the pericardial fluid.

Specific etiologic diagnosis in viral pericarditis is helpful in determining prognosis and in ruling out other more ominous diagnoses. Most definitive is isolation of a virus from pericardial fluid or tissues. Prompt delivery of the refrigerated (4°C) specimen to a viral diagnostic laboratory will give the greatest yield. If transport will take more than 24 hours, the specimen should be frozen and transported on solid CO_2. A viral diagnosis may also be suggested by isolation of a virus from respiratory or gastrointestinal tract secretions and demonstration of a fourfold or greater rise in antibodies to the isolate.

Prognosis

Viral pericarditis is a relatively benign illness that usually resolves in a few weeks. Approximately 20% of patients experience relapses that are also usually benign. When an associated myocarditis is prominent, it may lead to serious complications such as arrhythmias, myocardial failure, and rarely, to a late constrictive pericarditis.

Acute bacterial pericarditis continues to be a serious illness with an overall mortality rate of 50% to 70%. The observation that more than a third of patients are first diagnosed at autopsy indicates that late or missed diagnoses are still important factors leading to high mortality. Cardiac tamponade, myocardial abscess and general sepsis are early complications, whereas constrictive pericarditis may be a late complication in survivors.

Untreated tuberculous pericarditis is usually fatal. Overall, the case–fatality rate persists at 30% to 40% with most of the deaths occurring in patients who were undiagnosed and untreated. Congestive heart failure caused by cardiac tamponade or constrictive pericarditis are the major complications in both treated and untreated patients. Also, a subacute effusive–constrictive form of tuberculous pericarditis has been recognized.

Therapy

Acute viral pericarditis should be treated with bed rest because an associated myocarditis is usually present (see Chap. 133, Myocarditis). Pain can usually be controlled with salicylates or with other nonsteroidal anti-inflammatory agents. Glucosteroids are not recommended during the first two weeks of the illness; however, they may be useful in the occasional patient with persistent pain, progressing effusions or recurrent disease. An aggressive search for evidence of tuberculosis and fungal infection should be completed before glucosteroids are administered.

Successful therapy for acute bacterial pericarditis depends upon early identification of the etiologic agent by examination of the pericardial fluid, administration of appropriate antimicrobics, and prompt drainage of the pericardial effusion. It is not necessary to irrigate the pericardium with antimicrobial solutions because antimicrobics readily penetrate into the inflammed pericardial space. Antimicrobial therapy should be continued for 4 to 6 weeks. At the outset, drainage of pericardial fluid to relieve tamponade and obtain material for diagnosis is most rapidly accomplished by percutaneous needle aspiration. In most patients, however, surgical drainage is necessary. A pericardial window is usually satisfactory if the infection has been diagnosed and treated promptly. When the fluid is actually pus, or if adhesions and loculations are present, pericardiectomy is preferred to assure complete drainage and to prevent constrictive pericarditis.

Tuberculous pericarditis should be treated with antimicrobial agents (see Chap. 35, Extrapulmonary Tuberculosis). Glucosteroids, (*e.g.,* in dosages of 80 mg/day decreasing gradually to cessation of treatment in 6–8 weeks) appear to have a beneficial effect in reducing inflammation and associated arrhythmias, effusions, and scarring. When medical therapy fails to control effusions, or effusive–constrictive pericarditis develops in the first few months of therapy, pericardiectomy may be indicated. Early on, the pericardium peels relatively easily from the myocardium, whereas later, when constrictive pericarditis is overt, the operation is more difficult and more hazardous.

Prevention

The enteroviruses that are the principal causes of pericarditis are immunologically diverse, and the infections are so sporadic that immunization is unlikely to be practical. The apparent increasing incidence of acute purulent bacterial and fungal pericarditis is related to increasing numbers of patients at high risk because of cardiac surgery or an immunocompromised state. Mortality from pericarditis in these situations may be reduced by an increased awareness of the early signs of pericarditis.

Remaining Problems

Most diagnoses of viral pericarditis are made on clinical grounds, indicating a need for more aggressive searches for etiologic agents. Use of glucosteroids and other anti-inflammatory agents in viral and bacterial pericarditis is still controversial. Additional animal-model and clinical studies are needed to understand the processes involved in the pathogenesis and healing of infectious pericarditis and the potential role of anti-inflammatory agents in therapy.

Bibliography

Books

HURST JW, LOGUE RB, RACKLEY CE, SCHLANT RE, SONNENBLICK EH, WALLACE AG, WENGER NK (eds): The Heart, Arteries and Veins. 5th ed. New York, McGraw–Hill, 1982. pp 1363–1393.

SPODICK DH ed: Pericardial Diseases. Philadelphia, FA Davis, 1976. 297 pp.

Journals

AGNER RC, GALLIS HA: Pericarditis. Differential diagnostic considerations. Arch Intern Med 139:407–412, 1979

CHANDRARATNA AAN, ARONOW WS: Echocardiographic evaluation of pericardial disease. Compr Ther 5:55–63, 1979

CULLIFORD AT, LIPTON M, SPENCER FC: Operation for chronic constrictive pericarditis: Do the surgical approach and degree of pericardial resection influence the outcome significantly? Ann Thorac Surg 29:146–152, 1980

FELDMAN WE: Bacterial etiology and mortality of purulent pericarditis in pediatric patients. Am J Dis Child 133:641–644, 1979

FOWLER NO: Diseases of the pericardium. Curr Probl Cardiol 2:6–38, 1978

GABRIEL L, SHELBOURNE JC: "Acute" granulomatous pericarditis: A clinical and hemodynamic correlate. Chest 71:473–478, 1977

GOULD K, BARNETT JA, SANFORD JP: Purulent pericarditis in the antibiotic era. Arch Intern Med 134:923–927, 1974

HAGEMAN JH, D'ESOPO ND, GLENN WWL: Tuberculosis of the pericardium. N Engl J Med 270:327–332, 1964

KLACSMANN PG, BULKLEY B, HUTCHINS GM: The changed spectrum of purulent pericarditis: An 86 year autopsy experience in 200 patients. Am J Med 63:666–673, 1977

KRIKORIAN JG, HANCOCK EW: Pericardiocentesis. Am J Med 65:808–814, 1978

MANN T, BRODIE BR, GROSSMAN W, MCLAURIN R: Effusive-constrictive hemodynamic pattern due to neoplastic involvement of the pericardium. Am J Cardiol 41:781–786, 1978

MCGREGOR M: Pulsus paradoxus. N Engl J Med 301:480–482, 1979

MONTGOMERIE JZ, LEWIS AJ, FIALA M, LOCKS MO, YOSHIKAWA TT, TURNER JA: Pericarditis: Teaching conference, University of California, Los Angeles and Harbor General Hospital, Torrance (specialty conference). West J Med 122:295–309, 1975

ORTBALS DW, AVIOLI LV: Tuberculous pericarditis. Arch Intern Med 139:231–234, 1979

PONKA A: Carditis associated with *Mycoplasma pneumoniae* infection. Acta Med Scand 206:77–86, 1979

RUBIN RH, MOELLERING RC: Clinical, microbiologic and therapeutic aspects of purulent pericarditis. Am J Med 59:68–77, 1975

SHABETAI R: The pericardium: An essay on some recent developments. Am J Cardiol 42:1036–1043, 1978

SPODICK DH: Acoustic phenomena in pericardial disease. Am Heart J 81:114–124, 1971

TAN JC, HOLMES JC, FOWLER NO, MANSTSAS GT, PHAIR JP: Antibiotic levels in pericardial fluid. J Clin Invest 53:7–12, 1974

CHARLES B. SMITH

Myocarditis

133

Myocarditis—defined pathologically inflammation of the heart—is associated with a clinical spectrum that varies from asymptomatic to rapidly progressive myocardial failure. All kinds of infectious agents may be associated with myocarditis, and mechanisms for pathogenesis include direct toxicity of infectious agents for myocardial cells, indirect toxicity mediated by circulating microbial toxins, and inflammation secondary to infection-induced autoimmune phenomena.

Etiology

Although myocarditis has been reported to be caused by almost every kind of infectious agent, data substantiating the diagnosis of myocarditis or the associated infection have occasionally been tenuous. In particular, a diagnosis of myocarditis based entirely on nonspecific electrocardiographic S-T segment and T-wave changes is suspect because other abnormalities associated with infection such as fever, hypoxia, and electrolyte abnormalities may alter the electrocardiogram (ECG). Diagnosis of an associated infection that is based on a single elevated serum antibody titer should also be interpreted with caution. Conversely, pathological demonstration of myocardial necrosis and isolation of the infectious agent from the lesion clearly establishes the association. A comprehensive list of infectious agents reported to be associated with myocarditis is given in the list below. In the following discussion, emphasis will be placed on the infectious agents that are common and well documented causes of myocarditis.

Viruses are the most important infectious causes of myocarditis. Coxsackie B viruses (see Chap. 149, Coxsackievirus and Echovirus Infections) have been commonly associated with myocarditis, and other picornaviruses including Coxsackie A, ECHO, and polio viruses are also important etiologic agents. These viruses have all been isolated from inflammed myocardium, and laboratory studies indicate a particular tropism of some of the picornaviruses for myocardial cells. Influenza viruses are important causes of myocarditis, whereas other respiratory viruses appear to be rare causes. Several common viruses may occasionally cause myocarditis: EB virus (Chap. 137, Infectious Mononucleosis), the hepatitis viruses (Chap. 70, Hepatitis A; Chap. 71, Hepatitis B; Chap. 72, Non-A, Non-B Hepatitis), mumps (Chap. 74, Mumps), rubella (Chap. 87, Rubella), and cytomegalovirus (Chap. 75, Cytomegalovirus Infection). The fetal heart appears to be particularly susceptible to damage from rubella virus, and fetal mumps infection has been associated with endocardial fibroelastosis.

It is important to recognize that *Chlamydia psittaci* and *Mycoplasma pneumoniae* infections may be associated with myocarditis. Although these infections are typically manifest as nonbacterial pneumonias (Chap. 30, Nonbacterial Pneumonias), the causative agents are susceptible to antimicrobics and specific therapy may be helpful.

INFECTIOUS AGENTS OF MYOCARDITIS

Viral
- Enteroviruses (coxsackie, ECHO, polio)

Influenza A and B
- Mumps
- Rubella
- Rubeola
- Varicella-zoster
- Herpes simplex
- Epstein–Barr virus
- Cytomegalovirus
- Hepatitis viruses
- Vaccinia
- Rabies
- Adenoviruses

Lymphocytic choriomeningitis
Yellow fever
Dengue
Lassa virus
Chlamydial
Chlamydia psittaci
Rickettsial
Rickettsia tsutsugamushi
Rickettsia prowazekii
Rickettsia rickettsii
Coxiella burnetii
Mycoplasmal
Mycoplasma pneumoniae
Spirochetal
Leptospira interrogans
Treponema pallidum
Borrelia recurrentis
Bacterial
Corynebacterium diptheriae (toxinogenic strains)
Streptococcus pyogenes (group A)
Neisseria meningitidis et *gonorrhoeae*
Staphylococcus aureus
Streptoccocus pneumoniae
Haemophilus influenzae
Salmonella typhi; other *Salmonella* spp.
Pseudomonas pseudomallei
Brucella spp.
Clostridium perfringens
Yersinia spp.
Mycobacterium tuberculosis
Actinomyces israelii
Fungal
Coccidioides immitis
Histoplasma capsulatum
Blastomyces dermatitidis
Sporothrix schenckii
Candida spp.
Cryptococcus neoformans
Aspergillus spp.
Protozoal
Trypanosoma cruzi
Trypanosoma rhodesiense et *gambiense*
Toxoplasma gondii
Plasmodium spp.
Leishmania donovani
Balantidium coli
Naegleria spp.
Metazoal
Shistosoma spp.
Trichinella spiralis
Echinococcus granulosus
Loa loa
Strongyloides stercoralis
Paragonimus westermani
Taenia solium (cysts)
Ascaris lumbricoides
Toxocara canis et *cati*
Unclassified
Lyme disease agent
Whipples disease

The rickettsias attack vascular endothelial cells, and myocarditis is seen commonly in scrub typhus (Chap. 99, Scrub Typhus), and occasionally in Rocky Mountain spotted fever (Chap. 96, Spotted Fevers) and Q fever (Chap. 30, Nonbacterial Pneumonias). Myocarditis occurs in approximately 10% of patients with the newly described Lyme disease. Although no etiologic agent has been identified, the disease is tick transmitted and patients appear to respond to treatment with penicillin or tetracycline.

Diphtheria (Chap. 25, Diphtheria) is the best example of bacterial toxin-induced myocarditis. Cardiac involvement is a common complication, and myocardial failure is the major cause of death. The myocarditis of rheumatic fever, which follows group A streptococcal infections (Chap. 24, Streptococcal Diseases) is also indirect, occurring secondary to infection-induced autoimmunity directed at myocardial antigens (Chap. 5, Immunopathology of Infectious Diseases).

Acute myocarditis and myocardial diseases may occur in association with bacteremias caused by *Neisseria meningitidis* (Chap. 119, Bacterial Meningitis), *Staphylococcus aureus* (Chap. 100, Staphylococcal Skin Infections), *Salmonella* spp. (Chap. 63, Nontyphoidal Salmonelloses; Chap 64, Typhoid Fever), *Clostridium perfringens* (Chap. 156, Gas Gangrene), and other bacterial pathogens. Staphylococcal endocarditis is particularly likely to be associated with metastatic myocardial abscesses. The myocardium as well as the pericardium may be involved in patients with miliary tuberculosis (Chap. 34, Pulmonary Tuberculosis).

Disseminated fungal infections may be associated with diffuse miliary lesions or focal myocardial abscesses. Primary pathogens such as *Coccidioides immitis* (Chap. 41, Coccidioidomycosis) and *Histoplasma capsulatum* (Chap. 40, Histoplasmosis) may cause myocarditis, as may opportunistic fungi such as *Aspergillus* spp. (Chap. 44, Aspergillosis) and *Candida* spp. (Chap. 39, Candidosis).

In endemic areas *Trypanasoma cruzi* is an important protozoal cause of myocarditis (Chap. 136,

American Trypanosomiasis). Other blood-borne protozoa such as *Leishmania* spp. (Chap. 147, Leishmaniasis) and *Plasmodium* spp. (Chap. 145, Malaria) are less commonly associated with myocarditis. *Toxoplasma gondii* (Chap. 129, Toxoplasmosis) may cause myocarditis in both the congenital and acquired forms and is probably one of the most underdiagnosed protozoal causes of myocarditis in the United States.

Among helminthic infections, trichinosis (Chap. 150, Trichinosis) is most commonly associated with a myocarditis that is the major cause of fatalities. Other metazoal causes of myocarditis include schistosomiosis (Chap. 81, Schistosomiasis), echinococcosis (Chap. 78, Larval Cestodiasis) and visceral larval migrans (Chap. 78, Visceral Larva Migrans).

Epidemiology

In the United States, coxsackie and other enteroviruses are the leading causes of myocarditis. Rheumatic carditis continues to be a problem, particularly in underdeveloped countries. Chagas' disease is the major cause of myocarditis and heart disease in general in Central and South America.

The incidence of myocarditis in young adults examined at autopsy after accidental deaths ranges from 2% to 5%. Presumably the myocarditis was asymptomatic in most of these persons. In a different population—children who died of sudden, unexpected, nonaccidental causes—myocarditis was detected at autopsy in 15% to 20%; the myocarditis was a major cause of mortality. Except for occasional studies in which coxsackie viral antigens were detected in the myocardium, the assumption that pathological changes were viral in origin has been poorly defended.

Studies of the incidence of cardiac involvement in patients with viral infections have yielded rates of 20% to 30% as judged by nonspecific electrocardiographic abnormalities; rates are much lower when clinical evidence of myocardial damage is required for the diagnosis. Using strict criteria for diagnosis, myocarditis was present in 5% to 10% of persons infected with Group B coxsackievirus.

Studies of Group B coxsackieviral myocarditis in humans and in murine models have elucidated several host factors that predispose to myocarditis. Myocardial involvement is particularly common during the first year of life, uncommon during childhood, and common during adolescence and later life. Males of adolescent age or older appear to have greater susceptibility than females to cardiac involvement, with the exception that pregnancy may also be a risk factor. In mice, the severity of myocardial involvement is increased by exercise, malnutrition, and glucosteroids.

Pathogenesis and Pathology

Pathological changes in myocarditis vary with the nature of the infecting agent and with the mechanisms of pathogenesis. Diphtherial toxin inhibits cellular protein synthesis; it is directly toxic to myocardial cells and to the conducting system producing necrosis and secondary inflammatory infiltrates. Group A streptococci may be directly toxic for the heart during septicemic infections producing perivascular infiltrates and focal necrosis, whereas in post-streptococcal rheumatic fever, pericarditis with characteristic Aschoff lesions is apparently the product of infection-induced immune reaction to cardiac antigens (Chap. 5, Immunopathology of Infectious Diseases; Chap. 24, Streptococcal Diseases).

Most pathogens that cause myocarditis during septicemic infections are directly toxic to the myocardium and cause lesions that are similar to those found in other organs. Staphylococci may cause miliary microabscesses or single large abscesses in the myocardium. *Mycobacterium tuberculosis* may invade the heart directly from adjacent nodes or may seed the heart in a miliary pattern during lymphohematogenous dissemination; miliary or large nodular granulomas may result. A similar picture is seen when disseminated histoplasmosis or coccidioidomycosis involve the heart. Aspergillosis causes focal infarctions as the fungus invades through blood vessels. Rickettsias are associated with focal panvasculitis in the heart, which is similar to that seen in other organs.

Trypanosoma cruzi appear to have a particular tropism for the heart. In the acute phase, protozoa are found in myocardial cells in association with necrosis and inflammatory reactions. In the chronic phase of Chagas' disease there is extensive myocardial fibrosis and chronic inflammation, which is thought to be secondary to both humoral and cell-mediated immune reactions directed against the heart.

Pathologic changes associated with viral myocarditis are similar for most viruses. Necrosis of myofibers is seen initially, and this may be either patchy of diffuse. An acute inflammatory reaction with polymorphonuclear leukocytes may be seen during the first few days of infection, and this is promptly followed by a mononuclear cellular infiltrate by the end of the first week. Late changes include fibrosis and loss of myofibers.

Group B coxsackieviral myocarditis in mice resembles myocarditis in humans in many ways and has been used to study pathogenesis. Myocardial cell damage appears to occur in several ways. The Group B coxsackieviruses have a particular tropism for myofibers, and damage in the acute phase of the illness is probably the result of direct viral damage to myocardial cells. Inhibition of humoral and macrophage-mediated immunity early in the course of infection leads to more severe acute disease. However, the immune response may contribute to the pathogenesis of late changes in viral myocarditis. Depletion of T-cells capable of lysing virus-infected myofibers reduces the severity of myocarditis, and there is evidence that natural killer cells may be activated by viral infection to attack normal myofibers. Some investigators have suggested that chronic cardiomyopathies and valvulitis may be late sequelae of acute viral myocarditis.

Manifestations

The manifestations of myocarditis can be divided into those that relate to the general manifestations of the disease caused by the particular infectious agent and to specific manifestations attributable to cardiac involvement.

Typically, myocarditis results from infection with coxsackieviruses or other enteroviruses. In infants and young children, these infections are more fulminant, beginning with fever, tachycardia, and listlessness, progressing rapidly with signs and symptoms of central nervous system, gastrointestinal–hepatic, and myocardial involvement. Cardiac failure may be evident within a few days of onset of the illness.

In older children and adults, the illness usually progresses more slowly. Initially, general manifestations of the viral infection may be localized to the respiratory tract with moderate fever, coryza, and cough or to the abdomen with pain, nausea, and vomiting. Myocardial involvement often becomes manifest 1 or 2 weeks after the initial illness with fever, malaise, fatigue, dyspnea, and palpitations. An early clue to myocardial involvement is a tachycardia that is out of proportion to the height of the fever and general state of toxicity. At this stage the heart sounds may be muffled, and transient pericardial rubs may be heard. Chest pain is common in symptomatic myocarditis and may be pleural–pericardial, indicating an associated pericarditis, or ischemic, indicating myocardial damage. In more advanced cases, myocardial involvement is overt and associated with tachyarrhythmias or signs of heart failure including cardiomegaly, diastolic gallop rhythms, murmurs of mitral regurgitation, pulsus alternans, distended neck veins, edema, and pulmonary congestion.

The most common electrocardiographic changes in myocarditis are nonspecific S-T and T-wave changes. These may also be the result of infection-related anoxia, fever, or metabolic abnormalities and do not substantiate the diagnosis of myocarditis. Occasionally the appearance of Q waves and other changes indicating myocardial damage may appear. More nearly diagnostic are the appearance of new atrial or ventricular arrhythmias and conduction defects. Arrhythmias are presumed to be the etiology of the sudden death that occasionally results from myocarditis.

Laboratory abnormalities in patients with myocarditis include elevations in sedimentation rate and leukocyte count secondary to the inflammatory process. Elevations in specific myocardial isoenzymes may be helpful in documenting myocardial damage. Radiographic findings of cardiomegaly or pulmonary congestion may be the first signs of cardiac involvement.

Diagnosis

The clinician must answer three questions in evaluating myocarditis: (1) does the patient have myocarditis; (2) is the myocarditis infectious or noninfectious; (3) if infectious, what is the etiology?

The diagnosis of myocarditis is poorly substantiated in the patient who has only nonspecific S-T and T wave changes and tachycardia; it is obvious in a young person who develops progressive arrhythmias, conduction defects, and myocardial failure following a viral illness. In doubtful cases, newer noninvasive techniques such as echocardiography may be helpful in demonstrating ventricular enlargement without pericardial effusions and valvular abnormalities. Radionuclide myocardial imaging may reveal a focal area of necrosis suggestive of myocardial abscess, or more diffuse myocardial damage suggestive of viral myocarditis. ^{111}In-labeled leukocyte scans may be useful in locating an acute inflammatory reaction in the myocardium of patients with early bacterial myocarditis.

A very large number of noninfectious diseases and agents may damage the heart and produce a clinical picture similar to infectious myocarditis. These include inflammatory diseases such as systemic lupus erythematosus, vasculitis, and thrombotic thrombocytopenic purpura; infiltrative neoplastic diseases; toxins such as alcohol and other hydrocarbons; heavy metals; directly toxic therapeutic agents such as emetine and chloroquine; hypersensitivity reactions to drugs such as sulfonamides and tetracyclines; and physical agents including heat, cold, and radiation.

Often the evidence that the myocarditis is infectious in etiology is a strongly compatible clinical history; affirmation of an appropriate infection by isolation of an infectious agent or serologic data is helpful. When pericarditis with effusion is also present, pericardiocentesis may provide material that yields the etiologic infectious agent. Myocardial tissue may be obtained by venous catheter and transthoracic needle biopsy techniques. These procedures may be justified in the occasional patient with progressive myocarditis who has clinical evidence of a potentially treatable infectious etiology.

Prognosis

Viral myocarditis is typically a benign illness with only transient electrocardiographic changes. Even symptomatic viral myocarditis usually responds to a few weeks of bed rest. Because infants and young children are more likely to develop rapidly progressive cardiac failure, acute mortality is most common in this group. Occasionally, as a result of the propensity for involvement of the conduction system in viral myocarditis, patients with mild disease die suddenly of arrhythmias.

There are well-documented instances of patients with coxsackieviral myocarditis whose illness progressed slowly over periods of several months and eventually led to death. It is likely that some cases of so-called congestive cardiomyopathy may be the result of coxsackieviral infection.

On the other hand, the etiologies of most cases of congestive cardiomyopathy have not been established. Similarly, reports that Group B coxsackieviral myocarditis may induce valvular damage resembling rheumatic valvulitis are anecdotal.

Therapy

The treatment of bacterial, fungal, and protozoal myocarditis should be directed at the specific infectious agents. *Mycoplasma pneumoniae,* Q fever, and psittacosis may be associated with a viruslike myocarditis that should be treated with appropriate antimicrobics. To date, no antiviral drugs are effective against coxsackieviruses and other enteroviruses. Amantidine should be tried in acute influenza viral myocarditis.

Bed rest during the symptomatic stages of myocarditis continues to be an important part of therapy. Although its effectiveness has not been proven in controlled clinical trials, anecdotes have associated exacerbations and sudden worsening of failure with exercise early in the course of the illness. The best justification for bed rest is that studies of murine Group B coxsackieviral myocarditis clearly indicate that exercise or anoxia increase myocardial damage and mortality. Other supportive therapy should include maintenance of adequate ventilation and oxygenation and avoidance of fluid overload. Because of the frequency of arrhythmias and the potential for cardiac arrest, patients should be hospitalized and monitored during the active phase of illness. The pharmacologic methods for control of arrhythmias and failure are similar to those used in other cardiac diseases. Some patients may exhibit unusual sensitivity to the toxic effects of digitalis. Anti-coagulants are sometimes recommended because the damaged endocardium is more susceptible to the formation of thrombi, and the combination of failure plus bed rest increases the chances of peripheral venous thrombosis. Anticoagulants should probably be avoided in patients with concomitant acute pericarditis because of the increased risk of pericardial bleeding.

Glucosteroids administered during the acute phase of viral myocarditis have been associated with rapid clinical deterioration, and their deleterious effect has been clearly demonstrated during the acute phase of coxsackieviral myocarditis in mice. In nonhuman animals, it appears that immune mechanisms may be involved in the pathogenesis of the late myocardial cell damage of coxsackieviral myocarditis; however, because of the relative lack of understanding of the role and timing of immune pathogenic mechanisms in human disease, glucosteroids or other immunosuppressive therapy should be avoided in patients with viral myocarditis.

Prevention

Control of the major viruses that cause myocarditis awaits the development of antiviral-immunologic methods for the prevention of enteroviral infections. Diphtherial myocarditis can be prevented by maintenance of active immunity. Public health measures are critical to the control of rheumatic myocarditis, tuberculous myocarditis, trichinosis, and protozoal myocarditides.

Remaining Problems

Studies of Group B coxsackieviral myocarditis should continue to enhance our understanding of the role of viral, host, and immune factors in the pathogenesis of this disease and may lead to more effective therapy. The potential roles of interferon and other antiviral agents for treatment of viral myocarditis need to be studied in both nonhuman and human animals. Perhaps the greatest potential for important advances in this area is in more aggressive epidemiologic and etiologic studies of the role of viruses in the pathogenesis of coronary artery disease, chronic valvulitis, and the congestive cardiomyopathies.

Bibliography

Books

ABLEMANN WH: Clinical aspects of viral cardiomyopathy in myocardial diseases. In Fowler NO et al (eds): Myocardial Diseases. New York, Grune & Stratton, 1973. pp 253–279.

WYNNE J, BRAUNWALD E: The cardiomyopathies and myocarditides. In Braunwald E (ed): Heart Disease: A Textbook of Cardiovascular Medicine. Philadelphia, WB Saunders, 1980. pp 1437–1500.

Journals

LEVINE HP: Virus myocarditis: A critique of the literature from clinical, electrocardiographic and pathologic standpoints. Am J Med Sci 277:132–143, 1979

WALSH TJ, HUTCHINS GM, BULKLEY BH, MENDELSOHN G: Fungal infections of the heart: Analysis of 51 autopsy cases. Am J Cardiol 45:357–366, 1980

WENGER NK: Infectious myocarditis. Cardiovascular Clinics 4:168–185, 1972

WOODRUFF JF: Viral myocarditis. Am J Path 101:426–479, 1980

PAUL D. HOEPRICH
DAVID T. DURACK

Infective Endocarditis

134

Microorganisms can cause endocarditis in two ways: directly, by actually colonizing the endocardium, and indirectly, by inducing hypersensitivity, as in acute rheumatic fever (Chap. 24, Streptococcal Diseases). This chapter is limited to *infective endocarditis,* which is caused by microorganisms physically present in endocardial lesions known as vegetations. *Infective endarteritis,* such as may occur with a patent ductus arteriosus, is a condition very similar to infective endocarditis except in the location of vegetations.

Disease with an abrupt onset and short course (2 to 4 weeks or less before therapy) is termed *acute endocarditis.* Disease that begins insidiously and progresses over weeks and months is known as subacute or chronic endocarditis. These common terms imply more than simply the duration of illness. Acute endocarditis is usually caused by virulent, pyogenic bacteria, such as *Staphylococcus aureus,* whereas subacute or chronic disease is generally caused by relatively avirulent bacteria such as viridans group *Streptococcus* spp. Previously normal intracardiac surfaces may be invaded and severely damaged by acute endocarditis; the chronic form usually involves previously abnormal hearts. Acute endocarditis often follows seeding of the bloodstream by bacteria from an evident source, such as septic thrombophlebitis in a drug addict. Emboli arising from the vegetations of acute endocarditis are more likely to give rise to metastatic suppurative complications. Bacteriologic cure is easier to achieve in the subacute form of the disease; even with modern antimicrobics, the prognosis is worse for many forms of acute endocarditis.

Intermediate clinical forms of infective endocarditis are common, and the course of the disease is usually altered by specific chemotherapy. Therefore, the general designation infective endocarditis is frequently appropriate. The terms native valve endocarditis (NVE) and prosthetic valve endocarditis (PVE) are self-explanatory. To make the terminology more specific, the name of the etiologic agent should be given whenever it is known—for example, acute infective endocarditis caused by *Staphylococcus aureus,* or chronic prosthetic valve endocarditis caused by *Candida albicans.*

Etiology

Most of the bacteria and many of the fungi associated with human disease have been found to cause infective endocarditis on occasion. However, only a few species account for the great majority of cases. For example, streptococci and staphylococci together cause about four out of every five cases of NVE. The approximate frequencies with which various organisms cause endocarditis on native valves, on prosthetic valves, and in IV drug abusers are listed in Table 134-1.

Invasive, pathogenic bacteria may spread from a site of primary infection—for example, *Streptococcus pneumoniae* from lobar pneumonia—to the bloodstream and then colonize apparently normal heart valves. The widespread use of effective antibacterial agents for the treatment of common primary infections such as pneumonia and gonorrhea has significantly decreased the frequency of endocarditis caused by *S. pneumoniae* and *Neisseria gonorrhoeae.*

Relatively avirulent microorganisms derived from the normal flora of the body cause most cases of infective endocarditis. They gain access to the blood intermittently, apparently as a result of minor trauma to the mucosa of the oropharynx, gastrointestinal tract, or genitourinary tract. Such transient bacteremias usually occur without ill effects, but occasionally they lead to endocarditis or endarteritis in patients with an underlying cardiovascular lesion. Thus viridans group streptococci originating from the mouth flora constitute the most frequent cause of chronic bacterial endocarditis. Group D streptococci, which normally inhabit the bowel, cause 5% to 25% of cases. Almost half such isolates are nonenterococcal group D streptococci (primarily *Streptococcus bovis,* rarely *Streptococcus equinus*) which are usually fully susceptible to penicillin, whereas the enterococcal group D species (*Streptococcus faecalis, Streptococcus faecium* and *Streptococcus durans*) are resistant to penicillin.

Notably, bacterial endocarditis seldom follows the common bacteremias caused by aerobic gram-negative bacilli. For example, *Escherichia coli* rarely causes native valve endocarditis, and even prosthetic valve infection with this frequent cause of bacteremia is uncommon. It may be relevant to note that many kinds of gram-negative bacteria are susceptible to lysis by complement in the presence of specific antibody, whereas all gram-positive bacteria are resistant. For *Haemophilus* and *Brucella* spp., the disparity between the frequency of bacteremia and the rarity of endocarditis is less marked than for the enteric gram-negative bacilli.

Epidemiology

Infective endocarditis is relatively uncommon. The overall incidence of this disease in the United States is estimated to be about two cases per year per 100,000 population. Thus a physician in general practice might see only one patient with infective endocarditis in 5 to 10 years. The advent of effective therapy for other bacterial infections has caused a decrease in the frequency of some forms of bacterial endocarditis, whereas other therapeutic advances such as cardiovascular surgery have been associated with an increase in cases caused by gram-negative bacilli, fungi, and other previously unusual causes of endocarditis.

The etiologic agents of infective endocarditis are commonly drawn from the patient's resident microbiota. Hence, the association of viridans group *Streptococcus* spp. with dental manipulations and oropharyngeal surgery and of group D streptococci with procedures involving the urinary tract. Over one-half of the cases of infective endocarditis that complicate the IV self-administration drugs are caused by *Staphylococcus aureus;* the patients generally carry on their skin staphylococci of the same phage type that is responsible for their endocarditis.

There are striking geographic differences in the epidemiology of infective endocarditis, which may relate to regional variations in the frequency of predisposing cardiac diseases or to the size of the local population of drug addicts. Thus, if chronic rheumatic valvular heart disease is prevalent in a given area, infective endocarditis will be correspondingly common. Over the past 30 years, there has been a striking decline in the frequency of acute rheumatic fever in the United States and in most other developed countries. Over the same period, infective endocarditis engrafted upon rheumatic valvular disease has become less frequent, especially in the younger age groups. Meanwhile, the incidence in the elderly has steadily increased and the disease is now common in persons over 60 years in age. The growing frequency in the aged may reflect the longer survival of persons with organic cardiovascular diseases. The ratio of males to females is about 2:1 overall, with the preponderance of males more marked among patients over 60 years.

Pathogenesis and Pathology

Infectious agents must enter the bloodstream before they can cause endocardial or endarterial infection. The great majority originate from the gastrointestinal tract, the genitourinary tract, or the skin. However, the actual portal of entry into the blood can be identified in only about 20% of patients with chronic infective endocarditis, and in about 50% of acute cases. Of persons who undergo dental manipulations and oropharyngeal or maxillofacial surgery, 10% to 80% have associated transient bacteremias, often with species of streptococci. Instrumentation of the urinary tract results in transient bacteremia (often with enterococci) in 10% to 40% of patients even without an active urinary tract infection. The pathogenetic importance of these transient bacteremias is attested by numerous case reports citing a history of trauma to the upper respiratory or urinary tracts preceding onset of endocarditis and a predominance of streptococci among the etiologic organisms.

Theoretically, blood-borne microorganisms might colonize the endocardium from the capillary vessels of the endothelium or from the blood within the endocardial lumen. The location of most of the inciting microorganisms in the periphery of the vegetations of infective endocarditis argues for direct deposition of microorganisms from intracardiac blood. In addition, the localization of infectious agents on valvular prostheses could only come about through implantation from the bloodstream.

The leading conditions predisposing to infective endocarditis include congenital, rheumatic, and degenerative cardiac diseases; previous endocarditis; and cardiac surgery. The relative frequency of these

Table 134-1. *Frequency of Various Microorganisms That Cause Infective Endocarditis**

	NVE (%)	IV Drug Abusers (%)	Early PVE (%)	Late PVE (%)
Streptococcus spp.	65	15	10	35
viridans, α-hemolytic	35	5	<5	25
S. bovis (group D)	*15*	<5	<5	<5
S. fecalis (group D)	10	8	<5	<5
Other streptococci	<5	<5	<5	<5
Staphylococcus spp.	25	50	50	30
Coagulase-positive	23	50	20	10
Coagulase-negative	<5	<5	30	20
Gram-negative, aerobic bacilli	<5	15	20	15
Fungi	<5	5	10	5
Miscellaneous bacteria	<5	5	5	5
Diphtheroids, *Propionibacterium* spp.	<1	<5	5	<5
Other anaerobes	<1	<1	<1	<1
Coxiella burnetii	<1	<1	<1	<1
Chlamydia spp.	<1	<1	<1	<1
Polymicrobial infection	<1	5	5	5
Culture-negative endocarditis	5–10	5	<5	<5

*These are representative figures collated from several reports; wide local variations in frequency are to be expected.

(Hurst JW, Logue RB, Rackley CE, Schlant RC, Sonnenblick EH, Wallace AG, Wenger NK (eds): The Heart, Arteries, and Veins, 5th ed. New York, McGraw–Hill, 1982)

Table 134-2. *Approximate Frequency of the Major Preexisting Cardiac Lesions in Patients With Infective Endocarditis*

	Children Under 2 Years (%)	Children 2–15 Years (%)	Adults 15–50 Years (%)	Adults >50 Years (%)	Adults IV Drug Abusers (%)
No known heart disease	50–70	10–15	10–20	10	50–60
Congenital heart disease	30–50	70–80	20–30	10–20	10
Rheumatic heart disease	Rare	10–20	30–40	20–30	10
Degenerative heart disease	0	0	Rare	10–20	Rare
Previous cardiac surgery	5	10–15	10–20	10–20	10–20
Previous endocarditis	Rare	5	5	5–10	10–20

(Hurst JW, Logue RB, Rackley CE, Schlant RC, Sonnenblick EH, Wallace AG, Wenger NK (eds): The Heart, Arteries, and Veins, 5th ed. New York, McGraw–Hill, 1982)

Table 134-3. *Approximate Frequency of Anatomic Location of Vegetations in Subacute or Chronic, Acute, and IV Drug-Abuse-Associated Infective Endocarditis*

	Subacute or Chronic (%)	Acute (%)	IV Drug Abusers (%)
Left-sided valves	85	65	40
Aortic	15–26	18–25	25–30
Mitral	38–45	30–35	15–20
Aortic and mitral	23–30	15–20	13–20
Right-sided valves	5	20	50
Tricuspid	1–5	15	45–55
Pulmonary	1	Rare	2
Tricuspid and pulmonary	Rare	Rare	3
Left- and right-sided sites	Rare	5–10	5–10
Other sites (patent ductus, VSD, coarctation, jet lesions)	10	5	5

(Hurst JW, Logue RB, Rackley CE, Schlant RC, Sonnenblick EH, Wallace AG, Wenger NK (eds): The Heart, Arteries, and Veins, 5th ed. New York, McGraw–Hill, 1982)

broad categories among patients with infective endocarditis varies widely according to the age of onset (Table 134-2). However, some patients have no known heart disease before they develop infective endocarditis, especially IV drug abusers and infants. Most cases of endocarditis in children are associated with congenital heart disease.

Arranged in order of descending frequency, the anatomic sites at which valvular vegetations develop are mitral, aortic, combined mitral and aortic, tricuspid, and pulmonic (Table 134-3). This sequence correlates both with the leading sites of damage in rheumatic valvulitis and with the resting pressure and the magnitude of the pressure differential across each valve. The latter presumably determines the degree of stress and trauma borne by each of the valves during the cardiac cycle. When an IV drug user develops endocarditis, it is likely to involve the right side of the heart. Possible reasons include an unusually high inoculum of organisms passing through the heart as a bolus before dispersion in the vessels of the lung, and prior damage to the endothelium of the tricuspid valve by adulterated drugs containing impurities and particles.

Estimates of the relative risks for endocarditis incurred by various cardiac abnormalities are given in Table 134-4. Important congenital lesions include bicuspid aortic valve, ductus arteriosus, coarctation of the aorta, and pulmonary stenosis. Infective endocarditis rarely complicates atrial septal defects but is common with ventricular septal defects. Cyanotic congenital heart disease poses a relatively high risk, as do valvular prostheses. Since syphilitic cardiovascular disease is now uncommon, it rarely underlies infective endocarditis. Prolapsing mitral valves are now known to predispose to endocarditis; previously, rheumatic valvular disease would have been implicated in such patients.

With all such lesions, the vegetations usually form downstream. Even in patients presumed to have no abnormality of the heart valves before onset of infection and in patients with nonvalvular endocarditis (ventricular septal defects) or endarteritis (ductus arteriosus, coarctation of the aorta), the vegetations are found on the downstream side of the affected valves or underlying lesions. The rheologic mechanism involved is presumed to be the pressure changes across these anatomic structures, which cause turbulent blood flow and eddy currents. These abet localization of bacteria on the endothelium on the low pressure side of the system.

Preexisting endothelial damage leads to formation of small aggregates of platelets and fibrin known as nonbacterial thrombotic endocarditis (NBTE). Some of these sterile lesions grow large enough to form visible vegetations. Whether large or small, NBTE presents a sticky platelet–fibrin surface to which some organisms, especially streptococci and staphylococci, readily adhere. It is believed that NBTE is the predisposing lesion for most cases of chronic endocarditis. Whether NBTE plays a role in onset of acute endocarditis is uncertain. Sites where abnormal jets of blood strike the endothelium and damage it, as in the pulmonary artery when the ductus arteriosus is patent, are called jet lesions. These are also susceptible to infection.

The essential lesion of infective endocarditis is the vegetation (Fig. 134-1). Vegetations vary greatly in size, from tiny nubbins to masses large enough to occlude valve orifices. Often, they are rather soft and

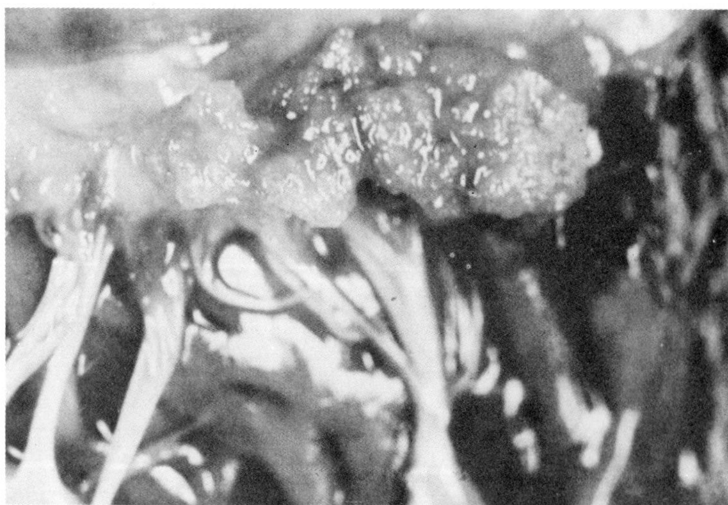

Fig. 134-1. Vegetations on the mitral valve. Acute bacterial endocarditis caused by *Staphylococcus aureus* in a 44-year-old woman; 12 days elapsed from clinical onset of illness to death. (Unstained, original magnification approximately × 3.5)

Table 134-4. *Estimates of the Relative Risk for Infective Endocarditis Posed by Various Cardiac Lesions*

Relatively High Risk	Intermediate Risk	Very Low or Negligible Risk
Prosthetic heart valves	Mitral valve prolapse	Atrial septal defects
Aortic valve disease	Pure mitral stenosis	Arteriosclerotic plaques
Mitral insufficiency	Tricuspid valve disease	Coronary artery disease
Patent ductus arteriosus	Pulmonary valve disease	Syphilitic aortitis
Ventricular septal defect	Previous infective endocarditis	Cardiac pacemakers
Coarctation of the aorta	Asymmetric septal hypertrophy	Surgically corrected cardiac lesions (without prosthetic implants, more than 6 months after operation)
Marfan's syndrome	Calcific aortic sclerosis	
Cyanotic congenital heart disease	Hyperalimentation or pressure-monitoring lines that reach the right atrium	
	Nonvalvular intracardiac prosthetic implants	

(Hurst JW, Logue RB, Rackley CE, Schlant RC, Sonnenblick EH, Wallace AG, Wenger NK (eds): The Heart, Arteries, and Veins, 5th ed. New York, McGraw–Hill, 1982)

Table 134-5. *Summary of the Major Clinical Manifestations of Infective Endocarditis*

	History	Examination	Investigations
Manifestations of systemic infection	Fever, chills, rigors, sweats, malaise, weakness, lethargy, delirium, headache, anorexia, weight loss, backache, arthralgia, myalgia Portal of entry: Oral, skin Urinary tract Drug addiction Nosocomial bacteremia	Fever Pallor Weight loss Asthenia Splenomegaly	Anemia Leukocytosis (variable) Raised ESR Blood cultures positive Abnormal CSF
Manifestations of intravascular lesion	Dyspnea, chest pain, focal weakness, stroke, abdominal pain, cold, and painful extremities	Murmurs Signs of cardiac failure Petechiae—skin, eye, mucosae Roth spots, Osler's nodes Janeway lesions Splinter hemorrhages Stroke Mycotic aneurysm Ischemia or infarction of viscera or extremities	Blood in urine Chest roentgenogram Echocardiography Arteriography Liver-spleen scan Lung scan, brain scan, CT scan Histology, culture of emboli
Manifestations of immunologic reactions	Arthralgia, myalgia, tenosynovitis	Arthritis Signs of uremia Vascular phenomena Finger clubbing	Proteinuria, hematuria, casts, uremia, acidosis Polyclonal increases in gamma globulins Rheumatoid factor, decreased complement, and immune complexes in serum Antistaphylococcal teichoic acid antibodies

(Hurst JW, Logue RB, Rackley CE, Schlant RC, Sonnenblick EH, Wallace AG, Wenger NK (eds): The Heart, Arteries, and Veins, 5th ed. New York, McGraw–Hill, 1982)

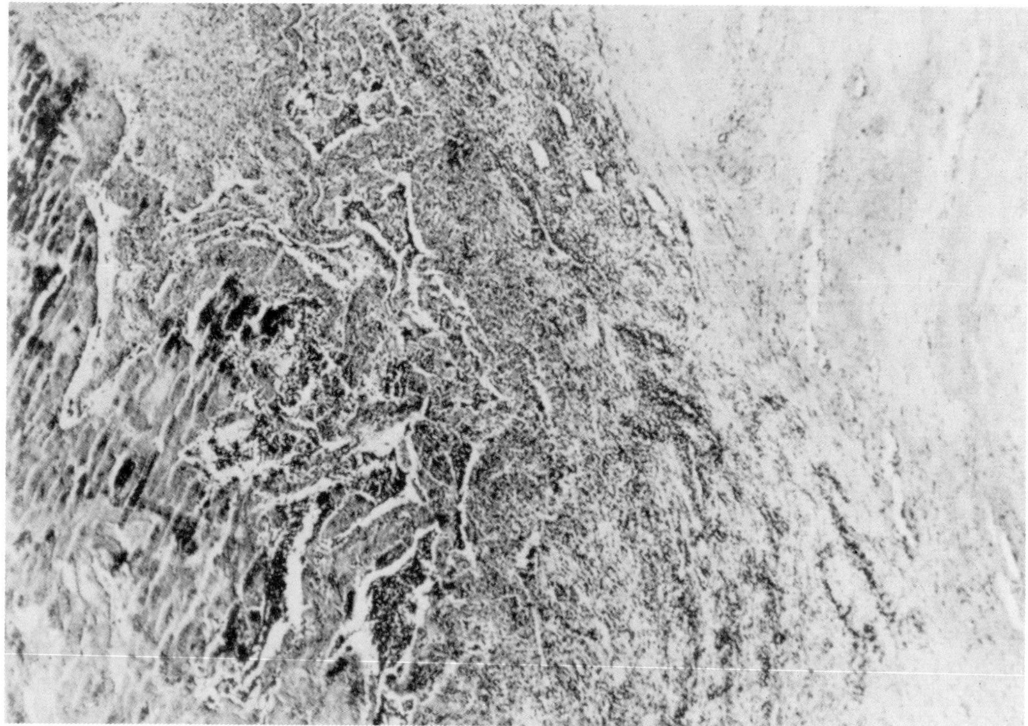

Fig. 134-2. Section through vegetation from a patient with chronic bacterial endocarditis caused by viridans group *Streptococcus* spp. The fibrotic mitral valve is at the right; a zone of granulation tissue and leukocytes abuts on the valve. Bacterial colonies lie under the fibrin covering on the left. (Original magnification approximately × 500) (Moore RA: J Lab Clin Med 3L:1279–1293, 1946)

friable, and only loosely attached to the valvular endothelium or to the endocardium. Thus, they break off easily to form arterial emboli. Fungal vegetations tend to be bulky, giving rise to large emboli. Apart from propensity to generate emboli, there is no reliable correlation between size of vegetations and severity or virulence of infective endocarditis.

The bulk of the vegetation is an amorphous mass of fibrin and platelets containing large colonies of microorganisms. There may or may not be a collection of inflammatory cells at the site of attachment of the vegetation to the endothelium—actual microabscesses in some acute cases. A layer of fibrin and platelets lies between these microorganisms and the circulating blood (Fig. 134-2).

There are four significant consequences to the anatomic nature of the vegetation. First, the sequestration of infecting microorganisms within the vegetation protects them from antibodies, complement, leukocytes, and other antibacterial factors in the blood. Second, in this sanctuary the organisms are often metabolically inactive, replicating at an unusually slow rate, rendering them relatively resistant to the action of many antimicrobics. Third, healing is slow because macrophages and fibroblasts must spread through the vegetation from its site of attachment, and endothelial cells must grow over the surface before organizaton is complete. Fourth, emboli are generated when bits of vegetation break off and are swept away by the passing bloodstream. Catastrophic infarctions may result, depending on the size and site of lodgment of these emboli. Numerous microemboli may be generated, causing nonspecific morbidity and distant manifestations such as petechiae in the kidneys, skin, and mucous membranes. Metastatic infection carried by emboli is uncommon, not because the emboli are sterile but because the microorganisms they bear are often of low virulence. Moreover, once lodged in a distant organ these organisms are exposed to the full onslaught of host defenses, which they had largely escaped while living in the vegetation.

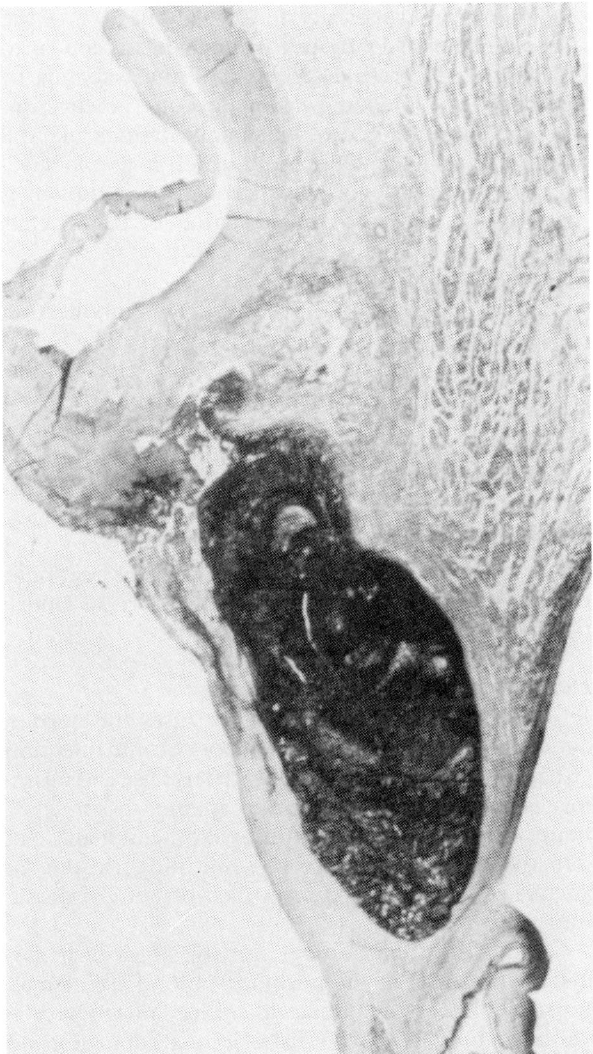

Fig. 134-3. Valve-ring abscess involving both aortic and mitral rings. The abscess has perforated the endocardium at the base of the aortic leaflet. (Phloxine-methylene blue, original magnification approximately × 6) (Sheldon WH, Golden A: Circulation 4:1–12, 1951)

Abscesses may develop by direct invasion of the valve rings of the heart near infected vegetations (Fig. 134-3). A development of ominous prognostic import, such abscesses occur most commonly during infections with the pyogenic cocci, and rarely with other microorganisms, unless a prosthetic valve is present. Thus, valve-ring abscesses have been demonstrated at necropsy in about half of the patients who die of acute bacterial endocarditis, and in a large majority of patients who die with prosthetic valve infections.

Manifestations

The manifestations of infective endocarditis are both numerous and diverse (Table 134-5). Many symptoms are the nonspecific results of a systemic infection: chills, fever, anemia, malaise, anorexia, asthenia, weight loss, myalgias, and arthralgias. The classic triad of fever, anemia, and murmur should always alert the physician to consider seriously the diagnosis of endocarditis.

Fever

Formerly, it was held that fever occurred in all patients with infective endocarditis. This is still generally true, but exceptions do occur; some patients are afebrile when first seen. Two temperature peaks within each 24-hour period are said to be characteristic of gonococcal endocarditis, which is now rare. Otherwise, there is no fever pattern that is characteristic of infective endocarditis.

Cardiac Manifestations

Any patient with a heart murmur indicating organic heart disease who develops a persistent fever must be suspected of having infective endocarditis. Of proven cases, virtually all have a murmur significant of pathology either at some time or throughout the course of the disease. However, up to 15% of patients lack a murmur *when first examined.* Change in the murmur has been overemphasized as a characteristic of infective endocarditis. Changing murmurs are most often related to variations in fever, anemia, position of patient, and respiration. However, the development of a *new* murmur, especially an aortic diastolic murmur, in any patient with a febrile illness, is a strong indication of infective endocarditis.

Preexisting, new, or worsening valvular damage, together with the stress of the infection, may lead to heart failure—the single most important complication of endocarditis. Although failure is not prominent among the initial manifestations of infective endocarditis, it may develop at any time during the course of the disease, even during or after successful treatment. However, the development of cardiac failure may indicate relapse or failure of treatment.

Embolic Manifestations

Multiple, clinically diverse manifestations result from emboli that originate from vegetations. The greater the duration of the disease without proper treatment, the more likely the occurrence of embolic manifestations. These emboli often contain bacteria, but they seldom cause metastatic infections, except in acute endocarditis caused by *Staphylococcus aureus.*

When extracardiac infections do occur, it is often impossible to tell whether they arose from the bacteremia or from septic emboli.

Embolic infarction of the spleen is quite common and is often announced by pain in the left upper quadrant of the abdomen. Local tenderness, left shoulder pain, left pleural effusion, and a friction rub, are additional manifestations.

Microemboli have been invoked in the pathogenesis of petechiae, splinter hemorrhages, Osler's nodes, and Janeway lesions. The characteristics of these lesions are summarized in Table 134-6. Although not specific for infective endocarditis, petechiae are common. They tend to appear in crops, often above the clavicles and on the lower neck, about the axillary skin folds, and at the beltline; other important sites where they are easy to detect are the conjunctivae and the oropharyngeal mucosa. Splinter hemorrhages—again nonspecific manifestations—are seen more often under the fingernails than under the toenails.

Osler's nodes are tender, reddish-purple pea-sized swellings that usually appear on the extremities, especially the pulp of the fingers. Although they are nearly pathognomonic of infective endocarditis, they are specific neither for the microorganism nor for the time course of the infection. The etiologic agent has sometimes been recovered by culture of aspirates of Osler's nodes; occasionally, they suppurate. Janeway lesions are small, reddish, macular lesions most frequently found on the palms and soles, suggesting an embolic rather than immunologic origin.

Clubbing of the fingers is now an uncommon manifestation of infective endocarditis. It is sometimes associated with the other features of hypertrophic pulmonary osteoarthropathy, and may occur in patients with infective endocarditis who do not have cardiac or pulmonary failure. Their pathogenesis is unclear.

Neurologic manifestations are extremely important in infective endocarditis. As initial signs of the disease, they may cause diagnostic confusion; also, they may determine morbidity and sequelae.

Acute staphylococcal endocarditis may cause a meningeal reaction with a moderate number of polymorphonuclear leukocytes and slightly increased protein in the cerebrospinal fluid (CSF), but normal glucose and negative cultures. Less commonly, true bacterial meningitis, cerebritis, or brain abscess may develop in association with acute endocarditis, either from septic emboli or from the bacteremia that initiated the infective endocarditis, perhaps continuing or resuming as the endocarditis progresses. Brain abscess is uncommon in chronic endocarditis.

Cerebrovascular lesions producing focal signs, including major strokes, account for about 50% of the neurologic manifestations; the mechanisms appear to be emboli to cerebral arteries causing ischemia or infarction, or bleeding from mycotic aneurysms. About 20% of the neurologic manifestations take the form of toxic encephalopathy, which may conceivably arise from showers of microemboli, although it may be a nonspecific manifestation of bacteremia.

Renal Manifestations

Ischemic infarctions of the kidney from embolization of vegetations are signaled by pain or gross hematuria; they are common, but fortunately seldom cause renal failure. Focal embolic glomerulonephritis is also a common renal lesion which seldom causes serious renal failure. Immune-complex glomerulonephritis is the most significant renal lesion of infective endocarditis. It is a diffuse process that occurs in 5% to 15% of patients and frequently causes mild to severe renal failure that usually resolves after successful treatment of the endocarditis. In a few cases, the renal failure persists and worsens despite cure.

Hematologic Changes

Infective endocarditis frequently causes the normocytic and normochromic anemia of chronic infection (Chap. 7, Manifestations of Infectious Diseases). Uremia is a contributing factor to anemia in some patients. The lassitude, weakness, pallor, and malaise of infective endocarditis are in some measure due to anemia as well as to the manifestations of a systemic infection.

Neither the total number nor the kinds of leukocytes circulating in the peripheral blood are characteristic in infective endocarditis. Large phagocytes—variously termed endothelial cells, macrophages, and circulatory histoid cells—have been found in the peripheral blood, particularly if obtained from the earlobes.

Diagnosis

Because the protean clinical features of infective endocarditis are often nonspecific, laboratory tests play a critical role in diagnosis. An exact etiologic diagnosis is necessary in order to select the best antimicrobics for treatment. The infecting microorganism can be isolated from venous blood in about 95% of cases when samples are drawn at intervals of 6 to 8 hours over 2 to 3 days before the application of antimicrobial therapy. The yield of successful isolations is somewhat lower when one or more of the following are present: age $\geq$ 50 years, disease of unusually

Table 134-6. *Cutaneous Lesions in Infective Endocarditis and Endarteritis*

	Petechiae	Splinter Hemorrhages	Osler's Nodes	Janeway Lesions	Clubbing
Incidence	Common	Common	Infrequent	Infrequent	Rare
Distribution	Anywhere, especially above clavicles	Distal third of nails (red when fresh, then brown or black)	Typically in thenar, hypothenar, palmar and fingertip areas; occasionally on flanks forearms, ankles, feet, and ears Red or blue nodules	Red macules	Fingers or toes
Pathology	Increased capillary permeability; emboli and bacteria are rare	Blood in avascular squamous epithelium under nail; emboli(?); increased capillary fragility(?)	Intracutaneous, local vasculitis; bacteria rarely found; occasional abscess formation or desquamation of overlying skin; ulceration rare Probably embolic in origin	Possibly embolic or allergic in origin	Soft tissue swellings occasionally periosteal new bone formation
Pain	None	None	Mild to moderate	None	None to moderate
Duration	Days	Weeks	Several days	Several hours to days	Weeks to months
Significance	Nonspecific	Nonspecific	Almost pathognomonic; rarely seen in bacteremia without endocarditis		Nonspecific
Notes	Found in acute rheumatic fever and many other disorders	In many normal people and in 44% of patients with mitral stenosis	Appear in crops; onset early or late in disease May also appear weeks to months after treatment and are then presumably embolic Very rare in congenital heart disease Commonest in subacute bacterial endocarditis	Commonest in acute bacterial endocarditis	In many cardiopulmonary disorders; can be congenital

long duration, or renal failure. Generally, no useful purpose is served by culturing arterial blood from an extremity, because the peripheral capillary bed has little capacity to clear organisms from the blood as it passes from the arteries to the veins.

Five to fifteen milliliters of venous blood should be drawn from the patient and inoculated immediately into bottles containing suitable broth mediums (Chap. 10, Clinical Specimens for Microbiologic Examinations). Incorporation of sodium polyanetholsulfonate to prevent clotting and to inactivate leukocytes and complement has been recommended. If penicillin therapy is already underway, penicillinase should be added to the culture medium.

Quantitative blood cultures may help to distinguish significant bacteremia from contamination. Persistently positive blood cultures with 10 to 200 colony-forming units of bacteria per milliliter of blood are typical of an intravascular infection. Occasionally, quantitative blood cultures may help to localize the site of infection: a real increase in the density of bacteremia or fungemia comparing blood samples aspirated from upstream and downstream sites identifies the valve between as the probable origin; however, the presence of another vegetation at another site is not thereby excluded.

When bacteria that proliferate within phagocytes are suspected (*e.g., Brucella* spp.), culture of bone marrow may yield the organism. Supplemented culture mediums may be necessary to isolate certain streptococci with special nutritional requirements. Hyperosmolar culture mediums need not be used routinely, because there is no proof that osmotically fragile, cell-wall-deficient bacteria play a role in infective endocarditis.

Serologic tests are occasionally useful in the diagnosis of infective endocarditis. About half of the patients with chronic endocarditis develop rheumatoid factor, sometimes in high titer, a finding that may provide a clue to the diagnosis. The titer usually falls after appropriate treatment for endocarditis is begun and disappears after cure.

Echocardiography is a noninvasive test that is most useful when a target consistent with a vegetation is identified. However, vegetations must be ≥ 2 mm in size to be detectable, and false-negative results are common. Infective endocarditis cannot be excluded solely on the basis of a negative echocardiogram.

Prognosis

It is doubtful that spontaneous cure of infective endocarditis ever occurs. With modern antimicrobial therapy a high proportion of patients can be cured, but this figure varies greatly according to the organism and cardiac lesion involved (Table 134-7). Few patients die because the infecting microorganism is resistant to available antimicrobial agents, that is, it is much easier to achieve bacteriologic cure than to eliminate morbidity and mortality. The most important factor working against cure is delay in diagnosis and institution of treatment, thus allowing cardiac failure and other complications to develop. It is in acute endocarditis that errors are most often made and delay is most costly. Thus, despite the availability of a number of potent bactericidal agents, about 50% of older patients with acute endocarditis caused by *Staphylococcus aureus* still die of their disease. Although much less common, infections with gram-negative bacilli, fungi, and rare organisms such as *Coxiella burnetii* are often fatal. Combined medical and surgical therapy offers the best hope for cure in these forms of endocarditis.

Cardiac failure is the single most important prognostic factor. The underlying cardiac lesion that predisposed the patient to infective endocarditis may worsen, leading to heart failure, which develops even while the infection is undergoing microbiologic cure. Myocarditis and embolic myocardial infarction may contribute to heart failure.

Emboli may arise from vegetations even after appropriate antimicrobial therapy has been applied. Indeed, until the vegetation is secured by organization, pieces may break off to cause infarctions; if vital organs such as the brain are involved, death may result.

Renal failure can be progressive if a glomerulonephritis is engendered by the infection. If nephrotoxic antimicrobics must be used, additional stress is placed on kidneys already compromised by the complications of infective endocarditis.

Relapse, as reinfection, carries a somewhat worse prognosis because it increases the chance of progressive valvular damage with worsening cardiac function, and increases the risk of complications.

Therapy

Cure of infective endocarditis requires sustained therapy with antimicrobial agents capable of killing the microorganisms responsible for the infection. The selection of antimicrobics appropriate for treatment of a given patient therefore depends on the isolation of the causative microorganism and the determination of the susceptibility of that isolate to antimicrobial agents. Tube dilution or microtiter methods (Chap. 12, Susceptibility Testing) are best for this

*Table 134-7. An Estimate of Bacteriologic Cure Rates for Various Forms of Endocarditis**

Native Valve Endocarditis	Antimicrobial Therapy Alone (%)	Antimicrobial Therapy Plus Surgery (%)
Streptococcus spp: viridans group, Group A, *S. bovis,* and *S. pneumoniae*	98	98
Neisseria gonorrhoeae		
Streptococcus fecalis	90	90
Staphylococcus aureus (in young drug addicts)	90	>90
Staphylococcus aureus (in elderly patients with chronic underlying diseases)	50	70
Gram-negative aerobic bacilli†	40	65
Fungi	5	50

Prosthetic Valve Endocarditis (PVE)	Early PVE	Late PVE	Early PVE	Late PVE
Streptococcus spp: viridans group, Group A, *S. bovis,* and *S. pneumoniae*	‡	80	‡	90
Neisseria gonorrhoeae				
Streptococcus fecalis	‡	60	‡	75
Staphylococcus aureus	25	40	50	60
Staphylococcus epidermidis	20	40	60	70
Gram-negative aerobic bacilli	<10	20	40	50
Fungi	<1	<1	30	40

*Morbidity and mortality is significantly greater than these figures indicate for bacteriologic cure.

†Excluding *Haemophilus* spp.

‡Insufficient data to estimate rate.

(Hurst JW, Logue RB, Rackley CE, Schlant RC, Sonnenblick EH, Wallace AG, Wenger NK (eds): The Heart, Arteries, and Veins, 5th ed. New York, McGraw–Hill, 1982)

purpose because they allow the definition of a lethal concentration, the testing of multiple concentrations of a variety of antimicrobics, and the assay of combinations of agents. Estimates of the overall *bacteriologic* cure rates for various types of infective endocarditis, with and without valve replacement, are listed in Table 134-7. Replacement of the affected valve improves the prognosis in many patients, especially those with significant cardiac failure. Therefore, surgery should not be delayed unduly, lest heart failure progress to the stage at which operation is no longer possible. Once the indications for surgery are clear, it is not necessary to wait for antimicrobial therapy to clear the organisms before valve replacement.

The success of every treatment regimen should be evaluated both at the bedside and in the laboratory. Determination, during treatment, of the highest dilution at which the patient's serum is still capable of killing the etiologic bacteria is useful. Treatment regimens causing the patient's serum to be lethal to the infecting bacteria at a dilution of 1:8 to 1:16 or higher is generally associated with cure. The blood should be cultured once or twice during therapy. To help prevent relapse, follow-up blood cultures should be obtained several times during the first month, with a final culture 2 to 3 months after treatment ends.

Subjective improvement—diminution of malaise, resolution of toxicity (including toxic encephalopathy), and return of appetite—may begin during the first week and is usual by the second week of appropriate therapy. Gain in weight and repair of anemia progress slowly. The erythrocyte sedimentation rate (ESR) falls slowly to normal over 4 or more weeks after cure, and may indicate failure of treatment if it remains elevated without other cause. Fever should resolve over the first week or two, but may take as long as 3 weeks when *Staphylococcus aureus* causes the infection, even if treatment is progressing satisfactorily. Fever may persist because of adverse reactions to antimicrobics—drug fever, and myositis or thrombophlebitis from injections—or because of complications such as infarctions or abscesses. Leukocytosis and raised ESR also may persist because of local reactions to emboli or to injections of antimicrobics. Regression in the size of the spleen is too slow to be useful in judging the appropriateness of treatment. Persistent enlargement, if associated with persistent tenderness, may indicate an abscess in the spleen. Changes in heart murmurs and serial echocardiograms are of little value in assessing the adequacy of therapy.

Empiric Therapy

It is sometimes necessary to begin antimicrobial therapy before the etiologic agent has been isolated or tested for susceptibility. In assessing the need for urgent therapy, the physician must weigh many factors, but especially the rate of progress, the severity, and the duration of the illness. The detection of a focus or source for the endocardial or endarterial infection is also helpful. For patients with the syndrome of acute endocarditis, antimicrobial therapy should be started as soon as three individual blood cultures have been obtained, without waiting for the results. Chronic endocarditis usually does not require immediate treatment, and antimicrobic therapy may be delayed for 2 to 3 days; if 5 to 6 blood cultures remain negative, empiric treatment may be given, provided bacterial endocarditis remains the leading diagnosis. If cultures yield an organism later, therapy should be modified accordingly.

Particular attention must be paid to clinical indicators of response once blind treatment is underway. The most difficult problems are posed by those patients whose blood cultures remain negative and who have not improved after 7 to 10 days of treatment. A painstaking review of history, physical findings, laboratory tests, and progress is mandatory, seeking clues to the infecting microorganism or to other diagnoses, including noninfectious conditions. If no new data become available, combined therapy should be tried. For subacute cases, the following regimen may be tried: ampicillin (or an acylureidopenicillin), 200 to 250 mg/kg/day, IV, as six equal portions 4-hourly, plus gentamicin, tobramycin, or netilmicin, 5 to 6 mg/kg/day, IV, as three equal portions, 8-hourly. In acute infective endocarditis, the following combination may be used: vancomycin 25 to 30 mg/kg/day, IV, as three equal portions, 8-hourly, plus ampicillin (or an acylureidopenicillin), 200 to 250 mg/kg/day, IV, as six equal portions, 4-hourly, plus gentamicin, tobramycin, or netilmicin, 5 to 6 mg/kg/day, IV, as three equal portions, 8-hourly. If the diagnosis of endocarditis is certain but the patient does not improve on maximal antimicrobic therapy, surgical excision of the affected valve(s) and replacement with prosthetic valve(s) is often necessary.

Culture-Negative Endocarditis

In 5% to 10% of patients with bacterial endocarditis, blood cultures do not yield the etiologic organism. In these difficult cases, the physician must be guided by less specific indicators, especially the history, repeated physical and laboratory examinations, and the course of the disease over time. For example, the patient with culture-negative infective endocarditis who has bacteriuria caused by enterococci should be treated empirically for presumed enterococcal endocarditis. Indeed, initial therapy for chronic infective endocarditis in which etiologic diagnosis has not been successful is reasonably directed against enterococci. Necropsy studies have shown that enterococci constitute one of the more frequent causes of abacteremic bacterial endocarditis. However, if the course has been acute, initial therapy should be directed against penicillinase-producing *Staphylococcus aureus* (Table 134-8).

Therapy After Etiologic Diagnosis

Suitable regimens for treatment of the more common kinds of bacterial endocarditis are presented in Table 134-8. The combination of an inhibitor of cell-wall synthesis with an aminocyclitol acts synergistically against many species that cause endocarditis, especially the gram-positive cocci. The best-known example is the importance of *in vitro* and *in vivo* synergy between penicillins and aminocyclitols against enterococci and viridans group streptococci. Synergy between antimicrobics can kill the infecting bacteria; it is therefore particularly valuable in treatment of bacterial endocarditis because leukocytes are often unable to reach and dispose of surviving organisms in vegetations.

Because β-lactam antimicrobics are established as effective in treatment of infective endocarditis, it is sometimes thought necessary to use one of them in spite of a history of hypersensitivity to penicillin. This is usually possible unless there is evidence that an anaphylactoid reaction will be provoked (*e.g.,* an immediate reaction by skin testing—Chap. 18, Antimicrobics and Anthelmintics for Systemic Therapy). Every facility must be mobilized in preparation for the treatment of a potentially serious reaction before the antimicrobic is administered. Nonanaphylactoid reactions may still occur, but they are seldom serious and usually can be suppressed with antihistamines or glucosteroids. Cefazolin may be used to replace the penicillin in these regimens, except for disease caused by enterococci and "methicillin"-

Table 134-8. *Treatment Regimens for Infective Endocarditis Caused by Gram-Positive Cocci*

Organism	Regimen	Comments
Viridans group *Streptococcus* spp.; *Streptococcus bovis*	1. Procaine penicillin G, 35–40 mg (0.05–0.06 megaU)/kg body wt/day, IM, as 3 equal portions, 8-hourly, for 2 weeks, *plus* streptomycin, 25–30 mg/kg body wt/day, IM, as 2 equal portions, 12-hourly, for 2 weeks *or*	1. For patients <65 years old without renal failure, eighth-nerve defects, or serious complications
	2. Penicillin G (K^+ salt), 65–70 mg (0.1 megaU)/kg body wt/day, IV, as 4 equal portions, 6-hourly for 4 weeks, *plus* streptomycin, 20 mg/kg/day, IM, as 2 equal portions, 12-hourly, for 2 weeks, *or*	2. For patients with complicated disease, *e.g.,* CNS involvement, shock, moderately penicillin-resistant organism, failed previous treatment
	3. Procaine penicillin G, 35–40 mg (0.05–0.06 megaU)/kg body wt/day, IM, as 3 equal portions, 8-hourly, for 4 weeks, *or*	3. For patients >65 years old with renal failure or eighth-nerve defect
	4. Cefazolin, 100 mg/kg body wt/day, IV, as 4 equal portions, 6-hourly, for 4 weeks, *or*	4. For patients allergic to penicillins
	5. Vancomycin, 25 mg/kg body wt/day, IV, as 3 equal portions, 8-hourly, for 4 weeks	5. For patients allergic to penicillins
Streptococcus pyogenes *Streptococcus pneumoniae*	1. Procaine penicillin G, 35–40 mg (0.05–0.06 megaU)/kg body wt/day, IM, as 3 equal portions, 8-hourly, for 2–4 weeks, *or*	1–3. These organisms are usually highly susceptible to penicillin; 2 weeks is adequate for most cases.
	2. Penicillin G (K^+ salt), 65–70 mg (0.1 megaU)/kg body wt/day, IV, as 4 equal portions, 6-hourly, for 2–4 weeks, *or*	
	3. Cefazolin, mg/kg body wt/day, IV, as 4 equal portions, 6-hourly, for 2–4 weeks	
Streptococcus fecalis and other penicillin-resistant *Streptococcus* spp.	1. Ampicillin (Na^+ salt) or an acylureidopenicillin, 200–300 mg/kg body wt/day, IV, as 6 equal portions, 4-hourly, for 4–6 weeks, *plus* gentamicin, tobramycin, or netilmicin 5–6 mg/kg body wt/day, IV, as 3 equal portions, 8-hourly, for 4–6 weeks	1. 4 weeks is adequate for most cases.
	2. Vancomycin, 25–30 mg/kg body wt/day, IV, as 3 equal portions, 8-hourly for 4–6 weeks, *plus* streptomycin, 30 mg/kg body wt/day, IM, as 2 equal portions, 12-hourly, for 4–6 weeks	2. 4 weeks is adequate for most cases.

Table 134-8. (continued) *Treatment Regimens for Infective Endocarditis Caused by Gram-Positive Cocci*

Organism	Regimen	Comments
Staphylococcus aureus	1. Nafcillin (Na^+ salt), 150–200 mg/kg body wt/day, IV, as 6 equal portions, 4-hourly, for 4 weeks after defervescence, *plus* gentamicin, tobramycin, or netilmicin 5–6 mg/kg body wt/day, IV, as 3 equal portions, 8-hourly, for 1 week or longer, *or*	1. Use to initiate therapy. Continue nafcillin if β-lactamase positive. Continue gentamicin or tobramycin if isolate tolerant to nafcillin.
	2. Penicillin G (K^+ salt), 200–400 mg (0.33–0.67 megaU)/kg body wt/day, IV, as 6 equal portions, 4-hourly, for 4 weeks after defervescence, *plus* gentamicin, tobramycin, or netilmicin 5–6 mg/kg body wt/day, IV, as 3 equal portions, 8-hourly, for 1 week or longer, *or*	2. Use only if isolate is proved to be β-lactamase negative. Continue gentamicin or tobramycin if isolate is tolerant to penicillin.
	3. Cefazolin, 100–150 mg/kg body wt/day, IV, as 4 equal portions, 6-hourly, for 4 weeks after defervescence, *plus* gentamicin, tobramycin, or netilmicin 5–6 mg/kg body wt/day, IV, as 3 equal portions, 8-hourly, for 1 week or longer, *or*	3. Use in patients allergic to penicillins. Continue gentamicin or tobramycin if isolate is tolerant to cefazolin.
	4. Vancomycin, 25–30 mg/kg body wt/day, IV, as 3 equal portions, 8-hourly, for 4 weeks after defervescence, *plus* gentamicin, tobramycin, or netilmicin 5–6 mg/kg body wt/day, IV, as 3 equal portions, 8-hourly, for 1 week or longer	4. Use in patients allergic to penicillins and cephalosporins and when isolate is resistant to alternatives. Since both drugs are both nephrotoxic and ototoxic, close surveillance is necessary.

(After Hurst JW, Logue RB, Rackley CE, Schlant RC, Sonnenblick EH, Wallace AG, Wenger NK (eds): The Heart, Arteries, and Veins, 5th ed. New York, McGraw–Hill, 1982)

resistant staphylococci, in which case vancomycin is the preferred alternative.

Probenecid is usually not necessary. Its effectiveness diminishes as the total dosage of the penicillin increases because the competitive advantage of probenecid for active tubular transport is overwhelmed, and at the same time the capacity for biliary excretion of ampicillin, the acylureidopenicillins, the isoxazolyl penicillins, and nafcillin increases. Moreover, probenecid itself can cause gastrointestinal disturbances and skin rashes.

Treatment for the many other microorganisms that only rarely cause endocarditis must be individualized using information from susceptibility tests. The penicillins are the mainstay of therapy for many of these less common bacteria, including *Haemophilus* spp., *Neisseria* spp., *Erysipelothrix rhusiopathiae, Listeria monocytogenes, Streptobacillus moniliformis,* and *Actinomyces israelii.* A second antimicrobic may be added according to the results of susceptibility testing, which should include assays for synergism and antagonism.

For the Enterobacteriaceae, it is usual to try a combination of a β-lactam antimicrobic and an aminocyclitol, again relying on *in vitro* tests for information as to potential synergism/antagonism. Most isolates

Table 134-9. Suggested Regimens for Prophylaxis of Endocarditis

Procedure	For Most Congenital Heart Disease, Acquired Valvular Heart Disease, Asymmetric Septal Hypertrophy, Mitral Valve Prolapse With Mitral Insufficiency	For Prosthetic Heart Valves
All dental procedures that are likely to result in gingival bleeding	Regimen A or B	Regimen B
Surgery in the oral cavity or upper respiratory tract	Regimen A or B	Regimen B
Surgery of genitourinary or gastrointestinal tracts, drainage of abscesses, incision of infected tissues	Regimen C	Regimen C
Cardiac surgery	Regimen D or E	Regimen D or E

Regimen A *or* Parenteral plus oral penicillin

Adults: Aqueous crystalline penicillin G 1 million units mixed with procaine penicillin G 600,000 units IM 30 min to 1 hour before procedure; then penicillin V 500 mg orally every 6 hours for 8 doses

Children: Aqueous crystalline penicillin G 30,000 units per kilogram mixed with procaine penicillin G 600,000 units IM; then penicillin V 500 mg (250 mg for children less than 60 lb) orally every 6 hours for 8 doses

or Oral penicillin

Adults: Penicillin V 2.0 g orally 30 min to 1 hour before the procedure; then 500 mg orally every 6 hours for 8 doses

Children:* For children weighing less than 60 lb, 1.0 g orally; then 250 mg orally every 6 hours for 8 doses (for children weighing over 60 lb use adult dose)

or For patients allergic to penicillin use either vancomycin (see Regimen B), *or*

Adults: Erythromycin 1.0 g orally 1 to 2 hours before the procedure; then 500 mg orally every 6 hours for 8 doses

Children:* Erythromycin 20 mg/kg orally; then 10 mg/kg every 6 hours for 8 doses

Regimen B

Adults:† Aqueous crystalline penicillin G 1 million units mixed with procaine penicillin G 600,000 units IM *plus* streptomycin 1 g IM 30 min to 1 hour before the procedure; then penicillin V 500 mg orally every 6 hours for 8 doses

Children:* Aqueous crystalline penicillin G 30,000 units per kilogram mixed with procaine penicillin G 600,000 units IM *plus* streptomycin 20 mg/kg IM; then penicillin V 250 mg every 6 hours for 8 doses

or For patients allergic to penicillin

Adults: Vancomycin 0.5 to 1.0 g IV infused slowly over 1 hour, starting 30 min to 1 hour before the procedure; then erythromycin 500 mg orally every 6 hours for 8 doses

Children:* Vancomycin 20 mg/kg IV infused slowly over 1 hour; then erythromycin 10 mg/kg orally

Regimen C

Adults:† Ampicillin (or an acylureidopenicillin) 1.0 g IM or IV *plus* gentamicin (or tobramycin or netilmicin) 1.5 mg/kg IM or IV 30 min to 1 hour before procedure; then repeated every 8 hours for 2 additional doses. If staphylococcal infection is present, substitute nafcillin for ampicillin.

Children:* Ampicillin (or an acylureidopenicillin) 50 mg/kg IM or IV plus gentamicin (or tobramycin or netilmicin) 2.0 mg/kg IM or IV

or For patients allergic to penicillin:

Adults:† Vancomycin 0.5 to 1.0 g IV infused slowly over 1 hour *plus* streptomycin 1.0 g IM given 30 min to 1 hour before the procedure. Both drugs may be repeated once 12 hours later.

Children:* Vancomycin 20 mg/kg IV infused slowly over 1 hour *plus* streptomycin 20 mg/kg IM

Regimen D

Adults: Cefazolin 2.0 g IM or IV 30 min before the operation, repeated every 8 hours for 5 additional doses

Children:* Cefazolin 30 mg/kg IM or IV

Regimen E

Adults: Cefazolin 2.0 g IM or IV plus gentamicin 1.5 mg/kg IM or IV. Give initial dose 30 min before the operation, then repeat both drugs every 8 hours for 5 additional doses.

Children:* Cefazolin 30 mg/kg IM or IV plus gentamicin 2.0 mg/kg IM or IV

*Timing and number of doses for children is the same as for adults.

†For brief procedures such as a single tooth extraction, change of urinary catheter, or cystoscopy, one dose of these combination regimens will probably suffice. Conversely, in the case of unusually prolonged or repeated procedures or delayed healing, several additional doses may be given.

(After Hurst JW, Logue RB, Rackley CE, Schlant RC, Sonnenblick EH, Wallace AG, Wenger NK (eds): The Heart, Arteries, and Veins, 5th ed. New York, McGraw–Hill, 1982)

of *Proteus mirabilis* are relatively susceptible to penicillin G, ampicillin, the acylureidopenicillins, and cefazolin. Penicillin G is preferable because it is generally effective, causes fewer adverse reactions, and costs less. Some strains of *Proteus mirabilis* produce penicillinase; with these, cefazolin is the agent of choice. The regimens given for *Staphylococcus aureus* in Table 134-8 are appropriate. For *Pseudomonas aeruginosa* and *Pseudomonas maltophilia,* gentamicin, tobramycin, or netilmicin 5 to 6 mg/kg body wt/day, IV, as three equal portions, 8-hourly, plus an acylureidopenicillin, 300 mg/kg body wt/day, IV, as six equal portions, 4-hourly, is the current best treatment. However, *Pseudomonas cepacia* are not susceptible to these agents; favorable responses to treatment with trimethoprin plus sulfamethoxazole combined with polymyxin B have been reported.

In infective endocarditis caused by fungi, amphotericin B has occasionally provided a cure, but surgical resection is nearly always required (Table 134-7). Presently available antimicrobial agents do not cure endocarditis caused by *C. burnetii;* surgical resection of the site of infection is necessary. Infective endocarditis and endarteritis caused by *Brucella* spp. may respond to tetracycline 25 mg/kg body wt/day, PO, as four equal portions, 6-hourly, plus streptomycin, 15mg/kg body wt/day, IM, as two equal portions, 12-hourly.

Therapy for Infected Prostheses

When an intracardiovascular prosthesis is the site of infection, removal of the infected prosthesis is often necessary to achieve cure. If the infecting microorganism is known, appropriate antimicrobial treatment should be given in full dosage before, during, and after surgical intervention. If the infecting microorganism is not known, empiric antimicrobial treatment should be applied similarly.

Nonspecific Therapy

Measures to relieve stress on the heart during treatment of infective endocarditis include rest, a low-salt diet, alleviation of congestive heart failure, control of fever, and transfusion to maintain a hematocrit close to 30%. The maintenance of fluid and electrolyte balance is important, and parenteral feeding is occasionally necessary to combat the catabolic state induced by infective endocarditis.

Anticoagulation with heparin is contraindicated. Cerebral embolism may be complicated by catastrophic hemorrhage when the blood is hypocoagulable. Furthermore, although vegetations are thrombotic in nature, antimicrobial therapy is not measurably aided by anticoagulation.

Prevention

When a medical procedure is likely to put microorganisms into the circulation of a person with a heart lesion that is susceptible to infection, it is standard practice to administer appropriate antimicrobics immediately before, during, and for a short span after the period of risk. It remains to be proved that such measures actually prevent endocardial colonization in humans, but endocarditis is such a serious disease that every effort should be made to prevent it (Chap. 19, Chemoprophylaxis of Infectious Diseases). Suggested regimens for prevention of endocarditis under various circumstances are listed in Table 134-9. Patients should be urged to report any symptoms suggesting infection following dental or other surgery.

Because barium enema, proctoscopy, and sigmoidoscopy seldom cause bacteremia, they are not indications for routine chemoprophylaxis unless biopsy or other surgical manipulation is contemplated. Even though the risk is low, chemoprophylaxis directed primarily against enterococci and anaerobic streptococci should then be given.

Remaining Problems

More information is required about how best to apply both old and new antimicrobics in the therapy of infective endocarditis, especially in cases caused by unusual organisms. The critical evaluation of preventive measures is yet to be accomplished. There remain many fascinating questions: exactly how and why do certain blood-borne microorganisms settle on heart valves? How critical is pre-existing endothelial and subendothelial inflammation? Must there be nonthrombotic endocarditis before there can be infective endocarditis? Is vaccination against endocarditis possible?

Bibliography

Books

BISNO AL (ed): Treatment of Infective Endocarditis, New York, Grune & Stratton, 1981. 340 pp.

DUMA RJ (ed): Infections of Prosthetic Heart Valves and Vascular Grafts, Baltimore, University Park Press, 1977. 352 pp.

DURACK DT: Ch. 54, Infective Endocarditis and Noninfective Endocarditis. In Hurst JW, Logue RB, Rackley CE, Schlant RC, Sonnenblick EH, Wallace AG, Wenger NK (eds): The Heart, Arteries and Veins, 5th ed. New York, McGraw–Hill, 1982. pp 1250–1277.

KAYE D (ed): Infective Endocarditis. Baltimore, University Park Press, 1976. 272 pp.

KAPLAN, EL, TARANTA AV (ed): Infective Endocarditis. Dallas, American Heart Association, Monograph No. 52, 1977. 99 pp.

KERR A JR: Subacute Bacterial Endocarditis. Springfield, Ill, Charles C. Thomas, 1955. 343 pp.

RAHIMTOOLA SH (ed): Infective Endocarditis. New York, Grune & Stratton, 1978. 386 pp.

Journals

ANGRIST AA, OKA M: Pathogenesis of bacterial endocarditis. JAMA 183:249–252, 1963

COHEN PS, MAGUIRE HJ, WEINSTEIN L: Infective endocarditis caused by gram-negative bacteria: A review of the literature, 1945–1977. Prog Cardiovasc Dis 22:205–242, 1980

KAPLAN EL, ANTHONY BF, BISNO A, DURACK D, HOUSER H, MILLARD HD, SANFORD J, SHULMAN ST, STILLERMAN M, TARANTA A, WENGER N: Prevention of bacterial endocarditis. Circulation 56:139A–143A, 1977

LEPESCHKIN E: On the relation between the site of valvular involvement in endocarditis and the blood pressure resting on the valve. Am J Med Sci 224:318–319, 1952

MOELLERING RC JR, WATSON BK, KUNZ LJ: Endocarditis due to Group D streptococci. Comparison of disease caused by *Streptococcus bovis* with that produced by the enterococci. Am J Med 57:239–250, 1974

PAZIN, GJ, PETERSON KL, GRIFF FW, SHAVER JA, HO M: Determination of site of infection in endocarditis. Ann Intern Med 82:746–750, 1975

PHAIR JP, CLARKE J: Immunology of infective endocarditis. Prog Cardiovasc Dis 22:137–144, 1977

PRUITT AA, RUBIN RH, KARCHMER AW, DUNCAN GW: Neurologic complications in bacterial endocarditis. Medicine 57:329–343, 1978

RODBARD S: Blood velocity and endocarditis. Circulation 27: 18–28, 1963.

ROSS RS, MCKUSICK VA, HARVEY JC: The problem of fever in patients with valvular heart disease. JAMA 165:1–7, 1957

STEWART JA, SILIMPERI D, HARRIS P, WISE NK, FRANKER TD, KISSLO J: Echocardiographic documentation of vegetative lesions in infective endocarditis: Clinical implications. Circulation 61:374–380, 1980

TUAZON CU, CARDELLA TA, SHEAGREN JN: Staphylococcal endocarditis in drug users: Clinical and microbiologic aspects. Arch Intern Med 135:1555–1561, 1975

RICHARD H. PARKER

135 Septic Thrombophlebitis

Septic or suppurative thrombophlebitis is characterized by inflammation of the walls of veins caused by infiltration with microorganisms; bacteremia and occlusion of veins are frequent consequences. In contrast, there is no suppuration of the walls of veins in association with bacteremias complicating the IV infusion of contaminated liquids or arising from infections of IV catheters.

Septic thrombophlebitis occurs in four clinical forms: superficial vein, pelvic vein, cerebral vein, and portal vein; the latter is discussed in Chapter 84, Pylephlebitis and Liver Abscess. In recent years, superficial septic thrombophlebitis has increased in frequency, keeping pace with the increased use of intravenous catheters. Intravenous catheterization is the most common factor associated with nosocomial bacteremias in the United States, and many patients who receive this treatment also have superficial septic thrombophlebitis.

Etiology

Precise data are not available regarding the microbial causes of septic thrombophlebitis. The classical causes of the three clinical forms under discussion are listed in Table 135-1. As with many other bacterial diseases, the probability that the Enterobacteriaceae, *Pseudomonas* spp., and fungi are involved increases if the disease occurs after prolonged hospitalization or use of extended-spectrum antimicrobial agents.

Epidemiology

At one time, superficial septic thrombophlebitis was usually associated with skin infections, but during the past three decades the frequency of association with devices indwelling in veins has increased steadily. It is a dangerous misconception to believe that this potentially lethal problem is linked only to the use of plastic catheters, although the risk may be approximately 40 times higher with plastic catheters than with scalp-vein needles. Intravenous therapy is very common in hospitalized patients and therefore it is not surprising that superficial septic thrombophlebitis may account for as much as 10% of all nosocomial infections. This disease has been a particular problem in patients with cancers and burn wounds. Indeed, septic thrombophlebitis may be the most common cause of infection-associated death in patients with burns.

Pelvic thrombophlebitis has been associated with parturition, surgery, abortion, and pelvic infection, especially pelvic abscesses. Hence, pelvic thrombophlebitis afflicts primarily 15- to 40-year-old women. The risk of this complication varies from 0.5% in septic abortion to 0.05% in parturition, with an intermediate risk of 0.13% in gynecologic surgery. The probability of the occurrence of pelvic thrombophlebitis is directly related to the extent of trauma to the pelvic tissues.

Cavernous sinus thrombophlebitis follows facial infections most frequently, but may also be caused by paranasal sinusitis or infection in the mouth.

Pathogenesis and Pathology

The pathogenesis of septic thrombophlebitis is not clear. Possibly, the initiating event is endothelial damage either from perivascular inflammation or intravascular insult (*e.g.,* caused by a catheter), which then leads to the deposition of fibrin and the formation of thrombi. Thrombi may serve as nidi for colonization and proliferation of microorganisms that subsequently invade the wall of the vein. In superficial septic thrombophlebitis, the source of the bacteria may be the patient's skin with migration between

Table 135-1. *Microorganisms Commonly Associated With Septic Thrombophlebitis*

Cerebral	Pelvic	Superficial
*Staphylococcus aureus**	*Bacteroides* spp.*	*Staphylococcus aureus**
Streptococcus spp., aerobic and anaerobic	Anaerobic streptococci*	*Staphylococcus epidermidis*†
Bacteroides spp.	Enterobacteriaceae	Enterobacteriaceae†
Fusobacterium spp.		*Pseudomonas* spp.†
Fungi		*Candida* spp.†

*Most frequently recovered microorganisms.
†Frequency increases in nosocomial setting.

the external surface of the catheter and perivascular tissues, contaminated intravenous fluids, or hematogenous spread from a remote, infected focus. In specific cases, it is often difficult to identify the exact origin of the infecting microorganisms.

Although any component of the pelvic venous system may be involved with thrombophlebitis, the veins draining the uterus, the ovarian veins, and the inferior vena cava are implicated most often. The augmented blood flow of the gravid uterus and the hypercoagulable state of parturition may be factors favoring pelvic thrombophlebitis. Microorganisms, representing the normal flora of the vaginal and perineal areas, infect the thrombosed veins through the regional blood or lymph vascular systems.

Enlarged, tortuous veins with thickened walls, perivascular suppuration, or hemorrhage are evident on inspection. The lumina of the veins may contain pus or thrombi. The thrombi often extend beyond the area of suppuration. Microscopic examination confirms endothelial damage with thickening and fibrinoid necrosis of the walls of the veins; there may be microabscesses in the wall of the vein with extension into the surrounding tissue. Septic pulmonary emboli with infarction and metastatic abscesses are present in approximately half of the fatal cases.

Manifestations

The manifestations of superficial and pelvic septic thrombophlebitis are often nonspecific, and systemic findings may dominate the clinical picture. In contrast, the findings in cerebral septic thrombophlebitis, particularly in the early stages, are primarily related to local abnormalities. Some of the characteristic symptoms and signs are listed in Table 135-2. Because of the paucity of local findings in many cases of superficial septic thrombophlebitis, the correct diagnosis is rendered antemortem in fewer than 50% of cases. Similarly, pelvic septic thrombophlebitis may be difficult to diagnose because the finds are nonspecific, mimicking pyelonephritis, perinephric abscess, ureteral obstruction, parametritis, endometritis, pelvic abscess, pelvic inflammatory disease, pelvic hematoma, twisted adnexal mass, sickle cell crisis, and many other intraabdominal and intrapelvic problems. Both septic thrombophlebitis and pelvic septic thrombophlebitis should be suspected in any patient with unexplained pulmonary emboli or metastatic abscesses, particularly when associated with rigors and hectic fevers.

Diagnosis

Specific diagnosis requires histologic examination of the vein. This is probably feasible only in certain cases of superficial thrombophlebitis. Most cases are diagnosed when clinical manifestations are supported by positive blood cultures. Bacteremia occurs in almost 90% of cases of superficial thrombophlebitis, 20% to 30% of cases of pelvic septic thrombophlebitis, and most cases of cerebral septic thrombophlebitis. The yield of positive blood cultures in pelvic thrombophlebitis depends upon use of techniques that assure isolation of obligate anaerobic microorganisms.

Table 135-2. *Signs and Symptoms Associated With Septic Thrombophlebitis*

Cerebral	Pelvic	Superficial
Edema of eyelids	Palpable tender pelvic vein	Fever
Periorbital edema	Normal pelvic exam	Tender vein
Papilledema		Warmth over vein
Conjunctival edema	Unexplained fever	Pulmonary emboli
Dilated, fixed pupil	Pulmonary emboli	No local signs of inflammation
Ocular palsies		
Exophthalmos		
Spread to opposite side		

Prognosis

The risk in allowing superficial-vein septic thrombophlebitis to go untreated is of bacteremia and the many ill consequences of blood-borne dissemination of bacteria. Appropriate medical therapy usually brings about resolution, although surgical excision may be required if abscesses have formed.

Failure of treatment of septic pelvic thrombophlebitis may also lead to bacteremia, with or without septic emboli. The latter may be lethal if vital organs are involved.

Untreated cerebral-vein septic thrombophlebitis is usually fatal. The infection may extend into the brain, orbit, or extracranial organs such as the lungs.

Therapy

The treatment of septic thrombophlebitis includes antimicrobial therapy, removal of intravenous devices, and surgery. Recommendations for initial antimicrobial therapy are listed in Table 135-3. Specific choice of agent should be based on knowledge of causative microorganisms peculiar to a given area and antimicrobial susceptibility patterns.

Superficial septic thrombophlebitis often requires surgery plus antimicrobial therapy in order to avert a fatal outcome. An exploratory venotomy should be carried out proximal to the probable site of infection. Following ligation of the vein proximal to the phlebitis, the vessel should be compressed moving distally to obtain material for microscopic examination and culture. The involved vein and all affected tributaries should be excised. Simple ligation, without excision, is followed by a high rate of relapse.

Medical therapy alone results in cures of approximately 90% of patients with pelvic septic thrombophlebitis. Patients who do not respond within 7 days should have an exploratory laparotomy for drainage of abscesses and ligation/excision of involved veins.

Appropriate antimicrobial therapy results in cure of about 90% of patients with cerebral-vein thrombophlebitis. However, residual cranial nerve deficits occur in 20% to 40% of patients.

Prevention

Cavernous sinus thrombophlebitis may possibly be prevented by prompt therapy of facial infections. Pelvic septic thrombophlebitis may possibly be prevented by reducing trauma to pelvic tissues and by prompt treatment of pelvic infections. In both of these kinds of septic thrombophlebitis it is doubtful that preventive measures are effective.

In contrast, the frequency of catheter-induced superficial septic thrombophlebitis is quite definitely reduced by (1) restricting the use of intravenous catheters and needles to absolutely necessary therapeutic or diagnostic maneuvers; (2) preferential use of stainless steel needles or cannulas, reserving plastic catheters for situations requiring a secure route for vascular access (with replacement of the catheter every 48–72 hours); (3) wearing a surgical mask and sterile gloves when placing cutdown and central-venous catheters, and washing hands thoroughly before percutaneous insertion of needles and cannulas; (4) eschewing the lower extremities, preferring always veins in the upper extremities; (5) paying meticulous attention to aseptic technique, scrubbing the site of insertion of a catheter with tincture of iodine, chlorhexidine, an iodophore, or 70% alcohol (hexachloroprene and aqueous quaternary ammonium compounds should never be used); (6) securely anchoring cannulas at the site of insertion and covering with a sterile dressing while leaving visible for daily inspection as much of the area as possible; (7) avoiding covering the wound with occlusive tape and recording the date of insertion on the dressing; (8) inspecting the site daily with palpation to detect tenderness or induration (either, especially if there is also fever, should prompt removal of the dressing and direct inspection of the site; (9) removing and replacing cannulas every 48 to 72 hours or, when prolonged use of a peripheral catheter or heparin-lock device is necessary, changing the dressing every 24 to 48 hours; (10) replacing all tubing used for IV administration every 24 to 48 hours; (11) discarding the entire system when there is any evidence of cellulitis, intravenous-therapy-related bacteremia, or septic thrombophlebitis; and (12) refraining from routine use of in-line filters for intravenous therapy.

Remaining Problems

The major problem is implementation of existing guidelines for prevention. The possible role of the newer antimicrobial agents in therapy also needs better definition.

Bibliography

Book

MAKI DG: Sepsis arising from extrinsic contamination of the infusion and measures for control. In Phillips I, Meers

Table 135-3. Therapy in Septic Thrombophlebitis

Therapy	Intracranial	Pelvic	Superficial
Primary antimicrobics	Nafcillin Loading dose—50 mg/kg body wt, (→0.11 mEq Na^+/kg body wt), IV in first hour Maintenance dose—200 mg/kg body wt/day (→0.45 mEq Na^+/kg body wt/day, IV, as 6 equal portions, 4-hourly Chloramphenicol, succinate derivative Loading dose—25 mg/kg body wt, IV, in first hour Maintenance dose—50–60 mg/kg body wt/day, IV, as 4 equal portions, 6-hourly	Penicillin G Loading dose—50 mg (~80,000 U)/kg body wt (→0.13 mEq K^+/kg body wt), IV, in first hour Maintenance dose—200 mg (~320,000 U)/kg body wt/day (→0.52 mEq K^+/kg body wt/day, IV, as 6 equal portions, 4-hourly Clindamycin phosphate Loading dose—7.5 mg/kg body wt, IV, in first hour Maintenance dose—30 mg/kg body wt/day, IV, as 4 equal portions, 6-hourly	Nafcillin Loading dose—50 mg/kg body wt (→0.11 mEq Na^+/kg body wt), IV, in first hour Maintenance dose—200 mg/kg body wt/day (→0.45 mEq Na^+/kg body wt/day), IV, as 6 equal portions, 4-hourly Tobramycin or gentamicin Loading dose—1–2 mg/kg body wt, IV, in first hour Maintenance dose—5–6 mg/kg body wtday, IV, as 3 equal portions, 8-hourly
Alternative antimicrobics	Moxalactam[‡] Loading dose—50 mg/kg body wt (→0.19 mEq Na^+/kg body wt), IV, in first hour Maintenance dose—150 mg/kg body wt/day, (→0.77 mEq Na^+/kg body wt/day), IV, as 3 equal portions, 8-hourly Metronidazole Loading dose—15 mg/kg body wt, IV, in first hour Maintenance dose—30 mg/kg body wt/day, IV, as 3 equal portions, 8-hourly Vancomycin* Loading dose—7.5 mg/kg body wt, IV, in first hour Maintenance dose—30 mg/kg body wt/day, IV, as 3 equal portions, 8-hourly	Chloramphenicol, succinate derivative Loading dose—25 mg/kg body wt, IV, in first hour Maintenance dose—50 mg/kg body wt/day, IV, as 4 equal portions, 6-hourly Metronidazole Loading dose—15 mg/kg body wt, IV, in first hour Maintenance dose—30 mg/kg body wt/day, IV, as 3 equal portions, 8-hourly	Moxalactam[‡] Loading dose—50 mg/kg body wt (→0.19 mEq Na^+/kg body wt), IV, in first hour Maintenance dose—150 mg/kg body wt/day, (→0.77 mEq Na^+/kg body wt/day, IV, as 3 equal portions,. 8-hourly Amikacin Loading dose—7.5 mg/kg body wt, IV, in first hour Maintenance dose—15 mg/kg body wt/day, IV, as 3 equal portions, 8-hourly
Other	Heparin[†] Loading dose—100 units/kg body wt, IV, in 5–10 minutes Maintenance dose—injections every 6 hours, IV, in a dose adequate to yield a predose activated coagulation time of whole blood of 150–180 seconds	Heparin[†] Loading dose—100 units/kg body wt, IV, in 5–10 minutes Maintenance dose—injections every 6 hours, IV, in a dose adequate to yield a predose activated coagulation time of whole blood of 150–180 seconds	Remove catheter

*Entry into the central nervous system/cerebrospinal fluid is variable.

[†]The value of anticoagulation treatment is not proved.

[‡]Depending on susceptibility test data and local custom, cefoperazone, cefotaxime, ceftizoxime, or ceftriaxone may be preferred alternatives.

PD, D'Arcy PF (eds): Microbiologic hazards of intravenous therapy. Lancaster, England, MTP Press Ltd, 1977. pp 99–141.

Journals

BENTLY DW, LEPPER MH: Septicemia related to indwelling venous catheter. JAMA 206:1749–1752, 1968

BROWN BJ, MACKOWIAK PA, SMITH JW: Care of veins during intravenous therapy: Incidence of phlebitis as related to knowledge and performance. Am J Inf Cont 8:107–112, 1980

JOSEY WE, STAGGERS SR JR: Heparin therapy in septic pelvic thrombophlebitis: A study of 46 cases. Am J Obstet Gynecol 120:228–233, 1974

MAKI DG, BAND JD: A comparative study of polyantibiotic and iodophor ointments in prevention of vascular catheter-related infection. Am J Med 70:739–744, 1981

MUNSTER AM: Septic thrombophlebitis: A surgical disorder. JAMA 230:1010–1011, 1974

STEIN JM, PRUITT BA JR: Suppurative thrombophlebitis: A lethal iatrogenic disease. N Engl J Med 282:1452–1455, 1970

SHAW R: Cavernous sinus thrombophlebitis: A review. Br J Surg 40:40-48, 1952

TULLY JL, FRIEDLAND GH, BALDINI LM, GOLDMAN DA: Complications of intravenous therapy with steel needles and Teflon catheters. Am J Med 70:702–706, 1981

ZINNER MJ, ZUIDEMA GD, LOWERY BD: Septic nonsuppurative thrombophlebitis. Arch Surg 111:122–125, 1976

KENNETH E. MOTT

American Trypanosomiasis

136

American trypanosomiasis, or Chagas' disease, is an acute and chronic infection caused by *Trypanosoma cruzi.* The chronic disease is manifested by cardiomyopathy, megaesophagus, and megacolon, which vary in frequency and severity in different geographic areas of Latin America. The parasite enters man through the skin or conjunctival mucosa after posterior station transmission from infected triatomine bugs. The disease was first described in central Brazil in 1909 by Carlos Chagas. In his unique monograph, he described the parasite, the disease it causes in humans, and the characteristics of infection in experimental animals, as well as the vector and its ecology. His studies of the clinical manifestations and electrocardiographic alterations of chronic Chagas' cardiomyopathy received little attention until the late 1940s.

Etiology

Trypanosoma cruzi (Schizotrypanum cruzi) is a flagellate protozoan (Fig. 136-1*A*) that undergoes intracellular transformation in vertebrate hosts to an oval or spherical nonflagellate form, the amastigote (Fig. 136-1*B*). Multiplication proceeds intracellularly; prior to cell rupture, the amastigotes transform into epimastigotes and subsequently into trypomastigotes. Thus, in its life cycle, *T. cruzi* is intermediate between the African trypanosomes, which have no tissue phase, (although a flagellate round form has recently been associated with *T. brucei*) and the *Leishmania* spp. which have no alternate blood form. The actively motile, circulating, trypomastigote measures 15 μm to 20 μm. The kinetoplast (the aggregation of extranuclear DNA lying anterior to the nucleus) and the nucleus are argentophilic, Feulgen positive, and stain red with Giemsa stain; the cytoplasm and undulating membrane stain light blue.

The metabolism of *T. cruzi* is not unlike that of its mammalian host. Bloodstream and culture forms of *T. cruzi* reoxidize NADH by a cytochrome system. The virulence of *T. cruzi* has been associated with high concentrations of NADP-glutamate dehydrogenase and NADP-dependent synthetase. *De novo* biosynthesis of pyrimidines, DNA synthesis, and the use of salvage pathways and interconversion of purines into RNA occur in all forms of *T. cruzi.* Incomplete aerobic glycolysis has been described. Choline and ethanolamine phosphoglycerides are synthesized and incorporated into complex lipids.

Isoenzyme mapping of trypanosomes enabled differentiation of strains that are now designated as zymodemes. The three major zymodemes described in Brazil are distinct from the common zymodemes of Venezuela. The pattern of restriction endonuclease products of kinetoplast DNA minicircles may also be used to identify strains of *T. cruzi.*

Semidefined mediums (Pan) are now available that consist of tissue culture mediums, trypticase, heme, and bovine fetal serum. *Trypanosoma* spp. grow well in tissue cell cultures, but the blood-base NNN medium (see Chap. 11, Diagnostic Methods for Protozoa and Helminths) is most commonly employed for isolation of *T. cruzi.* Its diagnostic efficacy is enhanced by overlaying with tissue culture medium. In NNN cultures, epimastigote forms predominate (Fig. 136-2*A*), although amastigotes may be grown under special conditions (Fig. 136-2*B*).

Tissue cultures of human diploid cells may be useful for isolation or production of trypomastigotes.

Trypanosoma cruzi are antigenically complex; however antigenic variation, such as occurs in African trypanosomiasis has not been observed. *Trypanosoma cruzi* antigens have been identified on the surfaces of infected and uninfected cells.

Antibodies directed against antigens on the surface of *T. cruzi* may immobilize trypomastigotes *in vitro.* However, in the blood, only a small portion of the

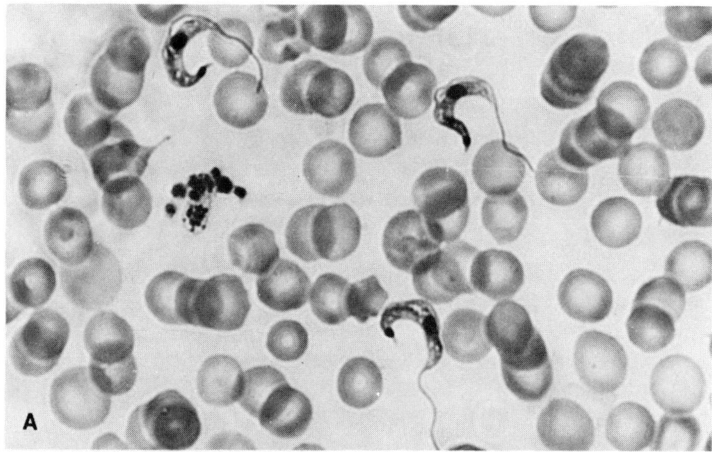

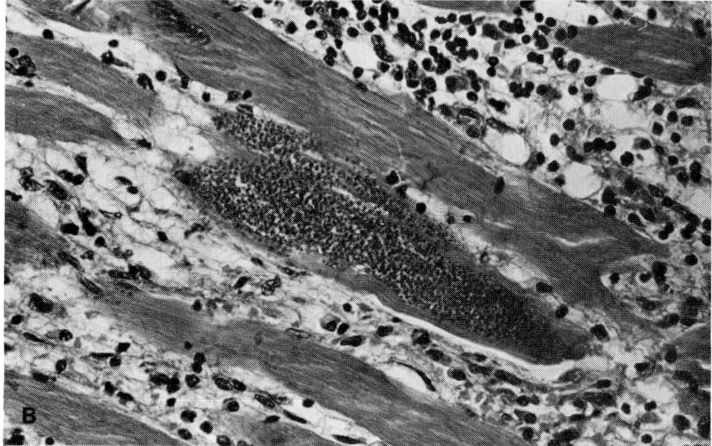

Fig. 136-1. (*A*) Trypomastigote form of *Trypanosoma cruzi* in peripheral blood of a mouse. (Original magnification approximately × 1200) (*B*) Amastigote pseudocyst of *Trypanosoma cruzi* in human myocardium with fibrosis, myocytolysis, and lymphohistiocytic inflammatory infiltrate. (Original magnification approximately × 300) (Courtesy of SC Pan, Harvard School of Public Health)

trypomastigotes are resistant to antibody-dependent cytotoxicity.

Although antibodies that cross-react between human myocardium and *T. cruzi* have been found, their relationship to pathogenesis is unknown. No specific protective antibody against *T. cruzi* infection has been demonstrated. Experimentally, partial protection to challenge with *T. cruzi* may occur between heterologous strains. IgM antibodies are present in the acute stage of infection and IgG antibodies are associated predominately with chronic infections.

Epidemiology

Chagas' disease is known to occur only in the Western hemisphere. More than 15 million persons living in the region from southern Argentina to Texas are infected with *T. cruzi.* The leading cause of cardiovascular death in South America is Chagas' cardiomyopathy; overall, in endemic areas, it is the most important cause of death among males between the ages of 25 and 44 years.

The principal domestic vectors of *T. cruzi* in most of Latin America are *Triatoma infestans* (Fig. 136-3*A*) and *Panstrongylus megistus. Rhodnius prolixus* (Fig. 136-3*B*) is the most important domestic vector in Venezuela. *Triatoma infestans* also maintains a sylvatic cycle and appears to be spreading into new areas in central and northeast Brazil. Infected sylvatic *Triatoma* species have been found in most states of the southern United States (Fig. 136-4).

Chagas' disease typically afflicts inhabitants of a specific ecologic environment. The woodstick, frame, and mud house of the interior of South America provides the ideal site for the triatomine vector to maintain its blood-dependent life cycle. The vector propagates best in a dry environment between 27°F and 30°C from sea level to 3000 feet. Dogs and cats are important domestic reservoirs, and the presence

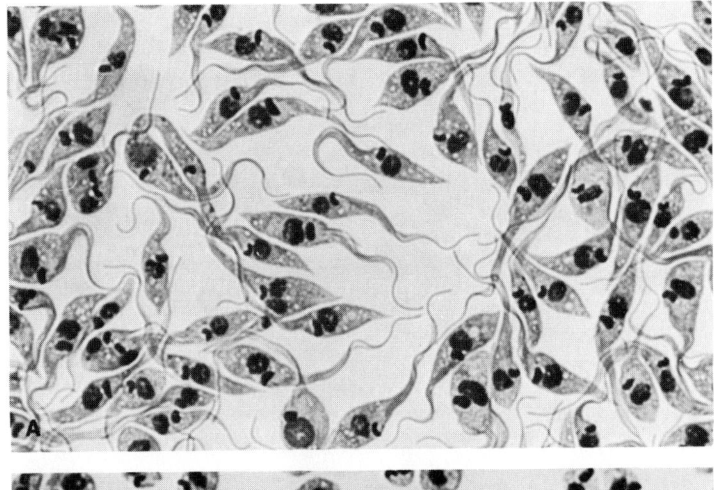

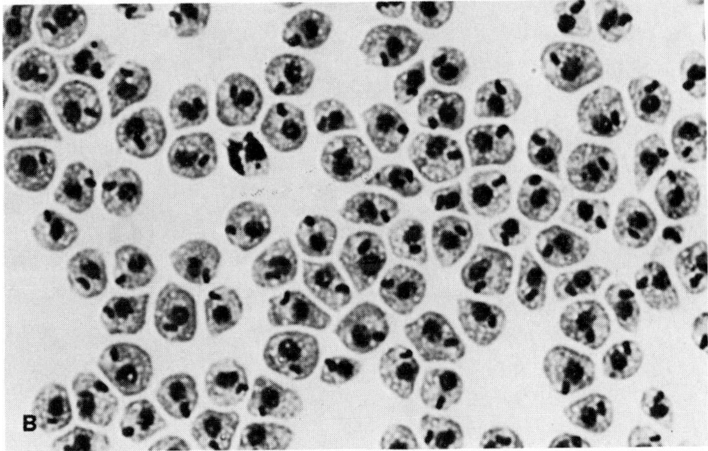

Fig. 136-2. (*A*) Epimastigote of *Trypanosoma cruzi* from F-69 culture medium. (Original magnification approximately × 1200). (*B*) Amastigotes of *Trypanosoma cruzi* from F-69 culture medium. (Original magnification approximately × 1200) (Courtesy of SC Pan, Harvard School of Public Health)

of an infected animal is an indication that there is probably seropositivity to *T. cruzi* among household members. Opossums, rats, armadillos, and native rodents are important sylvatic reservoirs.

Triatomines usually feed at night, and may remove up to 1.0 ml of blood per bug, depending upon the stage and species. During or after feedings, the vector usually defecates and the host is infected when the trypomastigotes in the feces penetrate the broken skin or conjunctival mucosa.

Pathogenesis and Pathology

Initially, after penetration into the human host, the trypomastigotes multiply in the reticuloendothelial system. Subsequently the myocardium, smooth and skeletal muscle, and at times, the central and autonomic nervous systems are invaded. The extent of destruction of these tissues in the acute phase of the disease is probably the most important determinant of the chronic state. Experimentally, lymphocytes activated by infection with *T. cruzi* may destroy myocardial cells *in vitro,* and a similar process may explain the progressive damage observed in chronic Chagas' cardiomyopathy.

In acute Chagas' cardiomyopathy, a diffuse polymorphonuclear and lymphocytic infitrate with marked myocytolysis and sometimes hemorrhage, occur in direct proportion to the intensity of invasion. Amastigote pseudocysts may be observed in the myocardium and most organs of the body in acute infections.

In chronic Chagas' cardiomyopathy, foci of lymphocytes and histiocytes, with few eosinophils, are associated with moderate fibrosis and myocytolysis (Fig. 136-1*B*). Rarely, the inflammatory infiltrate is diffuse. Degenerative lesions may be present in the intrinsic conduction system without adjacent parasites or inflammation. Perineural lymphocytic infil-

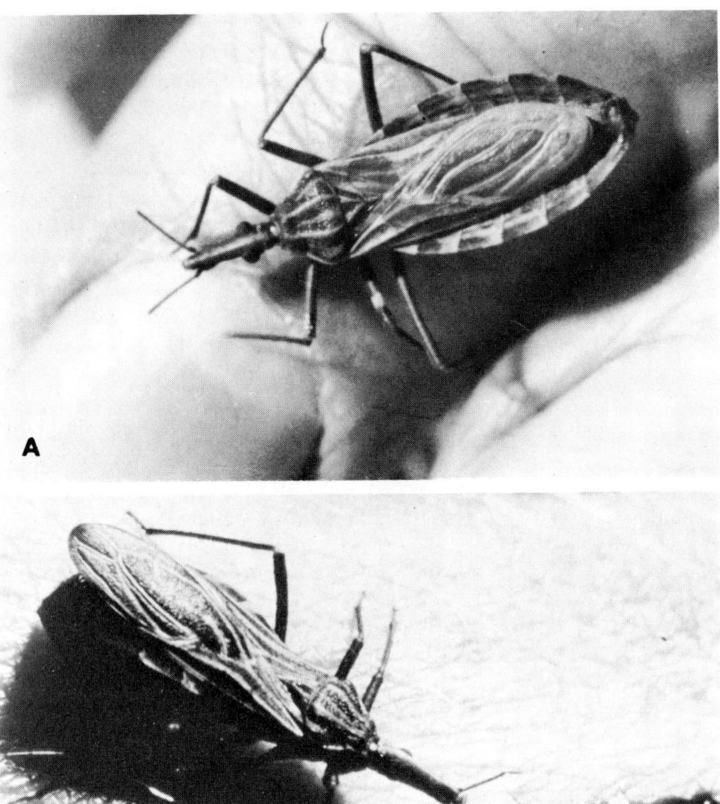

Fig. 136-3. (*A*) *Triatoma infestans* on the finger of a man. (Approximately life size) (*B*) *Rhodinus prolixus* beside recently deposited feces on the skin of a human. (Approximately life size) (Courtesy of PD Marsden, London School of Tropical Medicine)

trates and neuronophagia of the autonomic nerve ganglia of the heart may occur in acute and chronic infections. In Brazil, amastigote pseudocysts have been found in only 30% of autopsied patients with chronic cardiomyopathy attributed to infection with *T. cruzi.* On the other hand, in Venezuela, amastigotes were rarely seen in the myocardium, although *T. cruzi* were frequently isolated by xenodiagnosis from peripheral blood.

The heart in chronic Chagas' cardiomyopathy is flaccid and usually weighs more than 500 g. All the chambers are markedly enlarged, with prominent left ventricular hypertrophy. Endocardial thickening with mural thrombi in the right atrial appendage and the left ventricular apex (with or without a characteristic aneurysmal dilation) is frequent.

Destruction of the autonomic nerve plexuses and smooth muscle elements of the esophagus and colon results in the marked dilation of these organs characteristic of chronic involvement. In biopsy specimens taken from the rectums of patients with Chagas' megacolon, the nerves appear to be morphologically normal. However, there is a general decrease in the number of neurons, and the concentrations of neural and hormonal peptides is reduced.

Geographic strain differences in *T. cruzi* may be related to the isoenzyme patterns and have been cited as bases for (1) the rare occurrence of megaesophagus in Venezuela, (2) a predominance of gastrointestinal involvement in central Brazil compared to cardiac disease in northeast Brazil (3) a predominance of megacolon over megaesophagus with rare clinical cardiac disease in Chile, and (4) the high frequency of clinical acute disease in Argentina.

Manifestations

Acute Chagas' disease occurs 8 to 14 days after infection with *T. cruzi.* Frequently there are no signs of

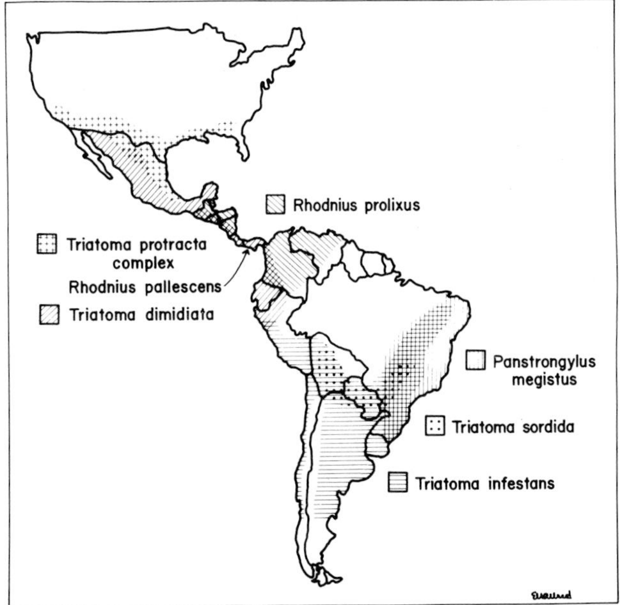

Fig. 136-4. Areas of principal vectors of *Trypanosoma cruzi.* The distribution of *Triatoma brasiliensis* is similar to that of *Triatoma sordida.* (Courtesy of Elizabeth Allred)

the portal of entry. Unilateral bipalpebral edema, often with conjunctivitis (Romaña's sign), is infrequent although pathognomonic of acute infection within endemic areas (Fig. 136-5). In some patients, a careful examination reveals an erythematous, desquamating, slightly indurated, macular area, measuring up to 4 cm in diameter (chagoma) at the site of penetration of the skin (Fig. 136-6). Fever is common and lasts 10 to 14 days or longer. The pattern may be either remitting or constant, but if the infection becomes severe, hypothermia may develop. Other complaints include malaise, irritability, anorexia, palpitations, convulsions, and watery diarrhea. The child or young adult is usually toxic and febrile with nontender, general lymphadenopathy. Tender hepatosplenomegaly, tachycardia with gallop rhythm, and general nonpitting edema may be present. Acute meningoencephalitis may occur and is usually fatal. A nephrotic syndrome is rarely associated with the acute infection. The electrocardiogram (ECG) shows slight prolongation of the P-R interval and nonspecific S-T and T-wave changes in the early stages of the disease. Leukocytosis with lymphocytosis, elevated serum glutamic and pyruvic transaminases, and bilirubin are commonly present. Elevations of IgG and IgM specific for *T. cruzi* are found in acute Chagas' disease. The cells, protein, and glucose of the cerebrospinal fluid are usually normal, although *T. cruzi* may be isolated by culture of the sediment in many acute cases.

The acute illness subsides spontaneously with gradual disappearance of *T. cruzi* from the blood in 90% of cases. The mortality among patients hospitalized with acute disease is about 10%.

After the acute infection has subsided and prior to the onset of clinical manifestations of chronic Chagas' disease, there may be persistence of antibodies to *T. cruzi* and parasitemia detected by culture or xenodiagnosis. In some patients between the ages of 15 and 25 years—usually postpartum women or active male laborers—congestive heart failure develops rapidly and is commonly fatal.

Chronic Chagas' cardiomyopathy, is manifest as palpitations, syncopal episodes, or recurrent congestive heart failure. In the most severely ill, there is an irregular pulse, marked cardiomegaly, right or left ventricular congestive heart failure, and depending on the degree of cardiac hypertrophy and dilation, a

Fig. 136-5. A child with Romaña's sign (unilateral bipalpebral edema, often with conjunctivitis), a manifestation of Chagas' disease. (Clinica de Doencas Tropicais, Federal University of Bahia, Prof Aluizio Prata)

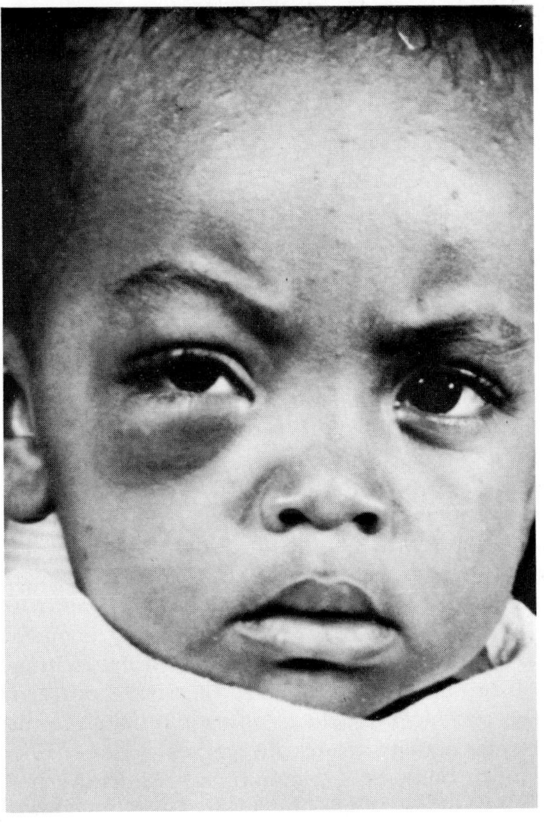

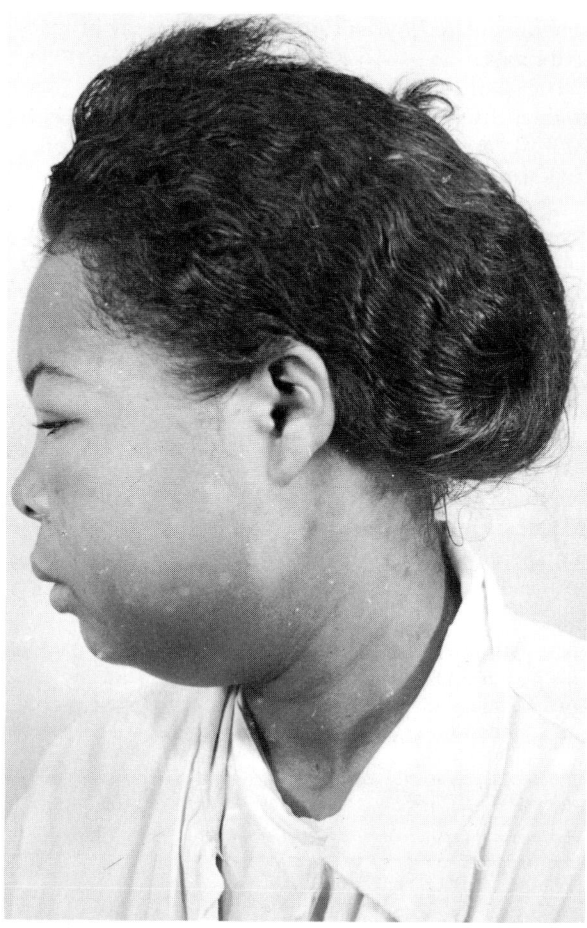

Fig. 136-6. An inoculation chagoma (irregular desquamating lesion with hypopigmentation) in a patient with acute Chagas' disease and nephrotic syndrome. (Clinica de Doencas Tropicais, Federal University of Bahia, Prof Aluizio Prata)

soft, low-grade holosystolic murmur heard over the entire precordium. The earliest asymptomatic electrocardiographic changes are a P-R interval ≥ 0.20 or, in the presence of sinus tachycardia, a P-R interval ≥ 0.17. Conduction defects, particularly bifascicular blocks (right bundle branch block with anterior fascicular block is most frequent) occur 10 to 15 years earlier than evidence of ventricular ectopic activity. Total AV block or trifascicular block may occur at any age. Left bundle branch block and atrial arrhythmias are rare. In the hospitalized patient, both ventricular conduction defects and multifocal ectopic ventricular activity are usually present.

Mural thrombosis is common and results in cerebral, renal, splenic, and pulmonary embolism in 80% of hospitalized patients. A single instance of rupture of a left ventricular apical aneurysm has been reported. Sudden death without previous symptoms is frequent in endemic areas and may result from an Adams–Stokes attack, ventricular tachycardia with fibrillation, or pulmonary embolism.

The insidious onset of dysphagia for solid foods, progressing to difficulty in swallowing liquids and regurgitation of retained food, is characteristic of megaesophagus. Peristalsis is abnormal and is accentuated by cholinergic agents. The lower esophageal spincter pressure may be elevated—frequently in early stages, and consistently in more advanced stages. Up to 40% of patients with megaesophagus also have overt cardiac disease. Persistent constipation is indicative of megacolon.

Congenital infection with *T. cruzi* is a known cause of abortion in the first trimester and neonatal morbidity in endemic areas. However, the frequency of occurrence and the specific maternal risk factors are unknown. The transmission of *T. cruzi* by the transfusion of whole blood may cause acute infection.

Diagnosis

In acute Chagas' disease, the trypomastigotes may be demonstrated by direct microscopic examination of the peripheral blood or the leukocyte layer of a capillary (microhematocrit) tube after centrifugation, or by xenodiagnosis. Xenodiagnosis involves the use of laboratory-bred triatomes (usually 5–10 fourth- or fifth-stage nymphs of *R. prolixus* or *T. infestans*), which are allowed to feed on the patient for 15 to 30 minutes. The feces or gut contents are then examined at 30 and 60 days for the presence of trypomastigotes. Local immediate and delayed hypersensitivity manifest by urticaria occurs frequently at the sites of the xenodiagnosis triatomine bites. Application of 1% hydrocortisone cream under plastic wrap reduces or eliminates this adverse reaction. Anaphylaxis during xenodiagnosis with *R. prolixus* has been reported in Venezuela.

Direct agglutination and precipitin tests become positive early in the acute infection, but are rarely used because the trypomastigotes are readily found in the blood.

The indirect immunofluorescence test (IFA), complement fixation test (CF), and enzyme-linked immunosorbent assay (ELISA) become positive within 30 days after onset of naturally acquired infection.

In chronic infections, antibodies specific for *T. cruzi* can be detected by CF, IFA, or ELISA tests.

Using reliable CF procedures and a protein epimastigote antigen (Hoechst–Behringwerke), titers of 1:4 or less are negative and titers of 1:8 or greater indicate infection. The specificity (≥ 95%) and sensitivity (≥ 98%) of CF and ELISA tests are comparable to those of syphilis serology. Specificity may be decreased in older patients with severe hypertension, coronary artery disease, or cardiomyopathy of unknown etiology; such patients frequently have low titers of antibody that cross-reacts with antigens from *T. cruzi.*

Cross-reactions occur with serums from patients with rheumatoid arthritis, acute infectious mononucleosis (Chap. 137, Infectious Mononucleosis), and leishmaniasis (Chap. 147, Leishmaniasis). The IFA test using epimastigotes from cultures or trypomastigotes from the blood is as sensitive and specific as the CF test and is advantageous in enabling the use of filter paper specimens and the testing of anticomplementary serums.

Many patients with a positive CF test and evidence of cardiomyopathy or megaesophagus also have *T. cruzi* in their blood. Repeated xenodiagnosis or cultures of whole blood in NNN medium with a tissue culture medium overlay, such as F-29, may be necessary to detect the blood-borne trypomastigotes.

Megaesophagus is best detected roentgenographically. The esophagus is narrowed at the esophagogastric junction and dilated proximally, and in extreme cases it may protrude into the right hemithorax. Esophageal motility studies using methacholine chloride (Mecholy) may be useful for diagnosis when classic changes are not present. A plain film of the abdomen may show a large fecaloma with megacolon.

In acute Chagas' disease, there is usually a fever of unknown origin with general lymphadenopathy and heptosplenomegaly that is not resolved until trypanosomes are demonstrated in the peripheral blood. Similar clinical manifestations also occur in infectious mononucleosis (Chap. 137, Infectious Mononucleosis), tuberculosis (Chap. 34, Pulmonary Tuberculosis), toxoplasmosis (Chap. 129, Toxoplasmosis), salmonellal infections (Chap. 63, Nontyphoidal Salmonelloses; Chap. 64, Typhoid Fever) rheumatoid arthritis, acute leukemia, and lymphoma.

Valvular disease on a rheumatic basis must be excluded as a cause of chronic cardiac disease. Rarely, rheumatic heart disease has been coincidental with Chagas' myocarditis. Coronary disease and hypertensive heart disease are infrequent in the age group afflicted with Chagas' myocarditis. Other causes of cardiomegaly should be considered, such as toxoplasmal myocarditis, endomyocardial fibrosis, alcoholic myocardiopathy, viral myocarditis, and idiopathic myocardiopathy. Definitive diagnosis is more often accomplished with Chagas' myocarditis.

The presence of megaesophagus does not exclude the possibility of idiopathic achalasia or esophageal carcinoma. Associated cardiac lesions or a history of residence in an endemic area help define the etiology. Megacolon of the entire large bowel is also seen in severely ill persons with toxic megacolon and ulcerative colitis.

Congenital syphilis (Chap. 59, Syphilis), listeriosis (Chap. 51, Listeriosis), toxoplasmosis (Chap. 129, Toxoplasmosis), and rubella (Chap. 87, Rubella) are also causes of abortion, stillbirth, and neonatal death.

Prognosis

The course of untreated acute or chronic Chagas' disease is unpredictable. In the acute disease, signs of meningeal involvement with convulsions, or congestive heart failure with ventricular conduction defects or ventricular ectopic activity, are associated with increased mortality. Of persons hospitalized with acute Chagas' disease 10% die of meningoencephalitis or myocarditis.

The prognosis of asymptomatic persons whose diagnosis rests solely on a positive serologic test for antibodies specific for *T. cruzi* is unknown. Conduction defects, as in coronary artery disease, may progress to total AV block. Total AV block with cardiac enlargement, recurrent palpitations, and congestive heart failure indicate a negative prognosis. The peak incidence of mortality attributable to Chagas' cardiomyopathy occurs between 25 and 44 years of age: the fatality rate is greater among males than among females.

Megaesophagus and megacolon carry no specific prognosis if unassociated with cardiac lesions. Aspiration pneumonia from the regurgitation of food, or lipoid pneumonia after the aspiration of mineral oil, occurs in the late stages of megaesophagus. Volvulus of the large bowel secondary to fecaloma with megacolon is common in endemic areas.

Although some degree of protective immunity has been observed experimentally, no protective immunity has been demonstrated in humans. The importance of reinfection is unknown.

Therapy

Acute Chagas' disease should be treated immediately after parasitological confirmation of the diagnosis. Either nifurtimox (Lampit) or benzonidazole

(Rochagan) may be used. In the United States, these drugs may be obtained from the Parasitic Disease Service, Centers for Disease Control, Atlanta, GA 30336. Weekly surveillance of their use should include complete blood counts, assessments of hepatic and renal functions, and monitoring of the parasitemia.

Nifurtimox acts by inhibiting *T. cruzi* through increased production of $\ddot{O}_2$ and H_2O_2 inside the protozoa. The dose in adults is 10 mg/kg body wt/day, PO, for 120 days. Children are given 25 mg/kg body wt/day, PO, for 14 days, followed by 15 mg/kg, PO, for 100 days. Adverse effects occur in fewer than 5% of patients and include nausea, vomiting, diarrhea, polyneuritis, and leukopenia; they reverse when the drug is stopped.

Benzonidazole is given in a dose of 5 mg/kg body wt/day, PO, for 60 days. Adverse effects develop in fewer than 5% of patients, and include polyneuritis, granulocytopenia, fever, and morbilliform rash; they disappear when the treatment is stopped.

Specific treatment is not recommended for chronic Chagas' disease as diagnosed by seroreactivity alone, without demonstration of *T. cruzi* in the blood either by culture or xenodiagnosis. The chronic cardiomyopathy of Chagas' disease is not reversed by chemotherapy.

Conservative treatment is most appropriate for patients with congestive failure from chronic Chagas' myocarditis. The judicious use of potassium salts, diuretics, and moderate salt restriction is recommended. Antiarrhythmic agents such as lidocaine and procainamide may be used in emergency situations. If digitalis is used, it must be given cautiously because of the extreme myocardial irritability, especially in the presence of hypokalemia.

In chronic Chagas' cardiomyopathy, total AV block and less severe defects of ventricular conduction appear to be indications for implanting a pacemaker if the arrhythmias are symptomatic, the heart is normal in size, and myocardial reserve is adequate as evaluated by cardiac catheterization. Dilation of the terminal esophagus is recommended in the early stages of megaesophagus. In later stages, surgical resection is widely used to alleviate retention. The formation of a fecaloma and subsequent volvulus can be avoided by the surgical resection of megacolon or megarectum.

Prevention

Chagas' disease is primarily a consequence of socioeconomic deprivation. The house of the occupant determines the initial infection and subsequent reexposure. The construction of solid-wall houses eliminates domestic habitats of the vector. Adequate data are now available that document the high cost of repeated spraying necessary to eliminate triatomine bugs permanently. Even if the domestic cycle were controlled, the zootic cycle would remain a potential source for infection of humans.

Transmission of *T. cruzi* infection through blood transfusion is an increasing public health problem. Persons who are seroreactive to *T. cruzi* by a valid immunodiagnostic test are not acceptable as blood donors. As many as 20% of the donors in endemic areas are seroreactive to *T. cruzi* antigens. In a major South American city, 30% of seroreactive urban residents were found to have received a blood transfusion. The risk of transmission of *T. cruzi* in whole blood may be reduced by adding gentian violet to a final concentration of 0.1 mg or amphotericin B.

In endemic areas, patients undergoing renal transplantation or receiving immunosuppressive chemotherapy should be screened for infection with *T. cruzi.*

Remaining Problems

The geographic variations in Chagas' disease may be epidemiologic evidences of the existence of many strains of *T. cruzi;* comparative immunologic, biochemical, and pathologic studies are needed. Longitudinal field studies of the natural history of Chagas' disease are needed to balance the many hospital-centered observations. Study of the ecology of the vector and nonhuman reservoirs may reveal ways of interrupting transmission of the disease to man. The mechanism(s) of persistence of *T. cruzi* for 20 to 30 years within the human host, despite the development of humoral and cellular immunity, is unexplained; is such persistence related to the development of cardiomyopathy and megaesophagus? Standardization of antigen for serologic tests for epidemiologic studies is necessary.

Bibliography

Books

BRENER Z, ANDRADE Z: Trypanosoma cruzi e Doenca de Chagas. Rio de Janeiro, Editora Guanabara Koogan SA, 1979. 463 pp.

SANTOS–BUCH CA: American trypanosomiasis: Chagas' disease. In Miescher PA (ed): Immunopathology, VIIth International Symposium. Basel, Schwabe & Co, 1976. pp 205–220.

Journals

BITTENCOURT AL: Congenital Chagas' Disease. Am J Dis Child 130:97–103, 1976

CHAGAS C: Nova Tripanozomiaze humana: Estudos sobre a morfologia e o ciclo evolutivo do Schizotrypanum cruzi n. gen., n. sp., agente etiolojico de nova entidade morbida do homen. Mem Inst Cruz 1:159–218, 1909

Enfermedad de Chagas. Medicina (Buenos Aires) 40 (Suppl 1):3–259, 1980

HOFF R, TEIXEIRA R, CARVALHO, JS, MOTT KE: *Trypanosoma cruzi* in the cerebrospinal fluid during the acute stage of Chagas' disease. N Engl J Med 298:604–606, 1978

LONG RG, Neural and hormonal peptides in rectal biopsy specimens from patients with Chagas' disease and chronic automonic failure. Lancet 1:559–562, 1980

MAGUIRE JH, MOTT KE, SOUZA JAA, ALMEIDA EC, RAMOS NB, GUIMARAES AC: Electrocardiographic classification and abbreviated lead system for population-based studies of Chagas' disease. Bull Pan Am Health Organ 16:47–58, 1982

MOTT KE, LEHMAN JS, HOFF R: The epidemiology and household distribution of seroreactivity to *Trypanosoma cruzi* in a rural community in Northeast Brazil. Am J Trop Med Hyg 25:552–562, 1976

PAN SC: *Trypanosoma cruzi* cultivation in macromolecule-free semisynthetic and synthetic media. Exp Parasitol 46:108–112, 1978

WOODY NC, WOODY HB: American trypanosomiasis. I. Clinical and epidemiological background of Chagas' disease in the United States. J Pediatr 58:568–580, 1961

Section XVIII

Infections of the Hematopoietic–Lymphoreticular System

Indigenous Microbiota of the Hematopoietic–Lymphoreticular System

(None)

JAMES C. NIEDERMAN

Infectious Mononucleosis

137

Infectious mononucleosis is an acute lymphoproliferative disease that is most common in children and young adults and is caused by the Epstein–Barr virus (EBV). Characteristic clinical features include: (1) fever, sore throat, and lymphadenopathy; (2) an associated absolute lymphocytosis including more than 10% atypical lymphocytes in the peripheral blood; (3) development of transient heterophile and persistent antibody responses against Epstein–Barr virus; and (4) abnormal liver function tests.

Etiology

EBV is one of the herpes viruses (Chap. 1, Attributes of Infectious Agents). It was first identified in 1964 in electron-microscopic studies of tumor cell lines derived from biopsies of Burkitt lymphoma that had been maintained in long-term cultures. Later, it was demonstrated by immunofluorescence and electron microscopy in cultures of peripheral blood leukocytes obtained from patients both during acute infectious mononucleosis and years thereafter. The virus is not readily discerned in fresh lymphocytes collected during the acute phase of disease; however, culture of peripheral blood leukocytes yields continuous cell lines in which each cell contains the EBV genome and expresses Epstein–Barr virus-determined nuclear antigen (EBNA).

In prospective clinical studies, specific EBV antibodies are regularly lacking before the onset of mononucleosis and develop during disease. As each biologic property of EBV has been discovered, it has been demonstrated that antibody responses to it are lacking before infectious mononucleosis and appear during the course of disease. These are usually measured by tests using immunofluorescence techniques for the demonstration of viral capsid, early, membrane, and nuclear antibodies. EBV-specific IgM is present in serums collected 1 to 6 weeks after onset and usually disappears in 3 to 6 months. On the other hand, EBV-specific IgG responses, also present during early illness, regularly persist and have been demonstrated as many as 52 years after clinical disease.

Transmission of EBV to antibody-negative humans by blood transfusion has been associated with acquisition of EBV antibody and occasionally with the development of heterophil-positive, clinical infectious mononucleosis.

EBV is present in saliva obtained from patients with acute infectious mononucleosis, and excretion of EBV from the oropharynx continues intermittently many months after the acute illness. Since the agent is invariably present in cell-free form in saliva and has been recovered in secretions from parotid gland orifices and ducts, the salivary glands appear to be sites of production of oropharyngeal EBV.

Epidemiology

Humans the world over are infected with EBV. The most nearly characteristic epidemiologic feature is occurrence of the disease among young adults, especially in the 15 to 25 year age group. Neither yearly nor seasonal variations occur in the general population; however, in college-age groups, early fall and early spring are periods of high frequency. In adolescence, females appear to develop clinical disease somewhat earlier than males. Among college-age susceptibles, the annual attack rate is approximately 12% per year, with a ratio of apparent to inapparent infections of 1:2 to 1:3.

Seroepidemiologic studies have demonstrated that the lack of EBV antibody correlates with susceptibility to the infection, whereas the presence of antibody corresponds to immunity. Prospective studies over periods of 4 to 8 years in more than 5000 children and young adults throughout the world support this relationship. Although EBV seroconversion developed in 29% of susceptibles, the clinical attack rate was 2% among the antibody-negative subjects.

Hygienic and background socioeconomic factors generally determine the age at which EBV infection occurs. In groups from tropical and developing areas, specific EBV antibodies are acquired early in life and high prevalence rates are found in young children. Among individuals living in more advantageous socioeconomic conditions, exposure to EBV is delayed, and only 50% to 60% of older children and young adults have demonstrable serum antibodies.

Pathogenesis and Pathology

EBV is present in saliva from patients with acute infectious mononucleosis, and excretion of virus from the oropharynx continues for many months after clinical disease—long after atypical lymphocytes and heterophil antibody have disappeared. Demonstration of the prolonged carrier state not only shed light on pathogenesis but also explained the moderate contagiousness and the difficulty in demonstrating case-to-case transmission. EBV has been detected in throat washings of approximately 20% of healthy, seropositive subjects who have no history of infectious mononucleosis, indicating that oropharyngeal excretion is also common after inapparent infection. Although EBV has been recovered from secretions from parotid gland orifices and ducts, the specificity of the producer cell is not known. Conceivably, low-level, long-term oropharyngeal production of EBV stimulates maintenance of specific antibodies.

In the usual nonfatal case of infectious mononucleosis, the sequence of events initiated by EBV is associated with a self-limited lymphoid response. Viremia presumably occurs inasmuch as the entire lymphoreticular system is involved. Lymphadenopathy, nasopharyngeal lymphoid hyperplasia and splenomegaly develop. Widespread focal and perivascular aggregates of mononuclear cells are present throughout the body. Nonlymphoid organs including liver, lungs, kidneys, heart, and central nervous system are sites of focal infiltrations that may be associated with functional abnormalities. The bone marrow shows marked generalized hyperplasia; in some cases, small granulomas are present. The lymphoproliferative reactions are due to activated or atypical T-lymphocytes, presumably responding to EBV-infected B cells in lymph nodes and peripheral blood.

Manifestations

In the adult, an incubation period of 30 to 50 days has been suggested on the basis of contact infections. Mononucleosis associated with the development of both heterophil and EBV antibodies has been reported in several cases 5 weeks after blood transfusions. It is thought that children may have a shorter (10–14 days) incubation period.

During a prodromal period of 4 to 5 days, dissemination of EBV throughout the body is associated with mild symptoms including headache, malaise and fatigue. The clinical features of the acute disease that follows are extremely variable in severity and include fever, sore throat, and cervical adenopathy in more than 80% of patients. Children may have little or no fever associated with infection, but in adults daily fluctuations in the range of 38°C to 39°C (101°F–102°F) during late afternoon and evening may continue for 7 to 10 days. In severe cases, temperature elevations to 40.6°C (105°F) may be present.

Sore throat is virtually a regular feature of infectious mononucleosis and develops during the first week of disease. Diffuse pharyngeal inflammation and edema are present and an exudative tonsillitis with a gray–white exudate occurs in approximately 50% of cases and persists for 7 to 10 days. At the end of the first week of illness, petechiae are present at the border of the hard and soft palates in about 30% of patients. This enanthem consists of 5 to 20 reddish, circumscribed petechiae and is suggestive, but not pathognomonic, of the disease.

Tender lymphadenopathy is a hallmark of infectious mononucleosis. Anterior and posterior cervical nodes are most frequently involved; however, generalized lymphadenopathy, including axillary, epitrochlear, mediastinal, and mesenteric nodes may occur. The nodes, usually 5 mm to 25 mm in diameter, are firm, tense, and discrete and may be enlarged singly or in clusters. Lymphadenopathy slowly subsides over several weeks, depending on the degree and extent of enlargement during acute disease.

Of patients with acute infectious mononucleosis, 50% develop splenomegaly, which is usually maximal during the second and third weeks of disease. Although rare, rupture of the spleen is one of the few potentially fatal complications; severe abdominal pain in infectious mononucleosis is unusual except in the presence of splenic rupture, a development necessitating immediate splenectomy.

Early in the disease, approximately 10% of patients develop a faint, erythematous, maculopapular eruption on the trunk and proximal extremities. The rash may simulate rubella, but may be hemorrhagic, urticarial, or scarlatiniform in appearance. Bilateral supraorbital edema may also be an early clinical feature.

Although hepatomegaly is detectable in only 10% of patients, liver function tests, especially serum transaminase values, are abnormal for several weeks in almost all cases. However, jaundice rarely develops in more than 5% of cases and is usually mild.

Infectious mononucleosis may be associated with pneumonia, pleuritis, and pleural effusion. No specific radiologic findings characterize the pneumonitis accompanying EBV infections, although the presence of hilar adenopathy has been emphasized. In childhood pneumonia, EBV may be a primary or secondary pathogen, or may be reactivated during pulmonary infection with other agents.

Fewer than 1% of patients, usually adults, develop syndromes referable to the central nervous system: aseptic meningitis, Bell's palsy, meningoencephalitis, transverse myelitis, Guillain–Barré syndrome, and acute cerebellar ataxia. Recovery is usually complete, although fatalities have been associated with encephalitis, and severe paralysis has been reported. Antibodies to EBV have been detected in the cerebrospinal fluid of patients with meningoencephalitis as the principal manifestation of mononucleosis. EBV has been found to be cell-associated in cerebrospinal fluid.

Diagnosis

The diagnosis of infectious mononucleosis is made on the basis of clinical manifestations and specific laboratory findings. The latter include a characteristic change in the blood and elevated titers of heterophil and EBV antibodies.

Laboratory Findings

Essential to the diagnosis is an increase in the relative and absolute number of lymphocytes and atypical lymphocytes. During disease, cells of the lymphocytic series may constitute 50% to 60% of peripheral blood leukocytes. Either the total leukocyte count is normal, or there is a slight leukopenia during the first week. During the second and third weeks of illness, the total count may increase to 20,000 with a relative and absolute lymphocytosis. Occasionally, the leukocytosis may range as high as 50,000 per mm^3.

Atypical lymphocytes, also known as Downey cells, glandular fever cells, and virocytes, usually represent at least 10% of the total leukocytes. They vary in size and staining qualities. The nucleus may be lobulated or indented and the cytoplasm is vacuolated and basophilic. B-lymphocytes in which EBV has multiplied and produced EBV nuclear antigen, constitute the majority of the early atypical lymphocytosis in infectious mononucleosis. During later stages of clinical disease, atypical lymphocytes are largely composed of T cells with an immunoregulatory function. Identical atypical cells have also been found in patients with acute viral hepatitis (Chap. 70, Hepatitis A; Chap. 71, Hepatitis B; Chap. 72, Non-A, Non-B Hepatitis), cytomegalovirus infection (Chap. 75, Cytomegalovirus Infections), rubella (Chap. 87, Rubella), rubeola (Chap. 86, Measles,), roseola (Chap. 88, Other Exanthems), mumps (Chap. 74, Mumps) and various other infectious and immunologic and lympho-proliferative disorders. In these conditions, however, the percentage of circulating atypical lymphocytes is usually less than 10%.

Anemia is rare in uncomplicated cases of infectious mononucleosis. Slight to moderate thrombocytopenia, usually asymptomatic, has been reported during the early weeks of disease.

Heterophil antibodies, that is, agglutinins for sheep erythrocytes, were first reported to be elevated in infectious mononucleosis by Paul and Bunnell in 1932. Although both the mechanism of heterophil antibody production and the source of heterophil antigen are unclear, the heterophil antibody of infectious mononucleosis is associated with IgM immunoglobulin and differs from other antibodies in human serums that also agglutinate sheep erythrocytes. The latter are found in relatively high titers in serum sickness and at lower levels in normal human serums (Forsmann agglutinins). Differentiation of these various heterophil antibodies is based on absorption techniques using guinea pig kidney tissue and beef erythrocytes (Table 137-1).

Sheep cell agglutinins usually develop during the first week of illness in adults, but occasionally their appearance is delayed. In one group of 166 patients, the heterophil antibody test was positive in 38% during the first week, 60% during the second week, and approximately 80% during the third week of illness. Heterophil antibodies persist for 3 to 6 months, but

Table 137-1. *Differentiation of the Heterophil Antibodies of Infectious Mononucleosis, Serum Sickness, and Normal Serum*

	Heterophil Antibody Titer		
		AFTER ABSORPTION WITH	
	NO TREATMENT	GUINEA PIG KIDNEY	BOVINE ERYTHROCYTES
Infectious mononucleosis	++	+	–
Serum sickness	++	–	–
Normal serum (Forssman)	+	–	+

rarely longer. In general, the higher the titer developed during the acute illness, the longer antibodies remain detectable during convalescence. However, in some cases clinically consistent with infectious mononucleosis, the heterophil antibody response is either transient or lacking. Development of EBV antibody has been demonstrated in these heterophil negative cases, which are common in infants and children.

Several qualitative tests for heterophil antibodies that use formalin-treated horse erythrocytes, beef red cells, or enzyme-treated and untreated sheep erythrocytes have been introduced. In the sheep or horse red cell agglutination tests, a titer of 1:40 or greater after absorption is considered diagnostic, and a rising titer indicates recent infection. The beef hemolysin test is highly specific, but usually becomes negative within 3 months after clinical illness. The horse red cell agglutination test is the most sensitive; elevated titers may persist over a year. It is useful in childhood infections, which may be heterophil negative by other tests. An immune adherence heterophil test of similar sensitivity has been developed.

Antibodies to EBV-associated antigens can be assayed by (1) immunofluorescence techniques that demonstrate viral capsid, early, membrane, and nuclear antigen (EBNA); (2) complement fixation; (3) immunodiffusion; (4) enzyme-linked immunosorbent assay; and (5) neutralization. The most widely used test is the immunofluorescence antibody technique demonstrating viral capsid antigen (VCA); in general, a titer of 1:40 to 1:160 develops during early disease, and significant increases in antibody are found in approximately 20% of cases.

EBV antibodies are lacking in pre-illness serums, but develop regularly during the course of infectious mononucleosis. The relationships between clinical symptoms, lymphocyte changes, and antibody levels in typical heterophil-positive cases are shown in Figure 137-1. Development of persistent VCA and neutralizing antibodies occurs early in disease, whereas EBNA antibodies arise one or more months after onset of disease. Viral-capsid-specific IgM and IgA antibodies appear during early infection, but like heterophil antibodies, they are transient responses and usually decline and disappear after several months. Responses to the D component of EBV-induced early antigens are observed in approximately 70% to 80% of patients during acute disease and persist for 3 to 6 months.

No correlation has been found between the levels of EBV and heterophil antibodies, or between the anti-EBV titer and the severity of symptoms. Heterophil antibody titers are highest during the first 4 weeks after onset; anti-EBV responses also reach peak titers within 2 to 4 weeks and persist for many years—probably for life. An EBV-VCA antibody titer of 1:40 has been demonstrated in serum collected 52 years after heterophil-positive infectious mononucleosis.

Clinical Aspects

Infectious mononucleosis may resemble a number of febrile illnesses, particularly those associated with lymphocytosis and atypical lymphocytes. Conditions frequently confused with acute-phase infectious mononucleosis include streptococcal pharyngitis and tonsillitis (Chap. 24, Streptococcal Diseases), nonbacterial exudative tonsillitis (Chap. 23, Nonbacterial Pharyngitis), diphtheria (Chap. 25, Diphtheria) and Vincent's angina. Differentiation may be accomplished by throat culture for bacteria, response to antimicrobics in the case of streptococcal disease, laboratory measurements of lymphatic and hepatic abnormalities, and assays for heterophil and EBV antibodies.

Blood dyscrasias and lymphoproliferative disorders must be considered when fever, lymphocytosis, lymphadenopathy, and splenomegaly are present. Laboratory studies, including bone marrow examination, and serologic tests are essential for establishing the proper diagnosis.

Infectious mononucleosis with jaundice may be confused with acute viral hepatitis infection (Chap. 70, Hepatitis A; Chap. 71, Hepatitis B; Chap. 72, Non-A, Non-B Hepatitis). During the preicteric febrile stages of acute hepatitis, there is often a transitory lymphocytosis; however, the hematologic changes in infectious mononucleosis are more persistent, and the percentage of atypical lymphocytes is usually higher. Demonstration of heterophil and EBV antibodies is helpful in differentiating these infections.

The prodromal stage of rubella (Chap. 87, Rubella) associated with fever, malaise, lymphadenopathy and lymphocytosis may be indistinguishable from infectious mononucleosis. The transient rash that develops in about 10% of patients with infectious mononucleosis is less extensive than rubella and is usually prominent only on the trunk and proximal extremities. Of greater value is the presence of large numbers of atypical lymphocytes and demonstration of rising or elevated titers of heterophil or EBV antibodies. Isolation of rubella virus from the throat and demonstration of a rise in rubella antibody titer confirms the diagnosis.

Cytomegalovirus mononucleosis usually involves an older age group than does infectious mononucleosis. Pharyngitis and cervical adenopathy are not char-

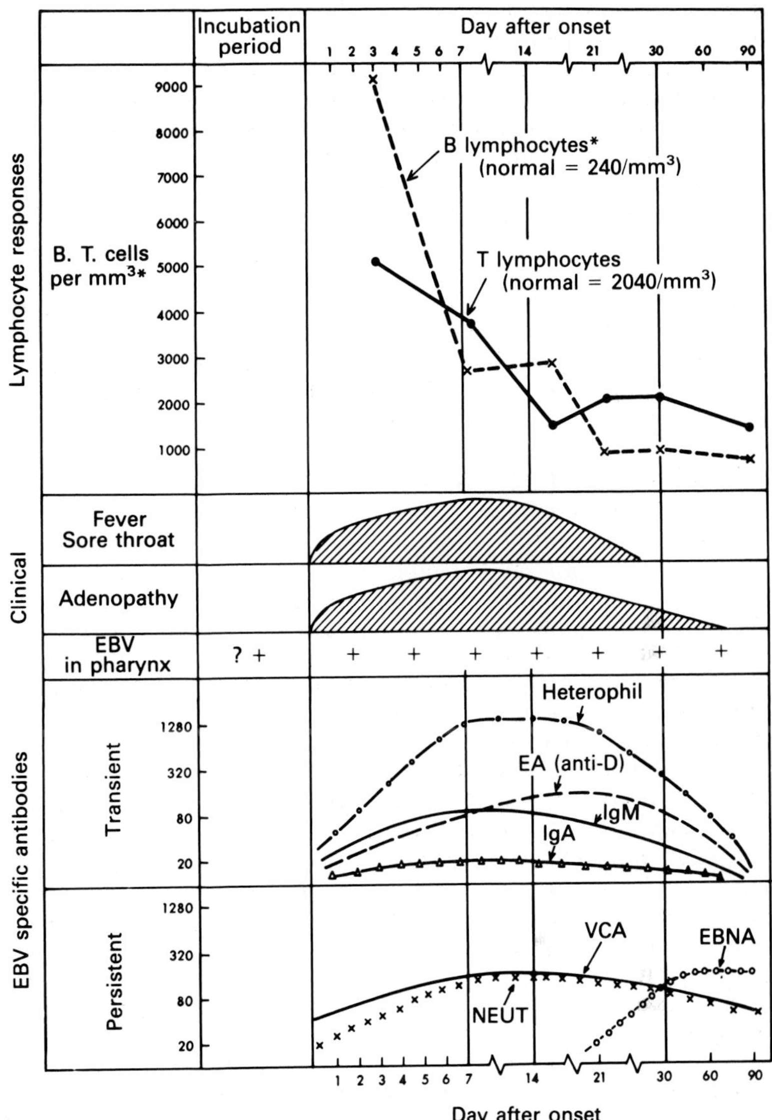

Fig. 137-1. Scheme of symptoms, lymphocyte responses, antibody production, and EBV oropharyngeal excretion in typical infectious mononucleosis.

acteristic, but splenomegaly, hepatic involvement and atypical lymphocytosis are common features of this infection (Chap. 75, Cytomegalovirus Infections). Cases may be sporadic or may follow multiple blood transfusions. The diagnosis may be made by isolation of cytomegalovirus from urine or detection of an antibody rise measured by indirect hemagglutination or immunofluorescence. Demonstration of CMV-IgM antibody by immunofluorescence techniques is consistent with current or recent infection.

Aseptic meningitis may be a presenting feature of early infectious mononucleosis, and the presence of antibodies to EBV-VCA has been demonstrated in cerebrospinal fluid. Serologic tests are required for differentiation of other forms of aseptic meningitis (Chap. 118, Viral Meningitis).

Acquired *Toxoplasma gondii* infections (Chap. 129, Toxoplasmosis) may be associated with fever, lymphadenopathy, and splenomegaly. Pharyngitis is rare, and liver function tests are normal. Definitive diagnosis is based on isolation of the agent from lymph node biopsy material; a high titer in the Sabin–Feldman dye test and the presence of toxoplasma IgM antibody by immunofluorescence are other specific diagnostic procedures.

Infectious lymphocytosis is a benign childhood disease of obscure etiology that may occur in epidemic form. Most patients have fever, upper respiratory symptoms, lymphadenopathy and occasionally diarrhea. The significant characteristic is a lymphocytosis consisting of small mature lymphocytes. This abnormal blood picture usually persists for 4 to 5 weeks, the heterophil antibody test is regularly negative, and no association with EBV infection has been demonstrated.

Prognosis

Most cases of infectious mononucleosis are mild or moderate in severity; the acute illness usually lasts 2 to 3 weeks, and patients recover uneventfully with resumption of their normal activities in 4 to 6 weeks. Rarely, symptoms persist for several months, and laboratory abnormalities resolve slowly.

Major complications are infrequent and occur in less than 5% of cases. Neurologic involvement may be associated with severe sequelae including the Guillain–Barré syndrome and toxic encephalopathy. EBV has been implicated in an X-linked recessive lymphoproliferative syndrome, and both lytic and proliferative manifestations have developed in one kindred. These include fatal infectious mononucleosis, malignant lymphoma, and agammaglobulinemia. Defects in humoral and cell-mediated immune responses to EBV or in production of interferon have been demonstrated in these cases.

Splenic rupture, associated with severe abdominal pain, may be fatal if the condition is not recognized and treated by transfusions and splenectomy.

Hemolytic anemia, agranulocytosis, and thrombocytopenia with hemorrhagic features have been reported, but are uncommon. Rarely, cardiac complications manifested by myocarditis or pericarditis have been observed, and minor electrocardiographic abnormalities have been described. Airway obstruction resulting from severe tonsillopharyngeal inflammation and edema requires prompt intubation or tracheostomy. A general skin rash associated with administration of ampicillin may occur in both EBV and cytomegalovirus mononucleosis.

Therapy

The treatment of infectious mononucleosis is supportive. Antimicrobial agents do not influence the course of EBV infection unless there is a concomitant tonsillopharyngeal beta-hemolytic streptococcal infection—as occurs in 20% of cases. During the acute febrile period, bed rest is advisable. Salicylates or other analgesics usually relieve the associated sore throat and headache; in severe cases, codeine or meperidine (Demerol) may be necessary. Gargling or throat irrigations with warm saline solutions often provide symptomatic relief of pharyngitis and stomatitis.

In patients who have severe pharyngotonsillitis with oropharyngeal edema and airway encroachment, a short course of treatment with glucosteroids is helpful through a prompt anti-inflammatory effect (40–60 mg of prednisone on the first day, decreasing the dose by 5 mg each day, terminating the treatment in 7–10 days). Pharmacologic doses of glucosteroids, (*e.g.,* prednisone, 1 mg/kg body wt/day) should be used in the management of other rare complications such as neurologic sequelae, thrombocytopenic purpura, hemolytic anemia, myocarditis, and pericarditis.

Glucosteroids should not be used in the treatment of the usual benign cases of infectious mononucleosis. Controlled studies of glucosteroid therapy in uncomplicated disease failed to demonstrate any effect on duration of clinical disease other than decreasing the febrile period.

Prevention

EBV infections occur in all human populations, and existing sociohygienic factors determine the age of acquisition of infection. There is no known way to prevent subclinical infection or the overt disease, since the lymphoproliferative changes are not caused by EBV-infected B cells, but rather result from activated T-lymphocytes responding to the virus itself or to virus-infected cells.

Remaining Problems

Further characterization of EBV-associated antigens and their corresponding antibodies would be of value to understanding the pathophysiology of infectious mononucleosis. Questions concerning EBV replication in cells other than B-lymphocytes persist. The demonstration of an EBV receptor and viral genome in nasopharyngeal carcinoma cells suggests that special epithelial cells elsewhere may be subject to infection. Investigations should be undertaken of possible sites of EBV persistence, including salivary gland, lymph node and splenic tissues, and peripheral blood.

Liberation of EBV from its restricted position in Burkitt lymphoma cells or lymphocytes from patients with EBV infections and adaptation of the virus for growth in non-neoplastic tissue culture systems are essential steps in future development of a vaccine.

Bibliography

Journals

EPSTEIN MA, ACHONG BG: Pathogenesis of infectious mononucleosis. Lancet 2:1270–1273, 1977

EPSTEIN MA, ACHONG BG: Recent progress in Epstein–Barr virus research. Ann Rev Microbiol 31:421–445, 1977

HENLE G, HENLE W, DIEHL V: Relation of Burkitt's tumor associated herpes-type virus to infectious mononucleosis. Proc Nat Acad Sci 59:94–101, 1968

MANGI RJ, NIEDERMAN JC, KELLEHER JE, DWYER JM, EVANS AS, KANTOR FS: Depression of cell-mediated immunity during acute infectious mononucleosis. N. Engl J Med 291:1149–1153, 1974

MILLER G: Epstein–Barr herpes virus and infectious mononucleosis. Prog Med Virol 20:84–112, 1975

MILLER G, NIEDERMAN JC, ANDREWS L: Prolonged oropharyngeal excretion of EB virus following infectious mononucleosis. N Engl J Med 288:229–232, 1973

MORGAN DG, NIEDERMAN JC, MILLER G, SMITH HW, DOWALIBY JM: Site of Epstein–Barr virus replication in the oropharynx. Lancet 2:1154–1157, 1979

NIEDERMAN JC, MCCOLLUM RW, HENLE G, HENLE W: Infectious mononucleosis: Clinical manifestations in relation to EB virus antibodies. JAMA 203:205–209, 1968

NIEDERMAN JC, EVANS AS, SUBRAMANYAN L, MCCOLLUM RW: Prevalence, incidence and persistence of EB virus antibody in young adults. N Engl J Med 282:361–365, 1970

NIEDERMAN JC, MILLER G, PEARSON HA, PAGANO JS, DOWALIBY JM: Infectious mononucleosis: EB virus shedding in saliva and the oropharynx. N Engl J Med 294:1355–1359, 1976

PURTILO DT: Epstein–Barr-virus-induced oncogenesis in immune deficient individuals. Lancet 1:300–303, 1980

PURTILO DT, BHAWAN J, HUTT LM, DENICOLA L, SZYMANSKI I, YANG JPS, BOTO M, THORLEY–LAWSON D: Epstein–Barr virus infections in the X-linked recessive lymphoproliferative syndrome. Lancet 1:798–801, 1978

PURTILO DT, HUTT L, BHAWAN J, YANG JPS, CASSELL C, ALLEGRO S, ROSEN FS: Immunodeficiency to the Epstein–Barr virus in the X-linked recessive lymphoproliferative syndrome. Clin Immunol Immunopathol 9:147–156, 1978

ROBINSON JE, BROWN N, ANDIMAN W, HALLIDAY K, FRANCKE U, ROBERT MF, ANDERSSON–ANVRET M, HORSTMANN D, MILLER G: Diffuse polyclonal B cell lymphoma during primary infection with Epstein–Barr virus. N Engl J Med 302:1293–1297, 1980

ROBINSON J, SMITH D, NIEDERMAN JC: Mitotic EBNA-positive lymphocytes in peripheral blood during infectious mononucleosis. Nature 287:334–335, 1980

ROBINSON J, SMITH D, NIEDERMAN J: Plasmacytic differentiation in circulating Epstein–Barr virus-infected B lymphocytes during acute infectious mononucleosis. J Exp Med 153:235–244, 1981

WENDELL H. HALL
MOHAMMED Y. KHAN

138 Brucellosis

Brucellosis is an infectious disease of nonhuman mammals that is contagious for man; it is caused by *Brucella* spp. Pregnant animals are particularly susceptible and often abort. In man, the acute infection is manifested by fever, chills, and weakness, usually without any localizing signs. Chronic infection may cause fever, weakness, anxiety, depression, and abscesses in the bones, spleen, liver, kidneys, or brain.

Etiology

The *Brucella* spp. classically infective for humans are *B. melitensis, B. suis, and B. abortus.* Of three newly recognized species (*B. ovis* in sheep and hares, *B. neotomae* in desert wood rats, and *B. canis* in dogs), *B. canis* may also cause disease in humans. All are gram-negative, small (0.5–0.7 μm × 0.6 μm to 1.5 μm), aerobic bacilli that are nonmotile and lack spores or capsules. They grow slowly, but optimally, in Albimi brucella broth at 37°C and a pH of 6.7. On solid mediums, *Brucella* spp. usually grow as smooth, translucent, blue–white to amber colonies. *Brucella canis* and *B. ovis* grow as rough, somewhat mucoid colonies. On primary isolation, *B. abortus* and *B. ovis* require an atmosphere of 10% carbon dioxide.

Differentiation of the *Brucella* spp. can be made by means of biochemical, metabolic, and immunologic tests (Table 138-1). Further differentiation within species on the basis of biochemical differences enables the distinction of nine biotypes of *B. abortus* three each of *B. suis* and *B. melitensis.* Most *Brucella* spp. are pathogenic for guinea pigs, rabbits, and mice, but not for rats and birds.

Epidemiology

Brucellosis in humans was first described in 1861 by Marston on the island of Malta. It was on that island in 1887 that Bruce first recovered the etiologic bacteria, a strain of *B. melitensis,* from the spleens of four patients. In 1905, Zammit detected the disease in goats and traced infection in humans to the drinking of raw goat's milk. Heating the milk destroyed the bacteria. In 1895, Bang (Denmark) found that contagious abortion in cattle was caused by infection with *B. abortus;* in 1914, Traum (United States) recovered *B. suis* from fetuses from aborting sows. In modern times, brucellosis is reported in humans most frequently in Russia, Africa, the Middle East, India, Europe, the United States, Mexico, and South America.

Brucellosis is commonly found in goats, dairy cattle, swine, sheep, and kennel-raised dogs (especially beagles). Infections are also found in horses, mules, wild buffalo, reindeer (caribou), deer, moose, hares, and desert wood rats. The placenta, fetus, milk, and semen of nonhuman animals with brucellosis may be infectious. Insects do not appear to be important in the spread of the disease. Brucellas may invade through the eye, nasopharynx, genital tract, and gut. Unbroken skin is resistant.

Most infections in humans are the result of direct contact with sick animals. Certain occupations, especially working in packing plants processing swine, dairy farming, veterinary surgery, and laboratory bacteriology, can lead to brucellosis.

Brucellas are distributed throughout the infected animal and may remain viable for 21 days in a refrigerated carcass. They may survive the curing of ham, but they are killed by smoking, cooking, and pasteurization.

Epidemics of brucellosis have been traced to the ingestion of unpasteurized milk, cream, butter, ice cream, or cheese from goats, cows, or sheep infected by *B. abortus, B. suis,* or *B. melitensis.* Normal gastric juice kills *Brucella* spp. *in vitro,* and most patients with active brucellosis have gastric achlorhydria. However, infections have been reported in patients with peptic ulcer taking antacids and a diet

Table 138-1. Differentiation of Species of Brucella

	***Brucella* species**					
	MELITENSIS	*SUIS*	*ABORTUS*	*CANIS*	*OVIS*	*NEOTOMAE*
Growth in the presence of						
Basic fuchsin	+	−	+	−	+	−
Thionin	+	+	−	+	+	−
Growth stimulation by						
Erythritol	+	+	+	−	−	
CO_2	−	−	+	−	+	−
H_2S production	−	+	+	+	−	+
Urease production	+	+	+	+	−	
Specific agglutinins	+	+	+	+	+	+
Lysis, anti-*abortus* phage	−	−	+	−	−	−

of raw milk. As a result of control measures in cattle and the compulsory pasteurization of milk in the United States, brucellosis in humans has declined from a peak of about 6000 cases in 1947 to a low of 172 in 1978. However, the incidence increased somewhat in 1974–1977 (Fig. 138-1*A* and *B*). The transmission of brucellosis through water has not been proved.

Epidemic brucellosis caused by *B. canis* has been recognized in the United States, West Germany, and Japan in kennel-raised beagles. The explanation for the apparently peculiar susceptibility of beagles to *B. canis* is unknown.

At present in the United States, brucellosis in humans occurs chiefly among workers in abattoirs and farmers. *Brucella abortus* is now the most common cause of the disease in humans in the United States.

The ratio of brucellosis in males to that in females in the United States is about 5 to 1. The usual age of patients is between 20 and 50 years. The disease is infrequent in children. Brucellosis is not spread from one human to another. Abortion may occur during the second trimester; congenital infections are unknown. No infections have been traced to human milk or excreta, although *Brucella* spp. have been isolated from the urine and the products of abortion.

Pathogenesis and Pathology

In a susceptible person, *Brucella* spp. quickly pass by way of the lymph to the regional nodes. Brucellas appear in the peripheral blood within a few hours and are engulfed by polymorphonuclear leukocytes and monocytes, which soon crowd the sinusoids of the lymph nodes, liver, spleen, and bone marrow. The bacilli lie in phagocytic vacuoles (phagosomes) in the leukocytes, and they multiply rapidly. The leukocytes soon burst, and the phagocytic reticuloendothelial (RE) cells lining the sinusoids ingest the brucellas. In these macrophages, brucellas may persist for weeks or months. In aborting cattle, *B. abortus* may crowd the cytoplasm of the fetal chorionic epithelial cells in the intercotyledonous areas of the placenta as a consequence of the presence of relatively high concentrations of erythritol, a carbohydrate that stimulates the growth of the bacteria. Erythritol is plentiful in the placenta of cattle, sheep, goats, and pigs, but not in the human. It is also found in the testes and seminal vesicles of susceptible animals.

Multiplication of the bacteria may end in the destruction of some phagocytic RE cells. In most intact RE cells, brucellas may be difficult to find. The fate of the tissue depends on the interplay of the brucellas and the defenses of the infected cells. In the phagocytes of immune animals, the brucellas are usually quickly destroyed. Bacteria in phagocytic cells are protected from serum antibodies and from some antimicrobics.

Infections caused by *B. abortus* produce granulomas containing clusters of epithelioid histiocytes and sprinkled with lymphocytes, monocytes, and plasma cells, plus a few neutrophils. There may be areas of central hyaline necrosis but no caseation necrosis; the granulomas thus resemble those of sarcoidosis. Langhans' and foreign-body giant cells are frequent. *Brucella melitensis,* and particularly *B. suis,* produce suppurative granulomas and abscesses. Peripheral fibrosis, central caseation, and calcification are common in abscesses caused by *B. suis.* These abscesses often persist for years, whereas small granulomas heal within months, leaving little residual fibrosis. In acute brucellosis caused by *B. abortus,* granulomas are

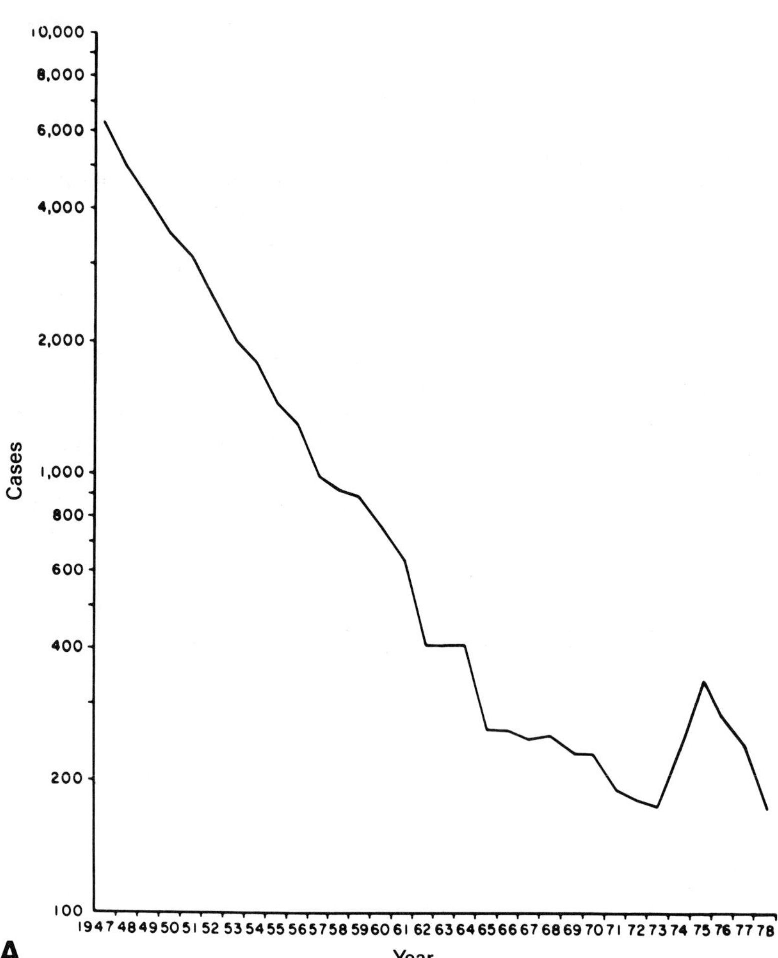

Fig. 138-1. Reported cases of brucellosis in the United States. (*A*) Cases per year, 1947–1978. (*B*) Cases by state in 1978 (Center for Disease Control, Brucellosis Surveillance)

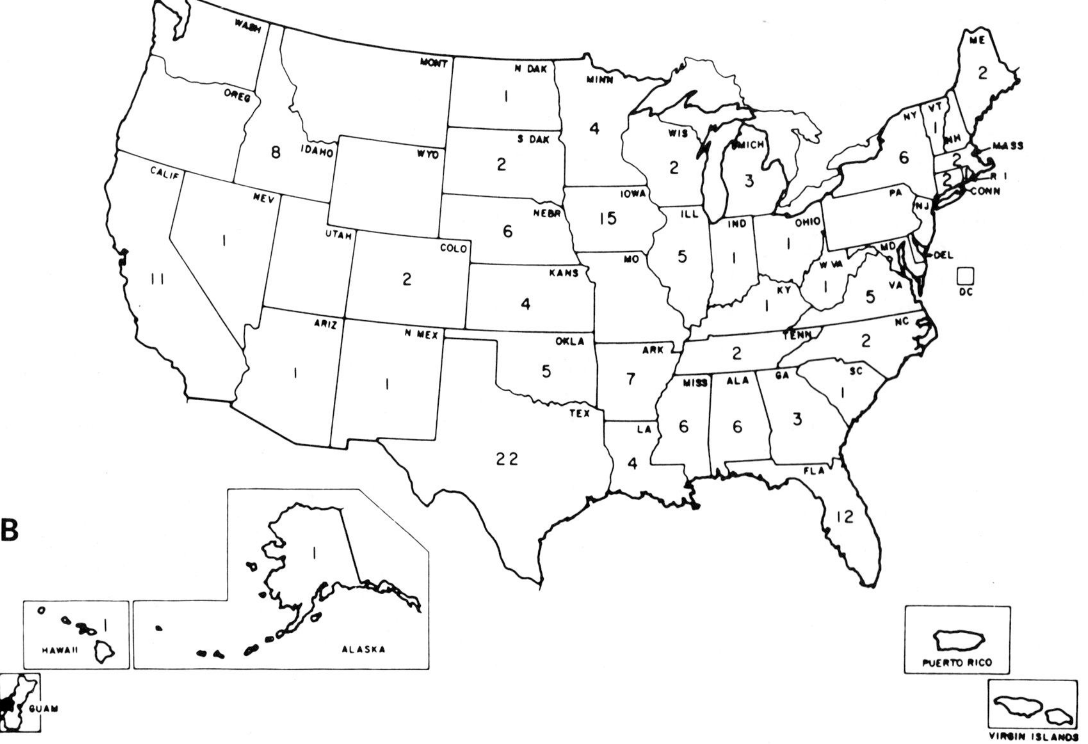

often found in biopsies of the liver (Fig. 138-2*A*), spleen, lymph nodes, and bone marrow (Fig. 138-2*B*). In chronic brucellosis, abscesses may occur in these organs and subcutaneous tissue, testis, epididymis, ovary, kidney, and brain. A granulomatous endophlebitis is occasionally observed in the liver, spleen, and legs. The latter may cause pulmonary emboli. With *B. melitensis* liver biopsies may show only nonspecific hepatitis and no granulomas. Pleural effusions and pulmonary granulomatous abscesses are rarely seen. Subacute hepatitis and, eventually, portal cirrhosis may develop. In fatal cases, perivascular foci of lymphocytes and plasma cells are often found in the brain, myocardium, testicles, and gallbladder.

Manifestations

The incubation period of natural brucellosis varies from a few days to several months. In accidental or experimental infection, the latent period is 5 to 35 days. The onset of the disease may be either sudden or insidious. The predominant symptoms are weakness, sweats, chills, malaise, headache, backache, and arthralgia. Usually, there are few physical abnormalities. Fever is present at some time in nearly all patients. Only a few patients have a true undulant fever; in some patients, even with bacteremia, fever may be transient, minimal, or even lacking. Many acutely ill patients have small, nontender cervical and axillary lymph nodes. Splenomegaly is observed in half the

Fig. 138-2. (*A*) Needle biopsy of liver in acute brucellosis caused by *Brucella abortus.* Note poorly organized granuloma in a portal area with numerous mononuclear cells and some epithelioid cells, but no necrosis. (Original magnification × 350) (J Clin Invest 31:958–968, 1952) (*B*) Trephine biopsy of bone marrow in acute brucellosis (*B. abortus*). Compact syncytium of epithelioid histiocytes between fat cells and sinusoids. There is no necrosis. Note resemblance to lesion of sarcoidosis. (Original magnification × 250)

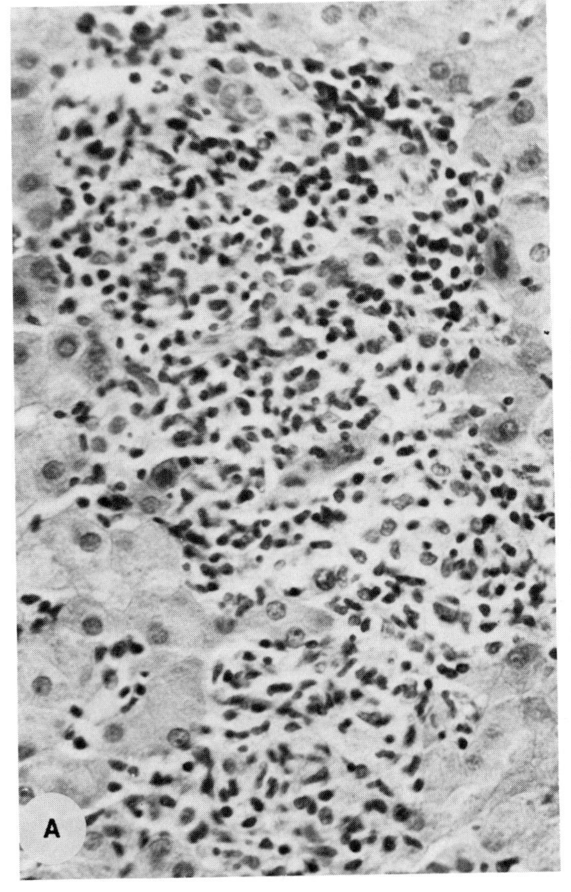

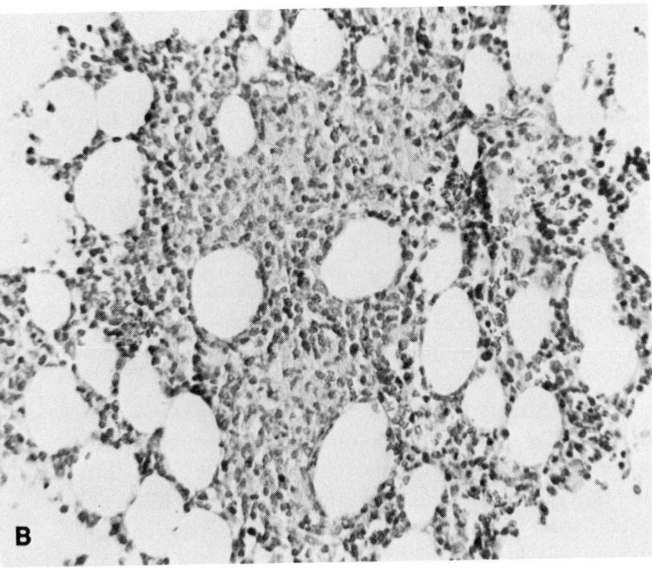

bacteremic patients, and moderate hepatomegaly is noted in 25%. Both organs may occasionally be tender.

In sensitized persons challenged with brucellas, chills and fever develop within minutes to hours and last 24 to 48 hours. Local reactions develop quickly at the site of inoculation.

Persons with chronic brucellosis may have malaise, headaches, sweating, recurrent depression, inertia, vague pains, sexual impotence, and insomnia. They may also develop abscesses in the liver, spleen, genitalia, spine, or long bones.

Diagnosis

Brucellosis should be suspected in a patient who has the typical manifestations and a history of exposure. The diagnosis can be proved only in the laboratory. The leukocyte count is usually normal or reduced, and there is a relative lymphocytosis. The erythrocyte sedimentation rate (ESR) is either normal or increased. Skin tests are rarely helpful. A positive test may persist long after infection has subsided, and false-negative tests may occur with anergy. Tests for brucellar serum antibodies are much more useful.

The standard method for the serodiagnosis of brucellosis is the agglutination test using serial dilutions of serum plus *B. abortus* antigen (prepared by the World Health Organization or the United States Department of Agriculture). Nearly all cases of acute brucellosis show an agglutinin titer of 1:160 or greater within 3 weeks. The agglutinin titer may rise with relapses, skin tests, or vaccine therapy. Specific antigens may show higher agglutinin titers in patients infected with brucellas other than *B. abortus,* for example, *B. canis.* The agglutinin titer tends to decline after 3 months or after chemotherapy, but often persists at low levels for months or years, especially with chronic infections. The prognosis of acute brucellosis may be predicted from the rate of fall of antibrucellar IgG (2-mercaptoethanol test), the antiglobulin (Coombs') agglutination test, or the complement-fixation test. Chronic brucellosis may perhaps be distinguished by persistent low titers of serum agglutinins, a high proportion of which may consist of either IgG or 7S immunoglobulins with blocking activity (either IgA or IgG). A negative 2-mercaptoethanol test will rule out chronic brucellosis. Healthy people exposed to *Brucella* spp., may develop low titers of serum agglutinins (asymptomatic infections?) consisting mainly of IgM. Opsonin and precipitin tests have not been useful or reliable for brucellosis. Cross-reacting antibodies for *Brucella* spp. may occur in infections caused by *Salmonella* spp., or *Yersinia enterocolitica,* and after vaccination for cholera or tularemia.

The isolation of *Brucella* spp. by culture is definitive. Blood cultures are most useful in acute disease. Cultures of infected tissues, biopsies of the RE system (*e.g.,* the bone marrow), and abscesses may also be helpful. The most convenient method employs the Castaneda double medium with both Albimi broth and an agar slant. Carbon dioxide must be added for the growth of *B. abortus* or *B. ovis.*

Acute brucellosis mimics influenza (Chap. 28, Influenza), malaria (Chap. 145, Malaria), typhoid fever (Chap. 64, Typhoid Fever), typhus (Chap. 98, Typhus Fevers), tularemia (Chap. 139, Tularemia), and miliary tuberculosis (Chap. 34, Pulmonary Tuberculosis). No single symptom or clinical feature is pathognomonic. Brucellosis may resemble infectious mononucleosis (Chap. 137, Infectious Mononucleosis) because of the lymphocytosis, lymphadenopathy, and splenomegaly; however, the titers of heterophil antibody are low or lacking, and antibodies to the Epstein–Barr virus are not found. Chronic brucellosis may be confused with lymphoma; splenic or liver calcifications should help to differentiate chronic suppurative brucellosis. It may be difficult to distinguish renal tuberculosis from renal brucellosis, but cultures and serologic tests are helpful.

Prognosis

The mortality rate in brucellosis was once about 3%. With antimicrobial therapy, however, death is rare. Without specific treatment, the duration of acute brucellosis is usually less than 6 months, and spontaneous recovery is frequently complete within weeks. In many patients, the acute illness is so mild that the disease may not be recognized. The disease occasionally persists for more than a year without localization. In patients with complications, it is likely to persist and cause prolonged disability. Relapses are also commonly seen. The incidence of serious complications and recurrences is decreased with adequate antimicrobial therapy.

A variety of complications may occur in 10% to 15% of patients with brucellosis, especially with *B. suis* and *B. melitensis.* Meningoencephalitis may lead to hearing and ocular disorders, aphasia, ataxia, intermittent coma, and hemiplegia. Chronic meningitis is rare. Intracranial hemorrhage can result from rupture of a mycotic aneurysm. Peripheral neuritis and arachnoiditis have also been seen.

Infective endocarditis is the most frequent cause of death in brucellosis. Either the aortic or the mitral valve may be involved, with microabscesses of the valve cusps leading to destruction of the valves and their commissures. Although previously existent valvular damage is not a necessary precondition, endocarditis is often associated with calcific, nodular stenosis of the aortic valve. Once established, brucellar endocarditis is often fatal; surgical replacement of the damaged valve with a prosthetic valve during treatment with bactericidal antimicrobics may be curative. Pericardial effusion and myocarditis are rare complications. Brucellosis may also be associated with arterial aneurysms and arteriovenous fistulas.

Pneumonitis, pleural effusion, or granulomatous lung abscess may be found. There are often diffuse hepatic and splenic granulomas, although usually without any serious sequelae. In *B. suis* infection, the liver and spleen may contain multiple abscesses that calcify and persist for years. Rarely, hepatic involvement may result in portal cirrhosis. In some patients, hypersplenism results in marked anemia, neutropenia, and thrombocytopenia. Acute cholecystitis is a rare complication.

Two forms of renal brucellosis exist: diffuse interstitial nephritis with azotemia, proteinuria, and hypertension; and abscesses and renal calcifications that mimic renal tuberculosis or chronic pyelonephritis. Ulceration of the renal pelvis, ureter, and urinary bladder also may occur. Routine urine cultures may be sterile, and the diagnosis is generally made only by serum agglutination tests and cultures of the excised kidney. Ovarian abscess, epididymitis, orchitis, and prostatitis may be seen occasionally.

Osteomyelitis is the most frequent complication in humans. The typical lesion is a suppurative spondylitis involving a disk and the adjacent vertebrae. Rarely, osteomyelitis of the pelvic bones or the shaft of a long bone may be seen.

Acute suppurative arthritis, bursitis, and intermittent joint effusion may be observed, but chronic destructive arthritis is rare. Other rare complications include iritis, choroiditis, keratitis, maculopapular rash, and subcutaneous abscesses.

Although relapses and chronic suppurative lesions occur in brucellosis, the disease does produce a substantial immunity to reinfection with *Brucella* spp. Immunity depends on both the specific serum antibodies and the enhanced bactericidal properties of phagocytic cells.

Therapy

Patients with brucellosis should rest in bed as long as they are febrile. Dehydrated patients should receive glucose and electrolyte solutions intravenously. The diet should be liberal in calories and carbohydrates to prevent starvation acidosis.

The keystone of therapy is the early use of specific antimicrobial agents. Active brucellosis—that is, fever, isolation of *Brucella* spp., high titers of serum antibody, local infeciton, and complications—is indication for treatment. Either tetracycline, oxytetracycline, or chlortetracycline should be given in a dose of 28 to 30 mg/kg body wt/day as four equal portions perorally, every 6 hours for 3 to 4 weeks. Adults with severe infections caused by *B. melitensis* may require 45 to 60 mg/kg body wt/day, as just described. Relapses of symptoms and bacteremia may occur in half the patients. If the larger daily doses of a tetracycline are given, or treatment with streptomycin is added to the regimen, relapses are less frequent. Relapses after treatment with a tetracycline are rarely due to actual bacterial resistance to tetracycline. A favorable clinical response usually follows a second course of treatment. Although streptomycin is not effective as the sole agent of therapy, it is valuable when given with tetracycline to seriously ill patients and those with abscesses. The dose of streptomycin should be 15 to 30 mg/kg body wt/day as two equal portions injected intramuscularly, 12-hourly, for 2 to 3 weeks. Rifampin is generally active against *B. melitensis,* but not always against *B. abortus.* It has been effective as a companion to tetracycline in a daily dose of 8 to 10 mg/kg body weight, perorally.

Patients who do not tolerate tetracycline may be treated with a combination of trimethoprim and sulfamethoxazole. The dose of trimethoprim is 5 to 10 mg/kg body wt/day, and of sulfamethoxazole, 25 to 50 mg/kg body wt/day, perorally, as 2 or 3 equal portions; 12- or 8-hourly, for 2 or 3 weeks.

Antimicrobics not recommended for treating brucellosis include all penicillins, all cephalosporins, chloramphenicol, novobiocin, cycloserine, erythromycin, neomycin, kanamycin, polymyxins B and E, and the sulfonamides. Treatment with blood transfusions, immune serum, brucella vaccines, and brucella phages is not recommended.

If possible, abscesses should be drained surgically. Abscesses of the spleen or of one kidney are cured by the removal of the organ. Spondylitis can be cured with appropriate antimicrobics, bed rest, and braces and without surgical drainage.

Antimicrobial therapy may initially provoke high fever, delirium, or shock. Such Herxheimer-like reactions can be prevented by the simultaneous administration of a glucosteroid. The recommended drug is either hydrocortisone, 5 mg/kg body wt/day, or prednisone, 1 mg/kg body wt/day, each as 3 equal portions, given 8-hourly perorally for 3 to 4 days. Glucosteroids should be given only together with adequate doses of a tetracycline.

Prevention

Brucellosis in humans can usually be traced to an animal source. Control of the disease therefore depends primarily on the elimination of animal reservoirs. Bang's disease has been largely eradicated in dairy cattle in the United States. Unfortunately, this has not been possible globally because of many social and economic factors. Furthermore, the disease has not been controlled in goats, sheep, and swine.

Pasteurization of milk and milk products is valuable in the control of brucellosis, but it does not eliminate the disease. Similarly, inspection of meat is useful but not sufficient.

The most effective plan for elimination of the disease in cattle is the detection of infected animals by periodic agglutination tests of milk and blood and the slaughter of positive reactors. If the disease is very widespread in cattle, an acceptable means of control is segregation of the infected cattle and vaccination of all calves at 4 to 8 months with live, avirulent brucella vaccine (strain 19). Adult cattle and pregnant heifers should not be vaccinated.

Brucellosis in sheep and goats poses a serious threat to the public health in many foreign countries. The vaccination and simultaneous serologic testing and slaughter of the infected animals might be a feasible approach to controlling the problem.

The prevention of brucellosis in high-risk occupational groups such as farmers, meat-packing plant workers, and veterinarians must depend on education, sanitation, and the eradication of infected animals. Efforts to eliminate the generation of infectious aerosols might be helpful. Because the available vaccines have been ineffective or unsafe, active immunization of personnel engaged in these occupations is not now practical.

Some degree of immunity may be induced by killed or attenuated/live vaccines. However, the current live vaccines have not been safe in humans. Attenuated/live vaccines have been effective in immunizing young, nonpregnant cows, goats, and sheep. There are as yet no effective vaccines for the prevention of *B. suis* infections in hogs. Wearing protective gloves and goggles might be preventive when heavy exposures can be anticipated.

Remaining Problems

A key problem is control of the infections in domestic and wild animals. The spread in domestic animals can be controlled by detection, slaughter, and immunization. Methods are needed for finding infected animals by serologic tests that can be used by untrained people in the field (*e.g.,* the card test).

New serologic methods for the diagnosis of brucellosis are especially needed for the detection of infections in hogs (*B. suis*).

The control of brucellosis in swine, sheep, goats, and heavily exposed human populations could be aided considerably by the development of effective vaccines similar to the *B. abortus* vaccines used in cattle. The use of attenuated *B. suis* vaccines seems to be a feasible approach to the immunization of swine. Attenuated *B. melitensis* vaccines are now available for use in goats and sheep.

We have little understanding of the basic mechanisms by which the symptoms of human brucellosis are produced. Most puzzling are the patients with chronic brucellosis who lack a demonstrable focus.

The intraphagocytic fate of brucellas in macrophages merits more exploration. Information is lacking on the membrane of the phagocytic vacuole. Poor penetration of the vacuole by tetracyclines may explain relapses of brucellosis after therapy. Therapeutic agents are needed that have fewer side-effects and are more often curative. Promising antimicrobics include rifampin, doxycycline, minocycline, and gentamicin.

Bibliography

Books

ALTON GG, JONES LM, PIETZ DE: Laboratory Techniques in Brucellosis. WHO Monograph No. 55, 2nd ed. New York, Columbia University Press, 1975. 163 pp.

HUDDLESON IF: Brucellosis in Man and Animals. New York, Commonwealth Fund, 1943. 379 pp.

SPINK WW: The Nature of Brucellosis. Minneapolis, University of Minnesota Press, 1956. 464 pp.

Journals

BERTRAND A, ROUX J, JANBON F, JOURDAN J, JONQUET O: Treatment of brucellosis with rifampin. Presse Med 8:3635–3639, 1979

BUCHANAN TM, FABER LC: 2-mercaptoethanol brucella agglutination test: Usefulness for predicting recovery from brucellosis. J Clin Microbiol 11:691–693, 1980

BUCHANAN TM, FABER LC, FELDMAN RA: Brucellosis in the United States, 1960–1972. Medicine 53:403–439, 1974

Centers for Disease Control: Brucellosis Surveillance, Annual Summary 1978, Issued June 1979

DAIKOS GK, PAPAPOLYZOS N, MARKETOS N, MOCHLAS S, KASTANAKIS S, PAPASTERIADIS E: Trimethoprim–sulfamethoxazole in Brucellosis. J Infect Dis 128:S731–S733, 1973

FARID Z, MIALE A, OMAR MS, VAN PEENEN PFD: Antibiotic treatment for acute brucellosis caused by *Brucella melitensis.* J Trop Med Hyg 64:157–163, 1961

HALL WH: Brucellosis in man: A study of 35 cases due to *Brucella abortus.* Minn Med 36:460–465, 1953

HALL WH, MANION RE: In vitro susceptibility of *Brucella* to various antibiotics. Appl Microbiol 20:600–604, 1970

KEPPIE J, WILLIAMS AE, WITT K, SMITH H: The role of erythritol in the tissue localization of the brucellae. Br J Exp Pathol 46:104–108, 1965

MACDONALD A, ELMSLIE WH: Serological investigations in suspected brucellosis. Lancet 1:380–382, 1967

MEYER ME, CAMERON HS: Metabolic characterization of the genus *Brucella.* J Bacteriol 82:387–410, 950–953, 1961

PRATT DS, TENNEY CM, RELLER LB: Successful treatment of *Brucella melitensis* endocarditis. Am J Med 64:897–900, 1978

REDDIN JL, ANDERSON RK, JENNESS R, SPINK WW: Significance of 7 S and macroglobulin brucella agglutinins in human brucellosis. N Engl J Med 272:1263–1268, 1965

ZINNEMAN HH, SEAL US, HALL WH: Some molecular characteristics of blocking antibodies in human brucellosis. J Immunol 93:993–1000, 1964

RICHARD B. HORNICK

139 Tularemia

Tularemia is a congeries of syndromes, all caused by *Francisella tularensis,* but each syndrome is conditioned in occurrence by the route of infection and the virulence of the infecting strain. An indolent, febrile disease manifested by a skin ulcer and tender enlargement of draining lymph nodes is the most common form of the disease—ulceroglandular tularemia. Pneumonic, typhoidal, and oculoglandular forms also occur.

Etiology

Francisella tularensis (Pasteurella tularensis) is a small, gram-negative coccobacillus (0.2 μm × 0.3 μm to 0.7 μm) that requires special culture mediums for isolation. The species name commemorates the original isolation of the microorganism in Tulare county, California, in 1911, from ground squirrels suffering from a plaguelike disease. The genus name *Francisella* is a tribute to Dr. Edward Francis, who derived much of the early bacteriologic and immunologic information about tularemia. *Francisella tularensis* has never been classified as *Brucella* spp. in the United States even though the genera share common antigens.

Although *F. tularensis* grows on glucose–cystine blood agar, selective mediums are often necessary to achieve separation from other bacterial species. For example, the addition of cycloheximide and penicillin G facilitates isolation by suppressing normal respiratory-tract flora or microorganisms simply resident in skin ulcers. The careful handling of laboratory cultures is needed. The use of contagion hoods with a filtered or incinerated exhaust system is recommended when cultures are manipulated to avoid accidental acquisition of the disease. The inoculation of laboratory animals for isolation or diagnosis is not generally recommended because of the high probability of precipitating an epizootic and infecting personnel.

All isolates of *F. tularensis* seem to be serologically homogeneous. However, in North America, two distinct varieties have been recognized. One variety is highly virulent for the common cottontail rabbit (*Oryctolagus*) and man (Jellison type A). It is found only in North America, is capable of fermenting glycerol, and is endowed with citrulline ureidase activity. The second variety is avirulent for the rabbit but capable of causing mild tularemia in man (Jellison type B). It is found in Europe and Asia, as well as in North America, but is is glycerol-negative and citrulline–ureidase-negative.

Killed or lysed *F. tularensis* displays pharmacologic activities identical with those associated with endotoxins derived from the enteric gram-negative bacilli.

Epidemiology

Man is very susceptible to infection with *F. tularensis.* In volunteer studies, fewer than 50 bacilli of Jellison type A cause disease, whether the route of infection is respiratory or intradermal. Although gastrointestinal infection has been described in man, the gut is a relatively refractory portal of entry. More than 10 million bacilli had to be given perorally to cause disease in volunteers. Larger numbers of type B *F. tularensis* are required to cause milder forms of unceroglandular or pneumonic infections than those evoked by type A bacteria.

Francisella tularensis normally parasitize approximately 100 kinds of nonhuman mammals and arthropod vectors. Type A bacteria are usually acquired from cottontail rabbits or the ticks (*Ixodes, Dermacentor*) that parasitize them. Type B strains are common in rodents (hares, moles, beaver, muskrats, squirrels, rats, mice), certain birds, and ticks. Tularemia bacilli can be spread by body lice (*Pediculus humanus* var. *corporis*). Infection may occasionally occur from the ingestion of contaminated water. Infection in man may follow bites or scratches from dogs, cats, skunks, coyotes, foxes, hogs, and bull snakes that are temporary oral or paw carriers from preying on infected rabbits or other rodents.

Rodent hosts, particularly rabbits, appear to be the major reservoir of *F. tularensis.* However, transovarial passage is said to occur in ticks. Other arthropod vectors (*e.g.,* deerflies) apparently acquire tularemia bacilli while feeding on infected mammals.

Humans of all races and ages and both sexes are uniformly susceptible and have become infected by many routes. Most commonly, the skin is the portal of entry through direct contact with infected tissues, body fluids, and pelts, or by the bites of infected or contaminated animals or arthropods. However, infection also occurs through inhalation of infected aerosols or droplet nuclei, transfer of *F. tularensis* into the conjunctival sac, and ingestion of improperly cooked meat or contaminated water. Tularemia is an occupational hazard for rabbit hunters, butchers, cooks, those who process pelts (*e.g.,* felt hat manufacturers) and frozen wild rabbit meat, agricultural workers, trappers, campers, sheep herders and shearers, mink ranchers, muskrat farmers, and laboratory technicians.

Small epidemics of tularemia have been reported in muskrat trappers, laborers bitten by deerflies (*Chrysops discalis*), and tick-infected troops on military maneuvers. The former two types of epidemics were probably caused by type B strains because the clinical manifestations were so mild. However, tularemia is a sporadic disease occurring in areas of high endemicity. Since 1939, there has been a steady decline in the incidence of tularemia in the United States (Fig. 139-1*A*).

In 1980, 234 cases were reported to the Centers for Disease Control. Most cases occurred in the Midwest (*e.g.,* Arkansas, 60; Missouri, 26; Oklahoma, 24; Tennessee, 8—Fig. 139-1*B*). The greatest frequency is in the summer, when ticks abound and have access to man. However, in the states east of the Mississippi River, tularemia is prevalent in the winter. The principal vector is the cottontail rabbit, and the number of infections increases during the hunting season.

Pathogenesis and Pathology

The livers of rabbits with tularemia may contain millions of *F. tularensis,* laboratory animals dying of the disease have thousands of bacilli per milliliter of blood. It is clear that evisceration of animals with tularemia provides ample opportunity for direct contamination of the skin. In addition, aerosols containing infective doses of *F. tularensis* may be generated.

Low resistance to infection with *F. tularensis* and accessibility to exposure mark the two most common portals of entry in man—the skin and the respiratory tract. *Francisella tularensis* is said to pass through unbroken skin. However, it is quite likely that entry is gained to the dermis through minute scratches or anatomic openings in the epidermis—for example, hair follicles and creases between skin fold and nail bed. Tularemia contracted by handling infected animals also leads to ulcers of the fingers or hands. Inoculation through bites (*e.g.,* by ticks) often yields lesions in the groin or axilla. Ulcers represent the final stage of pathologic changes set in motion by the multiplication of *F. tularensis.* About 48 hours after the bacilli gain entrance into the skin, a macular, erythematous lesion occurs that soon becomes papular, not unlike a positive tuberculin skin test. The papule is pruritic and enlarges, causing the skin to become taut, thin, shiny, and, rarely, fluctuant. Ulceration then occurs, some 96 hours after inoculation. The ulcer is distinguished by sharply demarcated edges and a depressed center. Fever is usually present by the time a nodule has appeared. As the ulcer develops, regional lymph nodes enlarge. In untreated patients, especially those infected with type A strains, the lymph nodes become caseous and form suppurating buboes. Immune persons develop only a small indurated papule at the site of infection. However, a site of ulceration at a previous infection may flare with sterile inflammation because the skin remains sensitized where *F. tularensis* has previously entered and multiplied.

Aerogenic infection accounts for pneumonic tularemia, the most serious form of the disease. Pneumonia seems to be initiated by an alveolar localization of minute infected particles that have been inhaled. An inflammatory reaction occurs around the site of deposition of the bacteria. Necrosis of alveolar walls enhances the leukoctye response (Fig. 139-2). Thus, it is possible to have many small areas of bronchopneumonia evident as patchy infiltrates throughout the lung fields. Although some areas may coalesce, consolidation is rare.

Pneumonia is not the invariable consequence of inhalation of *F. tularensis.* Alveolar macrophages ingest fine particles that penetrate to the distal reaches of the respiratory tract. More proximal localization may occur, as manifested by bronchitis and tracheitis. Thence, by way of hilar lymphatics, *F. tularensis* that was inhaled may gain access to the blood. In this way, a truly typhoidal form of tularemia results: toxemia, continuous fever without chills or sweats, myalgias, and severe headache. In some patients, a dry cough and retrosternal pain occur, providing the only clues to respiratory involvement.

The typhoidal form of tularemia was formerly

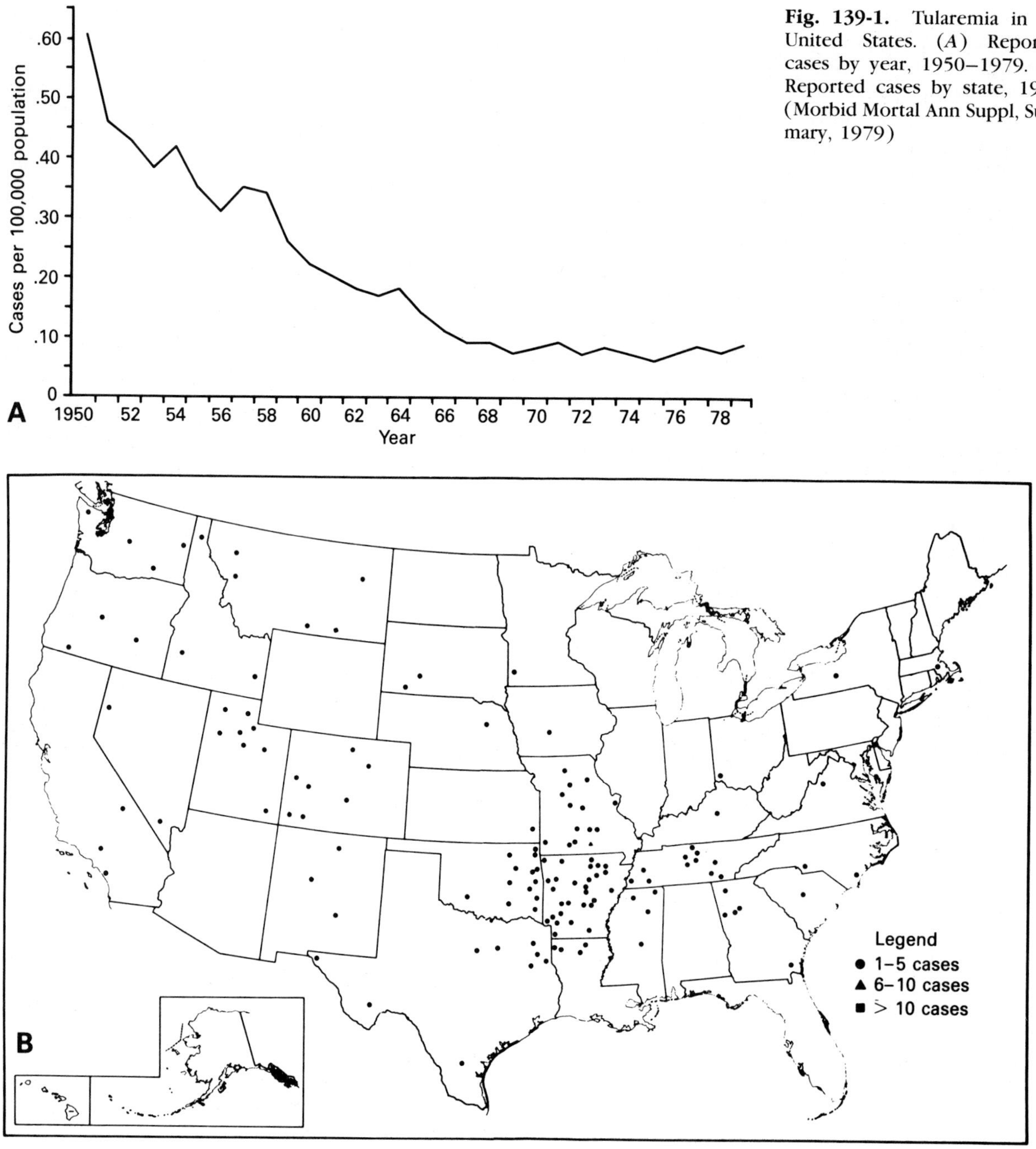

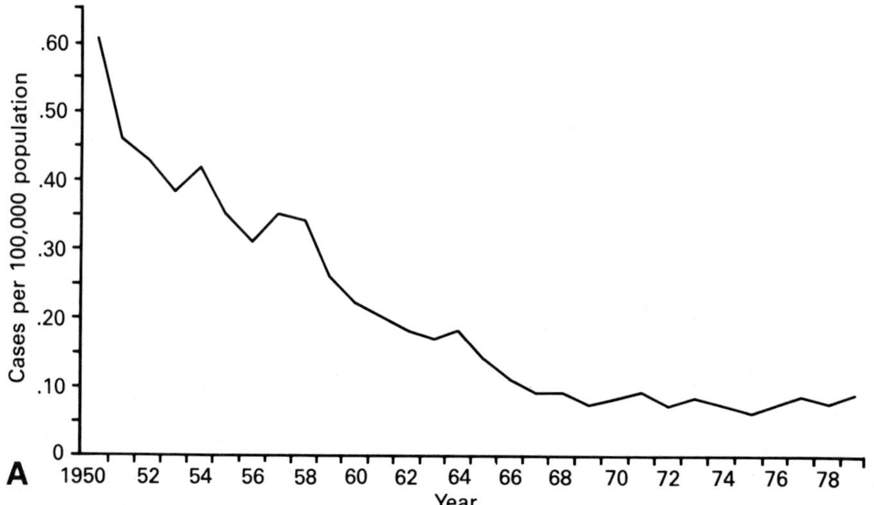

B

Legend
● 1–5 cases
▲ 6–10 cases
■ > 10 cases

Fig. 139-1. Tularemia in the United States. (*A*) Reported cases by year, 1950–1979. (*B*) Reported cases by state, 1979. (Morbid Mortal Ann Suppl, Summary, 1979)

thought to be consequent to the ingestion of *F. tularensis.* This view has not been supported by studies in volunteers, which have demonstrated the relative insusceptibility of humans to tularemia on enteric exposure. Only a few patients develop gastrointestinal tularemia if a large dose of *F. tularensis* is swallowed. Indeed, a major hazard to the ingestion of contaminated food apparently is aerogenic tularemia resulting from the inhalation of bacilli released by mastication. Direct invasion of the pharynx may also occur, producing fever, and tender and enlarged cervical lymph nodes with or without ulceration of pharyngeal mucosa.

Inoculation of the conjunctival sac follows wiping

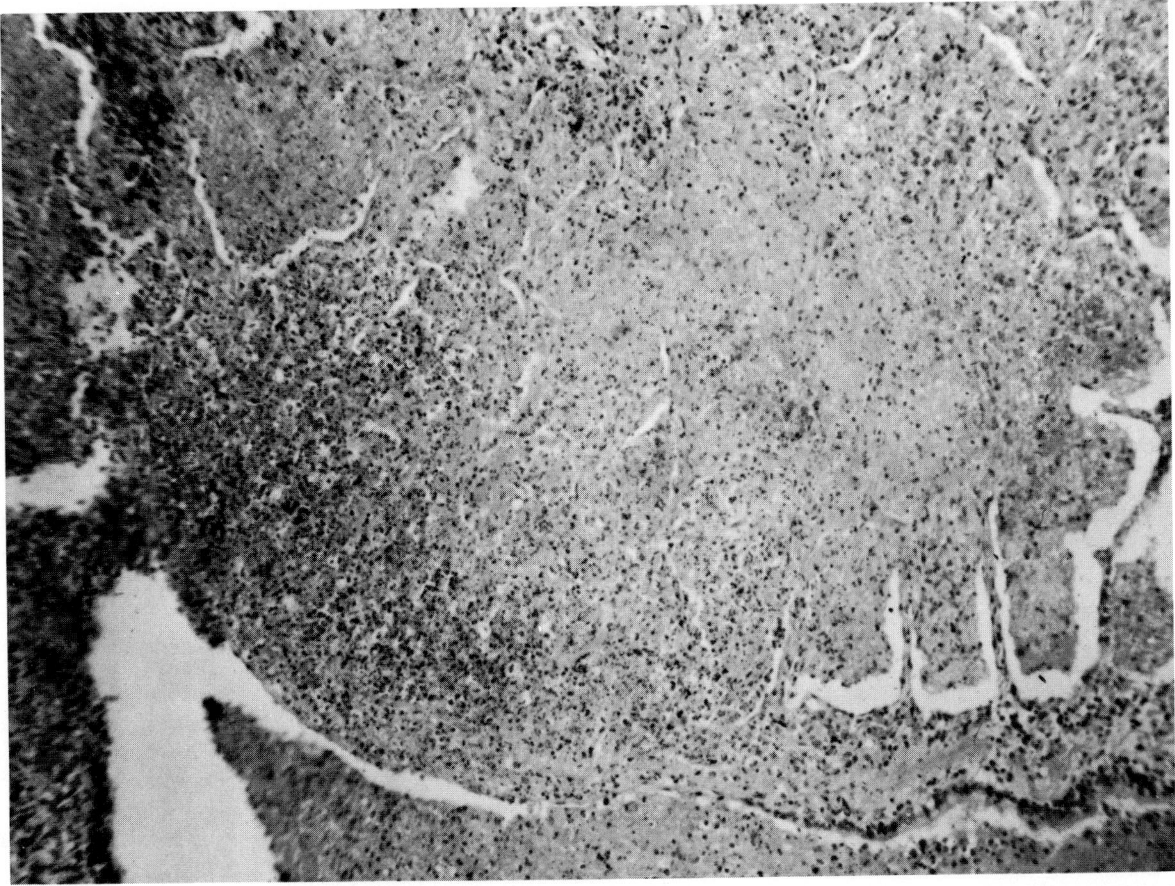

Fig. 139-2. Histopathology of pneumonic tularemia in man. Note the area of necrosis at the right. (H&E, original magnification approximately × 260)

the eyes with a contaminated hand or fingers. Other mechanisms rarely involved in oculoglandular tularemia include splashing infected liquids into the eye and ocular contact with infected aerosols.

Manifestations

The temperature course in patients with tularemia is characteristic. The fever begins abruptly and is often marked with rigors. A continuous or mildly remittent pattern with elevations of 40°C to 41°C (104–106°F) is usual. If the disease is untreated, fever will persist as long as a month. Hepatomegaly and splenomegaly can be detected in most patients; palpation usually causes pain.

Generalized headache is usual in tularemia and may be so severe that meningeal involvement is suspected. Occasionally, photophobia is also present.

Ulceroglandular tularemia is the most common form of the disease, accounting for more than four-fifths of the cases. The skin is ulcerated at the point of entrance of *F. tularensis,* and the regional lymph nodes are enlarged, usually without an intervening lymphangitis. The portal of entry is frequently so insignificant that it escapes attention, or it may be passed off as a paronychia. Generally lymphadenopathy may be present, but the nodes draining the ulcer are tender and particularly enlarged.

In severe infections, bacteremia occurs and may give rise to a secondary pneumonia. Physical findings are sparse in these patients; rhonchi may be the only indication of pulmonary disease. Radiographically, there are small patches of bronchopneumonia indistinct in outline and faint in density. Such infiltrates are difficult to visualize and may not be recognized until a series of chest films is reviewed.

Some patients develop a harassing, nonproductive

cough and a substernal burning or discomfort consistent with tracheobronchitis. Pleural effusions occur with or without evidence of an associated pneumonitis. In the latter circumstance, visceral pleural involvement with small granulomatous lesions, not unlike tubercles, is implicated. An indolent course with frequent relapses may result. The cellular response in the pleural fluid is predominantly mononuclear.

When lobar pneumonia occurs in tularemia, the mortality is greatly increased. There is severe respiratory distress with a debilitating, dry-hacking cough. Apprehension and toxicity are marked; shock is common. Hemoptysis is unusual, and abscess formation is rare. The chest findings are those of consolidation.

Oculoglandular tularemia accounts for less than 1% of cases. It is manifested by pain, photophobia, intense congestion, itching, lacrimation, chemosis, and a mucopurulent discharge. Small, yellowish granulomatous lesions may appear in the palpebral conjunctivae or cornea. Eventually, these may ulcerate, causing corneal perforation. Lymph nodes in the preauricular and cervical areas may enlarge and progress to suppuration.

Meningitis, osteomyelitis, and endocarditis are very unusual manifestations of tularemia.

Diagnosis

A thorough history is needed to aid in the diagnosis of tularemia. Contact with rabbits, ticks, or some of the vectors previously listed should alert one to the possibility of tularemia in a patient with an acute febrile illness. Lack of a history of contact with a vector does not eliminate the possibility of tularemia. In one large series of cases from Louisiana, the vector was not identified in 59% of patients. In the classic form of ulceroglandular disease, tularemia must be the diagnosis until excluded. However, with early papular lesions without significant lymph-node enlargement, a history of contact with a vector is essential to diagnosis. The location of the ulcers usually correlates with the kind of vector contacted—for example, on the fingers or hands from handling infected animals, and in the axilla or groin from tick bites. The seasonal prevalence of tularemia is a consequence of the regional means of transmission (tick bite or infected animals).

The severe forms of tularemia are even more difficult to diagnose. Of those patients with typhoidal tularemia, 80% may not have a history of vector contact. History taking must be thorough because the signs and symptoms of typhoidal tularemia are nonspecific. The headache, dry-hacking cough, substernal pain, myalgias, and severe malaise are hardly distinctive. The pneumonitis may be missed by both the physical and roentgenographic examinations of the chest. Infiltrates are usually ill-defined, and only infrequently is there an oval density that might bring tularemic pneumonia to mind.

Sputum examination by smear and Gram stain is usually unrewarding. Culture of the sputum, bronchial washings, and occasionally the blood yield *F. tularensis* if appropriate culture mediums are used. Routine culture mediums do not support the growth of tularemia bacilli from clinical specimens. When pulmonary infiltration is present, gastric washings collected early in the morning are an excellent source for the recovery of *F. tularensis.* The tube used to collect the specimen should be lubricated with water rather than mineral oil because the latter inhibits the growth of *F. tularensis.* Tularemia bacilli can be identified by inoculating guinea pigs intraperitoneally with sputum, bronchial and gastric washings, or pus from draining lymph nodes or blood. Death follows in 5 to 10 days, and *F. tularensis* can be isolated from the blood or spleen. In addition, the spleen and liver show characteristic granulomatous, noncaseous lesions. It must be emphasized that scrupulous care is mandatory in handling cultures of *F. tularensis* because of the danger of infecting laboratory personnel. Infected animals are even more hazardous. Only experienced personnel who have access to adequate facilities for isolation should carry out the inoculation of animals.

The agglutination test is a reliable, standard method for the diagnosis of tularemia. Agglutinins are first detectable from the tenth to fourteenth day of disease. The titer rises abruptly to a level of 1:640 or greater within the next week, reaching a maximum generally in excess of 1:1280 around the fourth to eighth week of illness. Some persons with no history of tularemia may possess low titer of antibody; a rising titer of agglutinins enables serodiagnosis to be made. Agglutinins for *Brucella* spp. may appear and increase during tularemia, but the titer of such cross-reacting antibody is generally one-fourth to one-sixth that of the tularemia titer. These cross-reacting antibodies are of the IgM class and decline in titer faster than tularemia antibodies. After a period of years following tularemia, agglutinins cannot be detected in the serum.

A skin test antigen derived by ether extraction from *F. tularensis* gives a positive reaction in more than 90% of patients within the first 7 days of the disease. Unfortunately, this product is not commercially available. It is a diagnostic reagent that can be obtained from the Centers for Disease Control, Atlanta, GA. In about 10% of patients, the skin test antigen may boost preexisting agglutinating antibody titers. Skin test reactivity has been shown to be associated with specially sensitized lymphocytes.

Hematologic studies are helpful to the extent that the leukocyte count is normal in the face of a high fever in a toxic patient. The sedimentation rate and C-reative protein (CRP) are elevated in direct proportion to the activity of the disease.

The diagnosis of ulceroglandular tularemia may at times be confused with cat-scratch fever (Chap. 166, Cat-Scratch Fever), sporotrichosis (Chap. 108, Sporotrichosis), infectious mononucleosis (Chap. 137, Infectious Mononucleosis), and lymphangitis secondary to an infected skin lesion. History of contact with cats, reaction to specific antigens, and lack of agglutinins for *F. tularensis* enables differentiation.

Sporotrichosis usually presents with multiple lesions that appear in centripetal sequence along the course of lymphatic drainage from the site of inoculation. Although the lesions may ulcerate, they are freely movable.

Infectious mononucleosis can be mistaken for glandular tularemia. Fever and cervical adenopathy may be the principal manifestations of oropharyngeal tularemia. The serologic manifestations of infectious mononucleosis plus the characteristic cellular response in the peripheral blood enable the two diseases to be distinguished.

Typhoid fever can mimic the severe, systemic form of tularemia (Chap. 64, Typhoid Fever). Failure to isolate *Salmonella typhi* in cultures of the blood, feces, or urine, and lack of abdominal pain suggest that the diagnosis is not typhoid.

The pneumonitis of tularemia can be mistaken for any of the nonbacterial pneumonias—for example, Q fever, atypical pneumonia, psittacosis (Chap. 30, Nonbacterial Pneumonias). All these conditions also respond to treatment with tetracyclines. Serologic diagnosis from paired serum samples enables a retrospective diagnosis to be made. Other causes of similar roentgenographic findings include histoplasmosis and coccidioidomycosis, diseases that can be acute in onset (Chaps. 40, Histoplasmosis and 41, Coccidioidomycosis). Serologic diagnosis is the surest method of differentiation. However, a careful history and physical examination often provide the clues necessary to arrive at a decision to institute therapy.

The mononuclear effusion seen in some cases of tularemia is similar to that found in tuberculosis. The history, serologic studies, and culture information are helpful in diagnosis (Chap. 34, Pulmonary Tuberculosis.

Finally, two very rare but potentially confusing conditions—melioidasis and glanders—exist in areas remote from the United States. However, both disorders are introduced into this country by returning servicemen and travelers. The cutaneous ulcers seen in these infections can mimic tularemia. The pneumonia of melioidosis is usually more severe than that of tularemia in the acute form, and the chronic form does not resemble tularemia (Chap. 141, Mediodosis).

Prognosis

Ulceroglandular tularemia without specific treatment has a fatality rate of approximately 5%. The disease lasts 2 to 4 weeks with a subsequent period of disability of 8 to 12 weeks. During this latter stage, the draining buboes heal slowly, and the ulcers gradually become covered by new skin. Mortality increases to 30% with pneumonia, whether primary or secondary to ulceroglandular tularemia.

Recovery from tularemia is associated with the development of immunity that seems to be lifelong. Second episodes of tularemia occur, but they are mild.

Therapy

Streptomycin is the agent of first choice for treatment. Fever usually responds within 24 to 36 hours unless suppurative lymph nodes are present. The recommended dosage is 30 to 40 mg/kg body wt/day, IM, as two equal portions, 12-hourly for 3 days, followed by half as much for an additional 3 days. Gentamicin (5–6 mg/kg body wt/day, IM as 3 equal portions, 8-hourly for 5 days) appears to be equally effective. The tetracyclines and chloramphenicol control the acute phase of tularemia, but these bacteriostatic agents fail to eradicate *F. tularensis,* and relapses occur. Daily therapy consisting of 50 to 60 mg/kg body wt/day, PO, as four equal portions, 6-hourly, for as long as 14 days has been tried. Relapses have occurred; reinstitution of the same regimen has brought about prompt clinical recovery—that is, resistance has not developed.

Prevention

Because of the high frequency of tularemia in rabbits, Moses' Law (see Leviticus 11:6, 7) should be invoked—that is, rabbits should be avoided as unclean. The interstate transfer of wild rabbits or frozen rabbit meat packaged for animal consumption should be prohibited. Rabbits that seem to be ill should be destroyed and buried without manipulation or direct handling. Rubber gloves should be worn by persons involved in the processing or handling of wild rabbits.

In tick-infested areas, tight wristbands and pants tucked into boots prevent the attachment of ticks. In addition, a careful search should be made for ticks, especially in the groin, axilla, and scalp as often as is practical. Ticks should be removed properly and the area of attachment wet thoroughly with 70% ethanol (Chap. 131, Tick Paralysis).

Vaccine prophylaxis of tularemia has been achieved. Previously, a formalin-killed suspension of tularemia bacilli was employed. It was apparent from the incidence of disease in vaccinated laboratory personnel that protection was incomplete. An attenuated, living strain of *F. tularensis* developed in Russia has been extensively evaluated in the United States. Administration is by acupuncture, as with vaccinia virus. Experimentally, both the respiratory and oral routes of administration have been effective. Reactions to the vaccine are minimal; a scar develops at the site of inoculation that is analogous to that in vaccinia. The protection offered by this vaccine is markedly superior to the killed vaccine and is complete against small numbers of *F. tularensis.* A moderate disease may develop when large doses of bacilli are inoculated. The duration of immunity has not been fully established, but revaccination can be accomplished safely. Until additional information is available the interval should be 3 to 5 years. Other than BCG, the live, attenuated tularemia vaccine is only live bacterial immunogen for use in man. Information gained from it will perhaps lead to better vaccines for preventing other serious bacterial infections.

The vaccine can be obtained for use in persons requiring protection against tularemia. The sponsor of the vaccine is the United States Army Medical Research Institute of Infectious Diseases, Fort Detrick, Maryland, 21701.

Mechanisms of immunity have not been elucidated. Circulating antibodies cannot be reliably correlated with resistance. Cellular immunity may be important, and sensitized macrophages are associated with resistance to infection in experimental animals.

Remaining Problems

As in many infections, the exact mechanisms of immunity in man are unknown. Tularemia has been induced in volunteers in order to evaluate an attenuated vaccine. If such studies are continued, modern methods for studying immunologic processes should be applied.

Bibliography

Journals

BELL JF: Ecology of tularemia in North America. J Jinsen Med 11:33–44, 1965

GIDDENS WR, WILSON JW JR, DIENST FT JR, HARGROVE MD: Tularemia. An analysis of one hundred forty-seven cases. J La Med Soc 109:93–98, 1967

LJUNG O: The intradermal test in tularemia with particular reference to reaction elicited in regions of different incidence of the disease. Acta Med Scand 160:135–148, 1958

LJUNG O: Intradermal agglutination test in tularemia, with particular regard to past infection. Acta Med Scand 160:149–154, 1958

MILLER RP, BATES JH: Pleuropulmonary tularemia: A review of 29 patients. Am Rev Respir Dis 99:31–41, 1969

JACK D. POLAND

Plague

140

Plague normally involves a three-way interaction between *Yersinia pestis,* wild rodents, and fleas parasitic on the rodents. *Yersinia pestis* gains entry into humans by accident; if infection occurs, it is virtually equivalent to disease—usually manifest as bubonic plague. Other clinical forms include pneumonic, septicemic, meningeal, and pharyngeal plague.

Etiology

Yersinia pestis is a plump (0.5 μm–0.8 μm × 1.5 μm–2 μm), gram-negative, nonmotile, nonsporulating, nonlactose-fermenting, pleomorphic bacillus. A bipolar or safety-pin appearance is best demonstrated in smears of infected animal tissues stained by Giemsa's or Wayson's method. This classic appearance is not dependably evident in preparations stained by Gram's method. The plague bacillus is identified by (1) its characteristic appearance in broth and agar cultures; (2) its staining characteristics; (3) lysis by specific bacteriophage; (4) the agglutination reaction; (5) fluorescent antibody (FA) staining; and (6) necropsy findings after inoculation into susceptible laboratory animals. Although biochemical reactions can be used to differentiate *Y. pestis* from *Yersinia pseudotuberculosis,* bacteriophage testing is highly specific and can be applied more rapidly.

Plague bacilli are aerobic and facultatively anaerobic. They are not fastidious and grow readily in most bacteriologic culture mediums. However, growth is slow even at the optimum temperature of 28°C and requires about 48 hours before colonies are readily discernible on plain agar; growth is satisfactory at 35°C to 37°C. Colonies are small (1 mm–3 mm in diameter) and grayish, with a granular or beaten-copper surface best seen with a 3- to 10-power lens. After 24 hours at 28°C in standard broth medium examined without shaking, plague bacilli exhibit a flocculent type of growth without turbidity.

The FA test is based on the presence of bacterial envelope fraction 1, which is produced most readily at 37°C but not at temperatures below 28°C. Consequently the FA test is best performed on smears of animal tissues, aspirates of exudates such as those from buboes, or cultures incubated at 37°C. This test makes possible the rapid presumptive identification of *Y. pestis.* Clinical specimens that were frozen or refrigerated after collection are suitable for immediate FA examination because bacterial growth is restricted. If growth has not been inhibited in transit, the specimen should be incubated at 37°C or inoculated into an appropriate laboratory animal to enhance production of envelope antigen fraction 1. Cross-reactions with *Y. pseudotuberculosis* have been recorded, and occasional strains of *Y. pestis* may not stain or may exhibit weak staining. If a positive FA test is supported by epidemiologic and clinical evidence, there is little doubt of the diagnosis.

Epidemiology

Owing to the great variety of mammalian hosts, fleas, and environmental conditions involved (Fig. 140-1), the ecology of plague is complex. The bacilli exist in nature in two broad and not entirely discrete ecologic forms: *enzootic plague* and *epizootic plague.*

Enzootic plague implies a stable rodent–flea infection cycle that is maintained in a relatively resistant host population without excessive host mortality. Enzootic foci serve effectively as long-term reservoirs of infection, but are inconspicuous and difficult to identify.

Epizootic plague occurs when plague bacilli are introduced into rodent or other small mammal populations that are moderately or highly susceptible to the lethal effects of the infection. Because mortality is high, such epizootics are often conspicous, especially among larger colonial rodents, such as prairie dogs. The risk of exposure is high whenever humans come

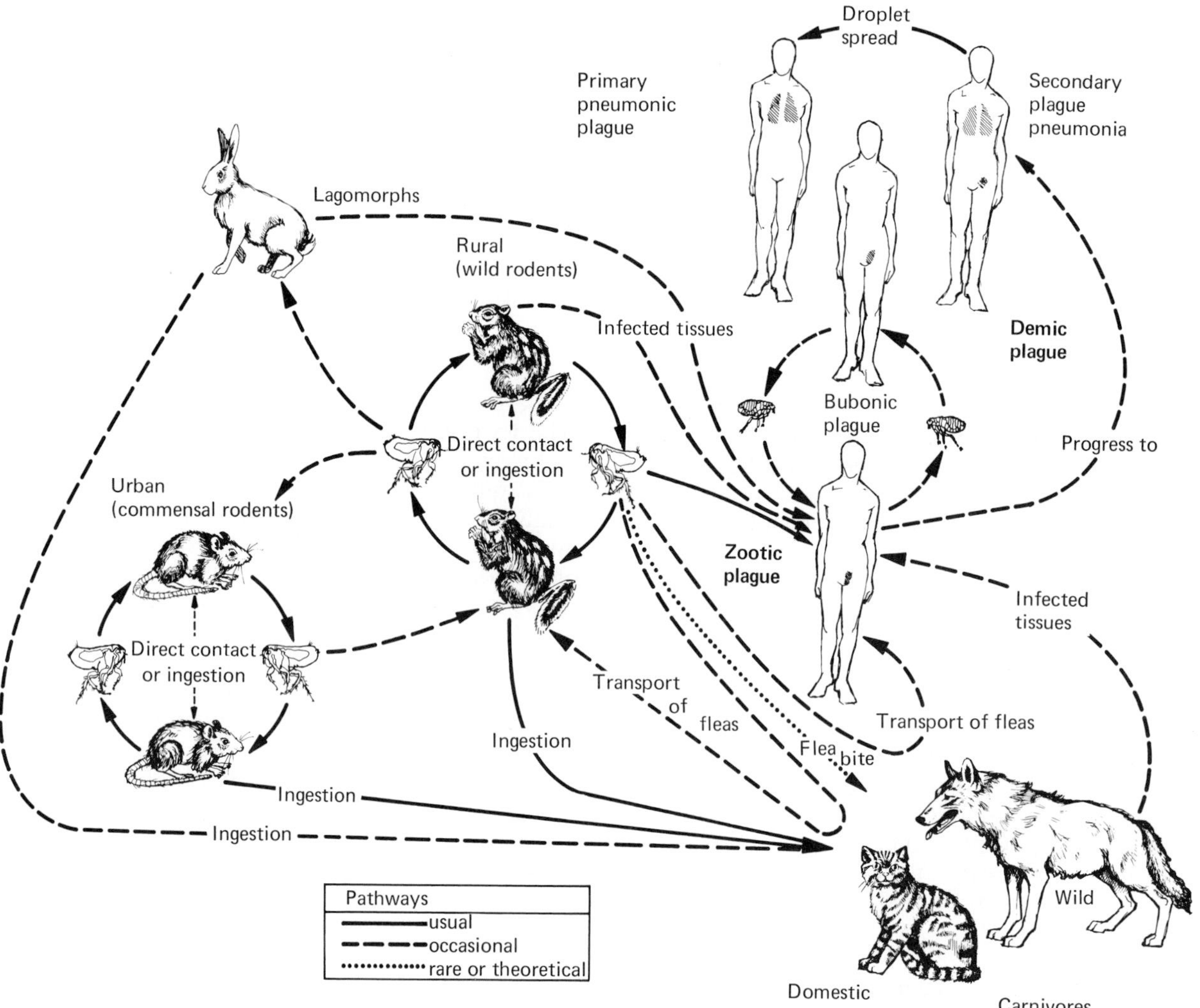

Fig. 140-1. Epidemiology of infection caused by *Yersinia pestis* in the United States. The cyclic nature of plague and some of the mechanisms responsible for its maintenance in nature are shown.

into contact with epizootic plague—for example, dwelling near ground squirrel populations, hunting, or camping. The transmission of *Y. pestis* from animal hosts to humans is referred to as *zootic plague;* transmission from man to man is *demic plague.*

Plague foci occur throughout the world. In the United States, *Y. pestis* is permanently established from the eastern slope of the Rocky Mountains westward. Periodic expansion has been detected as far east as the 98th parallel in Texas, the 100th parallel in the midwestern states, and into bordering Mexico and Alberta, Canada. During the first quarter of this century, zootic plague in the United States usually resulted from contact with domestic rats and their fleas. The hazard of rat-borne plague was reduced with the development of rat control programs and the application of higher standards of sanitation in urban areas and on ships. From 1925 to 1960, a yearly average of one case of plague resulted from rural exposures to small, wild mammals or their fleas. An annual average of three cases occurred in the 1960's, and eleven in the 1970's (Fig. 140-2). Of all cases since 1945, 87% have occurred in the Rocky Mountain states. Except for one urban case traced to a fox squirrel (*Sciurus niger*) in 1968, cases in the past 55 years have resulted from exposure in rural or suburban settings.

Males predominate both in frequency (55% of cases) and case fatality (23% compared to 14% in females—Fig. 140-3). Two-thirds of cases occur in

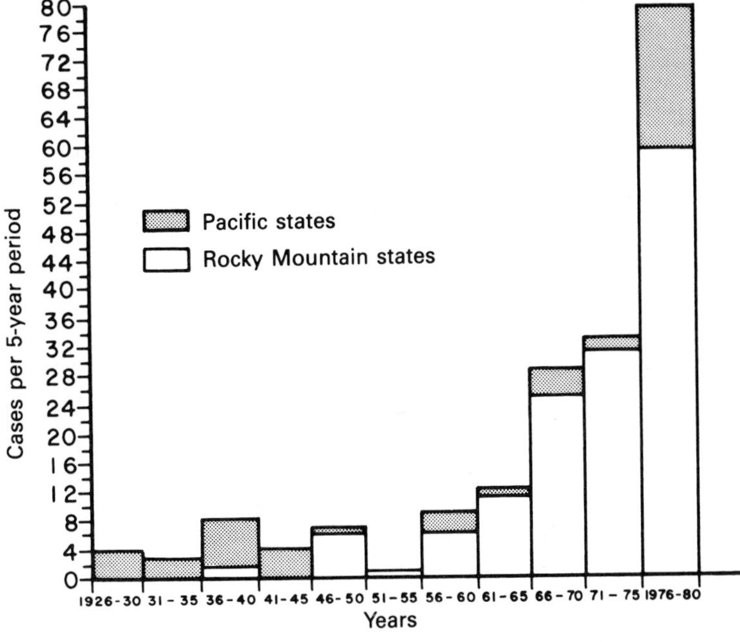

Fig. 140-2. Reported cases of plague in humans in the United States by 5-year periods, 1926–1980.

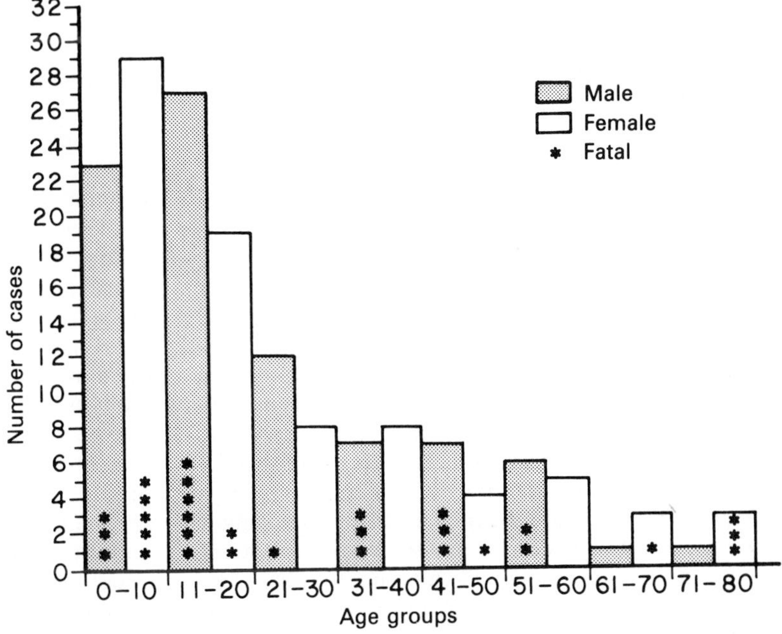

Fig. 140-3. Reported cases of plague in humans in the United States by 10-year age groups, 1950–1980.

persons under 25 years of age. During the decade 1970–1980, 53% of the patients were females, probably reflecting exposure in proximity to home environments rather than during field excursions. The principal sylvatic animals involved have been ground squirrels (*Spermophilus* spp.), prairie dogs (*Cynomys* spp.), chipmunks (*Eutamias* spp.), marmots (*Marmota* spp.), deer mice (*Peromyscus* spp.), wood rats (*Neotoma* spp.), rabbits (*Sylvilagus* spp.), and hares (*Lepus* spp.). In recent years, a strong association has been observed in the Rocky Mountain states between rock squirrels (*Spermophilus variegatus*) and human cases. Human infection from lagomorphs (rabbits and hares) usually results from tissue contact rather than flea bite, and it occurs predominantly in the fall and winter months. Voles (*Microtus* spp.), and deer mice are reservoirs of enzootic plague in the western United States, but have not often been associated with plague in humans.

Impact of Predators

Although predators, including carnivores, rapacious birds, and man, are essential neither to the natural perpetuation of plague nor to its classic transmission to humans, they have been implicated as significant determinants in plague epidemiology and undoubtedly are involved in ways not readily detected. Humans build both permanent and recreational residences in wilderness habitats where plague is enzootic and often alter the environment to favor increased populations of certain epizootic hosts such as rock squirrels, prairie dogs, other ground squirrels, pack rats, and deer mice.

Carnivorous mammals such as cats, dogs, coyotes, skunks, badgers, and raccoons are regularly seropositive for plague in areas of enzootic and epizootic plague activity. Serologic testing of these animals provides a more efficient means of plague surveillance than the monitoring of live-trapped rodents and their fleas. Laboratory studies have shown that seroconversion in carnivore species results from ingestion of plague-infected rodents. Except for felines, most carnivores develop neither illness nor septicemia and consequently do not appear to provide a mechanism for transmission of *Y. pestis* to other hosts through their natural ectoparasites.

Domestic cats and dogs have served as vehicles for human infection. They often transport infected wild rodents (caught or found dead) to a home environment, and infected fleas may be acquired during hunting forays and transported to the home environment. Rarely dogs and frequently cats (particularly kittens) become acutely ill following the ingestion of plague-infected rodents. They may then serve as a direct source for human exposure through purulent drainage of subcutaneous abscesses; respiratory tract secretions from animals developing a secondary pneumonia; mechanical transmission by biting, licking, or scratching; or oral secretions of animals with oropharyngeal colonization by *Y. pestis.*

From 1970–1980, carnivores were implicated as the source of infection for eight patients with plague. Two cases resulted from skinning plague-infected wild carnivores (a bobcat and a coyote); one patient was exposed by a domestic dog, four by house cats, and one by a house pet not specifically identified that was suspected to have plague. Only one of the house-cat associated patients (exposed by bites and scratches of an infected kitten) and the two wild-carnivore associated patients developed bubonic plague. The remaining five patients were apparently exposed to animals that had developed a secondary pulmonary infection. Three of these five developed primary plague pneumonia: one cat-associated case (fatal), one dog-associated (survived), and one for whom the infecting species was undetermined (fatal). One patient (who died) developed septicemic plague following exposure to a cat that succumbed with confirmed plague pneumonia, and one patient survived after developing pharyngeal plague from exposure to a plague-infected house cat with pneumonia and hemoptysis. The role of predators in the transport of plague-infected rodents or their fleas from one rodent population to another undoubtedly occurs but is difficult to document. Smaller carnivores with limited range may cause more localized dissemination; however, predatory birds or larger mammalian carnivores could conceivably transport plague-infected carcasses or fleas over long distances.

Incursion in Humans

Demic plague may result from pneumonic spread, human flea transmission, or spread by infected exudates. Human flea transmission is uncommon and has not been observed in the United States. Transmission by an infected exudate was noted in Indonesia when a child with classic bubonic plague (inguinal bubo) developed bilateral purulent dacryocystis (Fig. 140-4). *Yersinia pestis* was recovered from the pharynx of the boy's father, who did not develop an associated illness, presumably because of sulfonamide prophylaxis.

Primary pneumonic plague, the most serious form of demic plague, has its start from pulmonary involvement following bubonic or septicemic plague. Because *Y. pestis* is not effectively airborne, but rather is transmitted by droplets, the communicability of plague pneumonia is difficult to predict. Contact (droplet) transmission varies with environmental conditions and with the presence and nature of cough in the patients. Cough producing only thick, tenacious material is unlikely to produce tiny droplets (1μ to 5μ) that may be inhaled into the lower respiratory tract. Larger droplets may impinge on the upper respiratory tract, resulting in pharyngeal plague. Primary plague pneumonia occurs primarily in persons in close and prolonged contact with another person with pneumonic plague. Hence, respiratory transmission occurs most frequently to medical personnel or household contacts who are directly involved with the care of the patient.

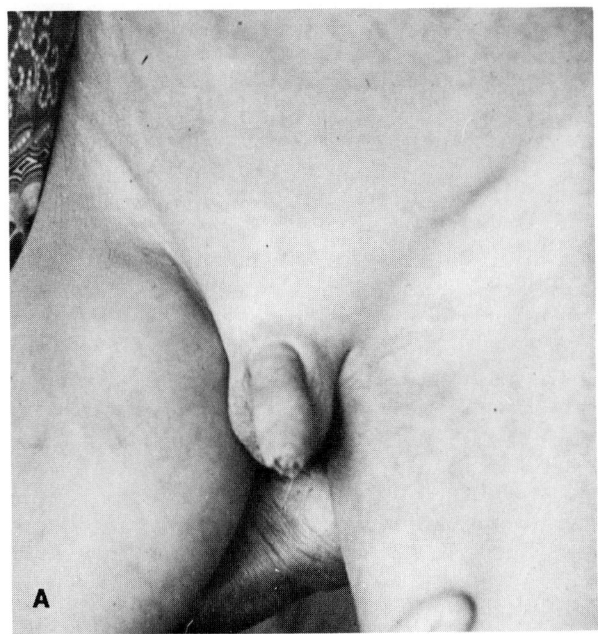

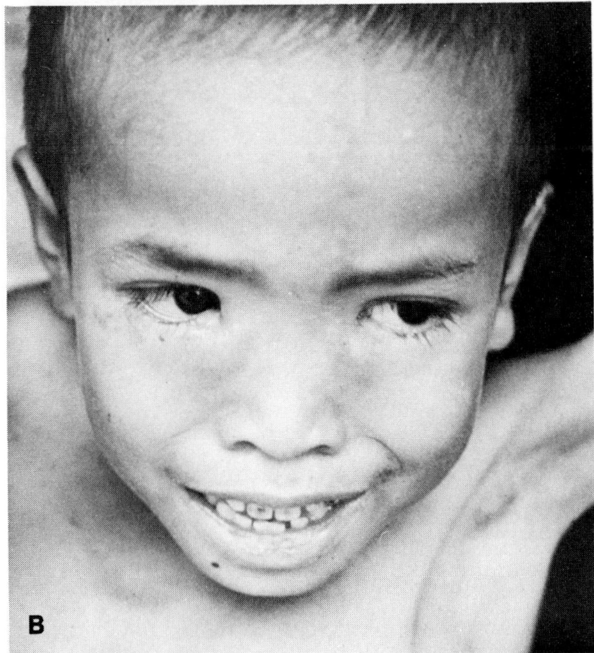

Fig. 140-4. Classic bubonic plague (right inguinal) complicated by disseminated lesions in a 7-year-old boy who recovered with streptomycin and sulfadiazine therapy. *Yersinia pestis* was isolated from the pharynx of the boy's father (holding the patient), who was presumably infected from purulent eye drainage. (*A*) Fluctuant, primary, right femoral bubo; left inguinal lymphadenitis evident by palpation. (*B*) Disseminated lesions in the same patient, including bilateral, purulent dacryocystitis and left axillary lymphadenitis. Conjunctivitis was not clinically evident. Right axillary, cervical, and left popliteal lymphadenitis were also present. All secondarily involved lymph nodes were nonfluctuant and smaller than the primary femoral node.

Plague pneumonia has been rare in the United States, and primary pneumonic plague in contacts has not been detected since 1925. However, from 1975 through 1980, 20 cases of confirmed plague with pneumonia have occurred and three of these appeared to be primary plague pneumonia acquired from domestic pets. During 1980, a 47-year-old woman with primary pneumonic plague had contact with about 180 persons before her 3-day course of illness ended fatally. Plague was diagnosed 4 days after her death. Although all contacts were placed on abortive therapy ("prophylaxis"), it appeared that pneumonic transmission had not occurred. The roentgenographic record of development of pneumonia secondary to bubonic plague in a patient who survived is shown in Figure 140-5. Of particular danger if plague pneumonia develops is the possibility of long distance travel prior to hospitalization. This has occurred in the United States: in 1957, exposure in Colorado—death, without premortem diagnosis or specific therapy, in eastern Texas; in 1961, exposure in New Mexico—death, without premortem diagnosis or specific therapy and with pneumonitis, in Massachusetts; and in 1975, exposure in New Mexico—death, with pneumonitis, in California.

Pathogenesis and Pathology

The development of *Y. pestis* in fleas involves the formation of masses of plague bacilli and fibrinoid material in the midgut. If blockage of the proventriculus (foregut) results, the flea cannot successfully ingest a blood meal. A blocked flea tends to dessicate and aggressively makes repreated attempts to feed; at each attempt, being unable to pass the blood meal past the blocked proventriculus, it regurgitates several thousand microorganisms into the site of the bite. Holding infected oriental rat fleas (*Xenopsylla cheopis*) in the laboratory at temperatures over 27°C (80°F) allows clearing of the proventricular blockage; a practical effect of this phenomenon is that plague epidemics have long been observed to subside spontaneously when ambient temperatures remain above 27°C to 30°C (80°F to 85°F).

Once *Y. pestis* is introduced into a human, a progressive infection generally results unless specific antimicrobial therapy is given. Nearly every organ and tissue of the body may be involved, with the production of acute or indolent signs and symptoms referable to a wide variety of organ systems. Depending on the length of survival, pyogenic, necrotic, infarctive, inflammatory, hemorrhagic, and edematous lesions are found in many tissues and organs, particu-

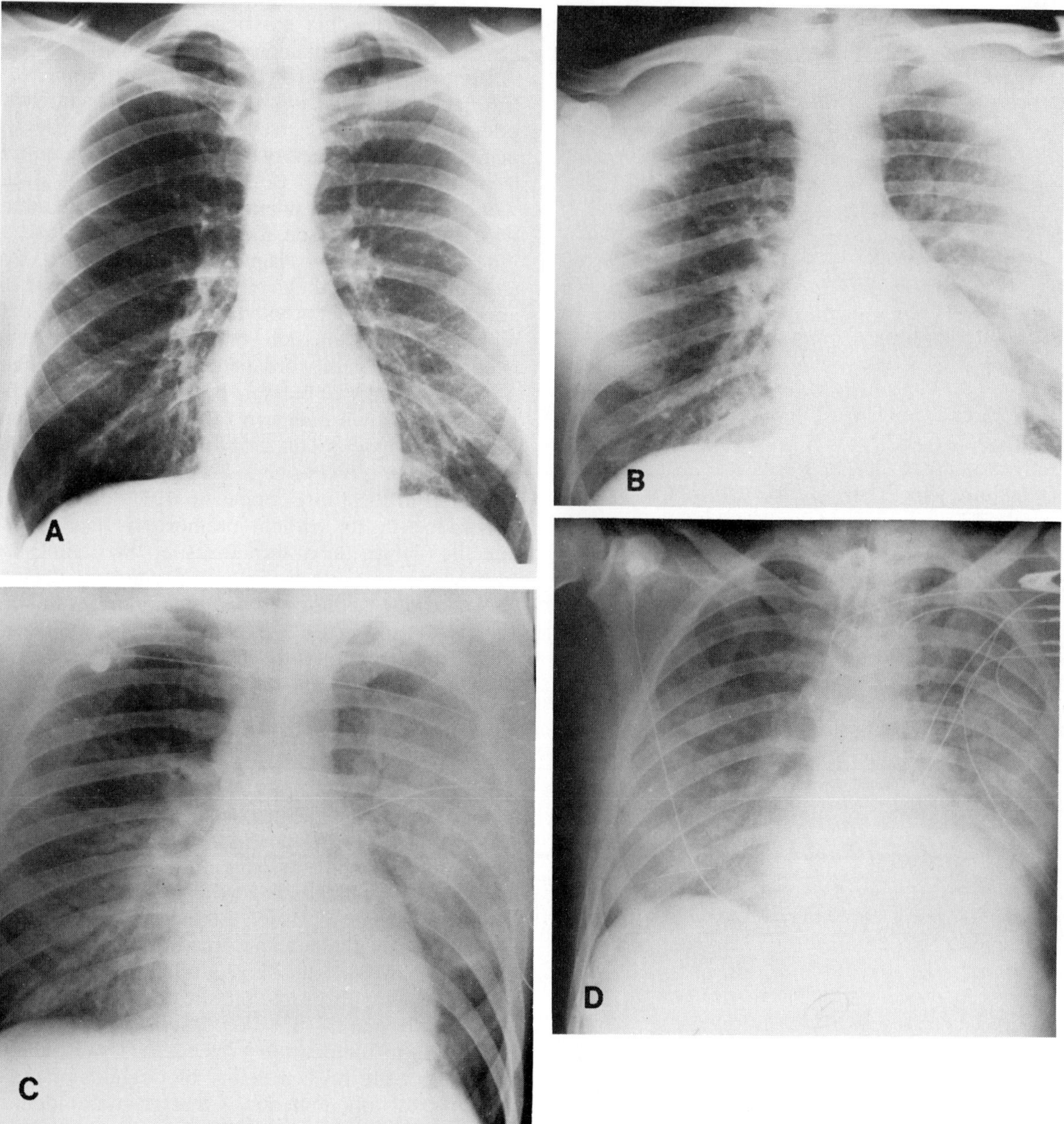

Fig. 140-5. Plague pneumonia secondary to bubonic plague. (*A*) Three days after onset and one day prior to clinical pneumonia. (*B*) Four days after onset and the day clinical pneumonitis became evident. (*C*) One day following onset of clinical pneumonia. (*D*) Two days after clinical pneumonia. Films over the 2 days subsequent to (*D*) were unchanged; rapid resolution of the infiltrates then followed. The patient subsequently recovered (owing to treatment with streptomycin and tetracycline) with no radiographic residua but with severe necrosis of the digits (see Fig. 140-6). (Courtesy of Dr. James Favata and the John C. Lincoln Hospital, Phoenix, Arizona)

larly the regional lymphatics, spleen, liver, lungs, skin, and mucous membranes. There may be circulatory collapse, a bleeding diathesis, and peripheral thrombotic phenomena similar to the reactions associated with the endotoxins of other gram-negative microorganisms. Toxemia may be progressive and result in death although the tissues are devoid of viable *Y. pestis* at necropsy—a paradox thought to result from vigorous bacteriolytic antimicrobial therapy, for example, with streptomycin. On the other hand, suboptimal antibacterial therapy favors the development of complications and possibly the establishment of resistant bacteria, for example, bacteria resistant to streptomycin. Progressive circulatory failure may develop in severe infections, and sudden death from cardiac failure has occurred even during convalescence.

On introduction into a human host, flea-borne *Y. pestis* is quite susceptible to phagocytosis. However, phagocyte-resistant bacilli persist and may give rise to septicemia, either after regional lymph nodes are involved (bubonic plague) or without apparent lymph node involvement (primary septicemic plague). Primary pneumonic plague is fulminant, resulting in severe prostration, respiratory distress, and death sometimes within hours after onset. The primary involvement of a vital organ (as the lungs) by direct inoculation with plague bacilli that are phagocyte-resistant from the outset probably contributes to the fulminant course of pneumonic plague.

Manifestations

The incubation period in bubonic plague is generally 2 to 6 days; in primary pulmonary plague it is 1 to 3 days. The severity at onset is variable. In the less malignant form, the initial manifestations are general malaise, fever, and pain or tenderness in an area of regional lymph nodes; there may be associated *buboes,* or lymph node enlargement. Buboes most often occur in the inguinal or axillary regions, but they may occur anywhere and in the past decade have been noted in supraclavicular, epitrochlear, cervical, postauricular, subpectoral, and popliteal sites. At this stage of the disease, toxicity may be minimal, but intermittent bacteremia occurs in most patients, as shown by the isolation of *Y. pestis* from at least one of a series of blood cultures. In more severe infections, or when treatment is delayed, the disease progresses rapidly to a septicemic phase: all blood cultures are positive for *Y. pestis* (ideally three or more), with the classic findings of toxicity, prostration, shock, and occasionally, hemorrhagic phenomena. The progression of infection can be extremely rapid—a patient appearing to be mildly ill, with complaints limited to fever and adenitis, may become moribund within hours.

In some patients, the onset of symptoms may be quite striking, with high, remittent fevers, chills, myalgias, headache, and severe malaise. Occasionally, buboes cannot be detected for several days after the onset of symptoms. Lack of early adenitis makes diagnosis difficult; clinical findings are not specific, and the clinician is not likely to consider obtaining a lymph node aspirate unless tenderness directs attention to a possible lymphadenitis. If bacteremia is present, the plague bacilli may sometimes be observed in a smear of peripheral blood—a grave prognostic sign. Less common symptoms include abdominal pain, nausea, vomiting, constipation followed by diarrhea (frequently bloody), skin mottling, petechiae, and circulatory collapse. Rarely, vesicular and pustular skin lesions occur. The gravity of the illness is indicated by varying degrees of restlessness, apathy, anxiety, apprehension, seizures, and coma.

The use of the term *pestis minor* to describe a mild form of bubonic plague should be abandoned, since it simply denotes a variation in the host response and not a variant of the infecting organism.

Diagnosis

The classic feature of plague contracted by cutaneous inoculation is an excruciatingly painful bubo. This finding in a patient with fever, prostration, and a history of possible exposure to rodents, rabbits,or fleas in the western United States should lead to the inclusion of plague in the differential diagnosis. Tularemia (Chap. 139, Tularemia) may mimic this clinical and epidemiologic picture; however therapy is the same for both diseases. In recent years bubonic plague has been diagnosed in cases ultimately found to have been adenitis caused by *Francisella tularensis* (Chap. 139, Tularemia), *Streptococcus* spp. (Chap. 24, Streptococcal Diseases), or *Staphylococcus aureus* (Chap. 101, Streptococcal Skin Infections and Glomerulonephritis); conversely, tularemia has often been diagnosed in cases subsequently confirmed as bubonic plague. Sporadic cases of primary septicemic plague are particularly difficult to recognize because there are no specific findings. Other comparably severe infectious diseases that may be confused with septicemic plague include meningococcemia (Chap. 119, Bacterial Meningitis), sepsis caused by enteric gram-negative bacteria, and certain rickettsioses (Chap. 96, Spotted Fevers and Chap. 98, Typhus Fevers). As soon as a diagnosis of suspected plague is made, local and state health officials must be notified so that epidemiologic investigation and control measures can be instituted. At least four blood cultures should be obtained; these can be taken over a period of 1 to 2 hours and need not inordinately delay initiation of specific therapy. Blood, bubo or parabubo aspirates, exudates, purulent drainage, and sputum should be examined by microscopy (smears stained with dyes and fluorescent antibody), culture (liquid and agar), and animal inoculation. Giemsa's or Wayson's methods of staining smears are particularly valuable for rapid, tentative diagnosis because bacteria morphologically consistent with *Y. pestis* are frequently demonstrable. Gram-stained preparations are less helpful because the characteristic bipolarity may not be readily discernible.

Buboes and abscesses should not be excised, or incised and drained, for diagnostic purposes. However, careful needle aspiration of an involved lymph node is essential to determine the microbial etiology of the lymphadenitis. The value of this procedure far exceeds the risk associated with judicious manipulation. The procedure should not be done until after blood cultures have been obtained; therapy may be started either concurrently with the aspiration or immediately after microscopic examination of stained smears of the aspirate. In the face of a negative smear examination, therapy may need to include drugs effective against gram-positive and gram-negative causes of lymphadenitis (including plague when the suspicion is reasonably well based). Most bacteria, with the exception of *Y. pestis,* other *Yersinia* spp., and *F. tularensis,* should grow readily within 24 hours. Negative cultures of aspirates at 24 hours should sharply increase the suspicion that plague or tularemia is the correct diagnosis. Acute and convalescent serums should be obtained from all patients suspected of having plague to enable an etiologic diagnosis in the event microorganisms cannot be isolated.

The several diagnostic efforts described permit cases of plague to be categorized as (1) *suspect plague*—appropriate clinical and epidemiologic findings or demonstration in stained smears of bacteria consistent with *Y. pestis;* (2) *presumptive plague*—FA-positive clinical specimens or a single, elevated antibody titer in an unvaccinated person with a plaguelike illness; (3) *confirmed plague*—isolation of *Y. pestis* from clinical materials or a fourfold rise or fall in specific antibody. Only presumptive and confirmed plague cases are officially reported in the United States because appropriate laboratory studies are readily available to exclude *Y. pestis* as the etiology in the dozens of samples submitted each year as suspect plague. However, if the diagnosis of suspect plague is supported by appropriate epidemiologic, ecologic, and clinical evidence, the case may be accepted for official reporting by the Plague Branch of the Centers for Disease Control (CDC).

Prognosis

Without treatment, the case–fatality ratio in bubonic plague is about 60%; in septicemic and pneumonic plague it is probably 100%. With early therapy, the mortality in bubonic plague should approach zero; however, the fatality rate of reported cases since 1950 has been 18%. The prognosis is poor in primary pneumonic plague if therapy is delayed more than 18 hours after the onset of symptoms. Age and general physical condition also affect survival in septicemic and pneumonic plague.

The immediate, life-threatening complications of plague are shock, hyperpyrexia, convulsions, and disseminated intravascular coagulation (DIC). In addition, hematogenous or lymphogenous dissemination may occur early in the disease. Antibacterial therapy that is inadequate or inappropriate (*e.g.,* use of ampicillin) appears to favor the development of metastatic infections such as plague meningitis, secondary pneumonia, endophthalmitis, and multiple lymph node involvement including intraabdominal and perihilar nodes.

Primary buboes may resolve slowly, despite appropriate chemotherapy, with pain and tenderness persisting for weeks. Necrosis and impending ulceration of a primary bubo may require incision and drainage; wound precautions should be instituted (personnel should wear masks and gloves when examining wounds and changing dressings; contaminated materials—exudates, gloves, soiled dressings, instruments—should be autoclaved or incinerated) because of remote, but definite, possibility that viable *Y. pestis* will persist in necrotic nodes.

Patients who have been severely ill should be observed for evidence of progressive cardiac failure, a rare but critical complication that may not occur until late in the recovery phase. The cardiac-active glycosides are effective.

In patients who survive severe septic shock, marked necrosis of peripheral tissues may occur (Fig. 140-6). Nursing care is vital to limit the amount of damage. Devices that further limit already compromised peripheral circulation to fingers and toes, for example, arm boards or other restraints, should be applied cautiously or not at all.

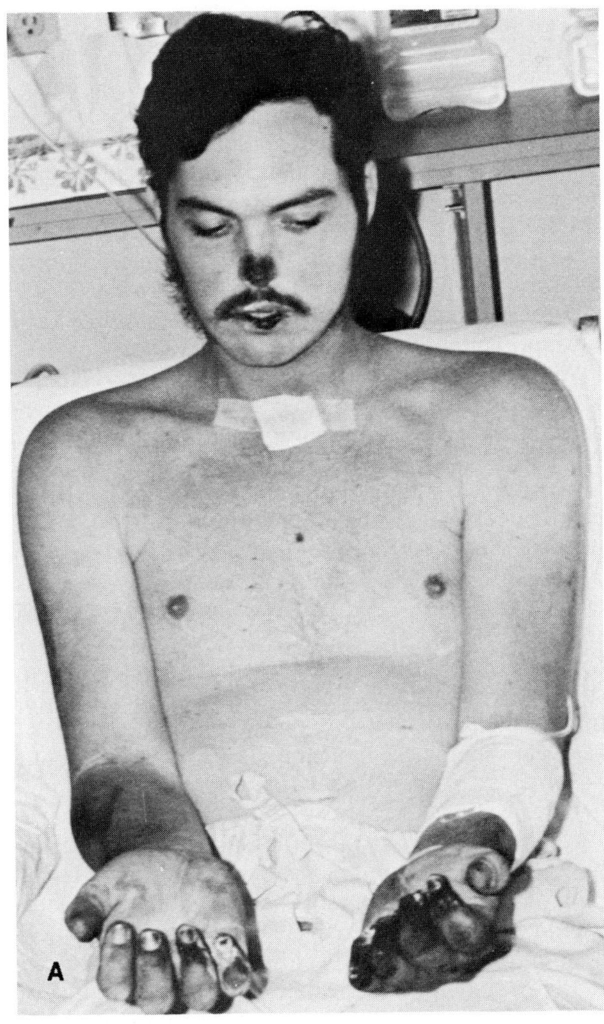

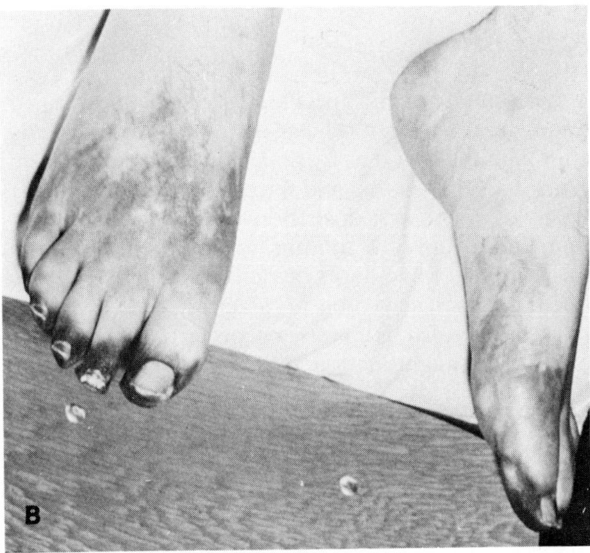

Prior to the availability of specific antimicrobial therapy, plague during pregnancy often resulted in abortion, although *Y. pestis* was not regularly present in the fetal tissues. With early therapy in the mother, the pregnancy should not be adversely affected. In cases in which delivery occurs within 48 hours after therapy is initiated in the mother, the newborn should be considered exposed to *Y. pestis* either by the transplacental route or (more likely) by contact with the mother's blood during delivery and should be treated.

Therapy

Because secondary plague pneumonia may already have developed, all patients with bubonic plague should be strictly isolated until 48 hours after specific therapy has been instituted. Isolation may be discontinued if respiratory symptoms or purulent drainage does not develop. Exudates or purulent discharges should be handled with rubber gloves. Face masks, including eye protection, are indispensable in caring for patients with pulmonary plague.

Nonspecific therapy consists of symptomatic and supportive management of complications such as shock, high fever, and convulsions. Fluid needs may require intravenous supplementation. Glucosteroids (*e.g.,* methylprednisolone, 30 mg/kg body wt/day by IV injection as a single dose for 2–3 days) should be considered in management of life-threatening toxemia and shock after specific antimicrobial therapy is instituted. Diazepam is beneficial in reducing apprehension and restlessness.

Antimicrobial therapy should be started promptly, without waiting for laboratory confirmation, after specimens have been obtained for diagnosis. The most effective drug against *Y. pestis* is streptomycin. Other effective drugs include kanamycin, chloramphenicol, the tetracyclines, and certain sulfonamides (*e.g.,* sulfadiazine). The penicillins are not effective in treating plague, although these drugs frequently

Fig. 140-6. Bubonic plague with secondary plague pneumonia (see Fig. 140-5) and resultant severe peripheral tissue necrosis (photographed during convalescence, 14 days after onset of illness). (*A*) Severe necrosis of fingers, nose, and lips. (*B*) Severe necrosis of toes; ecchymosis of the feet. Amputation of portions of all digits except the thumbs was necessary 3 months after the acute episode. Earlier in the disease, the nature and degree of blackened skin over the entire body was more profound and qualitatively different from simple cyanosis; it was reminiscent of the medieval epithet applied to plague—*the Black Death.*

show activity in *in vitro* testing. Gentamicin has been successful in treating plague in humans and in expериemental murine plague. Because of greater experience, it is still preferable to use streptomycin. Studies have not been done to determine the effectiveness of doxycycline in treating plague.

Because streptomycin is rapidly lethal to *Y. pestis,* it must be given circumspectly in the hope of avoiding a rapid and massive release of plague endotoxin, for example, 30 mg/kg body wt/day by IM injection of four equal portions, 6 hourly, for up to 10 days. If clinical considerations (*e.g.* potential for hearing loss in the elderly and patients with impaired renal function) predicate a shorter course, streptomycin may be given for 5 days. Ten days or more of total antibacterial therapy may be accomplished by overlapping an alternative to streptomycin for at least 24 hours before the streptomycin is stopped.

Alternative drugs include

1. Tetracycline: loading dose—15 mg/kg body wt (not to exceed 1 g) perorally, followed by 40–50 mg/kg body wt perorally as six equal portions, 4-hourly for the first day, and then 30 mg/kg body wt/day perorally as four equal portions, 6-hourly, for a total of 10–14 days; if peroral therapy is not tolerated, inject IV one-third of the calculated oral dosage until peroral treatment is accepted.
2. Chloramphenicol: loading dose—25 mg/kg body wt (not to exceed 3 g) perorally, followed by 50–75 mg/kg body wt/day perorally as four equal portions, 6 hourly, for a total of 10–14 days; if peroral therapy is not possible, inject 50 mg/kg body wt/day IV as four equal portions, 6 hourly, until peroral therapy is accepted.
3. Sulfadiazine, or preferably, trisulfapyrimidines: loading dose—25 mg/kg body wt perorally, followed by 75 mg/kg body wt/day perorally as four equal portions, 6-hourly, for a total of 10–14 days.

Tetracyline and chloramphenicol have been effective when used alone, but in patients with pneumonia or severely ill with plague, streptomycin is the preferred antimicrobic. The sulfonamides cannot be recommended when more effective and safer alternatives are available.

If there is meningitis or endophthalmitis, chloramphenicol should always be included in the regimen of therapy because of its relatively unrestricted entry into these areas.

Of available drugs, chloramphenicol offers the least hazard to the mother and her unborn child when it is necessary to treat a pregnant woman for plague. Streptomycin may be added for the first 3 to 4 days of therapy. The dosage given above are appropriate.

Newborns delivered during the potentially bacteremic phase of maternal plague should be treated either with kanamycin (15 mg/kg body wt/day injected IV or IM as four equal portions, 6-hourly) or streptomycin (10–20 mg/kg body wt/day injected IM as four equal portions, 6-hourly). Tetracyline (30 mg/kg body wt/day perorally as four equal portions, 6-hourly) and chloramphenicol (15–25 mg/kg body wt/day perorally as four equal portions, 6-hourly) are both potentially hazardous alternatives.

All contacts of patients with pulmonary involvement, whether primary or secondary, should be quarantined and given either tetracycline (30 mg/kg body wt/day perorally as four equal portions, 6-hourly) or trisulfapyrimidines (60–75 mg/kg body wt/day perorally as four equal portions, 6-hourly for 10 days). Other effective drugs that may be used for prophylaxis of contacts include chloramphenicol or sulfadiazine. Rapidly excreted sulfonamides, such as sulfisoxazole, should not be relied upon for prophylaxis. Close observation of pneumonic contacts should include bidaily measurement of temperature. If a febrile illness develops, hospitalization and streptomycin therapy are indicated. Paired serums should be obtained to establish whether infection with *Y. pestis* has occurred.

Chemoprophylaxis is not routinely indicated for household and community associates of patients with bubonic plague. Community and regional residents should be kept under surveillance for the detection of additional cases. Field studies must be undertaken to define and control the source of cases in humans.

Prevention

A heat-killed vaccine prepared from *Y. pesitis* produces humoral antibody in over 90% of recipients after administration as a primary series of three injections with the second and third doses given 4 and 16 weeks after the first dose. Booster injections are recommended every 6 months to maintain immunity. After a total of five doses of vaccine have been given, booster doses may then be given empirically at annual or biennial intervals, or preferably, when the passive hemagglutination antibody to fraction 1 of *Y. pestis* falls below 1:128.

Severe inflammatory reactions localized to the site of injection are frequent, and systemic reaction to the vaccine occurs occasionally. Active immunization is recommended only for persons at high risk—those engaged in military or other field operations and activities that must be carried out in areas endemic for plague or those in situations in which exposure to rodents and fleas cannot be controlled. Trained personnel using proper equipment in clinical laboratories or conducting plague investigations in field or laboratory fall into the high-risk group if they handle strains of *Y. pestis* that are resistant to antimicrobics or if aerosols of plague bacilli are produced. The general adequacy of standard bacteriologic procedures is attested by the fact that only four instances of laboratory plague infection in the United States have been reported since 1900.

Field exposures have resulted in human infections when sick or dead animals have been skinned and examined without appropriate precautions. Both infestation by the animals' ectoparasites and direct contact with tissues must be avoided.

The primary preventive or suppressive measures against urban plague consist of rigorous environmental sanitation aimed at reducing or eliminating commensal rodent populations, particularly rats and their fleas. In areas where enzootics or epizootics of plague are in progress, steps to reduce the host rodent population should be delayed until they can be undertaken concurrently with, or after, an effective flea control program. Rodent reduction alone would result in a massive release of infected fleas, increasing the potential for human exposure and further epizootic spread. In countries or areas where standards of sanitation are high and commensal rodents are few, plague should be uncommon. However, as long as plague continues to exist anywhere in the world, uncontrolled domestic rat populations are a hazard wherever they exist.

Remaining Problems

Identification of the toxic principle of *Y. pestis* that is responsible for the deadliness of severe infections is necessary to evaluate the therapeutic potential of antiserum. Antiserum could possibly modify the toxic reaction that results when *Y. pestis* is killed in the patient with plague who is treated with rapidly bactericidal agents. Such combined therapy would be most useful in patients who are desperately ill—precisely those patients in whom the diagnosis of plague is most difficult.

There are many questions related to the virulence of *Y. pestis* and the nature of the protective responses in man. Is the essential protective factor an immunoglobulin? If so, what component of *Y. pestis* is the antigenic determinant? Are there geographic or temporal virulence-oriented stain variants of *Y. pestis?* For example, does the increase of cases as well as the increase in those with secondary pneumonia since 1974 reflect a change in ecologic or strain factors? Can variants be defined by pathogenetic, biochemical, or immunologic methods? How frequently do "atypical" strains of plague bacilli infect humans, and is there an altered pathophysiology with such infections?

In order to improve methods of preventing the exposure of humans to plague, extensive field studies are needed to define more clearly the ecosystems that support enzootic and epizootic plague. Criteria should be developed and surveillance instituted so that periodic epizootic expansions can be anticipated and prevented or controlled.

Bibliography

Books

QUAN TJ, BARNES AM, POLAND JD: Yersinioses. In Ballows A, Hausler B (eds): Diagnostic Procedures for Bacterial, Mycotic and Parasitic Infections. Washington, DC American Public Health Association, 1981. pp. 221–243.

POLAND JD, BARNES AM: Plague. In Steele JH (ed): CRC Handbook Series in Zoonoses. Boca Raton CRC Press, 1979. pp. 515–597.

WHITE ME: Plague. In Conn HF (ed): Current Therapy. Philadelphia, W. B. Saunders, 1980. pp. 52–53.

Journals

CAVANAUGH DC: The specific effect of temperature upon the transmission of the plague bacillus by the oriental rat flea (*Xenopsylla cheopis*). Am J Trop Med Hyg 20:264–273, 1971

Compilation of recent work on plague immunology. J Infect Dis 129(Suppl), S1–S120 1974

FINDGOLD MJ: Pathogenesis of plague. Am J Med 45:549–554, 1968

POLLITZER R: Plague. WHO Monograph No. 22, 1954

WHITE ME, GORDON D, POLAND JD, BARNES AM: Recommendations for control of *Yersinia pestis* infections: recommendations from the CDC. Infection Control 1:324–329, 1980

WILLIAMS JE, HARRISON DN, QUAN JJ, MULLINS JS, BARNES AM, CAVANAUGH DC: Atypical plague bacilli isolated from rodents, fleas, and man. Am J Publ Health 68:262–264, 1978

CALDERON HOWE

141 Melioidosis

Melioidosis is a specific infectious disease of humans that resembles equine glanders in the spectrum of its clinical manifestations—that is, focal involvement of the lungs with a widespread suppurative process that is acute or chronic.

Etiology

The bacteria that cause glanders (*Pseudomonas mallei*) and melioidosis (*Pseudomonas pseudomallei*) together form the pseudomallei group of pseudomonads. They are gram-negative, nonsporulating, obligate aerobes exhibiting bipolar staining. *Pseudomonas pseudomallei* can be distinguished from other pseudomonads by agglutination or fluorescence with specific antibody and show cross-reactivity with *Legionella pneumophila* (Chap. 33, Legionnaires' Disease). Readily cultivable on blood and nutrient agar containing glycerol, *P. pseudomallei* dissociates in 3 to 5 days to give opaque, white, unpigmented colonies with a rough, corrugated, heaped-up appearance. Even though the organism does not ferment lactose, the colonies on MacConkey agar take up neutral red nonspecifically. The pseudomallei group is susceptible *in vitro* to commonly used broad-spectrum antimicrobics including the sulfonamides; *P. pseudomallei* are resistant to colistin and gentamicin.

Epidemiology

Sporadic cases of human glanders, caused by *P. mallei,* have long been recognized and associated with contact with diseased horses. Eradication of animal glanders through control measures and replacement of horse-drawn vehicles with mechanical contrivances have rendered the human disease a rarity in the western world. However, there has been a renaissance of interest in infections caused by *P. pseudomallei* because they have been seen in an appreciable number of persons returning from Southeast Asia.

This disease was first described in Malaya in 1913 as a severe, frequently fatal infection resembling equine glanders. The geographic distribution of recognized infection was once thought to be restricted to Southeast Asia. Sources of infection are now known to exist in Central and South America, the West Indies, Madagascar, Australia, and Guam. Although generally believed to be limited to tropical and subtropical climates, sporadic cases have also been reported from Turkey, Korea, and the Philippine Islands. The discovery of infection caused by *P. pseudomallei* in wild rodents and in domestic animals led to the earlier belief that rats might be a natural reservoir of infection. Only recently has it been concluded that (1) there is no natural animal reservoir, (2) the microorganism can be recovered directly from soil and water in regions where cases have been recognized, and (3) humans and many species of wild and domestic animals inhabiting these areas may show only serologic evidence of infection without overt disease. In short, *P. pseudomallei* is a normal inhabitant of soil and water, particularly in low-lying and rice-growing areas. Melioidosis therefore can no longer be regarded as a zoonosis; man-to-man transmission is unknown.

Pathogenesis and Pathology

Pseudomonas pseudomallei may be acquired directly from a contaminated environment through wounds or minor breaks in the skin. Ingestion and inhalation are other routes of infection. A wide spectrum of interaction with nonhuman and human hosts follows, ranging from inapparent infection (the usual result) to full-blown, even overwhelming, disease (a small minority of those infected).

Published autopsy reports obviously deal with patients of the less common kind. Multiple abscess formation in many organs is the outcome of massive hematogenous dissemination of bacteria.

A primary pneumonic form of melioidosis, without septicemia, may result in chronic, cavitary disease with calcification that resembles tuberculosis.

Foci of infection persistent for years may be consequent to any form of melioidosis. Pulmonary lesions, osteomyelitis, and soft-tissue abscesses are frequent localizations.

Manifestations

In addition to the rare, but frequently fatal, septicemic form, melioidosis may also be manifest as an acute or subacute pneumonitis or pneumonia. Chest pain, cough productive of purulent sputum, and hemoptysis are frequent. Signs of shock may develop and have been ascribed, in part at least, to endotoxins liberated from *P. pseudomallei.* Patients who were previously in good health generally do not develop septicemia. With adequate chemotherapy, recovery is usual.

Patients harboring latent infection may suffer reactivation and clinical relapse triggered by debilitation from any cause, whether it be malnutrition, major surgery, extensive burns, or wounds suffered in military action.

In most persons who contract melioidosis, the initial infection goes unnoticed, and only serologic evidence of contact with *P. pseudomallei* develops. In populations native to endemic areas, quite appreciable numbers of persons have been shown by serologic surveys to have high titers of antibodies to *P. pseudomallei* without clinical evidence of disease. Such persons may also harbor latent infection capable of reactivation under appropriate circumstances of stress.

Diagnosis

Because of protean manifestations and great variation in severity, melioidosis cannot be diagnosed with certainty on clinical grounds alone. The roentgenographic appearance of the lungs may resemble tuberculosis (Chap. 34, Pulmonary Tuberculosis) or any of the respiratory mycoses (Chaps. 39–45). A high index of suspicion should attend any patient with such roentgenographic changes who has recently returned from areas of the world in which *P. pseudomallei* is found in the environment. The specific diagnosis depends on isolation of *P. pseudomallei* and serologic evidence. For the latter, a passive hemagglutination reaction (*P. pseudomallei* polysaccharide absorbed to sheep erythrocytes) and the complement fixation (CF) reaction are most useful. Other laboratory data, particularly the leukocyte count, are so variable that they are of little diagnostic value.

Prognosis

Originally, melioidosis was described as a rare but usually fatal disease. With the application of serologic methods, it has become apparent that the usual outcome of infection of normal humans with *P. pseudomallei* is a subclinical infection that engenders a lasting protective immunity. The outlook for patients with overt clinical melioidosis, either primary or recrudescent, has been remarkedly improved by the availability of effective antimicrobial agents.

Therapy

Pseudomonas pseudomallei is generally susceptible to broad-spectrum antimicrobics, including the sulfonamides. A growing body of clinical experience supports the use of tetracycline supplemented with a sulfonamide, both in full dosage—that is, tetracyclyne, 50 to 65 mg/kg body wt PO every 24 hours as four equal portions, 6-hourly, and sufficient sulfonamide (*e.g.,* triple sulfapyrimidines), either IV or PO, to maintian a blood concentration of 10 to 15 mg/100 ml. *P. pseudomallei* are susceptible to trimethoprim and sulfamethoxazole, and the proprietary combination of these drugs has been advocated as effective primary therapy for melioidosis. In severe illness, chloramphenicol should be added in the same dose as tetracycline. Abscesses should be surgically drained after antimicrobial therapy has been instituted.

The effect of therapy must be judged by the amelioration of clinical signs and symptoms; it should be continued until lesions demonstrable by roentgenography have resolved. This may mean many weeks of therapy. Serologic evidence of infection mat persist long after subsidence of acute or overt clinical manifestations. The danger of relapse should be constantly borne in mind.

Prevention

There are no preventive measures except those based on good hygienic practices. Physicians examin-

Table 141-1. Differentiation of Pseudomallei Group From Other Pseudomonads

	P. mallei	*P. pseudomallei*	Other pseudomonads
Growth	Slow	Rapid	Rapid
Colonies	Cream, smooth	Cream, smooth to rough	
Motility	−	+	+
Pigment	None	None	Blue green
Susceptibility to pseudomallei bacteriophage	−	+	−
Phosphatase	Heat-stable	Heat-stable	Heat-labile
Susceptibility to colistin	Resistant	Resistant	Susceptible

ing returnees from Southeast Asia must be aware of the possibility of melioidosis in any unexplained pulmonary disease or febrile illness.

Bibliography

Journals

ASHDOWN LR: Identification of *Pseudomonas pseudomallei* in the clinical laboratory. J Clin Path (London) 32:500–504, 1979

ASHDOWN LR: An improved screening technique for isolation of *Pseudomonas pseudomallei* from clinical specimens. Pathology 11:293–297, 1979

CLAYTON AJ, LISELLA RS, MARTIN DG: Melioidosis: A serological survey in military personnel. Mil Surg 138:24–26, 1973

HOWE C, SAMPATH A, SPOTNITZ M: The Pseudomallei group: A review. J Infect Dis 124:598–606, 1971

VON GRAEVENITZ A: Clinical microbiology of unusual *Pseudomonas* species. Prog Clin Pathol 5:185–218, 1973

RICHARD H. PARKER

Rat-Bite Fever

142

Rat-bite fever is an acute febrile illness that is usually accompanied by a skin rash. It is caused by either *Streptobacillus moniliformis* or *Spirillum minor,* bacteria that generally infect humans as a result of the bite of a rat, mouse, or other rodent. Fever, skin rash, and lymphadenitis are associated with infection with either kind of bacteria. However, there are usually other clinical manifestations that allow differentiation of streptobacillary fever and spirillar fever. Clinically, either of these infections may mimic more common illnesses, such as secondary syphilis (Chap. 59, Syphilis) and Rocky Mountain spotted fever (Chap. 96, Spotted Fevers).

Streptobacillary Fever

Etiology

Streptobacillus moniliformis is a nonmotile, microaerophilic, gram-negative, non-acid-fast, pleomorphic bacillus that has been found in the nasal flora of both wild and laboratory rats. It has also been isolated from a wide variety of infections occurring in other nonhuman animals. In a liquid medium, such as trypticase soy broth enriched with 20% horse or rabbit serum, characteristic puffball-shaped colonies appear following 2 to 7 days' incubation under increased carbon dioxide tension. It is important that sodium polyanethol sulfonate not be present in the medium because this agent inhibits the growth of *S. moniliformis.* Cultures on agar mediums may spontaneously yield *L-forms,* a phenomenon that led to the first description of L-forms by Klieneberger. These cell-wall deficient forms differ in morphology from intact bacilli and are resistant to antimicrobics that interfere with cell-wall synthesis. The L-forms usually revert to the bacillary phase when subcultured.

Epidemiology

Information about the epidemiology of streptobacillary fever is limited because the disease is not reportable. However, data obtained from reported cases indicate that humans usually become infected in one of three ways: (1) bite or scratch of a wild animal (2) bite of a laboratory rat or (3) ingestion of milk contaminated by rat excrement.

Most cases of streptobacillary fever result from the bite of a wild rat, and approximately 50% of cases involve children under the age of 12 years. Because there is an association between problems of urbanization such as overcrowding or inadequate sanitation and high rat populations, the disease occurs frequently in cities. In addition, the disease may follow bites or scratches inflicted by mice, squirrels, weasles, dogs, or cats. Although *S. moniliformis* has been found in the nasopharynx of up to 50% of healthy wild rats, it is estimated that only 10% of people bitten by wild rats develop rat-bite fever. Laboratory rats harbor *S. moniliformis* as frequently as wild rats, and persons working with laboratory rats may acquire rat-bite fever.

When infection with *S. moniliformis* follows the ingestion of milk contaminated by rats, the resulting illness is known as *Haverhill fever.*

Pathogenesis and Pathology

Following a rat-bite there is minimal local inflammation with prompt healing of the wound and little, if any, regional lymphadenitis. If infection is not halted at the regional lymph nodes, bacteremia ensues and lesions distant from the bite appear 1 to 3 days after the bite. The incubation period of streptobacillary rat-bite fever is usually brief; however, occasionally it may be as long as 3 weeks after the bite. Seeding of the microorganisms in many tissue (*e.g.* soft tissue, brain, and myocardium) initiates a pyogenic response with the formation of abscesses. Microorganisms can usually be isolated from these lesions. Some of the manifestations of streptobacillary rat-bite fever are due to a nonpyogenic process, presumably an immunologically mediated inflammatory response. This is the explanation for the migratory polyarthritis and parotitis seen in some patients.

Manifestations

The onset of the disease is usually abrupt with intermittent fever, rigors, headaches, malaise, and myalgias. At this time the bite site may be completely healed or may be ulcerated with regional lymphadenopathy. These symptoms are followed shortly by the appearance of a generalized maculopapular or petechial skin rash that is most prominent on the extremities, especially on the palms and soles. The rash not only is similar in distribution to the rash of Rocky Mountain spotted fever but also may blanch under pressure and increase in intensity when the skin is warmed or a tourniquet is applied to the extremity. A nonsuppurative migratory polyarthritis occurs in approximately 50% of patients. This hallmark of the disease is a true arthritis and is unlike the arthralgia that may be a feature of Rocky Mountain spotted fever. In a few cases, the arthritis may progress to cause permanent restriction of joint function. Infants and children may suffer from severe weight loss and diarrhea. Rare complications include bronchopneumonia, endocarditis, parotitis, amnionitis, subglottic mass, and abscesses in the brain, myocardium, and subcutaneous tissue. The laboratory findings are consistent with acute bacterial infection, with the exception that 25% of cases may show a false-positive serologic test for syphilis.

Diagnosis

The triad of fever, regional lymphadenopathy, and rash involving the palms and soles should suggest the diagnosis of streptobacillary infection. A history of recent bite by a rodent or close association with rodents and the development of a migratory polyarthritis also favor disease caused by *S. moniliformis.* Definitive diagnosis demands either isolation of *S. moniliformis* (from the blood, the site of the bite, synovial fluid, or abscesses) or demonstration of an antibody response. Similar clinical illness may be associated with Coxsackie virus infection (Chap. 149, Coxsackie Virus and Echovirus Infections), Epstein–Barr virus infection (Chap. 137, Infectious Mononucleosis), streptococcal disease (Chap. 24, Streptococcal Diseases), leptospirosis (Chap. 76, Leptospirosis), Rocky Mountain spotted fever (Chap. 96, Spotted Fevers), and secondary syphilis (Chap. 59, Syphilis).

Prognosis

With specific therapy, death should be rare and morbidity shortened. However, the mortality of untreated streptobacillary infection has been as high as 10%. Fatality is usually associated with complications such as pneumonia, brain abscess, and endocarditis.

Therapy

Prevention of the infection may be accomplished by prompt cleaning of the bite wound with an antiseptic solution such as povidone-iodine solution and administration of phenoxymethylpenicillin (15 mg/kg body wt/day, PO, as 2 equal portions, 12-hourly, for 3 days). Because the value of antimicrobial therapy in prophylaxis has not been proven, the exposed person should be advised to report the occurrence of headache, joint pain, rash, or renewed inflammation at the site of the bite. The treatment of choice for streptobacillary fever is penicillin G. The usual dose is 5 to 10 mg (8,000–16,000 units) procaine penicillin G/kg body wt/day, IM, as two equal portions, 12-hourly, for 10 days.

Patients who are allergic to the penicillins may be treated for 10 days with tetracycline (30 mg/kg body wt/day, PO, as 4 equal portions, 6-hourly) and streptomycin (15 mg/kg body wt/day, IM, as 2 equal portions, 12-hourly).

Prevention

Prevention of rat-bite fever is best accomplished by eliminating or minimizing contact between humans and rodents. Laboratory personnel who must handle animals should be advised to seek medical attention following any rodent bite.

Spirillar Fever (Sodoku)

Etiology

Spirillum minor (previously known as *S. minus*) is gram-negative, measures 1.7 nm to 5 nm in length, displays 2 to 6 spirals, and is actively motile by means of bipolar flagellae. It has not been cultivated on artificial mediums. Laboratory diagnosis depends on detecting the characteristic microscopic appearance and demonstrating pathogenicity for mice and guinea pigs.

Epidemiology

Spirillar fever, like streptobacillary rat-bite fever, is associated with social and economic deprivation. The disease was first described in Japan, but cases have been diagnosed in Asia, Europe, and the United States. Infection usually follows the bite of a rat, mouse, or rodent-ingesting animal (*e.g.* a cat).

Pathogenesis and Pathology

There is a paucity of information about the pathogenesis and pathology of this disease in humans. The widespread tissue involvement demonstrated at necropsy supports hematogenous dissemination. In experimental animals, bacteremia has been demonstrated for several weeks.

Manifestations

During the incubation period of 7 to 21 days, the bite lesion heals. With the onset of illness, there is flaring of the initial wound with inflammation, induration, and occasionally a chancrelike ulceration. This is followed by paroxysms of chills and fever, lymphangitis, regional lymphadenitis, and the appearance of a maculopapular, erythematous, or dark purple eruption spreading from the initial lesion. The patient may complain of myalgias, but arthritis does not occur. There may be leukocytosis and a false-positive serologic test for syphilis. The illness may last 3 to 4 days and then subside, only to recur after a few days. Relapses have occurred weeks, months, or years after the initial illness.

Diagnosis

The diagnosis is most easily established by demonstrating the typical morphology and motility of *S minor* by darkfield examination of exudate from an infected site. Intraperitoneal inoculation of mice or guinea pigs with blood or exudate from the patient may result in spirillemia 5 to 15 days later. However, this examination is of value only if it has been demonstrated that the animals are not carriers of *S minor* by examination of their blood prior to inoculation.

Prognosis

In early reports of *S. minor* rat-bite fever from Japan, the mortality was about 10%; however, fatality from this infection is very unusual in the United States. Specific therapy and the lower incidence of infection are contributory factors.

Therapy

Spirillar rat-bite fever has been successfully treated with streptomycin and also with penicillin G.

Prevention

Improvement of socioeconomic conditions is the primary means of preventing this disease.

Remaining Problems

Development of a reliable method for cultivation of *S. minor* would improve the specific diagnosis of this infection.

Bibliography

Book

ROGOSA M: *Streptobacillus moniliformis* and *Spirillum minor.* In Lennette EH, Balows A, Haussler WJ Jr, Truant JP (eds) Manual of clinical microbiology, 3rd ed. American Society for Microbiology, Washington DC. pp 350–356.

Journals

BROWN TM, NUNEMAKER JC: Rat-bite fever: A review of the American cases with reevaluation of etiology: Report of cases. Bull Johns Hopkins Hosp 70:201–328, 1942

FARO S, WALKER C, PIERSON RL: Amnionitis with intact amniotic membranes involving *Streptobacillus moniliformis.* Obstet Gynecol 55 (Suppl):9S–11S, 1980

PORTNOY BL, SATTERWHITE TK, DYCKMAN JD: Rat-bite fever misdiagnosed as Rocky Mountain spotted fever. South Med J 72:607–609, 1979

RAFFIN BJ, FREEMARK M: Streptobacillary rat-bite fever: A pediatric problem. Pediatrics 64:214–217, 1979

PAUL M. SOUTHERN, JR.

143 Relapsing Fever

Relapsing fever, a disease characterized by recurrent pyrexial attacks, is caused by spirochetes of the genus *Borrelia,* which are transmitted to humans by lice or soft-bodied ticks. Synonyms include tick, fowl nest, cabin, and vagabond fever and bilious typhoid.

Etiology

All forms of relapsing fever are caused by spirochetes of the genus *Borrelia* (order Spirochaetales family Treponemataceae). These bacteria are 10 μm to 20 μm × 0.2 μm to 0.5 μm and have 3 to 30 loosely wound, coarse, irregular spirals per cell. *Borrelia* spp. are gram-negative, but stain well with combinations of aniline dyes (*e.g.,* the Giemsa stain) and metallic salts (*e.g.,* methenamine silver).

Louse-borne relapsing fever is caused by *Borrelia recurrentis;* it does not occur in the United States. The tick-borne disease does occur in the United States and is caused by several species of *Borrelia* each of which is closely identified with a particular tick—a relationship signalled in some cases by a shared species epithet: *Borrelia hermsii* with *Ornithodoros hermsi, B. parkerii* with *O. parkeri, B. turicatae* with *O. turicata* (Table 143-1).

Epidemiology

Body and head lice, *Pediculus humanus* var. *corporis* and *P. humanus* var. *capitis* (Chap. 114, Pediculosis), become infected by ingesting blood from a human spirochetemic with *B. recurrentis.* A few days later, infected lice can transmit borrelias; infection in lice is lifelong. Humans are inoculated when the infected blood and body fluids released from a crushed louse come into contact with bitten or otherwise abraded skin or mucous membranes. *Borrelia recurrentis* is not transmitted congenitally in lice; humans and nonhuman primates are the only reservoirs. Louse-borne relapsing fever occurs in epidemics under conditions favoring infestation with lice—crowding, deprivation, war, and migration. Recent outbreaks have occurred in Ethiopia and the Sudan. Louse-borne relapsing fever has not been recognized in the United States since approximately 1906.

The other species of *Borrelia* are transmitted during the bite of soft-bodied ticks of the genus *Ornithodoros.* Each species of *Borrelia* is believed to have a single natural tick vector (Table 143-1). The tick remains infected for the duration of its life, which may be several years; in some species, the infection is transmitted congenitally to succeeding generations. All developmental stages are capable of transmitting borrelias by contaminating bite wounds with saliva or coxal fluid containing borrelias. The bites of most *Ornithodoros* spp. are painless; thus, the victim may not be aware of the exposure (after feeding, the tick drops off the host).

Tick-borne relapsing fever occurs sporadically or in small outbreaks when humans are exposed through residence, occupation, or, more commonly in the United States, recreation. The incidence is higher during warmer seasons when ticks and their vertebrate hosts are more active and when humans may come into contact with ticks. However, an outbreak has occurred in cold weather among campers who slept in tick-infested, stove-heated log cabins. In the United States, relapsing fever is now acquired only in Western and Southwestern areas hospitable to certain species of ticks. *Ornithodoros hermsi* (Fig. 143-1) lives in mountainous areas, generally at altitudes above 3000 feet. Vertebrate hosts include chipmunks, various squirrels, and deer mice. Rodent nests, dead trees, and old wood buildings are infested. *Ornithodoros parkeri* lives in caves and burrows inhabited by ground squirrels, prairie dogs, and burrowing owls, but may occasionally feed on other rodents. *Ornithodoros turicata* is found in caves,

Table 143-1. Correlation of Relapsing Fever Borrelia *spp., Vectors, and Reservoirs*

Group	*Borrelia* spp.	Geographic Distribution	Vector	Reservoir
Louse-borne	*recurrentis*	Potentially cosmopolitan (epidemic in Ethiopia and Sudan)	*Pediculus humanus*	Humans, other primates
Tick-borne	*hispanica*	North Africa, Spain, Portugal, Middle East, East and West Africa	*Ornithodoros erraticus* ("large" form)	
	crocidurae group	Central Africa, Turkey Middle East, East and West Africa, Iran, Sahara, Dakar, Saudi Arabia	*O. erraticus* ("small" form)	Rodents
	duttonii	Tropical Africa, Senegal, Madagascar, Saudi Arabia	*O. moubata* *O. savignyi*	Rodents
	graingeri	Kenya	*O. graingeri*	
	persica	Central Asia, Middle East	*O. tholozani*	Rodents
	caucasica	Caucasus	*O. verrucosus*	Rodents
	latyschewii	Central Asia	*O. tartakovskyi*	Rodents, dogs
	venezuelensis	Central America, South America	*O. rudis*	Rodents
	mazzottii	Mexico, Central America, Texas	*O. talaje*	Rodents
	parkerii	Western United States Canada	*O. parkeri*	Rodents
	turicatae	Texas, southwest United States, Central and South America	*O. turicata*	Rodents
	hermsii	Western United States	*O. hermsi*	Rodents
	brasiliensis	South America	*O. brasiliensis*	Rodents
	dugesii	Mexico, Central America	*O. dugesi*	Rodents

(After Southern PM Jr: Relapsing fever. In Kelly VC (ed) Practice of Pediatrics. Philadelphia, Harper & Row, 1981)

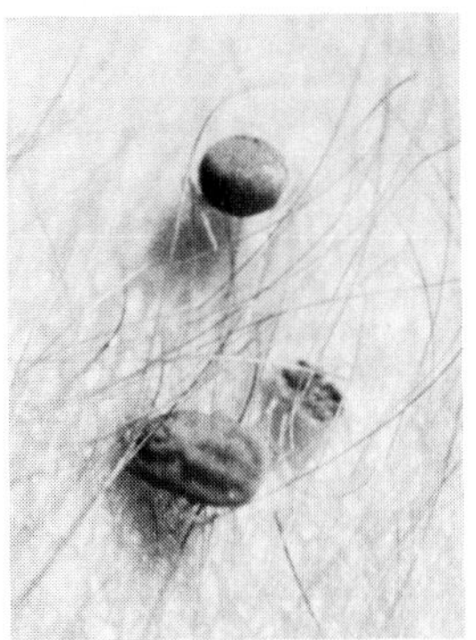

Fig. 143-1. *Ornithodoros hermsii.* Adult ticks in various stages of engorgement on the arm of a human. (Courtesy of Willy Burgdorfer)

burrows of field mice and other rodents, owls, and snakes, in huts, in animal barns, and under houses. *Ornithodoros talaje,* the carrier of *B. mazzotti* has occasionally been associated with relapsing fever in the Southwestern United States. It is usually found in caves, associated with rodents.

Congenital infection and transmission by contaminated blood have been reported.

Pathogenesis and Pathology

Borrelial spirochetemia is common during fever but is rare when there is no fever. During afebrile periods, borrelias may be found in the spleen, liver, bone marrow, and central nervous system (CNS).

Recovery and immunity in relapsing fever are thought to be largely dependent on humoral antibodies, rather than on cell-mediated immunity. The cyclic recurrence of attacks may reflect the emergence of antigenic variants of the infecting borrelias that were not destroyed by circulating antibody.

Autopsy data are available only from louse-borne relapsing fever. The spleen is heavily involved with miliary and necrotic lesions, microabscesses, and perisplenitis. Other lesions include hepatic congestion and focal necrosis, renal tubular congestion with red blood cell casts, pulmonary alveolar hemorrhages, and cerebral edema and congestion with focal cortical hemorrhages. Spirochetes are visible in myocardial blood vessels; spleen, liver, and renal tissues; renal tubular casts; and pulmonary blood vessels. Many of these lesions may be consequent on a Jarisch–Herxheimer-like reaction that occurs regularly after therapy of louse-borne relapsing fever and occasionally after treatment of the tick-borne disease. In severe cases, there is an increase in fibrin degradation products and a decrease in Hageman factor, plasma prekallikrein, and serum hemolytic complement activity. These findings, as well as the appearance of endotoxinlike activity in the plasma, have led to speculation that (1) disseminated intravascular coagulation (DIC) may be present in some patients before therapy and may be at least partly mediated by activation of Hageman factor and (2) activation of the complement system may play a role in adversely altering hemodynamics during the Jarisch–Herxheimer-like reaction after treatment. It is not known whether the endotoxinlike activity results from lysis of spirochetes, or whether altered hemodynamics permits the entry of products of enteric gram-negative bacilli into the circulation.

Manifestations

Despite minor differences in the clinical manifestations of relapsing fever, based on vector, parasite, and the immune status of the host, most episodes are remarkably similar. Tables 143-2 and 143-3 summarize clinical manifestations of relapsing fever based on a review of reported louse-borne and tick-borne cases.

Although patients in the United States acquire the tick-borne form of relapsing fever, there may be no history of tick bite. Patients seen in nonendemic areas should be queried for a history of travel and possible exposure in an endemic area. After an incubation period averaging 7 days there is a sudden onset of illness with chills, fever (40°C [104°F] or higher), and prostration. Headache, severe myalgias, and arthralgias are common. There may also be abdominal pain, vomiting, diarrhea, eye pain, cough, chest pain, and sore throat. The skin is hot and dry, tachycardia and tachypnea may be present and splenomegaly is common. There may also be hepatomegaly, muscle tenderness, lymphadenopathy, and lethargy with an altered sensorium. Some outbreaks have been associated with a macular rash over the torso.

The symptoms and signs usually subside 3 to 6 days after onset, at which time the temperature falls abruptly and there is profuse sweating. After an afebrile interval of variable length (commonly 3–6 days), a second febrile, symptomatic episode occurs. There are usually 2 to 4 relapses of progressively decreasing severity and duration separated by progressively lengthening intervals of relative well-being. In

Table 143-2. *Manifestations of Tick-Borne Relapsing Fever (Based on Review of 1143 Reported Cases)*

Manifestation	Mean Value or Incidence	Range
Sex incidence	Approximately 60% M:40% F	
Age incidence	Majority <20 years	Newborn–>50 years
Case–fatality rate	Approximately 2%–5% (>20% below 1 year of age)	0%–8% (overall)
Incubation period	Approximately 7 days	1 day–>18 days
Duration of primary febrile attack	3–4 days	12 hr–17 days
Duration of afebrile interval	5–7 days	1–63 days
Duration of relapses	1.5–3 days	12 hr–14 days
Number of relapses	2–4	0–13
Maximum temperature (primary attack)	Approximately 40.6°C (105°F)	
Splenomegaly	37% (of 216 cases)	
Hepatomegaly	17% (of 294 cases)	
Jaundice	7% (of 740 cases)	
Rash	24% (of 114 cases)	
Respiratory symptoms	16% (of 759 cases)	
CNS involvement	9% (of 613 cases)	

(Southern PM Jr: Relapsing fever. In Kelley, VC (ed): Practice of Pediatrics. Philadelphia, Harper & Row, 1981)

Table 143-3. Manifestations of Louse-Borne Relapsing Fever (Based on Review of 2565 Reported Cases)

Manifestation	Mean Value or Incidence	Range
Sex incidence	Approximately 50% M:50% F (of 2026 cases)	
Age incidence	Approximately 24% children (of 2026 cases)	0–90 years
Case–fatality rate	3.5%–5.5% treated, up to 40% untreated	
Duration of primary febrile attack	5.4 days (in 1980 cases)	2–12 days
Duration of afebrile interval	9.25 days (in 1668 cases)	3–27 days
Duration of relapses	1.9 days (in 1617 cases)	1–4 days
Number of relapses	Majority = 1 (in 2.008 cases), few = 2, rare = 3 or more	1–5
Maximum temperature	39°C–39.5°C (102.2°F–103.1°F)	37°C–40°C (98.6°F–104°F)
Splenomegaly	72% (of 2382 cases)	
Musculoskeletal pain	67% (of 2390 cases)	
Hepatomegaly	65% (of 2040 cases)	
Jaundice	38% (of 2382 cases)	
Cough	30% (of 2040 cases)	
CNS involvement	25% (of 2040 cases)	
Rash	6% (of 829 cases)	

(Southern PM, Jr: Relapsing fever. In Kelley VC (ed): Practice of Pediatrics. Philadelphia, Harper & Row, 1981)

louse-borne relapsing fever, there may be only one such recurrence.

Complications are uncommon in the United States, but have been described more frequently in Africa. These include iritis or iridocyclitis, meningitis, cranial nerve lesions, bronchitis, and pneumonia. If relapsing fever is acquired during pregnancy, there is a high rate of spontaneous abortion.

Diagnosis

Recognizing relapsing fever on clinical grounds is relatively simple in an endemic area of louse-borne disease. On the other hand, it can be extremely difficult in other circumstances, particularly in the United States.

Specific diagnosis is made by demonstrating spirochetes in smears of peripheral venous blood stained by either Giemsa's or Wright's method. During febrile periods, spirochetes will be found in such smears in approximately 70% of patients. Greater sensitivity is achieved by the demonstration of spirochetes in smears from the tail blood of young rats or mice 1 to 10 days after inoculation with blood or other tissues from the patient (Fig. 143-2). Spirochetes may be found in sputum, urine, cerebrospinal fluid (CSF), prostatic fluid, or tissues obtained by biopsy or at autopsy; they are most successfully demonstrated by inoculation of laboratory animals and are rarely seen on direct examination of stained smears.

Fig. 143-2. *Borrelia hermsii.* A Giemsa-stained smear of mouse blood. (Original magnification approximately × 2300) (Thompson RS, Burgdorfer W, Russell R, Francis BJ: JAMA 210:1045–1050, 1969. Copyright © 1969, American Medical Association)

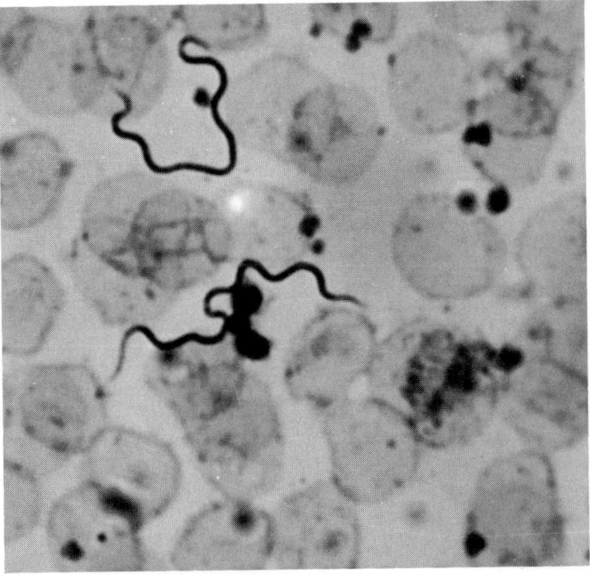

Table 143-4. *Summary of Laboratory Findings in Relapsing Fever (Based on Review of 3272 Cases)*

Examination	Mean Value	Range
Leukocyte count	8500/mm³	1600–25,000/mm³
Differential	60% PMN: ≥10% monocytes	Usually mild left shift of neutrophils and decrease in eosinophils
Hemoglobin	11.9 g/dl	6–16.5 g/dl
Erythrocyte count	4 million/mm³	Usually reduced
Erythrocyte sedimentation rate	65 mm/hr	3–145 mm/hr; frequently increased
Platelets: peripheral smear count	"Reduced" 90,000/mm³	Frequently reduced 30,000–220,000/mm³
Serologic tests for syphilis (blood)	4%–5% positive	0%–56% positive; includes FTA-ABS
Serologic tests for syphilis (CSF)	Rarely positive	
Proteus OX-K agglutinins		
Louse-borne	90% positive (≥1:40)	OX-19 may occasionally also become positive
	30% positive (≥1:100)	
Tick-borne	30%–35% positive (low titers)	OX-19 rarely positive
Complement fixation test (*Borrelia*)	Approximately 50% positive	
Serum borreliolysin test	Approximately 50%–60% positive	Titers of 1:100–1:20,000
Initial blood smears positive (for spirochetes)	Approximately 70%	
CSF (patients with signs of CNS involvement)		
Pressure	Elevated in 60%	
Cell count	950/mm³	15–2200/mm³
Protein	95 mg/dl	15–160 mg/dl; usually elevated
Glucose	75 mg/dl	50–100 mg/dl; usually normal
Spirochetes found (smear or inoculation)	Approximately 12%	

(Southern PM Jr: Relapsing fever. In Kelley VC (ed): Practice of Pediatrics. Philadelphia, Harper & Row, 1981)

The serologic diagnosis of relapsing fever is difficult at best, and the specific procedures are not generally available. Complement-fixing (CF), agglutinating, lysing, and immobilizing antibodies have been demonstrated. Many patients with louse-borne relapsing fever develop agglutinins to *Proteus* OX-K antigens, but rarely to *Proteus* OX-19 or OX-2. In areas where scrub typhus is endemic, the presence of *Proteus* OX-K antibodies should be interpreted with caution. Agglutinins to *Proteus* OX-K antigens occur infrequently in tick-borne relapsing fever. A summary of these and other laboratory findings appears in Table 143-4.

Before a remission–relapse cycle has been completed, the disease may resemble many other infections, some of which may later be distinguished either serologically or by isolation of an etiologic agent. The epidemiologic setting and some clinical aspects may assist in early differentiation. In nonendemic areas, the patient should be questioned about recent travel.

In Colorado tick fever, the febrile and afebrile periods are generally shorter; leukopenia is typical and thrombocytopenia may occur (Chap. 123, Colorado Tick Fever). Malaria (Chap. 145, Malaria) and dengue (Chap. 89, Dengue) also have shorter periods of fever. In malaria, sweating before defervescence is common.

Leptospirosis (Chap. 76, Leptospirosis) may follow contact with rodents or domestic animals, but results most commonly from exposure to water contaminated with excreta from these animals. Conjunctival suffusion and prominent involvement of the CNS or the liver are relatively common.

In rat-bite fever, there is usually a known bite or contact, and an inflammatory reaction at the site may be present; leukocytosis is typical (Chap. 142, Rat-Bite Fever).

The rickettsial infections may present problems in differential diagnosis in cases where the rash is mild and short-lived. However, the fever may fluctuate widely and does not alternate with periods of normal temperature except in trench fever. The rash of Rocky Mountain spotted fever (Chap. 96, Spotted Fevers) typically appears first on the limbs, involves the palms and soles, and becomes petechial within days. The rash of rickettsialpox (Chap. 97, Rickettsialpox) becomes vesicular, then pustular. Scrub typhus is characterized by an ulcerated eschar at the site of inoculation (Chap. 9, Scrub Typhus). Louse-borne typhus and flea-borne typhus (Chap 98, Typhus Fevers) in most cases have rashes of greater duration that are likely to become papular and sometimes hemorrhagic. Confusion and disorientation are often severe and may persist longer than the high fever.

Other considerations should include Q fever (Chap. 30, nonbacterial Pneumonias), meningococcemia (Chap. 119, Acute Bacterial Meningitis), enteric fever syndromes (Chap. 63, Nontyphoidal Salmonellosis, and 64, Typhoid Fever), and influenza (Chap. 30, Nonbacterial Pneumonias).

Prognosis

Ninety-five percent of patients recover with current treatment. Untreated louse-borne relapsing fever carries a high risk of fatality. Permanent sequelae are rare, but iritis and uveitis may lead to residual visual defects. Rare complications include respiratory ailments, nephritis, endocarditis, CNS dysfunctions, and hemorrhagic phenomena.

Therapy

The antimicrobic of choice for the treatment of relapsing fever is tetracycline. For adults, either 15 mg/kg body weight/day is given PO as four equal portions, 6-hourly, or 10 mg/kg/day is injected IV as three equal portions, 8-hourly; the duration of therapy is 4 to 5 days. In children, the appropriate dose is either 20 to 40 mg/kg/day, PO, or 10 to 20 mg/kg /day, IV (periodicity and duration of treatment as for adults). In infants and young children, chloramphenicol should probably be used in a dose of 25 or 100 mg/kg body weight/day (the lower dose for premature infants and neonates under 1 week old) given either PO or IV as four equal portions, 6-hourly, for 4 to 5 days.

Other regimens that have been associated with good results in louse-borne relapsing fever include (1) a single peroral dose of 100 mg of doxycycline and (2) a combination of 400,000 units of procaine penicillin G injected IM on the first day followed by tetracycline, 30 mg/kg body weight/day given PO in four equal portions, 6-hourly, for 7 days. The latter regimen was thought to reduce the severity of Jarisch–Herxheimer-like reactions while preventing relapses.

Jarisch–Herxheimer-like reactions occur commonly after the institution of antimicrobial therapy, particularly in the louse-borne disease. Such reactions are characteristic of the early phase of treatment of relapsing fever and should be anticipated by having at hand the capability for the prompt administration of oxygen, carefully controlled rehydration, and in some patients digoxin.

Prevention

Relapsing fever can be prevented by avoiding or eliminating the vectors involved. Louse control is discussed in Chapter 114, Pediculosis, and tick control in Chapter 131, Tick Paralysis. Prevention of contact with tick vectors in various endemic areas involves understanding the habits of *Ornithodoros* spp. Dwellings and other buildings in endemic areas must be built and maintained in such a way as to exclude animals that host ticks. Rotting wood, bark-covered logs, mud, and thatching should be avoided, and such materials should not be stored indoors.

In unsatisfactory buildings, partial protection may be obtained by spraying walls, floors, and ceilings with aqueous solutions of one of the following: 3% benzene hexachloride or pyrethrum, 1% aldrin, 0.5% dimpylate (Diazinon) or malathion, or 2% propoxur (Baygon). All cracks, joints, and surfaces should be covered with the spray.

Other precautions appropriate for visitors to potential habitants of soft-bodied ticks include protective clothing (cover as much skin as possible, with snug closures at the neck, wrists, and ankles); careful selection of sites for sleeping or resting; and use of insect repellants on skin, clothing, and bedding (Chap. 115, Thrombiculosis). Periodic inspection of the skin and removal of ticks may not prevent relapsing fever because of the feeding habits of ticks.

Bibliography

Books

FELSENFELD O: Borrelia: Strains, Vectors, Human and Animal Borreliosis. St Louis, Warren H. Green, 1971. 180 pp.

MOULTON FR (ED): A Symposium on Relapsing Fever in the Americas. Publication No. 18. Washington, D.C., American Association for the Advancement of Science, 1942. 130 pp.

Journals

ANNECKE S, QUIN P: Relapsing fever in South Africa: Its control. S Afr Med J 26:455–460, 1952

BOYER KM, MUNFORD RS, MAUPIN GO, PATTISON CP, FOX MD, BARNES AM, JONES WL, MAYNARD JE: Tick-borne relapsing fever: An interstate outbreak originating at Grand Canyon National Park. Am J Epidemiol 105:469–479, 1977

BRYCESON ADM, COOPER KE, WARRELL DA, PERINE PL, PARRY EHO: Studies of the mechanism of the Jarisch–Herxheimer reaction in louse-borne relapsing fever. Clin Sci 43:343–354, 1972

FELSENFELD O: Borreliae, human relapsing fever, and parasite–vector–host relationships. Bacteriol Rev 29:46–74, 1965

FUCHS PC, OYAMA AA: Neonatal relapsing fever due to transplacental transmission of *Borrelia.* JAMA 208:690–692, 1969

SALIH SY, MUSTAFA D, WAHAB SMA, AHMED MAM, OMER A: Louse-borne relapsing fever. I. A clinical and laboratory study of 363 cases in the Sudan. Trans R Soc Trop Med Hyg 71:43–48, 1977

SOUTHERN PM, SANFORD JP: Relapsing fever: A clinical and microbiological review. Medicine 48:129–149, 1969

THOMPSON RS, BURGDORFER W, RUSSELL R, FRANCIS BJ: Outbreak of tick-borne relapsing fever in Spokane County, Washington. JAMA 210:1045–1050, 1969

WARRELL DA, PERINE PL, BRYCESON ADM, PARRY EHO, POPE HM: Physiologic changes during the Jarisch–Herxheimer reaction in early syphilis: A comparison with louse-borne relapsing fever. Am J Med 51:176–185, 1971

RICHARD H. PARKER

Bartonellosis

144

Bartonellosis, or Carrion's disease, is typically a biphasic illness with a febrile hemolytic stage (Oroya fever) followed by development of cranberrylike tumors of the skin (verruga peruana). That one microorganism can sequentially cause two distinct clinical diseases was established by the experiment of Daniel Carrion, a Peruvian medical student. He injected himself with material obtained from a skin lesion of a patient with verruga peruana, and developed Oroya fever. He died of the disease, and the designation Carrion's disease is commemorative of his experiment.

Etiology

The agent of bartonellosis, *Bartonella bacilliformis,* was first described by Barton in 1909. It is a small, weakly-staining, gram-negative bacillus with a unipolar flagellum. In Giemsa-stained blood smears from infected patients, *B. bacilliformis* appears as red-violet rod or coccal forms situated on or in erythrocytes. It consists of obligate aerobes that grow at 28°C and 37°C but last longer at 28°C. Subsurface growth is obtained in semisolid agar containing 10% rabbit serum and 0.5% rabbit hemoglobin in 7 to 10 days. Identification is based on morphologic and culture characteristics. Human and nonhuman primates appear to be the only hosts that develop disease when infected.

Epidemiology

Humans are infected with *B. bacilliformis* by the bite of infected sandflies of the genus *Phlebotomus.* The habitat of these flies is confined to the river valleys of the Andes mountains at altitudes of 2000 to 8000 feet in Peru, Ecuador, and Colombia. Therefore, infection is confined to residents or persons traveling through this area. Because of the long incubation period, a patient may become symptomatic anywhere in the world after a visit to the endemic area. Within the endemic area, the disease may become epidemic if large numbers of susceptible persons are exposed to the night-biting vector, as has occurred during periods of major construction.

Pathogenesis and Pathology

When infected sandflies bite humans, *B. bacilliformis* is introduced into the bloodstream and infects endothelial cells where it proliferates in the cytoplasm for 2 to 3 weeks. After reentry of the microorganisms into the bloodstream, they adhere to and invade erythrocytes. The phagocytosis of infected erythrocytes by cells of the reticuloendothelial system results in a rapid and severe hemolytic anemia. The severity of the anemia is augmented by increased mechanical fragility of erythrocytes and decreased erythropoiesis. Tests for agglutinins and hemolysins, as well as the Coomb's test, are negative. This is the Oroya fever phase of bartonellosis, and recovery from it appears to be related to the development of immunity; that is, second episodes of Oroya fever are uncommon. With recovery, there is a progressive decrease in the number of microorganisms in the blood.

However, after a variable waiting period, in some patients the chronic, benign form of the disease called *verruga peruana* will develop. The hallmark of this form of the disease is hemangiomatous skin nodules consisting of newly formed small vessels with proliferation of endothelial cells that may contain *B. bacilliformis* within histiocytes. Fibrosis is characteristic of old skin lesions.

Manifestations

The febrile phase of bartonellosis follows an incubation period of approximately 3 weeks but which occasionally lasts as long as 4 months. The onset of symptoms may be either abrupt or insidious. The insidious form of the disease begins with prodromal symptoms of fever, myalgia, arthralgia, malaise, headache, and bone pain. The prodrome lasts for about 1 week. Occasionally, the disease ends with these influenzalike symptoms. More often, the disease either begins abruptly or progresses to a stage characterized by high fever, severe rigors, delirium, headaches, and severe diaphoresis. It is at this time that the severe anemia begins and the patient's skin becomes pale and jaundiced. Examination reveals nontender lymphadenopathy, petechiae, and ecchymoses. Signs of meningitis may be present in preterminal cases. Splenomegaly is not found in uncomplicated bartonellosis, and if present suggests the possibility of a complicating salmonellosis or malaria.

Peripheral blood leukocyte counts are variable, but there is usually a preponderance of immature neutrophils. Thrombocytopenia is present occasionally.

During recovery from Oroya fever, the patient may experience pains in bones, joints, and muscles. These symptoms are followed by the general nodular eruption of verruga peruana. The nontender reddish nodules develop over 1 to 2 months and may persist for months to years. They appear most frequently on the extremities, but can be found anywhere on the body, including the mucus membranes. During this stage of the disease the patient is afebrile and not anemic unless there is a complicating problem.

Diagnosis

The diagnosis of Bartonellosis should be suspected in patients who either reside in, or have traveled in, the endemic areas and who have the distinct syndrome of fever, headache, and a rapidly progressive hemolytic anemia. Confirmation of the diagnosis depends upon demonstration of the microorganism on the surface of erythrocytes or recovery of *B. bacilliformis* from blood cultures. The cutaneous disease should be suspected by its clinical appearance and proved by demonstration or culture of the microorganisms from the skin lesions.

In the United States, microorganisms resembling *B. bacilliformis* have been associated with cases of hemolytic–uremic syndromes. These microorganisms are considered closely related to members of the family Bartonellaceae.

Prognosis

There is a 40% mortality in humans who do not receive treatment for Oroya fever. Many of these deaths are caused by secondary salmonellosis and malaria. Verruga peruana may persist for months but is rarely fatal.

Therapy

Acute bartonellosis has been successfully treated with penicillin and streptomycin; however, chloramphenicol (40 mg/kg body wt/day, PO, as 4 equal portions, 6-hourly, for 10 days) is the treatment of choice. In patients too ill for peroral therapy, chloramphenicol may be given in the same dose by IV injection of the succinate derivative. Chloramphenicol offers an advantage over other possibly effective agents in its effectiveness in treatment of the frequent, complicating salmonellal infections. If transfusions of blood are needed for patients with severe anemia, it is preferable to obtain blood from patients who have recently survived bartonellosis, because the erythrocytes of such donors are usually more resistant to parasitism.

Tetracycline (30 mg/kg body wt/day, PO, as 4 equal portions, 6-hourly, for 10–14 days) may aid healing of the cutaneous lesions of verruga peruana.

Prevention

Prevention depends upon control of the sandfly. Environmental control consists in spraying the interiors and exteriors of dwellings with insecticides. Personal control includes use of insect repellents and protective clothing and avoidance of sandfly-infested areas.

Remaining Problems

Biologic factors determining the unique biphasic pattern of bartonellosis and the determinant of the enhanced susceptibility to intercurrent infection with both bacterial and protozoal parasites need clarification.

Bibliography

Journals

CUADRA MC: Salmonellosis complication in human Bartonellosis. Tex Rep Biol Med 14:97–113, 1956

DOOLEY JR: Haemotropic bacteria in man. Lancet 2:1237–1239, 1980

RECAVARREN S, LUMBRERAS H: Pathogenesis of the verruga of Carrion's disease. Am J Pathol 66:461–464, 1972

RICKETTS WE: Clinical manifestations of Carrion's disease. Arch Intern Med 84:751–781, 1949

SHULTZ MG: A history of Bartonellosis (Carrion's disease). Am J Trop Med Hyg 17:503–515, 1968

LOUIS H. MILLER

Malaria

145

Worldwide, malaria is one of the most common infectious diseases of man, causing much morbidity and significant mortality. In the United States, it is usually nonepidemic and protean. Accordingly, fever in a person who has either traveled in countries where malaria is endemic, received blood transfusions, or is a drug addict should alert the physician to the possibility of malaria.

Four species of *Plasmodium* infect man: *Plasmodium falciparum, Plasmodium vivax, Plasmodium ovale, and Plasmodium malariae.* Of these, *P. falciparum* most often causes serious morbidity and extensive mortality, and it provides a challenge because it is resistant to antimalarial drugs (*e.g.,* chloroquine). With *P. falciparum,* early therapy is essential, and its effectiveness depends on immediate diagnosis by examination of blood films.

Etiology

Of the four species pathogenic to man, *P. falciparum* and *P. vivax* occur most frequently. All have complex life cycles involving man and mosquitoes (Fig. 145-1). Infection is initiated in man when sporozoites are inoculated by female *Anopheles* spp. mosquitoes in the course of nocturnal feeding. Within 1 hour, the sporozites invade hepatic parenchymal cells, begin to grow, divide by exoerythrocytic (hepatic) schizogony, and develop into hepatic merozoites. One sporozoite of *P. falciparum* yields as many as 40,000 merozoites, each capable of invading an erythrocyte. In the other species, the merozoite yield per sporozoite is lower (Table 145-1). Hepatic parasites of *P. vivax* and *P. ovale* may persist for years in the liver (secondary exoerythrocytic schizogony), and as a consequence relapses may occur months to years after the initial infection.

The erythrocytic phase of malaria begins with invasion of erythrocytes by hepatic merozoites (Fig. 145-2). Development of the intraerythrocytic form of the parasite may follow one of the two pathways: an asexual, multinuclear schizont that contains 6 to 24 merozoites, depending on the species and sexual development to a male or female gametocyte. On release, erythrocytic merozoites invade other erythrocytes. Gametocytes are infectious only to anopheline mosquitoes.

Invasion of erythrocytes by merozoites is initiated at specific receptors on the erythrocyte surface. Human erythrocytes negative for the Duffy blood group (Fy Fy) are resistant to infection in culture by *Plasmodium knowlesi,* a cause of simian malaria, whereas Duffy-positive human erythrocytes are readily infected. The Duffy-negative genotype occurs in blacks and explains the absolute resistance of their erythrocytes to infection by *P. vivax.* That is, the Duffy blood group component may be an erythrocyte receptor for *P. vivax. Plasmodium falciparum* has a different receptor on the human erythrocyte, which may be an erythrocyte membrane sialoglycoprotein, glycophoran.

The remarkable high rate of reproduction of the asexual erythrocytic form of *P. falciparum* accounts, in part, for the high mortality of falciparum malaria. The merozoites of *P. falciparum* appear to enter erythroctyes more efficiently than the merozoites of the other malarias. *Plasmodium falciparum* is the only human malaria parasite found in erythrocytes of all ages, although it preferentially invades young red cells. In contrast, *P. vivax* primarily invades reticulocytes. Each cycle of *P. falciparum* produces more merozoites than does either *P. ovale* or *P. malariae.* Erythrocytes infected with *P. falciparum* develop electron-dense lesions and adhere to the venous endothelium of the heart and adipose tissue. The parasitized red cells are thus partially protected from destruction in the reticuloendothelial system.

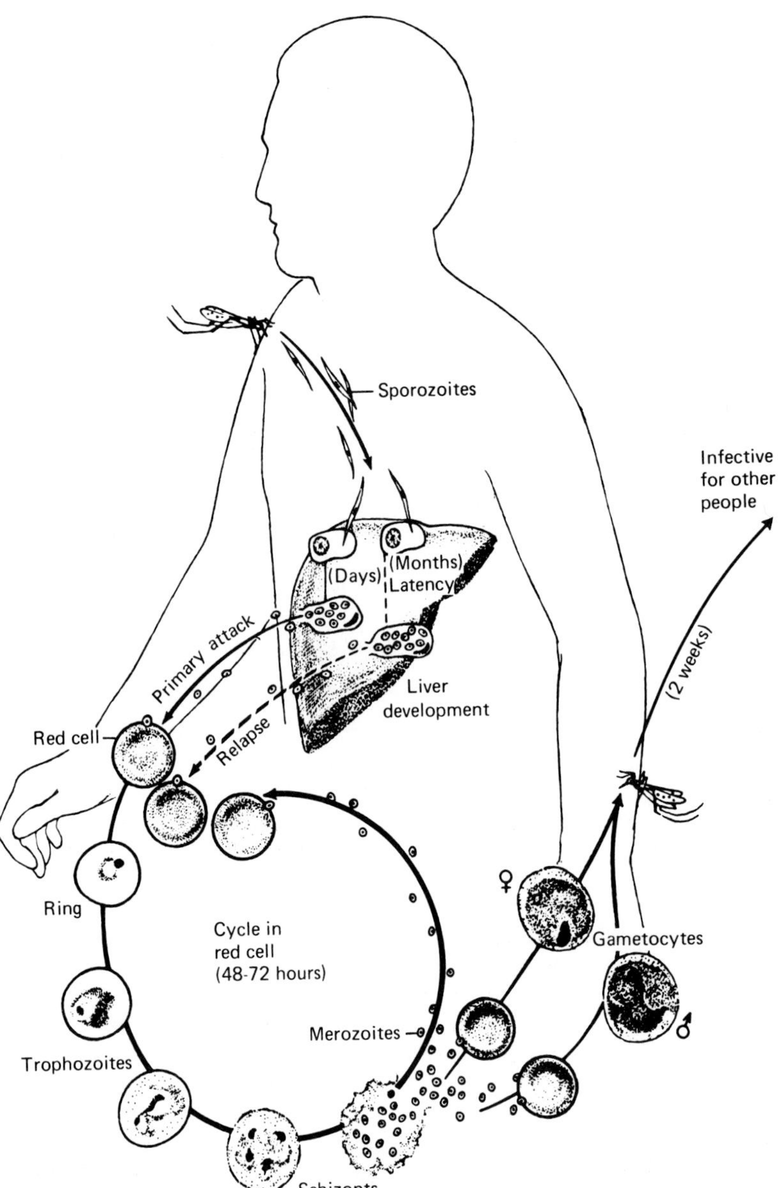

Fig. 145-1. Life cycle of malaria in man. (Miller LH: Transfusion malaria. In Greenwalt TJ, Jamieson CA (eds): Transmissible Diseases and Blood Transfusion. New York, Grune & Stratton, 1975)

Epidemiology

Most patients with malaria that are seen in the United States and in Europe have been infected while visiting in Asia, Africa, or Latin America. The impact of military importations and of control measures on the number of cases reported in the United States is shown in Fig. 145-3.

In the United States, the mosquito vectors capable of transmitting malaria are primarily *Anopheles quadrimaculatus* in the Southeast and *Anopheles freeborni* in the West. From 1964 to 1970, seven episodes of mosquito-transmitted malaria occurred in the United States; four of the seven outbreaks were near military installations.

Communal use of syringes by drug addicts can also serve to transmit malaria. From 1935 to 1940, the medical examiner of New York City reported 120 deaths among drug addicts caused by self-inoculation of *P. falciparum.* Recently, several epidemics of vivax malaria have occurred among drug addicts.

With the influx of veterans infected during the Vi-

Table 145-1. Summary of Important Characteristics of Malarias in Man

	P. falciparum	*P. vivax*	*P. ovale*	*P. malariae*
Incidence	Common	Common	Uncommon	Uncommon
Primary hepatic schizogony Sporozoite → merozoites	1 → 40,000 in 5.5–7 days	1 → 10,000 in 6–8 days	1 → 15,000 in 9 days	1 → 2000 in 13–16 days
Secondary hepatic schizogony Merozoite → merozoites	Lacking	Present	Present	Unknown
Erythrocytic schizogony Ring → merozoites	1 → 8–24 (Avg. 16) in 48 hr	1 → 12–24 (Avg. 16) in 48 hr	1 → 6–16 in 48 hr	1 → 6–12 (Avg. 8) in 72 hr
Incubation period*	8–25 days (Avg. 12)	8–27 days (Avg. 14) Occasionally months	9–17 days (Avg. 15)	15–30 days
Parasitemia	Very high (up to 60%)	Less than *P. falciparum* usually <1%	Usually low <<1%	Usually low <<1%
Mortality	High in nonimmunes	Uncommon	Rarely fatal	Rarely fatal

*Chemoprophylaxis may suppress for months an initial attack with *P. falciparum,* and for months to years with the non-*falciparum* species.

etnam War, the incidence of transfusion malaria increased; *P. falciparum,* rarely observed in the United States before 1964, was a frequent cause. Enforcement of the standards of the American Association of Blood Banking would prevent most cases of transfusion malaria, although in rare instances *P. malariae* would still be transmitted.

The congenital transmission of malaria has also been reported. However, infection in this way is rare.

Pathogenesis and Pathology

Disease in malaria is caused by the asexual erythrocytic cycle. The persistence of gametocytes after treatment with schizonticidal drugs is of no clinical significance. The rupture of infected erythrocytes at the completion of schizogony occurs every 48 hours with *P. falciparum, P. vivax, P. ovale,* and every 72 hours with *P. malariae,* producing fever, chills, and other nonspecific symptoms at 48- or 72-hour intervals (Fig. 145-4). However, synchronized schizogony and regular paroxysms of fever are uncommon with *P. falciparum* and are often lacking during the initial attack in other malarias.

Infected erythrocytes in malaria are ruptured by mature schizonts, and in heavy falciparum infections severe intravascular hemolysis causes marked anemia, hemoglobinemia, and hemoglobinuria. In many patients with malaria, the degree of anemia cannot be entirely explained by the level of parasitemia. Although autoimmune hemolytic anemia has been proposed to explain this observation, few instances of Coombs-positive hemolysis have been documented in malaria. Erythrophagocytosis by the reticuloendothelial system is common. Increased osmotic fragility develops. Bone marrow depression may also play a role in the anemia of malaria.

Some patients with falciparum malaria have a reduction in the number of blood platelets, a decrease in the concentration of plasma fibrinogen, and a prolongation in thrombin time, prothrombin time, and partial thromboplastin time. These findings are consistent with a diagnosis of disseminated intravascular coagulation (DIC; see Chap. 7, Manifestations of Infectious Diseases). Although several mechanisms may be operative in malaria, thromboplastins released by hemolysis can promote intravascular coagulation. Decreases in the numbers of platelets occur independent of DIC.

During the course of malaria, malarial antigens and immune complexes have been demonstrated in the cirulation and at the site of tissue damage (*e.g.,* the glomerulus). An increased turnover of C1q and decreased levels of C3 are observed in patients infected with *P. falciparum;* consumption of C1, C4, and C2, but not C3 and C6, occurs a few hours after schizont rupture in *P. vivax* malaria.

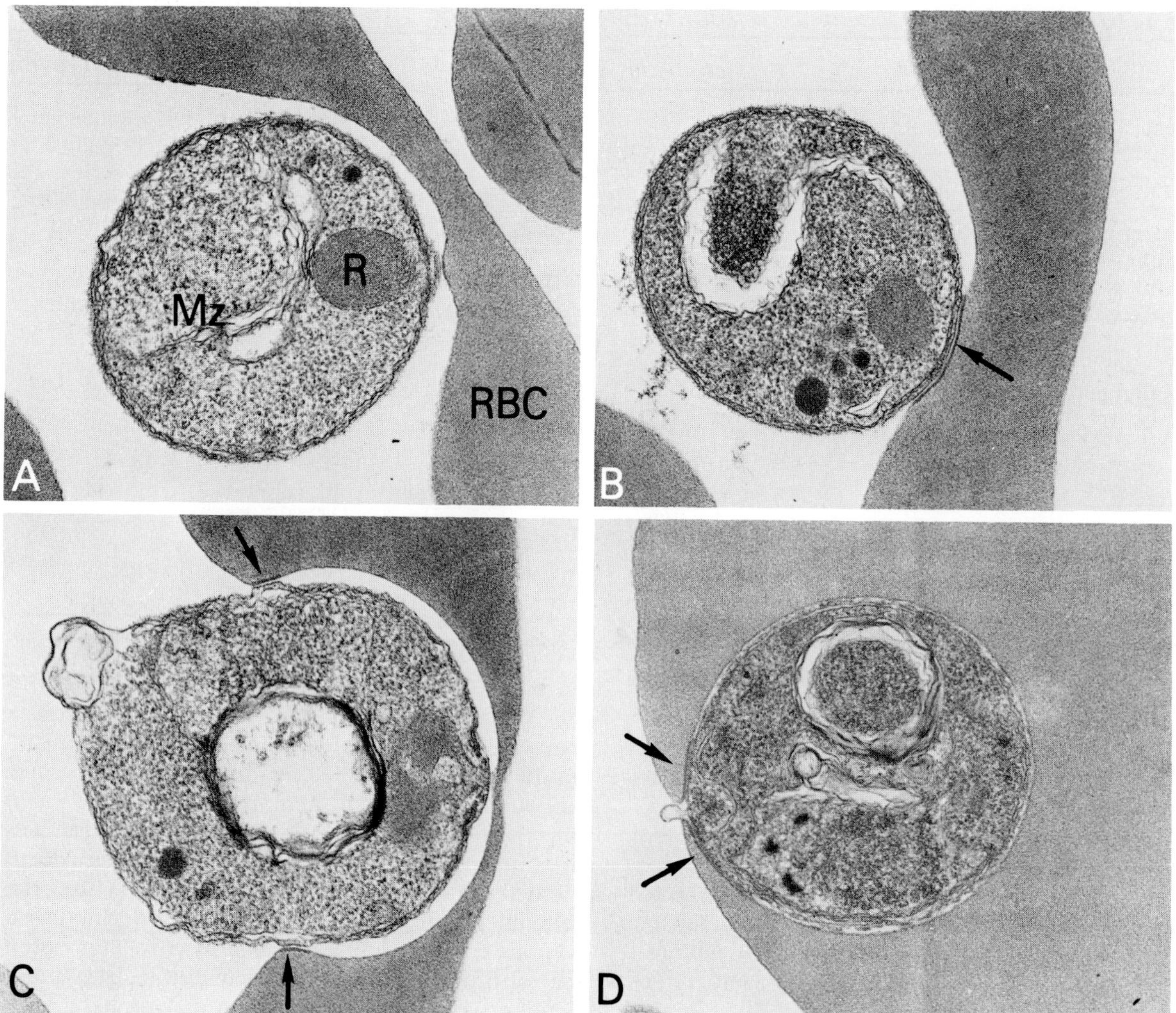

Fig. 145-2. The sequence of events during invasion of erythrocytes by malarial merozoites. The anterior end of the merozoite (M_z) attaches to the erythrocyte (RBC) by specific ligand-receptor interaction (*A*). This initiates two events: (1) junction formation between merozoite and erythrocyte (arrows) and (2) release of the contents of the merozoite rhoptries (*R*) onto the erythrocyte membrane. The junction that is initially at the apical end of the parasite (*B*) moves around the merozoite and remains attached to the erythrocyte at the orifice of the invaginated erythrocyte membrane (*C*). This moving junction brings the parasite within the erythrocyte invagination, and at completion of invasion (*D*) the membranes seal, leaving the parasite within a vacuole lined by erythrocyte membrane. (Aikawa M, Miller LH, Johnson J et al: Erythrocyte entry by malarial parasites. A moving junction between erythrocyte and parasite. J Cell Biol 77:72–82, 1978. Copyright 1978, The Rockefeller University Press)

Malaria is one of a long list of diseases that cause bilateral tubular necrosis of the kidney and centrilobular necrosis of the liver (Fig. 145-5*A*). In general, these serious complications are limited to falciparum malaria, possibly because other malarias do not attain such high levels of parasitemia. Much of the pathology is anoxic in origin and results from the severe anemia, reduced blood flow, and inhibition of oxidative phosphorylation. Symphathetically controlled splanchnic vasoconstriction decreases hepatic and renal blood flow. Organ perfusion may be further impaired by decreased deformability of infected

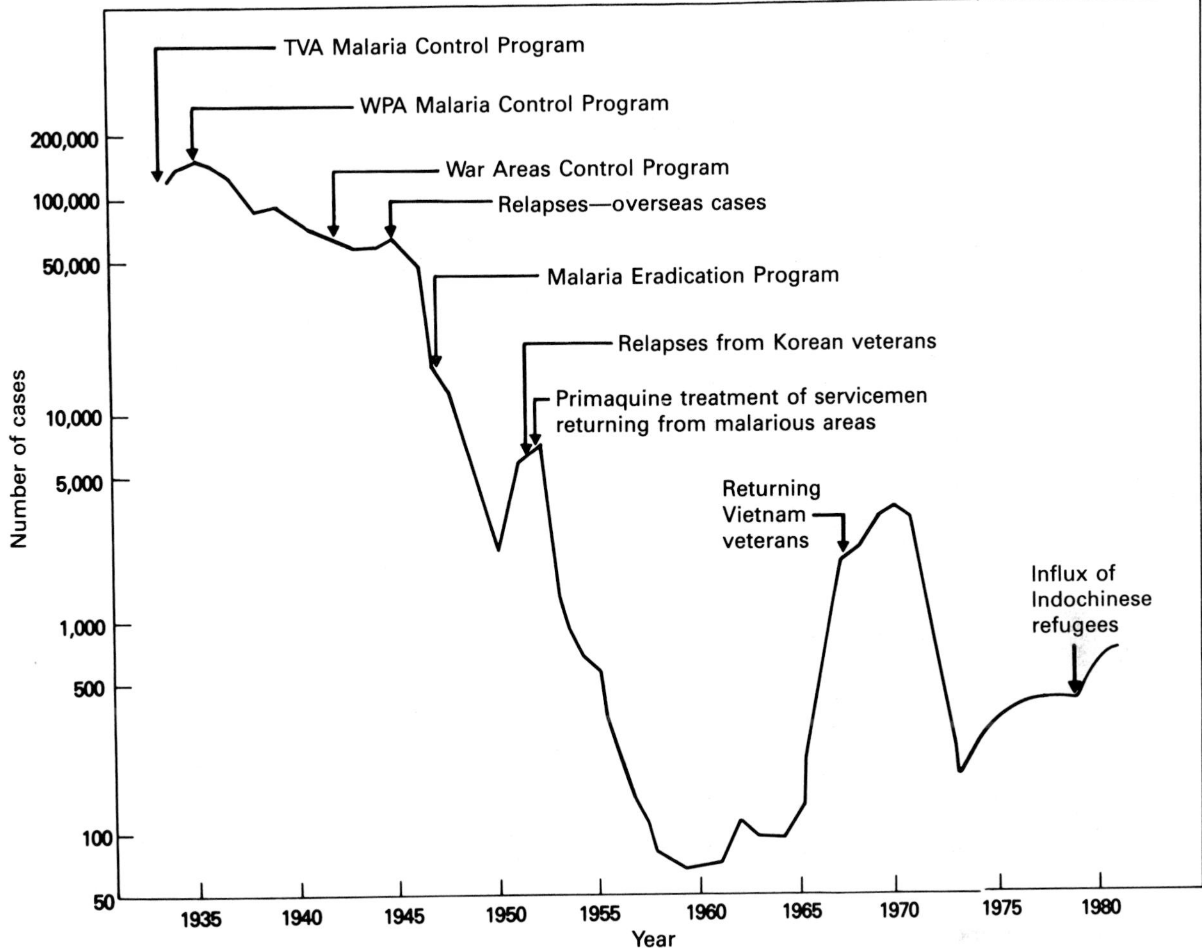

Fig. 145-3. Malaria cases in the United States by year of report. 1933–1980. The number of cases each year has fluctuated according to the application of control measures and military importations. (From Morbid Mortal Week Suppl, Summary, 1975)

erythrocytes, adhesion of red cells to endothelium, and DIC.

Metabolic derangements are common during malaria, although the exact mechanisms are unknown at present. Hyponatremia, one of the complications in seriously ill patients, is probably caused both by salt depletion and water retention. Within a few days after treatment, most patients again respond normally to a water load. Plasma volume and blood volume are usually expanded during the acute attack. A rare and serious complication of falciparum malaria is hypovolemic shock, which is associated with increased capillary permeability. The concentration of bradykinin is elevated. If pulmonary edema is associated with cerebral malaria and heavy parasitemia, it may reflect an increase in vascular permeability, although the possibility of left ventricular failure and fluid overload must always be considered. In fatal falciparum malaria in man, the venules and capillaries of the heart are jammed with parasitized erythrocytes; effective cornonary blood flow and cardiac function may be diminished in these patients.

The pathology in cerebral malaria is most striking. The capillaries and venules are filled with parasitized erythrocytes (Fig. 145-5*B*). Cerebral edema, ring hemorrhages (Fig. 145-5*C*), and necrosis around central veins (Fig. 145-5*D*) are observed throughout the brain. Changes in the cell membranes of infected erythrocytes may interfere with the movement of erythrocytes through the cerebral microcirculation. First, electron-dense, knoblike lesions on the erythrocyte membrane in falciparum malaria may cause the

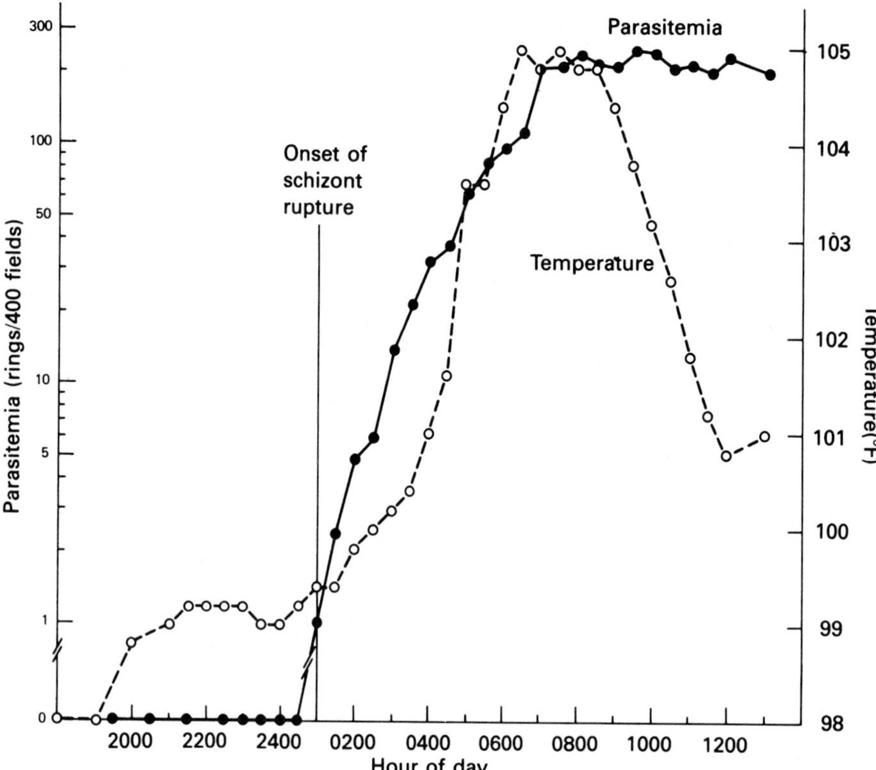

Fig. 145-4. Relation between schizont rupture (appearance of rings in erythrocytes) and fever. (Miller LH: Transfusion malaria. In Greenwalt TJ, Jamieson GA (eds): Transmissible Diseases and Blood Transfusion. New York, Grune & Stratton, 1975).

erythrocytes to be more sticky. Second, infected erythrocytes become spur-shaped and perhaps less deformable, thus becoming unable to move normally through the capillaries.

Manifestations

Acute Malaria

Symptoms usually occur 10 to 16 days after infection by mosquitoes. The incubation period is variable and tends to be longest with *P. malariae* (Table 145-1). After drug prophylaxis, the initial malarial attack may be suppressed for months in falciparum malaria and for months to years in other malarias.

Although no one sign or symptom is pathognomonic of malaria, a conjunction of features is usually sufficiently characteristic to lead to the diagnosis. Most patients have either synchronous or asynchronous episodes of chills, fever, headache, and myalgia. The pattern of paroxysmal illness interspersed with periods of relative well-being is the hallmark of benign malaria. Paroxysms frequently begin with bed-shaking chills that are followed by high fevers, sweating, headache, and myalgia. The symptomatic periods usually last less than 6 hours. Fever rises sharply, often to temperatures ranging from 40°C–41°C (104°F–106°F).

In malignant falciparum malaria, the fever and symptoms are usually more persistent. Headache is a consistent finding and may be associated with delirium. Myalgias, often involving the low back and thighs, are frequently present. Less common symptoms are thirst, nausea, and vomiting. The pulse rate is rapid, but it is usually not commensurate with the fever. Orthostatic hypotension is common in falciparum malaria, and weakness may persist for weeks after treatment. Labial herpes are often present. Splenomegaly occurs in about 50% of cases of acute malaria. Hepatomegaly is less common and is usually associated with splenomegaly. It is important to note that a lack of hepatosplenomegaly does not exclude the diagnosis of malaria. Skin rashes and lymphadenopathy are quite uncommon in malaria.

Anemia is usually mild in the uncomplicated infection. The total blood leukocyte count is rarely elevated and may be below 5000/mm^3. Thrombocytopenia is usually unassociated with a bleeding diathesis. Minimal proteinuria and occasional leukocytes in the urinary sediments are common and are

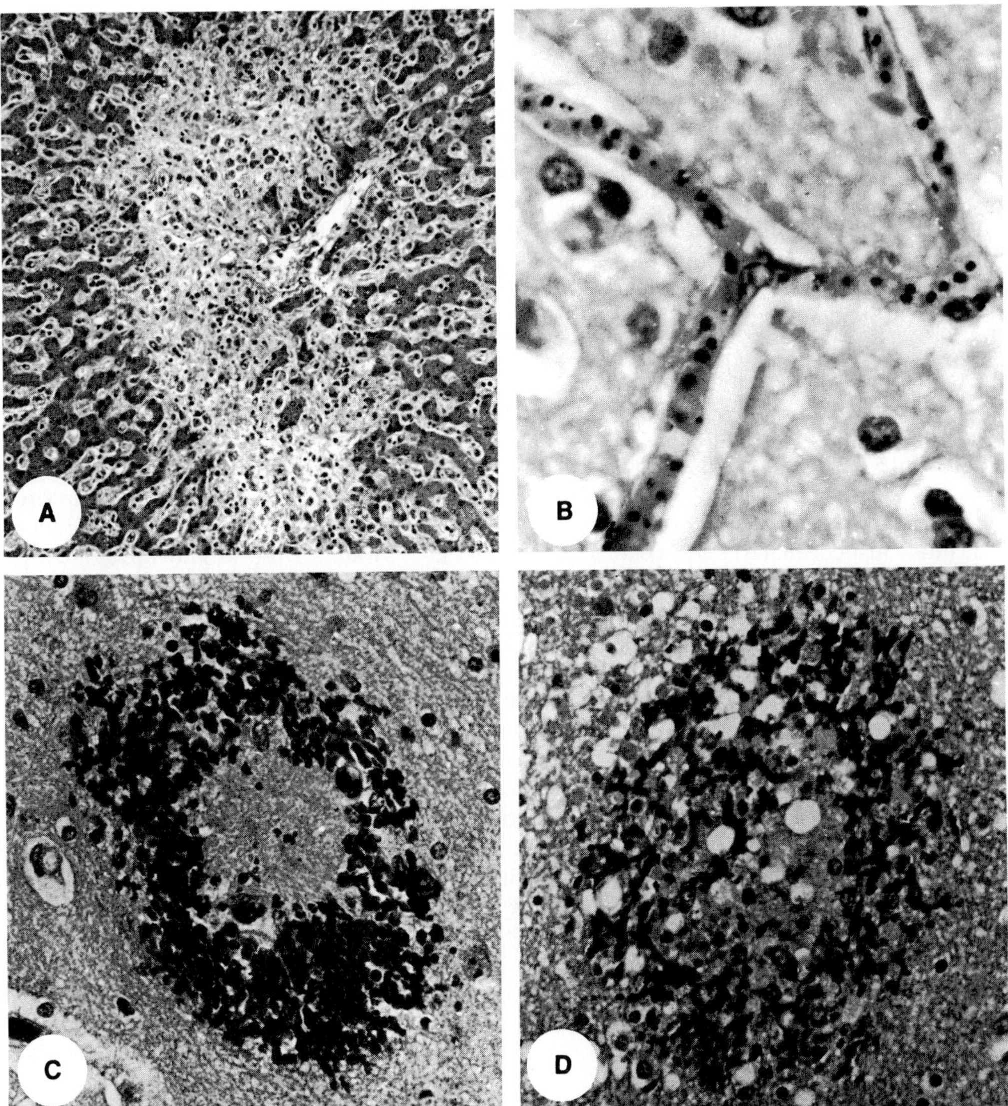

Fig. 145-5. Complications of severe falciparum malaria. (*A*) Centrilobular necrosis of liver. (Original magnification approximately × 90) (*B*) Cerebral vessels filled with parasitized erythrocytes. Note the edema. (Original magnification approximately × 900) (*C*) Ring hemorrhage in the brain. (Original magnification approximately × 370) (*D*) Hemorrhage and necrosis in the brain. (Original magnification approximately × 350)

probably consequent to fever. The serum gamma globulin is elevated. Although the serum albumin is depressed and elevations in transaminase levels are common, evidence of serious liver involvement is uncommon.

In nonendemic areas, such as the United States, the diagnosis of malaria is often missed. The physician must always consider malaria in a febrile patient who has received a transfusion a few weeks previously, or who has traveled in an endemic area. During early malaria, such patients may be thought to have influenza or some other viral illness with fever. Delay in the treatment of falciparum malaria may be disastrous.

Chronic Malaria

If malaria is untreated and complications do not ensue, patients develop humoral antibodies, cell-mediated immunity, and splenomegaly. Natural cure occurs within 1 year in falciparum malaria, although rarely the parasitemia may persist for longer. Relapses may occur over a 3-year period with *P. vivax* from exoerythrocytic schizonts in the liver and up to 53 years later with *P. malariae* from persistent erythrocytic infection.

Patients with chronic infections may have a low-grade parasitemia even though they are asymptomatic. Such patients might donate blood, unaware of the risk they pose to the recipient.

Diagnosis

The definitive diagnosis of malaria is made in the laboratory. Because malaria parasites may be overlooked in the course of a routine differential count, the clinician must suspect malaria and specifically order examination of blood smears for parasites. Thick and thin blood films (Chap. 11, Diagnostic Methods for Protozoa and Helminths) should be obtained immediately in a febrile patient who may have been exposed to malaria (Fig. 145-6). Blood examinations should be repeated at 6- to 12-hour intervals until a diagnosis is made. Thick smears should be examined for at least 5 minutes; if parasites are found, thin films must then be studied for species identification (Plate 145-1). When thick smears are negative, thin smears must still be examined. Ring forms (trophozoites) of *P. falciparum* often wash off thick smears in the course of staining, and only thin smears may be positive in a patient who has scanty parasitemia. Malaria pigment—hemozoin—in monocytes is an indication for therapy, even without parasites. If malaria is strongly suspected on clinical grounds in a patient with repeatedly negative smears, a therapeutic trial may be instituted.

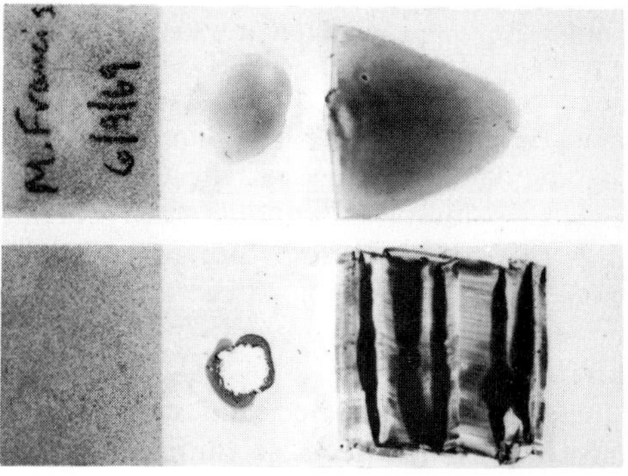

Fig. 145-6. Thick and thin malaria blood films. The upper slide is easy to read. The lower slide is unlabeled; the center of the thick smear has fallen off because too much blood was applied, and the thin smear is too thick and unevenly spread.

The indirect fluorescent antibody test for the serodiagnosis of malaria is available at the Centers for Disease Control, Atlanta, Georgia, for the identification of infected donors responsible for transfusion malaria. Serology, however, cannot replace blood films in the diagnosis of acute malaria because antibodies are usually not detectable until after the second week of infection.

Prognosis

Death from malaria is rare except in disease caused by *P. falciparum.* When parasitemia with *P. falciparum* rises above 100,000 infected erythrocytes per mm^3 of blood and the hematocrit falls below 30%, the patient is at grave risk of complications and death. Complications of *P. falciparum* include severe hemolytic anemia and involvement of the cerebral, renal, hepatic, pulmonary, and coagulation systems. It is not unusual for a patient to have a concurrent functional and pathologic derangement of many organs.

Cerebral malaria may occur at any time during the course of the disease, beginning most often with disturbances of consciousness that may then progress to coma. An acute organic psychosis, with confusion, disorientation, and intellectual deterioration may herald the onset of cerebral malaria. General convulsions may occur. In infants and young children, it is impossible to differentiate febrile convulsions from seizures secondary to cerebral malaria. Neurologic examination may demonstrate hyperreflexia and bilateral Babinski signs, but focal findings are uncommon because the pathology consists of a diffuse vascular involvement. Examination of the cerebrospinal fluid (CSF) is of little diagnostic value because the usual findings are an elevated pressure and concentration of protein, rarely accompanied by pleocytosis. Treatment by the parental administration of chloroquine and quinine results in the rapid recovery of most patients with cerebral malaria, although the possibility of sequelae has not been adequately studied.

The complication of blackwater fever—hemolytic anemia, hemoglobinuria, tubular damage, and acute renal failure—results from heavy parasitemia or other causes of massive intravascular hemolysis. Coombs-positive hemolytic anemia has been temporally related to quinine therapy and has been implicated in the etiology of blackwater fever. Drug-induced hemolytic anemia in patients with glucose-

6-phosphate dehydrogenase (G-6-PD) deficiency has been confused with blackwater fever. Hypersensitivity has been suggested as one of the causes—some patients with blackwater fever who have no history of quinine therapy, G-6-PD deficiency, or heavy parasitemia have become reinfected after immunity has waned. Renal failure may occur without hemolysis and in some cases may be associated with salt and water depletion and hypovolemia. Azotemia may not indicate renal failure but may reflect an increased catabolic rate.

Greatly elevated serum transaminase and bilirubin levels occur rarely in association with centrilobular necrosis of the liver. Ordinarily, hepatic damage is minimal. Pulmonary edema is another uncommon complication. In addition to anemia and disordered coagulation, there may be leukopenia.

Mortality from falciparum malaria is greatly reduced in blacks with sickle cell trait, although the susceptibility to infection is unchanged. The influence of G-6-PD deficiency on falciparum malaria is still controversial.

There is a growing body of evidence that chronic infections with *P. malariae* may produce chronic progressive nephritis that responds poorly to glucosteroids and antimalarials.

Rupture of the spleen is a rare complication of malaria that is usually associated with infections caused by *P. vivax.* Both the massive size of the spleen and the speed of enlargement are factors in rupture.

Therapy

Malaria caused by *P. falciparum* may be rapidly lethal. All patients with falciparum malaria should be hospitalized and treated as medical emergencies. Antimalarial agents that are active against the asexual, erythrocytic forms of *P. falciparum* (*e.g.,* the 4-aminoquinolines and quinine) must be given promptly to diminish morbidity and mortality. As in other infectious diseases, noninfectious abnormalities must also be cared for (*e.g.,* fluid and electrolyte balance). Because of the prevalence of drug-resistant strains of *P. falciparum,* the patient with malaria cannot be considered cured until he has remained asymptomatic and free of parasites at least 6 weeks. Persistence of gametocytes (sexual forms) is not an indication for further treatment.

Because exoerythrocytic (hepatic) schizogony persists for many years with *P. vivax* and *P. ovale,* treatment to eradicate the parasites in the liver must be instituted after the patient has recovered from the acute attack. In transfusion malaria, treatment should be directed solely against the erythrocytic phase because exoerythrocytic stages develop only after the inoculation of sporozoites by mosquitoes.

Immunity to malaria requires repeated infections over an extended period; it disappears when reinfection does not occur. Withholding chemotherapy to induce immunity is never justified, even in a patient who plans to return to an endemic area.

Specific Antimalarial Treatment

Some properties of several antimalarial agents used in the treatment and chemoprophylaxis of malaria are given in Table 145-2. In practice, combinations of agents are frequently used.

Erythrocytic Parasites. Chloroquine (a 4-aminoquinoline) has a rapid onset of action and is the chemotherapeutic agent of choice in all malarias except that caused by *P. falciparum* resistant to chloroquine. Within 24 hours after initiating therapy with chloroquine, the parasitemia decreases and the symptoms are improved. By the third to fourth day, the patient has usually recovered. The dosage schedule for oral treatment with chloroquine is outlined in Table 145-3. Intramuscular injection of chloroquine should be reserved for patients who are comatose or vomiting repeatedly and who are infected with strains of *P. falciparum* from areas known to be free of resistant strains. The recommended intramuscular dose is 300 mg base initially, repeated at 6 hours, not to exceed 900 mg in the first 24 hours. Toxic reactions to chloroquine include gastrointestinal symptoms, pruritus, headache, and visual disturbances, but they are uncommon.

If the patient is in shock or is comatose, quinine should be given by IV injection, as described below.

Chloroquine-resistant strains of *P. falciparum* are found in South America (Brazil, Colombia, Ecuador, Guyana, Surinam, and Venezuela), in Panama, throughout Asia (Bangladesh, Burma, Cambodia, eastern India, Indonesia, Malaysia, New Guinea, Philippines, Thailand and Vietnam) and in east Africa. All patients from these areas should be treated as if they were infected with chloroquine-resistant *P. falciparum.* Severe falciparum malaria resulting from blood transfusions should also be treated as though the parasite is chloroquine-resistant, unless it is certain that the infected donor acquired his infection in a region of the world free of resistant strains. If there is no response or if there is a recurrence after an adequate course of treatment with chloroquine, infection with a resistant strain should be assumed.

Of the many regimens advocated for the treatment of chloroquine-resistant malaria, the most widely ac-

Table 145-2. *Some Properties of Antimalarial Agents*

Agents	Class of Agent by Action	Site of Action	Therapeutic Use	Resistance	Toxicity
4-Aminoquinolines (chloroquine, amodiaquine)	Blood schizonticide*	Not definitely known; strongly bound to ferriprotoporphyrin, protein synthesis and glycolysis reduced	Acute attack, chemoprophylaxis	*P. falciparum* from Southeast Asia, South America	Minimal
Quinine§	Blood schizonticide*		Acute attack caused by chloroquine-resistant *P. falciparum*	Recrudescence in strains of *P. falciparum*	Cinchonism; immune hemolysis
Quinacrine	Blood schizonticide*		Nil—replaced by chloroquine	Cross-resistance with chloroquine—*P. falciparum*	Dermatitis
8-Aminoquinolines (primaquine, quinocide)	Hepatic schizonticide,† gametocide, sporontocide‡	Not definitely known; block glycolysis	Radical cure in *P. vivax, P. ovale;* chemoprophylaxis in combination with chloroquine	Strains of *P. vivax*	Hemolysis in G-6-PD deficiency
Chlorguanide Pyrimethamine Trimethoprim	Primary hepatic schizonticide, sporontocide‡	Block dihydrofolate reductase	Chemoprophylaxis; acute attack in chloroquine-resistant *P. falciparum*	Develop readily in all *Plasmodium* spp.	Minimal; thrombocytopenia with pyrimethamine
Sulfonamides Sulfones	Blood schizonticide	Block utilization of paraaminobenzoic acid	Acute attack in chloroquine-resistant *P. falciparum;* chemoprophylaxis	Develops readily in all *Plasmodium* spp.	Minimal; agranulocytosis (sulfones)

*A blood schizonticide that eradicates asexual erythrocytic forms.
†A hepatic schizonticide that eradicates exoerythrocytic (hepatic) schizonts and prevents relapses (radical cure).
‡A sporontocide that inhibits development of the form infectious for the mosquito.
§Quinidine, the D-enantiomorph of quinine, is at least as active as quinine, and may be effective in quinine-resistant malaria (30 mg/kg body wt/day, PO, as 3 equal portions, 8-hourly, for 7 days).

Table 145-3. *Peroral Chloroquine Treatment of Malaria*

Dosage Schedule	Dosage of Chloroquine Diphosphate (Chloroquine Base in Parentheses): ADULTS (OVER 15 YR) (MG)	CHILDREN* (MG/KG)
1st Dose	1000 (600)	17 (10)
2nd Dose (6 hours after 1st)	500 (300)	8.5 (5)
3rd Dose (24 hours after 1st)	500 (300)	8.5 (5)
4th Dose (48 hours after 1st)	500 (300)	8.5 (5)

*The dose for children should never exceed the adult dose.

cepted is quinine (640 mg PO three times per day for 10 days) combined with pyrimethamine (50 mg/day, PO, for the first 3 days) and a sulfonamide (*e.g.,* trisulfapyrimidines, 0.5 g every 6 hours for 5 days). This regimen takes advantage of the synergism between sulfonamides and 2,4-diaminopyrimidines (Chap. 18, Antimicrobics and Anthelmintics for Systemic Therapy).

The above regimen almost uniformly controls the infection, but some patients suffer a subsequent recrudescence. Recrudescent attacks of *P. falciparum* malaria may be treated either with a second course of the same regimen or, alternatively, with quinine (640 mg PO three times per day for 3 days) followed by tetracycline (250 mg four times per day PO for 10 days).

If quinine is not immediately available, treatment should be initiated with chloroquine combined with pyrimethamine and a sulfonamide, and later chloroquine can be replaced by quinine. Patients unable to take oral medication (*e.g.,* in cerebral malaria) should receive quinine dihydrochloride (600 mg diluted in 100 ml 5% glucose in water and administered by slow IV infusion). The dose may be repeated every 8 hours but should be replaced by oral therapy as early as possible.

Cinchonism (*i.e.,* nausea, vomiting, tinnitus, and vertigo) commonly results from treatment with quinine and is not a sufficient cause either to alter or to discontinue therapy. Coombs-positive hemolytic anemia, a rare complication of quinine therapy, is an indication for immediate withdrawal of the drug.

Hepatic Parasites. Primaquine, an 8-aminoquinoline antimalarial, is the only drug available in the United States that is active against the hepatic stage of the parasite. Accordingly, it prevents late relapses with *P. vivax* and *P. ovale.* Of two treatment schedules designed for adults (15 mg of the base PO per day for 14 days, or 45 mg of the base PO once a week for 8 weeks), the 14-day course is recommended because daily medication is easier to remember. For children, 0.25 mg/kg body wt/day should be given for 14 days. Relapses occur after primaquine therapy, but they are uncommon with most strains of *P. vivax.*

Primaquine is potentially toxic, causing the hemolysis of erythrocytes deficient in G-6-PD. Older erythrocytes are more susceptible to the drug. Because G-6-PD deficiency in American blacks is usually mild, hemolysis is self-limited and is usually not an indication for discontinuing primaquine at the dose recommended. Treatment should be monitored more closely in Asians or southern Europeans with a more severe G-6-PD deficiency. Primaquine should never be administered during the acute malarial attack, because aspirin, fever, and possibly other drugs may accentuate the hemolysis and provoke intravascular coagulaton.

Supportive Therapy

Headaches, muscular pain, and other symptoms of malaria are associated with high fever. The temperature can be brought below 39°C (102°F) by giving aspirin, sponging with tepid water, and fanning to increase evaporation. Orthostatic hypotension, usually observed early in falciparum malaria, is an indication for complete bed rest. Laboratory determinations in malaria caused by *P. falciparum* should include hematocrit, hemoglobin, electrolytes, blood volume, renal function studies (urine output, urine osmolality, and serum creatinine), and hepatic function studies (serum bilirubin, alkaline phosphatase, transaminases, total protein, and protein electrophoresis). Packed erythrocytes or whole blood should be infused slowly in severe anemia. The fluid balance of each patient must be individually appraised. Excessive water intake may accentuate dilutional hyponatremia and aggravate cerebral symptoms. Patients who have intravascular hemolysis and hemoglobinuria (blackwater fever) may be given a trial injection of mannitol or furosemide to prevent renal failure and oliguria. Large infusions of sodium chloride may precipitate pulmonary edema and are not recommended in most situations. An increase in catabolic rate and decreased efficiency of peritoneal dialysis complicate the management of acute renal failure. However, early institution of peritoneal dialysis can usually control the progress of uremia. Because quinine is excreted by the kidney and metabolized by the liver, the dosage should be decreased by at least half in patients with renal failure and hepatic disease. Ideally, the dose is adjusted on the basis of serial determinations of the blood concentration to attain 5 mg to 10 mg quinine per liter of plasma. Cerebral malaria is considered by many physicians an indication for glucosteroid administration, but there is no experimental basis for this recommendation. The rapid improvement in cerebral symptoms associated with use of antimalarials may in part be related to the anti-inflammatory properties of these agents.

Prevention

As in many infectious diseases for which there is no vaccine, the prevention of malaria depends primarily on the person. Contact with mosquitoes must be prevented. All of the following should be used in endemic areas: netting around sleeping areas, 18-mesh wire for screening houses, mosquito boots, insecticides, and mosquito repellents. *N, N*-diethyltoluamide (Off), a contact repellent that is effective for about 18 hours, is preferable to the shorter-acting odor repellents (6-12). However, mosquitoes attack any area not covered by the chemical. Clothing impregnated with *N, N*-diethyltoluamide provides effective protection for months.

Drug prophylaxis, although important in the prevention of malaria, does not supersede the foregoing recommendations. Because chloroquine and proguanil destroy only the asexual erythrocytic parasites and fail to interrupt hepatic persistence, relapses may occur at a later date with *P. vivax* and *P. ovale.* Proguanil and chloroquine are ineffective against chloroquine-resistant *P. falciparum.* The recommended doses of chloroquine are given in Table 145-4. Adjustments should be made for underweight children. A day of the week should be selected for dosage that breaks the ordinary, everyday routine (*e.g.,* Sunday). Travellers who were heavily exposed to malaria and are not G-6-PD deficient should receive primaquine (15 mg of the base per day, PO, for 14 days) on return from an endemic area to eliminate the hepatic forms of *P. vivax* and *P. ovale.*

Table 145-4. *Peroral Chloroquine Dosage for Chemoprophylaxis of Malaria*

Patient Age	Weekly Dose of Base (mg)
Adults	300.0
Infants	37.5
1–3 years	75.0
4–7	112.5
8–12 years	150.0
>12 years	300.0

*Chemoprophylaxis should begin 2 weeks before entry into, and continue 4 weeks after the departure from, an endemic area.

There is no antimalarial drug approved in the United States that is uniformly successful in preventing erythrocytic infection with multi-drug-resistant *P. falciparum.* Fansidar, a fixed drug combination of pyrimethamine, 25 mg, and sulfadoxine (a long-acting sulfonamide) 500 mg, is effective for prevention of chloroquine-resistant malaria and can be obtained outside the United States. The dose is one tablet a week, to be taken along with chloroquine, 300 mg (base) on the same day. However, resistance is frequent in Southeast Asia and will probably soon appear elsewhere.

In addition to giving instructions for the prevention of malaria, the physician should inform the patient that fever occurring weeks, months, and even years after exposure may be caused by malaria.

Remaining Problems

New drugs for treatment and for chemoprophylaxis against multi-drug-resistant strains of *P. falciparum* are needed. Efforts toward understanding the immune response in malaria (including immune suppression) and toward the development of a vaccine must continue. The problems of developing a practical vaccine are formidable, but recent successes have been a great stimulus to research: (1) volunteers were protected against mosquito-induced infection with *P. falciparum* and *P. vivax* by vaccination with irradiated sporozoites; (2) rhesus monkeys were protected against challenge with the blood forms of *P. knowelsi* by vaccination with merozoites in Freund's complete adjuvant; and (3) monoclonal antibodies produced by hybridomas block sporozoite infection of the liver, asexual development, and gamete fertilization, thereby identifying potential antigens for the development of a vaccine.

Bibliography

Books

BOYD MF (ED): Malariology. Philadelphia, WB Saunders, 1949. 1643 pp (2 vol).

Chemotherapy of Malaria. Geneva, World Health Organization Technical Report Series No. 375, 19. 91 pp.

COATNEY GR, COLLINS WE, WARREN MCW, CONTACOS PG: The Primate Malarias. Washington DC, U.S. Government Printing Office, 1971. 366 pp.

Developments in Malaria Immunology. Geneva, World Health Organization Technical Report Series No. 579, 1975. 68 pp.

GARNHAM PCC: Malaria Parasites and Other Haemosporidia, Oxford, Blackwell Scientific Publications, 1966. 1114 pp.

MILLER LH: Transfusion malaria. In Greenwalt TJ, Jamieson GA (eds): Transmissible Disease and Blood Transfusion. New York, Grune & Stratton, 1975. pp. 241–266.

PETERS W: Chemotherapy and Drug Resistance in Malaria. New York, Academic Press, 1970. 876 pp.

Journals

Chemoprophylaxis of malaria. Morbid Mortal Week Rep 27 (Suppl): 81–90, 1978

CLYDE DF, MCCARTHY VC, MILLER RM, WOODWARD WE: Immunization of man against falciparum and vivax malaria by use of attentuated sporozoites. Am J Trop Med Hyg 24:397–401, 1975

FREEMAN RR, TREJDOSIEWICZ AJ, CROSS G: Protective monoclonal antibodies recognizing stage-specific merozoite antigens of a rodent malaria parasite. Nature 284:366–368, 1980

HENDRICKSE RG, GLASGOW EF, ADENIYI A, WHITE RHR, EDINGTON GM, HOUBA V: Quartan malarial nephrotic syndrome: Collaborative clinicopathological study in Nigerian children. Lancet 1:1143–1149, 1972

Immunology of Malaria. Bull WHO 57 (Suppl 1):1–290, 1979

MILLER LH: Current prospects and problems for a malaria vaccine. J Infect Dis 135:855–864, 1977

MILLER LH, MASON SJ, DVORAK JA, MCGINNISS MH, ROTHMAN IK: Erythrocyte receptors for (*Plasmodium knowlesi*) malaria: The Duffy blood group determinants. Science 189:561–563, 1975

MITCHELL GH, BUTCHER GA, COHEN S: A merozoite vaccine effective against *Plasmodium knowlesi* malaria. Nature (Lond) 252:311–313, 1974

NEVA FA: Malaria: Recent progress and problems. N Engl J Med 277:1241–1252, 1967

RENER J, CARTER R, ROSENBERG Y, MILLER LH: Anti-gamete hybridoma antibodies synergistically block transmission of malaria. Proc Natl Acad Sci (USA) 77:6797–6799, 1980

SPITZ S: The pathology of acute falciparum malaria. Milit Surg 99:555–572, 1946

Workshops on the biology and *in vitro* cultivation of malaria parasites. Bull WHO 55:121–429, 1977

YOSHIDA N, NUSSENZWEIG RS, POTOCNJAK P, NUSSENZWEIG V, AIKAWA M: Hybridoma produces protective antibodies directed against the sporozoite stage of malaria parasite. Science 207:71–73, 1979

TRENTON K. RUEBUSH, II

Babesiosis

146

Babesiosis, or piroplasmosis, is a tick-borne protozoan disease of nonhuman animals that is occasionally transmitted to humans. It is characterized by fever, hemolytic anemia, jaundice, hemoglobinuria, and renal failure. Babesiosis is of historical interest because *Babesia bigemina,* the protozoan responsible for Texas cattle fever, was the first microorganism shown to be transmitted by an arthropod.

Etiology

Protozoa of the genus *Babesia* are intraerythrocytic parasites of many species of wild and domestic animals. They are transmitted by hard-bodied ticks (*Ixodid* spp.). On microscopic examination of stained smears of blood, *Babesia* spp. resemble *Plasmodium* spp.; however, there is no pigment in erythrocytes infected with babesias.

Approximately 70 species of *Babesia* have been described; however, in some cases apparently identical organisms carry several different names. Until recently, the identification of *Babesia* spp. was based primarily on the morphology of the organism in blood smears, and on the vertebrate host. This practice led to considerable confusion because babesial morphology may be different in different hosts, and the range of hosts for some species of *Babesia* is quite broad. The resolution of some of these taxonomic problems may be aided by characterizing *Babesia* spp. using biochemical techniques such as DNA boyant density and isoenzyme analysis.

Epidemiology

Babesial infections are common in both domestic and wild animals in many parts of the world, particularly the tropics and subtropics. In some areas, these infections are responsible for serious economic losses in livestock.

Ixodid ticks are the only known vectors of *Babesia* spp. Ticks are infected when they take a blood meal from a vertebrate with babesiosis; the ingested babesias then divide and spread throughout the body of the tick. There is evidence of a sexual stage of reproduction of babesias within the tick, but the details of this phase of the life cycle are not known. In some species of ticks, *Babesia* spp. enter the ovaries and are passed transovarially through the egg to the developing larva. Babesias are transmitted to another vertebrate host by way of salivary secretions when the tick next takes a blood meal. In other species of ticks, the babesias are ingested during one developmental stage and are transmitted at a subsequent stage when the tick feeds after molting (transtadial transfer). For transmission to occur, it appears that the tick must be attached and feed for several hours.

Babesiosis is a zoonotic disease. Humans are infected accidentally and probably play no role in the transmission and maintenance of the infection in nature.

Although babesial infections are widespread in nonhuman animals, the first published report of babesiosis in a human did not appear until 1957. Since then, more than 50 additional cases have been described. The majority of these infections were caused by *B. microti,* a parasite of rodents. They were acquired along the northeast coast of the United States in Massachusetts (Nantucket Island, Martha's Vineyard Island, and Cape Cod) and New York (Long Island and Shelter Island). *Ixodes dammini,* the tick responsible for transmission of *B. microti* among rodents, is thought to be the vector to humans. Only the nymphal stage of the tick appears to be capable of transmitting the infection. Most infections in humans are acquired during the summer months.

The reason for the limited geographic distribution of infections in humans caused by *B. microti* is unknown. The range of the tick vector includes most of the northeastern United States, and apparently identical parasites have been found in wild animals in upstate New York, Utah, California, England, and Germany.

Babesiosis in humans caused by *B. divergens* (a protozoan that normally parasitizes cattle and is probably identical to *Babesia bovis*) have been reported from Yugoslavia, France, Ireland, Scotland, and Russia. The probable vector is *Ixodes ricinus. Babesia divergens* differs from *B. microti* in that it appears to have a much narrower host range and, thus far, has been reported to cause disease only in persons who have undergone splenectomy. Apparently, lack of the spleen increases susceptibility to *B. divergens;* however, splenectomy is not a prerequisite to disease in humans with *B. microti.*

Human cases of babesiosis caused by organisms that could not be identified as to species have been reported from Georgia, California, and the Gulf Coast of Mexico.

Recently, several blood-transfusion-induced infections with *B. microti* have been documented in humans in the northeastern United States. This route of transmission may become more common in the future because of the tendency of *B. microti* to cause prolonged, asymptomatic parasitemia.

Pathogenesis

When *Babesia* spp. are inoculated into a vertebrate host by the bite of an infected tick, the protozoa apparently invade red blood cells directly without a preliminary exoerythrocytic stage such as occurs in malaria. Within the red cell, babesias multiply by budding, usually forming two or four daughter cells. When the infected cell ruptures, other erythrocytes are invaded and the cycle is repeated.

In nonhuman animals babesial infections may persist for many years following the acute illness. The prolonged parasitemia is probably due to the ability of these organisms to change their surface antigens in response to exposure to specific antibody (antigenic variation).

The spleen plays an important role in resistance to babesial infections. Persons who have had splenectomies tend to have higher levels of parasitemia and more severe illnesses than persons with functioning spleens. In monkeys infected with *B. microti,* splenectomy as long as 9 months after the initial infection can lead to a recurrence of parasitemia.

The age of the host also influences the response to a babesial infection. In most species of animals, babesial infections acquired early in life tend to be mild or asymptomatic with much lower mortality rates than those among older animals. A similar association between age and severity of infection has been noted in humans infected with *B. microti;* disease is more common in persons more than 40 years old, whereas younger persons usually have mild or subclinical infections. No such relationship has been observed in splenectomized patients infected with either *B. microti* or *B. divergens.*

Manifestations

The severity of babesiosis depends primarily on the species of *Babesia* causing the infection, but is also related to the presence or lack of the spleen and the age of the patient.

Babesia microti

Patients infected with *B. microti* usually recount a gradual onset of fever, chills, diaphoresis, general myalgia, and extreme fatigue. Although symptoms tend to fluctuate in severity, there is no periodicity as in malaria. Many patients do not recollect a tick bite. In those who do, the incubation period varies from 1 to 4 weeks. The acute illness may last from a few weeks to a month or more, and is often followed by persistence of malaise and fatigue for several months. The majority of patients infected with *B. microti* have no history of splenectomy. Patients who have had previous splenectomies tend to have a more severe illness.

The only constant abnormality on physical examination is fever. Mild hepatosplenomegaly is found occasionally. The total numbers of leukocytes and platelets are low to normal, and there is a mild to moderately severe hemolytic anemia. Hemoglobinuria is rare, although serum haptoglobin levels may be reduced. Slight elevations of serum glutamic-oxaloacetic acid transaminase (SGOT), alkaline phosphatase, and bilirubin are found in about half of the patients. Approximately 1% to 10% of the erythrocytes are parasitized. No clear relationship has been noted between the degree of parasitemia and the severity of the illness; however, splenectomized patients tend to have higher levels of parasitemia. Although asymptomatic parasitemia with *B. microti* persists in some patients for several months after clinical recovery, recurrences of symptoms have not been observed.

Based on serologic evidence, asymptomatic or mild infections with *B. microti* are quite common in persons more than 30 years old in areas from which parasitologically confirmed cases have been reported.

Babesia divergens

Disease in humans caused by *B. divergens* generally develops rapidly, with chills, high fever, jaundice, and dark or blood-stained urine. All of the patients have had prior splenectomies because of trauma, portal hypertension, surgical accidents, or Hodgkins' disease. Fever, hypotension, and jaundice are the major findings on physical examination. Anemia is severe, with elevated reticulocyte counts and nucleated red blood cells in smears of peripheral blood. The leukocyte counts vary from normal to more than 40,000, with an increase in band forms. Marked elevations of bilirubin, liver enzymes, urea nitrogen, and creatinine are found in most patients. The course of the illness is characterized by progressive anemia, jaundice, hemoglobinuria, and renal insufficiency.

Diagnosis

The diagnosis of babesiosis should be considered in any patient with fever and a history of a tick bite or exposure to ticks. The clinical manifestations of infections caused by *B. microti* are not specific and may mimic a variety of viral or bacterial illnesses. Anemia is usually present, but may not be severe.

The disease caused by *B. divergens* evolves so rapidly with severe anemia, jaundice, dark urine, and renal insufficiency that the diagnosis should be suspected. Although babesiosis in humans appears to be limited to Europe and North America, the diagnosis should be considered in persons from other areas because *Babesia* spp. infect nonhuman animals worldwide.

Babesia spp. are best recognized in thick or thin blood smears stained by Giemsa's method (Chap. 9, Microscopic Examinations). The protozoa vary in morphology and are often mistaken for malaria parasites. With *B. microti,* the most frequently observed form resembles a small ring form of *Plasmodium falciparum.* Round, ovoid, or pyriform organisms are more commonly seen with *B. divergens.* Dividing parasites usually consist of two or four daughter cells held together by a thin strand of cytoplasm. Unlike malaria parasites, *Babesia* spp. do not form pigment in parasitized erythrocytes.

Inoculation of a susceptible laboratory animal (hamster or gerbil) with blood from a patient with suspected babesiosis has been a useful technique in the diagnosis of *B. microti* infections in humans when organisms have been difficult to detect in blood smears. Infections usually appear in inoculated animals within 2 to 4 weeks.

Although not widely available, serologic tests may also be helpful in diagnosis. An indirect immunofluorescence test has been used as a diagnostic aid in many patients infected with *B. microti* and is available through the Centers for Disease Control, Atlanta, Georgia. Serum antibody titers rise within the first 2 to 4 weeks after the onset of illness and then gradually fall over a period of 6 to 12 months. Serologic cross-reactions with malaria occur occasionally, but the highest titers are generally those of the infecting *Babesia* spp.

Prognosis

Infections in humans caused by *B. microti* are usually self-limited. Although parasitemia, with or without malaise and fatigue, may persist for several months after the acute illness, no permanent sequelae have been observed. All patients have recovered, even those who had higher parasitemias and more severe illnesses because of a previous splenectomy. In contrast, the majority of patients infected with *B. divergens* have died in spite of aggressive therapy with blood transfusions, renal dialysis, and various antiprotozoal drugs.

Although little is known about the usefulness of the immune response of humans to infection with *Babesia* spp., infection of monkeys with *B. microti* provides strong protection against a subsequent challenge with the same organism. No cross-protection was found between *B. microti* and *Plasmodium fieldi,* a malaria parasite of monkeys.

Therapy

There are no completely effective drugs for the treatment of babesiosis in humans. Because infections caused by *B. microti* are usually self-limited, symptomatic therapy is recommended for all but the most severely ill patients. Although chloroquine has been used for the treatment of many patients infected with *B. microti,* it appears to have no activity against this organism. The slight improvement in fever and symptoms noted in some patients after starting treatment with chloroquine is probably attributable to its anti-inflammatory effect rather than to a direct antibabesial action.

In persons with severe infections caused by either *B. microti* or *B. divergens,* pentamidine isesthionate is a logical choice for therapy. It is effective against various species of *Babesia* in nonhuman animals, and it has been successfully in several patients infected with *B. microti;* however, the drug may simply reduce parasitemia without eliminating *B. microti.* It remains to be seen whether pentamidine will improve the prognosis in patients infected with *B. divergens.* In patients with life-threatening babesiosis, chemotherapy should be combined with aggressive supportive treatment including blood transfusions and renal dialysis.

Prevention

The only effective means of preventing infection with *Babesia* spp. is avoidance of tick-infested areas. Insect repellents may be of some value (Chaps. 115, Trombiculosis, and 123, Colorado Tick Fever). Because ticks appear to transmit babesias only after they have been feeding on a host for several hours, it may be possible to prevent infections by prompt removal of attached ticks.

Remaining Problems

Because infections caused by *Babesia* spp. are widespread in wild and domestic animals, infections in humans may be much more common than is appreciated at present. The species of *Babesia* that cause infections in humans and the geographic distribution of such infections should be determined. This is a problem of particular importance in malarious areas where *Babesia* spp. may easily be mistaken for *P. falciparum* on microscopic examination of blood smears. More effective and less toxic drugs are needed for the treatment of babesiosis n humans.

Bibliography

Journals

GARNHAM PCC: Human babesiosis: European aspects. Trans R Soc Trop Med Hyg 74:153–155, 1980

HOARE CA: Comparative aspects of human babesiosis. Trans R Soc Trop Med Hyg 74:143–148, 1980

RUEBUSH TK II: Human babesiosis in North America. Trans R Soc Trop Med Hyg 74:149–152, 1980

PHILLIP E. C. MANSON–BAHR

Leishmaniasis 147

Leishmaniasis in humans results from infection with protozoa of the genus *Leishmania,* which are normally parasites of canines and rodents. Transmission is effected by sandflies of the genera *Phlebotomus* in the Old World and *Lutzomyia* in the New World.

Etiology

Four species of *Leishmania* cause leishmaniasis in humans: *Leishmania tropica* and *Leishmania mexicana* are limited to the skin; *Leishmania braziliensis* metastasizes to the mucocutaneous areas of the body and other areas of the skin; and *Leishmania donovani* metastasizes throughout the reticuloendothelial system of the body causing the kala-azar syndrome.

In human, canine, and rodent hosts, the parasite lives intracellularly as a Leishman–Donovan body (amastigote), whereas in the insect host it is a flagellated microorganism or leptomonad (promastigote). The leishmania (amastigote), or Leishman–Donovan body, is ovoid or rounded, measuring about 2 μm to 3 μm in length. It lives intracellularly in monocytes, polymorphonuclear leukocytes, and endothelial cells. In preparations stained with Giemsa or Wright stain, the cytoplasm stains pale blue. The large, round nucleus is sometimes flattened on one side and is seen as a mass of red-staining granules. The characteristic kinetoplast, a rod-shaped body in the cytoplasm that points toward the nucleus, stains bright red or reddish purple.

The cultural or leptomonad forms (promastigotes) are pear-shaped or slender, spindle-shaped bodies 15 μm to 25 μm in length and 1.5 μm to 3.5 μm in width. The single flagellum may be 15 μm to 28 μm long.

Material such as skin, spleen pulp, sternal marrow, or blood may be cultured on NNN medium (a biphasic medium of agar and fresh rabbit blood—see Chap. 11, Diagnostic Methods for Protozoa and Helminths) or on Schneider's insect medium. Cultures are kept at 22°C and may show growth in 7 to 10 days but should not be discarded for 28 days. The leptomonad forms (promastigotes) are found in the water of condensation.

Hamsters are very susceptible to leishmaniasis, dying 3 to 6 months after the intraperitoneal inoculation of infected material. They are quite useful in testing biologic materials for the presence of leishmania (amastigotes).

Epidemiology

Leishmaniasis is essentially a zoonosis and may be found in an environment that varies from the humid rain forests of South and Central America to the dry savannahs of Africa south of the Sahara and the deserts of the Middle East. The actual reservoirs vary correspondingly, although transmission of leishmania to man occurs primarily by way of sandflies (excepting the rare instances of transmission of *L. donovani* by blood transfusion and the alleged coital transfer of the same parasite). These features are summarized in Table 147-1.

Sandflies (Fig. 147-1) are infected as they feed on mammals with leishmaniasis. The ingested amastigotes develop into promastigotes, the infective forms, in the anterior portion of the gut, and these move to the salivary glands in about 10 days. Inoculation of a susceptible mammal can then occur as the sandfly feeds.

Considerable moisture is needed to induce oviposition in the sandfly, and breeding places vary in different parts of the world. A humid microclimate with decomposing organic matter is usually needed. The life cycle of the sandfly lasts from 1½ to 2 months in the summer, but is extended in the winter months.

Table 147-1. *Epidemiology of Leishmaniasis*

Etiologic Agent	Sandfly Vector	Reservoir	Area	Remarks
Visceral leishmaniasis (kala-azar)				
Leishmania donovani	*Phlebotomus perniciosus, ariasi, major, longicuspis, simici, chinesis, argentipes, orientalis*	Dogs Foxes Dogs, foxes, jackals Dogs Humans Wild rodents *Arvicanthus niloticus* (grass rat); *Rattus rattus* (black rat); *Acomys albigena* Carnivores serval *(Felis phillipsi)*; genet *(Genetta senegalensis)*	Mediterranean Southern Europe Central Asia China India Sudan	Infantile kala-azar Acacia forest
	Phlebotomus martini *Lutzomyia longipalpis*	Humans Dogs, foxes	East Africa Central and South America	Termite hills Dry and semiarid country
Old World Cutaneous leishmaniasis (oriental sore)				
Leishmania tropica	*Phlebotomus sergenti, papatasii, perfiliewi, caucasicus, mongolensis, alexanderi, ansarii*	Giant gerbil, *Rhombomys opimus*; *Meriones libycus*; Fat mouse, *Psammomys obesus* Dogs, humans	Mediterranean Basin, Central Asia, and India	Two types, rural and urban
Leishmania tropica	*Phlebotomus dubosqui, bergeroti,*	Dogs, rodents	West Africa	
Leishmania aethiopica	*Phlebotomus longipes, pedifer, rossi*	Hyrax	East African highlands, above 2000 m (Ethiopia and Kenya); southwest Africa	

New world cutaneous leishmaniasis				
Leishmania mexicana complex				
mexicana mexicana (Chiclero ulcer)	*Lutzomyia olmeca*	Tree rats (*Orizomys capito, Ototylomis phyllotis*) *Heteromys desmaresteanus;* spiny pocket mouse (*Nycromys sumichrasti*)	Mexico, Guatemala	Zoonosis, an occupational hazard
mexicana amazonensis	*Lutzomyia flaviscutellata, panamensis*	*Orizomys capito, Orizomys macronelli, Nectomys squamipes; Neacomys* spp.	Central America, Amazonia	
Leishmania braziliensis complex				
braziliensis braziliensis (*espundia*)	*Psychodopygus wellcomei* *Lutzomyia pessoani, whitmani, mignoni*	Poorly known *Orizomys concolor,* paca (*Cuniculus paca*); agouti (*dasyprocta azarrae*)	Central and South America—Amazonia	Complex zoonosis in forest areas and bordering settlements
braziliensis panamensis	*Lutzomyia trapidoi* (major vector), *cruciata, pessoani, panamensis*	Two-toed sloth (*Choloepus hoffmani*) and three-toed sloth *Bradypus infuscatus*) main hosts. Spiny rat (*Hoplomys gymnurus*); marmoset (*Sanguineus goeffroyi*); kinkajou (*Potos flavus*)	Central America	
braziliensis guyanensis (Pian bois, bush yaws)	*Lutzomyia unbratilis*	Spiny rat (*Proechymis semispinosus*) Nine-banded armadillo (*Dasypus novemcinctus*	Guyana, Surinam (barren uplands—to 2800 m)	Multiple lesions, lymphatic spread
Leishmania peruviana (Uta)	*Lutzomyia verrucarum, peruensis*	Dog	Peru—western Andes (barren uplands—to 2800 m)	Single ulcer
Leishmania garnhami	*Lutzomyia townsendi*		Venezuela—eastern Andes (rain forest)	Single ulcer

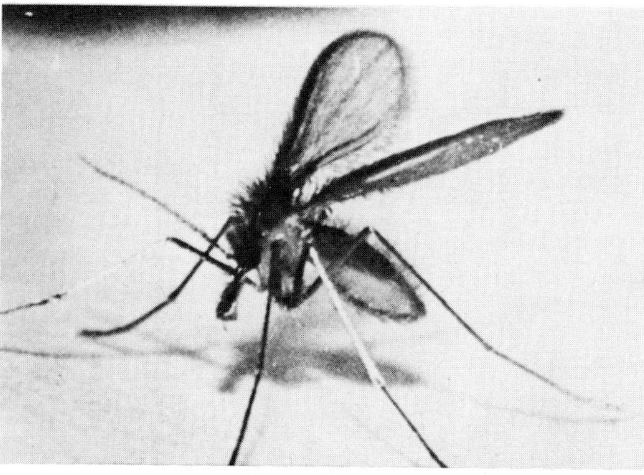

Fig. 147–1. Sandfly (*Phlebotomus longipes*).

Adults are normally nocturnal, but some sandflies bite during the day. Flight ranges vary from a few to hundreds of yards.

Leishmania tropica

Leishmania tropica, the cause of cutaneous leishmaniasis of the Old World, is parasitic to rodents, principally the giant gerbil *Rhombomys opimus,* and the *Meriones libycus.* These animals live in colonies in the semiarid parts of Asiatic Russia, Iran, Iraq, and other areas. A high percentage may exhibit leishmanial sores on the ears and tail (Fig. 147-2). Transmission by burrow sandflies (*Phlebotomus caucasicus*) is intense. However, anthropophagous sandflies (*P. papatasii*) also feed on these rodents and can transmit *L. tropica major* to man to yield moist or rural cutaneous leishmaniasis. In parts of the Middle East, the parasite, as it has become adapted to domestic dogs, is known as *L. tropica tropica;* it is transmitted from dogs to humans by *P. sergenti* and *P. papatasii* to cause the urban or dry form of cutaneous leishmaniasis. This is essentially a disease of children because most adults are immune.

Leishmania donovani

Leishmania donovani cause the kala-azar syndrome which is seen in southern Europe (France, Italy, Sicily), the eastern Mediterranean countries, North Africa, Sudan, East Africa, the Middle East (Iran, Iraq, Saudi Arabia, Oman), the USSR (Azerbaijan, Tadjikistan), India (Bengal, Assam), and northeast Brazil with pockets in Argentina, Colombia, Venezuela, Guatemala, and Mexico. Historically, *L. donovani* may first have been parasitic to rodents, adapting later to canids and then to humans. At present, the parasite circulates in primary foci in rodents, whereas secondary foci develop in canids and humans. Throughout most of its geographic range it infects humans only as a dead end maintaining itself in wild (fox, jackal) and domestic (dog) hosts. In India, humans are the only known host, and in the Sudan and East Africa human-to-human transmission is quite likely; no rodent host has yet been identified in East Africa.

Zoonotic Hosts

From isoenzyme studies, many leishmanias isolated from rodents are not actually *L. donovani;* only in the Sudan have true *L. donovani* been isolated from rodents. *Leishmania donovani* have been found in foxes (Europe, Brazil), jackals (USSR), dogs (the Mediterranean, Brazil, the Middle East, and East Africa).

MEDITERRANEAN

In North Africa and the nearby Mediterranean islands, the dog is the most important host. The disease is urban and sporadic, occurs mainly in infants (*ponos*—infantile kala-azar), and shows a seasonal pattern, appearing from April to October with infection having taken place in the previous fall. Following eradication of malaria, kala-azar became uncommon; however, in southern Europe, there has been a resurgence. The zoonotic host is the European fox (*Vulpes vulpes*); accordingly, the disease in this area is rural and sporadic, but there have been small epidemics in Italy where the majority of the infections were subclinical.

MIDDLE EAST

Kala-azar is found sporadically in Iran, Saudi Arabia, Oman, Yemen, and Aden. However, it has become almost epidemic on the outskirts of Baghdad, where jackals are probably the zoonotic host.

CENTRAL ASIA

Kala-azar is now confined to Azerbaijan and an area in Tadjikistan where jackals are the zoonotic host. It has largely disappeared from China.

INDIA

Kala-azar is epidemic in India, humans forming the only reservoir. In the last century epidemics devastated the Brahmaputra Valley and Assam, but the infection largely disappeared after the area was sprayed for malaria eradication. Lately it has returned in epidemic form. Periodic epidemics take place every 15 years and last 10 years. The maximum incidence is in the 10- to 14-year age group. It is a house disease—a disease that occurs with regularity in certain houses.

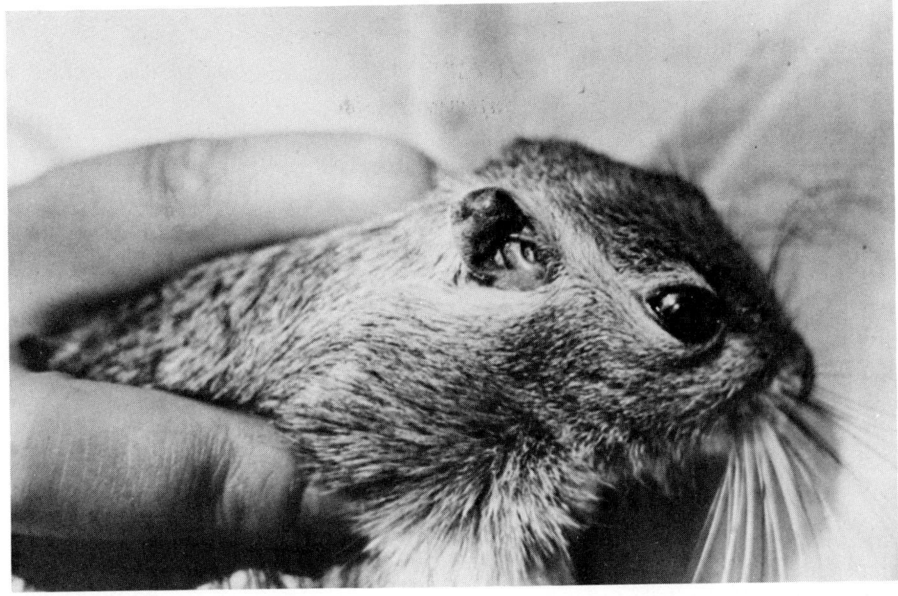

Fig. 147-2. Leishmanial nodule on ear of a giant gerbil, *Rhombomys opimus.*

AFRICA

African kala-azar is found from Lake Tchad eastward to the Sudan and Kenya in the Sahel zone. In the Sudan, where rodents may be hosts, the disease is sporadic, but epidemics lasting 10 years are separated by intervals of 15 years. Those affected are usually 10 to 14 years of age (sometimes older) and live in villages near acacia-balanites scrub growth. Similar epidemics take place in East Africa; although no rodent hosts have been identified, the disease occurs in microfoci in small homesteads situated near eroded termite hills. Early on, young adults are affected, but late in the course of epidemics young infants are also involved.

SOUTH AMERICA

In northeastern Brazil, kala-azar may be urban with a dog reservoir or rural with a fox reservoir. The disease affects children older than those who are affected in the Mediterranean.

Leishmania mexicana

Leishmania mexicana, the cause of cutaneous leishmaniasis (chicle ulcer) of the New World, is found in Central America, as far south as Panama. It is the only form of cutaneous leishmaniasis found in Mexico and Guatemala. In small forest rodents (the white-tailed mouse, spiny rats, and others; *Ototylomis phyllotis* in British Honduras), *L. mexicana* causes tiny, insignificant lesions on the tail, ears, and limbs. Relatively small enzootic foci are perpetuated in the humid rain forest areas of the Peten region of Guatemala and the Yucatan area of Mexico by *Lutzomyia flaviscutellata,* which feeds mainly on rodents. Transmission to humans is effected by anthropophilic species such as *Lutzomyia panamensis.* Humans are infected when they enter the forest to cut wood or collect gum (chicle). Thus, the disease has been called chicle ulcer.

Leishmania braziliensis

Leishmania braziliensis, the cause of mucocutaneous leishmaniasis (espundia) of the New World, is continuous in distribution with *L. mexicana* from Panama southward. The protozoan has been isolated from the paca, agouti, and small rodents in Amazonia. *Psychodopygus wellcomei* and *Lutzomyia pessoani, L. whitmani,* and *L. mignoni* are the vectors. Humans are infected when they enter the forest, as on military or police patrols, or as members of a construction camp. Because espundia is one of the main diseases affecting humans in construction camps and new settlements, it also affects development of the Amazon region.

Pathogenesis and Pathology

After the dermal inoculation of infective *Leishmania* spp., the parasites are engulfed by macrophage cells and elicit a reaction of round and plasma cells. These cells may eradicate the infection after the development of delayed hypersensitivity, as shown by the appearance of epithelioid and giant cells and leishmanin sensitivity. When the amastigotes in the skin have been eradicated, there is complete immunity to reinfection with homologous strains of *Leishmania* spp.

The immune response in leishmaniasis forms a spectrum ranging from self-healing to progressive disease. In diffuse, cutaneous leishmaniasis there is little or no cellular response, as in lepromatous leprosy, which it so closely resembles; in the non-self-healing kala-azar syndrome caused by *L. donovani,* there is immunosuppression until cure of the infection. In leishmaniasis recidiva and in espundia, the response is exaggerated (hyperergic) but does not eliminate the leishmanias. These variations in immune response result in variations in pathology. In the immunoresponsive cases, formation of granulomas is marked, there are few protozoa, and healing eventually takes place, as occurs with *L. tropica* and *L. mexicana* and in the self-healing infections with *L. donovani.* In nonresponsive cases, there are many leishmanias in macrophages with little or no cellular response, as occurs in diffuse cutaneous leishmaniasis and in the kala-azar syndrome—characterized also by an abnormal response consisting of the production of large amounts of nonprotective, polyclonal IgG.

Manifestations

Inapparent Infection

Not all persons infected with leishmanias develop disease. In fact, the number infected is probably far larger than the number diseased. Leishmanin skin testing in areas endemic for leishmaniasis has shown a high incidence of positive reactors; the percentage increases with increasing age. Conversion to positive may take place without any indication of overt infection such as a history of skin ulcers, presence of scars, or kala-azar. Furthermore, in an area where kala-azar appeared for the first time, it was shown that leishmanin conversion, humoral antibodies, and hepatic granulomas had developed without any illness.

Cutaneous Leishmaniasis of the Old World (Oriental Sore)

Two main kinds of clinical disease are caused by *L. tropica:* (1) *Leishmania tropica major* typically causes single or multiple skin lesions with a short incubation period, rapid growth, considerable tissue reaction with few parasites, and healing in less than 1 year (Fig. 147-3); (2) *Leishmania tropica minor* causes a single lesion with a longer incubation period, slower growth, less pronounced tissue reaction, and more parasites; healing takes longer than 1 year.

The incubation period is variously stated in days,

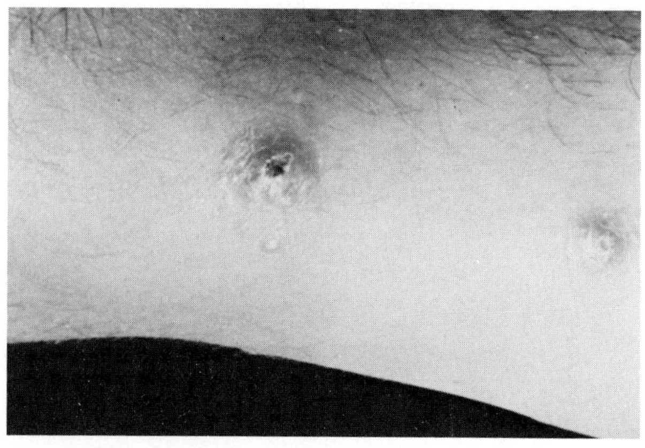

Fig. 147-3. Cutaneous leishmaniasis of the Old World. Note multiple sores, one showing satellite lesions.

weeks, or months, and it can last as long as 3 years.

The local lesion begins as a minute, itching papule that tends to expand as a shotty congested infiltration of the dermis. After a few days or weeks, the papule becomes covered with fine papery scales that later become moister, browner, and adherent.

In this way, a crust is formed that, on falling off or being scratched, uncovers a shallow ulcer. The sore, which is surrounded by an area of congestion, slowly extends by erosion of its edge. Subsidiary sores arise around the edge of the ulcer and merge with it. These sores are usually about 2 cm in diameter, and they may enlarge to occupy an area several cm across. After 2 or 3 to 12 months or more, healing sets in, often beginning at the center while the ulcer may be extending at the edge. Ultimately, a depressed white or pinkish scar forms (Fig. 147-4).

Contraction of the scar may cause unsightly deformity. Oriental sores may be single or multiple. Two or three are not uncommon, and in rare instances as many as 150 have been found on the same patient. Because ulcers correspond to the sites of inoculation, they are mostly situated on the face, hands, feet, arms, and legs, occasionally on the ears, tip of the nose, lower lip, tongue, and rarely, on the upper eyelids (ocular leishmaniasis). Sometimes the initial papule does not proceed to ulceration. Oriental sore does not cause death, but it is troublesome and unsightly. In many cities of the Middle East, most adults bear the typical scar of a healed sore.

American Cutaneous Leishmaniasis

Two main types of cutaneous leishmaniasis are found in the New World. *Leishmania mexicana* causes a single, nonmetastasizing skin lesion (chicle ulcer)

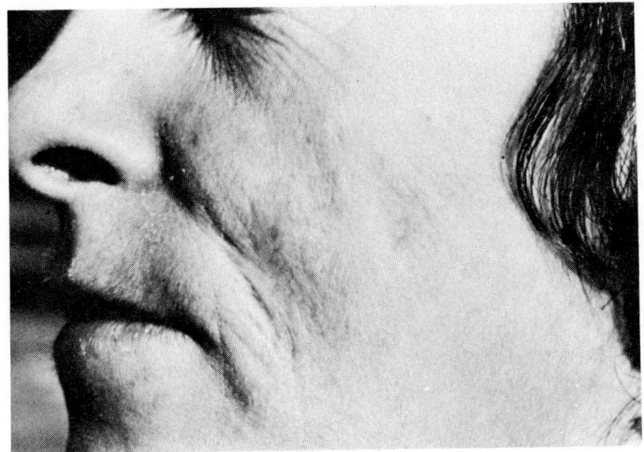

Fig. 147-4. Cutaneous leishmaniasis of Old World. Note typical fine papery scar on face.

that subsides spontaneously in about 6 months. *Leishmania braziliensis* causes a single sore or primary lesion (espundia). It may metastasize to other areas of the skin and mucous membranes, producing a disfiguring and sometimes fatal disease.

Chicle Ulcer (Bay Sore, Forest Yaws). The lesion is found on exposed areas of the body, usually the face, commonly on the ear, where it causes a very chronic ulcer that persists as long as 20 years and causes destruction of the pinna (chiclero's ear—Fig. 147-5). Elsewhere, the lesion is small and self-limiting, healing spontaneously in less than 6 months.

Espundia. The lesion begins as an ulcer on an exposed area of the skin or mucous membranes. It heals in a few months to years, leaving a charcteristic scar. After an interval of months or even years, secondary, intractable, fungating ulcers break out on the tongue and in the buccal or nasal cavities, destroying and obstructing them and leading to death from secondary infections and exhaustion after years of suffering (Fig. 147-6). The lymph nodes are often involved, but the viscera are spared. When a primary sore develops, it cannot be predicted whether it will metastasize or not—for example, the figures vary from 2% in Panama to 80% in Paraguay. Destruction of the nasal septum causes a characteristic disfigurement called *tapir nose*. Ulceration may extend to the larynx.

Unusual Forms of Cutaneous Leishmaniasis

Leishmaniasis Recidiva. In Iraq and Anatolia, a relapsing, tuberculoid form of leishmaniasis is found that closely resembles lupus vulgaris. Relapses occur after the original lesion heals, and they often take the form of nodules and papules situated at the periphery of the scar. Amastigotes are sparse in the apple jelly nodules, and the leishmanin skin test is strongly positive. Leishmaniasis recidiva is extremely resistant to all forms of treatment except irradiation with soft x-rays.

Diffuse Cutaneous Leishmaniasis. In parts of Venezuela and Ethiopia, a very chronic form of cutaneous leishmaniasis is found. The lesion begins in one area as a nodule that never ulcerates. Gradually, nodules spread all over the body, affecting the nose especially, but not destroying the nasal septum. Amastigotes are numerous in the lesions, but they stimulate

Fig. 147-5. Chiclero's ear. Chronic destructive lesion of pinna is visible.

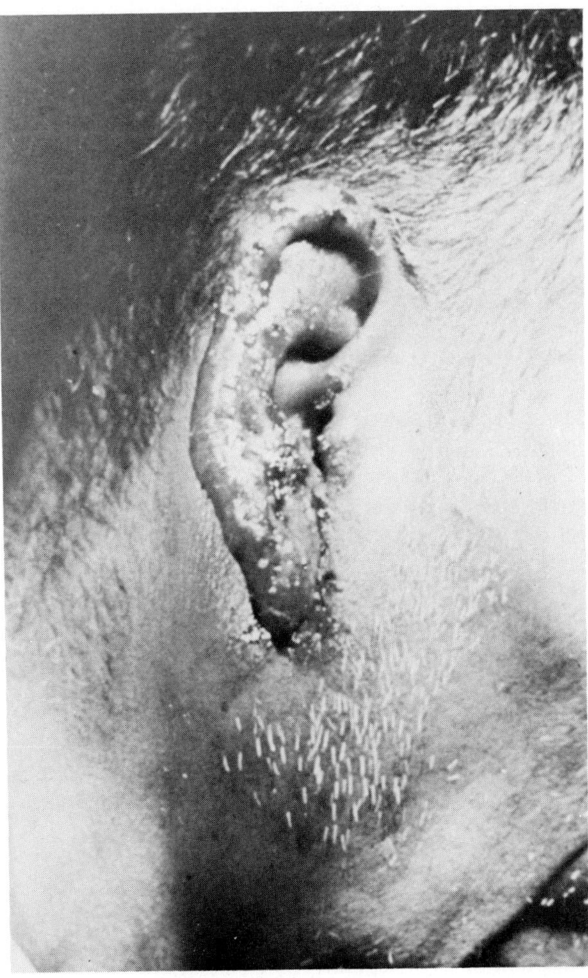

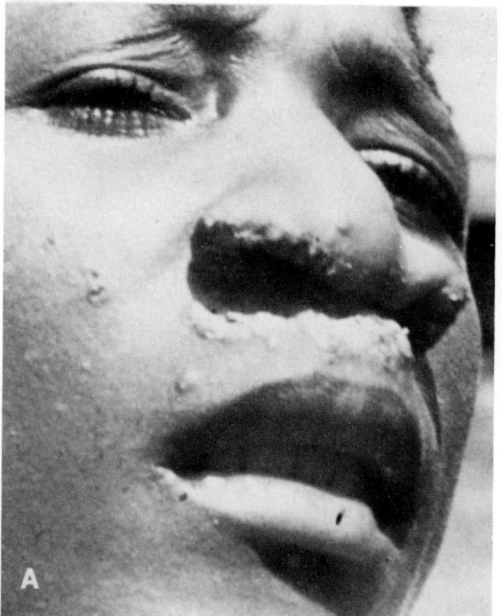

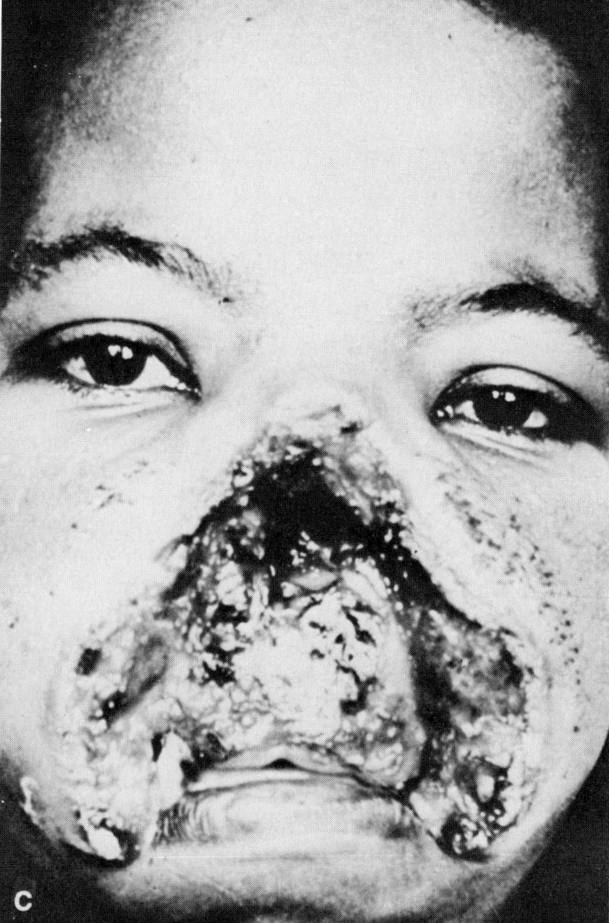

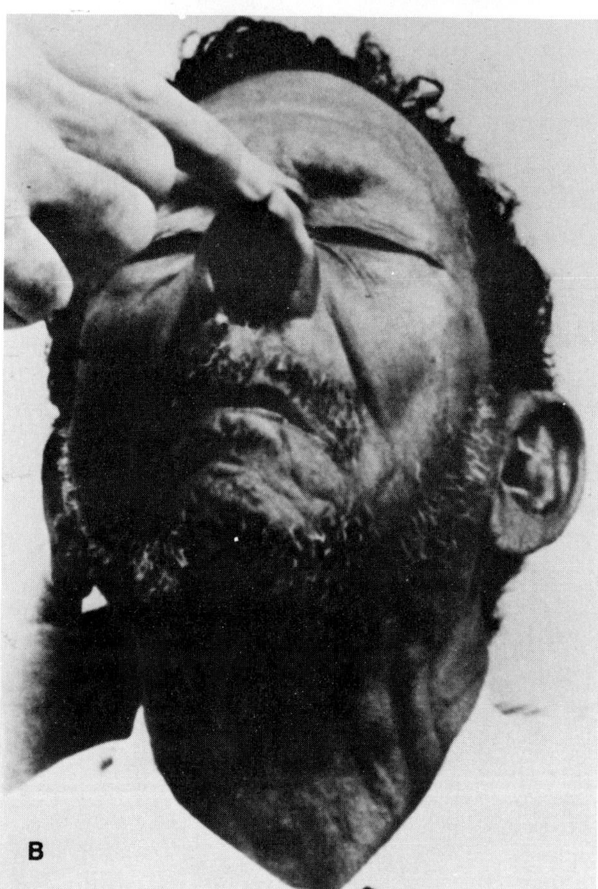

Fig. 147-6. Espundia. (*A*) Early oronasal lesion. (*B*) Destruction of nasal septum. (*C*) Gross destruction of nose and pharynx.

very little cellular reaction; the leishmanin skin test is persistently negative. There is failure of cell-mediated immunity, and the condition very closely resembles lepromatous leprosy. The course may extend 20 years or more. Treatment is difficult and involves prolonged application of pentamidine.

Visceral Leishmaniasis (Kala-Azar)

All the geographic forms of kala-azar are generally similar in their clinical manifestations. A primary skin lesion occurs in the African form, and amastigotes are found in the skin in the African, American, and Chinese forms. Post-kala-azar dermal leishmanoid (see Prognosis, below) is common in the Indian, less common in the African, and very rare in all the other forms.

The primary lesion at the site of the infective bite is usually so small that it cannot be distinguished. In the Sudan, more extensive lesions resembling epitheliomas have been described.

Infection without manifestations persists 4 to 6 months, even up to 10 years. When the protozoa invade the reticuloendothelial cells of the spleen, liver, bone marrow, and lymph nodes, disease is provoked.

The onset of symptoms may be abrupt, or as is common in the inhabitants of endemic areas, more insidious. Cough is frequent, and an attack of pneumonia may cause the patient to be admitted to the hospital. Diarrhea, even dysentery, and epistaxis with fever are also common. An insidious onset is marked by chronic, wasting disease. Pain beneath the left costal margin from an enlarging spleen is very characteristic.

In cases with an acute onset, the fever starts suddenly and may reach 104°F. Rarely, there is a characteristic pattern with two maxima during the day. In the more chronic cases, there is little or no fever. Characteristically, there is marked fever with little constitutional illness so that the patient is ambulant.

Moderate enlargement of the inguinal and femoral lymph nodes is typical and is especially notable in the African form. The spleen enlarges gradually so that eventually it may reach into the right iliac fossa. At first it is soft, but it soon becomes very hard. The liver also enlarges, but not as markedly. Jaundice occurs in the 10% of patients who are most severely ill. The concentrations of IgG in the serum may rise as high as 4 g/100 ml. A positive formol gel reaction is usual. Proteinuria is present in some patients, to a degree that is more marked than can be accounted for by the fever.

The progressive diminution in the number of polymorphonuclear leukocytes, thrombocytopenia, and normocytic normochromic anemia are part of an autoimmune phenomenon in which antibodies attack these elements and destroy them. The half-life of the red cells is greatly diminished, and they are destroyed in the spleen and elsewhere in the reticuloendothelial system.

Unusual Forms of Visceral Leishmaniasis

Tonsillar lesions with cervical lymph node enlargement resembling tuberculosis may occur in Mediterranean kala-azar. Severe toxic forms may be found in any area when there is a rapid increase in the number of infections, for example, hemorrhagic disease (often without splenic enlargement) or hepatic necrosis with death in 4 to 6 weeks. The diagnosis in such cases may be difficult and may only be achieved by serology because amastigotes may be scanty.

Diagnosis

The diagnosis of leishmaniasis is reliably made by the demonstration of the protozoa in smears and by isolation either in cultures or by animal inoculation. In cutaneous or mucocutaneous leishmaniasis, a specimen for examination is obtained by inserting a small needle under the ulcer, going through the skin peripheral to the lesion. In this way, relatively uncontaminated tissue juice can be obtained for the preparation of smears (staining by Giemsa's method), cultures (NNN medium, or Schneider's insect medium), or inoculation (hamsters). Amastigotes are abundant in Old World cutaneous leishmaniasis but are scanty in the New World form.

A full-thickness biopsy of the skin through the edge of a lesion may be especially useful in the diagnosis of New World leishmaniasis. Sections should be stained with hematoxylin and eosin and with Giemsa stain. The characteristic infiltration with lymphocytes and plasma cells—epithelioid and giant cells in chronic lesions—is helpful in diagnosis. However, the presence of amastigotes inside macrophages is the most useful finding. The absence of acid-fast bacilli is evidence against tuberculosis and leprosy, diseases it may not be possible to exclude on either clinical or other histopathologic grounds.

In kala-azar, specimens for examination, in descending order of usefulness, include spleen pulp, sternal marrow, liver tissue, and juice from lymph nodes. If the spleen is reasonably large and firm, and the prothrombin time is normal, splenic puncture is a safe procedure. An 18- or 20-g needle is used. The edge of the spleen is held in the left hand, and the needle is thrust into the edge and allowed to remain until some pulp has welled up in it. The hub is then blocked with the thumb, and the needle is withdrawn. A small amount of pulp is blown out onto a slide and stained (Fig. 147-7). The remaining material may be diluted with saline solution for culture and inoculation into a hamster. Use of a syringe for aspiration should be avoided because it would take up blood.

Splenic puncture is positive to a greater extent than any other method of diagnosis. Sternal puncture is safer in some hands, but it is not as often productive. Liver biopsy is also useful. Lymph node puncture is positive only in about 60% of cases.

The leishmanin skin test is used in the diagnosis of all forms of leishmaniasis. Leishmanin is a suspension of flagellate forms (promastigotes) obtained from cultures and suspended in 0.5% phenol in saline solution to a concentration of 10,000,000/mm^3. Some preparations now are standardized on the basis of nitrogen content. A dose of 0.1 ml to 0.2 ml is injected intradermally. A positive reaction is an area of induration greater than 5 mm in diameter 24 to 48 hours after injection. The test becomes positive in the first 6 weeks of infection with *L. mexicana* and after 3

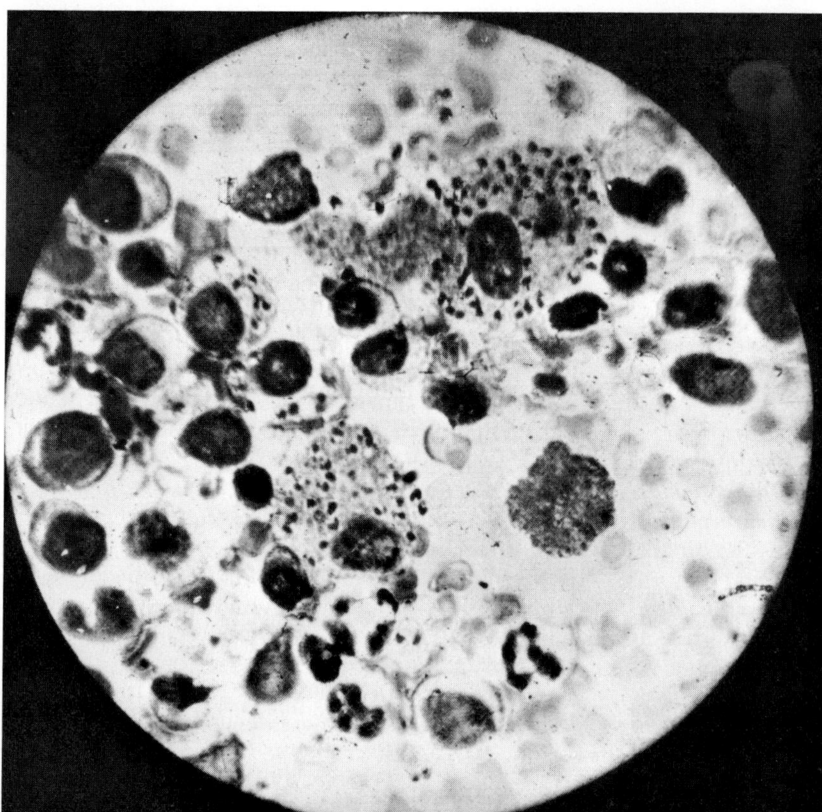

Fig. 147-7. Leishman–Donovan bodies in macrophages of spleen pulp (Original magnification approximately × 1000)

months with *L. tropica* and *L. braziliensis.* It remains positive for life after recovery. The test is negative in active kala-azar, and it only becomes positive 6 to 8 weeks after recovery; thus it is of no use in the diagnosis of active disease caused by *L. donovani.* Cross-reactions occur with certain forms of skin tuberculosis, but they are rare.

The susceptibility of serum to gelling by formalin is a function of the concentration of globulins. Because hyperglobulinemia is a hallmark of active visceral leishmaniasis, the formol gel test is useful in the diagnosis and evaluation of the treatment of kala-azar, but it is of no value in cutaneous and mucocutaneous leishmaniasis. Blood is allowed to clot, and the supernatant serum is drawn off. To 2 ml serum, 2 drops of 40% formalin is added. The mixture is shaken and allowed to stand for 20 min. The serum becomes solid with an opacity like the white of a hard-cooked egg in a positive reaction. The reaction becomes positive within the first 3 months of overt kala-azar and negative 6 months after cure.

Complement-fixing (CF) antibodies appear in the blood only in kala-azar. They appear early and are present while the disease is active, disappearing with cure. The antigen is prepared from an acid-fast bacillus (Kedrowsky's bacillus); titers of 1:20 or higher are significant. Cross-reactions occur with Chagas' disease and other forms of trypanosomiasis. There are no cross-reactions with tuberculosis or leprosy.

The indirect fluorescent antibody (IFAT) and the micro-enzyme-linked immunoabsorbent assay (micro-ELISA) tests are all useful in diagnosis. In kala-azar, significant IFAT titers (1:128) develop early and may reach 1:1200 or more before recovery begins. Although antibody is normally detected in recovered patients for up to 2 years, persistence of antibody may denote subclinical infection. Antibody titers are significantly elevated in espundia; cure is associated with a fall in titer, whereas persistence foretells metastasis from the cutaneous lesions. The IFAT test is negative in the purely cutaneous disease caused by *L. mexicana* and *L. tropica.* Cross-reactions are found with African and American trypanosomiasis (Chap. 130 and 136).

Cutaneous and mucocutaneous leishmaniasis must be differentiated from syphilis (Chap. 59, Syphilis), yaws (Chap. 106, Nonsyphilitic Treponematoses), chronic fungus infections (especially blastomycosis—Chap. 43, Blastomycosis), tuberculosis (Chap. 34, Pulmonary Tuberculosis), leprosy (Chap. 105, Leprosy), epithelioma, rhinoscleroma, and simple tropical ulcer. Amastigotes in smears and biopsy specimens and a positive leishmanin skin test enable the diagnosis of leishmaniasis to be made.

The differentiation of visceral leishmaniasis from other prolonged fevers of the tropics—malaria (Chap. 145, Malaria), typhoid (Chap. 64, Typhoid Fever), liver abscess (Chap. 84, Pylephlebitis and Liver Abscesses), brucellosis (Chap. 138, Brucellosis), disseminated histoplasmosis (Chap. 40, Histoplasmosis), and reticulosis—must be accomplished. In addition, the wasting may resemble that of starvation, pulmonary tuberculosis, or malignant disease. The diagnosis is made by isolating amastigotes from spleen, bone marrow, liver, or lymph node aspirates. The formol gel, CF, and fluorescent antibody (FA) tests are also quite useful. The splenomegaly must be distinguished from portal hypertension, schistosomiasis (*Schistosoma mansoni,* Chap. 81,) Schistosomiasis), myelogenous and lymphatic leukemias, and other severe anemias associated with splenomegaly.

Prognosis

Cutaneous leishmaniasis, whether caused by *L. tropica* or by *L. mexicana,* is a self-limited disease. Scarring is especially likely to be disfiguring if secondary bacterial infection has augmented tissue destruction.

The mucocutaneous lesions caused by *L. braziliensis* may not be self-limiting but may extend to secondary sites. Secondary infection is quite common. Death may ensue and is largely attributable to secondary bacterial pneumonias.

In untreated kala-azar, particularly in the African form, amastigotes may be widely distributed throughout the apparently normal skin. During and after recovery from the disease, a special form of dermal leishmaniasis appears which is known as post-kala-azar dermal leishmanoid. This condition appears during or shortly after treatment in the African form, but it may be delayed up to 2 years after treatment in the Indian form. There are two constituents of the eruption: (1) a macular, depigmented eruption found mainly on the face, arms and upper part of the trunk; and (2) a warty, papular eruption in which amastigotes can be found. When the rash is present, there are no longer any amastigotes in the internal organs. The condition must be differentiated from leprosy, which it closely resembles (Fig. 147-8).

Untreated kala-azar usually lasts several years, but African cases may run an acute course and terminate

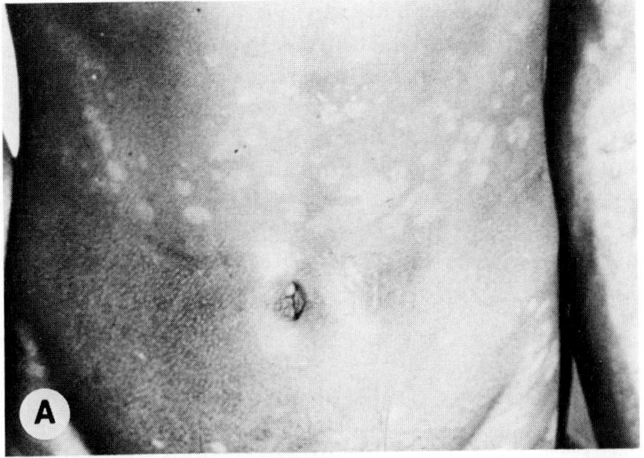

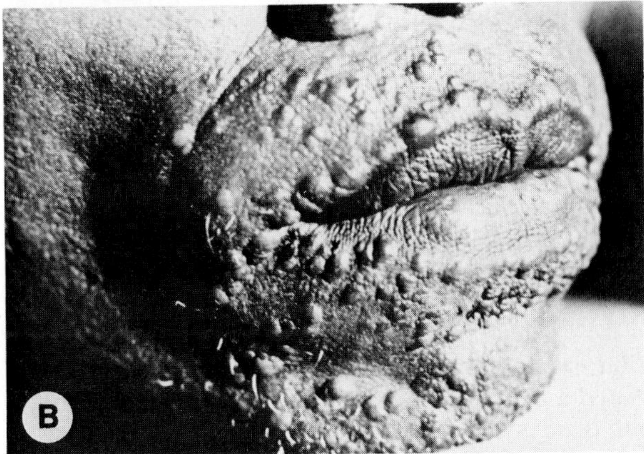

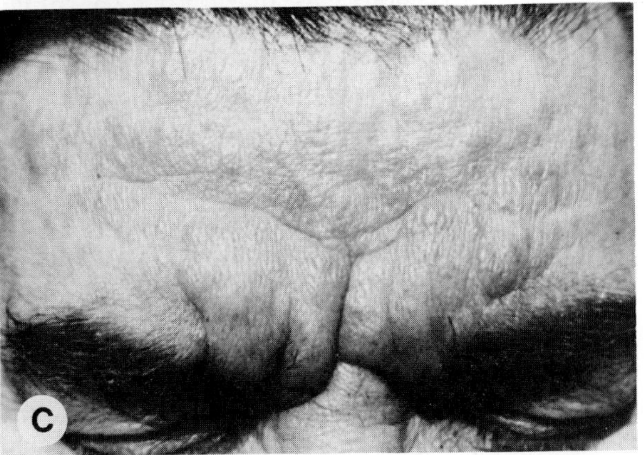

Fig. 147-8. Postkala-azar dermal leishmanoid. (*A*) Macular depigmented eruption. (*B*) Warty papular eruption. (*C*) Indurated rash on forehead resembling lepromatous leprosy.

within 5 months. In the terminal stages, ascites may develop from cirrhosis of the liver, hemic murmurs from severe anemia appear, and hemorrhages may occur from any part of the body. Death may result from several causes, for example exhaustion or intercurrent infections (dysentery or pneumonia). Noma is common in advanced cases. Common sequelae are cirrhosis of the liver, which is found in 10% of cases, and pulmonary tuberculosis. In advanced cases, amyloid disease appears with amyloid nephrosis.

Therapy

Most of the simple cutaneous lesions require no chemotherapy because they are self-healing. However, patients with metastasizing mucocutaneous and visceral leishmaniasis must be given specific therapy. Pentavalent antimony preparations, aromatic diamidines, and amphotercin B seem to be the most effective agents. The antifolic drugs, pyrimethamine (Daraprim) and cycloguanil pamoate (Camolar), are also useful in the treatment of American cutaneous leishmaniasis.

Sodium stibogluconate (Pentostam, Solustibosan) is given daily, by intravenous or intramuscular injection, as a solution containing the equivalent of 100 mg pentavalent antimony per milliliter. In adults, the dose is 10 mg/kg body wt for as long as 30 days. Although six injections cure Indian kala-azar, 30 injections are needed for all other forms of kala-azar. Ten injections are usualy sufficient for cutaneous leishmaniasis. The duration of therapy is unchanged for infants and children, but dosage is calculated at 15 mg/kg body wt. Glucantime (*N*-methylglucamine antimoniate) is used in exactly the same way.

Urea stibamine is compounded of urea with paraaminophenylstibonic acid. It is given intravenously in a dose of 3 mg/kg body wt/day for three courses of 10 days each, separated by 7 days of rest, in the treatment of non-Indian kala-azar. A total of six injections is sufficient for Indian kala-azar. Urea stibamine is not active in cutaneous, leishmaniasis. If there has been no response to antimony preparations, diamidine drugs must be used (they are of no use in cutaneous leishmaniasis).

Hydroxystilbamidine isethionate is given intravenously. The dose is 3 to 5 mg/kg body wt/day, as a single injection, for 10 days. Intervals of 10 days should separate the three courses necessary for all forms of kala-azar other than Indian kala-azar, for which one course is adequate. Administration of an antihistamine—for example, 10 mg promethazine hydrochloride (Phenergan) every 8 hours—is often helpful to avoid a drop in blood pressure.

If patients with either kala-azar or metastasizing mucocutaneous leishmaniasis do not respond to either pentavalent antimony or pentamidine isethionate, amphotericin B should be used (Chap. 39, Candidosis). A total dose of 2 g is sufficient. Splenectomy sometimes cures resistant kala-azar.

In American cutaneous leishmaniasis, a daily peroral dose of pyrimethamine (0.5 mg/kg body, as a single dose) for 21 days is usually effective. If necessary, after a rest of 12 days, the course can be repeated. Folinic acid and bakers' yeast may be required to combat bone marrow depression if treatment has to be prolonged (Chap. 129, Toxoplasmosis).

Cycloguanil pamoate has been used in the treatment of infection with *L. mexicana.* One injection of 5 mg/kg body wt is given intramuscularly; the dose may be repeated after 3 months.

Heat has been used successfully when applied locally to cutaneous lesions by means of close-fitting prostheses. The temperature in and beneath the lesion must be raised to 38°C to 40°C (101°F–104°F) and maintained for 12 hours. A series of such treatments may be necessary.

Prevention

Cutaneous leishmaniasis has been successfully controlled in southern Russia by destroying the wild rodent reservoir. Gerbil colonies were destroyed in their burrows with picrotoxin, and villages were situated more than 3 miles from any colonies.

In India, where humans are the only known reservoir, mass diagnosis and treatment of all cases of kala-azar achieved a fair degree of control before the appearance and use of residual insecticides enabled control of the vector.

Where the sandfly vectors live in close contact with humans, residual spraying with DDT has destroyed the sandflies and stopped transmission. The incursions of Indian kala-azar and urban cutaneous leishmaniasis in the Middle East were halted in this way. However, with cessation of residual spraying for malaria eradication in these areas sandflies have returned and the transmission of leishmaniasis has resumed, especially in the Middle East. Residual spraying at 6-month intervals is necessary to stop transmission permanently.

Inoculation with living promastigotes of *L. tropica major* to prevent later infection is practiced extensively with great success in the Middle East. A small lesion is produced on a covered area of the body. Evolution, without chemotherapy, that continues until healing occurs confers immunity that is apparently lifelong. Successful vaccination against American cutaneous leishmaniasis and kala-azar has not yet been achieved.

Leishmanin skin testing is valuable for surveillance. Skin testing of a population on an age basis shows the past and present incidence of infection. Testing can also be used to delineate foci of transmission as well as nonimmune populations that might suffer severely from the infection.

Remaining Problems

Leishmaniasis represents a unique immunologic problem because the immune response to *Leishmania* spp. is an example of pure cell-mediated immunity. Humoral antibodies are not involved, and the process of cell-mediated immunity and delayed hypersensitivity can be examined in animal models.

The immunity that develops in leishmaniasis is protective against reinfection with the homologous and some heterologous strains. It is unique in protozoal infections because it is complete and long-lasting and does not depend on a low-grade persisting infection to maintain it. One of the most important problems to be solved is finding strains of *Leishmania* spp. that cause a harmless cutaneous lesion and yet protect against the metastasizing strains of *L. braziliensis* and *L. donovani.* Solving this problem would make vaccination against these forms of leishmaniasis practical. This is a most important endeavor, because control of zoonoses is very difficult in the tropics.

Bibliography

Books

ADLER S: Leishmania, Vol. II. In Dawes B (ed): Advances in Parasitology. New York, Academic Press, 1964. pp. 35–96.

HERTIG M, FAIRCHILD GB, JOHNSON CM: Report of the Work and Operations of the Gorgas Memorial Laboratory, Washington DC, U.S. Government Printing Office, 1954

Journals

CAHILL KM: Leishmaniasis in American personnel. XXI. Infection in American personnel. Am J Trop Med Hyg 13:794–799, 1964

CONVIT J: Leishmaniasis tegumentaria diffusia. Rev Sanidad Asist Soc 1–28, 1958

HEISCH RB: Is there an animal reservoir of kala-azar in Kenya? East Afr Med J 40:359–362, 1963

HOARE CA: Cutaneous leishmaniasis. Trop Dis Bull 41:331–345, 1944

LAINSON R, SHAW JJ: Leishmanias and leishmaniasis of the New World, with particular reference to Brazil. Bull Pan Am Health Org 7:1–19, 1973

MANSON–BAHR PEC: Immunity in kala azar. Trans R Soc Trop Med Hyg 55:550–555, 1961

MANSON–BAHR PEC, SOUTHGATE BA: Recent research on kala azar in East Africa. J Trop Med Hyg 67:79–84, 1964

PAMPIGLIONE S, LA PLACA M, SCHLOCK G: Studies on Mediterranean leishmaniasis. I. An outbreak of visceral leishmaniasis in northern Italy. Trans R Soc Trop Med Hyg 68:349–359, 1974

PAMPIGLIONE S, MANSON–BAHR PEC, LA PLACA M, BORGATTI MA, MUSUMECI S: Studies in Mediterranean leishmaniasis. III. The leishmanin skin test in kala-azar. Trans R Soc Trop Med Hyg 69:60–68, 1975

PHILIP D. MARSDEN

148 Lymphoreticular Filariasis

Bancroft's filariasis is a classic lymphoreticular filariasis, and Malayan filariasis is similar. Recently, evidence has been offered supporting a filarial etiology for pulmonary tropical eosinophilia, implicating the same helminths.

Bancroftian Filariasis

The adult filarial *Wuchereria bancrofti* resides in the lymphatic system and produces recurrent lymphangitis with fibrosis and obstruction. Infective microfilariae are transmitted by several kinds of mosquitoes.

Etiology

The threadlike adult worms are 4 cm to 10 cm long and live for decades. The female worm is viviparous, producing microfilariae 130 μm to 320 μm long, which are found in the peripheral blood at night (nocturnal periodicity—Fig. 148-1). During the day, the microfilariae are in the lungs. At least two circadian rhythms are involved in this pattern: one in the microfilariae and the other a property of the physiologic rhythm of the host. The microfilariae live 3 to 6 months.

Microfilariae cannot cause filariasis if passed on to another human directly in blood by transfusion. However, if ingested by suitable mosquitoes, *Culex* spp., *Aedes* spp., and *Anopheles* spp., the microfilariae develop in the thoracic muscles of the insect and are present in its mouthparts after 2 weeks. They enter the skin of humans through the puncture wound when the mosquito next feeds, and they find their way to the lymphatics, where the males and females meet, mate, and mature. More than a year after infection, microfilariae appear in the peripheral blood.

Epidemiology

Humans are the only definitive host of this common tissue nematode. Periodic bancroftian filariasis is found throughout tropical Africa, North Africa, and on the tropical coastal borders of Asia and Queensland. It is endemic in the West Indies and the northern countries of South America. In the northern Pacific, bancroftian filariasis exhibits nocturnal periodicity. In the Pacific Islands east of longitude 160° (including New Caledonia, Fiji, Samoa, the Ellis and Cook Islands, Society Islands, and the Marquesas), the microfilariae are nonperiodic, being present in the peripheral blood throughout the day. The name *W. bancrofti* var. *pacifica* has been applied to this strain.

Pathogenesis and Pathology

The severity of the lesions probably depends on the load of adult worms, the site of infection, and the susceptibility of the host. Light infections are often asymptomatic, and microfilariae are detected accidentally during an examination of the blood. Maturing adults in the lymphatics are associated with endothelial thickening, fibrous deposition, and infiltration with eosinophils, histiocytes, and lymphocytes. Giant cells occur. Fibrotic and inflammatory changes tend to obstruct the lymphatics, and this process is exacerbated by the death of the worms, which may calcify. There is reactive hyperplasia in the lymph nodes, and small granulomas are seen. An eosinophilic endophlebitis of the small veins is present with evidence of chronic inflammation. Worms may not be present at the site of inflammation. Secretions of the worms, especially after molting, are thought to be responsible for some of these changes. As lymphatic obstruction becomes more extensive, chronic edema develops in the affected areas.

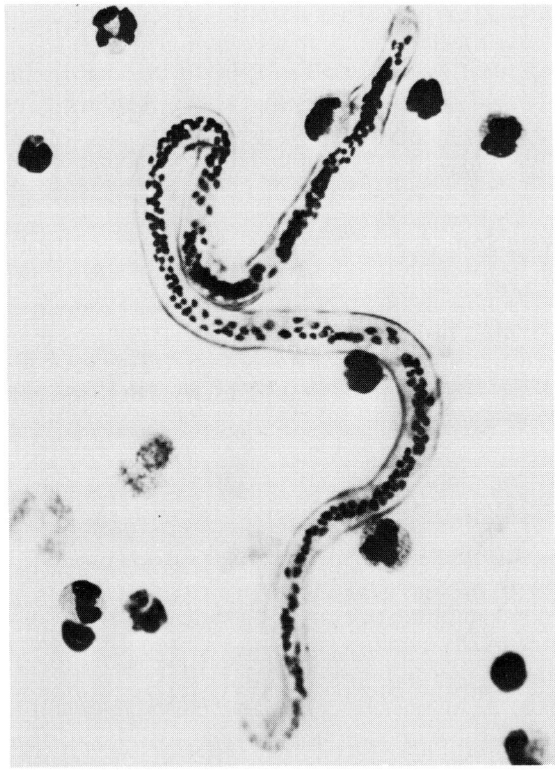

Fig. 148-1. Microfilaria of *Wucheria bancrofti* in thick film of blood. (Courtesy of the Wellcome Museum of Medical Science, London) (Giemsa, original magnification approximately × 750)

Manifestations

Attacks of fever, headache, and lymphadenopathy, sometimes associated with urticarial rashes, are known as filarial fever, and they occur in the acute phase of the disease. Often, however, no history of this early phase can be obtained. Epididymitis may occur as a lone lesion. The lymphatics most severely affected are those of the inguinal region, upper arm, and spermatic cord. Chronic lymphadenopathy is often the only sign of infection. Retrograde lymphangitis may be noted. In a few patients, lymphatic obstruction increases over the years, producing edema in all degrees of severity and affecting especially the lower limbs and scrotum. Initially, the edema is pitting, but as organization of the collagen occurs it becomes nonpitting. Eventually, the giant limbs of elephantiasis are produced in about 1% to 5% of patients who have been lifetime inhabitants of endemic areas. The skin over the affected part is smooth at first, but later it becomes scaly and fissured at points where the fascia is attached to the skin. Hyperkeratosis produces warts and nodules. Varicosities of the lymph nodes in the groin are the result of lymphatic dilation. Lymphedema of the scrotum is associated with the discharge of lymph from scrotal varices. Bacterial and mycotic infections may supervene in any of these lesions, with the formation of chronic discharging sinuses. Chronic inflammatory disease of the testicle and epididymis occurs, with or without hydrocele.

Chyluria may originate in the bladder or kidney, depending on the level at which a lymph varix communicates with the urinary tract. Cystoscopy and intravenous or retrograde pyelography may help to establish the site of communication.

Diagnosis

In the early stages, and when only lymphadenopathy is present, microfilariae are most likely to be found in smears of blood obtained at night; however, if a filtration–concentration technique is used (Chap. 11, Diagnostic Methods for Protozoa and Helminths), blood taken during the day will suffice. Although the motile microfilariae are easily seen in fresh films, staining is necessary for identification. Microfilariae may be lacking in the late stages of the disease. In one study, only 4% of patients with elephantiasis and 30% of patients with hydrocele had microfilariae in their blood. Concentration techniques that enable the detection of microfilariae in chylous urine or hydrocele fluid are available. Eosinophilia is not a constant finding. The filarial complement fixation (CF) test and skin tests, although only group specific, are useful in seeking the cause of lymphedema. Lymphangiography, which reveals the extent of the lymphatic obstruction, is useful preoperatively. The diagnostic excision of an enlarged lymph node to find adult *W. bancrofti* is rarely justified, and it may be harmful because the operation would further prejudice the lymphatic circulation. In endemic areas, surgeons frequently encounter adult filariae when operating on the groin.

The differential diagnosis must take into account other causes of lymphadenopathy (*e.g.*, other infections and neoplasms). Elephantiasis may be associated with congenital defects of the lymphatic drainage or tuberculous inguinal lymphadenitis. Tuberculosis, *Schistosoma haematobium,* and gonorrhea produce epididymitis (Chap. 35, Extra-Pulmonary Tuberculosis, Chap. 81, Schistosomiasis, and Chap. 56, Gonococcal Infection). Relatively few hydroceles are filarial in origin. Lymphatic obstruction owing to many other agents may produce lymphedema and chyluria. Chyluria may even be mimicked by adding milk to the urine after voiding.

Prognosis

An accurate appraisal of the course of untreated filariasis is difficult to make. However, multiple inoculations are almost certainly requisite to production of the disease. The mating of adult filariae may be a chance affair, and the microfilarial larvae produced in the human cannot mature there. The body burden of filariae tolerable to humans and the intensity of reaction mounted by a patient probably depend on many factors. Finally, when clinically significant filariasis develops, devolution into crippling affliction is certainly accelerated by secondary bacterial and fungal infections.

Even though chemotherapy is effective in eliminating *W. bancrofti,* structural changes may not be reversible.

Therapy

All patients with microfilaremia should be treated with diethylcarbamazine (Banocide, Hetrazan). Not only does this agent kill microfilariae, but it is also lethal to a large proportion of adult *W. bancrofti.*

Over a period of 4 days the dose, given PO, is increased from 3 mg/kg body wt to 12 mg/kg body wt/day—a dosage that is maintained for 14 days. Reactions are mild in comparison with onchocerciasis (Chap. 112, Cutaneous Filariasis), but fever, nausea, vomiting, and skin rashes may occur as with any drug. The arsenical Mel W and the antimonial Astiban (sodium antimony-αα-dimercaptosuccinate) kill adult *W. bancrofti,* but both are too toxic for general use.

The management of lymphedema depends on its severity. Patients with mild cases are best treated by elevating the foot of the bed and with elastic stockings. Careful instructions regarding foot care should be given because ascending streptococcal cellulitis in the edematous tissues is common and further prejudices the lymphatic circulation. Some workers believe the streptococci are more important in producing lymphangitis than the worms themselves. Any sepsis involving the feet requires early and vigorous treatment with appropriate antimicrobics. Tinea infections should be eradicated. Treatment with diethylcarbamazine is often given in elephantiasis on the grounds that it may prevent further lymphatic damage, but clinical improvement is seldom observed.

Surgical operations have been devised to remove the edematous subcutaneous tissue from the leg, scrotum, and breast. Success depends on the type of operation and the skill of the surgeon. In scrotal elephantiasis, care must be taken to preserve the testicles. Hydroceles can be treated by injecting sclerosing agents. Chyluria originating in the bladder can be terminated by fulgurating the leaking bladder lymphatics. Renal chyluria is best left alone. In the past, when kidneys were wrapped in cellophane, renal hypertension resulted.

Prevention

Diethylcarbamazine (3 mg/kg body wt taken PO once each month for 12–18 months) has been effective in mass prophylaxis. Residual DDT or dieldrin is effective against many of the mosquito vectors. The systematic destruction of mosquito breeding sites has also been successful.

Malayan Filariasis

A disease similar to bancroftian filariasis is produced by a closely related filarial worm, *Brugia malayi.* The sheathed microfilariae of this species have two distinct caudal nuclei (Fig. 148-2). Transmitted by

Fig. 148-2. Microfilaria of *Brugia malayi* in thick film of blood. (Giemsa, original magnification × 500) (Courtesy of the Wellcome Museum of Medical Science, London)

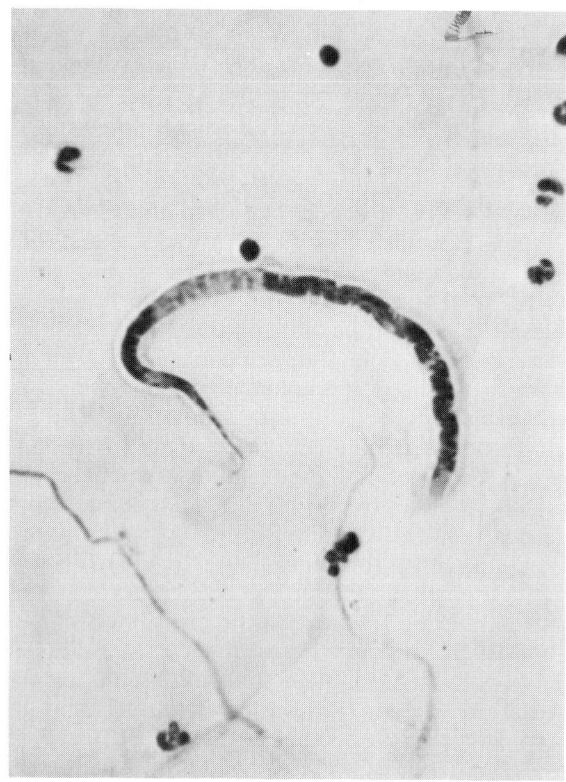

Mansonia spp. and *Anopheles* spp. of mosquitoes, this disease is the only filarial infection of humans in Malaya and Borneo, whereas in India, Ceylon, and tropical China it coexists with infection by *W. bancrofti. Brugia malayi* is responsible for only mild lymphedema in humans, usually located below the knee and associated with enlargement of the popliteal and femoral nodes. In contrast bancroftian filariasis, microfilaremia is quite frequent in children under 5 years of age. Again, there are *B. malayi* variants showing either nocturnal periodicity or a subperiodicity. The subperiodic variant is found in many nonhuman animals (primates, carnivores, rodents) and is a true zoonosis.

Pulmonary Tropical Eosinophilia (Eosinophilic Lung)

Pulmonary tropical eosinophilia is a well-recognized clinical entity common in India and Singapore. Recently, it has been attributed to an occult filarial infection, possibly with *W. bancrofti*. It is characterized by paroxysmal nocturnal asthma and cough, associated with a high eosinophilia, and relieved by diethylcarbamazine. There is a high titer of filarial antibodies in the blood. A similar syndrome has been induced in a volunteer using two *Brugia* species. Moreover, microfilariae have been demonstrated in the lungs of persons with this syndrome. Histologically, small eosinophilic granulomas, often containing portions of microfilariae, are found scattered throughout the lung. It has been shown that microfilariae disappear quickly from the circulation of immune animals. It is possible that the eosinophilic lung results from an alteration of host immunity to a filarial parasite, giving rise to allergic phenomena manifested by persistent hypereosinophilia and pulmonary symptoms.

Bibliography

Journals

GALINDO L, VON LICHTENBERG F, BALDISON C: Bancroftian filariasis in Puerto Rico: Infection pattern and tissue lesions. Am J Trop Med 11:739–748, 1962

LIE KJ: Occult filariasis and its relationship to pulmonary tropical eosinophilia. Am J Trop Med 11:646–652, 1962

NELSON GS: The pathology of filarial infections (abstr). Helminth 35:311–336, 1966

SCHACHER JF, SAHYOUN PF: A chronological study of the histopathology of filarial disease in cats and dogs caused by *Brugia phangi*. Trans R Soc Trop Med Hyg 61:234–243, 1967

TURNER JH: Studies in filariasis in Malaya: The clinical features of filariasis due to *Wuchereria malayi.* Trans R Soc Trop Med Hyg 55:107–134, 1961

Section | *XIX*

Muscle Infections

Indigenous Microbiota of the Skeletal Muscles

(None)

C. GEORGE RAY

Coxsackievirus and Echovirus Infections

149

Nonpolio enteroviruses comprise a major subgroup of small RNA viruses (picornaviruses) which readily infect and are shed from the lower digestive tract. These include the coxsackieviruses, echoviruses, and more recently discovered agents that are simply designated sequentially as enteroviruses, for example, enterovirus 70. Since the first discovery of coxsackieviruses in 1948 from patients in the village of Coxsackie, New York, the number of serotypes has grown to a total of at least 67, and more are likely to be found in the future.

Initially, it was believed that these agents were primarily causes of mild, acute aseptic meningitis syndromes, pleurodynia, exanthems, pericarditis, nonspecific febrile illness, and occasional fulminant encephalomyocarditis of the newborn. However, as more has been learned, it is apparent that the spectrum of disease is much broader and can lead to permanent sequelae, and that some infections may trigger chronic, active disease processes. This chapter deals primarily with the infections involving sites other than the central nervous system, because coxsackieviruses and echoviruses are also discussed in Chapter 118, Viral Meningitis.

Etiology

The picornaviruses as a group are extremely small (17 nm–28 nm in diameter), single-stranded RNA viruses of icosahedral symmetry. The enterovirus subgroup is resistant to ether, acid pH (4.0), and bile and displays cationic stability. In the presence of $MgSO_4$, the viruses become more resistant to thermal inactivation. They can survive for prolonged periods in sewage and even in chlorinated water if sufficient organic debris is present. Though some of the enteroviral serotypes share complement-fixing (CF) antigens, there are no significant serologic relationships between the classes listed in Table 149-1. Definitive identification of isolates usually requires neutralization tests, and serodiagnosis is also primarily based on determination of serum neutralizing antibodies.

The majority of these agents can be isolated in primate (human or simian) cell cultures, with the appearance of characteristic cytopathic effects. However, some strains, particularly several serotypes of Coxsackie A, grow poorly in cell cultures, and inoculation of newborn mice may be necessary for the detection of virus. The pathogenic effects of intracerebral inoculation of mice less than 24 hours old with observation for 2 to 12 days is in fact one basis for classifying Coxsackie A and B viruses. Coxsackie A viruses typically cause a widespread, inflammatory, necrotic effect on skeletal muscle, leading to flaccid paralysis and death, whereas Coxsackie B viruses cause encephalitis resulting in spasticity and occasionally convulsions. Other organs are variably affected, and histopathologic examination is sometimes helpful in distinguishing A from B. Echoviruses and polioviruses rarely have an adverse effect on mice, unless special adaptation procedures are first

Table 149-1. *Enteroviruses That Infect Humans*

Class	Number of Serotypes
Poliovirus	3
Coxsackievirus	
Group A	23*
Group B	6
Echovirus	31
Enterovirus	Types 68–71†

*Includes several subtypes; Coxsackievirus A_{23} is the same as echovirus 9.

†The classification of the more recently discovered enteroviruses is based on overlapping biologic characteristics. These enteroviruses are identified numerically. Also, echovirus 10 has been reclassified as reovirus 1; echovirus 28 is now rhinovirus 1A.

employed. The higher-numbered enteroviruses (types 68–71) have overlapping, variable growth and host characteristics, and have been classified separately.

Epidemiology

Frequency

The enteroviruses are distributed worldwide, and asymptomatic infection is common. Estimates of symptomatic-to-asymptomatic ratios vary from approximately 2% to 100%, depending upon the serotypes or strains involved and the ages of the patients. Secondary infections in households are common (40%–70%), depending upon factors such as family size, crowding, and sanitary conditions. The ubiquity of these agents is further demonstrated by data from serosurveys that have shown neutralizing antibody prevalences for one or more serotypes of Coxsackie B viruses in as many as 60% of adults, and similar or higher rates for selected serotypes of echoviruses.

Quite unpredictably, one or more serotypes emerge as dominant epidemic strains, then wane, only to reappear in epidemic fashion years later. For example, echovirus 16 was a major cause of outbreaks in the eastern United States in 1951 and did not appear again in high frequency in the same area until 1974. Coxsackie B_1 was common in 1963; echovirus 9 in 1962, 1965, 1968, and 1969; and echovirus 30 in 1968 and 1969.

Host Range

Humans are the only known natural host for the coxsackieviruses and echoviruses. There are other enteroviruses of nonhuman animals, such as the enteric cytopathic monkey orphan viruses (ecmoviruses) of monkeys and enteric cytopathic bovine orphan viruses (ecboviruses) of cattle, but these have a host range that is limited and does not appear to extend to humans. Conversely, viruses thought to be identical or related to the enteroviruses of humans have been isolated from dogs (coxsackieviruses B_1, B_3, and B_5, echoviruses 2, 6, and 19) and cats (echoviruses 16 and 19). Whether these agents cause disease in these animals is debatable, and there is no evidence of spread from animals to humans.

Factors in Transmission

A seasonal predilection is common for all enteroviruses, with epidemics most commonly observed during the summer and fall months. In subtropical and tropical climates, high rates of transmission sometimes extend further into the winter months. However, some serotypes, particularly coxsackie B viruses, appear sporadically throughout the year.

Direct or indirect fecal–oral transmission is considered the most common mode of spread. After infection, the virus persists in the oropharynx for 1 to 4 weeks, and can be shed in the feces for periods varying from 1 to 18 weeks. Thus, sewage-contaminated water, foods contaminated with feces, or insect carriers may occasionally be the source of infection. However, spread is usually direct, from person to person. Accordingly, the rates of infection are high among young children (because of poor hygiene) and in crowded households. Approximately two-thirds of all isolates are from children 9 years of age and younger.

The incubation periods may vary from 2 to 10 days, and illness is often seen concurrently in more than one family member. The clinical features vary within the household; for example, an infant may have a fever and exanthem, whereas an older child or parent may have an aseptic meningitis.

Pathogenesis and Pathology

The pathogenesis of enteroviral infections is assumed to be similar for all classes of enteroviruses, although relatively little investigative effort has been devoted to studying the sequence of events with the echoviruses. Following primary replication in the epithelial cells and paraepithelial lymphoid tissues in the gastrointestinal or upper respiratory tracts, viremic spread to other sites can occur. Potential target organs include the central nervous system, heart, vascular endothelium, liver, pancreas, lungs, gonads, skeletal muscles, synovium, skin and mucous membranes. The initial tissue damage is thought to result from the lytic cycle of virus replication; secondary spread to other sites may also ensue. Viremia is usually undetectable by the time symptoms appear, and the termination of virus replication appears to correlate with the appearance of neutralizing antibody, monocytes, and interferon. The early IgM antibody response wanes 4 to 6 weeks after onset as IgG antibodies rise in titer. The role of antibodies in termination of infection has been demonstrated in mouse models of coxsackie B virus infections and is supported by the observation of persistent echovirus and poliovirus replication in patients with antibody-deficiency diseases.

Although initial acute tissue damage may result from the lytic effects of virus on the cell, the chronic and secondary sequelae may be immunologically mediated. As with any infectious process, the disease and pathology will be determined by both the agent and the host response. Disseminated disease of the newborn, aseptic meningitis, encephalitis, and acute respiratory illnesses are thought to represent primary lytic infections and can usually be identified by employing routine methods of virus isolation and determination of changes in the titers of specific antibody.

However, other syndromes, such as nephritis, myositis, and, in adults, myopericarditis, have been associated with enteroviruses primarily by serologic and epidemiologic evidence. In many of these cases, viral isolation is the exception rather than the rule. The pathogenesis of these infections is not clear; however, it is noteworthy that the acute infectious phase in these disorders may be mild or subclinical and has often subsided by the time clinical illness becomes manifest. That is, the illness most likely represents an immunologic response by the host to tissue injury by the virus, or to viral or virus-induced antigens that persist in the affected tissues.

Experiments with coxsackie B viruses in mouse models tend to support this hypothesis. In experimental myocarditis, mononuclear inflammatory cells (monocytes) seemed to play a greater role than antibody does in terminating the infection, and the inflammation that persisted after disappearance of detectable virus or viral antigen appeared to be mediated by cytotoxic T-lymphocytes.

Reinfection by the same serotype has been reported, and is thought to result in subclinical or mild illness. There is no evidence that such repeated infections with identical serotypes or other serotypes that share similar antigens result in severe disease in a fashion similar to that postulated for the dengue shock syndrome (Chap. 89, Dengue); however, this possibility has not been explored.

Manifestations

Spectrum of Clinical Illness

Inapparent infection with enteroviruses is common, but varies with the infecting strain and the host involved. The range of manifestations of illness varies from mild to lethal and from acute to chronic. The major enterovirus-associated syndromes and the serotypes that are commonly involved with each syndrome are listed in Table 149-2. There is considerable overlap, and the one generalization that can be made is that the coxsackie B group appears to have the greatest latitude with regard to tissue tropism.

COXSACKIEVIRUSES

Herpangina Group A coxsackieviruses are the most common causes of herpangina. The highest incidence is among children 1 to 7 years old, but infection has also been described in neonates and older adults. There is usually an abrupt onset of fever associated with a sore throat, dysphagia, and malaise. One-quarter of the patients may have vomiting and abdominal pain. Early in the illness, gray-white vesicles, measuring 1 mm to 4 mm in diameter, appear over the posterior portion of the palate, uvula, tonsillar pillars, and, occasionally, on the oropharynx. These vesicles are discrete, surrounded by eythema, and usually fewer than twenty in number (Fig. 149-1). The vesicles usually rupture, leaving punched-out ulcers that may enlarge slightly, and new vesicles may appear. There may also be mild cervical adenopathy, headache, myalgia, arthralgia, and, rarely, parotitis or aseptic meningitis. Similar vesicles may sometimes appear on the vaginal mucosa. Coryza and other respiratory symptoms are lacking and clinical

Table 149-2. *Clinical Syndromes and Associated Enterovirus Serotypes**

Syndrome	Coxsackievirus GROUP A	Coxsackievirus GROUP B	Echovirus and Enterovirus (E)
Aseptic meningitis and encephalitis	2,4,7,9,*10	1,2,*3,*4,*5*	4,*6,*9,*11,*16,*30;* E70,E71
Muscle weakness and paralysis	7,*9*	2,3,4,5	2,4,6,9,11,30; E71
Cerebellar ataxia	2,4,9*	3,4	4,*6,*9*
Exanthems and enanthems	4,*5,*6,*9,*10,*16*	2,3,4,5	2,*4,*5,*6,*9,*11,*16,*18,*25*
Pericarditis and myocarditis	4,16	2,*3,*4,*5*	1,6,8,9,19
Epidemic myalgia and orchitis	9	1,2,*3,*4,*5*	1,6,9
Respiratory tract disease	9,16,21,*24	1,3,4,5	4,*9,*11,*20,25
Conjunctivitis	24*	1,5	7;*E70*
General disease in infants	—	1,2,*3,*4,*5*	3,6,9,11,14,17,19

*Serotypes most commonly associated with the syndrome.

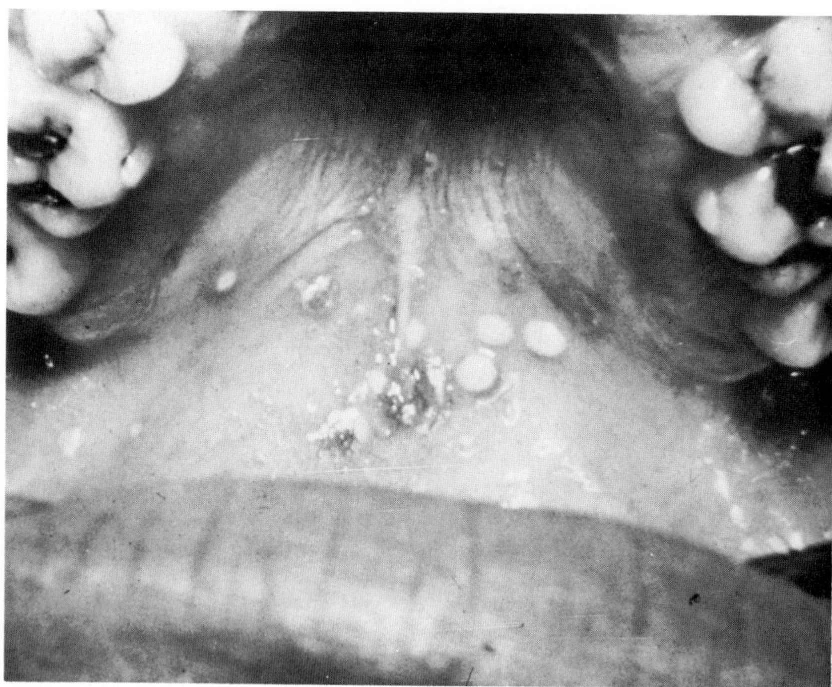

Fig. 149-1. Herpangina. (Smith DW (ed): Introduction to Clinical Pediatrics. Philadelphia. WB Saunders, 1977)

laboratory studies are usually normal. The fever lasts 1 to 4 days, local and systemic symptoms begin to improve in 4 to 5 days, and recovery is usually complete within a week of onset.

The manifestations of primary herpetic gingivostomatitis are similar to those of herpangina but differ in the greater number of lesions and the development of confluent ulcers over the gingiva, buccal mucosa, and tongue. Aphthous stomatitis, Koplik's spots in measles, streptococcal pharyngitis, Vincent's angina, diphtheria, infectious mononucleosis, and pharyngeal tularemia cause similar lesions, but are readily distinguished on other bases.

Lymphonodular pharyngitis Coxsackievirus A_{10} has been associated with a clinical syndrome that resembles herpangina. The characteristic lesions are raised, discrete, whitish to yellowish nodules surrounded by a zone of erythema 3 mm to 6 mm in diameter. The soft palate, tonsillar pillars, and pharynx are most often involved. Occasionally, similar lesions appear on the conjunctiva. Fever, headache, and myalgia are often present. The lesions usually appear as a single crop and do not ulcerate, and the illness resolves in 4 to 14 days without complications.

Hand-Foot-and-Mouth-Disease. Although hand-foot-and-mouth disease is one of the more common and unique syndromes associated with coxsackievirus A_{16}, other enteroviral causes include coxsackieviruses A_5, A_7, A_9, A_{10}, B_2 and B_5. In outbreaks, the highest attack rates are among children under 4 years of age, but adults are also frequently affected. The disease is usually mild and the onset is associated with a sore throat with or without a low-grade fever. Scattered vesicular lesions occur randomly on the oral structures, the pharynx, and the lips; these ulcerate readily, leaving shallow lesions with red aerolae. About 85% of patients also develop sparse grayish vesicles (3 mm–5 mm in diameter, surrounded by erythematous areolae) on the dorsum of the fingers, particularly in periungual areas, and on the margins of the heels. Occasionally, palmar, plantar, and groin lesions may appear, particularly in young children (Fig. 149-2). Rarely, the lesions take the form of a diffuse vesicular eruption and a maculopapular erythematous rash. The illness may last 4 to 8 days and is generally mild, but it can cause concern when the lesions appear to be pustular or hemorrhagic. Rarely, aseptic meningitis, paralytic disease, and fatal myocarditis with coagulopathy and pneumonia have been reported. The mouth lesions alone are not clinically diagnostic because herpes simplex (Chap. 91, Infec-

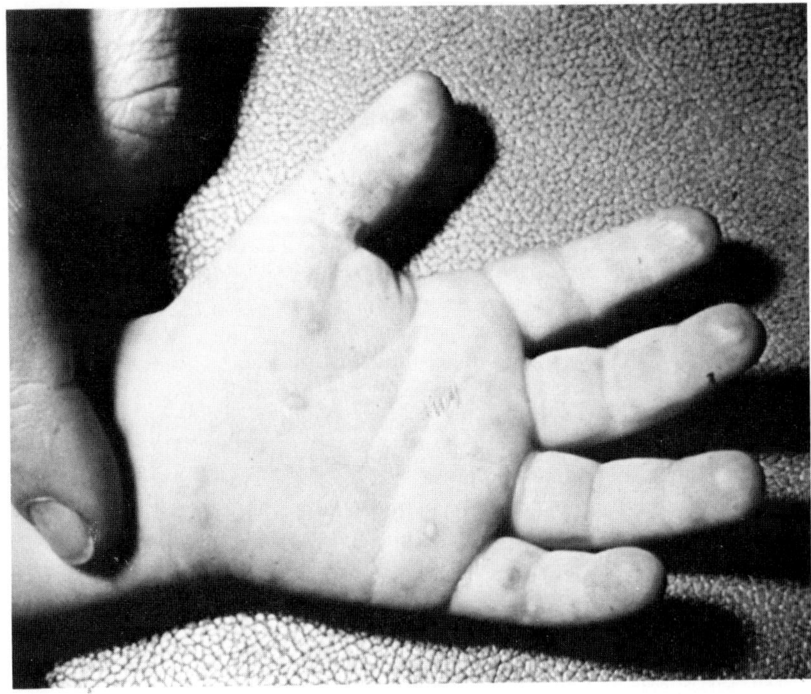

Fig. 149-2. Hand lesions in hand-foot-and-mouth disease.

tions Caused by Herpes Simplex Viruses), erythema multiforme, and rarely, herpangina may have a similar appearance. In addition, the peripheral lesions of gonococcemia (Chap. 56, Gonococcal Infections) may be confused with hand-foot-and-mouth disease.

Rhinopharyngitis. Though most common colds are caused by rhinoviruses, coronaviruses, adenoviruses, and paramyxoviruses (Chap. 21, The Common Cold), a number of coxsackieviruses and echoviruses have been implicated. One of the major causes of common cold syndromes in military recruits has been Coxsackievirus A_{21} (originally known as Coe virus). This and other enteroviruses have been associated with localized outbreaks, particularly in the military and among groups of young children.

Febrile Illness with Rash. Illnesses in infants and young children characterized by fever, and various rashes have been associated with at least 7 coxsackievirus A, 4 coxsackievirus B, and 17 echovirus serotypes. The clinical manifestations do not enable distinction as to which serotype is involved. Most commonly, a macular or maculopapular rash begins on the face and neck and descends to involve the trunk. As with most viral maculopapular eruptions, palmar and plantar involvement is usually minimal or lacking. Occasionally specific testing is required, particularly to exclude causes of rashes identical in appearance, for example, rubella (Chap. 7, Rubella), scarlet fever (Chap. 24, Streptococcal Diseases), adenoviruses (Chap. 30, Nonbacterial Pneumonias), infectious mononucleosis (Chap. 137, Infectious Mononucleosis), erythema infectiosum (Chap. 88, Other Exanthems), roseola infantum (Chap. 88, Other Exanthems), and drug eruptions.

Other, less common manifestations include vesicular or petechial rashes. Coxsackieviruses A_9, A_{16}, B_3, and B_4 have rarely caused a varicellalike eruption, which is differentiated from varicella by the tendency for lesions to occur in a single crop.

Pleurodynia (Epidemic Myalgia, Bornholm Disease, Devil's Grip) Various members of the group B coxsackieviruses (B_6 excepted) are the usual causes of pleurodynia; however, the disease may be caused by some group A coxsackieviruses as well as some echoviruses. Pleurodynia usually occurs sporadically, but epidemics have been reported. The incidene is highest in the summer and autumn, particularly among children and young adults. There is no sex predominance.

The onset is abrupt in about three-fourths of patients. However, about one-fourth have prodromal symptoms of headache, malaise, anorexia, and vague myalgia for 1 to 10 days. The major symptom is severe paroxysmal pain referred to the lower ribs or the sternum. Deep breathing, coughing, or other movement accentuate the pain, providing the syndrome with its misleading pseudonym; the pleura is not always involved. The pain is described as stabbing, knifelike, smothering, or catching; it may radiate to the shoulders, neck, or scapula, and is characteristically lacking between paroxysms. Abdominal pain occurs concomitantly in about one-half of the patients, but it may occur alone. Associated symptoms include fever, headache, cough, anorexia, nausea, vomiting, and diarrhea. Fever is usually about 38°C (100.4°F), but may vary from 37°C to 40°C (98.6°F to 104°F). The mean duration of the illness is 3½ days, varying from 1 to 14 days. A diphasic febrile course with recrudescence occurs in half the patients. The headache is typically frontal and moderately severe. The cough is usually nonproductive. If gastrointestinal symptoms occur, they come on during the prodrome or at the onset and are generally of short duration.

The pulse rate is usually proportional to the temperature. Muscle tenderness is ordinarily not prominent, but some patients experience marked cutaneous hyperesthesia over the affected areas. A pleural friction rub may be heard in 25% of patients. There may be splinting and tenderness on abdominal examination, more commonly in the upper abdominal and right periumbilical areas.

The laboratory findings, including chest roentgenography, are typically normal. Occasionally, pleural effusions occur, and coxsackievirus group B has been isolated from the pleural fluid.

Pleurodynia may occur concomitantly with aseptic meningitis (Chap. 118, Viral Meningitis). Pericarditis (Chap. 132, Pericarditis) with a typical pericardial friction rub and confirmatory electrocardiographic findings has been reported. In the rare patient with jaundice, liver biopsy may reveal cellular infiltration in the portal triads and cloudy swelling of the centrizonal liver parenchymal cells. Orchitis with or without epididymitis is a late complication, developing during the second week but occurring as late as the fourth week in 3% to 5% of males. In virtually all patients, the orchitis usually subsides within 2 to 6 days, leaving no sequelae, although a few cases of testicular atrophy have been ascribed to epididymoorchitis caused by coxsackievirus B_5.

The several manifestations of pleurodynia may lead to confusion with bacterial or mycoplasmal pneumonia (Chap. 31, Bacterial Pneumonias, and Chap. 30, Nonbacterial Pneumonias), idiopathic pleural effusion, pulmonary emboli with infarction, rib fractures, myocardial infarction, mediastinal emphysema, costochondritis (Tietze's syndrome), acute intraabdominal surgical conditions such as appendicitis, mesenteric lymphadenitis, perihepatitis (Fitz-Hugh–Curtis syndrome), and preeruptive herpes zoster (Chap. 93, Varicella and Herpes Zoster).

Gastroenteritis. Diarrhea, as well as vomiting, may occur as a minor feature of many enterovirus syndromes, especially in very young patients. However, neither coxsackieviruses or echoviruses have been epidemiologically implicated as important primary causes of acute gastroenteritis. The majority of the cases of viral gastrointestinal diseases are caused by rotaviruses, parvoviruses, certain adenoviruses, and possibly astroviruses, caliciviruses, and coronaviruses. Isolation of an enterovirus from the feces must be interpreted with caution, because it may represent asymptomatic carriage in a patient made ill by a noncultivable agent.

Coxsackie B viruses have been associated with acute abdominal pain and mesenteric adenitis syndromes, which can mimic acute appendicitis.

General Disease of the Newborn. Group B, coxsackieviruses and several echoviruses have been associated with a severe, sepsislike illness in the newborn, which is usually perinatally acquired. Frequently, there is a maternal history of an undifferentiated febrile illness within 2 weeks before onset of disease in the infant.

Typically, the illness begins suddenly within the first 2 weeks of life with anorexia, lethargy, and irritability. This may be followed by cough, vomiting, dyspnea, and cyanosis. The infant may improve for several days before signs of illness recur, or there may be continual worsening with seizures, cardiac failure, hepatic enlargement, jaundice, disseminated intravascular coagulation (DIC), circulatory collapse, and finally death. However, the disease is not uniformly fatal, and recovery may proceed as rapidly as illness developed.

The autopsy findings include evidence of encephalitis, hepatitis, myocarditis, and occasionally adrenal and renal necrosis. Virus can usually be isolated readily from the feces and throat swabs, as well as from postmortem tissues.

Central Nervous System Syndromes. Aseptic meningitis is the most common central nervous system manifestation of coxsackievirus and echovirus infections (Chap. 118, Viral Meningitis). In the past, these infections were considered to be brief, self-limited, and benign. However, it is now known that prolonged or recrudescent illness can occur for several weeks after the initial acute phase. In addition, permanent neurologic sequelae may result, particularly among infants who were less than 12 months of age when they became ill. Other central nervous system syndromes include encephalitis, polyneuritis, transverse myelitis, acute cerebellar ataxia, and mild paralytic disease resembling poliomyelitis. Coxsackievirus A_7 is considered an important cause of poliomyelitislike disease in outbreaks in Russia and Scotland. More recently, enterovirus 71 has also been implicated as a cause of outbreaks of aseptic meningitis—a 1975 Bulgarian epidemic was also associated with some severe cases of bulbar or spinal poliomyelitis-like disease.

Myocarditis and Pericarditis. Coxsackieviruses B_{2-5} are the most common enteroviruses associated with myopericarditis syndromes. These were first recognized as primary, lytic infections in newborn infants, and the lesions can be reproduced by inoculating these viruses into newborn mice. More recently, serologic studies have implicated these viruses in as many as 44% of older children and adults with sporadic myopericarditis. Interestingly, the virus is found by culture (throat, feces, tissue, or body liquids) in less than 5% of these cases, but the diagnosis is suggested by fourfold or greater rises in titer of antibody in comparison of acute and convalescent serums obtained 2 to 4 weeks apart. These observations are consistent with an immunologically mediated pathogenesis, a pathogenesis supported by animal studies. Cases may occur in any month of the year; in one study, the median age was 51 years, and 60% of the patients were men.

There is often a history of a preceding febrile or respiratory illness within 2 weeks of the onset of fever and precordial pain. Other findings may include a pericardial friction rub, pleural effusion, and serosanguineous pericardial effusions with cardiac tamponade; if myocarditis is present, arrhythmias and cardiac decompensation may also develop. Most patients have electrocardiographic abnormalities that include ST-T wave abnormalities. Laboratory tests may reveal a leukocytosis and elevations of the serum glutamic-oxaloacetic transaminase (SGOT).

Recovery is generally complete within 2 to 6 weeks. However, sudden death may result from ventricular arrhythmias, and congestive failure resulting from myocardial insufficiency or tamponade are concerns that may require aggressive therapy in the acute phase of illness. Such measures include pericardiocentesis, digitalis, and diuretics; in progressive, refractory cases, the use of glucosteroids may also be beneficial. Strict bed rest is recommended for patients during the acute phase of illness.

Occasionally, there have been patients with protracted illness, but the incidence of chronic or permanent heart damage is not known. Recurrent attacks have also been reported and appear to bode a poor prognosis.

Pneumonia. Coxsackievirus A_{21} occasionally produces a relatively mild pneumonitis, as well as the common cold syndrome. Less commonly, coxsackieviruses B_1, B_4, B_5 and echoviruses 19 and 20 have been associated with pneumonia in infants and children. The clinical manifestations of pneumonia caused by these agents include fever, hyperpnea, and cyanosis. The laboratory findings usually include a normal leukocyte count, although extreme leukocytosis is rarely encountered. Chest roentgenography may reveal perihilar infiltrates. Fatalities have occurred in infants and young children. Histopathologic study of the lungs has revealed thickening and infiltration of the alveolar septa, but no necrosis or giant cells. In adults, bronchopneumonia has been associated with coxsackievirus B_3 and echovirus 9. Echovirus 11 has been associated with subglottic croup.

Hepatitis. In addition to the occurrence of hepatitis as one aspect of general disease in the newborn, coxsackieviruses B_2, B_3, B_5, and A_9 have been associated with hepatitis in older children. In adults, coxsackieviruses B_3 and B_5 have been associated with hepatitis on rare occasions.

Acute Hemorrhagic Conjunctivitis. During the period 1969–1971, acute hemorrhagic conjunctivitis was pandemic in Asia and Africa. More than 60,000 cases occurred in Singapore alone in September and October 1970. An antigenic variant of coxsackievirus A_{24}, now classified as enterovirus 70 (prototype strain J670/71) was shown to be the responsible agent.

After an incubation period of about 24 hours, there was rapid onset of swelling of the eyelids with congestion, lacrimation, and pain in the eyes. A minority of patients developed characteristic subconjunctival hemorrhages—varying from petechiae to large blotches. Epithelial keratitis was common, but it was transient and was seldom followed by subepithelial opacities. Preauricular adenopathy was frequent. Occasionally, there was a mucopurulent discharge from the eyes. The illness was generally nonsystemic, although transient lumbar radiculomyelopathy was encountered Bombay, occurring 2 to 4 weeks after onset of the conjunctivitis; a poliomyelitislike illness was described in some cases in Thailand. Recovery was usually complete within 1 to 2 weeks of onset.

Other enteroviruses, including strains more closely related to coxsackievirus A_{24} and echovirus 7, have also been known to cause outbreaks of acute conjunctivitis or keratoconjunctivitis, usually without hemorrhagic manifestations.

Pancreatic Disease and Diabetes Mellitus. Given the wide range of organ tropism of coxsackieviruses, and the observation that lesions of pancreatic acini or islet cells can be produced by some strains in infected mice, it is not surprising that pancreatic disease might occur in humans. Acute pancreatitis associated with these viruses has been reported only rarely; however, there remains the intriguing possibility that group B coxsackieviruses may play a role in inducing insulin-dependent diabetes mellitus in genetically predisposed humans. This was first suggested by several seroepidemiologic studies, the significance of which has been debated. Recently, a type B_4 coxsackievirus was isolated from the pancreas of a 10-year-old boy with acute-onset diabetes mellitus. He developed a significant antibody response to the isolate, inflammation of the pancreatic islets was demonstrated, and the viral isolate was shown to be diabetogenic in susceptible mice.

Polymyositis/Dermatomyositis and Polyarthritis. As in insulin-dependent diabetes, it is primarily by serologic testing that coxsackievirus infections have been implicated in some cases of dermatomyositis, polymyositis, and acute rheumatoid arthritis syndromes. Picornaviruslike particles were seen in muscle biopsies of two patients, and coxsackievirus A_9 was isolated from the diaphragm of one patient with chronic, progressive polymyositis. Obviously, further studies will be necessary to define what role, if any, these viruses may have in the rheumatoid syndromes.

At present, it is clear that a variety of enteroviruses can cause acute, self-limited illnesses that include arthralgias, muscle weakness, and occasionally, overt arthritis. Experimentally, diffuse or localized polymyositis can also be produced in certain strains of mice with some group B coxsackievirus. The mouse model has also demonstrated that permanent sequelae may result from such infections.

Possible Associations. Coxsackieviruses, particularly the group B viruses, have been associated with a hemolytic–uremic syndrome, as well as acute oliguric renal failure and glomerulonephritis not due to group A β-hemolytic streptococcal infections. The evidence for infection was a significant rise in neutralizing antibody titer between acute and convalescent serums. Isolation or demonstration of coxsackieviruses in the tissues of these patients was rarely accomplished. The pathogenetic mechanisms by which coxsackieviruses may participate in these syndromes are unknown.

Coxsackieviruses have also been suggested as possible causes of congenital malformations, particularly involving the heart. However, further studies are necessary.

ECHOVIRUSES

For the most part, illnesses caused by echoviruses are similar to those described for the coxsackieviruses (Table 149-2). However, there have been several clinical manifestations that appear to be more frequently associated with echoviruses.

Boston Exanthem. Initially described during an epidemic of echovirus 16 infection in Boston in 1951, this disease reappeared in 1974. Both children and adults were affected. The illness in children was characterized by fever (38.3°C–38.9°C or 101°F–102°F), mild sore throat, headache, and gastrointestinal symptoms. Oral ulcers quite similar to those seen with herpangina occurred in about one-fourth of the children, along with minimal cervical lymphadenopathy. Defervescence occurred in 1 to 2 days. During or shortly after defervescence, a rash consisting of small, pink, maculopapular lesions appeared on the face and upper thorax, and occasionally became general—extending to involve the palms and soles. The rash lasted 1 to 5 days and subsided without complications.

In adults, the illness was more striking, with high fever, prostration, and signs of aseptic meningitis, but the rash was more fleeting or entirely lacking. The disease resembles exanthem subitum (roseola infantum—Chap. 88, Other Exanthems) with the occurrence of fever followed by defervescence, then the appearance of rash. However, unlike exanthem subitum, which occurs in young infants, the Boston exanthem involved children of all ages and even adults. The Boston exanthem differs clinically from rubella in the timing of the rash and in the lack of postauricular lymphadenopathy; however, it may be necessary to rule out rubella by serologic testing, because rubella may mimic many other exanthems (Chap. 87, Rubella).

Infection With Echovirus 9. Infection with echovirus 9 has occurred in epidemics and has been associated with a high incidence of aseptic meningitis. Multiple cases in a family unit occur in 25% to 35% of the families involved. In one-third of the patients, there is an initial phase with fever, anorexia, vomiting, and mild sore throat, which is followed by a short period without symptoms. This brief respite is followed by the abrupt onset of the major phase of illness. Fever occurs in all patients, and approximately one-third of patients have an associated rash that may occur concomitant with, or independent of, aseptic meningitis. Exanthems occur more frequently in children, especially those under 3 years of age. Characteristically, the rash begins on the malar prominences and neck, and descends rapidly within 6 to 8 hours to involve the thorax, abdomen, and extremities; rarely, it involves the palms and soles. Occasionally, an enanthem occurs that resembles Koplik's spots. The rash characteristically fades in 3 to 5 days. Petechial lesions, with or without maculopapular lesions, may occur, raising the possibility of meningococcemia (Chap. 119, Acute Bacterial Meningitis). Other diseases that must be considered include early roseola (Chap. 88, Other Exanthems), rubella (Chap. 87, Rubella), erythema infectiosum (Chap. 88, Other Exanthems), and infectious mononucleosis (Chap. 137, Infectious Mononucleosis).

Acute Hemangiomalike Lesions. In the course of surveillance of exanthematous disease, four children were observed who developed acute, transitory spider hemangioma-like lesions in association with infections caused by echovirus 25 and 32.

Infections in Immunodeficient Patients. Several patients, all with primary immunoglobulin deficiency states, have been observed to have chronic, progressive encephalitic disease, sometimes associated with dermatomyositis and hepatitis, which usually terminated fatally 8 to 15 months after onset. Echoviruses 5, 9, 11, 24, and 25 have been associated with these illnesses through repeated isolation from the cerebrospinal fluid and frequent isolation from the blood, bone marrow, and other organs. Pooled gamma globulin therapy did not alter the clinical course, whereas a few patients who were treated with repeated infusions of human plasma containing high titers of neutralizing antibody against the infecting echovirus serotype showed some clinical improvement before dying.

Miscellaneous Other Manifestations. Although reports of lower respiratory tract disease associated with enterovirus infections are uncommon, pneumonitis associated with echoviruses 9, 19, and 20 has been described, particularly in infants and children. In older children and adults, echoviruses 4 and 9 have been associated with acute hepatitis.

Diagnosis

The season of the year, the occurrence of other cases in the family or community, and the clinical manifestations are often sufficiently typical to enable diagnosis of many enteroviral diseases. Diagnoses are most readily confirmed by isolation of the responsible enterovirus from throat swabs, feces or rectal swabs, body liquids, and occasionally tissues. Viremia is usually undetectable by the time symptoms appear, and blood cultures are generally nonproductive. When there is central nervous system involvement, acute-phase cerebrospinal fluid cultures may be positive in 10% to 85% of cases, depending upon the stage of illness and the viral strain involved. When the virus is isolated directly from affected tissues or body liquids aspirated from enclosed spaces (*e.g.,* pleural, joint, pericardial, or cerebrospinal fluids), this usually confirms the diagnosis. The isolation of an enterovirus from the throat is highly suggestive of an etiologic association because the virus is usually detectable at this site for only 2 days to 4 weeks after infection. In contrast, the isolation of virus from fecal specimens only must be interpreted more cautiously because asymptomatic shedding from the bowel may persist for as long as 4 months. Clinical and epidemiologic judgment is required to decide on the significance of such findings.

The clinical diagnosis may also be supported by a fourfold or greater rise in titer of neutralizing antibody, comparing acute and convalescent serums. However, this is an expensive and cumbersome process because of the methods required and the number of serotypes involved. Serodiagnosis is generally reserved for special situations, for example, isolation of a virus solely from a peripheral source such as the feces, or suspicion of an illness such as myopericarditis, for which it is known that the yield on routine culture is low and there are a limited number of serotypes that might be expected to be involved. Quantitative interpretations of antibody titers on single serum samples are rarely helpful, because of the wide range of titers to different serotypes that can be found in healthy persons.

Prognosis

Overall, the prognosis in disease caused by coxsackieviruses, echoviruses, and enteroviruses is excellent. Protracted illness, death, or complications and sequelae are rare but may occur in central nervous system syndromes, myocarditis/pericarditis, pneumonitis, pancreatitis, and immunodeficiency disorders.

Therapy

None of the currently available antiviral agents have been shown to be effective in treatment of cosxackievirus or echovirus infections. Likewise, immune serum globulins, even those with high enteroviral antibody titers, have no therapeutic effect and are of questionable value in prophylaxis. Treatment is entirely symptomatic and supportive. Inasmuch as glucosteroids increase the quantity of virus and the extent of ensuing damage in experimental animals, their use is generally contraindicated. However, glucosteroids are sometimes employed in the management of established, severe pericarditis or myocarditis (Chap. 132, Pericarditis, and Chap. 133, Myocarditis).

Prevention

Although the proper disposal of feces and the practice of personal hygiene are recommended, the usual quarantine or isolation measures are relatively ineffective in controlling the spread of enteroviruses within family units or population groups. With at least 67 specific antigenic types known, the prospects for vaccine development appear to be remote.

Remaining Problems

With the decreasing prevalence of polioviruses in the population, it is possible that infections caused by the other enteroviruses may be increasing in number and significance. Awareness of their importance in disease in humans has increased as it has become clear that serious sequelae can result from infection and that the enteroviruses may cause a broad spectrum of acute, and possibly chronic, illnesses. Much remains to be learned about the host–virus interactions that determine disease expression, outcome, and immunity. From such studies, it may be possible to develop immunologic methods of prevention and treatment and to produce effective antiviral agents.

Bibliography

Book

WENNER HA, RAY CG: Diseases associated with coxsackieviruses and echoviruses. In Kelley VC (ed): Practice of Pediatrics, Vol. IV, Chap. 10. Philadelphia, Harper & Row, 1979

Journals

AUSTIN TW, RAY CG: Coxsackie virus group B infections and the hemolytic–uremic syndrome. J Inf Dis 127:698–701, 1973

BODENSTEINER JB, MORRIS HH, HOWELL JT, SCHOCHET SS: Chronic ECHO type 5 virus meningoencephalitis in X-linked hypogamma-globulinemia: Treatment with immune plasma. Neurology 29:815–819, 1979

BROWN GC, KARVNAS RS: Relationship of congenital anomalies and maternal infection with selected enteroviruses. Am J Epidemiol 95:207–217, 1972

CHERRY JD, BOBINSKI JE, HORVATH FL, COMERCI GD: Acute hemangioma-like lesions associated with Echo viral infections. Pediatrics 44:498–502, 1969

CHUMAKOV M, VOROSHIKOVA M, SHINDAROV L, LAVROVA I, GRACHEVA L, KOROLEVA G, VASILENKO S, BRODVAROVA I, NIKOLOVA M, GYUROVA S, GASHEVA M, MITOV G, NINOV N, TSYLKA E, ROBINSON I, FROLOVA M, BASHKIRTSEV V, MARTIYANOVA L, RODIN V: Enterovirus 71 isolated from cases of epidemic poliomyelitis-like disease in Bulgaria. Arch Virol 60:329–340, 1979

DALLDORF G, SICKLES GM: Unidentified, filterable agent isolated from feces of children with paralysis. Science 108:61–62, 1948

FINN JJ JR, WELLER TH, MORGAN HR: Epidemic pleurodynia: Clinical and etiologic studies based on one hundred and fourteen cases. Arch Intern Med 83:305–321, 1949

GRIST NR, BELL EJ: A six year study of coxsackievirus B infection in heart disease. J Hyg (Cambridge) 73:165–172, 1947

GYORKEY F, CABRAL GA, GYORKEY PK, URIBE—BOTERO G, DREESMAN GR, MELNICK JL: Coxsackie aggregates in muscle cells of a polymyositis patient. Intervirology 10:69–77, 1978

HUBER SA, JOB LP, WOODRUFF JF: Lysis of infected myofibers by Coxsackievirus B-3-immune T lymphocytes. Am J Pathol 98:681–684, 1980

KONO R: Appollo 11 disease or acute hemorrhagic conjunctivitis: A pandemic of a new enterovirus infection of the eye. Am J Epidemiol 101:383, 1975

KOONTZ CH, RAY CG: The role of coxsackie group B virus infections in sporadic myopericarditis. Am Heart J 82: 750–758, 1971

KROUS HF, DIETZMAN D, RAY CG: Fatal infections with echovirus types 6 and 11 in early infancy. Am J Dis Child 126:842–846, 1973

LAKE AM, LAUER BA, CLARK JC, WESENBERG RL, MCINTOSH K: Enterovirus infections in neonates. J Pediatr 89:787–791, 1976

LANSKY LL, KRUGMAN S, HUG G: Anicteric coxsackie B hepatitis: J Pediatr 94:64–65, 1979

MEADE RH, CHANG T–W: Zoster-like eruption due to echovirus 6. Am J Dis Child 133:283–284, 1979

MORGANTE O, WILKINSON D, BURCHAK EC, BRUCE M, RICHTER M: Outbreak of hand-foot-and-mouth disease among Indian and Eskimo children in a hospital. J Inf Dis 125:587–594, 1972

NAGINGTON J, WREGHITT TG, GANDY G, ROBERTON NRC, BERRY PJ: Fatal echovirus 11 infections in outbreak in special-care baby unit. Lancet 2:725–728, 1978

SANFORD JP, SULKIN SE: The clinical spectrum of ECHO virus infections. N Engl J Med 261:1113–1122, 1959

SELLS CJ, CARPENTER RL, RAY CG: Sequelae of central nervous system enterovirus infections. N Engl J Med 293:1–4, 1975

STEIGMAN AJ, LIPTON MM, BRASPENNICK H: Acute lymphonodular pharyngitis: A newly described condition due to Coxsackie A virus. J Pediatr 61:331–336, 1962

TANG TT, SEDMAK GV, SIEGERMUND KA, MCCREADIE SR: Chronic myopathy associated with coxsackievirus type A_9. N Engl J Med 292:608–611, 1975

WELLIVER RC, CHERRY JD: Aseptic meningitis and orchitis associated with echovirus 6 infection. J Pediatr 92:239–240, 1978

WILFERT CM, BUCKLEY RH, MOHANAKUNAR T, GRIFFITH JF, KATZ SL, WHISNANT JK, EGGLESTON PA, MOORE M, TREADWELL E, OMAN MN, ROSEN RS: Persistent and fatal central nervous system ECHO virus infections in patients with agammaglobulinemia. N Engl J Med 296:1485–1489, 1977

YOON J–W, AUSTIN M, ONODERA T, NOTKINS AL: Virus-induced diabetes mellitus: Isolation of a virus from the pancreas of a child with diabetic ketoacidosis. N Engl J Med 300:1173–1179, 1979

IRVING G. KAGAN

150 Trichinosis

Trichinosis is a helminthic disease caused by *Trichinella spiralis* ingested as larvae encysted in the striated muscles of an animal. In humans in the continental United States, exposure to the parasite results primarily from ingesting infected pork; however, persons have become parasitized by eating infected bear meat. In Alaska, the bear is the prime source of trichinosis in humans.

Etiology

The nematode parasite *T. spiralis* requires two hosts to complete its life cycle: it has no free-living stages. The definitive hosts for the parasite are flesh-eating mammals, of which at least 75 varieties are known. All mammals can serve as hosts for encysted larvae. *Trichinella spiralis* has both a sylvatic and a domesticated life cycle. Under sylvatic conditions, the cycle consists in direct transmission in wild carnivorous animals. In addition, there are probably secondary cycles through intermediate transport hosts such as necrophagous insects, crustaceans, amphipods, and fish—which may account for the prevalence of the parasite in insectivores and marine mammals. The domestic cycle depends primarily on the feeding of raw garbage and infected table scraps to swine. This is essentially a pig-to-pig cycle. The rat has been incriminated in this life history, but it probably plays a minor role in the transmission of the parasite.

Three subspecies of the parasite are recognized: *T. spiralis spiralis* (pig–man), *T. spiralis nativa* (an arctic strain that is resistant to cold), and *T. spiralis nelsoni* (wild pig–carnivore; found in East Africa). *Trichinella pseudospiralis* (a noncysting larval stage reported from Asia) may be a laboratory artifact.

Epidemiology

Because the ingestion of raw infected meat is essential to the survival of *T. spiralis,* trichinosis occurs in omnivorous man world-wide. Reports are sparse from tropical Africa and Central America, but the disease is endemic and epidemic in Europe and the United States.

In the United States, approximately 16% of samples from more than 5000 human diaphragms were positive for larvae of *T. spiralis* during the 1930s and early 1940s. A similar study was carried out between 1966 and 1968; only 4.2% of samples from 5000 diaphragms contained larvae of *T. spiralis,* documenting a rapid decline in the prevalence of trichinosis in the United States. The incidence of infections among persons 44 years old and under was only 1.6%. In addition, the intensity of infection was low because 80 of the 210 positive diaphragms contained less than 1 trichina per gram of material and only 13% had viable larvae, indicating that most of the infections were not of recent origin.

The decrease in the incidence of trichinosis in man is paralleled by a decrease in incidence in swine over the past 30 years. In grain-fed swine—that is, in 98.5% of the swine in the United States—infection has decreased from 9.5 per 1000 swine to 1.2 per 1000 swine. Laws that prevent the feeding of raw garbage to swine and the very successful programs to eradicate hog cholera and vesicular exanthema are contributory factors.

Frequently, an outbreak of trichinosis involves a pig that was fattened by a farm family on swill, including garbage and table scraps, before it was slaughtered for the production of sausage. If the sausage is eaten raw on the farm only, a family outbreak results.

Table 150-1 *Reported Cases of Trichinosis in the United States, 1947–1979*

Year	Cases	Deaths	Year	Cases	Deaths	Year	Cases	Deaths
1947	451	14	1958	176	4	1969	192	0
1948	487	15	1959	227	3	1970	109	3
1949	353	9	1960	160	3	1971	115	3
1950	327	9	1961	306	7	1972	96	1
1951	393	10	1962	194	1	1973	124	1
1952	367	10	1963	208	5	1974	141	0
1953	395	7	1964	198	1	1975	284	1
1954	277	1	1965	199	3	1976	96	0
1955	264	4	1966	115	3	1977	142	0
1956	262	5	1967	67	0	1978	91	0
1957	178	4	1968	84	1	1979	135	1

If the pig is sold to a meat market producing sausage, an outbreak involving many people may result. Most cases of trichinosis can be traced to the purchase and consumption of raw commercial pork products.

Trichinosis has been a reportable disease since 1947; however, formal surveillance to collect epidemiologic information was not initiated until 1967. The number of cases of trichinosis has declined from a high of 487 in 1948 to a low of 67 in 1967 (Table 150-1). Since then, the number of cases reported annually has varied from 84 to 284. In 1979, 135 cases were reported; the three states with the greatest number of cases were New Jersey (29), Alaska (27), and Louisiana (22). The one death that was reported occurred in an 82-year-old Laotian immigrant. The highest mean annual rates of occurrence for the 5-year period from 1975 to 1979 were observed in Alaska (4.8 cases/million population), Iowa (4.7), Connecticut (2.7), New Jersey (3.7), and Rhode Island (2.4). In 126 cases in which the probable source of infection was identified, 93 (73.8%) were from pork products and 33 (26.2%) were from nonpork products (walrus meat, 26—20.6%; bear meat, 2—1.6%; ground beef, 5—4.0%).

Pathogenesis and Pathology

On reaching the small intestine, the development of larval *T. spiralis* is very rapid. Worms become sexually mature in 24 to 48 hours, producing larvae in about 5 days. These larvae penetrate the mucosa of the small intestine and become dispersed throughout the body by the way of the blood or lymphatic system to begin invading striated muscles by the seventh day. The muscles of the diaphragm, chest, arms, and legs are those most commonly parasitized. During the second and third weeks of infection, larvae may be recovered from the feces. Infection by transmission of such larvae probably plays a minor role in the epidemiology of trichinosis, but it may account for the infection of pigs living under crowded conditions or wild animals feeding in pigpens.

After the third week of infection, larval migration diminishes and encystment of the larvae in the tissues begins. During this period, eosinophilia is the prominent sign. The involved muscles are pale and swollen, and they appear speckled with tiny red or white foci. As seen by microscopic examination, the typical coiled worm within a muscle fiber is surrounded by a zone of reaction consisting of edema and infiltration with lymphoctyes and eosinophils (Fig. 150-1).

Any organ may be involved in severe trichinosis; infection of either (or both) the heart or brain is potentially lethal. There may be petechiae, even ecchymoses in the pericardium, endocardium, and myocardium of a pale, flabby, dilated heart. The striking histopathologic differences from skeletal muscles is the lack of encysted worms in the heart muscle—the larvae are necrotic and scarcely recognizable. There is heavy infiltration with lymphocytes and occasional eosinophils throughout the myocardium (Fig. 150-2).

The brain is hyperemic. Meningeal infiltration with lymphocytes is typical. In the brain itself, foci of lymphocyte–glial cell reaction are intense about necrotic or living larvae.

Adult worms are usually eliminated after the third or fourth week of infection, and they may occasionally be found in the feces with larvae. It is at this point that serologic tests may become positive. The intradermal, complement fixation (CF), bentonite flocculation, fluorescent antibody (FA), and latex tests all become positive during the third to sixth week of infection in moderately infected persons.

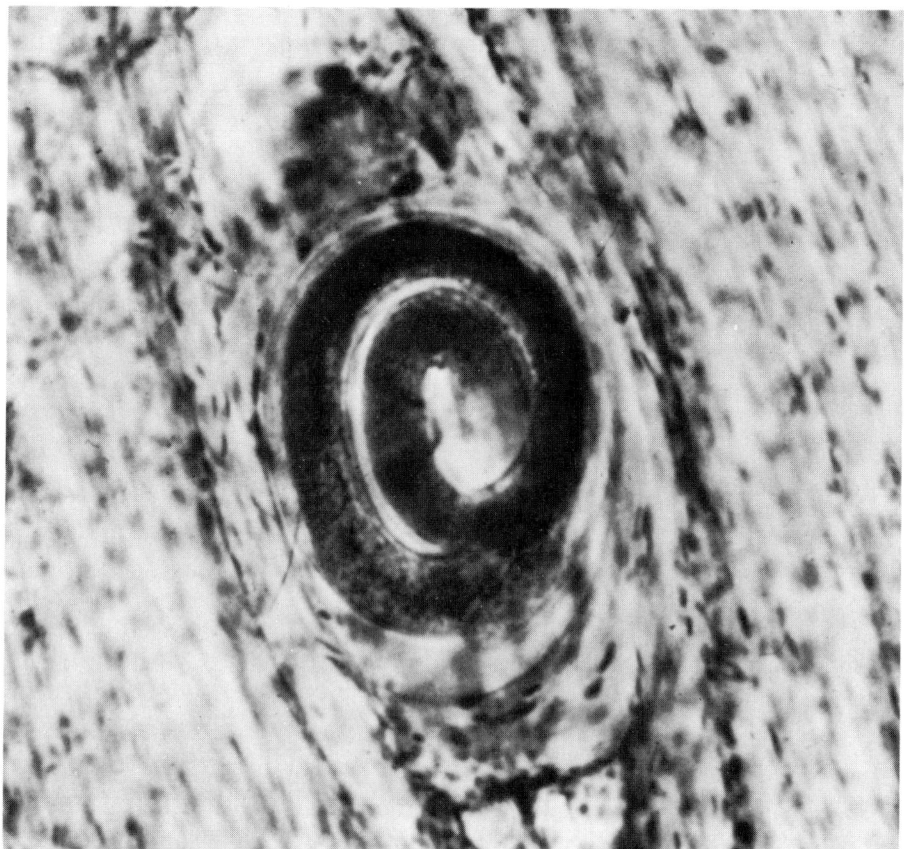

Fig. 150-1. Larva of *Trichinella spiralis* encysted in skeletal muscle.

Manifestations

Most patients with trichinosis in the United States are asymptomatic. When there is clinical illness, the manifestations can sometimes be correlated with stages in the life cycle of the parasite. Thus, early in the intestinal stage of the infection, abdominal pain with tenderness, cramping, diarrhea, and fever are the evidences of infection. Gastrointestinal symptoms may continue when larvae begin to penetrate the intestinal mucosa and migrate to striated muscles, but edema and myalgia become prominent. Neurologic symptoms may also occur because of invasion of the central nervous system (CNS). Overall, the kind and intensity of the symptoms and signs in a given patient with trichinosis are the result of the severity of the infection, the particular tissues invaded by the larvae, and the degree of hypersensitivity produced.

In the United States, most infections are light to moderate, and recognition of trichinosis is often difficult. Of some 75 symptoms and signs associated with trichinosis, the most important, in order of frequency of occurrence, are eosinophilia, periorbital edema, fever, and myalgia. Gastrointestinal symptoms, including diarrhea, nausea, rash, weakness, and neurologic signs and symptoms, are less frequently reported. In the chronic stage of the infection, neurologic, cardiac, and rheumatic symptoms are frequently attributed to trichinosis.

Diagnosis

The diagnosis of classical trichinosis is not difficult to substantiate if the disease is suspected. However, in the United States, most infections with *T. spiralis* result from light exposures, and clinical evidences of the infection may be lacking or minimal in the early stages. Because there are no eggs and few larvae in the feces or in body fluids, a diagnosis of trichinosis must be based on clinical findings, epidemiologic data, and laboratory tests. When gastrointestinal

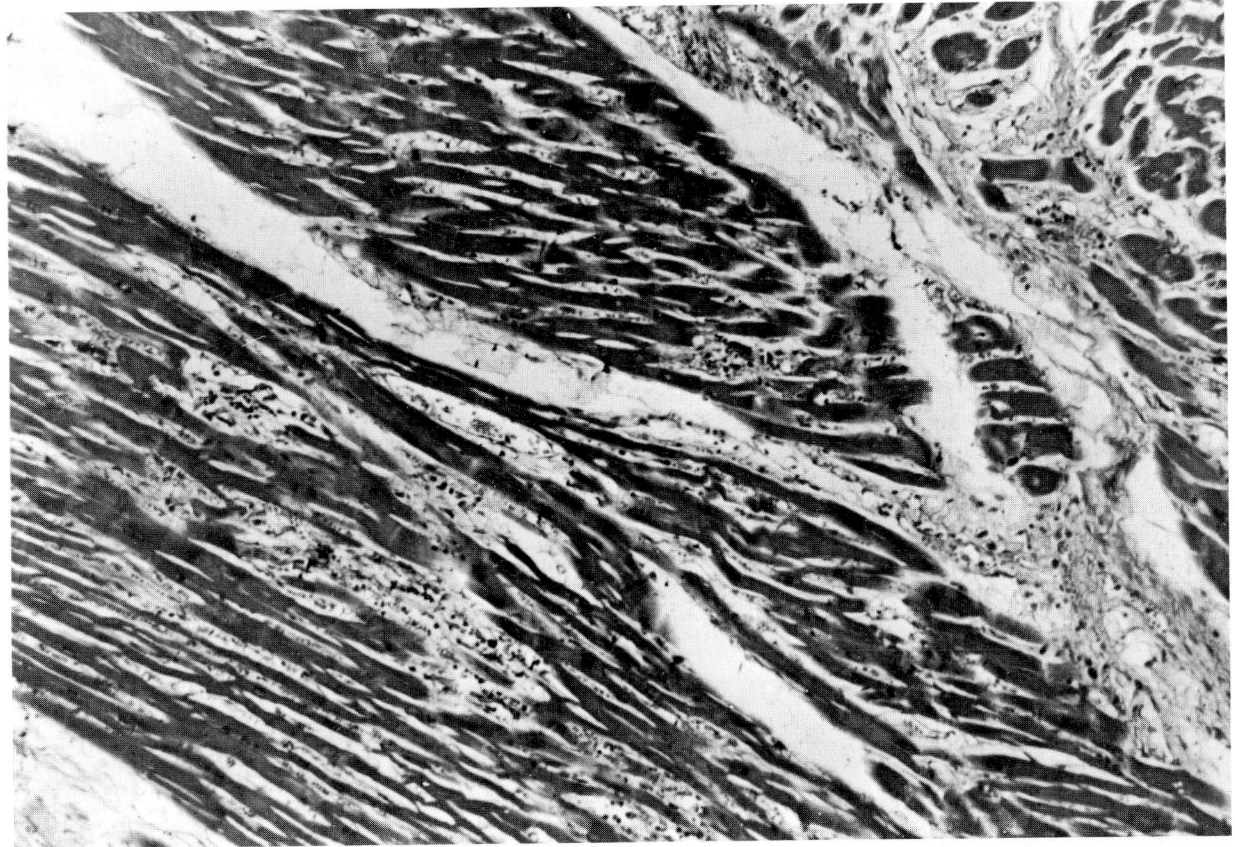

Fig. 150-2. Myocarditis in severe trichinosis. (Armed Forces Institute of Pathology, Neg. No. 55-20857 [143007])

symptoms occur early in the disease, they are frequently not associated with the infecting meal. Often, trichinosis is not suspected until several patients having similar symptoms report their problems to the physician.

The variety of symptoms manifested during the acute and chronic stages of infection mimic those of other diseases, making diagnosis based only on clinical data difficult. Indeed, many cases are diagnosed only after most of the common clinical disease entities such as food poisoning (Chap. 60, Gastroenterocolitis Syndromes; Chap. 61, Diarrheal Disease Caused by *Escherichia coli;* Chap. 63, Non-typhoidal Salmonelloses), typhoid fever (Chap. 64, Typhoid Fever), rheumatic fever (Chap. 24, Streptococcal Diseases), and other illnesses have been ruled out.

The use of press or digestion methods to examine meat samples suspected of causing an outbreak and tissues removed at autopsy gives reliable information that may confirm the diagnosis. The presence of freshly encysted larvae in muscle tissue removed by biopsy is positive identification of the infection. Unfortunately, larvae are quite difficult to find in biopsy specimens from patients with early and light infections.

Because evidence of parasitic infection with *T. spiralis* is not readily found in feces or body secretions, serologic and immunologic tests have been widely used to aid the diagnosis. Of the many serologic tests advocated, the flocculation tests presently in use apparently are the methods of choice for serodiagnosis. In most cases of clinical trichinosis, a period of at least 3 to 4 weeks is required for such antibodies to appear; in cases of light infection, a longer period may be necessary.

The skin test for trichinosis can be a valuable epidemiologic and diagnostic tool. The antigen employed must be carefully standardized and evaluated.

Reactivity is of the immediate, histaminic type, and it should be read 15 minutes after the intradermal injection of antigen. Because sensitivity may last at least 5 years after exposure, a positive reaction does not necessarily indicate current exposure to the larvae.

The serum enzymes—glutamic, oxaloacetic, and pyruvic transaminases—are elevated in the acute stage. Although several other enzymes may also be abnormally high, there has not been systematic, prospective evaluation of the usefulness of such tests.

The diagnosis of trichinosis in 119 cases in 1979 illustrates the combined use of epidemiologic information, clinical manifestations, muscle biopsy, skin testing, and serologic tests. The mean incubation period in 45 of 119 patients who recalled the date of consumption of the suspected meat was 14.7 days (range 1–45 days). Serums were collected from 104 of the 119 patients; in 85 (81.7%) there was serologic confirmation of the diagnosis. Muscle biopsies were performed on 34 patients; 26 (76.5%) were positive.

Prognosis

The prognosis in trichinosis is usually good. Most persons recover spontaneously after several weeks of illness when the larvae have encysted in the muscles. Calcification of the larvae begins approximately 1 year after infection. Trichina larvae were discovered in 1835 by a medical student who observed the calcified cysts in the cadaver he was dissecting dulled his scapel.

Sudden death from cardiac collapse may occur in a patient who has had moderate to severe disease and has been allowed out of bed too soon in convalescence. Bed rest must be continued after acute symptoms have abated to avoid a serious relapse and possible death.

Lasting protective immunity is apparently not acquired by humans through having had trichinosis. The humoral antibodies so evident in serologic tests play, at most, a minor role in elimination of worms in nonhuman animals with experimental infections. However, these experimental infections have yielded evidence that specific, delayed hypersensitivity is involved in the expulsion of adult *T. spiralis* from the intestinal tract on reinfection.

Therapy

The advisability of treatment and the nature of the treatment must be individualized on the basis of the severity of the infection, phase of the illness, tolerance to medication, and tendency toward allergic reactions. Mebendazole kills larvae encysted in the tissues of mice. The use of this drug in humans with trichinosis (5 mg/kg body weight/day, PO, as a single dose) has afforded prompt relief of symptoms, but it may cause nausea, vomiting, dizziness, dermatitis, and fever. It is clear that mebendazole is effective against the intestinal stages of the parasite, but its effectiveness against encysted larvae in man is still somewhat doubtful. Persons who suspect that they have ingested infected meat should be treated to rid the intestine of adult worms. Allergic side-effects of treatment require medication. Glucosteroids—for example, prednisone (0.5–1.0 mg/kg body wt/day, PO, reduced after 3 days and discontinued after 5 days)—usually bring about defervescence, diminution of myalgia, and amelioration of CNS manifestations.

Prevention

Trichinosis can be prevented by eating pork only after it has been thoroughly cooked. Trichina larvae are killed when heated to a minimum temperature of 131°F. Larvae may also be killed by freezing or curing. Larvae encysted in pork products held at −20°F for 6 to 12 days, −10°F for 10 to 20 days, or −5°F for 20 to 30 days are noninfective. Meat that has been salted or dried for long periods is safe for human consumption.

Every state in the continental United States has laws interdicting the feeding of raw garbage to swine. Enforcement of such laws would contribute to a further decline in the incidence of trichina in swine. At this time, there is no vaccine effective in preventing trichinosis. No inspection of carcasses at the time of slaughter (as is the rule in most European countries) has been made for over 50 years in the United States. A recent pilot study demonstrated both the sensitivity and economic feasibility of inspection by examining 20 pooled samples of swine diaphragms for larvae by a digestion method. Serologic testing of swine sera by the enzyme-linked immunosorbent assay (ELISA) method on a mass basis is routinely used in the Netherlands to detect infection in pigs.

Over the past 10 to 15 years, the incidence of trichinosis has stabilized in the United States. If additional laws are instituted to prevent the feeding of garbage in any form to swine or if serologic testing of slaughtered animals becomes routine, this helminthic infection could be virtually eliminated from humans in the United States.

Bibliography

Books

Centers for Disease Control: Trichinosis Surveillance. Annual Summary 1980, issued November, 1981. 10 pp.

GOULD, SE (ed): Trichinosis in Man and Animals. Springfield, Ill, Charles C Thomas, 1970. 540 pp.

KIM CW, PAWLOWSKI ZS (ed): Trichinellosis Proceedings of the Fourth International Conference on Trichinellosis. University Press of New England, 1978. 571 pp.

Journals

KAGAN IG: Trichinosis: A review of biologic, serologic, and immunologic aspects. J Infect Dis 107:65–93, 1960

STEELE JH, SCHULTZ MG: The epidemiology and control of trichinosis in the United States. J Parasitol 56:328–329, 1970

ZIMMERMANN WH, STEELE JH, KAGAN IG: The changing status of trichinosis in the U.S. population. Public Health Rep 83:957–966, 1968

Section | *XX*

Skeletal Infections

Indigenous Microbiota of the Skeleton

(None)

RICHARD H. PARKER

Septic Arthritis

151

Septic arthritis may be defined as the invasion of the synovial membrane by microorganisms, usually with extension into the joint space to produce a closed-space infection. Synonyms include suppurative arthritis, infectious arthritis, acute pyogenic arthritis, and pyarthrosis.

Although septic arthritis is usually not life-threatening, rapidity of diagnosis and therapy is mandatory if permanent damage to the joint and spread of the infection to contiguous bone and soft tissues is to be avoided. Without proper therapy, cartilage may be destroyed quickly, leaving the patient with a deformed, painful joint with a restricted range of motion.

Etiology

A clear-cut tropism for joints is not a striking characteristic of any one kind or group of microorganisms. Although a variety of infectious agents may infect the joint space, only a few genera are responsible for most cases of septic arthritis. Precise data are not available regarding the frequency with which different kinds of microorganisms cause septic arthritis. However, from reported cases, there seems to be a striking variation in the kinds of bacteria that cause infectious arthritis in different age groups (Table 151-1). These differences reflect primarily age-related differences in the causes of bacteremia. Gonococcal arthritis occurs in 1% to 3% of all cases of gonorrhea. Nongonococcal arthritis develops in more than 10% of patients with nongonococcal bacteremias—more than 15% of those caused by gram-positive bacteria as compared with about 5% of the bacteremias caused by gram-negative bacteria.

Epidemiology

Because bacteria are the common causes of septic arthritis and infectious agents usually reach the synovial membrane through the bloodstream, the epidemiology of septic arthritis is primarily the epidemiology of bacteremia. The age of the patient is a critical factor.

Children

Systemic infectious diseases such as pneumonia or meningitis are frequently present in children who have septic arthritis. The usual causes are *Staphylococcus aureus* (Chap. 100, Staphylococcal Skin Infections) *Streptococcus pyogenes* (group A) (Chap. 24, Streptococcal Diseases), *Streptococcus pneumoniae* (Chap. 31, Bacterial Pneumonias), and *Haemophilus influenzae* (Chap. 26, Epiglottitis, Laryngitis, and Laryngotracheobronchitis). Infectious arthritis caused by type b *H. influenzae* is seen almost exclusively in children under the age of 2 years. Gram-negative enteric bacilli (*Escherichia coli, Proteus* spp., *Pseudomonas* spp., *Salmonella* spp.) were once rare but are now more frequently identified as etiologic agents for septic arthritis in both infants and children.

Adults

The most common cause of septic arthritis in young adults is *Neisseria gonorrhoeae* (Chap. 56, Gonococcal Infections). Although gonococcal arthritis is most frequently observed in adults less than 30 years old, it may occur at any age. Before systemic antibacterial agents were available, gonococcal arthritis was more common in men than in women. However, more than 75% of cases of gonococcal arthritis now occur

Table 151-1. *Correlation of Bacterial Cause With Age of Patient in Septic Arthritis**

Microorganism	**Ages (years)** <2 (%)	**2–15 (%)**	**16–50 (%)**	**>50 (%)**
Staphylococcus aureus	30	40	15	75
Streptococcus pyogenes	15	25	5	5
Streptococcus pneumoniae	10	10	—	5
Hemophilus influenzae	30	2	—	—
Neisseria gonorrhoeae	—	5	75	—
Enterobacteriaceae and *Pseudomonas* spp.	13	15	5	10
Other	2	3	—	5

*The percentage of cases in each age group is a composite from several reports.

in females. The exact reason for this striking change in the sex incidence of gonococcal arthritis is not known. It may be that the increased incidence in women reflects a delay in recognizing gonorrhea in the female. About one-fourth of all cases of gonococcal arthritis are seen in pregnant women. It has been postulated that gonococci may be more easily disseminated during pregnancy because of the increased vascularity and movement of the internal genitalia.

Staphylococcus aureus is a major cause of septic arthritis in older adults, although infections caused by group A *Streptococcus pyogenes, Streptococcus pneumoniae,* and gram-negative bacilli are frequently seen in patients more than 60 years old. Septic arthritis of the aged is usually superimposed on some kind of chronic joint disease. Underlying rheumatoid arthritis is most common; it may be present in up to 50% of cases of infectious arthritis. However, infection also occurs in joints damaged by osteoarthritis, neuropathic joint disease (Charcot's arthritis), and ankylosing spondylitis.

Acute suppurative arthritis following instrumentation or surgery of either the urinary or the intestinal tract may be caused by gram-negative bacilli (Chap. 48, Urethritis and Cystitis). Gram-negative bacilli may also gain entry into the joint space during traumatic injury or arthrocentesis. Because bacteremia is often seen in salmonellosis, it is not surprising that salmonellal arthritis occasionally occurs. Salmonellal bacteremia in patients with sickle cell anemia is frequently associated with salmonellolal arthritis (Chap. 63, Nontyphoidal Salmonelloses). *Pseudomonas* and *Serratia* spp. have been recognized as common causes of septic arthritis complicating parenteral drug abuse. However, *Pseudomonas aeruginosa* has caused infection of the metatarsal phalangeal joint following puncture wounds, and *Serratia marcescens* may cause arthritis in nonparenteral drug abusers as a complication of nosocomial septicemia.

Two kinds of joint involvement may be seen in patients with meningococcemia. Polyarthralgias may occur during the first few days of meningococcal bacteremia. Afflicted joints show either no effusion or a small, sterile effusion. Starting about 5 days after onset of the illness, some patients with meningococcemia develop a typical monoarticular septic joint. The culture of synovial fluid in these patients yields *Neisseria meningitides* (Chap. 119, Bacterial Meningitis). Not only does meningococcal arthritis mimic gonococcal arthritis clinically, but also in recent years some cases of meningococcal infection appear to have been transmitted venereally.

Brucellosis may also be complicated by two kinds of joint disease. About one-third of patients with acute brucellosis have mild, transient arthralgias, often with a sterile joint effusion. Weeks or even months after the acute phase of brucellosis, about 10% of the patients have actual septic arthritis, and culture of the synovial fluid reveals *Brucella* spp. (Chap. 138, Brucellosis). Brucellar spondylitis is usually secondary to vertebral osteomyelitis.

Mycobacterium tuberculosis (Chap. 35, Extrapulmonary Tuberculosis) may cause suppurative arthritis, but this is usually associated with osteomyelitis. Nontuberculous *Mycobacterium* spp. (Chap. 36, Nontuberculous Mycobacterioses), frequently cause infectious arthritis involving the tendon sheaths of the wrist and hand; such infections often follow local trauma. All the fungi associated with deep mycotic infections (Chap. 39, Candidosis, Chap. 40, Histoplasmosis, Chap. 41, Coccidioidomycosis, Chap. 42, Paracoccidioidomycosis, Chap. 43, Blastomycosis, and Chap. 44, Aspergillosis) and *Sporotrichum schenckii* (Chap. 108, Sporotrichosis) may cause joint infections. *Actinomyces israelii (Chap. 38, Actinomycosis*) and the *Nocardia* spp. (Chap. 37, Nocardiosis) may also cause septic arthritis clinically similar to arthritis produced by *Mycobacterium* spp. and fungi.

Pathogenesis and Pathology

Microorganisms are brought to joints either by the blood (most common), by direct implantation (less common), or by extension from vicinal infections (least common). Virtually any kind of primary infection, such as pneumonia, gonorrhea, meningitis, bacterial endocarditis, and infected wounds, may be the source of microorganisms that are carried to the synovial membrane in the blood. Hematogenous infection of a joint may also occur without an identifiable primary focus of infection; for example, septic arthritis has been reported after endoscopy and after clean surgical procedures.

When joint infection occurs as a result of bacteremia, the initial growth of microorganisms is either in the synovial membrane or in the adjacent bone. In either case, an inflammatory reaction of the synovial membrane is quickly established and results in a marked increase in leukocytes in the synovial fluid, even though the fluid itself is sterile on culture. When the microorganisms have spread into the joint fluid, culture of the fluid usually reveals the etiology of the infection.

The direct implantation of microorganisms into the joint from an exogenous source may occur as a result of penetrating wounds or during the intraarticular infection of medications. In infants, septic arthritis of the hip has followed femoral venipuncture. Direct implantation is the primary route of infection for atypical *Mycobacterium* spp. *Sporotrichum schenckii, Actinomyces* spp., and many gram-negative bacilli.

Septic arthritis initiated by extension occurs when there is a spread of infection into the joint from adjacent osteomyelitis or cellulitis (*e.g.,* tuberculosis of the bone).

The pathologic findings of septic arthritis are varied and depend on the duration of the infection, the kind of microorganism, and the resistance of the host. Early in the infection, only inflammatory changes in the synovium are seen. Late in the course of untreated septic arthritis, destruction of joint structures is marked. Articular cartilage is particularly vulnerable because it is an avascular tissue.

In acute, pyogenic arthritis, the cartilage characteristically dissolves first at points of articular contact to expose the underlying bone. Extension of the infection into the bone does not occur. Once destroyed, the cartilage cannot regenerate, and proliferation of bone to repair the defect overshoots to cover the remaining peripheral cartilage. As destructive changes occur, several abnormalities appear in the synovial fluid that may contribute to (or result from) the process: increased pressure, low pH, low concentration of glucose, and the activation of proteolytic and other enzymes. Without treatment, about 25% of patients sustain permanent loss of function of the involved joint.

The nonpyogenic septic arthritides progress less rapidly, but they may cause even more severe destruction. Granulomas may involve all of the synovial membrane, proliferating to extend into the joint space, covering the articular cartilage with a pannus of granulation tissue. The subcartilaginous proliferation of granulation tissue loosens the cartilage, abetting the destruction contributed by pannus and direct involvement. Characteristically, the cartilage is first destroyed at the periphery, initially sparing the cartilage-to-cartilage portion. There is concomitant destruction of contiguous bone.

Manifestations

The clinical manifestations of septic arthritis are variable and related to many factors, including the kind of microorganism causing the infection, the joint involved, and the age of the patient.

Gonococcal Arthritis

Two clinical varieties of gonococcal arthritis occur. About 75% of patients have prominent prodromal symptoms of fever, chills, headache, anorexia, and malaise. Most of these patients also note migratory polyarthralgia or polyarthritis before there is localization of the infection in one or more joints. The occurrence of migratory polyarthralgias is an important clinical feature of gonococcal arthritis. Except for meningococcal infection, polyarthralgia is not seen in other infectious arthritides. The patients with striking prodromal symptoms often have skin lesions of gonococcemia and small joint effusions. Cultures of synovial fluid from these patients are usually sterile. This may represent an early stage of septic arthritis when the site of infection is still localized to the synovial membrane.

Other patients with gonococcal arthritis may have monoarthric involvement that has been present for several days. These patients deny prodromal symptoms and complain only of the sudden onset of a swollen, painful, tender, and hot joint. *Neisseria gonorrhoeae* is usually cultured from the synovial fluid of these patients.

In either kind of gonococcal arthritis, the large joints are usually infected. The knee is most often involved, followed by the wrists, ankles, and elbows. A striking feature in about one-third of patients is tenosynovitis.

Nongonococcal Arthritis

The clinical picture of nongonococcal septic arthritis is variable. At one extreme, the patient may complain of an acutely painful, swollen joint that is exquisitely tender and rigidly limited in range of motion, but have no manifestations of infection elsewhere. At the other extreme, the primary, nonarticular infection may so dominate the clinical picture that the signs of joint inflammation go unnoticed. Also, the patient with chronic inflammatory joint disease may have symptoms and signs that are indistinguishable from an exacerbation of the preexisting, noninfectious disease. Occasionally, joints are infected without any clear-cut signs of inflammation. Finally, inflammation in deep-seated joints, such as shoulders or hips, may be obscured by the overlying tissues.

Chronic Infectious Arthritis

Patients with chronic infectious arthritis usually complain of swelling, moderate pain, and limitation of motion. Tenderness and an increased temperature over the involved joint are uncommon. Examination of the synovial fluid often provides the first clues to joint infection.

Diagnosis

The diagnosis of septic arthritis cannot be established without examination of the synovial fluid. Using aseptic technique, the synovial fluid should be obtained by arthrocentesis and divided into three tubes as follows: (1) a sterile tube for cultures and serology, (2) a tube with anticoagulant for cell examination, and (3) a tube for chemical determinations. It is essential that blood be drawn at the time of arthrocentesis for the valid comparison of synovial fluid and blood glucose concentrations.

Septic arthritis provokes a brisk inflammatory reaction in the synovial fluid with more than 10,000 polymorphonuclear leukocytes per mm^3 and a decreased glucose concentration (Table 151-2). The diagnosis is confirmed by demonstration of the causative microorganisms in the synovial fluid (microscopic examination of a gram-stained smear, isolation of bacteria by culture, or identification of bacterial antigen using counterimmunoelectrophoresis [CIE]).

Microorganisms are not demonstrable in synovial fluid in all cases of septic arthritis. This is particularly true in gonococcal arthritis and when patients have received antimicrobial therapy prior to arthrocente-

Table 151-2. *Characteristics of Synovial Fluid in Septic Arthritis Compared With Synovial Fluid in Noninfectious Conditions*

Characteristic	**Septic Arthritis**	**Nonseptic Inflammatory Arthritis**	**Noninflammatory Effusions**
		(*e.g.,* rheumatoid arthritis)	(*e.g.,* traumatic hydroarthrosis)
Color	Yellow to green	Yellow	Colorless to pale yellow
Turbidity	Purulent, turbid	Turbid	Clear to slightly turbid
Mucin precipitate	Small, friable	Small, friable	Tight, ropy clump
Leukocytes/mm^3	>10,000	1000–50,000	<1000
Predominant cell	PMN*	PMN*	MONO†
Ratio of [glucose] synovial fluid/blood‡	<0.6	0.6–0.8	0.8–1
Protein (g/dl)	3–7	3–7	1–5
Lactic acid (mg/dl)	>65§	<65	<65

*PMN = polymorphonuclear leukocyte

†MONO = mononuclear leukocyte, either lymphocyte or monocyte.

‡Calculation of ratio is valid only if specimens were obtained simultaneously after at least 6 hours of fasting.

§Patients with gonococcal arthritis may not have elevated synovial fluid lactic acid.

sis. Before instituting antimicrobial therapy, blood cultures and cultures of other appropriate body fluids (*e.g.*, urine, cerebrospinal fluid, pleural fluid) and exudates should be obtained from all patients suspected of having septic arthritis. These cultures may yield growth, indicating the etiology of the infection even when the synovial fluid is sterile. Serologic studies are useful in determining the etiology of septic arthritis when paired serum specimens are obtained so that an increase in titer of antibodies can be demonstrated. The first serum specimen must be obtained at the time the diagnosis of septic arthritis is initially considered. Serologic studies are most useful in the diagnosis of salmonellosis, brucellosis, and coccidioidomycosis. Detection of bacterial antigen by CIE has been useful in the etiologic diagnosis of joint infections caused by *Streptococcus pneumoniae, H. influenzae, and Streptococcus pyogenes.* A positive Limulus assay for endotoxin is useful in recognizing septic arthritis caused by gram-negative bacteria, but is not found in infections caused by gram-positive microorganisms. The use of a hyperosmolar culture medium may aid in the isolation of a microorganism from the synovial fluids of patients who have already received antimicrobial therapy.

The clinical picture of patients with acute rheumatic fever, gout, rheumatoid arthritis, or trauma to a joint may mimic septic arthritis. Rheumatoid arthritis, rheumatic fever, and gout also cause an increase in the numbers of polymorphonuclear leukocytes in the synovial fluid. However, the concentration of glucose is usually normal in these conditions. In traumatic arthritis, there is bleeding into the synovial fluid. If bloody fluid is aspirated, the fluid must be examined completely if there is any doubt as to the etiology of the joint effusion. In many cases, it is impossible to ascertain whether septic arthritis is superimposed on underlying joint disease. Antimicrobial therapy should be given while awaiting the results of cultures and other diagnostic studies—a course particularly indicated when the manifestations of an acute infectious process might be dampened by the previous administration of glucosteroids.

Prognosis

When appropriate antimicrobial therapy is instituted within the first week after onset of the symptoms and signs, complete symptomatic recovery with little, if any, residual limitation of joint motion is the rule. In septic arthritis evident for more than 1 week before the insitution of medical treatment, recovery may be complete, or varying degrees of functional impairment, chronic effusion, or arthralgia may be the sequelae. Delays in institution of therapy also increase the possibility of local and systemic spread of the infection

Therapy

The successful treatment of septic arthritis requires both drainage and the prompt use of an effective antimicrobial agent. If treatment is instituted early in the course of the disease, repeated percutaneous needle aspirations provide effective drainage, and the patient is spared the morbidity associated with surgical drainage. To be effective, arthrocentesis may have to be repeated every day. Surgical drainage is mandatory when medical therapy is ineffective. Generally, this occurs when treatment is undertaken late in the course of the disease and the exudate has become loculated or too thick to be aspirated through a needle.

Antimicrobics should be administered systemically, regardless of whether synovial fluid is drained by repeated arthrocenteses or by surgery. There is no need from the intraarticular injection of antimicrobial agents unless systemically administered antimicrobics fail to enter the synovial fluid. Such an occurrence is rare, even with poorly diffusible drugs such as the polymyxins or amphotericin B. The antimicrobics of choice for the treatment of almost all cases of septic arthritis are the penicillins, cephalosporins, tetracyclines, chloramphenicol, and macrolide antimicrobics—agents that achieve effective concentrations in synovial fluid after systemic administration. Not only is the intraarticular injection of antimicrobial agents unnecessary, but it is also contraindicated because of the risk of secondary infection due to contamination at the time of arthrocentesis, and of synovitis caused by the high concentrations of antimicrobics injected into the synovial space. Specific recommendations for the use of antimicrobial agents in the treatment of septic arthritis are listed in Table 151-3.

Prevention

Because septic arthritis is usually a complication of bacteremia originating from a primary infection elsewhere in the body, prevention is not usually possible. However, many cases of septic arthritis caused by the direct implantation of microorganisms are preventable by avoiding the unnecessary injection of medication into joints and by the use of aseptic technique when intraarticular injection is absolutely necessary.

Table 151-3. *Antimicrobial Therapy of Septic Arthritis*

Primary Antimicrobic(s)	Alternative Antimicrobic(s)	Comments
Staphylococcus aureus, *penicillinase-producing*		
Nafcillin (or dicloxacillin or oxacillin) Loading dose—50 mg/kg body wt, IV, in 30–45 min Maintenance dose—150–200 mg/kg body wt/day, IV, as 6 equal portions, 4-hourly	Cefazolin Loading dose—15–25 mg/kg body wt, IV, in 30–45 min Maintenance dose—50–75 mg/kg body wt/day, IV, as 3 equal portions, 8-hourly	Continue antimicrobial therapy for at least 1 week after defervescence or cessation of effusion—preferably by IV injection. Peroral therapy is permissible only if assays of serums document adequate absorption. Change nafcillin to cloxacillin or dicloxacillin, cefazolin to cephalexin or cephradine—50–60 mg/kg body wt/day as 4 equal portions, 6-hourly; clindamycin—20–25 mg/kg body wt/day as 4 equal portions, 6-hourly.
	Clindamycin Loading dose—10 mg/kg body wt, IV, in 30–45 min Maintenance dose—20–25 mg/kg body wt/day, as 4 equal portions, 6-hourly	Clindamycin, either parenteral or peroral, may cause colitis. To avoid accumulation to toxic levels in patients with renal dysfunction, the doses of antimicrobics that are primarily excreted in the urine must be reduced to compensate for the diminished excretory capacity (Chap. 18, Antimicrobics and Anthelmintics for Systemic Therapy). Of the antimicrobics listed in this table, clindamycin and chloramphenicol are exceptions. With large doses of some antimicrobics, large quantities of Na^+ or K^{+*} may also be given. Dangerous accumulation of these cations may occur in patients with renal or cardiac failure. Procaine penicillin G and cephaloridine are exceptions.
Staphylococcus aureus, *nonpenicillinase-producing*		
Penicillin G Loading dose—50 mg (80,000 U)/kg body wt, IV, in 30–45 min Maintenance dose—150–200 mg (240,000–320,000 U)/kg body wt/day, IV, as 6 equal portions, 4-hourly	As for penicillinase-producing *S. aureus*	Susceptibility to penicillin G must be documented by *in vitro* testing before penicillin G is used. If IM injection is not contraindicated, the final week of treatment (see above) may be either procaine penicillin G, 0.75 g (1.2 million U), IM, 8-hourly; or penicillin V, 50–60 mg/kg body wt/day, PO, as 4 equal portions, 6-hourly. Cefazolin may be changed to either cephalexin or cephradine in the same peroral dose as penicillin V. The peroral dose for clindamycin is the same as the parenteral dose (either IV or IM).
Streptococcus pyogenes, Streptococcus pneumoniae, Neisseria gonorrhoeae		
Penicillin G Loading dose—25 mg (40,000 U)/kg body wt/IV, in 30–45 min Maintenance dose—60–75 mg (95,000–120,000 U) kg body wt/day, IV, as 6 equal portions, 4-hourly	Cefazolin Loading dose—10 mg/kg body wt, IV, in 30–45 min Maintenance dose—25–50 mg/kg body wt/day, IV, as 3 equal portions, 8-hourly	With *S. pyogenes* or *S. pneumoniae:* For final week of treatment (see above), penicillin G may be changed to either procaine penicillin G (0.4 g [600,000 U], IM, 8-hourly) or penicillin V (25–30 mg/kg body wt/day, PO, as 4 equal portions, 6-hourly); cefazolin may be changed to either cephalexin or cephradine in the same dose as penicillin V.

Table 151-3. (continued) *Antimicrobial Therapy of Septic Arthritis*

Primary Antimicrobic(s)	Alternative Antimicrobic(s)	Comments
	Clindamycin (not with *N. gonorrhoeae*): same as for nonpenicillinase-producing *S. aureus* Tetracycline (not with *S. pyogenes* or *S. pneumoniae*): Loading dose—10–15 mg/kg body wt/day, PO; Maintenance dose—25–30 mg/kg body wt/day, PO, as 4 equal portions, 6-hourly for 7 days	With *N. gonorrhoeae,* parenteral therapy for 3 days is generally sufficient. If clinical improvement is slow, additional treatment may be given: procaine penicillin G, as above, or amoxicillin, 50–60 mg/kg body wt/day, PO, as 4 equal portions, 6-hourly. If symptoms persist after a total of 10 days of treatment, complete reevaluation is necessary.
Haemophilus influenzae		
Ampicillin (or an acylureido-penicillin) Loading dose—50 mg/kg body wt, IV, in 30–45 min	Chloramphenicol (succinate) Loading dose—30 mg/kg body wt, IV, in 30–45 min	Susceptibility testing is essential because strains resistant to ampicillin have been isolated in many areas of the United States. For the final week of treatment, ampicillin may be changed to amoxicillin, 50–60 mg/kg body wt/day, PO, as 4 equal portions, 6-hourly. Chloramphenicol can often be given perorally from the outset, in the dose listed for IV injection; IM injection should not be used because absorption is unreliable.
Maintenance dose—150–200 mg/kg body wt/day, IV, as 6 equal portions, 4-hourly	Maintenance dose—30–50 mg/kg body wt/day, IV, as 4 equal portions, 6-hourly	Bone marrow suppression is a hazard to use of chloramphenicol (Chap. 18, Antimicrobics and Anthelmintics for Systemic Therapy). In premature and neonatal infants (less than 1 week of age) the dose of chloramphenicol should not exceed 25 mg/kg body wt/day.
Escherichia coli, Proteus mirabilis		
Ampicillin (or an acylureido-penicillin) As given previously	Cefazolin As given previously	In terms of safety and efficacy, there is little difference between these agents; cost should be considered. Some strains of *P. mirabilis* produce a β-lactamase that is active against penicillins, but relatively inactive against cephalosporins. When strains resistant to both penicillins and cephalosporins are encountered, gentamicin (tobramycin) and chloramphenicol may be useful in dosages as given.
Non*-mirabilis Proteus *spp.*, Klebsiella *spp.*, Enterobacter *spp.*, Serratia *spp.		
Gentamicin (tobramycin or netilmicin) Loading dose—1.7 mg/kg body wt, IV, in 30–45 min Maintenance dose—5–6 mg/kg body wt/day, IV or IM, as 3 equal portions, 8 hourly	Chloramphenicol As given previously	Although ticarcillin is usually active against the non-*mirabilis Proteus* spp., it is virtually never effective against klebsiellas, enterobacters, or serratias, unlike the acylureidopenicillins. Cefoxitin is often inactive against *Enterobacter* spp. Gentamicin, tobramycin and netilmicin are quite similar in antibacterial effectiveness and are virtually identical in pharmacokinetics. Both

Table 151-3. (continued) *Antimicrobial Therapy of Septic Arthritis*

Primary Antimicrobic(s)	Alternative Antimicrobic(s)	Comments
Ticarcillin or an acylureido-penicillin (non-*mirabilis* *Proteus* spp.) Loading dose—40 mg/kg body wt, IV, in 30–45 min Maintenance dose—200–250 mg/kg body wt/day, IV, as 6 equal portions, 4-hourly, or by continuous infusion		are potentially nephrotoxic and ototoxic; complications may be avoided by steady-state therapy, *i.e.,* doses yielding low–high concentrations in the serum of 3–8 μg/ml. Periodic assays of concentrations in the serum are desirable. Because the intraarticular penetration of aminocyclitols may not be adequate, the synovial fluid–exudate should be assayed; intraarticular administration may be necessary.
Salmonella *spp.*		
Chloramphenicol (succinate) As given previously	Ampicillin As given previously	With chloramphenicol-resistant *S. typhi;* high-dose therapy with ampicillin, *e.g.,* 200–300 mg/kg body wt/day, may be effective.
Pseudomonas aeruginosa		
Gentamicin (tobramycin or netilmicin) As given previously Ticarcillin or an acylureido-penicillin As given previously	Amikacin Loading dose—7.5 mg/kg body wt, IV, in 30 min Maintenance dose—15 mg/kg body wt/day, IV, as 3 equal portions, 8-hourly, not to exceed 1.5 g/day	There is generally cross-susceptibility–resistance between gentamicin and tobramycin; the exceptions may be therapeutically important. Amikacin is often active when neither gentamicin nor tobramycin is effective.
Bacteroides fragilis ***with or without other anaerobic bacteria***		
Chloramphenicol As given previously	Clindamycin As given previously	
Bacteroides melaninogenicus ***with or without other anaerobic bacteria***		
Penicillin G As for nonpenicillinase-producing *Staphylococcus aureus*	Chloramphenicol As given previously	Rare strains of *Fusobacterium* spp. are resistant to penicillin G

* Na^+; Penicillin G, 2.7 mEq/g (1.7 mEq/million U); cefazolin, 2.1 mEq/g; nafcillin, 1.2 mEq/g; dicloxacillin, 0.5 mEq/g; oxacillin, 2.5 mEq/g; ampicillin, 3.1 mEq/g; carbenicillin, 4.7 mEq/g; chloramphenicol succinate, 2.3 mEq/g K^+: Penicillin G, 2.7 mEq/g (1.7 mEq/million U)

Remaining Problems

The differentiation of gonococcal arthritis from the arthritis of Reiter's syndrome, rheumatic fever, and other inflammatory processes is a major problem. Gonococci are difficult to recover by culture of the synovial fluid or blood, even from patients who give an appropriate history and have typical manifestations of gonococcal arthritis. Development of rapid, specific techniques that identify either bacterial antigen or metabolic products are needed.

Bibliography

Journals

ARGEN RJ, WILSON CH JR, WOOD P: Suppurative arthritis. Arch Intern Med 117:661–666, 1966

GOLDENBERG DL, COHEN AS: Acute infectious arthritis. Am J Med 60:369–377, 1976

MANSHADY BM, THOMPSON GR, WEISS JJ: Septic arthritis in a general hospital 1966–1977. J Rheumatol 7:523–580, 1980

NELSON JD, KOONTZ WC: Septic arthritis in infants and children: A review of 117 cases. Pediatrics 38:966–971, 1966

PARKER RH: Transport and choice of antibiotics in septic arthritis. Mod Treat 6:1071–1080, 1969

Addendum

Lyme Disease

Lyme disease is an illness of uncertain etiology manifested by recurrent bouts of arthritis or arthralgia associated with erythema chronicum migrans (ECM) skin lesions. The suspected etiologic agent is a penicillin-susceptible microorganism (most likey a treponemalike spirochete) transmitted by *Ixodes* spp. ticks and perhaps by other vectors. In addition to the ECM and joint abnormalities (which may occur independently), the syndrome may include headaches and stiff neck, which are associated with meningitis; neurologic deficits consistent with encephalitis or pareses of cranial or spinal nerves; and disturbances of cardiac conduction with arrythmias and other electrocardiographic changes. Occasionally, patients may have chronic arthritis following the acute illness. The diagnosis is based on recognition of the typical ECM skin lesions; an association between neurologic, cardiac, or rheumatic abnormalities; and epidemiologic evidence. Although it was first recognized in Lyme, Connecticut, the disease has been reported from at least 14 other states, grouped in three geographic areas: the East (Connecticut, Delaware, Georgia, Maryland, Massachusetts, New Jersey, New York, Pennsylvania, Rhode Island); the Midwest (Minnesota, Wisconsin); and the West (California, Nevada, Oregon). Possibly, the disease will be discovered wherever there are *Ixodes* species ticks, for example, one case was reported from Arkansas. Moreover, the illness may become manifest after travel in an endemic area. The recommmended therapy is penicillin V, 15 mg/kg body wt/day, PO, as 4 equal portions, 6 hourly, for 7 to 10 days. Patients allergic to penicillins may be treated with tetracycline given in the same dose as that recommended for penicillin V. Erythromycin is of no benefit in the treatment of Lyme disease.

Bibliography

Journals

BURGDORFER W, BARBOUR AG, HAYES SF, BENACH JL, GRUNWALDT E, DAVIS JP: Lyme disease: A tick-borne spirochetosis? Science 216:1317–1319, 1982

Centers for Disease Control: Lyme disease: United States, 1980. Morbid Mortal Week Rep 30:489–497, 1981

Lyme disease. Morbid Mortal Week Rep 31:367–368, 1982

STEERE AC, MALAVISTA SE, HARDIN AJ, RUDDY S, ASKANASE PW, ANDIMAN WA: Erythema chronicum migrans and Lyme arthritis: The enlarging clinical spectrum. Ann Intern Med 86:685–698, 1977

STEERE AC, MALAVISTA SE: Cases of Lyme disease in the United States: Locations correlated with distribution of *Ixodes dammini*. Ann Intern Med 91:730–733, 1979

GEORGE F. BROOKS
VINCENT G. PONS

152 Osteomyelitis

Osteomyelitis is a purulent inflammation of bone caused most often by bacteria and occasionally by other microorganisms. It is often described as acute or chronic. However, distinguishing between acute osteomyelitis and the more refractory, chronic form of the disease by either clinical or histologic criteria is frequently difficult. Instead, clinicians should consider whether an initial episode or a recurrent or prolonged episode is involved when diagnosing and prescribing treatment for osteomyelitis. For diagnostic and therapeutic reasons, it is important to know whether the osteomyelitis is the result of hematogenous dissemination of microorganisms or the result of secondary spread from a contiguous source such as a soft tissue infection, wound infection, or an open fracture. Similarly, the anatomic site of infection, the presence of prosthetic devices, and multiple other host factors influence the spectrum of etiologic agents as well as therapy and prognosis.

Etiology

There is no single etiology of osteomyelitis. The relative frequency of occurrence of several bacterial causes of osteomyelitis is given in Table 152-1. Acute hematogenous osteomyelitis is most commonly caused by *Staphylococcus aureus* or *Streptococcus* spp. Other bacteria such as *Pseudomonas aeruginosa* and Enterobacteriaceae also cause hematogenous osteomyelitis, often in relation to specific epidemiologic settings. Blood cultures and cultures from nonosseous sites of overt infection are often diagnostically helpful. A specific bacterial etiology can be determined in 50% to 80% of patients with acute hematogenous osteomyelitis, depending upon the clinical–epidemiologic setting.

Osteomyelitis secondary to contiguous infections or trauma and chronic osteomyelitis yield *Staphylococcus aureus* in about 80% of patients. However, cultures frequently yield other aerobic or anaerobic bacteria, and mixed infections are common, particularly when anaerobes are present. Infections associated with prosthetic joints commonly yield *Staphylococcus aureus, Staphylococcus epidermidis,* and diphtheroids. However, gram-negative bacilli and many other organisms may also cause infection in this setting.

Epidemiology

Age is an important determinant of the etiology of osteomyelitis. Staphylococci are the most common causes of osteomyelitis in infants. However, infants are very susceptible to infections with gram-negative enteric bacilli and group B streptococci. Prior to 6 months of age bacteremia with these organisms followed by osteomyelitis is a common sequence of events. From infancy to about 5 years of age, *Haemophilus influenzae* commonly causes bacteremia but infrequently causes osteomyelitis.

Acute, hematogenous staphylococcal osteomyelitis occurs most frequently in late childhood and at the time of puberty (Fig. 152-1). In adults, acute hematogenous osteomyelitis caused by staphylococci is relatively uncommon when compared to the frequency of staphylococcal bacteremia. In about 50% of the patients with hematogenous staphylococcal osteomyelitis, there is a recognizable, preceding focus of infection, often furunculosis. The carrier state and other ecologic factors that affect staphylococcal epidemiology also may play a role in determining the incidence of osteomyelitis (Chap. 101, Staphylococcal Skin Infections and Glomerulonephritis). The common sources for bacteremias that lead to osteomyelitis are infections involving the skin, the respiratory tract, and the genitourinary tract.

In young adults, other epidemiologic factors are important. Persons who self-administer drugs by in-

Table 152-1. Relative Frequency of Bacterial Causes of Osteomyelitis

Aerobic Isolates	(%)	Anaerobic Isolates	(%)
Staphylococcus aureus	60	*Bacteroides* spp.	35–40
Streptococcus spp.	10	*B. melaninogenicus* (15)	
Enterobacteriaceae	20	*B. fragilis* (5–10)	
Proteus spp. (8)		Other *Bacteroides* spp. (15)	
Escherichia coli (6)		*Peptococcus* spp.	35–40
Klebsiella spp. (< 5)		*Peptostreptococcus* spp.	10
Enterobacter spp. (< 5)		*Fusobacterium* spp.	10
Salmonella spp. (< 5)		Others	10
Pseudomonas spp.	5		
Others	<5		

travenous injection are particularly prone to infections of the spine and sternoclavicular joint caused by *P. aeruginosa.* Sickle cell disease and sickle cell trait are conducive to salmonellal osteomyelitis. Puncture wounds of the feet are often associated with pseudomonal osteomyelitis.

Many factors other than age affect the development of osteomyelitis. Malignant neoplastic disease, particularly when the hematopoietic–lymphoreticular system is involved, is an example. Bacteremias occur more frequently in such immunocompromised hosts, and dissemination to bone increases correspondingly. Similarly, bone infections caused by *Aspergillus* and *Candida* spp. are increased in this group of patients. Infections of the genitourinary tract may spread to the spine through connecting venous plexuses. In patients with diabetes mellitus and peripheral vascular disease, osteomyelitis may occur in the distal extremities, though the infections are most often staphylococcal, there is also a high incidence of infection with the Enterobacteriaceae, particularly *Proteus* spp., and with anaerobic bacteria (Fig. 152-2). *Bacteroides melaninogenicus* and other anaerobes are frequently found in osteomyelitis of the mandible or other bones of the face or head, especially when the osteomyelitis is associated with oral or dental infections.

Early postsurgery prosthetic joint infections are generally complications of the surgical procedure, whereas late prosthetic infections are more likely to be associated with bacteremia. In the late infections, the cause of bacteremia frequently provides a clue to the etiology of the bone and prosthetic joint infection.

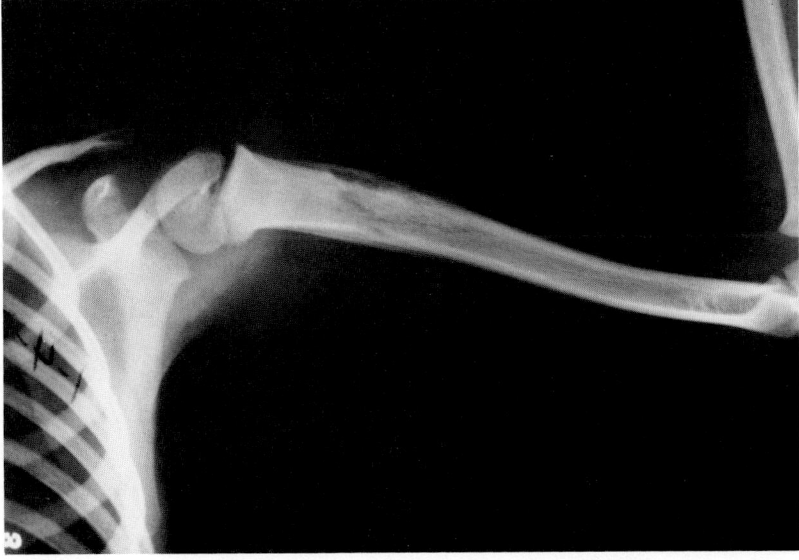

Fig. 152-1. Roentgenogram of the left humerus in an 11-year-old boy with chronic staphylococcal (*Staphylococcus aureus*) osteomyelitis from a hematogenous source. A permeative pattern of the diaphysis with laminated periostitis is present as well as a small sinus tract. (Courtesy of Clyde A. Helmes, M.D., Assistant Professor, Department of Radiology, University of California, San Francisco, CA)

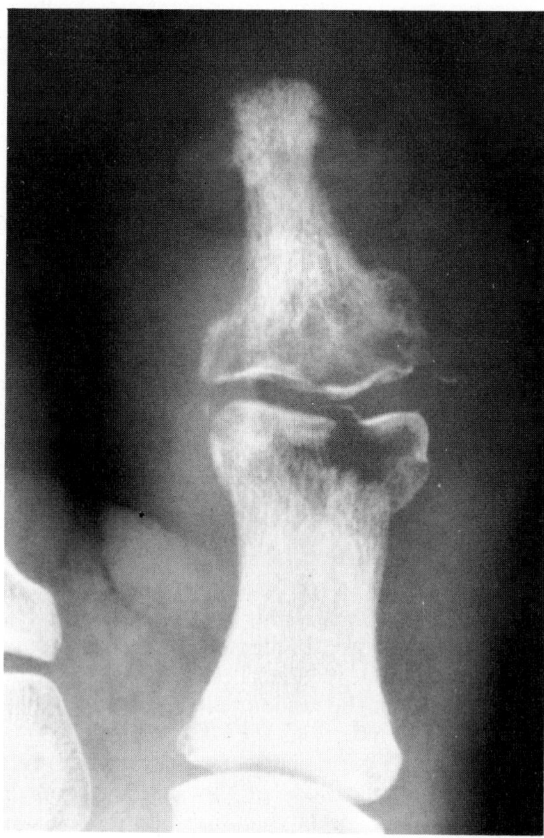

Fig. 152-2. Magnification roentgenogram of multiple organism osteomyelitis in the great toe of a 35-year-old woman with diabetes and ulceration of the foot. Soft-tissue swelling was present. Cortical destruction of bone and subarticular collapse of the joint are present. (Courtesy of Clyde A. Helmes, M.D., Assistant Professor, Department of Radiology, University of California, San Francisco, CA)

Overall, osteomyelitis occurs more often in males than in females by a 7:3 predominance. Characteristically, a single bone is involved; bones of the lower extremity are afflicted three times as often as those of the upper extremity (Fig. 152-3). There is a history of recent trauma to the area of infection in about 25% of the patients.

Pathogenesis and Pathology

Hematogenous osteomyelitis in children at or before puberty characteristically involves the metaphysis of a long bone. The nutrient arteries to the metaphysis enter into large sinusoids near the zone of epiphyseal growth. Here blood flow is sluggish, and the lining lacks functionally active phagocytic cells. Trauma may cause focal hemorrhage, further sheltering bacteria from the body's defense mechanisms. The host responds to the presence of bacteria with a local increase in vascular permeability, resulting in edema, increased vascularity, and the influx of polymorphonuclear leukocytes. Pressure increases as pus collects and is confined within rigid bone. Exudation through Volkman's canals and the haversian canal affords little relief, although the relatively inelastic periosteum may become elevated. The blood supply to the area of involvement is decreased secondary to the pressure; necrosis of the infected bone may result in the formation of a sequestrum. A protein-rich liquid containing inflammatory cells may collect in an adjacent joint. Such effusions are sterile. The actual extension of infection into the joint space is quite unusual because it requires dissection of pus under the periosteum into the joint space. The hip or the shoulder are the joints most frequently infected by extension of osteomyelitis.

After the vascular supply to the involved area has been interrupted and necrosis has occurred, the chronic phase of osteomyelitis is established. The residual dead bone acts as a foreign body, making the eradication of bacteria impossible until the sequestrum is removed.

If the affected area become well demarcated and the infection is contained, the acute inflammatory process may subside, leaving a subperiosteal accumulation of pus which may be discovered by tenderness on palpation. This relatively quiescent form of subperiosteal infection is called a Brodie's abscess (Fig. 152-4). After some time, there is deposition of new bone, the involucrum, under the elevated periosteum.

In osteomyelitis of the spine, infection most often involves the vertebral body. It spreads readily through the anastomotic venous system to adjacent ligaments and vertebral bodies. Thus, it is common for more than one vertebral body to be involved. Pus may accumulate between the vertebral periosteum and dura mater, forming an extradural abscess. Compression of the spinal cord may result, yielding a paraplegia. If a subdural abscess ruptures into the subarachnoid space, meningitis results.

Manifestations

Acute hematogenous osteomyelitis is often preceded by the signs and symptoms of bacteremia. This phase of the illness may last for several days, extending almost to the time that inflammation and pain in the bone appear. Anorexia, irritability, malaise, and fever

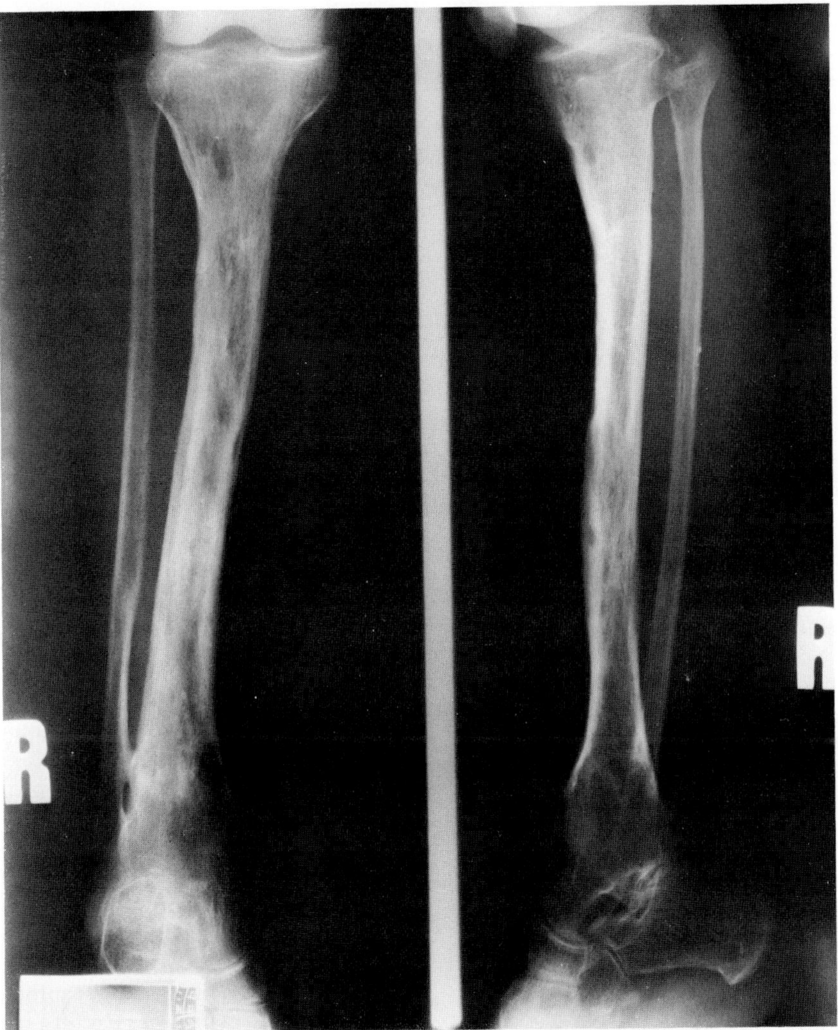

Fig. 152-3. Roentgenogram of a chronic osteomyelitis of the tibia in a 64-year-old woman demonstrating mixed lytic and sclerotic changes with benign thickened periostitis. The tibial-talar joint is fused. Numerous sinus tracts are present. The osteomyelitis developed as a consequence of a contiguous infection from a soft-tissue injury. (Courtesy of Clyde A. Helmes, M.D., Assistant Professor, Department of Radiology, University of California, San Francisco, CA)

that may be as high as 40.6°C (105°F) are present during the acute phase. In infants and children, the clinical onset of involvement of a bone may cause restricted motion of the extremity, resulting in pseudoparalysis. The soft tissue around the inflamed bone is hyperemic, warm, edematous, and tender to touch, but in the newborn there may be a paucity of clinical findings.

In older children and adults the constitutional symptoms often are not marked. Occasionally, the first manifestation of illness are the signs and symptoms of involvement of the bone. In patients with peripheral vascular disease and ulcers of the foot that extend to bone, osteomyelitis is common even when abnormalities of the bone are not apparent on roentgenograms. Osteomyelitis resulting from direct extension of a decubitus ulcer, wound infection, or open fracture may be difficult to detect clinically before the infection has become established as a chronic osteomyelitis. In patients with vertebral oste-

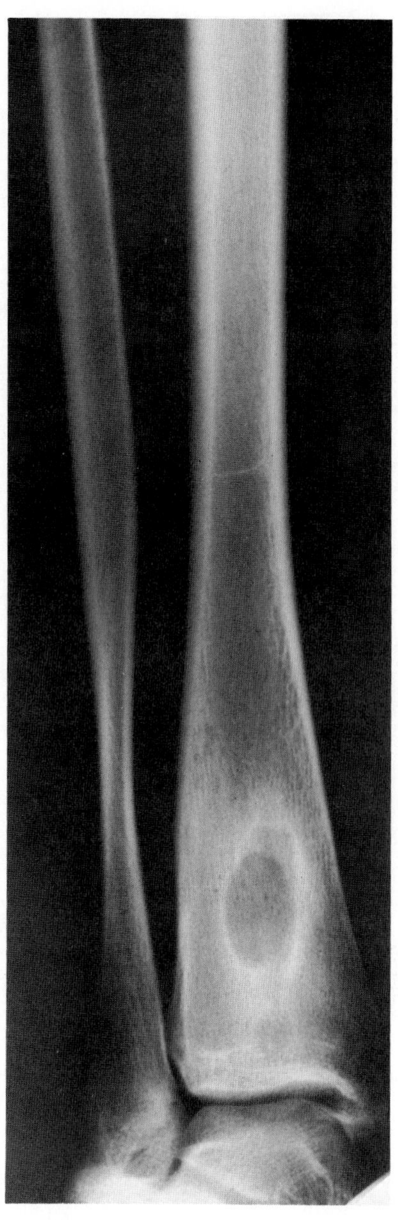

Fig. 152-4. Roentgenogram of the distal tibia in a 16-year-old woman demonstrating a lytic lesion with well-defined sclerotic margins characteristic of a Brodie's abscess. (Courtesy of Clyde A. Helmes, M.D., Assistant Professor, Department of Radiology, University of California, San Francisco, CA)

omyelitis, back pain is often the only manifestation. Fever, if present, is usually mild.

Tuberculous and fungal osteomyelitis are usually associated with a clinical course that is more insidious and chronic than that of acute bacterial osteomyelitis. Low-grade fever, weight loss, anorexia, and chronic pulmonary symptoms may be prominent. Tuberculosis may involve the vertebral column, with pathologic fractures of the affected vertebrae and angular kyphosis of the spine (Pott's disease).

Diagnosis

Early recognition of osteomyelitis, before the impairment of blood flow to the involved bone leads to chronic disease, is essential to improvement of the prognosis. Patients with clinical and laboratory evidence of infections must be examined carefully for the presence of bone pain, soft tissue swelling, and limited motions of the extremities. If roentgenographically diagnostic changes are awaited, the process will often have progressed to chronic osteomyelitis.

Febrile illnesses with bone, joint, or soft tissue manifestations may mimic osteomyelitis. Severe pain and limitation of the motion of joints may occur in rheumatic fever. However, there is no bone tenderness, in contrast to acute osteomyelitis. In acute monoarthric rheumatoid arthritis, the major swelling and tenderness is limited to the joint, without focal tenderness on palpation over the adjacent metaphysis. Tenderness of the bone in an apparently paralyzed extremity indicates osteomyelitis rather than another process such as poliomyelitis.

Joints affected by septic arthritis (Chap. 151, Septic Arthritis) are exquisitely tender and painful, whereas the swollen joint associated with osteomyelitis may be gently manipulated through a limited range of motion. Bacterial cellulitis causes warmth, erythema, pain, and edema of the soft tissue, but it is usually more clearly demarcated than the soft tissue reaction to underlying osteomyelitis. It may be difficult to distinguish osteomyelitis associated with sickle cell crisis from the underlying disease itself.

Roentgenographic abnormalities of the bone may be helpful in confirming the presence of infection. In children, the characteristic roentgenographic changes in the bone may be apparent as early as 5 to 6 days after onset. In adults, 2 to 3 weeks is the usual minimum period, although periosteal elevation may be detected somewhat earlier. Occasionally, a period of 1 to 2 months is required before changes are evident. As a result, it is often necessary to make a presumptive diagnosis of osteomyelitis when there is soft tissue infection or ulceration that in itself could be responsible for the clinical findings (pus, draining sinuses). In these circumstances, the diagnosis of infection of the bone may not be established until changes are evident in bone scans or roentgenograms. In granulomatous osteomyelitis as caused by tubercle bacilli and fungi, the roentgenographic evidence of osteomyelitis may provide the initial indication of bone infection. When several bones are apparently involved simultaneously, a specific etiology of the osteomyelitis such as *Salmonella* spp. or *Cryptococcus neoformans* must be strongly suspected.

Radionuclide bone scanning is more sensitive than conventional roentgenography in the early detection of osteomyelitis; it is also useful in detecting osteomyelitis at clinically unsuspected sites. Abnormalities of blood flow in osteomyelitis usually precede radiographically evident bone changes; however, similar changes in blood flow occur in soft tissue infections such as cellulitis, and when bones are involved with neoplasms, sickle cell disease, and Paget's disease. Comparison of scans taken immediately after injection of a radionuclide and later may help in differentiation or in determining whether chronic changes are caused by active or inactive infection of the bone. Computed tomographic (CT) scans may be especially useful in the detection of abscesses associated with osteomyelitis of the spine or other bones and may prove useful in defining the full extent of the disease. Additionally, ^{67}Ga scans may be useful diagnostic adjuncts. Figure 152-5 illustrates the use of roentgenograms and scans in the diagnosis of osteomyelitis.

In patients with signs suggestive of osteomyelitis and positive bone scans, with or without roentgenographic changes, a surgical procedure is often necessary to establish the correct diagnosis. Specimens for aerobic and anaerobic cultures should be collected and transported directly to the laboratory. Some neoplasms (*e.g.,* eosinophilic granuloma) may be difficult to differentiate from osteomyelitis at the time of surgery, illustrating the need for routine submission of portions of surgical specimens for both culture and histologic examination. In vertebral osteomyelitis and in possible disc space infections a needle aspiration and biopsy should be done for diagnosis.

In patients with chronic, recurrent osteomyelitis, antimicrobial therapy is dictated by the microorganisms present within the infected bone. Cultures of drainage from the sinus tracts often yield bacteria that are not present in the bone and also may fail to yield all of the causes of mixed infections. Thus, in patients with chronic osteomyelitis, cultures of superficial drainage should be used only as rough guidelines for initial therapy. Definitive antimicrobial therapy usually depends on the results of cultures of specimens of infected bone and exudate obtained by needle aspiration or surgical biopsy.

The erythrocyte sedimentation rate (ESR) is often very high in osteomyelitis, although it returns to normal with effective therapy. Therefore, it is not specifically helpful in diagnosis, but is useful in determining the activity of the infection. However, it should be recognized that the ESR may remain slightly elevated even when the osteomyelitis is cured.

The diagnosis of infection associated with a prosthetic joint may be difficult. In general, pain referred to the region of the joint is the primary clinical symptom. Fever and chills are usually lacking, although leukocytosis and an elevated ESR suggest the presence of active infection. The infected prostheses usually fail: loosening of both the femoral and acetabular components in total hip arthroplasties are often demonstrable. An arthrocentesis and arthrogram with smear and culture of the synovial fluid is essential. Purulent fluid wth microorganisms identified by gram stain or culture is diagnostic of infection. However, it must be noted that in many instances failure and loosening of prostheses are not due to infection. Moreover, there are instances when arthrocentesis does not yield a diagnosis of infection but infection is confirmed at the time of surgical revision of the failed arthroplasty. At surgical operation, specimens for culture and histopathology should include granulation tissue, joint capsule, synovial fluid, and bone.

Prognosis

If acute osteomyelitis is treated promptly with appropriate antimicrobics, the infection is usually eradicated with minimal or no residual deformity; surgery should not be necessary. If treatment is delayed, avascular necrosis of the bone may occur and provide a persistent focus of infection that often cannot be cured by long-term antimicrobial therapy alone.

The metaphyses of long bones are the most common sites of osteomyelitis, and damage to the epiphyseal growth centers may lead to a shortening of the affected extremity. In a young child with osteomyelitis, even when the epiphysis is apparently destroyed by the infectious process, it may regenerate with little interruption of linear growth, providing the epiphyseal cartilage is preserved. These variables make it very difficult to predict the extent of residual damage in individual patients with osteomyelitis.

Once chronic osteomyelitis is established, the draining sinuses and external evidences of infection may be controlled by antimicrobial therapy. However, when chemotherapy is interrupted, the process usually reactivates and external drainage resumes. Systemic symptoms are unusual in chronic, draining

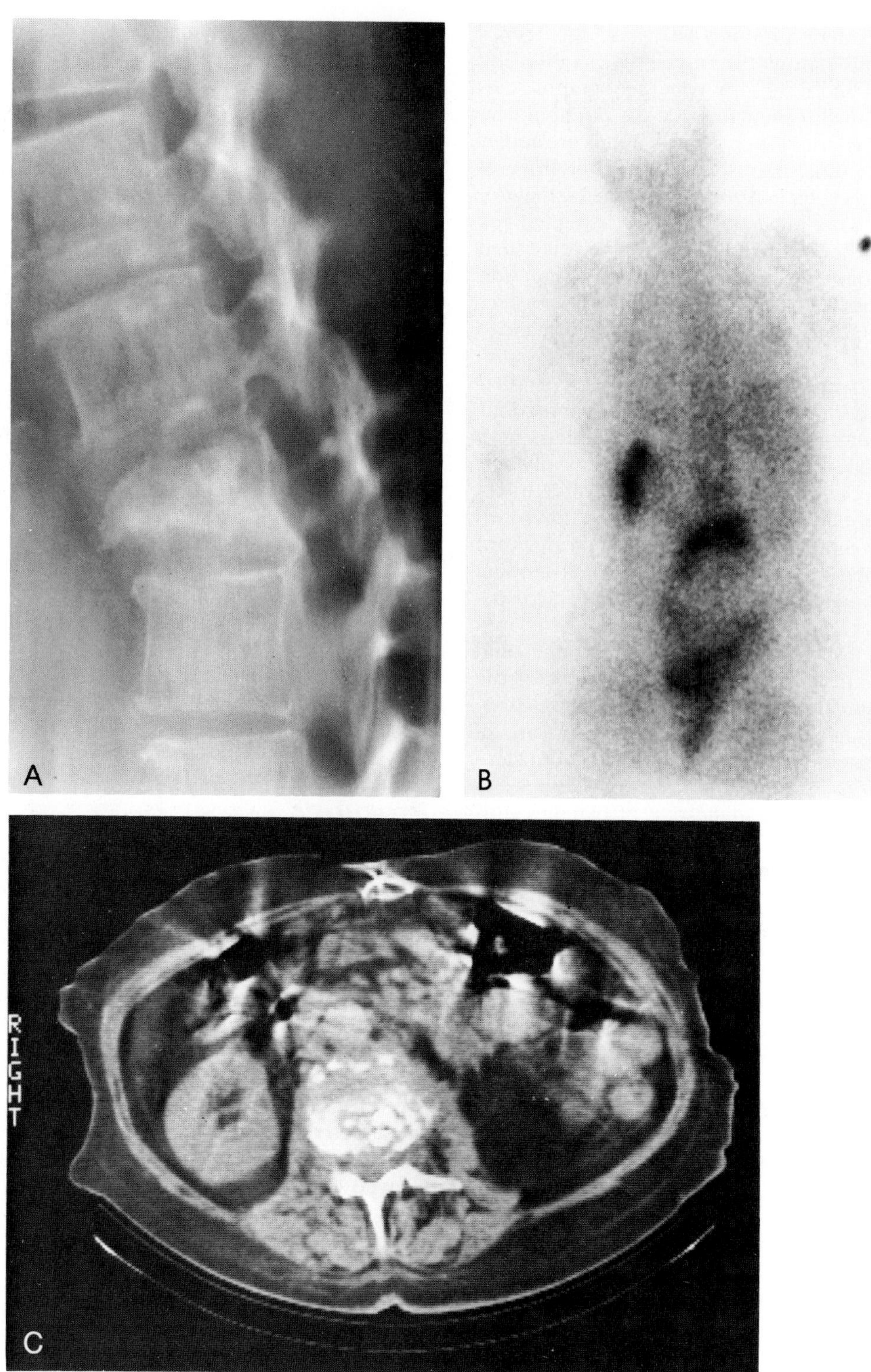
A
B
C
RIGHT

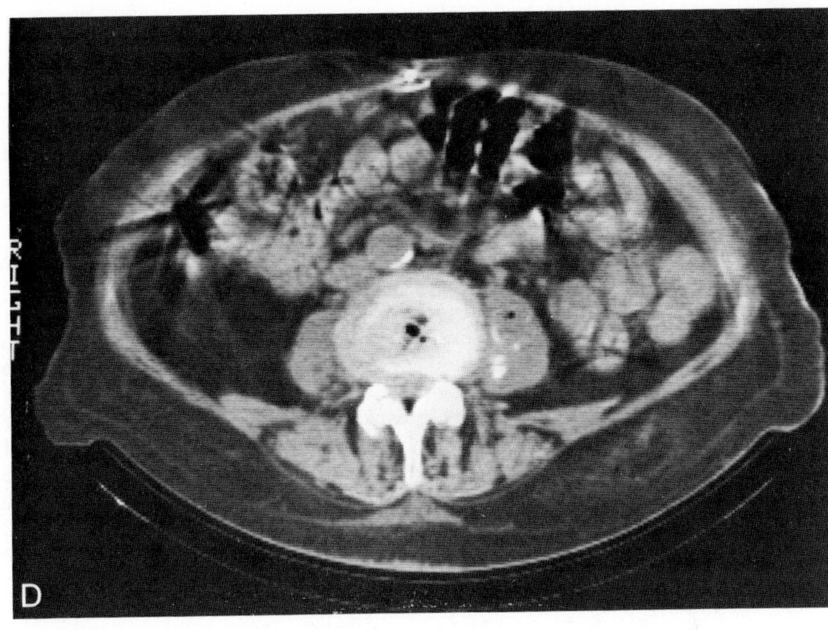

Fig. 152-5. Roentgenogram and scans from a 73-year old woman with a history highly suggestive of a recent urinary tract infection. She developed severe lumbar pain and fever. Blood cultures were positive for *Escherichia coli.* (*A*) Roentgenogram showing marked destruction of the second lumbar vertebra. (*B*) A ^{67}Ga scan showing normal activity in the colon, bone marrow, liver, and soft tissues. The area of intense activity at the L2-3 level extended to the left paraspinous area and was consistent with osteomyelitis and a paraspinous inflammatory mass. (*C*) CT body scan demonstrating marked destruction of the second lumbar vertebra. (*D*) CT body scan at the L3 level showing a left paraspinous-psoas mass containing fragment of bone and gas, consistent with destruction of bone and a gascontaining paraspinous abscess.

osteomyelitis, and metastatic spread to a new focus occurs only rarely after the chronic phase is established.

Carcinomas occasionally arise in the fistulous tracts accompanying chronic osteomyelitis, possibly as a response to chronic inflammation. This late complication of osteomyelitis should be considered whenever a soft tissue change compatible with neoplasia is noted.

Therapy

Medical

Acute bacterial osteomyelitis should be treated with parenterally administered antimicrobics. Only in this way can effective concentrations of the antimicrobial agent(s) be attained promptly and reliably in the site of the infection. Continued treatment with orally administered antimicrobics is possible and acceptable if therapeutic adequacy can be proved by assays of serum concentrations or by measuring serum bactericidal activity using the patient's infecting organism.

The appropriate duration of antimicrobial therapy cannot be determined by clinical criteria. Prompt subsidence of both systemic and local manifestations of infection is usual. The roentgenographic changes of healing osteomyelitis lag considerably behind the actual clinical situation and are of little aid in deciding when to terminate therapy. In acute osteomyelitis the continuation of antimicrobial therapy is recommended for a minimum of 4 weeks after defervescence, with surveillance during and after treatment by serial roentgenography, bone scans, and determinations of the ESR.

Acute hematogenous osteomyelitis is caused by *Staphylococcus aureus* in about 80% of patients, and cure results from the early, proper administration of an appropriate antistaphylococcal antimicrobic. Specific recommendations for the antimicrobial therapy of osteomyelitis caused by staphylococci (and other gram-positive cocci) are given in Table 152-2. Initially, a penicillinase-resistant, semisynthetic penicillin (*e.g.,* nafcillin) should be used. Subsequently, if the causative staphylococcus proves susceptible to penicillin G, therapy should be continued using penicillin G parenterally. Oral therapy with a semisynthetic penicillin or penicillin V, usually with probenicid, has been used successfully in patients in whom adequate serum bactericidal levels were obtained. Predose (trough or low-point) serum bactericidal titers of $\geq$ 1:2 and peak titers of at least 1:8 appear to correlate with effective therapy. The cephalosporanic acid derivates are the preferred alternatives in patients with hypersensitivity to penicillins. The role of oral cephalosporanic acid derivatives in the treatment of acute osteomyelitis has not been well defined. Alternatives to the β-lactam antimicrobics include vancomycin and possibly clindamycin. Bactericidal agents are preferable to bacteriostatic agents because areas of osteomyelitis are relatively

Table 152-2. Antimicrobic Therapy of Acute Osteomyelitis Caused by Gram-Positive Cocci

Primary Agent(s)	Alternate Agent(s)	Comments*
Staphylococcus aureus, *penicillinase-producing*		
Nafcillin (or oxacillin), 150–200 mg/kg body wt/day, IV, as 6 equal portions, 4-hourly (usual adult dosage, 8–12 g/day)	Cefazolin, 75–100 mg/kg body wt/day, IV, as 4 equal portions, 6-hourly (usual adult dosage, 3-6 g/day) Clindamycin, 15–20 mg/kg body wt/day, IV, as 4 equal portions, 6-hourly (usual adult dosage, 1.2–2.4 g/day) Vancomycin, 20–30 mg/kg body wt/day, IV, as 3 or 4 equal portions 8- or 6-hourly (usual adult dose 1.5–2.0 g/day)	Parenteral therapy for 4 weeks is recommended. If additional therapy is needed, the following antimicrobic regimen can be used: dicloxacillin (or cloxacillin) 50–60 mg/kg body wt/day, PO, as 4 equal portions, 6-hourly Cefazolin may be changed to cephalexin, cephradine, or cefaclor in the same dosage as that for dicloxacillin. Clindamycin may be given PO in the same dose as that given IV. Vancomycin is the drug of choice for nafcillin-resistent *S. aureus.* The dose should be adjusted to keep the concentrations in the blood between 10 μg and 30 μg/ml. With oral therapy and possibly with parenteral therapy, the lethal activity of the patient's serum for the patient's infecting bacterium should be monitored: peak serum killing dilutions of ≥1:8 and trough killing dilutions of ≥1:2 are desired. Probenecid, 25–40 mg/kg body wt/day, PO, may be used to increase antimicrobic concentrations in the serum and hence the serum bactericidal titer.
Staphylococcus aureus, *nonpenicillinase-producing*		
Penicillin G, 150–200 mg (240,000–320,000 U)/kg body wt/day, IV, as 6 equal doses, 4-hourly (usual adult dosage, 12–20 megaU)	Alternate agents as for penicillinase-producing *Staphylococcus aureus*	Following parenteral therapy if additional therapy is needed change penicillin G to penicillin V, 50–60 mg/kg body wt/day, PO, as 4 equal portions, 6-hourly.
Streptococcus pyogenes *(group A), Streptococcus pneumoniae*		
Penicillin G, 60–70 mg (95,000–120,000 U)/kg body wt/day, IV, as 6 equal portions, 4-hourly (usual adult dosage, 8–12,000,000 U/day)	Cefazolin, 25–50 mg/kg body wt/day, IV, as 4 equal portions, 6-hourly (usual adult dosage, 2–4 g/day) Clindamycin, as for nonpenicillinase-producing *Staphylococcus aureus*	IV therapy for 2–4 weeks is recommended. If an alternate route of therapy is needed, change penicillin G to either: procaine penicillin G, 0.4 g (600,000 U, IM, 8-hourly) or penicillin V, 25–30 mg/kg body wt, PO, as 4 equal doses. A total of 4 weeks of antimicrobic therapy is recommended. Cefazolin may be replaced with either cephalexin, cephradine, or cefaclor in the same dose as that for penicillin V. Clindamycin may be given PO in the same dose as that given IV.

*Loading doses of some antimicrobics should be given when patients are acutely ill and when patients have decreased renal function requiring reduced maintenance doses.

When large doses of some antimicrobics are given, large quantities of Na^+ or K^+ are also given, which may lead to dangerous accumulation in patients with renal or cardiac failure. The concentrations are as follows: Na^+—penicillin G, 2.7 mEq/g (1.7 mEq/million U); cefazolin, 2.1 mEq/g; nafcillin, 1.2 mEq/g; dicloxacillin, 0.5 mEq/g; oxacillin, 2.5 mEq/g. K^+—penicillin G, 2.7 mEq/g (1.7 mEq/million U).

isolated from phagocytes and other host defenses. Oral antimicrobic therapy has been used in the successful treatment of acute osteomyelitis in children; it is acceptable treatment only if based on documentation of attainment of adequate serum lethal activity against the patient's infecting organism.

The selection of antimicrobial agents for the treatment of osteomyelitis caused by gram-negative bacteria is more difficult. Initially, clues regarding the bacteria most likely to be responsible must be gleaned from preexisting illnesses, evident lesions, and the age of the patient. The regimen selected initially must be modified according to the results of cultures and susceptibility studies. The antimicrobial agents of preference and alternatives, according to specific bacteria, are listed in Table 152-3.

The specific treatment of tuberculous and fungal infections of the bone cannot be separated from a general approach to these infections (Chap. 34, Pulmonary Tuberculosis, and Chap. 39, Candidosis). Rickettsial osteomyelitis should respond to treatment with a tetracycline (Chap. 96, Spotted Fevers).

Nonspecific measures of treatment should not be neglected. Immobilization of the affected extremity by splinting or the application of a cast may afford relief from pain and protection from trauma. Disc space infections of the spine usually respond to antimicrobial therapy coupled with bed rest. Underlying noninfectious diseases such as diabetes mellitus may require treatment; debridement of decubitus ulcers and drainage of furuncles is often necessary.

Surgical Management

Successful management of chronic osteomyelitis requires the combination of surgical and antimicrobic therapy. The surgical considerations include full debridement and excision of all dead bone and necrotic tissue, a procedure commonly referred to as *sequestrectomy.* Depending upon the site and extent of the infection, the surgeon may either elect to leave the wound open and allow granulation to occur before covering with a split-thickness skin graft, or choose primary closure after filling the excavated space with a muscle flap or a skin flap. In general, the space resulting from excision of the infected bone should not be left open. Frequently, closed irrigation and suction of the operative site are provided by placing a sterile plastic tube system in dependent portions of the wound before closure. Antimicrobics are frequently included in the irrigation fluid. The tubes are usually

Table 152-3. *Antimicrobic Therapy of Acute Osteomyelitis Caused Gram-Negative Bacilli*

Primary Agent(s)	Alternate Agent(s)	Comments
Escherichia coli, Proteus mirablis		
Ampicillin or an acylureido-penicillin, 150–200 mg/kg body wt/day, IV, as 6 equal doses, 4-hourly (usual adult dosage, 6–9 g/day)	Cefazolin (moxalactam, cefotaxime, cefoperazone), 75–100 mg/kg body wt/day, IV, as 4 equal doses, 6-hourly (usual adult dosage, 3-6 g/day)	Parenteral therapy for at least 4 weeks minimum is recommended. If peroral therapy is to be used following parenteral therapy, the serum lethal activity should be monitored (Table 152-2). Other cephalosporins are equally effective. Factors of selection include cost, ease of administration, and adverse reactions. Some strains of *P. mirabilis* produce a β-lactamase that is active against penicillins, but relatively inactive against cephalosporins. When strains resistant to both penicillins and cefazolin are encountered, then one of the new cephalosporanic acid derivatives (*e.g.,* cefotaxime, moxalactam, cefoperazone), ureidopenicillins (*e.g.,* azlocillin), an aminocyclitol (gentamicin, tobramycin, amikacin), or chloramphenicol may be used. If peroral therapy is utilized, ampicillin or amoxicillin 50-60 mg/kg body wt/day, as 4 equal portions, 6-hourly is recommended. Cephalexin or cephradine may be used in the same dose.

Table 152-3. (continued) *Antimicrobic Therapy of Acute Osteomyelitis Caused Gram-Negative Bacilli*

Primary Agent(s)	Alternate Agent(s)	Comments
Providencia *spp.*, Klebsiella *spp.*, Enterobacter *spp.*, Serratia *spp.*		
Gentamicin, tobramycin, or netilmicin, loading dose, 2.0 mg/kg, IV, followed by 1.5–1.7 mg/kg body wt/every 8 hours *Possibly with* Ticarcillin or an acylureido-penicillin, 200–250 mg/kg/day, IV, as 6 equal portions, 4-hourly	Chloramphenicol, 50–75 mg/kg body wt/day, IV, or IM, as 4 equal portions, 6-hourly (usual adult dosage, 2–4 g/day) Cefoxitin (cefamandole, moxalactam, cefotaxime, cefoperazone), 50–100 mg/kg body wt/day, IV, as 4 equal portions, 6-hourly	Carbenicillin usually is not effective against *Klebsiella* spp. Addition of carbenicillin to an amino-cyclitol should take into account the clinical setting and laboratory evaluation of the synergistic or additive potential of the combination. Susceptibility testing of the infecting organism is essential to selection of antimicrobic(s) for therapy. Gentamicin and tobramycin are similar in antibacterial effectiveness and in pharmacokinetics. Potentially, both are nephrotoxic and ototoxic (as is amikacin). These complications may be reduced by periodically monitoring blood concentrations and giving doses that yield trough and peak serum concentrations of 2 and 10 μg/ml for gentamicin and tobramycin. Peroral chloramphenicol may be given in the same dose as injected. Bone marrow suppression is a hazard in the use of chloramphenicol. In prematures and infants under 1 week of age, the dose of chloramphenicol should not exceed 25 mg/kg body wt/day.
Salmonella *spp.*		
Chlorampenicol, dosage as above	Ampicillin, dosage as above. Trimethoprim–sulfamethoxazole, one tablet (400 mg SMZ, 80 mg TMP), PO, 6-hourly	The efficacy of chloramphenicol, ampicillin and trimethoprim–sulfamethoxazole for *Salmonella* spp. is very similar. The optimal drug should be picked using data from susceptibility tests, history of allergy, and consideration of side-effects of long-term therapy.
Pseudomonas Aeruginosa		
Gentamicin, tobramycin, or netilmicin dosage as above *Plus* Ticarcillin or an acylureido-pencillin, dosage as above	Amikacin, 7.5 mg/kg body wt, IV, as a loading dose followed by 5 mg/kg body wt, IV, every 12 hours Polymixin B, loading dose, 1 mg/kg body wt, IV, followed by 2.5 mg/kg body wt/day, as 3 equal portions, 8-hourly	Susceptibility tests should be done with *Pseudomonas aeruginosa* to assist in choice of the optimal drug(s) for therapy. Polymixin B should be given by slow injection, *e.g.,* about 4 hours/dose. Rapid administration may be associated with paresthesias.
Bacteroides fragilis, Bacteroides melaninogenicus		
Clindamycin, 15–20 mg/kg body wt/day, IV, as 4 equal portions, 6-hourly	Chloramphenicol, dosage as above Metronidazole, 20–40 mg/kg body wt/day, PO, as 4 equal portions, 6-hourly (usual adult dosage, 2 g/d)	Almost all strains of *B. fragilis* and as many as two-thirds of *B. melaninogenicus* produce β-lactamases and may not be killed by penicillin G.

left in place for 1 to 2 weeks after surgery, with irrigation–suction. This adjunctive therapy may increase the success in treatment of chronic osteomyelitis. Potential hazards of the tube system include superinfection and systemic absorption of toxic antimicrobics. Parenteral antimicrobics remain a mainstay of treatment. There are few data to indicate the optimal duration of parenteral therapy in chronic osteomyelitis after surgery has been completed. In general, at least 4 weeks of parenteral therapy is recommended, followed by several weeks to months of peroral therapy.

Management of osteomyelitis in the presence of internal devices used to stabilize a fractured bone is a difficult problem. In general, whenever an open fracture occurs, early debridement of the area, including the bone and any hardware or grafted bone used for the stabilization of the fracture, with prompt use of antimicrobics, should help to avoid the onset of deep wound infection. However, once deep infection is established, certain principles need to be followed in the approach to the therapy. Despite the presence of infection, stabilization of the fracture with bony union is the primary goal. Usually, metal plates, rods, or pins should be left in place until union occurs. The infection should be suppressed with appropriate antimicrobic therapy during this time. Later, once bony fusion has been established, the internal fixation devices may be removed and multiple cultures obtained. Debridement of infected tissue and definitive antimicrobic therapy for the infection may then be pursued. Use of a muscle flap may enhance the possibility of cure.

However, the presence of infection may impede the process of fusion. If fusion does not occur, if the internal fixation device does not provide adequate stabilization, or if evident sepsis persists despite antimicrobial therapy, the hardware should be removed and surgical debridement should be carried out. External fixation devices or a modified fracture stabilization device may be applied; antimicrobics (parenteral followed by peroral) should be given according to the results of cultures and susceptibility testing of isolates from the specimens taken at debridement.

Management of infections complicating prosthetic joints pose special problems. An early postoperative infection in the surgical wound or in a deep tissue space should be approached vigorously with debridement, excision of infected tissue, and in some cases closure over tubes for irrigation with antimicrobics and suction drainage. If infection becomes established in the prosthesis, joint space, and bone, there are several therapeutic alternatives. In gross infection associated with loosening of the prosthesis, especially with *Staphylococcus aureus* or gram-negative bacilli, total excision of the infected device and debridement of the bone are recommended. The wound is then closed over a tube irrigation–suction system. Prolonged intravenous antimicrobic therapy is given and followed by prolonged oral antimicrobial therapy for a total duration of several months. Replacement arthroplasty can be considered 6 to 12 months later, after completion of antimicrobic therapy and follow-up arthrocentesis with negative cultures. Infrequently, immediate replacement of the infected prosthesis is considered as a single-step procedure; however, the rate of relapse of infection is higher than that associated with the two-step procedure outlined above. The virulence of the infecting organism may be a major factor in the success of immediate replacement of an infected prosthesis. For example, the prognosis is better when *Staphylococcus epidermidis* or diphtheroids cause the infection. If infection of an arthroplasty is confirmed by arthrocentesis or at surgery but the components are not loose, it may be reasonable to leave the prosthesis in place, fully debride any infected tissue, and attempt salvage of the infected prosthesis by the use of the closed irrigation–suction system and prolonged antimicrobial therapy.

Prevention

The prevention of hematogenous osteomyelitis lies in the prevention of bacteremia. The adequate treatment of furunculosis and urinary tract infections should reduce the risk of dissemination of bacteria to the bones. The prophylactic use of antimicrobics may decrease the incidence of surgery-related osteomyelitis and arthritis to patients who require orthopedic surgery, particularly if prosthetic joints are installed.

In soft tissue infections or contaminated open fractures, local cleansing of the wound, debridement, drainage, and the use of antimicrobics also may help prevent subsequent osseous infections. If decubiti are treated effectively while still superficial, the complication of osteomyelitis should be entirely preventable.

Remaining Problems

Serologic tests have proved useful in the diagnosis of infections caused by *Staphylococcus aureus* and other organisms. However, most of these tests measure antibodies directed against the infecting agents, and therefore several weeks may pass after the onset of infection before the tests are positive. Also, the tests are not specific for the diagnosis of osteomyelitis, and careful clinical correlation is required to confirm a diagnosis.

Although the concentrations of antimicrobics in bone have been measured for many drugs, the results often do not correlate with clinical usefulness. Further investigation is warranted to overcome problems such as affinity of binding, extraction techniques, the presence of blood-borne drug, and the effect of polymorphonuclear cells.

Animal models that use the injection of sclerosing agents to support the development of chronic osteomyelitis are not directly comparable to human infections. However, the animal models of osteomyelitis allow the study of antimicrobial regimens, particularly combinations of drugs, and may rationalize the selection of regimens for clinical study in humans.

Hyperbaric oxygen may have a role in the treatment of osteomyelitis, but there is no definitive information in humans clearly indicating it is beneficial. In the animal model, hyperbaric oxygen alone has yielded as good a therapeutic success as antimicrobial therapy, an interesting observation, but not directly applicable to humans.

The therapy of osteomyelitis often requires prolonged administration of antimicrobics. The development of systems for the intravenous administration of antimicrobics to patients at home could provide improved therapy and prognosis at greatly reduced cost.

Bibliography

Book

WALDVOGEL, FA, MEDOFF G, SWARTZ MN: Osteomyelitis Springfield, Ill, Charles C Thomas, 1971, 110 pp.

Journals

BELL SM: Further observations on the value of oral penicillins in chronic staphylococcal osteomyelitis. Med J Aust 2:591–593, 1976

BURTON DS, SCHURMAN DJ: Salvage of infected total joint replacements. Arch Surg 112:574–578, 1977

CLAWSON DK, DAVIS FJ, HANSEN SJ JR.: Treatment of chronic osteomyelitis with emphasis on closed suction-irrigation technic. Clin Orthop 96:88–97, 1973

DICH VQ, NELSON JD, HALTALIN KC: Osteomyelitis in infants and children. Am J Dis Child 129:1273–1278, 1975

DUSZYNSKI DO, KUHN JP, AFSHANI E, RIDDLESBERGER MM: Early radionuclide diagnosis of acute osteomyelitis. Radiology 117:337–340, 1975

FITZGERALD RH, NOLAN DR, ILSTRUP DM, VAN SCOY RE, WASHINGTON JA, CONVENTRY MB: Deep wound sepsis following total hip arthroplasty. J Bone Joint Surg (Am) 59:847–855, 1977

HORWITZ T: Surgical treatment of chronic osteomyelitis complicating fractures: A study of 50 patients. Clin Orthop 96:118–128, 1973

HORWITZ T: Surgical treatment of chronic osteomyelitis complicating fractures: 6 year interim follow-up. Clin Orthop 114:207–208, 1976

HUNTER GA: The results of reinsertion of a total hip prosthesis after sepsis. J Bone Joint Surg (Br) 61:422–423, 1979

KELLY PJ, MARTIN WJ, CONVENTRY MB: Chronic osteomyelitis. II. Treatment with closed irrigation and suction. JAMA 213:1843–1848, 1970

LEWIS RP, SUTTER VL, FINEGOLD SM: Bone infections involving anaerobic bacteria. Medicine 57:279–305, 1978

MACAUSLAND WR, EATON RJ: The management of sepsis following intramedullary fixation of fractures of the femur. J Bone Joint Surg (Am) 45:1643–1653, 1963

MACKOWIACK PA, JONES SR, SMITH JW: Diagnostic value of sinus-tract cultures in chronic osteomyelitis. JAMA 239:2772–2775, 1978

MAY JW JR, GALLICO GG III, LUKASH FN: Microvascular transfer of free tissue for closure of bone wounds of the distal lower extremity. N. Engl J Med 306:253–257, 1982

MEYER S, WEILAND AJ, WILLENEGGER H: The treatment of infected non-union of fractures of long bones. J Bone Joint Surg (Am) 57:836–842, 1975

OVERTON LM, TULLY WP: Surgical treatment of chronic osteomyelitis in long bones. Am J Surg 126:736–741, 1973

PROBER CG, YEAGER AS: Use of the serum bactericidal titer to assess the adequacy of oral antibiotic therapy in the treatment of acute hematogenous osteomyelitis. J Pediatr 95:131–135, 1979

SAPICO FL, MONTGOMERIE JZ: Pyogenic vertebral osteomyelitis: Report of nine cases and review of the literature. Rev Infect Dis 1:754–776, 1979

SAPICO FL, MONTGOMERIE JZ: Vertebral osteomyelitis in intravenous drug abusers: Report of three cases and review of the literature. Rev Infect Dis 2:196–206, 1980

SHANNON JG, WOOLHOUSE FM, EISINGER PJ: The treatment of chronic osteomyelitis by saucerization and immediate skin grafting. Clin Orthop 96:98–107, 1973

SIMPSON MB, MERZ WG, KULINSKI JP, SOLOMON MH: Opportunistic mycotic osteomyelitis: Bone infections due to *Aspergillus* and *Candida* species. Medicine 56:475–482, 1977

TETZLAFF TR, MCCRACKEN GF, NELSON JD: Oral antibiotic therapy for skeletal infections of children. II. Therapy of osteomyelitis and suppurative arthritis. J Pediatr 92:485–490, 1978

WALDOVOGEL FA, MEDOFF G, SWARTZ MN: Osteomyelitis: A review of clinical features, therapeutic considerations and unusual aspects. N Engl J Med 282:198–206, 260–266, 316–322, 1970

WALDOVOGEL FA, VASEY H: Osteomyelitis: The past decade. N Engl J Med 303:360–370, 1980

WEST WF, KELLY PJ, MARTIN WJ: Chronic osteomyelitis. I. Factors affecting the results of treatment in 186 patients. JAMA 213:1837–1842, 1970

JOHN P. UTZ

153

Mycetoma

Mycetoma is a local, chronic, and progressive infectious disease of the skin, subcutaneous tissues, and bone. It is characterized by swelling that is often grotesque and disfiguring and by multiple sinus tracts that drain granule-containing pus. A variety of fungi and bacteria can cause mycetoma.

Etiology

At least 20 species of actinomycetes and higher fungi can cause mycetomas. Those most frequently encountered include bacteria of the order Actinomycetales, *Nocardia brasiliensis* and *Actinomadura (Nocardia) madurae* (Chap. 37), Nocardiosis), and the fungi *Madurella mycetomi, Phialophora jeanselmi,* and *Petriellidium boydii*. The latter microorganism is the most common cause of the disease in the United States. Recently, the dematophyte *Microsporin audouinii* was shown to be causative. Algae (*Prototheca* spp.) have also been implicated.

Petriellidium boydii grows on culture mediums as dark gray colonies. Microscopically, the identifying features are 5 μm × 10 μm spores (conidia) and oval, fruiting bodies (ascocarp) that are 100 μm long. The ascocarps rupture at maturity, releasing ascospores that are pointed at both ends and resemble conidia in size (Fig. 153-1).

Epidemiology

Mycetoma is worldwide in distribution, but the strikingly increased frequency and historic importance of the disease in Madura province, India, have resulted in the common use of *Madura foot* and *maduramycosis* as synonyms for the disease. However, the Sudan in Africa is apparently the area in which the greatest number of cases have been reported. In the Sudan, there is a rainy season of approximately 3 months and a dry season thereafter. Virtually all cases have been reported from tropic or temperate regions. *Petriellidium boydii* has been isolated frequently from soil in the eastern, central, and northern United States.

Pathogenesis and Pathology

The frequency of disease in the foot, the common custom of walking barefoot in tropic areas, and the recovery of so many of the causative microorganisms from the soil suggest that the disease is acquired from traumatic implantation in the skin. Such implantation is presumed to be followed by the multiplication and production in tissues of colonies (granules) of the etiologic agent. On microscopic examination, such granules are covered with an eosinophilic protein material, discernible most clearly at the periphery, which represents tissue reaction by the host. In the immediate area, the tissue reaction is characteristically suppurative, but at the periphery there may be granulomas and giant cells. Rarely, infection seems to spread through the lymphatics or bloodstream to other sites.

Manifestations

The most common site of involvement is the foot (Fig. 153-2). However, lesions are also seen on the shoulders of laborers who carry burdens or on the hand, buttocks, or back, where there is opportunity for implantation from soil or thorns. As indicated by the name of the disease, the characteristic findings are swelling and tumefaction. The deformity frequently results in some degree of disability, with hobbling or the need for crutches. A second characteristic is draining sinuses; the presence of granules in the pus is the third element of the triad of characteristics.

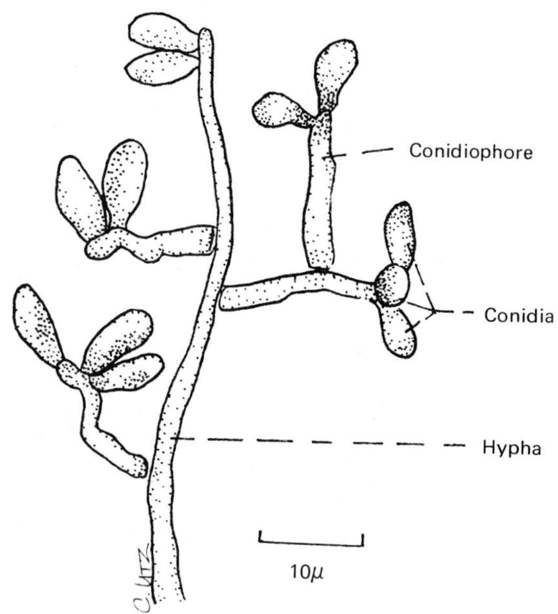

Fig. 153-1. Diagrammatic representation of the microscopic appearance of *Petriellidium boydii.*

It is surprising that in spite of subcutaneous and bone involvement, pain is relatively rare and characteristically transient. Such general manifestations of infection as fever, chills, sweats, and weight loss are rarely encountered. Lymphadenopathy is rare.

Diagnosis

The diagnosis is generally apparent from the appearance of the lesion itself. However, an etiologic diagnosis is usually established by finding granules in unstained tissue sections or in pus. The granules of *M. mycetomi, Madurella grisea, Phialophora jeanselmi* are brown to black, whereas those of *Petriellidium boydii, A. madurae,* and *N. brasiliensis* are white to yellow.

Biopsy material is preferred for culture because superficial scrapings or swabs are almost always contaminated with less pathogenic bacteria or fungi. Reliance solely on the use of culture mediums rendered selective by the addition of antimicrobics is not advisable. If cycloheximide is included, *Petriellidium boydii* will be inhibited, and if either chloramphenicol or neomycin is included, *N. brasiliensis* may be inhibited. However, in many instances it is difficult, if not impossible, to isolate a fungus unless some mediums are employed that include antibacterial agents.

Occasionally, lesions of the feet or other sites are encountered from which only bacteria (notably, *Staphylococcus* spp. and *Streptococcus* spp.) can be cultured. Such disease has occasionally been called by the atrocious term *botryomycosis.* On those rare occasions when lesions due to chronic filariasis (elephantiasis) become secondarily infected and drain transiently, this disease may mimic mycetoma.

Prognosis

The course of the disease is chronic and progressive. In late stages, the lesions may be partially disabling, but death from mycetoma alone is rare.

Therapy

The wide variety of microorganisms that is typically recovered precludes generalities about chemotherapy. *Petriellidium boydii* is generally resistant to amphotericin B, but there are reports of the efficacy of estrogens, both experimentally and in patients. *Nocardia* spp. are susceptible to sulfonamides. Some strains of *M. mycetomi* have been reported to be susceptible to concentrations of amphotericin B in the range that might be obtained in serum. Griseofulvin is somewhat less active *in vitro* and has been less successful in the few patients treated with it. Testing *in vitro* and limited, preliminary experience in humans suggest that ketoconazole may be helpful.

Excision or debridement is not usually efficacious. Radical measures, such as amputation, have been more successful.

Prevention

More widespread use of shoes or other protective clothing would logically seem to be important prophylactic measures in areas where disease is frequently encountered.

Control of the causative microorganisms in soil has not been shown to be either helpful or feasible. Because mycetoma can be caused by a wide variety of microorganisms, the development of vaccines would not be warranted, even if it were feasible.

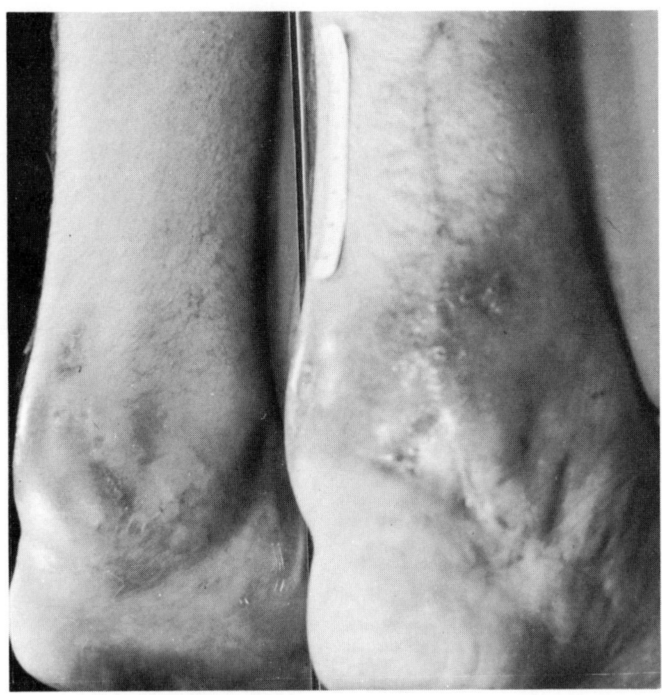

Fig. 153-2. Lateral, posterior, and medial aspects of mycetoma of the foot and ankle. On culture, *Petriellidium boydii* was isolated.

Remaining Problems

The frequency of occurrence and the disability from mycetoma in certain areas of the world warrant public health methods of prevention. However, the problems encountered in this regard seem to be socially and economically unsolvable at this time. Because virtually all children in the United States go barefoot out of doors for at least brief periods, it is reasonable to inquire why mycetoma occurs in few people in this country. The fact that a single microorganism can often be cultured consistently from mycetoma leads to the expectation that appropriate antimicrobial therapy, consistently applied for long periods, might be effective. A search for additional antifungal agents is imperative. The intriguing results obtained with estrogens experimentally and clinically need further study and confirmation.

Bibliography

Books

EMMONS CW, BINFORD CH, UTZ JP: Medical Mycology, 3rd ed. Philadelphia, Lea & Febiger, 1977. pp 389–418.

MURRAY JG: Laboratory aspects of mycetoma. In Systemic Mycoses. London, J & A Churchill, 1968. pp 78–95.

Journals

MOHR JA, MUCHMORE HG: Maduramycoses due to *Allescheria boydii.* JAMA 204:335–336, 1968

SEGRETAIN G, DESTOMBE SP: Recherche sur les mycetome à *Madurella grisea* et *Pyrenochaeta romeroi.* Sabouraudia 7:51–61, 1969

WEST BC, KWON–CHUNG KJ: Mycetoma caused by *Microsporum audouinii.* Am J Clin Pathol 73:447–454, 1980

WOLFE ID, SACKS HG, SAMORODIN CS, ROBINSON HM: Cutaneous protothecosis in a patient receiving immunosuppressive therapy. Arch Dermatol 112:824–832, 1976

Section | *XXI*

Wound Infections

Microbiota of Traumatic Wounds

Species or Group	
Bacteria	
Gram-positive cocci	**70–75***
Staphylococcus epidermidis	++; 1–7†
Staphylococcus aureus	±
Micrococcus spp.	+; 1–6
Streptococcus spp.	
viridans group	±
other, non-group A	±
Gram-positive bacilli	**65–75**
Lactobacillus spp.	± to 0
Aerobic *Corynebacterium* spp.	+; 1–7
Bacillus spp.	+; 1–7
Streptomyces spp.	± to 0
Propionobacterium acnes	± to 0
Propionobacterium spp.	+; 1–3
Clostridium perfringens	± to 0
Other *Clostridium* spp.	± to 0
Aerobic gram-negative bacilli	**20–22**
Escherichia coli	±
Enterobacter spp.	±
Serratia spp.	± to 0
Other Enterobactericeae	±
Pseudomonas spp. (not *aeruginosa*)	±
Fungi	**8–10**
non-albicans *Candida* spp.	±
Mucor spp.	± to 0
Dermatophytes	± to 0
Rhodotorula spp.	± to 0

± to 0, race; ±, irregular or uncertain (may be only pathologic); +, common; ++, prominent.

*Boldface values (*e.g.,* **30–60**) = range of incidence in percentage.

†Per gram of tissue excised at initial debridement.

F. WILLIAM BLAISDELL

Infections Following Blunt Trauma

154

Blunt trauma may result from blows, falls, crushing injuries, or accidents involving moving vehicles. Superficial abrasions, lacerations, avulsions, or the blowout of hollow organs may be produced. However, the most common result is contused injuries with tissue hemorrhage and necrosis. Largely as a consequence of our industrial society and our penchant for high-speed vehicular travel there are hundreds of thousands of cases of blunt trauma each year in the United States.

Pathogenesis and Pathology

Blunt injuries in themselves are not necessarily contaminated and therefore do not carry the same risk of infection as do penetrating injuries. However, the very nature of some injuries may facilitate the introduction of contamination. Compound fractures of the tibia and fibula secondary to a motorcycle accident are a classic example. Similarly, shearing forces in accidents can avulse or roll back the superficial layers of the skin or damage the subcutaneous tissues and may introduce foreign material and bacteria deep under the skin flap.

In most instances, blunt trauma produces relatively clean injuries in which the skin remains intact but in which there is secondary hemorrhage or devitalization of soft tissues. Blunt trauma to the head, neck, and chest rarely results in injuries that are contaminated or that are in themselves particularly vulnerable to infection. Blunt trauma to the abdomen most commonly produces injury to solid organs such as the liver, spleen, and kidneys in which there is minimal contamination; occasionally, however, disruption of loops of bowel and gross peritoneal or retroperitoneal contamination result from abdominal trauma as associated with sudden deceleration and compression of the abdomen.

Thus, in blunt injury there are two sources of bacterial contamination. The first consists of bacteria introduced from the environment. These are most often associated with disruption of the skin from shearing or avulsion injuries and compound fractures. They usually produce relatively simple infections caused by one predominant bacterium from the skin or the environment. Such infections are usually preventable.

The second source of contamination is the host—particularly, the hollow viscera of the abdomen. Most commonly, ruptures of the gastrointestinal tract are involved, and complex infections may result from both aerobic and anaerobic bowel flora. Prevention of such infections is virtually impossible, and all of the skills and judgment of the surgeon are required to minimize and contain the infection.

In addition, a new spectrum of infections complicating major injuries is emerging as better resuscitation measures and more definitive surgical treatment secures survival from previously lethal injuries. Major burn injuries and massive trauma with multi-system injuries are classic examples. These patients, despite the lack of overt contamination, develop serious infections and these infections emerge much earlier in the clinical course. It is apparent that patients are predisposed to these infections when the injury is of sufficient magnitude to overwhelm the natural defenses against infection. Despite overt contamination, diffuse peritoneal, or more commonly, pulmonary infections involving the local flora develop. The exact nature of this loss of immune competence has yet to be defined, but apparently it involves the loss of both humoral and cellular mechanisms; for example, there is loss of cutaneous reactivity to standard sensitins, depression of white cell function, and impairment of the macrophage system.

Manifestations

Manifestations of infections involving the skin and subcutaneous tissues are usually evident by the classic signs of inflammation. Streptococcal infections typically develop in the first 24 hours of injury; most remaining infections are not clinically evident for 3 to 5 days after the injury. Local signs include evidence of lymphangitis and cellulitis; systemic signs include fever and elevation of the white cell count. The onset of infections of the body cavities may be more subtle. Peritonitis secondary to a ruptured viscus usually becomes manifest within 6 to 12 hours of the loss of integrity of the gut by the development of progressive abdominal tenderness, ileus, leukocytosis, and fever. Characteristically, the patient looks extremely ill. Infections of the neck, pleural cavity, or mediastinum, although quite rare following blunt trauma, can usually be diagnosed by evidence of accumulation of pleural fluid in the chest roentgenogram and, in the case of mediastinitis, by mediastinal widening or mediastinal air. Cervical infections can be recognized by tenderness and crepitation in the tissues of the neck.

Infections in patients with critical injuries, particularly those associated with immune incompetence, may be extremely difficult to diagnose because the patient may not develop fever or leukocytosis. Inevitably, however, these infections produce local and systemic alterations in vascular permeability so that the patient manifests hypovolemia and requires increasing amounts of fluid to maintain peripheral perfusion and urine output. When a patient who has previously been in relatively stable fluid balance requires increased amounts of fluid, infection is the most likely cause, and the source must be established and specifically treated.

Diagnosis

The diagnosis of most infections complicating blunt trauma is readily made on the basis of the clinical manifestations. The early appearance of a diffuse cellulitis or lymphangitis is sufficiently characteristic of infection caused by *Streptococcus pyogenes* to provide assurance of control by treatment with penicillin G. When the wound itself is involved, exudate should be obtained from gram stain and culture. If there is evidence of a chest infection, a thoracentesis should be done to obtain intrapleural liquid for examination and culture. Peritoneal lavage or abdominal paracentesis is not usually productive because the peritoneal reaction seals loops of bowel together and obliterates the free peritoneal cavity. Also, there is the risk of damaging the distended bowel by paracentesis. With all infections, blood cultures should be taken at the time of a chill or ascent of fever; 3 to 4 blood cultures, one taken every 8 to 6 hours, is often sucessful in isolating the offending microorganism.

Therapy

The treatment of infections that develop secondary to blunt trauma is both medical and surgical. Antimicrobics, selected if possible on the basis of examination of smears of pertinent specimens, should be administered when the infection is first identified. Wounds infected with nonstreptococcal bacteria should be opened widely to ensure adequate drainage, evacuate hematomas, and remove any devitalized or necrotic tissue. If infection involves a movable part such as an extremity, this should be splinted and elevated. Moist dressings should be used to dress open wounds in order to prevent crusting and ensure drainage. Infections involving the pleural space or peritoneal cavity are usually treated only with appropriate antimicrobics at the outset. If there is failure of response, or if the infection localizes and becomes accessible, surgical therapy should be added. For example, tube thoracentesis should be used to drain empyemas.

Posterior drainage with or without a sump arrangement should be used for local abdominal collections that have failed to respond to medical management. A laparotomy is often required, although occasionally subhepatic collections can be identified and drained posteriorly without entering the peritoneal cavity—the optimal procedure, because transperitoneal drainage may result in further contamination of the peritoneal cavity and risk recurrence of the problem. General infections of the peritoneal cavity cannot be drained because drains, like other foreign materials, are promptly isolated and walled off as a normal peritoneal defense measure. When there is no overt communication between the bowel and the peritoneal space, peritonitis is managed conservatively.

The development of signs of acute peritoneal infection in a patient who has not had an exploratory laparotomy demands immediate surgical intervention because diffuse peritoneal infections are rare when none of the viscera are perforated. The peritoneum can handle a single episode of contamination, but cannot handle the continued contamination associated with injury of a hollow viscus.

Infections that occur in the immunosuppressed patient are often diffuse, infiltrating processes that are rarely amenable to surgical drainage. It is important that the cause be identified by blood cultures if possible so that specific antimicrobial therapy can be given. Initially, and in patients in whom an exact etiologic diagnosis is not made, a combination of gentamicin or tobramycin (5–6 mg/kg body weight/day as 3 equal portions, IV, 8-hourly; the dose should be modified according to measurements of concentrations in the blood) and clindamycin (15–30 mg/kg body weight/day as 4 equal portions, IV, 6-hourly).

Support of the immunosuppressed patient with infection usually requires intensive care with attention directed toward maintaining blood volume and supporting respiratory function with mechanical ventilation. It is usually necessary to provide nutritional support. The gastrointestinal tract should be used when possible for oral high-calorie supplements or for tube feeding. Usually, however, intravenous hyperalimentation is necessary to provide sufficient calories to carry the patient through the critical illness and infection. The malnourished patient suffers loss of humoral defenses as a result of decreased protein synthesis. The critically injured patient remains vulnerable to infection throughout the period of recovery. Caloric support appears to be especially effective in reducing morbidity and mortality due to infection in this group of patients.

Prevention

The prevention of injuries from blunt trauma involves fundamental surgical principles: the thorough debridement and extensive irrigation of superficial wounds, avulsion damage, and compound fractures. If at all possible, definitive surgical treatment should be instituted within the *golden period* of wounding, that is, within 6 to 8 hours of contamination. When a longer interval is allowed to transpire, the infection may have invaded the tissues, and local debridement and irrigation may not be sufficient to reducing the number of contaminating organisms below that likely to produce a clinically evident infection. Contaminated wounds treated after the golden period should, as a general rule, be left open unless they involve the face.

When there has been blunt trauma to the abdomen, close surveillance is necessary to recognize intraabdominal injury as soon as possible. If the possibility of abdominal injury exists, prompt surgical intervention is indicated. Exploratory laparotomy is the key to recognition of unsuspected bowel injuries and to prevention of lethal consequences.

When the injuries are clean and uncontaminated, prophylactic administration of antimicrobics has no place in the management of blunt trauma. Indeed, such treatment may be detrimental in altering the existing flora to ensure the dominance of resistant bacteria if a clinical infection develops. With contaminated injuries such as compound fractures, antimicrobial chemoprophylaxis is generally employed using a cepholosporin, for example, cefazolin 15 to 20 mg/kg of body weight, injected IV in the emergency room prior to surgery. If contamination is first recognized at operation, the same dose is given at that time. The treatment is continued in a dose of 60–80 mg/kg/day as 4 equal portions, IV, 6-hourly for 24 to 28 hours postoperatively. There is no evidence that there is any benefit after this period, and prolonged treatment runs the risk of infection with cefazolin-resistant bacteria.

Bibliography

Books

Committee on Trauma of the American College of Surgeons: *The Early Care of the Injured Patient.* Philadelphia, WB Saunders, 1976, 443 pp.

Journals

ALTMAN LC, KLEBANOFF SJ, CURRERI PW: Abnormalities of monocyte chemotaxis following thermal injury. J Surg Res 22:616–620, 1977

BRANSON HE, WYATT LL, SCHMER G: Complement consumption in acute DIC without antecedant immunopathology. Am J Clin Pathol 66:967–975, 1976

CHRISTOU NV, MCLEAN APH, MEAKINS JL: Host defense in blunt trauma: Interrelationships of kinetics of anergy and depressed neutrophil function, nutritional status and sepsis. J. Trauma 20:833–839, 1980

DOWNEY EC, CANTANZARO A, NINNEMANN JC, PETERS RM, SHACKFORD SR: Long term depressed immunocompetence of patients splenectomized for trauma. Surg Forum 31:41–42, 1980

EFFANY DJ, BLAISDELL FW, MCINTYRE KE, GRAZIANO CJ: The relationship between sepsis and intravascular coagulation. J Trauma 18:680–695, 1978

GRAZIANO C, MILLER, CL LIM RC JR: Role of monocyte function in alteration of the thrombofibrinolytic system after shock. Surg Forum 31:24–25, 1980

HIEBERT JM, MCGOUGH M, RODEHEAVER G, TOBIASEN J, EDGERTON MT, EDLICH RF: The influence of catabolism on immune competence in burned patients. Surgery 86:242–247, 1979

KAPLAN JE, SCOVILL WA, BERNARD H, SABA TM, GRAY V: Reticuloendothelial phagocytic response to bacterial challenge after traumatic shock. Circ Shock 4:1–12, 1977

MEAKINS JL, MCLEAN APH, KELLY R, BUBENIK O, PIETACH JB, MCLEAN LD: Delayed hypersensitivity and neutrophil chemotaxis: Effect of trauma. J Trauma 18:240–247, 1978

MILLER CL, TRUNKEY DD: Thermal injury: Defects in immune response induction. J Surg Res 22:621–625, 1977

F. WILLIAM BLAISDELL

155 Infections Following Penetrating Injuries

Penetrating injuries involve the skin and subcutaneous tissue and may extend deeply into fascia, muscle, hollow viscera, or body cavities. When the injuries do not involve a body cavity, the source of contamination can be presumed to be external and to relate to the organism or organisms that predominate on the skin or on the wounding object. If penetration of a body cavity occurs, the presumed infection is one consistent with the organ or organs that have been injured. This may involve organisms from the pharynx or esophagus, the upper respiratory tract, or the gastrointestinal tract, depending upon whether the neck, chest or peritoneal cavity has been transgressed.

Wounds may consist of open lacerations such as slashes from glass, sharp metal, or knives, or may be narrow and penetrating such as occur with shards of glass, knives, bullets, pins, splinters and nails.

Pathogenesis and Pathology

The risk of infection following any wound varies inversely with the local blood supply and related directly to the degree of contamination—that is, the concentration of organisms introduced, the amount of foreign material, the degree of tissue destruction, and associated factors such as formation of hematomas.

Surprisingly severe degrees of contamination can be handled by most tissues of the body without overt infection, provided no foreign material remains and the tissue injury is minimal. Thus, it is essential to ascertain whether the wound contains dirt, splinters of wood, or fragments of glass, clothing, or metal.

Another important factor is the degree of soft tissue injury. This relates to the amount of energy released into the tissues by the wounding object. Thus, high-velocity missiles deliver an explosive impact on tissues; extensive necrosis is the result. If the wounding object moves slowly, as a knife might, a simple shearing injury is produced; associated soft tissue damage is minimal. Therefore, in assessing penetrating wounds the entire tract of the wound must be taken into account, and the evaluation must start at the level of the skin.

Other factors that relate to the incidence of infection are hematomas and collections of serum in the wound. Both provide a favorable culture medium that is wet, warm, dark, and isolated from the host's protective mechanisms.

Normal, well-vascularized tissues are resistant to infection and only *Streptococcus pyogenes* need be feared in a relatively clean wound in which there is minimal tissue destruction, foreign material, and hematoma. Almost all other infections require some combination of factors that lower resistance in the wound. Anaerobic bacteria require dead or devitalized tissue, and the presence of facultative bacteria.

The organisms involved in penetrating wounds that do not involve hollow viscera are those introduced from the outside environment. Thus, a rusty nail from a barnyard is a classic instrument of penetrating injury that carries the risk of tetanus and other clostridial infections. On the other hand, a sharp piece of glass from a broken window is virtually bacteria-free and the most likely infecting bacteria are those carried into the wound from the skin. Anaerobic infections associated with the introduction of foreign material or with tissue damage carry the greatest risk of morbidity and mortality.

When the penetrating object enters a body cavity and a hollow viscus there is a high probability that there will be continuous contamination of the tract of the wound. Ordinarily, a single episode of contamination is handled by local defenses; however, continued soiling of tissues or body cavities with a gamut of aerobic and anaerobic bacteria sets the stage for a lethal infection.

Manifestations

When the injury is limited to the skin and subcutaneous tissues, the manifestations of infection consist in the classic evidences of inflammation. Erythema that develops rapidly with minimal induration is most consistent with streptococcal infection. Infections caused by other bacteria are associated with a latent period of at least a day or two before pain, tenderness, erythema, and induration appear.

Infections involving body cavities may be covert. Injuries of the neck that penetrate the pharynx or esophagus may at first cause only local discomfort; fever and leukocytosis may follow, with the development of tenderness and crepitation occurring subsequently. Because the infection is deep and subfascial, external signs of inflammation may be lacking. Infections of the thoracic cavity are relatively rare following penetrating trauma. The esophagus occupies a relatively small fraction of the chest cavity so that the incidence of injury is small. It is quite uncommon for penetrating injuries of the lung to be associated with infection. Major bronchial injuries typically give rise to emphysema and pneumothorax but have a low incidence of complicating infections. Mediastinal infections may develop from unsuspected injuries to the cervical portion of the esophagus and extend down into the mediastinum along the deep fascial structures common to the neck and the mediastinum.

Abdominal injuries with penetration of the bowel are usually signaled by peritoneal irritation, or are recognized when laparotomy is carried out. Because such injuries are usually identified early and are treated promptly there is a low incidence of complicating infections. Although the general rule states that all gunshot wounds that pass in or near the peritoneal cavity must be explored, many surgeons approach stab wounds conservatively. However, observation of patients with any kind of penetrating trauma may result in delayed recognition of injury, allowing infection to become established before definitive treatment is instituted.

Injury to a hollow viscus leads to increasing abdominal tenderness with evidence of muscle spasm and rebound. The temperature and the white count rise progressively over a period of hours. Within 6 to 8 hours infection is usually well established with invasion of the peritoneum and tissue planes; surgical operation at this time may not be successful in controlling the infectious process. Retroperitoneal injuries of the bowel often go undetected until infection is well established because there are no early signs analogous to peritonitis. These are extremely dangerous injuries for an additional reason, namely, the retroperitoneal tissues are far less resistant to infection than the peritoneum. Because the bowel has high concentrations of anaerobic and aerobic bacteria, rapid extension along fascial planes is favored by bacterial synergy. A clue to recognition is provided by systemic toxicity out of proportion to the local findings.

Diagnosis

The diagnosis of infection from penetrating wounds is relatively straightforward if the manifestations are noted and heeded. Once infection is suspected, exudate from the penetrating wound should be examined by smear and cultures. Signs of infection in the neck should lead to immediate surgical exploration. In some patients, injuries of the pharynx or esophagus may be detected preoperatively by laryngoscopy, esophagoscopy, or instillation of a water-soluble, radioopaque solution. These measures are appropriate whenever injury to the mediastinal esophagus is suspected because the injury may be difficult to localize at the time of operation in the presence of extensive mediastinitis. Infected abdominal injuries are usually clinically evident and rarely require specific diagnostic studies. Whenever there has been abdominal penetration followed by any sign of infection, laparotomy should be carried out without delay.

Therapy

The basic treatment of infected, penetrating wounds is a combination of both medical and surgical therapies. The only exceptions are wounds in which the infection is presumed to be streptococcal; these can be managed with penicillin and local treatment with moist heat. All other wounds in which infection is apparent should be opened widely. Devitalized tissue should be debrided, hematomas evacuated, and the wound packed open. Specimens should be obtained for smears and cultures with initial antimicrobial therapy based on the smear results and knowledge of the usual bacterial flora of the kind of wound under treatment. If the infection is not controlled, antimicrobial therapy should be modified according to the results of the cultures.

Penetrating wounds of the neck or the body cavities must be explored because injury to hollow viscera is likely to be present when cervical, intrathoracic or intraabdominal infections complicate such wounds. The body defenses cannot handle continuing contamination from such injuries. It is usually impossible to repair the hollow viscus when recognition of the injury is delayed; exteriorization or defunctionalization of the involved segment of the viscus is necessary. If the injury involves the large bowel, defunctionalization of the injury by proximal colostomy, resection with colostomy, or exteriorization of the injury are the choices. If the injury involves the small bowel, the injured segment can be exteriorized or can be excised with primary anastomosis. Resection must be generous so that the anastomosis will be distant from the site of infection.

When the pharynx is the source of the infection, external drainage is necessary. When the esophagus is the source, external drainage or defunctionalization is indicated.

Prevention

Adherence to fundamental surgical principles is critical to prevention of complicating infections. As soon as possible after wounding, the skin around the wound and the wound itself should be washed with a germicidal soap or detergent; depending upon the nature of the wounding object, the wound should either be explored to its depth or dressed. If there is reason to suspect foreign material was deposited in the wound or there is bleeding from the depths of the wound, the wound should be opened. Nonfacial wounds should be opened using an incision corresponding in length to the depth of the wound. All foreign material and blood clots should be evacuated and hemostasis should be attained.

When the wounding object may be presumed to be relatively clean, for example, a piece of glass or a sharp knife, the wound should be gently irrigated and then dressed. If the depths of a laceration can be seen, cleaned, and debrided adequately, and if the injury is treated within 6 to 8 hours of wounding (the *golden period*) it may be closed with sutures or tapes and should heal primarily. With the exception of the face and neck, all wounds seen after 6 to 8 hours should be presumed contaminated both on the surface and within. The choice here is between wide excision of the wound with closure (not usually done) and packing the wound open. The prophylactic administration of antimicrobics is rarely necessary if the wound has been well managed; penicillin G may be given if the wound is badly contaminated. The wound should be observed after 24 hours and 3 days later. Major contamination of wounds, for example, those associated with foreign bodies from the soil such as rusty nail wounds of the foot, must be considered tetanus prone. Either a booster dose of tetanal toxoid—if there is a history of immunization—or tetanal immune globulin plus toxoid—if the history of immunization is questionable—should be given. Penicillin G prophylaxis may be appropriate.

Prevention of serious infections involving body cavities involves a high index of suspicion and aggressive use of surgical exploration.

Bibliography

Books

American College of Surgeons: Manual on Control of Infection in Surgical Patients. Philadelphia, JB Lippincott, 1976. 280 pp.

FREY CF: Initial Management of the Trauma Patient. Philadelphia, Lea & Febiger, 1976. 498 pp.

SHIRES GT: Care of the Trauma Patient. New York, McGraw–Hill, 1979. 642 pp.

WALT AJ, WILSON WF: Management of Trauma: Pitfalls and Practice. Philadelphia, Lea & Febiger, 1975. 626 pp.

Journal

TRUNKEY DD, BLAISDELL FW: Trauma rounds: Penetrating abdominal wounds. West J Med 120:252–254, 1974

BRUCE M. WOLFE

Gas Gangrene

156

Gas gangrene classically refers to clostridial myonecrosis, a necrotizing anaerobic infection of skeletal muscle associated with severe systemic toxicity. Necrotizing clostridial infections of other soft tissues produce similar systemic toxicity, and necrotizing infections of muscle and other soft tissue may be caused by gas-forming bacteria other than clostridia. For purposes of definition, gas gangrene refers to necrotizing infection of soft tissues caused by *Clostridium* species.

Etiology

Clostridium species are large (0.5 μm × 1.5 μm), gram-positive, rod-shaped, usually motile, spore-forming obligate anaerobes. They are widely present in soil and clothing. In humans, their usual habitat is the intestinal tract and female genital tract, although they may also be present on the surface of the skin. Over 60 species have been recognized. *Clostridium perfringens* (capsulated, nonmotile) is recovered in about 80% of cases. Other *Clostridium* spp. commonly implicated as causes of gas gangrene in humans include *novyi, septicum,* and *sordelli* (noncapsulated, motile). As bacillary or vegetative forms, clostridia are destroyed by a variety of chemical and physical agents and are susceptible to penicillin G and other antimicrobics. As spores, they are resistant to heat, cold, sunlight, drying, and many chemical agents.

Epidemiology

Simple contamination of soft tissue wounds with clostridia is relatively common, since positive cultures may be obtained from 10% to 30% of nonmilitary traumatic wounds and up to 80% of war wounds. Gas gangrene was one of the major causes of postoperative infection and death in war injuries in the pre-Listerian era, but gas gangrene is now distinctly uncommon. The incidence is less than 0.1 per 100,000 population per year.

Pathogenesis and Pathology

Clostridia are obligate anaerobes that require a low oxidation-reduction (redox) potential for proliferation. There are several means by which tissue redox potentials may be diminished: impaired blood supply due to vascular occlusive disease, vascular injury, or pressure from edema in an extremity confined in a cast; direct tissue injury; and the presence of foreign bodies. Once the active infection is initiated, necrotizing toxins and local edema may impair circulation to adjacent tissue, enabling the anaerobic infection to spread rapidly. Carbon dioxide and hydrogen are liberated, and they contribute to the local edema and ischemia as well as opening fascial tissue planes, facilitating further spread of infection. The clostridia produce toxins that are largely responsible for the local and systemic manifestations. Five types of *C. perfrin-*

gens have been described on the basis of the toxins that are elaborated. All types produce α- toxin, a necrotizing, hemolytic exotoxin, which is a lecithinase. Other toxins that may be produced include hemolysin, collagenase, hyaluronidase, and deoxyribonuclease.

Manifestations

The manifestations of clostridial infections in humans may vary from simple asymptomatic contamination to rapidly fatal myonecrosis. The following classification is somewhat arbitrary, and considerable overlap between the types of clostridial infections may occur.

Simple Contamination

Cultures taken from traumatic wounds may reveal clostridia without clinical manifestations of infection. Providing standard principles of wound management are followed, such wounds heal without specific therapy for clostridia. Clostridial colonization may be clinically insignificant at other sites, including the gallbladder.

Suppurative Infection

A variety of clostridial species may be isolated as components of the bacterial flora from localized intraabdominal abscesses, pleural or pulmonary infections, and other mixed aerobic–anaerobic infections. There are no signs of myonecrosis or toxemia in these cases, and it is difficult to assign a pathogenetic role to the clostridia as opposed to the role of other organisms also present at the same location.

Localized Infection of Skin and Soft Tissue

Clostridial infections may be invasive and produce local necrosis without producing systemic signs of gas gangrene. Such infections are relatively indolent, spread slowly, and may involve skeletal muscle only locally. They may occur in a stump following amputation, in pararectal abscesses, or in diabetic ulcers of the lower extremities, and are commonly seen in heroin addicts. Crepitation may occur in these localized infections, but the amount of gas formed is slight, and it does not spread.

Diffuse Cellulitis

Rapidly spreading cellulitis associated with marked crepitation typically begins at a site rendered susceptible by injury or ischemia. The evidence of gas is followed by signs of cellulitis; spread is rapid above the deep fascia and through subcutaneous tissue planes, and may go from the extremities to the trunk. Systemic manifestations are highly variable—from surprisingly little systemic reaction to signs of overwhelming clostridial toxemia. Such signs include shock, renal failure, intravascular hemolysis, and jaundice. The patient may die within 48 to 72 hours after onset. Myonecrosis is not present in such cases, but the clostridia are present in the affected fascia or subcutaneous tissue. Diffuse clostridial cellulitis may occur without apparent injury or site of entry for the infection. If no local cause for clostridial cellulitis can be identified, a colonic source such as a perforation should be suspected. Hematogenous dissemination of *Clostridium* spp. originating in an enteric neoplasm is often the explanation for such otherwise unexplained cases.

Clostridial Myonecrosis Gas Gangrene

Clostridial myonecrosis (gas gangrene) begins in a wound, such as the operative wound of an ischemic extremity, or following trauma to soft tissues. The interval from injury or operation to the onset of symptoms varies from 6 hours to 3 days. Pain in the area of the wound that is not explained by the severity of the wound itself is the first manifestation. Swelling and tenderness of the area around the wound soon follow. The skin becomes tense as edema progresses and changes in appearance from an initially pale to dusky. Bullae form and may become hemorrhagic (Fig. 156-1); the skin around the wound becomes necrotic. Necrotic muscle may be apparent at the base of the wound. Crepitation is usually present, but may not be detectable. Profund toxemia typically occurs early and is characterized by marked tachycardia, hypotension, and tachypnea. Fever is low grade. Hemolysis with jaundice and oliguria and renal failure may follow. Delirium is usually present, although the patient may remain remarkably alert despite profound hypotension. A brown, seropurulent, foul-smelling exudate, often containing bubbles, oozes from the wound.

Clostridial Puerperal Sepsis

Clostridial sepsis following childbirth is rare, but uterine clostridial sepsis following gross contamination, as in criminal abortion, produces systemic manifestations identical to those of clostridial myonecrosis.

Diagnosis

The diagnosis of clostridial myonecrosis is based on (1) the presence of a wound with contamination, tis-

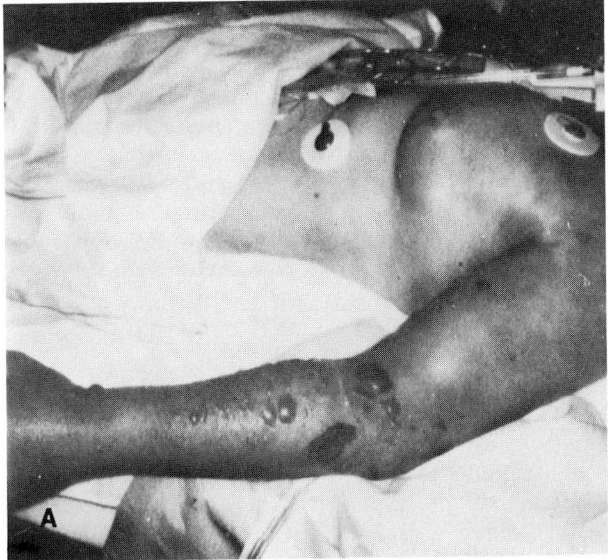

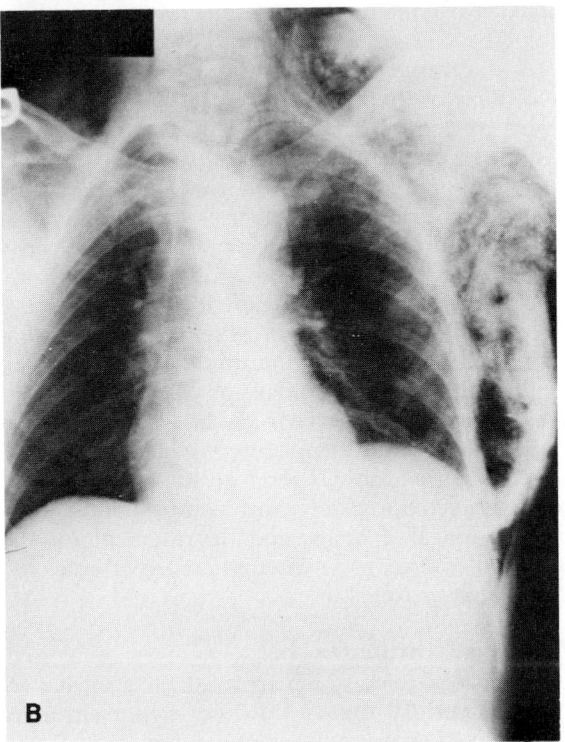

Fig. 156-1. Fatal gas gangrene (anaerobic myositis) that began in the left forearm (*A*) and rapidly extended to involve the chest wall (*B*). *Clostridium septicum* was isolated from the amputated forequarter; Fig. 31-1 *H* is a photomicrograph of a Gram-stained muscle imprint preparation. (Courtesy of Dr. Elliot Goldstein)

sue destruction, or ischemia; (2) the typical appearance of the wound, including edema, discoloration, and discharge; (3) excessive pain in the area of the wound; and (4) signs of systemic toxicity, including tachycardia and hypotension. Crepitation or evidence of the formation of gas is usually, but not always, present. Gram stains of the exudate from the wound or bullae show gram-positive rod-shaped bacteria and a paucity of white blood cells. The above criteria are adequate for the establishment of a clinical diagnosis of clostridial myonecrosis; when met, treatment should be initiated immediately. Specimens of the exudate from the wound and blood should be taken for culture, since many cases of myonecrosis prove to be caused by multiple organisms.

The diagnosis of suppurative intraabdominal infection or localized infection of the skin, subcutaneous tissue or muscle is based on gram stain and culture results from appropriate specimens. Clinical findings are the basis for distinguishing localized infection from rapidly progressive cellulitis or myonecrosis. The diagnosis of cellulitis with extensive formation of gas when there is no wound is more difficult. Identification of gram-positive rods on gram stain of edema fluid forms the basis of a clinical diagnosis. Cultures of wounds and blood in clostridial infections may be falsely negative because of the fastidious and anaerobic nature of these microorganisms.

Primary problems in the differential diagnosis of clostridial myonecrosis are identification of infection caused by nonclostridial gas-forming organisms and necrotizing fascitis caused by nonclostridial organisms. Several bacterial species may form gas as well as or more vigorously than the clostridial species. Both aerobic (*Escherichia coli*) and anaerobic (*Streptococcus* spp. and *Bacteroides* spp.) bacteria may produce larger amounts of gas in the tissues. Infections associated with gas in the extremities of diabetics with cutaneous ulcers or gangrenous lesions are usually caused by bacteria other than clostridia.

Necrotizing fascitis refers to a necrotizing infection of the subcutaneous tissue, fascia, and muscle. Such infections are associated with operative or traumatic wounds. This disease was formerly thought to be caused by a synergistic interaction of streptococcal and staphylococcal species, but other bacteria are usually isolated from such infections, for example, gram-negative, aerobic, and anaerobic bacteria. These nonclostridial infections may be responsible for severe systemic manifestations and death, but are generally less rapid in their progression than is clostridial myonecrosis.

Prognosis

Untreated clostridial myonecrosis, rapidly progressive cellulitis, and clostridial sepsis associated with septic abortion are fatal diseases. Delay in treatment may also lead to a fatal outcome, but with prompt, proper treatment the majority of patients with established gas gangrene should survive. Major morbidity may occur following amputation or debridement of involved tissue.

Therapy

The basic elements of treatment are surgical incision and debridement, antimicrobics, and hyperbaric oxygenation.

Surgical Therapy

Wide drainage of all wounds infected with clostridia (as well as other bacteria), must be accomplished. Decompressive fasciotomy must be done, particularly in extremities in which edema has impaired the blood supply. All devitalized tissue must be excised. Indiscriminate use of major amputation or chest or abdominal wall excision is unnecessary, particularly in localized infections. Surgical judgment is required to determine whether a given tissue is viable. Muscle that is pale or grey, is noncontractile, and shows no sign of bleeding should be excised. Multiple surgical debridements, done over a short period of time, may be necessary to assure complete excision of devitalized tissue without removing salvagable tissue in an unnecessarily radical excision at an initial, single procedure. Areas of widespread cellulitis do not require excision beyond the inciting wound or area of infection if the viability of the involved tissue is confirmed.

Clostridial sepsis originating in the uterus may require hysterectomy. Evacuation of the endometrial contents has been sufficient in properly selected cases—a decision requiring astute clinical judgment.

Antimicrobics

Penicillin G in a dose of 200 to 250 mg (320,000 U–400,000 U) /kg body wt/day by IV injection of 12 equal portions, 2-hourly (*i.e.,* 24–30 megaU/day in adults) should be administered as soon as the clinical diagnosis of clostridial myonecrosis or cellulitis is made. Patients with severe systemic manifestations are likely to have infection with multiple organisms, and additional therapy for staphylococcus (*e.g.,* nafcillin, 150–200 mg/kg body wt/day, IV, as 6 equal portions, 4-hourly) and gram-negative organisms (*e.g.,* tobramycin, 5–6 mg/kg body wt/day, IV, as 3 equal portions, 2-hourly (*i.e.,* 24–30 megaU/day in patient is allergic to penicillins, a cephalosporin may be used (*e.g.,* cefazolin, 100 mg/kg body wt/day, IV, as 4 equal portions, 6 hourly). The above measures, in addition to supportive measures including maintaining the circulatory volume and respiratory and cardiac function, should be instituted as rapidly as possible. A delay of several hours in accomplishing definitive surgical debridement may result in loss of limb or life.

Hyperbaric Oxygen

The role of hyperbaric oxygenation in the treatment of clostridial infections is controversial. In some, but not all, studies using nonhuman animals, there is a positive effect.

The patient is placed in a chamber containing 100% oxygen at an absolute pressure of 3 atmospheres for 90 minutes—3 times the first day and twice daily thereafter. Possible mechanisms of action of hyperbaric oxygenation include direct bactericidal action, decreased production of toxins by clostridia, inactivation of toxins, and increased oxygenation of the involved and surrounding tissue. Controlled clinical trials to evaluate the benefits of hyperbaric oxygen therapy have not been carried out, largely because of the small number of cases seen at individual institutions, the difficulty in categorizing the severity of cases, and ethical considerations of randomizing treatment in a group of critically ill patients. The use of hyperbaric oxygenation at centers where it is available is associated with low morbidity from the treatment itself (occasional convulsions) and is routine at such centers. Similar survival and limb salvage results have been reported from centers where hyperbaric oxygen is not available. Therefore, the patient should not be subjected to a delay in accomplishment of definitive surgical drainage and debridement for the purpose of transfer to a center where hyperbaric oxygen therapy is available.

Clostridial Antitoxin

Antitoxins of equine origin are available against a variety of clostridial toxins. However, hypersensitivity reactions and serum sickness may follow use of such antitoxins. Moreover, the antitoxins are of uncertain value and are not used clinically.

Prevention

The key to prevention of clostridial infections lie in the proper initial management of wounds: all foreign bodies must be removed and all devitalized tissue must be excised. Heavily contaminated wounds should not be closed primarily. Adequate anesthesia is required to accomplish adequate exploration of penetrating wounds.

Bibliography

Journals

ALTEMEIER WA, FULLEN WD: Prevention and treatment of gas gangrene. JAMA 217:806–813, 1971

BESSMAN AN, WAGNER W: Nonclostridial gas gangrene. JAMA 233:958–963, 1975

DEMELLO FJ, HAGLIN JJ, HITCHCOCK CR: Comparative study of experimental *Clostridium perfringens* infection in dogs treated with antibiotics, surgery and hyperbaric oxygen. Surgery 73:936–941, 1973

DRAKE SG, KING AM, SLACK WK: Gas gangrene and related infection: Classification, clinical features, and etiology, management and mortality. Br J Srg 64:104–112, 1977

GIULIANO A, LEWIS F, HADLEY K, BLAISDELL FW: Bacteriology of necrotizing fascitis. Am J Surg 134:52–57, 1977

HOLLAND JA, HILL GB, WOLFE WG, OSTERHOUT S, SALTZMAN HA, BROWN IW JR: Experimental and clinical experience with hyperbaric oxygen in the treatment of clostridial myonecrosis. Surgery 77:75–85, 1975

MACLENNAN JD: The histotoxic clostridial infections of man. Bacteriol Rev 26:177–276, 1962

ROBERT H. DEMLING

157 Infections Following Burns

Infection remains the leading cause of mortality in burned patients, accounting for approximately 80% of deaths. The major septic focus continues to be the burn wound. Burn wound infections not only cause mortality, but also increase morbidity by converting partial injury to full-thickness injury. Infection is also a stimulus to hypertrophic scarring in the healing wound. Although patients who have sustained thermal injuries may develop infections in sites other than burn wounds, prevalence alone dictates that the major concern of this chapter must be infections actually involving burn wounds.

Etiology

For a short period postburn, the surface of the burn wound is sterile unless there was an initial gross contamination. Usually after the second day, bacterial colonization of the wound begins. At first, the bacteria come from the patient's own endogenous flora: *Staphylococcus epidermidis* from the skin, *Staphylococcus aureus* and other gram-positive bacteria from the upper respiratory tract, and enteric bacilli from fecal flora. Of these, *S. aureus* predominates in the burn wound (Group A *Streptococcus pyogenes* is no longer a cause for burn wound sepsis).

After several weeks, or earlier depending on the magnitude of the burn injury, gram-negative bacilli begin to predominate. The most significant of these is *Pseudomonas aeruginosa.* Recently, however, *Providencia* spp. and *Serratia marcescens* have been recovered with increasing frequency. These three kinds of gram-negative bacilli are often resistant to most conventional antimicrobics. Since they are acquired from the hospital environment, they are agents of nosocomial infections.

Yeasts and filamentous fungi may also colonize the burn wound, and occasionally may cause sepsis. *Candida* spp. are most common with *Fusarium* spp., *Aspergillus* spp., and Zygomycetes seen less frequently.

Epidemiology

Burn wounds are colonized initially from the patient's own endogenous flora. However, exogenous bacteria that are indigenous in the hospital or in the burn units soon come to predominate. They are acquired primarily by direct contact, although a number of investigators assign importance to airborne transmission.

Pathogenesis and Pathology

The burned tissue or eschar is nonviable and is an excellent culture medium. Supraeschar colonization or multiplication of bacteria on the surface of the burn wound is of no major consequence. However, bacteria easily penetrate through the heat-denatured collagen to establish intraeschar colonization. It is only when bacteria begin to invade viable tissue beneath the burn eschar that the term burn wound infection or burn wound sepsis is used. This process of invasion correlates very well with the quantity of bacteria in the eschar. Invasion usually begins when bacteria exceed 10^5 per gram of full-thickness eschar. This number appears to overwhelm the defense mechanisms of the underlying viable tissue. When bacterial numbers approach 10^9 per gram of eschar, blood vessel invasion occurs and bacteremia results.

The burned patient is clearly an immunosuppressed host. The primary granulocyte functions of chemotaxis, phagocytosis, and bacterial killing are all depressed to a degree directly proportional to the total size of the burn. Chemotaxis is decreased by a heat-labile serum inhibitor released into the patient's plasma. Lymphocyte and macrophage function is impaired—in large part as a result of lymphocyte suppressor cell, especially T-suppressor cell, activity. The degree of impairment of lymphocyte function appears to be a useful predictor of the severity of sepsis.

The hypermetabolism of the postburn patient results in severe negative nitrogen balance. If protein catabolism goes unchecked, sepsis is favored.

Manifestations

Fever and leukocytosis are universally present in the burn patient with or without additional evidence of infection. Both may reflect severe stress or may result from the absorption of pyrogens from the eschar itself and from degenerating bacteria in the burn wound. Early symptoms of infection are often as subtle as a mild anorexia or increasing fatigue. A high index of suspicion is required in order to make the diagnosis. Deterioration of mental status and hemodynamic instability, including impaired perfusion of vital organs, (*e.g.,* oliguria and hypotension), are obvious but late signs of invasive burn wound sepsis.

Diagnosis

Documenting the presence of bacteria in the wound surface is not diagnostic of burn wound infection because all burns are colonized on the surface. Even when infection is present, standard clinical parameters remain unreliable. Only 50% of patients who die of fulminant burn sepsis have positive blood cultures. That is, death may be caused by the liberation of toxic bacterial byproducts, such as endotoxin, from the site of primary infection. Until the popularization of bacterial quantitation in burned tissue, the diagnosis of infection was a major dilemma. Quantitative biopsy of the burn eschar has now been shown to be a reliable diagnostic method. Briefly, the technique is as follows. Specimens are obtained by full-thickness biopsy of the washed burn wound eschar using a scalpel or punch biopsy instrument. Specimens are weighed immediately and then processed by maceration, suspension in 0.9% NaCl solution, and serial dilution before inoculation on appropriate culture mediums. Values are expressed as the number of bacteria per gram of burn tissue. The entire process requires about 24 hours. A more rapid slide technique has also been introduced that allows semiquantitation in less than 1 hour. The finding of $\geq 10^5$ bacteria per gram of tissue is diagnostic of burn wound infection. Because such high bacterial densities are attained in advance of clinical evidence of sepsis, early institution of specific therapy is possible. Quantitative biopsy-culture of thick eschar in extensively burned patients twice weekly is now standard procedure in burn centers.

Prognosis

Treatment of infections established in burn wounds is rendered difficult by (1) the avascular eschar—an excellent culture medium; (2) compromised cell-mediated host defenses; and (3) the catabolic, protein-losing state of the patient. For these reasons, the primary emphasis of burn care is aimed at improving host defenses in order to prevent severe infection rather than the more difficult task of eradicating an established infection. Although the treatment of burn infection has improved substantially in recent years, the impressive decrease in the burn mortality rate is due primarily to more aggressive measures to prevent infection.

Therapy

Because the burn eschar is essentially avascular, systemic antimicrobics are of little benefit in controlling infection until viable tissue becomes invaded. The mainstay of the control of bacteria in the burn wound is the topical application of antimicrobics that penetrate into the dead eschar from the surface and control colonization. Of several topical antimicrobics in current use, the most popular are silver sulfadiazine (Silvadine) and a methylated sulfonamide, mafenide (Sulfamylon). Silver nitrate in a 0.5% solution is now used sparingly. All of these compounds are quite active against gram-negative bacteria, but are only modestly active against gram-positive bacteria. Mafenide is the most effective antibacterial agent, and it penetrates the burn eschar into subjacent viable tissue. There are, however, two major disadvantages with its use. First, mafenide is a carbonic anhydrase inhibitor, which decreases bicarbonate resorption by the kidney, resulting in metabolic acidosis when applied to large burn surfaces. The acidosis usually is in part compensated for by an increased respiratory drive, often resulting in severe tachypnea and hyperpnea. The second problem is that many patients experience pain when mafenide is applied, particularly on partial-thickness burns. Because of these problems, mafenide is usually the second agent of choice, used primarily to treat burn wound infection not controlled by silver sulfadiazine—currently the most popular agent. Although silver sulfadiazine penetrates eschar less effectively, there is no major complication with its use. A transient neutropenia is occasionally seen in the first several days after application of silver sulfadiazine; because it reverses spontaneously, discontinuation of the drug is not necessary. There is rapid absorption of the antibacterial agents into the eschar; at least twice daily the cream residual on the surface of the eschar must be removed before reapplication of fresh drug. Because long-term use is associated with staphylococcal proliferation and the emergence of resistant gram-negative bacilli, change to other topical agents is frequently necessary.

Subeschar administration of antimicrobics may be used when topical agents fail to control infection. The aminocyclitols are most commonly applied. Maximum daily doses are administered by subcutaneous clysis with multiple needle infusions of approximately 200 ml solution per 100 to 200 cm^2 eschar. The appropriate antimicrobic is selected by susceptibility testing of the bacteria recovered from the quantitative biopsy. The total volume injected per day should be limited to approximately 2 liters in the adult.

Systemic antimicrobics are indicated when the diagnosis of wound infection (greater than 10^5 organisms) is made by quantitative cultures. Prophylactic administration should be avoided except possibly for use of penicillin G to prevent streptococcal infection. However, streptococcal burn wound infections are now so rare that most burn centers use no systemic chemoprophylaxis in the early postburn period. When systemic antimicrobics are indicated, monitoring of serum concentrations is necessary, particularly for the aminocyclitols because of a shortened drug half-life in many burn patients. A shorter dosage interval and an increased total daily dose are frequently necessary to maintain therapeutic concentrations. It has not yet been determined whether the shortened half-life represents loss of drug into burn dressings or an increased rate of metabolism.

Pseudomonas vaccine appeared, in early clinical studies, to be very beneficial; however, the vaccine has not been widely used. Pseudomonas antiserum has also been reported to be beneficial, although no controlled clinical trials have yet been completed.

Prevention

Surgical Excision of Burn Tissue

Because the dead burn eschar is the primary source of infection, early removal should diminish infection. Early excision in adults with full-thickness burns exceeding 65% of their total body surface resulted in a significant decrease in mortality. However, patients over 55 years of age frequently tolerate major excisions poorly, primarily because of the development of pulmonary complications. The greatest success in early excision therapy has been found in the pediatric age group. Proper patient selection is the key to success with this therapy.

Biologic Dressings

The most commonly used biologic dressings are homograft or cadaver skin, porcine heterograft or pigskin, and human amniotic membrane. These agents have clear, albeit undefined, antibacterial properties and are useful for decreasing the concentration of bacteria on a wound or controlling bacterial growth on a recently excised wound while waiting for autografts to become available. Occasionally, the biologic dressings themselves may be the source of bacterial growth, although current processing techniques are much improved over earlier techniques. Changing the dressing every 2 days, or more frequently if the wound becomes purulent, is recommended.

Supernutrition

Aggressive replacement of postburn calorie and protein losses promotes the restoration of immune competence, rapid healing of the open wound, and improved adherence of skin grafts. Accordingly, early institution of a vigorous nutritional program, preferably by the oral route, is now common practice in burn centers. Parenteral hyperalimentation is used if sufficient calories cannot be provided by the alimentary tract. Improved nutrition has clearly decreased mortality from burn wound sepsis.

Isolation Techniques

It is clear that patients who are at high risk for infection, or who already have an infection with a resistant organism, should be geographically isolated from other patients. However, despite what appear to be adequate isolation techniques, virulent strains of bacteria are passed from patient to patient in burn units. Two factors—overcrowding of patients and understaffing of burn care centers—result in frequent breaks in isolation technique and favor cross-contamination.

There is an increasing interest in the use of laminar airflow systems as an adjunct to spatial isolation. Although a decrease in the rate of cross-contamination has been reported with the use of laminar airflow isolators, the greater attention given to detail in the care of the wound and the improved nurse:patient ratio required with laminar airflow may be as responsible as the sterile airflow for the improved results.

Other Infections After Burn Injury

Pneumonia

Pneumonia is the second most common infection of burned patients. It usually begins in the second postburn week and is particularly prone to occur after inhalation injury. Impairments of immune defenses may play a major role in facilitating this complication. The cause of the pneumonia is usually the same as that found in the burn wound; a hematogenous source is responsible for about one-third of the cases. Early institution of vigorous pulmonary care and early ambulation are necessary to decrease the occurrence of pneumonia.

Suppurative Thrombophlebitis

Suppurative thrombophlebitis is the third most important life-threatening complication in burn patients. The duration of intravascular cannulation and the magnitude of the burn injury are the primary determinants of occurrence. Infection occurs most frequently in veins in the lower extremity. *Staphylococcus aureus* is the most common single cause, but gram-negative bacilli predominate overall. *Candida albicans* is the most common nonbacterial etiology. Successful treatment requires identification of the septic vein and surgical excision of the involved segment. Meticulous attention to aseptic technique in vascular cannulation and frequent changing of intravenous infusion sites are necessary. Peripheral intravenous catheters should be changed at least every 48 hours. Central catheters that do not pass through burned tissue may be changed less frequently if strict protocols for care are implemented.

Auricular Chondritis

The avascularity of the cartilage of the ear makes this tissue extremely vulnerable to infection after the overlying skin is injured by a burn. Auricular chondritis rarely leads to sepsis, but it is a major complication, for it may cause extreme pain and disfigurement. The infecting bacteria are the same as those present in the burn wound. Treatment requires the removal of the infected cartilage and, of less importance, the systemic administration of antimicrobics. Prevention involves avoiding any pressure on the burned ear from dressings or pillows and the frequent application of topical antimicrobics to any area of exposed cartilage.

Viremia

Life-threatening viral infections have been reported in burned patients, but the incidence is quite low. *Herpesvirus hominis* is the most common cause. Herpetic lesions are characteristically found in healing or recently healed burns of the nasolabial region, but vesicles have also been found in healing burns in other parts of the body.

Remaining Problems

Decreases in the rate of infection of the burn wound and other sites will come from a combination of meticulous care of the wound and aggressive augmentation of the patient's immune defenses. Antimicrobial agents are not the answer.

Bibliography

Books

ARTZ CP, MONCRIEF JA, PRUITT BA: Burns: A Team Approach. Philadelphia, WB Saunders, 1979. 583 pp.

POLK HC JR, STONE HH: Contemporary Burn Management. Boston, Little, Brown, 1971. 444 pp.

Journals

ALEXANDER JW, OGLE CK, STINNETT JD, MACMILLAN BF: A sequential, prospective analysis of immunologic abnormalities and infection following severe thermal injury. Ann Surg 188:809–816, 1978

BAXTER CR, CURRERI WP, MARVIN JA: The control of burn wound sepsis by the use of quantitative bacterial studies and subeschar clysis with antibiotics. Surg Clin North Am 53:1509–1539, 1973

BROMBERG BE, SONG FC: Skin substitutes, homo- and heterografts. Am J Surg 112:28, 1966

DOWLING JA, FOLEY FD. MONCRIEF JA: Chondritis in the burned ear. Plast Reconstr Surg 42:115, 1968

LOEBL EC, MARVIN JA, HECK EL, CURRERI PW, BAXTER CR: The method of quantitative burn-wound biopsy cultures and its routine use in the care of the burned patient. Am J Clin Pathol 60:20–24, 1973

ZASKE DE, SAWCHUK RJ, STRATE RG: The necessity of increased doses of amikacin in burn patients. Surgery 84:603–608, 1978

SEBASTIAN CONTI

158 Infections Following Surgical Operations

Infection following surgery was the rule rather than the exception prior to the Listerian antiseptic era, when mortality from deep or extensive wounds exceeded 75%. Although Lister's antiseptic technique markedly reduced the occurrence of infection, it soon became obvious that antisepsis alone was insufficient. Aseptic principles and practices, including the use of face masks, drapes, and rubber gloves, were adopted in the late 19th century and brought about a further reduction in the frequency of infection.

The rate of infection following surgical operations decreased again when antibacterial agents became available. However, the price paid was the emergence of bacteria (predominantly gram-negative bacteria) resistant to many antimicrobics. More recently, the use of antimicrobics to prevent wound infection has become popular (Chap. 19, Chemoprophylaxis of Infectious Diseases), but this practice has certainly not eliminated the problem. It may be that too much reliance is now placed on chemoprophylaxis and not enough on asepsis, surgical technique, and wound care. Whatever the reasons, the economic costs are enormous. The cost of postoperative wound infections in the United States may exceed 10 billion dollars annually.

Etiology

In a collaborative study performed by the National Research Council, the overall incidence of surgical wound infections was 7.5%. The frequency of recovery of the five most common bacteria causing wound infections was *Staphylococcus aureus,* 31.3%; other *Staphylococcus* spp., 31.5%; *Escherichia coli,* 22.3%; *Proteus* spp., 13.3%; and *Pseudomonas* spp., 13.3%. Whenever the gastrointestinal tract is entered during a surgical operation, gram-negative bacteria are the predominant organisms recovered from complicating wound infections.

Epidemiology

In most cases, the patient or operating room personnel act as the main source of wound contamination. The primary mode of transmission is direct contact from the source, which can be either endogenous (patient's skin or transected viscera) or exogenous (contaminated instruments or hands). Hematogenous contamination in patients with established infections in other parts of the body is more common than is generally realized. Lesions, that is, disease, caused by *S. aureus* constitute an important source, whereas simple carriage of staphylococci generally does not lead to infection. On the ward, an open, infected, draining wound is a major source of contamination. Inanimate objects such as food trays and linen do not pose risks.

Pathogenesis and Pathology

The development of a wound infection depends upon the virulence of the invading organism, the site of bacterial inoculation, and host resistance. Local and systemic factors that favor wound infection are listed on p. 1353. If host resistance is compromised, even avirulent and noninvasive bacteria or a small inoculum of virulent bacteria can cause an infection. Local factors are important as well. For example, a concentration of more than 10^7 *S. aureus* is required to produce an infection in a noncompromised host with an otherwise healthy, clean wound. A loose silk suture reduces the inoculum required to produce infection 10 thousand times. With the more virulent Group A *Streptococcus pyogenes,* only 10^2 bacteria deposited in a clean wound can initiate an infection.

FACTORS THAT FAVOR THE DEVELOPMENT OF WOUND INFECTIONS

Local	Presence of necrotic tissue, dead space, hematomas, seromas, foreign bodies
	Large inoculum of bacteria
	Reduced local blood supply
Systemic	Compromised host resistance due to malignancy, malnutrition, chemotherapy, diabetes, extremes of age, immunodeficiency diseases
	Remote infection
	Obesity
	Shock
	Prolonged treatment with broad spectrum antimicrobics
	Prolonged preoperative hospitalization

Manifestations

Wound infections caused by *S. aureus* and other pus-forming bacteria typically become manifest 5 to 7 days after operation and are heralded by an elevated pulse rate, lethargy, poor appetite, fever, and sweating. Initially, the wound may appear normal, but after a day or two, swelling, redness, tenderness, and fluctuance appear; if a suture is removed, pus is discovered.

Infections caused by *S. pyogenes* are manifested earlier, often within 48 hours. Fever, chills, tachycardia, and leukocytosis are present. The wound may appear normal, but if the infection is rapidly invasive, an area of cellulitis surrounds the wound; in fulminant cases, fascitis and even gangrene of the skin may be seen. Severe necrotizing infections may be caused by *Clostridium* spp., or by several kinds of bacteria acting in concert to produce a fulminant and often fatal course (Chap. 156, Gas Gangrene).

Diagnosis

The diagnosis of postoperative wound infection depends primarily on the clinical manifestations. Opening and inspecting the wound enables confirmation when the infection is caused by pyogenic bacteria. In doubtful cases, or in cases in which the infection is thought to be caused by *S. pyogenes,* needle aspiration lateral to the wound may yield an exudate that can be stained and cultured for identification of the infecting bacteria.

Therapy

Successful management of postoperative wound infections depends upon early diagnosis, accurate identification of the causative organism, judicious surgical intervention, appropriate general and local supportive care, and appropriate antimicrobic therapy. Wound infections caused by *S. aureus* or aerobic gram-negative bacilli are usually well localized and therefore adequately treated simply by opening the incision to provide drainage. The administration of antimicrobics is generally not indicated unless there are manifestations of systemic illness or the patient is immunologically incompentent. When infection complicates wounds in patients with cardiac valvular disease, prosthetic valves, or vascular grafts, and when the wound is located near the meninges or on the face, treatment with systemically administered antimicrobics is also necessary.

Wound infections caused by *S. pyogenes* are best treated by parenteral administration of penicillin G for 7 days after all signs of infection have subsided.

Prognosis

Treatment with drainage and antimicrobics, if indicated, usually results in prompt healing and a satisfactory cosmetic appearance. However, in some cases, considerable morbidity and even mortality may be caused by wound infection. For example, dehiscence of an abdominal wound may result in no more than an incisional hernia; but fascial disruption with evisceration of abdominal contents may cause major morbidity. A vascular graft that becomes infected poses not only a threat of hemorrhage but also the risk of loss of limb or life if the graft must be removed because of the infection.

Prevention

Adherence to time-honored principles of surgical asepsis and antisepsis, gentle handling of tissues, use of monofilament suture material, avoidance of undue tension during wound closure, removal of devitalized tissue and blood clots—in short, the practice of flawless surgical technique—is of paramount importance for the prevention of wound infection in clean operative cases. Where there is unavoidable contamination due to traumatic injuries, transection of viscera, or operations performed in an infected field, other considerations are necessary. The effectiveness of antimicrobics administered before, during, and for a short period after operations from which bacterial contamination is expected has clearly been established. Wound infections in cases in which bacterial contamination is substantial, as in fecal peritonitis, are best prevented by employing the principle of delayed primary closure. Quantitative cultures of wound biopsy tissue serve as a reliable guide in timing wound closure.

Bibliography

Journals

Ad Hoc Committee of the Committee on Trauma, Division of Medical Sciences, National Academy of Sciences–National Research Council: Postoperative wound infections: The influence of ultraviolet radiation of the operating room and of various other factors. Ann Surg (Suppl) 160:2, 1964

ALEXANDER WA: Nosocomial Infections. Curr Probl Surg, August, 1973. 54 pp.

DAVIS MC, COHEN J, RAO A: The incidence of surgical wound infection: A prospective study of 20,822 operations. Aust NZ J Surg 43:75–83, 1973

EDWARDS LD: The epidemiology of 2,056 remote site infections and 1,966 surgical wound infections occurring in 1,865 patients. Ann Surg 184:758–766, 1976

Section | *XXII*

Ophthalmic Infections

Indigenous Microbiota of the Eyes

Species or Group	Conjunctiva
Bacteria	
Gram-positive cocci	
Staphylococcus epidermidis	**37–94***
Staphylococcus aureus	**0–30**
Streptococcus mitis; undifferentiated α and γ streptococci	**0.3–1**
Streptococcus pyogenes (usually group A unless noted)	**0.3–2.5**
Streptococcus pneumoniae	**0–5**
Gram-negative cocci	
Branhamella catarrhalis	**2.3**
Gemella haemolysans	
Gram-positive bacilli	
Lactobacillus spp.	**3–83**
Aerobic *Corynebacterium* spp.	
Aerobic gram-negative bacilli	
Enterobacteriaceae	**2.1**
Klebsiella spp.	**0.1**
Proteus mirabilis, other *Proteus* spp.,	**0.4**
Morganella morganii,	
Providencia spp.	
Alcaligenes faecalis	±
Moraxella lacunata	±
Acinetobacter calcoaceticus	±
Haemophilus influenzae	**0.4–25**

± to 0, rare; ±, irregular or uncertain (may be only pathologic); +, common; ++, prominent.

*Boldface values (*e.g.,* **30–60**) = range of incidence in percentage, rounded, in different surveys.

MARIO L. TARIZZO*

Trachoma

159

Trachoma is a specific keratoconjunctivitis caused by a chlamydia. Severe and complicated cases often occur where the disease is endemic, and such cases may result in partial or total loss of vision. Trachoma is still the most important single cause of preventable blindness. It is estimated that 500 million people are affected and that 2 million have been blinded by it.

Etiology

From a taxonomic point of view, the agent of trachoma, *Chlamydia trachomatis,* belongs to the order *Chlamydiales,* family Chlamydiaceae. There is only one other species in the genus *Chlamydia,* namely, *psittaci.* The structure and metabolism of chlamydias are similar to those of bacteria: they contain both RNA and DNA. However, they are obligate intracellular parasites in that they depend on the host cell metabolism for precursors to nucleic acids and in part for energy production (Chap. 1, Attributes of Infectious Agents). As a consequence of their relatively complex metabolism, they are susceptible to the action of certain antimicrobics. The agent of trachoma shares a common complement-fixing (CF) group antigen with other chlamydias, which are responsible for lymphogranuloma venereum (LGV; Chap. 54, Lymphogranuloma Venereum), ornithosis (Chap. 30, Nonbacterial Pheumonias), and several infections of mammals and marsupials. Specific antigenic properties have been demonstrated by neutralization, hemagglutination, gel diffusion, immunoelectrophoresis, and immunofluorescence. Indirect immunofluorescence allows differentiation between different serotypes of *C. trachomatis* A through L; serotypes A, B, Ba, and C are associated with endemic trachoma, whereas serotypes D through L are those usually recovered from genital or oculogential infections. Three types of LGV strains have been described—L1, L2, and L3, all differing from the trachoma strains in their pathogenicity for both humans and experimental animals.

Individual particles or bodies are round, 200 nm to 400 nm in diameter, and easily visible under an ordinary microscope. With electron microscopy, individual bodies show a dense central nucleoid surrounded by a less dense periphery and by a limiting membrane. They are pink to purple with the Giemsa stain, red with Macchiavello and with Giménez stains, and dark blue with the Castaneda stain. With acridine orange and ultraviolet light, the early-phase, predominantly RNA-coated particles are brick red. The evolution to the infective phase, characterized by predominantly DNA-coated elementary bodies is marked by a gradual change to yellow and finally to yellowish green. Large aggregates of individual bodies or inclusions result from successive binary fissions. In trachoma, these inclusions may be observed most often in the perinuclear region of the cytoplasm of epithelialike cells in conjunctival scrapings or impression smears. The typical inclusion contains a carbohydrate matrix that stains reddish brown or purple with iodine.

The agent of trachoma may be cultivated in the laboratory in the yolk sac of embryonated eggs and in tissue cultures. Tissue culture methods are now preferred for the isolation of chlamydias because they are more rapid and sensitive and because they yield isolates for serotyping. Laboratory-grown strains can cause experimental trachoma in humans and a mild follicular keratoconjunctivitis in some nonhuman primate species. Although not normally pathogenic for laboratory animals, they are toxic to mice by intravenous inoculation.

*Died November 11, 1980.

Epidemiology

Trachoma occurs throughout the world, without definite relationship to either climate or race. Historically, trachoma was prevalent at one time or another in most regions of the world. It is only in the present century that it has disappeared as a severe disease from western Europe. Trachoma and its complications still represent a serious public health problem in parts of Africa, Asia, and Latin America. In the United States, the disease has been observed mainly in the Southwest, and a trachoma control program has been carried out by the United States Public Health Service, Division of Indian Health.

Spread of the disease in its classic form is essentially from eye to eye through direct or indirect contact with infected material. In countries where the disease is sporadic, extraocular localization occurs and is mainly genital; venereal transmission does take place. When the agent localizes in the cervix uteri, infection of the newborn may result, taking the form of inclusion conjunctivitis—a disease akin to trachoma that may also afflict adults.

In areas where trachoma is endemic, the severity may be influenced by the duration of the clinical manifestations and by the occurrence of relapses or reinfections. The association with bacteria such as *Haemophilus* spp. and *Moraxella* spp. often results in the aggravation of symptoms and may facilitate the development of complications.

In endemic areas, the age of onset of the disease tends to be inversely proportional to the degree of endemicity; complications may be observed even in very young persons. The use of common towels, eye cosmetics, and contaminated water for washing, and the presence of flies have been incriminated in the dissemination of the infection. The disease is more frequent and more severe when living conditions and sanitary or socioeconomic levels are unsatisfactory.

Pathogenesis and Pathology

On the palpebral conjunctiva, the process begins with diffuse hyperemia and infiltration that tends to become localized, resulting in the formation of vascular papillae and lymphoid follicles. Both upper and lower lids may be involved, but typically, the lesions are present in the area covering the upper tarsal plate. In later stages, cicatricial tissue develops either as a consequence of follicular necrosis or diffuse infiltration and fibrosis. Structural alterations in the lids may cause thickening and eventually deformation through retraction of the cicatricial tissue. This leads to trichiasis and entropion, which may lead to corneal damage with partial or total loss of vision.

In the cornea, infiltration and neovascularization of the upper limbus may extend downward and reach the pupillary area in cases of severe and long-standing activity. The corneal conjunctiva may also be affected, and follicles may develop at the upper limbus. A superficial keratitis may also occur. Resorption of infiltration at the limbus may lead to the formation of Herbert's pits—small circular excavations along the limbus, which are pathognomonic for trachoma; the keratitic involvement may lead to corneal opacification or, in very severe cases, to ulceration.

Manifestations

Symptoms of lacrimation and photophobia may be accompanied by seromucous or frankly purulent secretion. The disease tends to have a chronic evolution, and even without reinfections there may be spontaneous exacerbations and regressions. Mild cases usually evolve toward spontaneous cure.

Extraocular localizations of the agent are often symptomless, but may be accompanied in males by the signs and symptoms of nonspecific urethritis.

Diagnosis

In areas of endemicity, the presence of two of the typical signs—upper tarsal follicles, limbal follicles, or Herbert's pits; corneal infiltration and neovascularization (pannus); conjunctival scars of characteristic configuration—is sufficient for diagnosis. In mild cases, careful examination using a slit lamp and optical magnification is recommended.

Laboratory tests may confirm the clinical diagnosis by demonstrating the agent either by microscopic examination of conjunctival material stained by Giemsa, iodine, or immunofluorescence or by isolation in tissue culture. Immunofluorescence methods are recommended for detecting and measuring type-specific chlamydial antibodies in serum or tears.

Other forms of conjunctivitis must be differentiated (Chap. 161, Conjunctivitis and Scleritis). Infections with adenovirus, molluscum contagiosum virus, and *Haemophilus aegyptius* (Morax–Axenfeld bacillus) are examples. Chemical conjunctivitis such as may result from the chronic administration of physostigmine must be recognized.

Prognosis

The prognosis in individual cases reflects, to a certain extent, the severity of the disease in the community. Also, prolonged infection, relapses, reinfections, and association with bacteria all facilitate the occurrence of complications. There is some evidence that sensitization resulting from repeated exposure might play a role in the severity of the disease and in the development of complications. Infection does not result in protection against reinfection with homologous or heterologous strains.

Therapy

The course of trachoma is favorably influenced by the sulfonamides and certain other antimicrobics. Mass use of sulfonamides should be avoided, however, because there is a risk of toxic and allergic reactions. Under adequate supervision, particularly in the treatment of individual cases, sulfonamides may be preferred. Long-acting preparations may be convenient because an oral loading dose of 25 to 30 mg/kg body wt is followed by a weekly dosage of 15 mg/kg body wt for several weeks.

In areas of endemicity, the risk of loss of vision can be reduced by prolonged application of tetracyclines and erythromycin administered locally in the form of opthalmic ointments or oily suspensions. There are practically no contraindications to these agents, and they have been widely used in mass treatment campaigns. The efficacy of the treatment of trachoma with antimicrobics has been questioned, and it has been stated that they act mainly on the associated bacterial flora. This point has little more than theoretical significance where the disease is endemic. In any case, therapy reduces the risk of complications even if complete cure may be obtained only after prolonged treatment. It should be noted in this respect that the susceptibility of the trachoma agent *in vitro* closely corresponds to the results of antimicrobial therapy.

Prevention

Vaccination against trachoma has not yielded results warranting large-scale application. The killed vaccines used in these trials have induced, at best, temporary and partial protection. In some cases, they have also been used in the treatment of otherwise resistant cases. The rather unsatisfactory results obtained may reflect the poor antigenicity of the agent and the local nature of the disease. Experimental trials with live vaccines in animals have been discontinued because of the agent's tendency to spread.

Remaining Problems

Reduction in the loss of vision will result from adequate treatment of endemic, severe trachoma; improvements in public health; and betterment of socioeconomic conditions. Increased recognition of trachoma as a cause of preventable blindness should stimulate new research, lead to new knowledge of the basic properties of the agent, and result in practical applications in diagnosis, treatment, and prevention. Wider application of newly developed laboratory techniques should be useful in assessing changes in the degree of endemicity either as a consequence of, or independent of, control measures. The need for prolonged treatment and for repeated administration of presently available antimicrobics is a serious disadvantage that should be overcome by development of more rational and more effective therapeutic agents and methods of administration. Systemic administration of antimicrobics has been advocated as a possible alternative. Active immunization may become possible once the antigenic properties of the agent and its interrelationship with the host are more precisely defined.

The role of extraocular localizations of the trachoma agent also needs further clarification. Other problems to be solved include the interrelationship between different chlamydias of human and nonhuman origin and the possibility of an etiologic role in other conditions, such as urethritis and Reiter's syndrome (see also Chap. 55, Nongonococcal Urethritis).

Bibliography

Books

BIETTI GB, WERNER GH: Trachoma,; Prevention and Treatment. Springfield, Ill. Charles C Thomas, 1967. 227 pp.

Expert Committee on Trachoma, Third Report, Geneva, WHO Technical Report Series No. 234, 1962. 48 pp.

Fourth Scientific Group on Trachoma Research Report. Geneva, WHO Technical Report Series No. 330, 1966

Guide to the Laboratory Diagnosis of Trachoma. Geneva, World Health Organization, 1975. 38 pp.

Guide to Trachoma Control in Programmes for the Prevention of Blindness, Geneva, World Health Organization, 1981. 56 pp.

NATAF R: Le Trachome. Paris, Masson, 1952

NICHOLS RL (ed): Trachoma and Related Disorders Caused by Chlamydial Agents. Amsterdam, Excerpta Medica, 1971. 586 pp.

SOWA S, SOWA J, COLLIER LH, BLYTH W: Trachoma and Allied Infections in a Gambian Village, Special Report Series, London, Medical Research Council, 1965. 88 pp.

TARIZZO ML (ed): Field Methods for the Control of Trachoma. Geneva, 1973. 48 pp.

Journals

BECKER Y: The agent of trachoma. Recent studies of the biology, biochemistry and immunology of a prokaryotic obligate parasite of eukaryocytes. Monogr Virol 7:1–99, 1974

The biology of the trachoma agent, New York, May, 1961. Ann NY Acad Sci 98:1–382, 1962

Conference on trachoma and allied diseases, San Francisco–Asilomar, August, 1966. Am J Ophthalmol 63: 1027–1657, 1967

DAWSON CR, JONES BR, DAROUGAR S: Blinding and non-blinding trachoma: Assessment of intensity of upper tarsal inflammatory disease and disabling lesions. Bull WHO 52:279–282, 1975

DAWSON CR: Chlamydial infections of the eye: Trachoma and inclusion conjunctivitis. Contact Intraocular Lens Med J 6:217–226, 1980

JAWETZ E, THYGESON P: Tric viruses: Agents of trachoma and inclusion conjunctivitis. Ergeb Mikrobiol 48:55–95, 1964

JONES BR: Prevention of blindness from trachoma. Trans Ophthal Soc UK 95:16–33, 1975

TARIZZO ML, NATAF R: The treatment of trachoma. Rev Int Trach 46&47:7–48, 1970

H. BRUCE OSTLER
MASAO OKUMOTO

Infections of the Eyelids and Orbital Cellulitis

160

Infections of the Eyelids

Virtually any organism that infects the skin can also cause infections of the eyelids. These and other inflammatory diseases of the eyelids are commonly referred to as blepharitis. The most common type is marginal blepharitis, which is an infection or allergy of the margins of the eyelids.

Etiology

Bacteria

The most common causes of bacterial blepharitis are *Staphylococcus aureus* and *Moraxella nonliquefaciens.* Less common causes are *Moraxella lacunata* (the diplobacillus of Morax–Axenfeld, formerly common in California and possibly still common in Arizona and North Africa); gram-positive bacteria such as *Streptococcus pyogenes, Corynebacterium diphtheriae,* and *Bacillus anthracis;* gram-negative bacteria such as *Psudomonas aeruginosa, Proteus* spp, and *Pseudomonas mallei;* the acid-fast organisms *Mycobacterium tuberculosis* and *Mycobacterium leprae;* and some of the bacteria that cause venereal diseases—*Treponema pallidum, Haemophilus ducreyi,* and *Calymmatobacterium granulomatis.* Rarely, eyelid infections may be caused by anaerobic bacteria: *Clostridium* spp. and *Actinomyces israelii,* and by a mixture of *Peptococcus* spp., *Peptostreptococcus* spp., and *Bacteroides* spp.

The enteric organisms (coliforms, *Pseudomonas* spp. and *Proteus* spp.) infect the lid margins only in immunosuppressed patients.

Rickettsias

Infections of the eyelid caused by rickettsias are uncommon, but occasionally the primary lesion of scrub typhus occurs on the eyelid.

Fungi

The most common causes of fungal infections of the eyelids are *Candida* spp. and the dermatophytes. Other fungal agents include *Coccidioides immitis, Blastomyces dermatididis, Paracoccidioides brasiliensis, Sporothrix schenkii, Cryptococcus* spp., *Rhinosporidium* spp., and *Aspergillus fumigatus.* Two yeastlike organisms (*Pityrosporum ovale* and *orbiculare*) are often found in scrapings of the margins of eyelids, but are probably not related to disease.

Viruses

The eyelid is often infected by the viruses of herpes simplex, varicella zoster, verrucae, and molluscum contagiosum. Vaccinial lid infections are now rare, but before the eradication of smallpox this was not the case; at one time, both vaccinial and variolar infections were not uncommon. The eyelid is also occasionally infected by other viruses such as ecthyma contagiosum (the cause of orf).

Protozoa

Rarely, the etiologic agents of leishmaniasis may infect the eyelids.

Metazoa

Demodex folliculorum often infects the hair follicles of the eyelashes. Less commonly, *Phthirus pubis* may infect the lid margins. *Loa loa* may also infect the eyelid during its wandering throughout the body. Some of the platyhelminthes (*Schistosoma* spp., *Distoma ringeri, Spirometra* spp., *Echinococcus* spp., and larval *Taenia solium*) have been found embedded in thickened areas of the eyelid. Some of the roundworms (*Ascaris lumbricoides, Enterobius vermicularis, Ancylostoma duodenale, Necator americanus, Trichinella spiralis,* and *Dirofilaria immitis*) and the blood flukes (*Schistosoma* spp.)

may cause toxic or urticarial edema or nodular thickening of the eyelid.

Seborrhea

The most common cause of blepharitis is seborrhea, and it must be distinguished from infectious causes. It is accompanied characteristically by dandruff of the scalp, eyebrows, and external ears. Even more characteristic are the greasy scales (seborrheic scurf) between the lashes. A problem in management that occurs all too often is mixed seborrheic and staphylococcal blepharitis.

Epidemiology

Infections of the eyelids that are associated with systemic infections also share the epidemiology of that disease. Immunosuppression is frequently a contributing factor.

Bacteria

Staphylococcal blepharitis is usually caused by the same phage type of *Staphylococcus aureus* that colonizes the anterior nares, umbilicus, perineum, and axillae. *Moraxella nonliquefaciens* is a common commensal on the lid margins and in the anterior nares, especially in warm climates.

Fungi

Although candidosis of the lid is usually associated with a candidal infection elsewhere, the lid margins often become infected when there is local immunosuppression by treatment of the eye with topical glucosteroids or broadly active antimicrobics.

Rhinosporidiosis is uncommon in the United States; most cases are seen in India and South Africa. The primary lesions are usually in the anterior nares, the eyelids becoming involved as a result of autoinoculation.

Metazoa

Demodex folliculorum is found in the hair follicles of about 50% of the population and may play a role in staphylococcal infection by carrying staphylococci into the follicles of the eyelashes.

Pathogenesis and Pathology

In bacterial blepharitis the hair follicles and the glands of the eyelid (Zeis, Moll, and meibomian) are often infected. A chronic, nongranulomatous inflammatory reaction associated with acanthosis, hyperkeratosis, or parakeratosis of the epidermis may thicken the lid margins. Ulcerations with fibrinous exudate often occur in staphylococcal infections.

External hordeola (styes) arise from acute suppurative inflammations of the superficial glands (sweat glands of Moll, sebaceous glands) or of the follicles of the lashes. Histologically, there is an accumulation of polymorphonuclear leukocytes, edema, and vascular congestion centered around the hair follicles or infected glands.

Internal hordeola arise from an acute purulent inflammation of a meibomian gland in the tarsus. Histologically, the lesions differ from external hordeola only in their location.

A chalazion is a chronic inflammation of a meibomian gland. Histologically, it is a zonal granulomatous inflammatory reaction centered on the lipid material of the meibomian gland. Multinucleated giant cells may be in evidence, and the granulomatous reaction is surrounded by polymorphonuclear leukocytes, plasma cells, and lymphocytes.

Histologically, the pedunculated lesion of rhinosporidiosis contains large spherules filled with conidia and sometimes surrounded by a granulomatous or nongranulomatous reaction.

Manifestations

Bacteria

With the exception of infections caused by enteric bacteria, most bacterial infections of the eye are associated with discharge and hyperemia of the skin of the lid. With some etiologic agents, distinctive signs may serve as clues to the identification of the causal organism.

Staphylococcal blepharitis is characterized by one or more of the following signs: ulceration of the lid margin; collarettes (fibrinous scales wrapped around the eyelash—resembling round pieces of paper impaled on sticks); styes; whitening of individual eyelashes; sparse, misdirected, or broken eyelashes; multiple or recurrent chalazia; fine epithelial keratitis affecting the lower half of the cornea; and catarrhal corneal ulcers or infiltrates.

Morax–Axenfeld blepharitis is marked by fissuring and scaling at the external or internal canthus or both. There is usually also an associated angular conjunctivitis.

Blepharitis caused by coliform bacilli has no distinguishing characteristics.

A *hordeolum* (either internal or external) is a discrete, elevated, tender, erythematous papule on or near the margin of the lid.

A *chalazion* is a hard, painless nodule embedded in the eyelid away from the margin of the lid.

Fungi

Candidosis of the margins of the lids is often ulcerative, granulomatous, or both, with small granulomata appearing at the edges of the small ulcerations. In other cases, the infection may simulate ringworm.

Rhinosporidiosis of the lid margin resembles a papilloma in its early stages but becomes pedunculated or verrucous as it enlarges.

Viruses

A molluscum nodule in the lid is a benign, round, pearly white, waxy, noninflammatory lesion similar to molluscum nodules elsewhere. However, there may result a follicular conjunctivitis, subsequent conjunctival scarring, superior corneal pannus, and superior epithelial keratitis suggestive of trachoma.

Verruca vulgaris of the lid is a pedunculated or broad-based multilobulated lesion. When it occurs on the lid margin it may produce papillary conjunctivitis and, rarely, mild epithelial keratitis.

Metazoa

Infection of the margins of the eyelids by *Phthirus pubis* is associated with itching. The nits and adult organisms are distinctive, but can easily be missed. In the child, follicular conjunctivitis often accompanies the infection.

Demodex folliculorum may cause itching of the eyelid. The finding of sleeves (clear, tubelike processes that extend up over the base of the eyelash for 0.5 mm to 1.0 mm is characteristic. The organism is a microscopic, acarian parasite characterized by eight stubby legs and cross-striations on its abdomen.

Diagnosis

Although the manifestations of blepharitis often suggest a specific etiologic agent, verification should be sought by direct examination and culture of scrapings from the involved lid.

Prognosis

Staphylococcal blepharitis is often chronic; associated with recurrent conjunctivitis, keratitis, styes, and chalazia; and difficult to eradicate. With the exception of the complications of molluscum of the lid margin, fungal, viral, protozoan, and metazoan infections of the eyelid are usually benign and self-limited.

Therapy

Once an etiologic diagnosis has been made, specific antimicrobial treatment against the offending organism can be instituted and should be accompanied at least once a day by scrubbing the lid to remove the detritus and crusts. For this purpose, a mild soap (*e.g.,* Johnson's Baby Shampoo) and water can be rubbed gently on the lid margin and then rinsed off. After scrubbing, an antimicrobic-containing ointment (bacitracin, neomycin, erythromycin, or a sulfonamide—often selected on the basis of *in vitro* susceptibility testing) is then applied to the bases of the eyelashes. The topical treatment must be applied for at least 4 to 6 weeks and may have to be continued either periodically or indefinitely. The systemic administration of antimicrobics is sometimes necessary.

External or internal hordeola should be treated with hot packs until the papule developes a point, and then should be drained surgically.

The nodule of rhinosporidiosis should be excised at its base, and the patient should be kept under observation for recurrences.

The nits of *Phthirus pubis* should be removed from the lashes and the adult parasites smothered with a bland ointment. The pubic area should be treated with a suitable insecticide (Chap. 114, Pediculosis).

Demodex responds readily to scrubbing the eyelids with soap and water.

Seborrheic blepharitis can be controlled by (1) the use of antiseborrheic shampoos for the scalp, forehead, and eyebrows; and (2) nightly cleansing of the margins of the lids with a mild soap (*e.g.,* Johnson's Baby Shampoo), followed by application of an ointment that combines 1% salicylic acid and 1% ammoniated mercury in a white petrolatum base.

Prevention

Many cases of staphylococcal blepharitis follow staphylococcal conjunctivitis. Prompt, adequate therapy is important.

Remaining Problems

In spite of the best available treatment, chronic blepharitis often persists and may require very long-continued treatment. The entire pathophysiology of this disease needs better understanding so that eradication may become possible.

Orbital Cellulitis

Orbital cellulitis refers to inflammation of the tissues surrounding the eye within the orbit. The orbital process may reflect inflammatory disease of the contiguous paranasal sinuses.

Etiology

Bacteria

The most common bacterial causes of orbital cellulitis are *Staphylococcus aureus* and *Streptococcus pyogenes.* In children under three years of age, *Haemophilus influenzae* is also a common cause of orbital cellulitis. Less common are *Streptococcus pneumoniae,* the coliform bacilli (*Escherichia coli* and *Klebsiella* spp.), *Proteus* spp., and *Pseudomonas* spp. The fusiform bacteria may also cause orbital disease; *M. tuberculosis* and *Treponema pallidum* are not common causes.

Fungi

Zygomycosis commonly afflicts the orbit, whereas *A. fumigatus, B. dermatitidis, Sporothrix schenkii,* and *Histoplasma duboisii* are quite uncommon.

Metazoan

Uncommonly, the orbit may be infected with *Echinococcus granulosus,* larval *Taenia solium, Trichinella spiralis,* and *Loa loa.* The orbit may be invaded by the larvae of flies (orbital myiasis), especially of *Oestrus ovis* (sheep botfly), and by the larvae of *Diptera* spp., *Hypoderma bovis, Wohlfahrtia magnifica,* and *Caliphora vomitoria.*

Epidemiology

Suppurative orbital cellulitis is usually secondary to trauma or to an extension of endophthalmitis. Zygomycosis may cause suppurative orbital cellulitis and is usually associated with some underlying cause such as acidosis. Nonsuppurative orbital cellulitis commonly arises as an extension of an inflammation or infection of the paranasal sinuses.

The cause of chronic nongranulomatous and granulomatous inflammations of the orbit is often unknown, but may be a reaction to an infection already controlled by the host or a secondary reaction to the toxic products of tissue destruction. Granulomatous inflammation may be caused by tuberculosis, syphilis, fungi, protozoa, and metazoa.

Manifestations

The cardinal signs of orbital cellulitis are edema of the eyelids, chemosis of the conjunctiva, restriction of movement of the globe, and proptosis. The degree of proptosis and restriction of movement, and the direction of the proptosis, vary according to the location of the inflammation. For example, there is severe limitation of movement very early in the course of zygomycosis; subsequently, infection within the muscle cone causes severe axial proptosis, whereas infection of the subperiosteal area causes moderate proptosis directed away from the infection.

Chills, fever, malaise, and leukocytosis often accompany orbital cellulitis.

Diagnosis

Although the signs of orbital cellulitis do not vary substantially according to cause, it is important to determine the specific etiology. A clue may be obtained by determining the site of origin of the inflammation. Infections occurring within the muscle cone usually follow trauma or septicemia. Roentgenograms of the orbit for the detection of a foreign body, and cultures of the patient's blood and extraocular lesions may be very valuable. A cellulitis arising as a contiguous reaction from the paranasal sinuses begins in the area of the affected sinus; thus, investigation of the paranasal sinuses is often rewarding.

Tenonitis may simulate orbital cellulitis and is often associated with it. The proptosis is mild, and there is voluntary restriction of movement of the globe to prevent pain. Tenonitis may also be caused by *Trichinella spiralis,* and may also arise as an extension of endophthalmitis, or from metastatic lesions.

Specimens obtained by swabbing a draining orbital sinus, or preferably, by aspirating a fluctuant area within the orbit should be examined directly (with smears) and by culture.

Prognosis

Orbital cellulitis may be severe and may lead to corneal ulceration, cavernous-sinus thrombosis, and brain abscess. The infection must be evaluated carefully and treated promptly.

Therapy

Treatment of orbital cellulitis is directed against the underlying cause. Large doses of antimicrobics, as for the treatment of meningitis (Chap. 119, Acute Bacterial Meningitis), are often necessary. Surgical drainage of suppuration in the orbit and of blocked paranasal sinuses is necessary.

Zygomycosis of the orbit requires control of a predisposing acidosis, excision of the affected area, and administration of amphotericin B.

Prevention

Prevention of orbital cellulitis involves controlling or minimizing predisposing immunosuppression, and adequate treatment of infections of structures in, near, or surrounding the orbit.

Remaining Problems

As long as broadly immunosuppressive measures are necessary in medicine, the likelihood of occurrence of severe infections of the orbit will increase. Methods of controlling disease without the penalty of immunosuppression must be developed.

Bibliography

Books

FINEGOLD SM: Anaerobic Bacteria in Human Disease. New York, Academic Press, 1977. 110 pp.

YANOFF M, FINE BS: Ocular Pathology: A Text and Atlas. Philadelphia, Harper & Row, 1982, 916 pp.

JAWETZ E, MELNICK JL, ADELBERG EA: Review of Medical Microbiology. Los Altos, Lange Medical Publications, 1976. 542 pp.

Journals

OSTLER HB, OKUMOTO M, HALDE C: Dermatophytosis affecting the periorbital region. Am J Ophthalmol 72:934–938, 1971

OSTLER HB, THYGESON P, OKUMOTO M: Infectious diseases of the eye. J Continuing Educ Ophthalmol 39:13–25, 1978

THYGESON P: Etiology and treatment of blepharitis. Arch Ophthalmol 36: 445, 1946

H. BRUCE OSTLER
MASAO OKUMOTO

161 Conjunctivitis and Scleritis

Conjunctivitis

Conjunctivitis is an acute, subacute, or chronic inflammation of the conjunctiva that is associated with a serous, mucoid, or purulent exudate.

Etiology

Conjunctivitis may be caused by many kinds of infectious agents as well as by noninfectious processes such as allergy, irritation from noxious stimuli, and diminished secretion of tears.

Conjunctival infections are classified according to kind of exudate and etiology in Table 161-1. If the conjunctivitis persists without specific treatment for 1 to 2 weeks, it is acute; if longer than 2 weeks, it is chronic.

Epidemiology

Conjunctivitis occurs worldwide. It is especially common to technologically underdeveloped countries, where it often occurs in seasonal epidemics, and may be associated with vectors such as flies. In the Middle East, for example, conjunctivits caused by *Haemophilus aegyptius* becomes epidemic in the late spring and persists throughout the summer and into the early fall. In the same area, pneumococcal conjunctivitis becomes epidemic in the winter and persists until early spring.

Trachoma (Chap. 159, Trachoma) is the most common cause of blindness in the world; in developing countries, for example, in the Middle East and India, millions of people are infected. Acute hemorrhagic conjunctivitis, which occurs in epidemic form throughout most of the rest of the world, was recently reported in the United States and the rest of the American continents.

Pathogenesis and Pathology

Although the conjunctivae are exposed to many microorganisms, infection does not result unless the diluting and sluicing action of the tears and the growth-inhibiting action of lysozyme, betalysin, IgA, and IgG contained in the tears are overcome. A diminution of tears (*e.g.,* by keratoconjunctivitis sicca, occlusion of the nasolacrimal duct, or injudicious use of a dressing) may reduce these normal defense mechanisms and pave the way for infection. Foreign bodies (including contact lenses) in the conjunctival sac may also reduce resistance to infection.

Papillary hypertrophy is a fine, velvety hyperemia of the conjunctiva that occurs in all forms of conjunctivitis. By histologic examination, there is an accumulation of polymorphonuclear cells and a few lymphocytes lying between the fine fibrils that attach the conjunctival epithelium to the tarsus.

Follicular hypertrophy is characterized by white or gray, round, avascular structures on the tarsal conjunctiva. Such follicles are usually found in chlamydial and viral conjunctival infections; histologically, they consist of a central zone of reticuloendothelial cells surrounded by a peripheral zone of lymphocytes. In trachoma, the central cells often degenerate, become necrotic, and produce conjunctival scars.

Manifestations

The hallmark of purulent conjunctivitis is copious formation of pus. Typically, there is also severe edema of the eyelids, and corneal complications are frequent.

The membrane of membranous and pseudomembranous conjunctivitis is grayish-yellow and occurs either in patches or as a continuous sheet on the tarsal (or sometimes bulbar) conjunctiva. In the membranous disease, bleeding usually occurs when the

Table 161-1. Correlation of Exudative Response With Specific Etiology of Infectious Conjunctivitis

Exudative Response	Etiology
Viral	
Follicular	Adenovirus types 3, 7, and others (pharygoconjunctival fever); primary herpes simplex virus; varicella-zoster; Newcastle disease virus
Pseudomembranous	Adenovirus types 8 and 19 (epidemic kerato-conjunctivitis)
Acute hemorrhagic	Enterovirus type 70; coxsackievirus A-24
Keratoconjunctivitis	Measles; Newscastle disease
Blepharoconjunctivitis	Vaccinia; molluscum contagiosum
Chlamydial	
Follicular	*Chlamydia trachomatis*—trachoma, lymphogranuloma venereum;* inclusion conjunctivitis *Chlamydia psittaci*—psittacosis; feline pneumonitis
Rickettsial	
	All rickettsias pathogenic for humans (may be the portal of entry)
Bacterial	
Hyperacute purulent	Most common; *Neisseria gonorrhoeae, Neisseria meningitidis;* exceptionally, other bacteria, *e.g., pseudomonas* spp.
Acute mucopululent	*Staphylococcus aureus; Streptococcus pyogenes; Streptococcus pneumoniae; Haemophilus aegyptius, Haemophilus influenzae; Escherichia coli; Pseudomonas* spp.
Acute membranous and pseudomembranous	Most common, *Streptococcus pyogenes, Corynebacterium diphtheriae* Compromised hosts, *Staphylococcus aureus, Haemophilus aegyptius, Haemophilus influenzae, Escherichia coli, Shigella* spp., *Pseudomonas aeruginosa*
Subactue catarrhal	*Haemophilus influenzae*
Chronic catarrhal	Commonly, *Staphylococcus aureus* Warm climates, *Moraxella lacunata, Moraxella liquefaciens* Occasionally, *Escherichia coli, Proteus* spp.
Granulomatous*	*Mycobacterium tuberculosis; Mycobacterium leprae; Treponema pallidum; Francisella tularensis; Leptotrichia* spp.
Fungal	
Granulomatous*	Most Common, *Candida* spp. Also, *Sporothrix schenkii, Rhinosporidium seeberi, Coccidioides immitis*
Metazoal	
	Thelazia californiensis, Trichenella spiralis, Taenia solium, Schistosoma haematobium, Onchocerca volvulus, Loa loa Fly larvae, *e.g., Oestrus ovis*

* Parinaud's oculoglandular syndrome.

membrane is stripped from the underlying conjunctiva.

Acute catarrhal conjunctivitis begins with acute conjunctival hyperemia and a watery exudate that soon becomes mucopurulent. Petechial hemorrhages are usually present when either *Streptococcus pneumoniae* or *H. aegyptius* cause this form of conjunctivitis.

Subacute catarhhal conjunctivitis is characterized by a watery or flocculent exudate and mild hyperemia that is limited principally to the palpebral conjunctiva and fornices.

Chronic catarrhal conjunctivitis gives rise to the sensation of a foreign body and causes itching and burning of a severity that is out of proportion to the minimal mucoid exudate and mild to moderate hyperemia present.

Follicular conjunctivitis is typical of viral and chlamydial infections occurring in persons over 2 months of age. The conjunctiva does not develop an adenoid layer until the baby is 1.5 to 2 months of age; as a result, the newborn with inclusion conjunctivitis does not form follicles.

Granulomata appear as nodules or as polypoid or

sessile masses located in the fornix or on the tarsal or bulbar conjunctiva. They are found in many diseases, but when they are associated with a grossly visible preauricular node, they are classified as a feature of Parinaud's oculoglandular syndrome.

Diagnosis

Although the clinician can often differentiate the various forms of conjunctivitis on the basis of manifestations, the laboratory is frequently an invaluable adjunct in determining the etiologic agent. Conjunctival scrapings containing epithelial cells that underlie the exudate are most helpful. A predominantly polymorphonuclear inflammatory cell reaction is found in bacterial or chlamydial conjunctivitis, and in viral conjunctivitis when there is a pseudomembrane. In other cases of viral conjunctivitis, mononuclear cells predominate.

Bacterial conjunctivitis can be differentiated clinically from chlamydial conjunctivitis on the basis of follicles, which are characteristic of chlamydial infection. Because follicles do not occur in the very young, diagnosis in newborns depends on finding intracytoplasmic epithelial chlamydial inclusions.

Conjunctival scrapings containing multinucleated giant cells characterize the conjunctivitis of herpes simplex, herpes zoster, and measles.

The bacterial and fungal organisms causing conjunctivitis can usually be identified in gram-stained or Giemsa-stained preparations of conjunctival scrapings. Further identification is often made by culturing material collected from the conjunctiva, lid margin, or both.

Two important variants of noninfectious conjunctivitis are allergic conjunctivitis and keratoconjunctivitis sicca. Allergic conjunctivitis is characterized by intense itching and a milky appearance of the conjunctiva; scrapings usually contain eosinophils or extracellular eosinophilic granules. In keratoconjunctivitis sicca, the tear film is deficient; mucold strands often cling to the cornea, and the patient complains that the symptoms worsen as the day wears on.

Prognosis

Except for chronic catarrhal conjunctivitis and trachoma, infectious conjunctivitis is almost always self-limited. A purulent membranous or pseudomembranous conjunctivitis may ultimately affect the cornea and lead to its perforation and to loss of the eye; purulent, membranous, and pseudomembranous conjunctivitis and trachoma may cause scarring of the conjunctiva. The scarring is usually not severe, but the production of mucus by the conjunctival goblet cells may be reduced or lacking, and a dry eye may result. Trachoma may seriously reduce vision by producing a fibrovascular membrane (pannus) over the cornea.

Treatment

Purulent conjunctivitis, pseudomembranous and membranous conjunctivitis of bacterial origin, and chlamydial infections all require systemic therapy aimed at the specific etiologic agent. Topical medications are of secondary importance but are often used in conjunction with the systemic medications.

On the other hand, in other kinds of bacterial conjunctivitis, the topical use of suitable antimicrobics usually suffices. Topical bacitracin, erythromycin, and the sulfonamides are the medications of choice in acute catarrhal conjunctivitis. In subacute catarrhal conjunctivitis, topical chloramphenicol, sulfonamides, and erythromycin answer the purpose. The lid margins must also be treated in chronic catarrhal conjunctivitis (Chap. 160, Infections of the Eyelids and Periorbital Cellulitis).

The viral conjunctivitides are self-limited and do not respond to antiviral medications. Frequent irrigation of the eye with 0.9% NaCl solution, followed by cold packs, often gives the patient symptomatic relief.

Candidal conjunctivitis responds well to application of topical preparations containing either nystatin (100,000 u/g, a dermatological preparation) or amphotericin B (1.5–3.0 mg/ml).

The conjunctivitis and systemic disease associated with granulomata and a grossly visible preauricular node—Parinaud's oculoglandular syndrome—often respond rapidly to excisional biopsy of the granulomata; possibly, an antigenic mass that provokes the clinical manifestations is thereby removed.

Prevention

Prevention of ophthalmia neonatorum by use of the Crede procedure or by instillation of tetracycline or erythromycin is well established. Epidemic keratoconjunctivitis is often transmitted in the physician's office by way of contaminated eye solutions (especially fluorescein) or by the physician's fingers. Proper handwashing between patient examinations and sterilization of solutions and fomites used in or around the eye must be strictly maintained.

Remaining Problems

Although trachoma has been virtualy controlled in the industrially developed countries of the world, it remains a serious problem in many other countries. Control of trachoma and many of the types of conjunctivitis prevalent in developing countries calls for education, sanitation, and treatment.

Scleritis

Scleritis and episcleritis are acute or chronic inflammations of the sclera or episclera, respectively; both are usually associated with tearing and photophobia.

Etiology

Scleritis and episcleritis are rarely caused by infectious agents, and then only in association with a systemic infectious disease. Much more often, they are associated with noninfectious systemic diseases such as rheumatoid arthritis. Unfortunately, in too many cases the etiology is unknown.

Occasionally, simple episcleritis may accompany varicella-zoster or tuberculosis, and nodular episcleritis may accompany coccidioidomycosis or syphilis.

Diffuse anterior scleritis has been seen in active tuberculosis, syphilis, herpes zoster, onchocerciasis, and leprosy. Nodular scleritis may occur in herpes zoster, herpes simplex, *Staphylococcus aureus* infections, and syphilis. A severe form of nodular keratitis, often referred to as necrotizing scleritis, has been seen in both active tuberculosis and syphilis.

Epidemiology

The epidemiology of episcleritis and scleritis is the same as that of the underlying systemic infectious disease.

Pathogenesis and Pathology

Episcleritis may be diffuse or nodular. Diffuse episcleritis may afflict a large sector of the episcleral tissue in a nongranulomatous process characterized by widespread hyperemia, edema, and infiltration with lymphocytes and plasma cells. Nodular episcleritis occurs as elevated, well-circumscribed, slightly tender areas; in the center of the lesions, there are large mononuclear cells and some giant cells, with or without central necrosis and destruction of the scleral collagen fibers. The central area is surrounded by a zone of infiltration with lymphocytes or plasma cells.

Scleritis may also be diffuse or nodular. The reactive capacity of the sclera is similar to that of the tendons and tendon sheaths of the body: all are virtually avascular. However, histologic examination of the scleral tissue in scleritis usually shows an acute inflammatory reaction. Nodular scleritis may be associated with varying degrees of fragmentation of the collagenous connective tissue, which are usually less severe than the fragmentation and necrosis observed in necrotizing scleritis.

Manifestations

The symptoms of episcleritis, whether diffuse or nodular, are redness, photophobia, and tearing. The affected area is hyperemic and has a pink or purple color when viewed in the daylight. Tenderness is minimal, and the episcleral vessels blanch when epinephrine (1:1000) is instilled into the conjunctival sac. The episclera is always edematous, but this can be seen only with a slit-lamp.

Scleritis is characterized by redness, photophobia, tearing, tenderness, and pain. There is an intense violaceous discoloration that may be localized to a nodule or may be diffuse. When epinephrine is instilled, the deep, congested scleral vessels remain dilated and hyperemic. Edema of the sclera can be seen with a slit-lamp.

Diagnosis

The etiologic diagnosis of most cases of episcleritis and scleritis can be made on the basis of the association of the inflamed episcleral and scleral tissue with an infectious disease process, for example, with herpes zoster ophthalmicus. Another clue is the favorable response of the inflammation to treatment of the apparently causal disease, for example, coccidioidomycosis. Sometimes the episcleral or scleral tissues may have to be biopsied and the etiologic diagnosis made from histologic examination and the cultures of the specimen.

Both episcleritis and scleritis may be simulated by iritis, keratitis, or the congestive phase of closed-angle glaucoma. Iritis may accompany scleritis, but tends to be mild, whereas the iritis that simulates scleritis is usually severe and associated with a miotic pupil. The congestive phase of closed-angle glaucoma may simulate either episcleritis or scleritis and is usually associated with pupil dilation and severely elevated intraocular pressure. In the masquerading keratitis, the cornea is usually heavily infiltrated with white cells and has lost its brilliant luster.

Prognosis

Episcleritis is usually self-limited, and although it may recur, the complications, if any, are minimal. However, herpes zoster episcleritis sometimes progresses to scleritis.

Scleritis may cause thinning of the sclera, and a staphyloma may eventuate.

Therapy

When episcleritis and scleritis are caused by infectious agents, they usually respond moderately well to treatment of the systemic disease. In some cases, biopsy of the affected ocular tissue and removal of the major focus of infection may be necessary.

Bibliography

Books

HOGAN MJ, ZIMMERMAN LE: Opthalmic Pathology: An Atlas and Textbook. Philadelphia, WB Saunders, 1962. 797 pp.

WATSON PG, HAZELMAN BL: The Sclera and Systemic Disorders. Philadelphia, WB Saunders Co, 1976. 458 pp.

Journals

DAWSON CR: Epidemic Koch–Weeks conjunctivitis and trachoma. Am J Ophthalmol 49:801, 1960

FRIEDMAN AH, HENKIND P: Unusual causes of episcleritis. Trans Am Acad Ophthalmol Otolaryngol 78:890–895, 1974

OSTLER HB, BRALEY AE: Conjunctivitis: Its etiologic diagnosis and treatment. J Iowa Med Soc 44:427–436, 1954

OSTLER HB, THYGESON P, OKUMOTO M: Infectious diseases of the eye, Part II. J Continuing Educ Ophthalmol 11–32, May 1978

THYGESON P: Clinical signs of diagnostic importance in conjunctivitis. JAMA 33:437–441, 1947

H. BRUCE OSTLER
MASAO OKUMOTO

Corneal Infections

162

Many corneal infections are altogether preventable; in others, cicatricial sequelae and diminished vision may often be prevented if the etiologic agent is quickly determined and proper treatment is promptly instituted. Regardless of location at onset, most corneal infections spread toward the center of the cornea, away from the vascularized limbus. The ulcers that form are called *central corneal ulcers* or *hypopyon ulcers.* Although some corneal infections may remain peripheral for long periods, bacterial and fungal infections are usually progressive.

Etiology

Bacterial Infections

Although the pneumococcus is the one true bacterial pathogen of the cornea, in recent years the bacterial causes of central corneal ulcers have been (in order of decreasing frequency) *viridans* group *Streptococcus* spp., *Pseudomonas* spp., *Moraxella* spp., *Staphylococcus aureus, Staphylococcus epidermidis,* mixed bacterial infections, *Streptococcus pneumoniae, Nocardia* spp., and a miscellaneous group that includes hemolytic *Streptococcus* spp., *Peptostreptococcus* spp., *Branhamella* spp., nonhemolytic *Streptococcus* spp., and *Acinetobacter* spp.

Fungal Infections

Most fungal corneal ulcers are caused by five opportunistic fungi: *Candida* spp., *Fusarium* spp., *Aspergillus* spp., *Penicillium* spp., and *Cephalosporium* spp. But other opportunists—*Alternaria* spp., *Helminthosporium* spp., and *Rhizopus* spp.—occasionally infect the cornea.

Viral Infections

Herpes simplex viruses (HSVs) are by far the most common viral causes of infection of the cornea. However many other viruses may involve the cornea in connection with a viral conjunctivitis or some systemic viral infection such as rubeola, varicella-zoster, infectious mononucleosis, mumps, adenoviral disease, Newcastle disease conjunctivitis, and acute hemorrhagic conjunctivitis.

Epidemiology

Scarring of the cornea from infection is a major cause of reduced vision and blindness. It is important to recognize that corneal infections—bacterial, fungal, and viral—have been increasing in frequency and severity. In the developed countries of the world, corneal infections are most commonly caused by HSV, but bacterial infections are also common, and fungal infections, once rare, are now seen regularly.

The general increase in frequency and severity of corneal infections is largely traceable to the increasingly common use (especially the topical use) of immunosuppressive agents, for example, the glucosteroids, in the treatment of eye diseases. This can be inferred from the fact that in underdeveloped countries, the pneumococcus is by far the most common cause of bacterial corneal ulcers, whereas in developed countries, nonpneumococcal bacteria and fungi are most common. Similarly, in areas where heavy concentrations of bacteria or fungi tend to contaminate corneal abrasions and wounds, nonpneumococcal infections are most common.

Under normal circumstances, the corneal epithelium acts as a natural barrier that must be breached if bacteria and fungi are to cause infection. *Corynebacterium diphtheriae, Neisseria gonorrhoeae,* and *Haemophilus aegyptius* are exceptions, since they cause corneal infection by actually invading the epithelium.

Streptococcus pneumoniae is the only true stromal pathogen of the cornea. All that is required to produce a central corneal ulcer is a minimal epithelial breach and the introduction of a few capsulated (protected from phagocytosis) cocci. Other bacteria and fungi require either an overwhelming inoculum or an immunosuppressed cornea.

Once microorganisms reach the corneal stroma, the infection is resisted first by nonspecific factors, including phagocytosis, which participate in the acute inflammatory reaction. Later, humoral and cell-mediated immunity play a vital role. Stromal resistance is often reduced disastrously in immunosuppressed hosts such as alcoholics, diabetics, elderly or debilitated persons, patients with keratoconjunctivitis sicca or chronic dacryocystitis, and patients under treatment with immunosuppressants (e.g., glucosteroids, topical anesthetics, and idoxuridine).

Pathogenesis and Pathology

Central corneal ulcers almost always have a hypopyon and are commonly called hypopyon corneal ulcers. The hypopyon consists of a collection of inflammatory cells in the anterior chamber, most of which are neutrophils, with some mononuclear cells and macrophages. In bacterial corneal ulcers, the hypopyon is sterile as long as Descemet's membrane is intact; in fungal corneal ulcers, the hypopyon often contains fungal elements in spite of an intact Descemet's membrane. In smears prepared from material taken from the edges of the ulcer and stained properly (*e.g.,* with MacCallum's stain), the infecting microorganisms and many inflammatory cells may be seen.

A hypopyon may also occur in corneal infections caused by HSV if there is a necrotic focus that results in an axonal-reflex outpouring of leukocytes into the anterior chamber.

Histologic examination of bacterial and fungal corneal ulcers shows destruction of the corneal epithelium and of both the superficial and deep lamellae of the stroma. Because Descemet's membrane is relatively resistant to the enzymes produced by leukocytes and infecting organisms, it is often intact until late in the infection.

Histologic study of herpes simplex corneal ulcers reveals only epithelial necrosis unless the underlying stroma is affected. Virions may then be recognized in the keratocytes of the cornea by electron microscopy.

Manifestations

Bacterial Corneal Ulcers

The corneal ulcers caused by different kinds of bacteria are similar in appearance and differ only in severity. This close resemblance is particularly characteristic of the ulcers caused by opportunistic bacteria, for example, *viridans* group *Streptococcus* spp., *Staphylococcus aureus, Nocardia* spp., and *Mycobacterium fortuitum,* all of which tend to be indolent and to spread slowly and superficially. However, the following bacterial ulcers do have some distinctive clinical features.

PNEUMOCOCCAL CORNEAL ULCERS

Pneumococcal corneal ulcers may develop as early as 24 to 48 hours after the inoculation of a cornea with disturbed epithelium. Typically, the ulcer is well circumscribed and has a gray center; the surrounding cornea is often clear. The ulcer tends to progress centrally in an irregular fashion—the advancing border showing activity, the trailing edge tending to heal. By virtue of this peculiarity, the ulcer is often referred to as serpiginous. The superficial cornea is affected first, the deep cornea later. Early in the course of the infection, a typical hypopyon forms.

PSEUDOMONAL CORNEAL ULCERS

Pseudomonal corneal ulcers are often accompanied by severe pain. The ulcer begins as a gray or yellow corneal infiltrate at the point of entry of the organism. The developing ulcer spreads rapidly, facilitated by the proteolytic enzymes produced by the organism, remaining round and superficial during its early stages. The base of the ulcer and the exudate are sometimes greenish. There is typically a large hypopyon that tends to increase in size as the ulcer progresses.

MORAXELLA LIQUEFACIENS AND *MORAXELLA NONLIQUEFACIENS*

Moraxella liquefaciens and *nonliquefaciens* cause corneal ulcers that are characteristically indolent. They are usually located inferior to the pupil and progress toward the deep stroma over a period of days or weeks. The ulcer begins as a central, gray infiltrate with the rest of the stroma remaining clear. There is either no hypopyon or only a small one. Moraxellal ulcers occur principally in alcoholics, and also in patients debilitated from other causes such as diabetes.

OTHER BACTERIAL CORNEAL ULCERS

Other bacterial corneal ulcers generally have no distinguishing characteristics. However, ulcers caused by more virulent bacteria, for example, *Staphylococcus aureus, Streptococcus pyogenes,* and *Escherichia coli* usually provoke a more severe inflammatory reaction and hypopyon than *Staphylococcus epidermi-*

dis and *viridans* streptococci. The corneal ulcers caused by *Mycobacterium fortuitum* and *Nocardia asteroides* often resemble fungal ulcers and are usually accompanied by minimal inflammatory reactions.

Fungal Corneal Ulcers

Corneal ulcers caused by hyphate mould fungi usually display a number of the characteristics listed below. The most common of these are satellite lesions, hyphate edges, a firm, elevated base, and an endothelial plaque. When nonhyphate fungi, for example, *Candida* spp., cause corneal ulcers, the lesions generally resemble indolent bacterial corneal ulcers; in exceptional cases, the characteristics are those of hyphate fungal ulcers.

Viral Corneal Ulcers

HERPES SIMPLEX VIRUS CORNEAL INFECTION

Because corneal anesthesia occurs early in the course of corneal infection with HSV, the patient often has little or no pain and minimal photophobia. However, irritation and tearing are common complaints.

The characteristic epithelial corneal lesion of HSV is the dendritic ulcer—a linear lesion that tends to branch and ends with terminal bulbs. Other epithelial lesions caused by HSV are usually transitory and eventually become dendritic; they include blotchy epithelial keratitis, stellate epithelial keratitis, and filamentary keratitis. A dendritic ulcer may evolve into a geographic ulcer—a large, epithelial ulcer with angulated edges. Failure to heal because of the anesthetic cornea may result in a trophic ulcer—a round or oval lesion with slightly heaped-up edges.

Marginal keratitis is linear in form, and it may also be produced by HSV. In this disorder, an epithelial defect precedes the development of a subepithelial infiltrate; in contrast, a subepithelial infiltrate precedes the epithelial defect in the evolution of a catarrhal corneal ulcer.

Other corneal changes produced by HSV are disciform keratitis, focal avascular interstitial keratitis, and hypopyon central corneal ulcer. Disciform keratitis is a round lesion that affects most of the depth of the stroma and is usually located centrally. Characteristic also are fine to medium-sized white keratic precipitates that lie directly under the disciform lesion. In focal avascular interstitial keratitis, focal areas of stromal infiltration and edema are surrounded by clear areas; typically, there are no vessels. The HSV-induced corneal ulcer associated with hypopyon is usually central and indolent.

VARICELLA-ZOSTER VIRUS KERATOIRITIS

When the nasociliary branch of the ophthalmic division of the fifth cranial nerve is affected by varicella-zoster virus (VZV), corneal lesions result that consist of blotchy, amorphous, epithelial keratitis and an occasional pseudodendrite. This is a linear lesion with some tendency to branch, but it stains poorly and does not have terminal knobs. Stromal lesions in the form of round opacities with irregular edges may also occur in herpes zoster in all layers of the cornea. Disciform keratitis may develop, and as in HSV keratitis, corneal sensation is reduced or lacking.

OTHER VIRAL CORNEAL INFECTIONS

A fine epithelial keratitis may be associated with many other viral infections, for example, measles, mumps, rubella, infectious mononucleosis, acute hemorrhagic conjunctivitis, Newcastle disease conjunctivitis, and verruca of the lid margin. These lesions have no identifying features except that under high magnification they can be seen as small epithelial infiltrates grouped into larger, grossly visible lesions.

HISTORY AND SIGNS OF FUNGAL (HYPHATE-PRODUCING) CORNEAL ULCERS

- A history of the use of glucosteroids in the eye
- A history of ocular injury with introduction of organic material
- Severe inflammation of the anterior segment, especially if glucosteroids have been reduced in amount or discontinued
- Superficial ulceration
- An irregular, hyphate-edged infiltrate
- Satellite lesions distinct from the main lesion
- An immune ring
- A corneal abscess
- A firm ulcer bed, often elevated above the surface of the cornea
- An endothelial plaque directly under the corneal infiltrate
- A severe anterior-chamber reaction and hypopyon

Diagnosis

A central corneal ulcer not obviously caused by HSV should be considered an ocular emergency, and every effort should be made to determine the cause as quickly as possible. The cornea is anesthetized and scrapings are taken from the ulcer with a sterile platinum spatula or Bard–Parker knife. If the lesion is evolving rapidly, the advancing edge of the ulcer is scraped; if the ulcer is indolent, the base is scraped. Two scrapings are obtained: one for microscopic study and a second for culturing on blood agar, chocolate agar, Sabouraud's agar without inhibitors (Emmons' modification), and cooked meat broth. The Sabouraud's agar culture is incubated at 30°C, and the other cultures are maintained at 35°C to 37°C.

After gram or Giemsa staining, microscopic examination enables etiologic diagnosis in 75% of cases. If insufficient material is collected, the scraping procedure should be repeated.

Lack of corneal sensation and presence of a typical dendritic lesion is highly suggestive of HSV infection. Epithelial scrapings from the edge of herpetic ulcer contains multinucleated epithelial (giant) cells, and yield HSV readily in many cell lines.

Corneal lesions associated with other viral infections are usually identified from the manifestations of the accompanying systemic disease (*e.g.,* measles, mumps, rubella), or on the signs of the accompanying conjunctivitis (*e.g.,* adenoviral conjunctivitis).

Prognosis

The prognosis of a central corneal ulcer caused by bacteria or fungi is usually poor unless proper treatment is undertaken promptly. Even when this is the case, severe central corneal scarring may reduce vision, and vascularization, thinning, and perforation may supervene.

Corneal infections caused by HSV are usually self-limited and heal with minimal or no scarring. However, if immunosuppression has been induced locally or systemically, the disease may be prolonged and lead to severe scarring, severely reduced vision, and even loss of the eye.

Therapy

Nonspecific Therapy

Early in the course of a corneal infection, 1 drop of a cycloplegic, for example, Cyclogyl, 1% or 2%, should be instilled into the eye 4 times daily. Later, atropine, 1%, or scopolamine, 0.25%, instilled twice daily, may be substituted. If the pupil is not fully dilated, topically applied neosynephrine, 2.5% or 10%, should be added to the regimen as 4 instillations per day.

If there is a concomitant elevation of intraocular pressure, a carbonic anhydrase inhibitor, for example, Diamox, 0.25 g 4 times daily, should be given systemically along with a β-blocker such as timolol maleate (Timoptic), 0.25% or 0.5%, administered topically twice daily. If the pressure is still not controlled, topical epinephrine, 1.0%, may also be instilled into the eye twice daily. Miotics must not be used. (If a carbonic anhydrase inhibitor is used over a long period, a potassium supplement, for example, 10% or 20% potassium chloride solution, should also be given. Timolol maleate should not be used if there is a history of asthma, irregular heartbeat, or heart block.)

Specific Therapy

Treatment for central corneal ulcer must be instituted promptly, and adequate dosage must be given if the lesion is to heal. Systemic administration of antimicrobics is often unnecessary because high concentrations may be attained in the cornea from subconjunctival and topical application. If the ulcer is very severe, systemic as well as subconjunctival and topical administration may be helpful, since it is possible that higher concentrations of appropriate antimicrobics in the cornea may result, and two or more drugs may be given in the hope that an additive or synergistic effect will result.

Subconjunctival injections of antimicrobics should be repeated every 12 to 24 hours for a total of 3 to 6 doses. Topical instillation should be repeated every hour during the daytime and every 2 hours during the hours of sleep for 7 to 10 days. (If a penicillinlike drug and an aminocyclitol are injected subconjunctivally, they must not be mixed in the same syringe. However, they should be injected in the same conjunctival quadrant; if scarring occurs, it is then confined to one quadrant.) Systemic medications should be given for 5 to 7 days.

Antimicrobial therapy should be initiated according to the findings on microscopic examination of epithelial scrapings. The regimen should be modified as necessary, according to (1) the response of the cornea, (2) the culture reports, and (3) the susceptibility test reports (see Table 163-2 for the drugs of choice, routes of administration, and dosages).

Prevention

Bacterial corneal ulcers rarely occur unless the corneal epithelium has been breached. Abrasion of the cornea, as when ointment is instilled into the eye, may have unhappy consequences. The cornea should be protected against drying during general anesthesia. Any notching of the eyelid or any mechanical dysfunction of the eyelid that prevents adequate closure, should be corrected.

Fungal corneal ulcers arise all too often in patients

who are immunosuppressed. The physician should be aware of the potential consequences of the severe immunosuppression associated with topical use of glucosteroids.

Viral corneal infections other than herpes zoster and herpes simplex are usually self-limited. HSV infections may be set off by upper respiratory infections, fever, trauma, emotional stress, sunburn, exposure to sunlight, and onset of the menstrual cycle. Aspirin may be preventive with fever, upper respiratory infection, and onset of the menstrual cycle; sunburn, sunlight, stress, and trauma should be avoided.

Remaining Problems

Adequate delivery of antimicrobics to the ulcerated cornea remains a problem. Although most ulcers can be controlled if appropriate treatment is instituted promptly, corneal necrosis and scarring often eventuate and result in reduced vision. The general public and health care professionals need to be alerted to the dangers of using topical glucosteroids to treat nonspecific ocular inflammation.

Bibliography

Book

VAUGHAN D, ASBURY T: General Ophthalmology. Los Altos, Lange Medical Publications, 1980. 410 pp.

Journals

FEDUKOWICZ H, HORWICH H: The gram-negative diplobacillus in hypopyon keratitis. Arch Ophthalmol 49–202, 1953

OSTLER HB, OKUMOTO M, WILKEY C: The changing pattern of the etiology of central bacterial corneal (hypopyon) ulcer. Trans Pac Coast Otoophthalmol Soc 57:235–241, 1976

OSTLER HB, THYGESON P, OKUMOTO M: Infectious diseases of the eye. III Infections of the cornea. J Continuing Educ Ophthalmol pp. 13–25, September 1978

THYGESON P, OKUMOTO M: Keratomycosis: A preventable disease. Trans Am Acad Ophthalmol Otolaryngol 78:433–439, 1974

H. BRUCE OSTLER
MASAO OKUMOTO

163 Endophthalmitis

Endophthalmitis is an inflammatory disease involving one or more of the coats of the eye, and of the adjacent cavities. It must be distinguished from panophthalmitis, in which the inflammation has spread through the sclera into the adjacent soft tissues of the orbit.

Endophthalmitis may be classified as exogenous or endogenous in origin. Exogenous endophthalmitis results from (1) spread of an infection from the orbit, a sinus, or an eyelid to the inner eye; (2) spread of an infection from the cornea to the inner eye; or (3) a penetrating foreign body or other ocular wound, including a surgical wound. Endogenous endophthalmitis arises from (1) hematogenous spread of septic emboli to the inner eye; (2) an inflammatory process originating in the optic nerve; (3) necrosis of tissue within the eye, for example, tumor tissue; or (4) a severe immune reaction within the eye, as from a hypermature lens. The following discussion is focussed on infective endophthalmitis.

Etiology

Bacteria

Most endophthalmitis is caused by bacterial infection, and more than 50% of the invading bacteria are either *Staphylococcus aureus* or *Staphylococcus epidermidis.* Other gram-positive bacteria occur less frequently: *Streptococcus pneumoniae,* other *Streptococcus* spp., and *Bacillus* spp. *Pseudomonas aeruginosa* has been recovered from more than 25% of cases of bacterial endophthalmitis; other gram-negative bacteria are rarely implicated: *Klebsiella pneumoniae, Proteus* spp., *Escherichia coli,* and *Serratia marcescens.*

Metastatic bacterial endophthalmitis is rare but may be consequent on infection caused by *Neisseria meningitidis, Neisseria gonorrhoeae, Mycobacterium tuberculosis, Listeria monocytogenes, Streptococcus pneumoniae, Streptococcus pyogenes, viridans* group *Streptococcus* spp., and *Actinomyces israelii.*

Fungi

Opportunistic fungal endophthalmitis is most often caused by *Candida* spp., followed by *Aspergillus* spp. and other filamentous fungi. However, metastatic fungal endophthalmitis also occurs and is caused by more virulent fungi such as *Sporothrix schenkii Blastomyces dermatitidis* and *Coccidioides immitis.*

Epidemiology

Penetrating ocular injuries or intraocular surgery are the usual antecedents to infective endophthalmitis. The frequency of postoperative endophthalmitis varies from 0.06% to 0.5%. Metastatic endophthalmitis arising either from a distant focus of infection or from an intravenous inoculation is increasing in frequency as a consequence of the extended survival of immunocompromised patients, long-continued intravenous therapy, and intravenous self-administration of drugs.

Pathogenesis and Pathology

The sources of the infecting agent(s) of endophthalmitis secondary to penetrating ocular injuries or intraocular surgery are the eyelashes, eyelids, conjunctival sac, lacrimal sac, contaminated instruments, foreign bodies, or contaminated irrigating solutions. The surgeon may also be a source of infection. Sometimes the etiologic agent gains access to the interior of the eye in the postoperative period by way of a filtering bleb, a vitreous wick, or an externalized suture.

Metastatic endophthalmitis may arise from meningitis, endocarditis, prostatitis, otitis media, a severe dermatitis, or pulmonary infection. An intravenous catheter left in place unduly long not infrequently becomes colonized and is then a source for infection (*e.g., Candida albicans*).

When the lens–iris diaphragm of the eye is intact, the infection is usually confined to the anterior chamber or to the vitreous cavity until very late in the course of the disease. Most bacteria produce suppuration early in the course of endophthalmitis, although the infection may not be conspicuous for a period of weeks or months if the causal organism is of low virulence (e.g., *Staphylococcus epidermidis*). Fungal endophthalmitis is often slow in onset and is usually nonpurulent. Metastatic fungal endophthalmitis is usually confined to the retina and vitreous cavity.

Manifestations

Bacterial Endophthalmitis

The symptoms of bacterial endophthalmitis are pain, photophobia, redness (largely circumcorneal), and reduced vision. The severity and rapidity of onset of the symptoms vary according to the virulence of the infecting bacteria. Classically, the symptoms arise within 48 hours after trauma or surgery, but if the organism is of low virulence, the onset may be delayed for weeks or months. Patients with a metastatic bacterial endophthalmitis usually have blurred vision but little or no pain, photophobia, or redness.

The signs of bacterial endophthalmitis are edema of the eyelids, conjunctival injection, chemosis, loss of corneal luster, a moderate to severe anterior-chamber reaction, hypopyon, miosis, a severe anterior vitreous reaction, and loss of the red reflex. The signs of metastatic bacterial endophthalmitis are usually confined to the vitreous cavity and retina and consist of a vitreous reaction (clouding, haziness) and an underlying retinitis. If the patient is gravely ill with the underlying systemic disease, the signs and symptoms of the endophthalmitis may be missed until late in the course of the infection.

Fungal Endophthalmitis

Fungal endophthalmitis usually arises weeks or months after the precipitating trauma or surgery. The symptoms are usually less severe and the onset is less acute than in bacterial endophthalmitis, but the symptoms are identical: pain, redness, and reduced vision.

Early in the course of fungal endophthalmitis, gray-white puffball-like spherical bodies appear in the anterior vitreous. As they enlarge and approach the pupillary border, there is a severe inflammatory reaction. The pupillary aperture fills with a fibrinous exudate, and the anterior chamber gradually becomes more and more shallow until the eye is lost from a secondary glaucoma.

A metastatic fungal endophthalmitis may be missed in a comatose or extremely ill patient unless the fundus of the eye is examined frequently. An alert patient may complain of blurred vision. The typical sign is a white, elevated, retinal lesion with overlying inflammation in the vitreous. In fungal endophthalmitis—for example, coccidioidal endophthalmitis—there is also an anterior-chamber reaction consisting of keratic precipitates; cells and flare in the aqueous humor; large iris nodules; and posterior synechiae.

Diagnosis

It is sometimes extremely difficult to differentiate severe noninfectious inflammatory endophthalmitis from a true infection. Noninfectious postsurgical and traumatic inflammations tend to begin early (within hours) after the surgical or other trauma, quickly reach a maximum intensity, which may be maintained for a period or subside. A true infection, on the other hand, begins after a longer interval (usually more than 24 hours) and continues to worsen unless treated appropriately.

When the inflammation arises from necrotic ocular tissue, as that associated with retinoblastoma, the inflammatory cells in the anterior chamber are often clumped, resembling lumps of mashed potatoes.

Lens-induced uveitis may simulate infectious endophthalmitis. The reaction arises from the toxic or immunologic effects of lens protein liberated into the eye as a result of rupture of the lens capsule or leakage of small lens proteins through the lens capsule. The anterior-chamber reaction may be severe and mimic endophthalmitis, but it is most intense around the lens or lens fragments.

When infective endophthalmitis is suspected, the clinician must regard the situation as an emergency and must take immediate steps to determine the cause of the infection. Blind treatment may be inappropriate or inadequate; yet, delay for even a few hours, for example, waiting for an operating room where diagnostic studies can be done most conveniently, may affect the prognosis adversely. Etiologic diagnosis can be approached quickly in cooperative adults by aspirating both aqueous and vitreous in the office, at the bedside, or in the examining room.

Paracentesis of the Anterior Chamber

After the topical application of an anesthetic (*e.g.*, proparacaine), a lid speculum is inserted, and a small amount of xylocaine (1% or 2%) is injected under the conjunctiva in the area near the limbus where the conjunctiva is to be grasped. Once this area is adequately anesthetized, the conjunctiva is grasped with a small, toothed forceps and a 27-gauge disposable needle attached to a disposable 1-ml syringe is used to penetrate the cornea at an oblique angle 1 mm to 2 mm from the limbus. The needle readily penetrates the cornea, especially if it is gently rotated as it is inserted. As soon as the needle has entered the anterior chamber, 0.1 ml to 0.2 ml of fluid is aspirated for microscopic study and culture.

Aspiration of Vitreous

When the eye is aphakic, the vitreous face is entered through the pupil after aspiration of the aqueous. The needle is simply directed through the pupil into the vitreous face, and aspiration is carried out. Sometimes the vitreous is very viscous and the clinician may need to probe to find a pocket of liquid vitreous.

When the lens–iris diaphragm is intact, the vitreous is approached through the pars plana, about 4 mm behind the limbus and at either 1:30, 4:30, 7:30, or 10:30 to avoid the rectus muscles. After the conjunctiva has been anesthetized, a 20- or 18-gauge needle is inserted into the area.

Prognosis

Endophthalmitis is a devastating disease that results in loss of vision and often in loss of the eye. The earlier the etiologic agent is identified, the better the prognosis, because intensive administration of appropriate antimicrobics is still possible. If the cause is an opportunist (*e.g., Staphylococcus epidermidis*) the outlook is better than it is with a more virulent pathogen such as *Staphylococcus aureus.*

Therapy

The treatment of infective endophthalmitis by the intraocular injection of antimicrobics, with or without vitrectomy, is a matter of controversy. At the present time, it appears that the result is much the same with aggressive treatment as with conventional administration of antimicrobics systemically and conjunctivally. However, the recommended doses of antimicrobics for intravitreal injection are listed in Table 163-1.

Table 163-1. *Doses of Antimicrobics for Intravitreal Administration*

Agent	Dosage
Methicillin	2.0 mg
Ampicillin	0.5 mg
Carbenicillin	0.25 mg–2.0 mg
Cephaloridine	0.25 mg
Vancomycin	1.0 mg
Lincomycin	1.5 mg
Gentamicin	0.1 mg–0.4 mg
Tobramycin	0.1 mg–0.4 mg

Treatment is aimed first at sterilizing the infectious process, a goal that requires rapid application of appropriate specific therapy. Eliminating the inflammatory reaction is secondary but is also very important.

Immediate Treatment

Because delay in treatment is hazardous, gentamicin, 20 mg, and methicillin, 100 mg, should be injected subconjunctivally (using separate syringes) immediately after specimens have been collected for smear and culture, while the patient is still under the influence of the anesthetic agent. Penicillin G (200–400 mg/kg body weight/day, *i.e.,* 300,000 to 600,000 units/kg body weight/day) is given by IV injection of 6 equal portions, 4-hourly. In patients allergic to penicillin, cephaloridine (100 mg subconjunctivally, and 50 to 60 mg/kg body weight/day as 4 equal portions, 6-hourly by IV injection) or cefazolin (100 mg subconjunctivally, and 100 mg/kg body weight/day as 4 equal portions, 6-hourly by IV injection) may be substituted.

Treatment should be modified according to the results of smears of specimens taken from the eye, modified again when the results of cultures and clinical observations are correlated, and modified yet again when the results of susceptibility tests and clinical observations are correlated.

Antimicrobics of choice, alternatives, and dosages are listed in Table 163-2. In general, topical antimicrobics are given every 30 to 60 minutes during the day and every 1 to 2 hours during the patients' usual sleeping time; the subconjunctival injections are given every 12 to 24 hours for 3 to 5 days; and systemic administration is continued for 7 to 10 days.

Antiinflammatory Treatment

In all cases of nonfungal endophthalmitis, a cycloplegic (atropine 1%, or Cyclogyl 1% with phenylephrine 2.5%) should be instilled into the eye three or four times a day to help prevent the formation of

Table 163-2. Antimicrobial Treatment of Corneal Ulcers and Endophthalmitis According to Causal Microorganism

Microorganism	Drugs of Choice	Alternative Drugs
Gram-positive cocci (*e.g., Streptococcus pneumoniae)*	Topical	
	Erythromycin (5 mg/G)	Bacitracin (10,000 U/ml)
	Subconjunctival	
	Penicillin G (300 mg–600 mg—0.5 to 1.0 million U)	Cephaloridine (100 mg) or Cefazolin (100 mg)
	Systemic	
	Penicillin G (200 mg–400 mg—300,000–400,000 U/kg/day—as 6 equal doses, IV)	Cefazolin (100 mg/kg/day as 4 equal doses, IV)
Gram-positive cocci or bacilli other than pneumococcus; also Gram-negative cocci	Topical	
	Erythromycin (5 mg/G)	Bacitracin (10,000 U/ml)
	Subconjunctival	
	Methicillin (100 mg); gentamicin (20 mg–40 mg)	Cefazolin (100 mg) and Gentamicin (20 mg–40 mg) *or* Vancomycin (100 mg); Amikacin (40 mg–60 mg)
	Systemic	
	Nafcillin (200–400 mg/kg/day as 6 equal doses, IV)	Cefazolin (100 mg/kg/day as 4 equal doses, IV)
Gram-negative bacilli (*e.g., Pseudomonas* spp.)	Topical	
	Polymyxin B (17,000 U/ml)	Gentamicin (8–15 mg/ml)
	Subconjunctival	
	Tobramycin (20 mg–40 mg)	Gentamicin (20 mg–40 mg)
	Systemic (for endophthalmitis only)	
	Gentamicin 5–6 mg/kg/day as 3 equal doses, IV or IM) *and* carbenicillin (400–500 mg/kg/day as 6 equal doses, IV)	Amikacin (15–20 mg/kg/day as 3 equal doses, IV or IM) *and* Ticarcillin (300–500 mg/kg/day as 6 equal doses, IV)
Gram-negative bacilli (*e.g., Moraxella* spp.)	Topical	
	Gentamicin (8–15 mg/ml	Sodium sulfacetamide (10%–30%)
	Subconjunctival	
	Rarely necessary	
Other gram-negative bacilli (*e.g.,* enterics)	Topical	
	Gentamicin (8–15 mg/ml)	Carbenicillin (4 mg/ml)
	Subconjunctival	
	Gentamicin (20 mg–40 mg); Carbenicillin (100 mg)	Amikacin (40 mg–60 mg); Ticarcillin (100 mg)
	Systemic	
	Ampicillin (200–400 mg/kg/day as 6 equal doses, IV) *and* Gentamicin (5–6 mg/kg/day as 3 equal doses, IV or IM)	Cefazolin (100–150 mg/kg/day as 4 equal doses, IV) *and* Amikacin (15–20 mg/kg/day as 3 equal doses, IV or IM)

Table 163-2. (continued) *Antimicrobial Treatment of Corneal Ulcers and Endophthalmitis According to Causal Microorganism*

Microorganism	Drugs of Choice	Alternative Drugs
Gram-positive bacilli (*e.g., Mycobacterium fortuitum, Nocardia* spp., and *Actinomyces* spp.)	Topical Sodium sulfacetamide (10%–30%) Subconjunctival Streptomycin (40 mg–50 mg) Systemic Triple sulfonamides (70 mg/kg/day as 4 equal doses, PO) *with* Tetracycline (15–30 mg/kg/day as 4 equal doses, PO)	Streptomycin (50 mg/ml)
Yeastlike fungi (*e.g., Candida* spp.)	Topical Amphotericin B (1.5–3.0 mg/ml) *and* Flucytosine (1%) Subconjunctival Amphotericin B (750 μg/ml, on alternate days) Systemic (for endophthalmitis only) Flucytosine (200 mg/kg/day as 4 equal doses, PO)	Natmycin (5%) *and* Flucytosine (1%) Amphotericin B (see Chap. 39 for dosage and administration)
Hyphal fungi (*e.g., Aspergillus* spp.) identical regimens are used when no organism is identified but fungal infection is presumed on clinical grounds)	Topical Natamycin (5%) Subconjunctival Amphotericin B (750 μg/ml on alternate days) Systemic: Amphotericin B (see Chap. 39 for dosage and administration)	Amphotericin B (1.5–3.0 mg/ml)
None identified (but bacterial infection presumed on clinical grounds)	Topical Polymyxin B (17,000 U/ml) *and* Bacitracin (10,000 U/ml) Subconjunctival Gentamicin (20–40 mg) *and* Methicillin (100 mg) Systemic Nafcillin (200–400 mg/kg/day as 6 equal doses, IV) *and* Amikacin (15–20 mg/kg/day as 3 equal doses, IV, or IM)	Gentamicin (8–15 mg/ml) *and* Erythromycin (5 mg/G) Amikacin (40 mg–60 mg) *and* Penicillin G (300 mg–600 mg—0.5–1.0 million U) Penicillin G (200 mg–400 mg 300,000–400,000 U/kg/day as 6 equal doses, IV *and* Tobramycin (5.6 mg/kg/day as 3 equal doses, IV or IM)

synechia. Systemic glucosteroids should be withheld for 24 hours; as soon as the eye looks better, or at least has not worsened, prednisone 50 mg to 80 mg may be given systemically; the dose should then be reduced gradually over the next 7 to 10 days.

Surgical intervention with evisceration of the globe may be necessary in patients in whom the endophthalmitis is not controlled and panophthalmitis has supervened.

Prevention

Measures that prevent postoperative endophthalmitis are identical with those that prevent infections following general surgery (Chap. 158, Infections Following Surgical Operations). The duration of hospitalization should be limited to prevent colonizing the patient with resistant organisms. Systemic infections, for example, respiratory tract infections, should be controlled prior to surgery. Elective intraocular surgery should not be performed on patients with manifest ocular disease, for example, blepharitis, conjunctivitis, dacryocystitis, or keratitis.

Antimicrobic prophylaxis against bacterial contamination in connection with surgery may prevent infection but engenders the risk of toxic or allergic reactions and superinfections with resistant bacteria or fungi. Gentamicin and methicillin may be given just prior to surgery (subconjunctivally at the time of the preparation of the patient, or systemically 1 to 2 hours before surgery) to provide high concentrations in the surgical area at the time of the incision. Treatment may be continued for 24 hours.

Remaining Problems

The use of intraocular antimicrobics and vitreous surgery in the treatment of infective endophthalmitis is still highly controversial.

Bibliography

Journals

SACK RB: Prophylactic antibiotics? The individual versus the community. N Engl J Med 300:1107–1108, 1979

FORSTER RK, ZACHARY IG, COTTENGHAN AJ, NORTON EWD: Further observations on the diagnosis, course, and treatment of endophthalmitis. Am J Ophthalmol 81:52–56, 1976

ROBERTSON DM, RILEY FC, HERMANS PE: Endogenous *Candida* endophthalmitis. Report of two cases treated with flucytosine. Arch Ophthalmol 91:33–38, 1974

BAUM JL, PEYMAN GZ: Antibiotic administration in the treatment of bacterial endophthalmitis: Viewpoints. Surv Ophthalmol 21:332–346, 1977

CHRISTY NE, LALL P: Postoperative endophthalmitis following cataract surgery. Arch Ophthalmol 90:361–366, 1973

ALLEN HF, MANGIARACINE AB: Bacterial endophthalmitis after cataract extraction, II. Incidence in 36,000 consecutive operations with special reference to pre-operative topical antibiotics. Trans Am Acad Ophthalmol Otolaryngol 77:581–588, 1973

JENSEN AD, NAIDOFF MA: Bilateral meningococcal endophthalmitis. Arch Ophthalmol 90:396–398, 1973

Section XXIII

Otic Infections

Indigenous Microbiota of the Ears

Species or Group	External Auditory Canal
Bacteria	
Gram-positive cocci	
Staphylococcus epidermidis	**27–100***
Staphylococcus aureus	**12–20**
Anaerobic micrococci	
Streptococcus mitis;	
undifferentiated	**0.2–23**
α and γ streptococci	
Streptococcus pneumoniae	+
Gram-positive bacilli	
Lactobacillus spp.	**86**
Aerobic *Corynebacterium* spp.	
Aerobic gram-negative bacilli	
Enterobacteriaceae	**4–8**
Escherichia coli	
Enterobacter spp.	**0.1–0.4**
Klebsiella spp.	+
Proteus mirabilis, other *Proteus* spp.,	**0.2–1**
Morganella morganii,	
Providencia spp.	
Pseudomonas aeruginosa	**0–1.3**
Alcaligenes faecalis	**1.1–1.6**
Fungi	
nonalbicans *Candida* spp.	+

± to 0, rare; ±, irregular or uncertain (may be only pathologic); +, common; ++, prominent.

*Boldface values (*e.g.,* **30–60**) = range of incidence in percentages, rounded, in different surveys.

JOHN D. NELSON

Infections of the Ear

164

Inflammatory disease of the mucosal lining of the middle ear with exudation is one of the most common infections besetting children. Almost all children have at least one episode of otitis media with effusion (OME) and approximately one-third have repeated episodes of OME during infancy. Although antimicrobial therapy has markedly decreased the frequency of serious suppurative complications, it may have increased the frequency of recurrent or persistent, sterile middle ear effusions. Hearing deficits associated with such effusions may occur at critical times of speech and language development and may lead to learning disabilities with lifelong impact.

Etiology

Aspiration of liquid from the middle ear in the syndrome of acute OME yields a bacteriologically sterile fluid in about 10% of cases. Respiratory syncytial virus, influenza A, coxsackie, parainfluenza, and adenoviruses have, on occasion, been isolated from this liquid, but most attempts to isolate viruses or mycoplasmas have been unsuccessful. Anaerobic bacteria are not commonly isolated from acute or chronic effusions. Their role in pathogenesis has never been established and is considered unimportant by most investigators.

Streptococcus pneumoniae is the most common pathogen in OME of children or adults and is found in approximately 30% of cases. *Haemophilus influenzae* accounts for 25% of cases in infancy and for 20% of cases in older children and young adults. The isolates of *H. influenzae* are almost always noncapsulated; if capsulated and of type b, it is likely that there is an associated systemic disease such as meningitis.

Staphylococcus epidermidis and *Branhamella (Neisseria) catarrhalis* are frequently isolated from acute middle ear effusions, but their etiologic significance has not been clearly established.

Although pneumococcal and haemophilan rates of isolation are consistent, *Streptococcus pyogenes* appears to have geographic limitations. It is found in approximately 10% of cases in cold climes, but in only 2% of patients in warmer zones.

In infants under 6 weeks of age, coliform bacilli account for 5% to 20% of cases of OME and they may be found in older children and adults who are compromised hosts. *Staphylococcus aureus* is rare in initial attacks but becomes more prominent in recurrent otitis, especially when the tympanic membrane has been ruptured.

Tuberculous and diphtheritic otitis are rarely seen today.

In chronic otitis media, the spectrum of etiologic agents changes completely to the gram-negative bacillary genera—*Proteus, Klebsiella, Enterobacter,* and *Pseudomonas.* Episodic, acute exacerbations are rather common in the course of chronic disease and are caused by pneumococci, *H. influenzae,* or *Streptococcus pyogenes.*

Pneumococci, *S. aureus,* and group A streptococci, in that order, are the usual pathogens in acute mastoiditis. *Haemophilus* spp. rarely cause acute mastoiditis in spite of a high incidence in acute OME.

Acute diffuse external otitis is most commonly caused by streptococci or *Staphylococcus aureus*—also the cause of furuncles in the external auditory canal. *Pseudomonas aeruginosa* or other pseudomonads are characteristically isolated from patients with chronic external otitis, but fungi may also be involved.

Bullous myringitis was formerly attributed to infection caused by *Mycoplasma pneumoniae* infection; however, current opinion holds that bullous myringitis is merely one manifestation of OME caused by various nonmycoplasmal microorganisms.

Epidemiology

Nonhuman animals and vectors have no role in the transmission of the agents responsible for otitis media. Environmental factors are important in patients in whom allergy is the precipitating event and in cases of barotrauma. Geographic or environmental factors favoring frequent upper respiratory tract viral infections result in a higher incidence of otitis media.

OME is more common among the lower socioeconomic classes and is notoriously common in American Indians and Eskimos and perhaps other groups of Mongolian extraction. OME is less common in blacks than in whites.

Principally a disease of infancy, OME is more likely to recur the earlier in life it first occurred. Conversely, infants who escape otitis media in their first 2 years are likely to be spared or to have only a single episode. By 24 months of age, only 23% of children have not had OME and 34% have had 3 or more episodes. Males are affected slightly more often than females.

Pathogenesis and Pathology

The eustachian tube has three major functions: ventilation and pressure equilibration of the middle ear cleft, prevention of ingress of foreign material, and drainage of foreign matter and of the mucus normally produced by the middle ear. Malfunction of the eustachian tube is the primary event in the pathogenesis of OME. Formerly, clinical distinctions between acute suppurative otitis and serous otitis were made. The preferred term is now OME. This single term emphasizes the unitarian concept of pathogenesis and recognizes that the clinician cannot reliably distinguish between infected and noninfected fluid by viewing the tympanic membrane.

Obstruction of the eustachian tube leads to resorption of air in the middle ear cleft and to serous effusion—which may become purulent if bacteria proliferate in it. In Apache children, and presumably in other Amerindian children, the problem is reversed, namely, the eustachian tube is abnormally patent; OME results from reflux and insufflation rather than from obstruction.

Anatomy, immunologic virginity, and microbiologic inexperience conspire against the infant to produce a far greater frequency of otitis media in this age group than in older children and adults. The infant's eustachian tubes are oriented almost horizontally with resultant poor drainage. The orifice is relatively patulous and is surrounded by abundant lymphoid tissue. Cartilage is deficient in amount and is not compliant in the infant. With a succession of first exposures to a variety of infectious agents, mucosal swelling and adenoidal hypertrophy are nearly constant and favor the establishment in the middle ear of pathogenic bacteria normally resident in the nasopharynx. Because most upper respiratory tract infections are caused by viruses, the usual sequence begins with viral infection followed in 5 to 10 days by the onset of bacterial middle ear infection. This has long been recognized in the case of clinically obvious viral infections such as measles and has been documented in other viral infections identifiable only by laboratory tests. It is unusual for OME to complicate streptococcal sore throat. Allergens may initiate the same process in allergic persons, but this relationship has not been firmly established.

Anatomic abnormalities of the nasopharynx predispose to middle ear infection. For example, the infant with a cleft palate is strikingly vulnerable to recurrent otitis media.

"Bottle-propping" (letting an infant nurse from a bottle while lying supine) predisposes to recurrent otitis media. Radiographic studies have demonstrated that liquid may jet from the nasopharynx into the eustachian tubes in persons who swallow while supine.

The acute inflammatory response changes the thin cuboidal lining of the middle ear cavity into a structure two to three times its normal thickness. The neutrophils of the acute inflammatory response migrate into the cavity to render purulent the initially serous fluid; exudate accumulates. As pressure increases, not only does the tympanic membrane bulge outward, but also pus may be forced into pneumatized portions of the temporal bone with resulting acute mastoiditis. Relief of the pressure is critical to resolution of the process and may occur through rupture of the eardrum or drainage through the eustachian tube.

The liquid that does not drain out of the middle ear becomes a focus for organization leading to mucosal thickening. If perforation of the tympanic membrane persists, ingrowth of squamous epithelium from the external auditory canal may occur. Round cell infiltration and fibrosis of the middle ear mark chronic infection.

Cholesteatomas form as a result of retraction of a pocket of tympanic membrane consequent on chronic atelectasis without effusion in the middle ear cleft.

Effusions commonly persist for several weeks after antimicrobial therapy for acute OME. Clinical signs of inflammation are lacking, and the fluid is usually sterile. Although bacteria are recovered in approximately 20% of cases, their role in the persistence of effusion is unresolved. Similarly, little is known of the possible relationship of immunologic factors to persistence of effusions. The unabsorbed liquid becomes increasingly viscid (*glue ear*); eventually there is invasion by fibroblasts, which may lead to immobilization or destruction of the ossicles.

Subacute or chronic external otitis media is caused by factors that favor retention of moisutre in the external auditory canal. Such patients may have defective cerumen, partially obstructing lesions, or foreign bodies.

Manifestations

The onset of acute OME is typically abrupt with a feeling of fullness and pain in the ears. Sudden alleviation of the pain may signal the occurrence of spontaneous perforation of the tympanic membrane. Moderate fever and moderate leukocytosis are so characteristic that high fever and counts over 20,000 per mm^3 should prompt the physician to search for another focus of infection, such as a meningitis. Othei symptoms are generally those of the viral respiratory infection or the allergic reaction that preceded the middle ear infection.

In infancy, the major manifestations may be fever, irritability, vomiting, and loose stools. Bilateral otitis is twice as common as unilateral disease in infants, whereas unilateral OME is more common in adults. There is no regional lymphadenopathy in either children or adults.

Inspection reveals an opaque tympanic membrane with bulging and loss of normal landmarks. The bulging may be obvious only in Shrapnell's membrane, superiorly. When there is a question about the presence of effusion in the middle ear, pneumatic otoscopy is useful since liquid diminishes the movement of the tympanic membrane in response to external pressure. Tympanometry is helpful in questionable cases.

The physical signs are similar regardless of the etiology of acute OME, although the tympanic membrane is likely to be more opaque and the bulging greater if there is a suppurative effusion. Neither coloration of the membrane nor changes in the light reflex are clues to etiology. With persisting sterile effusion, the tympanic membrane often has a dull, bluish cast, and discrete blood vessels may be seen.

When there is atelectasis of the middle ear cleft, the tympanic membrane is retracted and the long process of the malleus is prominent. With pneumatic otoscopy there is no inward movement on positive pressure, but in the negative pressure phase the tympanic membranes moves outward.

Interpretation of the physical signs may be difficult in patients with recurrent otitis media. The tympanic membrane becomes thickened and is less likely to show either intense redness or obvious bulging.

Chronic otitis media is almost invariably associated with a central or anterior perforation and some degree of mastoid infection. Periodically, patients with chronic middle ear and mastoid disease have increased drainage and fever caused by infection with pyogenic bacteria. Cholesteatomas have the appearance of dirty, greasy masses of tissue.

When acute mastoiditis complicates OME, the patients usually become sicker. In infants, the mastoid process is not fully developed so the signs of inflammation are localized above and behind the ear and the upper pinna is pushed out. In older children and adults, the signs are principally behind and below the ear, and the earlobe may be elevated.

Acute external otitis is often associated with more severe pain than OME. There is fever and regional lymphadenopathy, and the canal is obstructed by inflammation. In subacute or chronic external otitis (*swimmer's ear*), the patient complains of itching, and there is a sticky, scant discharge. Fungus infection is manifested by dry, cheesy material in the canal.

Diagnosis

In acute OME, the diagnosis is established by physical examination and, when necessary, by tympanometry. The diagnosis of otitis media may be difficult in a febrile, crying infant in whom the normal tympanic membrane may appear flushed and bulging. Myringitis, that is, inflammation of the tympanic membrane, may occur without middle ear disease and accompanies many acute viral syndromes. The bony landmarks are still visible, and movement of the eardrum is normal with pneumatic otoscopy. Bullous myringitis is characterized by one or more serous fluid-filled blebs on the tympanic membrane.

Pain may be referred to the ear from disease in many parts of the head or neck, and this should be kept in mind when a patient complaining of pain in the ear has a tympanic membrane that appears normal.

Routine nasopharyngeal cultures are poorly predictive of the microflora of the middle ear and are not recommended. If there is pus in the ear canal, a swab specimen should be obtained for examination. Staphylococci and diphtheroids are normal flora in the external auditory canal—which must be allowed for when interpreting the smear and culture results. If the tympanic membrane is intact, a specimen of the middle ear effusion can be obtained either by needle aspiration or myringotomy. Needle aspiration is preferable because it is less traumatic and the specimen is less likely to be contaminated. Before either procedure, the canal and the surface of the tympanic membrane should be cleaned with 70% ethanol or povidone-iodine. With myringotomy, the specimen is the pus on the knife blade. The specimen should be inoculated in culture mediums appropriate to the isolation of the pathogens specific to otitis media.

In suspected acute mastoiditis, roentgenographic examination is diagnostic in older patients, but because of irregular and asymmetrical pneumatization, interpretation may be difficult in young children. The bacterial etiology is established by culture of middle ear fluid; if a subperiosteal abscess has formed, culture of pus aspirated from it will be diagnostic. Lumbar puncture should be carried out to investigate the possibility of a complicating meningitis.

The diagnosis of external otitis is made by inspection. The bacterial or fungal etiology is determined by culture of swab specimens.

Prognosis

Because the facial nerve passes near the middle ear, a transient facial nerve palsy occasionally accompanies otitis media and is more likely to occur with mastoiditis. Petrositis, labyrinthitis, lateral sinus thrombosis, and brain abscess are rare complications of OME or mastoiditis.

The relation of middle ear disease to meningitis is controversial. Certainly, the majority of cases of otitis media are not complicated by meningitis, but otitis is considered a major antecedent event in meningitis. From autopsy studies, virtually all cases of meningitis in infancy are associated with middle ear disease, even when it may not have been apparent clinically. Whether the infection proceeds directly through venous channels or by another, indirect mechanism is not known.

Impairment of hearing is a serious complication of recurrent, persistent, or chronic middle ear disease. Transient loss of hearing from persistent presence of middle ear fluid in young children may result in delayed development of speech and language skills. Permanent deafness from chronic disease is rare, but can occur in neglected cases.

Death is rare in acute mastoiditis if appropriate medical and surgical therapy are promptly instituted.

Swimmer's ear is a recurrent affliction over many years, but the frequency and severity of episodes can be ameliorated by appropriate preventive and therapeutic measures.

Therapy

Symptomatic relief of pain in acute OME can be achieved with analgesics or local heat, but the most dramatic relief of severe pain is obtained with myringotomy. Myringotomy is performed by making a semilunar incision in the inferior portion of the tympanic membrane after first cleansing the auditory canal and the surface of the membrane with an antiseptic solution. Anesthesia is not used in infants; for older patients, topical application of cocaine is adequate. Drainage of pus, essential to therapy in preantimicrobic times, is less important today. The period of acute morbidity is shortened by drainage, but it probably has no effect on the eventual outcome. Thus, persistent or recurrent otitis media is said to be no more frequent in patients treated with antimicrobics alone than it is in those treated with antimicrobics plus myringotomy. This position has been questioned recently, and the role of myringotomy in acute OME is being reevaluated. Myringotomy in acute suppurative otitis media is generally carried out for relief of severe pain, to obtain pus for culture when it is thought imperative for successful therapy, and to avoid spontaneous perforation when it is judged to be imminent. In addition, by providing drainage and material for culture and susceptibility testing, myringtomy or needle tympanocentesis benefits patients with recurrent otitis media and those who have failed to respond to a trial of antimicrobial therapy.

The therapeutic benefits of nasal decongestants as applied to OME are doubtful, but anyone with a stuffy nose is entitled to symptomatic relief. Antihistamines may be useful in allergic persons, but prescribing them to the usual patient not only is ineffectual, but also may burden the patient with uncomfortable side-effects. Decongestants or antihistamines have never been shown to have a beneficial effect on the rate of healing or eventual outcome in controlled clinical trials.

Selection of an antimicrobic is based on the anticipated etiologic agents: pneumococci, *H. influenzae*, or group A streptococci. The appearance of β-lactamase-producing strains of *H. influenzae* in the early 1970s diminished the effectiveness of ampicillin, amoxicillin, and cyclacillin. Cefaclor or erythromycin–sulfonamide combinations are effective against the usual pathogens, but trimethoprim–sulfamethoxazole is limited because of its ineffectiveness against group A streptococci. Penicillin V was formerly recommended for older children and adults because it was thought that haemophilan infections were rare beyond infancy. With the recognition that *H. influenzae* is almost as common in older patients with acute OME as in infants, it became clear that penicillin V is not suitable.

There is no general agreement on the drug of choice for acute OME. All antimicrobics have advantages or disadvantages regarding cost, antibacterial spectrum, adverse effects, or patient compliance (the bitter taste of suspensions of the penicillins and trimethoprim–sulfamethoxazole mitigates against their use).

The usual dosages of the above-mentioned antimicrobics are as follows: penicillin V, 30 to 40 mg/kg/day in 3 or 4 equal portions; ampicillin or cyclacillin, 75 to 100 mg/kg/day in 3 or 4 equal portions; cefaclor or amoxicillin, 40 mg/kg/day in 3 equal portions; erythromycin, 40 mg/kg/day, with sulfisoxazole, 120 mg/kg/day in 3 or 4 equal portions; and trimethoprim, 8 mg/kg/day, with sulfamethoxazole, 40 mg/kg/day in 2 equal portions.

Infants under 6 weeks of age may have coliform infection unresponsive to the usual antimicrobics prescribed for acute OME. Culture and susceptibility testing may be necessary to select appropriate drugs. Cefaclor or trimethoprim–sulfamethoxazole is effective against many coliform bacteria, but hospitalization for parenteral therapy with aminocyclitols is sometimes necessary.

After symptomatic improvement and subsidence of the signs of inflammation, persistence of middle ear effusion can be anticipated for several weeks in 30% to 50% of patients with acute OME. If the fluid has not drained or been resorbed after approximately 3 months, it has been common practice to perform myringotomy for suction removal of the viscous fluid and insertion of a ventilatory tube through the tympanic membrane. The possible advantage of tube placement over myringotomy and drainage alone has never been proved in controlled studies. Since long-term adverse sequellae of ventilatory tubes have been reported, the optimal surgical approach is questionable and requires investigation.

Acute supprative mastoiditis can often be managed with myringotomy drainage and antimicrobics. However, severe disease may require urgent surgical intervention for drainage of subperiosteal abscess or pus in the mastoid.

Chronic otitis media with perforation and low-grade mastoid infection is commonly treated with topical antimicrobic solutions—an ineffectual effort. Indeed, the addition of systemic antimicrobics is also of no avail except for the occasional acute exacerbations caused by pneumococci or *H. influenzae.* Ultimately, many patients with chronic middle ear and mastoid infection require mastoidectomy and tympanoplasty.

Acute external otitis is treated with systemic antimicrobics. Topical antimicrobical solutions on a wick may provide additional benefit. After acute inflammation subsides, one or more debridement procedures are necessary to remove necrotic material.

Swimmer's ear is best managed by preventive measures such as avoiding water or instilling topical water repellant solutions into the canal. Acetone or alcohol irrigations may be used to remove water if the patient has not avoided exposure. Antimicrobic ointments directed against *Pseudomonas* spp. are of little value unless the other measures are also employed. Fungal infection of the external auditory canal can be managed by irrigations with equal parts of alcohol and vinegar.

Prevention

Prevention of OME is virtually impossible because the antecedent viral infections, with the exceptions of measles and influenza, cannot be prevented by immunization. The possible hazards of bottle-propping can be pointed out to mothers. Good management of allergic problems decreases the incidence of OME if allergy is truly a predisposing factor. Giving decongestant medications to patients with upper respiratory tract infections has not been shown to prevent OME in controlled clinical trials.

In several controlled trials involving small numbers of children with histories of recurrent otitis media, continuous prophylaxis with a sulfonamide during the winter and spring months decreased the frequency of episodes of OME. However, the degree of protection was limited, and this approach is not practical or useful in most situations.

The value of prophylactic tonsillectomy and adenoidectomy or adenoidectomy alone has been disputed for years. A review of the subject reveals no proof that tonsillectomy and adenoidectomy have any preventive value.

Trials with capsular polysaccharide vaccines of type b *H. influenzae* and the pneumococcal serotypes commonly associated with OME have been disappointing for several reasons. Polysaccharide vaccines are poor immunogens in young infants. At least

90% of the strains of *H. influenzae* that cause OME are noncapsulated; hence, a vaccine prepared from polyribosphosphate capsular material should not be expected to prevent the occurence of OME. Finally, the basic pathophysiology of OME is dysfunction of the eustachian tubes, a defect unrelated to specific microorganisms.

Acute mastoiditis is prevented or aborted by effective antimicrobic therapy for acute OME.

Remaining Problems

Is persistent effusion after acute OME more common now than previously or is it merely recognized more often because of increased use of pneumatic otoscopy and tympanometry? If it is truly more common, is persistence a result of the comparative infrequency of myringotomy for acute OME or application of antimicrobics and decongestants? Is persistent effusion immunologically mediated?

Can OME be prevented by adenoidectomy, tonsillectomy, or both?

Do tympanostomy tubes provide any long-term benefit or only the short-term benefit of improved hearing? Do the long-term adverse effects of tympanostomy tubes outweigh the short-term benefits? Do ventilatory tubes increase the problem of reflux in children whose basic defect is abnormal patency of the eustachian tube rather than obstruction?

Can antimicrobic prophylaxis for OME in otitis-prone children be effective and practical?

Does the delay in speech and language development in infants with recurrent or persistent middle ear effusion lead to permanent learning disability or is there a catch-up phenomenon once hearing is restored?

Bibliography

Book

BLUESTONE CD, STOOL SE (eds): Pediatric Otolaryngology. Philadelphia, WB Saunders, 1982. 800 pp.

Journals

BEAUREGARD WB: Positional otitis media. J Pediatr 79:294–296, 1971

GINSBURG CM, RUDOY R, NELSON JD: Acute mastoiditis in infants and children. Clin Pediatr 19:549–553, 1980

HOWIE VM, PLOUSSARD JH: The "in vivo sensitivity test": Bacteriology of middle ear exudate during antimicrobial therapy in otitis media. Pediatrics 44:940–944, 1969

MCGOVERN JP, HAYWOOD TJ, FERNANDEZ AA: Allergy and secretory otitis media: An analysis of 512 cases. JAMA 200:124–128, 1967

OLSON AL, KLEIN SW, CHARNEY E, MACWHINNEY JB, MCINERNY TK, MILLER RL, NAZARIAN LF, CUNNINGHAM D: Prevention and therapy of serous otitis media by oral decongestant: A double-blind study in pediatric practice. Pediatrics 61:679–684, 1978

PARADISE JL: Otitis media in infants and children. Pediatrics 65:917–943, 1980

PARADISE JL, BLUESTONE CD: Early treatment of the universal otitis media of infants with cleft palate. Pediatrics 53:48–54, 1974.

PERRIN JM, CHARNEY E, MACWHINNEY JB JR, MCINERNY TK, MILLER RL, NAZARIAN LF: Sulfisoxazole as chemoprophylaxis for recurrent otitis media. N Engl J Med 291:664–667, 1974

ROBERTS DB: The etiology of bullous myringitis and the role of myoplasmas in ear disease: A review. Pediatrics 65:761–766, 1980

RODDY OF JR, EARLE R JR, HAGGERTY R: Myringotomy in acute otitis media: A controlled study. JAMA 198:849–853, 1966

SCHWARTZ R, RODRIGUEZ WJ, WAHEED NK, ROSS S: Acute purulent otitis media in children older than 5 years. JAMA 238:1032–1033, 1977

SHURIN PA, HOWIE VM, PELTON SI, PLOUSSARD JH, KLEIN JO: Bacterial etiology of otitis media during the first six weeks of life. Pediatrics 92:893–896, 1978

TETZLAFF TR, ASHWORTH C, NELSON JD: Otitis media in children less than 12 weeks of age. Pediatrics 59:827–832, 1977

VAN DISHOECK HAE, DERKS ACW, VOORHORST R: Bacteriology and treatment of acute otitis media in children. Acta Otolaryngol 50:250–261, 1959

Section | *XXIV*

Presumed or Possibly Infectious Diseases

MARIAN E. MELISCH

Kawasaki Syndrome

165

Kawasaki syndrome, or mucocutaneous lymph node syndrome (MLNS), is an acute febrile disease primarily affecting children that was first described in Japan in 1967. It was first described outside of Japan in 1974, and since that time Kawasaki syndrome has been reported to occur on all continents in people of all racial groups.

Etiology

The etiology of Kawasaki syndrome remains unknown. Extensive efforts to recover a bacterial or viral agent by standard microbiologic and cell culture techniques have been unrewarding. Early reports of detection of a rickettsialike agent by electron microscopy in skin biopsy material have not been confirmed. No viruslike agents were found in feces, serum, or throat washings by direct or immune electron microscopy. Limited animal inoculation studies failed to produce disease. Although an association with a specific infectious agent has been reported in a number of individual cases, testing of a larger number of cases has failed to confirm any unique association with any known agent.

Epidemiology

Kawasaki syndrome has an overwhelming predilection for young children. The peak age incidence is between 1 and 2 years, and more than 75% of cases occur before the age of 4 years. Cases are very rare beyond the age of 8 years. None of the cases reported in adults have met all diagnostic criteria, and most appear to represent toxic shock syndrome (Chap. 50, Infections of the Female Genital Tract). In Kawasaki syndrome, males are affected more often than females by a ratio of 1.6:1. The disease is generally endemic and nonseasonal. More than 18,000 cases have been reported in Japan and several nationwide surveys have revealed an incidence of 9 to 50 per 100,000 children under 4 years in age. There are no pronounced differences in incidence between urban and rural populations or among climatic zones within Japan. Community-wide epidemics have been reported in diverse locations including Ehime, Japan; Honolulu; New York City and Rochester; eastern Massachusetts; and Los Angeles. Epidemic outbreaks have occurred in winter and spring, whereas endemic cases appear to be rather evenly distributed throughout the year. As a result of study of three epidemics, it appears that (1) the disease is widely distributed geographically in the affected communities, (2) there is no evidence of person-to-person transmission beyond the family unit, and (3) no point source exposure is implicated. Therefore, except within the intimate confines of the family, Kawasaki syndrome does not appear to be very communicable.

A pronounced ethnic difference in susceptibility was noted in Hawaii and in a retrospective analysis of sporadic cases reported to the Centers for Disease Control (CDC) from diverse areas of the United States. Japanese children are overrepresented as compared to their share in the population, whereas white children are significantly underrepresented. In Hawaii, the incidence of Kawasaki syndrome among Japanese children is equal to that of most prefectures in Japan. It remains unclear whether this predilection for children of Japanese ancestry is related to a genetic susceptibility or to environmental influences. No unique relationship to human leukocyte antigen (HLA) was discovered, and no epidemiologic evidence was found of an ethnic-related environmental factor that predisposes to Kawasaki syndrome. Children of Japanese ancestry living in Hawaii are very much Americanized and therefore have a markedly different diet and life-style compared with their counterparts in Japan.

Pathogenesis and Pathology

More than 80% of the deaths from Kawasaki syndrome occur within 2 months of onset of illness. At autopsy, the major pathologic findings are multisystem vasculitis with a predilection for the coronary arteries. The cause of death is acute thrombosis of inflamed aneurysmal coronary arteries in more than 80% of the fatal cases. Rupture of coronary arteries, early pancarditis, and late myocardial infarction (MI) are also seen. Variable and scattered involvement of extracardiac vessels afflicts primarily the extraparenchymal portions of medium sized, muscular arteries. Lymph nodes, when enlarged, show only nonspecific lymphoid hypertrophy. The vasculitis of Kawasaki syndrome is acutely episodic rather than chronically progressive. Early lesions (less than 14 days duration) show intimal and perivascular infiltration with an acute polymorphonuclear infiltrate and involvement of arterial microvessels. In early subacute lesion (14–35 days) there is total involvement of the arterial wall with an infiltrate consisting of polymorphonuclear leukocytes, lymphocytes, and plasma cells. Aneurysmal dilation is seen at this stage with interruption of internal and external elastic lamina. Later subacute lesions (35–50 days) show decreased inflammation with formation of granulation tissue, and late lesions (more than 2 months from onset) show little or no inflammation but prominent scarring. The pathology of Kawasaki syndrome is indistinguishable from the previously described infantile periarteritis nodosa, a condition diagnosed only at autopsy. However, the pathologic and clinical features of fatal Kawasaki syndrome differ considerably from classic periarteritis nodosa, a chronic progressive vasculitis with a predilection for kidney, skin, and pulmonary tissues, which is seen primarily in adults.

PRINCIPAL DIAGNOSTIC CRITERIA FOR MUCOCUTANEOUS LYMPH NODE SYNDROME

- Fever persisting for more than 5 days
- Conjunctival injection
- Changes in the mouth
  - Erythema, fissuring, and crusting of the lips
  - Diffuse oropharyngeal erythema
  - Strawberry tongue
- Changes in the peripheral extremities
  - Induration of hands and feet
  - Erythema of palms and soles
  - Desquamation of fingertips and toetips approximately 2 weeks after onset
  - Transverse grooves across fingernails 2 to 3 months after onset
- Erythematous rash
- Enlarged lymph node mass measuring more than 1.5 cm in diameter

ASSOCIATED FEATURES (IN ORDER OF FREQUENCY)

1. Pyuria and urethritis
2. Arthralgia and arthritis
3. Aseptic meningitis
4. Diarrhea
5. Abdominal pain
6. Myocardiopathy
7. Pericardial effusion
8. Obstructive jaundice
9. Hydrops of gallbladder
10. Acute Mitral insufficiency
11. Myocardial infarction

Manifestations

Kawasaki syndrome is a distinctive clinical entity with a predictable clinical course. The principal and associated features of the disease are listed on p. 000. The fever is remittent with peak temperatures exceeding 39°C (104°F); it persists for an average of 11 days.

There is discrete vascular injection of the bulbar conjunctiva, and some patients also have a follicular palpebral conjunctivitis. Ocular discharge and corneal ulceration are not seen, thus distinguishing the conjunctivitis of Kawasaki syndrome from the purulent conjunctivitis of Stevens–Johnson syndrome.

Changes in the mouth consist of (1) eythema progressing to fissuring, cracking, and bleeding of the lips; (2) a strawberry tongue indistinguishable from that related to streptococcal scarlet fever; and (3) diffuse erythema of the oropharynx.

Changes in the hands and feet constitute the most distinctive feature of Kawasaki syndrome. In the acute phase, the hands and feet become firmly indurated and slightly swollen with stretched, shiny skin. The palms and soles are diffusely and deeply erythematous. These changes are followed by a distinctive pattern of desquamation in the subacute phase. The erythematous rash associated with Kawasaki syndrome may take several forms, most often as raised, deep red, pruritic plaques, or morbilliform erythematous papules. Occasionally, the skin shows diffuse scarlatiniform erythroderma or has an exanthem with characteristics of erythema marginatum.

Lymph node swelling is the least common feature of Kawasaki syndrome, occurring in slightly more than half the patients. It is usually unilateral and cervical. The enlarged mass of nodes measures more than 1.5 cm, is nonfluctuant, and is only moderately tender.

The associated features of Kawasaki syndrome attest to its multisystemic nature. Sterile pyuria reflecting urethritis is found in three-quarters of patients. Arthritis of major weight-bearing joints occurs in one-third. Gastrointestinal complaints including abdominal pain, severe diarrhea and nausea occur in approximately one-third during the early stages of the disease. Central nervous system (CNS) involvement with severe lethargy, semicoma, and aseptic meningitis occur in one-quarter of patients. Obstructive jaundice and acute gallbladder hydrops are seen in about 5% of patients.

The most important associated feature of Kawasaki syndrome is heart disease. Clinical cardiac disease occurs in approximately 20% and is most often manifest as pericarditis, myocarditis, congestive heart failure, and arrhythmias. Angiographic and two-dimensional echocardiographic studies performed on a routine basis 4 to 8 weeks after onset demonstrate coronary artery aneurysms in approximately 20% of patients. Although aneurysms may be found in asymptomatic children, they occur most often in male children less than 1 year of age who have clinical cardiac disease.

The clinical course of Kawasaki syndrome is illustrated in Figure 165-1. The acute febrile phase of the disease is marked by rash, conjunctival infection, strawberry tongue, edema and erythema of the hands and feet, lymphadenitis, aseptic meningitis, and hepatic dysfunction. After defervescence, these signs rapidly disappear, but the child remains irritable and anorectic. Arthritis and cardiac disease are likely to be found in the subacute phase of the illness, which is marked also by desquamation and thrombocytosis. This subacute period and the early convalescent period, the third and fourth weeks from onset, constitute the time of greatest risk for sudden death from acute coronary artery thrombosis.

Laboratory abnormalities in Kawasaki syndrome are quite nonspecific. In the acute phase, most patients show leukocytosis with abundant band-form neutrophils. Increased erythrocyte sedimentation rate (ESR) is a universal feature during the subacute period. The number of platelets is normal up to day 10, and then rises, peaking at a mean of 800,000 per mm^3 between days 14 and 25 of illness.

Diagnosis

The diagnosis of Kawasaki syndrome is based upon strict adherence to the principal diagnostic criteria together with rigid exclusion of other diseases that may mimic Kawasaki syndrome. In the acute phase, the presence of five of the six principal criteria is

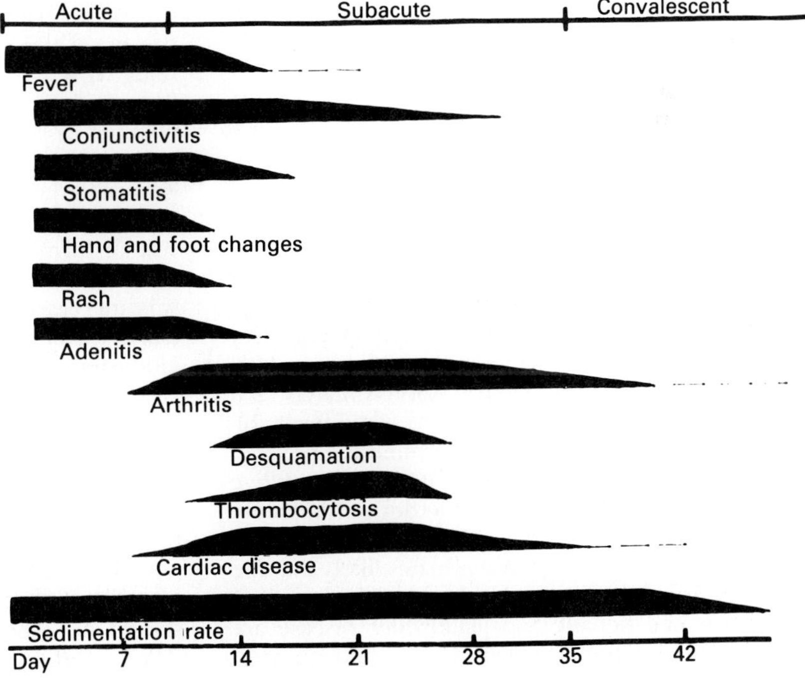

Fig. 165-1. Schematic representation of the clinical events in Kawasaki syndrome from time of onset of fever.

required for diagnosis. Group A β-hemolytic streptococcal scarlet fever (Chap. 24, Streptococcal Diseases) should be ruled out by throat culture or serology. Leptospirosis (Chap. 76, Leptospirosis) may mimic Kawasaki syndrome and should be excluded by culture or serology. Measles (Chap. 86, Measles) may also mimic Kawasaki syndrome; the patient's immunization history and local measles epidemiology should be considered. Rarely, Kawasaki syndrome may be misdiagnosed as Stevens–Johnson syndrome, primarily because of the eye and mouth changes together with the erythema multiformelike rash common to both syndromes. However, the conjunctivitis of Kawasaki syndrome is nonpurulent, and there are neither mucosal lesions nor bullae in the skin. Because treatment with glucosteroids is contraindicated in Kawasaki syndrome but is sometimes advocated for Stevens–Johnson syndrome, it is particularly important to make this distinction.

Toxic shock syndrome (TSS) may be confused with Kawasaki syndrome because of the abrupt onset, high fever, conjunctival suffusion, and peeling of the digits in convalescence. The major differences include (1) hypotension with progression to shock within 1 to 3 days of onset in TSS; (2) the severity of the vomiting and diarrhea is TSS; (3) presence of thrombocytopenia in acute TSS; (4) a strong association of TSS with menses and use of tampons or with focal staphylococcal infections; (5) the respective erythematous rashes—scarlatiniform erythroderma in TSS, urticarial or morbilliform in Kawasaki syndrome; and (6) the ages of the patients—7 years is the age of the youngest TSS patient, whereas Kawasaki syndrome is a disease of young children.

Prognosis

Kawasaki syndrome is primarily acute and self-limited, cardiac disease being the only important sequel. The cardiac damage may be manifest soon after onset or may not become apparent until years later. Approximately 20% of all patients develop coronary artery aneurysms detectable by angiogram or two-dimensional echocardiography. Approximately 2% of patients die of coronary disease. Long-term follow-up studies are needed to determine the prognosis of those with aneurysms as well as the incidence of coronary disease not detectable during the acute illness. Japanese studies have shown that regression of aneurysms may occur, but it remains likely that the coronary arteries are permanently damaged.

Arthritis and hepatic and gallbladder disease are not associated with permanent damage and are present for only 6 to 10 weeks.

Nothing is known about immunity. Second attacks appear to be rare, occurring within 4 months to 8 years in 3 of more than 150 patients.

Therapy

There is at present no specific therapy for Kawasaki syndrome. A thoughtfully designed program of supportive care and attentive follow-up is necessary to detect and manage complications. To this end, patients may be admitted to a hospital to facilitate diagnostic testing, provide stabilization during the distressing early febrile course, and enable education of the family regarding the disease. However, at parental request, milder cases may be managed entirely as outpatients.

Once Kawasaki syndrome has been diagnosed, treatment with aspirin should begin using a dose of 80 to 100 mg/kg body wt/day as 4 equal portions 6-hourly. The dose should be adjusted to maintain the concentrations of salicylate in the blood between 18 and 25 mg/dl. The fever will dissipate within 48 hours in two-thirds of patients. At this point, patients may be discharged from the hospital and followed as outpatients with complete clinical examinations twice a week until the fifth week of the illness.

When the fever has been controlled, the dose of aspirin should be reduced to 10 mg/kg body wt/day as 2 equal portions 12-hourly; this low dose is continued throughout the period of thrombocytosis and for several weeks until the ESR is normal. Reduction of the dose of aspirin is important because 10 mg/kg body wt/day provides adequate suppression of platelet aggregation without stimulating vascular thrombogenic factors, a problem with higher doses.

Treatment with glucosteroids is contraindicated in Kawaski syndrome. In a controlled trial, it was shown that glucosteroid therapy significantly increased the risk of formation of aneurysms. Also, according to uncontrolled observations in Japan, the mortality rate was increased by treatment with glucosteroids. Finally, thrombocytosis results from treatment with glucosteroids, whereas the adhesiveness of platelets is unaffected.

Monitoring for cardiovascular complications should begin when Kawasaki syndrome is diagnosed. Clinical evaluations, and serial chest roentgenograms and electrocardiograms enable detection of congestive heart failure and arrhythmias that can be treated with conventional drug therapies. Pericarditis and mitral insufficiency are generally self-limited, but should be observed in hospital until they resolve.

As a routine, M-mode and two-dimensional echocardiograms are obtained during the fourth week of illness. If the echocardiogram is normal, aspirin is continued until the ESR is normal; the patient is then discharged and seen in follow-up twice weekly through the fourth week after discharge and at successively longer intervals if all remains well.

If clinical cardiac disease develops, the patient is readmitted to the hospital for monitoring and intensive care. This regimen allows careful clinical follow-up throughout the period of highest risk while avoiding prolonged hospitalization.

If the echocardiogram obtained during the fourth week of illness reveals coronary aneurysms, the aspirin is continued indefinitely and the patient is monitored clinically and has follow-up echocardiograms and electrocardiograms every 3 months. In Japan, two-dimensional echocardiography has been demonstrated to be nearly as sensitive as angiography in detecting left coronary aneurysms, although it misses approximately one-third of right coronary lesions. Because aneurysms are bilateral and near the origin of the coronary arteries in most cases, the complete echocardiogram (M-mode plus biplanar studies) detects most aneurysmal lesions and provides information about ventricular contractility, chamber dimensions, valve function, and pericardial effusion. Angiography may therefore be reserved for special cases. Although coronary artery bypass surgery has been performed in a few patitients in the United States and Japan, the proper role of this therapy is unclear. At present it should probably be reserved for untreatable and progressive angina. Aneurysmal lesions tend to regress with time—two-thirds are no longer detectable by angiography after 1 year.

Once treatment with aspirin has been started, supportive care and careful monitoring to detect and manage complications are all that can be offered. Although often quite severe, arthritic, hepatic, and gastrointestinal involvement is self-limited and usually resolves within 2 weeks. If acute noncalculous gallbladder distention (hydrops) develops it can be diagnosed and followed by repeated abdominal ultrasound examinations.

Prevention

There are no known preventives of Kawasaki syndrome.

Remaining Problems

Determining the etiology and pathogenesis of Kawasaki syndrome is a prime objective because it should lead to rational treatment and prevention of the disease. Long-term studies of coronary artery disease in survivors of Kawasaki syndrome over at least two decades are urgently needed to determine the true morbidity of the syndrome.

Bibliography

Journals

DAVIS JP, CHESNEY PJ, LAVENTURE M: Toxic shock syndrome: Epidemiologic features, recurrence, risk factors and prevention. N Engl J Med 303:1429–1435, 1980

DEAN AD, MELISH ME, HICKS RM: An epidemic of Kawasaki syndrome in Hawaii.

FUJIWARA H, HAMASHIMA Y: Pathology of the heart in Kawaski disease. Pediatrics 61:100–107, 1978

KAWASAKI T, KOSAKI F, OKAWA S, SHIGEMATSU T, YANAGAWA H: A new infantile acute febrile mucocutaneous lymph node syndrome (MLNS) prevailing in Japan. Pediatrics 54:271–276, 1974

LANDING BH, LARSON EJ: Are infantile periarteritis nodosa with coronary artery involvement and fatal mucocutaneous lymph node syndrome the same? Pediatrics 59:651–662, 1977

MELISH ME, HICKS RM, MARCHETTS NJ: Endemic and epidemic Kawasaki syndrome. Clin Res 29:126A, 1981

MORENS DM, ANDERSON LJ, HURWITZ ES: National surveillance of Kawasaki disease. Pediatrics 65:21–25, 1980

HENRY G. CRAMBLETT

166 Cat-Scratch Fever

Cat-scratch fever (cat-scratch disease, benign lymphoreticulosis, nonbacterial regional lymphadenitis) occurs primarily in children. Characteristically, there is a slowly progressive and chronic enlargement of single or regional lymph nodes. Rarely, more serious disease with involvement of other organs may occur. The disease was first recognized as a clinical entity in the United States by Foshay in the early 1930s during the course of his studies on tularemia. An antigen he prepared from pus removed from affected lymph nodes produced a positive reaction on intradermal injection into human subjects. At about the same time in France, Debré recognized the occurrence of suppurative adenitis in children with negative tuberculin tests but with numerous scratches attributed to cats. With a supply of Foshay's antigen, Debré was able to study ill patients with positive skin tests, and this led to the first clinical description of the disease in 1950.

Etiology

The etiology of cat-scratch fever is unknown. Specimens of pus from patients with this disease have been studied intensively since 1950 by many investigators without recovering the responsible agent. Techniques have been used that are suitable for the recovery or demonstration of bacteria (including mycobacteria), fungi, viruses, chlamydias, rickettsias, and protozoa with negative results.

As is often the case, when an agent is not recovered from a disease that is probably infectious in origin, its cause is ascribed to a virus. Indeed, the pathologic lesion in lymph nodes is consistent with a viral etiologic agent.

Epidemiology

Cat-scratch fever is a major cause of regional or local lymphadenopathy of obscure cause. The frequency of the disease is unknown because there is no generally available means of diagnosis.

It is well established that the agent of the disease is usually transmitted from cats to humans by means of scratch. Two-thirds of the patients have a history of being scratched by a cat, and 90% give a history of contact with a cat. It has been suggested that contact with the excreta or saliva of cats may suffice for transmission without an actual scratch. More often than not, the cats are young and not fully grown. There is not evidence that the agent of cat-scratch disease produces infection or illness in the cat. The scratch or bite of other animals, such as dogs or monkeys, or even scratches by inanimate objects are said to have been responsible for spread of the agent to humans.

Cat-scratch fever occurs only in humans. Most cases are observed in late fall, winter, or early spring. Children are more commonly affected than are adults. It is not uncommon for more than one member of a family to have the disease (Fig. 166-1), and regional outbreaks have been reported. The incubation period, judged by the time interval between contact with cats and the development of lymphadenopathy, is 1 to 8 weeks.

Pathogenesis and Pathology

The essential components of the pathologic lesion in affected lymph nodes include hyperplasia, granuloma formation, and suppuration with central liquefaction necrosis (Fig. 166-2). The microscopic findings in

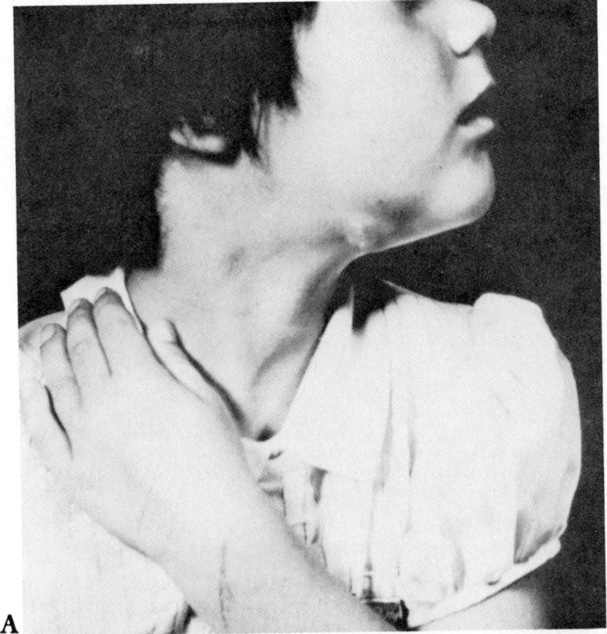

A

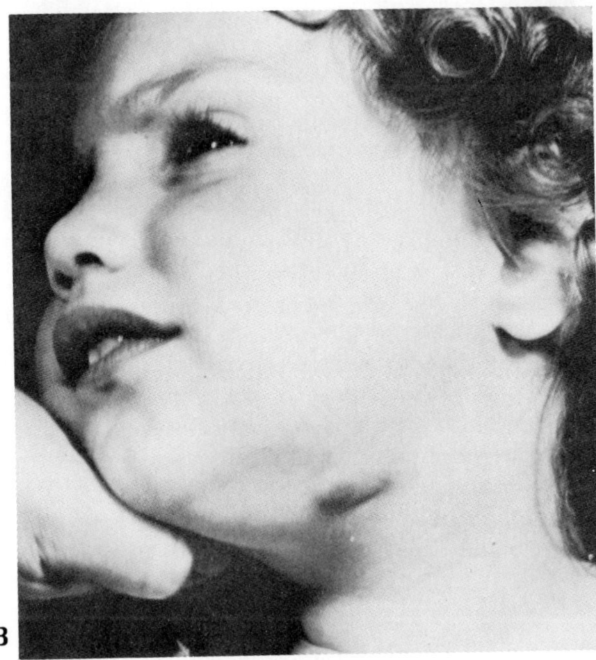

B

Fig. 166-1. Sisters with submandibular lymphadenitis. Both girls were scratched on numerous occasions by a 5-month-old cat. Excision of the lymph nodes was followed by rapid recovery. (*A*) The 5-year-old girl had lymphadenitis of 4 months' duration. Note scratches on the back of her hand. (*B*) The 3⅓-year-old girl had lymphadenitis of 5 months' duration.

nodes have been divided into early, intermediate, and late stages. In the early lesion, there is at most only a slight distortion of the architecture of the lymph node. The lymphoid follicles and their germinal centers are enlarged but not otherwise conspicuous. The reticulum cell predominates. The lesion may become stationary and then regress, or it may proceed to the next stage. In intermediate lesions, tuberculoid foci appear; multinucleated giant cells are rare. The capsule is often broken, and the architecture of the node is definitely distorted. In the late lesion, microabscesses and macroabscesses are present and commonly surrounded by epithelioid cells with a palisading arrangement.

Manifestations

A primary local lesion at the site of scratch or injury occurs in about 13 days in half the cases. Taking the form of a small papule, vesicle, or pustule, the primary lesion may be missed on cursory physical examination. Regional lymphadenopathy (more often consisting of single than multiple nodes) becomes evident within a few days to a few weeks (range, 3–50 days after the local lesion appears. The nodes are usually moderately tender and are freely movable. In 30% to 50% of cases, the nodes become suppurative. General lymphadenopathy or involvement of the lymph nodes of more than one region is unusual.

About one-third of patients have no signs or symptoms of illness other than lymphadenopathy. Mild fever and malaise occur in less than half the patients. Chills, general aching, and nausea are infrequently present. Occasionally, patients have conjunctivitis, implicating the eye as a portal of entry for the infectious agent. With conjunctivitis there is usually preauricular, tender lymphadenopathy—the oculoglandular syndrome of Parinaud.

Other much less common manifestations of cat-scratch disease include encephalitis, pneumonitis, erythema nodosum, thrombocytopenia, and osteolytic lesions.

Diagnosis

The diagnosis of cat-scratch disease should be considered in anyone with acute, subacute, or chronic lymphadenitis that is either regional or local. Support for this diagnosis is gained if the patient has been scratched or has had contact with a cat. In the presence of a compatible clinical picture, and after all other possible causes have been ruled out, the spe-

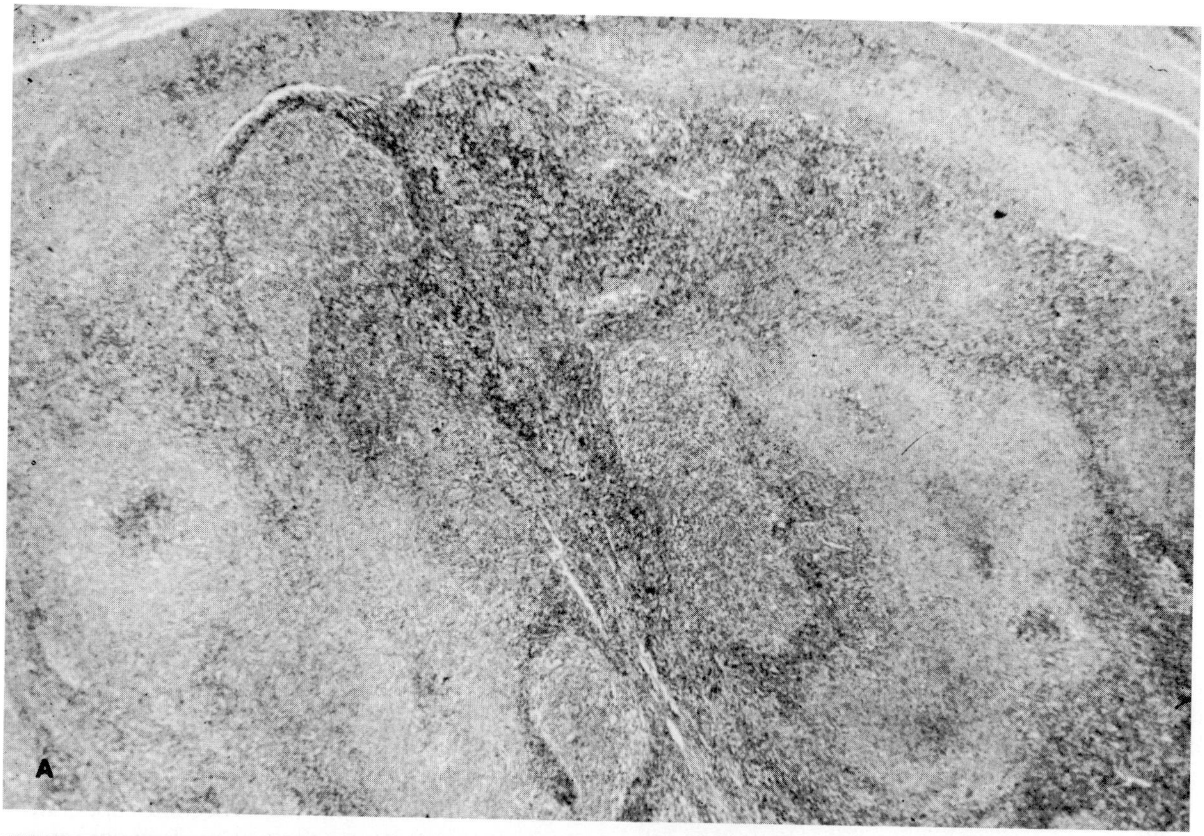

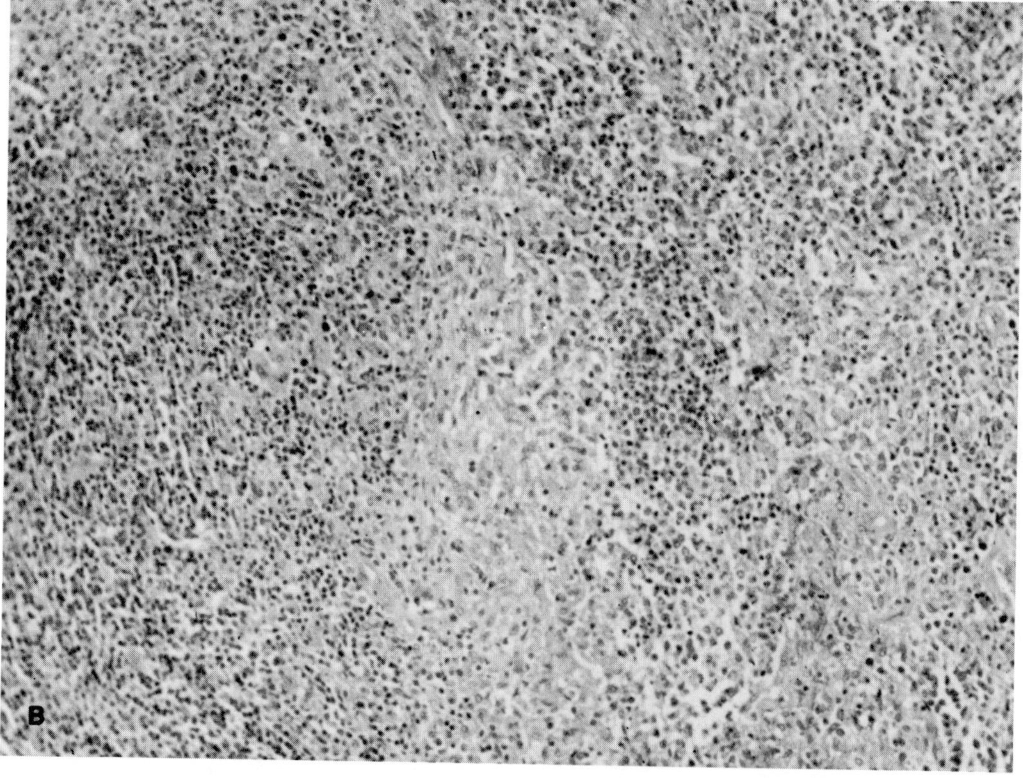
B

cific diagnosis can be made by demonstrating a positive skin test.

Preparation

The skin test antigen is prepared by obtaining purulent material from involved lymph nodes either by percutaneous aspiration or from surgically excised nodes. It is cultured for bacteria (aerobic and anaerobic), mycobacteria, fungi, and viruses. The material is then frozen at −70°C until further processing is performed.

First, heat inactivation must be sufficient to ensure complete inactivation of hepatitis virus, if it is present. Soulier showed that heating biologic preparations for 10 hours at 60°C may not kill all hepatitis B virus—resulting in one breakthrough in 11 cases. Subsequently, Schulkind demonstrated that heating pus from nodes obtained from a patient with cat-scratch disease at 60°C for 20 hours did not destroy its antigenicity. Accordingly, potential test material should be heated to 60°C for a minimum period of 20 hours. The material is next diluted 1:5 with 0.9% NaCl solution for injection, a portion is cultured for bacteria (aerobic and anaerobic), mycobacteria, fungi and viruses, and the remainder is frozen. When the cultures are reported as negative (4–6 weeks later), the antigen is dispensed into sterile vials in 0.15-ml amounts for individual tests and is frozen at −20°C until used. All new antigens must be tested in both known positive and known negative reactors to ensure specificity of the antigen. If desired, semiquantitation of the antigenicity can be accomplished by testing intradermal reactivity to further dilutions of the antigen.

Fig. 166-2. (*A*) Low-power photomicrograph of a section of lymph node from a patient with cat-scratch fever. There are several foci of necrosis with central neutrophilic infiltration, a lighter zone of histiocytic (epithelioid) cell reaction, and an outermost zone of small round-cell (lymphocytes and a few plasma cells) infiltration. Although the pattern is consistent with and suggestive of cat-scratch fever, it is not diagnostic. Other diseases that may produce a similar histologic pattern of reaction are lymphogranuloma venereum, histoplasmosis and other fungal lesions, tularemia, brucellosis, sarcoidosis, and tuberculosis H & E, original magnification × 60) (*B*) Higher magnification of section of (A) Multinucleated histiocytic giant cells vary greatly in numbers in different cases, but they are usually present. No inclusion bodies were identified. (H & E original magnification × 250) (Courtesy of CB Reiner, Department of Pathology, Ohio State University College of Medicine and Children's Hospital, Columbus, Ohio)

Performance

The test is performed by injecting 0.1 ml of the antigen intradermally. Often a flare reaction is observed shortly after the injection and is of no consequence. The test is read at 36 to 48 hours. A positive test is either an induration 5 mm or more in diameter with or without erythema or an erythema 10 mm or more in diameter if no induration is present. Although anaphylaxis has not been reported, epinephrine (1:1000 dilution) should be available for emergency use.

Differential Diagnosis

Cat-scratch disease must always be considered in the differential diagnosis of regional lymphadenopathy. Suppurative bacterial lymphadenitis may occur in association with obvious respiratory illness. Smears and cultures of node aspirates are helpful in the differentiation.

Lymphadenitis caused by atypical mycobacterial infection may cause similar disease (Chap. 36, Nontuberculous Mycobacterioses). Unfortunately, sensitins corresponding to atypical mycobacteria are not available commercially, and cross-reaction with standard tuberculin cannot be relied on for diagnosis. Smear or culture typically reveals acid-fast organisms. Other, less frequent causes of regional lymphadenopathy in children include tularemia (Chap. 139, Tularemia), toxoplasmosis (Chap. 129, Toxoplasmosis), infectious mononucleosis (Chap. 137, Infectious Mononucleosis), tumors, lymphogranuloma venereum (Chap. 54, Lymphogranuloma Venereum), and coccidioidomycosis (Chap. 41, Coccidioidomycosis).

Prognosis

The disease is usually self-limiting. Complications such as thrombocytopenic purpura, oculoglandular syndrome, osteolytic lesions, central nervous system involvement, erythema nodosum, and erythema multiforme are rare. There are no known sequelae. It is not known whether immunity is acquired form having had the disease.

Therapy

There is no specific therapy for this disease. The administration of antimicrobics has no effect on the course of the illness.

Surgical excision of the affected lymph nodes is indicated in selected instances in which the nodes have become large, tender, and fluctuant. Because the disease is self-limiting, nodes should only be removed when a good cosmetic result can be obtained. Pus may be removed by needle aspiration. With repeated aspiration, a sinus tract occasionally forms and chronic drainage ensues.

Prevention

There are no known means of prevention. Because the disease is so mild and self-limiting, it hardly seems justified to recommend avoidance of cats.

Remaining Problems

The etiologic agent of cat-scratch fever remains to be discovered.

Bibliography

Journals

Editorial: Cat scratch disease and Parinaud's oculoglandular syndrome. JAMA 152:1717, 1953

MARGILETH AM: Cat scratch disease: Nonbacterial regional lymphadenitis. Pediatrics 42:803–818, 1968

NAJI AF, CARBONELL F, BARKER HJ: Cat scratch disease. Am J Clin Pathol 38:513–521, 1962

SCHULKIND ML, AYOUB, EM: Cell mediated immunity in cat-scratch disease. J Pediatr 85:199–203, 1974

SMALL WT, SNIFFEN RC: Nonbacterial regional lymphadenitis ("cat-scratch fever"). N Engl J Med 255:1029–1033, 1956

SOULIER JP, BLATIX C, COUROUCE AM, BENAMON D, AMOUCH P, DROUET J: Prevention of virus B hepatitis (SH hepatitis). Am J Dis Child 123:429–434, 1972

WARWICK WJ: The cat-scratch syndrome: Many diseases or one disease? Prog Med Virol 9:256–301, 1967

FRED E. PITTMAN

Whipple's Disease

167

Whipple's disease (intestinal lidodystrophy) is probably an infectious disease. Not only are the clinical manifestations characteristic, but also there are identifying pathologic changes in the gut and in many other organs, including the brain and eyes. The usual course terminates in death from malnutrition unless the disease is recognized and treated with antimicrobics.

Etiology

In 1907, Whipple reported a previously undescribed, chronic wasting disease in a 36-year-old, male medical missionary. Death ensued 5½ years after onset. In a small mesenteric lymph node (Levaditi stain), Whipple found ". . . great numbers of a rod-shaped organism (?) . . . about the diameter of the spirochete of syphilis but not of the spiral shape and rarely exceeding 2 μm in length." He also isolated a ". . . bacillus belonging to the colon group . . ." from mesenteric nodes, but was reluctant to consider the disease infectious in origin. He proposed the name intestinal lipodystrophy because of the presence of large deposits of lipid in lymph nodes and in the mucosa and submucosa of the small intestine.

Although the material present in "foamy cells" described by Whipple was shown in 1949 to stain intensely dark red by the periodic acid-Schiff (PAS) method, that is, to be PAS-positive (contain glycoprotein), it was not until the late 1950's when electron microscopy was applied to jejunal mucosal biopsies that the PAS-positive material was discerned to be masses of tiny bacilliform structures characteristic of bacteria. In untreated patients, they are 0.25 μm to 0.30 μm wide × 1.5 μm to 2.5 μm long, appear to undergo fission, and occur extracellularly as well as intracellularly (Fig. 167-1).

There is little doubt that these microorganisms play a major causal role in Whipple's disease. They are invariably present in untreated patients, and antimicrobic therapy results in their disappearance. At the same time, the number of intestinal mucosal macrophages decreases, and the patient undergoes dramatic clinical remission. Several different kinds of bacteria have been isolated from biopsy specimens, including aerobic and anaerobic *Corneybacterium* spp., *Haemophilus* spp., brucellalike bacteria, and L-form streptococci. None has been proved to be related to the disease either by inoculation into experimental animals or by serology.

Epidemiology

Over 200 cases have been reported—mostly from the United States, the United Kingdom, and continental Europe, and a few from South America. The actual incidence of the disease is unknown, and it occurs sporadically.

The third and fourth decades of life are the ages of maximal incidence, although the span is 20 to 67 years. Approximately 90% of patients, have been white men, with only occasional reports in blacks, American Indians, and women. Occupation, social stratum, geographic location (whether urban or rural), and contact with livestock do not seem to be relevant. The disease has occurred in brothers, but in general it is not familial, and there is no firm evidence of communicability. The disease has not been reported in either wild or domesticated animals.

Pathogenesis and Pathology

Because duodenojejunal mucosal involvement is present in almost all reported cases, it has been suggested that the small bowel is the initial site of involvement. The primary support of this hypothesis is the fact that the histopathologic findings present in the small in-

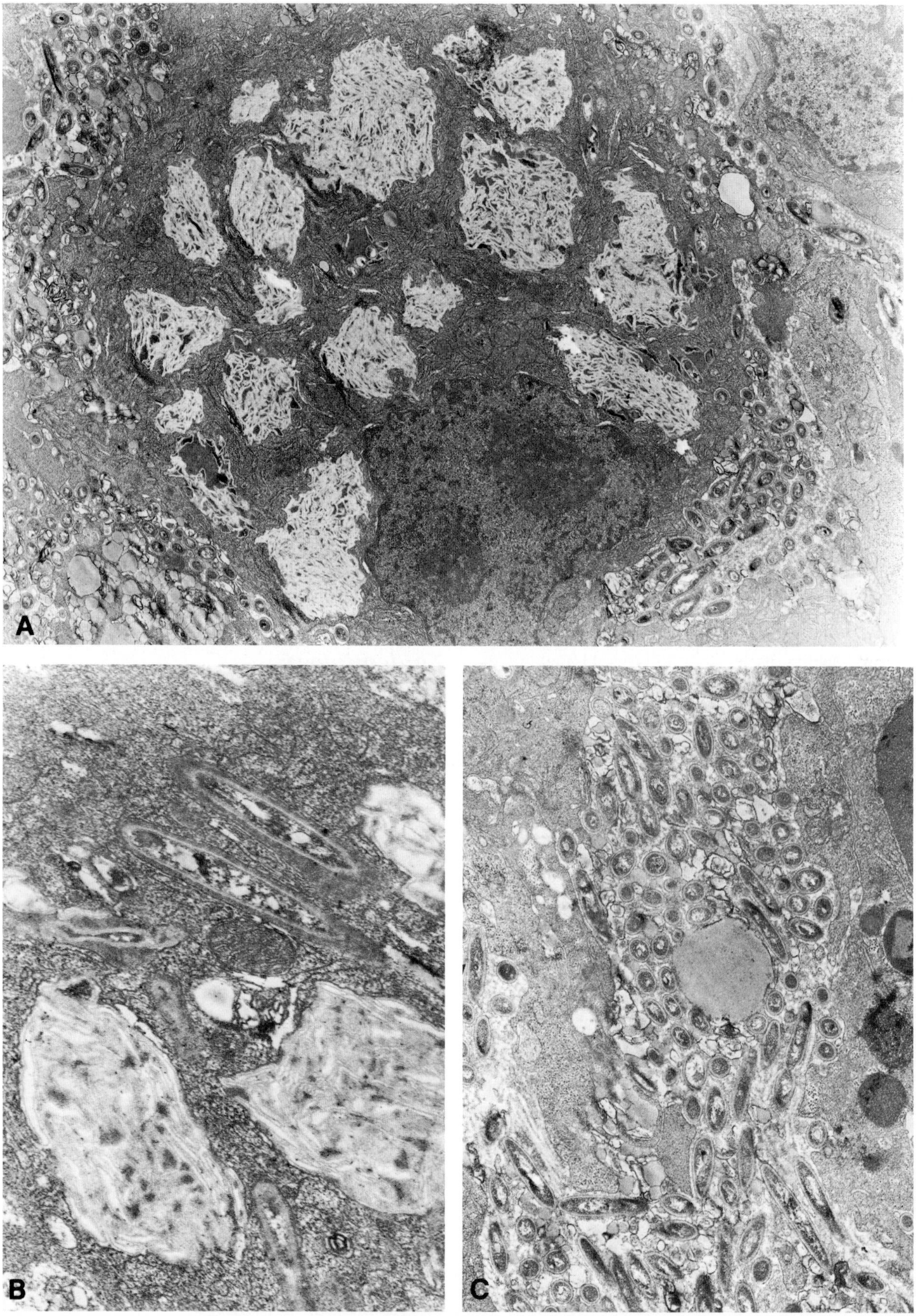

A

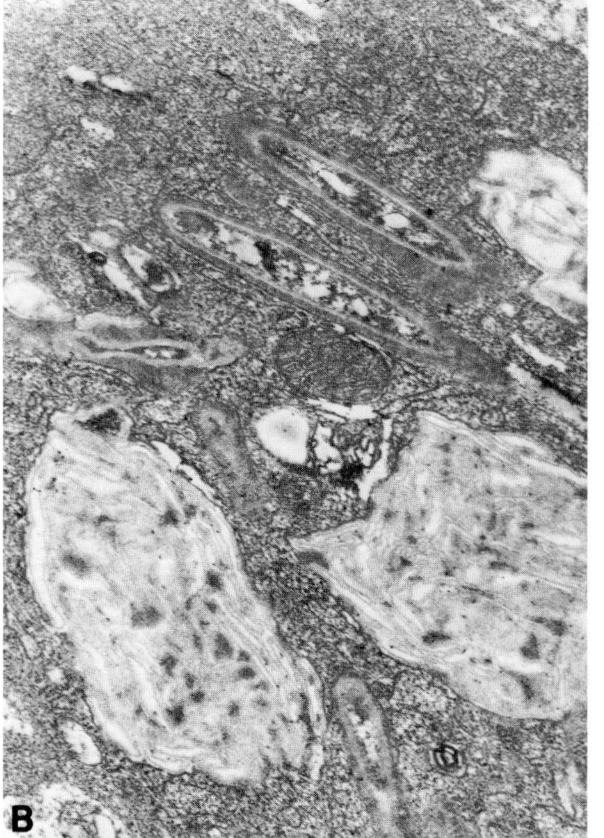

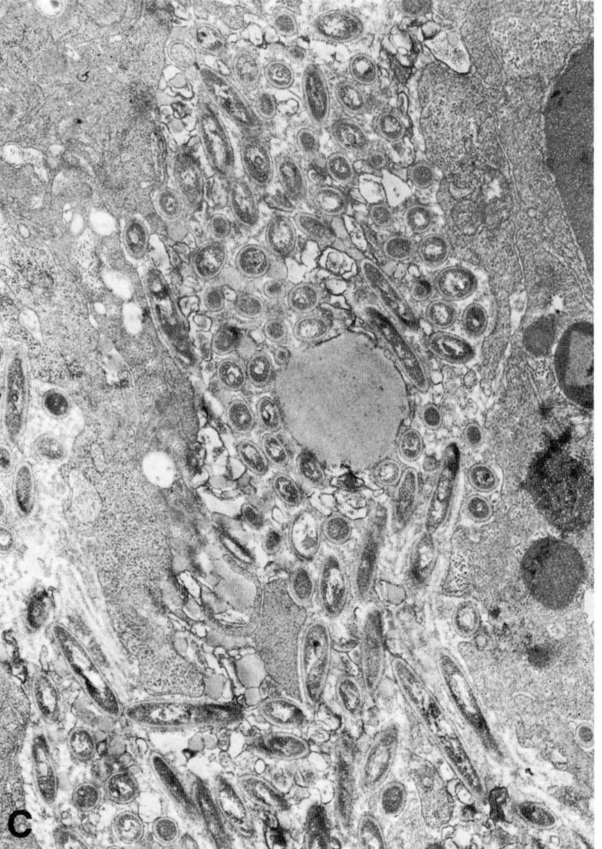

testine in virtually all untreated patients are most prevalent in the duodenum; gradually diminish in number progressing through the jejunum, upper ileum, and midileum; are usually lacking in the terminal ileum. However, the disease is widespread outside the gut, as has been shown by the finding of PAS-positive macrophages and bacilliform microorganisms in mesothelial cells of the pleura, peritoneum, pericardium; synovial lining cells; the liver; and mesenteric and peripheral nodes. The result is anemia, emaciation, lymphadenopathy, organizing peritonitis, pleuritis, pericarditis, and aortic endocarditis. Involvement of the central nervous system (CNS) may lead to ventricular dilation; chronic granular ependymitis with PAS-positive material in ependymal cells and in macrophages in periventricular cerebral tissue has been described.

It is not known how the organisms and the macrophages produce the enteric manifestations observed in the disease. For example, the electron microscopic appearance of the intestinal absorptive cells is usually normal, and only very occasionally have organisms been demonstrated within these cells. The extensive macrophage infiltration of the mucosal, submucosal, and mesenteric lymph nodes produces mechanical blockage with dilation of mucosal lymphatics similar to that seen in intestinal lymphangiectasia (Fig. 167-2). In both conditions, malabsorption of fat and protein-losing enteropathy may be profound. It is also possible that macrophages block transport of absorbed substances across the lamina propria to capillaries. Other pathophysiologic effects, such as release of toxic substances by the organisms or by the macrophages or direct injury by the organism, are also possible.

Except for decreased concentrations of IgM in some patients, the humoral immune system is normal. There are no abnormal deposits of complement or immunoglobulins within the intestinal mucosa, and there is no evidence for autoantibody production. Circulating immune complexes have been described, perhaps reflecting a defect of antigen exclusion in the disease.

Fig. 167-1 Electron micrographs of a jejunal mucosal biopsy from a patient with untreated Whipple's disease. (*A*) Jejunal mucosal macrophage and extracellular bacilli. (Original magnification approximately × 25,000) (*B*) Bacilli and membranous inclusions (presumably incompletely digested bacterial membranes) within macrophages. (Original magnification approximately × 48,000) (*C*) Bacilli surrounding a lipid-containing lymphatic channel in the subepithelial lamina propria. (Original magnification approximately × 48,000)

Immediate hypersensitivity reactions to cutaneous antigens are slightly depressed. There are conflicting reports of impairment of delayed cutaneous reactions dependent on cell-mediated immunity in untreated and treated patients. There appears to be a partial but irreversible disorder of cell-mediated immunity in some patients. It is postulated that this might predispose to bacterial invasion of the small bowel and allow proliferation with the development of a state of immunologic tolerance.

Manifestations

In many patients, the disease begins with nondeforming polyarthralgias or polyarthritides. Back pain from spondylitis may occur. Fever (low-grade, spiking, or sustained); malaise; and weight loss associated with anorexia are common early on and may occur with the joint symptoms several years before gastrointestinal or other manifestations are observed. Diarrhea is the most common gastrointestinal complaint and may be minimal or may be a major symptom. The feces may be watery or semiformed and, if malabsorption is present, may have the characteristics of steatorrhea. Usually, the feces contain no gross or occult blood, though hematochezia has been reported. Occasionally constipation is prominent. Bloating and abdominal cramps are not infrequent complaints. An ileuslike picture has been described. Although malabsorption may be significant in advanced cases, when it occurs with anorexia marked cachexia may result, leading to severe nutritional deficiencies such as those seen in far-advanced nontropical and tropical sprue. Hyperpigmentation of the skin has been reported.

Peripheral lymphadenopathy, with or without splenomegaly, may be present.

If serosal membranes are involved, there may be manifestations of pericarditis or congestive heart failure with or without cardiac valvular damage; pleuritis and pneumonia; and ascites. Peripheral edema is often seen.

Clinically apparent involvement of the CNS in Whipple's disease (with or without ocular disease) is unusual when gastrointestinal manifestations are prominent. Typical are personality changes; progressive dementia (memory loss, periods of confusion, inappropriate behavior, and apathy); myoclonus; supranuclear ophthalmoplegia; and ataxia. Papilledema, optic atrophy, and uveitis have also been reported. Less common are headaches, hearing loss, impotence, major motor seizures, and coma. CNS and ocular involvement may occur after treatment of the intestinal disease.

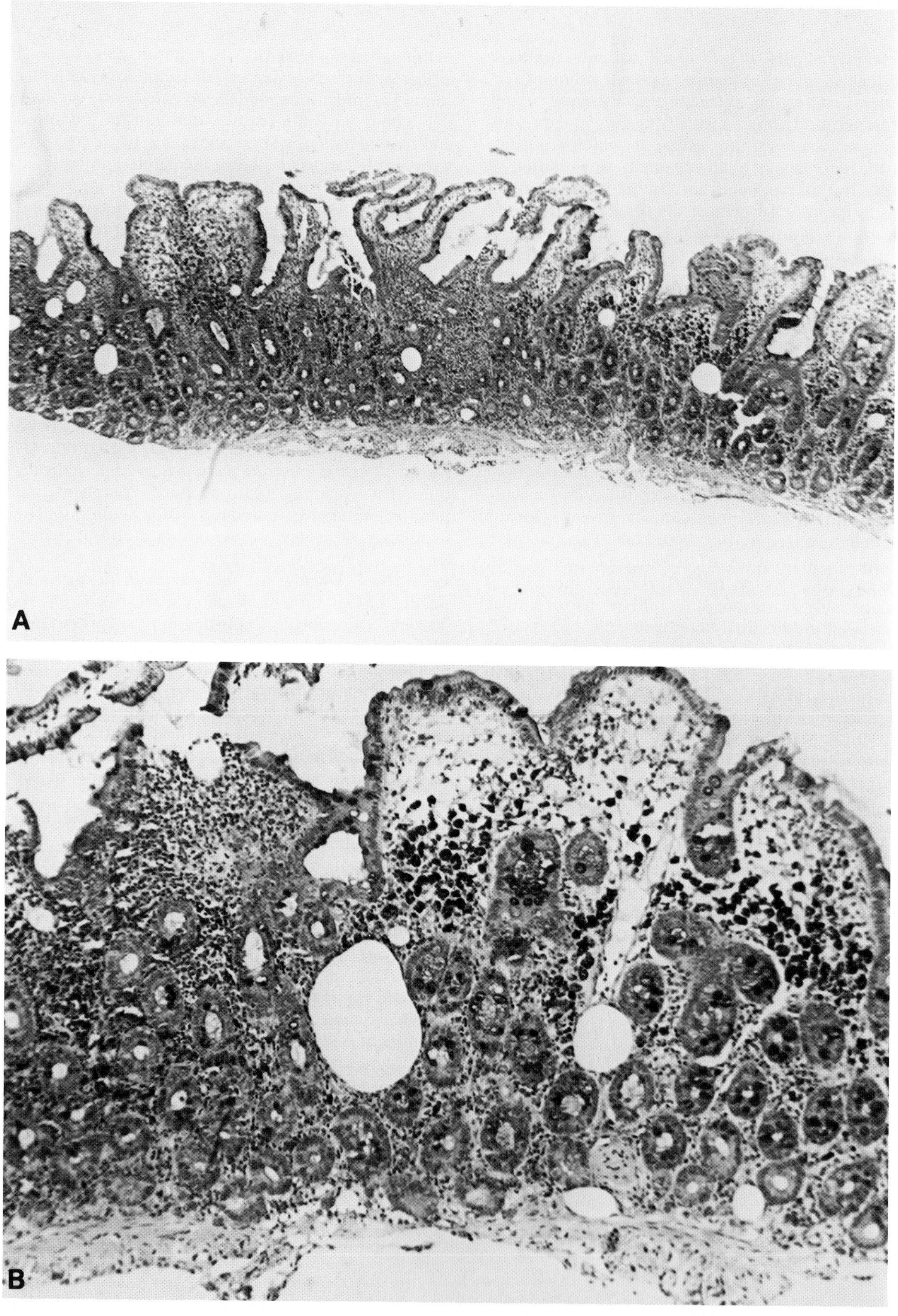

A

B

There may be a mild leukocytosis in febrile patients, but most abnormalities of laboratory tests are related to malnutrition and malabsorption. In severely ill patients, the usual tests of absorption, including quantitative fecal fat determination and the d-xylose absorption test, are abnormal. Tests of protein-losing enteropathy may be positive. Hypokalemia, hypocalcemia, hypomagnesemia, and hypoalbuminemia are often present. Iron deficiency or folate deficiency has been seen with either microcytic or macrocytic anemia. Thrombocytosis has been described.

Contrast radiographic examination of the upper intestinal tract reveals diffuse, nonspecific abnormalities such as dilation and loss of the normally delicate, feathery pattern due to thickening of the mucosal folds (Fig. 167-3). Radiologic diagnoses such as edema of the bowel, deficiency pattern, or malabsorption pattern are often reported. These radiographic abnormalities usually disappear following treatment. Cranial computed tomography (CT) may be abnormal if there is CNS involvement. CT may prove useful in evaluating patients with CNS findings and intestinal complaints and should be done for baseline evaluation of the CNS status in all new patients.

Diagnosis

Whipple's disease should be strongly suspected in any patient who has a long-standing history of arthritis or arthralgia and who later develops diarrhea with marked weight loss. In such cases, the demonstration of steatorrhea provides additional evidence for Whipple's disease. Clinically, the disease can be confused with any diffuse disease of the small bowel: sprue, regional enteritis, lymphoma, scleroderma, primary amyloidosis, tuberculosis (Chap. 34, Pulmonary Tuberculosis), lymphangiectasia, and mesenteric artery insufficiency.

The diagnosis of Whipple's disease is best established by PAS staining of histologic sections of duodenal or upper jejunal mucosa obtained by peroral biopsy. Presence of PAS-positive macrophages in the lamina propria accompanied by dilation of mucosal and submucosal lymphatics is diagnostic (Fig. 167-2). If such macrophages are not found, the disease should not be excluded on the basis of a single biopsy when Whipple's disease is strongly suspected. Duodenal or jejunal mucosa should be obtained from several sites; enlarged lymph nodes should be biopsied and examined after PAS-staining; biopsy of the bone marrow with PAS-staining may be helpful. Biopsies of rectal mucosa are not useful.

When the CNS is involved, PAS-positive macrophages may be detected in brain biopsy specimens even if other tissues fail to show such histopathology. Examination for PAS-positive cells in synovial fluid, synovial biopsy material, cerebrospinal fluid (CSF), and biopsy material or fluid from other potentially involved sites is worthwhile. Electron microscopy of duodenojejunal mucosal biopsies to document the presence of the bacilliform organisms characteristic of Whipple's disease (Fig. 167-1) is highly desirable.

Fig. 167-2. Transmitted light photomicrographs of jejunal mucosa in untreated Whipple's disease. Periodic acid-Schiff stain. (*A*) The villi are irregular and variably edematous. Dilated lymphatics are scattered throughout, as are PAS-positive macrophages. (Original magnification approximately × 40) (*B*) Extensive subepithelial edema is evident in several villi. It is probable that exudation of albumin-rich liquid occurs through breaks in the epithelium leading to the protein-losing enteropathy and hypoalbuminemia commonly seen in Whipple's disease. (Original magnification approximately × 125)

Prognosis

Patients with Whipple's disease who go untreated invariably die of malnutrition. With diagnosis and application of appropriate antimicrobial treatment, the prognosis is excellent unless there is involvement of the CNS. The treatment of Whipple's disease of the CNS has been disappointing.

Therapy

Nutritional deficiencies should be treated with appropriate replacements. Two regimens of antimicrobial therapy are equally effective in bringing about remission, which is rarely followed by relapse of non-CNS Whipple's disease: (1) procaine penicillin G, 12.5 mg (20,000 U)/kg body wt/day, IM, for 10 to 14 days, plus streptomycin, 15 mg/kg body wt/day, IM, as 2 equal portions, 12-hourly, for 10 to 14 days, and tetracycline, 15 mg/kg body wt/day, PO, as 4 equal portions, 6-hourly, for 1 year; or (2) procaine penicillin G, 37.5 mg (60,000 U)/kg body wt/day, IM, as 2 equal portions, 12-hourly, for 10 to 14 days, then penicillin V, 7 to 8 mg/kg body wt/day, PO, as 2 equal portions, 12-hourly, for 2 to 4 months (until histologic examination of the intestinal mucosa reveals return to normal). Since relapse of intestinal disease is frequent if tetracycline is used alone, or if short-

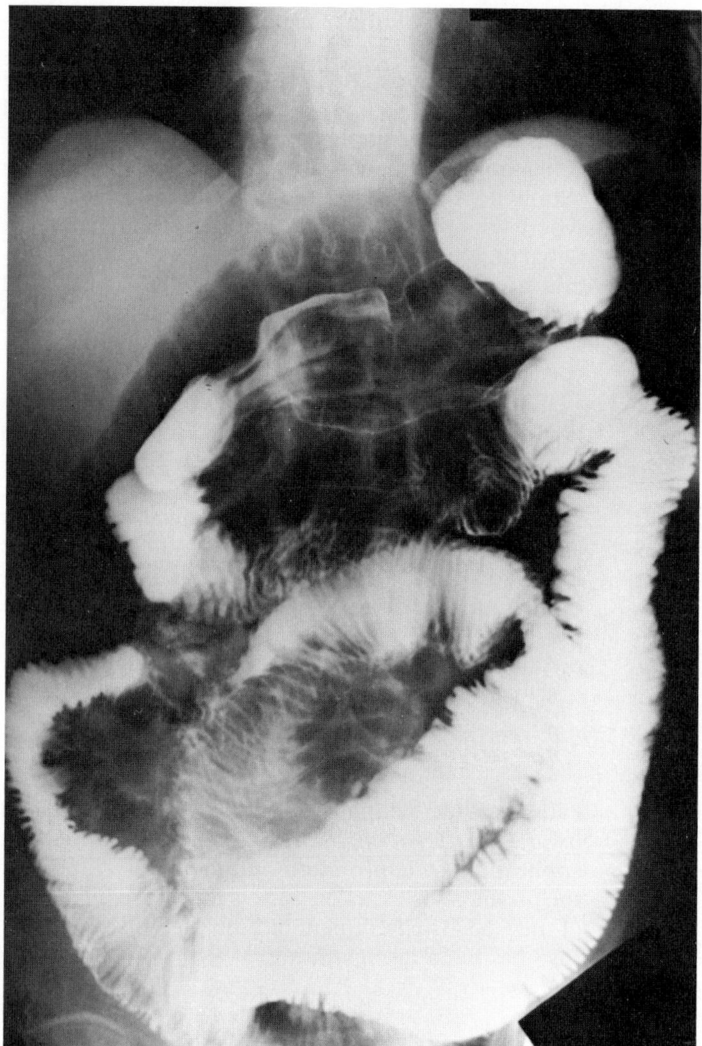

Fig. 167-3. Contrast roentgenogram of the small bowel in untreated Whipple's disease. The upper small intestine is dilated, and the mucosal folds are thickened with loss of the normal feathery pattern.

term therapy is prescribed, only the regimens given in (1) and (2) above are recommended. Patients must be followed at 9- to 12-month intervals for several years to detect relapses as early as possible.

Treatment of Whipple's disease of the CNS or eyes has not been satisfactory using the conventional regimens that are successful for intestinal disease. Possibly, poor ingress of antimicrobics into the CNS and ocular tissues is to blame, or possibly the damage from the disease is irreversible when treatment is begun. However, the fact that CNS/ocular involvement may become clinically apparent during successful treatment of intestinal Whipple's disease favors the former construction. Hence, it may be prudent to substitute trimethoprim–sulfamethoxazole, 80 mg + 400 mg, respectively (1 tablet), PO, 12-hourly, for tetracycline, since both components of the combination penetrate into the CNS and eyes. Chloramphenicol and rifampin may also be alternatives, since both enter the CNS and eyes sufficiently.

Prevention

Because it is not known how Whipple's disease is acquired, or why one person develops the disease and another in the same environment does not, preventive measures cannot be suggested. It is possible that prolonged treatment of Whipple's disease of the intestine with two or more antimicrobics that penetrate into the CNS may prevent the development of CNS disease.

Remaining Problems

It is not known whether Whipple's disease is the result of infection with an unusual organism or several different organisms. Isolation, identification, and propagation of Whipple's disease organisms from multiple cases and development of an animal model remain elusive but critical steps toward solving the mystery of the disease.

There remains a lack of understanding of pathogenetic mechanisms in Whipple's disease. Is altered susceptibility the major factor in the development of the disease?

What are the mechanisms of CNS and ocular damage, and how can they best be prevented?

Bibliography

Journals

BATTLE WM, KROOP HS, DIMARINO AJ JR, REDFIELD E: Relapse of Whipple's disease after short-term antibiotic treatment. J Med Soc NJ 77:194–196, 1980

BAYLESS TM: Whipple's disease: Newer concepts of therapy. Adv Intern Med 16:171–189, 1970

BLACK–SCHAFFER B: The tinctoral demonstration of a glycoprotein in Whipple's disease. Proc Soc Exp Biol Med 72:225–227, 1949

CHEARS WC, ASHWORTH CT: Electron microscopic study of the intestinal mucosa in Whipple's disease. Gastroenterol 41:129–138, 1961

DOBBINS WO: Is there an immune deficit in Whipple's disease? Dig Dis Sci 26:247–252, 1981

ELSBORG L, GRAVGAARD E, JACOBSEN NO: Treatment of Whipple's disease with sulphamethoxazole–trimethoprim. Acta Med Scand 198:141–143, 1975

FELDMAN M, HENDLER RS, MORRISON EB: Acute meningoencephalitis after withdrawal of antibiotics in Whipple's disease. Ann Intern Med 93:709–711, 1980

GROSSMAN RI, DAVIS KR, HALPERIN J: Case report: Cranial computed tomography in Whipple's disease. J Comp Assist Tomog 5(2):246–248, 1981

JOHNSON L, DIAMOND I: Cerebral Whipple's disease: Diagnosis by brain biopsy. Am J Clin Path 74:486–490, 1980

KENT SP, KIRKPATRICK PM: Whipple's disease: Immunological and histochemical studies of eight cases. Arch Pathol Lab Med 104:544–547, 1980

KNOX DL, BAYLESS TM, PITTMAN FE: Neurologic disease in patients with treated Whipple's disease. Medicine 55:467–476, 1976

PASTOR BM, GEERKEN RG: Whipple's disease presenting as pleuropericarditis. Am J Med 55:827–831, 1973

PITTMAN FE, SMITH WT, MIZRAHI A, BLANC WA, PITTMAN JC: Clinical, histochemical, and electron microscopic study of colonic histiocytosis. Gut 7:458–467, 1966

POWERS JM, RAWE SE: A neuropathologic study of Whipple's disease. Acta Neuropathol (Berl) 48:223–226, 1979

SCHMITT BP, RICHARDSON H, SMITH E, KAPLAN R: Encephalopathy complicating Whipple's disease. Ann Intern Med 94:51–52, 1981

SIERACKI JC, FINE G: Whipple's disease: Observations on systemic involvement. II. Gross and histologic observations. Arch Pathol 67:81–91, 1959

TAURIS P, MOESNER J: Whipple's disease: Clinical and histopathological changes during treatment with sulphamethoxazole–trimethoprim. Acta Med Scand 204:423–427, 1978

WHIPPLE GH: A hitherto undescribed disease characterized anatomically by deposits of fat and fatty acids in intestinal and mesenteric lymphatic tissues. Bull Johns Hopkins Hosp 18:382–391, 1907

D. GERAINT JAMES

168 Sarcoidosis

Sarcoidosis is a multisystem disorder of unknown etiology. It affects young adults most commonly; bilateral hilar lymphadenopathy, pulmonary infiltration or skin lesions are the most common manifestations. The diagnosis is established most securely when clinicoradiographic findings are supported by histologic evidence of widespread, noncaseating, epithelioid cell granulomas in more than one organ or by a positive Kveim–Siltzbach skin test. The skin test also reflects the activity of the disease. Immunologic features are depression of delayed hypersensitivity (T cell anergy) and raised serum immunoglobulins (B cell overactivity). There may also be hypercalciuria, with or without hypercalcemia. The course and prognosis correlate with the mode of onset; acute onset usually heralds a self-limiting course with spontaneous resolution, whereas insidious onset may be followed by relentless, progressive fibrosis. Glucosteroids relieve symptoms and suppress inflammation and the formation of granulomas.

Etiology

There are many well-recognized causes of granulomas (see list on p. 1411), but the cause of sarcoidosis is unknown. There have been numerous claims for various infectious agents, but none has been substantiated. Raised serum antibody titers for the Epstein–Barr, herpes simplex, rubella, measles, and parainfluenza viruses should not be misconstrued as evidence of yet another etiologic agent, but should be taken as a reflection of a widespread, nonspecific response to lymphoproliferation.

The occasional occurrence of familial sarcoidosis may reflect genetic influences. On observing sarcoidosis in 9 families involving 19 patients, sarcoidosis occurred most commonly in brother–sister or mother–offspring relations; it was not observed in any father–offspring relations. Thus, there appears to be a recessive mode of inheritance for susceptibility to sarcoidosis.

Another possible contributory factor is the immunologic derangement characteristic of sarcoidosis. An antigenic insult, whether by an infective agent or by chemical or even vegetable matter, is met by a reticuloendothelial response in which both thymus-derived (T) cells and bone-marrow-dependent (B) cells participate. The T cells are transformed, possibly by undergoing antigenic alteration on their cell surfaces and become depleted. Depletion may result not only from T cell transformation but also from T cell interaction against transformed T cells. Depletion results in depression of delayed hypersensitivity, which is recognized by cutaneous anergy and by lymphocyte transformation *in vitro* (Fig. 168-1*A*). At the same time, there is vigorous lymphoproliferation, and the B cell response is recognizable by an increase in circulating immunoglobulins (Fig. 168-1*B*). This phase of expansive lymphoproliferation may be a consequence of lack of suppressor control by the deficient, defective T cells. This T cell and B cell imbalance coincides with the phase of granuloma formation (Fig. 168-1*C*). The antigen responsible for T cell eclipse, lymphoproliferation, and granuloma formation almost certainly also resides in Kveim–Siltzbach antigen.

Epidemiology

Sarcoidosis is worldwide in distribution, but it is most frequently recognized in sophisticated communities with adequate diagnostic facilities (Table 168-1). Mass chest roentgenography reveals an overall prevalence of 20 per 100,000 population, rising to a figure of 120 per 100,000 for Irishmen and 200 per 100,000 for Irishwomen in London. Although the overall incidence is similar in men and women, it is twice as common in women of child bearing age.

SEVERAL CAUSES OF GRANULOMAS

Infections
Viral
  Cat-scratch agent(?)
Chlamydial
  Lymphogranuloma agent
Bacteria
  Brucella spp.
  Francisella tularensis
  Mycobacterium spp.
Spirochetes
  Treponema spp.
Fungi
  Blastomyces dermatitidis
  Coccidioides immitis
  Histoplasma capsulatum
  Sporotrichum schenkii
Protozoa
  Leishmania spp.
  Toxoplasma gondii
Metazoa
  Schistosoma spp.
  Toxocara spp.
Neoplastic
  Carcinoma
  Reticulosis
  Pinealoma
  Dysgerminoma
  Seminoma
  Reticulum cell sarcoma
  Malignant nasal granuloma
Chemical
  Beryllium
  Zirconium
  Silica
  Starch
Immunologic deficiency
  Sarcoidosis
  Crohn's disease
  Primary biliary cirrhosis
  Wegener's granulomatosis
  Giant cell arteritis
  Peyronie's disease
  Hypogammaglobulinemia
  Systemic lupus erythematosus
Leukocyte oxidase defect
  Chronic granulomatous disease of childhood
Extrinsic allergic alveolitis
  Farmer's lung
  Bird fancier's
  Mushroom worker's
  Suberosis (cork dust)
  Bagassosis
  Maple bark stripper's
  Paprika splitter's
  Coffee bean worker's
Other
  Pyrexia of unknown origin
  Radiotherapy
  Cancer chemotherapy
  Panniculitis
  Chalazion
  Sebaceous cyst
  Dermoid

In the United States, sarcoidosis is ten times more frequent among blacks than among whites, which immediately raises the problem of whether the same holds true in Africa and elsewhere. Sarcoidosis was found ten times more frequently in Bantus than in South African whites. Moreover, in Bantus it was a necrotizing, mutilating form of the disease, with lupus pernio and other chronic skin lesions, bone cysts, and nail dystrophies. Some of the patients were institutionalized in a leprosy sanitarium, and others failed to respond to antituberculous and antisyphilitic treatment before the true diagnosis of sarcoidosis was established.

Pathogenesis and Pathology

The sarcoid granuloma consists of focal collections of radially arranged large epithelioid cells that stain pink with eosin, a few multinucleate giant cells, and a surrounding rim of lymphocytes. Central necrosis is minimal. Schaumann, asteroid, and residual inclusion bodies may be present; none is diagnostic of sarcoidosis. Schaumann bodies are nonspecific, concentrically laminated, basophilic, conchoidal bodies that originate in epithelioid cells and giant cells. They are made up of calcium carbonate or phosphate and iron. Asteroid bodies are star-shaped lipoproteins with a central core and radiating, slightly curved spines. They are most commonly found in giant cells, occurring in only about 2% of patients with sarcoidosis. Residual bodies are cytoplasmic granules in epithelioid and giant cells; they are end products of activated lysosomes. As the lesion ages, reticulum becomes evident, progressing to fibrosis and hyalinization. When the lesion becomes completely hyalinized, it is difficult to distinguish from end-stage fibrosis due to other causes. Electron microscopy of sarcoid tissue shows many mitochondria, rough endoplasmic retic-

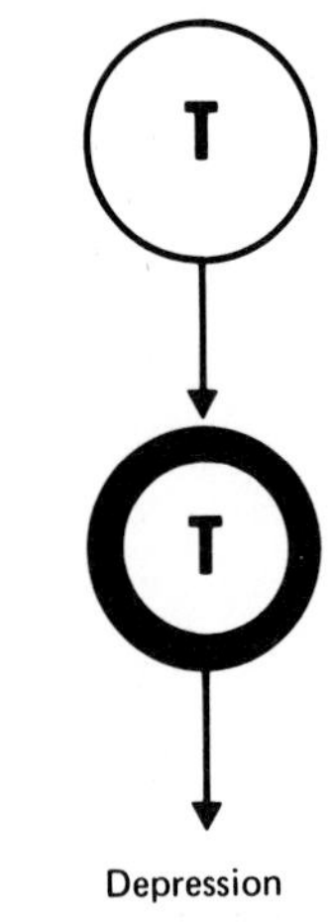

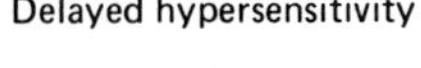

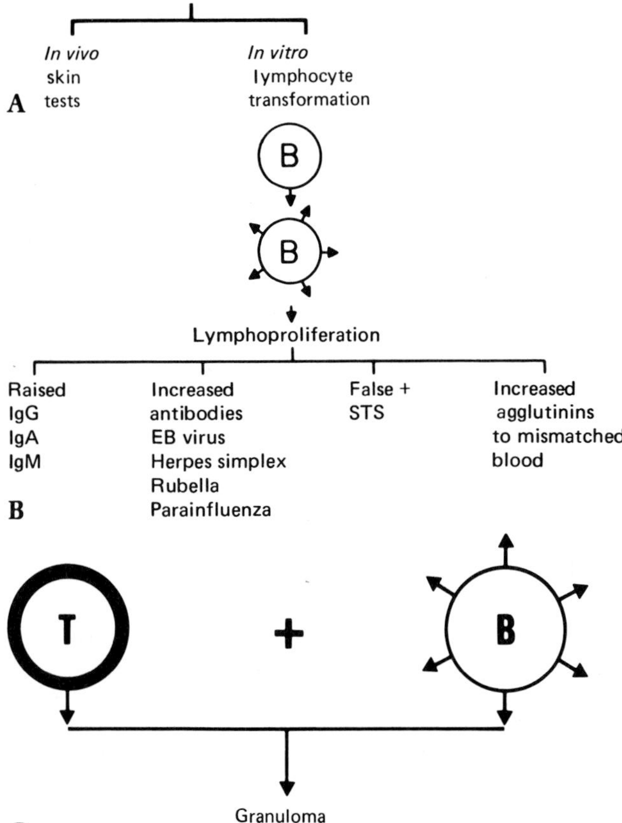

Fig. 168-1. (*A*) Defective T-lymphocytes result in depression of delayed hypersensitivity (recognized by cutaneous anergy) and impaired lymphocyte transformation *in vitro.* (*B*) The B-lymphocytes proliferate vigorously, yielding increased concentrations of serum immunoglobulins, raised serum antibody titers to viruses, false-positive reaginic tests for syphilis (STS), and increased levels of hemagglutinins. (*C*) At times of T cell waning and B cell waxing, granulomas form in all organ systems.

Table 168-1 *Incidence of Pulmonary Sarcoidosis per 100,000 of Population Examined*

Area	Prevalence	Area	Prevalence
Argentine	1–5	Leipzig	13
Australia	9	London	19
Brazil	0.2	New Zealand	6–24
Canada	10	North Ireland	10
Czechoslovakia	3	Norway	26
Eire	33	Poland	10
Finland	5–8	Portugal	0.2
France	10	Scotland	8
Holland	21	Sweden	55–64
Hungary	5	Switzerland	16
Israel	1.6	Uruguay	0.4
Italy	11	West Berlin	14
Japan	5.6	Yugoslavia	11

ulum, Golgi complex, and a number of vacuolar structures in the cytoplasm of the epithelioid cells. Giant cells have an ultrastructure similar to that of epithelioid cells, but they also contain many small, dense bodies and few or no clear vacuolar structures. All these features remain nonspecific.

Since aspiration needle biopsy has become commonplace, noncaseating liver granulomas have been reported with increasing frequency. Hepatic granulomas of widely differing causes may be confusingly similar; others have distinctive features—for example, the morphology of primary biliary cirrhosis, the caseation of tuberculosis, the rare finding of acid-fast bacilli, or the presence of a schistosome egg. Granulomas in sarcoidosis retain their reticulin network, unlike those of tuberculosis. Among 138 patients with miliary hepatic granulomas, 75 had sarcoidosis, 26 had primary biliary cirrhosis, 23 had miscellaneous recognizable disorders (cirrhosis, hepatitis, bile duct obstruction, cancer, Hodgkin's disease), and 14 remained undiagnosed.

Whereas the immediate type of hypersensitivity is normal, the delayed type of hypersensitivity is depressed because of hypoactive cellular antibodies. This phenomenon is restricted neither to sarcoidosis nor to tuberculin, since it is also evident when cutaneous tests are made with other antigens, including pertussis, mumps, trichophytin, oidiomycin, and even pine pollen. Whereas cellular antibodies are defective, circulating humoral antibodies are unimpaired. The response to typhoid–paratyphoid vaccine is normal, with the production of IgM after primary immunization and IgG after secondary booster inoculations.

*Table 168-2. Features of Sarcoidosis in a Worldwide Survey of 3676 Patients in 11 Cities**

City	Female	Presentation Under 40 Years of Age	Predominant Manifestations			Resolution of Chest X-Ray
			INTRATHORACIC	SKIN	OCULAR	
London	56	67	84	56	27	60
New York	68	71	92	30	20	38
Paris	45	72	94	18	11	73
Los Angeles	67	69	93	36	11	41
Tokyo	47	74	87	16	32	28
Reading	62	64	89	45	16	76
Lisbon	44	72	88	30	6	36
Edinburgh	64	72	94	40	11	80
Novi Sad	60	37	90	15	15	68
Naples	53	77	99	6	0	34
Geneva	47	79	97	17	12	54
Overall	57	68	87	26	15	54

*All figures are percentages of each series.

Manifestations

In a recent survey of 3676 patients attending 11 sarcoidosis clinics in 9 different countries, it was clear that the major presentations of sarcoidosis around the world are surprisingly similar (Table 168-2). Sarcoidosis has an equal sex distribution. Two-thirds of the patients are in the 20- to 40-year age group when they first consult a physician—usually with respiratory, skin, or ocular manifestations.

The general examination of the patient must be thorough. It is incomplete unless it includes a chest radiograph, slit lamp examination of the eyes, 24-hour urine calcium level, serum angiotensin-converting enzyme (SACE) determination, and histologic confirmation of the diagnosis. Sarcoidosis is characterized by multisystem involvement with intrathoracic involvement in nine-tenths of patients, and reticuloendothelial and ocular involvement and skin lesions in about one-quarter of patients (Table 168-3 and 168-4).

Diagnosis

The clinical diagnosis should be supported by histologic demonstration of sarcoid granulomas, which may be accomplished by biopsy. Bronchioles and lung tissue can be obtained in the majority of patients through the flexible fiberoptic bronchoscope with forceps. Hepatic granulomas are found in 67% of aspiration biopsies of the liver if serial sections are cut through the specimen. Biopsy of other tissues may be rewarding, because they are not uncommonly involved; these include skin, nasal mucosa, conjunctiva, spleen, muscle, minor salivary glands, and gum.

Two skin tests are useful. The Kviem–Siltzbach skin test is a reliable, safe, specific, and simple outpatient method for delineating multisystem sarcoidosis from the numerous other causes of nonspecific sarcoidlike tissue reactions. It is positive in about 80% of patients around the world. The standard tuberculin skin test (Chap. 15, Skin Tests, and Chap. 34, Pulmonary Tuberculosis) is negative in 67% of patients worldwide (Table 168-2). At the onset of acute sarcoidosis, a previously positive skin test becomes negative, and with cure it tends to revert to its previous responsiveness. Treatment with glucosteroids allows T cells to reassert themselves and tends to make the tuberculin skin test positive once again.

The concentration of SACE is elevated in about 60% of patients with sarcoidosis, and there is a false-positive rate of up to 10%. Because the enyzme appears to be generated by active metabolic turnover of epitheliod granulomas in the pulmonary capillary bed, SACE reflects the activity of the disease. The occurrence of false-positive results prevents measurement of SACE from being an absolutely reliable diagnostic test, but it serves a most useful role in monitoring the progress of treated sarcoidosis. Glucosteroids cause the concentration of SACE to fall to normal, where it remains with cure, but it rises again to herald a relapse. As a means of surveillance of activity of the disease, measurement of SACE offers the advantage over serial chest radiography of reduced irradiation; this is particularly important during pregnancy. Also, rising levels of SACE may be an indication for further glucosteroid therapy.

Table 168-3. *Investigations and Prognosis of Sarcoidosis in a Worldwide Survey of 3676 Patients in 11 Cities*

	Skin Tests		**Blood Tests**		**Treated With Steroids**	**Cause of Mortality**	
	NEGATIVE TUBERCULIN	POSITIVE KVEIM–SILTZBACH	HYPERGLOBULINEMIA	HYPERCALCEMIA		SARCOIDOSIS	OTHER CAUSES
London	55	82	34	24	34	5	1
New York	63	92	61	14	33	5	3
Paris	80	77	22	7	68	2	2
Los Angeles	85	72	86	11	65	4	1
Tokyo	62	54	25	9	68	>1	>1
Reading	52	81	40	14	25	>1	>1
Lisbon	93	78	65	28	47	8	0
Edinburgh	58	64	24	3	44	1	2
Novi Sad	43	81	46	6	92	>1	2
Naples	70	56	84	8	40	>1	>1
Geneva	73	84	34	3	45	2	4
Overall	64	78	44	11	47	2	1

*All figures are percentages of each series.

Table 168-4. Initial Manifestations of Sarcoidosis

Chest Physician	Dermatologist	Ophthalmologist
Breathlessness Bilateral hilar lymphadenopathy Pulmonary fibrosis Cor pulmonale	Erythema nodosum Lupus pernio Plaques, scars, keloids Maculopapular eruptions	Iridocyclitis Keratoconjunctivitis sicca Sjögren's syndrome Choroidoretinitis Glaucoma, cataract
Neurologist	**Gastroenterologist**	**Cardiologist**
Cranial nerve palsy Myopathy, neuropathy Space-occupying lesion Meningitis	Hepatic granulomas Splenomegaly Similarity to Crohn's disease	Cardiac arrhythmias Bundle-branch block Cardiomyopathy Complete heart block
General Physician	**Rheumatologist**	**Urologist**
Acute rheumatism Lymphadenopathy Parotid enlargement Peripheral lymphadenopathy	Polyarthralgia Bone cysts Dactylitis	Hypercalciuria Nephrocalcinosis Renal calculi Uremia

Hypercalcemia and hypercalciuria are such well-recognized components of sarcoidosis that they are included in the descriptive definition. In the world-wide survey, hypercalcemia was noted in 11% of patients examined (Table 168-2). Hypercalciuria was even more common; it may be present even when the serum calcium level is normal. On the contrary, when there is hypercalcemia there is always associated hypercalciuria.

The single-breath diffusing capacity and the vital capacity are useful, practical tests of respiratory function. In the early stage of hilar adenopathy, there may be a reduction in the diffusing capacity and also in the arterial oxygen tension. Later, when there is radiographic evidence of pulmonary involvement, there is also reduction of vital capacity, airway resistance, maximum midexpiratory flow, and arterial oxygen tension on exercise. The worse the pretreatment impairment, the higher the SACE level will be and the greater the immediate temporary response to glucosteroid therapy.

The differential diagnosis of sarcoidosis includes tuberculosis (Chap. 34, Pulmonary Tuberculosis), Hodgkin's disease, primary biliary cirrhosis, extrinsic allergic alveolitis, Crohn's regional ileitis, and other granulomatous disorders (see list on p. 1411).

The most predictable course is that of sarcoidosis with erythema nodosum. There is subsidence within a month of onset, and the accompanying hilar adenopathy regresses within the course of 1 year; recurrences and sequelae are rare.

Skin and pulmonary lesions are similar in course and in response to treatment. Transient skin lesions are usually associated with hilar adenopathy, whereas chronic skin lesions are more likely to be accompanied by pulmonary fibrosis. The transient skin lesions tend to clear without treatment. The chronic skin lesions fail to do so despite prolonged therapy. Resolution of all types of pulmonary sarcoidosis may be expected in 60% of patients, but it is less likely to occur in older patients and in those in whom there is accompanying extrathoracic disease, particularly bone and skin lesions. The combination of pulmonary and cutaneous sarcoidosis is the hallmark of chronicity, presumably because longstanding fibrosis has supervened. Clearing of the abnormal chest roentgenogram occurs in only 67% of patients with bone cysts, in 20% with skin lesions, and in only 17% of patients in whom bone and skin lesions accompany pulmonary sarcoidosis (Fig. 168-2).

Sarcoidosis would remain a relatively benign and unimportant disease but for the development of certain devastating complications: nephrocalcinosis and irreversible fibrosis in the lungs and eyes (Table 168-5). In assessing the prognosis, it is important to evaluate the degree of functional failure of lungs, heart, eyes, and kidneys. In the practical management of sarcoidosis, it is the physician's duty to diagnose the condition sufficiently early so that effective therapy may prevent these unfortunate sequelae.

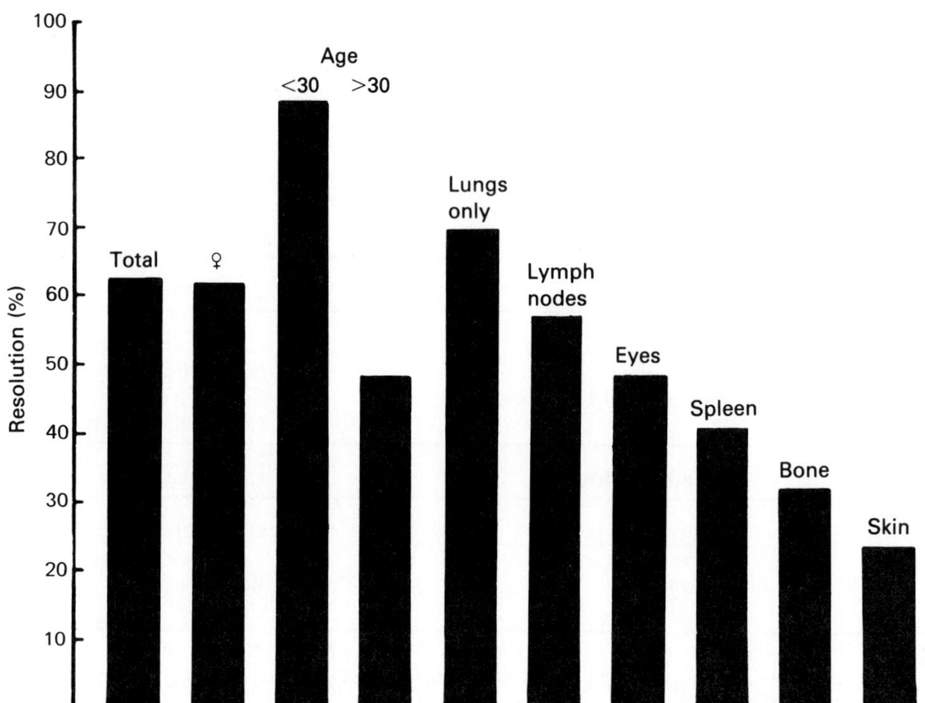

Fig. 168-2. Correlation of resolution of the abnormal chest roentgenogram with lesions in other organ systems. Bone and skin lesions constitute the hallmark of chronicity of pulmonary sarcoidosis.

Table 168-5. *Complications of Sarcoidosis*

Complication	Consequence	Clinical Result
Pulmonary fibrosis	Cor pulmonale	Cardiopulmonary failure
Chronic uveitis	Glaucoma; cataract	Blindness
Hypercalcemia, hypercalciuria	Nephrocalcinosis	Renal failure

Prognosis

There are two different types of sarcoidosis (Table 168-6). Acute sarcoidosis has an abrupt onset, acute inflammatory lesions, exudative histologic picture, hydroxyprolinuria, a positive Kveim–Siltzbach test, a high incidence of spontaneous remission within 2 years, good response to glucosteroids and to other antiinflammatory drugs, and a good prognosis. Chronic sarcoidosis has an insidious onset, a grumbling, relapsing course, a fibrotic histologic picture, a negative Kveim–Siltzbach test, and a poor prognosis despite treatment.

Therapy

Glucosteroids are recommended for treatment. Their use is particularly indicated for uveitis, worsening chest roentgenogram, breathlessness, persistent hypercalciuria, disfiguring skin lesions, myocardial and neurologic involvement, and involvement of salivary and lacrimal glands, and hypersplenism.

There are alternative treatments when glucosteroids are contraindicated or have proved ineffective, but the choice depends on whether it is acute or chronic sarcoidosis. Oxyphenbutazone controls acute exudative sarcoidosis, whereas chloroquine and potassium paraminobenzoate are indicated for chronic fibrotic sarcoidosis. Azathioprine may be considered for its temporary glucosteroid-sparing effect, especially when massive doses would be necessary.

Persistent hypercalciuria may require a low-calcium diet and drugs that chelate with calcium in the intestine, for example, sodium phytate and inorganic phosphate.

Certain treatments that were once popular but are now contraindicated include radiotherapy, calciferol, and antituberculous drugs.

Table 168-6. Differences Between Subacute (Transient) and Chronic (Persistent) Sarcoidosis

	Subacute-Transient	Chronic-Persistent
Age	Under 30 years	Over 30 years
Onset	Abrupt	Insidious
Skin	Erythema nodosum, maculopapular rash, vesicular eruptions	Lupus perino, placques, scars, keloids
Eyes	Conjunctivitis, acute iritis	Keratoconjunctivitis sicca, chronic uveitis, glaucoma, cataract
Lungs	Hilar adenopathy	Pulmonary mottling
Bone cysts	Lacking	Present
Parotitis		
Lymphadenopathy	Usually transient	Rarely permanent
Splenomegaly		
Bell's palsy		
Histology	Epithelioid and giant cells	Hyaline fibrosis
Calcium metabolism	Hypercalcemia, hypercalciuria	Nephrocalcinosis
Kveim–Siltzbach test	Positive	May be negative
Spontaneous remission	Frequent	Rare
Hydroxyproline excretion	Increased	Normal
Steroid therapy	Abortive effect	Symptomatic relief
Recurrence after steroid therapy	Rare	Frequent
Alternative treatment	Oxyphenbutazone	Chloroquine, paraaminobenzoate
Prognosis	Good	Poor

Prevention

There is no known preventive of sarcoidosis.

Remaining Problems

What is the cause of sarcoidosis? Is it an infection, an autoimmune disorder, or some hypersensitivity phenomenon? The clinical features of erythema nodosum, polyarthralgia, uveitis, and meningism are consistent with the occurrence of circulating immune complexes. Intensive studies of immune mechanisms in sarcoidosis are in progress, for they may provide a key to the cause not only of sarcoidosis, but also of other disorders associated with granulomas.

Further work is also needed on epidemiology. In the past there have been erroneous admissions of patients with sarcoidosis to tuberculosis sanatoriums; such patents are now seen in leprosariums. Where should the search turn next?

Because sarcoidosis seems to arise in the wake of tuberculosis, in the areas of the world where national efforts at eradication of tuberculosis are underway, follow-up studies should now be planned to detect emerging cases.

Bibliography

Books

JAMES DG: Sarcoidosis. In Beeson PB, McDermott W (eds): Textbook of Medicine, 14th ed. Philadelphia, WB Saunders, 1975. pp 164–174.

JAMES DG: Sarcoidosis: Disease-a-Month. Chicago, Year Book Medical Publishers, 1970. pp 3–43.

STUDDY PR, JAMES DG, BIRD R, SHERLOCK S, SILTZBACH LE, KRAKOF L, DORPH D, TEIRSTEIN AS, SHARMA OP, MIKAMI R, YOTSUMOTO H, KITAMURA S, TACHIBANA T, YAMAMOTO M, OKAMO H, IWAI K, IZUMI T, HOSODA Y, NIITU Y, NAGAYAMA H, HORIKAWA M, HASEGAWA S, KOMATSU S, SUETAKE, T, SUZAKI K, LIEBERMAN J, NOSAL E, SCHLEISSNER LA, KAEFFLER P, SANDRON D, LECOSSIER D, MOREAU F, BASSET G, BATTESTI JP, GRÖNHAGEN—RISKA C. FRÖSETH B, HELLSTRÖM P—E, WÄGNER G, SPRINCE NL, KAZEMI H, FANBURG BL, SELROOS O, TIITINEN H, FYHRQVIST F, KLOCKARS M: Serum angiotensin-converting enzyme (SACE): Experience in ten centres. Proceedings of the VIII Conference on Sarcoidosis. Cardiff, Alpha-Omega, 1980. pp 241–244.

Journals

JAMES DG, NEVILLE E, WALKER A: Immunology of sarcoidosis. Am J Med 59:388–394, 1975

JAMES DG, NEVILLE E, PIYASENA KHG, WALKER AN, HAMLYN AN: Possible genetic influences in familial sarcoidosis. Postgrad Med J 50:664, 1974

JAMES DG, NEVILLE E, SILTZBACH LE, TURIAF J, BATTESTI JP, SHARMA OP, HOSODA Y, MIKAMI R, ODAKA M, VILLAR TG, DJURIC B, DOUGLAS AC, MIDDLETON W, KARLISH A, BALSI A, OLIVERI D, PRESS P: A worldwide review of sarcoidosis. Ann NY Acad Sci 278:321–331, 1976

STUDDY PR, BIRD R, NEVILLE E, JAMES DG: Biochemical findings in sarcoidosis. J Clin Pathol 33:528–533, 1980

ARTHUR D. SCHWABE

Familial Mediterranean Fever

169

Familial Mediterranean fever (FMF) is an inherited disorder of unknown etiology that is characterized by irregularly recurring attacks of fever and inflammation of the peritoneal, pleural, or synovial membranes. Synonyms encountered in medical writings include periodic disease, Armenian disease, benign paroxysmal peritonitis, familial paroxysmal polyserositis, and recurrent polyserositis.

Etiology

An infectious origin in FMF might be suggested by the recurrent episodes of fever, inflammation, and leukocytosis. Moreover, increased numbers of polymorphonuclear leukocytes with marked phagocytic activity have been demonstrated in synovial aspirates and pleural and peritoneal exudates during attacks. However, exhaustive searches for viruses, bacteria, protozoa, and other pathogenic microorganisms have yielded negative results. Treatment with a variety of antibacterial, antimalarial, and amebicidal agents has been ineffective. These and other observations favor the concept that FMF is due to either an inborn error of metabolism or defective immunity.

Epidemiology

FMF is most commonly encountered in persons of Armenian, Jewish, and Arab origins, but it has occasionally been found in Turks, Italians, and others of Mediterranean background. Isolated cases have been reported in northern Europeans and Orientals.

There is a high familial incidence of FMF, and detailed genetic studies in non-Ashkenazic Jews strongly support inheritance of the disease as a single recessive autosomal trait. Spontaneous remissions lasting months or years have been observed, and complete remissions occur frequently during pregnancy.

Pathogenesis and Pathology

The lack of clear-cut information about the etiology is paralleled by a lack of knowledge of the pathogenesis of FMF.

The histology of peritoneal and synovial biopsies obtained during attacks is that of mild to moderate acute inflammation. During the rare, protracted episodes of FMF with arthritis, the changes of chronic synovial inflammation may be found. However, despite these pathologic changes, the inflammatory process usually subsides without leaving any residual damage. Chronic irreversible changes are most likely to occur in the hip joints.

At necropsy, generalized amyloidosis of the perireticulin type with marked renal involvement is commonly seen in non-Ashkenazic Jews, but rarely, if ever, in Armenians.

Manifestations

FMF usually becomes clinically evident in childhood, appearing before age 20 in more than 80% of cases. The characteristic attacks of fever, accompanied by peritonitis, pleuritis, or arthralgia, usually last for 12 to 72 hours and are followed by completely asymptomatic periods of varying duration.

Joint involvement is usually monarthric, afflicting a large joint, and it may assume a protracted course. Under these circumstances, a picture of a chronic monarthritis with swelling, synovial effusion, heat, and redness is seen. An erysipelaslike erythema is most commonly found on the lower extremities. It may occur with a short bout of fever or in association with an attack of arthralgia. Rarely, fever, which may rise as high as 104°F, may be the sole manifestation of FMF.

Diagnosis

The first attack, whether manifestly pleural, peritoneal, or synovial, is usually a diagnostic challenge. An attack of pleuritis, which may be accompanied by a transitory pleural effusion, may mimic a viral or bacterial infection. Attacks of abdominal pain may simulate acute pancreatitis, acute appendicitis, or a perforated viscus. Multiple surgical scars in some patients attest to the difficulty in arriving at the correct diagnosis. The erythrocyte sedimentation rate (ESR), plasma fibrinogen, C-reactive protein (CRP), haptoglobins, IgM, and lipoproteins are usually elevated, but these abnormalities are seen in many other disorders and have litle diagnostic value. The diagnosis at present is based entirely on the history of recurrent, self-limited attacks of fever and pain, and the physical findings of acute serosal inflammation in persons of Mediterranean ancestry. A set of criteria has been developed to facilitate arriving at the diagnosis (see list below). At least three of the major plus one of the minor criteria must be met by each case diagnosed as FMF.

DIAGNOSTIC CRITERIA FOR FAMILIAL MEDITERRANEAN FEVER

Major
- Recurrent fever (1–3 days)
- Recurrent attacks of peritonitis (1–3 days)
- Recurrent attacks of pleuritis (1–3 days)
- Recurrent arthritis (1–30 days)
- Recurrent erysipeloid erythema (1–3 days)
- Armenian, Jewish, or Arab ancestry
- Positive family history for FMF

Minor
- Recurrent arthralgias (1–30 days)
- Protracted, seronegative arthritis
- Recurrent abdominal pain without peritonitis (1–3 days)
- Onset of symptoms in childhood
- Remissions during pregnancy
- Favorable response to colchicine

Prognosis

The febrile paroxysms tend to recur at various intervals throughout the lifetimes of patients with FMF. The development of amyloidosis in patients at risk is insidious, and amyloid nephropathy, progressing from a preclinical stage through proteinuria, nephrosis, and uremia, is the usual cause of death, especially in non-Ashkenazic Jews.

Therapy

During an acute attack of FMF, supportive measures are employed to alleviate the symptoms of fever and inflammation. Pleural effusions are transient and require no specific treatment. Glucosteroids are ineffective and should not be used.

Prevention

The prophylactic use of colchicine has proved to be effective in suppressing attacks. On an oral dose of 0.6 mg colchicine 3 times a day the attacks may be prevented in approximately 70% of patients with FMF. Smaller doses may be effective in selected cases. Long-term follow-up for periods as long as 10 years indicates persistent benefit and a lack of significant side-effects from this form of treatment. In some patients, restricting dietary fat intake to 20 g or less a day prevents, or markedly reduces, the frequency of attacks.

Bibliography

Journals

DINARELLO CA, WOLFF SM, GOLDINGER SE, DALE DC, ALLING DW: Colchicine therapy for familial Mediterranean fever. N Engl J Med 291:934–937, 1974

GOLDSTEIN RC, SCHWABE AD: Prophylactic colchine therapy in familial Mediterranean fever. Ann Intern Med 81:792–794, 1974

SCHWABE AD, PETERS RC: Familial Mediterranean fever in Armenians: Analysis of 100 cases. Medicine 53:453–462, 1974

SIEGAL S: Familial paroxysmal polyserositis. Am J Med 36:893–918, 1964

SOHAR E, GAFNI J, PRAS M, HELLER H: Familial Mediterranean fever: A survey of 470 cases and review of the literature. Am J Med 43:227–253, 1967

ALEXIS SHELOKOV

Epidemic Neuromyasthenia

170

Epidemic neuromyasthenia (ENM), also called epidemic myalgic encephalomyelitis, is a puzzling and controversial, nonfatal clinical syndrome of unknown etiology. It has been reported from many parts of the world during the past 45 years. Severely affected patients characteristically complain of fatigability and muscle pain; if use of affected muscles continues, there may be progress to demonstrable weakness. Patients may also undergo striking behavioral changes: depression, emotional lability, and temporary deficits in intellection, especially memory. Also characteristically, convalescence may lapse into an unaccountably protracted and debilitating course. In some outbreaks, symptoms and signs compatible with encephalomyelitis dominate the clinical picture. Outbreaks occur either in the general population, or more dramatically, in closed population groups such as the nursing staff of a hospital; in both settings women are afflicted much more often than men. Undoubtedly, mild epidemic disease occurs commonly; sporadic cases have been recognized, but are difficult to diagnose when there is no epidemic.

Etiology

The etiology of ENM is unknown. On clinicoepidemiologic grounds, it is reasonable to presume it is an infectious disease caused by an unknown agent or group of related agents. It has been particularly tempting to invoke persistent or chronic viral infections. However, the limited studies so far conducted have failed to produce convincing evidence of viral causation. A bacterial etiology of ENM was dismissed long ago, but occasional references to an outbreak in which certain paracolon organisms were peripherally implicated still confuse matters. Toxic causes have been repeatedly sought, but without success.

In most outbreaks, the possibility that ENM is a manifestation of mass hysteria or psychoneurosis was considered and dismissed by the investigators. However, a so-called psychosocial hypothesis was popularized a decade ago by two psychiatrists who compared the published ENM data with their own observations during an outbreak of hysterical overbreathing in a girls' school. Their conclusion—that every known outbreak of ENM could be explained by hysterical overreaction either on the part of the subjects or on the part of the attending medical staff—has contributed to the disrepute of ENM as a clinical diagnosis.

A few provocative laboratory observations have been reported that have not yet been followed up. These include (1) a 1955 Australian report of reproducible histopathologic lesions in the nerve tissue of monkeys inoculated with feces from patients with ENM; (2) a 1959 South African report of an unknown toxic factor in the urine of patients convalescing from ENM; (3) several 1974 British findings: structures resembling antigen–antibody complexes in patients' serums; abnormally prolonged survival of cultured lymphocytes from some of the same patients; serum anticomplementarity that developed during convalescence in some patients; and false positivity of serums from many patients (48/58) by a Paul-Bunnell screening test for infectious mononucleosis, whereas the Epstein–Barr (EB) virus antibody titers were not elevated.

Epidemiology

Although students of ENM assume that the illness is common throughout the world, only 30 outbreaks have been reported during the past 45 years. The reports came from the United States, the British Isles, Europe, Iceland, Australia, and South Africa—that is, the more developed countries. There has not been a predictable epidemic pattern, but most outbreaks have occurred in the summer and fall months and in the past were often confused with poliomyelitis. Characteristic features include (1) concentration of clinical cases in young and middle-aged adults, although children and the elderly were not spared in some outbreaks; (2) increased frequency and severity of cases in women, (3) protracted convalescence with symptomatic relapses precipitated by exertion, stress, exposure to cold, changes in the weather (specificially including sudden drops in barometric pressure), and menses; and (4) a seeming predilection for closed populations, especially nursing and medical personnel. About one-half of the outbreaks were reported from hospitals, possibly as a result of investigations prompted by the sudden appearance of cases of a disabling illness among the nursing staff or of a greater risk in hospitals of frequent and close exposure to the agent(s).

Some outbreaks lasted for a few weeks, others for several months. The incubation period is estimated at 5 to 8 days for most outbreaks, but may be as long as 2 to 3 weeks. Sporadic nonepidemic cases must occur, but their recognition has been hampered by the lack of unequivocal diagnostic tests and of accepted definition of a case of ENM. The transmission of ENM remains unknown. The epidemic curves are consistent with patterns of an infectious disease spreading directly from person to person, but the possibility of spread from a common source exists, as the two following examples illustrate. 1. The classic 1938 study of ENM in a Los Angeles hospital concluded that infection was spread by personal contaact, but a recent review of the data was consistent with the late cases among physicians and nurses resulting from injections of a serum prepared from pooled bloods donated by convalescing colleagues. 2. A 1957 study of two closely spaced outbreaks of ENM suggested a food handler as being the source of infection not only with two antigenically distinct strains of paracolon bacteria, but also with the unknown agent of ENM.

Pathogenesis and Pathology

Practically nothing is known of the pathology of ENM or its pathogenesis. No deaths have ever been attributed to ENM, and the abnormal results obtained in the rare histologic and electron microscopic examinations of biopsied tissues are not conclusive. Early ideas about the nature of ENM were reflected in the original names: poliomyelitislike disease (United States, Iceland, and Europe), epidemic vegetative neuritis (Denmark), benign myalgic encephalomyelitis (United Kingdom), and epidemic neuromyasthenia (United States). Variations in the clinical picture from one outbreak to the next were viewed as the usual spectrum of a disease or considered a hint that the syndrome comprises two or more pathophysiologic entities that share common diagnostic features.

The cardinal manifestations of ENM point to the nervous or muscular system, although other organ systems, including the reticuloendothelial, may be affected. Some observers are convinced that the muscles are normal, and that the primary process lies in demyelination, possibly owing to an immunopathologic disorder similar to experimental autoallergic encephalomyelitis; other observers are convinced that damage to the muscle mitochondria best explains the characteristic fatigability and weakness; still others suggest dysfunction of the myoneural junction with a neurotransmission deficit analogous to myasthenia gravis, botulism, or Eaton–Lambert syndrome. A toxic metabolite has been detected in the urine of some patients; according to recent observations, the toxic substance may be released from the affected muscles *after* exercise, causing transient, general muscle weakness and encephalopathic changes.

Manifestations

The typical patient with ENM is a woman in the prime of life who reports that following a prodromal episode of viruslike respiratory or gastrointestinal illness, she developed headache, dizziness, malaise, lassitude, and tiredness. Localized muscle fatigability appeared in certain muscle groups, progressing to temporary paresis with repeated use; the muscles became painful, tender, and subject to fasciculation. Most patients also report some of the following symptoms: low-grade fever (more correctly, instability of body temperature, swinging from 35°C to 38°C in the course of the day); vasomotor instability (sometimes accompanied by striking facial pallor, transient cyanosis, and edema of limbs); paresthesias, peculiar proprioceptive disturbances, and other sensory changes; severe aching of the neck and back, and pleurodynialike chest pains. Patients find it hard to concentrate, to read and write, and to perform certain routine mechanical tasks. There may be odd lapses of memory, a disturbing alteration of dream patterns, increasing anxiety, and frightening depression, particularly as convalescence is interrupted by recurring relapses, which sometimes progress to a state of physical, mental, and emotional exhaustion.

In some well-studied outbreaks, these typical features were secondary to dramatic manifestations indicative of encephalomyelitis: cranial nerve disturbances (particularly ocular and facial palsies), diplopia, nystagmus, myoclonus, palatal paralysis, altered tendon reflexes, and extensor plantar responses. Few physical abnormalities are found outside of the neuromuscular systems; however, there may be an enlargement of lymph nodes, spleen, and liver.

Diagnosis

Mass hysteria afflicting a group of young women is often initially proposed to explain the outbreak because of the array of subjective complaints and the paucity of physical signs. However, the consistency of the epidemiologic and clinical findings and the lack of some of the essential features of hysteria eventually make this diagnosis untenable. Sporadic cases of ENM undoubtedly occur before, after, and in the absence of epidemics, but they are difficult or impossible to differentiate from psychoneurosis. The word epidemic was included in ENM to stress that both epidemiologic and clinical appraisal of cases is necessary until reliable tests become available to support the diagnosis.

Most students of ENM agree that abnormal muscle fatigability is the distinguishing clinical characteristic of this syndrome; characteristically, muscle complaints are accompanied by behavioral changes—depression, emotional lability, and odd deficits in intellection; also characteristically, convalescence is punctuated by disabling relapses. In some outbreaks, these features are overshadowed by findings diagnostic of encephalomyelitis.

At one time, ENM was described as being poliomyelitislike because of muscle weakness, seasonal occurrence, and community overreaction to a cluster of cases. Even today, enteroviral diseases, including meningoencephalomyelitis and epidemic myalgia, have to be ruled out. Various intoxications, including those associated with pesticides, should be considered; for example, in one community, an outbreak of ENM-like disease was apparently caused by exposure to organic mercury. Several epidemics of ENM were thought to be infectious mononucleosis because of the clinical picture and the finding of lymphadenopathy and atypical lymphocytes. When cases of ENM first come to a physician's attention, multiple sclerosis, myasthenia gravis, and polymyositis often have to be included in the differential diagnosis.

Routine laboratory findings are not very helpful in making the diagnosis of ENM. Several investigators have reported that the 24-hour excretion of creatine in the urine may be markedly elevated while the serum creatine phosphokinase level remains normal. Unfortunately, determinations of creatine in the urine are seldom carried out reliably. Hypoglycemia and abnormal glucose tolerance test results have been recorded; the significance of elevations in serum myoglobin and lactic dehydrogenase is a matter of controversy. Electromyography may disclose patterns of denervation potentials and widespread polyphasic activity in a plurisegmental distribution. On muscle biopsy, abnormalities interpreted as acute and chronic denervation, with or without atrophy, have been reported. Electroencephalographic abnormalities indicative of disturbed cerebral function may be present, but are of little value in differential diagnosis because they resemble changes seen in other disorders.

Prognosis

For several weeks or months, the recovery period of most patients is characterized by proneness to fatigue and emotional lability, with slow gradual recovery. Some clinically severe cases enter on a chronic relapsing course associated with exertion, inclement weather, menses, and stress. Eventually the patient, whether an epidemic or sporadic case, is likely to be told that the disorder is functional and should be treated accordingly, although psychiatrists find that ENM patients do not fit into any recognized psychiatric category. As the relapses recur, increasing apprehension, anxiety, depression, and hostility complicate the patient's response to the illness. Obviously, supportive and sympathetic management by the physician is critically important in helping the patient cope with the demoralizing outlook. The intriguing suggestion has been made that some forms of psychoneurosis may represent the residual deficits from epidemic or sporadic cases of ENM.

Therapy

There is no specific treatment. A variety of medications and therapeutic regimens have been tried; for brief periods, some seemed to be promising. It is most important to explain to the patient that physical rest is required to restore muscle power to the fatigued and aching muscles, and with it the sense of personal well-being. The period of rest may have to be measured in days rather than hours, depending on the severity of the relapse and the extent of involvement of muscles. It appears essential to elevate the affected leg during rest to assure recovery.

Glucosteroids have provided relief, but controlled studies of their effectiveness have not been done, and their use is not advised. Antidepressant and mood-elevating drugs are undoubtedly overprescribed. Acupuncture, carried out by qualified physicians practicing at reputable centers, deserves further evaluation in ameliorating relapses, although the very mention of acupuncture conjures visions of placebo-like therapy of functional disorders. Psychotherapy has been notably unsuccessful in helping typical patients with ENM to cope with their illness.

Remaining Problems

Some British investigators insist that changing the name to epidemic myalgic encephalomyelitis (EME) would better describe what they believe is the pathophysiologic process; others suggest that the name should be changed because it sounds like "neurasthenia." Whatever the name, the fact remains that this peculiar disorder, although subjectively disabling, does not visibly cripple or kill its victim. As a result, it has failed so far to arouse sufficient interest among members of the medical profession to generate adequate research support.

Bibliography

Books

GILLIAM AG: Epidemiological study of an epidemic, diagnosed as poliomyelitis, occurring among the personnel of the Los Angeles County General Hospital during the summer of 1934. Public Health Bulletin No. 240. Public Health Service. Washington DC, Government Printing Office, 1938. 90 pp.

Journals

ACHESON ED: The clinical syndrome variously called benign myalgic encephalomyelitis, Iceland disease and epidemic neuromyasthenia. Am J Med 26:569–595, 1959

DILLON MJ, MARSHALL WC, DUDGEON JA, STEIGMAN AJ: Epidemic neuromyasthenia: Outbreak among nurses at a children's hospital. Br Med J 1:301–305, 1974

HENDERSON DA, SHELOKOV A: Epidemic neuromyasthenia: Clinical syndrome? N Engl J Med 260:757–764, 814–818, 1959

HILL RCJ, CHEETHAM RWS, WALLACE HL: Epidemic myalgic encephalomyelopathy: The Durban outbreak. Lancet 1:689–693, 1959

LYLE WH, CHAMBERLAIN RN (eds): Epidemic neuromyasthenia 1934–1977: Current approaches. Postgrad Med J 54:705–774, 1978

MCEVEDY CP, BEARD AW: Concept of benign myalgic encephalomyelitis. Br Med J 1:11–15, 1970

PELLEW RAA, MILES JAR: Further investigations on a disease resembling poliomyelitis seen in Adelaide. Med J Aust 42:480–482, 1955

SHELOKOV A, HABEL K, VERDER E, WELSH W: Epidemic neuromyasthenia: An outbreak of poliomyelitislike illness in student nurses. N Engl J Med 257:345–355, 1957

Index

Numbers set in bold type, e.g., **92–1**, indicate color plates.

U